T0199979

Occupational Therapy *for* Physical Dysfunction

EIGHTH EDITION

Occupational Therapy *for* Physical Dysfunction

EIGHTH EDITION

EDITORS: **Diane Powers Dirette, PhD, OTL, FAOTA**
Editor-in-Chief *The Open Journal of Occupational Therapy*
Professor
Department of Occupational Therapy
Western Michigan University
Kalamazoo, Michigan

Sharon A. Gutman, PhD, OTR, FAOTA
Professor
Programs in Occupational Therapy
Department of Rehabilitation and Regenerative Medicine
Vagelos College of Physicians and Surgeons
Columbia University
New York, New York

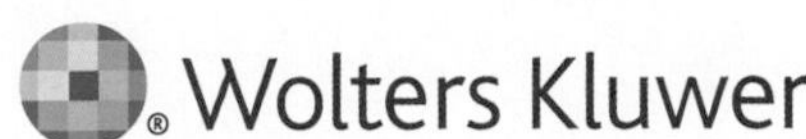

Philadelphia • Baltimore • New York • London
Buenos Aires • Hong Kong • Sydney • Tokyo

Acquisitions Editor: Matt Hauber
Senior Development Editor: Amy Millholen
Managing Editor: Laura Horowitz
Editorial Coordinator: Tim Rinehart
Marketing Manager: Shauna Kelly
Production Project Manager: Catherine Ott
Design Coordinator: Joseph Clark
Art Director, Illustration: Jennifer Clements
Manufacturing Coordinator: Margie Orzech
Prepress Vendor: S4Carlisle Publishing Services

Eighth edition

9 8 7 6 5 4 3 2

Printed in China

Library of Congress Cataloging-in-publication Data

ISBN-13: 978-1-975110-55-0

ISBN-10: 1-975110-55-2

Library of Congress Control Number: 2019917011

---

shop.lww.com

CCS0821

Dedication

We dedicate this book to Dr. Jim Hinojosa and Dr. Anne Mosey—two of the foremost influential scholars in the profession of occupational therapy. We were fortunate to have both as mentors in our pursuit to become scholars in the profession. We are eternally grateful for their scholarship, knowledge, and insight that helped shape our thinking, guided the occupational therapy program at New York University, and provided pioneering and innovative direction for the profession as a whole.

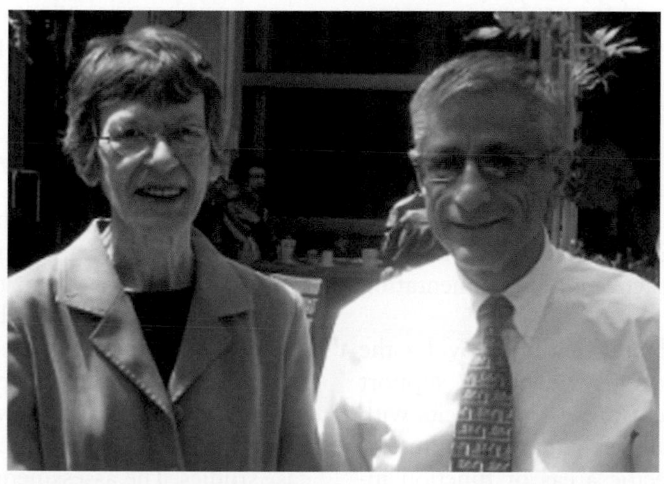

Preface

The eighth edition of *Occupational Therapy for Physical Dysfunction* integrates the foundational concepts developed by Dr. Catherine A. Trombly Latham and the work of Dr. Mary Vining Radomski with new evidence in the profession to guide occupational therapy practice for adults with physical disabilities. The intention of this text is to provide comprehensive and detailed instruction in best practice for occupational therapy assessment and intervention with this population.

Organization

The eighth edition of *Occupational Therapy for Physical Dysfunction* has six sections that guide the reader in the conceptual foundations of the profession, assessment and treatment of commonly presenting problems, the use of technology and frames of reference, and the treatment of specific diagnoses in physical rehabilitation as follows:

- **Section 1: Occupational Function** provides the reader with the basis of the profession of occupational therapy including the foundational concepts, philosophy, clinical reasoning, art of practice, and documentation guidance.
- **Section 2: Assessment and Intervention** provides the reader with detailed steps and evidence to support the assessment and treatment process of deficits with which adults with physical disabilities may present. This section covers 11 specific areas of function including vision, visual perception, cognition, sensation, motor function, motor control, balance, communication, swallowing and eating, cranial nerve function, and environmental modification.
- **Section 3: Rehabilitation Technology** guides the reader in the use and fabrication of orthoses and in the selection and use of physical agent modalities, wheelchairs, and assistive technology.
- **Section 4: Restoration of Independent and Community Living Roles** presents information about how to improve participation in activities of daily living, roles (family, parenting, social, home, community, work, and recreational), functional mobility, driving, and community mobility.
- **Section 5: Frames of Reference for Physical Disability Rehabilitation** provides the theoretical bases, function/dysfunction continua, indicators of function and dysfunction, and postulates regarding change for the Biomechanical, Rehabilitation, and Motor Learning and Task-Oriented Approaches. In addition, the functional uses of various neurological approaches including Brunnstrom, Neurodevelopmental Treatment (NDT), Rood, and Proprioceptive Neuromuscular Facilitation (PNF) frames of reference are discussed.
- **Section 6: Guidelines for Physical Dysfunction Diagnostic Categories** provides the reader with specific evaluations and interventions for 15 of the most common physical disability diagnoses with which adults present in occupational therapy practice. In addition, sleep disorders that may accompany these diagnoses and psychosocial adaptation to these physical disabilities are discussed to help guide occupational therapy assessment and intervention in these areas.

Features and Ancillaries

Many of the features of the seventh edition have been streamlined and integrated into the text in the eighth edition. Bulleted lists within the text provide information that had been provided in boxes, such as Procedures for Practice, in the previous edition. This edition includes several features to enhance learning and support occupational therapy practice with adults with physical dysfunction including assessment tables, evidence tables, and case studies. The assessment tables detail the description, administration time, validity, reliability, sensitivity, and strengths and weaknesses of the most commonly used measures. The evidence tables provide the most recent, best evidence to support intervention. These tables include a description of the intervention, participants, dosage, research design, level of evidence, and results of each study. The case studies assist the reader in understanding application of chapter content to a typical individual who may be treated by an occupational therapist using that particular intervention in an adult physical dysfunction setting. Each case study includes patient information, occupational therapy recommendations, summary of short-term goals, intervention, and progress.

There are also ancillaries for this edition including an instructor test bank for each chapter and audiovisual content. The test bank includes 10 to 20 multiple choice questions written by chapter contributors. The audiovisual content, which is available to students, can be accessed at thepoint.lww.com. This content includes audiovisual examples of how to conduct assessments and treatments for various problems with which adults present in physical dysfunction settings.

Terminology

In this edition, the term **occupational therapist** is used as an inclusive term and not as an exclusive term. Occupational therapists include those who have been educated in the use of occupation as a means of intervention to achieve occupational participation as the desired treatment outcome. This term includes all who participate in practice, education, or research in the occupational therapy profession. There has been a push in the profession of occupational therapy to use the term **occupational therapy practitioner**, but the term becomes cumbersome and exclusive in its use. To be concise and inclusive, the term **occupational therapist** is preferred by the authors.

The reader will also note the use of both of the terms **patient** and **client** to indicate the person who is participating in occupational therapy services. The term used in each chapter was chosen by the individual chapter authors to reflect the term that is most often used in that practice setting. For example, in Chapter 48, Burn Injuries, by Dr. Rebecca Ozelie, the term *patient* is used because the person participating in occupational therapy services is most often treated in a primary, acute care, or inpatient setting in which the participants are referred to as patients. In Chapter 31, Restoring Driving and Community Mobility by Dr. Sherrilene Classen and Dr. Beth Pfeiffer, however, the term *client* is used to reflect the outpatient or community-based setting in which the person is most often treated and in which participants are referred to as clients.

Throughout the text, terminologies from both the *Occupational Therapy Practice Framework: Domain and Process* (third edition) and the International Classification of Functioning from the World Health Organization are used based on congruence with common professional and interprofessional language in the practice settings addressed. The use of various terms and frameworks reflects the diverse ways occupational therapists communicate about our profession to various consumers, coworkers, and researchers. Just as with the use of the terms **patient** and **client**, the use of general terminology will often reflect the practice area. Individual chapter contributors were encouraged to use the terms that best reflected the terminology used in their practice areas.

Contributors

In this edition, we have 52 chapters authored by a total of 72 contributors with expertise as clinicians, researchers, and educators in the respective treatment areas discussed in each chapter. Each contributor provided a perspective that has a great depth of experience, but that is also clear, concise, and accessible to all readers including occupational therapy students who are learning the information for the first time, new occupational therapists who need detailed direction in their practice area, and experienced occupational therapists who desire information regarding the latest, evidence-based interventions. Each of the outstanding chapter authors has contributed to building this comprehensive resource that will help guide and shape occupational therapy practice for adults with physical dysfunction.

Diane Powers Dirette
Sharon A. Gutman

Acknowledgments

A textbook of this magnitude is compiled by the efforts of multiple professionals who are dedicated to the profession's advancement of knowledge and continued growth. Foremost, we thank Dr. Catherine A. Trombly Latham, who developed this seminal textbook in 1977 and edited editions 1 to 7, and Dr. Mary Vining Radomski who, along with Dr. Trombly Latham, edited editions 5 to 7. Their collective work on this book has both advanced the education of thousands of occupational therapists and promoted the science underlying assessment and intervention techniques. We are prodigiously grateful for their expert consultation on the eighth edition.

If not for the many expert chapter authors, who generously shared their high level of knowledge and skill in the compilation of the eighth edition, this textbook would not have reached the highest standard of knowledge dissemination. The chapter authors helped to create a textbook that is accessible, easy to understand, and replete with the latest evidence-based knowledge regarding occupational therapy practice for adults with physical dysfunction. We are exceedingly grateful for their willingness to share their expertise and mastery (see the list of current contributing authors). The eighth edition was constructed on the solid foundation of the many editions before it, and we are also immensely grateful for and acknowledge the scholarship of the contributing authors of all past editions (see the list of past contributing authors).

Working behind the scenes, but whose efforts were paramount in the development of this eighth edition are the following professionals, who although not occupational therapists have demonstrated dedication to the profession's continued advancement through their sustained work on this textbook: Laura Horowitz (managing editor), Matt Hauber (acquisitions editor), Amy Millholen (senior development editor), Jennifer Clements (art director), and Tim Rinehart (editorial coordinator). Because of their commitment and aptitude, the eighth edition exceeded the standards we hoped to attain. We are exceptionally grateful for these individuals' high level of skill and proficiency.

Lastly, we thank the many people whose assistance in the development of this textbook has gone without formal acknowledgment: those who served as photographic and video models; patients who allowed their images and stories to be presented in this edition; and colleagues, family, friends, and pets who provided support for and finessed the many details of this eighth edition. We are enormously grateful for the unseen but critically important contributions made by these individuals as well.

Diane Powers Dirette
Sharon A. Gutman

Contributing Authors of Past Editions

First Edition
Anna Deane Scott, MEd, OTR
Catherine Anne Trombly, MA, OTR
Hilda Versluys, MEd, OTR

Second Edition
Anne G. Fisher, MS, OTR
Beverly J. Myers, BS, OTR
Lillian Hoyle Parent, MA, OTR
Cynthia A. Philips, MA, OTR
Anna Deane Scott, MEd, OTR
Catherine Anne Trombly, MA, OTR
Hilda P. Versluys, MEd, OTR
Patricia L. Weber, MS, OTR

Third Edition
Patricia Weber Dow, MS, OTR
Anne G. Fisher, ScD, OTR
Beverly J. Myers, MHPE, OTR/L
Lillian Hoyle Parent, MA, OTR
Cynthia A. Philips, MA, OTR/L, ASHT
Lee Ann Quintana, MS, OTR
Anna Deane Scott, MEd, OTR
Catherine Anne Trombly, MA, OTR
Hilda Powers Versluys, MEd, OTR

Fourth Edition
M. Irma Alvarado, MA, OTR
Ben Atchinson, MEd, OTR
Julie Bass Haugen, PhD, OTR
Jane Bear-Lehman, MS, OTR
Karen Bentzel, MS, OTR
Bette R. Bonder, PhD, OTR/L
Felice Celikyol, MA, OTR
Barbara Cooper, PhD (abd), OT(C)
Wendy Coster, PhD, OTR
Jean Deitz, PhD, OTR/L
Glenn Digman, MSW, MA, OTR/L
Patricia Weber Dow, MS, OTR
Brian Dudgeon, MS, OTR/L
Maria Elena Echevarria, BS, OTR/L
Marilyn Ernest-Conibear, MA, OT(C)
Judy R. Feinberg, PhD, OTR
Glenn Goodman, MOT, OTR/L
Laura Devore Hollar, MSOT, OTR
Karen Jacobs, EdD, OTR/L, CPE
Lyn Jongbloed, PhD, OT(C)
Katherine A. Konosky, MS, OTR
Mary Law, PhD, OT(C)
Susan L. Lee, BS, OTR/L
Lori Letts, MA, OT(C)
Kathryn Levit, BS, OTR
Cheryl Linden, MS, OTR
Jaclyn Faglie Low, PhD, OTR
Colleen T. Lowe, MPH, OTR/L, CHT
Virgil Mathiowetz, PhD, OTR
Beverly J. Myers, MHPE, OTR
Elizabeth M. Newman, BS, OTR/L
Cynthia A. Philips, MA, OTR/L, ASHT
Janet L. Poole, MA, OTR
Robert E. Post, PhD, PT
Lee Ann Quintana, MS, OTR
Nancy Pearson Rees, MOT, OTR
Patricia Rigby, MHSc, OT(C)
Joyce Shapero Sabari, PhD, OTR
Anna Deane Scott, MEd, OTR
Cara Stewart, BS, OTR
Debra Stewart, BSc, OT(C)
Susan Strong, BSc, OT(C)
Dorie B. Syen, OTR, CHT
Linda Tickle-Degnen, PhD, OTR/L
Jeannette Tries, MS, OTR/L
Catherine A. Trombly, ScD, OTR/L
Hilda Powers Versluys, MEd, OTR/L
Anne M. Woodson, BS, OTR
Ruth Zemke, PhD, OTR

Fifth Edition
Jennifer Angelo, PhD, OTR, ATP
Michal S. Atkins, MA, OTR
Wendy Avery-Smith, MS, OTR/L
Julie Bass Haugen, PhD, OTR
Jane Bear-Lehman, PhD, OTR
Karen Bentzel, MS, OTR
Bette R. Bonder, PhD, OTR/L
Alfred G. Bracciano, EdD, OTR
Mary Ellen Buning, MS, OTR, ATP
Nancy Callinan, MA, OTR, CHT
Felice Gadaleta Celikyol, MA, OTR
Barbara Acheson Cooper, MHSc, PhD, OT(C)
Cynthia Cooper, MFA, MA, OTR/L, CHT
Lois F. Copperman, PhD, OTR/L
Elin Schold Davis, OTR/L, CDRS
Jean C. Deitz, PhD, OTR/L
Lisa Deshaies, OTR, CHT
Brian Dudgeon, PhD, OTR/L
Donald Earley, MA, OTR
Susan E. Fasoli, ScD, OTR/L
Nancy A. Flinn, MA, OTR, BCN
Susan Jane Forwell, MA, OT(C)
Glenn Goodman, PhD, OTR/L
Julie McLaughlin Gray, MA, OTR
Carolyn Schmidt Hanson, PhD, OTR
Lucinda L. Hugos, MS, PT
Nancy Huntley, OTR, CES
Jeanne Jackson, PhD, OTR
Douglas D. Jones, JD, MEd
Theodore I. King II, PhD, OT
Mary Law, PhD, OT(C)
Lori Letts, PhD (abd), OT(C)
Kathryn Levit, MA, OTR
Jaclyn Faglie Low, PhD, OTR
LTC Stephen Luster, MS, OTR/L, CHT
Virgil Mathiowetz, PhD, OTR
Amy C. Orroth, OTR/L, CHT
Monica Pessina, MEd, OTR
Susan L. Pierce, OTR, CDRS
Carolyn Robinson Podolski, MS, OTR/L
Lee Ann Quintana, MS, OTR
Mary Vining Radomski, MA, OTR
COL Valerie Rice, PhD, OTR/L, CPE
Patricia Rigby, MHSc, OT(C)
Joyce Shapero Sabari, PhD, OTR, BCN
Shoshana Shamberg, MSEd, OTR/L
Jo M. Solet, EdM, PhD, OTR/L
Debra Stewart, MSc, OT(C)
Susan Strong, MSc, OT(C)
Linda Tickle-Degnen, PhD, OTR/L

Catherine A. Trombly, ScD, OTR/L
Anne M. Woodson, BS, OTR
Y. Lynn Yasuda, MSEd, OTR
Ruth Zemke, PhD, OTR

Sixth Edition

Anne Armstrong, MA, OTR/L
Michal S. Atkins, MA, OTR/L
Wendy Avery, MS, OTR/L
Julie Bass-Haugen, PhD, OTR
Jane Bear-Lehman, PhD, OTR
Karen Bentzel, MS, OTR/L
Bette R. Bonder, PhD, OTR/L
Alfred G. Bracciano, EdD, OTR
Mary Ellen Buning, PhD, OTR, ATP
Nancy Callinan, MA, OTR/L, CHT
Cynthia Cooper, MFA, MA, OTR/L, CHT
Lois Copperman, PhD, OTR(L)
Elin Schold Davis, OTR/L, CDRS
Jean C. Deitz, PhD, OTR/L
Lisa Deshaies, OTR/L, CHT
Brian J. Dudgeon, PhD, OTR/L
Susan E. Fasoli, ScD, OTR/L
Nancy A. Flinn, PhD, OTR/L, BCN
Susan Forwell, PhD, OT(C)
Glenn Goodman, PhD, OTR/L
Julie McLaughlin Gray, PhD (candidate), OTR/L
Carolyn Schmidt Hanson, PhD, OTR/L
Lucinda L. Hugos, MS, PT
Nancy Huntley, OTR/L, CES
Jeanne Jackson, PhD, OTR
Anne Birge James, PhD, OTR/L
Sharon Kurfuerst, EdD, OTR/L
Lori Letts, PhD (abd), OT Reg (Ont)
Kathryn Levit, PhD, OTR/L
Joanna Bertness Lipoma, MOT, OTR
Jaclyn Faglie Low, PhD, OTR
Mandy Lowe, MSc, OT Reg (Ont)
Stephen Luster, MS, OTR/L, CHT
Colleen Maher, MS, OTR/L CHT, MLD
Virgil Mathiowetz, PhD, OTR/L
E. Stuart Oertli, MS, OTR
Karin J. Opacich, PhD, MHPE, OTR/L
Amy C. Orroth, OTR/L, CHT
Monica Pessina, PhD, MEd, OTR
Susan Lanier Pierce, OTR, CDRS, SCDCM
Carolyn Robinson Podolski, MA, OTR, SCDCM
Lee Ann Quintana, MS, OTR/L
Mary Vining Radomski, MA, OTR/L
Valerie Rice, PhD, OTR/L, CPE
Patricia Rigby, MHSc, OT Reg (Ont)
Pamela Roberts, MSHA, OTR/L, CPHQ
Kathy Longenecker Rust, MS, OT
Dory Sabata, OTD, OTR/L
Joyce Shapero Sabari, PhD, OTR, BCN
Shoshana Shamberg, MSEd, OTR/L
Margarette L. Shelton, PhD, OTR
Jo M. Solet, EdM, PhD, OTR/L
Debra Stewart, MSc, OT Reg (Ont)
Kathy Stubblefield, OTR/L
Linda Tickle-Degnen, PhD, OTR/L
Catherine A. Trombly Latham, ScD, OTR/L
Michael Williams, PhD
Anne M. Woodson, BS, OTR
Y. Lynn Yasuda, MSEd, OTR
Ruth Zemke, PhD, OTR

Seventh Edition

Khader A. Almhdawi, PhD, OT
Mattie Anheluk, MOT, OTR/L
Michal S. Atkins, MA, OTR/L
Wendy W. Avery, MS, OTR/L
Julie D. Bass, PhD, OTR/L, FAOTA
MAJ Priscillia D. Bejarano, MA, OTR/L, CHT
Karen Bentzel, MS, OTR/L
Bette R. Bonder, PhD, OTR/L, FAOTA
F. D. Blade Branham, PT, DPT, CHT
Mary Ellen Buning, PhD, OTR/L, ATP/SMS
Nettie Capasso, MA, OTR/L
Cynthia Cooper, MFA, MA, OTR/L, CHT
Lois F. Copperman, PhD, OTR
Oana Craciunoiu, MSc, OT Reg. (Ont.)
Jean C. Deitz, PhD, OTR, FAOTA
Lisa D. Deshaies, OTR/L, CHT
Margaret R. Dimpfel, MOT, OTR/L, ATP
Claire-Jehanne Dubouloz, PhD, OT Reg. (Ont.), FCAOT
Brian J. Dudgeon, PhD, OTR, FAOTA
Mary Y. Egan, PhD, OT Reg. (Ont.), FCAOT
LTC Andrew J. Fabrizio, MS, OTR/L, CHT
Susan E. Fasoli, ScD, OTR/L
Rachel Feld-Glazman, MS, OTR/L
Nancy A. Flinn, PhD, OTR/L
Susan J. Forwell, PhD, OT(C), FCAOT
Setareh Ghahari, PhD, MSc, BSc (OT)
Gordon Muir Giles, PhD, OTR/L, FAOTA
Glenn D. Goodman, PhD, OTR/L
Kim Grabe, MA, OTR/L
Alison Hammond, PhD, OT
Carolyn Schmidt Hanson, PhD, OTR
Shayne E. Hopkins, OTR/L
Lucinda L. Hugos, MS, PT
Nancy Huntley, OTR/L, CES
Anne Birge James, PhD, OTR/L
Jennifer Kaldenberg, MSA, OTR/L, SCLV, FAOTA
Kathryn Levit, PhD, OTR/L
Colleen Maher, OTD, OTR/L, CHT
Virgil G. Mathiowetz, PhD, OTR/L, FAOTA
MAJ Sarah Mitsch, OTR/L
M. Tracy Morrison, OTD, OTR/L
Karin J. Opacich, PhD, MHPE, OTR/L, FAOTA
Amy Clara Orroth, OTR/L, CHT
Monica Ann Pessina, OTR, MEd, PhD
Susan Pierce, OTR, SCDCM, CDRS
Catherine Verrier Piersol, PhD, OTR/L
Janet M. Powell, PhD, OTR/L, FAOTA
MAJ Charles D. Quick, MS, OTR/L, CHT
Mary Vining Radomski, PhD, OTR/L, FAOTA
MAJ Jose Rafols, OTD, MHSA, OTR/L
Valerie J. Berg Rice, PhD, MHA, MS, CPE, OTR/L, FAOTA
Patricia Rigby, PhD, MSc
Pamela Roberts, PhD, OTR/L, SCFES, FAOTA, CPHQ
Kathy Longenecker Rust, MS, OT
Joyce Shapero Sabari, PhD, OTR, FAOTA
Dory Sabata, OTD, OTR/L, SCEM
Jo M. Solet, MS, EdM, PhD, OTR/L
Jennifer L. Theis, MS, OTR/L
Linda Tickle-Degnen, PhD, OTR/L, FAOTA
Catherine A. Trombly Latham, ScD, OT(retired), FAOTA
Lisa Smurr Walters, MS, OTR/L, CHT
Orli M. Weisser-Pike, OTR/L, CLVT, SCLV
Lynsay R. Whelan, OTR/L
Christine M. Wietlisbach, OTD, OTR/L, CHT, MPA
Anne M. Woodson, OTR
MAJ(P) Kathleen E. Yancosek, PhD, OTR/L, CHT
Joette Zola, OTR/L, STAR-C

Contributing Authors of Eighth Edition

Debbie Amini, EdD, OTR/L, FAOTA
Director of Professional Development
American Occupational Therapy Association
Bethesda, Maryland

Mattie Anheluk, MOT, OTR/L
Occupational Therapist
Courage Kenny Comprehensive Outpatient Rehabilitation
Courage Kenny Rehabilitation Institute
Minneapolis, Minnesota

Wendy Avery, MS, OTR/L
Occupational Therapist
Amedisys Home Health
Bluffton, South Carolina

Christine P. Below, OTR/L
Adjunct Faculty
Department of Occupational Therapy
Western Michigan University
Kalamazoo, Michigan

Sue Berger, PhD, OTR/L, FAOTA
Clinical Associate Professor Emeritus
Department of Occupational Therapy
Sargent College of Health & Rehabilitation Sciences
Boston University
Boston, Massachusetts

Angela K. Boisselle, PhD, OTR, ATP
Utilization Management Therapy Supervisor
Cook Children's Health Care System
Fort Worth, Texas

Michael J. Borst, OTD, OTR, CHT
Associate Professor of Occupational Therapy
Concordia University Wisconsin
Mequon, Wisconsin

Alfred G. Bracciano, MSA, EdD, OTR/L, FAOTA
Professor
Department of Occupational Therapy
School of Pharmacy and Health Professions
Creighton University
Omaha, Nebraska

Deborah E. Budash, PhD, OTR/L
Assistant Professor
Department of Occupational Therapy
University of Scranton
Scranton, Pennsylvania

Anne Carney, MS, CCC-SLP
Lecturer
Department of Speech, Language & Hearing Sciences
Sargent College of Health & Rehabilitation Sciences
Boston University
Boston, Massachusetts

Ginger Carroll, MS, OT/L
Research Coordinator
Courage Kenny Research Center
Minneapolis, Minnesota

Kara Christy, MS, OTR/L, CBIS
Occupational Therapy Clinical Supervisor
Origami Brain Injury Rehabilitation Center
Mason, Michigan

Carrie Ciro, PhD, OTR/L, FAOTA
Associate Professor and Chair
Department of Occupational Therapy Education
School of Health Professions
The University of Kansas Medical Center
Kansas City, Kansas

Sherrilene Classen, PhD, MOH, OTR/L, FAOTA, FGSA
Chair and Professor
Department of Occupational Therapy
College of Public Health and Health Professions
University of Florida
Gainesville, Florida

Taliah Cook, OTD, OTR/L
Occupational Therapist
Bayada Home Care
Wilmington, Delaware

Anne Crites, OTR/L
Academic Fieldwork Coordinator, Associate Professor
Occupational Therapy Assistant Program
Division of Health Sciences
Mott Community College
Fenton, Michigan

Lori DeMott, OTD, OTR/L, CHT
Associate Faculty, Lecturer
Occupational Therapy Division
The Ohio State University Wexner Medical Center
Columbus, Ohio

Diane Powers Dirette, PhD, OTL, FAOTA
Editor-in-Chief *The Open Journal of Occupational Therapy*
Professor
Department of Occupational Therapy
Western Michigan University
Kalamazoo, Michigan

Rosanne DiZazzo-Miller, PhD, OTRL, CDP, FMiOTA
Associate Professor
Department of Occupational Therapy
Wayne State University
Eugene Applebaum College of Pharmacy & Health Sciences
Detroit, Michigan

Catherine Donnelly, PhD, OT
Associate Professor
School of Rehabilitation Therapy
Queen's University
Kingston, Ontario, Canada

Barbara M. Doucet, PhD, LOTR
Associate Professor
Department of Occupational Therapy
School of Allied Health Professions
Louisiana State University Health New Orleans
New Orleans, Louisiana

Anne Escher, OTD, OTR
Clinical Assistant Professor
Department of Occupational Therapy
Sargent College of Health & Rehabilitation Sciences
Boston University
Boston, Massachusetts

Jennifer Fortuna, MS, OTRL
Assistant Professor
Department of Occupational Science and Therapy
Grand Valley State University
Grand Rapids, Michigan

Susan J. Forwell, PhD, OT, FCAOT
Professor and Head
Department of Occupational Science and Occupational Therapy
Research Associate
MS-NMO Clinic, Division of Neurology, Department of Medicine
Faculty of Medicine
University of British Columbia
Vancouver, British Columbia, Canada

Kris M. Gellert, BS, C/NDT, OTR/L
Neurorehabilitation Supervisor
Occupational Rehabilitation
Cone Health System
Greensboro, North Carolina
Member, Board of Directors, Executive Committee
Neuro-Developmental Treatment Association
Laguna Beach, California

Patricia A. Gentile, DPS, OTR/L
Clinical Assistant Professor
Department of Occupational Therapy
Steinhardt School of Culture, Education, and Human Development
New York University
New York, New York

Setareh Ghahari, BSc, MSc, PhD, OT Reg. (Ont.)
Assistant Professor
Occupational Therapy Program, School of Rehabilitation Therapy
Queen's University
Kingston, Ontario, Canada

Gordon Muir Giles, PhD, OTR/L, FAOTA
Professor
Department of Occupational Therapy
Samuel Merritt University
Oakland, California
Director of Neurobehavioral Services
Crestwood Treatment Center
Fremont, California

Glen Gillen, EdD, OTR/L, FAOTA
Professor and Director, Programs in Occupational Therapy
Vice Chair, Department of Rehabilitation and Regenerative Medicine
Assistant Dean, Vagelos College of Physicians and Surgeons
Columbia University
New York, New York

Julie L. Grabanski, PhD, OTR/L
Associate Professor
Department of Occupational Therapy
School of Medicine and Health Sciences
University of North Dakota
Grand Forks, North Dakota

Lenin C. Grajo, PhD, EdM, OTR/L
Assistant Professor
Programs in Occupational Therapy
Department of Rehabilitation and Regenerative Medicine
Vagelos College of Physicians and Surgeons
Columbia University
New York, New York

Kimatha Oxford Grice, OTD, OTR, CHT
Associate Professor and Distinguished Teaching Professor
Department of Occupational Therapy
University of Texas Health Science Center
San Antonio, Texas

Sharon A. Gutman, PhD, OTR, FAOTA
Professor
Programs in Occupational Therapy
Department of Rehabilitation and Regenerative Medicine
Vagelos College of Physicians and Surgeons
Columbia University
New York, New York

Pamela Hewitt, MS, OTR/L
Clinical Assistant Professor
Department of Occupational Therapy
Quinnipiac University
Hamden, Connecticut

Mary W. Hildebrand, OTD, OTR/L
Associate Professor
Department of Occupational Therapy
MGH Institute of Health Professions
Boston, Massachusetts

Midge Hobbs, MA, OTR/L
IMPACT Course Coordinator/Adjunct Faculty
Center for Interprofessional Studies and Innovation
MGH Institute of Health Professions
Boston, Massachusetts

Nancy S. Hock, PhD (cand), MOT, OTRL, CHT
Master Faculty Specialist and Site Coordinator
Department of Occupational Therapy
Western Michigan University
Grand Rapids, Michigan

Natasha Huffine, MS, OTR/L, CBIS
Clinical Manager/Occupational Therapist
Origami Brain Injury Rehabilitation Center
Mason, Michigan

Lucinda L. Hugos, MS, PT
Associate Professor
Department of Neurology
Oregon Health & Science University
Portland, Oregon
Research Scientist
VA Portland Health Care System
Portland, Oregon

Sclinda L. Janssen, PhD, OTR/L, CLA
Associate Professor
Department of Occupational Therapy
School of Medicine and Health Sciences
University of North Dakota
Grand Forks, North Dakota

Michelle L. Lange, OTR/L, ABDA, ATP/SMS
Access to Independence, Inc.
Arvada, Colorado

Catherine A. Trombly Latham, Sc.D., OT (retired), FAOTA
Professor Emerita
Department of Occupational Therapy
College of Health and Rehabilitation Sciences: Sargent College
Boston University
Boston, Massachusetts

Kelly Lewis, MS, OTR/L
Adjunct Faculty
Department of Occupational Therapy
Western Michigan University
Kalamazoo, Michigan

Debra K. Lindstrom, PhD, OTR/L, FAOTA
Professor
Department of Occupational Therapy
Western Michigan University
Kalamazoo, Michigan

Alicia Flores Lohmann, OTD, MOT, OTR, CBIS, ATP
Neurologic Music Therapy Trained
Associate Clinical Professor
Texas Woman's University School of Occupational Therapy
Houston, Texas

Colleen Maher, OTD, OTR/L, CHT
Assistant Professor
Department of Occupational Therapy
Samson College of Health Sciences
University of the Sciences
Philadelphia, Pennsylvania

Cara Masselink, MS, OTR/L, ATP
Clinical Supervisor of Occupational Therapy
Department of Occupational Therapy
Western Michigan University
Kalamazoo, Michigan

Guy L. McCormack, PhD, OTR/L, FAOTA
Associate Professor
Department of Occupational Therapy
University of the Pacific
Sacramento, California
Professor Emeritus
Samuel Merritt University
Oakland, California

Rochelle J. Mendonca, PhD, OTR/L
Assistant Professor
Programs in Occupational Therapy
Department of Rehabilitation and Regenerative Medicine
Vagelos College of Physicians and Surgeons
Columbia University
New York, New York

Allison Chamberlain Miller, MS, OTR/L
Associate Editor
The Open Journal of Occupational Therapy
Clinical Faculty Specialist
Department of Occupational Therapy
Western Michigan University
Kalamazoo, Michigan

Marianne H. Mortera, PhD, OTR/L
Independent Health Care Provider
New York, New York

Dawn M. Nilsen, EdD, OTR/L, FAOTA
Associate Professor
Programs in Occupational Therapy
Department of Rehabilitation and Regenerative Medicine
Vagelos College of Physicians and Surgeons
Columbia University
New York, New York

Rebecca Ozelie, DHS, OTR/L
Associate Professor
Academic Fieldwork Coordinator
Occupational Therapy
Rush University
Chicago, Illinois

Anita Perr, PhD, OT/L, ATP, FAOTA
Clinical Associate Professor
Department of Occupational Therapy
New York University
New York, New York

Beth Pfeiffer, PhD, OTR/L, BCP, FAOTA
Associate Professor
Rehabilitation Sciences
Temple University
Philadelphia, Pennsylvania

Pat Precin, PhD, PsyaD, NCPsyA, LP, OTR/L, FAOTA
Assistant Professor
Programs in Occupational Therapy
Department of Rehabilitation and Regenerative Medicine
Vagelos College of Physicians and Surgeons
Columbia University
New York, New York

Karen Halliday Pulaski, MS, OTR/L
Staff Therapist
Cone Health Neurorehabilitation Center
Greensboro, North Carolina

Mary Vining Radomski, PhD, OTR/L, FAOTA
Senior Scientific Advisor
Courage Kenny Research Center
Minneapolis, Minnesota

Gayle J. Restall, OT Reg (MB), PhD
Associate Professor
Department of Occupational Therapy
College of Rehabilitation Sciences
University of Manitoba
Winnipeg, Manitoba, Canada

Veronica T. Rowe, PhD, OTR/L
Assistant Professor
Department of Occupational Therapy
University of Central Arkansas
Conway, Arkansas

Preethy S. Samuel, PhD, OTRL
Associate Professor of Occupational Therapy
Department of Health Care Sciences
Wayne State University
Detroit, Michigan

Martha J. Sanders, PhD, MSOSH, OTR/L, CPE
Professor
Department of Occupational Therapy
Quinnipiac University
Hamden, Connecticut

Susan Santalucia, MS, OTR/L
Occupational Therapist
Department of Occupational Therapy
Jefferson College of Rehabilitation
Thomas Jefferson University
Philadelphia, Pennsylvania

Brigette Vachon, PhD, OT
Associate Professor
Occupational Therapy Program, School of Rehabilitation, Faculty of Medicine
Université de Montréal
Montreal, Quebec, Canada

Tracy Van Oss, DHSc, MPH, OTR/L, FAOTA
Clinical Professor and Academic Coordinator
Department of Occupational Therapy
Quinnipiac University
Hamden, Connecticut

Laura VanPuymbrouck, PhD, OTR/L
Assistant Professor
Department of Occupational Therapy
Rush University
Chicago, Illinois

Asha K. Vas, PhD, OT, CBIST
Assistant Professor
School of Occupational Therapy
Texas Woman's University
Dallas, Texas

Lisa Smurr Walters, MS, OTR, CHT
Clinical Therapy Specialist—Upper Limb Prosthetics
Arm Dynamics
Houston, Texas

Lee Ann Westover, MS, OTR/L
Clinical Fieldwork Instructor
Programs in Occupational Therapy
Department of Rehabilitation and Regenerative Medicine
Vagelos College of Physicians and Surgeons
Columbia University
New York, New York

Sunny R. Winstead, EdD, OTR/L
Assistant Professor
Division of Occupational Therapy
Keuka College
Keuka Park, New York

Tracey L. Zeiner, OTD, OTR/L
Clinical Instructor
Department of Occupational Therapy
University of Central Arkansas
Conway, Arkansas

Joette Zola, OTR/L
Cancer Cognitive Impairment Team Lead
Courage Kenny Rehabilitation Institute
Minneapolis, Minnesota

User's Guide

Framework

The eighth edition uses the framework established by Catherine A. Trombly Latham, who also wrote the first two chapters. This new edition is clear, concise, and streamlined with the inclusion of the essential information for occupational therapists in the physical dysfunction setting.

Conceptual Foundations for Practice

Catherine A. Trombly Latham

Occupation: Philosophy and Concepts

Catherine A. Trombly Latham

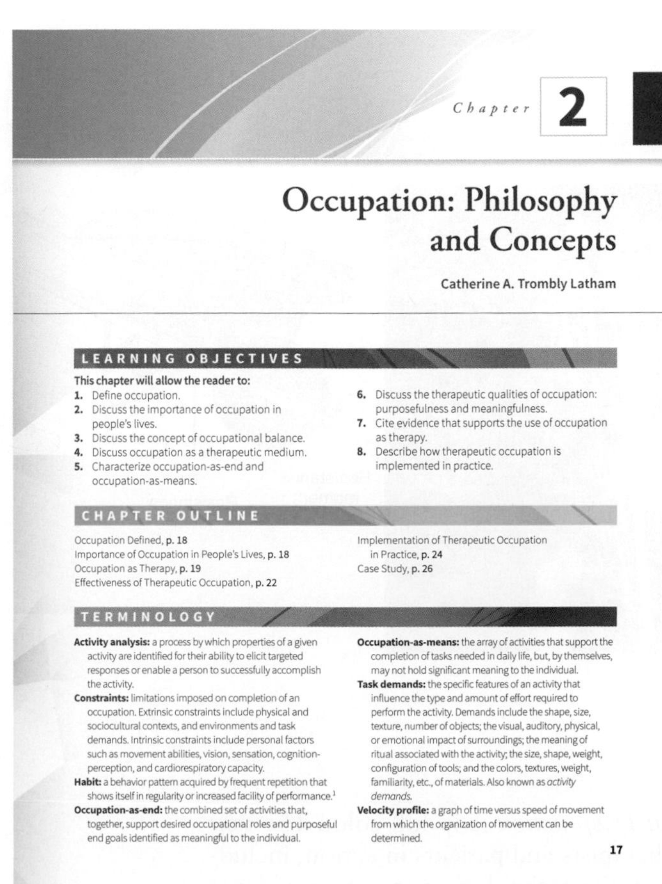

Chapter 2

Occupation: Philosophy and Concepts

Catherine A. Trombly Latham

LEARNING OBJECTIVES

This chapter will allow the reader to:

1. Define occupation.
2. Discuss the importance of occupation in people's lives.
3. Discuss the concept of occupational balance.
4. Discuss occupation as a therapeutic medium.
5. Characterize occupation-as-end and occupation-as-means.
6. Discuss the therapeutic qualities of occupation: purposefulness and meaningfulness.
7. Cite evidence that supports the use of occupation as therapy.
8. Describe how therapeutic occupation is implemented in practice.

CHAPTER OUTLINE

TERMINOLOGY

Activity analysis: a process by which properties of a given activity are identified for their ability to elicit targeted responses or enable a person to successfully accomplish the activity.

Constraints: limitations imposed on completion of an occupation. Extrinsic constraints include physical and sociocultural contexts, and environments and task demands. Intrinsic constraints include personal factors such as movement abilities, vision, sensation, cognition-perception, and cardiorespiratory capacity.

Habit: a behavior pattern acquired by frequent repetition that shows itself in regularity or increased facility of performance.[1]

Occupation-as-end: the combined set of activities that, together, support desired occupational roles and purposeful end goals identified as meaningful to the individual.

Occupation-as-means: the array of activities that support the completion of tasks needed in daily life, but, by themselves, may not hold significant meaning to the individual.

Task demands: the specific features of an activity that influence the type and amount of effort required to perform the activity. Demands include the shape, size, texture, number of objects; the visual, auditory, physical, or emotional impact of surroundings; the meaning of ritual associated with the activity; the size, shape, weight, configuration of tools; and the colors, textures, weight, familiarity, etc., of materials. Also known as *activity demands.*

Velocity profile: a graph of time versus speed of movement from which the organization of movement can be determined.

17

Learning Objectives, Chapter Outline, and Terminology

Each chapter begins with Learning Objectives that provide an overview of the content to follow. Chapter Outlines offer an overview of each chapter's content. Key terms and definitions for each chapter are presented in the Terminology list.

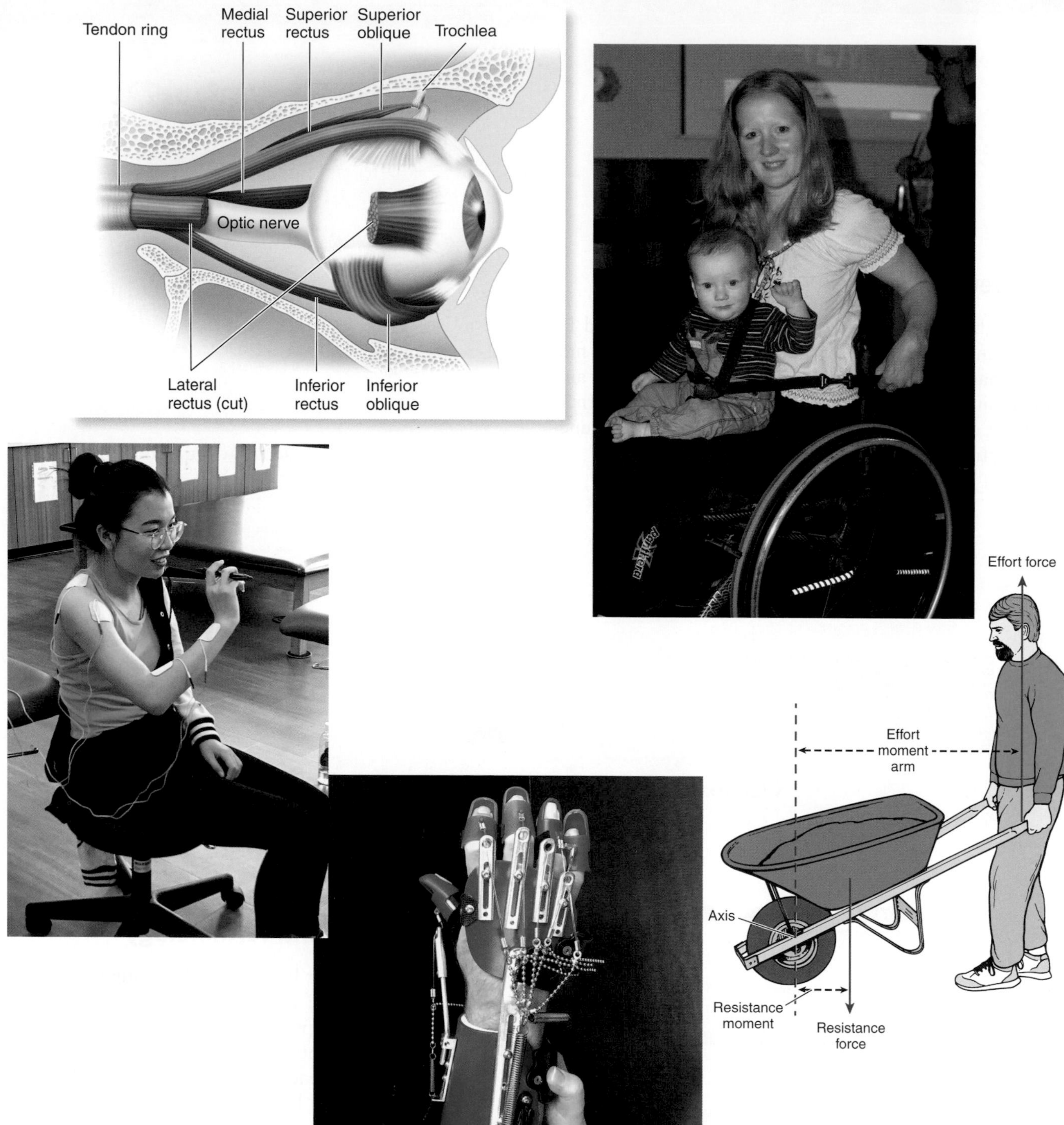

All New Full-Color Art Program

For the first time, *Occupational Therapy for Physical Dysfunction* is in full color. The text contains hundreds of photos showing occupational therapists and patients in action, including assessments, interventions, equipment, orthoses, assistive technology, restoration of function, and disease-specific conditions.

Case Study

Each chapter ends with a Case Study that addresses Patient Information, Assessment Process and Results, Occupational Therapy Problem List, Occupational Therapy Goal List, and Intervention.

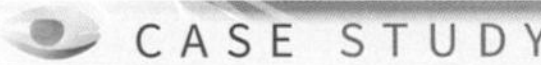

CASE STUDY

Patient Information

Gordon is a 78-year-old retired high school teacher, director of a high school vocational program, and carpenter who experienced a stroke related to carotid artery angioplasty with stenting. The stroke resulted in hemiparesis of his right, dominant side that affected balance, weight shift, and right UE strength and coordination. The emergency room doctor conducted the Mini-Mental State Examination (MMSE) where Gordon scored 20/30, which indicated mild cognitive impairment. He was in the hospital for 3 days and then returned home to independent living with his wife. While still in the hospital, Gordon lost his balance and fell in the bathroom while bending and rotating. He stated, "This stroke caused my right arm and hand to be a dish rag."

Assessment Process and Results

The occupational therapist met with Gordon for evaluation and intervention. One of the first things he told the occupational therapist was that he could not drive because he could not turn the key in the ignition or hold the steering wheel with his right hand. The occupational therapist used multiple tools for the assessment process, including patient interview, Activity Card Sort, the MMSE, biomechanical assessments (9-Hold Peg Test, power of grasp, tensiometer, ROM), and the Mini-Balance Evaluation Systems Test (Mini-BEST).

Results indicated that Gordon was also having difficulty brushing his teeth, buttoning his sleeve cuffs, and holding a spoon to scoop grapefruit pieces, which he reported eating daily to lower his cholesterol. He periodically verbalized concern about his inability to manipulate grapefruit pieces, suggesting that this was an important goal to target. Gordon was independent in all other self-care tasks. He additionally desired to complete his own home maintenance, such as lawn mowing. Gordon's occupational interests included carpentry, such as remodeling his daughter's basement, which required the ability to use tools such as a drill, trowel, and hammer; model airplane building and flying; and playing music with piano, guitar, and harmonica.

Since his initial hospitalization, Gordon's MMSE score improved to 28/30, indicating no cognitive impairment. Scores on the 9-Hole Peg Test were 50 seconds right and 30 seconds left UE. Scores for power of grasp were 10 lb on the right and 60 lb on the left. Scores for lateral grasp were 3 lb on the right and 20 lb on the left. ROM was within normal limits throughout both UEs but a slight movement delay was present in the right UE. Score for the Mini-BEST was 24/28 because of limitations in reactive postural control.

Occupational Therapy Problem List

- Difficulty feeding self with utensils, especially when scooping grapefruit because of right hand weakness and limited coordination
- Difficulty brushing teeth because of right hand weakness and limited coordination and postural instability
- Difficulty with home maintenance, such as lawn mowing, because of balance impairment and weak grasp to pull the mower starter cord
- Difficulty driving because of right hand weakness and limited coordination

Occupational Therapy Goal List

During selection of occupation-as-end activities, the therapist asked Gordon which activities were the most immediately important to him. He prioritized the following goals:

- Gordon will demonstrate modified independence in feeding himself with utensils, especially scooping grapefruit, with 10 lb lateral grasp, 15 lb power of grasp, and normal coordination within 2 weeks.
- Gordon will demonstrate independence in brushing teeth with 15 lb power of grasp, normal fine motor coordination, and intact reactive postural control with transitional movements to set up items needed within 1 month.
- Gordon will be able to start his lawn mower and mow his lawn with intact balance and weight shift within 1 month.
- Gordon will demonstrate independence in driving as evidenced by 10 lb of lateral grasp in order to turn the key in the car ignition within 1 month.

Intervention

To enhance performance of each occupation, it was important to target hand and finger strength, fine motor coordination, and balance with transitional movements. During the second visit, the therapist developed a bank of intervention activities that Gordon could perform within his natural environment including carpentry tasks, lawn mowing, brushing teeth, playing piano and guitar, and feeding himself grapefruit. The therapist used a neurodevelopmental treatment (NDT) frame of reference, while also integrating task-specific motor learning in which specific activity aspects were analyzed and modified to promote repetition, duration, specificity, and intensity.

The therapist initiated patient education during simulations of several meaningful activities that Gordon identified. For example, the therapist found a drill, screws, and wood from the maintenance department to show Gordon how to incorporate weight bearing on his affected, extended right UE. The drill handle was large, which facilitated Gordon's ability to grasp it. His grip strength, however, was too weak to hold the drill upright against gravity, as would be required to push screws into a wall. To grade the task to a lower challenge level, the therapist instructed Gordon to hold the drill downward so that gravity could assist when pushing the screw into the wood. With practice, Gordon gained the ability to activate the power switch with his right index finger. He used his left hand to precisely hold the screw when initially drilling it into the wood, followed by a two-handed method (both hands on the drill) to finish drilling the screw into the wood.

Evidence Tables

Many chapters include an Evidence table at the end that collects the best evidence for interventions in the topic area.

Evidence Table of Studies Involving Occupational Therapy Selection, Gradation, and Adaptation of Occupation

Intervention	Description	Participants	Dosage	Research Design and Evidence Level	Benefit	Statistical Significance and Effect Size
Comparative effectiveness of (1) combined therapeutic exercise and occupation-based activities and (2) therapeutic exercise alone[19]	Group #1: Picking up small everyday objects, typing on a keyboard, washing and wiping dishes in addition to therapeutic exercises in both hand therapy sessions and home program Group #2: Therapeutic exercises in both hand therapy sessions and home program	46 patients with UE injuries treated in outpatient hand occupational therapy clinic	10 weeks of therapy: supervised hand therapy 1-hour sessions, 2 times/week; and home exercise program 120 minutes, once a week	Randomized controlled trial. Level I	Combined intervention had better outcomes, including reduced pain, improved AAROM in fingers, subjective functional status, and subjective performance and satisfaction of performance	Combined intervention showed statistically significant improvement in outcome measures compared to therapeutic exercise group: DASH score ($p < 0.02$), total active motion ($p < 0.01$), neuropathic pain ($p < 0.02$), COPM performance ($p < 0.001$), COPM satisfaction ($p < 0.001$) Effect size not reported
Comparative effectiveness of occupation-based intervention and rote exercise[8]	Group #1: Immobilization of healthy hand using therapeutic occupations for intervention Group #2: Immobilization of healthy hand during rote exercise of affected hand Control Group #3: No immobilization of healthy hand while practicing different movements and activities	36 outpatients (22–55 years old)	Groups #1 and 2 received intervention 3 hours each day, 3 days/week, over 4 weeks	Randomized controlled trial. Level I	Compared to rote exercise, occupation-based group had better performance in objective and subjective measures, motivation, satisfaction with and perception of performance, and continued improvement at follow-up	Post hoc analyses revealed significant difference among all three groups with most increased mean change for occupation-based group ($p < 0.01$) Effect size not reported
Comparative effectiveness between combined (1) resistive exercises, functional exercises, and ADLs, and (2) resistive exercises[22]	Group #1: Combination of resistance exercise, functional exercise, and ADL exercise Group #2: Resistance exercise	52 older adults, mean age = 73 years	Measured at baseline, postintervention, and 6-months follow-up	Randomized controlled trial. Level I	Postintervention improvement was found within groups but not between groups. At 6-month follow-up, a decline in resistance exercise group was found. Combined exercise group continued to show improvement. More adverse events (soreness, pain) for resistance exercise group	Combined intervention group (mean change = 0.29, $p < 0.02$); resistance exercise group (mean change = 0.24, $p < 0.13$). At 6 months postintervention, combined intervention group showed within-group *mean change* of 0.37 ($p < 0.01$)
Comparative effectiveness between occupation-based intervention and repetitive task practice[20]	Group #1: Focused on performance of occupations with facilitation methods Group #2: Focused on 10–50 repetitions of each task	16 (21–69 years old) in chronic phase of stroke recovery	Measured at baseline and postintervention. Interventions were 55-minute sessions, 2 times/week for 4 weeks for both groups	Pilot randomized controlled trial comparative study with parallel group block design. Level I	Improvements in occupational performance and motor performance in both groups were similar. Authors suggested engagement greater and demand greater in occupation-based group because of meaningfulness and multijoint activities	Although within-group changes after intervention were found for both groups ($p < 0.0001$), no between-group differences were found. Effect size not reported

ADLs, activities of daily living; UE, upper extremity.

Most Commonly Used Standardized Assessments

Instrument and Reference	Intended Purpose	Administration Time	Validity	Reliability	Sensitivity	Strengths and Weaknesses
Baking Tray Task[25,26]	Used to assess for unilateral spatial neglect	<10 minutes	Found to detect more cases of neglect than the three-item Behavioral Inattention Test and is even more accurate when used in combination with the Line Bisection Test	Test–retest 0.87	Increased through combination with other tests; more sensitive than the three-item Behavioral Inattention Test	Easy to administer. Most sensitive single test to detect spatial neglect. Easy and cost-effective to create your own with the measurements provided. Not a lot of depth to the test or scoring. Assumed cognitive impairment if spatial neglect is not present.
Line Bisection Test[27]	Used to detect unilateral spatial neglect	<5 minutes	Convergent validity with Baking Tray Task: $r = -0.66$	Test–retest reliability: 0.97 Internal consistency: no evidence	Detects spatial neglect with 76.4% accuracy	Many versions; however, the procedures are rarely standardized.
Trail Making A and B[28–30]	Used to assess visual conceptual and visuomotor tracking conditions	5–10 minutes	Construct validity for rapid visual search and visual sequencing. Trails A: Visual perceptual abilities Trails B: working memory and task switching	Test–retest reliability: Test A: $r = 0.83$ Test B: $r = 0.90$	Functional MRI studies demonstrate activation of the ventral and dorsal visual processing streams	Public domain assessment is easy to administer and obtain. Some versions have therapist correct mistakes along the way.
Bell's Test[31,32]	Quick screen for visual neglect in the near extrapersonal space	<5 minutes	Criterion Validity: more likely to evidence left neglect than Albert's Test, Star Cancellation Test, Line Bisection Test, and Line Crossing Test	No evidence	No evidence	The Bell's Test requires no specialized training to administer and only minimal equipment is required (a pencil, a stopwatch, the test paper, and scoring sheet). The test is simple to score and interpret.
Motor-Free Visual Perception Test (MVPT-3)[10,33]	Widely used standardized test of visual perception, assessing visual perception independent of motor ability	20–30 minutes	Criterion related: 0.78 with the DTVP-2 and 0.73 with the DTVP	Internal consistency: 0.86–0.90 Test–retest: 0.92	General measure for motor-free visual perceptual components	Does not provide norms for separate subtests. Short and simple measure that is tolerated well by most clients.

Assessment Tables

The chapters focused on assessment include an Assessment table that collects the most commonly used standardized assessments for the topic area.

Contents

Chapter 1

Conceptual Foundations for Practice

Catherine A. Trombly Latham

LEARNING OBJECTIVES

This chapter will allow the reader to:

1. Describe the *Occupational Functioning Model* (OFM).
2. Relate the American Occupational Therapy Association's *Occupational Therapy Practice Framework* (OTPF) to the OFM.
3. Use the language of the *OFM* and the American Occupational Therapy Association's *OTPF* interchangeably.
4. Organize assessment and treatment planning according to the *OFM*.

CHAPTER OUTLINE

TERMINOLOGY

Ability: a general trait an individual brings to learning a new task.[1]

Activity (activities): in the *Occupational Functioning Model* (OFM), activities are considered small units of goal-directed behavior that make up tasks. The *Occupational Therapy Practice Framework* defines activity as a class of human actions that are goal directed; the term *occupation* encompasses activity.[2]

Activity analysis: the basic process used by occupational therapists to identify the properties inherent in a given occupation, task, or activity, as well as the skills, abilities, and capacities required to complete it. Activity analysis is used to analyze performance; to select occupations to remediate deficient capacities and abilities, or, knowing the person's skills, abilities, and capacities; to modify an activity or environment to ensure successful completion of the activity.

Adaptive therapy: an intervention that promotes a balance among a person's goals, capabilities, and environmental demands by use of assistive technology, adaptation of the environment or methods of accomplishing an activity, and/or redefinition of goals.

Augmented maturation: the therapeutic techniques that challenge further development of first-level capacities or developed capacities. Such techniques include controlled sensory stimulation and activities that promote responses in developmental postures or patterns.

Capacities: potential attributes that, once developed into abilities and skills, will contribute to occupational functioning. Capacities are the basis of performance.

Context: the interrelated conditions in which something exists or occurs.[3] Context is the personal, social, cultural, physical, temporal, and situational dimensions in which occupation occurs and may be fully understood.

Environment: the tangible objects, structures, or conditions by which one is surrounded and in which one's daily occupations occur. In the OFM, environment is considered the encompassing surround in which the person accomplishes the activities and tasks of his or her life.

Impairment: any significant deviation or loss of body structure or physiological or psychological function.

Occupation-as-end: occupation that is the functional goal (activity, task) to be learned or accomplished. Through repeated carrying out of an occupation ("task-specific training"), the patient will relearn the actions and routine of an activity, or through adaptation, the activity will be made possible for the person, given his or her current capacities and abilities.

Occupation-as-means: the therapeutic change agent to remediate impaired abilities or capacities.

Occupational balance: the distribution of occupations within a person's life. When the occupations are balanced, the person perceives him- or herself to be healthy or stress free; too much or too little of an occupation or type of occupation is unhealthy. The dimension through which satisfactory balance may be achieved differs for different people and at different times in a person's life. Dimensions identified to date are time (hours spent in self-care, play, work, and rest, for example), degree of difficulty (challenging occupation vs. relaxing occupation), and degree of self-focus (occupation is meaningful for the person vs. being meaningful for others; care of one's self vs. care of others).[4,5]

Occupational dysfunction: the inability to accomplish a necessary or desired occupational goal because of either impairment of abilities and skills or environmental barriers. Occupational dysfunction is the focus of occupational therapy.[4]

Occupational Functioning Model: a conceptual model that guides occupational therapy evaluation and treatment of persons with occupational dysfunction secondary to physical dysfunction. The particulars of the model are as follows: (1) To engage satisfactorily in a life role, a person must be able to do the tasks that, in his or her opinion, make up that role. (2) Tasks are composed of activities, which are smaller units of behavior. (3) To be able to do a given activity, one must have certain sensorimotor, cognitive, perceptual, emotional, and social abilities. (4) Abilities are developed from capacities that the person has gained through learning or maturation. (5) Developed capacities depend on first-level capacities that derive from a person's genetic endowment or spared organic substrate.[6,7]

Self-efficacy: the perceived capability to perform a behavior. It is the belief in personal competence.[8]

Skill: competence in doing.[3]

Introduction

Students may wonder how occupational therapists know what to do when a person with **occupational dysfunction** secondary to a disease or injury that results in physical **impairment** is referred to them. First, therapists have *specific knowledge* about what the diagnosis means in terms of limitations of bodily structure or function and subsequent probable limitation of occupational performance and they know the effectiveness of interventions available—the evidence base of practice. Second, they have *specific skills* for assessing and treating persons with occupational dysfunction secondary to physical impairment. Third, they know *how therapy is organized*—the conceptual foundation for practice. The organization or process of occupational therapy is found in various conceptual models of practice. An occupational therapy model of practice describes the interrelatedness of personal characteristics, environment, and occupational goals to guide assessment and intervention.

The American Occupational Therapy Association's (AOTA) *Occupational Therapy Practice Framework* (OTPF) is meant to be used in conjunction with conceptual models of practice. That framework describes the domain and process of the entire practice of occupational therapy.[2] The framework aims to standardize the language of the domain and process of occupational therapy. Because the framework is not a conceptual model, it is expected that occupational therapists will apply pertinent aspects of the framework through the particular conceptual model they choose to guide their practice. Therapists may choose from among many different conceptual models of practice in order to put the framework into practice. This textbook has chosen the **Occupational Functioning Model (OFM)** to conceptualize the process of occupational therapy for persons with physical dysfunction. How, then, do the *OTPF* and the OFM relate? What are their similarities and differences? The language and process of the two are comparable (Tables 1-1 and 1-2). They share some commonalities and differ on others (Table 1-3).

The Occupational Functioning Model

The OFM guides assessment and treatment of persons with physical dysfunction, leading to competence in occupational performance and subsequent feelings of self-empowerment. The OFM was derived from clinical

Table 1-1. The Domains of the Occupational Functioning Model and the Occupational Therapy Practice Framework

OCCUPATIONAL FUNCTIONING MODEL	OCCUPATIONAL THERAPY PRACTICE FRAMEWORK[2]
Competence and Satisfaction with Life Roles and Competence in the Performance of Tasks of Life Roles	**Occupations**
Life roles and the tasks that comprise them are defined by the patient or client. Generally, roles fall into one of the following three categories: *Self-maintenance roles*—These roles maintain self, family, pets, and home, including all BADLs and IADLs associated with self-care; all IADLs associated with care of family; and all IADLs associated with care of home, and other possessions	*BADLs*—Care of one's body including bathing and showering, bowel and bladder management, dressing, swallowing, eating, self-feeding, functional mobility, personal device care, personal hygiene and grooming, sexual activity, and toilet hygiene *IADLs*—Activities to support daily life in the home and community including care of others, child rearing, care of pets, communication management, community mobility, financial management, health management and maintenance, home establishment and management, meal preparation and cleanup, religious observance, safety and emergency maintenance, and shopping *Rest and sleep*—Rest, sleep, sleep preparation, and sleep participation
Self-advancement roles—These roles add to the person's skills, possessions, or other betterment	*Education*—Participation in formal or informal education; exploration of informal educational needs or interests *Work*—Employment interests and pursuits, employment seeking and acquisition, job performance, retirement preparation and adjustment, and volunteer exploration and participation
Self-enhancement roles—These roles contribute to personal accomplishment and enjoyment or sense of well-being and happiness	*Play*—Play exploration and participation *Leisure*—Leisure exploration and participation *Social participation*—Engaging in activities that result in successful interaction at the community, family, or peer/friend levels
Competence in the Performance of Activities and Habits of the Tasks of Life Roles	**Performance Patterns**
Activities—Smaller units of goal-directed behavior that comprise tasks *Habits*—Chains of action sequences acquired by frequent repetition that can be carried out with minimal attention. Therapy aims to sustain useful habits, release useless habits, and develop new habits	*Habits*—Automatic, consistent behavior carried out in familiar situations or environments. Habits can be useful, dominating, or impoverished and either support or interfere with performance in areas of occupation *Routines*—Patterns of behavior that provide structure for daily life *Rituals*—Symbolic actions that contribute to the client's identity and reinforce values and beliefs *Roles*—A set of behaviors expected by society, shaped by culture, and defined by the client
Abilities and Skills	**Performance Skills**
Abilities and skills that are basic to interaction with objects and physical and social environments including: *Motor*—Adequate strength, coordination, range of motion, dexterity, and muscular endurance *Sensory*—Abilities to adequately receive and interpret sensory stimuli to enable occupational performance *Cardiorespiratory*—Adequate cardiac and pulmonary function to sustain performance *Visual-perception*—Adequate visual acuity and ability to perceive and interpret sensory stimuli and to perceive self and objects in space to enable occupational performance *Cognitive*—Abilities and skills that are basic to interaction with the environment, to organizing life tasks, and to solving occupational problems; abilities include attention, memory, problem solving *Socioemotional*—Abilities and skills that enable occupational performance in a social context or environment	Observable elements of action having an implicit functional purpose *Motor skills*—Actions or behaviors used to move and physically interact with tasks, objects, contexts, and environments; includes reaches, bends, lifts, and manipulates. *Process skills*—Skills observed as a person utilizes tools and materials; carries out actions; modifies performance when problems are encountered. Includes attends, chooses, uses, and sequences. *Social interaction skills*—Skills observed during social exchanges. Includes approaches/starts, concludes/disengages, and empathizes.

(continued)

Table 1-1. The Domains of the Occupational Functioning Model and the Occupational Therapy Practice Framework (*continued*)

OCCUPATIONAL FUNCTIONING MODEL	OCCUPATIONAL THERAPY PRACTICE FRAMEWORK[2]
Developed Capacities	Client Factors
Voluntary responses that have developed from first-level capacities	*Body functions*—Includes mental functions; sensory functions; neuromusculoskeletal and movement-related functions.
First-Level Capacities	Client Factors
The reflexive subroutines of voluntary movement and behavior. These functional foundations for movement and behavior include sensorimotor, cognitive-perceptual, and socioemotional capacities	(as above)
Organic Substrate	Client Factors—Body Structures
Structural and physiological foundation for movement, cognition, perception, and emotions. The substrate includes central nervous system organization and the integrity of skeleton, muscles, peripheral nerves, heart, lungs, and skin	Those anatomical parts of the body that correspond to the functions mentioned earlier
Environment and Context	Context and Environment
Physical—Including the natural and built environments, objects and utensils, and the requirements that tools and utensils pose for use *Personal*—Including age, gender, activity history, sense of competency, and spirituality *Cultural*—Including norms, values, beliefs, and routines or rituals of the family, ethnic group, community, or religious group *Social*—Including therapeutic interaction and relationships with family members, peers and friends, and community *Temporal*—Including temporal demands of role tasks, activities, and habits; balance of activity types; and balance of activity and rest *Situational*—Including circumstances related to the setting or surroundings at a given moment	*Context* *Cultural*—Including ethnicity, beliefs, activity patterns, and behavior standards *Personal*—Including age, gender, socioeconomic status, and educational status *Temporal*—Including stage of life, time of year or day, duration, rhythm of activity, and history *Virtual*—Defined as the communication that occurs via airwaves or computers with an absence of physical contact *Environment* *Physical*—Including built and natural nonhuman environments and objects in them *Social*—Including relationships with individuals, groups, organizations, and systems

BADLs, basic activities of daily living; IADLs, instrumental activities of daily living.

practice with persons with physical impairments. The primary belief is that people who are competent in their life roles experience a sense of **self-efficacy**, self-esteem, and life satisfaction. Research indirectly supports the idea that competency is related to satisfaction or a positive quality of life.[9] Successful performance strengthens personal efficacy beliefs.[8,10,11] The goal of treatment, according to the OFM, is to enable competent engagement in valued roles whether by restored self-performance (personal agency) or by directing others (proxy agency).[11]

Another assumption of the OFM is that the **ability** to carry out one's roles, tasks, and activities of life depends on basic abilities and **capacities** (e.g., strength, perception, ability to sequence information). As with other systems, this hierarchical organization assumes that lower level capacities and abilities are related to higher level performance of everyday tasks and activities. This organization has been tangentially supported by research.[12–15] However, the relationship between impairments and performance is multifactorial.[13] Only part of the variance associated with performance is accounted for by any one ability or combination of abilities. For example, Rudhe and van Hedel[16] found a moderately strong ($r_s = 0.84$) relationship between scores of the self-care category of the SCIM III (Spinal Cord Independence Measure III)[17] and the scores of manual muscle testing and a moderate relationship ($r_s = 0.81$) between hand capacity tests and self-care scores. This outcome does indicate that sensorimotor control of the upper extremities is related to self-care, but because the variance (r^2) is only approximately 65% to 70% (0.81^2 or 0.84^2), other unidentified variables must account for the remaining approximately 35% variance associated with activities of daily living (ADLs). This makes sense because, in addition to upper extremity function, ADL independence requires such skills as sitting and standing balance, perception of positions of objects in space, ability to sequence steps of a procedure, environmental support, and so forth.

It appears that the relationship between two adjacent levels of performance (e.g., capacities and abilities) is stronger than between two nonadjacent levels (e.g., capacities and roles).[12,14,18,19] The relationship between levels is strong both at the low end of the model[14,20] and

Table 1-2. The Process of Occupational Therapy

PROCESS	OCCUPATIONAL FUNCTIONING MODEL	OCCUPATIONAL THERAPY PRACTICE FRAMEWORK[2]
Goal of therapy	Satisfactorily engage in self-identified, important life roles through which the person gains a sense of self-efficacy and self-esteem	Support health and participation in life through engagement in occupation
Evaluate to identify the problem(s)	• Identify roles, tasks, and activities the person wants to do or needs to do • Measure perceptions of self-efficacy regarding the tasks of identified goals • Assess occupational balance • Observe and analyze the person's performance, preferably within usual context • Identify inadequate performance • Identify impaired abilities or capacities that contribute to inadequate performance and assess level of impairment using valid, reliable assessment tools administered according to the standardized protocol • Identify environmental or contextual enablers or hindrances • Interpret assessment data to the patient and family and document in the patient's record	• *Occupational profile*—To understand the client's occupational history, patterns of daily living, occupational balance, interests, values, needs, problems with performance, and priorities • Analysis of occupational performance by observation within personally relevant context to specifically identify client's assets and problems that affect performance skills • Assess environment and context; activity and occupation demands; client factors; performance skills and patterns • Interpret assessment data to identify facilitators and barriers to performance • Develop hypotheses about what strengths and weaknesses the client brings to occupation
Plan intervention	• Plan in collaboration with the person or family, after presenting the current evidence, to determine whether the person wants to engage in either remediation of impaired abilities or capacities to enhance overall performance or restoration of occupational performance through relearning and/or adaptation of method or environment • With the patient, establish short-term goals that directly relate to the long-term goal of successful role functioning identified by the patient and that can be objectively and reliably measured • Select interventions that have evidence for effectiveness for the immediate goal	• With the client, develop a plan with objective, measurable goals and a time frame to guide action • Plan occupational therapy intervention based on theory and evidence • Select outcome measures • Consider discharge needs and plan • Refer to other professionals as needed
Implement the intervention	Use therapeutic mechanisms, as appropriate: *Occupation* • Occupation-as-end to restore occupational functioning • Occupation-as-means to optimize abilities or capacities *Therapeutic rapport* *Education*—Learning or relearning *Adjunctive therapies*—Therapies such as orthoses, technological aids, physical agent modalities, mobility aids used to facilitate performance *Contextual and environmental modification*—To facilitate performance	*Determine occupational therapy interventions* to be used and carry them out, such as • Therapeutic occupations and activities • Preparatory methods • Education and training • Advocacy • Group interventions Monitor and document client's response
Evaluate the result	**Assess patient outcomes** • Determine whether the short-term goals were achieved • Determine whether achievement of the short-term goals resulted in desired occupational performance • If not, reevaluate and modify the plan relative to achieving targeted outcomes • If yes, determine whether the person was satisfied with his or her achievement • Plan for the next level of therapy or plan for discharge and referral as appropriate	*Intervention review* • Determine success or progress toward achieving targeted outcomes • Modify the plan as needed • Determine need for continuation, discontinuation, or referral
Types of outcomes	• Satisfactory occupational performance to allow expected discharge success • Voiced, or otherwise indicated, sense of self-efficacy and self-esteem • Prevention of further disability through education and follow-up, if necessary	Occupational performance outcomes congruent with client goals

Table 1-3. The Similarities and Differences between the AOTA Occupational Therapy Practice Framework and the Occupational Functioning Model

	OCCUPATIONAL THERAPY PRACTICE FRAMEWORK[2]	OCCUPATIONAL FUNCTIONING MODEL
Central focus	Achieving health, well-being, and participation through engagement in occupation	Self-fulfillment through role competence
A conceptual model	No	Yes
Describes the relationships (dynamic interaction) among the terms and categories in the classification system	No[57]	Yes
Domain	Incorporates all aspects of occupational therapy practice	Limited to practice for those with physical dysfunction
Hierarchical	No[58]	Yes; successful performance of higher occupations depends on lower abilities, skills, and capacities
Clients include person, organization, society	Yes	No; limited to practice with individuals
End goal	Support health and participation in life through engagement in occupation	Satisfactorily engage in self-identified, important life roles through which the person gains a sense of self-efficacy and self-esteem
Process	Evaluation, planning, intervention, outcome monitoring	Evaluation, planning, treatment, reevaluation
Evaluation	Occupational profile and analysis of occupational performance, including factors that influence performance	Determination of client goals; assessment of role, task, and activity performance; measurement of skills, abilities, developed capacities, first-level capacities, and determination of organic substrate, as needed. Assessment of environmental and contextual influences on performance
Top-down evaluation process	Yes	Yes
Process of evaluating, planning, treating, and monitoring outcome is iterative, not sequenced	Yes	Yes
Process is collaborative, that is, client centered	Yes[59]	Yes
Key skill of occupational therapist	Analysis of occupational performance: observe, analyze, and interpret performance and detect the client, contextual, or environmental factors that enable successful performance or that impede that performance	Activity analysis: observe, analyze, and interpret performance and detect the clinically relevant impairment and/or the contextual-environmental enablers or barriers to performance
Interventions	Therapeutic use of occupation and purposeful activities Preparatory methods Education and training Advocacy Group interventions	Therapeutic rapport Therapeutic use of occupation as occupation-as-means and/or occupation-as-end Learning (education) Therapeutic technologies
Occupational therapy intervention approaches	Create, promote (health promotion) Establish, restore (remediation, restoration) Maintain Modify (compensation, adaptation) Prevent (disability prevention)	Collaborate Remediate skills and abilities by therapeutic use of occupation-as-means Restore activities, tasks, and role performance by relearning or adaptation or environmental or contextual modification

Table 1-3. The Similarities and Differences between the AOTA Occupational Therapy Practice Framework and the Occupational Functioning Model (*continued*)

	OCCUPATIONAL THERAPY PRACTICE FRAMEWORK[2]	OCCUPATIONAL FUNCTIONING MODEL
Evidential support	None offered[58]	Tangential supporting evidence, i.e., incidental evidence of the various assumptions, but not direct evidence for the model
Practical usefulness (usable and clinically relevant; use of everyday language)	No[57,59]	Yes

AOTA, American Occupational Therapy Association.

at the high end.[12,17] Pendlebury et al. found a strong (r = 0.90; r^2 = 81%) relationship between deficits in organic substrate and deficits of motor capacities and abilities.[20] In a large sample of persons with spinal cord injury, Dijkers found a moderate relationship (r = 0.24–0.42) between life satisfaction and roles related to social integration and occupation (work) but not between impairments and life satisfaction (r = 0.04–0.07).[12] He concluded that "these relationships suggest a causal chain [i.e., one link leading to the next]. . . . The impact of impairment on quality of life is almost entirely through its impact on disability, and the effect of disability is largely through its impact on handicap" (p. 874).[12] This research suggests that the relationship between low-level capacities and abilities and higher level tasks and roles is not direct. That is, having a particular ability, such as strength, does not ensure that a person can accomplish a given **activity** or task.[21] Likewise, the ability to accomplish a single activity does not account for role performance. Many capacities contribute to the development of one ability, and many abilities are needed to engage successfully in an activity. When one capacity or ability is impaired, occupational dysfunction does not automatically occur. A person may adaptively use other capacities and abilities to allow accomplishment of the activity.[22]

Another assumption of the OFM is that satisfactory occupational functioning occurs only within enabling **environments** and **contexts** particular to the individual.[23] True occupational functioning does not occur in a vacuum or in a controlled situation such as the clinic; occupational functioning is the successful interaction of the person with the objects, situations, and surroundings of his or her home, family, and community. Although the contexts of particular actions and occupations used to regain lost abilities and capacities may be controlled at first, therapy is not complete until generalization to the person's particular environment has occurred.[24]

Achievement of occupational functioning after injury or disease is accomplished through occupation as well as adjunctive therapies described in this textbook. In the OFM, occupation has two natures: **occupation-as-end** and **occupation-as-means.**[7] Occupation-as-end equates to the higher levels of the OFM, at which the person tries to accomplish a functional goal (an activity or task) by using whatever skills, abilities, habits, and capacities he or she has. Occupation-as-means, on the other hand, is *the therapy* used to bring about changes in impaired capacities and skills. Occupation-as-means is therapeutic because the goal presents challenges to impaired capacities and abilities, and the successful achievement of that goal results in improved organic or behavioral impairments.

The constructs of the OFM are described next.

Sense of Self-Efficacy and Self-Esteem

The goal of occupational therapy is the development of competence in the activities and tasks of one's cherished roles, which promotes a sense of self-efficacy and self-esteem. *Competence* is the effective interaction with the physical and social environments (Fig. 1-1). To be

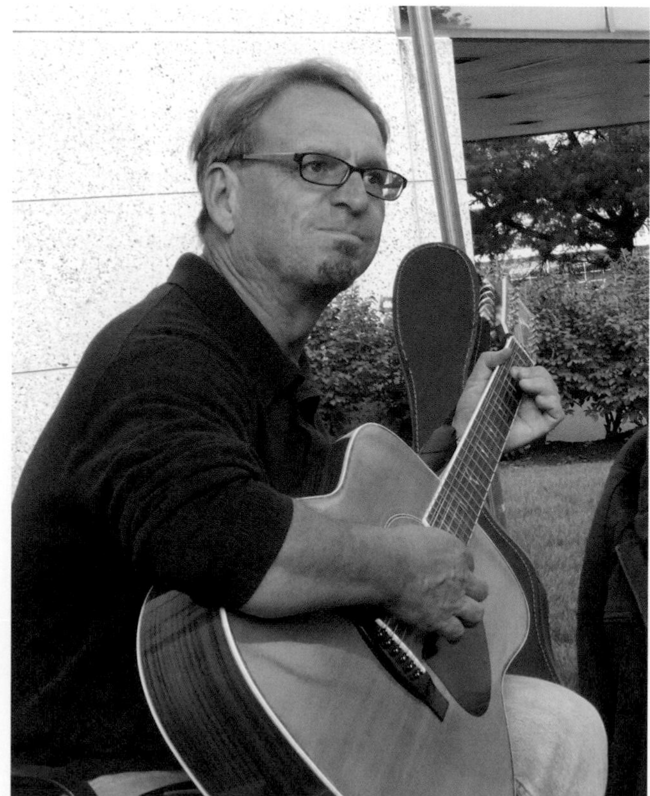

Figure 1-1. Competency of self-advancement role of musician.

competent means to have the skills that are sufficient or adequate to meet the demands of a situation or task.[25,26] It does not equate to excellence, normality, or the ability to do everything, and it recognizes that there are degrees of sufficiency and adequacy in people.[25,27]

Competence develops by enabling a person to engage in graduated, goal-directed activity that is accomplishable by that person and that produces a feeling of satisfaction.[26] Occupational therapists help people achieve competence through graded engagement in occupation, vicarious engagement in occupation (watching others), virtual engagement in occupation, developmental and instrumental learning with immediate and precise feedback, and therapeutic interaction with the therapist.[9,28]

When people feel competent, they have a sense of self-efficacy. The most powerful source of personal efficacy expectations is past accomplishments in similar situations. They have perceived their capability to perform a behavior. Self-efficacy is concerned not with the skills one possesses but with the judgments of what one can do with those skills. Perceived self-efficacy is influenced through an ongoing evaluation of success and failure with each task people participate in over the course of their lives.[29] Feelings of self-efficacy are likely to lead people to esteem themselves.[30]

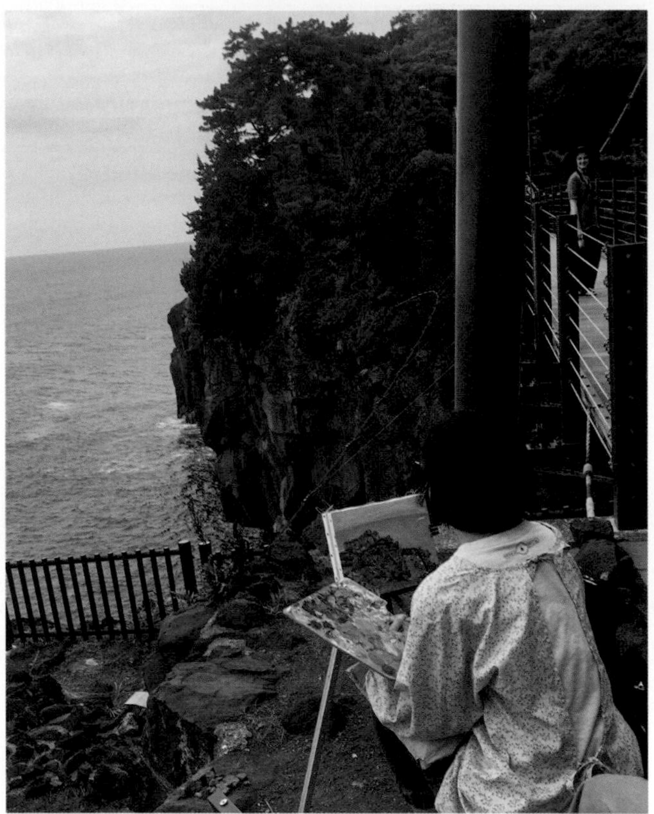

Figure 1-2. For this accomplished artist, painting a picture is a task of one of her self-advancement roles (worker). For another person for whom painting is a hobby, it would be classified as a task of self-enhancement role (hobbyist).

Satisfaction with Life Roles [Occupations]*

Being in control of one's life means being able to engage satisfyingly in one's life roles or to voluntarily reassign a role to another. Role performance is a vital component of productive, independent living and life satisfaction.[31] Various occupational therapy scholars have proposed taxonomies of roles. The OFM sorts roles into three domains related to aspects of self-definition: self-maintenance, self-advancement, and self-enhancement,[4,6,7] but recognizes that the assignment of roles to a particular category is not absolute. Some roles may be classified in one domain by one person but in another domain by another person, depending on the motivation or context (Fig. 1-2). For example, volunteering may be classified by one person as a self-advancement role because volunteering promotes skills that will be useful in a worker role. Another person may classify volunteering as self-enhancement because it promotes a sense of satisfaction without expectation of gain. The individuality of motivation underscores the importance of assessing each person from his or her own point of view, letting each define his or her roles and their meaning.[31] Assessment of individuality is a major aspect of client-centered therapy.

Self-Maintenance Roles [Activities of Daily Living, Instrumental Activities of Daily Living, and Rest and Sleep]

Self-maintenance roles are associated with care of the self, family, pets, and home. Examples of roles in this domain are independent person, grandparent, parent, son, daughter, homemaker (Fig. 1-3), home maintainer (Fig. 1-4), exerciser, cat owner, and caregiver.

Self-Advancement Roles [Work and Education]

Self-advancement roles are those that draw the person into productive activities that add to the person's skills, possessions, or other betterment. Examples of roles in the self-advancement role domain include worker (Figs. 1-1 and 1-5), student, intern, commuter, shopper, investor, manager, and voter.

Self-Enhancement Roles [Play, Leisure, Social Participation]

Self-enhancement roles contribute to the person's sense of accomplishment and enjoyment or sense of well-being and happiness (Figs. 1-2 and 1-6). Examples of roles in this domain include hobbyist, friend, club member, religious participant, vacationer, golfer, moviegoer, and violinist.

---

*The comparable *Occupational Therapy Practice Framework* language is added in brackets to assist the student in using the language interchangeably.

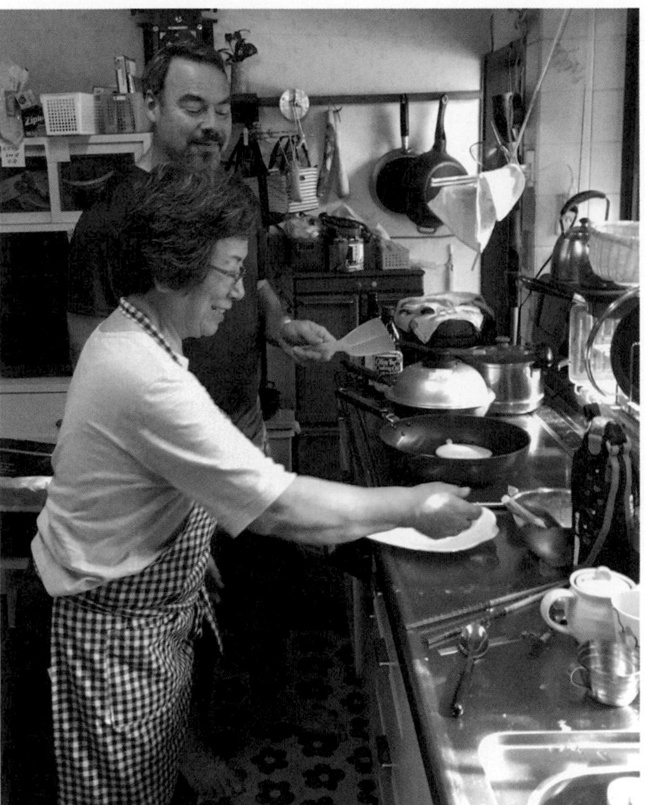

Figure 1-3. Self-maintenance role: homemaker; task: meal preparation; activity: making pancakes.

Competency in Tasks of Life Roles [Occupations]

Roles consist of constellations of tasks. For example, the role of homemaker may include the tasks of food preparation (Fig. 1-3) and service, housecleaning, laundry, and decorating (Fig. 1-4). The tasks identified for the same role by different people may be different.[6,7] The value ascribed to tasks varies among people of similar situations and may vary from what therapists consider important for patients. Because people have different values, each person must define his or her role by identifying the tasks that he or she believes are crucial to satisfactory engagement in that particular role. The therapist cannot assume that particular tasks are or are not important to a person's interpretation of a role.

Tasks consist of constellations of related activities and are therapeutically developed using occupation-as-end, which is practicing the activities constituting the task in normal temporal order and environmental demand, with or without assistive technology as required.

Activities and Habits [Occupations and Performance Patterns]

Activities, in the OFM, are smaller units of goal-directed behavior that, taken together, comprise tasks. Activities bring together abilities and skills within a functional context. For example, one task of the gardener is pest control. Activities that make up this task may include hanging

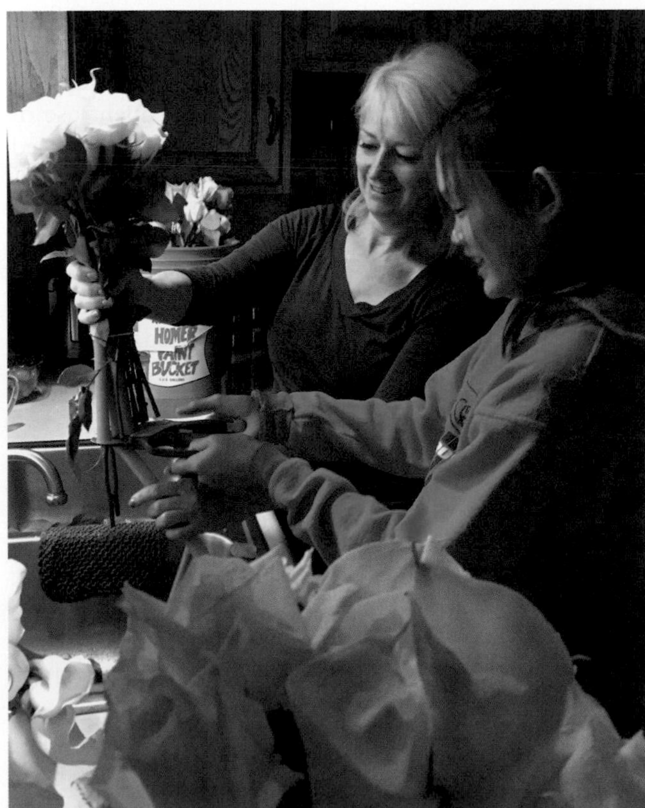

Figure 1-4. Self-maintenance role: home maintainer; task: gardening; activity: flower arrangement.

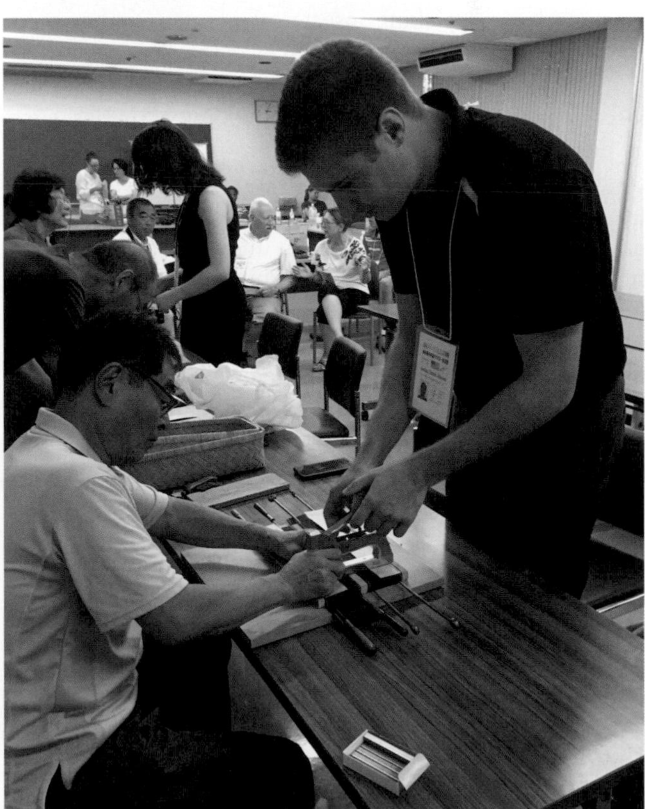

1-5. Self-advancement role: contractor; task: tatami mat construction; activity: stapling.

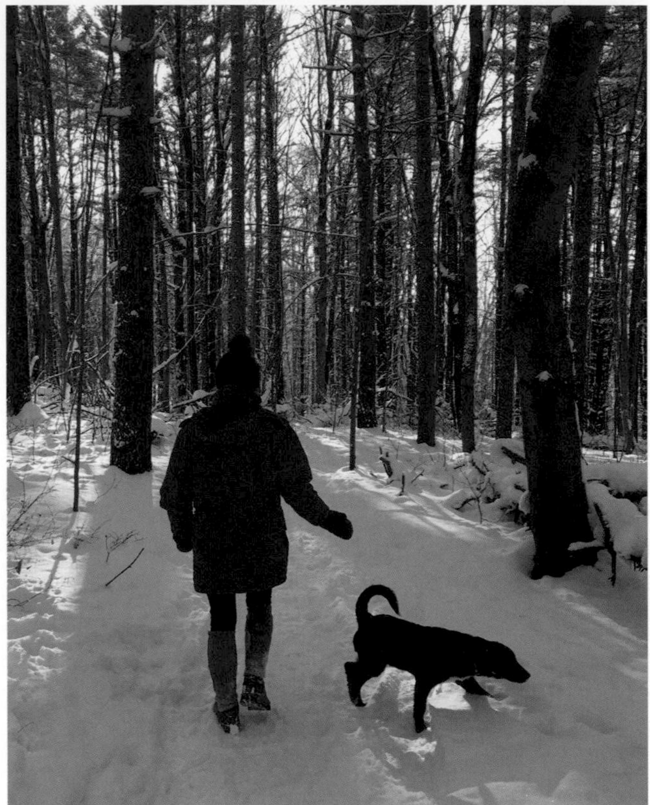

Figure 1-6. Self-enhancement role: pet owner; task: exercise dog; activity: walking.

lures, spreading granular insect killer, mixing and spraying liquids, and picking insects off plants. Furthermore, each of these activities consists of even smaller units of behavior, such as opening the package and pouring granular insect killer into a garden spreader. Some activities, such as picking insects off plants, require full attention. Others, called habits, do not. Habits are chains of action sequences that are so well learned that the person does not have to pay attention to do them under ordinary circumstances and in familiar contexts. Physical dysfunction disrupts habits, requiring attention to be paid to the simplest of ADLs. This adds to the fatigue experienced by many persons.[32] Using the OFM, occupational therapists seek to help the person sustain or relearn adaptive habits, let go of habits that are no longer adaptive, and develop new habits given the person's changed abilities and capacities.

Activities and habits are learned using occupation-as-end, that is, "task-specific training." In task-specific training, functional and meaningful activities are practiced over and over using assistive technology, adaptive methods, or adapted environment to enable performance, if necessary. See Chapter 2 for a discussion of the therapeutic use of occupation-as-end.

Abilities and Skills [Performance Skills]

Activities depend on more basic abilities.[1,33] A person with a great number of highly developed abilities can become proficient at a greater variety of activities. An ability is a general trait, such as muscle strength or memory, that individuals bring with them to a new task.[1] In the OFM, abilities are seen as a combination of endowed talents and acquired skills. A **skill** is the ability to use one's knowledge to effectively and readily execute performance.[3] Skill enables goal achievement under a wide variety of conditions with a degree of consistency and economy. Abilities and skills develop from one or more developed capacities. They are more voluntary and organized and evidence smoother execution than do developed capacities. The OFM identifies six categories of abilities and skills: motor, sensory, cognitive, perceptual, socioemotional, and cardiorespiratory.

To accomplish the activity of hanging lures in the previous example of the gardener, the person needs certain abilities, such as coordination, dexterity, and ability to follow directions. The person also needs to be able to translate these endowed talents into the skilled actions required to hang the lures. Carefully analyzed occupation-as-means is used to develop deficient abilities and skills. In the process of repeatedly accomplishing occupations that demand greater levels of the deficient ability or skill in varying contexts, the patient gains greater levels of that ability or skill. By varying the context, the therapist encourages more robust learning. See Chapter 2 for a more complete discussion of the therapeutic use of occupation-as-means.

Developed Capacities [Client Factors]

Developed capacities reflect the organization of first-level capacities into more mature, less reflexive, and more voluntary responses. For example, to support dexterity, an ability, a person needs independent use of fingers, graded release and pinch, which are developed capacities that derive from reflexive grasp and automatic release (first-level capacities). This organization is normally acquired through maturation. In therapy, occupation-as-means is used to develop these capacities. Therapeutic demands for gradually more mature and varied responses are made through repeated opportunities to engage in selected occupations.

First-Level Capacities [Client Factors—Body Functions]

First-level capacities are the functional foundation for movement, cognition, perception, and emotional life based on the integrity of the organic substrate. In the motor domain, first-level capacities are reflex-based motor responses that reflect the organization of primary visual, sensory, and motor systems. Examples include reflexive grasp, reflexive release, primitive reaching, kicking, and stepping. They are the subroutines that Bruner[34] described as underlying the development of all voluntary movement. The ability to recognize a connection between an instrumental, nonreflexive response given consistently within a particular perceptual situation is a first-level capacity of cognition and perception. The fascination of babies with human faces is a first-level capacity of the socioemotional domain.

Organic Substrate [Client Factors—Body Structure]

Organic substrate is the structural and physiological foundation for movement, cognition, perception, and emotions, including the primitive central nervous system (CNS) organization in the neonate; the CNS organization that is spared or recovers spontaneously after injury or illness; and the integrity of the brain, skeleton, muscles, sensory and motor nerves, heart, lungs, and skin. If the organic substrate is not present, therapy cannot generate it. If it exists at all, therapy attempts to develop it into first-level capacities through techniques classified as **augmented maturation** (see Chapter 34).

Environment and Context [Context and Environment]

The words *environment* and *context* are often used interchangeably. In current health care literature, the term *context* is used to encompass all that influences any aspect of human functioning, including physical, social, personal, temporal, and situational influences, as well as familial and cultural beliefs and practices that influence the life of an individual. Context is the interpretive dimension of the circumstances surrounding occupational engagement. Seemingly similar circumstances may result in different occupational behavior depending on the person's interpretation of the circumstances. It is this interpretive dimension of context that is important to the occupational therapist.

Environment is defined as the complex of external factors, circumstances, objects, structures, and social surround that inhibit or facilitate occupational functioning. Research has shown that familiarity of the environment positively affects daily functioning.[23,24]

Context in the OTPF refers to cultural, physical, social, personal, temporal, and virtual aspects of living. Similar to the OTPF, the OFM assumes that context and environment surround and permeate all levels of the occupational functioning hierarchy. However, the OFM distinguishes between the greater influence of context and environment at the higher levels of the hierarchy and the lesser influence at the lower levels. At the lower levels, the immediate physical and personal context and environment influence the actions. For example, organization of a reaching movement was shown to differ when actual, natural objects and utensils were used versus when simulated objects were used.[35,36] Cultural and social contexts pertain less to this level. At the higher levels of activities, tasks, and roles, however, all aspects of context and environment—personal, social, cultural, temporal, situational, and physical—interact with the person's abilities to yield occupational functioning for the particular person.

When the challenges of the environment exceed the capabilities of a person, that person is said to be disabled.[37] A person with impaired abilities and capacities, however, may be able to accomplish activities and tasks of his or her roles if the environment is adapted to enable that.[23] Therefore, occupational therapy treatment may focus on changing the environment or context rather than on remediating the person's impaired abilities or capacities.

The Process of Occupational Therapy for Persons with Physical Dysfunction

The process of occupational therapy follows the universal plan for problem solving: identify the problem, determine possible solutions, intervene, and evaluate the result. The occupational therapist, however, focuses only on problems related to the person's occupational life, including **occupational balance**. What a person needs to do, wants to do, and can do are identified. Discrepancy between what the person needs or wants to do and what he or she can do identifies the problem. The occupational therapist then uses various occupational, adaptive, and adjunctive therapies to intervene. Or the occupational therapist may detect dissatisfaction or stress caused by an occupational imbalance and intervene using educational therapies. The processes of the OFM and the OTPF are similar (Table 1-2). A discussion of the OFM process follows.

Assessment [Evaluation]

The hierarchical organization of the OFM indicates that higher level occupational functioning is established on a foundation of abilities and capacities. Assessment *always* follows a top-down approach. That is, the therapist determines what roles and tasks the person was responsible for in life before the accident or disease and what the person is expected to be, and wants to be, responsible for in postrehabilitation life, including the context and environment in which the person typically engaged in these valued roles and tasks.[6,7] The *AOTA Occupational Profile* guides discussion of clients' occupational history, goals, context, and environment; its use is a requirement of the CPT evaluation codes.[2] Other examples of assessments the therapist may use to gather more in-depth information are *The Role Checklist*,[38,39] the *Canadian Occupational Performance Measure* (COPM),[40] and the *Client-Oriented Role Evaluation*.[41]

The therapist may also measure the patient's sense of self-efficacy concerning the ability to do the tasks required to fulfill particular roles by having the patient assign a number on a visual analog scale that ranges from 0 (not at all confident) to 10 (absolutely certain) for each major task that defines a specific role. For example, "on a scale from 0 to 10, how confident are you that you can prepare your own lunch without help?" Other assessments of self-efficacy are the *Self-Efficacy for Functional Activities Scale*[42] and the *Self-Efficacy Gauge* designed especially for occupational therapists to measure the patient's current level of perceived self-efficacy and the change in perceived self-efficacy over time.[25]

Occupational balance, a person's perception of whether his or her life activities are in balance, can be assessed through careful interviewing or the use of an assessment such as the *Life Balance Inventory* that evaluates perceived balance between desired and actual time usage.[43]

When evaluating a patient's competence to accomplish the roles identified as important, the therapist observes the patient attempting to do the tasks and activities that the patient identifies as key to those roles in the most familiar context. The *Assessment of Motor and Process Skills* (AMPS),[44] the *Klein-Bell ADL Scale*,[45] the *Barthel Index*,[46,47] and the *Performance Assessment of Self-Care Skills* (PASS)[48] are examples of standardized observational assessments of tasks and activities. Using an assessment that structures observation of performance and having knowledge of the probabilities established by the diagnosis and age of the person, the therapist detects which of the myriad abilities and capacities assumed to be related to accomplishment of these activities are impaired (the process of **activity analysis** applied to assessment; see Chapter 3 for client-centered activity analysis procedure and example). The therapist then assesses these abilities and capacities more directly using assessments that have been validated and found reliable for the type of patient being evaluated. For example, if the patient's goal is to shave with an electric razor, but he appears to lack the grasp strength and endurance to do so, strength and endurance are assessed. A person whose abilities and capacities are found deficient may be treated to optimize them, allowing not only shaving but also other occupations.

Some therapists prefer to use a bottom-up evaluation procedure in which capacities, abilities, and skills are assessed before occupational performance.[49] This practice, however, often results in emphasizing these lower level factors without translation of the regained abilities to occupational performance. Furthermore, when this approach is used, the patient often fails to see the connection between therapy to optimize skills and abilities and achievement of his or her occupational goals.

The environment in which the patient will live, work, or play is assessed to determine whether it enables or hinders occupational functioning. Assessments of the home environment have been developed (e.g., *Safety Assessment of Function and the Environment for Rehabilitation* [SAFER][50] and *Home Occupational-Environmental Assessment*[51]), but assessments of other environments have not yet been developed. To assess the effects on occupational performance of other physical and social environments typical for the patient, the occupational therapist needs to observe performance under those conditions, using the process of client-environment fit activity analysis (see Chapter 3). In practice, this assessment usually occurs immediately before or after discharge from an inpatient rehabilitation setting.

Treatment [Intervention]

Treatment may focus on changing the environment,[24] changing the impaired skills and abilities of the person,[52] teaching specific tasks or activities using goal-directed training,[53] or teaching compensatory ways to accomplish activities and tasks. Treatment to improve occupational functioning, then, may start toward the bottom of the OFM hierarchy, focusing on optimizing abilities and capacities; or it may start higher, at the activity level of the hierarchy, focusing on restoring competence in doing the activities and tasks of valued roles that the patient has identified as concerns; or it may start peripheral to the person, focusing on modifying the context or environment. The starting point should acknowledge the problem that the patient has identified as an immediate concern, although treatment may not actually start there. For example, if the patient identified resuming fishing as the goal, the therapist may choose to teach adaptive methods to enable that. If, however, the evidence and the experience of the therapist indicated that it would be more effective to start treatment by regaining finger dexterity to enable various activities related to fishing (e.g., baiting the hook and removing the fish from the line), the therapist *must help the patient understand* how treatment of this lower level ability addresses the stated concern at the task level. In addition, the therapist *must ensure carryover* of any gained dexterity to the fishing task.

Optimizing impaired abilities and capacities is accomplished through remedial therapy in which a change in physiological structure, function, or organization is sought through occupation-as-means. If remediation of deficit abilities or capacities does not restore occupational functioning, if economic constraints prevent such thorough treatment, or if the patient is not committed to the extensive work required to recover abilities and capacities, a degree of competence can be restored using goal-specific training and/or adaptive therapy. **Adaptive therapy** seeks to find and promote a balance among the person's goals and environmental demands and his or her current capacities and abilities. In this type of therapy, the method of doing an activity may be modified, assistive technology may be used to enable completion of the activity, and/or the physical or social environments may be modified. The person may be counseled to reassess the need to accomplish a particularly difficult or time-consuming activity alone and opt to employ another to do it.

Optimizing Abilities and Capacities [Intervention]

As in the typical development of capacities and abilities, therapy engages the patient in circumscribed encounters with the environment using occupation-as-means. Occupation-as-means, that is, activities that provide stretch of soft tissues, active or passive movement to preserve and restore full range of motion, resistance and other stress to strengthen weak muscles, or graduated, increasing levels of aerobic exercise or time of engagement to improve endurance, is used to optimize motor abilities and capacities. Using the example of the man who wanted to shave, the therapist might start treatment by providing a cuff to hold the razor to eliminate the need for grasp (adaptive therapy) and let the patient shave as much as he could. Then the occupational therapist would finish the activity. Day by day, the patient's endurance for shaving would increase, and he would do more of the task on his own (occupation used as a means of remediation). Concurrently, the therapist would engage the patient in other activities that require increasingly greater grasp strength until the patient was able to hold the razor.

When impairment of the CNS results in the inability to move voluntarily to effect a desired change in the environment, a therapist may use occupation-as-means in conjunction with controlled sensory input and ontogenetic or recovery-based developmental postures or patterns (**augmented maturation**) to facilitate change in first-level and developed capacities of sensorimotor organization. Whereas some therapists have anecdotally reported success using controlled sensory stimulation and developmental movements or postures to develop motor control, there is little to no evidence in the literature to support these approaches. However, because some therapists do find aspects of these approaches clinically helpful, especially when there is a need to optimize first-level capacities, a chapter describing these approaches has been included in this textbook (see Chapter 34), while recognizing that the approaches lack an evidence base.

Alternatively, because of the preponderance of research that documents that neural reorganization occurs secondary to practice of goal-directed movements, the therapist may use motor learning principles in conjunction with occupation-as-end to bring about change in voluntary movement behavior.[53] This approach uses functional tasks to improve task performance, heeding the research findings on the effect of context on the organization of movement, which indicates that practicing a skill under simplified, non–context-specific conditions is different from practicing with an actual object in a context-specific situation.[36,54,55] The therapist arranges practice schedules and provides appropriate feedback to facilitate the learning process.

Restoring Competence [Intervention]

When activity, task, and role levels of the OFM are dysfunctional, treatment may aim at restoring occupational functioning in spite of any residual impairment. Competence in tasks and activities is synthesized through successful engagement with the environment. Occupational therapists are skilled in developing graduated encounters with objects and the surrounding physical and social environments to promote successful performance. They are also experts in teaching methods to compensate by reorganizing activity patterns or adapting techniques, equipment, or the environment. Some therapists use this compensatory approach exclusively; others believe that first optimizing the impaired abilities and capacities requires less compensation and produces more versatility of performance. There is no research to support one point of view over the other.

The goal is independence in activities and tasks of valued roles. People are considered independent when they perform tasks for themselves using assistive equipment, alternative methods, or adapted environments, as required, or when they appropriately oversee completion of activities by others on their own behalf. The therapist teaches the patient or caregiver the principles and concepts of adaptation so that the patient or caregiver can become an independent problem solver. Therapeutic mechanisms of change include occupation-as-end, teaching-learning, therapeutic rapport, and environmental and/or process modification.

Summary

This chapter describes one model, the OFM, to guide the process of occupational therapy for persons with occupational dysfunction secondary to physical impairments and relates that model to the *OTPF*, which is an official document of the AOTA concerning domain and process of the entire practice of occupational therapy. The framework needs an organizational model to guide assessment and intervention. That model can be the OFM, *the Model for Human Occupation* (MOHO),[33] the *Occupational Adaptation Model*,[56] or any number of other models that complement your way of thinking and analyzing problems and that facilitate your clinical reasoning.

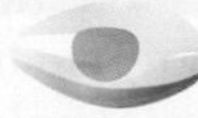

CASE STUDY

Patient Information

- ***Diagnosis.*** Mr. J has a fracture/dislocation of C6–7 vertebrae secondary to a diving accident. He is status post cervical laminectomy and fusion; medically stable; exhibits C6 functional level (see Chapter 38).
- ***Occupational Profile (abbreviated).*** Mr. J is a 24-year-old college graduate who lives with his parents in a second-floor apartment. His four older brothers live away. He was employed as a computer programmer and identifies keyboarding as a crucial task of this role. The company is holding his job for him. He has many friends and plays sports. The family is supportive but expects him to be independent in self-care and to resume work.

Assessment Process and Results

- ***Observation:*** He is unable to move his lower extremities and has poor sitting balance. Dependent in all basic activities of daily living (BADLs) and instrumental activities of daily living (IADLs).
- ***Measurement:*** Manual muscle testing revealed that Mr. J's proximal upper extremity musculature rated 4 to 5, with the exception of the triceps, which graded 2 (see Chapter 13, which describes muscle strength grading). Wrist extensors graded 3+ on the left and 4− on the right; wrist flexors and finger and thumb muscles graded 0 bilaterally.

Occupational Therapy Problem List

1. Paralyzed lower extremities; unable to walk or relieve ischial pressure
2. Weak upper extremities
3. Unable to grasp
4. Poor sitting balance
5. Dependent in tasks and activities of valued roles (independent person, computer programmer, sports)

Occupational Therapy Goal List

1. Develop beginning independence in basic self-care
2. Develop beginning wheelchair skills
3. Improve upper extremity strength
4. Develop tenodesis grasp
5. Develop habit of relieving pressure on skin to prevent decubiti
6. Explore adapted methods of computer use

Intervention

1. Collaborate with the physical therapist to order wheelchair
2. Engage in occupation-as-end to relearn basic ADL skills, learn to use wheelchair, learn to relieve ischial pressure to prevent decubiti, learn to solve problems by adapting methods or equipment to enable performance of tasks
3. Use occupation-as-means to increase strength of upper extremities
4. Group educational sessions for social, emotional, and practical problem solving with other persons with similar activity limitations

Outcome

1. Able to wheel 50 feet on flat carpeting
2. Proximal upper extremity musculature recovered to normal strength
3. Learned adaptive methods for relieving pressure to maintain skin integrity
4. Wrist extensor strength improved to 4+ bilaterally, which allowed a functional tenodesis grasp. This enabled showering, dressing, and bowel and bladder management.
5. He keyboards using universal cuffs with typing sticks tipped with rubber ends. He learned to adapt his computer to allow one-key depression for all operations and other adaptations.
6. He learned about the local wheelchair basketball team from the group that he plans to join.

Referrals

1. Outpatient occupational therapy to continue improving his strength, improving his IADLs, and have environmental evaluations at home and work executed
2. Occupational therapy driving specialist
3. Social worker to arrange for visiting nurse to supervise bowel and bladder care and ischial pressure relief until these becomes habitual; to arrange for handicapped accessible housing; to hire an in-home helper to help him achieve occupational balance
4. Organizer of the wheelchair basketball team

References

1. Fleishman EA. On the relation between ability, learning, and human performance. *Am Psychol.* 1972;27:1017–1032.
2. American Occupational Therapy Association. Occupational therapy practice framework: domain and process (3rd ed.). *Am J Occup Ther.* 2014;68(suppl 1):S1–S48. doi:10.5014/ajot.2014.682006.
3. Merriam-Webster Dictionary. Context. Springfield, MA: Merriam-Webster Inc. https://www.merriam-webster.com/dictionary/context. Accessed January 18, 2018.
4. Rogers JC. The foundation: why study human occupation? *Am J Occup Ther.* 1984;38:47–49. doi:10.5014/ajot.38.1.47.
5. Wagman P, Håkansson C, Björklund A. Occupational balance as used in occupational therapy: a concept analysis. *Scand J Occup Ther.* 2012;19:322–327. doi:10.3109/11038128.2011.596219.
6. Trombly C. Anticipating the future: assessment of occupational function. *Am J Occup Ther.* 1993;47:253–257. doi:10.5014/ajot.47.3.253
7. Trombly CA. Occupation: purposefulness and meaningfulness as therapeutic mechanisms. *Am J Occup Ther.* 1995;49:960–972. doi:10.5014/ajot.49.10.960.
8. Brock K, Black S, Cotton S, Kennedy G, Wilson S, Sutton E. Goal achievement in the six months after inpatient rehabilitation for stroke. *Disabil Rehabil.* 2009;31:880–886. doi:10.1080/09638280802356179.
9. Robinson-Smith G, Johnston MV, Allen J. Self-care self-efficacy, quality of life, and depression after stroke. *Arch Phys Med Rehabil.* 2000;81:460–464. doi:10.1053/mt.2000.3863.
10. Bandura A. Self-efficacy: toward a unifying theory of behavior change. *Psych Rev.* 1977;84:191–215.
11. Bandura A. Social cognitive theory: an agentic perspective. *Ann Rev Psychol.* 2001;52:1–26. doi:10.1146/annurev.psych.52.1.1.
12. Dijkers MPJM. Correlates of life satisfaction among persons with spinal cord injury. *Arch Phys Med Rehabil.* 1999;80:867–876. doi:10.1016/S0003-9993(99)90076-x.
13. Michielsen ME, de Niet M, Ribbers GM, Stam HJ, Bussmann JB. Evidence of a logarithmic relationship between motor capacity and actual performance in daily life of the paretic arm following stroke. *J Rehabil Med.* 2009;41:327–331. doi:10.2340/16501977-0351.
14. Pollard B, Johnston M, Dieppe P. Exploring the relationships between International Classification of Functioning, Disability and Health (ICF) constructs of impairment, activity limitation and participation restriction in people with osteoarthritis prior to joint replacement. *BMC Musculoskelet Disord.* 2011;12:97–104. http://www.biomedcentral.com/1471-2474/12/97.
15. Sveen U, Bautz-Holter E, Sødring KM, Wyller TB, Laake K. Association between impairments, self-care ability and social activities 1 year after stroke. *Disabil Rehabil.* 1999;21:372–377.
16. Rudhe C, Hubertus JA, van Hedel HJA. Upper extremity function in persons with tetraplegia: relationships between strength, capacity, and the spinal cord independence measure. *Neurorehabil Neural Repair.* 2009;23:413–421. doi:10.1177/1545968308331143.
17. Catz A, Itzkovich M, Agranov E, Ring H, Tamir A. SCIM—Spinal cord independence measure: a new disability scale for patients with spinal cord lesions. *Spinal Cord.* 1997;35;850–856.
18. Dijkers M. Quality of life after spinal cord injury: a meta-analysis of the effects of disablement components. *Spinal Cord.* 1997;35:829–840.
19. Yozbatiran N, Keser Z, Hasan K, et al. White matter changes in corticospinal tract associated with improvement in arm and hand functions in incomplete cervical spinal cord injury: pilot case series. *Spinal Cord Ser Cases.* 2017;3:17028. doi:10.1038/scsandc.2017.28.
20. Pendlebury ST, Blamire AM, Lee MA, Styles P, Matthews PM. Axonal injury in the internal capsule correlates with motor impairment after stroke. *Stroke.* 1999;30:956–962.
21. Dagfinrud H, Kjeken I, Mowinckel P, Hagen KB, Kvien TK. Impact of functional impairment in ankylosing spondylitis: impairment, activity limitation, and participation restrictions. *J Rheumatol.* 2005;32:516–523. www.jrheum.org. Accessed January 21, 2018.
22. May-Lisowski TL, King PM. Effect of wearing a static wrist orthosis on shoulder movement during feeding. *Am J Occup Ther.* 2008;62:438–445. doi:10.5014/ajot.62.4.438.
23. Geusgens CA, van Heugten CM, Hagedoren E, Jolles J, van den Heuvel WJ. Environmental effects in the performance of daily tasks in healthy adults. *Am J Occup Ther.* 2010;64:935–940. doi:10.5014/ajot.2010.07171.
24. Raina KD, Rogers JC, Holm MB. Influence of the environment on activity performance in older women with heart failure. *Disabil Rehabil.* 2007;29:545–557. doi:10.1080/09638280600845514.
25. Gage M, Noh S, Polatajko HJ, Kaspar V. Measuring perceived self-efficacy in occupational therapy. *Am J Occup Ther.* 1994;48:783–790. doi:10.5014/ajot.48.9.783.
26. White RW. Motivation reconsidered: the concept of competence. *Psychol Rev.* 1959;66:297–333.
27. White RW. The urge towards competence. *Am J Occup Ther.* 1971;25:271–274.
28. Radomski MV. Self-efficacy: improving occupational therapy outcomes by helping patients say "I can.". *Phys Disabil Spec Interest Sect Q.* 2000;23:1–3.
29. Gage M, Polatajko H. Enhancing occupational performance through an understanding of perceived self-efficacy. *Am J Occup Ther.* 1994;48:452–461. doi:10.5014/ajot.48.5.452.
30. Hughes A, Galbraith D, White D. Perceived competence: a common core for self-efficacy and self-concept? *J Pers Assess.* 2011;93:278–289. doi:10.1080/00223891.2011.559390.
31. Juengst SB, Adams LM, Bogner JA, et al. Trajectories of life satisfaction after TBI: influence of life roles, age, cognitive disability, and depressive symptoms. *Rehabil Psychol.* 2015;60:353–364. doi:10.1037/rep0000056.
32. Wallenbert I, Jonsson H. Waiting to get better: a dilemma regarding habits in daily occupations after stroke. *Am J Occup Ther.* 2005;59:218–224. doi:10.5014/ajot.59.2.218.
33. Kielhofner G. *Model of Human Occupation: Theory and Application.* 4th ed. Philadelphia, PA: Lippincott Williams & Wilkins; 2008.

34. Bruner J. Organization of early skilled action. *Child Dev.* 1973;44:1–11.
35. Ma H-I, Trombly CA, Robinson-Podolski C. The effect of context on skill acquisition and transfer. *Am J Occup Ther.* 1999;53:138–144. doi:10.5014/ajot.53.2.138.
36. Wu C-Y, Trombly C, Lin K-C, Tickle-Degnen L. Effects of object affordances on reaching performance in person with and without cerebrovascular accident. *Am J Occup Ther.* 1998;52:447–456. doi:10.5014/ajot.52.6.447.
37. Field MJ, Jette AM, eds; Institute of Medicine (US) Committee on Disability in America. *The Future of Disability in America.* Washington, DC: National Academy Press; 2007.
38. Oakley F, Kielhofner G, Barris R, Reichler R. The role checklist: development and empirical assessment of reliability. *OTJR (Thorofare N J).* 1986;6:157–170.
39. Barris R, Oakley F, Kielhofner G. The role checklist. In: Hemphill BJ, ed. *Mental Health Assessment in Occupational Therapy.* Thorofare, NJ: Slack, Inc.; 1988:73–91.
40. Law M, Baptiste S, Carswell A, McColl M, Polatajko H, Pollack N. *Canadian Occupational Performance Measure.* 5th ed. Ottawa, Canada: CAOT Publications; 2014.
41. Toal-Sullivan D, Henderson PR. Client-Oriented Role Evaluation (CORE): the development of a clinical rehabilitation instrument to assess role change associated with disability. *Am J Occup Ther.* 2004;58:211–220. doi:10.5014/ajot.58.2.211.
42. Resnick B. Reliability and validity testing of the self-efficacy for functional activities scale. *J Nurs Meas.* 1999;7:5–20.
43. Matuska K. Description and development of the Life Balance Inventory. *OTJR (Thorofare N J).* 2012;32:220–228. doi:10.3928/15394492-20110610-01.
44. Fisher AG, Bray-Jones K. *The Assessment of Motor and Process Skills.* 7th ed. Fort Collins, CO: Three Star Press; 2010.
45. Klein RM, Bell B. Self-care skills: behavioral measurement with Klein-Bell ADL Scale. *Arch Phys Med Rehabil.* 1982;63:335–338.
46. Della Pietra GL, Savio K, Oddone F, Reggiani M, Monaco F, Leone MA. Validity and reliability of the Barthel Index administered by telephone. *Stroke.* 2011;42:2077–2079. doi:10.1161/STROKEEAHA.111.613521.
47. Mahoney FI, Barthel DW. Functional evaluation: the Barthel index. *Md State Med J.* 1965;14:61–65.
48. Holm MB, Rogers JC. Functional assessment: the Performance Assessment of Self-Care Skills (PASS). In: Hemphill BJ, ed. *Assessments in Occupational Therapy Mental Health: An Integrative Approach.* Thorofare, NJ: Slack Inc; 1999:117–124.
49. Weinstock-Zlotnick G, Hinojosa J. Bottom-up or top-down evaluation: is one better than the other? *Am J Occup Ther.* 2004;58:594–599. doi:10.5014/ajot.58.5.594.
50. Chui T, Oliver R, Marshall L, Letts L. *Safety Assessment of Function and the Environment for Rehabilitation Tool Manual.* Toronto, Canada: COTA Comprehensive Rehabilitation and Mental Health Services; 2002.
51. Baum CM, Edwards DF. *Guide for the Home Occupational-Environmental Assessment.* St. Louis, MO: Washington University Program in Occupational Therapy; 1998.
52. Lum PS, Mulroy S, Amdur RL, Requejo P, Prilutsky BI, Dromerick AW. Gains in upper extremity function after stroke via recovery or compensation: potential differential effects on amount of real-world limb use. *Top Stroke Rehabil.* 2009;16:237–253. doi:10.1310/tsr1604-237.
53. Mastos M, Miller K, Eliasson AC, Imms C. Goal-directed training: linking theories of treatment to clinical practice for improved functional activities in daily life. *Clin Rehabil.* 2007;21:47–55. doi:10.1177/0269215506073494.
54. Mathiowetz V, Wade MG. Task constraints and functional motor performance of individuals with and without multiple sclerosis. *Ecol Psychol.* 1995;7:99–123.
55. Trombly CA, Wu C-Y. Effect of rehabilitation tasks on organization of movement after stroke. *Am J Occup Ther.* 1999;53:333–344. doi:10.5014/ajot.53.4.333.
56. Jack J, Estes RI. Documenting progress: hand therapy treatment shift from biomechanical to occupational adaptation. *Am J Occup Ther.* 2010;64:82–87. doi:10.5014/ajot.64.1.82.
57. Nelson DL. Critiquing the logic of the domain section of the occupational therapy practice framework: domain and process. *Am J Occup Ther.* 2006;60:511–523. doi:10.5014/ajot.60.5.511.
58. Roley SS, Delany J. Improving the occupational therapy practice framework: domain & process. *OT Pract.* 2009;14:9–12.
59. Gutman SA, Mortera MH, Hinojosa J, Kramer P. The issue is: revision of the occupational therapy practice framework. *Am J Occup Ther.* 2007;61:119–126. doi:10.5014/ajot.61.1.119.

Chapter 2

Occupation: Philosophy and Concepts

Catherine A. Trombly Latham

LEARNING OBJECTIVES

This chapter will allow the reader to:

1. Define occupation.
2. Discuss the importance of occupation in people's lives.
3. Discuss the concept of occupational balance.
4. Discuss occupation as a therapeutic medium.
5. Characterize occupation-as-end and occupation-as-means.
6. Discuss the therapeutic qualities of occupation: purposefulness and meaningfulness.
7. Cite evidence that supports the use of occupation as therapy.
8. Describe how therapeutic occupation is implemented in practice.

CHAPTER OUTLINE

TERMINOLOGY

Activity analysis: a process by which properties of a given activity are identified for their ability to elicit targeted responses or enable a person to successfully accomplish the activity.

Constraints: limitations imposed on completion of an occupation. Extrinsic constraints include physical and sociocultural contexts, and environments and task demands. Intrinsic constraints include personal factors such as movement abilities, vision, sensation, cognition-perception, and cardiorespiratory capacity.

Habit: a behavior pattern acquired by frequent repetition that shows itself in regularity or increased facility of performance.[1]

Occupation-as-end: the combined set of activities that, together, support desired occupational roles and purposeful end goals identified as meaningful to the individual.

Occupation-as-means: the array of activities that support the completion of tasks needed in daily life, but, by themselves, may not hold significant meaning to the individual.

Task demands: the specific features of an activity that influence the type and amount of effort required to perform the activity. Demands include the shape, size, texture, number of objects; the visual, auditory, physical, or emotional impact of surroundings; the meaning of ritual associated with the activity; the size, shape, weight, configuration of tools; and the colors, textures, weight, familiarity, etc., of materials. Also known as *activity demands*.

Velocity profile: a graph of time versus speed of movement from which the organization of movement can be determined.

Occupation Defined

Occupation is both the center of human experience and the core of our profession.[2] Occupation is the unique therapeutic medium of occupational therapy[3] as well as outcome.[4] Occupation is "everything people do to occupy themselves, including looking after themselves, enjoying life, and contributing to the social and economic fabric of their communities."

Although the terms *occupation* and *purposeful activity* have been used interchangeably, they are distinct in meaning. The key difference is that occupations are central to a person's identity and influence how one spends time and makes decisions, whereas purposeful activity is a class of human actions that are goal directed and allow a person to develop skills that enhance occupational engagement but do not assume a place of central importance or meaning to a person's life. Each occupation is composed of several purposeful activities.[5] Purposeful activity is circumscribed, demands specific responses within particular contexts, and is used therapeutically to facilitate change in impairments and functional limitations. In this text, **occupation-as-end** is equated to occupation, and **occupation-as-means** is equated to purposeful activity.

Importance of Occupation in People's Lives

Occupational engagement contributes to the experience of a life worth living.[6,7] Engagement in positive occupations (e.g., care of self, others, property, and creative or productive endeavors), for which a person has both the capability and desire, regulates the rhythm of personal and community life. Such occupations absorb attention and evoke creativity, promote feelings of satisfaction with achievement, and contribute to a sense of self-esteem and self-efficacy (Fig. 2-1). These occupations are potentially therapeutic. In the absence of social and productive occupation (as occurs, e.g., early in retirement, in the acute stage of motor disability, or immediately after a profound loss[8]), a person may experience a sense of disorganization, depression, and lost sense of self-worth.

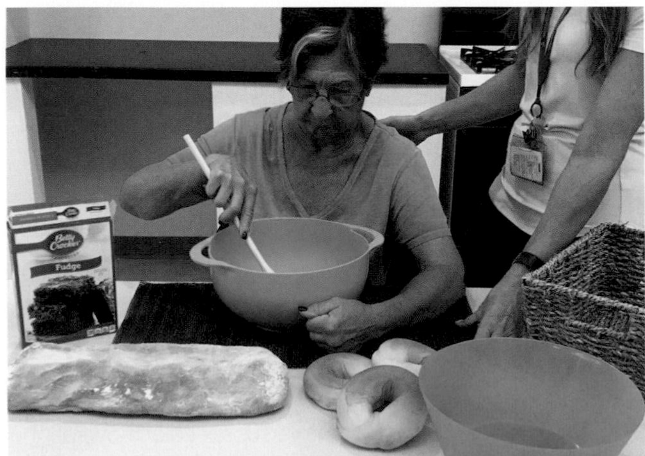

Figure 2-1. Occupation-as-end. Baking again under new circumstances after stroke.

Not all occupation is beneficial. Attempts to engage in occupations beyond one's capabilities can lead to frustration, anxiety, and depression.[9] Engagement in negative occupation (e.g., crime and destruction) disrupts personal and community life. Doing the same activity repetitively beyond the requirements of the task, as seen in obsessive-compulsive disorder (OCD), reinforces pathology. Imposition of unsuitable, negatively meaningful activities (e.g., children's games used as therapy for elderly patients) fails to build a sense of self-esteem and satisfaction. These types of occupation are not therapeutic. Therapeutic occupation, a special type of occupation, is defined as the use of positive, relevant, meaningful, and purposive activities to improve a person's ability to participate in life, or to improve abilities and capacities to enable improved occupational functioning.

Occupational Balance

Occupational therapy subscribes to the belief that the balance of engagement in life occupations, including rest, is basic to health and wellness.[10,11] The ideal configuration of this balance is individually defined, consisting of occupations that are meaningful to a particular person and that promote wellness.[12,13] As part of the occupational profile interview, therapists can ascertain whether patients feel that they are in occupational balance and on what basis each person defines that balance.

Balance may be defined on the basis of challenging versus relaxing occupations, activities meaningful to the individual versus those meaningful to society, or activities intended to care for oneself versus those intended to care for others.[12] Other gradients on which balance is established include allotment of time among physical, mental, social, and rest occupations, or mixing physically taxing occupations with light, relaxing occupations (also called pacing).

If balance is skewed toward one end of the gradient, then occupational dysfunction can occur. For example, if too much time is spent in self-enhancement activities (e.g., video gaming) to the detriment of other roles, then the person's work, social life, and/or self-care suffers, and he or she is occupationally "out of balance." If the person engages in mentally challenging occupations without balance with rest or lesser challenging occupations, then the person becomes stressed ("burned out"), unhealthy, and ineffective in other life areas. If the person engages in physically stressful occupations or movements without rest, damage occurs to involved body structures (e.g., cumulative trauma).[14]

Occupation as Therapy

Occupational therapists work with people who have experienced, or are in danger of experiencing, significant occupational dysfunction secondary to changes in their physical, cognitive, emotional, or social well-being, or to their environments. It is the role of the occupational therapist to help patients grieve losses and reconstruct acceptable occupational identities.[15]

Occupation is used to create or promote health, to remediate impairments or restore an ability or skill, to modify or adapt performance, to maintain performance capabilities, or to prevent disability.[5] The appropriate occupation results in the participant's sense of mastery.[16] Occupational intervention becomes therapeutic when it is guided by theory. In this text, the theoretical guideline is the Occupational Functioning Model (Chapter 1), but therapists may choose to use other guidelines or frames of reference.

What about occupation that maintains or restores health? That question is still debated, but one suggestion is that occupation is therapeutic when it has meaning for the patient, when it makes demands on the system needing improvement, and when it fulfills a purpose in the person's life.[17] The notion that purpose is necessary for a therapeutic effect has persisted throughout the history of therapeutic occupation, whereas the idea that occupation should be meaningful was temporarily lost after World War II, during the biomechanical era of occupational therapy. At that time, occupational therapists, in an attempt to mirror the medical model, promoted exercise using the motions of an activity—thereby "preserving" meaningfulness—without true meaning (e.g., "weaving" on a floor loom for exercise without thread on the loom).[16] Another aspect of therapeutic occupation is the just right challenge, the optimal fit between demands of the occupation and the skills of the person.[2,9] An occupation is therapeutic when it requires effort for the patient but is possible to accomplish. By accomplishing the occupation, the patient improves the impaired ability or capacity being challenged. By succeeding in the challenge, the patient is motivated to continue or repeat the experience.[9] A successful therapeutic occupation results in feelings of self-efficacy, self-esteem, and self-satisfaction, as well as improved occupational functioning.

Occupational therapists help people achieve satisfying occupational competence in several ways. One way is to adapt methods of accomplishing activities; another is to adapt the environment or tools and teach the person how to use these contextual adaptations.[18] In this case, occupation is both the treatment and the end goal (occupation-as-end). Occupation-as-end may remediate impairments, but this benefit is serendipitous, and the occupation is not chosen for that purpose. A second way is to remediate impaired capacities and abilities that prevent successful performance of activities and tasks required of a patient's roles.[18] In this case, occupation is the means to remediate impairment (occupation-as-means) (Fig. 2-2). The occupation used may actually be the same, for instance, chopping apples to make a pie. If the goal is to relearn how to make an apple pie, then it is considered occupation-as-end. If the goal is to improve grasp strength to enable multiple other life occupations, then chopping apples is considered occupation-as-means.

The key skill of the occupational therapist is the ability to analyze activities in terms of the required skills, abilities, and capacities; what influence the social and physical environments have on the likelihood of successful occupational performance; and what abilities and capacities the person brings to the therapeutic encounter. Analysis allows selection, gradation, and adaptation of activities to promote a therapeutic outcome (as described in Chapter 3).[19]

Occupation-as-End

Occupation-as-end is the complex of activities and tasks that comprise roles (Fig. 2-3). It is a person's functional goal that he or she tries to accomplish in a given environment using the abilities and capacities he or she has, and any adaptations that may be necessary. The occupational therapist uses a person-environment-occupation focused analysis to evaluate and plan therapy. Successful intervention involves a match among the client's goals and abilities, the task itself, the client's perception of the task's challenges, the client's sense of self-efficacy regarding the task,[20] and the environment in which the task is to be carried out.

Purposeful occupation-as-end organizes a person's behavior, day, and life. Occupation-as-end is purposeful by virtue of its focus on accomplishing valued activity goals. Occupation-as-end is not only purposeful but also meaningful because it is the performance of activities that a person perceives as important. Meaning is

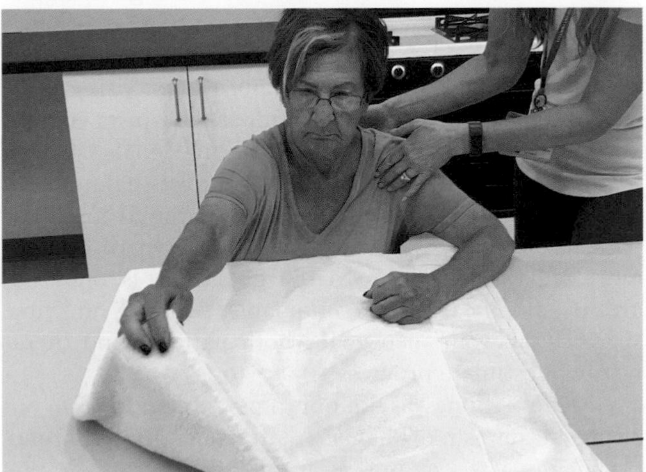

Figure 2-2. Occupation-as-means. Folding towels to improve sitting balance after stroke.

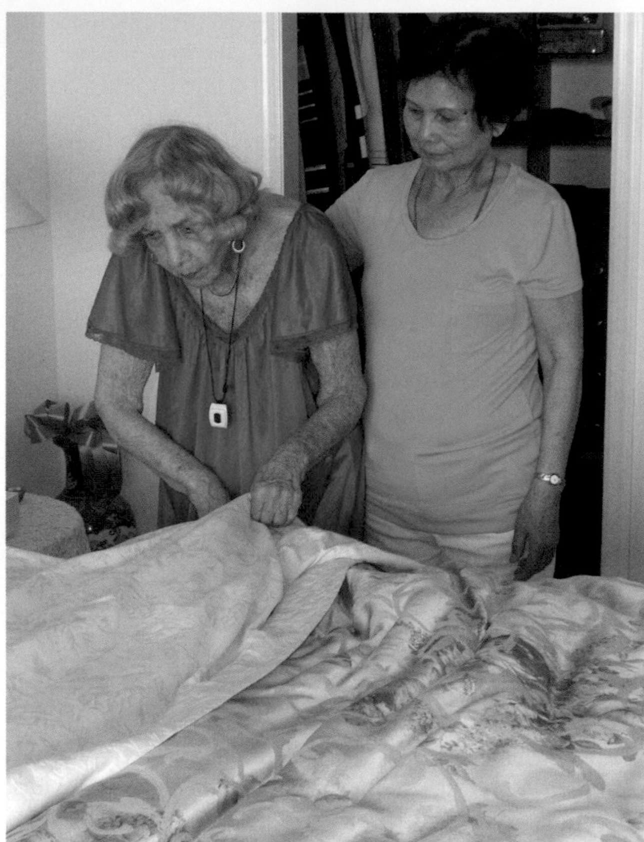

Figure 2-3. Occupation-as-end. Relearning to make bed after stroke.

individual, and although the occupational therapist can speculate about what may be meaningful to the patient based on the person's life history, the therapist must verify with each patient that the particular occupation *is* meaningful to that person *now* and verify that the person perceives value in relearning it. What a person finds meaningful may not only relate to his or her occupational history but also be a function of the person's stage in the recovery trajectory. That is, even if someone has an occupational history of enjoying cooking, she may not be ready emotionally to assume cooking tasks after a devastating injury because engaging in that occupation would force her to confront her loss and therefore would not be positively meaningful to her. Using a client-centered approach, occupational therapists encourage patients to choose the occupational goals of most importance at the present time. Therapists cannot substitute their own estimation of occupational goals for patients. However, patients may need help to develop more general goals into SMART goals, that is, ones that are *s*pecific, *m*easureable, *a*ttainable, *r*ealistic, and *t*ime specified.[21] From such goals, both patients and therapists can estimate progress.

Meaningfulness is not only a psychological term but also a mechanism of change. It affects neurological functioning, as was seen in a positron emission tomography (PET) study by Decety et al.[22] who discovered that brain activation differed with the meaning of an action regardless of subjects' strategies. Newman-Norlund et al.[23] also discovered, using functional magnetic resonance imaging (fMRI), that certain neurons in the brain distinguish between meaningful and meaningless actions.

Habits and Routines as Components of Occupation-as-End

Most self-maintenance and many self-advancement and self-enhancement roles depend on habits and routines. **Habits** are behavior patterns performed automatically. Routines are performance patterns that give life order.[5,24] Both habits and routines are carried out without conscious thought until they are disrupted by change in the environment or to a person's capabilities, at which time they fail to accomplish a specified goal requiring the person to pay attention and modify actions. Injury, disease, environmental change, and significant life changes disrupt useful routines and habits that may cause occupational dysfunction.

Habits may be preserved after brain injury. If a patient with brain injury is placed in a familiar context that provides the cues needed to perform habitual actions, he or she may be able to engage in formerly important, albeit automatic, occupations, even when he or she may not be able to learn new methods. Therapists would be interested in determining whether such habits were preserved in patients with brain injury by setting the context to trigger habitual responses.

When habits or routines are disturbed, for example, as occurs when moving to a nursing home or after a sudden trauma, life suddenly becomes chaotic and confusing, unlike the orderliness of familiar routines that contributed to an efficient and goal-directed life prior to the change.[24] The therapist will acknowledge this loss with the patient and prepare to develop new habits and routines, given the new circumstances. Habits and routines are learned through repetition of an action under particular cue conditions that result in a reward (successful completion of an activity). In the beginning, the person must focus on the action, but with repetition and consistency of context, little to no attention is necessary.

In a study of Swedish adults who experienced stroke, Wallenbert and Jonsson[25] learned that although patients were frustrated in their daily occupations because of impairments, they resisted developing new habits because they feared that doing so would diminish possible gains they could make by struggling to regain lost skills. They perceived development of new habits as detrimental. Resistance to change should be explored with patients to better understand the benefits of learning new habits.

Some habits or routines are not health promoting and need to be changed, for example, sitting for prolonged periods without relieving pressure on compromised skin regions. In this case, therapists should attempt to interrupt the habitual aspect of the action by (1) changing the cues (environment/context) and/or (2) changing the reward, that is, ensuring that the habitual action does not accomplish the goal the person expected. For example, a switch could be installed beneath a wheelchair cushion that would turn a computer or TV off if skin pressure was not relieved after an allotted time period.

Occupation-as-Means

Occupation-as-means is the use of occupation as a treatment to improve a person's impaired capacities and abilities to enable eventual occupational functioning. Occupation-as-means refers to occupation acting as the therapeutic change agent. An occupational therapist uses a client-focused **activity analysis** (see Chapter 3) when prescribing therapeutic occupation. It is important to remember that although the linkage between occupation-as-means and the remedial goal is obvious to the therapist, it is likely not to the patient. Therefore, when using occupation-as-means, the therapist must *repeatedly* and clearly explain why a given activity is recommended or used in therapy. Various arts, crafts, games, sports, exercise routines (Figs. 2-4 and 2-5), and daily activities that are systematically selected and tailored to each individual are used as occupation-as-means.

Occupation-as-means is therapeutic when the activity has a purpose or goal that challenges the patient's capacities and abilities needing improvement, yet has a prospect for success ("just right challenge") and engages the person *repeatedly* in the action.[26] Because the central nervous system (CNS) is organized to accomplish goals,[27] the goal or purpose seems to organize the most efficient response, given the **constraints** of person and context.[28] Furthermore, if an activity has meaning and relevance to the individual requiring change, it is more likely to motivate the patient's will to learn and improve.

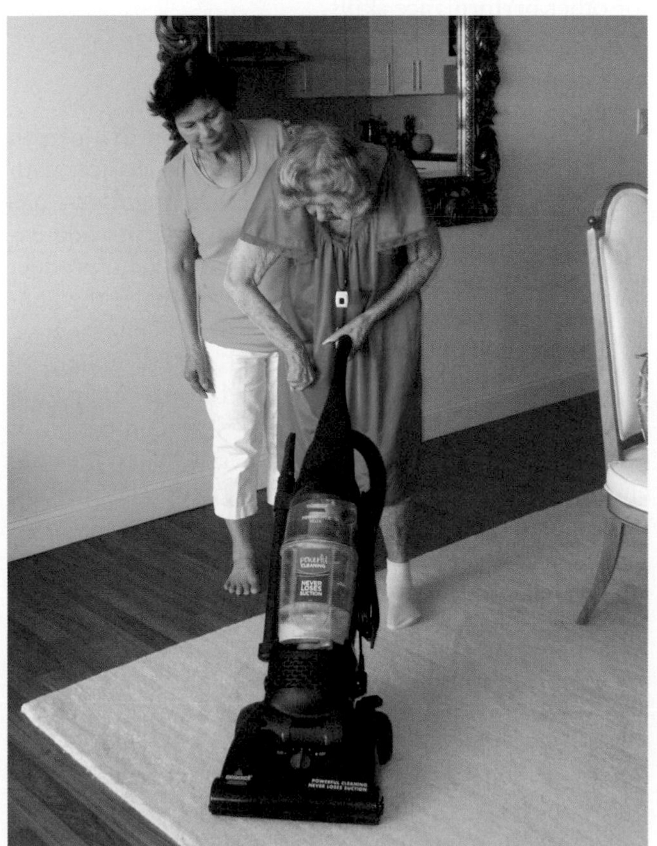

Figure 2-4. Occupation-as-end. Relearning to vacuum after stroke.

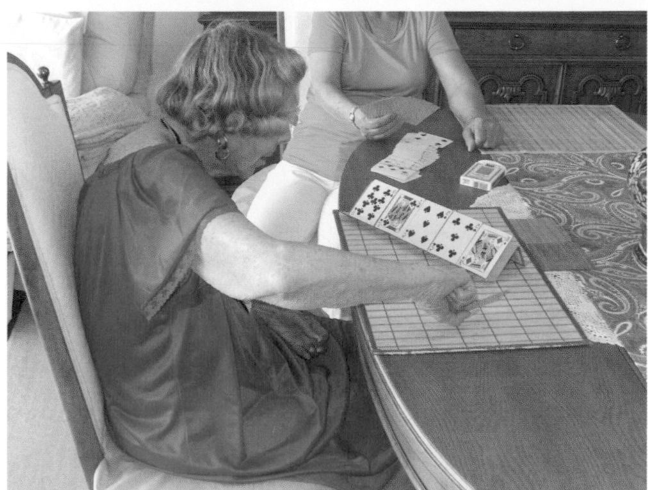

Figure 2-5. Occupation-as-means. Playing cards using an adapted card tray to improve coordination.

Meaningfulness in the sense of occupation-as-means has an immediate aspect. Choosing to participate in an activity at the moment is based on immediate motivation that is guided by currently perceived needs, feelings, and desires that may or may not be related to life goals. The meaningful aspect of occupation-as-means may be the emotional value that an interesting and creative experience offers the patient.[29] Meaningfulness may also stem from familiarity with the occupation, its power to arouse positive associations, the likelihood that completion of it will elicit approval from others who are respected and admired, its value in learning a prized skill, or its potential to contribute to recovery. Thus, the therapeutic aspects of occupation used as a means to change impairments are purposefulness and meaningfulness.

Evidence that Occupation-as-Means Organizes Responses

Evidence of changes in organization of emotions, cognition, and perceptions secondary to engagement in occupation or activity having the therapeutic quality of purposefulness is not easily obtained. However, evidence concerning the organization of movement can be easily gained using kinematic instruments to track the spatial–temporal aspects of movement. Movement organization can be detected from the shape of the **velocity profile** (Fig. 2-6),[30] which is a graph of time versus speed of movement. Different velocity profiles, which indicate differences in movement organization and CNS control, emerge for particular goals or purposes.[31]

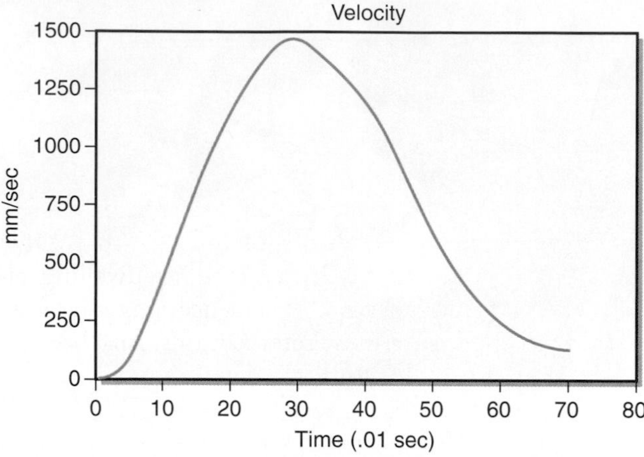

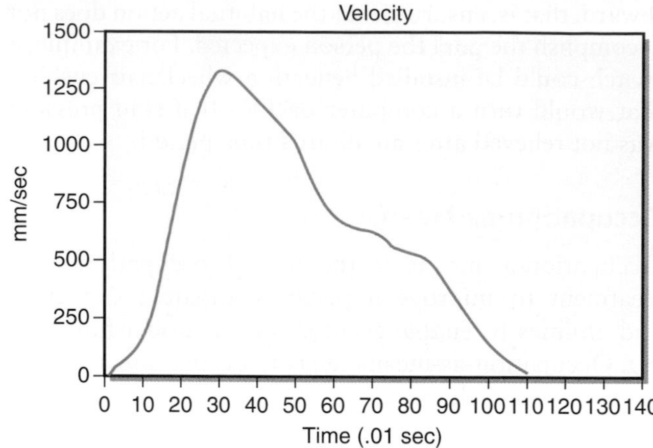

Figure 2-6. Velocity profiles of two reaches showing different movement organizations. The profile on the left is symmetrical and bell-shaped, which is commonly seen in preplanned, or programmed, reach. This organization may be seen in reaching to a stationary large target, to a familiar object, or to accomplish an automatic goal such as throwing the object. The peak of the velocity profile, which is the end of the acceleration phase of the reach, occurs roughly mid-reach. The profile on the right is left-shifted, which is commonly seen in guided reach to a small or imaginary target or to accomplish a precise goal such as putting a coin in a slot. The peak velocity occurs early in the reach and the deceleration phase is extended as the person guides the hand to the target.

Examples of evidence that goal-directed or purposeful occupation-as-means organizes movement responses are reported here and in the Evidence table.

In 1987, Marteniuk et al.[32] demonstrated for the first time the effect of goal on the organization of movement as detected from velocity profiles. They found that five university students organized movement differently when they reached for the same object for different purposes. One goal was to pick up a 4-cm disk and *place it* into a slot. The other goal was to pick up the disk and *throw it* into a basket. They measured the reach *to* the disk, not the placing or throwing motion. The distance and biomechanical demands were exactly the same under both conditions. Only the intent after reach was different. The two goals produced different velocity profiles for reaching for the disk, indicating different movement organizations.

Goal or purpose is generated from the patient's own intention, from the therapist's directions,[33,34] or from the context, including which objects are available, the relevance of the objects, and what the objects afford the person in terms of action. We are familiar with generation of goals by the person or by the therapist, but contextual indication of goals may be unfamiliar. High object affordance (e.g., presence of real functional objects as opposed to imagined, absent, or substitute objects) promotes optimal motor performance according to a systematic review of 35 studies by Hétu and Mercier[35]; this finding implies that the goal, as defined by the object, organizes movement. Filippi et al.[36] mapped gray matter volume changes associated with motor learning of goal-directed motor sequences and nonpurposeful motor actions in 31 healthy subjects. The researchers concluded that motor learning results in structural brain changes, with specific areas affected depending on whether learning involves a goal. In terms of motor responses, then, purposiveness, as transmitted by instruction or context, appears to organize behavior and may affect brain structure and function. Further study is required to verify these ideas and confirm them to be true for other performance skills.

Evidence that Occupation-as-Means Motivates Participation

Although the meaningfulness of occupation to a person must be determined by interview and discussion with that person, for research purposes, *meaningfulness* has been operationalized in four ways: to (1) provide enjoyment[37,38]; (2) offer choice[39]; (3) offer an end product that can be kept[40]; and (4) enhance or make the context more applicable to the person's life.[41] The response, *motivation*, is operationally defined as the number of repetitions or length of time engaged in the occupation or the amount of effort expended.[42,43] Examination of the studies cited here as well as others leads to the conclusion that meaningfulness appears to motivate continued performance, although further research is needed.

Effectiveness of Therapeutic Occupation

Based on personal experience and observation, occupational therapists have historically believed, before evidence was established, that occupation maintained or restored mental health and gave meaning and quality to one's life through its organizational and attention-demanding aspects.[3,16] Later, on the basis of deductive reasoning and anecdotal accounts, that belief was extended to include restoration of physical function through the biomechanical aspects of engagement in occupation. Occupational therapy began as a philosophically based profession and is now becoming a scientific, evidence-based profession.[16,44] The research efforts of occupational therapists and other scientists have begun to establish a solid basis for the health-regaining action of occupation. For example, advances in technology have enabled examination of brain function of humans engaged in occupations. Such research has resulted in remarkable advances in knowledge demonstrating that the cortex is functionally and structurally plastic throughout life and that engaging—or not engaging—in occupation modifies the brain's topography and physiology.[45] There is, however, an urgent need to experimentally verify the effects of occupation to cause particular changes[46] and to determine the key therapeutic mechanisms underlying *how* occupational interventions cause therapeutic change.[47]

Evidence that Occupation Restores a Sense of Self-Efficacy or Self-Esteem

Very few studies address the association between self-efficacy and self-esteem. A qualitative study by Rebeiro and Cook[48] provides some evidence that engagement in occupation restores one's sense of efficacy and self-worth. The participants were eight long-time members of an outpatient women's group at a mental health facility who engaged in a cooperative occupational project—making a quilt. On interview after 25 weeks of participation, the participants reported that engagement in the occupation gave them a sense of self-confidence and competency because of their accomplishment, which they did not have before the introduction of occupation to the group. Another is a pretest–posttest, three-group design by Landa-Gonzalez and Molnar[49] who evaluated the effectiveness of occupation-based intervention (10–15 minutes of preparatory activities followed by 30 minutes of occupation-based activities 2 times/week for 4 weeks) versus enabling/preparatory intervention (30 minutes of preparatory activities followed by 10–15 minutes of occupation-based activities for the same frequency and duration) versus no treatment (social visiting at same frequency and duration) on improving self-care skills, perceived performance, satisfaction, role function, and self-esteem/self-efficacy of 29 community-dwelling elders with osteoarthritis who were randomly assigned to the group. Both intervention groups scored significantly ($p = 0.012$) higher than the control group on measures of self-esteem/self-efficacy; however, there was no significant difference between intervention groups on these measures. Contamination of the independent variable (both groups received occupation-based activities in different amounts) may have influenced this outcome. Therefore, further research is needed to confirm that occupation restores a sense of self-efficacy or self-esteem.

Evidence that Occupation-as-End Restores Self-Maintenance, Self-Enhancement, and Self-Advancement Roles

Orellano et al.[46] reviewed 38 studies, of which 82% offered Level I evidence, to determine the effectiveness of occupation- and activity-based interventions on performance of instrumental activities of daily living (IADLs) basic to role engagement by community-dwelling elders. They concluded that the evidence was moderate to strong in support of these interventions. Another systematic analysis of 15 studies[50] determined that there was a 16% greater success rate for improved IADL and a 30% greater success rate for improved basic activities of daily living (BADLs; self-care) as a result of home-based, task-specific, occupation-based training than occurred due to control conditions. Wolf et al.[51] reviewed 39 studies published between 2003 and 2012, of which 21 addressed activities of daily living (ADLs) performance of stroke patients. They found strong evidence to support the use of occupation-based interventions to improve BADL performance. However, they also found that too few studies addressed IADLs, leisure, or social participation to draw conclusions regarding these domains. Trombly et al.[52] studied the achievement of valued IADL goals in persons with mild to moderate brain injury and found that goal-directed, occupation-based therapy resulted in achievement of 81% of all goals named by participants. A thorough systematic review and meta-analysis, with 14,593 possible studies narrowed down to 9 well-controlled randomized trials that met inclusion criteria, concluded that patients who received occupational therapy that focused on improving ADLs after stroke were significantly ($p = 0.01$) more independent in personal ADL as compared to control.[53] But not all patients benefited and the authors stated the need to define who are most likely to benefit.

Evidence that Occupation-as-Means Remediates Impairments

Studies of the effects of occupation-as-means on persons with particular physical impairments are few and scattered. One systematic review of 29 studies on the effects of occupational therapy on psychosocial, cognitive-perceptual, and sensorimotor impairments post-stroke concluded that engaging in homemaking tasks resulted in greater improvement in cognitive ability than paper-and-pencil drills and that practice of movement to achieve a specific action goal had small to moderate positive effects ($r = 0.27$) compared with control conditions.[54] Another review of 149 studies conducted to determine the effectiveness of interventions to improve occupational performance in people with motor impairments after stroke found that there are a variety of effective occupation-as-means-type interventions.

The commonalities among the effective ones were goal-directed (purposeful), individualized (meaningful) activities that promoted *high repetition* of task-specific movements.[26] Clearly, much more research is needed.

Implementation of Therapeutic Occupation in Practice

Occupation-as-end is implemented by teaching the activity or task directly, using whatever abilities the patient has and/or by providing whatever adaptations are necessary to enable performance. Because occupation occurs within a person-task-environment interaction, change in any one of these variables may result in successful performance. Implementation of occupation-as-end focuses on changing the **task demands** and/or the environment, whereas occupation-as-means focuses on changing the person. Therapeutic principles for application of occupation-as-end derive from cognitive information processing and learning theories. Such therapeutic principles are referred to as the rehabilitative approach. In this approach, occupations are analyzed to ensure that they are within the capabilities of the patient, but are not used to bring about change in these capabilities per se. The patient learns the skill with the help of the therapist as teacher and adaptor of task demands and context. In the therapeutic encounter, the therapist:

- determines the patient's occupational goals
- analyzes the task and environment to determine whether the task is within the person's capabilities in that environment
- organizes or modifies the environment or task demands to facilitate success
- organizes the subtasks to be learned so the person will succeed
- provides clear instructions
- provides feedback to promote successful outcome
- structures the practice to ensure continued improvement

To implement occupation-as-means, occupations of interest are analyzed to determine that they demand particular responses from the person and that the responses demanded are slightly more challenging than what the person can easily produce. The therapist provides the opportunity to engage in the potentially therapeutic occupation repeatedly, and as the person makes the effort and succeeds, the particular impairment—which the occupation-as-means was chosen to remediate—is reduced. In the therapeutic encounter, the therapist:

- ascertains the patient's interests
- selects occupations that reflect those interests
- analyzes the occupations to determine which would provide the correct challenge to impaired abilities
- lets the patient choose from among several offered occupations
- explains to the person how engaging in this activity should improve his or her ability and how that relates to achieving the person's overall goal
- instructs the patient in the correct procedure for doing the activity to derive the most therapeutic benefit
- grades the occupation to increase the challenge as the patient improves

Lyons et al.[55] described ways they organized one clinic to efficiently use occupation therapeutically. The treatment areas in the clinic were rearranged to resemble a homelike environment (e.g., bedroom, living room, and nursery). The therapists prepared "occupation kits," which were large plastic boxes containing all the props necessary to engage in an occupation. Occupation kits were made for gardening, letter writing, pet care, fishing, scrapbooking, and car care, which were the most commonly named activities by their clients. Furthermore, therapists in this clinic were encouraged to work with patients in the various areas of the hospital campus and surrounding environment, the larger community, and the client's own community (e.g., barbershop, market, or place of worship) to provide meaningful occupation-based interventions in natural contexts.

The processes involved in using occupation therapeutically are activity analysis, selection and gradation, and adaptation. Guidelines for these processes are presented in Chapter 3.

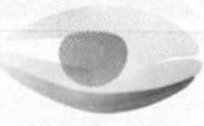

CASE STUDY

Patient Information

Chesa is a 65-year-old, right-handed woman who sustained a left cerebral vascular accident (LCVA) resulting in hemiparesis of her dominant side. She is depressed because she fears the loss of important roles and occupations. She was originally from the Philippines, where she worked as a schoolteacher. Now she is retired, living in the United States with one of her daughters.

Assessment Process and Results

Using the *Occupational Profile*, a description of a typical day in chronological sequence revealed that her routine consisted of cooking breakfast for her granddaughters, participating in housework, playing with her grandchildren, going to church in the evening, and sending text messages to her friends in the Philippines.

Evaluation of impairments included assessments of muscle tone and strength, voluntary control of movement, sensation of the affected upper extremity (UE), and standing balance. The speech pathologist reported recovering motor aphasia. The results were (1) decreased motor control and strength but development of volitional movement in her right arm, (2) impaired sensation, (3) slight spasticity in the right side of her body, (4) ability to stand for short periods of time, and (5) impaired but improving expressive language.

Occupational Therapy Problem List

- Inability to carry out BADLs independently
- Inability to prepare light meals
- Inability to participate in home management tasks such as laundry and vacuuming
- Loss of habitual computer skills
- Impaired proprioceptive sensation of the affected UE
- Weakness in affected UE
- Impaired motor control of the affected UE
- Impaired standing balance
- Depression

Occupational Therapy Goal List

Goal setting was accomplished using the COPM (Canadian Occupational Performance Measure[56]). Chesa's goals included the following most valued occupations:

- care for own BADLs
- prepare light meals
- engage in play with grandchildren
- send e-mails to friends
- participate in church

Intervention

Therapy included occupation-as-end and occupation-as-means. Occupation-as-means to improve strength and motor control involved incorporating Chesa's right arm into activity completion. While standing, she used the light meal preparation occupation kit to practice handling implements and packaging, which promoted motor skills and standing balance as well as prepared her for light meal preparation. Occupation-as-end involved daily morning practice of dressing and grooming skills using familiar clothing and utensils in her room. Other intervention sessions were held in the kitchen to learn safe and adapted methods of making sandwiches, soup, and cookies, and in a simulated living room where her daughter and two children visited. At first, the granddaughters did not know how to play with Chesa as they had before. But Chesa used her teaching skills to explain her new participation level and started a therapist-suggested game to play with her grandchildren. Occupation-based treatment involved developing Chesa's new view of herself as someone who could now continue to participate in her roles, which lightened her depression.

Outcome

At discharge from inpatient rehabilitation, Chesa's status was as follows:

- Affected UE strength and motor control recovered enough to permit independence in BADL, light kitchen work, use of the computer, and handling of prayer books.
- Standing balance recovered to allow working in her kitchen, walking into the church, and participation in the women's group.
- Confidence in her abilities allowed her to adopt a creative approach to playing with her grandchildren.

Referrals

1. Outpatient occupational therapy to continue improvement of IADLs
2. Occupational therapy driver specialist

Adapted with permission from Lyons A, Phipps SC, Berro M. Using occupation in the clinic. *OT Practice*. 2004;9(26):11–15.

Examples of Evidence Regarding Effectiveness of Therapeutic Occupation

Intervention	Description	Participants	Dosage	Research Design and Evidence Level	Benefit	Statistical Significance and Effect Size
Occupation-as-end: Goal-specific training to achieve valued occupational goals[57]	Valued ADLs goals were worked toward via a series of written contracts that specified interim and short-term goals. Carried out in homes, day centers, and workplace. Control: Booklet that listed resources with those particular to what the participant highlighted	110 (75.5% male) community-dwelling persons with moderate to severe TBI aged 16–65 years, in acute to chronic stages of recovery. Randomized to group. 94 (85%) available at 2-year follow-up, but only 75 (68%) available for analysis of BICRO-39a	2–6 hours/week for a mean of 27 weeks for experimental group; one visit for control group. The independent variable was compromised because some of the patients in the control group received up to 1 month of experimental treatment before randomization.	Randomized controlled trial. Level I	Practice of valued goal activities in a community setting yielded benefits to persons with severe TBI that outlived the active treatment period by at least 18 months.	35% of experimental group vs. 20% of control group improved significantly ($p < 0.05$) from baseline to follow-up on the Barthel Index. The experimental group scored significantly ($p < 0.05$) better at posttest than the control on the total BICRO-39 score and self-organization and psychological well-being subscales. Effect sizes could not be calculated from data provided.
Occupation-as-end: Group-based and individual task-specific dressing retraining[58]	Group-based retraining for outer garment dressing supervised by two occupational therapists and individual training for underclothing and particular dressing problems. Multiple repetitions were encouraged.	Consecutive cohort of 119 patients; ~2 weeks poststroke, medically stable	Group: 1 hour twice weekly MEAN = 4.0, 1-hour group sessions. No record of number of individual treatments	Pretest–posttest design; retrospective analysis of data. Level III	Yes. Task-specific practice of dressing made a clinically important difference to dressing performance.	Three subgroups: upper body dressing, lower body dressing, and both upper and lower body dressing. All groups improved significantly ($p = 0.0001$) on the questions relating to dressing on the FIM. The effect size was estimated to be small ($r = 0.34$).
Occupation-as-means: Hand Dance Pro gaming system to reduce UE impairment and improve function[59]	High repetitions ($M = 1{,}118$ per session) of unilateral and bilateral reaching to targets coordinated to music and visual prompts with immediate feedback. The target buttons aligned with affected shoulder and placed to encourage maximum elbow extension. Trunk restrained to prevent substitution.	Nine persons post-stroke, categorized by FMA UE subtest to mild (>50/66; $n = 3$), moderate (26–50/66; $n = 5$), or severe (<26/66); $n = 1$. All able to actively raise the involved arm from side (0°) to 45° in any plane[b]	Fifteen 2-minute songs per session with at least 1-minute rest between songs; 18 sessions over 6 weeks	Single-group cohort pretest–posttest design. Level II	The gaming intervention improved UE movement kinematics, but not clinical measures in this group. The subjects enjoyed playing the game and were motivated to improve scores. Carryover of kinematic improvements to functional tasks may require concurrent practice of those tasks.	Significant ($p < 0.05$) improvements and medium to large effect sizes in kinematic measures of movement duration ($d = 0.67$),[c] velocity ($d = 0.97$), and elbow excursion ($d = 0.45$). Some subjects improved in performance time, grip strength, and hand function, but not scores of Wolf Motor Function Test ($d = 0.04$–0.17) or Stroke Impact Scale ($d = 0.08$–0.34).
Occupation-as-means: Activities in a modified C-IMT[60]	Practice of purposeful activities at high repetitions in clinic and at home while wearing a mitt constraint on unaffected hand. Resisted exercise, stretching, and weight bearing were used in preparation.	52-year-old female violinist 4 years after ischemic stroke affecting right side of body with returning voluntary movement of right UE	3 hours/day, 5 days/week, for 4 weeks plus 5–6 hours/day outside of therapy for 4 weeks	Case report. Level V	She improved in gross and fine motor coordination, UE strength, and spontaneous use of the UE. Able to play her violin to her satisfaction and rejoin the community symphony orchestra, as was her goal.	NA

[a] BICRO-39 is the Brain Injury Community Rehabilitation Outcome-39, a self-report that measures level of activity, participation, and psychological aspects of functioning in the community.
[b] Some voluntary movement at the outset is a prerequisite for regaining voluntary control through therapy.
[c] d, Cohen's d effect size; small, 0.20, medium, 0.50, and large, 0.80.

References

1. Merriam-Webster Dictionary. Habit. Springfield, MA: Merriam-Webster Inc. https://www.merriam-webster.com/dictionary/habit. Accessed January 28, 2018.
2. Law M. Participation in the occupations of everyday life. *Am J Occup Ther*. 2002;56:640–649. doi:10.5014/ajot.56.6.640.
3. Reilly M. Occupation can be one of the great ideas of 20th century medicine. *Am J Occup Ther*. 1962;16:1–9.
4. Trombly CA. Occupation: purposefulness and meaningfulness as therapeutic mechanisms. *Am J Occup Ther*. 1995;49:960–972. doi:10.5014/ajot.49.10.960.
5. American Occupational Therapy Association. Occupational therapy practice framework: domain and process (3rd ed.). *Am J Occup Ther*. 2014;68(suppl 1):S1–S48. doi:10.5014/ajot.2014.682006.
6. Bar MA, Jarus T. The effect of engagement in everyday occupations, role overload and social support on health and life satisfaction among mothers. *Int J Environ Res Public Health*. 2015;12:6045–6065. doi:10.3390/ijerph120606045.
7. Hammell KW. Dimensions of meaning in the occupations of daily life. *Can J Occup Ther*. 2004;71:296–305. doi:10.1177/000841740407100509.
8. Hoppes S. When a child dies the world should stop spinning: an autoethnography exploring the impact of family loss on occupation. *Am J Occup Ther*. 2005;59:78–87. doi:10.5014/ajot.59.1.78.
9. Rebeiro KL, Polgar JM. Enabling occupational performance: optimal experiences in therapy. *Can J Occup Ther*. 1999;66:14–22. doi:10.1177/000841749906600102.
10. Meyer A. The philosophy of occupational therapy. *Arch Occup Ther*. 1922/1977;1:1–10. (Reprinted in *Am J Occup Ther*. 1977;31:639–642.)
11. Rogers JC. Why study human occupation? *Am J Occup Ther*. 1984;38:47–49. doi:10.5014/ajot.38.1.47.
12. Stamm T, Lovelock L, Stew G, et al. I have a disease but I am not ill: a narrative study of occupational balance in people with rheumatoid arthritis. *OTJR (Thorofare N J)*. 2009;29:32–39.
13. Wagman P, Håkansson C, Björklund A. Occupational balance as used in occupational therapy: a concept analysis. *Scand J Occup Ther*. 2012;19:322–327. doi:10.3109/11038128.2011.596219.
14. Barcenilla A, March LM, Chen JS, Sambrook PN. Carpal tunnel syndrome and its relationship to occupation: a meta-analysis. *Rheumatology (Oxford)*. 2012;51:250–261. doi:10.1093/rheumatology/ker108.
15. Unruh AM. Reflections on: "So . . . what do you do?" occupation and the construct of identity. *Can J Occup Ther*. 2004;71:290–295. doi:10.1177/000841740407100508.
16. Laws J. Crackpots and basket-cases: a history of therapeutic work and occupation. *Hist Human Sci*. 2011;24(3):65–81. doi:10.1177/0952695111399677.
17. Dooley NR. Application of activities in practice. In: Hinojosa J, Blount M-L, eds. *The Texture of Life: Purposeful Activities in Context of Occupation*. 3rd ed. Bethesda, MD: AOTA Press; 2009:229–252.
18. Moyers PA, Dale LM. *The Guide to Occupational Therapy Practice*. 2nd ed. Bethesda, MD: AOTA Press; 2007.
19. Watson DE, Wilson SA. *Task Analysis: An Individual and Population Approach*. 2nd ed. Bethesda, MD: AOTA Press; 2003.
20. Lowenstein N, Tickle-Degnen L. Developing an occupational therapy home program for patients with Parkinson's disease. In: Trail M, Protas EJ, Lai C, eds. *Neurorehabilitation in Parkinson's Disease: An Evidence-Based Treatment Model*. Thorofare, NJ: Slack; 2008:231–243.
21. Mastos M, Miller K, Eliasson AC, Imms C. Goal-directed training: linking theories of treatment to clinical practice for improved functional activities in daily life. *Clin Rehabil*. 2007;21:47–55. doi:10.1177/026921550607394.
22. Decety J, Grezes J, Costes N, et al. Brain activity during observation of actions: influence of action content and subject's strategy. *Brain*. 1997;120;1763–1777. doi:10.1093/brain/120.10.1763.
23. Newman-Norlund R, van Schie HT, van Hoek ME, Cuijpers RH, Bekkering H. The role of inferior frontal and parietal areas in differentiating meaningful and meaningless object-directed actions. *Brain Res*. 2010;1315:63–74. doi:10.1016/j.brainres.2009.11.065.
24. Segal R. Family routines and rituals: a context for occupational therapy interventions. *Am J Occup Ther*. 2004;58:499–508. doi:10.5014/ajot.58.5.499.
25. Wallenbert I, Jonsson H. Waiting to get better: a dilemma regarding habits in daily occupations after stroke. *Am J Occup Ther*. 2005;59:218–224. doi:10.5014/ajot.59.2.218.
26. Nilsen DM, Gillen G, Geller D, Hreha K, Osei E, Saleem GT. Effectiveness of interventions to improve occupational performance of people with motor impairments after stroke: an evidence-based review. *Am J Occup Ther*. 2015;69(1):6901180030p1–6901180030p9. doi:10.5014/ajot.2015.011965.
27. Granit R. *The Purposive Brain*. Cambridge, MA: MIT; 1977.
28. Wu C, Trombly CA, Lin K, Tickle-Degnen L. A kinematic study of contextual effects on reaching performance in persons with and without stroke: influences of object availability. *Arch Phys Med Rehabil*. 2000;81:95–101.
29. Ayres AJ. Basic concepts of clinical practice in physical disabilities. *Am J Occup Ther*. 1958;12:300–302, 311.
30. Georgopoulos AP. On reaching. *Annu Rev Neurosci*. 1986;9:147–170.
31. Jeannerod M. *The Neural and Behavioral Organization of Goal-Directed Movements*. Oxford, UK: Clarendon; 1988.
32. Marteniuk RG, MacKenzie CL, Jeannerod M, Athenes S, Dugas C. Constraints on human arm movement trajectories. *Can J Psychol*. 1987;41:365–378.
33. Lin KC, Wu CY, Lin KH, Chang CW. Effects of task instructions and target location on reaching kinematics in people with and without cerebrovascular accident: a study of the less-affected arm. *Am J Occup Ther*. 2008;62:456–465. doi:10.5014/ajot.62.4.456.
34. Massie CL, Malcolm MP. Instructions emphasizing speed improves hemiparetic arm kinematics during reaching in stroke. *NeuroRehabilitation*. 2012;30:341–350. doi:10.3233/NRE-2012-0765.
35. Hétu S, Mercier C. Using purposeful tasks to improve motor performance: does object affordance matter? *Br J Occup Ther*. 2012;75:367–376. doi:10.4276/030802212X13433105374314.

36. Filippi M, Ceccarelli A, Pagani E, et al. Motor learning in healthy humans is associated to gray matter changes: a tensor-based morphometry study. *PLoS One*. 2010;5:e10198. doi:10.1371/journal.pone.0010198.
37. Melchert-McKearnan K, Dietz J, Engel M, White O. Children with burn injuries: purposeful activity versus rote exercise. *Am J Occup Ther*. 2000;54:381–390. doi:10.5014/ajot.54.4.381.
38. Omar MTA, Hegazy FA, Mokashi SP. Influences of purposeful activity versus rote exercise on improving pain and hand function in pediatric burn. *Burns*. 2012;38:261–268. doi:10.1016/burns.2011.08.004.
39. Tasky KK, Rudrud EH, Schulze KA, Rapp JT. Using choice to increase on-task behavior in individuals with traumatic brain injury. *J Appl Behav Anal*. 2008;41:261–265. doi:10.1901/jaba.2008.41-261.
40. Murphy S, Trombly CA, Tickle-Degnen L, Jacobs K. The effect of keeping an end-product on intrinsic motivation. *Am J Occup Ther*. 1999;53:153–158. doi:10.5014/ajot.53.2.153.
41. Lang EM, Nelson DL, Bush MA. Comparison of performance in materials-based occupation, imagery-based occupation, and rote exercise in nursing home residents. *Am J Occup Ther*. 1992;46:607–611. doi:10.5014/ajot.46.7.607.
42. Bloch MW, Smith DA, Nelson DL. Heart rate, activity, duration, and affect in added-purpose versus single-purpose jumping activities. *Am J Occup Ther*. 1989;43:25–30. doi:10.5014/ajot.43.1.25.
43. Kircher MA. Motivation as a factor of perceived exertion in purposeful versus nonpurposeful activity. *Am J Occup Ther*. 1984;38:165–170. doi:10.5014/ajot.38.3.165.
44. Holm MB. Our mandate for the new millennium: evidence-based practice. *Am J Occup Ther*. 2000;54:575–585. doi:10.5014/ajot.54.6.575.
45. Nudo RJ. The role of skill versus use in the recovery of motor function after stroke. *OTJR (Thorofare N J)*. 2007;27 (suppl 1):24S–32S.
46. Orellano E, Colón WI, Arbesman M. Effect of occupation- and activity-based interventions on instrumental activities of daily living performance among community-dwelling older adults: a systematic review. *Am J Occup Ther*. 2012;66:292–300. doi:10.5014/ajot.2012.003053.
47. Stav WB, Hallenen T, Lane J, Arbesman M. Systematic review of occupational engagement and health outcomes among community-dwelling older adults. *Am J Occup Ther*. 2012;66:301–310. doi:10.5014/ajot.2012.003707.
48. Rebeiro KL, Cook JV. Opportunity, not prescription: an exploratory study of the experience of occupational engagement. *Can J Occup Ther*. 1999;66:176–187. doi:10.1177/000841749906600405.
49. Landa-Gonzalez B, Molnar D. Occupational therapy intervention: effects on self-care, performance, satisfaction, self-esteem/self-efficacy, and role functioning of older Hispanic females with arthritis. *Occup Ther Health Care*. 2012;26:109–119. doi:10.3109/07380577.2011.644624.
50. Trombly CA, Ma H-I. A synthesis of the effects of occupational therapy for persons with stroke: Part I. Restoration of roles, tasks and activities. *Am J Occup Ther*. 2002;56:250–259. doi:10.5014/ajot.56.3.250.
51. Wolf TJ, Chuh A, Floyd T, McInnis K, Williams E. Effectiveness of occupation-based interventions to improve areas of occupation and social participation after stroke: an evidence-based review. *Am J Occup Ther*. 2015;69:6901180060p1–6901180060p11. doi:1.5014/ajot.2015.012195.
52. Trombly CA, Radomski MV, Trexel C, Burnett-Smith SE. Occupational therapy and achievement of self-identified goals by adults with acquired brain injury: phase II. *Am J Occup Ther*. 2002;56:489–498. doi:10.5014/ajot.56.5.489.
53. Legg L, Drummond A, Leonardi-Bee J, et al. Occupational therapy for patients with problems in personal activities of daily living after stroke: systematic review of randomised trials. *Br Med J*. 2007;335:922–929. doi:10.1136/bmj.39343.466863.55.
54. Ma, HI, Trombly CA. A synthesis of the effects of occupational therapy for persons with stroke: Part II. Remediation of impairments. *Am J Occup Ther*. 2002;56:260–274. doi:10.5014/ajot.56.3.260.
55. Lyons A, Phipps SC, Berro M. Using occupation in the clinic. *OT Practice*. 2004;9:11–15.
56. Law M, Baptiste S, Carswell A, McColl M., Polatajko H, Pollack N. *Canadian Occupational Performance Measure*. 5th ed. Ottawa, Canada: CAOT Publications; 2014.
57. Powell J, Heslin J, Greenwood R. Community based rehabilitation after severe traumatic brain injury: a randomized controlled trial. *J Neurol Neurosurg Psychiatry*. 2002;72:193–202. doi:1.1136/jnnp.72.2.193.
58. Christie L, Bedford R, McCluskey A. Task-specific practice of dressing tasks in a hospital setting improved dressing performance post-stroke: a feasibility study. *Aust Occup Ther J*. 2011;58:364–369. doi:10.1111/j.1440-1630.2011.00945.
59. Combs SA, Finley MA, Henss M, Himmler S, Lapota K, Stillwell D. Effects of a repetitive gaming intervention on upper extremity impairments and function in persons with chronic stroke: a preliminary study. *Disabil Rehabil*. 2012;34:1291–1298. doi:10.3109/09638288.2011.641660.
60. Earley D, Herlache E, Skelton DR. Use of occupations and activities in a modified constraint-induced movement therapy program: a musician's triumphs over chronic hemiparesis from stroke. *Am J Occup Ther*. 2010;64:735–744. doi:10.5014/ajot.2010.08073.

Chapter 3

Occupational Selection, Analysis, Gradation, and Adaptation

Julie L. Grabanski and Sclinda L. Janssen

LEARNING OBJECTIVES

This chapter will allow the reader to:

1. Select occupations based on patient self-reported meaning, desired participation, and ability to promote client-centered therapeutic outcomes.
2. Analyze occupations by examining how the activity, patient abilities and limitations, and environmental characteristics affect occupational participation.
3. Analyze occupations to determine whether they are within patient capabilities and identify specific impediments to participation.
4. Grade occupations to challenge the patient's abilities and improve occupational performance.
5. Adapt occupations to enhance the patient's participation in desired roles.

CHAPTER OUTLINE

TERMINOLOGY

Activity analysis: a systematic process through which occupations are analyzed to understand their component parts, their meaning to patients, and their therapeutic potential.[1]

Activity demands (also called task demands): the specific physical, cognitive, and psychosocial skills required to carry out and complete desired occupations.

Learning: a change in behavior (including knowledge, attitudes, and skills) that can be observed or measured, and that occurs as a result of exposure to internal and external environmental stimuli.[2]

Occupation-as-end: the activities that collectively support the roles of a given individual.[3,4]

Occupation-as-means: the client-centered activities that therapists select to remediate specific skill deficits and impairments.[3,4]

Task analysis: a similar process to activity analysis that is primarily used in relation to work assessment (ergonomics) and refers to an analysis of the dynamic relationship among a patient, an occupation, and the environment.[5]

Therapeutic grading: the modification of activity demands to reduce or increase the activity's challenge level.

Introduction

Participation in desired occupations is central to an individual's identity, self-efficacy, and life meaning.[6] As described in Chapter 2, occupation is the therapeutic medium of occupational therapy and should be used to facilitate patient health and life participation.[6] Therapists must select appropriate occupations that will help to remediate specific patient skill deficits (occupation-as-means) and facilitate the performance of patient-valued occupational roles (occupation-as-end).[3] To select appropriate occupations, therapists must be able to perform activity analysis. To improve decreased abilities, selected occupations must appropriately challenge impaired abilities and be continually adjusted as the patient's performance changes. Therapists control the challenge level of all occupations by grading activities along a therapeutic continuum and by adapting occupations to match the patient's abilities. When the patient's impairments and limitations prevent usual engagement in an occupation, therapists adapt activity demands, activity properties, and environmental contexts to enable performance of desired occupations. This chapter describes how to select, analyze, grade, and adapt occupations.

Activity Selection

Using occupation as a means of therapy is the core of occupational therapy practice.[6] Occupation is used to promote the functional performance of a person's roles and routines, thereby supporting self-esteem and meaning.[3] The benefits of using occupation as therapy are well supported in the literature.[7] Although rote exercise interventions are valuable for targeting specific skill limitations, the use of occupation as therapy has broader, long-term benefits for overall occupational functioning.[8] Use of occupation as therapy fosters motivation toward performance by selecting interventions that are meaningful to the patient and that are able to remediate skill deficits. Occupation as therapy also promotes a broader range of improvement through the simultaneous recruitment of multiple and synchronized skills needed to perform an activity.

Selection of Occupation-as-End Activities

Occupation-as-end activities are those that support the patient's life roles and routines. The therapist and patient identify key occupations that enable him or her to engage in desired roles within particular environmental contexts. Through activity analysis, the therapist matches a patient's skills to the demand level of a specific occupation. Comparison between activity demands within the usual environmental context and the patient's skills determines whether the patient will be able to perform the activity independently, with adaptation, or not at all.[7,8] Self-efficacy and mastery are fostered when patient skills match the situational challenges posed by the activity.

Selection of Occupation-as-Means Activities

The patient's occupational goals help to determine the activities that should be used in intervention to promote the restoration of impaired patient abilities, referred to as occupation-as-means. Activities used to restore impaired skills must not only be within the patient's capacity, but also challenge the patient's ability level so that improved performance can be facilitated through effort and practice. Some specific characteristics of the goals commonly addressed by occupational therapists who treat patients with physical disabilities include increased range of motion (ROM), strength, coordination, memory, and attention. When therapists select contrived methods of therapy—for example, using pegs and cones to increase strength and ROM—instead of the patient's self-identified, real-life, daily activities, the value of therapy is often diminished. Contrived methods also require the patient to focus directly on the process of activity, rather than the end goal, further undermining therapeutic value. An example of the appropriate selection of occupation for a musician whose end goal is to restore hand function after injury would involve intervention activities related to playing a patient-specific musical instrument, such as the piano or violin. Inappropriate examples of occupational selection would include the singular use of pegboards, putty, elastic bands, and weights.

Activity Analysis

Activity analysis, or **task analysis**, is a fundamental skill of occupational therapists. Occupational therapists analyze activities to determine (1) whether a patient with specific abilities can be expected to perform an activity and (2) how an activity can be adapted to facilitate improved occupational performance. Activity analysis enables therapists to understand an activity's components and skill requirements.[6] Therapists begin activity analysis by identifying **activity demands**, that is, the essential skills required for participation. Activity analysis also requires the identification of patient skill limitations that may impede performance. Some activity demands to be considered are the size and type of tools, the placement of selected tools and equipment in relation to the patient, the speed at which the activity is to be performed, the complexity of the activity, and the physical and/or social environment in which the activity will be carried out. Changes in any of these variables alter activity demands and may impact patient performance. The prerequisite abilities needed to accomplish an activity should be identified. If a patient is lacking these prerequisite abilities, and the goal is to participate in the activity to support a specific patient-desired role (occupation-as-end), the activity must then be modified to promote the patient's participation. Modification may involve the adaptation of one or more specific activity demands to reduce challenge level so that the patient can complete some components of the activity (occupation-as-means)—for example, practicing the maintenance of balance while sitting upright at a piano using a bench with an adapted backrest.

Although activities require particular performance skills and abilities, identification of these factors is a high-level skill that requires practice under supervision. Activity analysis involves three primary components: analysis of (1) the activity, (2) patient performance, and (3) environmental supports and barriers influencing activity participation.

Analysis of the Activity

Using an analytical approach, the therapist examines an occupation to determine its components and required skill level (see Table 3-1). Activity analysis can be used to select activities for remediation, match a patient's skills with the demands of the activity, or modify the activity to enhance patient participation. All analyses should occur within some conceptual framework to give them direction, coherence, and meaning.[9] For example, planting a tulip bulb in a container can be analyzed

Table 3-1. Activity Analysis

STEPS OF ANALYSIS	ACTIVITY (BANK OF IDEAS)	PATIENT (OCCUPATION-AS-MEANS)	ENVIRONMENT (OCCUPATION-AS-END)
1. Identify the activity, patient capabilities, and context	Describe activity	Identify primary goals that the activity is intended to enhance through patient performance.	Identify the environment(s) in which the patient wants or needs to perform a given activity.
2. Identify aspects to target	Activity demands, e.g.: • objects used • environmental demands • social demands • sequencing and timing • activity steps • prerequisite capabilities • safety precautions	Identify the primary patient abilities the activity is intended to challenge, e.g.: • ROM • strength • motor performance • sensation • visual-perception • cognition • praxis	Identify the environmental demands of the activity, e.g.: • space demands • equipment height • work space surface area • standing/sitting demands • floor surface demands • visual contrast of foreground/background • social demands • noise level • lighting • temperature
3. Identify therapeutic aspects and value as related to desired performance	Adapt activity demands to align with therapy goals.	Evaluate the activity's therapeutic value based on patient characteristics, e.g.: • meaningfulness • within patient's capabilities • repetitive • gradable	Evaluate how environmental demands can be modified to meet/challenge the patient's performance level.
4. Calibrate difficulty level to promote performance	Modify activity demands, e.g.: • objects used • space demands • social demands • contextual demands • sequencing and timing • activity steps • needed skills level • safety precautions	Specify activity parameters for patient performance, e.g.: • instructional method • nature and level of cuing • social and environmental demands • required performance skills	Implement environmental modifications to promote performance.
Example: Patient with CVA, right dominant hemiparesis; enjoys painting	1. Activity: Brushing teeth, painting activities 2. Toothbrush, social demand of good hygiene, intact proximal stability and fine motor coordination 3. Built-up handle, sitting in wheelchair 4. Gradually decrease size of handle and progress toward standing	1. Patient will brush teeth independently while standing at sink 2. Patient challenge: stability and right hand fine motor coordination 3. Patient enjoys painting; skills transfer to patient goal of brushing teeth 4. Built-up handles to paint and brush teeth. Grade from sitting to supported standing. Decrease size of handles as patient skills emerge	1. Brush teeth independently at home 2. Evaluate bathroom at home 3. Narrow space that prevents use of wheelchair; stable bathroom vanity for proprioceptive input (e.g., resting hand on surface) 4. Decrease fall risks; remove clutter from vanity surface

CVA, cerebrovascular accident; ROM, range of motion.

using various frames of reference. The biomechanical approach prompts the therapist to examine the physical requirements of an activity such as grasp, coordination, and ROM, whereas the cognitive-perceptual approach is used to examine the activity according to its cognitive or perceptual demands, such as attention, problem solving, and spatial requirements.

The first step of an activity analysis is to compile a detailed description of activity demands, followed by the activity's therapeutic aspects, and finally the gradations to activity demands that can calibrate the level of difficulty or challenge. Activities selected to restore motor function must take into account the person's physical status, cognitive and visual-perceptual skills, emotional status, cultural background, and interests. An analysis of the cognitive functions required for an activity should include the number and complexity of the steps involved in performing the activity, the requirements for organizing and sequencing the steps, the amount of concentration and memory required, and the ability to follow verbal or written instructions. Visual-perceptual factors include whether the activity requires the patient to distinguish figure from ground, determine position in space, construct a two- or three-dimensional object, or interpret topographical orientation. Psychosocial aspects of an activity that may be important to patients include whether the activity must be done alone or in a group, requires verbal and/or nonverbal interaction, involves the sharing of materials with others, is likely to cause frustration, requires insight and emotional regulation, and offers the likelihood of producing a satisfying outcome.

Some therapists maintain files of activity analyses, which they can adapt to specific patients. Over the years, activity analyses have been published for general use by therapists including Hi-Q game,[10] macramé,[11] planting a small garden,[12] and bilateral inclined sanding.[13] An activity analysis form[5] was published based on the American Occupational Therapy Association's Occupational Therapy Practice Framework.

Analysis of Patient Performance

When evaluating whether a patient possesses needed skills to perform a desired occupation, therapists should consider (1) the patient's sensory and motor, visual-perceptual, cognitive, and psychosocial functions; and (2) whether these underlying skills are at a level sufficient to support occupational participation. When deficits in these underlying skills impede desired occupational participation, therapists must select occupation-as-means activities to remediate skills, adapt activity demands to promote patient engagement, or use compensatory strategies and devices that substitute for a patient's deficient skills.

As a first step, the therapist should observe the patient's performance of role-related occupations to determine whether the patient can accomplish desired roles in accordance with self-identified needs and expectations.[14] If not, the patient should identify the activities within the role that are not accomplished to his or her standards. Observing the patient's attempt to perform an activity provides the therapist with clues about which abilities and capacities may need further evaluation and treatment.

The performance analysis proposed by Fisher and Bray Jones[14] involves observational evaluation of the "transaction between the client and the environment as the client performs a task that is familiar, meaningful, purposeful, and relevant" (p. 517). To accomplish this, Fisher uses a standardized performance analysis, the Assessment of Motor and Process Skills (AMPS),[14] although analysis can also be completed through informal observation. The quality of patient performance, rather than the patient's underlying capacities, is graded, although patient capacities are considered when interpreting outcome and planning treatment.

Analysis of the Environment

When therapists analyze the environment in which an activity is performed, they analyze the person–environment fit—in other words, how well the environment supports or impedes a patient's occupational participation. Environmental analysis is an essential component of activity analysis because any subtle change in environmental conditions can significantly affect a patient's performance level. For example, a patient may easily be able to self-propel a wheelchair on a clinic tile floor, but may struggle to self-propel it at home on a carpeted floor. A patient's dynamic balance may be sufficient for ambulation across the therapy gym, but may deteriorate on unlevel sidewalks in the community.

In addition to the physical environment, therapists must also address the patient's social contexts and financial resources. For example, a practitioner may complete a home evaluation with recommendations for installation of shower grab bars and toilet handrails. Although such equipment would enhance a patient's safe self-care performance and reduce possible falls, the patient may not have the financial resources to purchase the equipment or employ a contractor to install them. In such cases, the therapist must identify needed community resources such as organizations that provide used, restored durable medical equipment at low or no cost, and contractors who provide services to economically compromised groups for a minimal fee.

Similarly, a therapist may wish to provide a home therapy program to a patient who sustained a cerebrovascular accident (CVA). The home therapy program may incorporate the use of modified constraint-induced movement therapy (mCIMT) in which a restraining mitt is placed on the unaffected upper extremity (UE) to promote use of the affected extremity in daily activities. Although mCIMT has been shown to increase motor performance of the affected limb in patients with CVA, mCIMT requires the presence of a caregiver who can secure the mitt onto the patient's affected extremity and monitor the patient's use throughout the day. Patients who live alone or in facilities without this level of social support would not be able to benefit from home therapy programs incorporating mCIMT, and therapists would then be required to develop home programs with less demand from the patient's social environment.

Gradation

Therapeutic grading is the modification of activity demands to reduce or increase the activity's challenge level. Grading is used to change activity demands to promote psychomotor **learning,** leading to increased occupational performance. Multiple dimensions of an activity can be graded to increase or reduce challenge level. Some examples of commonly graded activity dimensions include ROM, weight, resistance, speed, position, surface height, texture, size, duration, repetition, complexity, number of steps, cognitive demand, and assistance level. When more than one dimension is identified for gradation, the therapist should be careful to grade one or two dimensions at a time so that change in each dimension can be assessed. The best activities for remediation are those that demand a specific response requiring skills targeted for improvement, and that allow incremental gradations beginning at the level at which the patient can be successful (see Table 3-2).

Adaptation

Activity adaptation is the process of modifying an activity of daily living to enable performance, prevent cumulative trauma injury, or accomplish a therapeutic goal. There are four reasons to adapt an activity in the treatment of patients with physical disabilities. One is to modify the activity to make it therapeutic when it would not be so otherwise. For example, while washing windows

Table 3-2. Selecting and Grading Occupation-as-Means Activities

REMEDIATION GOAL	KEY DIMENSIONS OF THE ACTIVITY
To retrain sensory awareness and/or discrimination	Offer various textures, sizes, shapes. Grade from diverse to similar, coarse to smooth, large to small.
To decrease hypersensitivity	Offer various textures and degrees of hardness or softness. Grade from acceptable to barely tolerable.
To relearn skilled voluntary movement	Require patient-desired, purposeful movement; allow feedback. Grade from simple to complex movements.
To increase coordination and dexterity	Require skilled motor actions that the patient can control. Grade from slow, gross movement involving limited number of joints to fast, precise movement involving a greater number of joints.
To increase active ROM	Require repeated movement to the limits of joint range. Grade to demand greater amounts of movement.
To increase passive ROM or elongate soft tissue contracture	Provide controlled stretch or traction. Grade from lesser to greater ROM.
To increase strength	Require movement or holding against resistance. Grade from lesser to greater resistance or from slow to fast movement.
To increase cardiopulmonary endurance	Use activities rated at the patient's current MET level. Grade by increasing duration, frequency, then intensity (METs).
To increase muscular endurance	Require repetitive movement or holding against 50% or less of maximal strength. Grade by increasing repetitions or duration.
To decrease edema	Allow use of the extremity in an elevated position and require isotonic contraction.
To improve perceptual impairments	Perform activities that require perceptual processing at the patient's highest current skill. Grade by complexity of stimuli.
To increase attention	Practice activities that are graded from less distracting to more distracting, and from less time demand to more time demand.
To increase memory	Practice activities that are graded from simple to complex in terms of demand on the patient's ability to remember.
To improve problem solving	Practice activities that are graded from simple (one step) to complex (multiple steps), concrete to abstract, and familiar to unfamiliar. Higher level activities should include unexpected challenge.

MET, metabolic equivalent; ROM, range of motion.

with a patient who has limited shoulder strength, the occupational therapist can add a weight to the patient's wrist to make the activity more therapeutic.

A second reason for adaptation is to grade the amount and type of exercise offered by an activity along a therapeutic continuum to accomplish goals. For example, to increase coordination, an activity should be graded along a continuum from gross-imprecise to fine-accurate movement. Checkers and other board games lend themselves easily to such gradations. For example, checker and cribbage boards, and their pieces can be changed in size so that the patient can engage in self-identified leisure activities while continuing to benefit therapeutically.

A third reason for adapting activities is to enable a person with physical impairments to perform an activity for which he or she would be otherwise unable. For example, after sustaining a CVA causing hemiparesis (weakness of one UE), a patient can learn one-handed dressing methods. Similarly, the environment in which a favorite activity is accomplished can be modified to allow engagement. For example, a gardener who undergoes bilateral lower extremity amputation secondary to diabetes can continue to garden from a wheelchair using raised planting beds.

A fourth reason for adapting activities, particularly work activities in which people participate for long periods, is to prevent cumulative trauma injury. Examples of such adaptation include changing table height to reduce back and UE strain, or performing the activity while seated to reduce lower back stress.

As with all therapeutic techniques, it is vital for the patient to understand the reason why an activity is adapted. For patients with cognitive impairment, it is important to determine their cognitive capacity to process complex and abstract information, and explain the reason for activity participation using understandable language.[15]

Parameters Used to Adapt or Modify Activities

There are multiple characteristics of beneficial adaptations. First, adaptations should promote normal movements, body postures, and motor patterns. It is also essential that adaptations be safe. Adaptations should additionally demand a specific automatic response upon which the client does not have to concentrate. Finally, adaptations should support, rather than detract from the meaningfulness of the activity.

Activity Demand: Required Body Functions

This group of adaptations focus on specific body functions that support the actions used to perform activities (e.g., muscle strength and standing balance).

Positioning the Activity Relative to the Person

The position of the person relative to the activity to be accomplished dictates all required movements and the specific muscle groups that must be used. Poor positioning of activity equipment relative to the patient's size may result in musculoskeletal discomfort or repeated stress injuries.[16] Adaptive positioning of the activity in relation to the patient refers to changes in work surface height and incline, work equipment location, and equipment item placement to require specific body movements.

Activities that are commonly performed on a flat surface, such as painting, board games, and sanding wood, can be made more or less resistive by changing the surface incline. For example, resistance is provided to shoulder extension and elbow flexion when the surface is inclined downward and away from the patient. Resistance is provided to shoulder flexion and elbow extension when the surface is inclined upward and toward the patient (Fig. 3-1).

Similarly, the standard horizontal work surface can be raised or lowered to make demands on specific muscle

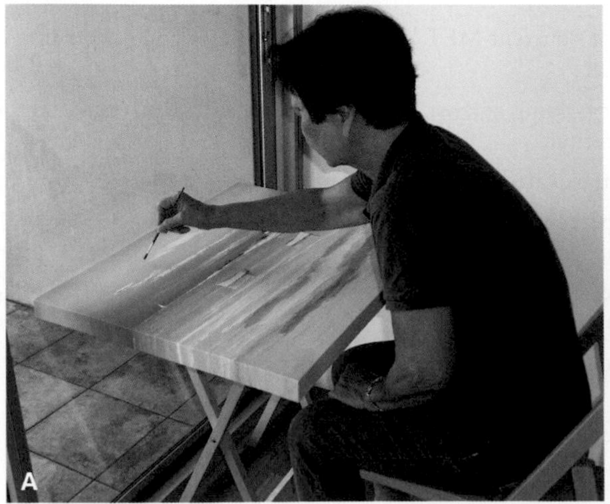

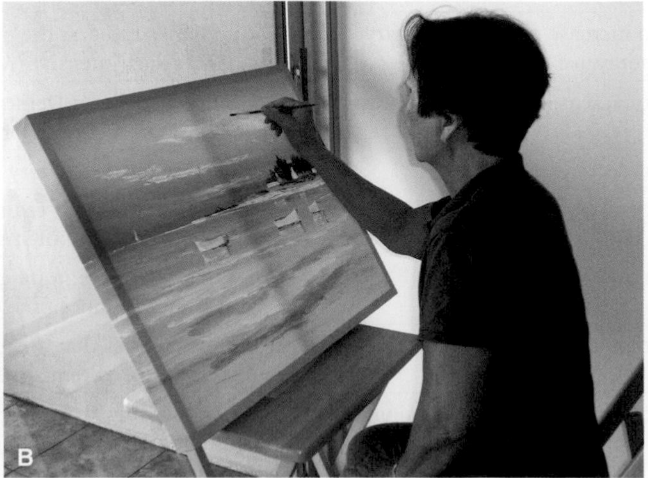

Figure 3-1. A. Resistance is provided to shoulder extension and elbow flexion when the surface is inclined downward and away from the patient. **B.** Resistance is provided to shoulder flexion and elbow extension when the surface is inclined upward and toward the patient.

groups or to alter the effect of gravity. For example, a table raised to axilla height allows flexion and extension of the elbow on a gravity-eliminated plane and may enable a person with grade 3+ muscles to eat independently. These positional changes serve to increase joint strength and ROM, and promote performance.

Placing items—such as nails, mosaic tiles, yarn, beads, darts, beanbags, and paintbrushes—in various locations changes the movements required to reach and retrieve them. Placement may be high to encourage shoulder flexion or abduction; lateral to encourage shoulder rotation, trunk rotation, or horizontal motion; or low to encourage trunk flexion or lateral trunk flexion. All of these placements would encourage improvement in dynamic balance.

Arranging Objects Relative to Each Other

To grade an activity for improving perceptual skill deficits (e.g., poor figure-ground discrimination, unilateral neglect), the arrangement of objects and the amount of page print can be graded from sparse to dense (e.g., fewer objects or words with space between vs. many objects or words with little or no space between). Placing game pieces on the right side of a game board encourages use of the right hand, whereas placement on the left encourages use of the left hand. Arrangement of ingredients on a kitchen counter across the room from the mixing bowl encourages walking that would not occur if all supplies were placed together. On the other hand, placing all objects needed for an activity together reduces the energy required to perform the task.

Modifying Lever Arm Length

The amount of work that a muscle or muscle group expends depends on the resistance. Resistance is determined by the pull of gravity on a limb and the equipment used by the patient, which together act as the resistance lever arm. The effect of a given amount of resistance can be altered by lengthening or shortening the resistance arm. The longer the resistance arm, the greater the force required to counterbalance it. The resistance arm can be altered by shortening or lengthening the limb. For example, flexing the knee, which shortens the limb, offers less resistance to hip extension than if the knee was extended. Another example involves carrying an object close to the body, which requires less involvement of back muscles than if the object was carried at arm's length. On the other hand, increasing the length of the force lever arm decreases the muscle activity needed to accomplish a task (Fig. 3-2).

Attention to lever arm length is important both to adapt an activity's required body movements to make the activity more therapeutic and to adapt object weight for patients with decreased strength. The adaptation of lever arm length guides workers in methods of lifting and handling to avoid musculoskeletal injuries on the jobsite.

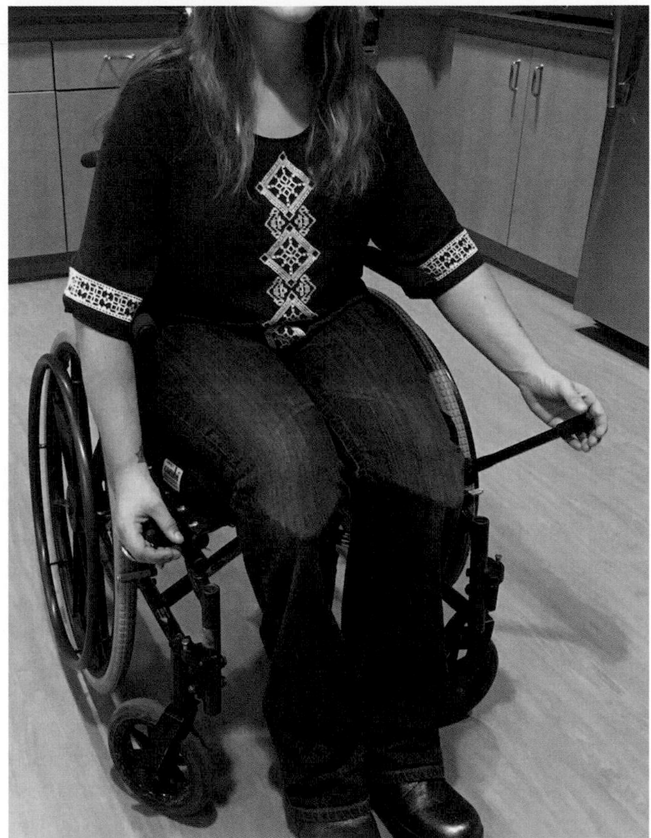

Figure 3-2. Patient sitting in a wheelchair using an extended brake handle to increase leverage.

Activity Demand: Required Actions and Performance Skills

This group of adaptations focuses on methods used to adapt the actions and skills required to carry out an activity.

Modifying Performance Method and Physical Context

Modifying the performance method is used both for **occupation-as-means** and **occupation-as-end** activities. Such compensatory adaptation allows the performance of an activity that would be impossible otherwise because of a patient's disability. Bowling, basketball, and many other sports can be accomplished while seated instead of standing. A change of rules adapts some sports, such as track and field events, to match the activity limitations of physical impairment. Sewing and needlework, typically bilateral activities, can be made unilateral by adaptations that hold the material steady for the working hand. Books, laptop computers, and other tools can be transported via a rolling backpack or rolling table instead of carrying them.

By altering the physical context, individuals are able to perform an activity more optimally.[17] For example, if a patient cannot flex his shoulder against gravity, placing him in a side-lying position will minimize the effects of gravity, allowing the desired movement. Movement organization in a gravity-eliminated plane, however, differs from movement in an against-gravity context, requiring different muscle recruitment. Movement organization is also atypical in simulated contexts using contrived objects, as compared to movement patterns executed in natural contexts with real-life objects.[8,18–20] Because movement organization is sensitive to contextual changes,[17] some rehabilitation centers are now designed with manufactured "real" environments that allow patients to practice in realistic contexts to facilitate best performance and carryover to real-life contexts (Fig. 3-3).

Modifying Level of Difficulty

Patterns for craft activities, game rules, number of steps, and creativity level can be downgraded to enable patient success or upgraded to demand higher performance level. Modifying an activity's difficulty level can entail changing the number of pieces and instructions that must be navigated, changing the problem-solving level from concrete to abstract reasoning, and changing the directions from specific to general. For example, a patient with traumatic brain injury may be unable to write a check if the desktop is cluttered with papers, but may be able to manage if one bill is presented on a cleared desk surface. A patient with low cardiopulmonary endurance may not be able to stand for long periods in the kitchen to prepare a simple meal, but could complete a kitchen activity while seated on a stool. As endurance increases, difficulty level can be increased to include standing positions during activity portions.

Activity Demand: Objects and Their Properties

This next group of adaptations focuses on the adaptation of the tools, materials, and equipment used to perform an activity.

Modifying Materials and Textures

To change an activity's level of resistance, gradation along the strengthening continuum may be accomplished through the selection of materials by type, texture, and density. For example, resistance can be changed by beginning a project requiring scissor cutting first with tissue paper and then progressing to heavier materials. Metal tooling can be graded for resistance by choosing materials in grades from thin aluminum to thick copper. Sandpaper is graded from extra fine to coarse, and resistance increases as the grade coarsens. Mixing ingredients can be graded along a continuum from making gelatin dessert, to scrambled eggs, and finally to biscuit batter. If materials are graded in the opposite direction—that is, from heavy to light—the activity demands increased coordination from the patient. Weaving may begin using thicker material, such as rug roving yarn, and be graded toward fine linen threads as the patient progresses in coordination. Cutaneous stimulation changes with the amount of object and surface texture. By making balls from yarn or terrycloth toweling, carpeting the surfaces upon which a patient works, and padding handles with textured material, the therapist adapts the activity to increase sensory stimulation.

Modifying Tool and Utensil Handles

Padding the handles of utensils and tools with high-density foam or other firm but soft material reduces stress on painful finger joints and enhances use by patients with poor grip strength. For example, patients with rheumatoid arthritis often benefit from foam tubing placed on toothbrushes, pens, hairbrushes, and eating utensils to provide a larger grip area that reduces pain and promotes motor control (Fig. 3-4). Other modifications to tool handles include using weighted-handled eating utensils to decrease tremors for patients with Parkinson disease.

Modifying Object Size and Shape

Therapists can adapt the size and shape of board game pieces to offer a therapeutic benefit that would not be possible with standard objects. For example, checkers,

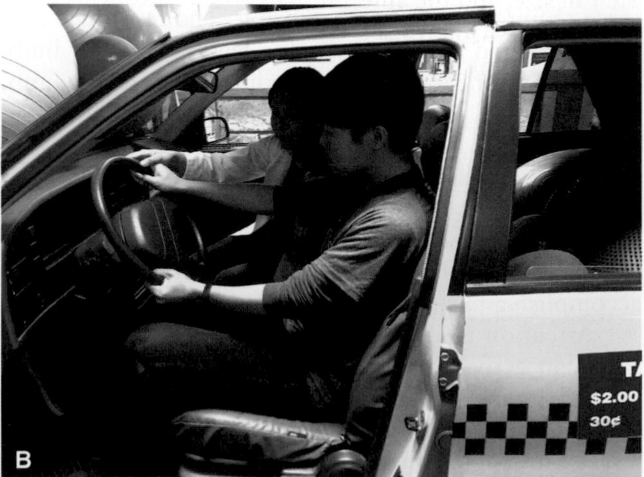

Figure 3-3. **A.** Patient using a simulated grocery store in a clinical setting. **B.** Patient relearning to drive in a simulated clinic vehicle.

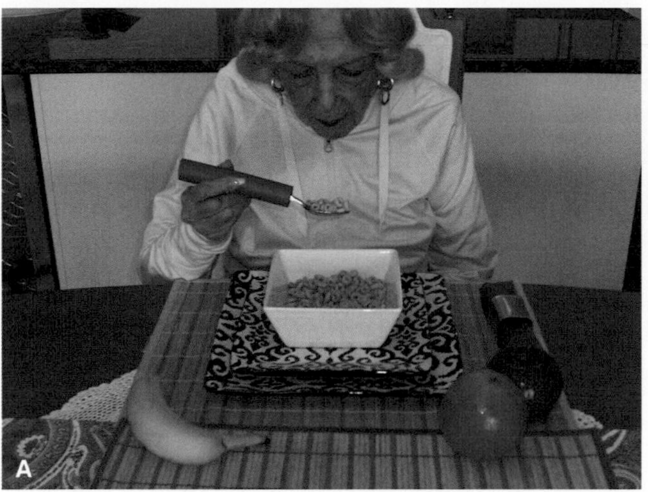

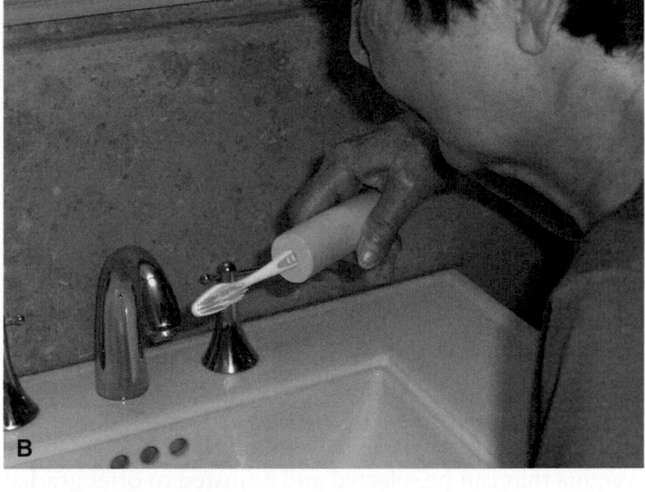

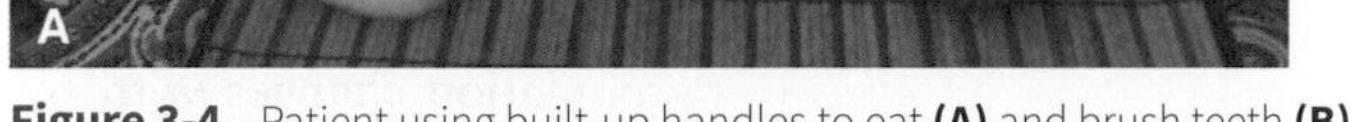
Figure 3-4. Patient using built-up handles to eat **(A)** and brush teeth **(B)**.

which are usually flat pieces approximately 2.5 cm in diameter, can be replaced by cylinders, squares, cubes, or spheres; can range in size from tiny to as large as a person's grasp permits; and can be adapted with handles for easier retrieval.

Reducing the size or changing the shape of an activity's objects and pieces facilitates the goals of increased dexterity and fine motor coordination. Therapists creatively change the size of craft materials (e.g., weaving thread, tiles, paint-by-number guidelines, and ceramic pieces) and recreational materials (e.g., puzzle pieces, chess pieces, and target games) to increase coordination. Tools and utensils can be adapted by changing the length, diameter, or shape of their handles, or by adding handles to tools that do not typically possess them. The actual size of a tool can be selected to offer greater or lesser resistance. For example, saws range in size from small coping saws and hacksaws to large cross-cut and rip saws. The resistance of saws can also be graded by the number of teeth per inch on a blade—the fewer the teeth, the greater the resistance. Woodworking planes vary in size, and the amount of exposed blade can be adjusted to provide resistance. The size of scissors, screwdrivers, stirring spoons, and other tools and utensils can also be varied.

Modifying Color Contrast between Objects

Figure-ground discrimination[10] can be facilitated by changing background and foreground objects from similar to increasingly contrasting colors. For example, patients with visual-perceptual deficits may have difficulty distinguishing light-colored foods (e.g., mashed potatoes and sliced chicken) against white plates, and white bars of soap against white bathroom sinks. In such cases, it would be beneficial to place foods against plates with a distinctly contrasting color background. Similarly, the color of toothpaste brushes and tubes, lotions, and hairbrushes can be modified by adhering brightly colored tape to these items to provide contrast against a white bathroom countertop (Fig. 3-5).

Modifying or Using Supplemental Tools and Utensils

Using tools when none are typically used or modifying tools and utensils enables a patient to accomplish activities and tasks that he or she would not be able to perform otherwise. For example, toast can be retrieved from a toaster using a wooden, spring-hinged clothespin when sensory precautions are in effect. Angling the handles on carving knives allows a person with rheumatoid arthritis to cut meat or vegetables without placing deforming forces on the wrist and fingers. Changing keyboard or mouse designs can prevent carpal tunnel syndrome. Including the tool in a specially designed splint can reduce symptoms caused by prolonged holding. Although manufacturers offer tools and household

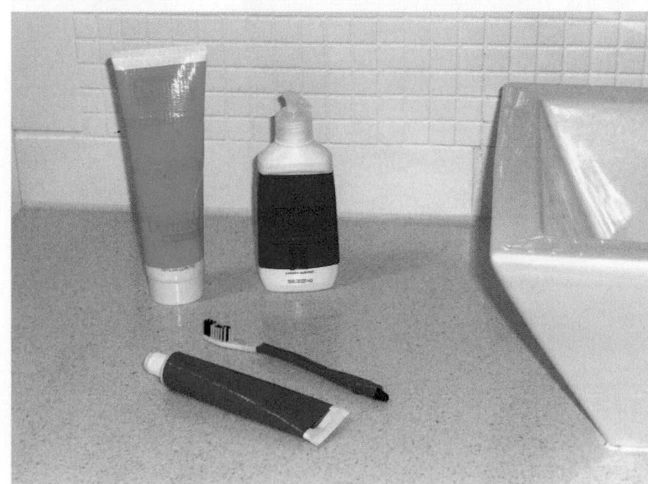
Figure 3-5. The color of toothpaste tubes, soaps, and lotions can be modified by adhering brightly colored tape to these items to provide contrast against a white bathroom countertop.

utensils designed to enable patients with weak grasp or arthritic pain to use them comfortably, therapists must not assume that tools labeled "ergonomic" offer better positioning or less discomfort than nonadapted tools. Patients' perceived comfort and ease of use must guide the selection of all tools and utensils.[21]

Adding Weights

The addition of weights adapts an activity to meet such goals as an increase of strength, promotion of muscular co-contraction, and an increase of passive ROM by stretch. Some nonresistive activities can be made resistive by adding weights directly to the apparatus or by using pulleys. Others may be made resistive by adding weights to the person using weighted cuffs. Tools also are weights that can be selected and adjusted to offer graded resistance (Fig. 3-6). For instance, hammers range from lightweight tack hammers to heavy claw hammers.

Adding Springs or Rubber Bands

Springs and rubber bands are a means of adapting activity to increase strength through resistance, to assist a weak muscle, or to stretch a muscle and other soft tissues to increase passive ROM. When offering resistance, the spring or rubber band is positioned so that its pull is opposite to the pull of motion of the target muscle group. If used for assistance, the spring or rubber band is set to pull in the same direction as the contracting muscle group. Springs and rubber bands applied for the purpose of stretching are placed so that the pull is against the tissue to be stretched. Springs of graduated tensions may be applied directly to larger pieces of equipment. Rubber bands can be added to smaller pieces of equipment and can be graded from thin with light tension to thick with heavy tension. For example, a rubber band can be wrapped around the pincer end of a spring-type clothespin to add resistance when it is used in games involving the retrieval of small pieces.

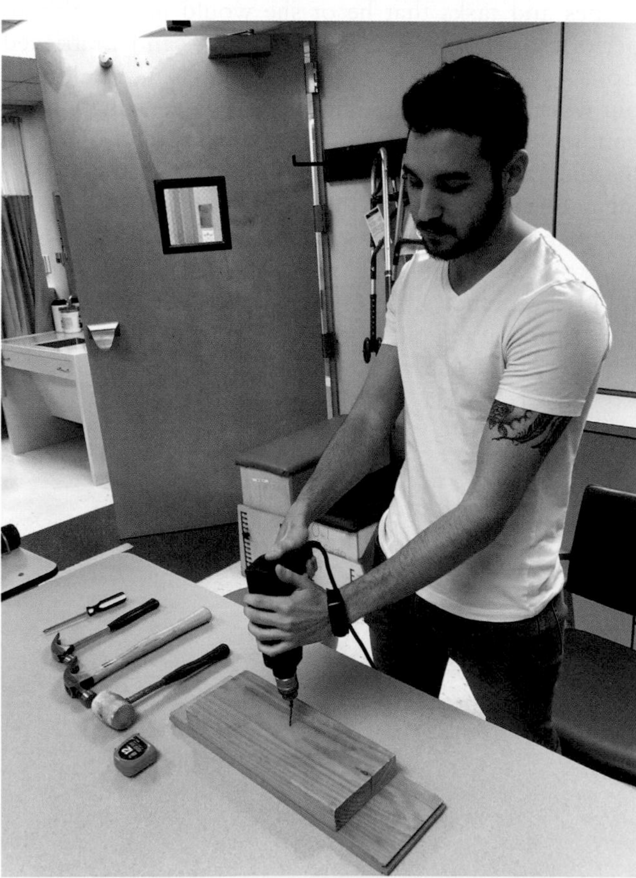

Figure 3-6. Tools are weights that can be selected and adjusted to offer graded resistance.

Activity Demand: Sequence and Timing

This final group of adaptations involves changing demands related to the steps involved in an activity including the sequence of steps and the time required to complete the steps.

Modifying Steps

An activity can be modified by increasing the number of steps to complete the activity. Grading the number of steps from one to two steps to multiple steps can be used to increase attention, concentration, and memory. For example, the activity of "brushing teeth" can be graded from two steps: (1) brush teeth and (2) rinse mouth; to five steps: (1) get supplies from cabinet, (2) put toothpaste on brush, (3) brush teeth, (4) rinse mouth, and (5) return supplies to cabinet.

To address memory deficits, an activity can be adapted to include a sequential checklist of the steps needed to perform the activity. Depending on the person's cognitive ability, the checklist can be written or pictorial. Using the same example above, a written checklist for the steps involved in brushing teeth could be posted on a mirror in the bathroom. Conversely, the patient may receive a singular instruction to complete a multistep task (such as prepare and clean up a light lunch within 30 minutes) to facilitate decision-making and problem-solving skills.

Modifying Time

Changing and monitoring the length of time needed to complete the individual steps of an activity, or the entire activity, can be used to enhance patient attention and concentration skills. For example, making a peanut butter and jelly sandwich can be graded by increasing the required time to make one or more sandwiches. Devices can be used to promote a therapeutic goal or enable performance such as the use of a kitchen timer or alarm clock.

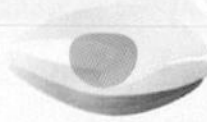

CASE STUDY

Patient Information

Gordon is a 78-year-old retired high school teacher, director of a high school vocational program, and carpenter who experienced a stroke related to carotid artery angioplasty with stenting. The stroke resulted in hemiparesis of his right, dominant side that affected balance, weight shift, and right UE strength and coordination. The emergency room doctor conducted the Mini-Mental State Examination (MMSE) where Gordon scored 20/30, which indicated mild cognitive impairment. He was in the hospital for 3 days and then returned home to independent living with his wife. While still in the hospital, Gordon lost his balance and fell in the bathroom while bending and rotating. He stated, "This stroke caused my right arm and hand to be a dish rag."

Assessment Process and Results

The occupational therapist met with Gordon for evaluation and intervention. One of the first things he told the occupational therapist was that he could not drive because he could not turn the key in the ignition or hold the steering wheel with his right hand. The occupational therapist used multiple tools for the assessment process, including patient interview, Activity Card Sort, the MMSE, biomechanical assessments (9-Hold Peg Test, power of grasp, tensiometer, ROM), and the Mini-Balance Evaluation Systems Test (Mini-BEST).

Results indicated that Gordon was also having difficulty brushing his teeth, buttoning his sleeve cuffs, and holding a spoon to scoop grapefruit pieces, which he reported eating daily to lower his cholesterol. He periodically verbalized concern about his inability to manipulate grapefruit pieces, suggesting that this was an important goal to target. Gordon was independent in all other self-care tasks. He additionally desired to complete his own home maintenance, such as lawn mowing. Gordon's occupational interests included carpentry, such as remodeling his daughter's basement, which required the ability to use tools such as a drill, trowel, and hammer; model airplane building and flying; and playing music with piano, guitar, and harmonica.

Since his initial hospitalization, Gordon's MMSE score improved to 28/30, indicating no cognitive impairment. Scores on the 9-Hole Peg Test were 50 seconds right and 30 seconds left UE. Scores for power of grasp were 10 lb on the right and 60 lb on the left. Scores for lateral grasp were 3 lb on the right and 20 lb on the left. ROM was within normal limits throughout both UEs but a slight movement delay was present in the right UE. Score for the Mini-BEST was 24/28 because of limitations in reactive postural control.

Occupational Therapy Problem List

- Difficulty feeding self with utensils, especially when scooping grapefruit because of right hand weakness and limited coordination
- Difficulty brushing teeth because of right hand weakness and limited coordination and postural instability
- Difficulty with home maintenance, such as lawn mowing, because of balance impairment and weak grasp to pull the mower starter cord
- Difficulty driving because of right hand weakness and limited coordination

Occupational Therapy Goal List

During selection of occupation-as-end activities, the therapist asked Gordon which activities were the most immediately important to him. He prioritized the following goals:

- Gordon will demonstrate modified independence in feeding himself with utensils, especially scooping grapefruit, with 10 lb lateral grasp, 15 lb power of grasp, and normal coordination within 2 weeks.
- Gordon will demonstrate independence in brushing teeth with 15 lb power of grasp, normal fine motor coordination, and intact reactive postural control with transitional movements to set up items needed within 1 month.
- Gordon will be able to start his lawn mower and mow his lawn with intact balance and weight shift within 1 month.
- Gordon will demonstrate independence in driving as evidenced by 10 lb of lateral grasp in order to turn the key in the car ignition within 1 month.

Intervention

To enhance performance of each occupation, it was important to target hand and finger strength, fine motor coordination, and balance with transitional movements. During the second visit, the therapist developed a bank of intervention activities that Gordon could perform within his natural environment including carpentry tasks, lawn mowing, brushing teeth, playing piano and guitar, and feeding himself grapefruit. The therapist used a neurodevelopmental treatment (NDT) frame of reference, while also integrating task-specific motor learning in which specific activity aspects were analyzed and modified to promote repetition, duration, specificity, and intensity.

The therapist initiated patient education during simulations of several meaningful activities that Gordon identified. For example, the therapist found a drill, screws, and wood from the maintenance department to show Gordon how to incorporate weight bearing on his affected, extended right UE. The drill handle was large, which facilitated Gordon's ability to grasp it. His grip strength, however, was too weak to hold the drill upright against gravity, as would be required to push screws into a wall. To grade the task to a lower challenge level, the therapist instructed Gordon to hold the drill downward so that gravity could assist when pushing the screw into the wood. With practice, Gordon gained the ability to activate the power switch with his right index finger. He used his left hand to precisely hold the screw when initially drilling it into the wood, followed by a two-handed method (both hands on the drill) to finish drilling the screw into the wood.

(continued)

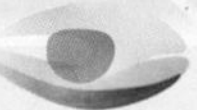

CASE STUDY *(continued)*

Gordon and his therapist also addressed the difficulty he was experiencing scooping grapefruit with a spoon. He reported that it felt like "there was oil on my spoon handle." The therapist adapted his grapefruit spoon and toothbrush by placing 2-inch foam tubes onto both handles to make them larger and easier to grasp. She also gave Gordon 1-inch tubes to replace the 2-inch ones, as his hand strength and coordination progressively improved.

In his third visit, Gordon brought carpentry tools and a list of tasks he needed to complete to remodel his daughter's basement. The use of these tools was meaningful, within his capabilities, repetitive, and gradable in nature. The therapist and Gordon initially practiced each activity in a simulated manner, primarily using Gordon's right hand as a stabilizer with the intent to improve grip strength. Two-handed techniques were then used to improve coordination. Gordon and the therapist continued to grade the activity by gradually increasing key elements such as range, resistance, speed, and surface height. The therapist concurrently used restorative NDT with activity-specific techniques and precautions for balance. Demonstration and return demonstration were used as teaching and learning strategies.

The fourth visit took place in Gordon's home in order to observe his activity performance in his natural environment. Gordon pointed out the tall, uncut lawn grass and was highly motivated to mow the lawn. The therapist examined Gordon's ability to operate the lawn mower (activity analysis), attend to uneven lawn surfaces (environmental analysis), and maintain his stability while pushing and turning the mower (analysis of patient abilities). Mowing stimulated bilateral hand use and repetitive, activity-specific movement patterns (stepping, crossing midline, turning, and weight shifting) over an extended duration of time. Gordon initially practiced with the mower off, but turned it on once his motions were safe. The handle of the mower served as a stabilizing element for his balance and he gradually, and safely, increased his speed.

Gordon said that he felt ready to start work on his daughter's basement over the next month, including tasks such as pounding nails into and finishing sheetrock walls. These carpentry activities offered inherent gradation to further challenge strength, coordination, and balance. Gordon's strength improved, enabling him to hold the drill upright against gravity to drill screws into walls.

During another session, the therapist and Gordon attempted piano playing to facilitate fine motor coordination. Although he improved within 15 minutes of playing, he acknowledged that it was still too frustrating for him and he did not wish to continue. This activity was not a good therapeutic selection because of the mismatch between the activity challenge level and Gordon's personal abilities and standards.

Gordon spent the next month engaged in "his therapy," as he described to friends and family, by remodeling his daughter's basement and by participating in additional therapeutic exercises. After 2 months, he regained strength, balance, and most fine motor coordination, with limitations in his third, fourth, and fifth digits. Gordon demonstrated modified independence with dressing, using a buttonhook as an adaptation. He regained independence in driving, mowing his lawn, brushing his teeth, and eating with utensils, including scooping grapefruit. Finally, he regained sufficient fine motor coordination to build model airplanes and play the harmonica. Gordon reported being satisfied with his recovery from stroke because he was able to perform meaningful occupations that supported his roles as a father and carpenter. He now enjoys describing his therapy to others by stating that, "I did all of my therapy in my daughter's basement."

Evidence Table of Studies Involving Occupational Therapy Selection, Gradation, and Adaptation of Occupation

Intervention	Description	Participants	Dosage	Research Design and Evidence Level	Benefit	Statistical Significance and Effect Size
Comparative effectiveness of (1) combined therapeutic exercise and occupation-based activities and (2) therapeutic exercise alone[19]	Group #1: Picking up small everyday objects, typing on a keyboard, washing and wiping dishes in addition to therapeutic exercises in both hand therapy sessions and home program Group #2: Therapeutic exercises in both hand therapy sessions and home program	46 patients with UE injuries treated in outpatient hand occupational therapy clinic	10 weeks of therapy: supervised hand therapy 1-hour sessions, 2 times/week; and home exercise program 120 minutes, once a week	Randomized controlled trial. Level I	Combined intervention had better outcomes, including reduced pain, improved AAROM in fingers, subjective functional status, and subjective performance and satisfaction of performance.	Combined intervention showed statistically significant improvement in outcome measures compared to therapeutic exercise group: DASH score ($p < 0.02$), total active motion ($p < 0.01$), neuropathic pain ($p < 0.02$), COPM performance ($p < 0.001$), COPM satisfaction ($p < 0.001$) Effect size not reported.
Comparative effectiveness of occupation-based intervention and rote exercise[8]	Group #1: Immobilization of healthy hand using therapeutic occupations for intervention Group #2: Immobilization of healthy hand during rote exercise of affected hand Control Group #3: No immobilization of healthy hand while practicing different movements and activities	36 outpatients (22–55 years old)	Groups #1 and 2 received intervention 3 hours each day, 3 days/week, over 4 weeks	Randomized controlled trial. Level I	Compared to rote exercise, occupation-based group had better performance in objective and subjective measures, motivation, satisfaction with and perception of performance, and continued improvement at follow-up.	Post hoc analyses revealed significant difference among all three groups with most increased mean change for occupation-based group ($p < 0.01$) Effect size not reported.
Comparative effectiveness between combined (1) resistive exercises, functional exercises, and ADLs, and (2) resistive exercises[22]	Group #1: Combination of resistance exercise, functional exercise, and ADL exercise Group #2: Resistance exercise	52 older adults, mean age = 73 years	Measured at baseline, postintervention, and 6-months follow-up	Randomized controlled trial. Level I	Postintervention improvement was found within groups but not between groups. At 6-month follow-up, a decline in resistance exercise group was found. Combined exercise group continued to show improvement. More adverse events (soreness, pain) for resistance exercise group.	Combined intervention group (mean change = 0.29, $p < 0.02$); resistance exercise group (mean change = 0.24, $p < 0.13$). At 6 months postintervention, combined intervention group showed within-group *mean change* of 0.37 ($p < 0.01$).
Comparative effectiveness between occupation-based intervention and repetitive task practice[20]	Group #1: Focused on performance of occupations with facilitation methods Group #2: Focused on 10–50 repetitions of each task	16 (21–69 years old) in chronic phase of stroke recovery	Measured at baseline and postintervention. Interventions were 55-minute sessions, 2 times/week for 4 weeks for both groups	Pilot randomized controlled trial comparative study with parallel group block design. Level I	Improvements in occupational performance and motor performance in both groups were similar. Authors suggested engagement greater and demand greater in occupation-based group because of meaningfulness and multijoint activities.	Although within-group changes after intervention were found for both groups ($p < 0.0001$), no between-group differences were found. Effect size not reported.

ADLs, activities of daily living; UE, upper extremity; AAROM, active assistive range of motion; DASH, disabilities of the arm, shoulder, and hand questionnaire; COPM, Canadian occupational performance measure.

References

1. Crepeau EB, Schell BAB. Analyzing occupations and activity. In: *Willard and Spackman's Occupational Therapy*. 11th ed. Philadelphia, PA: Lippincott Williams & Wilkins; 2009:359–374.
2. Bastable S, Gramet P, Jacobs K. *Health Professional as Educator: Principles of Teaching and Learning*. Burlington, MA: Jones & Bartlett Learning; 2010.
3. Trombly CA. Occupation: purposefulness and meaningfulness as therapeutic mechanism. *Am J Occup Ther*. 1995;49;960–972. doi:10.5014/ajot.49.10.906.
4. Padilla CR, Griffiths Y. *A Professional Legacy: The Eleanor Clarke Slagle Lectures in Occupational Therapy, 1955-2010*. Bethesda, MD: American Occupational Therapy Association; 2011.
5. Watson DE, Wilson SA. *Task Analysis: An Individual and Population Approach*. Bethesda, MD: AOTA Press; 2003.
6. American Occupational Therapy Association. Occupational therapy practice framework: domain and process (3rd ed.). *Am J Occup Ther*. 2014;68(suppl 1):S1–S48. doi:10.5014/ajot.2014.682006.
7. Wolf TJ, Chuh A, Floyd T, McInnis K, Williams E. Effectiveness of occupation-based interventions to improve areas of occupation and social participation after stroke: an evidence-based review. *Am J Occup Ther*. 2015;69(1):6901180060 doi:10.5014/ajot/2015.012195.
8. Rostami HR, Akbarfahimi M, Hassani Mehraban A, Akbarinia AR, Samani S. Occupation-based intervention versus rote exercise in modified constraint-induced movement therapy for patients with median and ulnar nerve injuries: a randomized controlled trial. *Clin Rehabil*. 2017;31(8):1087–1097. doi:10.1177/0269215516672276.
9. Mosey AC. *Occupational Therapy: Configuration of a Profession*. New York, NY: Raven Press; 1981.
10. Neistadt ME, McAuley D, Zecha D, Shannon R. An analysis of a board game as a treatment activity. *Am J Occup Ther*. 1993;47(2):154–160. doi:10.5014/ajot.47.2.154.
11. Chandani A, Hill C. What really is therapeutic activity? *Br J Occup Ther*. 1990;53(1):15–18. https://doi.org/10.1177/030802269005300106.
12. Nelson DL. Occupation: form and performance. *Am J Occup Ther*. 1988;42(10):633–641. doi:10.5014/ajot.42.10.633.
13. Spaulding SJ, Robinson KL. Electromyographic study of the upper extremity during bilateral sanding: unresisted and resisted conditions. *Am J Occup Ther*. 1984;38(4):258–262. doi:10.5014/ajot.38.4.258.
14. Fisher AG, Jones KB. *Assessment of Motor and Process Skills: Development, Standardization, and Administration Manual*. Vol. 1. Fort Collins, CO: Three Star Press Inc.; 2003.
15. McCraith DB, Austin SL, Earhart CA. The cognitive disabilities model in 2011. In: Katz N, ed. *Cognition, Occupation, and Participation Across the Lifespan: Neuroscience, Neurorehabilitation, and Models of Intervention in Occupational Therapy*. 3rd ed. Bethesda, MD: American Occupational Therapy Association; 2011:374–406.
16. Sung CY, Ho KK, Lam RM, Lee AH, Chan CC. Physical and psychosocial factors in display screen equipment assessment. *Hong Kong J Occup Ther*. 2003;13(1):2–10.
17. Nilsen DM, Kaminski TR, Gordon AM. The effect of body orientation on a point-to-point movement in healthy elderly persons. *Am J Occup Ther*. 2003;57(1):99–107. doi:10.5014/ajot.57.1.99.
18. Dunn W, Brown C, McGuigan A. The ecology of human performance: a framework for considering the effect of context. *Am J Occup Ther*. 1994;48(7):595–607. doi:10.5014/ajot.48.7.595.
19. Che Daud AZ, Yau MK, Barnett F, Judd J, Jones RE, Nawawi RF. Integration of occupation based intervention in hand injury rehabilitation: a randomized controlled trial. *J Hand Ther*. 2016;29(1):30–40. doi:10/1016/j.jht.2015.09.004.
20. Skubik-Peplaski C, Custer M, Powell E, Westgate PM, Sawaki L. Comparing occupation-based and repetitive task practice interventions for optimal stroke recovery: a pilot randomized trial. *Phys Occup Ther Geriatr*. 2017;35(3–4):156–168. doi:10.1080/02703181.2017.1342734.
21. Tebben AB, Thomas JJ. Trowels labeled ergonomic versus standard design: preferences and effects on wrist range of motion during a gardening occupation. *Am J Occup Ther*. 2004;58(3):317–323. doi:10.5014/ajot.58.3.317.
22. Liu CJ, Xu H, Keith NR, Clark DO. Promoting ADL independence in vulnerable, community-dwelling older adults: a pilot RCT comparing 3-step workout for life versus resistance exercise. *Clin Interv Aging*. 2017;12:1141. doi:10.2147/CIA.S136678.

Acknowledgments

We thank Devon Olson and Marilyn Klug for their assistance in chapter preparation. We also thank "Gordon" for sharing how occupation as therapy was used during his recovery from a stroke.

Chapter 4

The Teaching and Learning Process

Lenin C. Grajo and Angela K. Boisselle

LEARNING OBJECTIVES

This chapter will allow the reader to:

1. Describe the teaching and learning process within occupational therapy practice.
2. Define the stages of learning according to Dreyfus: acquisition, retention, transfer, and generalization.
3. Describe Meichenbaum's model of mastery: global learning strategies and metacognition mastery.
4. Assess the learning capacities of patients to optimize the therapeutic relationship.
5. Apply various teaching and learning principles during assessment and intervention.

CHAPTER OUTLINE

TERMINOLOGY

Acquisition: is a process of learning a new skill involving the development of strategies and skill completion.

Domain-specific strategies: are cognitive techniques that facilitate or improve performance that is task-, child-, or situation-specific.

Functional literacy: is the ability to interpret common written materials needed to effectively carry out basic daily life skills and participate in meaningful occupations and social roles.

Generalization: is the ability to take a newly learned skill and apply it to a real-life situation.

Global strategies: are methods that focus on increasing metacognitive awareness through training the patient to self-monitor and self-evaluate.

Health literacy: is the ability to obtain, process, and understand the basic health information and services that patients need to make appropriate health decisions.

Metacognition: is the awareness of one's cognitive level and ability to control one's thoughts.

Occupational profile: is a summary of gathered information about the patient's occupational participation and needs.

Retention: is a process of learning that involves storage of information for later use.

Transfer of skills: is the application of previously learned skills to a new task or activity.

The Occupational Therapist as a Facilitator of Learning

Facilitating teaching and learning is a continuous process embedded within occupational therapy evaluation and intervention. Occupational therapists work with patients who need to either acquire new skills or relearn lost skills secondary to illness, disability, or atypical human development. From the first encounter with patients, occupational therapists employ a variety of teaching and learning strategies in an array of therapeutic contexts. The methods through which occupational therapists employ teaching and learning approaches may facilitate or hinder successful therapeutic relationships. This chapter provides an overview of teaching and learning contexts, theories, and principles to help occupational therapists maximize the therapeutic context when supporting patients.

Contexts for Teaching and Learning within the Occupational Therapy Process

First, six different contexts for teaching and learning within the occupational therapy process are introduced. Later in this chapter, these contexts are applied as practical principles that can be employed in the therapeutic relationship.

Assessment as a Teaching and Learning Context

During the screening and/or formal evaluation of a patient, the occupational therapist both gathers information about the patients' occupational needs and uses this opportunity to educate the patient about the role of occupational therapy. Such education both supports the patient's understanding and helps to develop a mutually beneficial therapeutic relationship. A later section of this chapter describes how teaching and learning can be optimized when gathering data to produce a patient occupational profile.

Establishing a Therapeutic Relationship

Occupational therapists and the patients they work with all have varying teaching and learning styles. The right match between a therapists' teaching approach and a patient's learning style can significantly impact the therapeutic relationship. Some patients make greater therapeutic progress when paired with a more directive and hands-on occupational therapist, whereas other patients may require a more supportive and guiding therapist.

Skill Development, Strategy Generation, and Enhancing Occupational Participation

Appropriate teaching and learning processes not only influence the therapeutic relationship but also determine how well patient skills develop and strategies are generated, and occupational participation is enhanced. No one teaching-learning context is similar. Some teaching approaches may work for patients with specific learning styles and at distinct stages of readiness for change in the recovery process, whereas other approaches may not work. The teaching and learning process must be understood as an ongoing and continuously evolving process that is facilitated by the patient and shaped by the therapist's abilities. The teaching and learning process must also be viewed as mutually beneficial: both the patient and therapist facilitate each other's learning as they explore various strategies to best reach the patient's rehabilitation goals. Embedded within the teaching-learning process is problem identification, problem solving, and outcome assessment that unfolds as therapy progresses.

Modifying, Adapting, and Choosing Appropriate Environments

Teaching and learning is also employed as the occupational therapist and patient modify and adapt selected environments and contexts to support the patient's desired occupational participation. As much as possible, learning should occur in the natural environment. Although use of natural contexts may not always be possible in all practice settings, the occupational therapist should spend a reasonable amount of time creating realistic and occupation-based activities to help foster contextual learning.

Collaborative Relationship with Families, Caregivers, Interprofessional Team, and Social Networks

Teaching and learning approaches are used within a variety of therapeutic contexts with patients, family members, caregivers, and interprofessional team members. The occupational therapist must both teach others and learn from the perspectives of families, caregivers, and interprofessional team members about how to best apply patients' newly learned skills to enhance occupational participation in the home and community. Therapists must also collaboratively discuss challenges and opportunities for skill transfer and generalization within the patient's desired social networks. Oftentimes, this collaborative relationship requires education about the roles of the occupational therapist, identifying ways to embed the patient's typical daily routines while in the clinical setting, and strategizing methods to co-manage the patient's clinical condition. In certain cases, the occupational therapist may also need to collaborate with the patient's employers, school, and community infrastructures (e.g., neighborhood grocery store, spiritual organizations, community wellness facilities) to teach and learn ways to help the patient reintegrate into, resume, or newly assume desired occupational roles.

Health and Wellness Promotion and Disability Prevention

Occupational therapists must also use teaching and learning approaches not only when working with individual patients, but when working with patient groups and populations to teach health and wellness promotion and disability prevention strategies. Occupational therapists also engage in teaching and learning with patient stakeholders (e.g., insurers, community leaders, policy makers) that may directly or indirectly impact occupational therapy provision for specific patient groups. For example, if patients are denied therapy services by their health care insurers, therapists should take an active role in documenting the client's occupational performance and participation needs to justify the medical necessity of occupational therapy services. Therapists should also provide third-party payers with high-quality evidence supporting the effectiveness and value of occupational therapy interventions specific to the patient.

Stages of Learning: Acquisition, Retention, Transfer, and Generalization

Occupational therapists use a combination of cognitive and motor learning approaches when considering the manner through which patients learn. Both approaches are discussed in greater detail in Chapters 10, 11, 15, and 16. Educational philosopher John Dewey contended that learning is not merely a cognitive act of absorbing theoretical ideas; nor is it based simply on the physical act of doing.[1] In addition to cognitive and motor learning strategies, learning involves the value and meaning that patients place upon the activities in which they participate. To better understand learning from a cognitive and motor perspective, it is important to first explore stages of learning. Although there are several theories describing learning stages across various disciplines, the acquisition, retention, transfer, and generalization stages as they relate to occupational therapy practice are the focus of this chapter.

Acquisition

Acquisition occurs when patients learn new skills, develop strategies for learning (either consciously or unconsciously), and apply new learning in desired, natural contexts. Acquisition begins when information is stored in memory.[2] In the Dreyfus Model,[3] one of the most recognizable learning theories related to skill acquisition, it is theorized that learning occurs on a continuum of five levels: novice, advanced beginner, competent, proficient, and expert. The novice learner requires specific and clearly defined directions. The advanced beginner learner possesses some acquired knowledge and can rudimentarily apply learning to real-life situations. The competent learner emerges as a person gains skill proficiency based on exposure to multiple experiences and begins to build a repertoire of skills that can be used in problem identification and resolution. The proficient learner uses a solid foundation of previously learned concepts and can intuitively apply acquired knowledge to similar contexts. The master/expert has a vast storage of implicit and explicit knowledge and is intuitively able to engage in problem identification and resolution without a formal set of guidelines or instructions.[4] Consider a patient with an above-elbow amputation of the dominant right arm who has been fitted with a myoelectric arm prosthesis. The patient is now learning to use the device in daily functional tasks. The novice learner begins by first learning to control electrodes within the device to flex and extend the elbow, wrist, and fingers. As the patient learns to use the prosthetic arm to perform tasks with more refined motor movements, such as grabbing and releasing an empty glass, the patient becomes an advanced beginner learner. With repetitive and varied practice in different contexts, the patient gains competency in prosthetic arm use. Proficiency develops as the patient learns to grab, lift, and transfer a water glass from table to mouth, and drink from the glass with minimal spillage. The patient may be considered an expert when he or she learns to use the prosthetic arm in more refined tasks such as using a fork to stabilize meat on a plate while the right hand slices pieces with a knife.

Overall, the learning of new skills initially requires greater attention and intention because of a lack of experience, but eventually becomes automatic, requiring less execution time. In the beginning stages of learning a new skill, the individual is focused on learning concrete steps (e.g., controlling the prosthetic device to flex and extend the elbow; using the prosthetic device to retrieve a coin from a desk), rather than on the contexts where learning transpires (e.g., using the prosthetic arm to complete computer tasks at work). Learning and relearning occur frequently for all patients throughout life as skill levels change and are impacted by aging, injury, and the progression of disability or disease. An example of the need to relearn previously acquired skills occurs when a patient fractures a dominant arm. The patient may need to relearn desired daily life activities such as writing, eating, buttoning clothing, and driving using different strategies and skills than those previously learned. Strategies for acquiring a new or modified skill may be intuitive, but in cases of difficulty require the skilled intervention of an occupational therapist. The therapist helps the patient focus on areas that are identified as meaningful and supports the development of strategic plans to problem solve and develop new methods to perform tasks.[5]

Retention

Retention of learning involves the storage of information for later use in familiar situations. To retain learning, retrieval practice is used to promote long-term retention of learned information. Retrieval or skill practice requires several processes[6]: monitoring of learning, cumulative learning, and strategy development and utilization. Monitoring of newly learned information is a repetitive process in which the patient identifies whether the desired performance skill is being enhanced. Cumulative learning is the solidification of knowledge by practicing new skills in familiar and novel situations. Strategy development and utilization involve the generation and application of tools and cues to enhance desired performance skills.

Transfer

Transfer of skills is the application of previously learned knowledge to a new task or activity.[5] An example of skill transfer occurs when an older adult with memory problems attempts to learn use of a new microwave whose control panel is similar to an older model that no longer works. Because most of the new microwave panel functions are the same as those on her old microwave, she is able to transfer her previously learned skills more easily. Another example involves a young adult with traumatic brain injury who attempts to learn tablet and touch screen computer use. Because the patient has already learned the performance skills of pinching, swiping, and double tapping needed to use a smartphone, he can transfer those skills when learning digital tablet and touchscreen computer use.

Generalization

Generalization refers to the ability to take a newly learned skill and apply it to a variety of real-life situations.[7] One example of generalization occurs when a patient who experienced a spinal cord injury attempts to relearn driving using adaptive vehicle equipment. The patient often begins training in a clinical setting, perhaps with a virtual platform. Once motor skills required for adaptive driving are learned in the clinical setting, the patient must then apply these skills while behind the wheel of a real adapted automobile. The patient will typically begin to drive the adapted vehicle in a minimized setting such as a parking lot. Once preliminary skills are mastered, the patient then begins driving on roads with lesser traffic before attempting heavily trafficked roads. Similarly, a patient with a traumatic brain injury learning strategies for self-administration of medication may begin by sorting multiple medicines into a medication container, then progress to identifying and sorting her own medicine with supervision, and finally to sorting medications independently while at home. It is not sufficient for patients to learn segregated components of a task in contrived environments. Patients must practice and apply newly learned performance skills in real-life occupations and settings.

Applying Teaching and Learning Theories in Occupational Therapy

This section addresses the application of specific teaching-learning theories in greater depth and relates them to occupational therapy practice.

Model of Mastery

Using a constructivist approach, Meichenbaum, a cognitive psychologist, developed a model of mastery that has been widely used in cognitive behavioral training and theoretically influenced the development of the Cognitive Orientation to daily Occupational Performance[8] (CO-OP) approach in occupational therapy. The model of mastery[9] states that as part of human development, an individual must learn new skills and concepts, sets of strategies to apply the skills and concepts, and strategies to accomplish tasks independently. As a highest order in the model of mastery, Meichenbaum[9] asserted that task learning involves:

1. Specification of the goal
2. Developing a plan of actions or procedures
3. Actual implementation of a task
4. Evaluation of the outcome's success

This four-step process of task performance was adapted as the Goal-Plan-Do-Check[8] global problem-solving strategies in the CO-OP approach. This teaching-learning process involves a facilitative and iterative process of:

1. Specifying the goal (Goal)
2. Creating a plan of action (Plan)
3. Implementing the task (Do)
4. Evaluating the outcome (Check)

For example, using the four-step process, a therapist teaches a patient with right-sided arm weakness to relearn how to trim nails with a nail clipper (see Fig. 4-1). The therapist facilitates the patient to:

1. Identify the task-specific goal: "I will trim the nails of my left hand using my weak right hand."
2. Create a plan to complete the task: "I will use the three strategies of (a) an adapted nail clipper that is stabilized on a counter; (b) positioning my right arm,

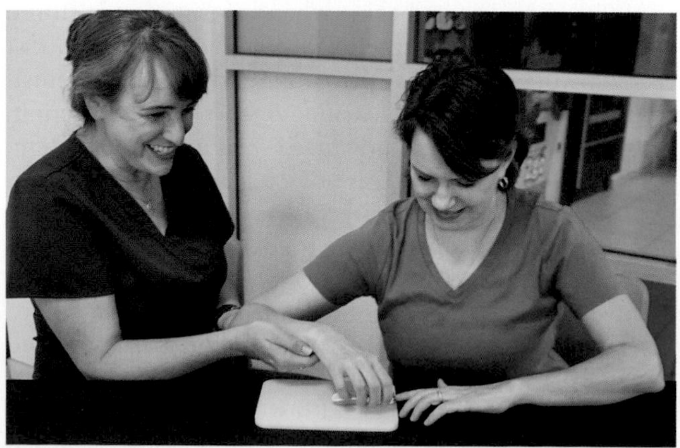

Figure 4-1. A therapist teaches a patient with right-sided arm weakness to relearn nail trimming with a clipper.

forearm, and hand appropriately for the task; and (c) adjusting my left hand finger position as my nails are being trimmed."

3. Perform the task following the plan: "I will now complete the task using all three strategies."
4. a. Evaluate the outcome: "I was able to clip the nails of my left hand in 25 minutes but feel extremely tired afterward," and
   b. Generate opportunities for learning task performance more efficiently: "I may need to choose a counter with a better height. I need to reposition the distance of the stabilized clipper so that it is closer to me. I need to learn a different right hand grip to help with clipping. I need to take a quick hand stretching break."

According to the model of mastery, a skill has been mastered when the individual demonstrates the ability to perform the skills, incorporates the skills when planning and implementing new tasks, and solves problems that may arise in the course of using the skills in various tasks.

Teaching Thinking: Facilitating Metacognition

Within the teaching-learning process, it is important that patients become agents of change in the therapeutic context. Instead of merely becoming passive participants in the therapeutic process, patients should take an active role in treatment. Occupational therapists must use facilitative rather than instructive techniques to help patients problem solve and transfer learned skills to a variety of occupational participation contexts. To be able to assume the role of change agents, occupational therapists may need to facilitate **metacognition** in the patients and families they serve. Meichenbaum[10] defined metacognition as the individual's awareness of his or her own level of cognition—in other words, the conscious awareness of one's thinking processes and the ability to relate to these processes in some way. Metacognition also involves the ability to control one's cognitions—for example, planning cognitive tasks, developing strategies to learn cognitive tasks, and monitoring the quality of task performance. Meichenbaum developed guiding principles for teaching thinking skills, which are adapted below for use in the therapeutic context.[10]

Learning Is a Sustained, In-depth Process that Occurs Over Time and Requires Feedback

Learning new skills or relearning previously learned skills is an iterative process that requires time and ongoing feedback. Both the occupational therapist and the patient must appreciate progress in small increments and understand that certain skills require longer time for mastery. To ensure motivation and facilitate a sense of mastery and competence, the occupational therapist must use occupational analysis to break down tasks and skills into smaller components so that mastery is achieved.

The Patient Is a Collaborator in the Process of Change

The patient is a collaborator and the central agent of change in the therapeutic process. The occupational therapist must learn to master facilitation instead of directly teaching patients skills and concepts. The patient must learn to develop and modify strategies to master a skill and use both strategies and skills in a variety of contexts.

Learning of Strategies Must First Be General in Nature and Can Be Applied in Various Contexts

Begin the learning process with the use of **global strategies** that are more general, before using more **domain-specific strategies** that are specialized.[8] Global strategies are an array of cognitive strategies that focus on facilitating or improving performance that is task-, patient-, or situation-specific.[8] For example, when teaching a patient how to chop vegetables, the occupational therapist first facilitates global learning strategies such as identifying proper safety precautions, awareness of body positioning relative to materials and tools, and self-monitoring the speed needed for chopping (see Fig. 4-2). Once global strategies are comprehended, the therapist can

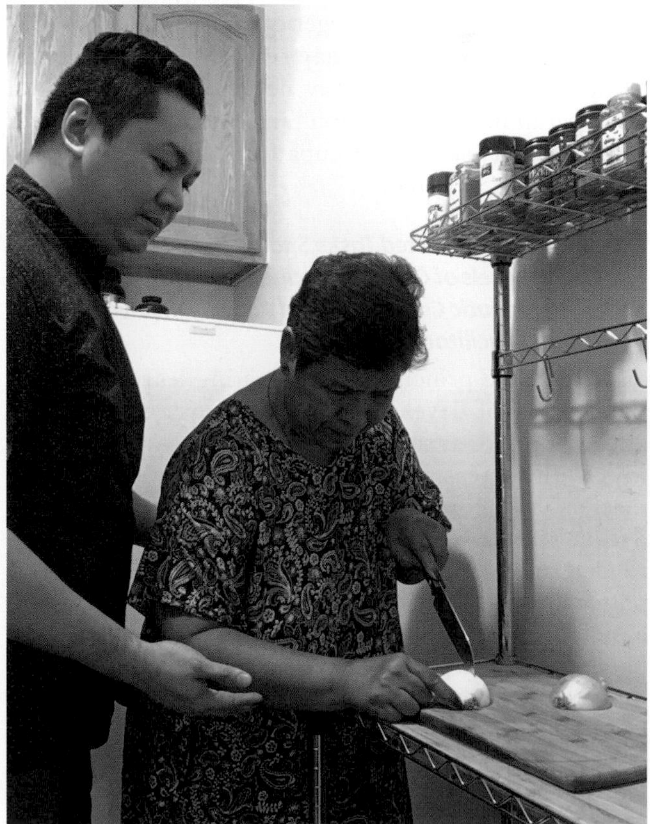

Figure 4-2. A patient learns the use of global strategies such as proper and safe positioning when chopping vegetables.

then facilitate the learning of domain-specific strategies—for example, how to chop distinct types of vegetables, use various kinds of knives, and employ different styles of chopping.

Learning Is Facilitated through a Reflective Process

Meichenbaum suggests using a coping approach[10] when teaching thinking, learning, and relearning skills. A coping approach involves the facilitation of a patient's awareness of perceived thoughts and feelings during task performance. In the therapeutic context, for example, the therapist can ask about the patient's perception of the task's difficulty level, the quality of task performance, how performance can be improved, what supports the patient's need to enhance performance, and the patient's performance satisfaction level.

Learning Must Be Integrated within the Patient's Recovery and/or Development Process

When learning complex skills and tasks, the occupational therapist must integrate the teaching-learning process within the patient's developmental process or recovery. For example, for a youth with developmental delays, it may be necessary to develop prerequisite in-hand manipulation and fine motor integration skills before he or she will be able to manage buttons and different fastener types during dressing tasks. For an adult who had multiple surgeries after a vehicular accident, using activities that may require several steps and complex cognitive skills may need to be delayed until postoperation disorientation and memory difficulties subside. Here, skills in occupational analysis and task gradation are required.

Use of Carefully Selected Tasks Should Be Graded with Increasing Levels of Complexity and Difficulty; Tasks Used in the Therapeutic Context Should Actively Involve the Patient and Facilitate Learning

Similar to the principle of integrating learning within the context of development and recovery, the patient and occupational therapist must carefully select activities with increasing levels of complexity to facilitate mastery and competence. Activity selection and gradation require an iterative problem-solving approach to determine the just-right challenge. Depending on patient needs, some situations might require slightly easier or slightly more difficult activities to keep the patient engaged and motivated to participate in the therapeutic context. The occupational therapist must also make sure that activities are not selected for the patient, but rather involve the patient in the selection and grading of activities. The occupational therapist can use facilitative prompts such as "You did that activity really well. What can you do to make that a little more challenging?"

Training Must Use Natural and Multiple Contexts

To facilitate transfer and generalization of learned skills and concepts, the occupational therapist must allow for practice of skills through the use of various activities, natural contexts, and multiple scenarios. Although it may be difficult to use natural contexts in certain practice settings such as acute care facilities and outpatient clinics, the occupational therapist must use similar or actual items used by the patient in daily life. For example, the occupational therapist can use the patient's actual clothes for buttoning or managing fasteners; use the patient's actual self-care products for grooming; and incorporate the patient's family members and friends in social occupations (such as cooking or recreation). Allowing patients to use their own materials, tools, and social support members can facilitate better transfer and generalization of learning, than merely using simulated activities and contrived contexts.

Assessing Patient Learning Capacities

Because every patient is unique, it is critical to understand each patient's distinct learning needs in order to successfully teach targeted skills in a therapeutic setting that enable occupational participation in real-life contexts. Occupational therapists formally and informally assess the learning capacities and needs of patients throughout the evaluation and treatment process. Therapeutic decisions are made through continuous appraisal of patients' psychological engagement with the therapeutic activity and context.

When analyzing learning capacity, one must take into account daily human dynamics that influence learning. Moment-to-moment learning processes can be positively or negatively impacted by a myriad of factors such as biological, psychological, and situational.[2] For example, a patient with multiple sclerosis may experience an increase in muscular weakness because of illness, weather, or a new environment demanding changes in muscle recruitment and endurance. Performance during a treatment session may be impacted by things seemingly unrelated to the learning activities at hand. The therapist should, whenever possible, attempt to explore confounding factors when the execution of learning seems to be more challenging than expected.

Learning with Disability

Assessment of the learning abilities of patients with varying degrees of disability can be a complicated process. In some cases, the patient may have motor and/or communication limitations that make it difficult to assess whether the patient is learning the concepts taught in therapy. The occupational therapist must collaborate with the patient, family members, caregivers, and health care team members to determine the most appropriate ways to assess the manner in which the patient learns. Informal and formal assessment of learning during the treatment and evaluation processes may occur through a variety of methods including the artful practice of functional observation and occupational analysis, assessing performance during standardized tests, and using patient or caregiver interviews.

Functional Observation

The occupational therapist can assess patient learning capacities during functional observation in various tasks or occupations. The therapist can use familiar and novel tasks to evaluate the patient's capacity to problem solve; learn simple or complex skills; perform simple or multistep tasks; learn tasks in familiar or novel environments or using familiar or novel tools; and generate, use, or modify strategies to solve occupational performance challenges. The therapist should also take note of how the patient responds to the therapist's prompts, verbal and nonverbal language styles, the pace and tone when giving instructions, and the level of questions (simple vs. longer sentences) that the patient can process.

Performance in Standardized Assessments

Determining how the patient learns can be facilitated by carefully constructed questions and standardized instruments. Assessments such as the Canadian Occupational Performance Measure[11] (COPM) and Goal Attainment Scaling[12] (GAS) may help facilitate a conversation about learning styles. Some noted advantages of these types of instruments include their focus on occupation, patient-centered perspective and applicability to all levels of patient function.[13,14]

The occupational therapist can also observe how the patient responds to the level and complexity of questions in standardized assessments. Because standardized instruments have been developed using uniform protocols and carefully studied sets of instructions, the manner by which the patient participates in these tests can provide information about the types of cues and prompts the patient needs to process information. This information can be very helpful in the teaching and learning process.

Patient, Family, and Caregiver Interview

The occupational therapist begins the teaching-learning assessment and process by understanding the patient's background, interests, and occupational needs. The occupational therapist generally begins by creating an occupational profile (see below). When it is not possible to gather information from the patient secondary to disability level, the occupational therapist may gather and use information from an immediate caregiver. It is important, however, to emphasize to the caregiver that in order for skills learned in occupational therapy to be generalized and transferred to the natural context, the patient must assume an active role in therapy.[7] When gathering information from families and caregivers, the occupational therapist can inquire about the most and least effective ways to communicate with the patient, ways to motivate the patient, and contexts that are most conducive for teaching and learning (e.g., time of day, kinds of prompts, physical environments).

Using Teaching-Learning Principles in the Therapy Process

In this section, all concepts from the chapter are synthesized as six essential principles to be considered in the teaching and learning process within the therapeutic context.

Identification of Patient's Meaningful Occupational Goals

As stated earlier in this chapter, the first context for teaching and learning within the therapy process occurs during screening and formal evaluation. During this process, the occupational therapist and patient discuss occupational needs and goals by developing an occupational profile. An **occupational profile** is an initial step in the therapy process needed to gather information about the patient's activity participation and needs.[15] The occupational profile is an important first step to determine what kinds of formal and nonstandardized assessments the therapist can use during the formal evaluation process.[16] Creating an occupational profile is also an important first step in establishing a teaching and learning relationship with the patient. Table 4-1 provides a summary of questions to ask as part of the occupational profile and illustrates how this information can facilitate the teaching and learning process.

Selection of Teaching-Learning Modes Compatible with Patients' Learning Capacities

Once the occupational therapist has assessed the patient's learning capacities, the therapist can then select appropriate teaching-learning modes within the therapeutic context. The following provides a summary of commonly used teaching-learning modes with examples.

Instructional Modes

Instructional modes refer to the types of media through which teaching can occur and includes visual (e.g., gestural cues, written and pictorial instructions), auditory (e.g., verbal instructions, alerting signals and alarms), tactile (e.g., cues delivered through touch, hand-over-hand guidance), and multimodal (e.g., combined verbal

Table 4-1. The Occupational Profile and Teaching-Learning Process

QUESTIONS AS PART OF AN OCCUPATIONAL PROFILE[15]	OPPORTUNITIES FOR TEACHING AND LEARNING WITHIN THE THERAPEUTIC CONTEXT
Why is the patient seeking occupational therapy services? What are the patient's concerns regarding occupational participation?	Information gathered can facilitate discussion about the role and distinct value of occupational therapy and clarify misconceptions about what occupational therapists do. Information gathered can open conversation about the therapy process, which activities may be done during therapy, what to expect during sessions, and how the patient and important others are involved in the process.
What are strengths and barriers affecting occupational performance?	Information gathered can help the therapist understand patient skills and capacities for learning and guide the development of therapeutic instructional materials (e.g., home program instructions, activity logs, health-related monitoring/tracking sheets).
What are the patient's interests and values? What are the patient's routine, roles, habits, and patterns of occupational participation?	Information can help the therapist understand ways to facilitate patient interests and motivation during therapy, and development and selection of therapy materials and tools to help reestablish habits, roles, and routines.
How is occupational participation impacted by the patient's contexts and environments?	Information can help the therapist (1) facilitate the patient's contexts (e.g., social networks) and involve them in the teaching-learning process; (2) understand how physical environments and cultural, temporal, and virtual contexts can promote understanding about how to develop instructional materials (e.g., suggestions for home and tool modifications, time-management worksheets, how to simplify activities using apps and technologies).

explanation and visual demonstration). The therapist must determine through which instructional modes patients learn best. It should be noted that a patient's preferred learning style may be compromised as a result of disability, prompting the need for alternative strategies.

Reinforcement

Reinforcement is the provision of reward or encouragement in response to patient performance and can be offered in a variety of forms including verbal (e.g., praise, redirection), visual (e.g., use of a checkmark system, smiling, positive physical gestures), and tactile or physical (e.g., pat on back, handshake). Therapists should continually reevaluate reinforcement types and frequencies that best facilitate learning for each patient.

Facilitative Prompts

Facilitative prompts are words, phrases, sentences, and questions that provide guidance when patients encounter difficulties or challenges. Such prompts are intended to promote awareness of the need to modify task performance. For example, to promote a patient's awareness of his or her need to modify grasp during an activity, therapists may use word prompts (e.g., "grip"), phrases (e.g., "check your grip"), and questions (e.g., "How well are you holding your glass?"). Therapists should continually reevaluate the types of facilitative prompts to which patients best respond when experiencing task difficulties.

Self-Monitoring Aids

Self-monitoring aids are methods that can be used to facilitate the patient's awareness of the need to regularly check the status of health and/or behavioral changes. Self-monitoring aids allow patients to assess health and behavioral change over time and are particularly useful for patients with memory problems. Examples include technology-based aids (e.g., using smartphone reminders to cue patients to perform blood sugar level tests or engage in periodic and scheduled movement to prevent physical complications) and activity logs (e.g., using a journal or chart to record the performance of needed activity such as self-administering medication). Therapists should continually reevaluate the types of self-monitoring materials that best facilitate carryover in clients' natural contexts (i.e., home, school, work, community).

Guidance

Guidance refers to the provision of instruction intended to help patients modify activity performance to promote optimal function and includes modeling, verbal cues, and physical assistance. Modeling occurs when a therapist demonstrates how to perform a specific activity such as proper body mechanics when lifting boxes from the floor. Verbal cues involve the offering of short words to guide and shape behavior, such as verbally reminding the patient to bend his or her knees when lifting boxes. Physical assistance is the provision of physical cues to shape behavior, such as tapping the patient on the knees to remind him or her to bend them when lifting boxes. Therapists should continually reevaluate the types of guidance that best facilitate learning and task adaptation.

Motivational Cues

Motivational cues are prompts that the therapist offers to patients as encouragement during challenging tasks and are intended to promote perseverance: "You are doing so well, keep going!" "That seemed easy for you! Good work!" "You can do it, you're almost there." Therapists should continually reevaluate the kinds of motivational cues to which patients best respond when experiencing frustration or lack of interest during therapy sessions.

Therapist Support

Therapist support refers to the roles that therapists assume in the teaching and learning process. Two common roles are (1) supportive-facilitative in which the therapist avoids direct teaching and allows the patient to assume greater active control over the teaching-learning context and (2) directive-instructive in which the therapist uses an instructor approach to actively convey specific information designed to be received by the patient. When selecting supportive or directive roles, therapists should determine a patient's readiness for change and receptivity to new information.

Addressing Patient's Health and Reading Literacy

There are multiple accepted ideas regarding the defining, assessing, and addressing of health literacy.[17] The U.S. Institute of Medicine defines **health literacy** as the degree to which individuals can obtain, process, and understand the basic health information and services needed to make appropriate health decisions. Health literacy is a process that depends on patient capacities, skills, preferences, and expectations of health information and care providers.[18] Other researchers have expanded definitions of health literacy with a multidimensional component to include:

- **functional literacy** (i.e., basic reading, writing, and numeracy skills)
- knowing when to seek health information (i.e., self-identification of the necessity to seek health care services)
- knowing where to seek health information (i.e., navigating health systems)
- verbal communication skills (i.e., the ability to describe one's health issues and understand information provided by health professionals)
- retaining and processing information skills (i.e., the ability to understand and make decisions based on health information)
- assertiveness (i.e., the ability to advocate for health needs and information)
- application skills (i.e., the ability to follow instructions and address health issues)[19]

Within the domain of occupational therapy, Grajo and Gutman have proposed a definition of functional literacy[20] that is rooted in the American Occupational Therapy Association definition of functional cognition (i.e., the thinking and processing skills needed to accomplish complex everyday activities such as home, financial, and medication management; work, school, and volunteer activities; and driving and community navigation).[21] Functional literacy is the ability to interpret common written materials needed to effectively carry out basic daily life skills and participate in meaningful occupations and social roles.[20] Grajo and Gutman assert that functional literacy must be part of occupational therapy evaluation and intervention.

To optimize the teaching and learning process, occupational therapists must assess the patient's functional and health literacy skills. Various quantitative and mixed-methods assessments are available for health care professionals to assess patient health literacy. A systematic review details different assessments including[22]:

- Short Assessment of Health Literacy—Spanish and English (SAHL-SE)[23]: a 32-item reading test in Spanish and English.
- All Aspects of Health Literacy Scale (AALS)[24]: addresses four items on functional health literacy, three items on communicative health literacy, four items on critical health literacy, and three empowerment items.
- Medical Term Recognition Test (METER)[25]: contains 40 medical words and 40 nonmedical words.
- Rapid Estimate of Adult Literacy[26]: contains 125 medical terms taken from printed patient education materials; regarded as one of the most widely used health literacy assessments.
- Test of Functional Health Literacy in Adults (TOFHLA)[27]: a 50-item reading comprehension and 17-item numerical ability test using actual hospital materials; regarded as one of the most widely used health literacy assessments.

Table 4-2 provides an overview of how occupational therapists can seize teaching and learning opportunities within the therapeutic context based on formal and informal assessments of patients' functional and health literacy.

Assessing Patient's Readiness for Behavioral and Lifestyle Change

Another important consideration in optimizing the teaching and learning process within the therapeutic relationship is assessing the patient's readiness for health behavior and lifestyle change. Motivation is a critical dimension in influencing patients to seek, comply with, and complete treatment.[28] Change, just like recovery, is a process. One model of change commonly used in rehabilitation is the Transtheoretical Model of Change.[29] Prochaska's model specifies four stages:

1. ***Precontemplation:*** the stage in which the individual is not intending to take action in the foreseeable future.
2. ***Contemplation:*** the stage in which people are intending to take action in the next 6 months; a stage marked by considerable ambivalence.

Table 4-2. Teaching and Learning Opportunities after Assessment of Patient Health and Functional Literacy

HEALTH AND FUNCTIONAL LITERACY COMPONENTS[19,20]	IMPLICATIONS ON THE THERAPEUTIC TEACHING-LEARNING PROCESS
Functional literacy	The occupational therapist can support development of and teach functional literacy skills as they relate to basic and instrumental activities of daily living and community participation.
Knowing when to seek health information	Within the context of health promotion and disability prevention, the occupational therapist can teach the client, family, and caregivers about causes and symptoms of illness or disability and how to gather information using online and community health resources.
Knowing where to seek health information	The occupational therapist can teach the client, family, and caregivers about different roles of the health care team and what kinds of questions to ask their health care team related to one's condition.
Verbal communication skills, retaining and processing health information skills, assertiveness with health professionals	The occupational therapist can teach the patient assertiveness and self-advocacy skills to facilitate skills in navigating the health care system, knowing how to ask the right questions related to health and well-being, and how to seek more information about one's health.
Application skills	The occupational therapist can teach the patient how to follow health care instructions and learn to embed health care practices into one's habits and routines (e.g., learning to schedule regular doctor's appointments; learning to include a healthy balance of exercise, leisure, and rest within a work week).

3. ***Preparation:*** the stage in which an individual intends to take action in the immediate future.
4. ***Action:*** the stage in which the individual has made specific, overt modifications in his or her behavior within the preceding 6 months.

Illness, disease, and disability are marked by life-altering changes that require adaptation.[30] Assessing the patient's readiness to change health behaviors is an iterative process that has direct implications for the ways through which therapists must use teaching and learning approaches. One evidence-based approach that can be integrated in the teaching-learning process is the use of motivational interviewing. Motivational interviewing is a client-centered counseling style designed to elicit behavioral change by assisting patients to explore and resolve ambivalence to desired change.[31] A systematic review and meta-analysis found that motivational interviewing in clinical settings effectively helped patients change their behavior and outperformed traditional advice-giving in approximately 80% ($n = 72$) of studies.[32] Essential components and principles of motivational interviewing include the following[31]:

- The patient's intrinsic values and goals should be identified to facilitate behavior change.
- Motivation to change should be elicited from the patient and must not be imposed.
- The patient should receive assistance to better understand the perceived benefits and costs of health behavior change by eliciting, clarifying, and resolving his or her ambivalence to change.
- Readiness to change is not a patient trait, but a fluctuating product of interpersonal interaction.
- Resistance and "denial" may signify the need to modify motivational and teaching strategies.
- Central in health behavior change is eliciting and reinforcing the patient's belief in his or her ability to succeed.
- The therapeutic relationship is a partnership based on respect for patient autonomy and must be patient centered.

Structuring the Environment to Facilitate Learning

The patient's physical and social environments, and various occupational performance contexts, may significantly influence the teaching and learning process. This process may involve the following aspects, among many others:

1. ***Identification of sensory qualities needed to best facilitate occupational performance in specific environments*** (e.g., the patient may work best in a room that is not too cold and has natural lighting and limited distraction)
2. ***Use of social and temporal contexts*** (e.g., the activity is best performed in the morning with the patient's significant other)
3. ***Modifying and adapting features of the physical environment*** (e.g., the patient's bathroom door entrance needs to be widened to accommodate the patient's permanent need for a wheelchair)

Feedback and Practice

Feedback and practice are essential components of teaching and learning in occupational therapy. Feedback provides patients with information needed to correct errors on subsequent practice trials. Therapists select specific feedback types and schedules when shaping a patient's learning experience. This section presents an overview of definitions and examples of feedback and practice using different paradigms. A more in-depth discussion of feedback and practice as it relates to motor learning is discussed in Chapters 15 and 16.

Feedback Based on Availability to Learner

- *Intrinsic feedback* is information that is available to the patient based on his or her own sensory systems. For example, the patient observes the position of her arm and hand while holding the spoon and bringing it to her mouth.[33]
- *Extrinsic feedback* is information that is supplemental to intrinsic feedback. For example, the therapist verbally cues the patient to visually monitor her arm movement when using the spoon during feeding.[33]
- *Knowledge of results* is a form of extrinsic feedback in which the outcome of the movement serves as feedback. For example, the patient observes the placement of the spoon relative to her mouth when her shoulder is abducted and internally rotated.[33]

Feedback Based on Sensory Modes

- *Visual feedback* is information derived from the visual-perceptual senses.[34]
- *Auditory feedback* is information derived from the auditory senses.[34]
- *Haptic feedback* is information derived from a combination of physical assistance and guidance (tactile, proprioceptive, kinesthetic).[34]
- *Multimodal feedback* is information derived from a combination of visual, auditory, and multimodal feedback.[34]

Various Definitions of Practice

- *Massed versus distributed practice* refers to the differences in practice time and rest time. In massed practice, patient practice time during trials is greater than rest time. In distributed practice, rest time between practice trials is equal to or greater than the amount of time for the entire trial.[33]
- *Constant versus variable practice* refers to practice in which training conditions (e.g., speed, number of repetitions) are either constant or variable.[33]
- *Random versus blocked practice* refers to practice in which the order of tasks is constant and ordered (blocked), or occurs in irregular patterns (random).[33]
- *Whole versus part training* refers to practice in which the activity is completed fully (whole) or is broken down into smaller steps (part).[33]
- *Mental practice* is the performance of a skill using imagination with no action involved.[33]

Summary

Teaching and learning are essential components of daily occupational therapy practice. The teaching-learning process is a collaborative process that is patient centered and involves the patient's important social networks and interprofessional health care team members. Teaching and learning approaches are driven by patient characteristics and needs, rather than assuming a one-size-fits-all approach. The teaching and learning process must integrate various information gathered throughout the therapeutic context such as the patient's occupational profile; health and functional literacy; patient, family, and caregiver learning modes; and feedback from the patient's occupational contexts and environments.

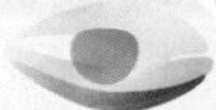

CASE STUDY

Patient Information

Dereque is a 22-year-old African American male with mixed quadriplegia (spasticity with dystonia) who participates in a day program at a community center for adults with cerebral palsy. The program houses an assistive technology center that is staffed by an occupational therapist and offers specialized training in assistive technology for greater home and community independence. Dereque's mother, Anelia, is his legal representative and provided medical information during the occupational therapy evaluation. Dereque uses a manual wheelchair pushed by a family member to access his home and community. Previous neuropsychological testing from high school revealed that Dereque has an IQ of 84, which is within the low-average range.

Assessment Process and Results

Dereque attended the initial evaluation while in his manual wheelchair, pushed by his mother. His occupational therapist began the assessment by developing an occupational profile. The therapist remained seated to maintain eye-level contact with Dereque. When his response was difficult to understand, Anelia answered for him. The therapist asked for Dereque's permission to obtain his medical history from his mother; Dereque nodded in agreement. Anelia explained that Dereque understands all spoken words, but has difficulty clearly forming words because of dysarthria. Anelia stated that as a result, people often do not wait for Dereque's answers and have habitually made decisions for him. This feedback signified to the therapist that she should facilitate learning situations during treatment in which Dereque would have the opportunity to direct the activities and select relevant goals.

Several assessment methods were used including range of motion (ROM) measurements, the Modified Ashworth Scale[36] (MAS) to measure upper extremity tone, the Modified Tardieu Scale[37] to measure velocity-dependent spasticity, and the COPM to aid in goal setting. Although Dereque responded well during testing, he

(continued)

CASE STUDY *(continued)*

demonstrated a startle reflex when touched for ROM without a verbal warning from the therapist. The therapist learned that she needed to provide prewarning prompts before touching him.

During information gathering for the occupational profile, the therapist learned of several factors that may hinder occupational engagement:

- *Physical:* Dereque was unable to independently access his home and community because of his current wheelchair.
- *Social:* Because he depends on his family for all activities of daily living (ADLs) and environmental access, participation in peer activities was limited.
- *Personal:* Dereque's opinion or preferences were often overlooked because of insufficient means to communicate. Peers often perceived him to have intellectual impairment because of dysarthria.

Occupational Therapy Goal List

Dereque and his mother developed goals using the COPM.[11] They discussed specifics about his daily routines and interests, including identifying his favorite activities of watching football and television with his siblings. Dereque stated that he also enjoys Friday dances at the community center with his girlfriend. Among other identified goals, Dereque's main priorities included (1) beginning classes at the local community college and (2) hosting a college football game watch party with his siblings and closest friends.

Interventions

Intervention 1

Anelia mentioned that Dereque was once independent with a power wheelchair, but it was now in disrepair and he had outgrown it 4 years ago. Dereque acknowledged that he missed his power wheelchair because it allowed him to access more places at home and in the community without help. In collaboration with his neurologist and durable medical equipment (DME) provider, all agreed that it was advantageous to pursue obtaining another power wheelchair.

When Dereque's power wheelchair was delivered, Anelia attended each session to understand how to grade the activity. Because Dereque was essentially relearning how to drive a power wheelchair, the occupational therapist broke the task into small parts during the learning acquisition phase. She used a multimodal instructional approach that included visual, auditory, and tactile feedback. Dereque first learned to propel forward and backward, and left and right using a head array drive system (i.e., drive controls operated by pressure sensors in the headrest). The learning approach was initially introduced as constant and blocked practice, and later modified with increasing complexity of varied wheelchair speeds with random directional commands from the therapist. Anelia was taught how to manage the different wheelchair drive controls and how to engage/disengage the batteries.

After approximately 2 weeks, the occupational therapist accompanied Dereque on community outings. This provided Dereque with the opportunity to transfer skills from the clinic to the community and included navigation of the college campus. The therapist also provided verbal and written instructions of practice activities for wheelchair use in the community and home.

Intervention 2

Dereque used a touch screen augmentative communication device (ACD) provided several years earlier by his high school. He had limited carryover at home because his family was not familiar with the steps needed to program the device, and many of the activities were related to high school coursework rather than daily activities. Additionally, Dereque often became frustrated with the device because he would miss the target picture needed to communicate a specific need. He also was not particularly interested in most of the items on the device (e.g., course subjects from high school), which further limited carryover at home. The occupational therapist and Dereque jointly problem solved to identify the best method to access the device by trialing a variety of methods. They discovered that touch using his fingers was not the best option. Integrating the device controls into his wheelchair head array was also cumbersome because it was difficult for Dereque to process the multiple steps required to navigate between the wheelchair drive controls and the communication device controls. After several trial-and error periods, the occupational therapist and Dereque discovered that eye gaze (using his eyes to select the target picture) was the best option. Dereque initially appeared to be unclear about various steps needed to use eye gaze control. The therapist worked with Dereque to clarify ambiguous steps and discussed the importance of making more challenging steps with each session. She often asked for his feedback about how he perceived his level of satisfaction by asking questions such as "How do you think you did?" and "Was that easy for you?"

Additionally, the therapist and Dereque used COPM results to guide the selection of activity options for the device, such as music, television channels, and favorite restaurant choices. Dereque's family members were also trained in the steps to add new choices as needed. A digital page was created in the device for Dereque's medical needs, such as medication times and doctor appointments, so that Dereque could begin self-advocating his health care needs.

Although Dereque was discharged from occupational therapy services, he continued to go to the community center and often visited the assistive technology lab to participate in adaptive gaming with several friends. He was proud to show that his device was now programmed (by his father) to control Dereque's television controls and bedroom and bathroom lights. Dereque was also consistently using the device and his power wheelchair to independently access his home and participate in community activities. He plans to begin college in the following fall semester.

Evidence Table for Interventions Using a Strategy Training Teaching-Learning Approach

Intervention	Intervention Description	Participants	Dosage	Research Design And Evidence Level	Benefit	Statistical Significance And Effect Size
Occupation-based strategy training to improve occupational performance of adults with traumatic brain injury[38]	Adapted intervention of the CO-OP	Thirteen adults with traumatic brain injury (7 = treatment group; 6 = control group)	Two 1-hour sessions for 10 weeks	Partially randomized controlled trial. Level I	Increased performance and satisfaction in identified occupational goals and transfer of learned skills in real-world environments	Treatment group reported increased performance on occupational goals ($t = 2.36$; $p = 0.04$); increased satisfaction with occupational performance ($t = 2.67$; $p = 0.03$).
Strategy training and behavioral intervention to improve occupational performance and reduce apathy in adults with stroke in inpatient rehabilitation[39]	Occupation-based training with use of the Goal-Plan-Do-Check strategy training approach	Thirty adults with stroke (15 = strategy training; 15 = reflective listening approach)	One session per day, five times a week in addition to regular inpatient rehabilitation	Secondary analysis of a randomized controlled trial. Level I	Decreased level of poststroke apathy for participants	A significant group time interaction ($F = 3.61, p = 0.040$) indicated that changes in apathy symptom levels differed between groups over time. The magnitude of group differences in change scores was large ($d = 0.99$, $t = 2.64, p = 0.013$) at month 3 and moderate to large ($d = 0.70, t = 1.86$, $p = 0.073$) at month 6.
Use of cognitive interventions to improve executive functions during daily task performance[40]	Two interventions were compared: use of strategy training using the CO-OP approach and computer-based executive function training	Nine adults with stroke (5 = CO-OP training; 4 = computer training)	Sixteen training sessions for 1 hour each	Randomized controlled trial. Level I	Increased performance and satisfaction in occupational performance with transfer of skills learned in real-world settings; increased self-efficacy was higher in CO-OP group	Both treatment groups showed large improvements in self and significant other rated performance and satisfaction with performance on their occupational goals immediately postintervention and at follow-up (CO-OP: ES = 1.6–3.5; COMPUTER: ES = 0.9–4.0), with statistically significant within-group differences in CO-OP ($p = 0.05$).
Cognitive strategy and task-specific training to improve cognitive flexibility, upper extremity use, and reduce stroke impact in adults with stroke[41]	Use of the Goal-Plan-Do-Check strategy of the CO-OP approach during occupational performance	Twenty-six adults with stroke (14 = CO-OP training; 12 = usual care)	Varied; data monitored when participants were discharged or received 10 sessions	Exploratory single-blind randomized controlled trial. Level I	Improved performance, cognitive skills, and arm movement in participants who received CO-OP training over usual care	At time 3, there was a medium effect for SIS Hand Function ($d = 0.6$) and the D-KEFS Trail Making subtest ($d = 0.5$).

CO-OP, Cognitive Orientation to daily Occupational Performance; ES, effect size; SIS, stroke impact scale; D-KEFS, delis-Kaplan executive function system.

References

1. McDermott JJ. *The Philosophy of John Dewey: Volume 1. The Structure of Experience. Volume 2: The Lived Experience*. Chicago, IL: University of Chicago Press; 1981.
2. Merriam SB, Caffarella RS, Baumgartner LM. *Learning in Adulthood: A Comprehensive Guide*. San Francisco, CA: John Wiley & Sons Inc; 2012.
3. Dreyfus H. The Dreyfus model of skill acquisition. In: Burke J, ed. *Competency Based Education and Training*. London, England: Falmer Press; 1989:181–183.
4. Peña A. The Dreyfus model of clinical problem-solving skills acquisition: a critical perspective. *Med Educ Online*. 2010;15(1):4846. doi:10.1177/0270467604265023.
5. McEwen SE, Polatajko HJ, Huijbregts MP, Ryan JD. Inter-task transfer of meaningful, functional skills following a cognitive-based treatment: results of three multiple baseline design experiments in adults with chronic stroke. *Neuropsychol Rehabil*. 2010;20(4):541–561. doi:10.1080/09602011003638194.
6. Karpicke JD, Roediger HL. The critical importance of retrieval for learning. *Science*. 2008;319(5865):966–968. doi:10.1126/science.1152408.
7. McEwen SE, Houldin A. Generalization and transfer in the CO-OP Approach. In: Dawson D, McEwen SE, Polatajko H, eds. *Cognitive Orientation to Daily Occupational Performance in Occupational Therapy: Using the CO-OP Approach to Enable Participation Across the Lifespan*. Bethesda, MD: AOTA Press; 2017.
8. Polatajko HJ, Mandich AD, Missiuna C, et al. Cognitive orientation to daily occupational performance (CO-OP) part III-the protocol in brief. *Phys Occup Ther Pediatr*. 2001;20(2–3):107–123. doi:10.1080/J006v20n02_07.
9. Meichenbaum D, Biemiller A. *Nurturing Independent Learners: Helping Students Take Charge of Their Learning*. Newton, MA: ERIC; 1998.
10. Meichenbaum D. *The Evolution of Cognitive Behavior Therapy: A Personal and Professional Journey with Don Meichenbaum*. New York, NY: Taylor & Francis; 2017.
11. Law M, Baptiste S, Carswell A, McColl MA, Polatajko H, Pollock N. *Canadian Occupational Performance Measure (COPM)*. Ottawa, ON:CAOT Publications; 2014.
12. Kiresuk TJ, Smith A, Cardillo JE. *Goal Attainment Scaling: Applications, Theory, and Measurement*. London, England: Psychology Press; 2014.
13. McDougall J, King G. *Goal Attainment Scaling: Description, Utility, and Applications in Pediatric Therapy Services*. London, ON: Thames Valley Children's Centre. 2007.
14. Parker DM, Sykes CH. A systematic review of the Canadian Occupational Performance Measure: a clinical practice perspective. *Br J Occup Ther*. 2006;69(4):150–160. doi:10.1177/030802260606900402.
15. American Occupational Therapy Association. Occupational therapy practice framework: domain and process (3rd ed.). *Am J Occup Ther*. 2014;68(suppl 1):S1–S48. doi:10.5014/ajot.2014.682006.
16. Royeen C, Grajo L, Luebben A. Nonstandardized testing. In: Hinojosa J, Kramer P, eds. *Evaluation in Occupational Therapy: Obtaining and Interpreting Data*. 4th ed. Bethesda, MD: AOTA Press; 2014.
17. Frisch A-L, Camerini L, Diviani N, Schulz PJ. Defining and measuring health literacy: how can we profit from other literacy domains? *Health Promot Int*. 2011;27(1):117–126. doi:10.1093/heapro/dar043.
18. Kindig DA, Panzer AM, Nielsen-Bohlman L. *Health Literacy: A Prescription to End Confusion*. Washington, DC: National Academies Press; 2004. https://www.ncbi.nlm.nih.gov/books/NBK216035/
19. Jordan JE, Buchbinder R, Osborne RH. Conceptualising health literacy from the patient perspective. *Patient Educ Couns*. 2010;79(1):36–42. doi:10.1016/j.pec.2009.10.001.
20. Grajo L, Gutman, S. The role of occupational therapy in functional literacy. *Open J Occup Ther*. 2019. doi:10.15453/2168-6408.1511.
21. American Occupational Therapy Association. *Role of Occupational Therapy in Assessing Functional Cognition*. 2016. https://www.aota.org/Advocacy-Policy/Federal-Reg-Affairs/Medicare/Guidance/role-OT-assessing-functional-cognition.aspx
22. Altin SV, Finke I, Kautz-Freimuth S, Stock S. The evolution of health literacy assessment tools: a systematic review. *BMC Public Health*. 2014;14(1):1207. doi:10.1186/1471-2458-14-1207.
23. Lee SYD, Stucky BD, Lee JY, Rozier RG, Bender DE. Short assessment of health literacy—Spanish and English: a comparable test of health literacy for Spanish and English speakers. *Health Serv Res*. 2010;45(4):1105–1120. doi:10.1111/j.1475-6773.2010.01119.x.
24. Chinn D, McCarthy C. All Aspects of Health Literacy Scale (AAHLS): developing a tool to measure functional, communicative and critical health literacy in primary healthcare settings. *Patient Educ Couns*. 2013;90(2):247–253. doi:10.1016/j.pec.2012.10.019.
25. Rawson KA, Gunstad J, Hughes J, et al. The METER: a brief, self-administered measure of health literacy. *J Gen Intern Med*. 2010;25(1):67–71. doi:10.1007/s11606-009-1158-7.
26. Davis TC, Crouch M, Long SW, et al. Rapid assessment of literacy levels of adult primary care patients. *Fam Med*. 1991;23(6):433–435.
27. Parker RM, Baker DW, Williams MV, Nurss JR. The test of functional health literacy in adults. *J Gen Intern Med*. 1995;10(10):537–541. doi:10.1007/bf02640361.
28. DiClemente CC, Bellino LE, Neavins TM. Motivation for change and alcoholism treatment. *Alcohol Res Health*. 1999;23(2):87–92. https://pubs.niaaa.nih.gov/publications/arh23-2/086-92.pdf
29. Prochaska JO. Decision making in the transtheoretical model of behavior change. *Med Decis Making*. 2008;28(6):845–849. doi:10.1177/0272989X08327068.
30. Grajo L, Boisselle A, DaLomba E. Occupational adaptation as a construct: a scoping review of literature. *Open J Occup Ther*. 2018;6(1):2. doi:10.15453/2168-6408.1400.
31. Miller WR, Rollnick S. *Motivational Interviewing: Preparing People for Change*. New York, NY: The Guilford Press; 2002.
32. Rubak S, Sandbæk A, Lauritzen T, Christensen B. Motivational interviewing: a systematic review and meta-analysis. *Br J Gen Pract*. 2005;55(513):305–312. https://www.ncbi.nlm.nih.gov/pmc/articles/PMC1463134/

33. Shumway-Cook A, Woollacott, M. *Motor Control: Translating Research into Clinical Practice*. 5th ed. Philadelphia, PA: Lippincott Williams & Wilkins; 2017.
34. Sigrist R, Rauter G, Riener R, Wolf P. Augmented visual, auditory, haptic, and multimodal feedback in motor learning: a review. *Psychon Bull Rev.* 2013;20(1):21–53. doi:10.3758/s13423-012-0333-8.
35. Bohannon RW, Larkin PA, Smith MB, Horton MG. Relationship between static muscle strength deficits and spasticity in stroke patients with hemiparesis. *Phys Ther.* 1987;67(7):1068–1071. doi:10.1093/ptj/67.7.1068.
36. Mackey AH, Walt SE, Lobb G, Stott NS. Intraobserver reliability of the modified Tardieu scale in the upper limb of children with hemiplegia. *Dev Med Child Neurol.* 2004;46(4):267–272. doi:10.1017/S0012162204000428.
37. Dawson DR, Binns MA, Hunt A, Lemsky C, Polatajko HJ. Occupation-based strategy training for adults with traumatic brain injury: a pilot study. *Arch Phys Med Rehabil.* 2013;94(10):1959–1963. doi:10.1016/j.apmr.2013.05.021.
38. Skidmore ER, Whyte EM, Butters MA, Terhorst L, Reynolds CF. Strategy training during inpatient rehabilitation may prevent apathy symptoms after acute stroke. *PM&R.* 2015;7(6):562–570. doi:10.1016/j.pmrj.2014.12.010.
39. Poulin V, Korner-Bitensky N, Bherer L, Lussier M, Dawson DR. Comparison of two cognitive interventions for adults experiencing executive dysfunction post-stroke: a pilot study. *Disabil Rehabil.* 2017;39(1):1–13. doi:10.3109/09638288.2015.1123303.
40. Wolf TJ, Polatajko H, Baum C, et al. Combined cognitive-strategy and task-specific training affects cognition and upper-extremity function in subacute stroke: an exploratory randomized controlled trial. *Am J Occup Ther.* 2016;70(2):7002290010p1–7002290010p10. doi:10.5014/ajot.2016.017293.

Chapter 5

Clinical Reasoning and the Art of Practice

Laura VanPuymbrouck

LEARNING OBJECTIVES

This chapter will allow the reader to:

1. Define and differentiate the reasoning processes used by occupational therapists.
2. Describe the historic rationale for why the American Occupational Therapy Association (AOTA) and the American Occupational Therapy Foundation (AOTF) implemented and supported the Clinical Reasoning Study.
3. Identify the reasoning styles that distinguish a novice from an expert therapist.
4. Describe the elements of occupational therapy approaches to evaluation and intervention that make practice an art.
5. Describe and differentiate between problem-based and experiential learning.
6. Understand how problem-based and experiential learning facilitate professional reasoning in occupational therapists.

CHAPTER OUTLINE

TERMINOLOGY

Clinical reasoning: the thinking processes used by occupational therapists when planning, conducting, and reflecting on their practice.[1]

Decision making: the cognitive process by which one makes a choice among two or more alternatives.[2]

Judgment: the cognitive process by which a person appraises a situation and determines the best course of action to take.[2]

Problem solving: the cognitive process by which one sequentially identifies a problem, interprets aspects of the situation, and selects a method to alleviate the problem.[2]

Professional reasoning: the thinking process used by occupational therapists inclusive of occupational therapy practices that extend beyond traditional settings to include those based in nonclinical settings such as schools, workplaces, or community programs targeting occupational performance; highlighting the overarching occupational lens used in reasoning unique to the profession.[3]

Reasoning strategies: methods or approaches to reasoning or the selection of a structure or organization for one's reasoning process.[2]

Introduction

During therapeutic evaluation and intervention, a therapist must identify and frame problems and make immediate choices based on the client's needs and the specific context of the interaction.[4] How does an occupational therapist analyze the person, the environment, and the task to make the many clinical decisions that will result in the best outcomes for clients? This question has been the basis of inquiry in the profession since Joan Rogers highlighted the concept of clinical reasoning in her Eleanor Clarke Slagle lecture in 1983.[1] In this lecture, Rogers emphasized the importance of understanding the artistic as well as the scientific and ethical dimensions of clinical reasoning that distinguish occupational therapy from other medical and allied health professionals.[1] This, plus seminal work from Schon[4] examining the tacit knowing of therapists, ignited excitement and interest in the profession for research exploring these dimensions and ultimately drove the impetus for the Clinical Reasoning Study[5] sponsored by the American Occupational Therapy Association (AOTA) and the American Occupational Therapy Foundation (AOTF). This effort resulted in a special issue in the *American Journal of Occupational Therapy* (AJOT) in 1991 that included articles describing the findings of the study. This special issue provided the basis for much of the profession's understanding of therapists' clinical reasoning and laid the groundwork for subsequent research. This body of work recognized the symbiotic qualities from both science and art as they guide our professional ethos[6] and have evolved to define and describe our commitment to client-centered and client-driven occupation-based evaluations and interventions. However, fully understanding how therapist reasoning impacts the development and maintenance of a client-centered therapeutic relationship that optimizes client outcomes continues to be an area of necessary research exploration.[7,8,9]

History and Background of Clinical Reasoning in Occupational Therapy

What Is Clinical Reasoning?

Allied health professions' clinical reasoning research has traditionally been medically oriented with a focus on understanding the logic and cognitive processes of a therapist informed by scientific knowledge of diagnostic pathways and procedures with evidence base that align with the profession's purpose.[10] The Occupational Therapy Practice Framework (OTPF)[11] defines the occupational therapy profession's **clinical reasoning** as "the process used by therapists to plan, direct, perform and reflect on care."[12] The framework further emphasizes clinical reasoning as a key component to developing and managing the therapeutic relationship as the therapist works to help clients process, make sense, and invest in the therapeutic experience.[11,13] Clinical reasoning is described as a core element of practice that includes scientific knowledge, reflection, and intuition that links professional research with clinical practice[14] and a necessary skill in order for an occupational therapist to be successful.[15] However, the processes therapists use can be heavily informed by temporal and spatial influences of the current conditions in which the profession exists.[16] Naming clinical reasoning as **professional reasoning** extends the reasoning that occupational therapists use to include those contexts outside the clinical environment such as community-based practices.[17] Whatever the clinical context, the fundamental processes that occupational therapists move through during assessment, analysis of information from the client, problem identification, and selection of intervention design specific to the client are clinical and professional reasoning distinctive to occupational therapy.[15] Understanding these distinct elements is vital to supporting their development for the individual therapist and more broadly for the profession as a whole.

Historically, occupational therapy has grappled with the challenges of weaving scientific biomedical evidence-based knowledge and social, humanistic, clinically acquired knowledge that explains all aspects of a therapist's clinical reasoning.[14] Efforts to embrace a professional identity that moves beyond biomedical and impairment-based **problem solving** to client-centered practice demand therapists use knowledge informed by more than a scientific medical model evidence base in their decision-making strategies. One of the primary purposes of the Clinical Reasoning Study was to identify and distinguish the unique processes of reasoning used by occupational therapists compared to health professions informed by more of a purely biomedical stance.[2]

Clinical Reasoning in Occupational Therapy

Rogers states in her seminal Slagle lecture, "The goal of clinical reasoning is to make treatment recommendations according to the best interests of a client."[1] Rogers further describes the process therapists move through as being grounded by their own conceptual frame of reference that guides how they perceive the client, the environment, and client occupations. Her description highlights how therapists' individualism informs their choice of tools for crafting their own therapeutic approach. This individuality allows for the personal background, culture, beliefs, and assumptions of the therapist to have a determinant effect on the outcomes of the clinical reasoning process.[18] These influences can shape what the therapist identifies as important, affect the meaning they are given, and inform the decisions made for evaluations and interventions.[17] Broader perspectives and past experiences clearly contribute to what the therapist brings to the reasoning process as well as extends appreciation for the influences of the therapist's theoretical stance and appreciation for ethical influences. So, what are the perspectives and experiences that contribute to developing a therapist's broader worldview that might promote expertise in clinical reasoning and optimize therapeutic outcomes?

On a daily basis, occupational therapists make clinical decisions regarding the clients' needs during therapy, the clients' outcome potential, and how to make recommendations to enhance occupation. Scientific reasoning is the foundation of many medical and health professional diagnostic and problem-based decision making. However, occupational therapy has a unique clinical or profession-based reasoning described by the findings of the Clinical Reasoning Study[5] as relying on several sources of cognitive reasoning processes. These include: procedural, interactive, conditional[5] and pragmatic[19] modes of thinking used by a therapist when attending to client and contextual factors. Fleming[2] extended clinical reasoning from these more cognitive-based processes to embrace a narrative story line that includes contextual factors therapists use to influence interactions with clients.

Research describes that procedural, interactive, and conditional modes of reasoning account for the majority of thinking processes used by therapists.[20] However, the focus of the therapist whether it be a more biomedical lens or psychosocial lens appears to inform the mode of reasoning.[2,20] Occupational therapy scholars suggest different preferences for modes of thinking and clinical reasoning may be dependent on the exposure to different academic stances during the educational process as well as during clinical learning experiences.[8] Seven different modes of thinking (scientific, procedural, interactive, conditional, narrative, pragmatic, and ethical) and their specific process characteristics are described in the following sections of this text and summarized in Table 5-1.

Definitions and Descriptions of Clinical Reasoning in Occupational Therapy

Scientific Reasoning

Scientific reasoning is a cognitive process of problem solving that involves "critical thinking in relation to content, procedural, and epistemic knowledge."[21] It is a fluid process embedded from the onset of an occupational therapy referral, throughout evaluation and intervention and during discharge planning. Because of the increasing emphasis on evidence-based practice in all disciplines of medicine and allied health professions, it is also described as an essential skill for a therapist to develop over the course of his or her professional education.[2] Scientific reasoning is typically only one part of a therapist's reasoning process because it does not include factors that ultimately influence decisions such as client factors or therapist experience. This approach to clinical problem solving is associated with focusing strictly on the biomedical diagnosis of a client using a hypothetical-deductive model of reasoning.[22] Scientific reasoning explores the context of a problem including the state of the identified issue of concern, the end goal, the means

Table 5-1. Definitions of Reasoning Approaches

REASONING APPROACH	DEFINITION
Scientific Reasoning	A cognitive process of problem solving that involves critical thinking in relation to content, procedural, and epistemic knowledge.[21] Uses diagnosis, impairment, and evidence-based approaches to inform decision making.
Procedural	A process of reasoning informed by clinical pathways or routines traditionally used by a therapist to improve function. Procedural reasoning stems from the scientific knowledge and evidence-based practice patterns that provide generalizable approach strategies for a client with a specific diagnostic presentation.
Interactive	Recognizes the client as expert in their own lived experiences and as such produces a process of interactive reasoning to collect critical information on the contexts of their lives and occupations of importance.
Conditional	Multifaceted and multiperspective reasoning process used to understand clients' needs to address potential shifts in identity because of changes in functional capacity.[2] Reasoning that incorporates flexibility in responding to the client's ever-changing upstream as well as downstream concerns.
Narrative	"Narrative thinking is the primary way of making sense of human experience."[63] Reasoning informed by knowledge gathered through listening to, reflecting on, and empathizing with the client to paint the picture for developing a client-centered intervention plan.
Pragmatic	Decision making that works within the parameters of the clinical as well as the social restriction of the context, the client, and therapist that includes time, place, and availability of resources. Can create dilemmas in clinical reasoning that force "underground" practices.[5]
Ethical	In the moment or bigger picture knowledge that creates a conundrum in reasoning among client-centered care, social justice, and administrative or structural barriers.

to the end, and the action steps required to move from the current state to the goal state.[23]

Occupational therapists evaluate the many client factors that impact a given occupational role and use scientific reasoning to understand action steps necessary to achieve the identified goals. At times, the logic and evidence of scientific reasoning may suffice in directing clinical decision making, although more often than not occupational therapists take additional steps to understand more holistically how client factors define an occupational diagnosis.[10] The research findings of the Clinical Reasoning Study highlighted that clinical reasoning processes of occupational therapy do indeed extend beyond the hypothetical-deductive lines of logic described in the scientific reasoning literature from other medical professions to incorporate a shift that attends to occupational engagement.[16]

Procedural Reasoning

Procedural reasoning stems from the scientific knowledge and evidence-based practice patterns that provide generalizable approach strategies in intervention design on what to do and when to do it with a client with a specific diagnostic presentation. This vein of reasoning is in fact closely linked to scientific reasoning processes.[19] A therapist identifies a problem and considers what to do and how to design or approach the intervention. It is often considered to be the reasoning approach novice therapists gravitate toward as procedural reasoning provides a more concrete strategy for analysis, synthesis, and decision making based on the disease or disability of the individual client.[24] However, in the early findings from the Clinical Reasoning Study, Fleming[2] describes how procedural reasoning is used as well by experienced therapists. This form of thinking is based on an "if this is the case, then this is what I need to do" scenario. As a result, the more experiences from which a therapist has to draw, the possibility of procedural reasoning may occur more frequently as well as automatically. Procedural reasoning was linked by Fleming[2] to be associated less with experience and more by concrete, tangible, or biomedical aspects of working with clients with similar diagnoses that can be woven into processes that also integrate more abstract, psychosocioemotional aspects that may require attention. Factors such as client habits, culture, and support systems as well as therapists' experiences with the given context move the therapist from strict scientific processes that guide decisions in intervention to incorporate the intersections of scientific and experiential knowledge. For example, procedural reasoning can be more rote decision making of a therapist based on experience such as the decision of whether to use a gait belt during a client transfer. A novice therapist's procedural reasoning for gait belt use may be to incorporate it with each client in every session. This procedural strategy for making this choice is grounded in the lack of experiential knowledge as well as documented procedural strategies for safety in client handling and mobility. The more experienced therapist may recognize client factors that inform a clinical decision that a gait belt may not be necessary (e.g., the client who is fully independent in all areas of functional mobility).

Interactive Reasoning

Prior to the Clinical Reasoning Study,[5] the primary clinical reasoning discourse in occupational therapy aligned predominantly with the scientific, hypothetical-deductive model used by the medical professions. The rise and increased commitment to client-centered practice in occupational therapy that demands consideration of the psychosocioeconomic factors of a client led to an appreciation for those strategies in problem identification and resolution that were different. Interactive reasoning is a process the therapist uses to understand the dynamics of the context, the client, and the diagnosis in order to develop a therapeutic relationship unique to each client. This form of thinking occurs during face-to-face encounters and is bolstered when the therapist works to create a collaborative and empathetic understanding of the client's experience. The strategies experienced therapists use in interactive reasoning processes include: (1) providing clients with choices; (2) individualizing treatment; (3) structuring the context to maximize success; (4) extending the therapeutic role to include "doing extra" for the client; (5) sharing personal experience with a client; and (6) collaborating on problem solving.[25] However, other researchers suggest that a highly complex process of varying strategies of interaction exists for successful interactive reasoning, potentially highly influenced by values and belief systems that might inform the process of thinking itself.[2] Reflective appreciation by therapists to understand how their own thinking informs their **judgments** and interactions in a therapeutic relationship has been suggested as a fundamental method for developing a refined interactive reasoning process.[19]

Developing efficacy for these strategies of interactive reasoning requires that occupational therapy students and novice therapists have the opportunity to practice engaging in collaborative and meaningful ways with clients to attend to the professional commitment to client-centered care. Skills of interactive reasoning depend on a therapist's basic skills of communication such as active listening and interpreting the body language of the client.[15] Curricula that rely heavily on scientific and procedural reasoning, promoting a more reductionist approach to interactions with clients, may overlook clients' contexts and understanding the meaningfulness of their occupations.[26] Often, interactive reasoning opportunities present themselves for the first time to a student during fieldwork experiences, later in the second year of occupational therapy education,[24] and this is one potential explanation for why interactive reasoning is observed more often in therapists with increased experience.[19]

Narrative Reasoning

Interactive reasoning, while valuable and critical to establishing rapport with a client, still only considers the client's impairment in the here and now. When a therapist considers the clients' perspectives, including their culture, motives, beliefs, and values, of the meaning of the illness or disability experience, a narrative approach to understanding occurs. Narrative reasoning is described by Mattingly and Fleming as "fundamental to the thinking of occupational therapists."[5] This narrative process is one of story-making that contextualizes the client's lived experience and offers the therapist an avenue to develop a phenomenological appreciation of the impact of the impairment or illness. Phenomenology explores the meaning of an experience, informed by the manner a person interprets a given event, at a given time.[27] Narrative reasoning also involves a reciprocal process of the therapist making sense through narrative exploration of a client's scenario with other therapists. Finally, this process can include narrative meaning making of therapeutic stories cocreated with the client to evoke motivation and investment of the client in the therapeutic process. Digging deeper through narrative reasoning provides a tool for therapists to link the client diagnosis and clinical observation to the heart of what's most meaningful and motivating to a client.

Narrative reasoning is critical to understanding in two ways: (1) it helps the therapist explore the possible ways a client is making sense of the experiences of disability and of the therapy experience, foreign to the client but familiar to the therapist; and (2) it helps the therapist examine the contextual and personal factors of the client as they might relate to their past client experiences as well as from experiences of the team of therapists around them.[5] Therapists using narrative reasoning take what they know of the general conditions of an illness or diagnosis but work to understand how this version of the experience translates to impact the people who are their clients. There is an essential synthesis of the scientific (e.g., diagnostic, prognostic) and procedural knowledge of a therapist from professional training and clinical experiences (including exposure to practice models or frames of references) with knowledge gathered by listening to, reflecting on, and empathizing with the client to paint the picture for developing a client-centered intervention plan. This, in essence, is the foundation for developing an art of practice as it blends with science to shape a clinical reasoning that is distinct to the profession of occupational therapy.

Conditional Reasoning

Conditional reasoning extends from narrative as the therapist moves beyond the person to explore the social, temporal, and material contexts of everyday life.[28] This is a higher level of expert reasoning identified as being employed by the therapists from the Clinical Reasoning Study. It is a multifaceted and multiperspective reasoning process that is used to understand clients' needs to address potential shifts in identity, priorities, and approaches to occupation, because of changes in functional capacity.[2] This might translate to understanding how changes in occupational performance because of life transitions or environmental (including social, attitudinal, informational) alterations challenge the participation strategies and patterns to which a person is accustomed. This type of reasoning involves logical and nonlogical schemes of thinking[19] by the therapist to conceive of the impact of the experience of disability and therapy on the client and how different treatment choices might shape outcomes of participation and function. Conditional reasoning in combination with narrative reasoning may push the assumptions and presumptions of the therapist if they attend to understanding the meaning and implications of impairment based on their "social context, personal priorities and resources."[29] By upholding the professional commitment to client-centered care, this may dictate that the therapist redirects intervention to attend solely on assisting the person in achieving full participation versus on reducing impairment.[30]

Fleming discussed how the term *conditional* is linked to three different meanings: the entirety of the client's condition, the changeability of the person's condition (physical, social, financial, etc.), and the conditional agreement that must be made for "by-in" and participation by the client of the chosen therapeutic approach.[2] The therapist is challenged to creatively or artfully imagine the outcome for the client when deliberating on an approach to care, bringing into the process everything the therapist can gather about the client's physical and social world blended with the therapist's "clinical experience and expertise."[31] Conditional reasoning occurs because with each iteration of therapy, the client's worlds may have changed.

Pragmatic Reasoning

The therapist's focus and efforts are directed at optimizing a clinical experience to achieve the greatest gains for a client in prioritized and meaningful occupations. However, the contextual factors of the clinical environment, as well as the personal factors of the therapist, to a lesser or greater degree play a role in the possible decisions that are made and therefore must factor into clinical reasoning. These influences were recognized and described by Schell and Cervero[19] as the pragmatic considerations therapists attend to while processing clinical decisions. In later research, Unsworth[20] describes pragmatic reasoning such as reimbursement or the availability of community resources in a client's discharge environment as being distinct from other reasoning processes therapists take into consideration. The demands of the administrative realities of therapy produce constraints and barriers that at times conflict with the tenets of client-centeredness and present conundrums that the therapists must include in their decision-making strategies. The organizational and structural components of providing care are recognized as having a significant influence that challenge therapists' choices.[32,33]

Pragmatic reasoning approaches consider how therapists think given their personal factors such as their values, beliefs, spirituality, and personality. These are understood to tint the worldview of a therapist by informing assumptions about clients and influencing the decisions a therapist makes regarding therapy. This worldview offers a foundation for the styles or modes a therapist may also prefer in developing a therapeutic relationship.[25] In fact, it has been suggested that clinical practice is largely informed by the individual preferences for approaches to care influenced by sociocultural factors.[32] Unsworth[20] suggests that these preferences may be too implicit to understand how they shape a therapist's decisions, but critical to acknowledge in understanding professional reasoning processes. A therapist's worldview is overarching and sets the stage for how thinking, even thinking about thinking, occurs and shapes the content that is valid and reasonable for consideration in clinical decision making and how the processes of reasoning emerge, are validated, used, and reused in daily practice. Research by Unsworth[20] describes a subcategory of reasoning labeled "generalized reasoning" that is based on a therapist's experience and knowledge and informs or influences each of the other modes of reasoning. The knowledge and general experiences of a therapist create a reciprocal relationship between their worldview and how thinking occurs. See Figure 5-1 for a visual image of how the worldview of a therapist encompasses, influences, and is influenced by the various forms of clinical reasoning.

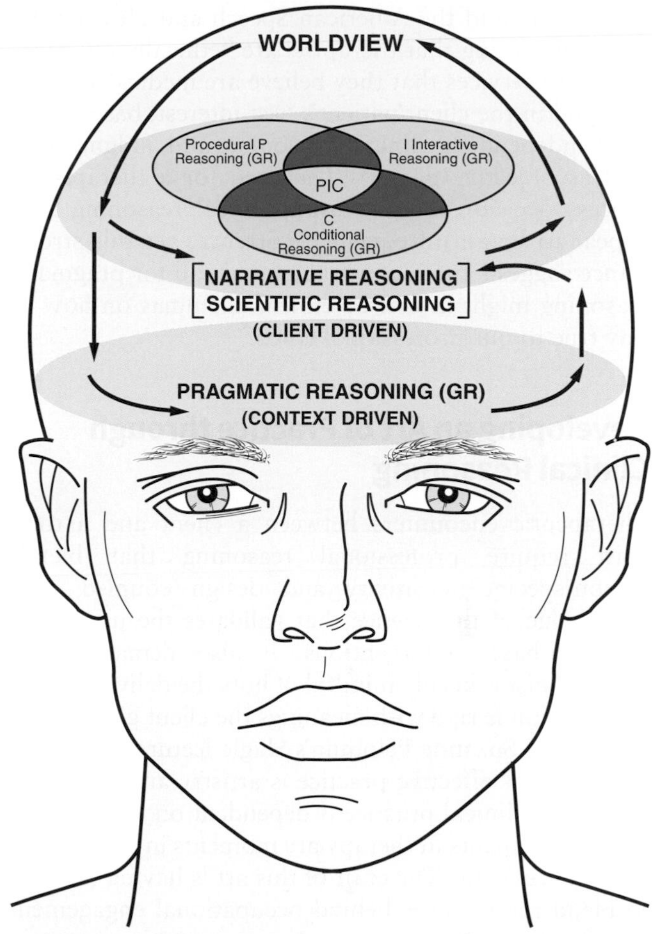

Figure 5-1. Clinical reasoning in client-centered occupational therapy by Unsworth. Note: Generalization reasoning (GR) is a subcategory of each type of reasoning in the model. (Reprinted with permission from Unsworth CA. Clinical reasoning: how do pragmatic reasoning, worldview and client-centeredness fit? *Br J Occup Ther*. 2004;67:17.)

Ethical Reasoning

Ethical reasoning is defined as "the frequently made decisions regarding moral, political and economic dilemmas that therapists regularly confront."[34] Ethical reasoning may occur in the moment for a therapist or emerge following a clinical experience when a therapist ponders the client's narrative story and potential futures. Ethical **decision making** in occupational therapy is grounded in professional commitments to client-centeredness, autonomy, beneficence and nonmaleficence,[35] and social justice.[36] Ethical reasoning can stem from knowledge that emerges through the narrative, interactive, and conditional processes as they intersect with scientific, procedural, and pragmatic reasoning to inform collaborative decision making. The professional commitment to client-centered care challenges therapists to attend to the broader contextual factors of clients' everyday environments and how they enable or disable participation, and as such stimulates ethical considerations of equity and justice.[37]

Critiques such as those that occupational therapists are confined to make clinical decisions based on the client's insurance plan[38] expose an ethical dilemma that can present itself in climates in which productivity and quotas supplant clinical judgment of what's best for a client. AOTA recognized this and put forth a Consensus Statement on Clinical Judgment in Health Care Setting (retrieved at: https://www.aota.org/Practice/Ethics/Consensus-Statement-AOTA-APTA-ASHA.aspx) in conjunction with the American Physical Therapy

Association and the American Speech and Hearing Association stating that therapists are "ethically obligated to deliver services that they believe are medically necessary and in the client/patient's best interest, based upon their independent clinical reasoning and judgment as well as objective data."[11] The need for a therapist to process decision making using ethical reasoning may appear to be an infrequent occurrence, yet this strong stance suggests those constraints that call for pragmatic reasoning might in fact be ethical dilemmas on how to stay true to our professional ethos.[6]

Developing an Art of Practice through Clinical Reasoning

Therapeutic encounters between a client and a therapist require professional reasoning that blends person-specific sensitivity and design coupled with knowledge of the science that validates the use of occupation-based interventions. It also demands that the therapist is keenly mindful of how the delivery of the intervention is ripe with meanings the client gives to the context. In Suzanne Peloquin's Slagle lecture she definitively states "effective practice is artistry and science."[6] The art of clinical practice is dependent on understanding that moments in therapy are moments in the journey of the client's life. The craft of this art is having the skill to blend the sciences behind occupational engagement that facilitate, educate, coach, empathize, encourage, and promote to empower and enable versus disable the client's self-determined desire to achieve identified goals. In defining an art of practice, Rogers claims "artistry involves the orchestration of broad strategies for grappling effectively with the uncertainties inherent in clinical practice."[1] This requires that the therapist not only be informed by but also look beyond the science of occupation-based interventions to embrace and embolden the spirit and the knowledge of the client. It also requires a therapist to move beyond scientific/diagnostic and procedural reasoning and incorporate narrative, conditional, pragmatic as well as ethical reasoning in their professional reasoning repertoire of practice.

Gary Kielhofner highlighted the challenges occupational therapists have as therapists in the scientific medicalized world of allied health professions by our commitment to combining scientific knowledge and judgment with artful approaches to intervention design.[39] He emphasized in his own model of practice, The Model of Human Occupation,[40] the inadequacies of a typical approach in medical models for supporting the foundation of what occupational therapy professes as its unique contribution to client care. In fact, this unique contribution has recently been identified as having a statistically significant association on maintaining health and wellness compared to other services provided in acute hospitalizations.[41]

How does this skillful blend of knowledge and creativity develop in a therapist? Understanding the art of practice provides a foundation for exploring the means of nurturing its development in oneself as well as in others. One of the founding theorists for clinical reasoning, Donald Schön, describes that the art of practice might be taught to all therapists if it were tangible and constant, but it is neither.[4] Fleming[31] describes expert therapists as they readily shift among procedural, interactive, and conditional thinking styles without losing site of the bigger perspective of the client scenario in a manner that invokes images of an artist mixing colors to achieve the image they and their client have conceived of in their minds. Unsworth and Baker's description is analogous to a dance as "professional reasoning involves all the thinking processes of the clinician as s/he moves into, through and out of the therapeutic relationship and therapy process with a client."[3] This blending especially calls for the reasoning processes that allow therapists to artistically and creatively work with clients to cultivate an image and then outcomes of participation in meaningful occupations. Intentional decisions that therapists make based on their understanding of the impact of their own verbal and nonverbal communication on achieving optimal client outcomes are skills necessary for this level of professional reasoning.

Therapeutic Use of Self in Clinical Reasoning Approaches

Deliberately responding to a client in a manner that will facilitate occupational participation and performance requires reflection by the therapist on how his or her own behaviors can be used to promote this change.[26] Deliberate or intentional selection of behaviors demands a thorough assessment of how the client may react in the therapeutic encounter and to the therapeutic relationship, as well as a grounded knowledge of therapists' characteristics and communication styles used during therapeutic exchanges. The Intentional Relationship Model (IRM)[25] is a conceptual practice model of strategies a therapist can use to enhance the client–therapist therapeutic relationship in order to optimize a client's occupational engagement. This model encourages therapists to explore predispositions to communication styles with suggestions for nurturing strengths and the development of less utilized interpersonal skills that facilitate an understanding of the intentional use of self as part of clinical reasoning.[15] Developing this understanding hones and evolves a therapist toward mastering the artistry of the therapeutic relationship.

The IRM reinforces that therapists must purposely reason and make decisions on how they might respond appropriately to the client during interpersonal events in order to develop a positive relationship and foster a therapeutic experience with the client. This intentionality requires preparedness by the therapists to understand their clients' perspectives and select manners of relating to clients, or modes of interaction, informed by the contexts of the experiences. The IRM identifies six interpersonal modes therapists might consider when preparing to address the needs of a client: advocating, collaborating, empathizing, encouraging, instructing, and problem solving.[25] Part of the preparedness of the therapist draws upon merging clinical reasoning, based on factors from the client and context, with the knowledge on how different modes of interacting may result in different responses of the client while engaged in therapy. Therefore, therapeutic use of self crisscrosses with clinical reasoning while in preparation for therapeutic experiences but also is used flexibly in response to a client's reaction to the context of a therapeutic event. This skillful, thoughtful, and flexible use of self is a method for weaving interpersonal **reasoning strategies** into the clinical decision making of an intervention to facilitate a client's occupational engagement.

Influence of Theories and Frames of Reference

The evidence-based approach to occupational therapy is grounded in the theories that support our profession,[16] but artful clinical reasoning requires that therapists have the ability for reflection, imagination, and creativity as well as beliefs that value and respect client choice. The type of clinical reasoning that a therapist uses can be influenced by exposure in professional training to theoretical frameworks and models of practice.[24] Many theories that provide an organizing foundation to the professional framework of practice have common features that represent the profession's commitment to the need for an artful element in our interventions.[42] The biomedical, restorative, or rehabilitative frames of reference may be necessary to understand the person–environment fit[43] and provide support to interventions to enhance functional performance, but often only require a therapist to use scientific or procedural reasoning.

Frameworks or models of practice emerging from dynamic systems theories, such as the Person-Environment-Occupation model,[44] Model of Human Occupation,[41] and Person-Environment-Occupation-Performance[45] align with a more comprehensive biopsychosocial model approach to analysis and support reasoning strategies with more phenomenological modes of thinking and reflection on the client–therapist relationship. These models share in common the resolute need to look at the person, the environment, and the occupation during problem identification and decision making in interventions and because of this may stimulate the development of more advanced clinical reasoning. However, the leaders in exploring clinical reasoning recognize that having a theory, model, or frame of reference itself is insufficient to help a student learn how to judge the context and make decisions.[46]

Developing and Advancing Professional Reasoning

Unsworth and Baker in a systematic review of occupational therapy literature on clinical reasoning describe that "it is only through examining the often tacit knowledge of specialists in the field that the skill and artistry of these experts can be identified, elucidated and, potentially learned and assimilated by others."[3] The challenge for students and novice therapists is identifying methods for recognizing and translating a master clinician's knowledge in a manner that fosters existing reasoning skills and strategies and funnel these toward the more complex models of reasoning used by skillful occupational therapists.

Research supports that clinical reasoning in occupational therapy moves through five stages: novice, advanced beginner, competent, proficient, and expert.[47] In the past, it was expected that entry-level therapists would continue to develop competencies in the more advanced stages of reasoning and achieve expert reasoning with experience.[48] However, there is a professional commitment[11] as well as probable expectations that therapists with clinical doctorate degrees enter the workforce with more fully developed strategies in advanced clinical reasoning skills and therefore a necessary focus for professional curricula.

Occupational therapy curricula are mandated by the Accreditation Council for Occupational Therapy Education (ACOTE) (available at: https://acote.aota.org) to focus on the development of students' clinical reasoning as part of the critical skill set necessary for good client-centered intervention design. Students learn to attend to the three levels as defined by Fleming[31] by developing skills in: assessing impairment, understanding and empathizing with the client, and examining the client's environmental world.[20] Becoming a well-rounded therapist that can deftly move between and within different problem-solving and reasoning strategies requires exposure to the basic concepts of clinical reasoning as well as to the process components[10] of professional reasoning. Much of the content knowledge will promote the development of scientific and procedural reasoning while process components demand that therapists use reflection, intuition, and awareness of self and others to develop the capacity for therapeutic use of self[25] in order to become experts in the art of professional reasoning.

One well-recognized approach that can be used to facilitating clinical reasoning is using a case-based method of real-life client scenarios with guided intervention assistance from an instructor.[49] Different formats for delivering these cases include written, videotape, simulated or standardized patients, and clients who identify as having lived experiences of different disabilities.[50] Traditionally, students work to identify impairment or problems within the case and apply knowledge from the curriculum to develop strategies for intervention design. This mode of reasoning is grounded in biomedical, impairment concerns and initiates scientific and procedural reasoning strategies. Using case-based scenarios that include more than a medical model perspective of a client, such as incorporating contexts from the client's social environment, client stories have been used to promote more client-centered and advanced clinical reasoning strategy development.[49] Researchers suggest that case scenarios with a more comprehensive format, including triggers that produce narrative or conditional thinking strategies, can be used successfully in the context of a traditional classroom setting.[49]

Advancing Professional Reasoning

It is clear that a therapist's advanced repertoire for reasoning supports a mastery of the art of clinical practice. Case scenarios focusing on problem-based learning (PBL) strategies through experiential learning appear to be growing as a popular approach for advancing clinical reasoning in occupational therapy curricula.[51] PBL is an adult learning approach that uses active participation and places learning responsibility on the student as a means for acquisition of new knowledge.[52] Advanced clinical and professional reasoning strategy development has been shown to occur with the dedicated inclusion of PBL that focuses on synthesizing knowledge for practice and increasing exposure to direct client contact.[24]

Hands-on experiential learning has long been embraced and identified as advancing clinical reasoning and critical thinking skills in students and novice therapists.[53] Professional training in occupational therapy has always incorporated a philosophical commitment to the necessity and importance of fieldwork education as a critical piece to developing advanced clinical reasoning skills in students.[46] This affords students an opportunity to learn from modeling master therapists with more advanced reasoning styles as they observe critical thinking in the moment and synthesize observations with guided reflection.

Schell has developed a model[17] of contextual teaching for professional reasoning, describing the interaction between student and teacher or master therapist as they interact to co-construct knowledge and engage in critical reflection to understand the meaning and significance of new knowledge (see Fig. 5-2). This process can occur in a preclinical narrative or written assessment or within an authentic context of learning that may require in the moment reflection superimposed during a guided and supervised clinical encounter.

In order to consider the best practice options that may be used, the "reflective therapist"4 uses both in the moment contemplation to direct clinical decisions and critical thinking to examine assumptions leading to clinical decisions. Schön[4] describes this process as reflection-in-action where the therapist "allows himself to experience surprise, puzzlement or confusion in a situation… and become a researcher in the practice context." Reflection is another valuable tool recognized for advancing clinical reasoning in the student, working therapist, as well as professional education experiences.[54] Using reflection[55] and models such as the IRM[25] has been suggested by researchers as an area in need of further study in understanding advancing skills in clinical reasoning.[3] These suggestions position the therapist to challenge themselves to explore why they know what they know, why they think what they think, as well as why they act the way they do in interactions with clients, assessing their own assumptions and clinical reasoning modes of thinking.

Recognizing Clinical Reasoning Strengths and Areas in Need of Development

There are measures and tools for students to use in recognizing their own skill sets and development in clinical reasoning. Although not a measure per se of clinical reasoning skills, the Dreyfus and Dreyfus Model of Skill Acquisition[56] provides a framework for the development of student and staff clinical reasoning that include stages of: novice, advanced beginner, competent, proficient, and expert. Research shows the model to be predictive and descriptive of skills development from one stage to the next.[57] Developers of this model recommend that to transition from a more novice entry-level therapist to a more advanced one demands that therapists remain open to experiential learning opportunities as they occur in the clinical world. For example, exposure to real-world problems with real-world solutions provides a basis for therapists to extend their hypotheses for conditional reasoning as well as offer alternatives in pragmatic reasoning. This suggestion encourages and supports pathways for students and novice therapists to seek out mentors in order to learn those tacit skills and multiple layers of professional reasoning through observing and modeling behaviors.

The Self-Assessment of Clinical Reflection and Reasoning (SACRR) by Royeen et al.[58] is a tool developed to assess students' perceptions of their clinical reflection and reasoning[52] as impacted by different methods of instruction. It consists of 26 self-report items related to student reflection and reasoning as measured by a 5-point Likert-type scale.[59] Although it was developed to assess students from all allied health professions,

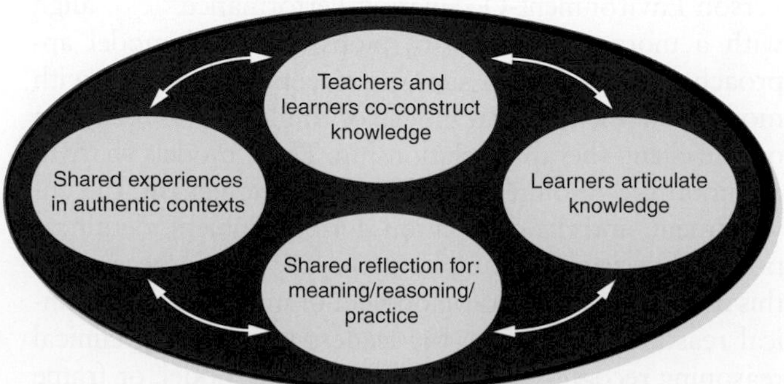

Figure 5-2. John Schell's model of contextual teaching for professional reasoning.

it has primarily been used in occupational therapy.[52,58,60] According to Royeen et al.,[58] a limitation of this instrument is that it relies on the subject's self-perception of clinical reasoning skills and behaviors rather than an objective measure of clinical reasoning performance. However, this may have value if used by a student or therapist as a tool for self-reflection and personal development. It was recently used as one measure in a study exploring the effect of using a student-run free clinic on interprofessional attitudes and clinical reasoning skills.[59] In this study, the SACRR showed a statistically significant change in occupational therapy, physical therapy, physician's assistant, medical, and pharmacy student perceptions of clinical reasoning skills when exposed to an interprofessional service learning course and student-run free clinic.[60] The Watson-Glaser Critical Thinking Appraisal (WGCTA)[61] was also used in this study. It is an objective tool that measures the critical thinking skills of attitudes of inquiry; inferences, abstractions, and generalizations; and skills in employing/applying these attitudes and knowledge.[61] In this study the WGCTA found that OT students compared to PT students had statistically greater increases in critical reasoning, causing the researchers to conclude that this might be due to OT curricula incorporating more activities where critical thinking processes were identified.[61]

These measurement tools and reported studies have explored how clinical reasoning is impacted by problem-based or experiential learning or specific points within the student learning process. Unsworth describes that, "Although many studies on clinical reasoning have been undertaken, most explore discrete areas of practice or types of reasoning."[20] What we know is that more holistic reasoning styles such as conditional reasoning are used more often by experienced therapists and procedural modes by novice therapists.[24] Research also points to how vital fieldwork practicums are, as they are the major channel through which occupational therapy students integrate knowledge into practice and advance their clinical reasoning styles.[24]

Areas for Future Study

Research from over a decade ago suggests that the profession consider alternatives for understanding the master therapist's intuitive reasoning using methods informed by judgment analysis.[62] This research recognized that clinical reasoning is influenced by what a therapist recognizes and prioritizes as the key factors that lead to occupational dysfunction. The prioritized factors become the lens that the therapist uses to design intervention. If the factors that lead to occupational dysfunction are physical impairment, the therapist's clinical reasoning dictates remediation of impairment through various biomechanical frames of reference.

In the recently published systematic review of the occupational therapy literature, Unsworth and Baker's findings show a dense amount of literature on understanding what "professional reasoning is" but a dearth on examining the differences between novice and expert therapist reasoning pathways, including a need for assessment tools.[3] To develop therapists that can master the art of practice, occupational therapy research recommendations point to extending problem-based and experiential learning to include and at times prioritize the contextual environments that influence occupational engagement beyond the clinical contexts.

Conclusion

Understanding how a therapist becomes an expert in clinical reasoning and artful practice that result in high levels of satisfaction from the clients served is useful for informing professional education, mentoring novice therapists, and advancing mastery with experience. Understanding relevance to the client demands dialogue and engagement with the client in the therapy process. It also demands reflective assessment from the therapist on their inner beliefs and assumptions.[7] A therapist must use science, ethics, and artistry to guide their clinical reasoning and ultimately the clinical decisions they make.[1] Artistry is a process that results in a unique outcome because of the uniquely individual attributes that the artist contributes. The art of practicing occupational therapy lies in blending experience and knowledge and including therapeutic use of self[25] to optimize opportunities for clients to engage in the occupations that they identify as being at the core of expressing who they are through engaging and participating in them. Considering the client and engaging the client dialectically in assessing their performance, the effectiveness of the intervention, and including subjective feedback on how the clinical process is impacting satisfaction with occupational performance are vital to the reasoning process. Client engagement in the exchange of reasoning processes offers optimal client-centered care as well as client ownership of the therapy journey. This process targets outcomes that address priorities for participation in a manner and style crafted to the client's needs together in partnership. This partnership is a therapist–client team that works collaboratively, inductively, and recursively to establish and achieve the therapy goals.

Occupational therapy straddles the worlds of a client's biomedical and psychosocial environmental concerns. The intersections between these two worlds requires professional reasoning simultaneously grounded in scientific and procedural theory and evidence, as well as is phenomenologically reflective and imaginative.[10] The heart of the art of practice is grounded in collaborative reflection to identify what is meaningful to a client and how occupation can be used as a means to evaluate and intervene in a way that addresses prioritized needs and promotes full participation and enablement in all of a society's culturally relevant occupations.

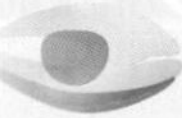

CASE STUDY

Scientific Reasoning

Adam works in an acute care hospital and has just received an order for an occupational therapy evaluation and treatment of Eve, a 49-year-old woman with a diagnosis of C7 spinal cord injury (SCI). Upon review of the medical records, he identifies that she acquired the SCI years ago when she was 23 and is currently in the acute hospital for bacterial pneumonia and general deconditioning. He immediately understands from scientific and diagnostic processes of reasoning what musculature would likely have been impacted as a result of central nervous system damage and how this might translate into functional performance. He also considers how her new illness might influence her overall functioning and uses this reasoning as a baseline prior to beginning his occupational therapy evaluation.

Procedural Reasoning

Adam begins his evaluation of Eve using his knowledge on what musculature he would expect her to have functional use of because of her level of SCI. His approach strategy is also influenced by his overarching knowledge of adaptive strategies and equipment she is likely to incorporate into her activities of daily living (ADLs). During the evaluation, Adam notes that Eve does present with the motor and sensory functional impairments that align with a diagnosis of a complete C7 SCI, although all of her innervated upper extremity (UE) musculature is weaker than anticipated. She also reports that she is having more difficulty in performing the UE dressing and grooming tasks than she was prior to the acute hospitalization.

Interactive Reasoning

During the initial evaluation, Eve confirms that she has lost "tons of strength" in both her arms and hand function. During the occupational profile, Adam identifies that Eve lives in her own apartment with a personal assistant who works for Eve daily to provide assistance with ADLs and instrumental activities of daily living (IADLs). During the evaluation, Adam uses processes of interactive reasoning to explore with Eve what she prioritizes for her occupational therapy sessions. Adam understands that Eve is an expert in living and managing her SCI as she has managed and lived with the disability for almost 26 years. Adam identifies that a strength and conditioning approach is necessary to increase ADL and IADL concerns but instead of immediately establishing an intervention course focusing on Eve's diagnosis targeting these client factors, he collaborates with Eve using interactive reasoning to identify her priorities for the sessions she will receive while in the acute hospital. Including Eve as an active partner to collaboratively identify her areas of concern is at the core of an occupational therapy client-centered approach to clinical reasoning in intervention design.

Narrative Reasoning

Adam is intrigued by the knowledge Eve has of how to manage her health and wellness, her organized manner of supervising and managing her personal assistant hours, and her adaptive approaches to performing ADLs and IADLs. He discusses some of her strategies for managing her ADLs with collogues and the conversation shifts to how well she has managed her health living with SCI for 26 years. He begins to question what factors led her to acquire the pneumonia and his expert judgment compels him to pose this question to her during a morning therapy session. Adam's narrative reasoning that emerged through conversations with his peers informed him that this question may be an important one from an occupational perspective for working with her to manage her health and wellness.

Conditional Reasoning

In narrative exploration, Eve explains her perspective of her recent health crisis. She explained to Adam that for years she has been fortunate to have physicians, dentists, pharmacists, and other wellness providers that had an understanding of the accommodation needs of people with disabilities. However, when her dentist retired she was at a loss of how to locate an accessible dental clinic. She had been referred to a dentist by a friend but the visit was a negative experience for her as she had her teeth cleaned while seated in her straight back wheelchair because of the inability for the clinic to offer her a transfer into an accessible dental examination chair. Eve illustrated what a painful experience this was both psychologically and physically, describing she "felt like a burden" to the staff at the clinic. She described how this experience influenced her decision not to get the routine dental care she had been so diligent about in the past. She developed tender gums and periodontal disease which she later learned increased her risk for lung infections, and she believes resulted in her recent health crisis. Adam began to understand how the environment and context of a provider office might negatively impact Eve's participation in her occupation of health management, one of her most vital ADLs. Despite knowledge and insights of strategies and approaches for managing her health and wellness, Eve's knowledge and strategies for how to self-advocate in primary care for accommodations were underdeveloped. He envisioned how this type of barrier would continue to supersede her self-management strategies and impact her health negatively. He made a clinical decision to discuss with Eve learning strategies and approaches for accessing community resources and services.

Pragmatic Reasoning

Adam and Eve are both invested in working to develop a "toolkit" for strategies in community resource seeking and utilization for her remaining occupational therapy sessions, as well as basic knowledge on her specific accommodation needs.

CASE STUDY *(continued)*

Adam had earlier anticipated 5 more days of work with Eve; however, a change in her medical plan occurred and now she had only 2 days left in the acute hospital before a transfer to a subacute rehabilitation facility. Adam's pragmatic reasoning allowed him to realize that the limited time with Eve constrained the ability to directly work on skill acquisition on resource seeking and utilization and demanded he provide resources for Eve directly. He reviewed with her the names and numbers of her local Center for Independent Living as well as a basic introduction to the Americans with Disabilities Act, reviewing her right to equitable health care services. Their discussion included basic methods for effectively communicating her needs when making a provider appointment. Adam understood that this approach failed to address Eve's larger issue of developing skills for community resource seeking and placed this recommendation in her discharge evaluation, hopeful the next occupational therapist might address this need. With this clinical experience, Adam had developed a new worldview on how access barriers can directly impact meaningful and vital occupational participation.

Ethical Reasoning

Adam's ethical reasoning that informed his clinical decision to work with Eve on strategies for accessing resources was grounded in his knowledge of occupational therapy's scope of practice. He understood that at times therapists are in positions to work on self-advocacy strategies with clients as described in the OTPF: "By understanding and addressing the specific justice issues within a client's discharge environment, occupational therapists promote therapy outcomes that address empowerment and self-advocacy."[11] His dilemma spurred his ethical reasoning on steps he might take to advocate for clients, also a scope of practice outlined in the OTPF: "Occupational therapists can indirectly affect the lives of clients through advocacy. Common examples of advocacy include talking to legislators about improving transportation for older adults or improving services for people with mental or physical disabilities to support their living and working in the community of their choice."[11] As a result, Adam joined a local disability advocacy group working on state health care policies impacting people with disabilities.

References

1. Rogers J. Eleanor Clarke Slagle Lectureship: clinical reasoning: the ethics, science and art. *Am J Occup Ther.* 1983;37:601–616.
2. Fleming MH. Clinical reasoning in medicine compared with clinical reasoning in occupational therapy. *Am J Occup Ther*. 1991;45(11):988–996.
3. Unsworth CA, Baker A. A systematic review of professional reasoning literature in occupational therapy. *Br J Occup Ther.* 2016;79(1):5–16. doi:10.1177/0308022615599994.
4. Schön D. *The Reflective Practitioner: How Professionals Think in Action*. New York, NY: Basic Books; 1983.
5. Mattingly C, Fleming M. *Clinical Reasoning: Forms of Inquiry in a Therapeutic Practice*. Philadelphia, PA: FA Davis Company; 1994.
6. Peloquin SM. The 2005 Eleanor Clarke Slagle Lecture—Embracing our ethos, reclaiming our heart. *Am J Occup Ther*. 2005;59:611–625.
7. Henderson W, Coppard B, Qi Y. Identifying instructional methods for development of clinical reasoning in entry-level occupational therapy education: a mixed methods design. *J Occup Ther Educ.* 2017;1(2):1–20. doi:10.26681/jote.2017.010201.
8. Knecht-Sabres L. Experiential learning in occupational therapy: can it enhance readiness for clinical practice? *J Exp Educ.* 2013;36(1):22–36. doi:10.1177/1053825913481584.
9. Unsworth CA. Clinical reasoning: how do pragmatic reasoning, worldview and client-centredness fit? *Br J Occup Ther.* 2004;67(1):10–19. doi:10.1177/030802260406700103.
10. Leicht S, Dickerson A. Clinical reasoning, looking back. *Occup Ther Health Care.* 2002;14(3–4):105–130. doi:10.1080/J003v14n03_07.
11. American Occupational Therapy Association. *Occupational Therapy Practice Framework: Domain and Process.* 3rd ed. Bethesda, MD: AOTA Press/American Occupational Therapy Association; 2014.
12. Schell B. Professional reasoning in practice. In: Schell P, Gillen G, Scaffa M, Cohn E, eds. *Willard & Spackman's Occupational Therapy.* Baltimore, MD: Lippincott Williams & Wilkins; 2014:384–397.
13. Taylor R, VanPuymbrouck L. Therapeutic use of self: applying the intentional relationship model in group therapy. In: O'Brien JC, Solomon JW, eds. *Occupational Analysis and Group Process.* St. Louis, MO: Elsevier; 2013:36–52.
14. Kristensen HK, Petersen KS. Occupational science: an important contributor to occupational therapists' clinical reasoning. *Scand J Occup Ther*. 2016;23(3):240–243.
15. Chapparo C, Ranka J. Clinical reasoning in occupational therapy. In: Higgs J, Jones M, Loftus S, Christensen N, eds. *Clinical Reasoning in Health Professions*. Philadelphia, PA: Elsevier; 2008:265–278.
16. Turpin M, Iwama MK. *Using Occupational Therapy Models in Practice: A Fieldguide*. London, England: Elsevier Health Sciences; 2013.
17. Schell B, Schell J. *Clinical and Professional Reasoning in Occupational Therapy.* Baltimore, MD: Lippincott Williams & Wilkins; 2008.
18. Kielhofner G, Barrett L. Meaning and misunderstanding in occupational forms: a study of therapeutic goal setting. *Am J Occup Ther.* 1998;52(5):345–353.

19. Schell BA, Cervero RM. Clinical reasoning in occupational therapy: an integrative review. *Am J Occup Ther.* 1993;47:605–610.
20. Unsworth CA. Using a head-mounted video camera to explore current conceptualizations of clinical reasoning in occupational therapy. *Am J Occup Ther.* 2005;59:31–40. doi:10.5014/ajot.59.1.31.
21. Barz DL, Achimas-Cadariu A. The development of scientific reasoning in medical education: a psychological perspective. *Clujul Med.* 2016;89(1):32–37. doi:10.15386/cjmed-530.
22. Higgs J, Jones MA, Titchen A. Knowledge, reasoning and evidence for practice. In: Higgs J, Jones MA, Loftus S, Christensen N, eds. *Clinical Reasoning in the Health Professions.* 3rd ed. Amsterdam: Butterworth-Heinemann; 2000:151–162.
23. Simon HA, Newell A. Human problem solving: the state of the theory in 1970. *Am Psychol.* 1971;26(2):145–159.
24. Liu KP, Chan CC, Hui-Chan CW. Clinical reasoning and the occupational therapy curriculum. *Occup Ther Int.* 2000;7(3):173–183.
25. Taylor R. *The Intentional Relationship: Outpatient Therapy and Use of Self.* Philadelphia, PA: FA Davis Company; 2008.
26. VanPuymbrouck L, Heffron, JL, Sheth AJ, Lee D. Experiential learning: critical analysis of standardized patient and disability simulation. *J Occup Ther Educ.* 2017;1(3):1–13.
27. Van Manen M. *Researching Lived Experience.* New York, NY: New York State University; 1990.
28. Arntzen C. An embodied and intersubjective practice of occupational therapy. *OTJR.* 2017;38(3):173–180. doi:10.1177/1539449217727470.
29. Reynolds F. Two-way communication. In: Swain J, Clark J, Parry K, et al., eds. *Enabling Relationships in Health and Social Care.* Oxford, England: Butterworth-Heinemann; 2004:109–130.
30. Hammell K. *Perspectives on Disability and Rehabilitation: Contesting Assumptions; Challenging Practice.* Philadelphia, PA: Elsevier; 2006.
31. Fleming MH. The therapist with the three-track mind. *Am J Occup Ther.* 1991;45(11):1007–1014.
32. Hooper B. Between pretheoretical assumptions and clinical reasoning. *Am J Occup Ther.* 1997;51(5):328–338.
33. Peloquin S. The patient-therapist relationship: beliefs that shape care. *Am J Occup Ther.* 1993;47(10):935–942.
34. Higgs J, Jones M. Clinical decision making and multiple problem spaces. In: Higgs J, Jones M, Loftus S, Christensen N, eds. *Clinical Reasoning in Health Professions.* Philadelphia, PA: Elsevier; 2008:3–18.
35. Kanny E, Slater D. Ethical reasoning. In Schell B, Schell J, eds. *Clinical Reasoning in Occupational Therapy.* Baltimore, MD: Lippincott Williams & Wilkins; 2008:188–208.
36. Wilcock AA, Townsend E. Occupational terminology interactive dialogue: occupational justice. *J Occup Sci.* 2000;7:84–86.
37. Braveman B, Suarez-Balcazar Y. Social justice and resource utilization in a community-based organization: a case illustration of the role of the occupational therapist. *Am J Occup Ther.* 2009;63:13–23.
38. Gupta J, Taff S. The illusion of client-centred practice. *Scand J Occup Ther.* 2015;22:244–251. doi:10.3109/11038128.2015.1020866.
39. Kielhofner G. *Conceptual Foundations of Occupational Therapy.* Philadelphia, PA: F. A. Davis Company; 1997.
40. Kielhofner G. *A Model of Human Occupation: Theory and Application.* 3rd ed. Baltimore, MD: Lippincott Williams & Wilkins; 2002.
41. Rogers AT, Bai G, Lavin RA, Anderson GF. Higher hospital spending on occupational therapy is associated with lower readmission rates. *Med Care Res Rev.* 2016:1–19. doi:10.1177/1077558716666981.
42. Hinojosa J, Kramer P, Royeen C. *Perspectives on Human Occupation: Theories Underlying Practice.* 2nd ed. Philadelphia, PA: FA Davis Company; 2017.
43. Edwards JR, Cable DM, Williamson IO, Lambert LS, Shipp AJ. The phenomenology of fit: linking the person and environment to the subjective experience of person-environment fit. *J Appl Psychol.* 2006;91:802–827.
44. Law M, Cooper B, Strong S, Stewart D, Rigby P, Letts L. The person-environment-occupation model: a transactive approach to occupational performance. *Can J Occup Ther.* 1996;63(1):9–23.
45. Christiansen C, Baum CM, eds. *Occupational Therapy: Enabling Function and Well-Being.* Thorofare, NJ: Slack; 1997.
46. Cohn ES. Fieldwork education: shaping a foundation for clinical reasoning. *Am J Occup Ther.* 1989;43(4):240–244.
47. Unsworth CA. Clinical reasoning of novice and expert occupational therapists. *Am J Occup Ther.* 2001;55:582–588. doi:10.1080/110381201317166522.
48. Henderson W, Coppard B, Qi Y. Identifying instructional methods for development of clinical reasoning in entry-level occupational therapy education: a mixed methods design. *J Occup Ther Educ.* 2017;1(2):1–20.
49. Lysaght R, Bent M. A comparative analysis of case presentation modalities used in clinical reasoning coursework in occupational therapy. *Am J Occup Ther.* 2005;59:314–324. doi:10.5014/ajot.59.3.314.
50. Murphy LF, Stav WB. The impact of online video cases on clinical reasoning in occupational therapy education: a quantitative analysis. *Open J Occup Ther.* 2018;6(3):1–11. doi:10.15453/2168-6408.1494.
51. Hooper B, King R, Wood W, Bilics A, Gupta J. An international systematic mapping review of educational approaches and teaching methods in occupational therapy. *Br J Occup Ther.* 2013;76(1):9–22. doi:10.4276/030803313X13576469254612.
52. Scaffa M, Wooster D. Brief report—effects of problem-based learning on clinical reasoning in occupational therapy. *Am J Occup Ther.* 2004;58:333–336. doi:10.5014/ajot.58.3.333.
53. Coker P. Effects of an experiential learning program on the clinical reasoning and critical thinking skills of occupational therapy students. *J Allied Health.* 2010;39(4):280–286.
54. Gibson D, Velde B, Hoff T, Kvashay D, Manross PL, Moreau V. Clinical reasoning of a novice versus an experienced occupational therapist: a qualitative study. *Occup Ther Health Care.* 2000;12(4):15–31. doi:10.1080/J003v12n04_02.
55. Bazyk S, Glorioso M, Gordon R, Haines J, Percaciante M. Service learning: the process of doing and becoming an occupational therapist. *Occup Ther Health Care.* 2010;24(2):171–187.

56. Dreyfus H, Dreyfus S. *Mind over Machine: The Power of Human Intuition and Expertise in the Era of the Computer.* New York, NY: Simon and Schuster; 2000.
57. Benner P. Using the Dreyfus model of skill acquisition to describe and interpret skill acquisition and clinical judgment in nursing practice and education. *Bull Sci Technol Soc.* 2004;24(3):188–199. doi:10.1177/0270467604265061.
58. Royeen C, Mu K, Barrett L, Luebben A. Pilot investigation: evaluation of a clinical reflection and reasoning before and after workshop intervention. In Crist P, ed. *Innovations in Occupational Therapy Education.* Bethesda, MD: American Occupational Therapy Association; 2001:107–114.
59. Vogel KA, Geelhoed M, Grice KO, Murphy D. Do occupational therapy and physical therapy curricula teach critical thinking skills? *J Allied Health.* 2009;38(3):152–157.
60. Seif G, Coker-Bolt P, Kraft S, Gonsalves W, Simpson K, Johnson E. The development of clinical reasoning and interprofessional behaviors: service-learning at a student-run free clinic. *J Interprof Care.* 2014;28(6):559–564. doi:10.3109/13561820.2014.921899.
61. Bauwens EE, Gerhard GG. The use of the Watson-Glaser Critical Thinking Appraisal to predict success in a baccalaureate nursing program. *J Nurs Edu.* 1987;26(7):278–281.
62. Harries PA, Harries C. Studying clinical reasoning, part 2: applying social judgement theory. *Br J Occup Ther.* 2001;64(6):285–292.
63. Mattingly C. The narrative nature of clinical reasoning. *Am J Occup Ther.* 1994;45(11):998–1005.

Chapter 6

Documentation of Occupational Therapy Services

Patricia A. Gentile

LEARNING OBJECTIVES

This chapter will allow the reader to:

1. Understand the importance of clinical documentation from a professional and legal standpoint.
2. Describe types and formats of documentation used in clinical settings.
3. Utilize accepted principles of documentation throughout the service delivery process.
4. Recognize the importance of documenting medically necessary and skilled occupational therapy services.
5. Be familiar with legal and ethical issues associated with clinical documentation.

CHAPTER OUTLINE

TERMINOLOGY

Authentication: the process of showing authorship and responsibility for something documented in the medical record.

Documentation: the recording of patient observations and the health care services provided, which is used to track a patient's status and communicate the health care provider's actions and thoughts to other members of the care team.

Fraudulent billing: to purposely bill for services that were never given or to bill for a service that has a higher reimbursement than the service produced.

Health Insurance Portability and Accountability Act (HIPAA): a federal mandate for individual rights in health information that imposes restrictions on uses and disclosures of individually identifiable health information and provides for civil and criminal penalties for violations.

Medical record: the chronological written or electronic document that includes a written account of a patient's medical and health history and complaints, physical findings, tests, interventions, and treatment outcomes.

Medically necessary: services that are needed to treat an illness, injury, condition, disease, or its symptoms and that meet accepted standards of care.

Protected Patient Health Information: individually identifiable health data, including demographic information, that are created or received by a health care provider that relate to an the individual's past, present, or future physical or mental health or conditions; the provision of health care to the individual; or the past, present, or future payment for the provision of health care to the individual.

Skilled services: services that, because of the patient's condition, require the skills, expertise, clinical reasoning, and judgment of a qualified therapist to ensure the effectiveness of the treatment goals and ensure medical safety.

State Practice Act: a state law that governs a profession.

Third-party payer: an entity (other than the patient or the health care provider) that reimburses and manages health care expenses. Third-party payers include insurance companies, governmental agencies such as Medicare or Medicaid, and employers.

Introduction

Observe, record, tabulate, communicate[1]

Documentation is an essential tool used in the delivery of health care services. It is the recording of patient observations and the services provided; it is used to track a patient's status and communicate a provider's actions and thoughts to other members of the care team.[2] Documentation provides a means to plan, evaluate, and communicate a patient's treatment. In occupational therapy (OT), documentation is an important part of daily clinical practice. It provides a record of the reason for referral, offers a summary of the patient's occupational history and evaluation, outlines patient and therapist treatment goals and plans, and records interventions and the patient's responses to those interventions.[2,3] In addition, documentation serves to substantiate coding used for billing, demonstrate compliance with regulations, provide data for quality improvement activities and utilization review, facilitate research, and offer evidence in medical–legal matters, including those involving malpractice lawsuits and professional discipline complaints.[2–4]

Documentation should be completed whenever professional services are provided to a patient.[5] There is no one single method for documenting OT services. Methods of documentation can vary in their mechanism (e.g., paper vs. electronic), format (e.g., narrative vs. template), and frequency (e.g., daily vs. weekly). The method used is established by the individual practice setting and is designed to meet all regulatory, accrediting, and payer requirements.[5] According to the American Occupational Therapy Association (AOTA) Standards of Practice for Occupational Therapy, occupational therapists are required to be knowledgeable of and comply with "the time frames, formats, and standards established by the practice settings, agencies, external accreditation programs, state and federal law, and other regulatory and payer requirements."[6] In settings that employ OT assistants, the occupational therapist is responsible for all aspects of OT service delivery.[7] Therefore, in these settings, it is the responsibility of the occupational therapist to review and verify all documentation completed by the OT assistant.

Purpose of OT Documentation

The major purpose of OT documentation is to provide chronological, timely, accurate, and complete information about all services provided.[2,3,8] Documentation should include the occupational therapist's observations, assessment, and intervention, as well as the patient's response to these interventions.[2,3,8] It should reflect the decision-making process used during the delivery of care.[9] Effective documentation also allows occupational therapists to articulate the profession's distinct value.[6,10,11]

Documentation in the **medical record** provides an important mechanism for the occupational therapist to communicate with other health care providers. This communication is essential to facilitate patient safety and continuity of care. This is especially true when a patient is treated jointly by an occupational therapist and OT assistant, or as a patient moves from one treatment setting to another.[3]

AOTA[7] has outlined several purposes of OT documentation. These purposes are to:

- articulate the rationale for provision of OT services and the relationship of this service to the client's outcomes
- reflect the occupational therapist's clinical reasoning and professional judgment
- communicate information about the client from the OT perspective
- create a chronological record of client status, OT services provided to the client, and client outcomes

It is important to keep in mind that information documented in the medical record is also used for other purposes and read by a variety of audiences (Table 6-1). It should be noted that these audiences can include patients, who under the **Health Insurance Portability and Accountability Act (HIPAA)**, are allowed access to their medical records.[12] Occupational therapists should keep all of these potential audiences in mind when recording their encounters.

Formats of Documentation

Formats for documentation differ and fall into three major categories: narrative, template, and acronym.[13,14] The format selected by the occupational therapist may vary depending on the practice setting and institutional policy.

Narrative Format

Narrative notes describe the sequence of events that occurred in the therapy encounter. Narrative notes are written in a free text format and can be organized in a

Table 6-1. Purpose of Documentation and Potential Audiences

PURPOSE OF DOCUMENTATION	PRIMARY AUDIENCE
Patient care information	Health care providers, patients
Reimbursement	Third-party payers
Quality improvement and utilization review	Case managers, third-party payers
Regulatory	Federal, state, and local regulatory bodies (e.g., The Center for Medicare and Medicaid, state health departments)
Accreditation	Accrediting bodies, including The Joint Commission and Commission on Accreditation of Rehabilitation Facilities
Research	Researchers, students
Legal	Risk management officers, attorneys

variety of ways, but should always be specific, concise, and clear. Narrative notes provide descriptive information that may not be captured when documenting via a form or when using a checklist.[13] The major advantage of narrative documentation is that it allows the occupational therapist to "tell the story" of the patient and the therapy encounter. Major disadvantages are that writing narrative notes can be time-consuming, the notes themselves tend to be lengthy, and because of the lack of structure, there is a risk of inadvertently omitting important information.[13,14] The use of an outline can address these issues by reminding the writer of key areas not to be missed in the note-writing process.[13] An additional disadvantage when using narrative formats is that it can be cumbersome to gather information for utilization review or when collecting data for research.

Template Format

Templates provide formats that outline all required and relevant information that should be recorded as part of an OT encounter. When using a template, the occupational therapist generally fills in empty data fields manually or, if using an electronic charting system, selects items from a drop-down menu.[15] Templates are useful because they are efficient and provide for standardization.[3,14] However, the use of templates alone may not provide a full picture of a patient's condition or performance.[13,15] If using templates, it is recommended that there be a space built into the template for the occupational therapist to add comments and observations.

Acronym Format

Documentation using acronym formats is highly structured and requires that information be recorded in the order of the acronym's initials.[8,13] The "SOAP" note is the most common example of acronym documentation.[8] The SOAP note is an acronym for subjective, objective, assessment, and plan[8] (see Box 6-1).

Box 6-1

SOAP Note Components

Subjective

Patient's view on his condition or treatment in his own words. May include the patient's chief complaint and goals for therapy

Example: *Patient reports pain in right hand has decreased since last therapy session*

Objective

The reason and purpose for therapy. Includes a summary of the interventions provided as well as a summary of the patient's response to treatment. Observations, tests, and assessment results should be recorded here

Example: *Patients continues to attend OT twice a week for pain management and ROM following right carpal tunnel release. Pain decreased to 5 to 1 to 10 scale; AROM wrist flexion 0° to 20° and wrist extension 0° to 15°. BADL improved; patient able to hold hairbrush to style hair now*

Assessment

The interpretation and analysis of all subjective and objective information, including their impact on functional performance. A projection of patient's potential for improvement and progress toward goals should be made here

Example: *Patient remains motivated and actively participates in therapy. She demonstrates improvements in AROM of right wrist; pain is decreased, and as a result, patient is using right hand more during grooming activities. Patient is progressing toward goals and is compliant with her home exercise program*

Plan

A summary of planned interventions and follow-up, including the provision of any home program and referrals to other providers

Example: *Continue therapy twice a week as per MD order; begin gentle resistive activities next session. Home program was reviewed and updated to include grasp strengthening*

The SOAP note format is applicable for use across practice settings and can easily be incorporated into both paper and electronic documentation systems.[8] SOAP notes can provide a helpful guide to structure narrative notes and documentation templates. They can also be used to set up all types of documentation reports, including evaluations, re-evaluations, progress notes, and discharge summaries.

Types of Documentation

Occupational therapists need to be familiar with and comply with all professional, institutional, accrediting, regulatory, and **third-party payer** requirements when documenting in a patient's medical record.[2,3] The AOTA has provided Guidelines for Documentation,[5] which outline and provide information about typical documentation reports in OT service provision. These reports are categorized divided into three phases of service delivery: evaluation phase, intervention phase, and discharge phase. A summary of the reports used throughout these phases can be found in Box 6-2. Although the specific types of documentation requirements and reports may vary depending on the practice settings,[5] these AOTA guidelines can be helpful to all occupational therapists to document their services.[5]

The Electronic Medical Record

The shift in health care from paper charts to electronic medical records (EMRs) (e.g., digital version of a medical record) is the result of the belief that the use of an EMR will improve patient care, enhance patient safety, increase quality of care, improve efficiency, and reduce costs.[16] The proliferation of EMR use by health care providers is a direct result of the passage of the Health Information Technology for Economic and Clinical Health (HITECH) Act,[17] which provided extensive funding to encourage adoption of EMR systems. Occupational therapists working in hospitals in particular will find themselves using EMRs because it has been reported that that 99% of hospitals in the United States are using electronic documentation systems.[18] It is important that any occupational therapist using an EMR ensure that the system use formats that have all the elements needed to accurately record all best practices.[14]

The use of good documentation practices extends to the EMR, especially in regard to the timeliness and accuracy of note writing. Unlike paper charts, when using an EMR, each entry is automatically time-stamped, indicating the date and time of the entry. Therefore, it is essential that documentation be completed during or shortly after the provision of services. EMR documentation shortcuts, such as reusing previous entries by "cutting and pasting" or using prepopulating fields, should be avoided as the information carried forward may not be accurate or up to date.[19]

Occupational therapists documenting in EMRs should be assigned a digital signature to link them to their documentation entries. A digital signature links the provider to a unique password or identification number and is used to authenticate the contents of electronic documents.[20]

EMR documentation is often done at the "point of service" (i.e., at the time of the delivery of clinical care). Point-of-service documentation is believed to improve the efficiency and accuracy of note writing. However, it can divert the provider's attention away from the patient, making the patient feel disconnected.[14,21] To prevent this,

Box 6-2

Types of Occupational Therapy Documentation Reports

Evaluation Phase

- ***Screening:*** Brief assessment to determine whether patient could benefit from full evaluation
- ***Evaluation:*** Data gathered through the assessment process. Should include an occupational profile, an analysis of occupational performance, and identification of patient's functional deficits and strengths. Treatment goal and plans should be recorded here
- ***Reevaluation Report:*** A summary of the findings from the reassessment process; should include modification of treatment goals and plans goals based on these findings

Intervention Phase

- ***Intervention Plan:*** Based on evaluation and revelation findings, the establishment of treatment goals, and planned interventions to achieve patient goals. Should include documentation of any home program or instruction provided and any referrals to other providers
- ***Contact Note:*** A record of interaction between the patient and therapist, including the types of intervention provided and patient's response. May also be used to document telephone contacts, participation in team meetings and consultations with other health care providers
- ***Progress Report/Note:*** Summarizes the therapy process and notes patient's progress toward goals achievement. As needed, records new assessment information, and the modification and updates to treatment goals and plans. Offers support for continuation of therapy services or the need to discontinue/discharge
- ***Transition Plan:*** Provides information to the next provider as patient moves from one treatment setting to another; provides "hand-off" information to next provider

Discharge Phase

- ***Discharge/Discontinuation Note:*** Summarizes therapy services provided and the reason for discharge/discontinuation; indicates if outcomes were met

Adapted from American Occupational Therapy Association. Guidelines for documentation of occupational therapy. *Am J Occup Ther*. 2013;67(6 suppl):S32–S38. doi:10.5014/ajot.2013.67S32.

it important to keep the focus on patient throughout the therapy session, even when entering information into the EMR.[14] This can be accomplished by[21–23]:

- Informing the patient at the beginning of the encounter that notes will be taken and entered into the EMR during the therapy session
- When reviewing patient's history that was previously entered, reading that information out loud and asking the patient to verify
- Sharing the screen to show patient his or her progress during revaluations (e.g., improvements in goniometric measurements)
- Using the screen to provide and reinforce patient education materials

General Principles of OT Documentation

Documentation can be written in a paper medical record or entered directly into an EMR. Regardless of the format of the medical record, the basic general principles of good OT documentation should be adhered to (i.e., entries should be timely, comprehensive, objective, and accurate).[3] General guiding principles to help achieve these objectives include:

- Being objective and factual
- Being accurate and concise
- Using correct grammar and spelling
- Avoiding jargon and slang
- Using only approved abbreviations
- Writing legibly and clearly
- Recording entries promptly
- Being sure to date, time, and sign all entries
- Reflecting individualized, patient-centered care
- Being professional; avoid disparaging remarks or comments about patient or other health care providers
- Never erasing or removing entries from the record; if changes or corrections need to be make after an entry is made, follow institution's correction or addendum policy

Medicare, who is the largest payer for OT services,[24] requires that OT documentation reflects the provision of medically necessary and skilled services[25] and includes goals focused on the improvement of impairments or functional limitations.[26]

Medically necessary services are those services that are "needed to treat an illness, injury, condition, disease, or its symptoms and meet accepted standards of care."[25] To demonstrate medically necessary services, the occupational therapist should document the reason the patient is being referred for services, include why the patient's diagnosis or condition warrants the need for therapy, and adequately assess the patient in order to identify his or her impairments and functional deficits.[26]

Skilled services are those services that, "because of the patient's condition, require the skills, expertise, clinical reasoning and judgment of a qualified therapist to ensure the effectiveness of the treatment goals and ensure medical safety."[25] Treatment is regarded as "skilled" only if it is at a level of complexity and sophistication that requires the services of an occupational therapist or an OT assistant supervised by a therapist.[25,26] To demonstrate skilled service, the OT notes must support the need for, or the continuation of, skilled services. This can be accomplished by[26]:

- Providing clear descriptions of skilled treatment and avoiding any indication that the patient is simply performing repetitive tasks
- Specifying any changes or adaptions made to interventions that are based on ongoing assessment of the patient's function and status
- Revising the treatment plan based on the occupational therapist's clinical reasoning and judgment, to move the patient toward the next more complex level or a more difficult task

To illustrate, during a treatment session focusing on upper extremity (UE) dressing with a patient who has left-sided inattention, the occupational therapist provides tactile cuing to increase patient's awareness of left side and to promote the use of left UE in the activity. These interventions need to be documented to show skilled service was provided. Therefore, rather than documenting that the patient "practiced UE dressing with cuing" (non-skilled), the occupational therapist should document that "due to left sided inattention, the therapist provided tactical cues to promote bilateral integration while donning a front-closure garment" (skilled).

Because most other third-party payers follow Medicare guidelines, it is recommended that OT documentation follow Medicare requirements for all payers.[2,4]

To demonstrate and help other health care providers, reviewers, and third-party payers understand the unique focus and emphasis of the OT treatment process, OT documentation should reflect the distinct value of the profession.[6,10,11, 27, 28] One way to achieve this is by incorporating an occupational profile and an analysis of a patient's occupational performance into the documentation process.[29] Regarding the inclusion of an occupational profile, occupational therapists should be aware that its use may be required in order to use certain evaluation billing codes.[30]

Because a client-centered approach is an essential principle of OT,[29] it is important that documentation reflects this.[8,31] This will demonstrate a partnership with and involvement of patients receiving OT services.[31] To do this, the occupational therapists should continually record patients' priorities for treatment and their active participation in the goal-setting and treatment planning process.

Legal and Ethical Issues

The Medical Record

The medical record is a legal document. Documentation contained within the medical record becomes part of this legal document.[32,33] The medical record may be handwritten, typed, or electronic. Regardless of its format, what the occupational therapist documents in the medical record needs to be a complete, accurate, and current account of all services provided and the outcome of these services.[33]

Medical records may be subpoenaed as evidence for a variety of purposes, including lawsuits, malpractice cases, and reimbursement claims review.[14,33] Occupational therapists need to be familiar with all federal and state guidelines regarding ownership, privacy, and retention of medical records[33,34] (see Box 6-3) and what constitutes **protected patient health information**[35] before releasing any medical record information.

Legal Considerations

Occupational therapists need to be familiar with their individual **state practice act** to ensure that what they are documenting is consistent with the legal definition of OT practice for that state.[32] For example, if a particular state's OT practice act does not include the use of physical agent modalities and the occupational therapist documents the provision of these modalities, it would mean that he or she is providing services outside the scope of OT.

Documentation is regarded as an essential part of the health care process[36]; in the legal process, a health care provider's failure to document properly can be considered a breach of the standard of care.[36] Documentation by the occupational therapist provides evidence of services provided as well as the reasoning behind the provision of these services.[34,36] In the event of a lawsuit, what is (and is not) documented in the medical record will form the basis for the plaintiff's case and or the health care provider's or facility's defense.[34] This evidence may be used to defend against lawsuits, malpractice cases, or claims by third-party payers of **fraudulent billing.**[13] Consequently, it is important that occupational therapists be aware and comply with key legal aspects of documentation related to legibility, timeliness, completeness, accuracy, and **authentication.**[13,33,34]

- *Legibility:* All handwritten notes must be legible. Notes that are illegible may be misread or misinterpreted.
- *Timeliness:* Documentation should be up to date and written during or on the day of the patient encounter. All notes should contain date and time. Documenting in advance is never acceptable nor is backdating a note. If, for some reason, a note cannot be written on the day service was provided, it should be entered as a late entry.
- *Completeness:* All information documented about the service provided should be complete (i.e., include what was done and how, justification for service provided, and the patient's responses).
- *Accurate:* All information should be documented and should be correct, truthful, and reflect the actual services provided.
- *Authentication:* Authentication refers to the process of showing authorship and responsibility for something documented in the medical record.[33,34] All documentation should be signed by the provider who delivered the service and should include the provider's credentials. In cases where an EMR is being used, a digital signature can be used for authentication.[33,34] By authenticating (e.g., signing) his or her note, the occupational therapist is verifying what was done and is taking responsibility for the entry.[33,34]

Occupational therapists need to be aware that depending on the state practice act or their specific institutional policy, they may be required to co-sign any notes written by OT students and OT assistants.[7] By co-signing these notes, the occupational therapist is verifying that supervision is being providing and is taking responsibility for what is written.[2] It is important that the occupational therapist reviews these notes carefully and clarifies any questions he or she may have before co-signing.

In the event of a lawsuit, what is (and is not) documented in the medical record will form the basis for the plaintiff's case and or the health care provider or facility's defense.[33,34] Therefore, it is essential that occupational therapists follow good documentation practices should they have to defend themselves in a lawsuit.

Box 6-3

Legal Considerations Regarding the Medical Record

- ***Ownership:*** The facility or practice generating the patient's medical record is the owner; however, all information documented in the medical record belongs to both the patient and the health care provider
- ***Privacy and Confidentiality:*** HIPAA regulations protect the privacy and confidentiality of protected patient health information. Health care facilities or practices should develop and implement policies and procedures to ensure compliance with these regulations
- ***Retention:*** State laws regarding how long medical records should be retained vary. Health care facilities and providers need to be adhere to their individual state's requirements

Ethical Considerations

Occupational therapists should follow standards of practice and ethical principles when documenting. The AOTA Occupational Therapy Code of Ethics[37] stresses the need for occupational therapists to be honest, accurate, and timely when documenting and to comply with all applicable regulations. Ethical challenges related to documentation often arise when occupational therapists are asked to document false or erroneous information in order to insure reimbursement.[38] Some examples of these ethical challenges might include:

- An administrator directs an occupational therapist to document that a patient is receiving 60 minutes of therapy, even though the patient is easily fatigued and can only tolerate 45 minutes.
- An occupational therapist is assigned to co-sign notes written by an OT assistant he or she is not supervising.
- A supervisor requests that an occupational therapist reword a treatment note so that a higher paying code can be assigned to a billing claim.

It is important that occupational therapists remember that documenting services that were not provided, using wrong billing codes, or co-signing notes without providing proper supervision are all serious infractions and could possibly result in legal and professional sanctions.[4,32,38]

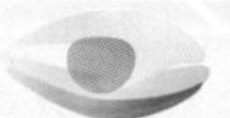

CASE STUDY

Case Scenario

Juana is a left-hand dominant, 75-year-old female. Two weeks ago, while running to catch the subway, Juana tripped and fell onto her left shoulder. Juana was seen in the emergency room immediately after her fall; radiographic studies revealed a left nondisplaced midshaft humeral fracture. A sling was applied to immobilize Juana's left shoulder. She was seen in orthopedic care 1 week later, and at that time, the sling was removed. Juana was then referred to outpatient OT for twice a week (BIW) therapy for pain management, gentle active and active-assistive range of motion (AROM), and activities of daily living (ADLs) training.

Juana is a retired secretary who lives alone and was independent in all basic activities of daily living (BADLs) and instrumental activities of daily living (IADLs) prior to her fall. She is active in her community and was volunteering in her local church's food bank prior to her injury. Her goal is to return to independence and to resume her volunteer work. She has been attending OT for 2 weeks, is motivated, and appears compliant with her home exercise program.

Sample Treatment Contact Note: SOAP Format

- ***S (subjective):*** Patient reports continued stiffness in left shoulder and reports a "4" on the 1 to 10 pain scale. She states she continues to have difficulty washing her hair while in the shower and putting on a blouse but is using her left arm more during these activities.
- ***O(objective):*** Patient actively participated in the 30-minute OT session with focus on left shoulder AROM to increase ability to raise arm overhead to facilitate grooming and overhead dressing activities. Goniometric measurements taken of left shoulder at start of session: AROM: flexion 0° to 100° (increase 8°); extension 0° to 15° abduction 0° to 80° (increase 10°); external rotation 0° to 60° (increase 10°); and internal rotation 0° to 45° (increase 5°).

  Patient performed multiple repetitions of left upper extremity (LUE) AROM forward and overhead reaching activities; she required occasional (<4) tactile cues to avoid trunk substitution when reaching above 90°. Trunk substitutions during reaching noted to increase as she fatigued. No complaint of increased pain reported; at end of activity, patient stated her shoulder "felt looser." Following AROM, ADL training performed for UE dressing; patient needed an initial verbal cue for correct placement of LUE into overhead garment. Patient was reeducated on home exercises program and was independent with return demonstration.
- ***A (assessment):*** Patient is demonstrating progress in UE AROM and functional use since last session. Reports of pain have decreased and improvements noted in AROM as per goniometric revaluation. She is progressing toward goals. Patient can benefit from continued skilled OT to further improve ROM and functional use. Potential for return to independent function is good, and she is please with her progress.
- ***P (plan):*** Continue OT BIW for ROM, pain management and ADL training, and home program. As per telephone conversation with orthopedic surgeon, patient is cleared to begin gentle resistive exercise at the next visit.

References

1. Silverman M, Murrary TJ, Bryan CS, eds. *The Quotable Osler*. Revised paperback ed./Edition 1. Philadelphia, PA: American College of Physicians; 2007.
2. Morreale MJ. Documentation of occupational therapy. In: Jacobs K, McCormack GL, eds. *The Occupational Therapy Manager.* 5th ed. Bethesda, MD: American Occupational Therapy Association; 2011: 367–384.
3. Sames KM. *Documenting Occupational Therapy Practice.* 3rd ed. Upper Saddle River, NJ: Pearson Education; 2015.
4. Braveman, B. *Leading and Managing Occupational Therapy Services: An Evidence Based Approach.* 2nd ed. Philadelphia, PA: FA Davis; 2016.
5. American Occupational Therapy Association. Guidelines for documentation of occupational therapy. *Am J Occup Ther.* 2013;67(6 suppl):S32–S38. doi:10.5014/ajot.2013.67s32.

6. American Occupational Therapy Association. Standards of practice for occupational therapy. *Am J Occup Ther*. 2015;69(suppl 3):6913410057. doi:10.5014/ajot.2015.696S06.
7. American Occupational Therapy Association. Guidelines for supervision, roles, and responsibilities during the delivery of occupational therapy services. *Am J Occup Ther*. 2014; 68:S16–S22. doi:10.5014/ajot.2014.686S03.
8. Gateley, CA, Borcherding. S. *Documentation Manual for Occupational Therapy: Writing SOAP Notes*. 4th ed. Thorofare, NJ: Slack; 2017.
9. Erickson, ML. Reasons for documenting in physical therapy. In: Erickson ML, Utzman RR, McKnight R, eds. *Physical Therapy Documentation: From Examination to Outcome*. 2nd ed. Thorofare, NJ: Slack; 2014:13–21.
10. Yamkovenko, S. *How to Be More Effective with Documentation: Q&A with Cathy Brennan*. American Occupational Therapy Association. Retrieved from https://www.aota.org/Publications-News/AOTANews/2014/QA-Cathy-Brennan-Effective-Documentation.aspx. Published 2014. Accessed June 1, 2018
11. Boyt Schell BA, Scaffa MR, Gillen G, Cohn ES. Contemporary occupational therapy practice. In: Boyt BA, Gillen G, Cohn ES, eds. *Willard & Spackman's Occupational Therapy*. 12th ed. Philadelphia, PA: Lippincott Williams and Wilkins; 2014:47–58.
12. Health Insurance Portability and Accountability Act. §164.524—Access of individuals to protected health information. https://www.gpo.gov/fdsys/pkg/FR-2000-12-28/pdf/00-32678.pdf. Published 2000. Accessed June 9, 2018
13. Quinn L, Gordon J. Essentials of documentation In: Quinn L, Gordon J, eds. *Documentation for Rehabilitation: A Guide to Clinical Decision Making*. 3rd ed. Maryland Heights, MO: Elsevier; 2016:8–20.
14. Scott RW. *Legal, Ethical, and Practical Aspects of Patient Care Documentation: A Guide for Rehabilitation Professionals*. 4th ed. Burlington, MA: Jones and Bartlett; 2013.
15. Brookstone A. *Data Entry Strategies: Using Templates*. American EMR Website. http://www.americanehr.com/blog/2011/05/data-entry-strategies-using-templates/. Published May 11, 2017. Accessed May 30, 2018.
16. What are the advantages of electronic health records? The Office of the National Coordinator for Health Information Technology Website. https://www.healthit.gov/faq/what-are-advantages-electronic-health-records. Last Reviewed March 21, 2018. Accessed June 1, 2018.
17. Health Information Technology for Economic and Clinical Health Act. https://www.hhs.gov/sites/default/files/ocr/privacy/hipaa/understanding/coveredentities/hitechact.pdf. Accessed May 30, 2018.
18. Pedersen, CA, Schneider, PJ, Scheckelhoff, DL. ASHP national survey of pharmacy practice in hospital settings: prescribing and transcribing—2016. *American Journal of Health-System Pharmacy*. doi:10.2146/ajhp170228.
19. Sulmasy LS, López AM, Horwitch C A. Ethical implications of the electronic health record: in the service of the patient. *J Gen Intern Med*. 2017;32(8):935–939. doi:10.1007/s11606-017-4030-1.
20. Christensson, P. (2009, May 29). *Digital Signature Definition*. Retrieved from https://techterms.com/definition/digitalsignature. Accessed June 19, 2018.
21. Lee WW, Alkureishi ML. The impact of EMRs on communication within the doctor-patient relationship. In: Papadakos P, Bertman S, eds. *Distracted Doctoring*. New York, NY: Springer, Cham; 2017:101–121.
22. Waite A. Record time: point-of-service documentation strategies help practitioners beat the time crunch. *OT Practice*. 2012;17(1):9–12. https://www.aota.org/~/media/corporate/files/secure/publications/otp/2012-issues/otp%20vol%2017%20issue%201.pdf. Accessed May 30, 2018.
23. Duke P, Frankel RM, Reis S. How to integrate the electronic health record and patient-centered communication into the medical visit: a skills-based approach. *Teach Learn Med*. 2013;25(4):358–365. doi:10.1080/10401334.2013.827981.
24. *Coverage by payer*. American Occupational Therapy Association Website. https://www.aota.org/Advocacy-Policy/Federal-Reg-Affairs/Pay.aspx. Accessed May 30, 2018.
25. Center for Medicare and Medicaid. *Medicare Benefit Policy Manual*. Chapter 15, Section 220. https://www.cms.gov/Regulations-and-Guidance/Guidance/Manuals/downloads/bp102c15.pdf. Revised February 2, 2018. Accessed June 9, 2018.
26. Center for Medicare and Medicaid Office of Financial Management. *Physical, Occupational and Speech Therapy Services*. https://www.cms.gov/Research-Statistics-Data-and-Systems/Monitoring-Programs/Medical-Review/Downloads/TherapyCapSlidesv10_09052012.pdf. September 5, 2012. Accessed May 30, 2018.
27. Fisher G, Frieseman J. Health policy perspectives—implications of the affordable care act for occupational therapy practitioners providing services to Medicare recipients. *Am J Occup Ther*. 2013;67(5):502–506. doi:10.5014/ajot.2013.675002.
28. *Improve your documentation with AOTA's occupational profile template*. American Occupational Therapy Association Website. https://www.aota.org/Practice/Manage/Reimb/occupational-profile-document-value-ot.aspx. Accessed June 3, 2018.
29. American Occupational Therapy Association. Occupational therapy practice framework: domain and process. 3rd ed. *Am J Occup Ther*. 2014;68(suppl 1):S1–S48. doi:10.5014/ajot.2014.682006.
30. American Medical Association. *CPT® 2017 Professional Edition*. Chicago, IL: American Medical Association; 2017.
31. Hammell KR. Client-centred practice in occupational therapy: critical reflections, *Scand J Occup Ther*. 2012;20(3):174–181. doi:10.3109/11038128.2012.752032.
32. Fearon HM, Levine SM. Legal aspects of documentation. In: Quinn L, Gordon J, eds. *Documentation for Rehabilitation: A Guide to Clinical Decision Making*. 3rd ed. Maryland Heights, MO; 2016:21–27.
33. Roach, WH, Hoban RR, Broccolo BM, Roth AB, Blanchard, TP. *Medical Records and the Law*. 4th ed. Sudbury, MA: Jones and Bartlett; 2006.
34. Levin BJ, Iyer P, eds. *Medical Legal Aspects of Medical Records: Volume I: Foundations of Medical Records*. 2nd ed. Tucson, AZ: Lawyers & Judges Publishing; 2010.
35. *Summary of the HIPAA privacy rule*. US Department of Health and Human Services Website. https://www.hhs.

gov/hipaa/for-professionals/privacy/laws-regulations/index.html. Last reviewed July 26, 2016. Accessed June 25, 2018.

36. Gutheil TG. Fundamentals of medical record documentation. *Psychiatry (Edgmont)*. 2004;1(3):26–28.
37. American Occupational Therapy Association. Occupational therapy code of ethics. *Am J Occup Ther*. 2015;69(suppl 3):6913410030. doi:10.5014/ajot.2015.696S03.
38. American Occupational Therapy Association. *The American Occupational Therapy Association advisory opinion for the ethics commission ethical considerations for productivity, billing, and reimbursement*. American Occupational Therapy Association Website. https://www.aota.org/~/media/Corporate/Files/Practice/Ethics/Advisory/reimbursement-productivity.pdf. Published 2016. Accessed June 10, 2018.

Chapter 7

Visual Function Assessment

Diane Powers Dirette and Jennifer Fortuna

LEARNING OBJECTIVES

This chapter will allow the reader to:

1. Define the key terms related to visual function.
2. Determine the impact of visual deficits in populations as well as for individual clients.
3. Connect underlying neurological and physiological impairments to the resulting visual deficits.
4. Describe screening techniques for visual acuity, visual fields, and oculomotor control.
5. Identify commonly used standardized visual assessments and their value for use in assessing visual function.

CHAPTER OUTLINE

TERMINOLOGY

Contrast sensitivity: the visual ability to distinguish the edges of objects against backgrounds of similar color or saturation.

Convergence: the oculomotor ability to move two eyes nasally simultaneously (the opposite is divergence).

Fixation: the oculomotor ability to maintain focus on an object in central vision.

Oculomotor: the ability to purposefully contract the muscles of the eyes to produce coordinated movement.

Saccades: the oculomotor ability to perform quick movements of the eyes from one target to another and focus the target in clear, central vision.

Scanning: the oculomotor ability of visually searching the environment.

Tracking/pursuits: the oculomotor ability to smoothly follow a slow moving target and keep it in the central vision.

Visual acuity: the level of clear central vision.

Visual fields: the span of vision that one sees while looking straight ahead. While the eyes are fixated straight ahead, the visual field is approximately 90° from center to the right and to the left sides, 70° inferiorly, and 60° superiorly.

Visual range of motion: the amount of movement of the eyes in all planes of movement vertically, horizontally, and diagonally.

Visual Function and Impairment in Daily Occupation

Visual function is the integrity of the visual system and includes visual acuity, oculomotor abilities, contrast sensitivity, pupillary function, and visual fields, which are all integral to the performance of daily occupations. Occupational performance problems can occur when a deficit arises in any of these components. Visual function is also the basis of many other client factors including visual perception, cognition, eye-hand coordination, balance, and mobility. Because vision underlies these other factors, a visual deficit can impact these factors that are also necessary for the performance of daily occupations. Visual deficits, therefore, can impact all aspects of a person's ability to perform activities of daily living (ADLs) and instrumental activities of daily living (IADLs).

Warren Model of Visual Functioning

Warren[1] described a visual perceptual hierarchy in adults (Fig. 7-1). This model suggests that higher level skills (such as visual attention and visual memory) are built on the foundations of **visual acuity, visual fields,** and **oculomotor** control (e.g. **fixation, saccades, visual range of motion**). The components in the hierarchy are as follows:

1. Oculomotor control, visual fields, visual acuity
2. Visual attention and alertness
3. Visual scanning
4. Pattern recognition
5. Visual memory
6. Visual cognition
7. Adaptation through vision

Table 7-1. Levels of Visual Impairment

LEVEL OF VISUAL IMPAIRMENT	DEFINITION
Moderate	Best-corrected visual acuity is less than 20/60.
Severe	Best-corrected visual acuity is less than 20/160, or visual field is 20° or less (legal blindness).
Profound	Best-corrected visual acuity is less than 20/400, or visual field is 10° or less (moderate blindness).
Near-total	Best-corrected visual acuity is less than 20/1,000, or visual field is 5° or less (severe blindness).
Total	No light perception (total blindness).

Source: Centers for Medicare & Medicaid Services. *Transmittal AB-02-078*. Department of Health and Human Services. Retrieved from https://www.cms.gov/transmittals/downloads/AB02078.pdf

Populations and Vision Impairments

Worldwide, an estimated 253 million people have vision impairments, with 36 million classified as blind and 217 million classified as moderately to severely visually impaired.[2] Table 7-1 shows the levels of visual impairment. Visual impairments are especially prevalent in the aging population, with 81% of people, aged 50 years and older, who are blind or have moderate or severe visual impairment.[2] Low vision is the third most common cause of impaired function among the elderly, and low vision disorders not only impair a person's ability to function but also increase a person's risk of depression, social isolation, falls, and a general decline in health.[3]

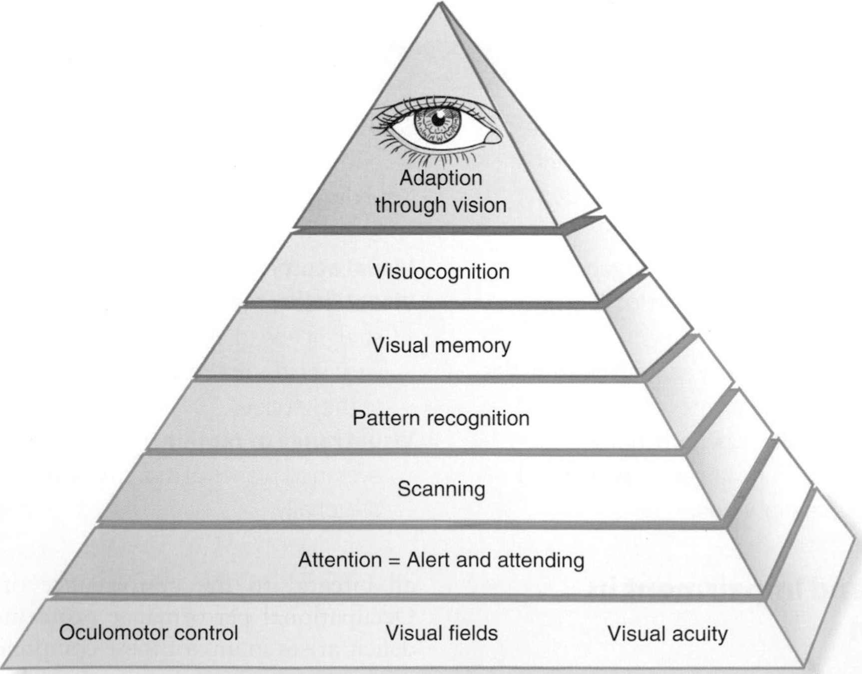

Figure 7-1. Hierarchy of visual perception. (Adapted from Warren M. A hierarchical model for evaluation for evaluation and treatment of visual perceptual dysfunction in adult acquired brain injury, Part 1. *Am J Occup Ther.* 1993;47:43. Copyright 1993 by the American Occupational Therapy Association, Inc. Reprinted with permission.)

The most common low vision disorders include macular degeneration, diabetic retinopathy, glaucoma, and cataracts.[4] Because of the aging of the global population, it is estimated that the number of people with visual impairment could triple by 2050 with 115 million people who are blind, up from 38.5 million in 2020.[2]

Beyond age-related vision loss and impairments, many clients experience vision problems because of neurologically based disability or illness. In a study of 328 patients who suffered a stroke, over 90% had visual problems in eye alignment, visual fields, and visual attention.[5] Many service members with blast-related brain injuries also receive occupational therapy screening for vision problems.[6–8]

Neurological and Physiological Basis of Visual Function

Visual Acuity

Clear central vision begins with light entering the lens of the eye, passing through the pupil, and being processed by the photoreceptors cells of the retina[9] (Fig. 7-2). The photoreceptor cells of the retina, the rod and cone cells, convert the light into neural signals.[10] The rod cells specialize in low levels of light intensity, such as night vision, and the cone cells specialize in higher levels of light intensity, such as color vision.[9] The cone cells are most highly concentrated in a small region of the retina, the fovea, where visual acuity is the greatest. Rod cells are evenly distributed in the retina, but are not present in the fovea.

From the retina, the neural signals are conveyed via axons in the optic nerve (cranial nerve [CN] II) to the optic chiasm, to the optic tract and then to the lateral geniculate nucleus. From the lateral geniculate nucleus, the visual information is sent via optic radiations to the primary visual cortex in the occipital lobes.[9]

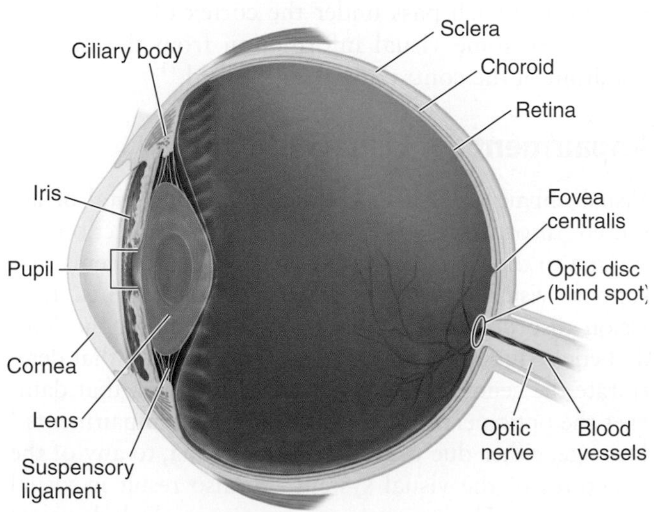

Figure 7-2. Anatomy of the eye.

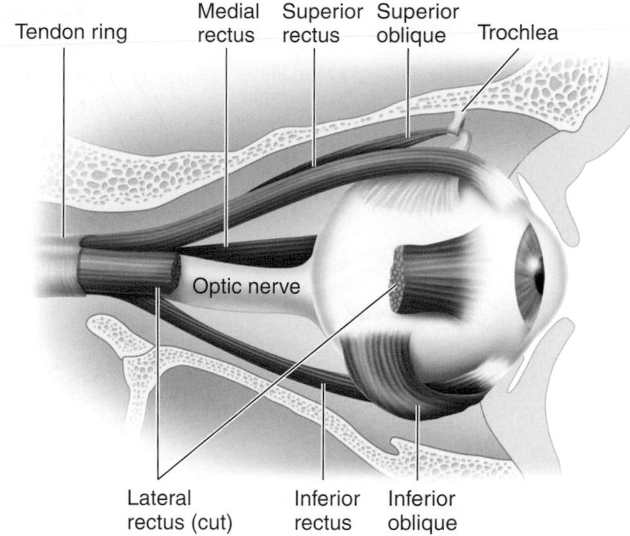

Figure 7-3. Muscles of the eye.

Oculomotor

Smooth, controlled eye movements are necessary for clear and accurate vision. Eye movements are controlled by the muscles of the eyes and the CNs that innervate them (Fig. 7-3). The muscles and the movements of the eyes that they control include the following[10]:

- Levator palpebrae superioris—Lifts the eyelid
- Superior rectus—Moves the eye upward
- Medial rectus—Moves the eye medially (nasally)
- Inferior oblique—Rotates the eye in and up
- Superior oblique—Rotates the eye down and out
- Lateral rectus—Moves the eye laterally (temporally)

CN II is responsible for transporting the image that comes in through the retina, but CNs III, IV, and VI are responsible for the movements of the eye (Fig. 7-4). CN III: Oculomotor innervates all of the muscles of the eye, except the superior oblique that is innervated by CN IV: Trochlear and the lateral rectus muscle that is innervated by CN VI: Abducens.

Constriction and dilation of the pupil are also oculomotor functions of the eye. The muscles that control pupillary functions are the sphincter pupillae muscle and ciliary muscle, which are both innervated by CN III. Accommodation, an increase in the curvature of the lens to focus on near objects, is also controlled by the ciliary muscle.

Visual Fields

Although it would logically seem as if the right eye would perceive the right visual field and the left eye the left visual field, that is not how the visual system functions. Each visual field is perceived and processed by half of each eye[9] (Fig. 7-5). For each eye, the optic nerve (CN II) is divided into half and wraps around the back of the eye. The left visual field is perceived by the nasal half of CN II in the

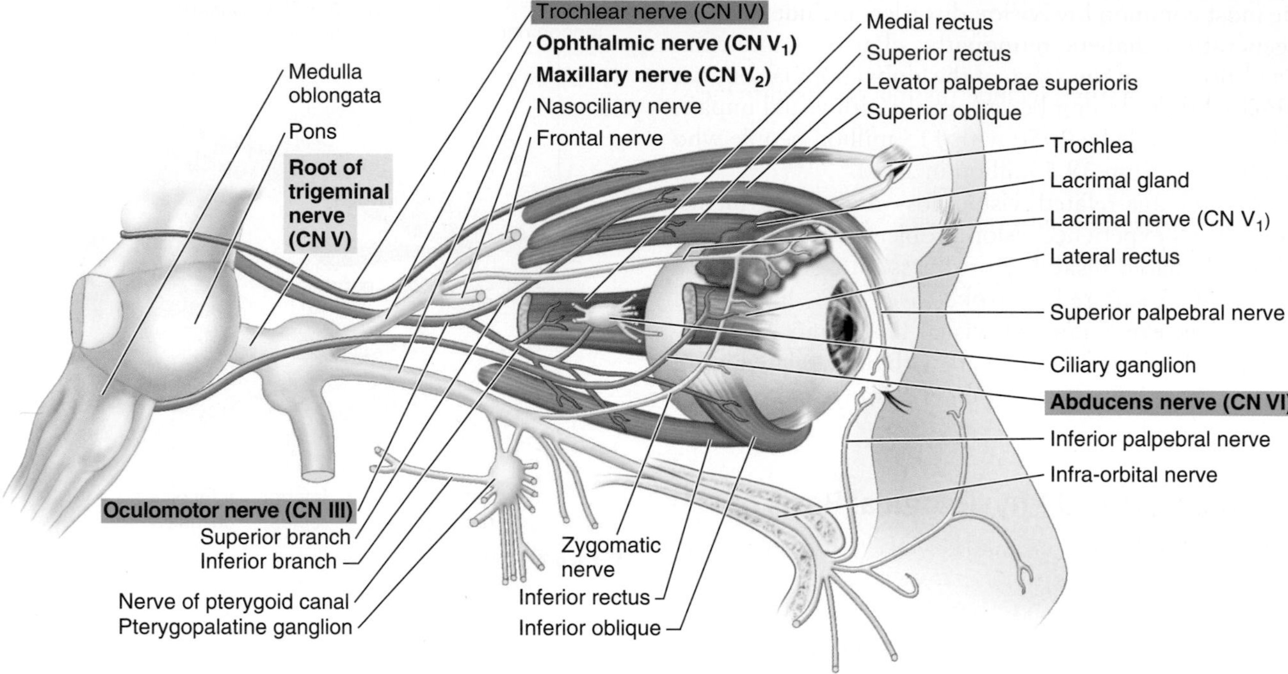

Figure 7-4. Innervation of the eye muscles. *CN, cranial nerve.*

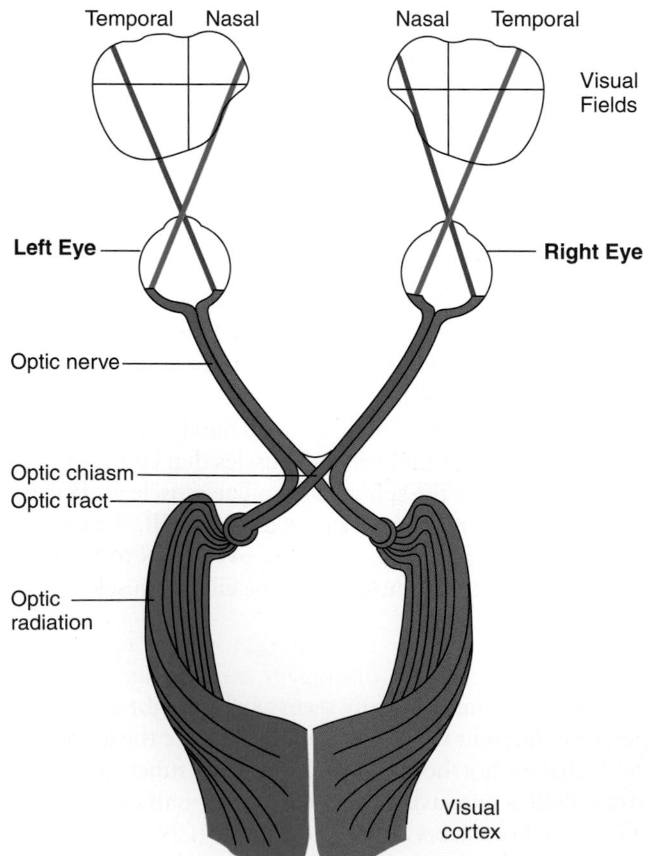

Figure 7-5. Model of visual pathway.

left eye and the temporal half of CN II in the right eye. The right visual field is perceived by the temporal half of CN II in the left eye and the nasal half of CN II in the right eye. Visual information from the nasal halves of the retina crosses over at the optic chiasm and is transmitted and processed on the contralateral half of the visual cortex. Visual information from the temporal halves of the retina, however, continues to the ipsilateral half and is processed on the same side of the visual cortex.[10]

Anterior to the lateral geniculate nucleus, some of the optic radiations carry visual information to the temporal lobes (Meyer's loop). Meyer's loop carries some of the visual information from the superior quadrant of the contralateral visual field. More medial parts of the optic radiations, which pass under the cortex of the parietal lobe, carry some visual information from the inferior quadrant of the contralateral visual field.[11]

Impairments of Visual Function

Visual impairments may be caused by congenital or acquired disorders. Low vision disorders, infection, or trauma to the visual system or neurological systems that support vision can result in visual impairments. Low vision disorders, such as cataracts that cloud the lens; diabetic retinopathy and macular degeneration that deteriorate the center of the retina; and glaucoma that damages the optic nerve can all result in visual impairments.[4] Damage, either due to infection or trauma, to any of the structures of the visual system can also result in visual impairments. These visual impairments can include visual acuity, oculomotor, and visual field dysfunction.

Visual Acuity

Refractive errors, in which the image is not accurately focused on the retina, include myopia (nearsightedness), hyperopia (farsightedness), and astigmatism (asymmetrical or distorted vision at any distance). In myopic vision, the image falls short of an exact focus on the eye because the eye is too long. The person can focus accurately on images that are near, but not on those that are far away. The opposite is true for hyperopia in which the image overshoots the retina. The person with hyperopia is farsighted, meaning that images that are far are clear, but those that are close are blurry. Astigmatism is caused by a curvature of the eye or the lens that then bends the light as it enters causing a distortion of the image on the retina.

As with the rest of the body, aging will impact the muscles and fluid of the eye and may cause presbyopia. Presbyopia is a loss of accommodation of the lens and a shortening of the eye caused by loss of aqueous fluid, resulting in the hyperopia in which the image overshoots the retina and the person becomes farsighted. This typically begins around 40 years of age.

Contrast sensitivity can also be impaired and typically declines with age. An inability to perceive contrast may be a combination of factors such as decreased acuity that result from refractive disorders, reduced pupillary function that regulates the input of light on the retina, and impaired accommodation of the lens.[12]

Visual scotomas, holes in visual acuity, can also occur. Scotomas can be caused by diseases or trauma that degenerate the macula or the retina, demyelinate or damage the optic nerve, or reduce the vasculature to the eye. They may also be caused by small lesions in the visual cortex.[9]

Oculomotor

Several oculomotor deficits may also be noted as follows:

- Strabismus: a misalignment of the eyes (e.g., esotropia: turned in, exotropia: turned out, hypertropia: one eye turned up)[12]
- Reduced ability to move one or both eyes through full range of motion
- An inability to smoothly and accurately track or pursue a target
- Nystagmus: small, involuntary, and repetitive movements of the eyes (sometimes elicited during attempts to perform saccadic eye movements)
- Convergence or divergence insufficiencies

Convergence and divergence are needed to bring objects into focus with both eyes. Binocular vision allows us to blend the two slightly different images from each eye into a singular image containing volume and depth (Fig. 7-6). Binocular vision depends on good eye alignment and the ability of the two eyes to work together. Binocular disparity is the visual difference in angles of the view of an object from two eyes when the eyes converge on an object. Binocular disparity is especially useful for perceiving depth and distance.

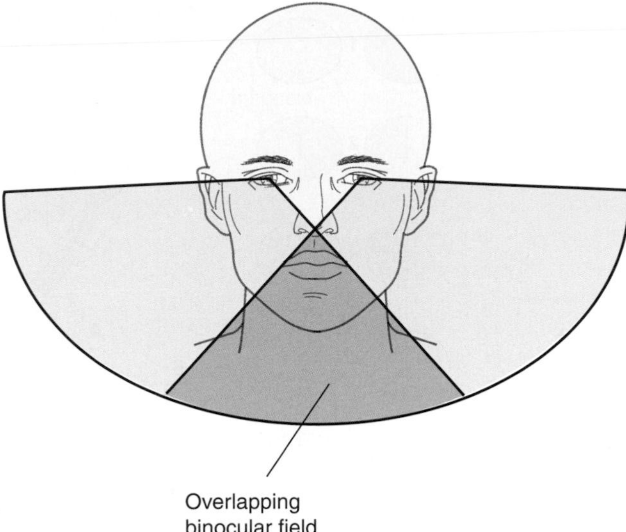

Figure 7-6. Binocular vision.

Visual Fields

Damage to the eye, optic nerves, or visual pathways may result in visual field losses (Fig. 7-7). Hemianopic visual field defects are loss of half of the visual field and are caused by damage to the visual pathways. Damage to the structures of the visual pathway posterior to the optic chiasm typically results in homonymous visual field deficits (loss of the same field in each eye). The visual field loss can be homonymous hemianopia, loss of the entire half of the visual field, or homonymous quadrantanopia, loss of one-quarter of each visual field. The loss is corresponding in each eye, which means that if the person loses the vision from the nasal half of the retina in the right eye, the vision from the temporal half of the retina in the left eye is lost. In this case, the visual loss would be a right homonymous hemianopia with a loss of vision for the right half of the visual field. This could be due to damage to the optic tract, the lateral geniculate nucleus, the optic radiations, or the visual cortex on the left side of the visual pathway. Damage on the right side of the visual pathway posterior to the optic chiasm would result in left hemianopic deficits.

Homonymous quadrantanopia could also be caused by damage to parts of the temporal lobe (Meyer's loop), resulting in a superior homonymous quadrantanopia, or damage to the optic radiation underlying the parietal cortex, resulting in an inferior homonymous quadrantanopia.[11]

Damage to the visual pathway posterior to the lateral geniculate nucleus may result in macular sparing.[11] Macular sparing is preserved input and processing of information from the fovea so that central, acute vision remains intact. The cause of this phenomenon is unknown.

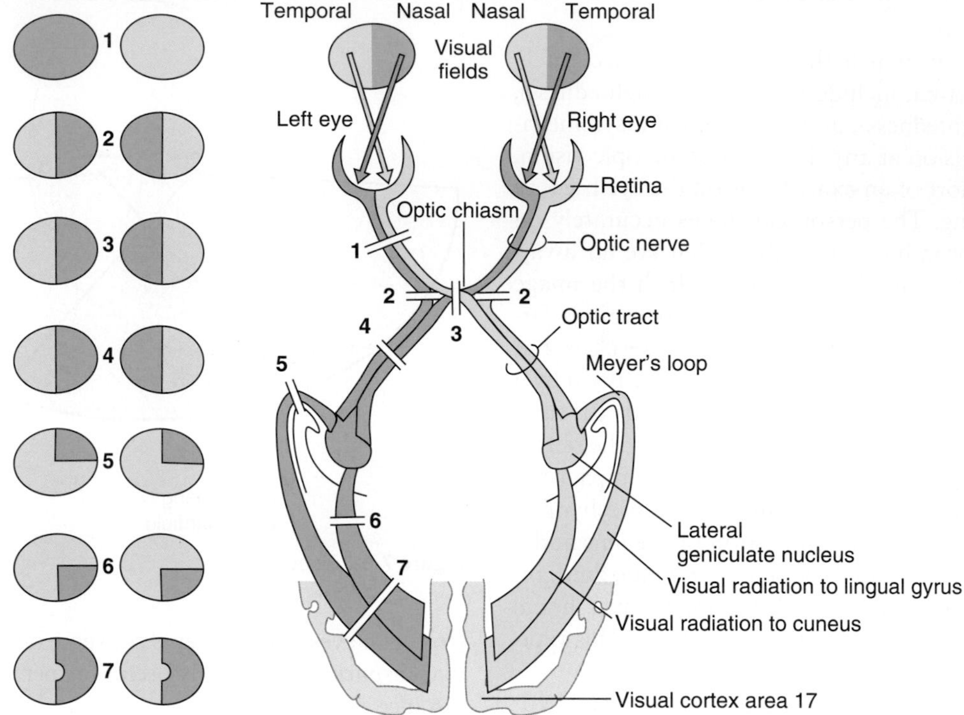

Figure 7-7. Visual fields deficits.

Screening of Visual Skills

The occupational therapist should perform a screening of visual deficits with each client with whom he or she works. The screening can be completed in 5 to 15 minutes and should be completed before any testing of visual perception, cognition, and ADLs. Occupational therapists are not ophthalmologists or optometrists and, therefore, are not licensed to make diagnoses related to visual acuity, low vision disorders, or underlying neurological pathologies that may cause other visual deficits. The role of the occupational therapist is to screen visual function, make referrals as needed, and provide remediation, compensation, or adaptations to support function.

The occupational therapy assessment of vision includes a basic eye history; interviews with the client and/or family about subjective complaints (e.g., difficulty concentrating, double vision, eye strain, and bumping into objects on one side); and screening of visual acuity, oculomotor functions, and visual fields. If a deficit is noted during the screening, the therapist may elect to further assess the deficit using a standardized assessment. The Assessment table at the end of this chapter describes and summarizes the psychometric properties of various occupational therapy vision assessments.

Visual acuity, oculomotor control, and visual fields form the foundations for visual function. Although deficits in any of these visual functions can affect client performance, clients may not complain of any problems, or they may make complaints that appear unrelated to vision. Therefore, it is important to screen the foundations of visual function even if the client denies visual difficulties.

Setup and Procedure

Lighting

All testing should be done in a room with even, ambient lighting from overhead sources, windows, or lamps. Check for glare on testing surfaces and provide direct, task lighting if the ambient sources are not sufficient to illuminate testing materials.

Positioning and Process

Unless otherwise noted, conduct all testing sitting face-to-face with the client at the same height to directly observe the client's eyes. Confrontation testing, which is conducted to screen visual fields, should be completed as a two-person test with the therapist standing behind the client and an assistant in front to observe any eye movements.

Because functional vision and occupational performance are performed with both eyes, the screening should begin by assessing visual function with both eyes being used. If a problem is noted, one eye at a time should be occluded to determine the location of the problem, either in one eye or in both.[12]

A visual screening checklist can be used to guide the screening. See Figure 7-8 for an example visual screening form.

VISUAL SCREENING

Name: ____ Date: _________
DOB: ______ Dx: ____________ Dominant Hand: ______ Lenses: _______

1. Visual Acuity:
   - Distance- Both eyes- intact _____ impaired _____
     - Right eye- intact _____ impaired _____
     - Left eye- intact _____ impaired _____
   - Near- Both eyes- intact _____ impaired _____
     - Right eye- intact _____ impaired _____
     - Left eye- intact _____ impaired _____
2. Contrast Sensitivity: intact _____ limited _____
3. Ocular Motor:
   - Fixation- Both eyes- middle _____ left _____ right _____
     - Right eye- middle _____ left _____ right _____
     - Left eye- middle _____ left _____ right _____
   - ROM- Both eyes- intact _____ limited _____
     - Right eye- intact _____ limited _____
     - Left eye- intact _____ limited _____
   - Pursuits/tracking- Both eyes- intact _____ impaired _____
     - Right eye- intact _____ impaired _____
     - Left eye- intact _____ impaired _____
   - Convergence- Intact _____ Impaired _____
     - Near point _____ Recovery point _____
   - Saccades- Accurate _____
     - Over/undershoots _____
     - Head/body movement _____
     - Nystagmus _____
4. Pupillary Functions:
   - Right eye- Responsive _____ Associated reaction _____
   - Left eye- Responsive _____ Associated reaction _____
5. Visual Fields:
   - Confrontation-
     - Two examiner single field- Intact _____ Reduced _____ Location _____
     - Simultaneous presentation- Intact _____ Reduced _____ R/L
   - Computerized perimetry- Intact _____ Reduced _____
   - Cancellation/scanning- Accuracy _____ Speed _____ Pattern _____
     - Accuracy _____ Speed _____ Pattern _____
   - Line bisection- Accurate _____ Lateralization _____ R/L
   - Figure Drawing/Copying- Accurate _____ Lateralization _____ R/L

Figure 7-8. Visual screening checklist. *L/R, left/right; ROM, range of motion.*

Equipment

Screening of visual abilities can be completed with a simple set of equipment, most of which is readily available in settings in which occupational therapists practice (Fig. 7-9). The following is a recommended list.

- Reading materials such as a newspaper or magazine
- Ruler or dowel marked at 4 and 16 inches
- Contrast sensitivity chart
- Two pens, one with a red cap and one with a green or blue cap
- Penlight
- Scanning sheets
- Line bisection sheet
- Blank paper

Step 1: Visual History and Observation

Interview

Begin the screening by asking the client or the caregiver if the client is experiencing any difficulty with vision. Keep in mind that visual deficits may not be apparent to the client or caregiver or that the client may have reduced awareness of deficits as a result of an injury. Some specific complaints should be indicated to the therapist that a problem might exist. For example, a client may complain about sensitivity to bright lights, which may indicate a problem with pupillary function; about double vision, which may indicate misalignment or reduced convergence; or about difficulty focusing during eye movement, which may indicate impaired tracking or nystagmus. People with loss of central visual acuity commonly refer to their vision as being blurry or veiled; common complaints include reading difficulties and inability to distinguish facial features.

Next, ask the client about his or her current eyewear usage for near and distant vision. If the glasses are prescribed, ask how long it has been since the prescription has been renewed. All testing, except for confrontations, should be conducted using the most current eyewear. If glasses are not available, the client can view the visual acuity testing materials through a small pinhole punched into an index card.[13] The pinhole method is a quick screen to determine whether visual acuity can be improved with eyeglasses or contact lenses, which can only be prescribed by an ophthalmologist or optometrist.

The therapist should also obtain a history of eye injury, deficits, and treatment. If available, a medical chart may contain some of this information, but ask the client or family member to confirm or add to any information about his or her visual history.

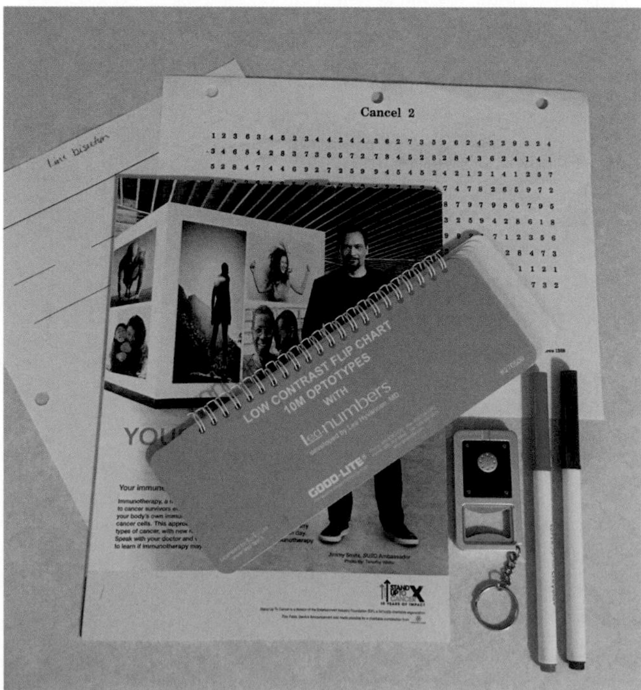

Figure 7-9. Basic screening equipment.

Observation

During the interview, the therapist observes the positioning of the client's body, head, and eyes. People typically hold their bodies in a neutral midline position and freely move their heads about as the environment is scanned or hold their heads directly facing objects or people on which they are focused. Deviations from midline with the head held to one side, tilted, pushed forward, or held facing slightly inferior or superior should be noted. For example, people with a left homonymous hemianopia may hold their heads slightly toward the left side to attempt to center the remaining visual field in front of their bodies.

During testing, the therapist should observe any attempts to compensate for visual loss. Clients may squint their eyes, move object closer or farther away, or turn materials sideways. They may also try to move their head instead of their eyes or blink excessively.

Eye Alignment

Observation of the resting position of the eyes should be noted before other oculomotor impairments are assessed (Fig. 7-10). Misalignment of the eyes may occur when there is an imbalance in the eye muscles or a fracture to the orbital socket. Note any inward, outward, upward, or downward deviations in one or both eyes.

Eye alignment is objectively measured by observation of the light reflected off of the corneas with both eyes at the same time. The client should wear glasses or corrective lenses if typically worn. The therapist asks the seated client to gaze at a target at least 20 feet away so that the eyes are in the position of primary gaze. The therapist holds a penlight centered approximately 16 inches away from the client's eyes. The therapist observes the light reflection in each eye; the reflection should be in the same position in both

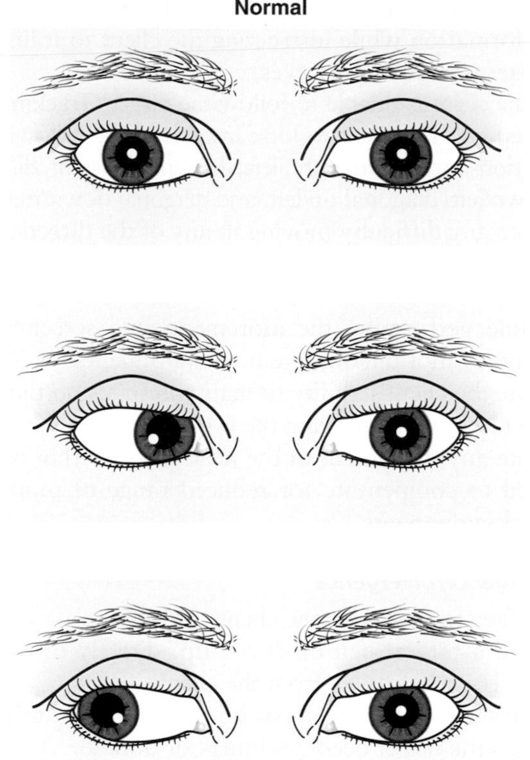

Figure 7-10. Eye alignment.

eyes (Fig. 7-10). Discrepancies in positions of the reflections are noted.[14]

Step 2: Visual Acuity Function

Distance Acuity

- Assure that the client is wearing prescribed eyewear.
- Point to three to five objects that are >10 feet away and ask the client to read or describe the image. Some examples can be wall clocks, paintings, or bulletin boards.
- Observe and record any difficulty with accuracy and observe any squinting or change is posture.

Near Acuity

- Assure that the client is wearing prescribed eyewear.
- Hold a newspaper or magazine 16 inches from the client's eyes (Fig. 7-11).
- Ask the client to read headline print, subheadings, and then fine print such as paragraph text.
- Observe and record any difficulties with accuracy at each of those levels and observe any squinting or change is posture or positioning of the text.

Step 3: Contrast Sensitivity

- Assure that there is sufficient lighting, but no glare.
- Have the client read the letters or numbers on a contrast sensitivity test, such as The Pelli-Robson contrast sensitivity chart, Vistech VCTS 6000 and 6500 Contrast Sensitivity Tests, or Hamilton-Veale Contrast Sensitivity Test (Fig. 7-12).
- Note the level of contrast sensitivity and any deficits.

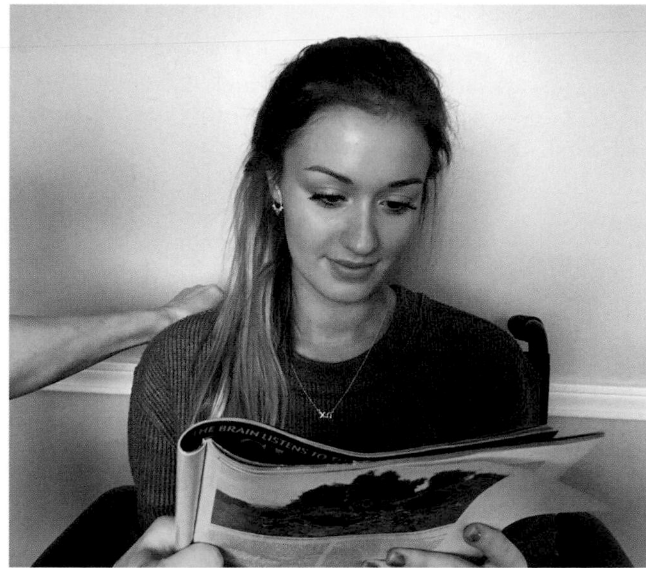

Figure 7-11. Visual acuity testing.

Step 4: Oculomotor

Fixation Testing

- Sit face-to-face with the client.
- Hold a target (pen or dowel tip) directly in front of and 16 inches away from the client's face (Fig. 7-13).
- Ask the client to focus on the object while the therapist counts for 5 seconds.
- Move the target horizontally 45° into the left visual field.
- Ask the client to look at the object, but to move only his or her eyes and not the head.
- Ask the client to maintain focus on the object while the therapist counts for 5 seconds.

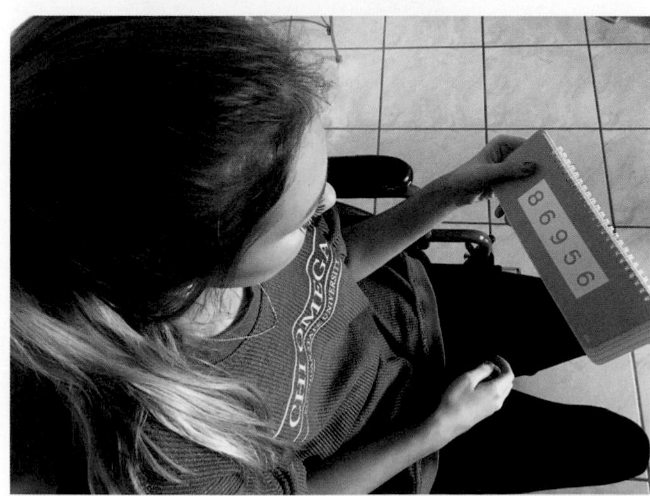

Figure 7-12. Contrast sensitivity testing.

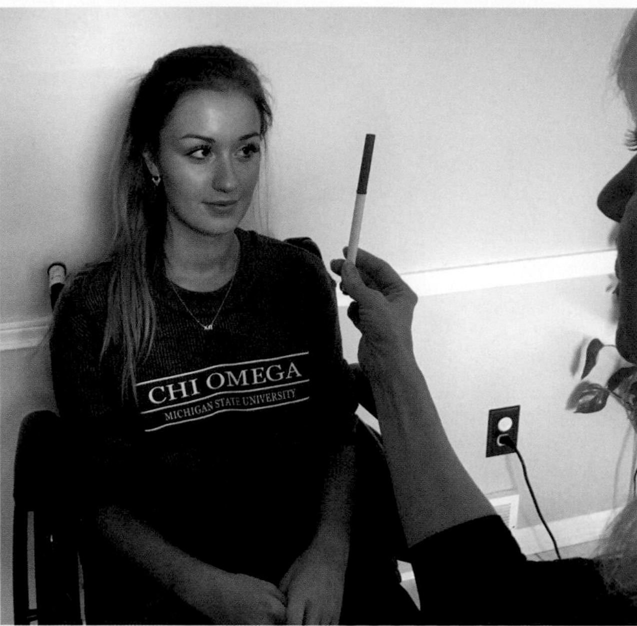

Figure 7-13. Fixation testing.

- Repeat this in the right visual field.
- Note any difficulty maintaining fixation on the object.

Range of Motion

- Sit face-to-face with the client.
- Hold a target (pen or dowel tip) directly in front of and 16 inches away from the client's face (Fig. 7-14).
- Instruct client to hold his or her head still and move only the eyes.
- Move the target in a large capital H formation and an O formation while instructing the client to follow the target with his or her eyes.
- If the client is unable to follow the target (**Tracking/Pursuits**), ask the client to look in each of the following directions: up, down, right, left, diagonal up/right, diagonal down/left, diagonal up/left, and diagonal down/right.
- Note any difficulty moving in any of the directions.

Tracking/Pursuits

- While performing the aforementioned screening for range of motion, observe tracking/pursuits.
- Note the client's ability to maintain focus on the moving target while moving the eyes smoothly.
- Note any movement of the head or body that may be used to compensate for reduced range of motion or tracking/pursuits.

Convergence/Divergence

- Sit face-to-face with the client.
- Hold a target (pen or dowel tip) directly in front of and 16 inches away from the client's face.
- Instruct the client to focus on the target and to report when the target becomes blurry or double.
- Slowly move the target toward the client's nose and slowly back out to 16 inches (Fig. 7-15).
- Note the client's ability to bring two eyes together nasally and back apart.

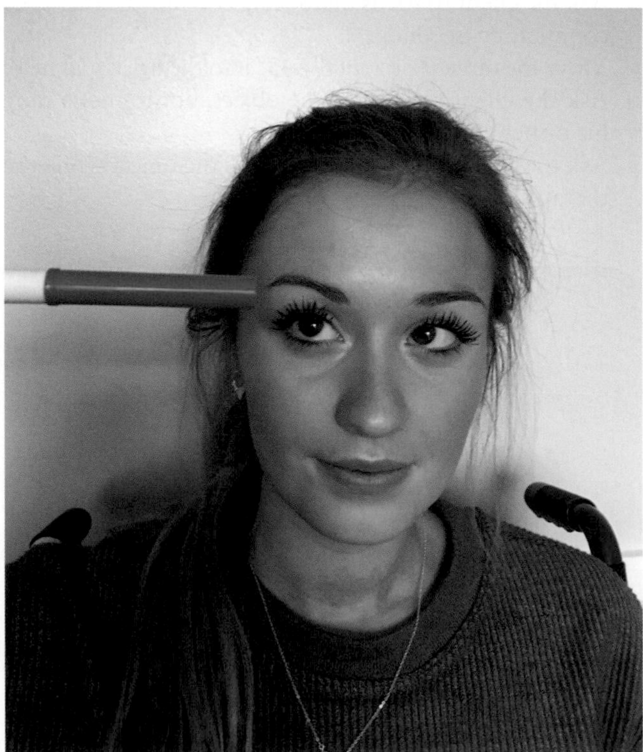

Figure 7-14. Range of motion and tracking/pursuits testing.

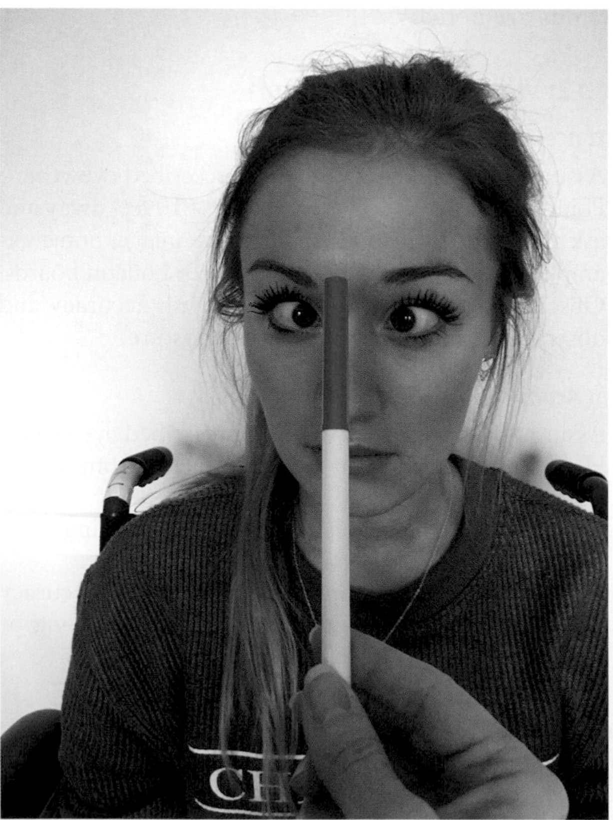

Figure 7-15. Convergence testing.

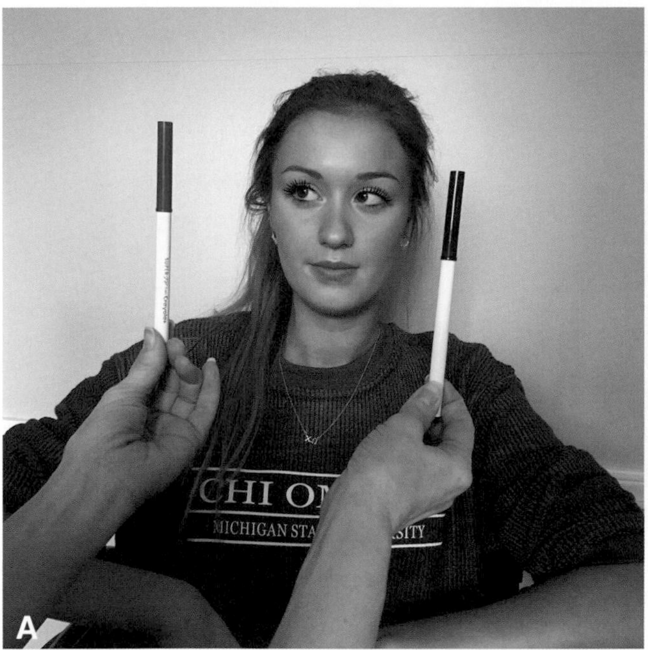

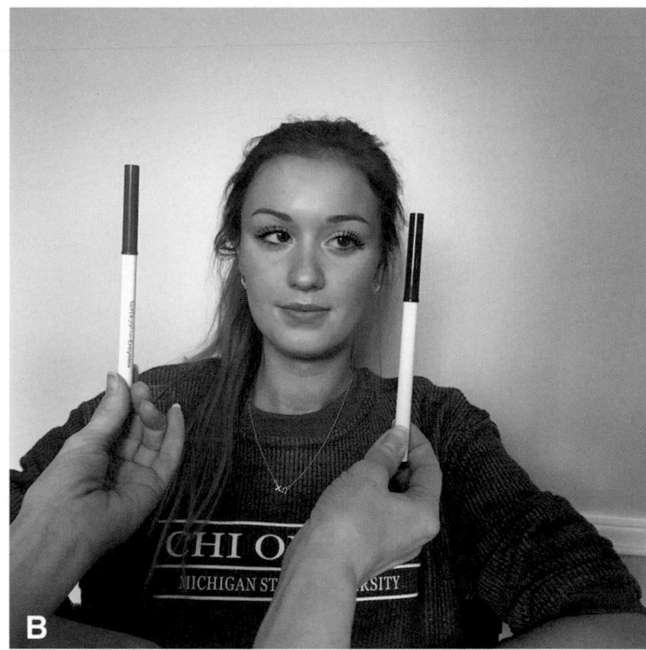

Figure 7-16. A. Saccades testing with shift to the right. **B.** Saccades testing with quick shift to the left.

- The client should report that the target becomes blurry at about 4 inches from the nose. Failure of the target to become blurry may be an indication of suppression of vision from one eye.
- Observe any drifting or deviations from the target in one or both eyes.

Saccades

- Sit face-to-face with the client.
- Hold a target (pen or dowel tip) in each hand. Each target should be of a different color (e.g., red and blue) and held approximately 16 inches away from the client's face and approximately 8 inches apart from each other.
- Instruct the client to hold his or her head still and look at one of the colored targets.
- Tell the client, "Look at the red target when I say red. Look at the blue target when I say blue, and remember to wait until I say to look."
- Instruct the client to look back and forth at the target for five to six times and then begin to move the targets farther apart. Instruct the client to keep shifting targets.
- When the targets are 12 to 14 inches apart, start to move them up and down and then cross them over each other and back three to four times while continuing to have the client switch focus on the targets.
- Observe the client's ability to maintain a focus on the target without over or undershooting it or moving the head or body. Also note any nystagmus that may be elicited during saccadic movements of the eyes (Fig. 7-16).

Pupillary Function

- Sit face-to-face with the client.
- Hold a pen light or small flashlight on the temporal side of the client's head.
- Slowly move the light in front of the client's eye and then repeat on the other side (Fig. 7-17).
- Observe the constriction of the pupil in response to the light.

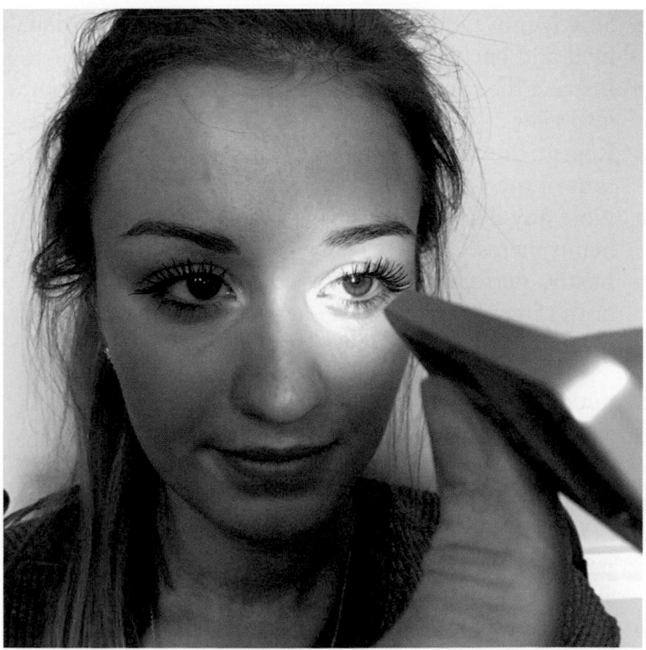

Figure 7-17. Pupillary function testing.

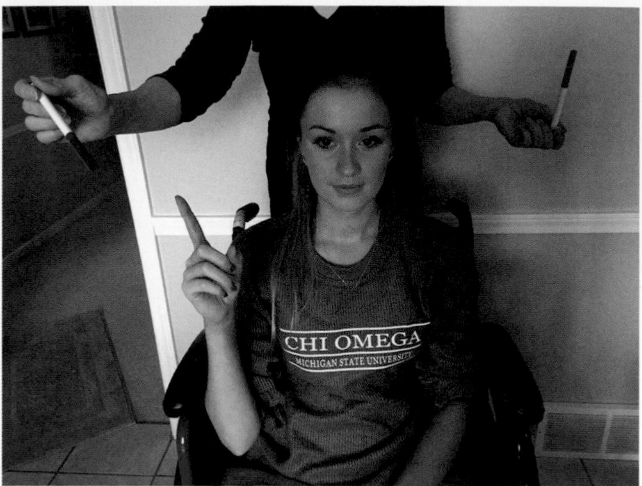

Figure 7-18. Visual field testing: confrontations.

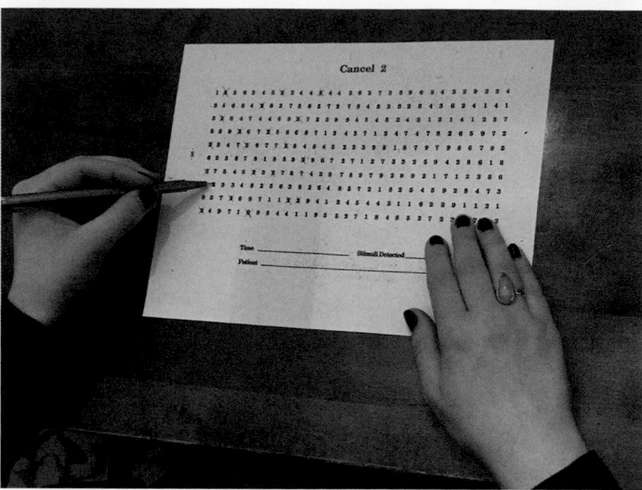

Figure 7-19. Sample of scanning sheet performance with right homonymous hemianopia.

- Note any associated reactions (constriction of the contralateral pupil) because this in an indicator of intact communication between the cerebral hemispheres.
- If a pen light or flashlight is not available, the therapist can use an object such as a pen to elicit pupillary constriction that accompanies accommodation. The pen should be moved directly toward the pupil to elicit constriction.

Step 5: Visual Fields

Confrontations

- Stand behind the client with another therapist in front to watch for any eye movement.
- Hold a target (pen or dowel tip) in each hand.
- Instruct the client to look straight ahead and fixate on a target.
- Slowly move one target at a time into the client's visual field and back out (Fig. 7-18).
- Instruct the client to point at each target when it comes into view.
- Repeat the movement of the targets into each quadrant of the visual fields.
- Note any delay in response in any of the quadrants or hemispheres.
- Lastly, perform a simultaneous presentation. Move both targets in at eye level at the same time. Note any delay in response on one side.

Scanning

- The client should be seated in front of a hard surface, such as a table or a desk. Give the client a pen.
- Place a scanning sheet at the client's midline squarely in front of the body. If the person attempts to move the paper to one side or turn the paper, tape the scanning sheet to the table in the correct position.
- Instruct the client to mark or cancel all of the targeted letters, numbers, or symbols on the sheet as quickly as possible (Fig. 7-19).
- Observe the scanning pattern. Left to right and zigzag (left to right, then right to left) are the most common scanning patterns for people from Western societies in which they learn to read in a horizontal pattern. Other patterns are vertical or random. A vertical pattern may indicate reduced visual fields, and a random pattern may indicate deficits in attention.
- Measure the speed of scanning. Slowed speed may be used to compensate for deficits in scanning. Most scanning sheets can be completed in 1 to 2 minutes.
- Check the accuracy of the cancellations and note any patterns of errors. Missing targets in specific hemispheres or quadrants may indicate hemianopic visual field deficits.

Line Bisection

- The client should be seated in front of a hard surface, such as a table or a desk. Give the client a pen.
- Place a line bisection sheet at the client's midline squarely in front of the body. If the person attempts to move the paper to one side or turn the paper, tape the scanning sheet to the table in the correct position.
- Instruct the client to mark the middle or cut into half each line on the sheet (Fig. 7-20).
- Check the accuracy of the marks. If the line is marked toward one side on each line or if lines are missed on one side of the paper, it may indicate hemianopic visual field deficits. For example, a client who marks all of the lines toward the left side may be having difficulty seeing the right side of the lines, and therefore, the center is skewed.

Drawings

- The client should be seated in front of a hard surface, such as a table or a desk.
- Place a blank piece of paper in front of the client and give the client a pen.
- Instruct the client to draw a clock with the time at 9:15. You may also instruct the client to draw a person or draw a flower.

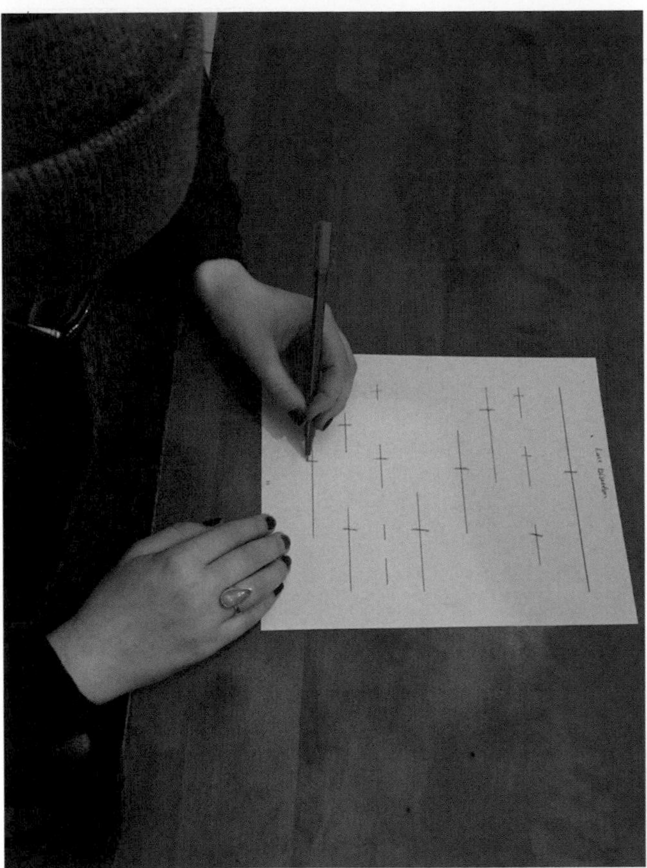

Figure 7-20. Line bisection sheet.

- If the person is having difficulty, this test can be graded by providing a line drawing to copy or a partially drawn figure.
- Note the accuracy of the figures and any lateralization, such as not drawing one side of the figure or drawing all of the parts of the figure on one half. These types of errors may indicate hemianopic visual field deficits (Fig. 7-21).

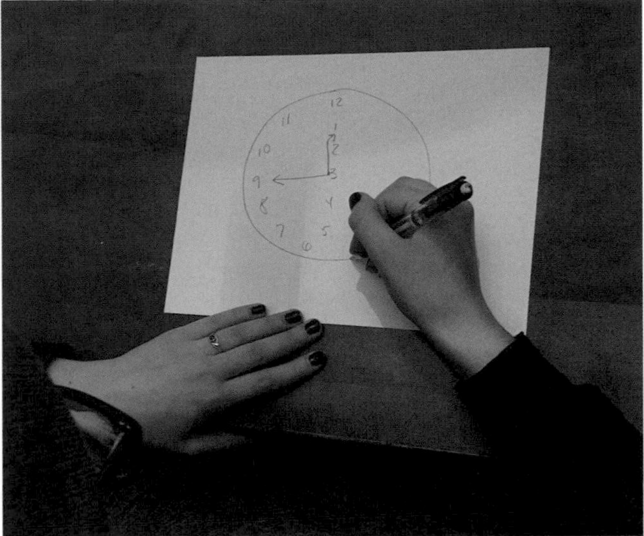

Figure 7-21. Example of figure drawing.

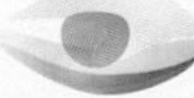

CASE STUDY

Patient Information

Quinn is a 43-year-old male who works full time as a project manager at a large technology firm. He was recently involved in a motor vehicle accident when driving home from work. As Quinn entered an intersection, another car ran a red light and struck his passenger side door at a high rate of speed. His car was totaled on impact. Quinn was sent to the hospital by ambulance for evaluation. He did not have any obvious head injuries and was discharged home the same evening. The next morning, Quinn's wife drove him to work. During the short 3-mile commute, Quinn experienced nausea and dizziness as a passenger in the car. While at the office, Quinn experienced headaches, dizziness, and sensitivity to light. He could not tolerate looking at his computer screen for more than a few minutes at a time. Quinn made an appointment with his primary care provider. He was diagnosed with a concussion, or mild traumatic brain injury (mTBI), and referred to occupational therapy for further evaluation. Prior to the accident, Quinn lived with his wife Sophie and two young daughters. He was independent in all ADLs and IADLs. Quinn maintained a very busy social life and active lifestyle.

Assessment Process

Prior to the initial evaluation, Quinn's OTR completed a chart review to create an occupational profile. During the client interview, the OTR asked open-ended questions to gain greater understanding of what a typical day is like for Quinn, what is important to him, and what he hopes to gain from occupational therapy intervention. The OTR summarized this information to create treatment goals with Quinn and Sophie. Next, the OTR administered the interviewer version of the National Eye Institute Visual Function Questionnaire-25 (NEI VFQ-25) to examine Quinn's vision-targeted health status. At the same time, Sophie completed the self-administered version of the assessment in the waiting room. Comparing the results of both assessments would provide insight into Quinn's current level of self-awareness, as well as the functional impact of visual impairment on his health-related quality of life.

The OTR completed a basic vision screening to assess Quinn's visual acuity, visual fields, oculomotor function (pursuits, saccades, convergence), and binocular vision. A standard vision chart was used to measure Quinn's visual acuity at near and far distances. A gross measurement of Quinn's visual fields was obtained through confrontation testing. Prior to screening Quinn's oculomotor function, the OTR assessed for misalignment of his eyes with a penlight. To assess smooth pursuits, the OTR instructed Quinn to follow a moving target in clockwise and counterclockwise motions, for two rotations in each direction. To assess saccadic eye movements, the OTR instructed Quinn to rapidly alternate his gaze between

(*continued*)

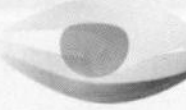

CASE STUDY *(continued)*

two stationary targets for five round trips, or a total of 10 fixations. To screen for deficits in convergence and divergence, the OTR instructed Quinn to fixate on a moving target as it moved slowly toward, and away from the bridge of his nose. Should Quinn's vision screening indicate signs of visual impairment, the OTR would administer standardized assessments to gather additional information. Finally, functional task observations will be used to determine whether and how Quinn's visual impairment may be affecting his functional performance. The findings from Quinn's visual screening will assist the OTR when selecting adaptations and modifications to promote enhanced participation.

Assessment Results

Quinn's chart review revealed no significant medical history prior to the accident. During the client interview, Quinn's subjective complaints included headaches, dizziness, and sensitivity to light. He also reported blurred vision after brief periods of reading and difficulty keeping his place on the page. Sophie indicated increased irritability and fatigue because of disturbed sleep patterns. At baseline, Quinn had a love of books and was an avid reader. He enjoyed an active lifestyle as a mountain biking enthusiast and dedicated member of an amateur cycling team. Quinn also reported looking forward to coaching his daughter's soccer team next season.

Results from the NEI VFQ-25 identified role limitations, difficulty with near vision activities, and dependency on others because of vision. More specifically, Quinn reported extreme difficulty driving, reading ordinary print, and noticing objects off to the side when walking. He also reported accomplishing less at work and feeling limited in how long he can tolerate work because of his vision. Screening for specific visual deficits would help the OTR to explain these functional limitations.

During the interview, the OTR noted that although Quinn's body was in a neutral midline position, his head was held with a slight turn to the left. This posture was indicative of visual field loss. During confrontation testing, the OTR presented targets at the 2, 4, 6, 8, and 10 o'clock positions. Quinn had difficulty finding targets in the 8 and 10 o'clock positions (i.e., left peripheral visual field). Quinn's performance provided the OTR cause to "rule-in" the possibility of a visual field deficit.

Findings from Quinn's visual screening indicated oculomotor dysfunction; therefore, further examination with standardized assessments was warranted. The Northeastern State College of Optometry (NSUCO) Oculomotor Test was administered to evaluate Quinn's oculomotor function. As Quinn followed the target for smooth pursuits, he was observed to refixate four different times over four rotations. During the saccadic eye movement subtest, Quinn reported feeling nausea and dizziness after three round trips. The OTR observed moderate overshooting of targets on two occasions, as well as compensatory head movements >50% of the time. These results warrant a more comprehensive examination by a qualified eye care professional.

When assessing convergence and divergence, Quinn was unable to converge his eyes while fixating on a target positioned approximately 6 inches from the bridge of his nose. The OTR administered the convergence Insufficiency Symptom Survey (CISS) to quantify the severity of symptoms that may be associated with convergence insufficiency. Quinn's score of 30 on the CISS was indicative of convergence insufficiency. Functional observations confirmed that Quinn was having difficulty completing tasks at near point. Quinn was able to perform all ADLs and IADLs independently, except for driving, with minimal difficulty when given extra time. The results of Quinn's occupational therapy evaluation justified establishing a plan of care and making a referral to a neuro-optometrist for a more comprehensive evaluation.

Occupational Therapy Problem List

ADLs/IADLs:

- Client is dependent on his wife for community mobility due to visual impairment.
- Overall participation in daily activities has decreased due to irritability and fatigue.

Rest and Sleep:

- Sleep disturbances make falling and staying asleep difficult.

Work:

- Productivity at work is limited by constant headaches and fatigue.
- Sensitivity to light limits the client's ability to use a computer for extended periods of time.

Social Participation:

- Difficulty following moving objects hinders the client's ability to fulfill his role as soccer coach.

Leisure:

- Decreased tolerance for visual motion limits the client's ability to engage in physical activities such as mountain biking.
- Inability to converge the eyes at near point impacts the client's ability to read.

Most Commonly Used Standardized Assessments

Instrument and Reference	Intended Purpose	Administration Time	Validity	Reliability	Sensitivity	Strengths and Weaknesses
Brain Injury Visual Assessment Battery for Adults (biVABA)[14]	A battery of objective tests to evaluate visual processing skills following brain injury.	Individual subtests take between 3 and 5 minutes to administer. The entire test battery may take up to 60 minutes.	Not reported	Not reported	Not reported	*Strengths*: Comprehensive, includes detailed guidelines for administration and interpretation; can be used to evaluate clients with brain injury and low vision. *Weaknesses*: No psychometric data available. Only the visual search subtest has been empirically tested; however, most of the subtests have been accepted by ophthalmologists as valid and reliable assessment tools.
Revised-Self-Report Assessment of Functional Visual Performance (R-SRAFVP)[15]	An objective assessment comprised of 33 vision-dependent ADL and IADL tasks that older adults with age-related eye disease most often report as being difficult due to vision loss.	Assessment takes approximately 20 minutes to administer.	Content Validity Index score of 0.9 demonstrates adequate evidence to evaluate the ability of older adults with vision impairment[16,17]	Internal consistency reliability coefficients for individual components (r range = 0.72–0.84); overall score ($r = 0.92$) (95% CI = 0.89–0.94)[16,17]	Not reported	*Strengths:* Revised to reflect activities completed by older adults in the digital age; available online, free of charge; provides detailed guidelines for administration and interpretation; toolkit spreadsheet automatically calculates composite score, percent disability, and G-code level. *Weaknesses:* Requires copyright permissions from the authors.
National Eye Institute Visual Function Questionnaire-25 (NEI VFQ-25)[18]	A self-report survey of vision-targeted health status that measures the influence of visual impairment on health-related quality of life.	Administration of the interviewer format takes approximately 10 minutes.	Significant correlations between NEI VFQ-25 total score and SF-36 variables ($r = 0.06$, $p < 0.05$); best-corrected visual acuity (BCVA) for the better- and-worse seeing eyes ($r = 0.68$, $p < 0.0001$); contrast sensitivity (r range = 0.06–0.56, p = 0.05–0.0001)[19]	Internal consistency reliability coefficients for multi-item subscales (r range = 0.62–0.91); total score ($r = 0.96$)[19]	Not reported	*Strengths*: Available online, free of charge; interviewer administered or self-administered formats; a robust predictor of future health and mortality in population-based studies. *Weaknesses*: Scores do not translate to a specific level of visual acuity or visual field impairment.

(*continued*)

Most Commonly Used Standardized Assessments (*continued*)

Instrument and Reference	Intended Purpose	Administration Time	Validity	Reliability	Sensitivity	Strengths and Weaknesses
Catherine Bergego Scale (CBS)[20]	A standardized checklist that detects the presence and degree of unilateral behavioral neglect and self-awareness of neglect (anosognosia) during self-care activities.	Administration may take approximately 15–45 minutes, depending on severity.	Significant correlation between CBS total score and performance on five conventional paper-and-pencil tests (r range = 0.49–0.77, $p < 0.0001$). Anosognosia correlated significantly with neglect severity ($r = 0.82$, $p = 0.0001$).[21,22] Significant correlation with line bisection subtest on the BIT ($r = 0.54$, $p < 0.05$).[23]	Good inter-rater reliability (r range = 0.59–0.99). Internal consistency reliability coefficients between individual question scores and CBS total score (r range = 0.58–0.88).[22] No studies have reported the test–retest reliability of the CBS.	The CBS was more sensitive to detecting the presence of spatial neglect than conventional paper-and-pencil tests.[22]	*Strengths*: Involves direct observation of performance during self-care activities; provides client insight into disabilities; clinician administered checklist and patient administered questionnaire formats. Normative data for adults.[24] *Weaknesses*: No manual: for instructions on administration and scoring, see the Kessler Foundation Neglect Assessment Process (KF-NAP).[25] May not be appropriate for some clients as test items require upper and lower limb movements in various testing positions.
Behavioral Inattention Test (BIT)[26]	A standardized assessment battery that detects the presence and extent of visual neglect. Versions include the Conventional (BITC) and Behavioral (BITB).	Administration takes approximately 30–40 minutes.	Significant correlations between BIT scores and Occupational Therapy Checklist ($r = -0.65$), the Rivermead Activities of Daily Living Assessment ($r = 0.55$),[27] and the Barthel Index ($r = 0.65$).[28]	Excellent test–retest reliability ($r = 0.89$ BITC; $r = 0.97$ BITB). Inter-rater reliability ($r = 0.99$ BITC; $r = 0.99$ BITB).[27]	The BITB was the single best predictor of poor functional outcomes at 3, 6, and 12-month follow-ups after stroke.[29]	*Strengths*: Involves observation during everyday tasks. Detects different forms of visual neglect. Normative data for adults.[27] *Weaknesses*: Measures neglect in peripersonal space only. Unable to distinguish between sensory and motor neglect. Should not be used with clients who have difficulty communicating (e.g., apraxia or aphasia).
Convergence Insufficiency Symptom Survey (CISS)[30]	A standardized self-report survey designed to quantify the severity of symptoms associated with convergence insufficiency.	Administration takes approximately 10 minutes.	Significant correlations between the responses of adults (0.88) and children (0.77).[31]	The mean difference in CISS scores between the first and second administration (0.68 points, SD = 4.2) indicates minimum bias.[31]	The CISS demonstrates excellent discrimination (sensitivity = 97.8%, and specificity = 87%).[31]	*Strengths*: Available online, free of charge; clinician administered or self-administered formats; Normative data available for children aged 9–18[30] and adults aged 19–30.[31]

Mars Letter Contrast Sensitivity Chart[32]	An objective screening to determine the lowest contrast level that can be detected.	Administration takes approximately 1 minute on average.	Mean contrast sensitivity scores on the Mars test and the Pelli-Robson test did not differ significantly for the group as a whole, for subgroups, or between age groups.[33]	The Mars test shows good agreement with the Pelli-Robson test and similar test–retest repeatability.[33]	Not reported	*Strengths*: Hand-held, durable, and portable; easy to illuminate evenly, greater accuracy than wall charts due to finer contrast decrements and scoring procedure.
Useful Field of View (UFOV) Test[34]	A standardized assessment designed to estimate the spatial extent of the useful visual field of view.	Administration takes approximately 15 minutes.	Scores on the UFOV were highly correlated when using either a touch screen or mouse to respond ($r = 0.916$, $p = 0.001$).[35]	The UFOV has good test–retest reliability when using a mouse ($r = 0.88$) or touch screen ($r = 0.73$).[35] Internal consistency reliability coefficients between three UFOV subtests (r range = 0.72–0.80) and composite score ($r = 0.88$).[36]	The UFOV showed better sensitivity and specificity as compared to standard perimetry testing and crash risk as compared to conventional neuropsychological measures.[37,38]	*Strengths*: Strong predictor of fitness to drive and motor vehicle crashes in older adults. Normative data for older adults aged 65–94.[37] *Weakness*: The extent of usable field may not be constant across testing parameters and spatial range.
Developmental Eye Movement (DEM) Test[39]	A standardized assessment of the quality, speed, and accuracy of saccadic eye movements.	Administration takes <5 minutes.	All DEM subtests except for ratio had significant negative correlations with the Wide Range Achievement Test (WRAT): vertical time ($r = -0.79$, $p < 0.001$); horizontal time ($r = -0.78$, $p < 0.001$).[39]	The DEM has good test–retest reliability for vertical time ($r = 0.89$, $p < 0.001$) and horizontal time ($r = 0.86$, $p < 0.001$). Medium test–retest reliability for ratio ($r = 0.57$, $p < 0.01$). Internal consistency reliability coefficients between all subtests were significant ($p < 0.001$), except vertical time and ratio score ($r = -0.5$).[39]	Not reported	*Strengths*: Useful for patients with poor attention and concentration. Normative data for children aged 6–13[39] and youth and adults aged 14–68.[40] *Weaknesses*: The visual-verbal format requires reading numbers; therefore, it is not useful with nonverbal individuals.
Northeastern State College of Optometry (NSUCO) Oculomotor Test[41]	A standardized assessment that uses direct observation to assess visual saccades and pursuits.	Administration time is <5 minutes.	Significant correlations between the oculomotor behavior of above average and below average readers on a standardized reading assessment ($p < 0.05$).[42]	Good test–retest reliability ($r = 0.87$, $p < 0.05$).[43] Inter-rater reliability pursuits ($r = 0.73$); saccades ($r = 0.75$).[41] Internal consistency has not been reported.	Not reported	*Strengths*: Requires limited verbal interaction. Examiner can make objective observations of performance to decide whether referral to a vision specialist is needed. Normative data for ages 5 to 14+.[43] *Weaknesses*: Has not been formally tested on adults with acquired brain injury.

ADL, activities of daily living; IADL, instrumental activities of daily living; CI, confidence interval; SD, standard deviation.

References

1. Warren M. Intervention for adults with vision impairment from acquired brain injury. In: Warren M, Barstow E, eds. *Occupational Therapy Interventions for Adults with Low Vision*. Bethesda, MD: AOTA; 2011:403–448.
2. Bourne RRA, Flaxman SR, Braithwaite T, et al. Magnitude, temporal trends, and projections of the global prevalence of blindness and distance and near vision impairment: a systematic review and meta-analysis. *Lancet Glob Health*. 2017;5:e888–e897. doi:10.1016/S2214-109X(17)30293-0.
3. Rosenberg EA, Sperazza LC. The visually impaired patient. *Am Fam Physician*. 2008;77:1431–1438.
4. Dirette DP. Low vision disorders. In: Atchison B, Dirette DP, eds. *Conditions in Occupational Therapy: Effect on Occupational Performance*. 5th ed. Philadelphia, PA: Wolters Kluwer; 2017:499–511.
5. Rowe F, Brand D, Jackson CA, Price A, et al. Visual impairment following stroke: do stroke patients require vision assessment? *Age Ageing*. 2009;38:188–193. doi:10.1093/ageing/afn230.
6. Brahm K, Wilgenburg H, Kirby J, Ingalla S. Visual impairment and dysfunction in combat-injured service members with traumatic brain injury. *Optom Vis Sci*. 2009;86:817–825. doi:10.1097/OPX.0b013e3181adff2d.
7. Cockerham G, Goodrich G, Weichel E, et al. Eye and visual function in traumatic brain injury. *J Rehabil Res Dev*. 2009;46:811–818. doi:10.1682/JRRD.2008.08.0109.
8. Dougherty A, MacGregor A, Han P, Heltemes KJ, Galarneau MR. Visual dysfunction following blast-related traumatic brain injury from the battlefield. *Brain Inj* 2010;25:8–13. doi:10.3109/02699052.2010.536195.
9. Ward J. *The Student's Guide to Cognitive Neuroscience*. 3rd ed. London, England/New York, NY: Psychology Press; 2015.
10. Lundy-Ekman L. *Neuroscience: Fundamentals for Rehabilitation*. 3rd ed. Philadelphia, PA: W.B. Saunders; 2007.
11. Purves D, Augustine GJ, Fitzpatrick D, et al. *Neuroscience*. 3rd ed. Sunderland, MA: Sinauer Associates; 2004.
12. Scheiman M. *Understanding and Managing Vision Deficits: A Guide for Occupational Therapists*. 3rd ed. Thorofare, NJ: Slack; 2011.
13. Scheiman M, Scheiman M, Whittaker S. *Low Vision Rehabilitation: A Practical Guide for Occupational Therapists*. Thorofare, NJ: Slack; 2007.
14. Warren M. *Brain Injury Assessment Battery for Adults: Test Manual*. Birmingham, AL: visABILITIES Rehab Services, Inc; 1998.
15. Warren M, Bachelder J, Velozo C, Hicks E. *The Self-Report Assessment of Functional Visual Performance*. Birmingham, AL: Occupational Therapy Departments at University of Alabama at Birmingham and University of Florida at Gainesville; 2008.
16. Zemina CL, Warren M, Yuen HK. Revised Self-Report Assessment of Functional Visual Performance (R-SRAFVP)—Part I: content validation. *Am J Occup Therapy*. 2018;72:1–7. doi:10.5014/ajot.2018.030197.
17. Snow M, Warren M, Yuen HK. Revised Self-Report Assessment of Functional Visual Performance (R-SRAFVP)—Part II: construct validation. *Am J Occup Therapy*. 2018;72:1–8. doi:10.5014/ajot.2018.030205.
18. Mangione C, Lee PP, Gutierrez, PR, Spritzer K. Development of the 25-item National Eye Institute Visual Function Questionnaire (VFQ-25). *Arch Ophthalmol*. 2001;119:1050–1058. doi:10.1001/archopht.119.7.1050.
19. Revicki DA, Rentz AM, Harnam N, Thomas VS. Reliability and validity of the National Eye Institute Visual Function Questionnaire-25 in patients with age-related macular degeneration. *Invest Ophthalmol Vis Sci*. 2010;51:712–717. doi:10.1167/iovs.09-3766.
20. Azouvi P, Marchal F, Samuel C, et al. Functional consequences and awareness of unilateral neglect: A study of evaluation scale. *Neuropsychol Rehabil*. 1996;6:133–150. doi:10.1080/713755501.
21. Azouvi P, Samuel C, Louis-Dreyfus A, et al. Sensitivity of clinical and behavioural tests of spatial neglect after right hemisphere stroke. *J Neurol Neurosurg Psychiatry*. 2002;73:160–166. doi:10.1136/jnnp.73.2.160.
22. Azouvi P, Olivier S, de Montety G, Samuel C, Louis-Dreyfus A, Tesio L. Behavioral assessment of unilateral neglect: study of the psychometric properties of the Catherine Bergego Scale. *Arch Phys Med Rehabil*. 2003;84:51–57. doi:10.1053/apmr.2003.50062.
23. Luukkainen-Markkula R, Tarkka IM, Pitkanen K, Sivenius J. Comparison of the Behavioral Inattention Test and the Catherine Bergego Scale in assessment of hemispatial neglect. *Neuropsychol Rehabil*. 2011;21:103–116. doi:10.1080/09602011.2010.531619.
24. Goedert KM, Chen P, Botticello A, Masmela JR. Psychometric evaluation of neglect assessment reveals motor-explanatory predictor of functional disability in acute-stage spatial neglect. *Arch Phys Med Rehabil*. 2012;93:137–142. doi:10.1016/j.apmr.2011.06.036.
25. Chen P, Hreha K, Fortis P, Goedert KM. Functional assessment of spatial neglect: a review of the Catherine Bergego Scale and an introduction of the Kessler Foundation neglect assessment process. *Top Stroke Rehabil*. 2012;19:423–435. doi:10.1310/tsr1905-423.
26. Wilson B, Cockburn J, Halligan P. Development of a behavioral test of visuospatial neglect. *Arch Phys Med Rehabil*. 1987;68:98–102.
27. Halligan PW, Cockburn J, Wilson BA. The behavioral assessment of visual neglect. *Neuropsychol Rehabil*. 1991;1:3–32. doi:10.1080/09602019108401377.
28. Cassidy TP, Bruce DW, Lewis S, Gray CS. The association of visual field deficits and visuospatial neglect in acute right-hemisphere stroke patients. *Age Ageing*. 1999;28:257–260. doi:10.1093/ageing/28.3.257.
29. Jehkonen M, Ahonen JP, Dastidar P, et al. Visual neglect as a predictor of functional outcome one year after stroke. *Acta Neurol Scand*. 2000;101:195–201. doi:10.1034/j.16000404.2000.101003195.x.
30. Borsting EJ, Rouse MW, Mitchell GL, et al. Validity and reliability of the revised convergence insufficiency symptom survey in children ages 9–18 years. *Optom Vis Sci*. 2003;80:832–838. doi:10.1097/OPX.0b013e3181989252.
31. Rouse MW, Borsting EJ, Mitchell GL, et al. Validity and reliability of the revised convergence insufficiency symptom survey in adults. *Opthalmic Physiol Opt*. 2004;24:384–390. doi:10.1111/j.1475-1313.2004.00202.x.
32. Arditi A. Improving the design of the letter contrast sensitivity test. *Invest Ophthalmol Vis Sci*. 2005;46:2225–2229. doi:10.1167/iovs.04-1198.

33. Dougherty BE, Flom RE, Bullimore MA. An evaluation of the Mars Letter Contrast Sensitivity Test. *Optom Vis Sci.* 2005;82:970–975. doi:10.1097/01.opx.0000187844.27025.ea.
34. Ball K, Owsley C. The useful field of view test: a new technique for evaluating age-related declines in visual function. *J Am Optom Assoc.* 1993;64:71–79.
35. Edwards JD, Vance DE, Wadley VG, et al. Reliability and validity of useful field of view test scores as administered by personal computer. *J Clin Exp Neuropsychol.* 2005;27:529–543. doi:10.1080/13803390490515432.
36. Visual Awareness Research Group, Inc. *UFOV User's Guide.* Version 6.1.4. Punta Gorda, FL; 2009.
37. Edwards JD, Ross LA, Wadley VG, et al. The useful field of view test: normative data for older adults. *Arch Clin Neuropsychol.* 2006;21:275–286. doi:10.1016/j.acn.2006.03.001.
38. Owsley C, Ball K, McGwin G, et al. Predicting future crash involvement in older drivers: who is at risk? *JAMA.* 1998;279:1083–1088.
39. Garzia RP, Richman JE, Nicholson SB, Gaines CS. A new visual-verbal saccade test: the developmental eye movement test (DEM). *J Am Optom Assoc.* 1990;61: 124–135.
40. Sampedro AG, Richman JE, Sanchez Pardo M. The adult developmental eye movement test (A-DEM) a tool for saccadic evaluation in adults. *J Behav Optom.* 2003; 14;1–5.
41. Maples WC, Ficklin TW. Inter–rater and test–rater reliability of pursuits and saccades. *J Am Optom Assoc.* 1988;59:549–552.
42. Maples WC, Ficklin TW. Comparison of eye movement skills between above average and below average readers. *J Behav Optom.* 1990;1:87–91.
43. Maples WC, Atchley J, Ficklin TW. Northeastern State University College of Optometry's oculomotor norms. *J Behav Optom.* 1992;3:143–150.

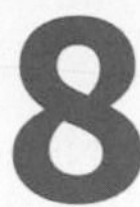

Chapter 8

Visual Function Intervention

Christine P. Below and Kelly Lewis

LEARNING OBJECTIVES

This chapter will allow the reader to:

1. Identify and describe specific treatment strategies for low vision (LV) and visual deficits related to neurological conditions.
2. Identify and describe treatment approaches for visual field defects.
3. Describe the functional implications of LV diagnoses and visual deficits resulting from neurological injury.
4. Apply understanding of best intervention when providing treatment for clients with visual dysfunction.

CHAPTER OUTLINE

TERMINOLOGY

Anchor: a visual or tactile cue on the side of visual field deficit to indicate starting position and facilitate scanning.

Central vision: the portion of the visual field, which is the inner 30° of vision and central fixation.

Eccentric viewing (EV): a visual compensatory technique in which a person looks slightly away from the subject in order to view it peripherally with another area of the macula/retina.

Fresnel prism: a compensatory lens that is applied to glasses to shift an image from the nonseeing area into the intact visual field, typically used with individuals with homonymous hemianopsia.

Peripheral visual field: the portion of vision that is outside the center gaze, and it is the largest portion of the visual field.

Preferred retinal loci (PRL): a spot on the retina just outside the damaged area that allows a person to see using his or her best vision during EV.

Relative distance magnification: a nonoptical enlargement strategy achieved by decreasing the distance between the desired stimulus and the eye.

Relative size magnification: an enlargement strategy in which the actual size of the object is increased, thereby increasing the retinal image with either optical or nonoptical devices.

Vision therapy: an organized therapeutic regimen used to treat a number of neuromuscular, neurophysiological, and neurosensory conditions that interfere with visual function.

Visual efficiency: the visual system's ability to clearly, efficiently, and comfortably gather visual information at school, work, or play. The various component skills that are important in this process are called visual efficiency skills and include the subcategories of accommodation, binocular vision, and ocular motility.

Visual integrity: the visual system's ability to see clearly at all distances and have a healthy optical system and eye.

Introduction

Occupational therapists address visual impairments in adults following neurological injury and age-related eye conditions. Persons with visual impairments that have resulted from injuries or age-related eye diseases may experience decreased ability to use their vision to participate in daily occupations. Reading, writing, and driving are almost completely dependent on vision, and many other functional activities may be negatively impacted by a decline in vision. Occupational therapists need to understand how vision is related to activity demands, and the impact of vision loss on a person's occupational performance to provide effective treatment to maximize safety, independence, and confidence for completing daily functional activities. Occupational therapists need to also be aware of the various health care professionals that are involved in treatment of visual deficits. A preferred model of treatment for visual impairments whether related to low vision (LV) conditions or neurological conditions includes a team of practitioners who may include, but is not limited to, ophthalmology, optometry, vision rehabilitation therapists, orientation and mobility specialists, and occupational therapists.

Neurological causes of vision disorder include traumatic brain injury (TBI), stroke, and concussions; and diseases such as Parkinson, multiple sclerosis, and Alzheimer dementia.[1] According to Warren's hierarchy of visual perception, visual foundation skills, including acuity, visual fields (VFs), and oculomotor function, should be addressed before high-level perceptual skills.[2] While some visual impairments following neurological injury may be remediated, most LV conditions are progressive and will be addressed using compensatory and adaptive strategies. This chapter focuses on treatment of visual foundation skills of acuity, oculomotor, and visual field deficits (VFD).

Conceptual Foundation Underlying Interventions for Visual Impairment

A functional definition of LV is uncorrectable vision loss that interferes with daily activities. It is better defined in terms of function, rather than numerical test results.[3] In other words, LV is not enough vision to do whatever it is you need to do, which can vary from person to person.

Many LV conditions cannot be corrected with surgery, leaving the individual with permanent vision loss. It is the occupational therapist's job to instruct and educate these individuals in techniques that will allow safe functioning at the highest level of independence possible in all activities of daily living (ADLs) and instrumental activities of daily living (IADLs).

An occupational therapist must use his or her best clinical judgment to choose treatments involving remediation, compensation, and/or adaptation. Each eye condition has its own set of symptoms, and each individual has a unique set of functional challenges relating to his or her eye condition. Therefore, it is important to know which strategies to use for the best functional outcome.

Remediation

Often, remediation is the preferred first treatment to address the underlying cause. Remediation, however, is only possible for some oculomotor conditions caused by muscle weakness or cranial nerve involvement. Each oculomotor issue has its own set of remediation strategies. Scanning and tracking exercises can be initiated to increase the strength of the eye muscles involved. Generally, scanning exercises start small and then advance to cover a larger area. For saccades, exercises are started at a greater distance, which requires less precision when changing focus from one object to another. As control is gained, near exercises are introduced, which require more precise control. For some oculomotor issues, a referral to an optometrist or ophthalmologist is advised because **vision therapy** may be indicated. This is true for binocular vision deficits.

In some cases, remediation has been shown to be not effective. For decreased acuity, remediation is not possible, so adaptation and compensation techniques are initiated to immediately impact safety and function, as well as a referral to an optometrist or ophthalmologist. Although controversy exists regarding the ability to remediate VFD, an occupational therapist will introduce compensation and adaptation strategies. In a situation when safety is at risk, compensation and adaptation strategies are introduced immediately to minimize safety risks during functional activities. Compensation and adaptation strategies may need to be implemented prior to remediation in this case.

Compensation

Compensation is the use of internal and/or external strategies to improve performance on a desired activity. This involves using a top-down approach to maximize safety and independence immediately. Examples of compensation include moving an object closer to the eye for better viewing, pacing techniques, organizational strategies, organized scanning patterns, line guides, and **anchors** to name a few.

Each condition requires its own set of compensatory strategies. For example, for poor oculomotor control that affects keeping one's place while reading, a line guide or using a finger to keep one's place may be taught. Having a bright-colored anchor at the left and/or right side of the page to encourage full scanning of the page may be helpful for those with decreased scanning abilities and/or VFD. Decreasing clutter in the environment may assist a person in finding an item when scanning ability is compromised. By teaching an individual about an organized scanning pattern, he or she is more likely to find an item when searching a busy cupboard or drawer. These strategies are taught to the individual with the goal of being used independently to maximize function and safety.

Adaptation

Adaptation is the process of using changes in the environment or changing the demands of a task to increase safety and function. Like compensation, adaptation is a top-down approach, and it can be used when treating all aspects of LV. The most common forms of adaptation for an individual with decreased vision are adjusting placement and intensity of lighting, increasing contrast between items, and adjusting print size to one that can be easily seen. Audible devices such as a talking thermometer and other sensory substitutions such as use of bump dots are common adaptation strategies.

Depending on the cause of decreased visual function, it may be appropriate to begin with remediation and then advance to compensation and adaptation if progress is not made following remediation efforts. Monitoring for progress and safety must be constant when deciding which type of treatment to use.

LV Disorders

Major causes of LV include cataracts, macular degeneration, glaucoma, and diabetic retinopathy (Fig. 8-1). In general, older adults with LV are approximately two times more likely to fall than those without vision loss.[4] The underlying cause of each LV condition is different; however, the end goal of treatment is the same: to facilitate safe functional performance in ADLs and IADLs. Unfortunately, the underlying cause of many LV eye conditions cannot be remediated. An occupational therapist must look at each functional activity that is affected and determine the most appropriate treatment approach. There are many ways to adapt activities and compensatory strategies that can be taught and implemented to assist individuals with LV so that they can function at the highest level possible.

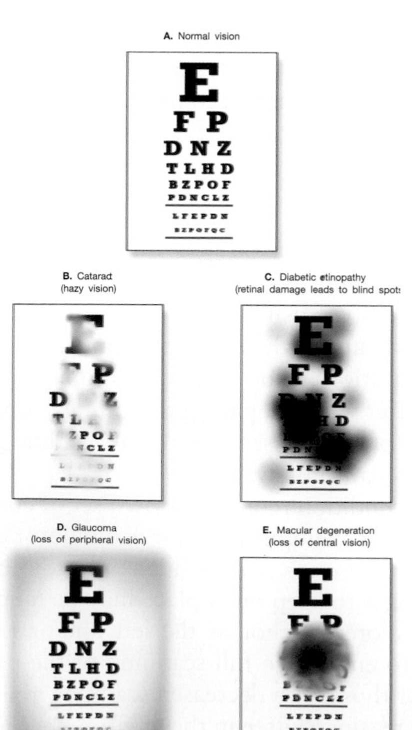

Figure 8-1. Simulated vision loss for most common low vision conditions.

Cataracts

- Functional Impact
  - Decreased visual acuity
  - Decreased contrast sensitivity
  - Difficulty with night driving
  - Diplopia
- Occupational therapy (OT) intervention
  - Color and contrast enhancement
  - Magnification
  - Management of lighting
  - Sensory substitution
  - Organizational strategies

Glaucoma

- Functional impact
  - Difficulty with night vision
  - Difficulty with mobility because of limited peripheral vision
  - End stage:
    - Difficulty with facial recognition
    - Difficulty with reading owing to central field involvement
- OT intervention
  - Education on VF impairment
  - Color and contrast enhancement
  - Glare control
  - Sensory substitution
  - Visual skills training
  - Organizational strategies
  - Magnification

Diabetic Retinopathy

- Functional impact
  - Can affect central and peripheral VFs
  - Development of scotomas
  - Decreased contrast and color discrimination
  - Decreased night vision
  - General visual fluctuations
- OT intervention
  - Color and contrast enhancement
  - Glare control
  - Magnification
  - Lighting enhancement
  - Visual skills training

- Sensory substitution
- Organizational strategies

Age-Related Macular Degeneration

- Functional impact
  - Decreased visual acuity, especially central vision
    - Creates scotomas (blind spots) in central vision, causing individual to miss pieces of the whole picture
  - Decreased contrast sensitivity
  - Difficulty with night driving and diplopia
- OT intervention
  - Color and contrast enhancement
  - Magnification
  - Management of lighting
  - Sensory substitution
  - Organizational strategies
  - Teach eccentric viewing (EV) strategies
  - Safety education

Psychosocial Aspects of LV

Individuals with LV can experience a variety of psychosocial challenges. It is estimated that between 10% and 30% of patients with macular degeneration develop clinically significant depression.[5] Deemer et al. report that depression in those with macular degeneration is associated with "a decline in visual function and greater levels of disability, medical costs, and mortality rates."[5] More than one-third of individuals with LV report not getting as much social interaction as they would like, compared with one-fifth of those without vision impairment.[6] Social relationships can be uncomfortable for the person with LV because of the difficulty interpreting visual social cues and decreased understanding by others.[6] Anxiety can also impact a person challenged with LV. One study found that persons with visual impairment were more than twice as likely to be diagnosed with a major depressive and/or anxiety disorder than their normally sighted peers.[7] By being aware of this correlation and making necessary referrals as needed, occupational therapists can help with these psychosocial aspects of vision loss. It is also important for the occupational therapist to educate his or her client about the potential for depression and anxiety and encourage participation in activities that can combat social isolation, depression, and anxiety.

Neurological Vision Disorders

Clients who have experienced a neurological event, such as a cerebrovascular accident (CVA) or a TBI, may experience a variety of vision-related problems, including decreased acuity and refractive disorders, oculomotor dysfunction, and VFD. An injury to the brain may impact **visual integrity** (visual acuity, refraction, and eye health), **visual efficiency** skills (accommodation, binocular vision, and ocular motor dysfunction), and VFs (homonymous hemianopsia or homonymous quadranopsia).

In order to help clients regain complex functions, treatment of visual dysfunction should be started at the basic processing level and proceed through the hierarchy of skills according to Warren's visual perceptual hierarchy. It is crucial that the occupational therapist performs a vision screen, makes appropriate referrals to the eye care physician, and communicates the functional impact of vision deficits to other therapy team members in order to maximize the individual's rehabilitation potential.

When referring to an eye care physician, it is important that the eye care professional practices with a full appreciation of the complexity of vision and preferably has extensive experience in vision rehabilitation and functional vision care. If possible, it is beneficial to refer the client with neurological visual deficits to a physician associated with the College of Optometrists in Vision Development.

Specific Interventions for Visual Impairments

Decreased Acuity and Refractive Errors

Occupational therapists take on a supportive role when treating clients with decreased acuity and refractive errors. Individuals with LV experience acuity levels of 20/70 and worse.[8] It is important to refer a client to his or her optometrist or ophthalmologist if refractive errors are suspected for correct diagnosis of potential problems and/or correction with prescription lenses if applicable. Decreased acuity can impact many aspects of ADLs and IADLs, including all self-care activities, reading and writing, home management, leisure and work activities, driving, and safety.

Accommodative Disorders

A client with accommodative insufficiency will have difficulty focusing on targets at various distances and may complain of blurred vision, headaches, eye strain, difficulty reading, fatigue, movement of print when reading, and difficulty with ADLs requiring sustained close work, or he or she may avoid close work altogether. Accommodative deficiencies occur in 20% to 30% of clients after TBI.[9]

One of the most effective tools for treatment of accommodative disorders is the use of lenses.[10] Similar to adults over 40 years of age who have presbyopia, lenses can be used to compensate for impaired accommodation. The occupational therapist may take on a supportive role by facilitating optometric treatment recommendations and helping to ensure that the client follows the recommendations during therapy and during other functional activities. This may involve making sure that the patient wears the prescribed glasses or prisms in the appropriate manner.

Treatment for Visual Acuity/Refractive Disorders

Remediation

- Cannot be remediated by OT. Refer to eye care professional.

Compensation

- Move items closer
- Move items farther away
- Use tactile substitutions
- Organize personal spaces

Adaptation

- Increased lighting
- Increased contrast
- Wear corrective lenses prescribed by eye care professional
- Magnifiers
- Glare filters
- Increased size of print
- Audible and/or tactile substitution

Oculomotor Dysfunction

Individuals living with LV may experience difficulty with fixation, tracking/pursuits, and saccades all of which impact visual function. Without good fixation, an individual may not be able to input information about an object or a scene correctly and thoroughly. Tracking/pursuits and saccades involve following a moving object and switching back and forth between two objects, respectively. If an individual's vision is impaired, all three of these visual skills may be affected, therefore impacting the person's ability to read and complete ADLs/IADLs.

Oculomotor dysfunction, including decreased fixation, saccades, and tracking/pursuits, can also occur following a neurological injury and is commonly treated by occupational therapists. Ocular motility disorders affect a person's ability to perform functional tasks such as reading, writing, and driving. The therapist may observe excessive head movements, and the client may complain of frequently losing their place and/or skipping lines when reading. Impaired oculomotor skills can also reduce visual scanning ability, which may result in disruption of high-level visual cognitive skills.

A referral should be made to ensure best optical correction of refractive problems and accommodative and binocular vision disorders. Although the occupational therapist may take on a more supportive role when treating acuity and refractive disorders, they are able to address eye movement disorders without specialized training.

It is important to begin working within the capabilities of the patient to achieve some early success. The occupational therapist will emphasize accuracy first and then speed when treating saccadic or eye pursuit movements. For saccades, the therapist will start with gross (large) eye movements and progress to fine (small) eye movements. For pursuits, the sequence is opposite, from fine (small) to gross (large) eye movements. The therapist will want to eliminate head movements during both tracking/pursuit and saccadic eye movements that can be reasonably accomplished without head movement. As the client progresses, increase the complexity of the task to facilitate more reflexive, automated pursuits and saccades. Examples include adding a metronome, a balance board, or simple cognitive tasks during any ocular motility task.[11] There are also several computer programs and apps that address ocular motor skills. Vision therapy activities should be used by the occupational therapist in conjunction with functional activities that address tracking/pursuits and saccadic eye movements.

Binocular Vision Disorders

Binocular vision disorders are characterized as either strabismic or nonstrabismic, can occur after stroke, and are the most common vision problem following TBI.[12] Binocular vision disorders are often caused by damage to the cranial nerves 3, 4, or 6; midbrain injury; or injury to the oculomotor nuclei. With strabismus, the eyes are not aligned, and it is characterized by the eyes turning in (esotropia), out (exotropia), up (hypertropia), or down (hypotropia). A hallmark symptom of binocular vision is double vision or diplopia, which can greatly interfere with a client's ability to participate in functional tasks. Other visual symptoms may include blurred vision, headaches, eye strain, reading problems, avoidance of reading or other near tasks, and difficulty with ADLs that require stereopsis (driving, reaching for objects, pouring liquids).

Occupational therapists treating a client with binocular vision deficits should do so with guidance from an ophthalmologist or optometrist. If double vision is occurring, increasing the visual comfort of a client should be addressed first to increase his or her ability to participate in rehabilitation. Similar to accommodative disorders, occupational therapists in an inpatient rehabilitation setting may take on a supportive role when treating a client with binocular vision disorders. The therapist may implement the use of compensatory strategies or adaptations, such as using larger print and limiting time spent on tasks, which cause discomfort. The occupational therapist may also have the client perform ocular calisthenics to improve eye muscle function and prevent contractures of the involved muscles. An example of an activity involves the client looking all the way to the right, then all the way left, then up, and then down while holding each position for several seconds. This would be repeated two to three times a day for a few minutes at a time.[12] An occupational therapist who specializes in vision therapy and often works under the direct supervision of an ophthalmologist or optometrist may use advanced vision therapy techniques including computer programs and use of virtual reality systems to target binocular vision disorders.

Convergence Insufficiency

Convergence insufficiency is a nonstrabismic binocular vision disorder in which a person's eyes have difficulty converging on a near object. A person with convergence insufficiency may experience difficulty with sustained near tasks, complain of headaches, and/or avoid close work. Impaired depth perception is often associated with convergence insufficiency. A referral to an optometrist is recommended if the occupational therapist suspects convergence impairments, as glasses and/or prisms may be necessary. Vision therapy procedures may also be used for convergence issues. The Brock string exercise (Fig. 8-2) involves a string either 6 or 12 feet long with different color beads. The client is asked to change his or her gaze from one bead to the next to practice convergence and divergence skills.

Treatment for Oculomotor Dysfunction

Remediation

- Scanning exercises
- Tracking exercises
- Range of motion exercises
- Computer programs
- Dynavision
- Brock string exercises

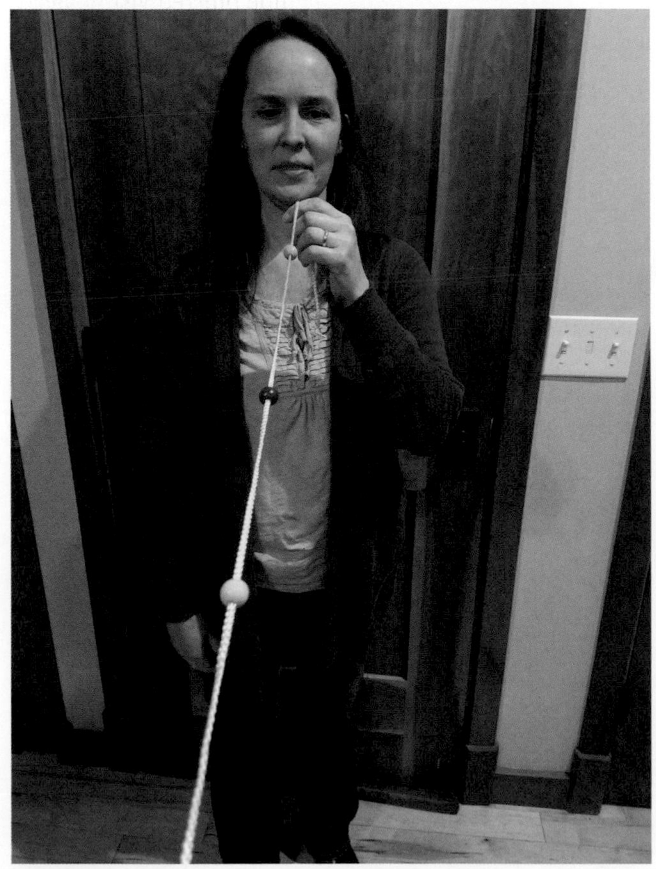

Figure 8-2. Brock string exercise.

Compensation

- Use visual anchors and line guides
- Use pacing strategies
- Increase awareness of deficit
- Head movements
- Teach systematic scanning

Adaptation

- Large print materials
- Prism glasses
- Increase lighting
- Increase contrast
- Eliminate visual clutter

Visual Fields

VFD associated with CVA or TBI include hemianopsia or quadrantanopia. This occurs due to a lesion along the visual pathways at some point from the optic nerve to the visual cortex. The right hemisphere of the brain carries information for the left half of the VF in both eyes, and the left hemisphere carries information from the right half of the VF in both eyes. VFD occur in 36% of people with right stroke and 25% of those with left stroke.[9]

An important aspect of VFD for occupational therapists to consider is perceptual completion. The visual system is automatic, and the brain tends to fill in any gaps caused by VFD. Because our brain can naturally and unconsciously complete a picture, patients with VFD will not necessarily recognize that they are missing part of the picture. Although a client with VFD may not recognize part of the picture is missing, he or she may complain of difficulty in mobility or ADLs. If visual inattention coexists with VFD, the rehabilitation process can be complicated by the client's difficulty implementing visual scanning strategies.

Education to create awareness and training for compensatory strategies is critical. Intact **peripheral VFs** play a large role in safety with ambulation and as our alerting system to make us aware of approaching danger. When the peripheral fields are affected, scanning strategies are an essential piece of the treatment plan. Peripheral VF loss may cause a person to not see drop-offs, obstacles, pets, or people because of a limited field of view.[13] Safe ambulation is often impacted by decreased peripheral VF.

Visual scanning is the ability to efficiently, quickly, and actively look for information relevant to your environment.[11] It is important for individuals with VF loss to use their remaining vision efficiently by quickly scanning for obstacles in the environment when walking around their homes or in the community. Individuals with peripheral vision involvement need to use organized patterns for scanning to compensate for the missing areas of vision.[13] A horizontal search pattern, vertical, or combined pattern can be used depending on situation. Field expansion devices such as prisms and telescopes used in reverse may be also beneficial.

Central VF Loss

Central field loss is a primary symptom of macular degeneration. Central field scotomas may interfere with reading, identifying objects, and clearly seeing a person's face. The scotoma may be relative or absolute in nature. Dense scotomas, or absolute scotomas, are insensitive to very bright objects, often making a black spot in the VF. Relative scotomas may create an effect of blur or fog over the image being looked at.[14] Ring scotomas are circular VF defects centered on fixation. Central ring scotomas are most often found within the central 10°.[15] Individuals with central field scotomas may complain of things disappearing and then reappearing when they shift their point of fixation.

Treatment for VFD

Remediation

- VFD are not effectively remediated

Compensation

- Use of organized scanning strategies
- Use of line guides
- Use of anchors
- Turning head to affected side
- Increase awareness

Adaptation

- High-contrast visual anchors placed on affected side
- Prism glasses
- Increased contrast
- Place items on unaffected side
- Increased organization of client's environment

Remediation of Visual Deficits

Vision therapy may also be referred to as orthoptics, vision training, visual training, or eye training. It is an organized therapeutic regimen used to treat various vision disorders that interfere with visual functioning (Fig. 8-3). Most commonly binocular dysfunction, accommodative dysfunction, and oculomotor dysfunction can be treated with vision therapy. There are some optometrists and therapists who specialize in vision therapy, and an overlap can be seen between the role of an occupational therapist and vision therapist for clients with neurological injury. Because of an occupational therapist's role in a rehabilitation setting, he or she is well positioned to screen and determine the need for a referral to an eye physician. If vision therapy is recommended, the occupational therapist may be best suited to provide vision rehabilitation or a vision therapist may need to be consulted. Any vision therapy provided should be done so with direct supervision and guidance by the optometrist. The occupational therapist may perform daily therapy techniques prescribed by the optometrist and, most importantly, can help the patient generalize visual skills into ADLs as well as assist with integration of compensatory and adaptive techniques.[16] The general guidelines for vision therapy from an optometric perspective are outlined in the subsequent section. These principles are in line with our framework as occupational therapists and demonstrate the similarities between the way occupational therapists and functional optometrists practice.

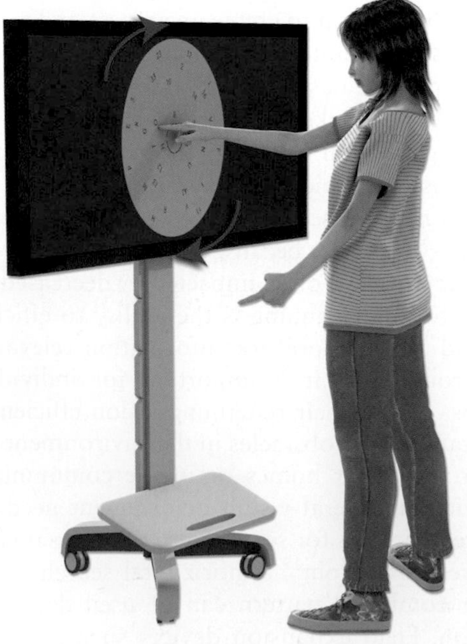

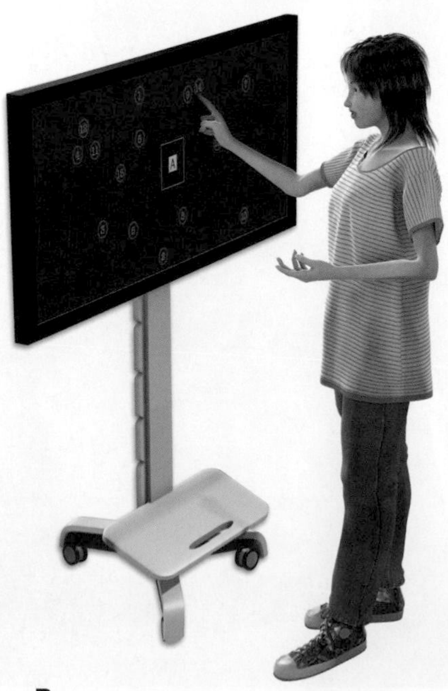

Figure 8-3. Examples of computerized tracking/pursuits (**A**) and saccadic vision therapy activities (**B**).

GENERAL GUIDELINES AND PRINCIPLES FOR VISION THERAPY

- Determine a level at which the patient can perform easily
- Be aware of the patient's frustration level
- Use positive reinforcement
- Maintain an effective training level
- Make the patient aware of vision therapy
- Set realistic therapy objectives and maintain flexibility with these objectives or endpoints[11]

Vision Therapy Activities

- Hart chart saccades
- Symbol tracking
- Letter tracking
- Visual tracing
- Rotator-type instruments
- Flashlight tag

Compensatory Strategies for Visual Deficits

Many individuals with visual deficits can be taught to use compensatory strategies that will help them independently function in their desired ADLs and IADLs. For visual deficits that cannot be remediated or for safety reasons, this may be the starting point of intervention for the occupational therapist.

Preferred Retinal Loci Training

To maximize vision when dealing with a central field scotoma, a person must learn to "move" the scotoma out of the way and use an alternative spot on the macula not affected by the degeneration. This strategy is called **eccentric viewing** (**EV**), and the position on the macula is the **preferred retinal loci** (**PRL**). Once learned, an individual can use his or her PRL to view close or distant objects. Some clients may have identified and be using a PRL without training. However, to make sure he or she is using the best and most efficient PRL, education with exercises should be initiated and practiced, making the use of the most effective PRL habitual for best results. Exercises to maintain oculomotor control, fixation stability, and skills to refixate on an object are necessary to maximize independence with reading and other functional tasks involving **central vision**.

Scanning Training

Visual scanning training is one of the most common interventions that occupational therapists use for VFD and oculomotor deficits. Scanning training may be remedial in nature when used for increased range of motion, accuracy, and/or speed of eye movements. When used for VFD, the goal of compensatory training is to establish an effective search strategy and to facilitate use of a systematic organized visual search of the environment (left to right, top to bottom). Warren[17] outlines the following components of an effective search strategy:

- Initiation of wide head turn toward the blind field
- An increase in the number of head and eye movements toward the blind field
- Execution of an organized and efficient search pattern that begins on the blind side
- Attention to and detection of visual detail on the blind side
- Ability to quickly shift attention and search between the central VF and the peripheral VF on the blind side

The occupational therapist will have the client complete visual scanning activities in personal, peripersonal, and extrapersonal space to address various tasks that require efficient scanning. Training may include paper-and-pencil tasks, computer programs, scanning in a functional setting, and use of specialized equipment, such as the Dynavision. Although the initial focus of visual scanning training is accuracy, as the client progresses, the speed of scanning will be emphasized and integrating movement during scanning is used to improve visual motor integration. Addressing visual scanning during mobility will help maximize safety during functional mobility tasks. If a client demonstrates good awareness of his or her VFD, visual scanning training can often be completed quickly, with the client demonstrating immediate use of search strategies.

Clients with VFD often have difficulty with reading tasks. With right VFD, the client must look into their field impairment as they read across the line. They may lose their place reading along or have difficulty identifying the end of the line. They may also have errors in word identification, such as with compound words; they may read foot when the word is football. Individuals with left VFD may have difficulty finding the beginning of the reading materials. In order to compensate for his or her VFD, the client must be aware of the problem and how it is affecting functional abilities. The occupational therapist may provide various types of cueing to facilitate effective scanning to the impaired VF. Use of an anchor (supplying a cue on the impaired side to indicate starting position) can assist the client in focusing attention back to the side of VFD. An "L" shaped marker can be used as an anchor, or a ruler or straight edge can assist the client with maintaining his or her spot when reading. Figure 8-4 illustrates reorientation of the reading materials as an effective strategy for reading with VFD.[18] It may be necessary to add adaptations to the environment such as contrasting color to objects such as door frames and furniture to help the client be able to locate them and to maximize safety.

Organization

Being organized is one of the most important strategies for someone with visual deficits to adopt. Keeping an

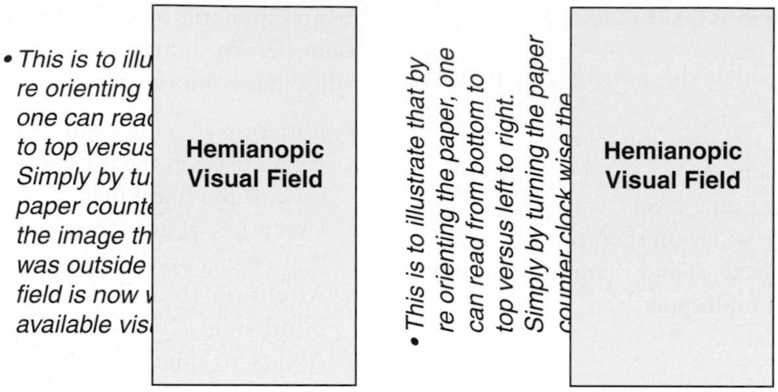

• This is to illu
re orienting
one can rea
to top versus
Simply by tu
paper count
the image th
was outside
field is now
available vis
Hemianopic Visual Field
• This is to illustrate that by
re orienting the paper, one
can read from bottom to
top versus left to right.
Simply by turning the paper
Hemianopic Visual Field

Figure 8-4. Example of compensatory strategy for reading with right hemianopsia.

item in a consistent place allows the individual to find it with less difficulty. Organizing money, items in the pantry or refrigerator, toiletries, and clothing in a way that makes sense to each individual is very beneficial. This can decrease frustration and the potential for mistakes or injury. If the individual is unable to use this strategy independently, it is important to educate family members in maintaining organization for their loved one's success and safety.

Sensory Substitution

People who have LV rely more heavily on tactile and audible strategies. These strategies are often simple, cost-effective, and easy to incorporate into everyday activities. For example, many microwaves have flat control panels with poor contrast for numbers and other desired settings. By placing a high-contrast, tactile bump dot on a frequently used control, an individual can locate and press with improved accuracy and decreased frustration. By placing a rust-proof safety pin on the tag of black pants, an individual can identify black pants from pants of another color. Pouring salt into the palm of the hand and then adding a pinch is a tactile way to apply the desired amount.

Talking clocks, books, bathroom scales, timers, screen readers, thermostats, and other audible devices assist individuals in hearing information versus reading it when vision is impacted. The pitch, speed, and volume of talking devices can often be changed to accommodate for individual preference or need. As with any condition, it is important to look at the individual's abilities and limitations to best determine intervention strategies.

Adaptations for Visual Deficits

Environmental adaptations are often necessary to maximize independence and safety for those with visual deficits. Lighting, glare, and contrast can be controlled or modified for maximizing performance during ADL and IADL tasks.

Lighting

Changes to the number of photoreceptors (rods) in the retina, hardening of the lens of the eye, presence of floaters, decrease in the pupil size, and common eye diseases like cataracts and glaucoma can reduce the amount of light that the eye can use and increase how sensitive the eye is to glare.[19] For some tasks, an individual aged 60 years may need 10 times the amount of light that a 20-year-old person would need.[19] With the large variety of lighting sources available today, it is important to educate individuals on the options and the reason older adults, especially those with LV, need more light and what type can be most helpful. Task lighting is lighting that can be adjusted to shine directly on a person's work (Fig. 8-5). Many individuals report that the natural light from the outdoors is the most beneficial. Therefore, the daylight light-emitting diode (LED) bulbs are often preferred for simulating the natural light of outdoors most closely. Positioning of light is also important to consider when completing tabletop tasks.

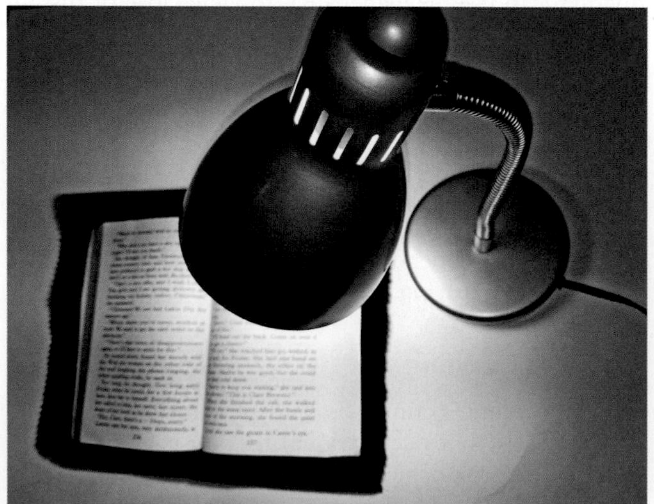

Figure 8-5. Example of a task light with good contrast of book on dark placemat.

Lighting Strategies

- Task lighting: Adjustable lamp placed to shine directly on work area for near activities. Recommended: an opaque shade positioned below eye level, LED daylight bulb (800 Lumens)
  - When increasing brightness, be aware of glare. Use of filters to manage glare with increased lighting can provide increased comfort and function.
  - Use LED flashlights for "spot-lighting"
  - Use under cabinet LED lighting in kitchens to brighten workspaces
- Ambient lighting is important for safety. LED daylight bulbs can be used to simulate natural sunlight.
  - Use nightlights in hallways, bathrooms
- Strip lighting along the floor in hallways to use as guidance

Glare Management

When making lighting adjustments, it is important to consider how glare can affect the eye. Sensitivity to glare is associated with many visual deficits. When in the sun or even when a person is sitting in the shade, sun can reflect from surfaces producing uncomfortable glare. By wearing a special filter with a polarized lens, glare is decreased (Fig. 8-6). Less glare can result in increased clarity and visibility. Reduced glare also lessens eye fatigue.[20]

Colored glare filters can be worn to enhance contrast when viewing a computer screen or television. Each individual may have different preferences regarding tint of these glasses. It is, therefore, beneficial to try a variety of colors to determine which is most effective.

Contrast Enhancement

People with LV disorders and visual dysfunction due to neurological injury may experience decreased contrast sensitivity. Decreased contrast sensitivity can significantly impact a person's ability to function. Difficulty seeing where to plug in an electrical appliance into an outlet, seeing the level of dark coffee poured into a black cup, being able to see an unpainted curb, or safely navigate a flight of stairs are all examples of functional issues. Education can assist in helping the individual know the potential safety implications of decreased contrast sensitivity. By applying a high contrasting color with tape or paint to the object/situation that presents difficulty, an individual may regain some independence in function and safety. For example, applying bright orange tape around the holes of a white electrical outlet located on a white wall or applying a bright-colored strip of paint/tape on each step of a staircase, or just to the top and bottom step to create more contrast can impact the individual's safety.

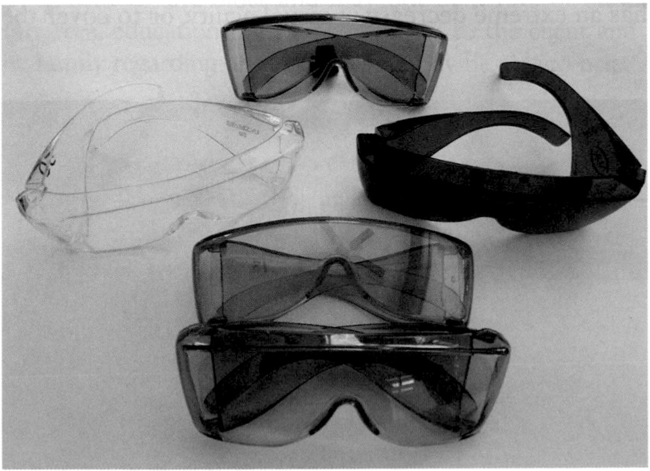

Figure 8-6. Colored fit over glare filters in a variety of colors.

Magnification

Adults with visual deficits often benefit from using magnification. There are two main types of magnification that an individual can use: relative distance magnification and relative size magnification. **Relative distance magnification** is decreasing the distance from the person to the item that he or she is trying to see. An example of this is moving closer to the TV screen or bringing a paper closer to read the writing. **Relative size magnification** is achieved using large print-written material or a magnifier. Many items are available in large print: books, magazines, bills, clocks/watches, telephones, and kitchen timers are just a few of the many large print items available. Computers are often equipped with accessibility features to enlarge print for websites and e-mail programs. An individual may need additional magnification from an optical device. There are many types of magnifiers: hands-free, stand- and handheld, electronic (both desktop and portable), spectacles, and telescopes (see Figs. 8-7 and 8-8). Each type of magnification has benefits and challenges. Regardless of which type of magnification that is used, it is critical to communicate with an optometrist or other eye care professional for recommendations and to then complete education and training for best use and success with the magnifier during functional activities.

Useful Information about Magnifiers

- Bigger is not always better!
- Greater magnification = smaller field of view.
- Educate on client on correct distance to hold magnifier from material (working distance).
- Use handheld and stand magnifiers for "spot reading" only—it is often fatiguing for continuous reading activities.
- Desktop electronic magnifiers are best for continuous reading activities and can be used for writing tasks, also.
- Hands-free magnifiers can be used for crafts, managing insulin pumps and other tasks that require two hands.

Best Evidence for Vision Interventions Used in Occupational Therapy (*continued*)

Intervention	Description	Participants	Dosage	Research Design and Evidence Level	Benefit	Statistical Significance
Short-term persistence of oculomotor rehabilitative changes following oculomotor therapy (OMT).[24]	Examined the short-term persistence of previously obtained positive OMT findings at 3 and 6 months following completion of OMT.	Eight participants with mild traumatic brain injury who had completed OMT training (1 male, 7 females)	Thirteen clinical measures were evaluated at 3 and 6 months after oculomotor-based vision rehabilitation. Measures were evaluated over two separate sessions. Measures included: near point of convergence, accommodative amplitudes, reading rates, and a subjective rating using the Convergence Insufficiency Symptom Score.	Pilot study reassessing clinical oculomotor parameters at 3- and 6-month periods. Level IV	The improvement in near point of convergence break and recovery and monocular and binocular accommodative amplitudes after OMT persisted during follow-up. Reading rate improvements persisted during follow-up. The number of fixations per 100 words and grade-level efficiency significantly improved at the 6-month follow-up.	Statistical analyses that compared clinical measures before OMT, immediately after OMT, and 3- and 6-months following completion of OMT found significant changes in clinical measures. More than 90% of the original abnormal baseline oculomotor parameters either significantly improved, after 9 hours of intense OMT.
The effect of visual training for patients with visual field defects due to brain damage: a systematic review.[25]	Studies were selected if they met the following entry criteria: (1) inclusion of only patients with HVFDs due to postchiasmatic lesions of the visual system after brain injury, documented by computed tomography/magnetic resonance imaging scans, and patients with left or right field defects ranging from homonymous quadrantanopia to complete homonymous hemianopia, with and without macular sparing; (2) applying the intervention of vision restoration therapy (VRT) or of compensatory saccadic eye movements and visual search strategies, that is, scanning compensatory therapy (SCT); (3) using the outcome measures of VF size, visual search field, reading time, and reading error, and subjective measures of questionnaires; (4) using the design of randomized controlled trial (RCT), controlled clinical trial, retrospective studies, or repeated measures design (RMD) studies;	Fourteen studies	Dosage of training varied in different studies.	Systematic review of 2 RCTs and 12 within-subject RMD. Level I	Five studies reported a significant effect of the VRT, whereas two studies reported no effect using scanning laser ophthalmoscopy or Goldmann perimetry as outcome measure. All authors of the studies on SCT found a significant effect of up to 30° visual search field, a significant increase in reading speed, or decrease in reading errors.	The effect of the restoration therapy needs to be further evaluated; visual search therapy is recommended.

Technology learning and use among older adults with late-life vision impairments[26]	How do older adults who experience severe late-life vision impairments use technology to communicate and seek information? What challenges do these older adults face in learning and using accessible information and communication technologies (ICTs)?	Fifteen older adults (aged 60–99; $M = 76.71$, $SD = 12.51$; 6 females) who had an acquired, severe vision impairment (e.g., blindness, low vision).	Participants were encouraged to demonstrate how they used various devices (e.g., phones, desktop/laptop computers, tablet computers) and services (e.g., phone operator service, phone voicemail, screen readers, search engines, e-mail) as a way to help them.	In-depth interviews were conducted with older adults in their homes or in a private conference-type room within their residential community. Level VI	Training resources for older adults with late-life vision impairments should focus on one-on-one support while enabling ways of receiving support remotely.	Late-life vision impairment is not a static condition and requires ongoing training and customization of access technologies.
Safety with visual field loss. Effects of acute peripheral/central visual field loss on standing balance.[27]	This study used a custom-made contact lens model to occlude the peripheral or central VFs in healthy adults compared with older adults with VF loss to improve our understanding of the etiology of balance impairments that may lead to an increased fall risk in patients with VF loss.	Nine young (aged 27.8 ± 2.1 years, 4 females) and 11 older adults (aged 72.2 ± 5.1 years, 7 females) were recruited.	Two visits were required to complete the study; the first visit consisted of screening procedures and the second included the experimental dynamic posturography session.	Within-subject approach. Level IV	Support to the functional sensitivity hypothesis that postulates central and peripheral VFs play different but necessary roles in postural control and stability/safety (especially in older adults).	VF occlusion had a significant effect on center of pressure (COP) displacement, but only in older adults. This finding holds true both when the floor is fixed ($p = 0.03$, $F = 3.89$, Table 3) and sway-referenced ($p = 0.05$, $F = 3.39$, Table 3). Postural control system is most sensitive to motion-related visual cues from the peripheral VF—both central and peripheral visions are important to maintaining balance, but peripheral vision in particular may be more sensitive to motion.

HVFD, homonymous visual field defects.

References

1. Dutton G. Cognitive vision, its disorders and differential diagnosis in adults and children: knowing where and what things are. *Eye*. 2003;17(3):289–304. https://www.ncbi.nlm.nih.gov/pubmed/12724689. Accessed June 25, 2018.
2. Warren MA. Hierarchical model for evaluation and treatment of visual perceptual dysfunction in adult acquired brain injury, part 1. *Am J Occup Ther*. 1993;47:42–54.
3. Massoff R, Lidoff L. *Issues in Low Vision Rehabilitation: Service, Delivery, Policy, and Funding*. New York, NY: AFB Press; 2001.
4. Crews JE, Chou CF, Stevens JA, Saaddine JB. Falls among persons aged ≥65 years with and without severe vision impairment—United States, 2014. *MMWR Morb Mortal Wkly Rep*. 2016;65(17):433–437. https://search-proquest-com.libproxy.library.wmich.edu/docview/1795938355?accountid=15099&rfr_id=info%3Axri%2Fsid%3Aprimo.
5. Deemer AD, Massof RW, Rovner BW, Casten RJ, Piersol C. Functional outcomes of the low vision depression prevention trial in age-related macular degeneration. *Invest Ophthalmol Vis Sci*. 2017;58(3):1514–1520. doi:10.1167/iovs.16-20001.
6. Coyle C, Steinman BA, Chen J. Visual acuity and self-reported vision status: their associations with social isolation in older adults. *J Aging Health*. 2017;29(1):128–148. doi:10.1177/0898264315624909.
7. van der Aa H, Comijs HC, Penninx BWJH, van Rens GHMB, van Nispen RMA. Major depressive and anxiety disorders in visually impaired older adults. *Invest Ophthalmol Vis Sci*. 2015;56(2):849–854.
8. Duffy M. Low vision and legal blindness terms and conditions. VisionAware Website. http://www.visionaware.org/info/your-eye-condition/eye-health/what-is-legal-blindness/125. Accessed December 11, 2018.
9. Stelmack J. Visual function in patients followed at a Veterans Affairs polytrauma network site: an electronic medical record review. *Optometry*. 2009;80:419–424.
10. Suchoff I, Gianutsos R. Rehabilitative optometric interventions for the adult with acquired brain injury. In: Grabois M, Garrison SJ, Hart KA, Lemkuhl LD, eds. *Physical Medicine and Rehabilitation*. Malden, MA: Blackwall Science; 2000:608–621.
11. Scheiman, M. Visual rehabilitation for patients with brain injury. In: Scheiman M, ed. *Understanding and Managing Vision Deficits: A Guide for Occupational Therapists*. 3rd ed. Thorofare, NJ: Slack; 2011:201–231.
12. Scheiman M. Understanding and managing visual deficits after acquired brain injury: a guide for therapists. Oral presentation at: Vision Education Seminars; January 2015; San Diego, CA.
13. Riddering A. Scanning efficiently for activities of daily living. Vision Aware. http://www.visionaware.org/info/your-eye-condition/eye-health/low-vision/scanning-efficiently-for-activities-of-daily-living/1235. Published 2018.
14. Fletcher DC, Schuchard RA, Watson G. Relative locations of macular scotomas near the PRL: effect on low vision reading. *J Rehabil Res Dev*. 1999;36(4):356–364.
15. Kerrison JB, Pollock SC, Biousse V, Newman NJ. Coffee and doughnut maculopathy: a cause of acute central ring scotomas. *Br J Ophthalmol*. 2000;84:158–164.
16. Scheiman M. Management of refractive, visual efficiency, and visual information processing disorders. In: Scheiman M, ed. *Understanding and Managing Vision Deficits: A Guide for Occupational Therapists*. 3rd ed. Thorofare, NJ: Slack; 2011:119–176.
17. Warren, M. Evaluation and treatment of visual deficits. In: Pedretti L, ed. *Occupational Therapy: Practice Skills for Physical Dysfunction*. St. Louis, MO: Mosby Inc; 2001.
18. Pambakian A, Currie J, Kennard C. Rehabilitation strategies for patients with homonymous visual field defects. *J Neuroophthalmol*. 2005;25:136–142.
19. Lewis B. Is glare light good for elderly people? How to light your home for changing vision. The Spruce Website. https://www.thespruce.com/lighting-for-aging-eyes-2175153. Updated April 16, 2018. Accessed June 19, 2018.
20. Enhanced Vision. Sunglasses for those with macular degeneration. Enhanced Vision Website. https://www.enhancedvision.com/low-vision-info/eye-health/sunglasses-for-those-with-macular-degeneration.html. Accessed June 16, 2018.
21. Bowers AR, Keeney K, Peli E. Community-based trial of a peripheral prism visual field expansion device for hemianopia. *Arch Ophthalmol*. 2008;126:657–664.
22. Giorgi RG, Woods RL, Peli E. Clinical and laboratory of evaluation of peripheral glasses for hemianopia. *Optom Vis Sci*. 2009;86:492–502.
23. Be My Eyes. Getting started: a guide for blind and low vision users. https://www.bemyeyes.com/. Accessed June 19, 2018.
24. Thiagarajan P, Ciuffreda J. Short-term persistence of oculomotor rehabilitatative changes in mild traumatic brain injury (mTBI): a pilot study of clinical effects. *Brain Inj*. 2015;29(12):1475–1479. doi:10.3109/02699052.2015.1070905.
25. Bouwmeester L, Joost H, Cees L. The effect of visual training for patients with visual field defects due to brain damage: a systematic review. *J Neurol Neurosurg Psychiatry*. 2007;78(6):555. doi:10.1136/jnnp.2006.103853.
26. Piper AM, Brewer R, Cornejo R. Technology learning and use among older adults with late-life vision impairments. *Univers Access Inf Soc*. 2017;16:699–711. doi:10.1007/s10209-016-0500-1.
27. O'Connel C, Mahboobin A, Drexler S, et al. Effects of acute peripheral/central visual field loss on standing balance. *Exp Brain Res*. 2017;235:3261–3270. doi:10.1007/s00221-017-5045-x.

Chapter 9

Visual Perceptual Assessment and Intervention

Kara Christy and Natasha Huffine

LEARNING OBJECTIVES

This chapter will allow the reader to:

1. Describe various visual perceptual impairments and the impact on daily occupation and function.
2. Understand the neurological and physiological basis for visual perception.
3. Identify appropriate screening procedures and standardized evaluations for visual perceptual impairments.
4. Understand the conceptual foundation underlying interventions for visual perceptual impairment.
5. Describe the difference between a remediation approach, compensatory approach, and adaptations for treatment of visual perceptual impairments.
6. Identify specific interventions for visual perceptual impairments.

CHAPTER OUTLINE

TERMINOLOGY

Depth perception: the visual ability to perceive relative distance of objects

Figure ground perception: the visual ability to distinguish foreground from background

Form constancy: the visual perceptual ability to identify objects despite their variation of size, color, shape, position, or texture

Pattern recognition: a perceptual process of matching incoming visual stimuli with stored visual memories

Spatial orientation: the visual ability to recognize the position of one's self or objects in relation to opposing positions, directions, movement, and environmental locations

Unilateral inattention: a phenomenon that causes one to experience an inability to orient and respond to one side of the environmental information

Visual closure: the ability to accurately identify objects that are partially covered or missing

Visual memory: the ability to take in a visual stimulus, retain its details, and store it for later retrieval

Visual organization: the ability to group objects on the basis of their identifying properties

Visual perception: the ability to interpret, understand, and define incoming visual information

Introduction

Visual perception is a dominant sense with which we gather information from our peripersonal (within arm's reach) and extrapersonal (beyond arm's reach) environments in order to use it for activities of daily living.[1] It is important that we are able to process this information accurately and efficiently for satisfactory engagement in daily occupations. The Occupational Therapy Practice Framework cites perception as a mental function under client factors, which influences performance in occupations.[2] Thus, it should be at the forefront of occupational therapist's evaluation and intervention process in both objective and subjective information gathering.

Visual Perceptual Function and Impairment in Daily Occupation

Warren developed a hierarchy describing the different levels of visual processing and visuocognition in relation to function. Simply stated, the impact of vision at each skill level of this hierarchy influences the overall integration of the visual environment. As seen in Figure 9-1, the foundation includes oculomotor control, visual fields, and visual acuity. These are the basic visual skills required to perceive information accurately from our visual world. Without these basic-level skills, the ability to attend to the incoming information is impacted. Unilateral inattention is represented in this second level, and this deficit would complicate our ability to properly scan and attend to incoming visual information. Decreased visual scanning would present difficulties in pattern recognition, which includes (1) from constancy, (2) figure ground perception, (3) visual closure, (4) visual organization, and (5) spatial orientation. Moreover, the optimal functioning of pattern recognition skills is necessary for our ability to retain visual information, also known as **visual memory**. The highest skill level of this hierarchy is visuocognition, with which we are able to integrate visual perceptual information with other sensory input in order to complete executive functioning tasks, such as planning, problem solving, and decision making. Without knowledge of where a deficit is located along this hierarchy, it is difficult to develop appropriate evaluation and treatment protocols.[3]

Dysfunction in these visual perceptual skill areas can severely compromise our ability to engage safely and independently in an array of performance components and activities of daily living associated with self-care, productivity, and play/leisure occupations.[4,5] See Table 9-1 for examples of common diagnoses and associated functional implications to consider.

Neurological and Physiological Basis of Visual Perceptual Function

Developmentally, vision is ever evolving in the brain from a neonatal state through adulthood. Vision and visual

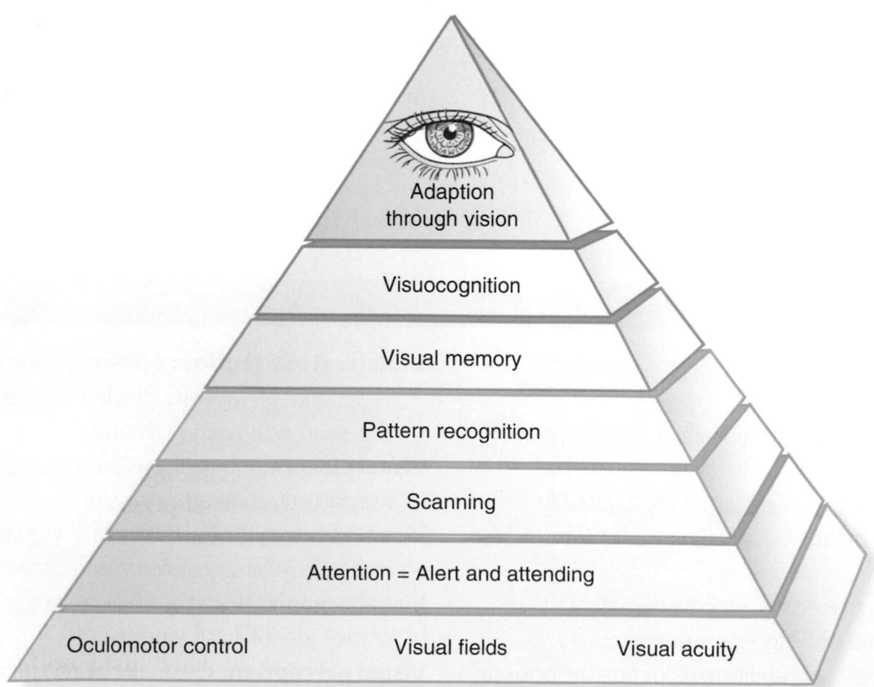

Figure 9-1. Hierarchy of visual perceptual skill development. (Adapted from Warren M. A hierarchical model for evaluation for evaluation and treatment of visual perceptual dysfunction in adult acquired brain injury, part 1. *Am J Occup Ther.* 1993;47:43. Copyright 1993 by the American Occupational Therapy Association, Inc. Reprinted with permission.)

Table 9-1. Diagnoses, Areas of Deficit, and Impairments in Daily Occupation

DIAGNOSIS	AREA OF DEFICIT	IMPAIRMENT IN DAILY OCCUPATION

Traumatic brain injury	• Binocularity
	• Ocular motility
	• Visual field deficits/neglect
	• Depth perception
	• Pattern recognition
	  • Form constancy
	  • Figure ground perception
	  • Visual closure
	  • Visual organization
	  • Spatial orientation
	• Visual memory
	• Visuocognition
		• Negotiating stairs and busy environments
		• Pouring liquids/foods into containers
		• Packing medications
		• Safety with driving and ambulating in parking lots
		• Recognizing traffic signs
		• Sorting laundry
		• Locating items in the grocery store
		• Reading
		• Remembering the location of a locker or school desk

CVA/acquired brain injury	• Unilateral inattention/neglect • Visual agnosia • Visuocognition • Visual midline shift	• Safety in self-care activities • Navigating personal environment • Recognizing utensils and measurements for cooking/ baking • Locating offices for medical appointments • Floor and walls appear tilted, causing a lean in posture
Progressive neurological disorders: Parkinson disease/multiple sclerosis	• Ocular motility • Pattern recognition • Depth perception • Visual field deficits/neglect • Contrast/color sensitivity	• Dressing • Home management • Navigation • Reading • Recognizing traffic signals • Navigating intersections while driving
Cerebral palsy	• Visual acuity • Reduced visual fields • Ocular motility • Pattern recognition • Visuocognition	• Tying shoes • Playing board games • Handwriting • Navigating a playground • Learning letters
Dementia	• Depth perception • Pattern recognition • Contrast sensitivity	• Navigating steps, curbs, and pavement cracks (falls) • Avoiding obstacles in the home
Sensory processing disorders: autism/low birth weight/attention-deficit hyperactivity disorder	• Visual matching • Visual memory • Pattern recognition • Laterality • Visual crowding	• Academic performance • Matching shapes and objects • Recognizing similar letters or words • Reversing letters in spelling • Difficulties in interpreting charts and graphs • Handwriting • Reduced performance in sports

CVA, cerebrovascular accident.

Source: Brown T, Elliott S, Bourne R, Sutton E, Wigg S, Morgan DD. The discriminative validity of three visual perception tests. *N Z J Occup Ther*. 2011;58(2):14–22. Accessed May 8, 2018; Brown T, Elliot S, Bourne R, et al. The convergent validity of the Developmental Test of Visual Perception–Adolescent and Adult, Motor-Free Visual Perception Test–Third Edition and Test of Visual Perception Skills (Nonmotor)–Third Edition when used with adults. *Br J Occup Ther*. 2012;75(3):134–143. doi:10.4276/030802212X13311219571783; Jung H, Woo Y, Kang J, Choi Y, Kim K. Visual perception of ADHD children with sensory processing disorder. *Psychiatry Investig*. 2014;11(2):119–123. doi:10.4306/pi.2014.11.2.119; Cooke DM, McKenna K, Flemming J. Development of a standardized occupational therapy screening tool for visual perception in adults. *Scand J Occup Ther*. 2005;12(2):59–71. doi:10.1080/11038120410020683-1; Geldof C, Wassenaer AV, Kieviet JD, Kok J, Oosterlaan J. Visual perception and visual-motor integration in very preterm and/or very-low-birth-weight children: a meta-analysis. *Res Dev Disabil*. 2012;33(2):726–736. doi:10.1016/j.ridd.2011.08.025; Menon-Nair A, Korner-Bitensky N, Ogourtsova T. Occupational therapists' identification, assessment, and treatment of unilateral spatial neglect during stroke rehabilitation in Canada. *Stroke*. 2007;38(9):2556–2562. doi:10.1161/STROKEAHA.107.484857; Pieker I, David N, Schneider TR, Nolte G, Schottle D, Engel AK. Perceptual integration deficits in autism spectrum disorders are associated with reduced interhemispheric gamma-band coherence. *J Neurosci*. 2015;35(50):16352–16361. doi:10.1523/jneurosci.1442-15.2015; Poole JL, Nakamoto T, McNulty T, et al. Dexterity, visual perception, and activities of daily living in persons with multiple sclerosis. *Occup Ther Health Care*. 2010;24(2):159–170. doi:10.3109/07380571003681202; Ego A, Lidzba K, Brovedani P, et al. Visual-perceptual impairment in children with cerebral palsy: a systematic review. *Dev Med Child Neurol*. 2015;57(2):46–51. doi:10.1111/dmcn.12687.

perception are processed globally throughout the brain. The right hemisphere is responsible for completing the initial processing of visual-spatial information. The left hemisphere is better at resolving detail of the visual-spatial array and carries out the fine processing needed to extract differences between objects. Both hemispheres are needed to ensure accurate identification of an object and deficits in visual cognition. More specifically, the parietal lobe is responsible for the localization of objects and their relationship to each other. The temporal lobe analyzes the visual information for details of color, form, and size. The occipital lobe is the primary visual cortex and analyzes visual information for position, movement, and orientation. The frontal lobe houses the prefrontal cortex in which we attend to and use the visual information for organization, planning, and sequencing of activities.[3] Visual information coming from the occipital cortex to the prefrontal cortex can take either the dorsal stream or the ventral stream. The dorsal stream, known as the "where zone," travels through the parietal cortex and is responsible for transforming information about location and size of objects, which facilitates actions. This stream is also responsible for distance and depth perception with the integration of these diverse cues. The ventral stream, known as the "what zone," travels through the temporal cortex is responsible for identifying the object and its location by recognizing size, location, shape, and orientation in relation to other objects and surfaces, as well as past experiences using visual memory. Difficulties with processing visual perception occurs when there is an asymmetry between these tracts.[1,6,7]

Screening of Visual Perceptual Skills

Before we can discuss formal evaluation of visual perceptual skills, it is imperative that we screen for the foundational visual skills outlined in the hierarchical model of visual perceptual dysfunction. Interpretation of higher level visual perceptual skills would not be accurate without first completing a thorough evaluation of these aforementioned foundational skills. Chapter 7 of this book can serve as a reference for specific details and instructions for screening measures. The advantage of applying a visual hierarchy framework to this process is that it provides a rationale for the selection of screening and evaluation tools that focus on the underlying causes of observed deficiencies.[3]

Visual perceptual deficits can often go unnoticed by clients and occupational therapists until they are evaluated directly. Diagnoses such as acquired brain injury, neurodegenerative diseases (multiple sclerosis, dementia, Alzheimer disease), autism, cerebrovascular accident, neuropsychiatric disorders (schizophrenia), and cerebral palsy are all commonly associated with visual perceptual changes.[5,8–14] Clients may be able to compensate for visual perceptual deficits during basic activities of daily living (ADLs) and instrumental activities of daily living (IADLs) by drawing upon other strengths. Thus, it is essential to have reliable, valid, and sensitive evaluation tools that determine whether visual perceptual deficits exist.[5] It is suggested that health care professionals recognize the importance of formally assessing visual perceptual abilities; however, this has been identified as one of the most difficult areas of evaluation.[15] Assessments can range from brief tabletop screening tasks involving writing, copying, and matching items to behavioral observations during functional tasks, through to complex standardized batteries of tabletop evaluations. The limitations of nonstandardized screening approaches, observations of performance components, and occupational task performance include difficulty defining, documenting, and communicating results, changes, and outcomes. Using standardized evaluations implies uniform procedures for administration and scoring.[16] In addition, standardized evaluations can be used to document current status, progress in therapy, and prioritize treatment goals.[17]

This process should begin with a clinical interview including a historical review of premorbid visual conditions as well as gathering the client and/or family complaints and symptoms. Following this, completion of clinical observation during functional activities and the use of screening tools can be a way for occupational therapists to quickly determine the presence of possible visual perceptual impairments. Clinical observation and screening can vary in depth depending on the facility and team members caring for the client. For example, in the school setting a therapist may need to rely solely on classroom observations due to limited communication with family members and eye care professionals. In contrast, an occupational therapist working in inpatient rehabilitation may be addressing an array of functional skills in collaboration with an interdisciplinary team and onsite eye care professionals, giving ample opportunity for observation and clinical discussion of visual skills.

Visual Perceptual Screening Procedures

Form Constancy

Form constancy plays a primary role in visual perception, relying on distinguishing various types of forms by color, orientation, edge, motion, and shape cues. Difficulties with form constancy are thought to emerge from damage or underdevelopment of the parietal and temporal lobes; however, there is evidence to suggest this involves multiple visual areas of the brain along the ventral stream.[6,10]

Screening Procedures

Form constancy can quickly be screened during various functional activities, determining if the client has difficulty with recognizing familiar items with various forms, such as kitchen utensils or food items at the grocery store. The following is an example of functional screening procedures:

- Have the client seated or standing in a well-lit area.
- Lay out various types and forms of kitchen utensils on a tabletop or countertop in a nonlinear array.
- Ask the client to identify the various kitchen utensils displayed.
- Observe for spatial neglect, perseveration, poor scanning patterns, and comprehension (see Fig. 9-2).

Assessing Impact on Daily Function

A client with decreased form constancy would likely experience difficulties with reading and writing, navigating and locating items in his or her personal environment, and recognizing various types of clothing for dressing. Subtle variations to form are difficult for a client to distinguish in recognition tasks, such as recognizing various pens and pencils as similar tools for writing. Various observations can be made in ADL and IADL tasks, such as experiencing difficulties with following directions with pictures on recipes or furniture instructions, problems with reading various types of handwriting or fonts, discriminating similar letters or words (b/d, was/saw), or difficulty recognizing people wearing different clothing or with a varied hair style.

Figure Ground Perception

Figure ground perception is the ability to distinguish a figure (foreground) from the background. The figure can be described at the primary focus of the individual at any given time. The separation of figure from background is established by differences in features such as color, depth, orientation, texture, and motion. There is contrasting evidence and theories determining if figure ground perception or object recognition occurs first developmentally, and this can incorporate both the dorsal and ventral streams through the visual loop.[6,10]

Screening Procedures

Figure ground perception can quickly be screened during various functional activities, determining if the client has difficulty with identifying items from a background on the basis of subtle or salient features. The following is an example of functional screening procedures:

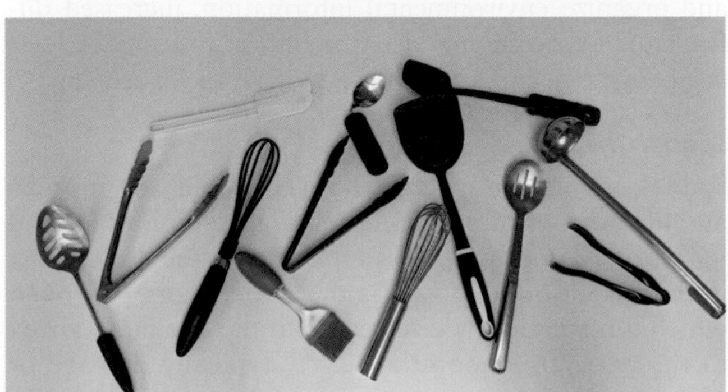

Figure 9-2. Example of functional screening with commonly used kitchen utensils for form constancy.

- Ask the client to locate specific coins from various options placed in his or her hand.
- Ask the client to locate items in a pencil box (glue stick, colored pencil, and eraser) or silverware in a cluttered drawer.
- Ask the client to identify road signs while escorting on an outing through a busy city environment.
- Observe for poor acuity, spatial neglect, perseveration, poor scanning patterns, agnosia, and comprehension.

Assessing Impact on Daily Function

A client with decreased figure ground perception is going to have difficulties in everyday occupations and activities that require identifying or locating objects from a busy or similar background. This can create difficulties with basic self-care tasks with locating the buttons or sleeves of a solid colored shirt or locating the towel hanging on the white wall. This expands into accessing the community to difficulties in locating signs for directions or road rules, finding items in cluttered drawers or shelves, or navigating aisles in a grocery store.

Visual Closure

Visual closure is the ability to visualize a complete whole when provided with fragmented pictures or incomplete information. When lines or pieces are placed close together, such as partially incomplete written letters or numbers, the client should be able to visualize closure of these lines to complete the whole image. If there are portions of an object missing or covered up, or large gaps are present such as attempting to identify a road sign partially covered by a tree branch, visual closure and visual memory are required to identify the object.[18] This is known to be a primary process of the ventral stream through the temporal lobe for object identification.[6] Deficits with visual closure can be identified frequently in individuals through handwriting difficulties, when there are incomplete words or letters. Furthermore, handwriting difficulties are often perceived as a reflection of low intelligence when visual perceptual difficulties are overlooked.[19] See Figure 9-3 for screening examples of handwriting before and after visual perceptual intervention.

Screening Procedures

Visual closure can quickly be screened for during various functional activities, determining if he or she has difficulty with recognizing objects, drawings, or portions of an environment when partially occluded or with missing information. Following are examples of functional screening procedures:

- Ask the client to complete a partially drawn picture or stencil, or to identify the whole image from a partially drawn form.

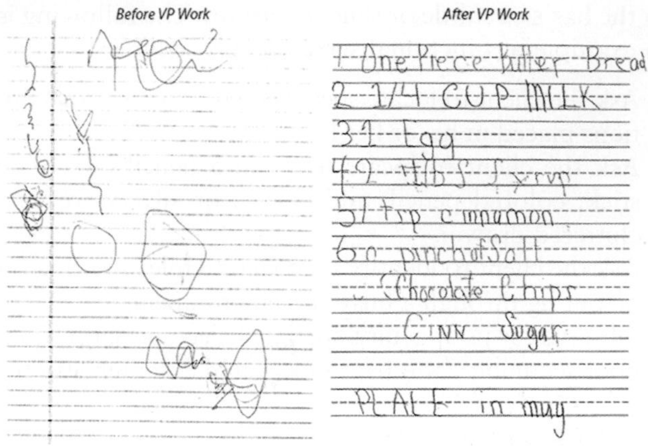

Figure 9-3. Handwriting screening examples before and after visual perceptual intervention.

- Have the client correctly identify 10 common objects from an array of 30 overlapping items.
- Write out a word or draw a simple image on a dry erase board, and erase a portion of this, asking the client to identify said word or image.

Assessing Impact on Daily Function

An individual with decreased visual closure skills will likely encounter difficulties with new learning tasks, handwriting skills, home management tasks, and community integration. If items are partially occluded due to clutter or due to overlapping within the visual field, accurate identification of objects is going to be difficult. For example, if a client is driving, and a stop sign is partially covered by another vehicle, the client would not be able to identify the sign accurately and make a safe decision. A face may become unrecognizable to the client with the eyes missing or covered. Providing opportunities for exposure to this deficit area, along with time for feedback, will aid in overall assessment of functional impact as well as additional chances for building awareness.

Visual Organization

Visual organization is a fundamental property of visual perception form discrimination. This visual perceptual skill is complex and requires dynamic integration of neural activity both within and between cortical areas of the visual loop. It requires the use of visual skills throughout the visual hierarchy and relies on notions of symmetry, continuity, and proximity for grouping visual information.[20,21] Grouping principles include the following qualities: proximity, color, size, orientation, common fate, symmetry, parallelism, continuity, closure, and common region.[13]

Screening Procedures

In addition to functional task completion for observation, the Leuven Perceptual Organization Test (L-POST) can provide quick and valuable information for mid-level visual perceptual abilities. Several of these subtests are useful for identifying visual organization difficulties.[14] The primary goal for this screening tool is to be a quick screen for possible mid-level visual perceptual deficits using digital technology.

- L-POST[14]
  - Visit L-POST testing site at www.gestaltrevision.be/tests.
  - Follow appropriate links to take the screening tool in your client's preferred language.
  - Complete the neglect pretest to rule out visual inattention for use of the computer screen. If inattention appears to be present, items will be presented vertically rather than horizontally.
  - Complete the 15 subtests, which takes a total of 15 to 20 minutes.
  - Scoring is completed electronically and automatically and saved under your account for comparison.
  - Norms are available for all subtests, along with image examples for comparison.
- Functional screening examples
  - Provide client with an array of similar and dissimilar items and ask him or her to sort into groups by various principals (color, size, texture, shape, etc.).
  - Provide client with two images and ask what is different and what is the same.
  - Provide client with visual images of a familiar task (e.g., cooking, grooming, playing a game) and ask him or her to put the images in sequential order.

Assessing Impact on Daily Function

Decreased visual organization creates difficulties in making sense of the extrapersonal and intrapersonal visual environments. Deficits in this area create increased difficulties with figure ground perception and visuoconstructional skills, where one would have to separate and group items in the foreground from the background, or organize visual pieces of information into a whole for two- and three-dimensional imagery.[16,13] Uhlhaas also discusses how this type of impairment is highly correlated with facial recognition.[21] If a client is unable to visually group and organize environmental information, increased difficulty is expected for visual memory and higher level visuocognitive and attention tasks such as sequencing.

Spatial Orientation

Spatial orientation includes both the ability to appreciate the location of objects in relation to each other and in respect to oneself. This is a function of the dorsal tract in the visual loop, known as the "where zone" through which information is directed from the occipital cortex to the parietal-temporal zone.[3,6,7] Typically damage or underdevelopment of the parietal lobe, particularly the right side, is associated with deficits in spatial orientation. Information used to create a sense of relations and orientation is multisensory and includes visual, somatic, proprioceptive, and auditory signals and is interpreted in relation to an ever-changing body scheme. This further requires intact attention skills, visual memory, and visual-motor for possible object manipulation.[7,10]

Screening Procedures

Using a simple Cross Test can be a quick and easy screen for concerns with visual-spatial relations. The procedures are outlined below:[10]

- Provide the client with a card with various cross markings drawn or printed. Start with two crosses as a practice.
- Ask the client to draw the crosses on a blank card as exactly as possible. If he or she does not understand, demonstrate this practice for him or her.
- Provide feedback with a transparent guide to show any disparities in the spatial relations.
- Complete this with three additional cards with five to six crosses in various arrays.
- Scoring is nonstandardized, but can be measured in total number of centimeters of discrepancy between the model and client reproduction. If a cross is missing, this should be scored as half of the width of the card.
    - Intact: score of 0 to 300 cm
    - Impaired: score of 300 to 600 cm
    - Severely impaired: score of >600 cm

In addition to quick paper/pencil screens such as the Cross Test, observations can be made from functional activities as a screen for visual orientation deficits. Following are some examples:

- While in a therapy gym, classroom, or the client's home ask him or her to describe various orientations with visible objects in relation to other objects and in relation to the client. For example, ask "what is directly in front of the treadmill?" or "are the books to your right or to your left?"
- Complete a navigation activity: ask the client to follow a route either through a therapy/school environment or as the passenger of a car in an active passenger activity, and then have the client retrace his or her steps or follow a return route. Another variation is to provide a map and have the client provide verbal directions from point A to point B using spatial references.
- Have the client point to a particular target, such as a clock on the wall, and then have the client move to another part of the room or into the hallway and then point to where that target is. For more advanced screening including visual memory in spatial orientation, have the second location in a position where the initial target is no longer visible.
- Have the client reproduce an arrangement of objects, first in the same orientation and at the client's midline, and then rotated in a different direction and not in midline.

Assessing Impact on Daily Function

Deficits with visual-spatial orientation create functional difficulties in general awareness of oneself and of objects in the interpersonal and extrapersonal environments. This presents as difficulties with basic self-care, such as aligning buttons on a shirt or recognizing which side of a shirt is the front versus the back. Furthermore, more complex concerns include difficulties learning new routes in a rehabilitation facility, or following a navigation system while participating in driver rehabilitation.[10,22]

Unilateral Inattention

Unilateral inattention is a decreased awareness of the body and spatial environment on the side contralateral to the brain lesion. It can occur in the peripersonal and extrapersonal environments[9] and often occurs without a sensory deficit. In the most severe cases, it is as if that side of the environment or world does not exist to the person. This does not have to be a co-requisite of visual field loss, rather a neglect and possible midline shift of the environment. In a visual midline shift, the visual environment is perceived to be shifted away from the affected side, causing a feeling of a tilted environment.[23] Visual inattention is most commonly experienced following a right hemispheric lesion, where left-sided-body-specific inattention is seen with frontal lesions and left-sided environmental neglect is seen with parietal lesions. Recent research has explored the impact of sustained attention skills on patterns of unilateral inattention.[7]

Screening Procedures

There are several readily available and quick screens that can be used in a clinical setting to determine possible unilateral inattention. Unfortunately, according to Menon-Nair, standardized assessments or screens are not readily used at intake and discharge in inpatient rehabilitation settings in the United States, where 61% of positive cases of unilateral inattention had not been detected in admission assessments.[9] The most commonly used screens in practice are the Bell's Test, Clock Drawing Test, Single Letter Cancellation Test, Star Cancellation Test, Comb and Razor Test, the Line Bisection Test, and the Rivermead Behavioral Inattention Test, among several other standardized evaluations. The screening procedures for the Clock Drawing Test and the Comb and Razor Test are outlined here. The procedures for the remaining screens are readily available online and are typically free assessment tools.

- Clock Drawing Test
    - Free Drawn: Provide the client with a blank sheet of paper and ask him or her to draw a clock set to a specific time (e.g., 10 after 11 o'clock). The 10-after-11-o'clock time setting requires visual attention to the left visual field, as well as cognitive skills such as transferring the 2 on the clock to 10 minutes.

- Predrawn: Provide the client with a sheet of paper with a circle predrawn, and ask him or her to draw the face of the clock and set to a specific time.
- There are several scoring guidelines available for the clock drawing test; with unilateral inattention, however, the therapist should screen for omitting numbers, missing hands on the clock, missing the left border of the clock or a presentation of an oblong clock face, or numbers crowding on one side of the clock (see, e.g., Fig. 9-4).

■ Comb and Razor Test
- For all clients, provide them with a comb and ask them to comb their hair. Time the client for 30 seconds and count number of right, left, and ambiguous strokes within the 30 seconds.
- For clients identifying as a male, provide the client with a razor with a shield and ask him to shave his face and continue until you say stop. Time this action for 30 seconds and count number of strokes on the right side, left side, and ambiguous strokes.
- For clients identifying as a female, provide the client with a powder compact and ask her to apply the powder until you ask her to stop. Time for 30 seconds and count the number of touches on the right side and left side as well as ambiguous touches.
- For the most updated scoring methods, apply the following calculation: % bias = (right – strokes)/(left + ambiguous + right strokes) × 100. The % bias formula yields a score between −1 (total left neglect) and +1 (total right neglect), with symmetrical performance at 0.[23]

Assessing Impact on Daily Function

Depending on the severity of unilateral inattention, the functional implications can be vast and possibly hazardous. This could be as minimal as difficulties with reading and writing, or as concerning as missing information while operating a motor vehicle or navigating a grocery store parking lot. These are typically more concerning than with clients experiencing a visual field loss as there is not awareness that this visual perceptual change exists. Clinical observations may include experiences such as missing food on the left side of a plate, running into door jambs on the left side, missing items on the left side of a grocery aisle shelf, or washing only one side of the body or hair in the shower.

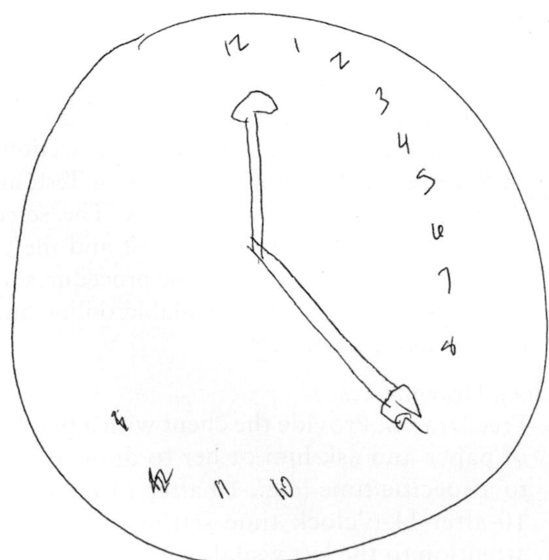

Figure 9-4. Example of a Clock Drawing Test following traumatic brain injury.

Depth Perception

Depth perception is a form of visual perception using coordination of both binocular cues and binocular disparity and the integration of monocular cues such as shading, texture, and linear perspective. When binocularity is intact, true depth perception is acquired through fusion of information from each eye on a horizontal plane, also known as stereopsis.[10] Depth perception has been found to be processed in the inferior parietal regions of the brain for peripersonal space, and in the ventral premotor, middle frontal, and superior temporal areas of the brain for extrapersonal space.[1] Depth perception is a developmental skill that does not typically need to be taught. Deficits with depth perception can arise when there is a strabismus of one eye causing suppression of that eye, and in turn a lack of binocularity.

Screening Procedures

Two screens that are available to occupational therapists that are widely used to detect deficits in stereopsis are the Lang Stereo Test and the Titmus Test.[24] The Lang Stereo Test 1 is found to have the highest sensitivity for stereopsis at 89.9%, and it does not require any additional cross-polarized lenses. The Titmus Test is sensitive 83.3% of the time in detecting stereopsis difficulties for depth perception and requires the use of cross-polarized lenses. Both test plates are to be held at 16 inches by the evaluator, thus testing depth in the peripersonal space. See procedures below for both.[24] These stereopsis screens in additional to functional activity observations can be useful in detecting deficits in depth perception.

■ Lang Stereo Test 1
- Hold test plate at 16 inches (40 cm) from the client at 90°.
- Ask the client to scan the card and identify what he or she may see. Observe eye movements. The client should report a cat, star, and a car.
- Test failure is incorrectly naming or omitting objects.

■ Titmus Test (see Fig. 9-5).
- Have the client wear cross-polarized lenses. Hold the test plate at 16 inches (40 cm) from the client in a well-lit room.
- In rows A, B, and C, have the client identify which animals appear to have depth.

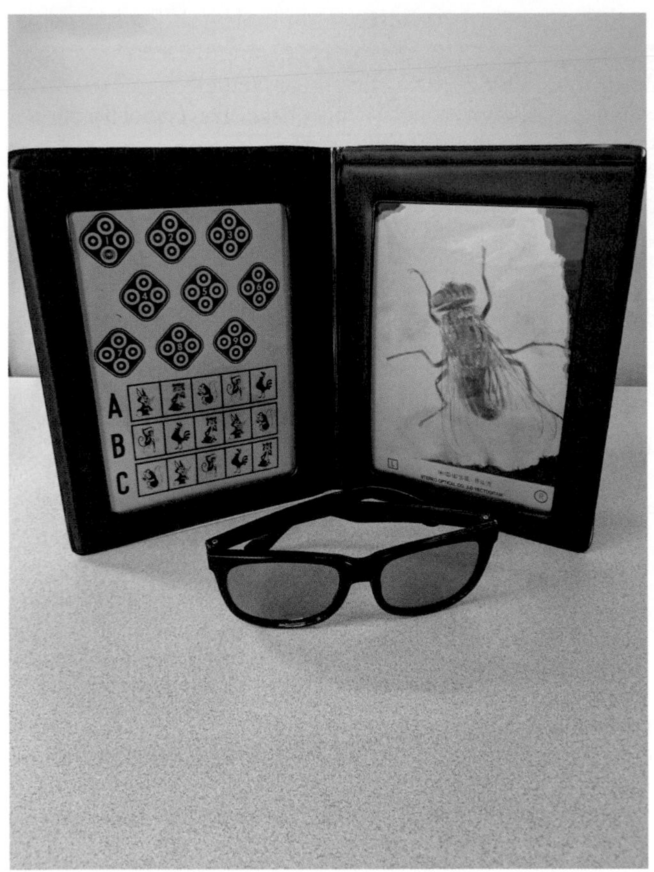

Figure 9-5. Stereo Fly Test for depth perception screening.

  - In areas 1 to 9, have the client identify which button appears raised (top, bottom, left, or right).
  - Answers are included on the back of the testing book. Test failure is inability to identify accurate animals for A, B, or C, as well as incorrectly identifying raised dots for items 5 to 9.
- Functional Screening Examples:
  - Have the client seated at a table with glasses in various heights and at varying distance from the client. Ask the client to pour water from a pitcher into each of these glasses.
  - Ask the client to position his or her wheelchair in the safest location for a transfer into a chair or a bed. Determine if distance from the transfer surface is adequate and safe.
  - Place an object on the table in front of the client and ask him or her to pick it up. Move the object into various locations in space, within arm's reach, and ask the client to grab the object.

Assessing Impact on Daily Function

Assessing and using depth perception through binocular or monocular cues is imperative for safety in navigating our extrapersonal environment. Impacts on depth perception can create frustrating situations such as difficulties with putting on socks, putting toothpaste on a toothbrush, or putting on makeup. It can also create hazardous situations when the depth of curbs or steps cannot be detected accurately. Following a screen of foundational visual skills, it should be common practice to ask clients and their support systems if the client is experiencing situations such as tripping over uneven surfaces, bumping into things, stopping at unsafe distances while driving, or spilling during meal preparation to get a better idea of functional concerns. See Table 9-2 for screening tools and observations for visual perceptual deficits.

Evaluation of Visual Perception

When further and more complex evaluation is warranted for visual perception, there are several factors that need to be considered before selecting your evaluation tool. Factors to consider include age, language abilities, education level, physical impairments, cognitive impairments, and environment. Based on goals and subjective information gathered, it should be determined whether testing should encompass motor reduced, visual-motor integration, or the combination of the two. Also to be considered is the validity, reliability, and temporal constructs of the evaluation tool.[5] Typical visual perceptual assessments include multiple subtests to assess the following visual skills: visual discrimination, visual memory, visual-spatial relationships, form constancy, visual sequential relationships, figure ground, visual-motor integration, and visual closure.[6] See the most commonly used standardized assessments at the end of the chapter.[25–37]

Conceptual Foundation Underlying Interventions for Visual Perceptual Impairment

Following screening and evaluation, proper treatment should consider both remedial and compensatory approaches. According to Warren, effective intervention should include three principals.[3] First, remove or minimize sensory deficits of foundational skills. Second, provide consistent education to increase awareness of deficits; for accurate compensation to occur, clients must be aware that deficits exist and experience the decreased reliability of these senses. Last, incorporate consistent training to both remediate and develop compensation strategies for the deficit areas, promoting overlearning to ensure consistency. The more complex the task, the more the deficit must be practiced for adequate skill acquisition.[3]

A remediation approach uses activities that challenge current abilities with a therapist providing opportunities for practice using graded tasks in controlled therapeutic settings. This type of approach is based on theories of neuroplasticity. Neuroimaging studies have documented changes in brain activation and connectivity during

Table 9-2. Screening Tools and Observations for Visual Perceptual Deficits

DEFICIT AREA	CLIENT COMPLAINTS	CLINICAL OBSERVATION	SCREENING
Form constancy	Difficulty reading Can't find personal belongings Difficulty with dressing, cooking, bathing, grocery shopping	Difficulty following directions with pictures such as a recipe, building furniture, or learning a new board game. Problems recognizing unfamiliar handwriting or new fonts. Recognizing people wearing different clothing. Difficulty in mastering the alphabet and numbers	Occupational Therapy Adult Perceptual Screening Test (OT-APST) Functional Exercise: • Locating various brands and sizes of items on a grocery store shelf • Locating utensils and correct size bowls for baking tasks • Reading directions to a game when words are in different fonts and colors
Figure ground perception	Trouble with laundry Unsafe driving Only plays with one toy	Unable to sort and match socks while folding laundry Difficulty locating clothing in drawers during ADLs Missing road signs or vehicles when driving Unable to locate toys in a toybox	Bells Test Occupational Therapy Adult Perceptual Screening Test (OT-APST) Star Cancellation Test Functional Exercise: • Locating correct change during a money management activity • Locating puzzle pieces during a jigsaw puzzle activity • Locating classroom objects in a pencil box (i.e., Glue stick, eraser, blue crayon, paper clip, etc.)
Visual closure	Unsafe driving Trouble cooking Difficulty playing cards	Cannot identify traffic signs that are partially hidden behind a tree or other vehicle Difficulty locating items in the refrigerator that are partially covered	Functional exercise: • Completing partially drawn pictures or stencils • Identifying 10 common objects in an overlapping array of 30 items
Spatial orientation	Difficulty reading and writing	Letter and number reversals Difficulty with spacing and organization of written school work	Occupational Therapy Adult Perceptual Screening Test (OT-APST) Baking Tray Test
Unilateral inattention	Falling Misplacing items People honking their horns at me Floor appears tilted	Applying makeup or shaving only half of the face Walking into furniture, doorways, and other objects Eating food from half of the tray Leaning or weight bearing to the unaffected side	Occupational Therapy Adult Perceptual Screening Test (OT-APST) Clock Drawing Test Line Bisection Test Bell's Test Star Cancellation Test Albert's Test Comb and Razor Test Baking Tray Task Visual Midline Shift Test
Depth perception	Spilling Tripping/clumsy Running into objects Decreased abilities in sports	Misjudging distances while pouring liquids Fender-bender auto accidents, running stop signs Difficulty with grooming, putting in contacts, placement of makeup Difficulty with catching a ball	Titmus Fly Stereotest Randot Stereotest Cover/Uncover Test Functional exercise: • Navigating a therapy gym, hallway, or playground with obstacles • Estimating common distances (i.e., from person to a fixed-distance point, such as a car) • Pouring liquids into measuring cups
Visual memory	Difficulty spelling and reading Difficulty remembering routes Loses or misplaces items (keys, wallet, etc.)	Cannot remember sight words Often transposes common words Gets lost in familiar routes or newly learned routes Difficulty remembering faces or new people	Clock Drawing Test Scenery Picture Memory Test (SPMT) Spot the Difference for Cognitive Decline (SDCD) Functional Exercise: • Study a photograph for 30 seconds, and describe the photo and items included • Display an array of items or words, remove visual and report as many items as they can remember

Table 9-2. Screening Tools and Observations for Visual Perceptual Deficits (*continued*)

Visual-motor integration	Clumsiness Different handwriting/ signature Difficulty with typing	Difficulty with letter formation and handwriting Decreased participation in sports Decreased ability to complete a puzzle or construction of an object with pictorial instructions	Occupational Therapy Adult Perceptual Screening Test (OT-APST) Clock Drawing Test Trail Making A and B Functional exercise: • Write name or copy a sentence on paper • Copy simple line drawings • Scissor along various dotted lines
Visuocognition (planning and organization)	Disorganized Decreased reading comprehension	Difficulty sorting and organizing personal belongings Difficulty sequencing and planning for an activity or game Difficulty making sense of typed or written words and sequencing a story	Trail Making A and B Functional exercise: • Sequence a recipe on the basis of pictorial steps • Sequence a grooming task with displayed items (i.e., toothpaste, toothbrush, faucet, towel, cup)

ADLs, activities of daily livings.

visual-spatial, visual attention, and perceptual organization after completing training. Tasks should be initially rudimentary and become more complex following success with a strong emphasis on repeated practice, mastery of skills, and the reacquisition of confidence. A remediation approach may be considered when clients show a potential for improvement, awareness of current limitations, and the ability to receive feedback.[38] A bottom-up approach should be used for reacquisition of foundational skills before adding complexity into treatment.

Once the client has achieved maximal benefit from remediation approaches, the therapist's next step could include practicing under a compensatory approach and using top-down treatment methods using strategies.[16] This approach may teach strategies for functional skill completion, such as upper body dressing, and would not assess for and treat the underlying task components such as primary visual skills and perceptual abilities.

Remedial and compensatory approaches should be incorporated into a variety of contexts to ensure carryover and application with ADL and IADL abilities. A mastery of skills cannot be accomplished without the ability to transfer these abilities into functional settings. In addition, one may consider an adaptive approach, which places emphasis on changing the environment or activity to meet the needs of the client. This is typically introduced once remedial and compensatory approaches have reached maximal potential or for safety reasons.[38]

Specific Interventions for Visual Perceptual Skill Dysfunction

There is evidence in the literature that supports the remediation of visual perceptual deficits, highlighting the importance of visual perceptual training occurring within functional context.[39] The theoretical approaches that should guide this treatment are both developmental and neurophysiological in nature. See the evidence table of intervention studies at the end of the chapter.[40–44] Occupational therapists should consider using various types of therapeutic activities to improve visual perceptual functions (see Table 9-3).[41] It is within an occupational therapists skillset to utilize activity analysis to identify appropriate treatment techniques and activities to remediate, compensate, and adapt for visual perceptual deficits.

The remedial or developmental approach is typically initiated on the basis of the premise that the brain can acquire or reacquire function through environmental stimulation. Reacquisition of skills should follow the original path of development, a hierarchical approach to the remediation of perceptual deficits used in treatment. In Piaget's model of cognitive development, the lower level performance components are acquired before more advanced cognitive skills. Treatment activities should place initial emphasis on foundational skills, regardless of the individual's level of functioning, in order to ensure that the foundation is solid before advancing to higher level cognitive skills.[39,45] Toglia emphasized the importance of practice drills and grading within treatment for direct remediation of observed deficits.[45] With that being said, repetition over a period of weeks should be implemented when using these various treatment approaches or modalities. Choosing activities that have multiple levels of difficulty and the ability to alter speed requirements and offer the opportunity to adjust levels of attention complexity are important to consider for grading activities up or down to foster meeting the client's goals while considering his or her just right challenge. Examples of grading activities up to maximize potential gains could include increasing environmental distractions by listening to music, podcasts, or news stations while participating in the visual perceptual activity. The therapist could also add time constraints, require recall of activity instructions, and implement categorization tasks or other cognitive loading activities while maintaining the expected accuracy and efficiency of the visual perceptual skill (see Table 9-4). To ensure continued appropriateness of a remediation approach, a therapist should

Table 9-3. Commonly Used Therapeutic Activities Related to Visual Perceptual Performance Areas

ACTIVITY	EXAMPLES	DEFICIT AREA
Card games	Mattel BLINK Set/Set Jr Nertz/Peanuts/Dutch Blitz Spot It! Carl's Cards Fast Flip! Uno Mattel Skip-Bo Swish On the Line/On the Dot Fluxx	Form constancy Figure ground perception Visual closure Visual organization Spatial orientation Unilateral inattention/neglect Depth perception
Board games	Qwirkle Q-Bitz IQ Twist I Trax Acuity Aztack Gravity Maze NMBR9 Avalanche Fruit Stand Wonky Connect 4 Guess Who Kerplunk Sequence/Sequence Jr Eye Found It Cribbage	Form constancy Figure ground perception Visual closure Visual organization Spatial orientation Unilateral inattention/neglect Depth perception
Yard games	Ladder ball Bean bag toss Washers Can Jam Horse Shoes Yard Darts Putt Putt golf Archery Catch Table tennis	Form constancy Figure ground perception Visual closure Visual organization Spatial orientation Unilateral inattention/neglect Depth perception
Tabletop activities	Pixy Cubes Labarynth Find It Beading Color By Number Sand Art Tan Knitting/Crocheting Cross Stitch Where's Waldo/Eye Spy Books Bingo Tactile Kinesthetic Pegboard	Form constancy Figure ground perception Visual closure Visual organization Spatial orientation Unilateral inattention/neglect Depth perception
Tablet exercises	Subway Surfers Cooking Fever Candy Crush Bejewled	Form constancy Figure ground perception Visual closure

ACTIVITY	EXAMPLES	DEFICIT AREA
	Temple Run/Minion Rush Look Again! Fruit Ninja Glowburst Minecraft Find It—Match It Vision Tap Tap the Frog iSays Monster Hunt Cut the Rope Flow Free Unblock Me	Visual organization Spatial orientation Unilateral inattention/neglect Depth perception
Gaming systems	Nintendo Wii • Big Brain Academy—Wii Degree • Wii Sports • Guitar Hero • Wii Play • Wii Fit • Band Hero X Box Kinect/360 • Fruit Ninja • Dance Dance Revolution • Deca Sports Freedom • Kinect Sports	Form constancy Figure ground perception Visual closure Visual organization Spatial orientation Unilateral inattention/neglect Depth perception
Computer exercises	Hidden picture/highlights hidden pictures Picture differences Word finds Mahjong Solitaire Mavis Beacon	Form constancy Figure ground perception Visual closure Visual organization Spatial orientation Unilateral inattention/neglect Depth perception
Other visual-spatial modalities	Vision coach/Dynavision Trunk rotation training Scrolling text Neck muscle stimulation Video feedback training Prism therapy Neurovisual Postural Training (NVPT) Virtual reality	Unilateral inattention/neglect Spatial orientation Visual-motor integration
Functional activities	Grocery shopping Complex cooking Sorting laundry Handwriting Grooming Reading the newspaper Driving	Form constancy Figure ground perception Visual closure Visual organization Spatial orientation Unilateral inattention/neglect Depth perception

Source: Menon-Nair A, Korner-Bitensky N, Ogourtsova T. Occupational therapists' identification, assessment, and treatment of unilateral spatial neglect during stroke rehabilitation in Canada. *Stroke.* 2007;38(9):2556–2562. doi:10.1161/STROKEAHA.107.484857; Christy K, Huffine N, Hannah T, DeLeion M. Outcomes after cognitive perceptual motor retraining (CPM) of patients with acquired brain injury (ABI). *Open J Occup Ther.* 2016;4(1). doi:10.15453/2168-6408.1076.

Table 9-4. Cognitive Loading Examples

COGNITIVE LOADING	EXAMPLES
Active listening for recall of information	Music Podcasts News stories How to videos on YouTube
Simplistic question and answer or categorical naming	Trivia cards or applications Fitz It Joe Name It Respond cards
Alternating between multiple tasks	Following a sequential key Self-timing transitions or following alarms Self-structure or structure the therapy hour activity

complete periodic retesting for objective measures for comparison.

Compensation is a treatment approach that aims to maximize existing visual function by providing strategies to enhance the client's ability to assimilate visual information efficiently. A compensatory approach should also place emphasis on understanding underlying difficulties in visual perception in order to learn when to initiate the use of strategies to overcome limitations. Rather than focusing on one task-specific skill, the client should gain the ability to use the learned strategies in various situations.[45] Warren supports the use of practicing strategies for visual perceptual deficits within context to ensure carryover of application to ADLs.[3]

Pattern Recognition

Pattern recognition is the perceptual process of matching incoming visual stimuli with stored visual memories. Although research is limited on the effectiveness of the use of computers, tablets, gaming systems, and tabletop exercises for the remediation of pattern recognition skills; it is common practice to utilize these modalities in treatment. Following this approach, compensation and adaptation for pattern recognition then requires personal and environmental alterations for deficits in the following skills: form constancy, figure ground perception, visual closure, visual organization, and spatial orientation. In general, these can include reducing visual stimulation and overlapping of objects, changing spatial arrangements into categorized or linear arrays, slowing down processing times for accuracy, forming proper scanning patterns, and incorporating multisensory techniques for visual perceptual input.[45] These strategies and adaptations can be used in both therapeutic activities and functional tasks. For example, during a laundry sorting task one could form piles of clothing to create categories by type to compensate for visual figure ground and form constancy. The clothing could also be sorted by color, and it could be unfolded to show its full form as a strategy for form constancy. While searching for a particular piece of clothing, one could start scanning in the top left portion of the pile moving to the right and then top to bottom to practice accurate and efficient scanning patterns. The person could then verbalize what is seen for further processing purposes, too.

Unilateral Inattention

When treatment planning for unilateral inattention, the therapist must consider the personal context that the client is impacted in. This can include impairments and inattention within personal, peripersonal, and extrapersonal space. Typically someone with unilateral inattention will also present with disrupted scanning patterns and poor awareness of the decreased visual input. According to Tham et al., unilateral inattention typically presents as disorientation to objects in the left half of a client's extrapersonal space, and clients typically are unable to wash or dress the left half of their bodies.[46] This can be compensated for by using prisms, attention training, scrolling text, audiovisual stimulation, video feedback training, learning new scanning patterns with anchors and guides, and lighthouse scanning to the affected side to enhance awareness of the visual field.[9,47,48] In order to master compensatory strategies, one should practice these in a variety of settings within the office, home, and community. An occupational therapist should also be sure to practice these strategies in all ADL and IADL contexts to ensure automaticity and habit formation, as well as to build awareness of this deficit.

Prisms

Those with unilateral inattention oftentimes develop poor habits with visual scanning and motor movements. Optometrists, occupational therapists, and physical therapists can work collaboratively to stimulate neuroplasticity through prism adjustments, feedback, and gross motor integration. Multisensory approaches teach new visual patterns through the integration of proprioception, vestibular skills, and peripheral vision. While the use of prisms sometimes is automatically integrated, other clients will need guidance from the therapist to attend to visual information and improve posture. Prisms are easily integrated into functional tasks and therefore make them an ideal therapy tool.[49] However, the research on this can be controversial for self-care.[50]

An optometrist will fit the client with the optimal size and type of prism through the use of objective balance and movement measures. The base end of the prism will be positioned on the same direction as the paretic side and visual inattention if there is a visual midline shift. Prisms yoked in this fashion have an effect of countering the expansion and compression of space, with the apex expanding space and the base compressing space.[23] An occupational therapist will use this tool during therapeutic scanning and functional activities (see Fig. 9-6). The therapist can first work with a client in the controlled environment to scan for signs, people, or objects on the affected side. To grade the task, the client will work up to busy environments and uneven walking surfaces in the community.[51]

Sustained Attention Training

It has been theorized that unilateral inattention could be due to decreased cognitive attention, and improving overall sustained attention and awareness can improve this deficit area. Facilitating activation of the sustained attention system is a strategy that has been discussed to decrease unilateral spatial inattention.[52] This is based on the premise that in the sustained attention system, one needs to anticipate a response in the absence of external stimuli.[53] A study integrated sustained attention training during a sorting task, first starting with an unpredictable auditory reminder with knocking and a verbal cue to "attend!" This was then graded to patient-driven auditory commands, and then to internal mental reminders, with encouragement to utilize this strategy in other daily tasks. The study concluded that this type of treatment program improved the patients' ability to sustain attention and reduced the effects of unilateral inattention.[53] This is further supported by the development of an awareness training program as described by Tham et al., upon the assumption that having an increased awareness of a deficit is a prerequisite to be able to learn and effectively use compensatory strategies.[46] They found that with training in awareness of a unilateral inattention deficit paired with sustained attention training, improvements were seen in overall occupational performance and a reduction in unilateral spatial neglect.

Scanning

Visual scanning training is a frequently used therapeutic approach for compensating for unilateral spatial inattention. This can include paper-and-pencil tasks, computer and tablet activities, and functional tasks such as scanning for items at a grocery store. Another modality that can be used for scanning training would be the use of a Vision Coach, Dynavision, or Wayne Saccadic Fixator (see Fig. 9-7). This type of training has been shown to be effective; however, it is typically not generalized beyond that situation.[52] For example, visual scanning training for a cooking task should be practiced in a kitchen environment, and developing scanning strategies for reading should be practiced with paper/pencil or tabletop activities. With that

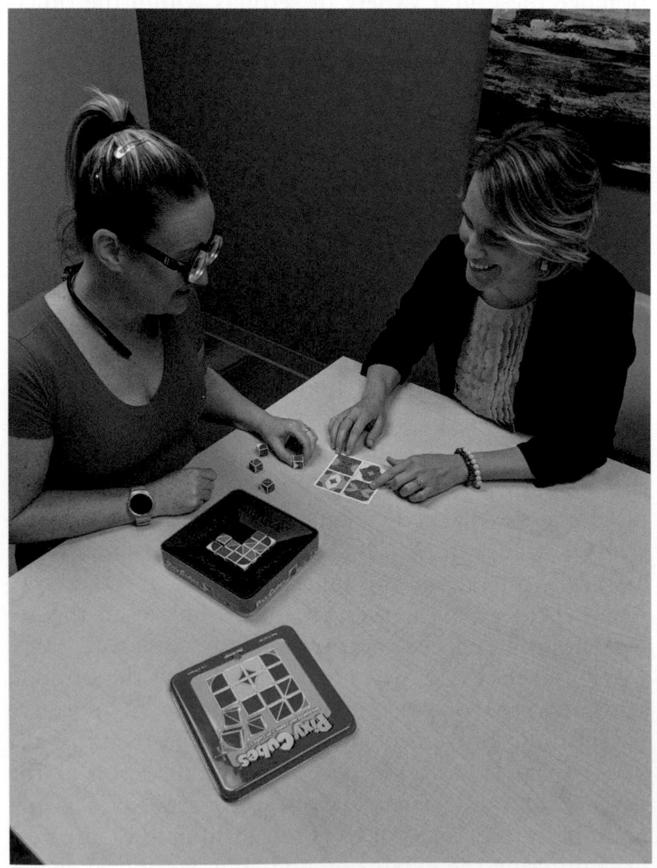

Figure 9-6. Therapist and client working on a visual scanning and pattern recognition task with yoked prisms.

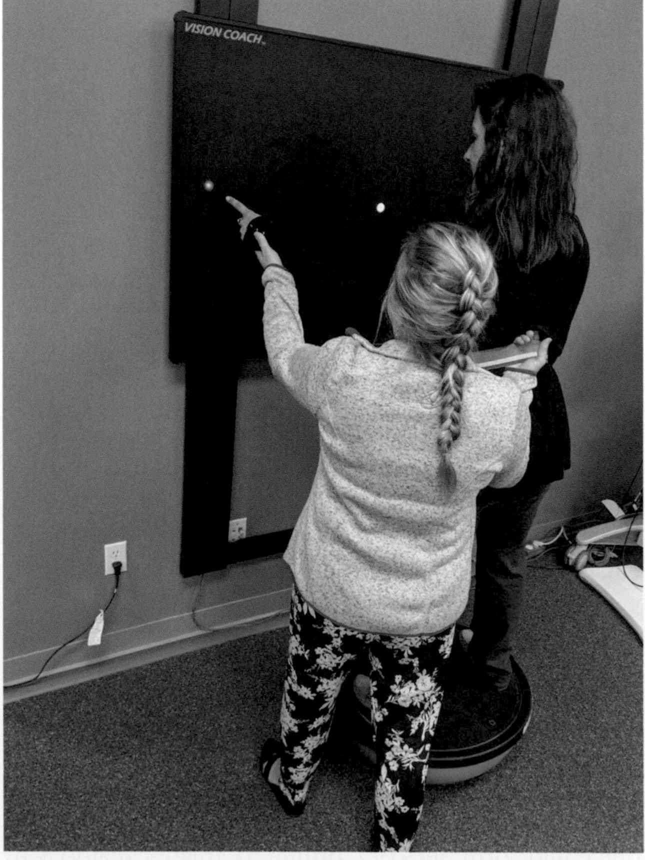

Figure 9-7. Use of the Vision Coach for a visual scanning activity with balance compromised.

being said, a combination of scanning training, sensory awareness, and spatial organizational training has been found to be effective for treatment for patients with right hemisphere damage.[53]

Quintana discusses both lighthouse scanning techniques, or imagining oneself as a lighthouse and using the eyes to sweep the environment, and using visual anchors to help bring attention back to the neglected side as effective strategies for unilateral inattention.[52] This type of approach can further be graded by the therapist by increasing or decreasing the complexity of the array of information to be scanned, reducing or increasing the location and type of visual anchor, and providing additional cueing as needed to ensure thorough scanning of the visual environment. Again, these strategies should be practiced in a variety of tasks and settings so the client is not task-specific learning, and so that the strategy can be carried over for functional use.

Patching

Patching can be a quick, effective, and inexpensive therapeutic tool for decreasing unilateral inattention that can be used across disciplines. There is research to support the use of patching for unilateral spatial inattention in that in individuals without disruption to the nervous system, retinal input is strongest to the contralateral superior colliculus.[53] Visual stimulation to one side (right) of the superior colliculus generates saccadic movements to the contralateral side (leftward). There is an assumption that by patching an entire eye, visual stimulation follows the stronger pathway and would facilitate attention and visual saccades to the contralateral side. A study by Butter and Kirsch found that patching an entire eye demonstrated improvements in a standard battery for inattention; however, the results did not translate to function once the patch was removed.[54] Furthermore, an additional study found no difference between a test group and control group with monocular eye patching.[55] In fact, patching a monocular side is considered a contraindication for clients following brain injury and can worsen spatial judgments with left neglect.[56] Best practice in utilizing patching is seen with research in using hemifield patching as compared with a control group without patching and when compared with monocular patching. Patients who donned right hemifield patches demonstrated improvements in functional independence measure scoring, pencil-and-paper tasks, and right eye movements in the left field.[52,53]

Audiovisual Stimulation

Multisensory treatment techniques have been shown to be an effective method for retraining visual perceptual function. Audiovisual stimulation provides opportunities for task grading with three types of stimulation integrating the audio and visual systems. As discussed in Tinelli et al.[57] and Frassinetti et al.,[58] these conditions include a unimodal visual condition with presentation of only visual stimuli, a unimodal acoustic condition with stimuli presented as only an acoustic cue, and a bimodal audiovisual condition, with audio and visual stimuli together. These can either be congruent or incongruent by location. The patients are cued to focus on a central focal point and shift their gaze (without head movements) to the visual target when detected, while pressing a response button. This type of treatment is shown to be effective through Telehealth services in facilitating the recovery of visual orientation skills.[57] Although research is limited on functional carryover of skills, bimodal multisensory integration with stimulation presented on the relative side improved awareness into the neglected visual region.[58]

Depth Perception

When depth perception cannot be remediated due to decreased binocularity and eye teaming, or with a malalignment of the eyes allowing for reacquisition of stereo depth perception, environmental contextual cues can be used. Typically, our visual system performs size estimations efficiently and effortlessly. When this is not the case, learning to interpret visual illusions and monocular cues can be taught as a compensatory strategy. Understanding shadowing and texture gradation, line of parallax or size cues, and recognizing superimposition of objects can be learned strategies for depth.[59] For examples of these environmental cues, see Table 9-5.

Table 9-5. Monocular Depth Cues

ENVIRONMENTAL CUE	EXPLANATION	IMAGE
Shadowing	Highlights and shadows can provide information about an object's dimensions and depth. Our visual system assumes light comes from above	

(continued)

Table 9-5. Monocular Depth Cues (*continued*)

ENVIRONMENTAL CUE	EXPLANATION	IMAGE
Line of parallax	Has to do with angles along line of sight. Nearby objects have a larger parallax than more distant objects	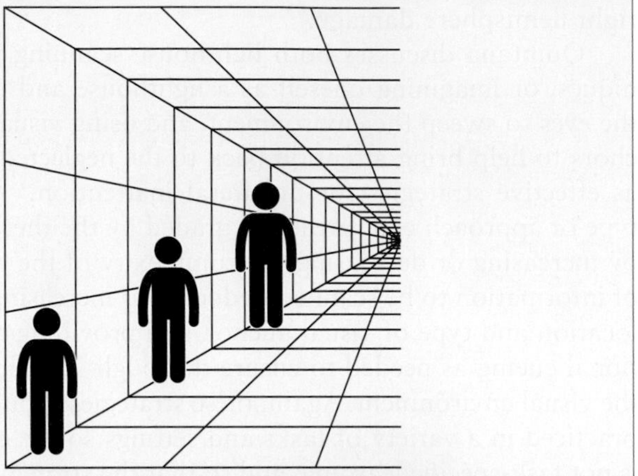
Superimposition	When there are two overlapping objects, the overlapped object is considered further away	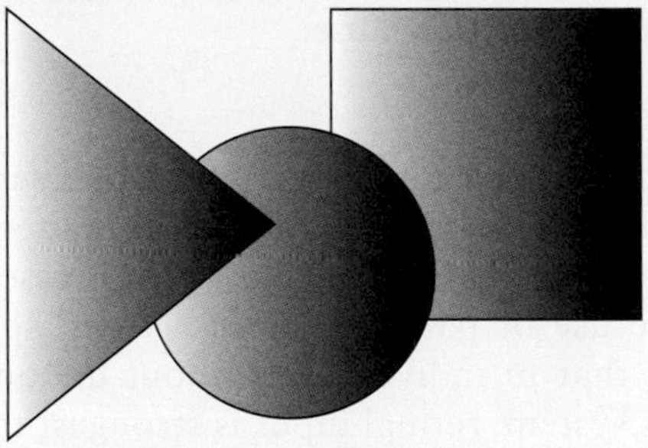
Size illusions	Ebbinghaus illusion	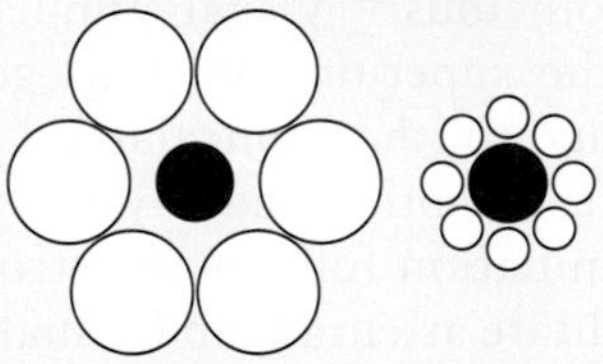
	Delboeuf illusion	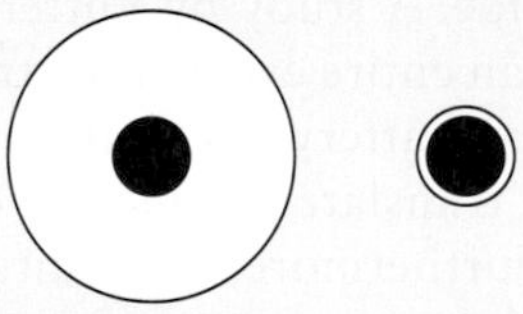
	Mueller-Lyer illusion	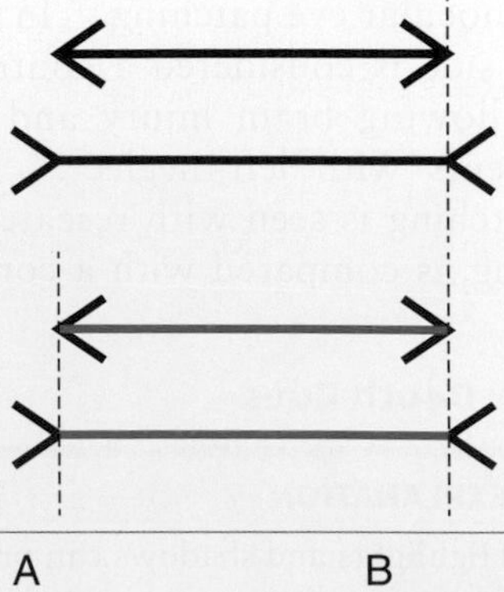
	Oppel-Kundt illusion	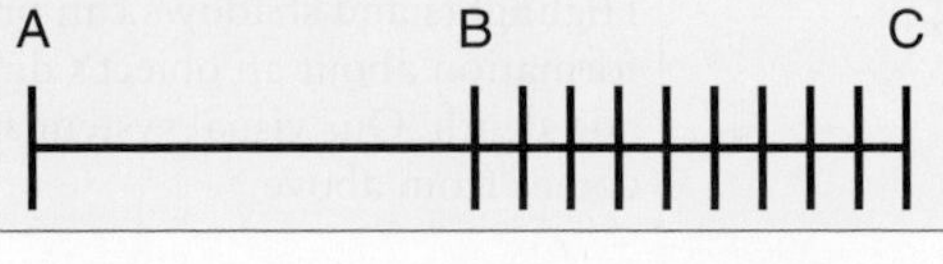

CASE STUDY

Patient Information

Jaden is a 17-year-old high school senior who prefers not to use gender-based pronouns and was involved in a motor vehicle accident. Jaden received inpatient rehabilitation immediately following the accident and was recently discharged to outpatient therapy. Jaden was employed as a restaurant host and busboy before their injury. They currently live at home with their parents and two brothers and have a strong network of friends, all of whom are supportive of Jaden's recovery process. Jaden is highly motivated to return to driving and normal life at school. However, they demonstrate limited acceptance and awareness of their brain injury and related changes and therefore does not understand the purpose of therapy in enabling them to return to these meaningful activities. Jaden is often disrespectful to therapists and distracted during sessions.

Assessment Process and Results

Upon admission to outpatient rehabilitation, Jaden participated in a full physical and cognitive occupational therapy evaluation. Their muscle tone, gross sensation and perception, range of motion, and strength was found to be within functional limits. Jaden's orientation and time management skills were also found to be intact, and psychosocial skills were appropriate for the environment. Jaden's visual screen indicated diplopia and deficits with ocular range of motion, saccadic movement, and pursuits. Jaden's visual deficits combined with difficulty with memory and slowed information processing speed led the occupational therapist to suspect that Jaden's visual perceptual skills had been affected in the accident. The occupational therapist administered the Developmental Test of Visual Perception–Adult Version. Jaden ranked in the fourth percentile for the Motor Reduced Visual Perceptual subtests with a *z*-score indicating mild impairment in this skill area. Within this skillset, figure ground perception and visual closure were most difficult for Jaden. Jaden's performance on the visual-motor integration earned them a percentile rank of less than one and a *z*-score representing borderline severe impairment in this skill area. Jaden especially struggled with the Visual Motor Search And Copying subtests, indicating difficulties with motor planning, visuoconstructional skills, and motor speed in response to visual input (see Fig. 9-8 for the Copying subtest). The occupational therapist also administered Trailmaking A and B to determine if visual cognitive skills were impaired, in which they scored within the severe impairment range. Jaden's performance on the variety of evaluations administered by the occupational therapist indicated deficits with visual perceptual skills.

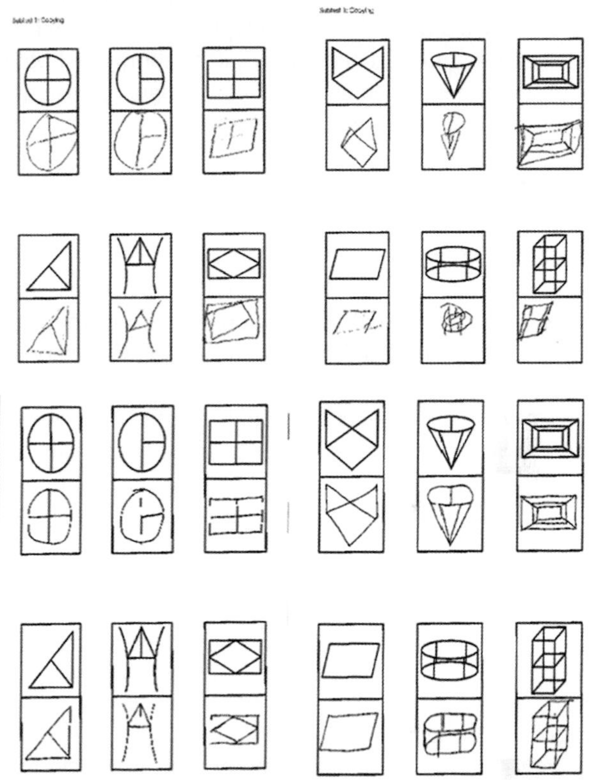

Figure 9-8. Copying subtest of the DTVP-A before and after Cognitive Perceptual Motor Remediation intervention.

Occupational Therapy Problem List

Based on the skill deficits revealed by Jaden's performance on the perceptual evaluations along with observations of functional tasks, the occupational therapist compiled a list of visual perceptual deficits to address with Jaden during their sessions.

- Difficulty identifying objects in a busy background, such as road signs or pedestrians within a city or town.
- Trouble identifying objects that may be partially covered or missing, such as the remote control sitting partially underneath a throw pillow.
- Difficulty alternating between two or more tasks efficiently and accurately, which is required for homework, driving, meal preparation, etc.
- Trouble managing controls in a motor vehicle while driving, difficulties typing or handwriting at an efficient speed, and/or difficulties with everyday tasks such as preparing food and playing sports.

(continued)

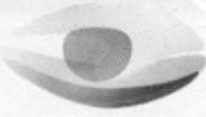

CASE STUDY *(continued)*

- Difficulties with independent use of the hands without visual assistance, such as using a blinker while driving, taking notes from a projector screen, or typing on a computer.
- Challenges comprehending new information in school or a productive employment setting secondary to decreased information processing speeds.

Occupational Therapy Goal List

Short-Term Goals:

- Jaden will improve visual scanning, visual anchoring, figure ground perception, eye/hand coordination, visual-motor integration, and visual information processing speeds to within-average ranges through participation in therapeutic activities.
- Jaden will improve visual perceptual skills to within-average ranges while participating in therapeutic activities with cognitive loading including focused/shifting visual attention, selective visual attention, sequencing, organization, and divided attention.
- Jaden will demonstrate independence in IADLs through the use of compensatory strategies for visual figure ground perception, visual scanning, visual anchoring, visual-motor integration, and visual information processing speeds.

Long-Term Goals:

- Improve visual-spatial, visual-motor, and executive functions to within-average ranges ($Z = -0.4$ to 0.4) on standardized testing measures to maximize safety, independence, and efficiency in the home, workplace, and community.
- Implement compensatory strategies 90% to 100% of the time independently to improve accuracy and efficiency in all IADLs.

Intervention

Based on findings from the evaluation, the occupational therapist determined that Jaden's significant visual and cognitive perceptual difficulties would best be addressed through a treatment method referred to as Cognitive Perceptual Motor Remediation (CPM). This therapy utilizes client-centered activities that require divided attention skills, quick information processing speeds, and visual perceptual skills such as form constancy and visual-motor integration. Jaden's typical sessions included many iPad application activities because these activities could be easily graded to their current level and increased in difficulty as skills progressed. Use of the iPad applications also allowed the occupational therapist to obtain quantifiable data on Jaden's performance to quickly assess skill progression. In early sessions, these applications required Jaden to interpret visual information and quickly respond with a motor output, as well as solve visual information problems and recognize the foreground versus the background. The activities also drew on Jaden's alternating and divided attention skills, which are necessary prerequisites for driving. The occupational therapist's short-term goals for each application accounted for Jaden's baseline performance and where it was determined Jaden's skills could be at discharge. After 3 months of therapy focusing on these applications with grading as necessary, Jaden had met four activity objectives with noted improvement on visual sequencing, visual-motor speed, and information processing speed.

With progress noted, Jaden was soon engaging in activities requiring increased visual memory skills, as well as increased eye–hand coordination and independent use of each hand. The occupational therapist graded her own level of co-participation in these activities to challenge Jaden, yet still provide them with a sense of achievement. For example, the occupational therapist would engage in an activity at 75% capacity when it was first introduced to Jaden to avoid causing them to feel frustrated and discouraged when comparing their skills with those of the occupational therapist.

By March, 6 months after beginning therapy, Jaden had met all their visual perception goals. The occupational therapist readministered the assessments initially used to evaluate Jaden's skills. Their scores improved to the mild impairment to average ranges. As an example of progress, Jaden's improvement on the Copying subtest of the DVTP-A is illustrated in Figure 9-8. Occupational therapy services continued, but the focus on visual perceptual skills shifted to task-specific training sessions. Jaden was pleased with the progress they had made despite the frequent frustrations throughout the months of intervention.

Most Commonly Used Standardized Assessments

Instrument and Reference	Intended Purpose	Administration Time	Validity	Reliability	Sensitivity	Strengths and Weaknesses
Baking Tray Task[25,26]	Used to assess for unilateral spatial neglect	<10 minutes	Found to detect more cases of neglect than the three-item Behavioral Inattention Test and is even more accurate when used in combination with the Line Bisection Test	Test–retest 0.87	Increased through combination with other tests; more sensitive than the three-item Behavioral Inattention Test	Easy to administer. Most sensitive single test to detect spatial neglect. Easy and cost-effective to create your own with the measurements provided. Not a lot of depth to the test or scoring. Assumed cognitive impairment if spatial neglect is not present.
Line Bisection Test[27]	Used to detect unilateral spatial neglect	<5 minutes	Convergent validity with Baking Tray Task: $r = -0.66$	Test–retest reliability: 0.97 Internal consistency: no evidence	Detects spatial neglect with 76.4% accuracy	Many versions; however, the procedures are rarely standardized.
Trail Making A and B[28–30]	Used to assess visual conceptual and visuomotor tracking conditions	5–10 minutes	Construct validity for rapid visual search and visual sequencing. Trails A: Visual perceptual abilities Trails B: working memory and task switching	Test–retest reliability: Test A: $r = 0.83$ Test B: $r = 0.90$	Functional MRI studies demonstrate activation of the ventral and dorsal visual processing streams	Public domain assessment is easy to administer and obtain. Some versions have therapist correct mistakes along the way.
Bell's Test[31,32]	Quick screen for visual neglect in the near extrapersonal space	<5 minutes	Criterion Validity: more likely to evidence left neglect than Albert's Test, Star Cancellation Test, Line Bisection Test, and Line Crossing Test	No evidence	No evidence	The Bell's Test requires no specialized training to administer and only minimal equipment is required (a pencil, a stopwatch, the test paper, and scoring sheet). The test is simple to score and interpret.
Motor-Free Visual Perception Test (MVPT-3)[10,33]	Widely used standardized test of visual perception, assessing visual perception independent of motor ability	20–30 minutes	Criterion related: 0.78 with the DTVP-2 and 0.73 with the DTVP	Internal consistency: 0.86–0.90 Test–retest: 0.92	General measure for motor-free visual perceptual components	Does not provide norms for separate subtests. Short and simple measure that is tolerated well by most clients.

(continued)

Most Commonly Used Standardized Assessments (*continued*)

Instrument and Reference	Intended Purpose	Administration Time	Validity	Reliability	Sensitivity	Strengths and Weaknesses
Test of Visual Perceptual Skills (TVPS-4)[4–6,17]	Visual Perception Test to use with children	25 minutes	Discriminative validity is significant for testing participants with and without neurological impairments for all subtests ($p < 0.001$).	Reliability was found in testing outlined skills within subtests using Spearman Rho Correlations. Significant Correlation with figure ground perception (0.306), spatial relations (0.193), and form constancy (0.465) between the DTVP-2 and TVPS-R.	Not established for most recent fourth edition	Simple to administer, able to use with students/clients with motor impairments. Test designs are bold, and verbal responses are not required.
Developmental Test of Visual Perception Adolescent and Adult (DTVP-A) (DTVP-2)[4,5,10]	Comprehensive assessment with subtests for motor reduced visual perception and visual-motor integration	20–30 minutes	Discriminative validity is significant for testing participants with and without neurological impairments for motor-free subtests ($p < 0.001$). Motor portions of the DTVP-2 were valid with subtests of the TVPS-4.	Interrater: 0.94–0.99 Test–retest: 0.70–0.84	The DTVP-A measures potential visual perceptual deficits for adults with diagnosed neurological impairment.	Able to standardize scores on the basis of age for all subtests and to separate out visual-motor integration and motor reduced visual perception. Ceilings for all subtests.
The Occupational Therapy Adult Perceptual Screening Test (OT-APST)[16,34–36]	Designed as a quick screening tool of 25 items for occupational therapists to assess for presence of visual perceptual impairment in the main constructs of visual perception and apraxia	20–25 minutes	Concurrent Criterion Validity for neglect: $p = 0.006$ (moderate correlation) Concurrent Criterion Validity for agnosia: $p \leq 0.001$ (moderate correlation)	Interrater reliability ranged from 0.66 to 1.0 for all subtests. Intrarater reliability ranged from 0.64 to 1.0 for all subtests. Test–retest reliability ranged from 0.76 to 1.0.	In comparison with the LOTCA sensitivity for agnosia is 85.7% and neglect is 69.2%.	Quick and easy-to-administer screening tool for visual perception and apraxia, paired with functional observations. Required to screen for primary visual functions before completing the OT-APST.
Rivermead Perceptual Assessment Battery (RPAB)[16,37]	Tests for 16 performance areas in visual perceptual skills	60–120 minutes	Reported content criterion and construct validity	Reported Interrater and test–retest reliability	RPAB is a significant predictor of functional outcomes in stroke patients.	Simple instructions to administer, including demonstrations. Longer assessment to administer, however, is designed to help with treatment planning.
Loewenstein Occupational Therapy Cognitive Assessment (LOTCA)[10]	Assessment in six different areas for orientation, visual perception, spatial perception, praxis, visuomotor organization, and thinking operations	45 minutes	Overlapping Figures Subtest: Administration of entire LOTCA is recommended versus administering subtests.	Interrater reliability: 0.82 to 0.97 for all subtests Internal consistency of Visual Identification of Objects: 0.87	No evidence	Lengthy assessment, however, can be completed over multiple sessions. Can be used to set therapeutic goals and to monitor cognitive status over time.

Evidence Table of Intervention Studies

Intervention	Description	Participants	Dosage	Research Design and Evidence Level	Benefit	Statistical Significance and Effect Size
Cognitive Perceptual Motor Remediation (CPM)[40]	A remedial approach for deficits in cognitive, perceptual motor, and sensory-motor functioning following a brain injury. It is hierarchical in nature, using a bottom-up approach and repetition. This approach uses computerized activities, paper/pencil tasks, manipulation of objects, and other tabletop activities, beginning with sensory-motor and perceptual tasks that precede cognition.	This study reviewed records of a total of 53 clients in which 30 identified as male and 23 identified as female. The mean age was 35.8 years. 43% were classified as severe traumatic brain injury, 19% as moderate traumatic brain injury, and 38% as mild.	CPM is typically prescribed 3 hours/week for therapy sessions. Additional home exercise programs can be recommended. In this study duration included 4 participants 12 weeks or less, 19 participants at 13–24 weeks, 18 participants for 25–36 weeks, 11 participants at 37–52 weeks, and 1 participant at more than 1 year.	This was a retrospective study, reviewing records from 1998 to 2009. The main outcome measures were objective changes in evaluation test scores. The tests of visual-spatial perception included Figure Ground Subtest of the Southern California Visual Perception Test, Cancellation of *H*, Alternating dot to dot, and Minnesota Spatial Relations Test. This was an evidence level of III.	Improvements in CPM-enabled clients to participate in more challenging therapies, such as vocational rehabilitation, and at discharge more than half of the participants were engaged in productive activity. Also, more than half of the participants returned to living at home independently or with initial supervision levels.	$p \le 0.000$ for all four subtests. *r* (effect size) Figure ground = 0.431 Cancellation of $H = 0.335$ Alternating Dot to Dot = 0.471 Minnesota Spatial Relations Test = 0.557
Computer-Aided Cognitive Rehabilitation (CACR)[42]	CACR uses standardized and structured training tasks that allow users to grade tasks on the basis of cognitive levels, focusing on visual reaction, visual scanning, attention, information processing speed, memory, and problem-solving abilities. It is objective and provides immediate feedback to clients. The tasks focus on ADLs such as driving, functional math, remembering names and faces, and other functional tasks.	Subjects were 30 individuals between the ages of 65 and 80 years in Korea. They were randomly and equally distributed to either a training group or a balance group.	CACR was used three times per week, 15 minutes each, for a total of 6 weeks.	This was a randomized control trial, evidence level I study. Pre- and posttest scores were reviewed using the Motor-Free Visual Perception Test (MVPT).	There were benefits in visual perceptual skills in both the CACR and the balance groups.	$p \le 0.05$ for MVPT scores, but no statistical significance between the test group and balance group postintervention. MVPT *t*-value test group: $t = -2.46$ Balance group: $t = -4.253$

(*continued*)

Evidence Table of Intervention Studies (*continued*)

Intervention	Description	Participants	Dosage	Research Design and Evidence Level	Benefit	Statistical Significance and Effect Size
Visual Feedback Training (VFT)[42]	VFT training using a force plate based on a computer game was used to allow clients to check their positions and posture for center of gravity in real time. For this study VFT was used in sitting to see effects on sitting balance and visual perception.	Participants included 26 individuals with chronic stroke from Korea. They were included if they could sit independently for 30 minutes, had no other orthopedic injuries, had a score >21 on the Korean Mini-Mental State Exam, and had not participated in any other balance training programs in the last 6 months. They were randomly assigned to either an experimental group or control group. Four total participants withdrew due to discharge.	Participants in the control group participated in standard physical therapy 5 days a week for 4 weeks, 60-minute sessions. Participants in the experimental group participated in the standard PT in addition to VFT sessions for 30-minute sessions, 5 days per week for 4 weeks.	This was a randomized control trial, evidence level I study. Pre- and posttest scores were reviewed using the MVPT.	This study, in addition to previous studies, shows improvements in visual perception, as well as static and dynamic sitting balance, in patients with chronic stroke using VFT methods.	Improvements were significant from pre- to posttesting using the MVPT between the two groups ($p < 0.05$).
Virtual Reality–based Rehabilitation[43]	The Interactive Rehabilitation and Exercise System (IREX) was used. Six virtual reality (VR) games were utilized (bird and balls, coconuts, drums, juggler, conveyer, and soccer).	Participants included 29 individuals following a stroke in Korea.	Both groups received traditional therapy in 30-minute sessions, 3 times a week for 4 weeks. The experimental group also received the IREX training for 60-minute sessions, 5 times per week for 4 weeks.	This was a randomized control trial, evidence level I study. Pre- and posttest scores were reviewed using the MVPT.	VR-based rehabilitation can have a positive impact on visual perceptual skills and ADLs. Significant improvements were noted specifically for visual discrimination and figure ground perception.	MVPT total score: $p < 0.001$ Visual Discrimination: $p < 0.01$ Figure Ground Perception: $p < 0.05$

138

Table Tennis Training (TTT)[41]	Table tennis is a racket sport that has different spatial and temporal demands. TTT includes motor skill learning, numerous repetition, and multisensory feedback. Table tennis is part of the school physical education curriculum in Taiwan, where this study took place.	Participants were 91 children age 6–12 years from Taiwan for the TTT and Standard OT (SOT) groups, and 41 participants were randomly assigned to a control group. 48% had mild intellectual disability, and 52% had borderline intellectual functioning.	The TTT group had three 60-minute sessions per week for 16 weeks. Dosing was the same for the SOT group.	This was a randomized control trial, evidence level I study. Pre- and posttest scores were reviewed using the Test of Visual Perceptual Skill–Third Edition (TVPS-3).	There were improvements in visual perception and executive functions with the TTT group compared with the SOT group and the control group. The treatment was motivating for students and is a feasible modality. The moderate level of exercise required also had positive impacts on the students.	Effect size was strong (>0.8) measured on the TVPS-3 for all subtests compared with the control group and was strong for spatial relations, visual closure, and the total raw score when compared with the SOT group ($p < 0.003$).
Visual Scanning Training (VST), Limb Activation Treatment (LAT), Prism Adaptation (PA) for Left Neglect[44]	**VST:** training to actively explore the contralesional side in various functional tasks; guided by visual stimulus cues and feedback. **LAT:** perform voluntary movements with contralesional limb, paired with visual cues. **PA:** wear prism goggles to shift stimuli along the horizontal plane with tasks involving visual targets into the contralesional side.	Thirty-one patients ranging in age from 41 to 86 years, with right hemisphere damage and left neglect from a neuropsychology department in Italy. All patients had unilateral lesions because of first stroke.	Four assessments completed with 2 weeks of training (20 sessions each) between assessments two and three. The first two assessments were to verify left neglect and the second two assessments were to verify effectiveness of treatment and lasting effects.	This was a randomized control trial, evidence level I study. Pre- and posttest scores were reviewed using the following outcome measures: the Comb and Razor Test, the Fluff Test, Picture scanning, Menu Reading, Coin Sorting, and the Catherine Bergego Scale.	All three treatments can be considered valid interventions for left neglect and the effects lasted for at least 2 weeks. However, this study did not include a control group.	The effect size was significant following intervention according to the following assessments: Picture Scanning Subtest, Menu Reading Subtest, Serving Tea Subtest, The Card Dealing Subtest, and The Catherine Bergego Scale.

References

1. Berryhill ME, Fendrich R, Olson, IR. Impaired distance perception and size constancy following bilateral occipitoparietal damage. *Exp Brain Res*. 2009;194(3):381–393. doi:10.1007/s00221-009-1707-7.
2. American Occupational Therapy Association. *Occupational Therapy Practice Framework: Domain and Process*. 3rd ed. Bethesda, MD: American Occupational Therapy Association; 2014.
3. Warren M. A hierarchical model for evaluation and treatment of visual perceptual dysfunction in adult acquired brain injury, part 1. *Am J Occup Ther*. 1993;47(1):42–54. doi:10.5014/ajot.47.1.42.
4. Brown T, Elliott S, Bourne R, Sutton E, Wigg S, Morgan DD. The discriminative validity of three visual perception tests. *N Z J Occup Ther*. 2011;58(2):14–22. Accessed May 8, 2018.
5. Brown T, Elliot S, Bourne R, et al. The convergent validity of the developmental test of visual perception-adolescent and adult, motor-free visual perception test-third edition and test of visual perception skills (non-motor)-third edition when used with adults. *Br J Occup Ther*. 2012;75(3):134–143. doi:10.4276/0308 02212X13311219571783.
6. Auld M, Boyd R, Moseley G, Johnston L. Seeing the gaps: a systematic review of visual perception tools for children with hemiplegia. *Disabil Rehabil*. 2003;33(19):1854–1865. doi:10.3109/19638288.549896.
7. Vasileva N. Dynamics of the complex forms of visual perception in children of pre-school age (a neuropsychological analysis). *J Spec Educ Rehabil*. 2015;16(3–4):52–70. doi:10.1515/JSER-2015-0011.
8. Jung H, Woo Y, Kang J, Choi Y, Kim K. Visual perception of ADHD children with sensory processing disorder. *Psychiatry Investig*. 2014;11(2):119–123. doi:10.4306/pi.2014.11.2.119.
9. Menon-Nair A, Korner-Bitensky N, Ogourtsova T. Occupational therapists' identification, assessment, and treatment of unilateral spatial neglect during stroke rehabilitation in Canada. *Stroke*. 2007;38(9):2556–2562. doi:10.1161/STROKEAHA.107.484857.
10. Zoltan B. *Vision, Perception, and Cognition*. 4th ed. Thorofare, NJ: SLACK Incorporated; 2007.
11. Brown GT, Gaboury I. The measurement properties and factor structure of the test of visual-perceptual skills-revised: implication for occupational therapy assessment and practice. *Am J Occup Ther*. 2006;60(2):182–193. doi:10.5014/ajot.60.2.182.
12. Possin K. Visual spatial cognition in neurodegenerative disease. *Neurocase*. 2010;16(6):466–487. doi:10.1080/13554791003730600.
13. Wagemans J, Elder J, Kubovy M, et al. A century of Gestalt psychology in visual perception: I. Perceptual grouping and figure-ground organization. *Psychol Bull*. 2012;138(6):1172–1217. doi:10.1037/a0029333.
14. Torfs K, Vancleef K, Lafosse C, Wagemans J, De-Wit L. The Leuven perceptual organization screening test (L-POST), an online test to assess mid-level visual perception. *Beh Res Methods*. 2014;46:472–487. doi:10.3758/s13428-013-0382-6.
15. Reynolds CR, Pearson NA, Voress JK. *Developmental Test of Visual Perception Adolescent and Adult Examiners Manual*. Austin, TX: Pro-Ed; 2002.
16. Cooke DM, McKenna K, Flemming J. Development of a standardized occupational therapy screening tool for visual perception in adults. *Scand J Occup Ther*. 2005;12(2):59–71. doi:10.1080/11038120410020683-1.
17. Richmond J, Holland K. Correlating the developmental test of visual perception-2 (DTVP-2) and the test of visual perceptual skills revised (TVPS-R) as assessment tools for learners with learning difficulties. *S Afr J Occup Ther*. 2011;41(1):33–37. Accessed April 11, 2018.
18. Cote CA. Levels of processing in visual perception tasks. *Am J Occup Ther*. 2011;18(3). Accessed May 10, 2018.
19. FederK,MajnemerA.Handwritingdevelopment,competency, and intervention. *Dev Med Child Neurol*. 2007;49(4):312–317. doi:10.1111/j.1469-8749.2007.00312.x.
20. Blake R, Rizzo M, McEnvoy S. Aging and perception of visual form from temporal structure. *Psychol Aging*. 2008;23(1):181–189. doi:10:10.1037/0882-7974.23.1.181.
21. Uhlhaas P, Pantel J, Lanfermann H, et al. Visual perceptual organization deficits in Alzheimer's dementia. *Dement Geriatr Cog Disord*. 2008;25:465–475. doi:10.1159/0000125671.
22. Duquette J. Spatial orientation in adolescents with visual impairment: related factors and avenues for assessment. *Institut Nazareth et Louis-Braille*. 2012. Accessed April 11, 2018.
23. Padula W, Munitz R, Magrun M. *Neuro-Visual Processing Rehabilitation: An Interdisciplinary Approach*. Santa Ana, CA: Optometric Extension Program Foundation, Inc.; 2012.
24. Ancona C, Stoppani M, Odazio V, La Spina C, Corradetti G, Bandello F. Stereo tests as a screening tool for strabismus: which is the best choice? *Clin Ophthal*. 2014;8:2221–2227. doi:10.2147/OPTH.S67488.
25. Gillen G. *Cognitive and Perceptual Rehabilitation: Optimizing Function*. St. Louis, MO: Mosby/Elsevier; 2009.
26. Appelros P, Karlsson GM, Thorwalls A, Tham K, Nydevik I. Unilateral neglect: further validation of the baking tray task. *J Rehabil Med*. 2004;36(6):258–261. doi:10.1080/16501970410029852. Accessed September 7, 2018.
27. Bailey M, Riddoch J, Crome P. Test-retest stability of three tests for unilateral visual neglect in patients with stroke: Star Cancellation, Line Bisection, and Baking Tray Task. *Neurospychol Rehabil*. 2004;14(4):403–419. doi:10.1080/09602010343000282.
28. Allen D, Thaler N, Ringdahl EN, Mayfield J. Comprehensive trail making test performance in children and adolescents with traumatic brain injury. *Psychol Assess*. 2011;24:556–564. doi:10.1037/a0026263.
29. Desrosiers G, Kavanagh D. Cognitive assessment in closed head injury: stability, validity, and parallel forms for two neuropsychological measures of recovery. *Int J Clin Neuorpsychol*. 1987;9(4):162–173. Accessed July 26, 2018.
30. Sanchez-Cubillo I, Perianez J, Adrover-Roig D, et al. Construct validity of the Trail Making Test: role of task-switching, working memory, inhibition/interference

control, and visuomotor abilities. *J Int Neuropsychol Soc.* 2009;15(3):438. doi:10.1017/S1355617709090626.
31. Gauthier L, Dehaut F, Joanette Y. The Bells Test: a quantitative and qualitative test for visual neglect. *Int J Clin Neuropsychol.* 1989;11:49–54. Accessed July 26, 2018.
32. Ferber S, Karnath HO. How to assess spatial neglect–Line Bisection or Cancellation Tests? *J Clin Expl Neuropsychol.* 2001;23:599–607. doi:10.1076/jcen.23.5.599.1243.
33. Brown TG, Rodger S, Davis A. Motor-Free Visual Perception Test—revised: an overview and critique. *Br J Occup Ther.* 2003;66(4):159–167. doi:10.1177/030802260306600405.
34. McKenna K, Cooke D, Fleming J, Jefferson A, Ogden S. The incidence of visual perceptual impairment in patients with severe traumatic brain injury. *Brain Inj.* 2006;20(5):507–518. doi:10.1080/02699050600664368.
35. Cooke DM, McKenna K, Fleming J, Darnell R. Criterion validity of the Occupational Therapy Adult Perceptual Screening Test (OT-APST). *Scand J Occup Ther.* 2006;13(1):38–48. doi:10.1080/11038120500363006.
36. Cooke DM, McKenna K, Fleming J, Darnell R. Australian normative data for the occupational therapy adult perceptual screening test. *Aust Occup Ther J.* 2006;53:325–336. doi:10.1111/j.1440-1630.2006.00597.x.
37. Friedman PJ, Leong L. The rivermead perceptual assessment battery in acute stroke. *Br J Occup Ther.* 1992;55(6): 233–237. doi:10.1177/030802269205500608 43.
38. Westfall T, Moore K, Bernardo de Leon M, Kulkarni M, Cook E. Cognitive perceptual motor retraining: remediation of deficits following brain injury. *J Cog Rehabil.* 2005;5–11. Accessed April 11, 2018.
39. Deutsch J, Borbely M, Filler J, Huhn K, Guarrera-Bowlby P. Use of a low-cost, commercially available gaming console (Wii) for rehabilitation of an adolescent with cerebral palsy. *Phys Ther.* 2008;88(10):1196–1207. doi:10.2522/ptj.20080062.
40. Christy K, Huffine N, Hannah T, DeLeion M. Outcomes after cognitive perceptual motor retraining (CPM) of patients with acquired brain injury (ABI). *Open J Occup Ther.* 2016;4(1). doi:10.15453/2168-6408.1076.
41. Chen M, Tsai H, Wang C, Wuang Y. The effectiveness of racket-sport intervention on visual perception and executive functions in children with mild intellectual disabilities and borderline intellectual disabilities. *Neuropsychiatr Dis Treat.* 2015;11:2287–2297. doi:209.133.111.226.
42. Lee Y, Lee C, Hwang B. Effects of computer-aided cognitive rehabilitation training and balance exercise on cognitive and visual perception ability of the elderly. *J Phys Ther Sci.* 2012;24(9):885–887. Accessed April 11, 2018.
43. Jo K, Yu J, Jung J. Effects of virtual reality-based rehabilitation on upper extremity function and visual perception in stroke patients: a randomized clinical trial. *J Phys Ther Sci.* 2012;14(11):1205–1208. Accessed September 7, 2018.
44. Prifitis K, Passarini L, Pilosia C, Meneghello F, Pitteri M. Visual scanning training, limb activation treatment, and prism adaptation for rehabilitation left neglect: who is the winner? *Front Hum Neurosci.* 2013;360(7):1–12. doi:10.3389/fnhum.2013.00360.
45. Toglia J. Visual perception of objects: an approach to assessment and intervention. *Am J Occup Ther.* 1989;43(9): 587–595. doi:10.5014/ajot.43.9.587.
46. Tham K, Ginsburg E, Fisher A, Tegner R. Training to improve awareness of disabilities in clients with unilateral neglect. *Am J Occup Ther.* 2001;55(1):46–54. doi:10.5014/ajot.55.1.46.
47. Berger S, Kaldenberg J, Selmane R, Carlo S. Effectiveness of interventions to address visual and visual-perceptual impairments to improve occupational performance in adults with traumatic brain injury: a systematic review. *Am J Occup Ther.* 2016;70(3):1–15. doi:10.5014/ajot.2016.020875.
48. Bailey MJ, Riddoch MJ, Crome P. Treatment of visual neglect in elderly patients with stroke: a single-subject series using either a scanning and cueing strategy or a left-limb activation strategy. *Phys Ther.* 2002;82:782–797. doi:10.1093/ptj/82.8.782.
49. Fox R. A rationale for the use of prisms in the vision therapy room. *J Behav Opt.* 2011;22(5):126–129. Accessed April 11, 2018.
50. Kortte KB, Hillis AE. Recent trends in rehabilitation interventions for visual neglect and anosognosia for hemiplegia following right hemisphere stroke. *Future Neruol.* 2011;6(1):33–43. doi:10.2217/fnl.10.79.
51. Wilcox D, Chronister C, Savage M. Methods for prism placement for hemianopic visual field loss in adults with low vision. *J Vis Impair Blind.* 2016;110(4):276. Accessed April 11, 2018.
52. Quintana L. Optimizing vision, visual perception, and praxis abilities. In: Radomski MV, Trombly Latham C, eds. *Occupational Therapy for Physical Dysfunction.* 6th ed. Baltimore, MD/Philadelphia, PA: Lippincott Williams & Wilkins; 2008:728–747.
53. Swan L. Unilateral spatial neglect. *Phys Ther.* 2001;81(9): 1572–1580. Accessed April 11, 2018.
54. Butter CM, Kirsch N. Combined and separate effects of eye patching and visual stimulation on unilateral neglect following stroke. *Arch Phys Med Rehabil.* 1992;73(12): 1133–1139. Accessed September 7, 2018.
55. Walker R, Young AW, Lincoln NB. Eye patching and the rehabilitation of visual neglect. *Neuropsycho Rehabil.* 1996;6(3):219–231. doi:10.1080/713755508.
56. Houston KE, Barrett AM. Patching for diplopia contraindicated in patients with brain injury? *Optom Vis Sci.* 2017;94(1):120. doi:10.1097/OPX.0000000000000976.
57. Tinelli F, Cioni G, Purpura G. Development and implementation of a new telerehabilitation system for audiovisual stimulation training in hemianopia. *Front Neurol.* 2017; 8(621):1–10. doi:10.3389/fneur.2017.00621.
58. Frassinetti F, Bolognini N, Bottari D, Bonora A, Ladavas E. Audiovisual integration in patients with visual deficit. *J Cogn Neurosci.* 2005;17(9):1442–1452. doi:10.1162/0898929054985446.
59. Makovski T. The open-object illusion: size perception is greatly influenced by object boundaries. *Atten Percept Psychophys.* 2017;79:1282–1289. doi:10.3758/s13414-017-1326-5.
60. Geldof C, Wassenaer AV, Kieviet JD, Kok J, Oosterlaan J. Visual perception and visual-motor integration in very preterm and/or very low birth weight children: a meta-analysis. *Res Dev Disabil.* 2012;33(2):726–736. doi:10.1016/j.ridd.2011.08.025.
61. Pieker I, David N, Schneider TR, Nolte G, Schottle D, Engel AK. Perceptual integration deficits in autism spectrum

disorders are associated with reduced interhemispheric gamma-band coherence. *J Neurosci.* 2015;35(50):16352–16361. doi:10.1523/jneurosci.1442-15.2015.
62. Poole JL, Nakamoto T, McNulty T, et al. Dexterity, visual perception, and activities of daily living in persons with multiple sclerosis. *Occup Ther Health Care.* 2010;24(2):159–170. doi:10.3109/07380571003681202.
63. Ego A, Lidzba K, Brovedani P, et al. Visual-perceptual impairment in children with cerebral palsy: a systematic review. *Dev Med Child Neurol.* 2015;57(2):46–51. doi:10.1111/dmcn.12687.
64. Cho M, Kim D, Yang Y. Effects of visual perceptual intervention on visual-motor integration and activities of daily living performance of children with cerebral palsy. *J Phys Ther Sci.* 2015;27(2):411–413. doi:10.1589/jpts.27.411.

Acknowledgment

We would like to acknowledge our level II fieldwork student, Colette Chapp, for her hard work on the Case Study.

Chapter 10

Cognitive Assessment

Diane Powers Dirette and Guy L. McCormack

LEARNING OBJECTIVES

This chapter will allow the reader to:

1. Describe specific cognitive abilities and how they are used in daily occupation.
2. Analyze the occupational dysfunction that occurs as a result of cognitive impairment.
3. Identify the neurological and physiological basis of cognitive function.
4. Determine how to screen for basic cognitive abilities.
5. Select cognitive assessment methods and tools based on individual clients' characteristics and the properties of various measures.
6. Anticipate and describe factors that should be considered in interpreting the results of cognitive assessments.

CHAPTER OUTLINE

TERMINOLOGY

Attention: the cognitive ability to direct mental processes toward information. Subtypes from lowest to highest functioning include focused attention, selective attention, sustained attention, alternating attention, and divided attention.

Cognition: the mental action or process of acquiring knowledge and understanding through thought, experience, and the senses.

Executive Functions: the cognitive skills required for high-level thinking. Some examples include planning, problem solving, organization, judgment, self-regulation, flexibility, categorization, sequencing, abstract reasoning, divergent thinking, and conceptualization.

Immediate recall/sensory register: the cognitive ability to recall information without any lapse in time from processing.

Long-term memory: the cognitive ability to recall information that is stored relatively permanently.[1]

Memory: the mental storage of information and the processes involved in the acquisition, retention, and retrieval of that information. Subtypes of memory include immediate recall/sensory register, working memory, long-term memory, episodic memory, procedural memory, semantic/declarative memory, prospective memory, and topographical memory.

Orientation: the cognitive ability to understand oneself and one's surroundings and circumstances. Examples include understanding person, place, time, and date.

Processing: the cognitive ability to quickly and accurately decode elements of information into meaningful terms.

Self-awareness: the cognitive ability to know one's own capacities, skills, limitations, and level of function.

Working memory: the cognitive ability to use information that is currently held "in mind."[1]

Cognitive Function and Impairment in Daily Occupation

Cognition is the mental process of understanding, acquiring, and knowing information, and it is essential for all aspects of daily occupation. Being alert, attentive, and processing information are the basis of cognition and are necessary to take in the world around us. In order to learn from the environment, **memory** is used for immediate, short-term, or long-term recall. **Executive functions** use the information that is gained to initiate, plan, problem solve, organize, categorize, sequence, judge, reason, and conceptualize actions for successful daily function. **Self-awareness** is used to determine, monitor, and adjust actions and behaviors to improve daily functions. Self-awareness makes it possible for people to form mental representations and concepts of themselves and to regulate their own behavior. In particular, self-awareness typically involves comparing oneself to goals, ideals, norms, other people, and various other standards.

When cognition is impaired, occupational dysfunction can occur in any area of daily function. The ability to perform any activity from the time a person wakes in the morning until he or she goes to sleep at night can be impacted by a cognitive impairment. The ability to get out of bed, perform self-care, prepare meals, drive or take transportation to the destination, follow a schedule, perform work or school activities, learn new tasks, participate in leisure activities, socialize with others, and maintain a home all rely on varied and integrated aspects of cognition. For example, a person who is a highly functional college student relies on cognition to perform home, school, work, leisure, and social activities. But if he or she sustains a brain injury that results in damage to the frontal lobes of the brain creating executive dysfunction, his or her ability to plan the day, problem solve what to wear or where to go and how to get there may all be limited. He or she may struggle to understand abstract concepts presented in the classroom or have difficulty with categorization and integration of the information that was presented. All aspects of his or her performance of daily activities rely on cognitive abilities.

Occupational therapists assess cognition because many people seeking occupational therapy services are likely to have some degree of cognitive impairment that influences their ability to perform daily activities.[2] Cognitive changes can be temporary, relatively static, or progressive. Many survivors of brain injury experience deficits in information processing, attention, memory, and executive functions that persist for months or years post injury.[3] A significant number of persons who sustain a spinal cord injury also have a concurrent brain injury with similar implications for cognition.[4] Cognitive changes may also be experienced by individuals with chronic conditions, including multiple sclerosis,[5] Parkinson disease,[6] cancer,[7] epilepsy,[8] pain,[9] systemic lupus erythematosus,[10] and human immunodeficiency virus/acquired immunodeficiency syndrome.[11] Even individuals with mild stroke who are independent in activities of daily living (ADL) may have memory deficits and executive dysfunction that impacts their ability to work, drive, and engage in recreational activities.[12]

Neuroplasticity

Neuroplasticity is the brain's ability to change its structure and function throughout the life span. Following an injury, such as an acquired brain injury including trauma, stroke, or brain tumor, an occupational therapist will ascertain cognitive function with the intent to provide cognitive rehabilitation focused on enhancing the recovery of deficits in cognitive function through remedial training techniques to enhance neural recovery and compensatory training to teach strategies using intact cognitive functions. There is emerging evidence that cognitive rehabilitation approaches enhance neuroplasticity.[13] The potential benefits of cognitive rehabilitation for enhancing neuroplasticity have been found for people with stroke,[14] Parkinson disease,[15] schizophrenia,[16] and aging adults,[17] including those with Alzheimer disease.[18]

Cognitive Hierarchy

Cognitive abilities are conceptualized in a hierarchy with arousal, orientation, attention, and processing at the base, the varied types of memory next, and executive functions and self-awareness at the top of the hierarchy (see Fig. 10-1). The cognitive skills at each level rely on the skills below.[19] For example, a person who has impaired attention and processing will not have intact working memory for learning new information, because the person will not be able to remember information that was never perceived or processed. The hierarchy continues with all the cognitive skills that underlie executive

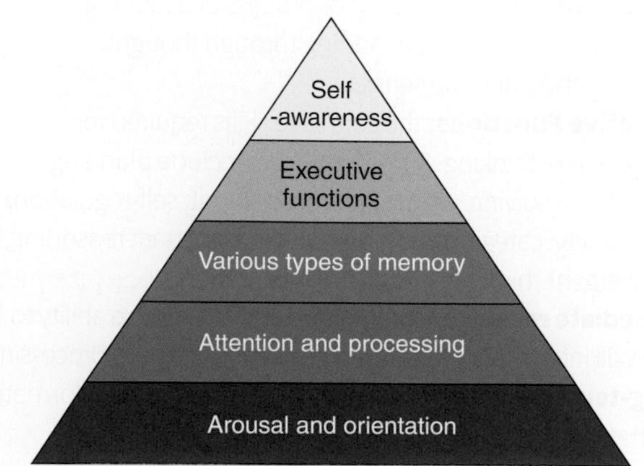

Figure 10-1. Cognitive hierarchy.

functions. If a person is unable to attend, process, or remember information, the person will not be able to work with that information to plan, problem solve, and organize an activity involving that information. Each cognitive skill relies on the one below to support cognitive function.

Integration of Cognitive Processes

In addition to the hierarchy of cognitive abilities, there is also an integration of cognitive processes.[20] Whereas executive functions rely on intact lower order cognitive abilities, such as attention and memory, executive functions are also integrated with attention and memory to regulate cognitive processes. When performing a task, executive functions are involved in focusing attention on relevant information and inhibiting irrelevant information, thereby regulating information that is available for working memory. Executive functions also monitor the acquisition of the contents of the information to be remembered; plan the sequence of subtasks on which to focus, process, and remember; and categorize the information that is being learned.

Attention, memory, and executive functions are also integrated with self-awareness. Attention and memory are used to comprehend the self in relation to the others and the environment. Self-regulation, planning, and problem solving are used in a feedback loop with self-awareness to improve the person's sense of self. Self-awareness and memory are used to compare the self to a given standard. If the self-awareness notes an unwanted discrepancy, the executive functions are used to initiate some action to remedy this by regulating actions, planning for differing behaviors, and problem-solving ways to make that change.[20]

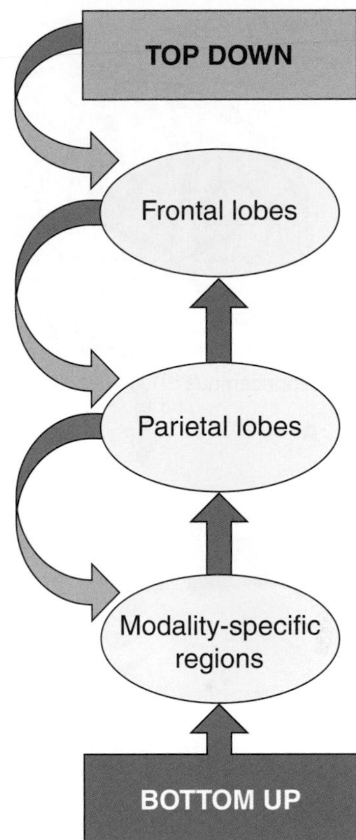

Figure 10-2. Model of attention and processing.

Neurological and Physiological Basis of Cognitive Function

Attention and Processing

Attention and processing can be described as either top down or bottom up (see Fig. 10-2). In top-down attention and processing, the person is aware of the need to attend and process information and uses the frontal lobes to modulate input, which includes focusing, selecting, sustaining, alternating, and dividing attention as needed. Conversely, when the person is engaged in bottom-up attention and processing, information is first perceived through the primary areas, including the occipital, temporal, and sensory motor areas.[1] Information is then filtered through the parietal lobes, which act as an interface between these primary areas and the frontal lobes.[21]

In bottom-up attention, the incoming information may not be conscious. For example, a person may be reading a page of text, get to the bottom of the page, and be unaware of the information that was in the text. Even when reading aloud, a person may attend to the text, but not actually process the information. Processing of information requires the interface of parietal lobes and awareness through the engagement of the frontal lobes.

Memory

There are several neurological correlates related to memory. Information that has been attended to and processed is relayed to the hippocampus and regions of the medial temporal lobes, including the entorhinal cortex, the perirhinal cortex, and the parahippocampal cortex[22] (see Fig. 10-3). The right hippocampus is specific to spatial memory, and the left hippocampus is specific to memory for contextual details.[23] The parahippocampal cortex is specific to location of objects, and the perirhinal cortex is involved in the memory of object features.[1]

Specified areas of the frontal lobes are involved in encoding information. The left ventrolateral prefrontal cortex is associated with verbal encoding, and the right ventrolateral prefrontal cortex with visual encoding. The dorsolateral prefrontal cortex (PFC) is related to the organization of information during encoding and the monitoring of the retrieval of information from **long-term memory**. Long-term memory is stored in specific posterior brain regions related to the type of information that is stored. For example, visual information is

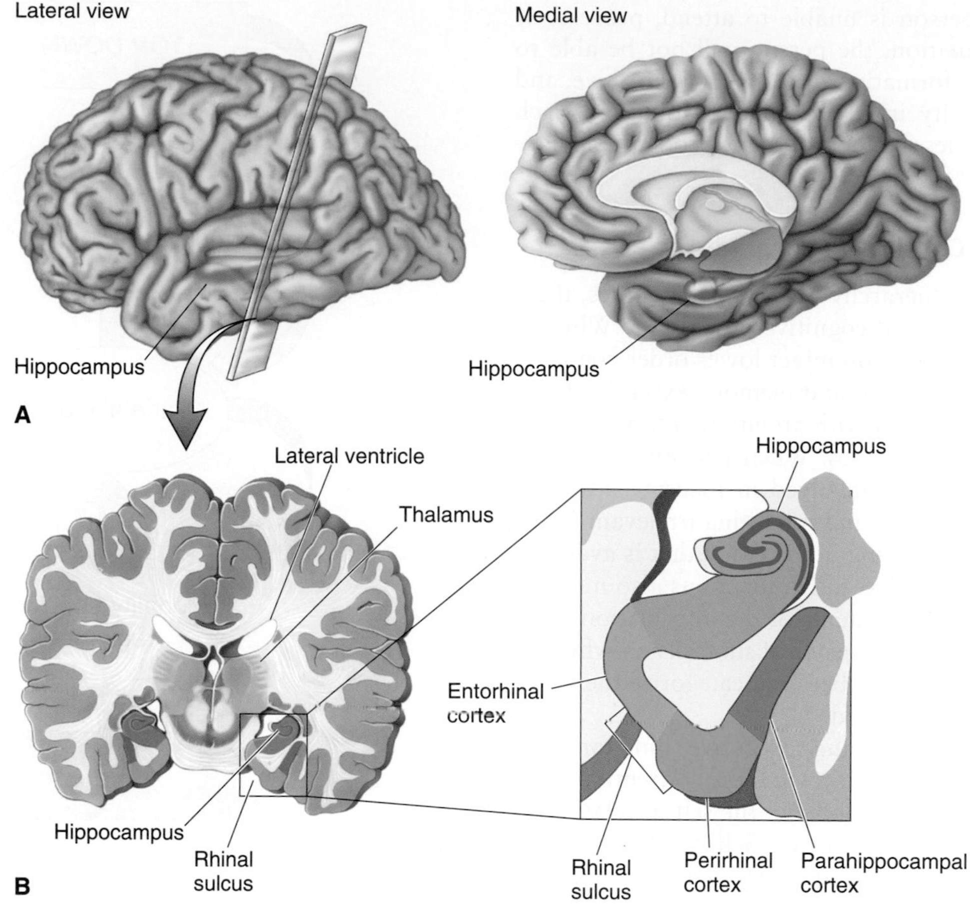

Figure 10-3. Memory cortices. **A,** Memory cortices lateral bisection; **B,** Memory cortices frontal bisection.

stored in the occipital lobes, and language information is stored in the left temporal lobes.

The PFC is also crucial for keeping information active for **working memory**. The dorsolateral PFC is involved in manipulating and monitoring information, whereas the ventrolateral PFC is involved in maintaining and retrieving information from long-term storage.[1]

Executive Functions

The neurological correlates for executive functions lie mostly in various regions of the PFC[20,22,24] (see Fig. 10-4). Various types of executive functions have been correlated with different, lateralized, and integrated regions of the PFC.[1] Planning that is unstructured is typically located in the right PFC, and planning that is structured in the left PFC.[20] The dorsolateral PFC is involved in formulation of plans, whereas the medial ventral PFC is involved in the execution of a plan. In addition, the anterior ventral lateral PFC is correlated with semantic planning, whereas the posterior ventral lateral PFC is correlated with motor planning.[25] Problem solving is correlated with the left dorsolateral PFC, especially for open-ended verbal problem solving.[26] Inhibition and monitoring of performance are correlated with the medial PFC, anterior cingulate cortex, and the presupplementary motor area, and slowed performance is noted with damage to the right lateral PFC.[1,26] Decision making is correlated with the dorsolateral PFC, with connections to the dorsal regions of the anterior cingulate, which functions in error detection and motivation. The dorsal regions of the anterior cingulate connect with the dorsolateral PFC, parietal lobes, premotor areas, and the supplementary motor cortex to monitor cognitive responses, and the anterior regions of the anterior cingulate connect with the limbic system and orbital frontal areas to monitor affective responses. The ability to multitask has been correlated with the anterior PFC, frontal pole, and the rostral PFC.[1]

Self-Awareness

Self-awareness of cognitive functions and self-awareness of psychosocial functions are located in different areas of the PFC. Awareness of one's own cognitive functions is correlated with the ventrolateral areas of the PFC.[27] Awareness of one's own psychosocial functions, however, are correlated with the anterior medial PFC, the posterior cingulate cortex,[28] and the ventromedial PFC,[27] especially on the right side.[29] A person who has

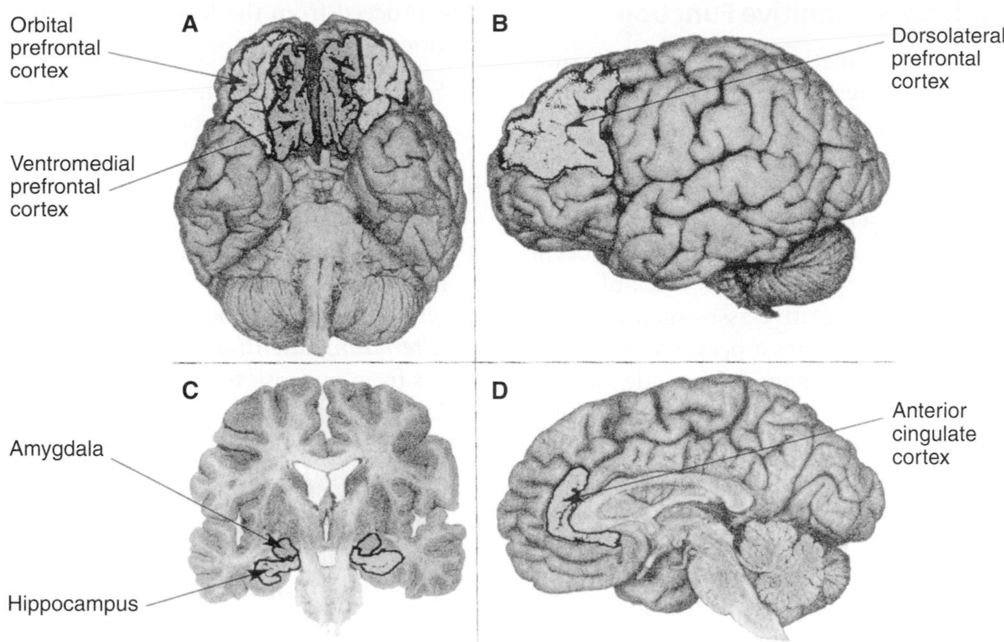

Figure 10-4. Executive cortices. **A,** Executive cotices; **B,** Orbital prefrontal cortex; **C** and **D,** ventromedial prefrontal cortex.

damage to both areas may have reduced self-awareness for both cognitive and psychosocial function.

Screening of Cognitive Skills

The Process of Cognitive Assessment

The cognitive assessment process can be categorized as either top down or bottom up, but most occupational therapists will integrate the two approaches to assess the occupational performance of the client (top down) while attempting to discover the specific underlying cognitive deficits that may be causing difficulty with task completion (bottom up).[19] Assessments in both top-down and bottom-up categories may be either nonstandardized or standardized. Nonstandardized assessments typically include informal observation of task performance or cognitive skills or a screening that combines observation with parts of standardized assessments. Standardized assessments are used to formally assess occupational performance or cognitive skills using a specified protocol for administration and scoring that may help reduce therapist bias. The method of administration of nonstandardized or standardized assessments can vary and may include self-report measures, dynamic assessments, functional assessments, or performance-based assessments.

Occupational therapists will typically perform a cognitive screening to ascertain occupational performance and basic cognitive functions. An occupational therapist may first have the person perform functional tasks that require cognition (e.g., planning and preparing a meal) as a top-down screening and also perform a quick screening of underlying cognitive deficits that may be impacting function as a bottom-up screening. For example, the therapist might use the Montreal Cognitive Assessment (MoCA) as a quick 10-minute screening before doing more in-depth screening and standardized testing (see Fig. 10-5). When a person demonstrates a deficit during the screening process, the person's occupational performance or cognitive skills will be tested further, sometimes with standardized assessments, to provide a more in-depth understanding of the deficits.

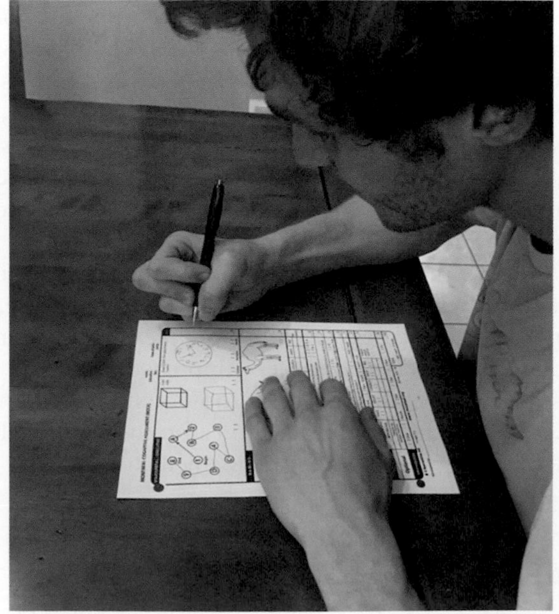

Figure 10-5. Client performing the Montreal Cognitive Assessment.

Factors That Influence Cognitive Function

An individual's cognitive function at any point in time is determined by many interacting variables, including affective, education, task, and environmental influences. Changes in any of these domains may improve or detract from a person's cognitive function and thereby his or her occupational performance. Therefore, to effectively assess cognition and interpret findings, occupational therapists must appreciate how variables can affect performance during cognitive assessment.

A person's emotional state has a pervasive influence on cognitive function.[30] Some examples include anxiety, depression, pain, and fatigue.[31] Anxiety is linked to difficulty with attention and working memory.[32] Depression is linked to memory deficits and executive functions.[33] Pain and fatigue (especially mental fatigue) interfere with working memory by occupying attention that is therefore unavailable to incoming data.[34] Under such circumstances, the occupational therapist may defer cognitive assessment to another time or, at a minimum, consider the influence of these factors when interpreting the assessment results.

A person's level of education may also influence the results of cognitive testing. In a study involving a random sample of age-stratified healthy older adults, younger age and higher education were associated with better performance on cognitive testing.[35] Because they are more familiar with testing processes, persons with higher education may score within normal limits on cognitive tests, even with decrements in their functioning, and/or persons with lower education who perform poorly on cognitive assessments may, in fact, be cognitively intact.

A person's familiarity with tasks may also influence cognitive performance. Tasks that are well-known to a person may be performed with relative ease because attention, memory, and executive functions are not as greatly taxed in familiar activities when compared with tasks that are new.[36] For example, if a person is asked to perform a leather lacing task by learning a stitch, the person who is already familiar with leather lacing, sewing, knitting, or crocheting may perform these stitches automatically using cerebellar pathways and motor habits that do not tax the higher cortical areas.

Finally, the environment can influence cognitive function. Variability in the structure, lighting, noise, familiarity, and presence of other people in the environment may all serve to either support or decrease the person's performance on both top-down or bottom-up assessments. The therapist will need to note all of these factors during the cognitive assessment.

Screening of Orientation, Attention, and Processing.

Orientation, **attention**, and **processing** are defined in the key terms, but there are also specific types of attention that proceed from the lowest to the highest level of attention as follows:

- ***Focused attention:*** The cognitive ability to be responsive to stimuli. This type of attention is also known as arousal.
- ***Selective attention:*** The cognitive ability to maintain focus on one stimulus despite distractions.
- ***Sustained attention:*** The cognitive ability to maintain focus over time. This type of attention is sometimes referred to as vigilance.
- ***Alternating attention:*** The cognitive ability to shift focus from one task to another.
- ***Divided attention:*** The cognitive ability to attend to two or more stimuli simultaneously.

Observation of a client with deficits in orientation, and lower level attention and processing may note confusion regarding person, place, and time; an inability to focus on visual or auditory stimuli; and slowed speed of processing with delays in response time during occupational performance.[37] As a person improves, he or she may be able to respond to stimuli and resolve some confusion regarding person, place, and time, but may have stimulus-bound attention with a need to respond to all stimuli and an inability to filter out distractions. For example, the person may respond to everything he or she sees or hears in a room or while walking down a hallway; this condition is clinically identified as stimulus-bound attention. With progress, the person will be able to focus, select, and sustain attention over time. Simultaneous improvement in the speed and accuracy of processing usually occurs through this progression. At the higher levels, the person will be able to alternate his or her attention between tasks and then ultimately divide attention between two different stimuli simultaneously (e.g., listening to a lecture and taking notes). It should be noted that divided attention is never expected for two of the same modes of attention. For example, a person cannot listen to two conversations at the same time or focus on two different visual stimuli (e.g., watching the road and a cell phone screen).

Screening of orientation, attention, and processing skills also can be completed through specific tasks as follows:

- To screen orientation and focused attention, use face-to-face positioning with observation of eye movements and focus, and questions regarding person, place, and time as appropriate to the level of communication. If the person is unable to communicate, observe the response to his or her name and the ability to appropriately use tools such as a spoon or toothbrush, keeping in mind that vision and visual perception should be evaluated before cognitive skills.
- To screen processing and selective attention, use a cancellation task. Ask the person to cancel a letter, number, or symbol on a sheet of paper. Observe the speed

and accuracy of processing and the pattern of cancellation. A random pattern of cancellation may indicate deficits in attention and warrant standardized testing.

- To screen selective and sustained attention, use digit span numbers and letters (auditory, visual, and motor). Present a series of numbers, letters, or same color blocks, starting with a series of three and progressing to nine. Ask the person to repeat the series in the same order. Repeat the tasks starting with three and progressing to seven, asking the person to repeat the series backward.
- To screen alternating attention, use a Trail Making Test or the modified trail making test developed by Joan Toglia and Betty Abreu. Ask the person to draw a line, without removing the pen from the paper, which connects the numbers in order. Next, ask the person to repeat this with alteration between letters and numbers, each in order (see Fig. 10-6).
- To assess divided attention, use the Stroop Color and Word Test.[38] Following the standardized approach to the task, have the person perform all three sheets in order.

Screening of Memory

The terms **memory**, **immediate recall/sensory register**, **working memory**, and **long-term memory** are all defined in the key terms. Memory, however, can also be subdivided according to the type of information that is being recalled and the time at which the information was obtained. Memory for specific types of information can be immediate, working, or long-term and is categorized as follows:

- ***Episodic memory:*** recall of information that is related to time.
- ***Procedural memory:*** recall of how to perform tasks.
- ***Semantic/declarative memory:*** recall of word-based information (i.e., knowledge about the meanings of words, objects, and events).
- ***Prospective memory:*** recall of information for upcoming events (e.g., appointments).
- ***Topographical memory:*** recall of a spatial representation or physical layout.

The time at which the information was obtained is divided into two categories, retrograde and anterograde, as follows:

- ***Retrograde memory:*** recall of information obtained prior to an injury. The term remote memory is also used for this concept. Some examples include word finding, ability to recognize people, and semantic/declarative knowledge.
- ***Anterograde memory:*** recall of information obtained after an injury. The terms recent memory and new learning are also used for this concept.

Screening of the various types of memory in different time frames (immediate recall, working memory, and long-term) can be adequately completed using some specific tasks and subtests from the Rivermead Behavioral Memory Test (RBMT).[39] The RBMT assesses visual, auditory, and motor recall in the various types of memory and in the categories of retrograde and anterograde memory (see Figure 10-7). If clinical time does not allow for completion of the entire standardized test, subtests,

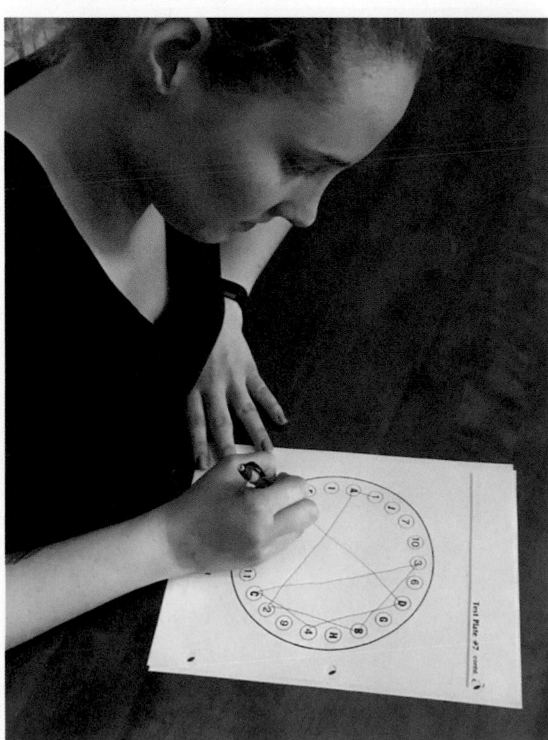

Figure 10-6. Client performing a modified Trail Making Test.

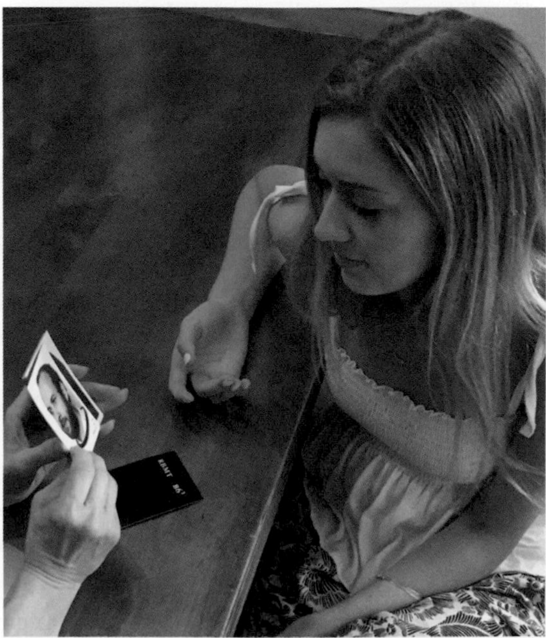

Figure 10-7. Client performing the Rivermead Behavioral Memory Test.

such as first and second names, belonging, and appointment, can be selected and incorporated throughout the screening process to screen the specific types of memory as follows:

- To screen episodic memory, use the orientation and date sections.
- To screen procedural memory, use the route and message sections.
- To screen semantic/declarative memory, use the name, story, and orientation sections.
- To screen prospective memory, use the belonging and appointment sections.
- To screen topographical memory, use the route and belonging sections.
- To screen retrograde memory, use the orientation section.
- To screen anterograde memory, use the name, pictures, story, faces, route, and message sections.

Screening of Executive Functions

Executive functions can be subdivided into the following types: planning, problem solving, organization, judgment, self-regulation, flexibility, categorization, sequencing, abstract reasoning, divergent thinking, and conceptualization. The definitions are as follows:

- ***Planning:*** developing a proposal for doing or achieving something
- ***Problem solving:*** the process of working through an issue to find a solution
- ***Organization:*** the act or process of putting the different parts of something in a certain order
- ***Judgment:*** the ability to make considered decisions or come to sensible conclusions
- ***Self-regulation:*** control of one's behavior, such as inhibition and initiation of responses
- ***Flexibility:*** the ability to change ideas or to compromise
- ***Categorization:*** the ability to sort objects or ideas according to common attributes
- ***Sequencing:*** placing items or performing tasks in the order in which they should happen
- ***Abstract reasoning:*** the ability to understand subjects on a complex level
- ***Divergent thinking:*** a thought process or method used to generate creative ideas by exploring many possible solutions
- ***Conceptualization:*** the ability to invent or formulate an idea

Most functional activities that involve executive functions will require a combination of these types of cognitive skills. The full range of executive functions can be screened using the following tools:

- To screen planning, problem solving, judgment, self-regulation, and sequencing, use the physical or virtual Tower of London Task[40] (see Fig. 10-8). Although there are various forms of the test, the typical test has three rods and seven to nine disks that can be used to grade the test to make it more difficult (see Figure 10-8). Start with four disks for the screening. The objective of the test is to restack the original stack on a different rod in the order of large to small in the smallest number of moves possible using the following rules: (a) only move one disk at a time from the top of a stack, (b) a larger disk can never be placed on a smaller disk.
- To screen organization, categorization, abstract reasoning, and conceptualization, use a grocery list task. The person is given a list of the following 30 grocery items and told to organize them into six categories that fit with the different sections of his or her grocery store, with one category being miscellaneous. The items include eggs, doughnuts, hamburgers, popsicles, milk, olives, creamer, bagels, apples, frozen peas, bread, chewing gum, yogurt, chicken, lettuce, apple juice, ice cream, muffins, hot dogs, potatoes, fish sticks, cheese, sausage, rolls, frozen pizza, strawberries, boxed noodles, carrots, turkey, and dog food. The categories are not given to them, but they should generate categories such as dairy, bakery, frozen, produce, meat, and miscellaneous. There will be five items in each category. To adapt the activity, the categories can be provided.
- To screen abstract reasoning, flexibility, conceptualization, and divergent thinking, use the Alternative Uses Test. Developed by J. P. Guilford in 1967, the

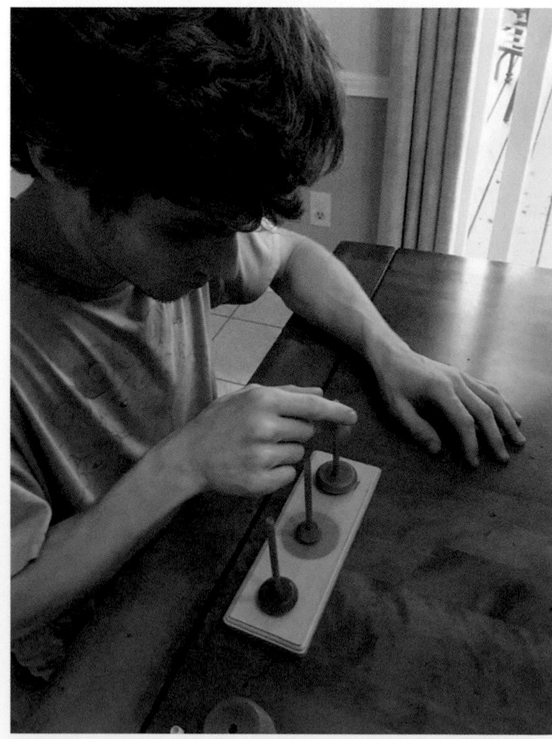

Figure 10-8. Client performing the Tower of London Task.

Alternative Uses Test challenges these areas of executive functions by asking the person to think of as many uses as possible for an everyday object like a chair, coffee mug, or brick, each in 2 minutes. The person should be able to generate four to six unique uses for each object.

Screening of Self-Awareness

Self-awareness is the cognitive ability to know one's own capacities, skills, limitations, and level of function. The categories of self-awareness include sensorimotor, cognitive, and psychosocial self-awareness. In general, a person will have a better awareness of his or her sensorimotor function than of more abstract cognitive and psychosocial functions, although deficits such as homonymous hemianopia and unilateral inattention are also abstract and may result in a lack of self-awareness. The Awareness Questionnaire is a good quick screen of self-awareness, but the therapist should categorize the questions according to those three areas to gain an understanding of the categories of self-awareness that are lacking.[41] On the Awareness Questionnaire, numbers 1 and 5 are general functional questions; 6 to 9 are sensorimotor questions; 2, 4, and 10 to 15 are cognitive questions; and 3, 16, and 17 are psychosocial questions. Keep in mind that people with impaired self-awareness may minimize problems on self-reports. Discrepancies among the person's self-report and that of a significant other or therapist are used to indicate the level of self-awareness,[42] with large discrepancies indicating more impaired self-awareness.

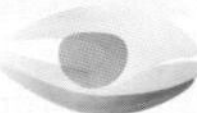

CASE STUDY

Patient Information

Santiago, a 22-year-old male of Mexican American descent, was attending graduate school to study foreign languages. The first one in his family to receive a college degree, his goal in life was to master foreign languages so he could teach abroad. He also loved music and singing karaoke in bars in different dialects. After "partying" with his friends, he drove home "under the influence" and skidded off the road on a rainy night and hit a tree "head-on." He was hospitalized and sustained a brain injury in the motor vehicle accident. Most of the damage was to his right hemisphere. He also had multiple basilar skull fractures, a small subarachnoid hemorrhage, and a disruption of his maxillary sinuses. The neurologist medically induced a coma for 3 weeks.

When Santiago first awoke, he was highly agitated and swore profusely. The vulgar language he used was uncharacteristic of him, given his education and working vocabulary for English. His friends and parents say he did not curse in public before the accident. His conversational language gradually returned, but he continued to have trouble remembering the names of common household items and had a loss of memory for events that occurred after the accident (anterograde amnesia). The neurologist used imaging studies, which suggested that the right-side temporal lobe damage may have affected his hippocampus, which is important in learning, memory, and navigation of the environment.[23] His loss of memory and damage to the right-side brain damage has caused some hemispatial inattention (also called unilateral neglect) on his left side. In addition, he also experienced sensory deficits involving auditory and visual memory challenges and a shortened sustained attention span. He may have some mild visual field impairment and hearing loss in the right ear. His medical insurance was dropped early in the process, forcing him to go on Medicare. Fortunately, the Bipartisan Budget Act of 2018 repealed the cap on Medicare Part B outpatient services for occupational therapy as long as the services were deemed medically necessary. The occupational therapist was able to see him in the clinic during the acute care phase, and later on she was able to visit him at home through the hospital's home health agency.

Assessment Process

The occupational therapist first evaluated his functional cognitive skills from a top-down perspective to see if he could carry out routine daily activities related to living independently and assessed whether he could dress himself, prepare meals, and take his medications independently.[43] He expressed the desire to go back to graduate school where he was maintaining a 3.60 GPA in foreign languages and taking education courses to earn a teaching certificate. Unfortunately, after his injury, he had to withdraw from graduate school and was unable to continue his work study job at the university. He needed some source of employment to earn an income and to obtain student loans for college. His initial mood swings such as feelings of sadness and emotional outbursts made it difficult to maintain friendships and the romantic relationships he had in the past. His executive functions such as mood regulation, social behavior, planning, and decision making were impaired, as observed in simulated work hardening activities of routine tasks in occupational therapy. The therapist conducted a screening of vision, visual perception, and cognition; then completed standardized assessments as indicated; and conducted a home visit. The patient had to move back home in the local community because he could no longer manage living in an apartment independently.

Assessment Results

To establish a baseline, the therapist conducted the Canadian Occupational Performance Measure (COPM) to obtain information about his executive function and ascertain his

(continued)

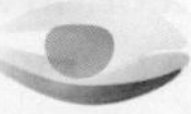

CASE STUDY (continued)

self-awareness and the degree of his cognitive problems. The COPM is an evidence-based outcome measure designed to evaluate the patient's self-perception of performance in everyday living, over time. Using this semistructured systematic interview, therapists engage the client in identifying daily occupations of importance that they want, need, or are expected to do but are unable to accomplish. The problems were identified by rating the importance of each of the occupations to his life using a 10-point rating scale. The client chose five of the most important problems: (1) Feelings of sadness or depression, (2) Lack of concentration to complete tasks, (3) Forgetting names and word-finding problems, (4) Reading comprehension, (5) Communicating effectively and controlling his emotions. The therapist entered the chosen problems and their importance ratings in the scoring section and calculated an average COPM performance score and satisfaction score.

The therapist also administered the MoCA to screen for attention and concentration, executive functions, memory, language, visuoconstructional skills, conceptual thinking, calculations, and orientation. The MoCA assessed different types of cognitive abilities, including orientation, short-term memory, executive function, language abilities, attention, and visuospatial ability. The assessment indicated that the patient had trouble with attention, working memory, and concentration.

More in-depth testing was completed to assess attention and memory. The digit span test, modified Trail Making Test, and the Stroop Color and Word Test were completed. Santiago was able to recall seven digits forward, but struggled with digit span backward. He also demonstrated slowed speed of processing for alternating numbers and letters in the Trail Making Test, part B, and the color/word section of the Stroop. The RBMT was used to assess memory functions. Santiago performed at a screening level of 7, indicating moderate memory impairments. Difficulties were noted on naming common objects, delayed recall of names, paragraph recall, and topographical memory.

The Executive Function Performance Test (EFPT) was used to assess top-down performance-based executive functioning of four basic tasks associated with self-maintenance: simple cooking, telephone use, managing medications, and paying bills. This assessment revealed that the patient had trouble managing medications and writing checks for bills.

The Brief Neuropsychological Cognitive Examination (BNCE) evaluated major cognitive functions in one short session, yielding a general cognitive profile in about 30 minutes. Specifically, the BNCE assesses working memory, gnosis (word cognition), praxis (inability to carry out planned movements), language, orientation, attention, and executive functions. It reveals specific cognitive abnormalities that may warrant more detailed evaluation. The advantage of using this assessment is that it provides a score that calibrates a validity index and a total score that determines whether the person can live independently. The patient's sore was 22 in the mild range of impairment, suggesting he was not yet able to live independently.

The Awareness Questionnaire (AQ) was completed by Santiago, his mother, and his occupational therapist. Discrepancies in the scores among the three questionnaires were noted on numbers 3 and 10 to 17, indicating reduced awareness of cognition and psychosocial functions.

Occupational Therapy Problem List

This problem list is the result of triangulation of clinical functional observation and standardized assessments.

- Attention problems (sustained, alternating, and divided)
- Difficulty in word finding or forgetting names for common objects
- Reduced topographical memory
- Feelings of sadness or depression
- Poor interpersonal communication
- Poor reasoning and judgment in managing daily living skills
- Poor medication management
- Mood dysregulation and agitation
- Reduced self-awareness

Most Commonly Used Standardized Assessments for Cognitive Function

Instrument and Reference	Intended Purpose	Administration Time	Validity	Reliability	Sensitivity	Strengths and Weaknesses
The Montreal Cognitive Assessment (MoCA)[44] www.mocatest.org/pdf_files/test/MoCA-Test-English_7_1.pdf	The MoCA is a brief 30-question test that takes around 10–12 minutes to complete. It was published in 2005 by a group at McGill University working for several years at memory clinics in Montreal. This is a screening tool developed to measure mild cognitive impairment. The MoCA screens attention and concentration, executive functions, memory, language, visuoconstructional skills, conceptual thinking, calculations, and orientation.	Approximately 10 minutes. The test is made freely available to any clinician, and its international use allows it to be administered in 35 different languages. The total possible score is 30, with any score higher than 25 considered normal. Any score of 25 or less is considered to be an indication of some form of cognitive impairment, which can predict or identify the onset of dementia in patients.	The MoCA has been validated on a range of patients, including those with stroke, Parkinson disease, and traumatic brain injury (TBI). Excellent concurrent validity among patients with mild Alzheimer disease ($r = 0.87$).[44] Also discriminant validity established on a variety of diagnostic groups with neurological impairments.[45] A MoCA test validation study by Nasreddine in 2005 showed that the MoCA was a promising tool for detecting MCI and early Alzheimer disease compared with the well-known Mini-Mental State Examination (MMSE).[46]	Very good reliability internal consistency ($\alpha = 0.83$); excellent test–retest reliability ($r = 0.92$)[44]	Sensitivity is good (0.97), but specificity is poor.[47] Using a cutoff of a raw value of 26 participants to identify MCI.	Strengths: Highly sensitive to mild cognitive impairment (MCI) in many populations; user-friendly with normative values; best used as a screening tool; found to be more sensitive to cognitive impairment after mild stroke than the MMSE and a better predictor of outcome of acute rehabilitation.[48] Weaknesses: May be overly sensitive with current published cutoff values (potentially suggesting impairment where there is none). Therapists should be cautious in determining MCI based only on the MoCA as an evaluation tool.
Cognistat (Neurobehavioral Cognitive Status Examination)[49]	Cognistat (Neurobehavioral Cognitive Status Examination) is a screening tool that is an efficient and metric approach that streamlines the testing process. Cognistat is available in three different formats: Cognistat Assessment System (CAS-II): a web-based, computer-assisted format with electronic data records (EDR). Cognistat Paper: the original Cognistat paper-and-pencil test. Cognistat Active Form: a new computerized PDF format that does not require web access. https://www.cognistat.com/	Test takes 12–15 minutes	Discriminant analysis: Wilcoxon analysis suggested that four of the subtests have discriminated between elderly persons with stroke and healthy independent elderly[50] statistically significant differences in mean scores for healthy controls, persons with dementia. Nabors and colleagues[51] retrospectively examined the concurrent validity of the Cognistat compared with standard neuropsychological measures. The results indicated that the Cognistat is useful in detecting cognitive impairment in the adult TBI population.	Lannin and Scarcia[52] evaluated the concurrent and incremental reliability of five different cognitive assessments. The Cognistat was the most sensitive tool for detecting cognitive impairment; if used with the Cognitive Assessment of Minnesota, specificity increases.	Found to be more sensitive than MMSE with neurosurgical patients.[53] Screen and Metric approach may not be sensitive to subtle or mild impairment; may yield false negative results in these cases.[54,55]	The test scores as average, mild, moderate, or severe impairment and is presented in a profile of performance in each domain; normative data available for healthy elderly persons.[56] Some test items (e.g. construction subtest) may be too difficult for both patients with stroke and healthy elderly persons.[57]; not appropriate for geriatric or psychiatric.

(continued)

Most Commonly Used Standardized Assessments for Cognitive Function (*continued*)

Instrument and Reference	Intended Purpose	Administration Time	Validity	Reliability	Sensitivity	Strengths and Weaknesses
Loewenstein Occupational Therapy Cognitive Assessment (LOTCA).[58] The LOTCA battery was developed as a measure of basic cognitive skills and visual perception in older adults with neurological impairment.	Microbattery consisting of 20 subtests in four areas: orientation, perception, visuomotor operations, and thinking operations.	Approximately 30–45 minutes. The LOTCA provides an in-depth assessment of basic cognitive abilities and can also be used in treatment planning and review of progress over time.	Discriminant validity: All subtests, except identification of objects, differentiated between patients with craniocerebral injury and healthy controls and stroke patients and health.[58] Katz et al. conducted a factor analysis to determine the construct validity of the original LOTCA, using two groups of patients with traumatic head injury or stroke ($n = 96$), and healthy adults ($n = 55$). The study found good validity measures.	Katz et al.[58] reported excellent interrater reliability for subtests of the LOTCA, with strong interrater reliability (Spearman's rank correlation coefficient ranged from 0.82 to 0.97 for various subtests).	No studies have examined the sensitivity of the LOTCA. Katz et al. observed improved test scores between test scores at admission and after 2 months for TBI and stroke patients.[59]	Strengths: The LOTCA permits use of domain-specific scores rather than just a global score, allowing for assessment of many aspects of the client's cognitive and perceptual abilities. Weaknesses: The LOTCA has been described as time-consuming because it takes more than several sessions to be completed.
Cognitive Assessment of Minnesota (CAM)[60] https://health.utah.edu/occupational-recreational-therapies/docs/...reviews/cam+.pdf	This test is designed to be used for adult clients who have cognitive impairments due to a cerebrovascular accident (CVA) or a TBI (Level IV through Level VII on the Rancho Los Amigos Scale of Cognitive Functioning). The CAM is a screening tool that assesses a wide range of cognitive skills. It is arranged in a hierarchy from simple to complex. The hierarchy is divided into four areas: store of knowledge, manipulation of old knowledge, social awareness and judgment, and abstract thinking.	Administered either as a 40-minute session, or two 20-minute sessions.	Validity: Concurrent, construct validity of the Cognitive Assessment of Minnesota in older adults was evaluated by Pearson product-moment correlations were calculated for total scores of the two cognitive measures (CAM and MMSE). The investigators determined the overall level of agreement of these screening measures to be valid for a group of older adults.	Reliability: Test– retest, internal consistency, interrater reliability has been performed. The CAM appears to be a promising measure for use with older adults with cognitive impairment, especially when investigators are interested in functional capacity recommendations. More research is necessary for exploring the psychometric properties of the CAM to explore its full utility with diverse populations. Previously, only one small study has examined the psychometric properties of the CAM using the MMSE as a comparison. Rustad and colleagues[60] found a moderate correlation ($r = 0.44, p = 0.05$); however, the sample size reported in this study was small ($n = 16$), and additional examinations are needed to determine whether this relationship will exist in other samples.	Not available	Strengths: The directions are clear and easy to follow, and can be found in both the examiner's guide and the quick reference subtest sheets. Weaknesses: Requires items not included in the kit that need to be gathered and/or purchased. Worksheets have to be copied for each administration.

Trail Making Test The Trail Making Test was originally part of the Army Individual Test Battery from 1944 and was then incorporated into the Halstead–Reitan Battery in 1985.	Today, the Trail Making Test is one of the most popular neuropsychological tests. The test can provide information about visual search speed, scanning, speed of processing, mental flexibility, as well as executive functioning (prefrontal lobe).	Trail A takes 29 seconds to complete; Trail B takes 75 seconds.	It is difficult to find validity scores for this assessment. Although trail making tests are very simple, they have been hypothesized to reflect a wide variety of cognitive processes, including attention, visual search, and scanning, sequencing and shifting, psychomotor speed, abstraction, flexibility, ability to execute and modify a plan of action, and ability to maintain two trains of thought simultaneously.[61] Cognitive imaging may confirm this claim.	In one study, significant differences were found between groups for Trails A and all Stroop tasks, but in another study, the only difference between participants with left and right frontal trauma was on the Stroop Color-Word task. Potential reasons why Trails A and the Stroop Test are sensitive to frontal lobe damage are discussed, such as novelty and processing speed.[62]	Three studies have examined the known groups validity of the Trail Making Test and found that it was able to differentiate between patients with and without brain damage; however, it was not sensitive to differentiating between front and non-frontal brain damage.[62]	Strengths: Easy to administer. Weakness: It is not a stand-alone measure of cognition.
STROOP Color and Word Test The Stroop effect is named after John Ridley Stroop, who first published the effect in English in 1935. The effect had previously been published in Germany in 1929 by other authors. When the name of a color (e.g., "red" "blue," or "green") is printed in a color that is not denoted by the name (e.g., the word "red" printed in blue ink instead of red ink), naming the color of the word takes longer and is more prone to errors than when the color of the ink matches the name of the color.	The standardized version of the Stroop consists of two parts. In the Color Task, the individual reads aloud a list of 112 color names in which no name is printed in its matching color. In the Color-Word Task, the individual names the color of ink in which the color names are printed.	Estimates suggest it takes 5 minutes to administer, but it depends on the cognitive ability of the patient. The **Stroop** Interference **Test**, originally developed in 1935 by **Stroop** to **measure** selective attention and cognitive flexibility, may take 10 minutes to administer.	Discriminant validity is supported by studies on patients with MCI and dementia, postconcussion syndrome and severe TBI, ADHD (treated and untreated), and depression (treated and untreated). Pearson's r was calculated for all of the tests except those that were not normally distributed, for which Spearman's rho was used. The correlation coefficients are given for the individual tests and the domain scores.[63] Reliability and validity of a computerized neurocognitive test battery, CNS Vital Signs Impaired performance of the Stroop task may be indicative of an underlying neurological disorder related to frontal lobe dysfunction; poor performance is not sufficient for a diagnosis of ADHD.	For most versions of the Stroop test, there are no available estimations of reliability.	The test is sensitive to malingerers and patients with conversion disorders. This test is considered to measure selective attention, cognitive flexibility and processing speed, and it is used as a tool in the evaluation of executive functions. An increased interference effect is found in disorders such as brain damage, dementias, and other neurodegenerative diseases, attention-deficit hyperactivity disorder, or a variety of mental disorders such as schizophrenia, addictions, and depression.	Strengths: It serves as an indicator of further testing if the participant does not perform well. Weaknesses: It is difficult to obtain exact values of validity and reliability.

(*continued*)

Most Commonly Used Standardized Assessments for Cognitive Function (*continued*)

Instrument and Reference	Intended Purpose	Administration Time	Validity	Reliability	Sensitivity	Strengths and Weaknesses
Rivermead Behavioral Memory Test (RBMT)[64]	Assesses working memory needed for daily living skills such as remembering appointments, travel routes around town, names, and faces.	Approximately 30–45 minutes	Wilson et al.[64] found statistically significant differences between healthy subjects and persons with brain injury ($p < 0.001$).	Interrater reliability: 100% agreement when 40 subjects with brain injury were scored separately but simultaneously by two raters.[64] Reliability was good with Cronbach's $\alpha = 0.84$ and PSI = 0.85 at admission. Fit to the Rasch model showed that one item (faces) deviated from model expectation. External construct validity was supported by expected correlations.[65] These scales show good test–retest reliability and adequate external construct validity.	The test proved sensitive ($t = 4.87$, $p < 0.0001$), and free of ceiling and floor effects in an elderly group of normal participants, who were expected to show modest differences in memory performance. The subtests varied in their sensitivity to this small age difference, but the RBMT was sensitive when performance was assessed the scaled scores that allowed calculation of an overall combined measure of memory.	Strengths: Subtests are similar to everyday tasks; useful in the characterization of memory disorders for a wide range of diagnostic groups.[61] Weaknesses: The test requires intact visual and verbal skills.
Executive Function Performance Test (EFPT)[66]	A standardized top-down performance-based measure of executive functioning. The EFPT examines the execution of four basic tasks associated with self-maintenance: simple cooking, telephone use, bill paying, and medication management.	Approximately 30–45 minutes	A cross-sectional study recently found the alternate, Internet-based form of the bill-paying task of the EFPT to be reliable and have construct validity for assessing executive function with people who have subacute stroke.[67] No significant differences were found between participants who performed the Internet-based version first ($t = -1.3$, $p = 0.187$) and those who did it second ($t = 0.3$, $p = 0.76$). Differences were also not found for the telephone-use total scores or time between participants who performed the Internet-based version first ($t = -1.4$, $p = 0.16$) and those who did it second ($t = 0.56$, $p = 0.57$). Criterion validity was also established for both tasks. Concurrent validity was established ($p = 0.61$) with the Assessment of Motor and Process Skills.[68] Construct validity was established by Baum et al.[69] with control EFPT total scores significantly ($p \leq 0.05$) lower (better) than mild stroke scores and moderate	Not available.	It is difficult to determine sensitivity or specificity. As such, no studies have reported on specificity of the EFPT in a stroke population.	Strengths: The EFPT is comprised of real-world tasks. The tool can be administered to individuals of varying ability owing to the flexibility to provide a hierarchy of cues as required. The tool is simple to administer, and guidelines are clearly stipulated in the test manual.

			stroke scores ($p \leq 0.0001$). Mild stroke scores were also significantly lower than moderate stroke scores ($p \leq 0.0001$). Construct validity was verified for bill paying, but not for telephone use. Criterion validity was verified for both tasks.			
Awareness Questionnaire (AQ) The AQ was developed by Sherer et al.[70] The initial version of the AQ, as well as the results of a factor analysis that resulted in the current version of the AQ, were published in 1998.	The AQ was developed as a measure of impaired self-awareness after TBI because patients with traumatic brain injuries often show impaired awareness of their deficits.	Approximately 20–30 minutes	The AQ was developed based on previous studies of impaired awareness and the clinical experience of the authors to assure patient awareness of functioning in physical, cognitive, and behavioral domains in community activities.	Because of the nature of self-awareness, it is difficult to obtain accurate reliability measures.	Criterion validity has been demonstrated as client vs. family/significant other differences, and the direct clinician rating of accuracy of self-awareness has been shown to be predictive of eventual productivity outcome for persons with TBI.[41] These two measures accounted for 31% of variance in productivity outcome in a sample of 66 persons with TBI.	One of few standardized performance-based measures and the only performance-based measure that provides clinicians with guidance on the level of cues needed to support clients' functional abilities; excellent reliability and validity.
Arnadottir OT-ADL Neurobehavioral Evaluation (A-ONE) The A-ONE consists of two parts: an A-ONE ADL scale and an A-ONE Neurobehavioral (NB) scale. The occupational therapist scores 22 test items based on the level of assistance needed to do ADL task as well as underlying neurobehavioral impairments impacting that performance.	The A-ONE is intended to be used only with clients with neurobehavioral disorders (e.g., stroke, brain injury, dementia). Research is ongoing to extend its application to children. The Assessment of Motor Process Skills (AMPS) is intended to be used with persons 3 to over 100 years of age, from all diagnostic groups. The A-ONE consists of two parts: an A-ONE ADL scale and an A-ONE NB scale. The occupational therapist scores 22 test items based on the level of assistance needed to do ADL tasks as well as underlying neurobehavioral impairments impacting that performance.	Approximately 75 minutes	Steultjens71 examined the concurrent validity of the A-ONE. Comparison of the A-ONE ADL scale with the Barthel Index and comparison of NB scores with the MMSE revealed excellent correlations ($r = 0.70$ and 0.85, respectively). The results provide minimal support for the construct validity of the A-ONE related to differentiating between ADL performance of persons with left and right CVA.[72]	The Mann Whitney U test and chi-square test were used to explore possible differences between the performance of participants with left and right CVA. Descriptive statistics were calculated for demographic data and for items on the Functional Independence Scale (FIS) and the Neurobehavioral Specific Impairment Subscale (NSIS). The level of significance was set at $p < 0.05$.	The assessment discriminated at a statistically significant level.	Requires a full hour; cannot be used as an outcome tool without test–retest reliability established

CAM, Cognitive Assessment of Minnesota.

References

1. Ward J. *The Student's Guide to Cognitive Neuroscience.* 3rd ed. New York, NY: Psychology Press; 2015.
2. Skidmore ER, Whyte EM, Holm MB, et al. Cognitive and affective predictors of rehabilitation participation after stroke. *Arch Phys Med Rehabil.* 2010;91:203–207. doi:10.1016/j.apmr.2009.10.026.
3. Skandsen T, Finnanger TG, Andersson S, Lydersen S, Brunner JF, Vik A. Cognitive impairment 3 months after moderate and severe traumatic brain injury: a prospective follow-up study. *Arch Phys Med Rehabil.* 2010;91:1904–1913. doi:10.1016/j.apmr.2010.08.021.
4. Macciocchi S, Seel RT, Thompson N, Byams R, Bowman B. Spinal cord injury and co-occurring traumatic brain injury: assessment and incidence. *Arch Phys Med Rehabil.* 2008;89:1350–1357. doi:10.1016/j.apmr.2007.11.055.
5. Rogers JM, Panegyres PK. Cognitive impairment in multiple sclerosis: evidence-based analysis and recommendations. *J Clin Neurosci.* 2007;14:919–927. doi:10.1016/j.jocn.2007.02.006.
6. Dirette DP. Progressive neurodegenerative disorders. In: Atchison BJ, Dirette DK, eds. *Conditions in Occupational Therapy: Effect on Occupational Performance.* 5th ed. Philadelphia, PA: Wolters Kluwer; 2017:403–422.
7. Conti GE. Acquired brain injury. In: Atchison BJ, Dirette DK, eds. *Conditions in Occupational Therapy: Effect on Occupational Performance.* 5th ed. Philadelphia, PA: Wolters Kluwer; 2017:363–386.
8. Helmstaedter C, Kurthen M, Lux S, Reuber M, Elger CE. Chronic epilepsy and cognition: a longitudinal study in temporal lobe epilepsy. *Ann Neurol.* 2003;54:425–432.
9. Urban MJ. Somatic symptoms and related disorders. In: Atchison BJ, Dirette DK, eds. *Conditions in Occupational Therapy: Effect on Occupational Performance.* 5th ed. Philadelphia, PA: Wolters Kluwer; 2017:229–240.
10. McLaurin EY, Holliday SL, Williams P, Brey RL. Predictors of cognitive dysfunction in patients with systemic lupus erythematosus. *Neurology.* 2005;64:297–303. doi:10.1212/01.WNL.0000149640.78684.EA.
11. Heaton RK, Marcotte TD, Rivera Mindt M, et al; The HNRC Group. The impact of HIV-associated neuropsychological impairment on everyday functioning. *J Int Neuropsychol Soc.* 2004;10:317–331. doi:10.1093/infdis/jis326.
12. Schriner M, Delahunt JZ. Cerebral vascular accident. In: Atchison BJ, Dirette DK, eds. *Conditions in Occupational Therapy: Effect on Occupational Performance.* 5th ed. Philadelphia, PA: Wolters Kluwer; 2017:291–327.
13. Chang Y. Reorganization and plastic changes of the brain associated with skill training and expertise. *Front Hum Neurosci.* 2014;8:35. doi:3389/fnhum201.00035.
14. Cumming TB, Marshall RS, Lazar RM. Stroke, cognitive deficits, and rehabilitation: still an incomplete picture. *Int J Stroke.* 2013;8(1):38–45. doi:10.1111/j.1747-4949.2012.00972.x.
15. Foster ER, Bedekar M, Tickle-Degnen L. Systematic review of the effectiveness of occupational therapy-related interventions for people with Parkinson's disease. *Am J Occup Ther.* 2014;68(1):39–49. doi:10.5014/ajot.2014.008706.
16. Fisher M, Holland C, Subramaniam K, Vinogradov S. Neuroplasticity-based cognitive training in schizophrenia: an interim report on the effects 6 months later. *Schizophr Bull.* 2010;36(4):869–879. doi:10.1093/schbul/sbn170.
17. Bherer L. Cognitive plasticity in older adults: effects of cognitive training and physical exercise. *Ann N Y Acad Sci.* 2015;1337:1–6. doi:10.1111/nyas.12682.
18. Herholz SC, Herholz RS, Herholz K. Non-pharmacological interventions and neuroplasticity in early stage Alzheimer's disease. *Expert Rev Neurother.* 2013;13(11):1235–1245. doi:10.1586/14737175.2013.845086.
19. Gillen G. *Cognitive and Perceptual Rehabilitation: Optimizing Function.* St. Louis, MO: Mosby; 2009.
20. Nadel L. *Encyclopedia of Neuroscience.* Hoboken, NJ: Wiley; 2005.
21. Posner MI. Attentional networks and consciousness. *Front Psychol.* 2012;3:64. doi:10.3389/fpsyg.2012.00064.
22. Lundy-Ekman L *Neuroscience: Fundamentals for Rehabilitation.* 3rd ed. Philadelphia, PA: W.B. Saunders; 2007.
23. Lambert KG, Kinsley C. *Clinical Neuroscience: Psychopathology and the Brain.* 2nd ed. New York, NY: Oxford University Press; 2011.
24. Yuan P, Raz N. Prefrontal cortex and executive functions in healthy adults: a meta-analysis of structural neuroimaging studies. *Neurosci Biobehav Rev.* 2014;42:180–192. doi:10.1016/j.neubiorev.2014.02.005.
25. Badre D, D'Esposito M. Is the rostro-caudal axis of the frontal lobe hierarchical? *Nat Rev Neurosci.* 2009;10(9):659–669. doi:10.1038/nrn2667.
26. Stuss DT, Alexander MP, Shallice T, et al. Multiple frontal systems controlling response speed. *Neuropsychologia.* 2005;43(3):396–417. doi:10.1016/j.neuropsychologia.2004.06.010.
27. Amodio DM, Frith CD. Meeting of minds: the medial frontal cortex and social cognition. *Nat Rev Neurosci.* 2006;7:268–277. doi:10.1038/nrn1884.
28. Johnson SC, Baxter LC, Wilder, LS, Pipe JG, Heiserman JE, Prigatano GP. Neural correlates of self-reflection. *Brain.* 2002;125:1808–1814.
29. Stuss DT, Levine B. Adult clinical neuropsychology: lessons from studies of the frontal lobes. *Ann Rev Psychol.* 2002;53:401–433. doi:10.1146/annurev.psych.53.100901.135220.
30. Ponsford J, Bayley M, Wiseman-Hakes C, et al. INCOG Recommendations for management of cognition following traumatic brain injury. Part II: Attention and information processing speed. *J Head Trauma Rehabil.* 2014;29(4):321–337. doi:10.1097/HTR.0000000000000072.
31. Spitz G, Schönberger M, Ponsford J. The relations among cognitive impairment, coping style, and emotional adjustment following traumatic brain injury. *J Head Trauma Rehabil.* 2013;28(2):116–125. doi:10.1097/HTR.0b013e3182452f4f.
32. Beaudreau SA, O'Hara R. The association of anxiety and depressive symptoms with cognitive performance in community-dwelling older adults. *Psychol Aging.* 2009;24:507–512. doi:10.1037/a0016035.
33. Lambert KG. Rising rates of depression in today's society: consideration of the roles of effort-based rewards and enhanced resilience in day-to-day functioning. *Neurosci Biobehav Rev.* 2006;30(4):497–510.

34. Dick BD, Rashiq S. Disruption of attention and working memory traces in individuals with chronic pain. *Anesth Analg*. 2007;104:1223–1229. doi:10.1213/01.ane.0000263280.49786.f5.
35. Ganguli M, Snitz BE, Lee CW, Vanderbilt J, Saxton JA, Chang CC. Age and education effects and norms on a cognitive test battery from a population-based cohort: the Monongahela-Youghiogheny Healthy Aging Team. *Aging Ment Health*. 2010;14:100–107. doi:10.1080/13607860903071014.
36. Gauvain M, Perez S. Cognitive development and culture. In: Lerner RM, Liben LS, Muller U, eds. *Handbook of Child Psychology and Development*. 7th ed. Hoboken, NJ: Wiley; 2015:854–896.
37. Takeuchi H, Kawashima R. Effects of processing speed training on cognitive functions and neural systems. *Rev Neurosci*. 2012;23(3):289–301. doi:10.1515/revneuro-2012-0035.
38. Goldman CJ, Freshwater SM. *Stroop Color and Word Test: A Manual for Clinical and Experimental Uses*. Los Angeles, CA: Western Psychological Services; 2002.
39. Wilson BA, Cockburn J, Baddeley A. *The Rivermead Behavioural Memory Test*. Reading, UK: Thames Valley Test; 1985.
40. Phillips LH, Wynn VE, McPherson S, Gilhooly KJ. Mental planning and the Tower of London task. *Q J Exp Psychol A*. 2001;54(2):579–597. doi:10.1080/713755977.
41. Sherer M, Bergloff P, Boake C, High W Jr, Levin E. The awareness questionnaire: factor structure and internal consistency. *Brain Inj*. 1998;12(1):63–68.
42. O'Keeffe F, Dockree P, Moloney P, Carton S, Robertson IH. Awareness of deficits in traumatic brain injury: a multidimensional approach to assessing metacognitive knowledge and online-awareness. *J Int Neuropsychol Soc*. 2007;13:38–49. doi:10.1017/S1355617707070075.
43. Corcoran, MY, Giles, GM. *Neurocognitive Disorder Interventions to Support Occupational Performance*. Bethesda, MD: AOTA Press, The American Occupational Therapy Association; 2014. *Neurorehabilitation in Occupational Therapy Series*; vol 1.
44. Nasreddine ZS, Phillips NA, Bédirian V, et al. The Montreal Cognitive Assessment (MoCA): a brief screening tool for mild cognitive impairment. *J Am Geriatr Soc*. 2005;53:695–699. doi:10.1111/j.1532-5415.2005.53221.x.
45. Nasreddine Z. The Montreal Cognitive Assessment (MoCA). 2013. http://www.mocatest.org/default.asp. Accessed April 24, 2018.
46. Luis CA, Keegan AP, Mullan M. Cross validation of the Montreal Cognitive Assessment in community dwelling older adults residing in the Southeastern US. *Int J Geriatr Psychiatry*. 2009;24(2):197–201. doi:10.1002/gps.2101.
47. Nasreddine ZS, Collin I, Chertkow H, Phillips N, Bergman H, Whitehead V. Sensitivity and specificity of the Montreal Cognitive Assessment (MoCA) for detection of mild cognitive deficits. *Can J Neurol Sci*. 2003;30:S2, 30. Presented at Canadian Congress of Neurological Sciences Meeting; June 2003; Québec City, Québec.
48. Toglia J, Fitzgerald KA, O'Dell MW, Mastrogiovanni AR, Lin CD. The Mini-Mental State Examination and Montreal Cognitive Assessment in persons with mild subacute stroke: relationship to functional outcome. *Arch Phys Med Rehabil*. 2011;92:792–798. doi:10.1016/j.apmr.2010.12.034.
49. Kiernan RJ, Mueller J, Langston JW, Van Dyke C. The Neurobehavioral Cognitive Status Examination: a brief but differentiated approach to cognitive assessment. *Ann Intern Med*. 1987;107:481–485.
50. Katz N, Elazar B, Itzkovich M. Validity of the Neurobehavioral Cognitive Status Examination (COGNISTAT) in assessing patients post CVA and healthy elderly in Israel. *Israel J Occup Ther*. 1996;5:E185–E198.
51. Nabors N, Rosenthal, M. Use of the neurobehavioral cognitive status examination (Cognistat) in traumatic brain Injury. *J Head Trauma Rehabil*. 1997;12(3):79–84. doi:10.1097/00001199-199706000-00008.
52. Lannin N, Scarcia M. The cognistat is a sensitive measure for screening and identifying people with cognitive impairment following ABI in acute hospital settings. *J Cognit Rehabil*. 2004:19–25. https://www.neuropsychonline.com/loni/jcrarchives/vol22/V22I4Lannin.pdf.
53. Schwamm LH, Van Dyke C, Kiernan RJ, Merrin E, Mueller J. The Neurobehavioral Cognitive Status Examination: comparison with the NCSE and MMSE in a neurosurgical population. *Ann Intern Med*. 1987;107:486–491. doi:10.7326/0003-4819-107-4-486.
54. Nokleby K, Boland E, Bergersen H, et al. Screening for cognitive deficits after stroke: a comparison of three screening tools. *Clin Rehabil*. 2008;22(12):1095–1104. doi:10.1177/0269215508094711.
55. Oehlert ME, Hass SD, Freeman MR, Williams MD, Ryan JJ, Sumerall SW. The neurobehavioral cognitive status examination: accuracy of the "screen-metric" approach in a clinical sample. *J Clin Psychol*. 1997;53(7):733–737.
56. Eisenstein N, Engelhart CI, Johnson V, Wolf J, Williamson J, Losonczy MB. Normative data for healthy elderly persons with the neurobehavioral cognitive status exam (Cognistat). *Appl Neuropsychol*. 2002;9(2):110–113. doi:10.1207/S15324826AN0902_6.
57. Osmon DC, Smet LC, Winegarden B, Gandhawadi B. Neurobehavioral cognitive status examination: its use with unilateral stroke patients in a rehabilitation setting. *Arch Phys Med Rehabil*. 1992;73:414–418.
58. Katz N, Itzkovich M, Averbuch S, Elazar B. Loewenstein Occupational Therapy Cognitive Assessment (LOTCA) battery for brain-injured patients: reliability and validity. *Am J Occup Ther*. 1989;43:184–192.
59. Katz N, Champagne D, Cermak S. Comparison of the performance of younger and older adults on three versions of a puzzle reproduction task. *Am J Occup Ther*. 1997;51:562–568. doi:10.5014/ajot.51.7.562.
60. Rustad RA, DeGroot TL, Jungkunz ML, Freeberg KS, Borowick LG, Wanttie A. *The Cognitive Assessment of Minnesota: Examiner's Guide*. San Antonio, TX: The Psychological Corp.; 1993.
61. Lezak MD, Howieson DB, Loring DW, Hannay HJ, Fischer JS. *Neuropsychological Assessment*. 4th ed. New York, NY: Oxford University Press; 2004.
62. Demakis G. Frontal lobe damage and tests of executive processing: a meta-analysis of the Category Test, Stroop Test, and Trail-Making Test. *J Clin Exp Neuropsychol*. 2004;26(3):441–450. doi:10.1080/13803390490510149.

63. Gualtieri CT, Johnson LG. Reliability and validity of a computerized neurocognitive test battery, CNS vital signs. *Arch Clin Neuropsychol.* 2006;21(7):623–643.
64. Wilson BA, Cockburn J, Baddeley A, Hiorns R. The development and validation of a test battery for detecting and monitoring everyday memory problems. *J Clin Exp Neuropsychol.* 1989;11:855–870.
65. Kutlay S, Küçükdeveci AA, Elhan AH, Tennant A. Validation of the Behavioural Inattention Test (BIT) in patients with acquired brain injury in Turkey. *Neuropsychol Rehabil.* 2009;19(3):461–475. doi:10.1080/09602010802445421.
66. Baum CM, Morrison T, Hahn M, Edwards DF. *Test Manual: Executive Function Performance Test.* St. Louis, MO: Washington University; 2003.
67. Rand D, Ben-Halm KL, Malka R, Portnoy S. Development of internet-based tasks for executive function performance test. *Am J Occup Ther.* 2018;72:720220560pi–7202205060p7. doi:10.5014/ajot.2018.023598.
68. Cederfeldt M, Widell Y, Andersson EE, Dahlin-Ivanoff S, Gosman-Hedstrom G. Concurrent validity of the executive function performance test in people with mild stroke. *Br J Occup Ther.* 2011;74:443–449.
69. Baum CM, Connor LT, Morrison T, Hahn M, Dromerick AW, Edwards DF. Reliability, validity, and clinical utility of the executive function performance test: a measure of executive function in a sample of people with stroke. *Am J Occup Ther.* 2008;62:446–455.
70. Sherer M, Hart T, Nick TG. Measurement of impaired self-awareness after traumatic brain injury: a comparison of the patient competency rating scale and the awareness questionnaire. *Brain Inj.* 2003;17(1):25–37.
71. Steultjens MPM, Dekker J, van Baar ME, et al. Internal consistency and validity of an observational method for assessing disability in mobility in patients with osteoarthritis. *Arthritis Care Res.* 1998;12:19–25.
72. Gardarsdóttir S, Kaplan S. Validity of the Árnadóttir OT-ADL Neurobehavioral Evaluation (A-ONE): performance in activities of daily living and neurobehavioral impairments of persons with left and right hemisphere damage. *Am J Occup Ther.* 2002;56:499–508. doi:10.5014/ajot.56.5.499.

Chapter 11

Cognitive Intervention

Mary Vining Radomski and Gordon Muir Giles

LEARNING OBJECTIVES

This chapter will allow the reader to:

1. Discuss the field of cognitive rehabilitation in general.
2. Distinguish cognitive rehabilitation approaches used by occupational therapists from those provided by other professions.
3. Describe theoretical approaches to occupational therapy cognitive intervention.
4. Employ specific clinical interventions that are supported by theory and evidence.

CHAPTER OUTLINE

TERMINOLOGY

Automaticity: initiation and execution of a behavior with minimal conscious decision-making in response to a stimulus; when a behavior is automatic conscious effort is required if the response is to be inhibited.[1]

Chaining: a method for training task performance in which tasks are broken down into component steps; a functional task can be thought of as a stimulus–response chain in which the completion of each activity acts as the stimulus for the next step in the chain.[2]

Cognitive rehabilitation: a wide range of therapeutic interventions designed to address neurocognitive impairment in one or more cognitive domain (e.g., attention, memory, or executive functions) and as a result to improve an individual's functioning in everyday life.

Compensatory cognitive strategies: tools or methods that are used by clients to help them overcome, circumvent, or minimize the load placed on an impaired cognitive domain, such as using alarm prompts on a smartphone to keep track of time-critical activities.[3]

Errorless learning: a method of learning in which errors are prevented and sufficient cueing is provided to achieve correct performance on each occasion a task is practiced.[4]

Functional cognition: how people use and integrate their thinking and processing skills to perform everyday activities in clinical and community settings.[5]

Metacognitive strategy instruction (MSI): direct instruction to teach clients to regulate their own behavior by using internal thinking procedures that are applicable to many realms of everyday functioning such as specifying goals, breaking tasks into steps, self-monitoring, modifying behavior if upon reflection, the goal is not met.[6]

Post-traumatic amnesia (PTA): the period following trauma in which the acquisition of new declarative knowledge is severely impaired; PTA is said to be resolved when continuous memory for ongoing events is restored.[7]

Press: aspects of the person's physical or social environment that influence the challenge of an activity (activity demand); reducing the press can make an activity easier to perform.

Routines: semiautomatic sequences of activities that are prompted by physical context and are fairly consistent for each individual on a day-to-day basis (e.g., a person's morning activities of daily living [ADL] routine).

Self-awareness: the ability to perceive one's strengths, weaknesses, and vulnerabilities with relative objectivity.[8]

Conceptual Foundation Underlying Interventions for Cognitive Dysfunction

As introduced in Chapter 10, many people who are referred to occupational therapy experience permanent, temporary, and/or progressive cognitive impairment or inefficiency that interferes with their occupational performance. Cognitive dysfunction may be associated with the person's primary diagnosis (including traumatic brain injury [TBI],[9] stroke,[10] multiple sclerosis,[11] Parkinson disease,[12] and major neurocognitive disorder [dementia][13]) or occur secondary to concurrent problems with pain,[14] anxiety, and depression.[15] Therefore, helping clients optimize their cognitive functioning is often a primary or secondary focus of occupational therapy intervention.

The central aim of this chapter is to advance evidence-informed cognitive intervention that reflects occupational therapists' focus on occupational performance. To that end, we first provide context relative to the broader cognitive rehabilitation field and then describe theory and practices associated with occupation-oriented cognitive intervention. Note that for simplicity, we use the term *client* when referring to the individual receiving occupational therapy. However, traditionally, the term *patient* is used in acute or inpatient rehabilitation medical settings, which underscores their medical and psychological vulnerability. We advise readers to use terminology that optimizes clear communication within their local practice context.

Cognitive Rehabilitation

Interest in the possibility of "reeducating" persons with a damaged brain dates back to the 1800s,[16] with wars of the 20th century giving rise to worldwide research and interventions to improve cognition after penetrating brain injuries. Most notably, the needs of veterans with brain injury sustained in the 1973 Yom Kippur War led to the development of an intensive, interdisciplinary rehabilitation program in Israel that focused on patients' cognitive and behavioral disabilities.[17] Similar programs were developed in the United States, ultimately legitimizing cognitive impairment as a primary focus of rehabilitation. **Cognitive rehabilitation** remains an interdisciplinary enterprise, typically involving occupational therapists, speech language pathologists, and neuropsychologists.[18] As such, there is the potential for complementary, overlapping, or conflicting roles among professions.

Cognitive intervention provided by occupational therapists has a distinct focus on functional cognition. **Functional cognition** has been defined as the ability to integrate thinking and performance skills to accomplish complex everyday activities.[19] This focus on functional cognition suggests two central features of cognitive intervention in occupational therapy. First, cognitive dysfunction is always addressed within the context of the client's broader capacities, concerns, resources, and relevant environments. For example, occupational therapy during inpatient rehabilitation for a young man with a moderate TBI addresses both cognitive and mobility limitations that interfere with his ability to perform ADLs and be discharged to home. Second, improvement in occupational performance is always the intended outcome of cognitive intervention within a given episode of care. For example, during outpatient occupational therapy, a woman with cancer-related cognitive dysfunction ("chemobrain") learns to use cognitive strategies applied to work-related activities so that she will experience a decrease in the frequency of memory failures in her job as a financial manager. Occupational therapists have the education and training to provide cognitive intervention and are accountable to their clients and the profession to employ occupation-focused, evidence-based approaches and to invest in ongoing learning in this important area of rehabilitation.

Approaches to Cognitive Intervention in Occupational Therapy

In this chapter, we describe three cognitive intervention approaches that occupational therapists use to help clients improve occupational performance: skill–habit training, cognitive strategy training, and environmental modification/adaptation. Multiple approaches are often employed to help clients meet their goals. Before implementing any approach, the therapist does the following:

- collaborates with the client (and family care partner, if available/appropriate) to identify the real-life scenarios in which cognitive impairments or inefficiencies are most problematic;

- uses assessment findings to determine the cognitive focus area and the client's current level of self-awareness;
- ascertains the client's preferences and requirements;
- considers the outcome expectations, and anticipated intensity and duration of therapy within the context of a given episode of care (see Table 11-1).

Addressing Client Self-Awareness across Intervention Approaches

Many clients who are referred to occupational therapy for cognitive intervention are not fully aware of the cognitive problems that interfere with their performance. Clients who are hospitalized with sudden-onset neurological conditions (such as stroke or TBI from motor vehicle accidents) may have injuries to the brain's frontoparietal control network that contribute to impaired **self-awareness**,[25] and the regimens and safety policies of the hospital setting rarely offer clients real-life feedback about the presence or consequences of cognitive impairments. Because impaired self-awareness is associated with poorer rehabilitation outcomes,[26] occupational therapists try to use a variety of techniques to help clients become more aware of their cognitive strengths and weaknesses throughout the intervention process.

- Appreciate the difference between neurologically based unawareness and adjustment-based denial. Furthermore, make an effort to determine what aspect of self-awareness may be impaired (metacognitive awareness, anticipatory awareness, error monitoring, self-regulation).[26,27]
- Create opportunities for clients to (1) predict how well they'll perform challenging tasks, (2) monitor their performance, (3) analyze the results of their efforts, and (4) determine what to continue or do differently next time.
- Introduce therapeutic structured failure when appropriate. That is, do not interfere with the natural consequences of the cognitive impairment during selected supervised activities. For example, if the client fails to initiate a cognitive compensatory strategy (such as use of a memory aid), do not provide further instruction, but rather create an opportunity for the client to observe what happens when the strategy is not used.
- Offer noncritical feedback in real time regarding observations of performance or behavior. Point out strengths and evidence of improvement as well.
- Collaborate with family members to provide feedback. In some cases, family members should focus on maintaining harmony in the household and appropriately

Table 11-1. Key Features of Four Cognitive Intervention Approaches

COGNITIVE INTERVENTION APPROACH	CHARACTERISTICS OF CLIENTS	OUTCOME EXPECTATIONS	EXAMPLES OF INTENSITY AND DURATION BASED ON STUDIES DEMONSTRATING INTERVENTION EFFICACY OR EFFECTIVENESS
Skill–habit training	Individuals with a wide range of cognitive capacities can benefit, including those with major neurocognitive disorder and moderate-to-severe TBI.	The client learns a set of procedures that enable him or her to competently perform a selected task. Training on one task is not expected to transfer to competence with another.	Daily application of errorless learning principles during post-traumatic amnesia following TBI for 3–4 weeks of training accelerates recovery and may shorten rehabilitation LOS.[20]
Cognitive strategy training	Clients must be aware of their limitations and sufficiently motivated in order to learn and employ new techniques.	The client learns how to perform a technique, use a tool or internal thinking procedure that can be applied to improve performance in a variety of tasks, roles, and settings.	Adults with TBI received two, 1-hour, individual weekly sessions for 10 weeks of metacognitive strategy instruction based on CO-OP.[21] Adults with TBI received training to use their smartphone as a memory aid over a 6-week period (one individual session and five group sessions that were each 1.5 hours).[22]
Environmental modification/ Adaptation	At a minimum, clients must have care partners available to modify the environment on clients' behalf.	The care partner implements changes in the home that helps a person with progressive cognitive dysfunction maintain his or her level of functioning in the home, reduces family care partner burden, and improves their quality of life.	Use of a daily routine and regular exercise helps maintain occupational performance in persons with Alzheimer disease.[23] Educating the care partner about how to modify the physical and social environment increases self-efficacy and reduces burden among care partners.[24]

CO-OP, Cognitive Orientation to Daily Occupational Performance; LOS, length of stay; TBI, traumatic brain injury.

prefer that the therapist assumes the responsibility of providing any feedback about performance problems to the client. In other cases, family members or coworkers are so afraid of offending or discouraging clients that they insulate them from any and all challenges or avoid mentioning errors and, as a result, deprive them of information that might improve self-awareness.

- Respect the clients' readiness to participate in therapy. Avoid badgering clients into improved awareness of deficits by maintaining a therapeutic partnership so that they will want to return for services in the future.

Skill–Habit Training

It is widely accepted that human beings have two systems for the control and execution of behavior: a conscious, controlled, slow, effortful, and deliberative cognitive system used when people are engaged in problem-solving, and a rapid, relatively effortless, habitual, or automatic system that supports frequently performed skills, tasks, and habits.[28,29] Solving novel problems constitutes a relatively small part of a person's life, and most of human behavior is automatic.[30,31] Automatic habits and **routines** enable people to perform complex skills and carry out everyday tasks with little or no mental energy. For example, most people employ relatively consistent procedures for daily activities, such as showering, brushing teeth, crossing the street, and getting to work. Practice increases the availability of target responses, such that conscious decision-making is replaced by the implementation of automatic action sequences.[32] When a skill becomes automatic, it becomes the easiest behavior to initiate from an array of possible behaviors, reduces interference error, and is experienced by the individual as effortless.

Helping clients develop new habits and routines that improve specific skills/behaviors (sometimes called specific skill or task-specific training)[33] is a potentially potent means of advancing occupational performance for people with cognitive impairments.[3,20,34] Skill–habit training addresses the disruption in long-standing habits and routines that may accompany disability and neurological impairments.[35] Following TBI or stroke or in the context of cognitive decline, what were once automatic skills for tasks performance (e.g., street crossing, doing laundry) can lead to insurmountable challenges and loss of self-esteem for a person with newly acquired deficits in planning, problem-solving, and decision-making. The lost competence in what were once effortless skills can have a profound impact on that individual's energy level and sense of continuity, competence, and self.[36]

The skill–habit training approach is intended to improve an individual's ability to perform a particular skill or task, but generalization to other skills is not expected. It has been suggested that improved functional competence improves self-confidence and willingness to engage in further training, but there is no expectation that skills other than the ones taught will improve. It is, therefore, important to look for areas with the client and family care partner for which improved functioning will have important outcomes for the individual. Skill–habit training, which relies on procedural and **errorless learning**, is often used with persons with severe impairment of memory or self-awareness, and/or those who have problems with ADL or simple instrumental ADL (IADL).[3,37] However, the relevance of skill–habit training is not limited to those with disabilities because most people rely on habits to a greater or lesser extent.

Implementing This Approach in Occupational Therapy Practice

- Guided by the client (and family care partner where appropriate), the therapist selects a key skill that becomes the target of intervention.[3,38]
- The therapist analyzes the physical and social context in which the routine or sequence is expected to occur to identify environmentally available cues or determine where to create new cues. Because routines and habit sequences are thought to be context specific, training is most effective if it occurs in the environment in which the routines will ultimately be performed.[3]
- A task analysis is performed that is specific to each client on the targeted skill.[3] Task analysis involves breaking the skill down into discrete steps so that when each step is performed in a **chain** until the target state (e.g., bathing dressing, making a cup of coffee) is achieved. A checklist may be created to assure that the steps are practiced in a consistent sequence (see Fig. 11-1).
- The client must then practice the task. The therapist or family care partner cues the client through the task performance so that it is performed without errors. The number of times that the client must practice the task depends on the task's complexity and the severity of the client's impairments, but some evidence of learning is usually apparent within days to weeks. As the client consistently performs the task, learning occurs and steps begin to "chunk" together so that gradually the client goes directly into the next step in the sequence without being cued and cues can be combined and the program can be shortened.[3] For some clients who have relatively intact initiation skills, once a program is established, a checklist can be used as the client checks each completed step.

Skill–habit training is a recommended, occupation-oriented approach to rehabilitation for individuals with moderate-to-severe memory or executive function impairments and for those with impaired self-awareness or who are in **PTA**. Unfortunately, skills training has often been undervalued by occupational therapists despite its alignment with occupational therapy theory and goals.

Morning planning checklist

Directions: each step after it is completed.

	Su	M	T	W	Th	F	Sa
1. After breakfast, open planner to yesterday's page.							
2. Check off all of the tasks you completed yesterday.							
3. Draw an arrow in front of undone or incomplete tasks.							
4. Re-write these tasks on today's page.							
5. Move the bookmark to today's planner page.							
6. Review today's schedule.							
7. Ask your wife if there are any tasks or appointments that you should write down for today.							
8. Make notes about at least things you would like to do today.							
9. Turn to tomorrow's page and make a note to remind yourself to do this checklist again.							

Wind-down checklist

Directions: each step after it is completed.

	Su	M	T	W	Th	F	Sa
1. When your phone alarm sounds at 9 pm, stop your current activity.							
2. Make notes about where you left off on your project.							
3. Put on your pajamas.							
4. Brush your teeth.							
5. Wash your face.							
6. Gather your magazines and go to your recliner.							
7. Set your alarm on your phone for 30 minutes and enjoy your magazines.							
8. When the alarm sounds, go to bed.							

Figure 11-1. Checklists like these are used to help clients re-establish task–habit sequences.

Compensatory Cognitive Strategy Training

People with neurocognitive impairment who use **compensatory cognitive strategies** experience improved cognitive functioning, confidence, and perseverance.[39] The therapist collaborates with the client (and family care partner, if available/appropriate) to ascertain the client's preferences and requirements for strategy use and then implements a training regimen. Sohlberg and Turkstra[40] proposed that cognitive strategy training is organized around three training phases, which are summarized as follows. Note that the case example in this chapter illustrates these phases of strategy training.

1. *Acquisition:* The therapist teaches the client about the selected cognitive strategy and how to use it. The client then practices strategy procedures, first with coaching from the therapist to minimize procedural errors. Next, the therapist provides practice opportunities to assure that the client can independently perform the strategy in response to a cue or trigger. Ideally, with the support of family care partners, clients identify opportunities to practice using the strategy at home.
2. *Mastery and generalization:* The therapist and client continue to identify contexts in which the new

strategy could optimize performance and the related cues that could trigger strategy implementation. The therapist creates strategy practice opportunities with varying cues, stimuli, and contexts. The therapist's feedback becomes less immediate and directive and more general and delayed (e.g., from "you forgot to set your alarm prompt" to "is there anything else you need to do to make sure you remember to take your medication at 2 pm?").[40]

3. ***Maintenance:*** It typically takes more time and repetition for a newly learned strategy to become automatic than are available during an episode of care. Therefore, the therapist sets up supports to minimize the possibility that the client will abandon the strategy when therapy is discontinued such as the following: (1) the client is scheduled for a follow-up or "booster" session a month or so after discharge; (2) the client is asked to periodically check in via email about ways in which he or she is using the new strategy after discharge; (3) the therapist identifies key people in the client's natural environment who are willing to support continued strategy use.

In this chapter, we provide an overview of two categories of compensatory cognitive strategies: memory-related strategies and metacognitive strategies, and recommend Haskins[41] for descriptions of other attention-management and executive functions-related strategies.

Memory Strategies

In this section, we discuss the use of internal and external memory strategies to advance occupational performance.

Internal Memory Strategies

Internal strategies are methods of mentally manipulating information so as to increase its depth of coding and likelihood of later recall (e.g., see Table 11-2).[42] O'Neil-Pirozzi and colleagues[43] reported positive outcomes of teaching internal memory strategies to participants with TBI who were already using external memory strategies. In general, internal memory strategies are considered effortful to learn and employ and may be best used as a complement to external strategies for memory tasks that cannot be practically managed by jotting or inputting a note (such as remembering name–face associations). Use of internal strategies tends to be most effective for people who have mild-to-moderate impairments and/or some preservation of executive functions.[44]

External Memory Strategies

External memory strategies are environmental supports or devices that optimize a person's recall and/or follow-through on tasks or appointments by providing prompts and/or information.

- ***Checklists:*** A client with severe memory impairment may not remember performing a task or the sequence for doing so, resulting in either a repeat of the activity or nonengagement in the activity in the mistaken belief that it has already been performed. Being taught to mark off each instruction or activity on a checklist as it is performed may help clients successfully perform new procedures (see Fig. 11-1).
- ***Timetables and Memory Books:*** Many inpatient programs use timetables and/or memory books to help clients remain oriented to the events of the day. A timetable is a simplified version of a personal schedule. The timetable may include time to wake up, wash and dress, eat meals, do chores, and regularly scheduled individual and group therapy times. A memory book is typically composed of sections with orientation information (e.g., a page with information about where the client is and why) and daily log sheets, on which the client, family, or staff write down what occurs on an hour-by-hour basis. Timetables and memory books are particularly helpful to clients with severe memory impairment. Staff and family use these tools to interact

Table 11-2. Examples of Internal Compensatory Strategies

TECHNIQUE	DESCRIPTION
Rehearsal	Client repeats the information to be remembered out loud or to self.
Visual imagery	Client consolidates information to be remembered by making a mental picture that includes the information (e.g., to remember the name *Barbara*, the client pictures a barber holding the letter A).
First-letter mnemonics	The **NAME** mnemonic adds rules to observing features and drawing associations when remembering names: **N**otice the person with whom you speak. **A**sk the person to repeat his or her name. **M**ention the name in conversation. **E**xaggerate some special feature. The **PQRST** method (**P**review, **Q**uestion, **R**ead, **S**tate, **T**est) can be used in academic contexts for recall of more complex verbal and written information.

Based on information from Parenté R, Herrmann D. *Retraining Cognition: Techniques and Applications*. 2nd ed. Austin, TX: Pro-ed; 2002.

with the client around orienting information, often cueing the client to look up information in the memory book or timetable. As clients recover, it becomes possible for them to review information spontaneously and make entries about ongoing events and/or progress to using a day planner/organizer.

- *Day Planners/Organizers:* Individuals with mild cognitive inefficiencies (such as those with concussion/mild TBI) or neurodegenerative conditions such as multiple sclerosis (MS) and those who are recovering from moderate-to-severe TBI are often taught to use a day planner or cognitive assistive technology (CAT) as a "memory prosthesis" to improve their functioning in daily life.[45,46] To do this successfully, clients must be taught to recognize the type of information that is pertinent for them in real time, initiate entry of the material into the planner or device, take or input notes accurately, and establish daily procedures and/or employ alarm prompts for referring to needed information in a timely manner. As with memory books, many day planners have function-specific sections that may include daily schedule/to-do lists, checklists pertaining to frequently performed procedures, notes about projects in process, reference information about medical providers or family members, and contact information. Use of commercially available systems offers a variety of sizes and formats (see Fig. 11-2), enables clients to customize and maintain their system on a long-term basis, and minimizes the stigma of needing to write things down.
- *CATs:* Clients may need or prefer to use some form of CAT as either a replacement for or complement to a planner/organizer. In fact, CAT may offer benefits to those with neurocognitive impairment over and above that derived from day planners.[47] CAT ranges from off-the-shelf smartphones to technologies developed especially for individuals with cognitive impairment, such as NeuroPage. Smartphones may have particular appeal because of their low cost and wide acceptance as a memory aid by people with and without neurocognitive impairment. Adults with acquired brain injury value the audible and visible smartphone reminders and having an all-in-one memory device but worry about losing it.[48] Despite the widespread use of smartphones in everyday life, clients with neurocognitive deficits cannot be expected to spontaneously adopt these devices or learn their use via a simple Tip Sheet. They need training to correctly perform key procedures and apply key apps to everyday life situations and assistance to set up Cloud-based synchronization on their devices in order to back up contacts, calendar, and tasks.[22,48] NeuroPage uses radio paging or SMS (text messaging) technology to send reminders of things to do to people with significant memory impairment. It is operated out of the Oliver Zangwill Centre for Neuropsychological Rehabilitation (the United Kingdom). The client wears an ordinary pager or mobile phone. He or she provides NeuroPage operators with a list of required date/time-specific prompts and then the system automatically sends out reminders for things like task initiation, taking medications, and sending birthday cards. NeuroPage has been studied extensively, demonstrating improved day-to-day functioning in the postacute period after TBI[49] and for people with cognitive limitations associated with MS.[39]

Tuesday
July 17, 2018
Daily planning
Call dentist
Do arm exercises
O.T. Homework
O.T.
Speech
Visit Carroll
Notes
1. Dr. K. said I need 6 more weeks of
2. CBS News
on service dogs

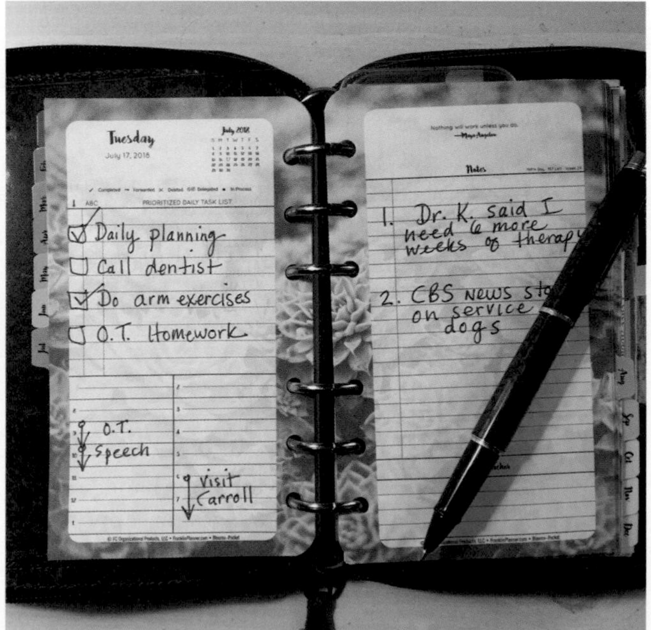

Figure 11-2. Use of function-specific sections of the planner page helps the client organize notes about the day.

Metacognitive Strategies

Metacognition refers to self-awareness and monitoring of a person's own cognitive processes. **MSI** involves teaching clients how to regulate their behavior by identifying problems, setting goals, evaluating possible solutions, and monitoring and modifying the solutions that they implement.[6] This approach is often used to address problems with executive functions.[6] Two MSI approaches developed with an occupation focus are Cognitive Orientation to Daily Occupational Performance (CO-OP)[50] and the multicontext approach for promoting transfer of strategy use,[3,51] which is summarized in Table 11-3.

Cognitive Orientation to Daily Occupations

The CO-OP approach teaches a global strategy (goal, plan, do, check) in a process of "guided discovery" so that clients can develop their own domain-specific strategies to solve personally relevant, specific performance problems.[52] CO-OP has been demonstrated to improve occupational performance for adults with TBI,[21] stroke,[53] and cancer-related cognitive dysfunction.[54]

Table 11-3. Components of the Multicontext Treatment Approach

COMPONENT	DEFINITION	EXAMPLE
Interventions to enhance self-monitoring and self-awareness	Methods designed to enhance the client's understanding of his or her strengths and limitations that are incorporated into every treatment session	• Asking the client to anticipate and identify specific challenges or obstacles that might occur in performance of a therapy task • Instructing the client to watch the therapist perform a task during which client-relevant errors are demonstrated (such as distractibility). Asking the client to identify problems and recommend strategies
Strategy self-generation and training	Internal or external cognitive techniques that contribute to the effectiveness of performance	• Mental repetition, visual imagery (i.e., internal processing strategies) • Memory notebooks, alarm cueing devices, use of checklists (i.e., external processing strategies) • Breaking projects into a list of substeps
Therapist uses task analysis to facilitate client experiences that enhance transfer	Identifying, manipulating, and/or stabilizing salient activity parameters (e.g., physical features, number of items, number of steps or choices involved in the task)	Helping client establish consistent procedures for using a checklist (read a step, do the step, check it off, read the next step, etc.) by first implementing a five-step morning hygiene checklist and then implementing a five-step breakfast preparation checklist
Promoting strategy transfer "sideways" across the continuum form near to far transfer	The therapist identifies a series of tasks that decrease in degrees of physical and conceptual similarity to the original task Near transfer: only one or two surface characteristics changed Intermediate transfer: three to six surface characteristics change; tasks share some physical similarities Far transfer: tasks are conceptually similar; surface characteristics are different or only one surface characteristic is similar Very far transfer: generalization, spontaneous application of what is learned in treatment to everyday life	Task: donning a pullover T-shirt in the therapy area Donning a pullover sweater (color and texture different from T-shirt) Donning a button-down cotton shirt in the client's room (type of clothing, color and texture, fine motor requirements, and environment changed) Donning outerwear (coat, jacket), pajamas, undershirt, or camisole (different types of upper body clothing) Donning pants (strategy of dressing affected side first remains the same for lower body dressing). The appearance of the task changes but utilizes the same strategy
Practice in multiple environments	Strategies are used in diverse situations (e.g., tasks and locations) to demonstrate their applicability and use to the client	Practicing of left-to-right scanning on letter cancellation tasks in the clinic and then used to locate items in a medicine cabinet or in the clients local grocery store

Adapted from Toglia J. The dynamic interactional model and the multicontext approach. In: Katz N, Toglia J, eds. *Cognition, Occupation, and Participation across the Lifespan*. 4th ed. Bethesda, MD: AOTA Press; 2018:355–385.

The following exemplifies the CO-OP training process, with the therapist–client interaction distilled into key features, such as "One thing at a time"; "Ask, don't tell"; "Coach, don't adjust"; and "Make it obvious."[52]

1. The client sets the goals that he or she wishes to work on and then the therapist teaches the global strategy of Goal, Plan, Do, Check.
2. The client is guided in dynamic performance analysis in which he or she identifies the performance problems that interfere with goal achievement.
3. The client is further guided to identify potential strategies that may solve his or her problems. The client then implements the strategy to solve the real-world functional problem and checks to see whether it worked. The implementation of the domain-specific strategy may or may not be done in the presence of the therapist, depending on the treatment context, stage of training, and other factors.

Cognitive strategy training relies on the implementation of conscious thinking procedures and is typically applied to persons with mild-to-moderate impairment and relatively intact self-awareness.

Environmental Modification/Adaptation

Occupational performance is affected by changes in the demands of the task itself or challenges or supports associated with the environment. Therapists can advise or train family care partners to make task or environmental changes that lower the cognitive demands placed on the client (see Fig. 11-3). This type of intervention can extend to the interpersonal environment, and family

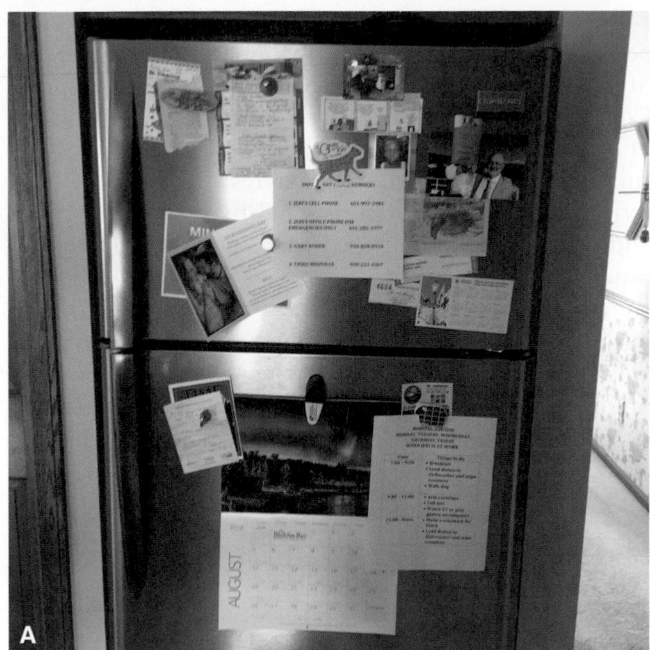

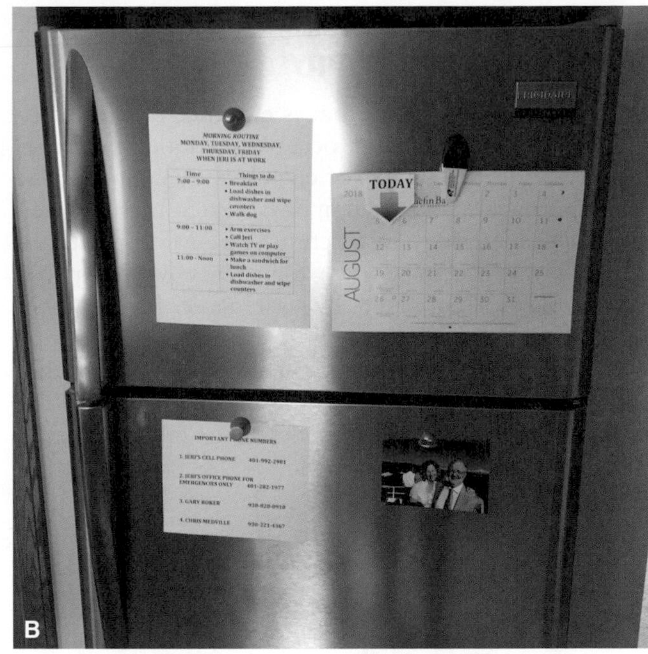

Figure 11-3. Simple changes in the kitchen lower the cognitive demands, making it easier for a person with cognitive limitations to find relevant information. **A.** High cognitive demand. **B.** Low cognitive demand.

care partners can be trained to use new ways of interacting with the client. In this approach, the client is not expected to learn or change, but the **press** of the task, social dynamics, and/or environment are changed to reduce the complexity of the behavior required for successful performance. In learning theory terms, this is antecedent control where the situational or other cues that are available to the person increase the chances that an appropriate behavior will be emitted. This approach is particularly appropriate for persons with major neurocognitive disorder or severe neurocognitive deficits from other causes (e.g., TBI, encephalitis, anoxia) where changes in learning and memory or executive functioning are particularly marked.

Implementing This Approach in Occupational Therapy Practice

Environmental modification/adaptation can be used both to address occupational performance and to decrease some of the negative behaviors that can occur when an individual's cognitive capacity is insufficient for the environmental demands that he or she needs to manage. The approach is informed by the competence-environmental press framework.[55] This framework suggests that the client's excess disability and/or negative behaviors is caused by the misalignment between the client's declining cognitive ability and the unchanged demands of the physical and social environment. The client's functional performance and behavioral control may be optimized as task, and environmental demands are matched to his or her capacities.[56,57] Simple interventions such as labeling clothing draws, preselecting clothing, removing excess clothes from closets, or laying clothes out for dressing reduce the decision-making requirement of dressing. Clothing itself can be simplified, such as having elastic waist bands on clothing rather than button-fastening jeans reducing the complexity of the task. Providing an organizational structure of the day by building in routine activities can reduce confusion in cognitively impaired clients. The client may not recognize the routine consciously, but a structure to the day maintained by the family care partner can reduce behavioral dysregulation and improves occupational performance. Occupational therapists can provide training to family care partners to reduce burden and delay institutionalization and to can also provide training to caregivers in institutional settings, such as assisted living and skilled nursing facilities. The extent to which family care partners who receive training in how to match cognitive demands to clients' capabilities are able to transfer or generalize this training to new problems or situations is not known. However, it appears that the effects of this training are time limited, and booster sessions may be needed.[57,58]

Environmental modification/adaptation is intended to address the needs of individuals with severe impairments and is not restorative or curative. It is often, though not exclusively, used in the context of individuals with progressive major neurocognitive disorders and with those who are going to require ongoing careful management to maintain safety and some degree of functional independence. As the proportion of the population who is over 65 years old continues to grow, occupational therapy expertise in environmental modification/adaptation will remain of critical importance.

Evidence-Informed Cognitive Intervention in Occupational Therapy

Provision of intervention that is evidence based is considered critical to ethical occupational therapy practice.[59] Within the context of cognitive intervention, the three approaches presented in this chapter are supported by evidence. Strategy instruction (e.g., MSI and use of compensatory memory aids) for clients with acquired brain injury is endorsed by systematic reviews, meta-analyses, and guidelines.[6,44,60–63] Skill–habit training and environmental modification/adaptation approaches are supported by numerous randomized controlled trials (RCTs), some of which are described in the Evidence table at the end of this chapter.

Beyond understanding what approaches are supported by evidence, it is equally imperative to be aware of what approaches do not have empirical support. Cognitive retraining exercises, often taking the form of drill and practice workbooks or computer games or simulations, that are intended to restore impaired cognitive abilities are not supported by evidence[44,60,63,64] and thus not recommended for occupational therapy practice.

This chapter serves as a primer for evidence-informed cognitive intervention for occupational therapists. Further study and attentiveness to the emergence of new evidence are necessary for assuring competence in this important dimension of occupational therapy practice.

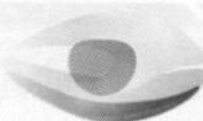

CASE STUDY

Client Information

Trevor is a 26-year-old single male who sustained a moderate TBI as a result of a motor vehicle accident. Records indicate that he lost consciousness for approximately 35 minutes. He also fractured his left radius. Trevor participated in inpatient rehabilitation for 2 weeks. Trevor graduated from college with a degree in law enforcement and worked in a rural community as a police officer at the time of his injury. Unable to return to his own apartment because of concerns about safety, Trevor was discharged from the inpatient rehabilitation unit to his brother's home.

Reason for Occupational Therapy Referral

Trevor was referred to outpatient occupational therapy at the time of his discharge from inpatient rehabilitation in order to continue his recovery and improve his independence.

Assessment Process and Results

The occupational therapist accessed *at-discharge* documents in the medical record, which indicated that Trevor could perform ADLs and simple IADL (light meal preparation) with supervision. The *Cognistat*,[65] administered near the time of discharge from inpatient rehabilitation, suggested performance within the average range for orientation, comprehension, naming, construction; mild impairment in similarities, judgment, calculations, repetition; and mild-moderate impairment in attention and memory.

At the initial outpatient session, Trevor appeared motivated to participate in therapy as a means of ultimately getting his own apartment; he did not appear distracted by pain or emotional distress. He reported that he used his iPhone to keep track of contacts and appointments and wanted to continue to do so.

The therapist administered the *Canadian Occupational Performance Measure (COPM)*[66] to obtain information about the client's perceived problems and priorities and conducted an interview with his brother, Carson.

- ***COPM:*** Trevor indicated that his ability to function independently was limited due to casted left forearm and radial fracture. He identified the following primary concerns: inability to drive (Performance 6; Satisfaction 1); slowness with which he dressed himself (Performance 4; Satisfaction 2); poor stamina because of his inability to workout (Performance 3; Satisfaction 1); and being unable to do previously enjoyed recreational activities (Performance 4; Satisfaction 2). When queried about known dependence on family members to take medications and his lack of initiation of everyday tasks, Trevor quickly dismissed these reports as awkwardness associated with being a guest in their home.
- ***Interview with Carson:*** Carson reported that Trevor seemed to have more skills that he actively used on a given day. For example, Carson observed that Trevor had the ability to perform all of his self-care tasks and even make his own light breakfast and lunch but didn't do any of these activities unless specifically instructed. Carson seemed to interpret Trevor's reticence to initiate as laziness, even though it was dramatically different from Trevor's premorbid nature. Carson seemed most interested in seeing Trevor advance to the point where he could manage his day at

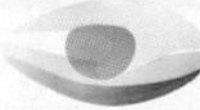

CASE STUDY *(continued)*

home safely without supervision while Carson was at work. Carson indicated a willingness to provide transportation to appointments and to attend at least weekly.

Occupational Therapy Problem List

- Cueing required for ADL and IADL likely due to problems with initiation associated with executive dysfunction
- Limited repertoire of exercise and avocational options
- Memory inefficiency and inadequate repertoire of memory compensation strategies

Occupational Therapy Goal List

The occupational therapist recommended one to two treatment sessions per week for 4 to 6 weeks to address the following goals:

- Trevor will independently initiate and carry out all self-care and selected light housekeeping tasks;
- Trevor will increase his level of productive activity at home such that he initiates an exercise program and avocational activities at least three times per week;
- Trevor will follow through on intended tasks at least 85% of the time through use of external memory aids and strategies.

The occupational therapist also requested that the physician refer Trevor for a psychological evaluation to rule out depression and determine needs for psychological support.

Intervention

The occupational therapist hypothesized that more frequent use of memory prompts would be central to Trevor's goal achievement, both in terms of initiation and task follow-through. Therefore, helping Trevor expand the use of his iPhone was the first priority of therapy (*cognitive strategy training intervention approach*). Trevor was instructed in how to set alarm prompts coupled with "appointments" as a means of remembering to perform tasks at certain times (*Acquisition*). Therapy homework provided opportunities for Trevor to practice these procedures. For example, he was assigned to call and leave a message for the therapist at preassigned dates/times. The therapist recommended creating a checklist to help Trevor establish a consistent sequence for his morning routine, which would be prompted by a recurring alarm/appointment (*skill-habit training intervention approach*). The establishment of a consistent routine would ultimately enhance **automaticity** of the ADL procedures, decrease performance time (important to Trevor), and enable Trevor to initiate these tasks without reminders (important to Carson). The occupational therapist asked Trevor to set his iPhone time/appointment alarm to prompt him to refer to his checklist, which was posted in his bathroom, at a routine time each morning. The occupational therapist brainstormed about other everyday activities that were important to Trevor and how he might use his iPhone time/appointment alarm to remind him about evening medications, performing his physical therapy exercise program, calling his mother on Sunday afternoons, and syncing his phone with his laptop every Saturday morning to back it up on the iCloud (*Mastery and Generalization*). Carson was supportive of this approach and worked with Trevor to consider other tasks for which he might use his iPhone reminders (*Maintenance*).

Checklists and iPhone alarm prompts were also used to help Trevor increase his productivity during the day while Carson was at work. The occupational therapist collaborated with Trevor's physical therapist to facilitate his performance of his exercise/fitness routine. Trevor started preparing simple meals for dinner, using a checklist to establish procedures that included cleaning up after himself and the alarm prompt to remember to start meal preparation. Trevor continued to use his iPhone to input reminders to complete his occupational therapy homework, which included a series of tasks aimed at exploring at-home avocational activities. These efforts were informed by the multicontext approach to advance transfer of learning.

Over the course of 6 weeks (and eight occupational therapy sessions), Trevor made substantive progress toward his goals. After approximately 3 weeks of therapy, he no longer required prompts for ADL or IADL or the morning routine checklist. In addition to preparing a simple dinner for his brother at least twice per week, Trevor did his own laundry, ordered groceries online, and scheduled his own appointments. Although Trevor was unable to afford to move into his own apartment, he and Carson were comfortable remaining roommates as Trevor shifted his focus toward returning to work. Prior to his discharge from occupational therapy, Carson helped Trevor obtain a volunteer job at a local animal shelter. Trevor, Carson, and the occupational therapist identified ways in which Trevor could apply his cognitive strategies to his volunteer responsibilities, which primarily involved performing routine cleaning tasks. The occupational therapist also helped them connect with a vocational counselor. They developed a plan wherein Trevor would increase his work hours over the course of the next month, and once he could manage 20 hours per week, they would begin to work with the vocational counselor to establish a longer term return to work plan. At the therapist's request, the physician also ordered an occupational therapy follow-up session in 2 months.

Evidence Table of Intervention Studies for Cognitive Impairments

Intervention	Description	Participants	Dosage	Research Design and Evidence Level	Benefit	Statistical Significance and Effect Size
Skill–habit training[20]	Training using neurofunctional principles of ADL and basic IADLs during PTA	One hundred four participants with severe PTA who remained in PTA >7 days	Daily from baseline to PTA emergence	Level I, RCT, manualized intervention comparing the neurofunctional approach to treatment as usual	Intervention group had greater improvement on Functional Independence Measure (FIM) scores from baseline to PTA emergence, with no increase in agitation than treatment as usual group	Differences were significant at emergence from PTA ($p = 0.001$) with moderate effect size $d = 0.70$; 95% confidence interval (CI; 1.09–0.30), and at inpatient rehabilitation discharge ($p = 0.001$) CI ($d = 0.74$; 95% CI, 1.14–0.34)
Skill–habit training[67]	Individualized goal-setting, task-specific training, environmental or task adaptation, and use of assistive devices	Twenty-six individuals (median age 65) who were ≥1 year poststroke and who were attending a community rehabilitation center	Twelve weeks of neurofunctional intervention with individualized goal-setting average number of treatment sessions 9 (range 2–20)	Level I, RCT with crossover	Significant differences were obtained on measures of occupational performance using the COPM after treatment, but not on quality-of-life measures. Nontargeted goals did not improve	Differences were significant at the $p = 0.001$ level, with large effect sizes 1.9–2.35
Metacognitive strategy instruction[21]	Occupation-based strategy instruction, an adapted version of CO-OP	Adults with chronic TBI ($n = 13$, 7 in experimental group; 6 in control group; age range 24–60 years; time since injury range 2.6–18.8 years)	CO-OP (experimental condition)—20 hours of training (two, 1-hour sessions/week) that focused on participants' top three concerns as identified via COPM interview. Control condition—no treatment	Level II, partially, pilot RCT	While there were no group differences in performance and satisfaction ratings on the three most problematic issues, there were group differences in terms of post-test ratings of performance and satisfaction of untrained goal areas, evidence of far transfer of training	Between-group differences in satisfaction ($p = 0.03$) and performance ($p = 0.04$) for untrained goal areas with large effect sizes (Cohen's d 1.53 and 1.33, respectively)
Training in a memory aid[39]	Training in use of a NeuroPage, a paging system that sends provides audio/vibrating prompts and SMS text messages	Adults with MS who had been diagnosed at least 12 months prior to study enrollment (Group 1, $n = 17$; Group 2, $n = 21$; age range 28–72; primarily women)	At one session, all participants received instructions about the messaging system. During the treatment arm, participants received prompts for self-selected problem areas for a 2-month period. During the control arm, participants received non–memory-related text messages	Level I, single, blind, crossover RCT	There were no group differences on the Everyday Memory Questionnaire, but those in the NeuroPage condition reported fewer everyday forgetting errors and less psychological distress than those in the control condition	Group differences: General Health Questionnaire ($p = 0.001$); anxiety-depression ($p = 0.04$); percentage of daily forgetting errors ($p = 0.01$) with moderate-to-large effect sizes (Cohen's d −0.47 to −0.84)
Task–environment modification training[57]	Tailored Activity Program	Veterans with motor neurone disease (MND) and their family care partners ($N = 160$ client/caregiver dyads)	Dyads received eight sessions to customize activities to the interests and abilities of the client and educate their care partners about use of customized activity in care for major neurocognitive disorder	Level I, RCT	At 4-month outcome assessment, the intervention group showed significant reduction in the number and severity of behavioral symptoms and in the number of activities with which the client needed assistance. Intervention group superiority was not maintained at 8 months	Differences in behavioral symptoms were change from baseline to 4 months = 0.68, 95% CI = 1.23–0.13, $p = 0.02$) and for reduction in need for assistance with functional activities (difference = 0.80, 95% CI = 1.41–0.20, $p = 0.009$)

References

1. Giles GM. A neurofunctional approach to rehabilitation following brain injury. In: Katz N, ed. *Cognition, Occupation and Participation Across the Life Span*. 3rd ed. Bethesda, MD: AOTA Press; 2011:351–381.
2. Kazdin AE. *Behavior Modification in Applied Settings*. 7th ed. Long Grove, IL: Waveland Press, Inc.; 2012.
3. Giles GM. Neurofunctional approach to rehabilitation after severe brain injury. In: Katz N, Toglia J, eds. *Cognition, Occupation, and Participation Across the Lifespan*. 4th ed. Bethesda, MD: AOTA Press; 2018:419–441.
4. Haslam C, Kessels RPC, eds. *Errorless Learning in Neuropsychological Rehabilitation: Mechanisms, efficacy, and Application*. New York, NY: Routledge; 2018.
5. Association AOT. Role of occupational therapy in assessing functional cognition. 2017. https://www.aota.org/Advocacy-Policy/Federal-Reg-Affairs/Medicare/Guidance/role-OT-assessing-functional-cognition.aspx. Accessed August 2, 2018.
6. Kennedy MR, Coelho C, Turkstra L, et al. Intervention for executive functions after traumatic brain injury: a systematic review, meta-analysis and clinical recommendations. *Neuropsychol Rehabil*. 2008;18(3):257–299. doi:10.1080/09602010701748644.
7. Lezak MD, Howieson DB, Bigler ED, Tranel D. *Neuropsychological Assessment*. 5th ed. New York, NY: Oxford University Press; 2012.
8. Prigatano GP, Schacter DL. *Awareness of Deficit After Brain Injury: Clinical and Theoretical Issues*. New York, NY: Oxford University Press; 1991.
9. Skandsen T, Finnanger TG, Andersson S, Lydersen S, Brunner JF, Vik A. Cognitive impairment 3 months after moderate and severe traumatic brain injury: a prospective follow-up study. *Arch Phys Med Rehabil*. 2010;91(12):1904–1913. doi:10.1016/j.apmr.2010.08.021.
10. Sun JH, Tan L, Yu JT. Post-stroke cognitive impairment: epidemiology, mechanisms and management. *Ann Transl Med*. 2014;2(8):80. doi:10.3978/j.issn.2305-5839.2014.08.05.
11. Chiaravalloti ND, DeLuca J. Cognitive impairment in multiple sclerosis. *Lancet Neurol*. 2008;7(12):1139–1151. doi:10.1016/S1474-4422(08)70259-X.
12. Watson GS, Leverenz JB. Profile of cognitive impairment in Parkinson's disease. *Brain Pathol*. 2010;20(3):640–645. doi:10.1111/j.1750-3639.2010.00373.x.
13. Hugo J, Ganguli M. Dementia and cognitive impairment: epidemiology, diagnosis, and treatment. *Clin Geriatr Med*. 2014;30(3):421–442. doi:10.1016/j.cger.2014.04.001.
14. Moriarty O, McGuire BE, Finn DP. The effect of pain on cognitive function: a review of clinical and preclinical research. *Prog Neurobiol*. 2011;93(3):385–404. doi:10.1016/j.pneurobio.2011.01.002.
15. Carelli L, Solca F, Faini A, et al. The complex interplay between depression/anxiety and executive functioning: insights from the ECAS in a large ALS population. *Front Psychol*. 2018;9:450. doi:10.3389/fpsyg.2018.00450.
16. Finger S. *Origins of Neuroscience: A History of Explorations into Brain Function*. New York, NY: Oxford University Press; 1994.
17. Boake C. History of cognitive rehabilitation following head injury. In: Kreutzer JS, Wehman PH, eds. *Cognitive Rehabilitation for Persons with Traumatic Brain Injury: A Functional Approach*. Baltimore, MD: Paul H. Brookes; 1991.
18. Medicine Io. *Cognitive Rehabilitation Therapy for Traumatic Brain Injury: Evaluating the Evidence*. Washington, DC: National Academies Press; 2011.
19. Giles GM, Edwards DF, Morrison MT, Baum C, Wolf TJ. Health policy perspectives—screening for functional cognition in postacute care and the Improving Medicare Post-Acute Care Transformation (IMPACT) Act of 2014. *Am J Occup Ther*. 2017;71(5):7105090010p1–7105090010p6. doi:10.5014/ajot.2017715001.
20. Trevena-Peters J, McKay A, Spitz G, Suda R, Renison B, Ponsford J. Efficacy of activities of daily living retraining during post-traumatic amnesia: a randomised controlled trial. *Arch Phys Med Rehabil*. 2018;99(2):329–337. doi:10.1016/j.apmr.2017.08.486.
21. Dawson DR, Binns MA, Hunt A, Lemsky C, Polatajko HJ. Occupation-based strategy training for adults with traumatic brain injury: a pilot study. *Arch Phys Med Rehabil*. 2013;94(10):1959–1963. doi:10.1016/j.apmr.2013.05.021.
22. Evald L. Prospective memory rehabilitation using smartphones in patients with TBI. *Disabil Rehabil*. 2018;40:2250–2259. doi:10.1080/09638288.2017.1333633.
23. Smallfield S, Heckenlaible C. Effectiveness of occupational therapy interventions to enhance occupational performance for adults with Alzheimer's disease and related major neurocognitive disorders: a systematic review. *Am J Occup Ther*. 2017;71:7105180010–7105180010p9. doi:10.5014/ajot.2017.024752.
24. Piersol CV, Canton K, Connor SE, Giller I, Lipman S, Sager S. Effectiveness of interventions for caregivers of people with Alzheimer's disease and related major neurocognitive disorders: a systematic review. *Am J Occup Ther*. 2017;71:7105180020p1–7105180020p10. doi:10.5014/ajot.2017.027581.
25. Ham TE, Bonnelle V, Hellyer P, et al. The neural basis of impaired self-awareness after traumatic brain injury. *Brain*. 2014;137(pt 2):586–597. doi:10.1093/brain/awt350.
26. Robertson K, Schmitter-Edgecombe M. Self-awareness and traumatic brain injury outcome. *Brain Inj*. 2015;29(7–8):848–858. doi:10.3109/02699052.2015.1005135.
27. Toglia J, Kirk U. Understanding awareness deficits following brain injury. *NeuroRehabilitation*. 2000;15(1):57–70.
28. Schneider W, Shiffrin RM. Controlled and automatic human information processing: I. Detection, search, and attention. *Psychol Rev*. 1977;84(1):1–66. doi:10.1037/0033-295X.84.1.1.
29. Birnboim S. The automatic and controlled information-processing dissociation: is it still relevant? *Neuropsychol Rev*. 2003;13(1):19–31. doi:10.1023/A:1022348506064.
30. Wood W, Neal DT. A new look at habits and the habit-goal interface. *Psychol Rev*. 2007;114(4):843–863. doi:10.1037/0033-295X.114,843.
31. Wood W, Rünger D. Psychology of habit. *Ann Rev Psychol*. 2016;67:289–314. doi:10.1146/annurev-psych-122414-033417.
32. Kramer AF, Strayer DL, Buckley J. Development and transfer or automatic processing. *J Exp Psychol Hum Percept Perform*. 1990;16(3):505–522.

33. Mastos M, Miller K, Eliasson AC, Imms C. Goal-directed training: linking theories of treatment to clinical practice for improved functional activities in daily life. *Clin Rehabil.* 2007;21(1):47–55. doi:10.1177/0269215506073494.
34. Clark-Wilson J, Baxter D, Giles GM. Revisiting the neurofunctional approach: conceptualising the essential components for the rehabilitation of everyday living skills. *Brain Inj.* 2014;28(13/14):1646–1656. doi:10.3109/02699052.2014.946449.
35. Wallenbert I, Jonsson H. Waiting to get better: a dilemma regarding habits in daily occupations after stroke. *Am J Occup Ther.* 2005;59(2):218–224.
36. Charmaz K. The self as habit: the reconstruction of self in chronic illness. *Occup Ther J Res.* 2002;22(suppl 1):31S–41S.
37. Giles GM. Cognitive versus functional approaches to rehabilitation after traumatic brain injury: commentary on a randomized controlled trial. *Am J Occup Ther.* 2010;64:182–185. doi:10.5014/ajot.64.1.182.
38. Parish L, Oddy M. Efficacy of rehabilitation for functional skills more than 10 years after extremely severe brain injury. *Neuropsychol Rehabil.* 2007;17(2):230–243. doi:10.1080/09602010600750675.
39. Goodwin RA, Lincoln NB, das Nair R, Bateman A. Evaluation of NeuroPage as a memory aid for people with multiple sclerosis: a randomised controlled trial. *Neuropsychol Rehabil.* 2018:1–17. doi:10.1080/09602011.2018.1447973.
40. Sohlberg MM, Turkstra L. *Optimizing Cognitive Rehabilitation: Effective Instructional Methods.* New York, NY: Guilford Press; 2011.
41. Haskins EC. *Cognitive Rehabilitation Manual: Translating Evidence-Based Recommendations into Practice.* Reston, VA: American Congress of Rehabilitation Medicine; 2011.
42. Kheirzadeh S, Pakzadian SS. Depth of processing and age differences. *J Psycholinguist Res.* 2016;45(5):1137–1149. doi:10.1007/s10936-015-9395.
43. O'Neil-Pirozzi TM, Strangman GE, Goldstein R, et al. A controlled treatment study of internal memory strategies (I-MEMS) following traumatic brain injury. *J Head Trauma Rehabil.* 2010;25(1):43–51. doi:10.1097/HTR.0b013e3181bf24b1.
44. Velikonja D, Tate R, Ponsford J, et al. INCOG recommendations for management of cognition following traumatic brain injury. Part V: Memory. *J Head Trauma Rehabil.* 2014;29(4):369–386. doi:10.1097/HTR.0000000000000069.
45. Gentry T. PDAs as cognitive aids for people with multiple sclerosis. *Am J Occup Ther.* 2008;62(1):18–27 doi:10.5014/ajot.62.1.18.
46. Gentry T, Wallace J, Kvarfordt C, Lynch KB. Personal digital assistants as cognitive aids for individuals with severe traumatic brain injury: a community-based trial. *Brain Inj.* 2008;22(1):19–24. doi:10.1080/02699050701810688.
47. Bos HR, Babbage DR, Leathem JM. Efficacy of memory aids after traumatic brain injury: a single case series. *NeuroRehabilitation.* 2017;41(2):463–481. doi:10.3233/NRE-151528.
48. Evald L. Prospective memory rehabilitation using smartphones in patients with TBI: what do participants report? *Neuropsychol Rehabil.* 2015;25(2):283–297. doi:10.1080/09602011.2014.970557.
49. Wilson BA, Emslie H, Quirk K, Evans J, Watson P. A randomized control trial to evaluate a paging system for people with traumatic brain injury. *Brain Inj.* 2005;19(11):891–894.
50. Polatajko H, Mandich A. *Enabling Occupation in Children: The Cognitive Orientation to Daily Occupational Performance.* Ottawa, ON: CAOT Publications; 2004.
51. Toglia J, Johnston MV, Goverover Y, Dain B. A multicontext approach to promoting transfer of strategy use and self regulation after brain injury: an exploratory study. *Brain Inj.* 2010;24(4):664–677. doi:10.3109/02699051003610474.
52. Polatajko H, Mandich A, McEwen S. Cognitive orientation to daily occupational performance (CO-OP): a cognitive-based intervention for children and adults. In: Katz N, ed. *Cognition and Occupation Across the Life Span.* Bethesda, MD: AOTA Press; 2011:299–321.
53. Wolf TJ, Polatajko H, Baum C, et al. Combined cognitive-strategy and task-specific training affects cognition and upper-extremity function in subacute stroke: an exploratory randomized controlled trial. *Am J Occup Ther.* 2016;70(2):7002290010p1–7002290010p10. doi:10.5014/ajot.2016.017293.
54. Wolf TJ, Doherty M, Kallogjeri D, et al. The feasibility of using metacognitive strategy training to improve cognitive performance and neural connectivity in women with chemotherapy-induced cognitive impairment. *Oncology.* 2016;91(3):143–152. doi:10.1159/000447744.
55. Lawton MP, Nahemow LE. Ecology and the aging process. In: Eisdorfer C, Lawton MP, eds. *The Psychology of Adult Development and Aging.* Washington, DC: American Psychological Association; 1973:619–674.
56. Gitlin LN, Winter L, Burke J, Chernett N, Dennis MP, Hauck WW. Tailored activities to manage neuropsychiatric behaviors in persons with dementia and reduce caregiver burden: a randomized pilot study. *Am J Geriatr Psychiatr.* 2008;16(3):229–239. doi:10.1097/JGP.0b013e318160da72.
57. Gitlin LN, Arthur P, Piersol C, et al. Targeting behavioral symptoms and functional decline in dementia: a randomized clinical trial. *J Am Geriatr Soc.* 2018;66(2):339–345. doi:10.1111/jgs.15194.
58. Gitlin LN, Corcoran M. *An Occupational Therapy Guide to Helping Caregivers of Persons with Dementia: The Home-Environment Skill-Building Program.* Baltimore, MD: American Journal of Occupational Therapy Press; 2005.
59. American Occupational Therapy Association. Occupational therapy code of ethics. *Am J Occup Ther.* 2015;69 (suppl 3):6913410030p1–6913410030p8. doi:10.5014/ajot.2015.696S03.
60. Cicerone KD, Langenbahn DM, Braden C, et al. Evidence-based cognitive rehabilitation: updated review of the literature from 2003 through 2008. *Arch Phys Med Rehabil.* 2011;92(4):519–530. doi:10.1016/j.apmr.2010.11.015.
61. Tate R, Kennedy M, Ponsford J, et al. INCOG recommendations for management of cognition following traumatic brain injury. Part III: Executive function and self-awareness. *J Head Trauma Rehabil.* 2014;29(4):338–352. doi:10.1097/HTR.0000000000000068.

62. Gillen G, Nilsen DM, Attridge J, et al. Effectiveness of interventions to improve occupational performance of people with cognitive impairments after stroke: an evidence-based review. *Am J Occup Ther.* 2015;69(1):6901180040p1–6901180040p9. doi:10.5014/ajot.2015.012138.
63. Radomski MV, Anheluk M, Bartzen MP, Zola J. Effectiveness of interventions to address cognitive impairments and improve occupational performance after traumatic brain injury: a systematic review. *Am J Occup Ther.* 2016;70(3):7003180050p1–7003180050p9. doi:10.5014/ajot.2016.020776.
64. Bahar-Fuchs A, Clare L, Woods B. Cognitive training and cognitive rehabilitation for persons with mild to moderate dementia of the Alzheimer's or vascular type: a review. *Alzheimers Res Ther.* 2013;5(4):35. doi:10.1186/alzrt189.
65. Kiernan RJ, Mueller J, Langston JW, Van Dyke C. The neurobehavioral cognitive status examination, a brief but differentiated approach to cognitive assessment. *Ann Intern Med.* 1987;107:481–485.
66. Law M, Baptiste S, Carswell As, McColl MA, Polatajko H, Pollock N. *Canadian Occupational Performance Measure.* 5th ed. Ottawa, ON: CAOT Publications ACE; 2014.
67. Rotenberg-Shpigelman S, Erez AB, Nahaloni I, Maeir A. Neurofunctional treatment targeting participation among chronic stroke survivors: a pilot randomised controlled study. *Neuropsychol Rehabil.* 2012;22(4):532–549. doi:10.1080/09602011.2012.665610.

Acknowledgments

Joette Zola, OTR/L of the Courage Kenny Rehabilitation Institute, provided expert guidance on the case example and we are most grateful.

Chapter 12

Sensory Assessment and Intervention

Carrie Ciro and Barbara M. Doucet

LEARNING OBJECTIVES

This chapter will allow the reader to:

1. Explain the neurological mechanisms of sensory perception and processing.
2. Describe a variety of occupations that might show impairment because of deficient sensation.
3. Select appropriate sensory assessment and interventions for patients.
4. Explain the rationale for sensory reeducation and desensitization.
5. Demonstrate a variety of sensory reeducation and desensitization strategies for patients following peripheral nerve injury or repair.
6. Name several mechanisms of damage to skin areas that result in diminished protective sensation and describe related compensatory strategies to prevent injury.
7. Demonstrate a variety of active and passive sensory training strategies for patients with sensory impairment following centrally mediated or peripheral sensory deficits.

CHAPTER OUTLINE

TERMINOLOGY

Allodynia: a type of hypersensitivity characterized by the perception of pain in response to a non-painful stimulus.

Centrally mediated sensation: sensation controlled primarily by the brain and spinal cord, such as stereognosis.

Desensitization intervention: a type of sensory intervention that involves the application of standardized and sequential textures to relieve hypersensitivity.

Exteroceptive sensation (or superficial sensation): a type of peripherally mediated sensation perceived locally by sensory receptors in the skin and mucous membranes and consists of touch, pain, and temperature awareness.

Haptic perception: a type of centrally mediated sensation characterized by identifying and perceiving object features achieved by active exploration of the object.

Hypersensitivity: a response to sensory information in which ordinary stimuli produce exaggerated or unpleasant sensations.

Hyperesthesia: a type of hypersensitivity characterized by heightened sensitivity to tactile stimuli.

Peripherally mediated sensation: is sensation controlled primarily by sensory receptors in the skin, such as light touch.

Quantitative sensory testing (QST): type of assessment; is the standardized application of a stimulus followed by an interpretation of the patient's response in quantitative measures, such as percentage of correct responses.

Sensibility: a person's sensitivity to sensory stimulation; considered a patient factor in occupational therapy.

Sensory reeducation: a type of sensory intervention in which therapists guide the process of reteaching the brain how to feel and interpret sensory stimulation.

Sensory Function in Daily Occupation

The ability to sense, feel, see, hear, taste, and process all that we daily encounter and experience is a remarkable function of our central nervous system. Occupational therapists frequently encounter individuals who exhibit sensory impairment due to injury or disease. For example, a person with diabetes can lose sensation in the hands and feet; older adults often experience primary sensory loss in the form of low vision, reduced hearing, and impaired balance; and a brachial plexus injury to an infant during childbirth can affect upper extremity (UE) function and sensation. Therefore, a comprehensive understanding of strategies for assessment and intervention is necessary. This chapter describes the neurological basis of sensation, discusses the functional impact of sensory dysfunction on occupational performance, and provides resources for occupational therapy evaluation and intervention. The chapter content focuses on both peripheral and centrally mediated sensory processes.

Sensory function, also known as **sensibility**, is subsumed under the client factor and body function categories in the Occupational Therapy Practice Framework.[1] Sensory dysfunction can influence other body processes, including joint and muscle movement as well as mental functions—all of which, when impaired, potentially disrupt a person's habits, routines, and roles. Challenges across all aspects of task performance in daily occupations, activities of daily living (ADLs), and instrumental activities of daily living (IADLs) will typically result.

Peripheral sensation includes touch and pressure awareness, temperature, pain, and two-point discrimination. For example, a person with carpal tunnel syndrome (CTS), in which the peripheral sensory processes are affected, commonly experiences sensory loss in the thumb and digits, impairing the ability to form and maintain functional grip and pinch patterns. Alternative grasp patterns that are weak and ineffective are usually employed, which can result in further injury. Sensory loss of this type in a carpenter with CTS would create safety concerns for grasping and manipulating tools. Following a wrist fracture, motor and sensory loss in the hand typically results, creating difficulty with in-hand manipulation of fine motor activities such as buttoning or writing.

Centrally mediated sensation, involving brain and spinal cord processes, has a varying presentation and usually involves loss of proprioception (position sense) and stereognosis (blinded object awareness), and may include diminished awareness of touch or pressure in the affected UE. A person who has experienced a stroke may exhibit inattention or unawareness of the affected UE due to cortical lesion disruption of motor and sensory processing. A person with this type of centrally mediated sensory loss may fail to position the arm safely away from walls and doorframes when navigating a wheelchair, or away from stove burners when performing a cooking activity. A young mother with a degenerative disease such as multiple sclerosis, experiencing pain, numbness, and hypersensitivity throughout the trunk and extremities would have difficulty caring for an infant or performing cooking activities.

A large-scale study indicated that 94% of older adults have age-related deficits in at least one of the five primary senses—audition, vision, olfaction, touch, and gustation—and that this dysfunction can be predictive of physical and mental decline and mortality.[2] Job settings, exposure to environmental toxins, and even drug interactions can deteriorate auditory function, leading to hearing loss. Additionally, inner ear pathology can result in vestibular difficulty and balance deficits creating fall risks, especially in older adults.[3] Although certain daily tasks are completed without vision—such as finding a key in a purse, retrieving coins from a pocket, or fastening a necklace—vision is a central sensation and the one most often used to compensate for other sensory deficits. In conditions such as diabetes, multiple sclerosis, and stroke, visual deficits are common and can profoundly impair navigation in crowded environments, or vending and automated bank teller machine use. Olfactory processes can also be impacted by disease or neurological conditions. Recent research suggests that olfactory loss can be a subclinical sign or predisposing factor for dementia,[4] Parkinson disease (PD),[5] and amyotrophic lateral sclerosis (ALS).[6] Similarly, gustation loss may occur in persons with chronic kidney disease[7] and in neurodegenerative diseases including PD and ALS.[8]

Haptic perception, or active touch, is one of the more critical senses needed for successful and safe performance of daily activities. Without the sense of touch, the amount of force needed to grip an object can be inadequate or inappropriate, resulting in objects being dropped or crushed; excessive grip forces can also create muscular fatigue in the hands from overactivity.[9] When grip force feedback is absent, individuals compensate with stronger grips that adversely influence object manipulation accuracy.[10]

Neurological and Physiological Basis of Sensory Function

The human sensory system operates through the skin, muscles, and joint receptors—each specialized to receive various types of stimulation, such as touch, temperature, or pain. Table 12-1 describes the ascending neural pathways of sensory stimuli received from the periphery that travel to the cortical sensorimotor area (located in the postcentral gyrus of the parietal lobe). There is redundancy in the sensory receptor system, because each sensory neuron, and the skin area it serves, overlaps with other sensory receptor areas. A single stimulus will, therefore, activate several adjacent sensory receptor

Table 12-1. Neural Pathways of Sensory Stimuli

TYPE OF SENSATION	SENSORY RECEPTOR	TYPE OF AFFERENT NEURON	PATHWAY	TERMINATION OF PATHWAY
Constant touch or pressure	Merkel's cell Ruffini's end organ	Type A-β slowly adapting I and II myelinated neurons	Ascend in dorsal column and medial lemniscus of the spinal cord in posterior pyramidal tract, cross to opposite side in medulla	Thalamus and somatosensory cortex
Moving touch or vibration	Meissner's corpuscles Pacinian corpuscles Hair follicles	Type A-β rapidly adapting I and II myelinated neurons		
Proprioception and kinesthesia	Same as both moving and constant touch or vibration plus touch receptors found in skin and joint structures	Same as for moving touch or vibration plus A-α myelinated neurons	Same as for moving touch or vibration plus spinocerebellar tract	Same as for moving touch or vibration plus cerebellum
	Muscle spindles			
	Golgi tendon organs			
Pain (pinprick)	Free nerve endings	Type A-δ myelinated neurons	Immediately cross to opposite side and pass upward in anterior spinothalamic tracts of spinal cord	Brainstem, thalamus, and somatosensory cortex
Pain (chronic)	Free nerve endings	Type C unmyelinated fibers		
Temperature	Free nerve endings Warm receptors Cold receptors	Type A-δ myelinated neurons and type C unmyelinated fibers		

Dellon AL. *Somatosensory Testing and Rehabilitation*. Baltimore, MD: The Institute for Peripheral Nerve Surgery; 2010; Chapman CE, Tremblay F, Ageranioti-Bélanger A. Role of primary somatosensory cortex in active and passive touch. In: Wing AM, Haggard P, Flanagan JR, eds. *Hand and Brain: The Neurophysiology and Psychology of Hand Movements*. San Diego, CA: Academic; 1996:329–347; Fredericks CM. Basic sensory mechanisms and the somatosensory system. In: Fredericks CM, Saladin LK, eds. *Pathophysiology of the Motor Systems: Principles and Clinical Presentations*. Philadelphia, PA: F. A. Davis; 1996.

fields. Innervation density refers to the number of sensory units (sensory neurons and terminations) within a given area. Areas with high innervation densities such as the face, hand, and fingers are more sensitive to incoming stimuli and have a proportionately larger representation in the somatosensory cortex.[11] Figure 12-1 shows the sensory homunculus, a representation of sensory receptors across the sensorimotor cortex.

The sensorimotor cortex (S1) receives incoming impulses from peripheral sensory receptors that transmit electrical impulses through a variety of neural tracts ascending to S1. These neural tracts create the connection from the external environment to our internal cortical awareness and response. In S1, impulses are decoded and processed, while additional neural transmissions occur to surrounding areas serving motor (behavioral response) and cognitive awareness (perception). For example, Meissner's corpuscles are among the most sensitive receptors with a very low threshold of response to light touch; these receptors are typically located in skin areas where awareness of light touch is paramount (e.g., fingertips, hands, lips).[12] The corpuscles activate C fibers from the periphery when very light touch is sensed, such as snowflakes falling on the skin or feathers brushed across the hand. The cell bodies of these fibers are located in the dorsal root ganglion positioned just outside the spinal cord. Impulses travel along afferent neural pathways of varying diameter and morphology: large-diameter, myelinated axons transmit peripheral impulses to the cortex more quickly; smaller-diameter unmyelinated afferents transmit less rapidly. These signals travel to the dorsal root ganglion at the cervical spinal cord level, synapse on interneurons in the white matter, and then cross midline into the dorsal horn, traveling cortically by route of the spinothalamic tract on the contralateral side. The spinothalamic tract carries the impulse through the medulla, pons, and midbrain, and finally through the thalamus to the sensorimotor cortex. From there, the appropriate response to the stimulus is generated through cognitive awareness and a motor response.[13]

Sensory receptors are responsive to varying types of incoming stimuli. Chemoreceptors respond to neurotransmitters or other chemical substances in the body and translate these into electrical signals that can be carried to the central nervous system for interpretation and

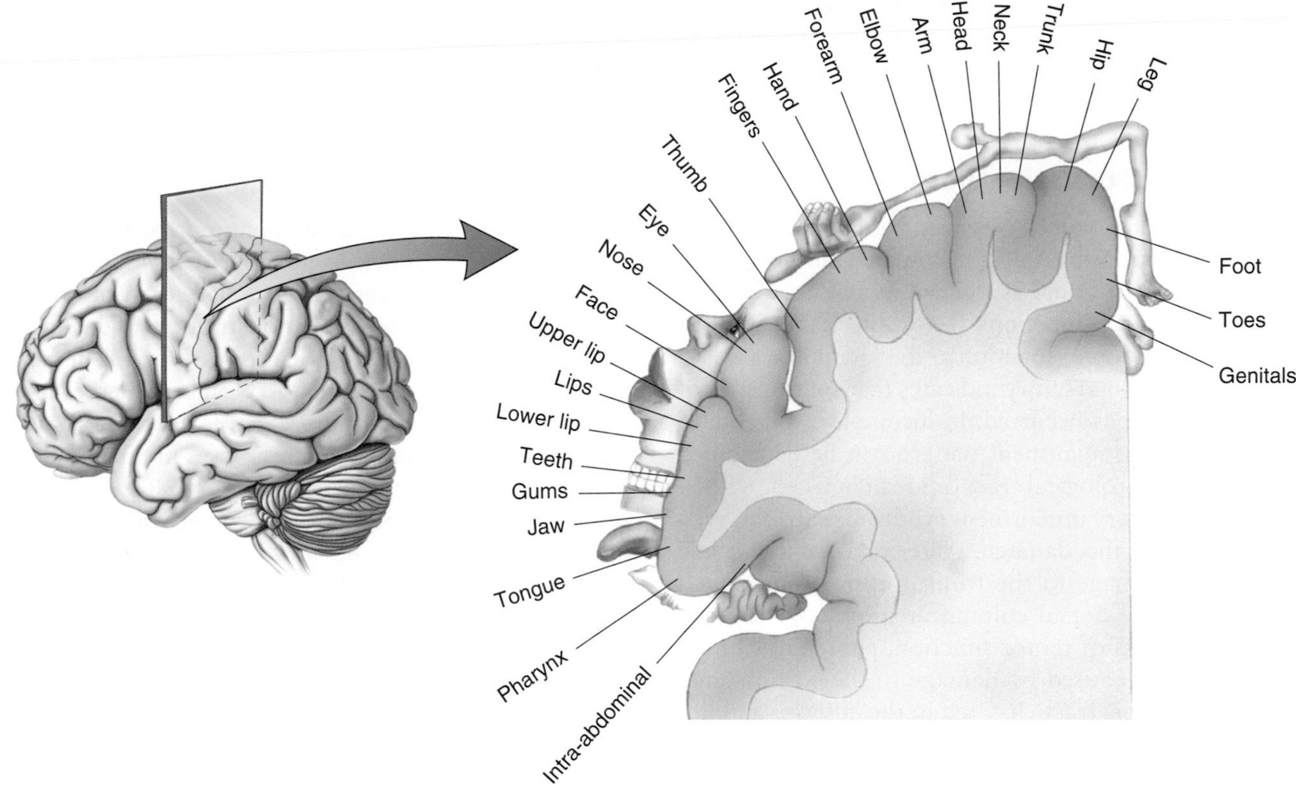

Figure 12-1. Sensory homunculus.

response. Chemoreceptors respond to chemical releases that occur when cells are damaged or during normal cellular processes, such as when tongue taste buds respond to ingested foods and liquids. Mechanoreceptors are activated with mechanical movement, such as when hair cells in the inner ear bend in response to sound waves. Nociceptors react to painful stimuli, and thermoreceptors detect changes in temperature.

Any interruption along the ascending sensory pathway or in the cortical sensory areas can lead to decreased or lost sensation. The extent and severity of sensory deficits can generally be predicted in accordance with the lesion or injury mechanism and location. Sensory impairment patterns are directly related to the involved neuroanatomical structures, which could be located anywhere in the central or peripheral nervous system. Somatosensory and perceptual impairments contribute to poor motor control and may impact a patient's rehabilitation participation.[14]

Despite neurological injury, the central nervous system can respond to damage or pathology through the process of neuroplasticity, whereby a reorganization of axonal and dendritic structure occurs, creating new avenues of transmission and communication. Research related to neuroplasticity in the cortex poststroke demonstrates that neurophysiological adaptations occur in both damaged and perilesional tissues and that behavioral and functional changes can result from targeted interventions.[15]

Impairment of Centrally Mediated Sensation

Cortical Impairment

Cerebrovascular accidents (CVAs) or strokes, acquired brain injuries, and other pathology affecting cortical structures can impair sensation. Rehabilitation efforts following stroke traditionally concentrate on motor deficits, with less attention to sensory impairment.[16] Strong associations have been found between sensory impairment poststroke and functional outcomes. Persons with significant sensory deficits, visual inattention, or neglect were found to have longer inpatient rehabilitation lengths of stay and decreased probabilities of returning home after discharge.[17] Although many clinicians report assessing sensory skills poststroke, assessment is often limited to light touch and proprioception and is not completed with standardized instruments.[18] Disruption of the anterior cerebral artery more commonly results in sensory loss in the contralateral leg than in the arm or face.[19] Lesions to the posterior thalamus can result in impaired cold and pain sensation, and in body orientation awareness deficits or "pusher" syndrome.[20] Sensory loss following stroke has been shown to reduce participation in desired activities.[21] For patients with brain injury, perception of fine touch and proprioception are most affected, temperature sensation is less affected, and pain sensibility is least affected.[22] Patterns of sensory loss following head injury are less predictable because of the more diffuse areas of brain damage associated with this condition.[23]

Impairment of the Spinal Cord

Spinal cord injuries can be classified by the American Spinal Injury Association (ASIA) as complete or incomplete. A complete spinal injury is defined as one in which all motor and sensory functions below the lesion are lost and no preservation of function at the sacral levels exists. An incomplete spinal injury indicates that some degree of sensory sparing has occurred. In incomplete spinal injuries, the sensory impairment pattern can be determined based on the neurological tract or area damaged.

Typical sensory impairment syndromes are observed with region-specific damage. Anterior cord syndrome results from damage to the front portion of the spinal cord, leaving the dorsal column area intact. There can be a variable loss of motor function, pain, and temperature sensation, caused by damage to the corticospinal and spinothalamic tracts located in the anterior and lateral cord aspects. Touch, vibration, and proprioception remain intact below the lesion due to dorsal column sparing. Likewise, injuries to the dorsal spinal cord area result in loss of touch, vibration, and proprioception, but pain and temperature remain mostly intact. Pathology or injury that impacts the central cord results in central cord syndrome, where pain and temperature below the lesion level are lost as these fibers pass through the center of the cord to the ipsilateral side upon entering. An asymmetric cord injury often produces a Brown-Séquard syndrome presentation involving loss of touch, vibration, and proprioception on the lesion side, and loss of pain and temperature on the side opposite to the lesion. This presentation occurs because pain and temperature fibers cross to the opposite side, whereas the dorsal columns ascend to the medulla oblongata in the brainstem before crossing to the opposite side.

Sensory recovery after spinal injury typically occurs within the first year, especially in the first 3 to 6 months for those with incomplete injuries.[24] The following sensory areas should be assessed in patients with spinal injury: pain, light touch, temperature, and vibration (see procedures in the "Sensory Evaluation" section). These results will inform the clinician about the patient's overall sensory awareness and assist in determining precise spinal-level function. Following incomplete spinal injury, return of sensation is dependent on several factors; however, two-thirds of individuals with sensory sparing and responsiveness to pain and pinprick in the lower extremities (LEs) following cervical injury were ambulating after a year, but less than 15% of those who showed responsiveness to light touch in the LEs regained ambulatory skills.[25] The ASIA motor scores for the quadriceps and gastrocnemius/soleus muscles, along with light touch scores for the L3 and S1 dermatomes, have been shown to accurately discriminate between potential walkers and nonwalkers after spinal injury.[26]

Impairment with Loss of Limb

Following loss of limb or amputation, cortical sensory maps have been shown to adapt and remodel.[27] Cortical somatosensory areas that lie adjacent to the cortical amputated sensory areas demonstrate remodeling and branching that can result in phantom sensations or pain.[28] Similarly, changes to the damaged peripheral nerve's axons and roots can be seen at the spinal level; these resultant changes alter pain and motor responses in the amputated limb. A common phenomenon after limb loss is phantom limb pain or phantom limb syndrome, which occurs in approximately 50% to 80% of individuals.[29] Symptoms can vary, but most individuals report pain in the removed limb area or a sensation of the limb's continued presence. Various interventions, including mirror therapy, transcutaneous electrical nerve stimulation (TENS), and graded motor imagery, have been proposed to relieve pain or decrease uncomfortable sensations; however, empirical evidence for intervention effectiveness is limited.[30]

Impairment of Peripheral Sensation

When peripheral nerves are damaged, symptoms correspond to the area of neural distribution, or dermatome. Impairment of a single spinal cord nerve root will impact sensation on the ipsilateral side of the body over the corresponding area served by that nerve root (Fig. 12-2, dermatomal distributions). For example, in CTS, compression of the median nerve within the carpal tunnel produces numbness and tingling in the thumb, index, middle, and half of the ring finger, following the median nerve distribution. Light touch, vibration, and two-point discrimination can also be impaired in CTS.[31] If nerve compression continues, hand function—particularly grasp and dexterity—can become impaired, and permanent sensory loss can occur. Both conservative intervention and surgery, however, can provide benefit and relief.[32] Typical conservative intervention for CTS includes splinting the wrist in a neutral position or 15° of extension to decompress the median nerve. Patients are usually advised to wear the splint at night to eliminate typical nocturnal numbness and tingling, but splints can also be worn during daily activities to prevent additional pain. Conservative treatment also includes patient education to avoid activities that exacerbate pain and to reduce repetitive movements that can inflame the median nerve, such as prolonged periods of wrist flexion. Sensory recovery and return to normal activity is typical if nerve compression is brief and relieved through conservative or surgical means.

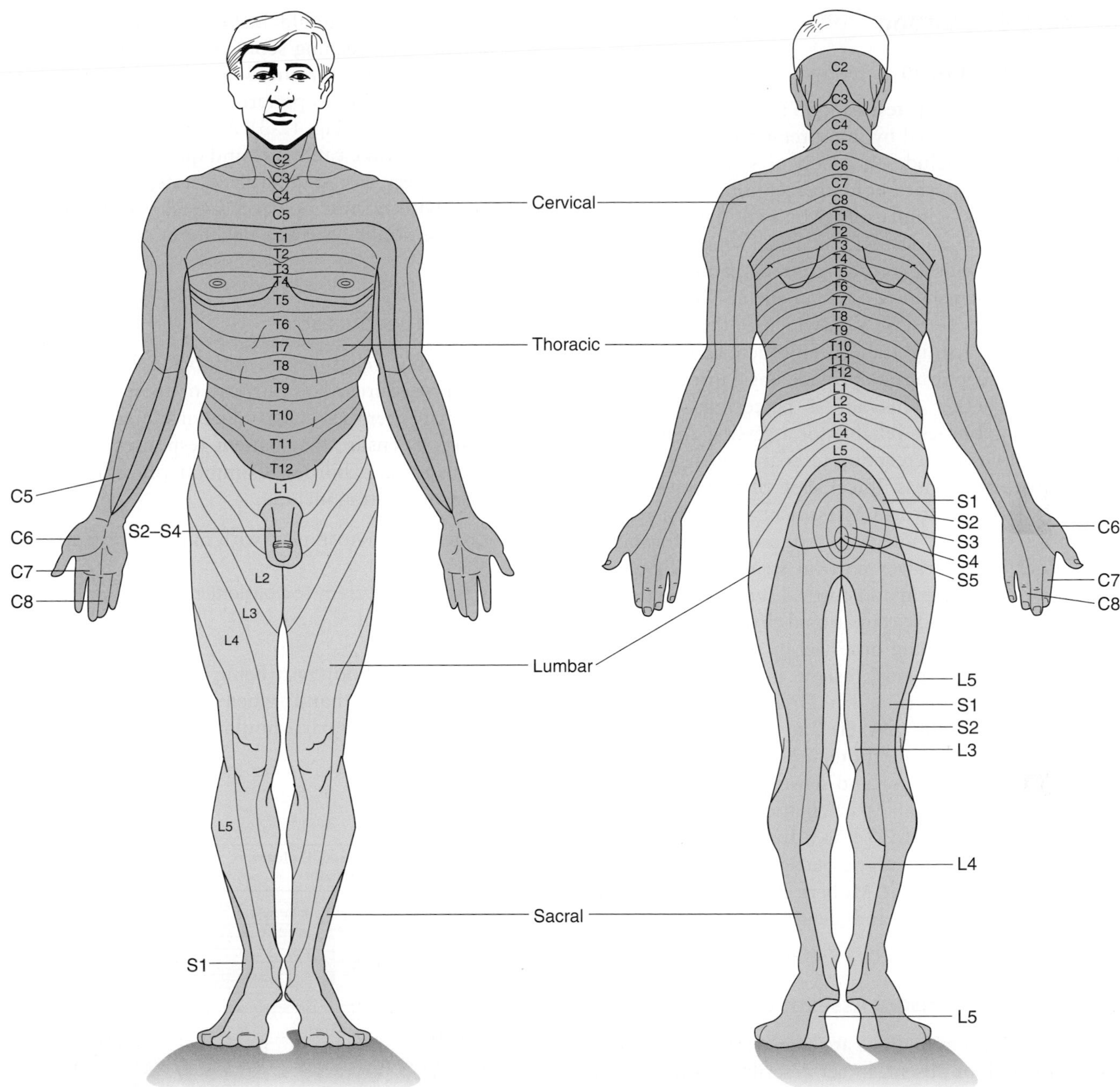

Figure 12-2. Dermatomes.

A peripheral nerve that has been completely transected has the capacity to regrow and reinnervate with surgical intervention. Typical regrowth rates average approximately 1.08 mm per day for pain fibers and 0.78 mm per day for touch fibers.[33] Sensory return typically follows a specific sequence, in which pain and temperature occur first, followed by moving touch sensation, light touch, and, finally, touch localization.[34] In chronic conditions such as diabetes mellitus, chronic regional pain syndrome, acquired immunodeficiency syndrome (AIDS), alcoholism, and smoking, peripheral nerve conduction and sensory responsivity can be impacted. A common glove and stocking distribution can occur, whereby sensation gradually diminishes in the feet and hands and spreads proximally, causing pain and increased mortality.[35] Sensory loss can also occur in conjunction with orthopedic fractures or traumatic crush/avulsion injuries and in patients receiving certain types of chemotherapy for cancer treatment.

Assessment of peripheral nerve injury should always prioritize delineation of protective sensation to insure patient safety and prevent further injury. Clinicians should strive to create an accurate map of intact and impaired sensory areas using the sensory evaluation techniques that follow.

Sensory Evaluation

Types of Evaluation

Quantitative sensory testing (QST) is the application of a stimulus followed by interpretation of the patient's response. QST includes a group of sensory tests that examine minimal threshold, perception, and integration of sensory stimulation. Minimal threshold tests can detect the smallest point at which sensation can be perceived. The most clinically utilized example of this is the Semmes-Weinstein Monofilament or Weinstein Enhanced Sensory Test (WEST), which both detect minimal thresholds for light and deep touch, and protective sensation. Perception tests provide basic information to determine whether sensation is perceived—important for screening, but less reliable for assessing change over time. Examples of perception tests are touch, pain, and temperature awareness. Integration of sensory stimulation is examined through assessments that first require perception and then integration of sensory information with other peripheral or cortical structures. Examples include proprioception and cortical sensory function.

Also available to occupational therapists are standardized tests examining observed or self-reported hand function, which provide insight into combined motor and sensory function. The Disabilities of the Arm, Shoulder, and Hand (DASH) and Quick DASH Outcome Measures are questionnaires designed to examine changes in UE motor and sensory function through self-reported activity and participation.[36] The Hand Active Sensation Test (HASTe) is a functional instrument designed to assess the haptic perception of people who sustained a stroke.[37] The Moberg Pick-up Test involves the picking up, holding, and identification of day-to-day objects.[38,39]

Documenting Sensory Assessment Results

Sensory evaluation findings are often summarized as intact, impaired, or absent. Intact describes normal sensation. Sensation is impaired when the patient is able to detect some but not all of the stimuli, or when perception of the stimulus differs from that of an intact skin area. Absent describes a total loss of sensation or inability to detect a specific sensory modality.

Unless otherwise indicated, the screening score is the number of correct responses divided by the number of applied stimuli. The expected score is 100%. When applicable, impairment should be recorded by peripheral nerve distribution, or dermatome, as relevant to the diagnosis. If a screening indicates impairment, the therapist may perform or recommend further testing. For both standardized and nonstandardized tests, results from the patient's affected area can be compared with results from the corresponding, contralateral unaffected area to determine the individual's "norms."

Documentation should include the test type, skin area tested, and screening score response. An easy way to document touch threshold testing with monofilaments is to use color or pattern codes on a drawing of the body part tested (Fig. 12-3). A series of sensory maps completed over time can easily and quickly demonstrate sensory recovery. For standardized tests, results can be compared with norms; however, age should be considered because studies show a decline in sensation with age.[40,41]

Common Procedures

Sensory testing reliability is optimized by following common procedures. The purpose of these procedures is to eliminate therapist cues and environmental/sensory distractions to ensure that patient responses accurately reflect sensory capabilities. Common procedures used across sensory testing include:

1. Choosing an environment with minimal distractions.
2. Developing a system for patient response, either verbal or nonverbal.
3. Stabilizing the body part being tested on a towel or in the therapist's hand (when pushed down with a stimulus, the body part should not move).

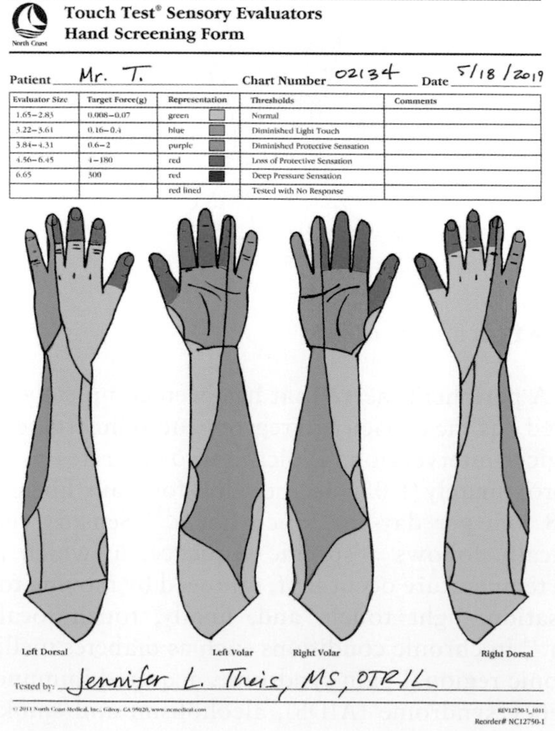

North Coast

Touch Test® Sensory Evaluators
Hand Screening Form

Patient Mr. T. Chart Number 02134 Date 5/18/2019

Evaluator Size	Target Force(g)	Representation	Thresholds	Comments
1.65–2.83	0.008–0.07	green	Normal	
3.22–3.61	0.16–0.4	blue	Diminished Light Touch	
3.84–4.31	0.6–2	purple	Diminished Protective Sensation	
4.56–6.45	4–180	red	Loss of Protective Sensation	
6.65	300	red	Deep Pressure Sensation	
		red lined	Tested with No Response	

Tested by: Jennifer L. Theis, MS, OTR/L

© 2011 North Coast Medical, Inc., Gilroy, CA 95020, www.ncmedical.com

REV12750-1_1011
Reorder# NC12750-1

Figure 12-3. Documentation of touch threshold with color or pattern code.

4. Noting differences in skin callouses on areas being tested, which can cause decreased sensation.

5. Demonstrating the test on the unaffected limb to ensure understanding of directions and elicitation of the correct response.

6. Occluding patient vision either by having patients close their eyes or hold a file to block vision.

7. Applying stimuli at uneven intervals or inserting times when no stimulus is given.

8. Avoiding giving inadvertent cues, such as auditory, visual, or facial cues.

9. Carefully observing the correctness, confidence, and promptness of each response.

10. Observing the patient for any discomfort relating to the stimuli that may signal hypersensitivity (exaggerated or unpleasant sensation).[34,42]

Nonstandardized Assessment: Quantitative Sensory Testing and Skilled Observation within Occupational Performance

Occupational therapists screen sensory skills to consider how sensory absence or impairment impact occupational performance. Screening may occur as part of a typical evaluation. Alternatively, skilled observations during occupational performance may lead therapists to suspect sensory function problems that warrant structured screenings. This section provides an explanation of sensory skills, skilled observations that demonstrate the need to screen, and full screening procedures. An example of moving into a two-story apartment will be used throughout to illustrate how sensory skills support occupational performance.

Exteroceptive Sensation

Exteroceptive sensation, or *superficial sensation,* is perceived locally by sensory receptors in the skin and mucous membranes and consists of touch, pain, and temperature awareness.

Touch Awareness (the ability to feel light and deep touch input)

1. Specific screening instructions:
   - Gather testing instruments needed for the assessment. For touch awareness, use common items such as a cotton ball, fingertip, and pencil eraser.
   - Direct the patient to respond "yes" or make an agreed-upon nonverbal signal each time the patient feels the stimulus.
   - Next, have the patient close the eyes and apply an object lightly to the skin; wait for his or her response (Fig. 12-4 and Video 12-1).

2. Examples of skilled observations indicating dysfunction in daily occupations:
   - The therapist may observe examples of touch impairment such as difficultly feeling a button when dressing or being unaware that one's arm is stuck in the hospital bed rail.
3. How light/deep touch support occupational performance:
   - Light and deep touch are used to appreciate the weight and pressure of a box. People use touch awareness, with other senses, to gauge the amount of force needed to pick up a box.

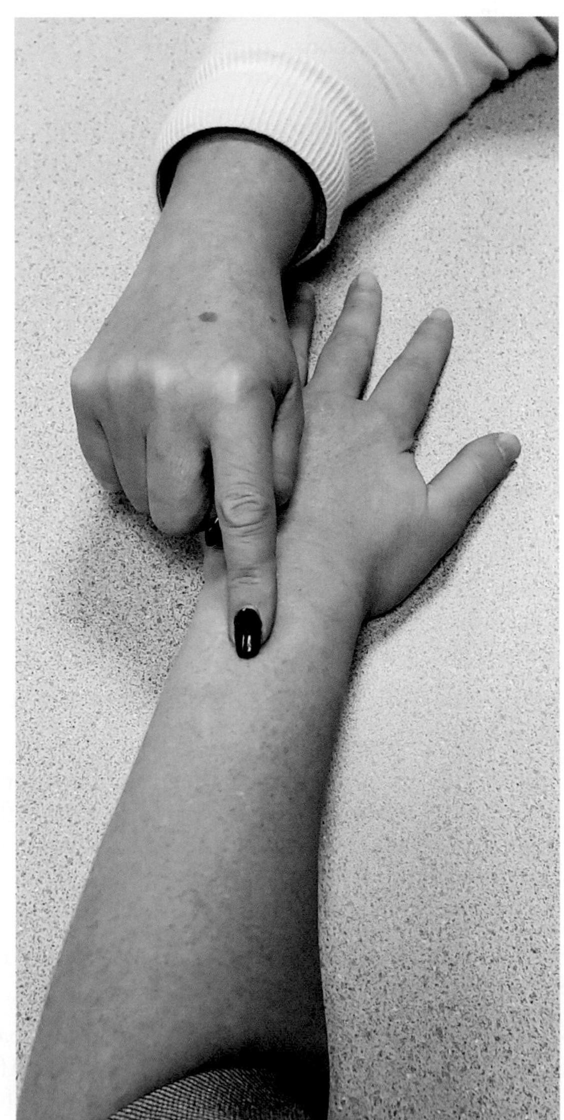

Figure 12-4. Screening for touch awareness.

Pain Awareness (the ability to feel topical pain)

1. Specific screening instructions:
   - All testing instruments needed for the assessment. An object with a sharp and dull side, such as a safety pin, works well for screening.
   - Direct the patient to respond "sharp" or "dull" after each stimulus.
   - Next, have the patient close the eyes and then randomly apply sharp and blunt safety pin ends, perpendicular to the skin, at the pressure that was necessary to elicit a correct response on the uninvolved body side. The therapist should allow adequate time for a response (Video 12-2).
2. Examples of skilled observations indicating dysfunction in daily occupations:
   - The therapist observes impairment in pain awareness when the patient is unable to feel a sharp knife blade as it slices the skin while cutting vegetables, or shows no response to the skin being pinched during activity.
3. How pain awareness supports occupational performance:
   - While moving to an apartment, pain awareness alerts a person carrying a box that it has a sharp corner, causing the person to shift the box and avoid skin injury.

Temperature Awareness (the ability to feel warm and cool temperatures)

1. Specific screening instructions:
   - First, gather a specific hot and cold discrimination kit or glass test tubes filled with warm (115°F–120°F) and cool (40°F) water.
   - Direct the patient to respond "hot" or "cold" after each stimulus.
   - Alternate applying hot and cold to the patient's skin and wait for a response (Video 12-3).
2. Skilled observations indicating dysfunction in daily occupations:
   - The therapist observes impairment in temperature awareness when the patient has difficulty differentiating water temperature for a shower or understanding that his or her hand is close to a hot stove burner.
3. How temperature awareness supports occupational performance:
   - After a long day of moving furniture to an apartment, the mover decides to take a shower. After running the water, he checks it with his hand before getting in, perceives that it is too hot, and lowers the temperature to avoid scalding.

Proprioceptive Sensation

Proprioceptive sensation, or deep sensation, is perceived locally in the muscles, tendons, ligaments, and joint structures and consists of joint position, movement, and vibration awareness.

Joint Position Awareness (the ability to understand joint position with vision occluded)

1. Specific screening instructions:
   - Hold the patient's body segment (e.g., arm, elbow, wrist, hand, fingers) on the lateral surface and move the part into different positions; follow by holding the position. If the patient can maintain the position, remove your support. If the patient cannot maintain the position, hold the position for the patient to complete the next step.
   - Ask the patient to mirror the position with the opposite extremity (Video 12-4).

2. Example of skilled observation indicating dysfunction in daily occupations:
   - The therapist may observe impaired joint awareness when the patient bumps his feet and legs on the bathtub wall while transferring out the tub. The patient with impaired or absent joint awareness is at risk for falls.[43]
3. How proprioception supports occupational performance:
   - The mover in our scenario is walking through a tight doorway with a box. Because of proprioception, he knows where his hands are placed on the box and visually checks to make sure that he can clear the door opening to avoid skin injury.

Movement Awareness (kinesthesia; the ability to sense the direction of joint motion, e.g., up, down, left, right)

1. Specific screening instructions:
   - Hold the patient's body segment (e.g., arm, elbow, wrist, hand, fingers) on the lateral surface and move the part into different positions; follow by holding the position. If the patient can maintain the position, remove your support. If the patient cannot maintain the position, hold the position for the patient to complete the next step.
   - Ask the patient to report whether the body part is moved up, down, left, or right (Video 12-5).

2. Examples of skilled observations indicating dysfunction in daily occupations:
   - The therapist may observe impairment in kinesthesia when the patient has difficulty recognizing whether he or she is moving in the correct direction. For

example, the therapist asks a patient to reach down to put socks on and the patient does not reach far enough or reaches up when he needs to reach down.

3. How kinesthesia supports occupational performance:
   - A mover walks upstairs with a heavy box and partially lands on the next step. His hips and knees perceive his center of gravity moving backward and self-corrects forward in part due to kinesthesia.

Vibration Awareness (the ability to feel different ranges of vibration)

1. Specific screening instructions:
   - Gather two tuning forks, one which vibrates at 30 cycles per second and the other at 256 cycles per second.
   - Ask the patient to close the eyes and then strike the tuning fork against your hand with enough force to cause vibration.
   - Place the prong tangentially to the fingertip of the affected and then unaffected hand and ask the patient, "Does this feel the same or different?"
   - Scoring is normal if stimuli to both hands feel the same and altered if stimuli feel different. The 30 cycles per second tuning fork is used to test the Meissner afferents, and the 256 cycles per second tuning fork is used to test the Pacinian afferents (Fig. 12-5 and Video 12-6).
2. Examples of skilled observations indicating dysfunction in daily occupations:
   - The therapist may observe impairment in vibration awareness if a patient has difficulty sensing a

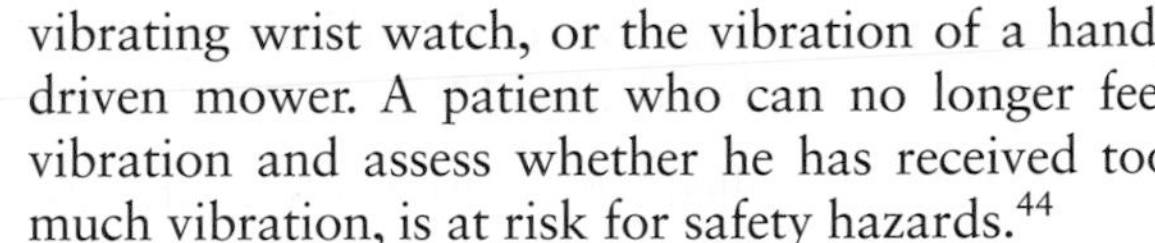

vibrating wrist watch, or the vibration of a hand-driven mower. A patient who can no longer feel vibration and assess whether he has received too much vibration, is at risk for safety hazards.[44]

3. How vibration awareness supports occupational performance:
   - A mover accidentally packed his cell phone, which is on vibration mode, in one of three boxes. He has his friend call his number and locates the phone by feeling the boxes through vibration awareness.

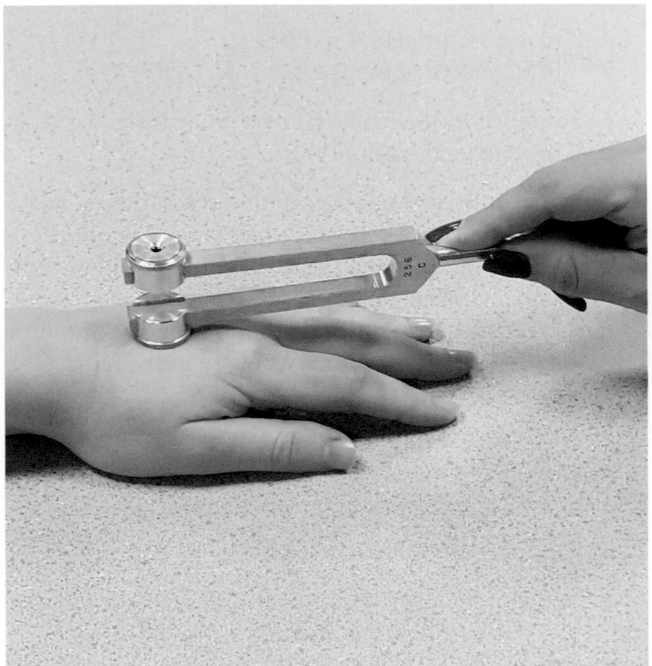

Figure 12-5. Screening for vibration awareness.

Cortical Sensory Function

Cortical sensory function requires the parietal lobe to discriminate between different stimuli provided through individual sensory inputs (e.g., touch).

Stereognosis (blinded object awareness; the ability to discern an object without looking at it)

The absence of stereognosis is called *astereognosis*.

1. Specific screening instructions:
   - Gather commonly used objects such as a quarter, pen, and a safety pin. Show the objects to the patient before testing.
   - With the patient's vision occluded, place an object in the hand to be tested.
   - Ask the patient to manipulate the item in the hand and name the object (Video 12-7).

2. Example of skilled observation indicating dysfunction in daily occupations:
   - A therapist may observe impairment in stereognosis when a patient has difficulty finding an object at the bottom of a purse or backpack when not looking directly into the bag.
3. How stereognosis supports occupational performance:
   - At the end of the move, the mover asks the patron to sign a billing statement. The mover reaches into his backpack and tries to locate a pen by feel through stereognosis.

Graphesthesia (ability to recognize symbols written on the skin)

The absence of graphesthesia is called *graphanesthesia*.

1. Specific screening instructions:
   - Gather a blunt object such as an eraser on a pencil or tongue depressor.
   - Instruct the patient that you will draw a number or letter on the patient's palm and will disclose the number or letter orientation. For example, "The number will be right side up," in accordance with the patient's orientation.
   - With the patient's vision occluded, draw the numbers or letters on the hand to be tested.

- Give the patient two trials to identify the correct letter or number (Video 12-8).

2. Example of skilled observation indicating dysfunction in daily occupations:
   - Graphesthesia is difficult to tie to specific foundations for occupational performance and appears to be important diagnostically. Impairments in graphesthesia indicate parietal lobe damage opposite of the hand being tested and has been hypothesized to be an early indicator of Alzheimer disease.[45]

Two-Point Discrimination (ability to recognize simultaneous stimulation by two different points either statically or dynamically)

Testing is most reliable on the fingers and hand.

STATIC TWO-POINT DISCRIMINATION

1. Specific screening instructions:
   - Gather the Disk-Criminator or Aesthesiometer.
   - Testing begins with a 5-mm separation of points. Lightly (just to the point of blanching) apply one or two points (randomly sequenced) in a transverse or longitudinal orientation on the hand.
   - Hold the pressure for at least 3 seconds or until the patient responds. Gradually adjust separation distance to find the least distance at which the patient can correctly perceive two points.
   - Direct the patient to respond by saying, "one," "two," or "I can't tell."
   - The final score is the smallest distance at which the perception of one or two points is better than chance. When the patient's responses become hesitant or inaccurate, require 2 of 3, 4 of 7, or 7 of 10 correct responses (Fig. 12-6 and Video 12-9).

2. Norms:
   - 3 to 5 mm on the fingertips for ages 18 to 70 years[46]; 5 to 6 mm on the fingertips for ages 70+.[40]
   - 5 to 9 mm on the middle and proximal phalanges in adults 18 to 60 years; 0 to 12 mm on the middle and proximal phalanges for ages 60+.[47]

DYNAMIC TWO-POINT DISCRIMINATION

1. Specific screening instructions:
   - Gather the Disk-Criminator or Aesthesiometer.
   - Testing begins with a 5 to 8 mm separation of points. Apply moving pressure of one or two points randomly from proximal to distal on the distal phalanx with points side-by-side and parallel to the long axis of the finger. Apply just enough pressure for the patient to appreciate the stimulus.
   - Hold the pressure for at least 3 seconds or until the patient responds. Then gradually adjust the separation distance to find the least distance at which the patient can correctly perceive two points.
   - Direct the patient to respond by saying, "one," "two," or "I can't tell."
   - The final score is the smallest distance at which perception of one or two points is better than chance. When the patient's responses become hesitant or inaccurate, require 2 of 3, 4 of 7, or 7 of 10 correct responses.

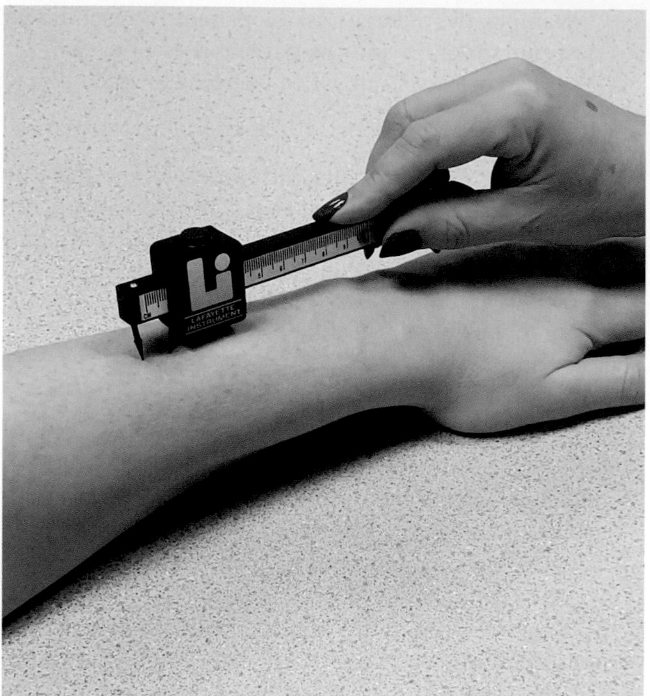

Figure 12-6. Screening for two-point discrimination.

2. Norms:
   - 2 to 4 mm for ages 4 to 60.[48]
   - 4 to 6 mm for ages 60+.[40,48]
3. Example of skilled observation indicating dysfunction in daily occupations:
   - Static and dynamic two-point discrimination are difficult to connect to specific foundations for occupational performance and appear to be important as a contributor to other sensory skills (e.g., localization and spatial discrimination) and to monitor the progression of neural recovery in the hand.[49]

Touch Localization (ability to localize where stimuli is "placed" on the body)

The absence of touch localization is topagnosia.

1. Specific screening instructions:
   - Gather a Semmes-Weinstein monofilament number 4.17, pen, or pencil eraser.
   - Apply touch to the patient's skin with vision occluded.

- Ask the patient to remember the stimulus location. With vision no longer occluded, instruct the patient to use the index finger to point to the spot just touched.
- The score is the measured distance in millimeters between stimulus and response locations.
- Normal response is approximately 3 to 4 mm on digit tips, 7 to 10 mm on palm, and 15 to 18 mm on forearm[50,51] (Fig. 12-7 and Video 12-10).

2. Examples of skilled observations indicating dysfunction:
   - A therapist may observe impairment in touch localization when a patient has difficulty understanding where his or her elbow grazed the wall when using a wheelchair.
3. How touch localization supports occupational performance:
   - While unpacking a box, a mover feels something crawling on his arm. He quickly swipes the area using touch localization.

Conceptual Foundation Underlying Intervention for Sensory Impairment

Choosing an Intervention Strategy

The selection of interventions for sensory impairment is based on diagnosis, prognosis, and evaluation findings. Diminished or lost protective sensation, the inability to feel pain in response to potentially damaging stimuli, suggests a need to teach patients and/or caregivers compensatory interventions to prevent injury. Findings of discomfort associated with touch (**hypersensitivity**) suggest a need for **desensitization intervention. Sensory reeducation** interventions (passive and active sensory training) are provided for patients who have some sensation and the potential for improved sensation or interpretation of sensory information. The following is a review of interventions designed to compensate for or improve sensory abilities.

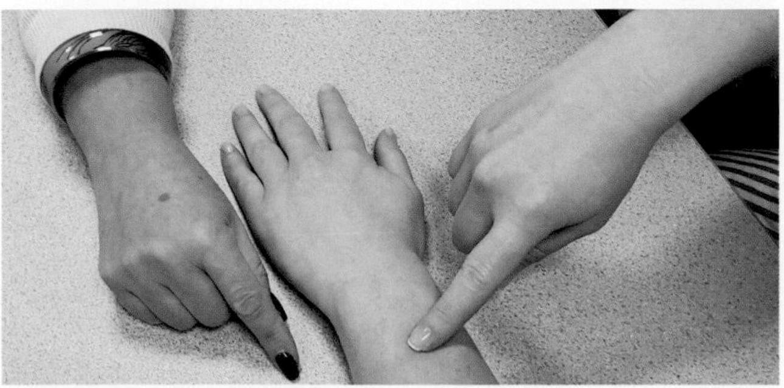

Figure 12-7. Screening for touch localization.

Compensatory Intervention

The primary goal of treatment for patients with diminished or absent protective sensation is to educate to avoid injury. Protective sensations are pain and temperature extremes that signal tissue damage threat. When the brain receives this message, the normal response is to move the body part away from the stimulus source. Without this message, tissue damage can quickly occur. Treatment consists of teaching the patient and/or the caregiver precautions necessary to prevent injury to any body part with compromised protective sensations.

The secondary goal of treatment is to teach the patient how to compensate for absent sensation. The therapist should teach the patient compensation strategies, such as (1) using vision to compensate for lack of sensation; (2) learning to use the sensate hand for tasks that require temperature or pain detection; (3) checking the insensate body part for abrasions, cuts, or burns; (4) wearing protective garments that prevent injury; and (5) modifying the task to avoid injury.

Desensitization Intervention

Desensitization is used when sensory evaluation reveals an area of hypersensitivity, in which ordinary stimuli produce exaggerated or unpleasant sensations.[52] Hypersensitivity includes **allodynia**, which is the perception of pain in response to a non-painful stimulus, and **hyperesthesia**, which is a heightened sensitivity to tactile stimuli. Desensitization intervention is designed to decrease discomfort associated with touch in the hypersensitive area. Desensitization programs generally include repetitive stimulation of the hypersensitive skin region with items that provide a variety of sensory experiences, such as textures ranging from soft to coarse.[53]

Sensory Reeducation Intervention

Because of recent research evidence regarding brain reorganization in response to lack of stimuli, repetitive stimuli, and problem-solving, sensory training currently consists of two approaches: passive sensory training and active sensory training. Sensory reeducation is an appropriate and commonly used treatment for a variety of peripheral nerve injuries, including nerve lacerations, and neural compressions and injuries, resulting in replantation, toe-to-thumb grafting, and skin grafting.[54] Sensory reeducation is also used for diminished or distorted sensation secondary to cerebral insults, such as stroke and traumatic brain injury. The techniques for both interventions are similar but different based on the nuances of retraining peripheral versus cortical structures.

Rationale for Sensory Reeducation after Peripheral or Cortical Injury

Hand representation in the somatosensory cortex has been found to reorganize as a result of peripheral nerve and cortical injuries.[54–56] In children, this reorganization is sufficient for return of normal sensory interpretation without sensory retraining. In adults, neural reorganization requires sensory reeducation.[54,57,58]

The return of sensation following hand injury or insult is a complex process. In peripheral nerve injuries, recovery involves both peripheral reinnervation and cortical somatosensory reorganization. Following nerve laceration and surgical repair, some sensory fibers, given sufficient time, regenerate. Peripheral nerves regenerate at a rate of 1 mm per day or 1 inch per month.[54] Sensory return is limited by scar tissue production along axonal sheaths and misdirection of growing fibers. Fibers usually do not regrow to innervate the same sensory receptors that they innervated preinjury.[57,59] This results in sensory coverage gaps in areas not fully reinnervated.

Conversely, peripheral nervous system structures, such as axons and sensory receptors, remain intact after cortical injury. Impaired neural structures lead to changes in the way the body appropriately interprets stimuli and withdrawals from danger. Lack of sensation, as in peripheral nerve injury, results in shrinkage of corresponding sensory homunculus regions. The return of sensation following cortical insult requires interventions that expand sensory cortical representation. Because sensation and motor use of the hand are highly correlated, functional use of the UE with reduced sensation is possible, but spontaneous use is limited. Without training, there is a tendency to refrain from using the extremity; learned nonuse leads to further loss of sensory and motor abilities and disrupted cortical representation.[60,61] Therapists may alter the cortical map by directing the sensory experiences of the patient.[62]

Sensory Reeducation Intervention Procedures

In the past, sensory reeducation was delayed until adequate sensation had returned.[63] However, in newer approaches, based on current knowledge of neuroplasticity, sensory reeducation is begun immediately through two sequential phases. Phase 1 (passive) focuses on maintaining sensory cortical representation by either providing directed sensory stimulation or by making the brain believe that no sensory changes have occurred.[57,63] Phase 2 (active) occurs when patients can appreciate some sensation and can learn to differentiate between sensation types. At first, in phase 2 of reeducation, patients learn to match their tactile perception of stimuli with their visual or auditory perception. Alternative senses, vision and hearing, are used to retrain sensation and improve tactile discrimination.[63] After time, when reinnervation allows for the perception of light nonmoving touch with good touch localization, the focus of intervention changes to more functional tasks, such as object identification through touch.[54]

Phase 1: Intervention

During phase 1, the formerly innervated body part is without sensation, and cortical representation undergoes rapid remodeling. The passive treatment techniques used in phase 1 are intended to maintain cortical hand representation.[63,64]

Mirror Visual Feedback Therapy

Mirror visual feedback (MVF) therapy was first proposed as a means to relieve amputee phantom limb pain in the 1990s. Therapists have increasingly used it to treat a range of other chronic pain conditions and as a means to reeducate sensorimotor abilities in patients with peripheral and central nerve injury.[65] MVF therapy is thought to work by improving sensory perception of the affected limb through false but congruent visual feedback of the unaffected limb, thereby restoring the normal sensory feedback–motor intention linkage. A mirror box is placed in front of the patient, and the sensory-deprived hand is hidden within it (Fig. 12-8). The reflection of the unaffected hand is visible in the mirror and appears as if it was the affected hand. Touching the unaffected hand provides the illusion that the affected hand has been touched. MVF protocols instruct the patient to (1) look at and perceive the reflected image to be the affected hand; (2) perform small then larger movements with the affected hand, and perceive the reflected image to be the affected hand; and (3) move both hands bilaterally while the affected hand remains occluded. Therapists can also address sensation by applying different textures to the unaffected hand as it is reflected in the mirror and by instructing the patient to perceive the sensation as if it was occurring to the affected hand. There is promising evidence that sensation improves through MVF protocols.[66]

Phase 2: Techniques

Active sensory reeducation is the process of involving patients in activities designed to facilitate detection of

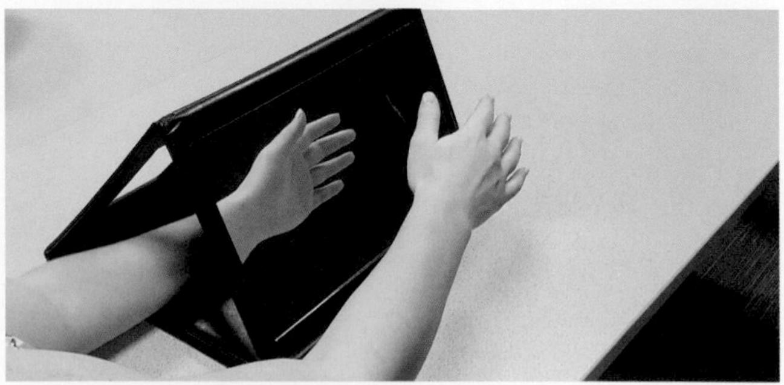

Figure 12-8. Mirror visual feedback therapy.

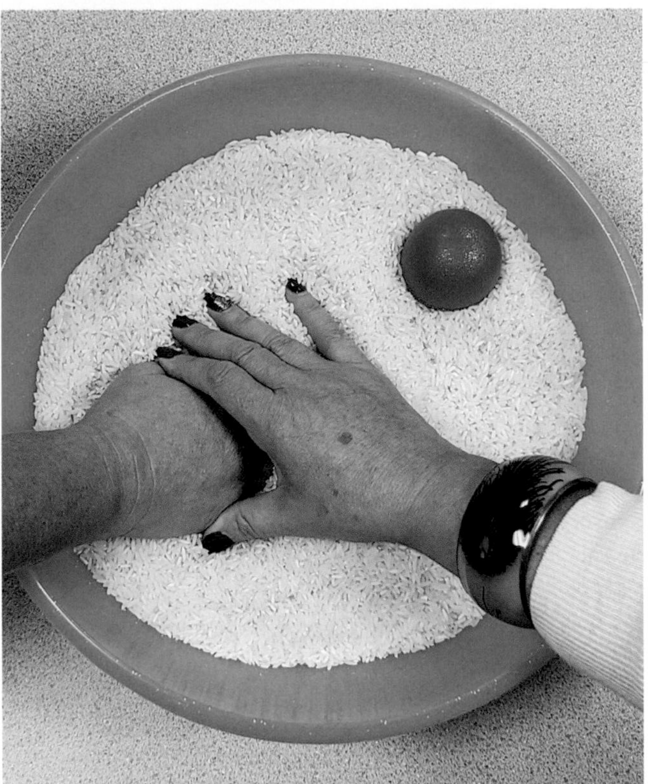

Figure 12-9. Active sensory reeducation. Patient feels for objects in containers filled with sand or rice.

and discrimination between sensory inputs.[54] The perception of moving touch is needed to begin phase 2, and steps occur sequentially after each preceding skill is achieved by the patient. First, the therapist develops a moving and constant touch sequence in which the patient must identify touch type with eyes closed, followed by eyes open, and concluding with eyes closed. Smaller and lighter stimuli should be used as the patient improves, with a goal of touch localization that is near the light touch threshold. Next, the therapist should present activities that force discrimination of similar and different textures using sandpaper, fabrics, and coin edges. The patient should touch various textures and discriminate between each, then advance to being touched by various textures, and finally identify each texture and area of localization. Progression in the active sensory reeducation sequence leads the patient to practice shape or letter block identification with vision occluded.

In later training stages, patients feel for objects buried in containers filled with sand or rice and identify objects by touch before using visual feedback (Fig. 12-9). Finally, patients practice daily living activities, particularly those in which the hand is visually occluded. A number of different active sensory reeducation protocols exist with varying levels of evidence (see the Evidence table at the end of this chapter).

Task-Specific Sensory Training

Sensory reeducation after CVA is less well defined than protocols described for peripheral injuries. Carr and Shepherd, in their book *Neurological Rehabilitation* (2010),[67] emphasize that task-specific sensory training should occur concurrently with motor learning. They advocate for the use of meaningful and relevant sensory and motor experiences very early in rehabilitation. Use of the more involved hand in bimanual tasks, such as opening jars and using eating utensils, is recommended. They suggest that patients be cued to attend to both task goals and object tactile qualities (e.g., weight, texture, slipperiness, temperature). Therapists should carefully structure therapy to include a variety of sensory inputs within occupational activities. For example, a therapist may ask a patient to remove items from the refrigerator having different tactile qualities, such as a stick of butter, a full milk gallon, and a jelly jar. Each object provides the opportunity for patients to express and feel differences across objects. Task-specific sensory training can be applied across varying occupations and contexts.

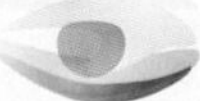

CASE STUDY

Patient Information

Dolores is a 55-year-old, left-handed African-American female admitted to an in-patient rehabilitation unit 3 days following right parietal lobe stroke. Past medical history includes right carpal tunnel surgery (1-year post) and hypertension.

Assessment Process and Results

Occupational Profile

Dolores has been married to her husband Ed for 30 years. They have two grown daughters who live close by. Their oldest daughter, Maya, has one son Alex who is 9. Dolores works as an elementary school teacher. Her work involves grading papers and standing at the front of the class to write on the board. She hopes to work until age 65. At home, Dolores is responsible for laundry, cleaning, and yard work and enjoys playing with Alex.

Occupational Performance

Objective Functional Independence Measure (FIM) Scores: Feeding, Dressing, Toileting, Grooming, and Bathing: (4/7) Minimal Assist/cues. Toilet, shower and bed transfers: (4/7) and Ambulation (4/7) with 4-point cane.

Subjective Report of Occupational Performance: The therapist used the Canadian Occupational Performance Measure (COPM) to identify Dolores' priority goals during rehabilitation and report her performance and satisfaction in each area.

(continued)

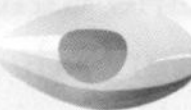

CASE STUDY *(continued)*

Top Priority Areas	Performance (1–10)	Satisfaction with Performance (1–10)
Write on dry-erase board with left hand	3	1
Play simple board games with grandson	4	1
Feed self without assistance	4	1
Complete full ADL routine prior to work	6	1

Patient Factor Screening and Assessments

Cognitive Screening: Scored 30/30 on the Montreal Cognitive Assessment indicating no signs of dementia or mild cognitive impairment. In ADLs, she can initiate, sustain, and complete tasks independently.

Psychosocial Screening: Scored 13/15 on the Geriatric Depression Scale (Short Form) indicating very few depressive symptoms.

Visual Perception Assessment: Dolores demonstrated below average abilities in visual perception using the Motor Free Visual Perception Test–Revised. Visual memory is a strength, and areas of concern include visual figure ground, closure, discrimination, and spatial relations.

Sensory Screening: Dolores demonstrated mild-moderate deficits in sensation as evidenced by the following sensory screening assessments.

Sensory Awareness	Norms	Results (R)	Results (L)	Observation during Occupation
Touch	Perceives 100% of stimuli correctly	80%	20%	Squeezing too hard or too little resulting in grasp difficulty; doesn't always feel object in hand such as fork, dry-erase marker.
Pain	Perceives 100% of stimuli correctly	80%	40%	Does not feel pain when hand/arm in compromised position
Temperature	Perceives 100% of stimuli correctly	80%	20%	Difficulty sensing difference in hot/cold water temps for shower
Joint position	Perceives 100% of stimuli correctly	100%	20%	Over and under reaches for objects; can visually correct if watching arm
Kinesthesia	Perceives 100% of stimuli correctly	100%	20%	
Stereognosis	Perceives 100% of stimuli correctly	80%	10%	Has to look for objects when reaching into her purse
Two-point discrimination	3–5 mm on the fingertips for ages 18–70 years; 5–6 mm on the fingertips for ages 70+	6 mm on fingertips	8 mm on fingertips	

Notes: Patient has history of right carpal tunnel release, which may explain mild impairment on unaffected right side.

Joint Range of Motion (ROM): Passive ROM is within normal limits in bilateral UE and LE.

Muscle Strength:

	Right (Unaffected Side)	Left (Affected Side and Dominant Hand)
Shoulder (all movements)	5/5	3−/5
Elbow flexion/extension	5/5	3−/5
Forearm pronation/supination	4/5	3−/5
Wrist flexion/extension	4/5	3−/5
Grip strength	Average of three trials: 56#	Average of three trials: 25#
Pinch	Tip: 8# Lateral: 10# Tripod: 11#	Tip: 2# Lateral: 5# Tripod: 5#

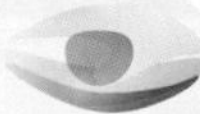

CASE STUDY *(continued)*

Occupational Therapy Strengths and Problems List

Strengths That Support Performance	Problems That Are Barriers to Performance
• Motivation for independence • Intact cognition • No signs of clinical depression • Supportive family system and personal resources	• Visual perception skills • Impairment in protective sensation • Impairment in sensory discrimination • Mild weakness in dominant UE • Mild balance deficits

Occupational Therapy Goal List

Occupational therapy goals were developed based on Dolores' priority areas determined through the COPM.

Long-Term Goals:

1. Dolores will complete ADLs with modified independence.
2. Dolores will perform activities that support the occupation of teaching with modified independence.

Short-Term Goals:

1. Dolores will complete her morning routine with SBA using modifications, adaptive equipment, and techniques.
2. Dolores will write on a dry-erase board in standing using her left hand/arm with SBA using modifications, adaptive equipment, and techniques.
3. Dolores will play Connect Four using her left hand with verbal cues on the use of sensory and visual compensatory techniques.

Intervention

Choice of intervention strategies included sensory interventions as part of a holistic treatment plan for Dolores after her stroke.

To address impairment in protective sensation, the therapist chose compensatory strategies. Using an educational approach, strategies were taught to protect Dolores' arm from harm. For example, when addressing showering, the therapist facilitated the integration of interventions such as checking water temperature with her right hand, improving shower transfers, visually locating the correct objects for washing hair, and scrubbing with the left hand.

To address impairments in interpretation of sensory stimulation, the therapist chose a sensory reeducation approach. In the passive phase of sensory reeducation, the therapist used MVF therapy to prevent loss of cortical sensory representation that also supported improvement in motor skills. In the active phase of sensory reeducation, the therapist began by addressing tactile discrimination. Preparatory methods and activities included identifying textures and shapes with the Dolores' eyes closed. Using an occupation-based intervention, the therapist addressed Dolores' ability to write on the dry-erase board by reaching for the dry-erase pen with vision occluded (as she might do when paying attention to students), standing at the board, encouraging use of the left hand and arm, and staying within dotted lines to write legibly.

These examples illustrate that sensory interventions can be delivered through preparatory methods, activities, and occupation-based practice. When appropriate for the level of recovery, embedding sensory interventions into occupation-based interventions provides patients with effective and personally meaningful care.

Most Commonly Used Standardized Assessment

Instrument Name	Intended Purpose	Administration Time	Validity	Reliability	Sensitivity	Strengths and Weaknesses
Semmes-Weinstein Monofilaments or Weinstein Enhanced Sensory Test (WEST)	Measure of threshold of light touch sensation[46]	Typically 10–15 minutes; may be variable depending on the extent of assessment needed	For construct validity, low correlation ($r = 0.17$) between pressure sensitivity and threshold	Inter-observer reliability—$ICC = 0.965$ (0.934)[72]	81%–82% sensitivity has been reported when filament 2.83 used as upper limit of normality[73]	Strengths: Inexpensive, easy to use, portable Weaknesses: Practice needed to administer effectively and interpret results
Modified Pick-Up Test[74]	Dellon's modification of the Moberg Pick-Up Test measures the interpretation of sensation in the distribution of the median nerve	Approximately 5–10 minutes	Discriminative validity between healthy and young, middle-aged, and elderly persons with CTS showed significant differences ($p = 0.06$, $p < 0.1$, and $p < 0.05$, respectively)	Test–retest reliability, 0.91 in patients with CTS; Inter-rater $p = 0.67$ for eyes open, 0.80 eyes closed[39]	No sensitivity data available	Strengths: Inexpensive, easy to use, portable Weaknesses: Ceiling effect, sensitivity may be limited
Erasmus MC–Revised Nottingham Sensory Assessment[75]	Quantitative functional measure of sensation after stroke. Sensations assessed include light touch, pinprick, pressure, two-point discrimination, and proprioception	10–15 minutes	No validity data available	Inter-tester reliability $k > 0.75$; Test–retest reliability, $k > 0.75$[75]	No sensitivity data available	Strengths: Establishes protocol/systematic procedure for tactile sensation measures; hierarchical Weaknesses: Administration time can vary
Fugl-Meyer Upper Extremity Sensory Subsection[76,77]	Assessment for persons with stroke; also measures motor function, balance, and joint movement	Approximately 30 minutes	Concurrent validity with Motor Assessment Scale ($r = 0.06$)	Inter-rater reliability ($r = 0.98$–0.99)	No sensitivity data available; however, responsiveness at 14–180 days (SRM = 0.67) and MDC at 90 days, 3.2 pts, have been reported	Strengths: Rates quality of specific movement patterns Weaknesses: Lengthy; Sensation subsection less suited for this instrument
Graded and Redefined Assessment of Strength, Sensibility and Prehension (GRASSP)[77,78]	Assessment for cervical tetraplegic population; also measures motor and prehensile skills	45 minutes	Concurrent validity with Spinal Cord Independence Measure sensation subtest (0.74)	Test/retest ($ICC = 0.86$–0.98); Inter-rater ($ICC = 0.84$–0.96)	No sensitivity data available	Strengths: Specific sensory testing for spinal injured Weaknesses: Length

CTS, carpal tunnel syndrome; DPN, diabetic peripheral neuropathy; ICC, intraclass correlation coefficient; MDC, minimal detectable change; SRM, standard response mean.

Evidence Table of Studies Supporting Interventions for Disorders of Sensation

Intervention	Intervention Description	Participants	Dosage	Research Design and Evidence Level	Benefit and Statistical Significance
Electrical stimulation[68]	Explored whether electrical stimulation (ES) improved peripheral nerve regeneration following nerve transection	Thirty-six patients following peripheral nerve transection	Fine wire electrodes were implanted following nerve transection surgery; patients randomized to receiving 1 hour of 20 Hz continuous ES or sham stimulation over 6 months	Level I: Randomized controlled trial	Patients receiving ES showed significant improvement in cold detection ($p < 0.001$) and tactile discrimination and pressure detection ($p < 0.001$); functional improvements were noted, but not significant. Subcutaneous ES delivered following peripheral nerve transection can improve sensibility.
Mirror therapy combined with TENS[69]	Investigated whether mirror therapy and TENS improved phantom limb pain (PLP)	Twenty-six participants with PLP	Patients with PLP randomized to either a mirror therapy group (Grp I) or TENS group (Grp II) for 4 days of treatment	Level I: Randomized controlled trial	Both groups showed significant decreases in pain on VAS (I—p = 0.003, II—$p = 0.003$) and UPS (I—$p = 0.001$, II—$p = 0.002$); no difference between groups. Mirror therapy and TENS can improve patient perceptions of PLP.
Perceptual learning-based sensory program[70]	Explored whether a perceptual learning-based sensory program was more effective than passive repeated sensory exposure for improving hand function after stroke	Fifty poststroke patients with UE sensory deficits	Two groups randomized to receive somatosensory discrimination program (SENSe) or repeated sensory exposure for ten 1-hour sessions; measured change in SSD index after intervention and at 6 weeks and 6 months	Level II Evidence: Two group randomized design with between-group comparisons	Significantly greater improvement in sensory capacity in sensory discrimination group ($p = 0.004$) with a mean change 11.1 SSD index; improvements maintained at 6-weeks and 6-months follow-up. Findings provide support for effectiveness of SENSe program for rehabilitation of sensory issues after stroke.
Self-massage and graded texture presentation[53]	Investigated whether self-massage and graded texture presentation was effective for reducing hypersensitivity after surgery	Thirty-nine patients after hand surgery	Patients experiencing pain in scar area from hand surgery massaged area 3×/day with textured material 2–5 minutes. Pain assessed with VAS; size of painful area measured in mm; OP measured with COPM	Level III: Single group, pretest–posttest design	Significant improvement in pain level, size of pain area, and higher OP scores on COPM after intervention. Further research with larger group needed to confirm findings.
Sensory reeducation training tool[71]	Studied whether hollow tubes made of various materials with 12 tactile stimulation elements of varying textures improved sensory deficits of the UE in persons with MS	Twenty-five persons with relapsing-remitting MS who report sensory deficits in UE	After a 7 week control baseline period, participants practiced with the tool for 20 minutes/day, 5 days/week for 3 weeks	Level III: Single group, pretest–posttest design	Participants demonstrated an improvement in the Nine-Hole Peg (26.8 vs 22.6 [SD = 3.2]); mean difference ($p = 0.03$) and functional dexterity tests (38.6 vs 33.8 [SD = 4.9]); mean difference ($p = 0.02$) at the end of the sensory reeducation phase. No differences were observed as to the monofilaments and two-point discrimination tests.

COPM, Canadian Occupational Performance Measure; ES, electrical stimulation; MS, multiple sclerosis; OP, occupational performance; PLP, phantom limb pain; SSD, somatosensory deficit index; TENS, transcutaneous electrical nerve stimulation; UE, upper extremity; UPS, universal pain score; VAS, visual analog scale.

References

1. American Occupational Therapy Association. Occupational therapy practice framework, 3rd ed. *Am J Occup Ther*. 2014;68:S1–S48.
2. Pinto JM, Wroblewski KE, Huisingh-Scheetz M, et al. Global sensory impairment predicts morbidity and mortality in older U.S. adults. *J Am Geriatr Soc*. 2017;65(12):2587–2595. doi:10.1111/jgs.15031.
3. Gauvin DV, Yoder JD, Tapp RL, Baird TJ. Small compartment toxicity: CN VIII and quality of life: hearing loss, tinnitus, and balance disorders. *Int J Toxicol*. 2017;36:8–20. doi:1091581816648905.
4. Adams DR, Kern DW, Wroblewski KE, McClintock MK, Dale W, Pinto JM. Olfactory dysfunction predicts subsequent dementia in older U.S. adults. *J Am Geriatr Soc*. 2018;66(1):140–144. doi:10.1111/jgs.15048.
5. Haehner A, Schopf V, Loureiro A, et al. Substantia nigra fractional anisotropy changes confirm the PD at-risk status of patients with idiopathic smell loss. *Parkinsonism Relat Disord*. 2018;50:113–116. doi:S1353-8020(18) 30076-2.
6. Gunther R, Schrempf W, Hahner A, et al. Impairment in respiratory function contributes to olfactory impairment in amyotrophic lateral sclerosis. *Front Neurol*. 2018;9:79. doi:10.3389/fneur.2018.00079.
7. Konstantinova D, Nenova-Nogalcheva A, Pancheva R, Alexandrova Y, Pechalova P. Taste disorders in patients with end-stage chronic kidney disease. *Italian J Nephrol*. 2017;34(3):54–60.
8. DeVere R. Disorders of taste and smell. *Continuum (Minneap Minn)*. 2017;23(2, Selected Topics in Outpatient Neurology):421–446. doi:10.1212/CON.0000000000000463.
9. Johansson RS. Sensory control of dexterous manipulation in humans. In: Wing AM, Haggard P, Flanagan JR, eds. *Hand and Brain: The Neurophysiology and Psychology of Hand Movements*. San Diego, CA: Academic; 1996.
10. Gibo TL, Bastian AJ, Okamura AM. Grip force control during virtual object interaction: effect of force feedback, accuracy demands, and training. *IEEE Trans Haptics*. 2014;7(1):37–47. doi:10.1109/TOH.2013.60.
11. Bear MF, Connors BW, Paradiso MA. *Neuroscience: Exploring the Brain*. Philadelphia, PA: Lippincott Williams & Wilkins; 2007.
12. Martini FH, Bartholomew EF. *Essentials of Anatomy and Physiology*. 6th ed. Washington, DC: Pearson Benjamin Cummings; 2013.
13. Swenson RH. *Review of Clinical and Functional Neuroscience*. Hanover, NH: Dartmouth Medical School; 2006.
14. Carr JH, Shepherd RB. *Neurological Rehabilitation: Optimizing Motor Performance*. 2nd ed. New York, NY: Churchill Livingstone; 2010.
15. Nudo RJ. Functional and structural plasticity in motor cortex: implications for stroke recovery. *Phys Med Rehabil Clin N Am*. 2003;14(1)(suppl):S57–S76. doi:S1047-9651(02)00054-2.
16. Kato H, Izumiyama M. Impaired motor control due to proprioceptive sensory loss in a patient with cerebral infarction localized to the postcentral gyrus. *J Rehabil Med*. 2015;47(2):187–190. doi:10.2340/16501977-1900.
17. Wee JY, Hopman WM. Stroke impairment predictors of discharge function, length of stay, and discharge destination in stroke rehabilitation. *Am J Phys Med Rehabil*. 2005;84(8):604–612.
18. Pumpa LU, Cahill LS, Carey LM. Somatosensory assessment and treatment after stroke: an evidence-practice gap. *Aust Occup Ther J*. 2015;62(2):93–104. doi:10.1111/1440-1630.12170.
19. Stein J, Brandstater M, Frontera W. *Delisa's Physical Medicine and Rehabilitation Medicine: Principles and Practice*. Philadelphia, PA: Lippincott Williams & Wilkins; 2010.
20. Karnath HO, Johannsen L, Broetz D, Kuker W. Posterior thalamic hemorrhage induces "pusher syndrome." *Neurology*. 2005;64(6):1014–1019. doi:10.1212/01.WNL.0000154527.72841.4A.
21. Carey LM, Matyas TA, Baum C. Effects of somatosensory impairment on participation after stroke. *Am J Occup Ther*. 2018;72(3):7203205100p1–7203205100p10. doi:10.5014/ajot.2018.025114.
22. Fredericks CM. Disorders of the peripheral nervous system: the peripheral neuropathies. In: Fredericks CM, Saladin LK, eds. *Pathophysiology of the Motor Systems: Principles and Clinical Presentations*. Philadelphia, PA: FA Davis; 1996:346–372.
23. Saladin LK. Traumatic brain injury. In: Fredericks CM, Saladin LK, eds. *Pathophysiology of the Motor Systems: Principles and Clinical Presentations*. Philadelphia, PA: FA Davis; 1996:467–485.
24. Kirshblum S, Millis S, McKinley W, Tulsky D. Late neurologic recovery after traumatic spinal cord injury. *Arch Phys Med Rehabil*. 2004;85(11):1811–1817. doi:10.1016/j.apmr.2004.03.015.
25. Craig Hospital. Incomplete spinal cord injuries: the early days. 2015. https://craighospital.org/uploads/Educational-PDFs/735.IncompleteEarlyDaysNOD.pdf.
26. van Middendorp JJ, Hosman AJF, Donders ART, et al. A clinical prediction rule for ambulation outcomes after traumatic spinal cord injury: a longitudinal cohort study. *Lancet*. 2011;377:1004–1010.
27. Yao J, Chen A, Kuiken T, Carmona C, Dewald J. Sensory cortical re-mapping following upper-limb amputation and subsequent targeted reinnervation: a case report. *Neuroimage Clin*. 2015;8:329–336. doi:10.1016/j.nicl.2015.01.010.
28. Limakatso K, Corten L, Parker R. The effects of graded motor imagery and its components on phantom limb pain and disability in upper and lower limb amputees: a systematic review protocol. *Syst Rev*. 2016;5(1):145. doi:10.1186/s13643-016-0322-5.
29. Richardson C, Kulkarni J. A review of the management of phantom limb pain: challenges and solutions. *J Pain Res*. 2017;10:1861–1870. doi:10.2147/JPR.S124664.
30. Barbin J, Seetha V, Casillas JM, Paysant J, Pérennou D. The effects of mirror therapy on pain and motor control of phantom limb in amputees: a systematic review. *Ann Phys Rehabil Med*. 2016;59(4):270–275. doi:10.1016/j.rehab.2016.04.001.
31. Tucker AT, White PD, Kosek E, et al. Comparison of vibration perception thresholds in individuals with diffuse upper limb pain and carpal tunnel syndrome. *Pain*. 2007;127(3):263–269. doi:10.1016/j.pain.2006.08.024.

32. Shi Q, Bobos P, Lalone EA, Warren L, MacDermid JC. Comparison of the short-term and long-term effects of surgery and nonsurgical intervention in treating carpal tunnel syndrome: a systematic review and meta-analysis. *Hand (N Y)*. 2018:1558944718787892. doi:10.1177/1558944718787892.
33. Waylett-Rendall J. Sensibility evaluation and rehabilitation. *Orthop Clin North Am*. 1988;19(1):43–56.
34. Callahan AD. Sensibility assessment for nerve lesions in-continuity and nerve lacerations. In: Mackin EJ, Callahan TM, Skirven LH, Osterman, AL, Hunter JM, eds. *Rehabilitation of the Hand and Upper Extremity*. 5th ed. St. Louis, MO: Mosby, Inc.; 2011.
35. Iqbal Z, Azmi S, Yadav R, et al. Diabetic peripheral neuropathy: epidemiology, diagnosis, and pharmacotherapy. *Clin Ther*. 2018;40(6):828–849. doi:10.1016/j.clinthera.2018.04.001.
36. Institute for Work & Health. The quick DASH outcome measure. www.dash.iwh.on.ca. Published 2006. Updated October 2, 2011. Accessed April 30, 2018.
37. Williams PS, Basso DM, Case-Smith J, Nichols-Larsen DS. Development of the hand active sensation test: reliability and validity. *Arch Phys Med Rehabil*. 2006;87(11):1471–1477. doi:10.1016/j.apmr.2006.08.019.
38. Amirjani N, Ashworth NL, Olson JL. Discriminative validity and test–retest reliability of the Dellon-modified Moberg pick-up test in carpal tunnel syndrome patients. *J Peripher Nerv Syst*. 2011;16:51–58.
39. Ng CL, Ho DD, Chow SP. The Moberg pickup test: results of testing with a standard protocol. *J Hand Ther*. 1999;12(4):309–312.
40. Desrosiers J, Hebert R, Bravo G, Dutil E. Hand sensibility of healthy older people. *J Am Geriatr Soc*. 1996;44(8):974–978.
41. Norman JF, Kappers AM, Beers AM, Scott AK, Norman HF, Koenderink JJ. Aging and the haptic perception of 3D surface shape. *Atten Percept Psychophys*. 2011;73(3):908–918. doi:10.3758/s13414-010-0053-y.
42. Reese NB. *Muscle and Sensory Testing*. 3rd ed. Philadelphia, PA: Saunders/Elsevier Health Sciences Division; 2011.
43. Ribeiro F, Oliveira J. Aging effects on joint proprioception: the role of physical activity in proprioception preservation. *Euro Rev Aging Phys Act*. 2007;4:71.
44. Buhaug K, Moen BE, Irgens A. Upper limb disability in Norwegian workers with hand-arm vibration syndrome. *J Occup Med Toxicol*. 2014;9:5.
45. McNamara D. Impaired graphesthesia may flag early Alzheimer's. *Intern Med News*. 2005;38(12):43.
46. Bell-Krotoski JA. Sensibility testing: history, instrumentation, and clinical procedures. In: Skirven TM, Osterman JM, Fedorczyk JM, Amadio PC, eds. *Rehabilitation of the Hand and Upper Extremity*. 6th ed. St. Louis, MO: Mosby; 2011.
47. Shimokata H, Kuzuya F. Two-point discrimination test of the skin as an index of sensory aging. *Gerontology*. 1995;41(5):267–272. doi:10.1159/000213693.
48. Dellon AL. *Somatosensory Testing and Rehabilitation*. Baltimore, MD: The Institute for Peripheral Nerve Surgery; 2010.
49. Won SY, Kim HK, Kim ME, Kim KS. Two-point discrimination values vary depending on test site, sex and test modality in the orofacial region: a preliminary study. *J Appl Oral Sci*. 2017;25(4):427–435. doi:10.1590/1678-7757-2016-0462.
50. Schady W. Locognosia: normal precision and changes after peripheral nerve injury. In: Boivie J, Hansson P, Lindblom U, eds. *Touch, Temperature, and Pain in Health and Disease: Mechanisms and Assessment*. Seattle, WA: IASP; 1994:143–150.
51. Sieg K, Williams, W. Preliminary report of a methodology for determining tactile location in adults. *Occup Ther J Res*. 1986;6:195–206.
52. Pillet J, Didierjean-Pillet A, Holcombe LK. Aesthetic hand prosthesis: its psychological and functional potential. In: Skirven TM, Osterman AL, Fedorczyk JM, Amadio PC, eds. *Rehabilitation of the Hand and Upper Extremity*. 6th ed. Philadelphia, PA: Mosby, Inc./Elsevier; 2010:1282–1292.
53. Göransson I, Cederlund R. A study of the effect of desensitization on hyperaesthesia in the hand and upper extremity after injury or surgery. *Hand Ther*. 2011;16:12–18.
54. Dellon AL. Diagnosis and treatment of ulnar nerve compression at the elbow. *Tech Hand Up Extrem Surg*. 2000;4(2):127–136.
55. Lundborg G, Rosen B. Hand function after nerve repair. *Acta Physiol (Oxf)*. 2007;189(2):207–217. doi:10.1111/j.1748-1716.2006.01653.x.
56. Merzenich MM, Jenkins WM. Reorganization of cortical representations of the hand following alterations of skin inputs induced by nerve injury, skin island transfers, and experience. *J Hand Ther*. 1993;6(2):89–104.
57. Rosén B, Lundborg G. Sensory reeducation. In: Skirven TM Osterman JM, Fedorczyk, JM Amadio PC, eds. *Rehabilitation of the Hand and Upper Extremity*. 6th ed. Philadelphia, PA: Mosby, Inc./Elsevier; 2010.
58. Rosén B, Lundborg G, Dahlin LB, Holmberg J, Karlson B. Nerve repair: correlation of restitution of functional sensibility with specific cognitive capacities. *J Hand Surg Br*. 1994;19(4):452–458.
59. Callahan AD. Methods of compensation and reeducation for sensory dysfunction. In: Hunter J, Scheider E, Mackin A, Callahan A, eds. *Rehabilitation of the Hand: Surgery and Therapy*. 4th ed. St. Louis, MO: Mosby, Inc; 2010.
60. Dannenbaum RM, Dykes RW. Sensory loss in the hand after sensory stroke: therapeutic rationale. *Arch Phys Med Rehabil*. 1988;69(10):833–839.
61. Sabari JS, Lieberman D. *Occupational Therapy Practice Guidelines for Adults with Stroke*. Bethesda, MD: American Occupational Therapy Association Press; 2008.
62. Nelles G, Spiekermann G, Jueptner M, et al. Reorganization of sensory and motor systems in hemiplegic stroke patients. a positron emission tomography study. *Stroke*. 1999;30(8):1510–1516.
63. Lundborg G, Bjorkman A, Rosen B. Enhanced sensory relearning after nerve repair by using repeated forearm anaesthesia: aspects on time dynamics of treatment. *Acta Neurochir Suppl*. 2007;100:121–126.
64. Rosen B, Vikstrom P, Turner S, et al. Enhanced early sensory outcome after nerve repair as a result of immediate post-operative re-learning: a randomized controlled trial. *J Hand Surg Eur Vol*. 2015;40:598–606. doi:10.1177/1753193414553163.

65. McCabe C. Mirror visual feedback therapy. A practical approach. *J Hand Ther*. 2011;24(2):170–178; quiz 179. doi:10.1016/j.jht.2010.08.003.
66. Wu CY, Huang PC, Chen YT, Lin KC, Yang HW. Effects of mirror therapy on motor and sensory recovery in chronic stroke: a randomized controlled trial. *Arch Phys Med Rehabil*. 2013;94(6):1023–1030. doi:10.1016/j.apmr.2013.02.007.
67. Carr J, Shepherd R. *Neurological Rehabilitation: Optimizing Motor Performance*. 2nd ed. Baltimore, MD: Churchill Livingstone; 2010.
68. Wong JN, Olson JL, Morhart MJ, Chan KM. Electrical stimulation enhances sensory recovery: a randomized controlled trial. *Ann Neurol*. 2015;77(6):996–1006. doi:10.1002/ana.24397.
69. Tilak M, Isaac SA, Fletcher J, et al. Mirror therapy and transcutaneous electrical nerve stimulation for management of phantom limb pain in amputees—a single blinded randomized controlled trial. *Physiother Res Int*. 2016;21(2):109–115. doi:10.1002/pri.1626.
70. Carey L, Macdonell R, Matyas TA. SENSe: Study of the Effectiveness of neurorehabilitation on sensation: a randomized controlled trial. *Neurorehabil Neural Repair*. 2011;25(4):304–313. doi:10.1177/1545968310397705.
71. Kalron A, Greenberg-Abrahami M, Gelav S, Achiron A. Effects of a new sensory re-education training tool on hand sensibility and manual dexterity in people with multiple sclerosis. *NeuroRehabilitation*. 2013;32(4):943–948. doi:10.3233/NRE-130917.
72. 72.Novak CB, Mackinnon SE, Kelly L. Correlation of two-point discrimination and hand function following median nerve injury. *Ann Plast Surg*. 1993;31(6):495–498.
73. MacDermid JC, Kramer JF, Roth JH. Decision making in detecting abnormal Semmes-Weinstein monofilament thresholds in carpal tunnel syndrome. *J Hand Ther*. 1994;7(3):158–162.
74. Dellon AL. A cause for optimism in diabetic neuropathy. *Ann Plast Surg*. 1988;20(2):103–105.
75. Stolk-Hornsveld F, Crow JL, Hendriks EP, van der Baan R, Harmeling-van der Wel BC. The Erasmus MC modifications to the (revised) Nottingham Sensory Assessment: a reliable somatosensory assessment measure for patients with intracranial disorders. *Clin Rehabil*. 2006;20(2):160–172.
76. Fugl-Meyer AR, Jaasko L, Leyman I, Olsson S, Steglind S. The post-stroke hemiplegic patient: a method for evaluation of physical performance. *Scand J Rehabil Med*. 1975;7(1):13–31.
77. Shirley Ryan Ability Lab. Rehabilitation measures database. https://www.sralab.org/rehabilitation-measures. Published 2018. Accessed September 17, 2018.
78. Kalsi-Ryan S, Beaton D, Curt A, et al. The graded redefined assessment of strength sensibility and prehension (GRASSP): reliability and validity. *J Neurotrauma*. 2012;29(5):905–914. doi:10.1089/neu.2010.1504.

Chapter 13

Motor Function Assessment: Range of Motion, Strength, and Endurance

Veronica T. Rowe and Tracey L. Zeiner

LEARNING OBJECTIVES

This chapter will allow the reader to:

1. Determine when evaluation of motion, strength, and endurance is appropriate and the best methods for obtaining such data.
2. Evaluate range of motion of the upper extremity using a goniometer.
3. Evaluate underlying causes of decreased motion and strength including edema, scar tissue, and pain.
4. Perform a manual muscle test to evaluate strength of the upper extremity.
5. Determine functional endurance level.
6. Interpret the findings of the evaluations described in this chapter.

CHAPTER OUTLINE

TERMINOLOGY

Cardiorespiratory endurance: the ability of the circulatory and respiratory system to supply oxygen during a time period while performing a task.

Dynamometer: a measure of applied force converted to a moment of force by multiplying by the perpendicular distance from the force to the axis of the lever.

End-feel: the resistance in the joint that the therapist feels at the end range of the passive limits of motion.

Goniometer: common instrument used for measuring limb joint motion, which has a protractor, an axis, and two arms.

Manual muscle testing: procedure for the evaluation of the strength of muscles depending on the performance of a movement in relation to the forces of gravity and manual resistance.

Maximum voluntary contraction (MVC): the greatest amount of tension a muscle can generate and hold only for a moment, such as in muscle testing.

Volumetric: measurement that documents changes in the mass of a body part by use of water displacement.

Within functional limits (WFL): represents capacities that may be less than normal limits, but sufficient for the client to participate in meaningful occupations to his or her own satisfaction.

Within normal limits (WNL): represents capacities that fall in the range of what has been determined to be normal depending on mean average ranges.

Functional Upper Extremity Screening

Depending on the reason for the referral to occupational therapy services, a preliminary screening of motion and functional strength may be more appropriate than an in-depth evaluation of individual measurements at each joint and muscle. It is often appropriate to screen some areas while taking formal measurements of others, which is why therapists will often begin with a functional screening. For example, a client may be referred to therapy following a distal radius fracture. When individuals have a cast on their wrist, they may lose motion at the shoulder and elbow as well because of nonuse and protective posturing. It would be appropriate to screen the shoulder and elbow and compare bilaterally to ensure motion is **within functional limits** (**WFL**) and then do specific range of motion (ROM) measurements at the wrist and hand. If deficits are noted during the screen at the shoulder or elbow, then it would also be appropriate to complete specific measurements of the joints where the limitations are noted.

Similarly, a gross screening of upper extremity (UE) strength may be more appropriate than testing individual muscles. This screening is often appropriate in inpatient and rehabilitation settings in which the client may be experiencing gross motor weakness from debilitation. During the screening, if the therapist determines any patterns such as weakness in one specific nerve distribution, he or she may wish to then do more specific **manual muscle testing** (**MMT**) of muscles innervated by that nerve.

The following instructions can be used as a functional screening of ROM and strength of the UE (see Video 13-1):

- The client should be seated, if possible.
- The client should perform the motions bilaterally, if possible. If not, the unimpaired or least impaired side should move first to set a baseline for normal for this person.
- Observe for complete movements, symmetry of movements, and timing of movements.
- Demonstrate the movements if the client has a language barrier or cognitive deficits.
- To estimate the amount of active movement and strength in the following motions, give instructions to the client, as shown in Box 13-1.

Box 13-1

Client Instructions for Functional Screening of ROM and Strength of Upper Extremity

- ***Shoulder flexion:*** Lift your arms straight up in front of you and reach toward the ceiling. Now, with your arms straight in front of you, do not let me push your arms down.
- ***Shoulder abduction:*** Move your arms out to the side. Now reach over your head. Next, with your arms straight out, do not let me push your arms down.
- ***Shoulder horizontal abduction and adduction:*** Raise your arms forward to shoulder height. Move each arm out to the side, and then back again while keeping your arm level. Push your arms against mine in both directions.
- ***External rotation:*** Touch the back of your head with your hand like you are washing your hair. Now push against me like you were going to throw a ball overhand.
- ***Internal rotation:*** Touch the small of your back with your hand like you are tucking in your shirt. Now push against my hand.
- ***Elbow flexion and extension:*** Start with your arms straight down by your sides. Now bend your elbows so your hands touch your shoulders. Push and pull against me starting with your arm flexed like you are making a muscle.
- ***Forearm supination and pronation:*** With your arms at your side and your elbows flexed to 90°, rotate your forearms so the palms of your hands face the floor and then the ceiling. Now, like we are shaking hands, resist my motion.
- ***Wrist flexion and extension:*** Move your wrists up and down. Now, resist my pressure.
- ***Finger flexion and extension:*** Make a fist, and then open your fingers. Squeeze my hands (ensure your hand is interlocked in the web space to avoid injury of your own hand).
- ***Finger opposition:*** Touch your thumb to the tip of each finger one at a time. Now, try to hold your thumb to your index finger and small finger without letting me break the circle.

Functional Lower Extremity Screening

Physical therapists typically complete any needed formal measurements of ROM and strength of the lower extremities (LEs). However, there is a role for occupational therapists in the functional assessment of the LEs insofar as they are commonly consulted regarding return to independence in activities of daily living (ADL) and instrumental activities of daily living (IADL) for clients with; for example, various orthopedic, neurological, and other debilitating conditions. In these cases, evaluation of LE function is typically done with the demonstration of ADL/IADL tasks and functional transfers. Occupational therapists are more interested in whether motion allows the individual to transfer to and from a toilet or complete dressing independently and safely, for example, rather than the exact degree of motion at the hip, knee, or ankle.

Instructions as outlined in Box 13-2 can be used as a functional screening of ROM and strength of the LE.

Impact of Motor Function on Occupational Performance

The assessments presented in this chapter are appropriate for clients who are unable to do or are restricted in doing the occupational tasks and activities important to them because of range of joint motion, strength, or endurance impairments. For the completion of most occupational tasks, it is essential to be able to move with adequate mobility and ROM, have enough strength to use extremities against resistance, and to be able to maintain

Box 13-2

Client Instructions for Functional Screening of ROM and Strength of Lower Extremity

- ***Hip:*** Show me how you would move from lying down to sitting on the edge of the bed.
  How would you get on and off the commode?
  Show me how you would get in and out of the tub.
  How would you get something from a bottom shelf?
- ***Knee:*** Show me how you would put on your socks.
  How would you get on and off the commode?
  How would you get something from a bottom shelf?
- ***Ankle:*** Show me how you will wash your feet.
  Show me how you would put on your socks.
- ***Functional transfers:*** Show me how you would get in and out of bed (assess bed mobility, supine to sit, sit to stand, stand to sit, and sit to supine).
  Show me how you would sit on the commode (assess stand to sit and sit to stand with toilet or bedside commode transfers).
  Show me how you will get in and out of the shower (assess shower bench or transfer bench or safety in getting in and out of tub or walk-in shower as appropriate to client).
  Show me how you will get in and out of the car (use real or simulated car).
  Show me how you will get up from this chair (cushioned seating vs. solid chair).

endurance for an extended period of time. For example, a person who cannot fully flex the elbow, is too weak to lift a spoon to the mouth, or is too fatigued to lift a utensil repeatedly cannot eat a meal independently. Because deficits in these abilities and capacities may lead to impaired occupational functioning, it is within the realm of occupational therapy to assess them. Keep in mind that occupational therapy assessments of mobility, strength, and endurance focus on how deficits in these areas impact occupational functioning. Occupational therapists also consider other variables in the overall evaluation, including environmental and contextual constraints that contribute to performance ability. The majority of this chapter focuses on evaluating limitations that impact UE function and occupational performance.

Additional underlying causes can affect motor function. These may include bony blocks to motion, capsular tightness around the joint, tightness of the muscle–tendon unit, edema, contractures, or extensive scar tissue. Changes in tone can also significantly limit motor function, especially ROM. Hypertonicity and hypotonicity from neurological impairments affect how one is able to complete a functional task. Distinguishing the difference in the effects of upper motor neurons and lower motor neurons is also important. Although insults to both types of neurons may affect ROM, muscle strength should be assessed appropriately with MMT for deficits from lower motor neuron injury, and tone should be assessed for deficits resulting from upper motor neuron injuries. A manual muscle test following an upper motor neuron insult would yield inconclusive results because of changes in tone, not necessarily in muscle strength. Therefore, MMT is inappropriate following a neurological event with resultant changes in tone.

Use of the assessments described in this chapter allows for the establishment of the client's baseline abilities. Reassessments at later dates allow documentation of progress or lack thereof as well as return to function **within normal limits** (WNL) or WFL. With the demands for efficiency in health care delivery, it is essential that occupational therapists be skilled in their evaluations of clients to justify continuation or discharge of therapy services.

Range of Motion Measurement

Measurement of joint range may be done actively or passively. Passive range of motion (PROM) is the amount of motion at a given joint when the joint is moved by an outside force. Typically, the outside force comes from the therapist or therapeutic equipment. Active range of motion (AROM) is the amount of motion at a given joint achieved when the client contracts the muscles that control the desired motion. Additional types of ROM include self-range of motion, where the client performs ROM on one side using the opposite side, and active assistive range of motion where the therapist, the client, or another caregiver may provide support during active motion to allow the client to move beyond the current AROM limits. These are not typically measured in an evaluation but may be used in treatment to improve deficits in ROM. It is normal to have slightly more PROM than AROM; however, if AROM is significantly less than PROM, there is a problem with how the underlying structures are functioning.

If limitations in AROM are observed, they are formally measured and documented. If there are no contraindications, the therapist then attempts to move the joint through its full PROM. If the joint is free to move to the end range, the problem is with active motion. If the end range cannot be attained when the therapist moves the limb, the problem is with passive motion, and the PROM limitation is measured and recorded.

Precautions to note in the evaluation of AROM and PROM:

- Carefully review consult/referral to therapy and note any contraindications to motion or restrictions in motion by the referring provider.
- Limited motion protocols may require that motion only be tested within the limits prescribed even if the client feels he or she can move beyond these limits. For example, following tendon repair, the surgeon may prescribe a limited arc of motion to avoid overstressing the repair during the healing process.
- Avoid pushing PROM when the underlying cause of the limitation is unknown, particularly with trauma.

- Avoid increasing edema or pain for the sake of a measurement. For example, immediately following casting, the therapist would expect tightness of the tissues that have been immobilized, and AROM measurements may be all that is needed to set baseline goals. It may be appropriate to try a heat modality (if edema does not contraindicate this) and then remeasure AROM to see whether increasing the extensibility of the soft tissues helps improve ROM.

End-Feel

When recording PROM, the therapist should also note any abnormal **end-feel**. Cyriax,[1] Kaltenborn,[2] and Paris[3] are three different classification systems of end-feel. All three require more research into the reliability of the classifications, but in general have found good intrarater and poor interrater reliability.[4,5] Commonly used terms for end-feel, mostly based on the Cyriax[1] and Kaltenborn[2] systems, include the following:

- ***Bone-to-bone hard end-feel*** is a stop in movement as the bony surfaces meet (normal for elbow and knee extension).
- ***Soft-tissue approximation*** is a stop in movement due to soft tissue (normal for elbow and knee flexion).
- ***Capsular end-feel*** is a movement that is somewhat firm or leathery but has some give (normal for shoulder external rotation and hip internal rotation).
- ***Spasm end-feel*** is a tissue response with a harsh movement in the opposite direction; passive movement stresses a fracture or inflamed joint (always abnormal).
- ***Springy end-feel*** is some hard rebound at the end ROM (always abnormal).
- ***Empty end-feel*** is no "feel," but rather the client asks to stop because of pain (always abnormal).

Although some of these may be a normal end-feel, it is important to note when they are abnormal. For example, a bony end-feel before full wrist extension may indicate underlying pathology, or a capsular end-feel during elbow extension when the elbow is at 30° may be the result of capsular tightness from immobilization. When pain occurs during PROM, the classification of end-feel is more difficult to determine.[5]

Goniometry

A **goniometer** is the most common tool used for measuring joint motion of the UE. Most goniometers are plastic or metal and come in many shapes and sizes. Every goniometer has a protractor, an axis, and two arms. The stationary arm extends from the protractor, on which the degrees are marked. The movable arm has a center line, or pointer, to indicate angle measurement. The axis is the point at which these two arms are riveted together. A full-circle goniometer, which measures 360°, or 0° to 180° in each direction, permits motion measurement in both directions, such as flexion and extension, without repositioning the tool. When using an opaque half-circle goniometer (such as one made of metal), the protractor must be positioned opposite to the direction of motion so that the indicator remains on the face of the protractor. A transparent, half-circle goniometer (such as one that is plastic), allows the examiner to read the pointer or the center line in either direction. A finger goniometer is designed with a shorter movable arm and flat surfaces to fit comfortably over the finger joints. Figure 13-1 shows examples of these types of goniometers. It is important to match the size of the goniometer to the size of the joint (e.g., use a larger goniometer for the shoulder and a smaller goniometer for the wrist and digits).

Some clinics use a manual or electronic inclinometer rather than a goniometer to measure ROM. These devices use gravity rather than the therapist's visual skills to determine the starting position for measurement and, therefore, can improve accuracy, particularly in more complex motions such as compound spine motions.[6–8] It is important to note that the position of the individual being measured may need to change with the use of an inclinometer because gravity is used to obtain the starting position. Applications for the smartphone can become inclinometers using the device's built-in tilt-sensitive systems.[9,10] These easily accessible electronic applications increase the clinical utility of inclinometers.

Another potential tool is the electrogoniometer. This tool can offer continuous, dynamic joint measurement of ROM once positioned and calibrated.[11] This may be particularly helpful in work- and industry-type settings where repetitive work tasks and ergonomic impact are being assessed.[12] When using the electrogoniometer, the therapist should calibrate the instrument for the task being performed to decrease errors often seen at angles greater than 45°.[13] With the advancement in technology

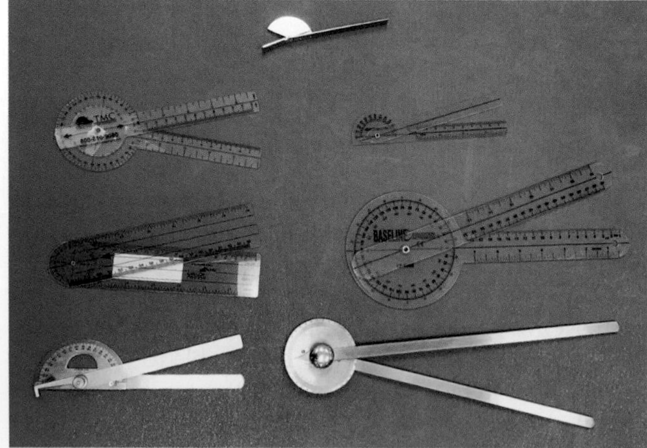

Figure 13-1. Types of goniometers. The small finger goniometer (*top*) has flat arms that fit over the fingers. The small half-circle goniometers are used to measure small joints, such as the wrist. The small and large full-circle goniometers are used to measure with the 360° method and for larger joints.

and access to digital cameras, photography-based goniometry has also been found to be an accurate and reliable measure of clinical goniometry for measuring ROM.[14–16]

Three-dimensional (3D) motion analysis is another way in which ROM can be measured. A benefit of 3D motion analysis is the capturing of dynamic movements in real time. With this type of analysis, both static joint position and the dynamic course of movement from a joint can be assessed.[17] Optical systems with reflective markers are the most common technique.[18] Because the goniometer is most commonly used in occupational therapy practice and the general principles apply to the alignment of other instruments, the figures depicting ROM measurement in this chapter include standard goniometers.

General principles to follow when using the goniometer include the following:

- Place the axis of the goniometer over the axis of motion. The axis of motion for some joints coincides with bony landmarks, but for others it must be found by observing movement and finding the point around which the movement occurs. In that case, the axis of motion can change position during movement, so it is acceptable for the goniometer to be repositioned at the end of range. When the two arms of the goniometer are placed correctly, they intersect at the axis of motion, so it is more important to have the arms line up correctly. The axis placement then automatically falls in line.
- Position the stationary arm parallel to the longitudinal axis of the body segment proximal to the joint being measured, although there are some exceptions.
- Position the movable arm parallel to the longitudinal axis of the body segment distal to the joint being measured, with some exceptions.

Range of Motion of the Upper Extremity

For the measurements given here, unless otherwise noted, the client is seated with trunk erect against the back of an armless straight chair, although the measurements can be taken with the client standing or supine, if necessary. This procedure can be done actively or passively. For active movement, take special care to ensure that there are no substitutions of movement. A substitution or compensatory movement is the use of an alternate muscle or position to complete a motion, possibly preventing measurement of the true limits of motion. To avoid this error, the therapist should watch the individual as the motion is completed rather than focusing too intently on the goniometer. For PROM, the tester supports both the body part and the goniometer proximal and distal to the joint, leaving the joint free to move. Comfortable handling of the goniometer together with the movable body segment may require practice.

On the pages that follow, the reader will find narrative and pictorial descriptions to help in understanding and practicing measurement of UE ROM. The narrative descriptions frequently use the sagittal, transverse, and frontal planes of motion to describe the motion being measured (see Fig. 13-2 for pictorial clarification of these planes of motion).

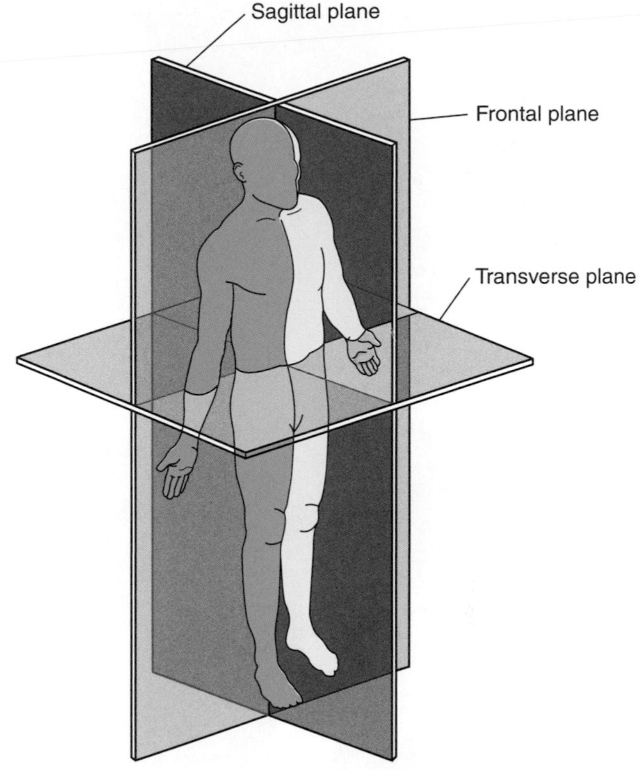

Figure 13-2. Planes of motion of the body.

Shoulder Flexion (0°–180°)

Movement of the humerus anteriorly in the sagittal plane, which represents both glenohumeral and axioscapular motion (Figs. 13-3 and 13-4).

Goniometer Placement

- *Axis:* A point through the lateral aspect of the glenohumeral joint; at the start of motion, it lies approximately 1 inch below the acromion process with arm in neutral rotation. At the end position, the axis has moved, and the goniometer must be repositioned to align with the center of the humeral head.
- *Stationary arm:* Parallel to the lateral midline of the trunk.
- *Movable arm:* Parallel to the longitudinal axis of the humerus on the lateral aspect.

Possible Substitutions

- Trunk extension and shoulder abduction.

Shoulder Extension (0°–60°)

Movement of the humerus posteriorly in the sagittal plane with the arm in neutral (Figs. 13-5 and 13-6).

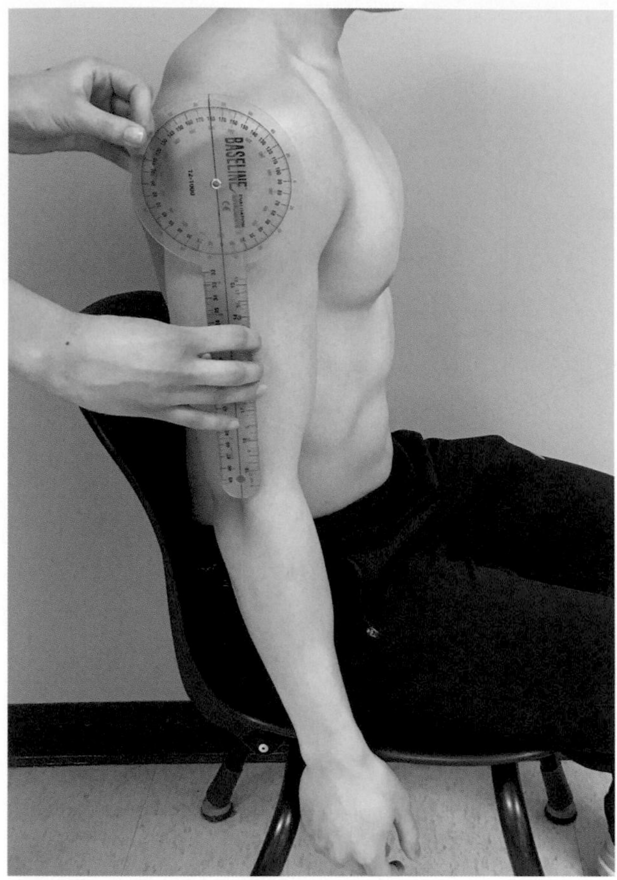

Figure 13-3. Shoulder flexion, start position.

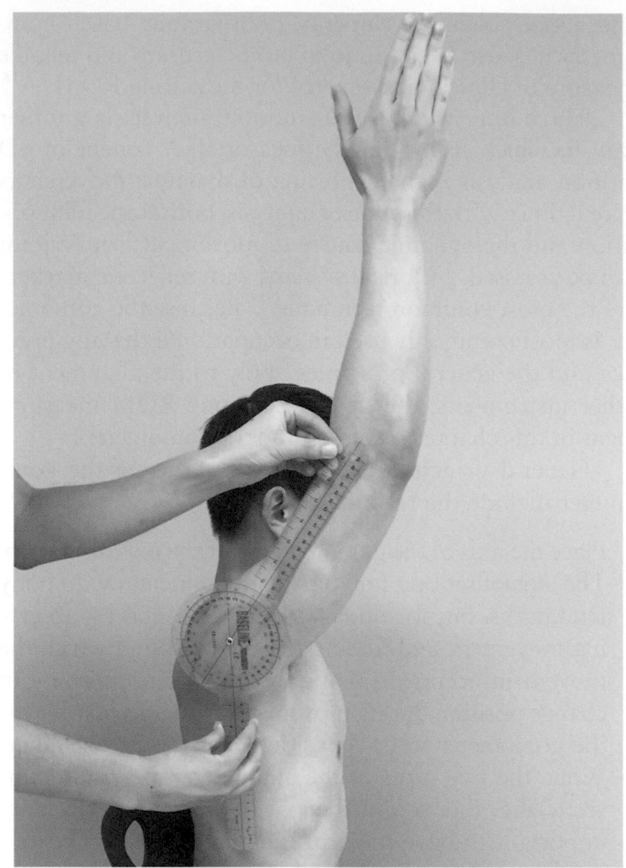

Figure 13-4. Shoulder flexion, end position.

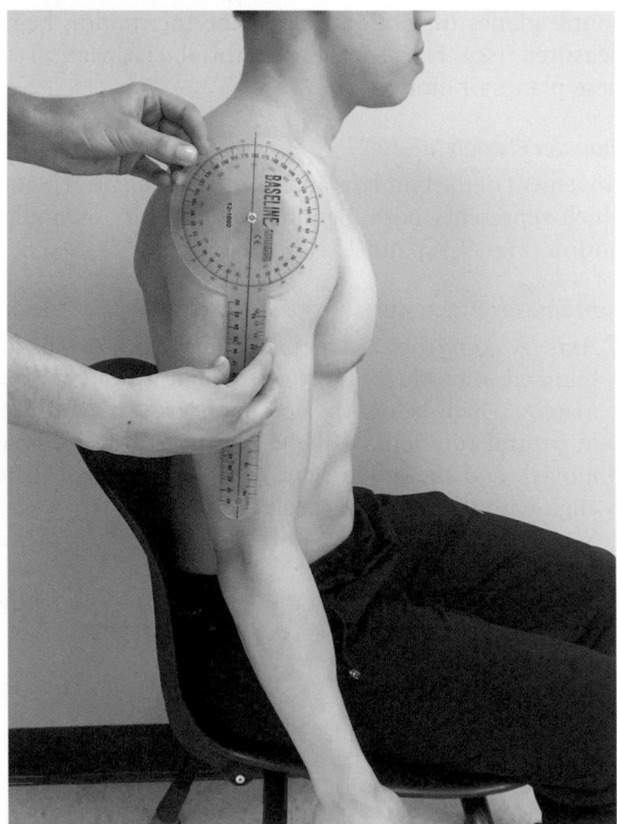

Figure 13-5. Shoulder extension, start position.

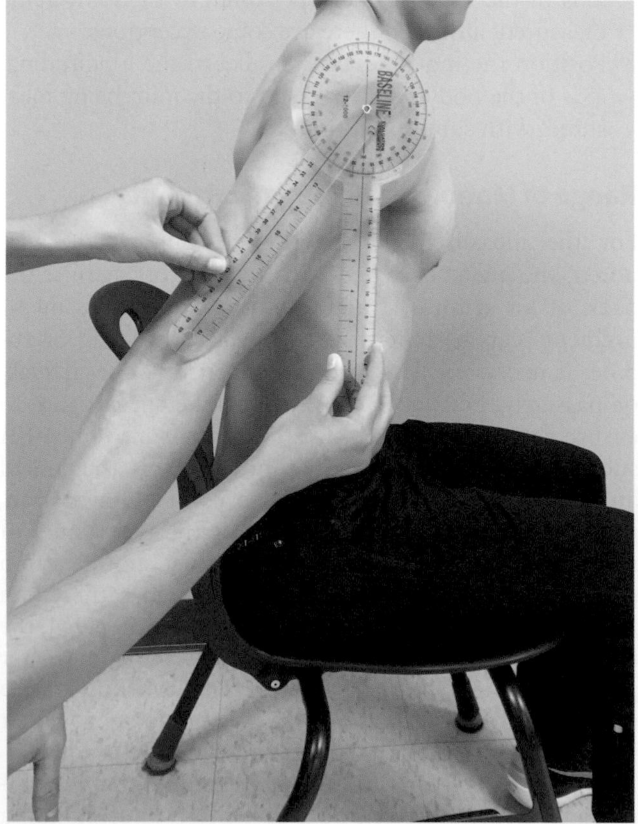

Figure 13-6. Shoulder extension, end position.

Goniometer Placement

- *Axis:* A point through the lateral aspect of the glenohumeral joint approximately 1 inch below the acromion process.
- *Stationary arm:* Parallel to the lateral midline of the trunk.
- *Movable arm:* Parallel to the longitudinal axis of the humerus on the lateral aspect.

Possible Substitutions

- Trunk flexion, excessive scapular elevation and downward rotation, and shoulder abduction.

Shoulder Abduction (0°–180°)

Movement of the humerus laterally in the frontal plane, which represents both glenohumeral and axioscapular motion (Figs. 13-7 and 13-8).

Goniometer Placement

- *Axis:* A point through the anterior or posterior aspect of the glenohumeral joint approximately 1 inch below the acromion process.
- *Stationary arm:* Along the trunk, parallel to the spine.
- *Movable arm:* Parallel to the longitudinal axis of the humerus.

Possible Substitutions

- Lateral flexion of trunk, scapular elevation, and shoulder flexion or extension. If excessive lateral flexion of the trunk is noted, the arm not being actively tested may be stabilized at 90° of abduction against a wall or other stable object to prevent trunk motion.

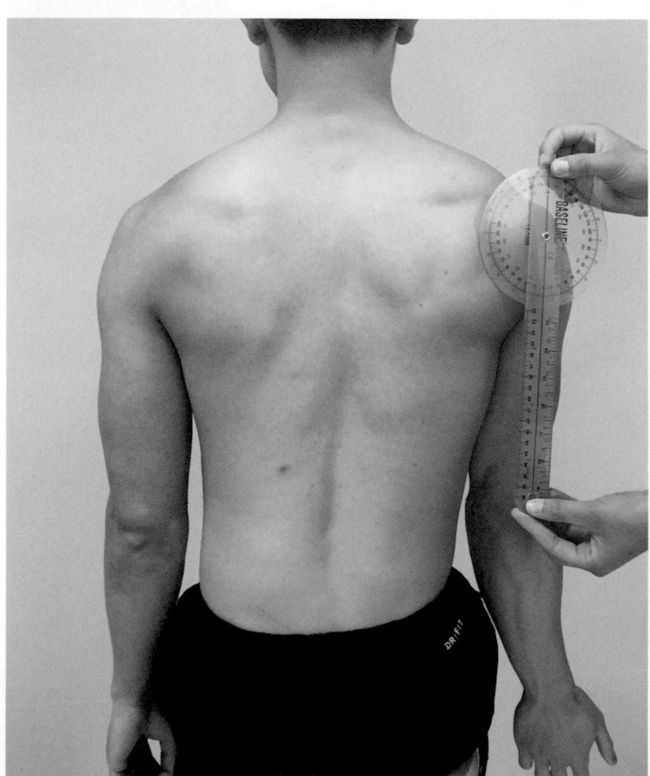

Figure 13-7. Shoulder abduction, start position.

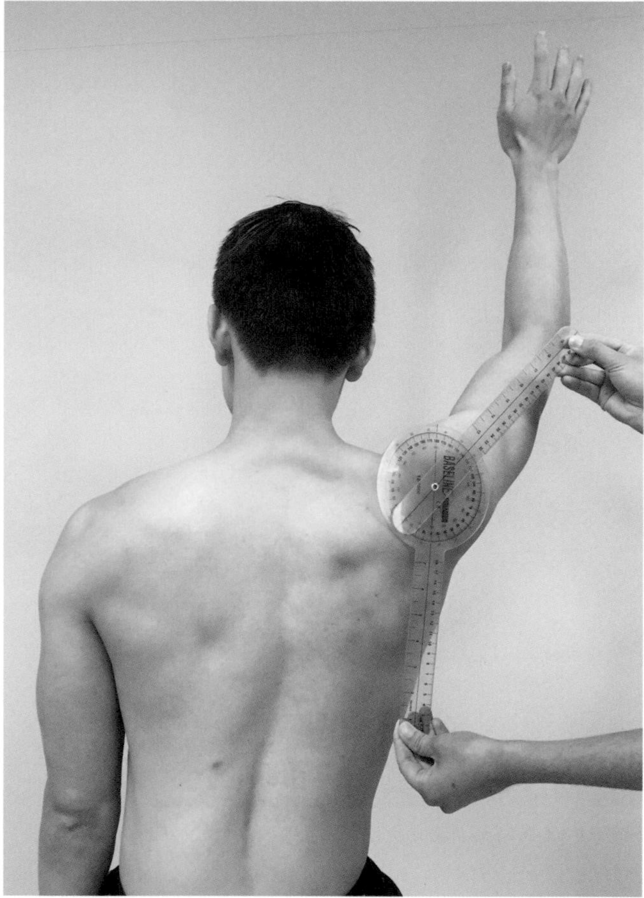

Figure 13-8. Shoulder abduction, end position.

Horizontal Abduction (0°–45°)

Movement of the humerus posteriorly on a horizontal (transverse) plane from 90° of shoulder abduction (Figs. 13-9 and 13-10).

Goniometer Placement

- *Axis:* On top of the acromion process.
- *Stationary arm:* To start, the stationary arm is parallel to the shaft of the humerus on the superior aspect and remains perpendicular to the body as the humerus moves posteriorly.
- *Movable arm:* Parallel to the longitudinal axis of the humerus on the superior aspect.

Possible Substitutions

- Trunk rotation and scapular motion.

Horizontal Adduction (0°–140°)

Movement of the humerus anteriorly on a horizontal (transverse) plane from 90° of shoulder abduction through 90° of shoulder flexion, across the trunk to the limit of motion (Figs. 13-11 and 13-12).

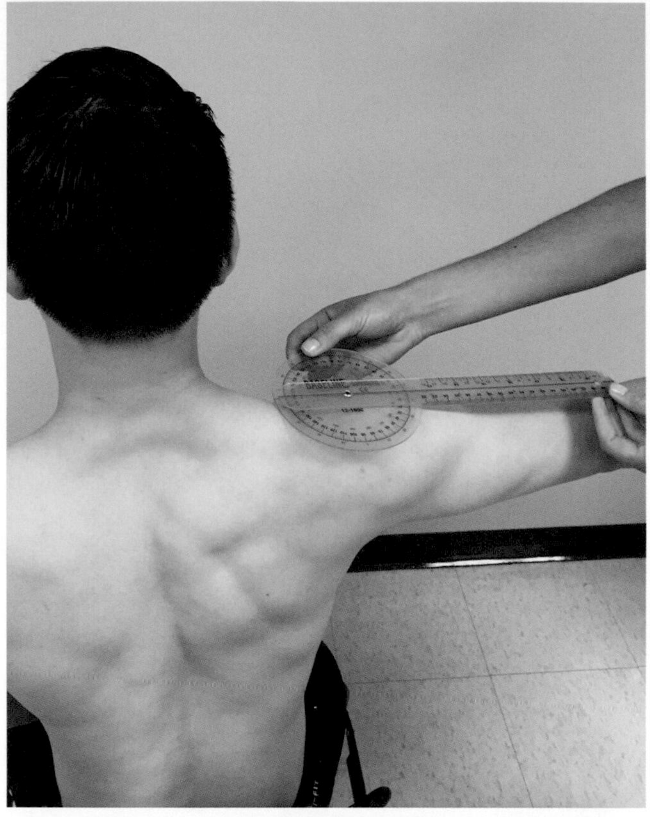
Figure 13-9. Shoulder horizontal abduction, start position.

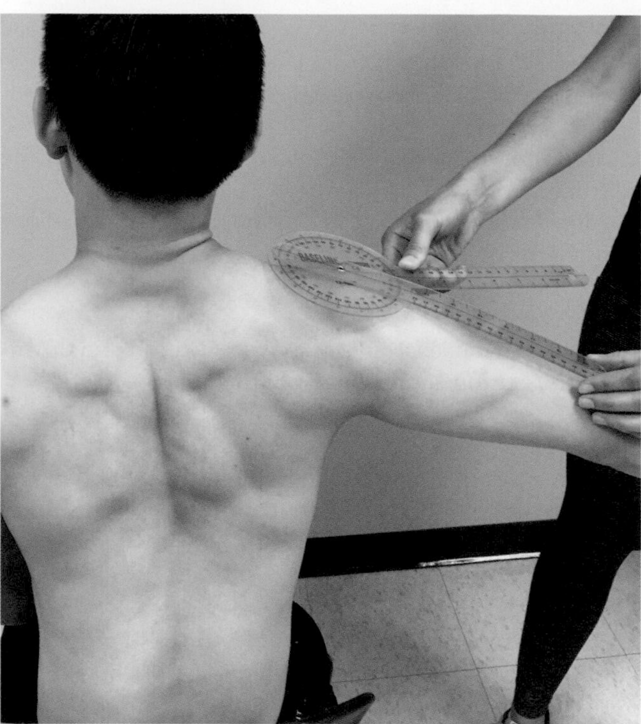
Figure 13-10. Shoulder horizontal abduction, end position.

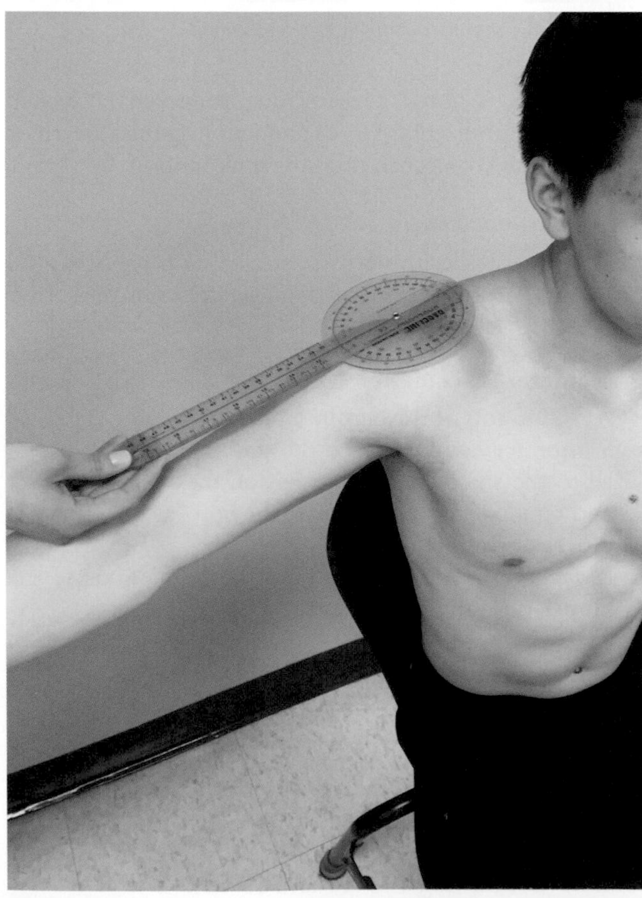
Figure 13-11. Shoulder horizontal adduction, start position.

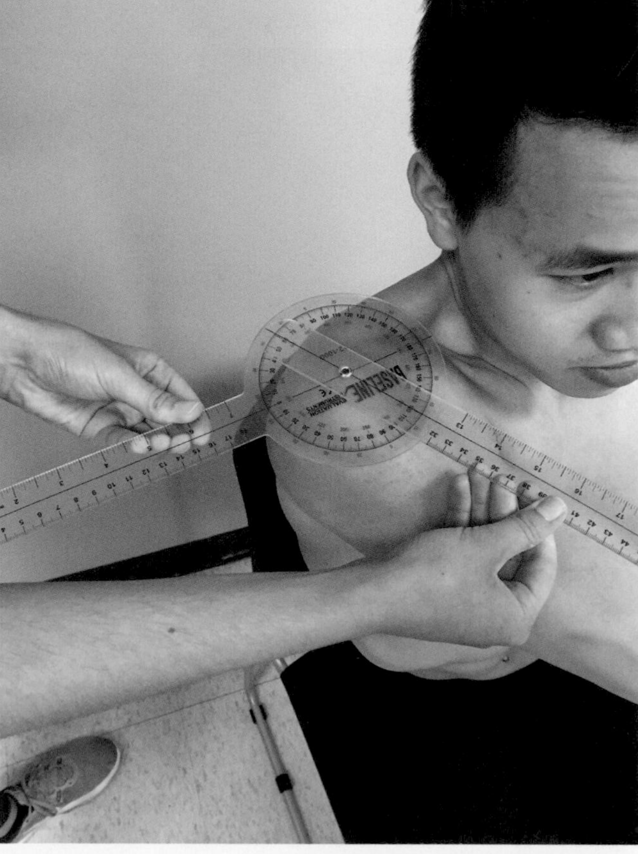
Figure 13-12. Shoulder horizontal adduction, end position.

Goniometer Placement

- *Axis:* On top of the acromion process.
- *Stationary arm:* To start, the stationary arm is parallel to the longitudinal axis of the humerus on the superior aspect and remains perpendicular to the body as the humerus moves anteriorly.
- *Movable arm:* Parallel to the longitudinal axis of the humerus on the superior aspect.

Possible Substitution

- Trunk rotation and scapular motion.

Internal Rotation (0°–70°)

Rotational movement of the humerus medially or downward toward the ground in the 90° abducted start position around the longitudinal axis of the humerus (Figs. 13-13 and 13-14). Preferably, the zero start position is with the arm abducted to 90° and elbow flexed at 90° with the forearm moving toward the floor from this starting position.

Goniometer Placement

- *Axis:* Olecranon process of the ulna.
- *Stationary arm:* Perpendicular to the floor, which will be parallel to the lateral trunk if the client is sitting up straight with hips at 90°.
- *Movable arm:* Parallel to the longitudinal axis of the ulna.

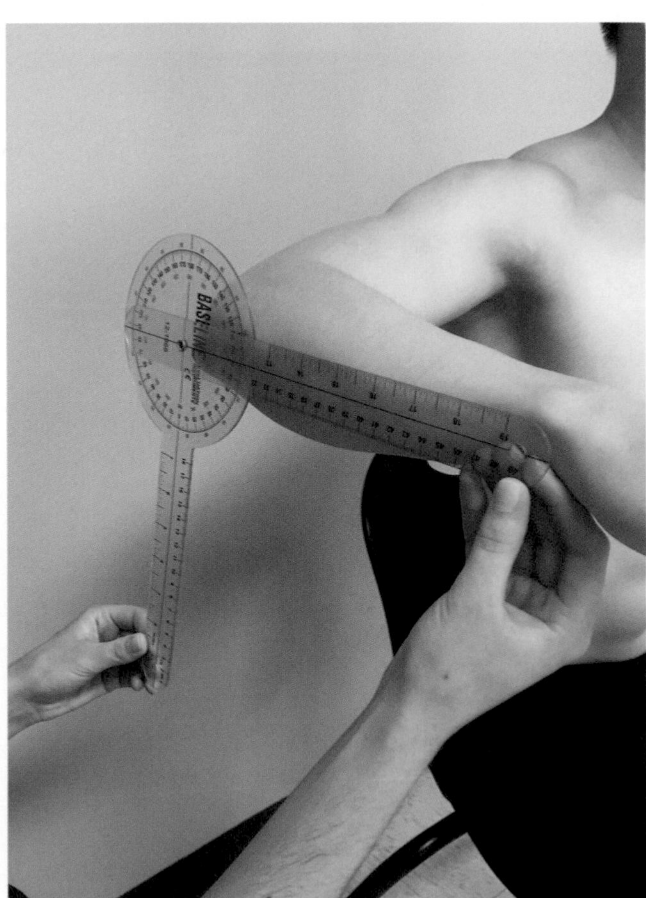

Figure 13-13. Shoulder internal rotation, start position.

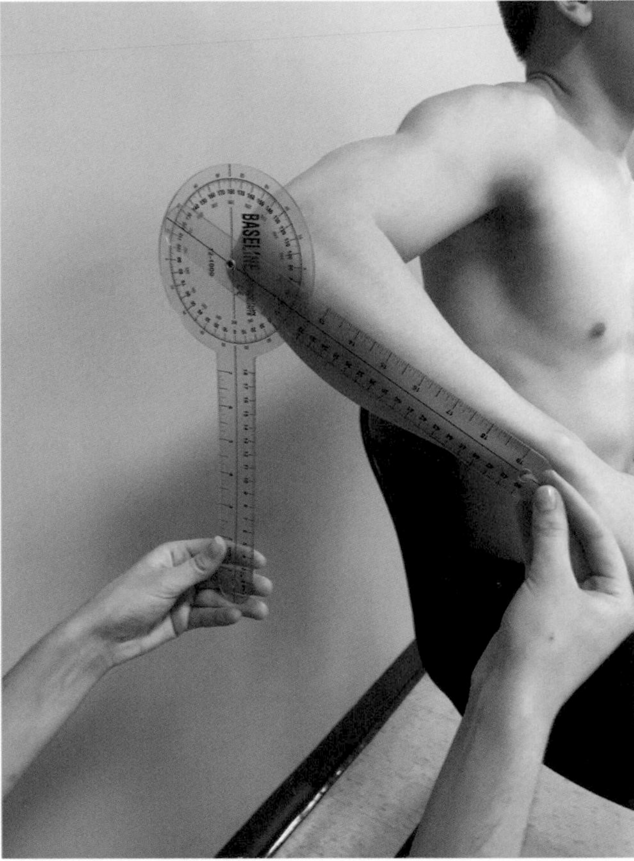

Figure 13-14. Shoulder internal rotation, end position.

Possible Substitutions

- Scapular elevation and downward rotation, trunk flexion, and elbow extension.

External Rotation (0°–90°)

Rotational movement of the humerus laterally or upward from the ground in the 90° abducted start position around the longitudinal axis of the humerus (Figs. 13-15 and 13-16). Preferably, the zero start position is with the arm abducted to 90° and elbow flexed at 90° with the forearm moving away from the floor from this starting position.

Goniometer Placement

- *Axis:* Olecranon process of the ulna.
- *Stationary arm:* Perpendicular to the floor, which will be parallel to the lateral trunk if the client is sitting up straight with hips at 90°.
- *Movable arm:* Parallel to the longitudinal axis of the ulna.

Possible Substitutions

- Scapular depression and upward rotation, trunk extension, and elbow extension.

Internal and External Rotation: Alternative Method

If shoulder limitation prevents positioning for the previously described method, the client may be seated with the humerus adducted to the side and elbow flexed to 90° with forearm in neutral (Figs. 13-17 to 13-19). The American

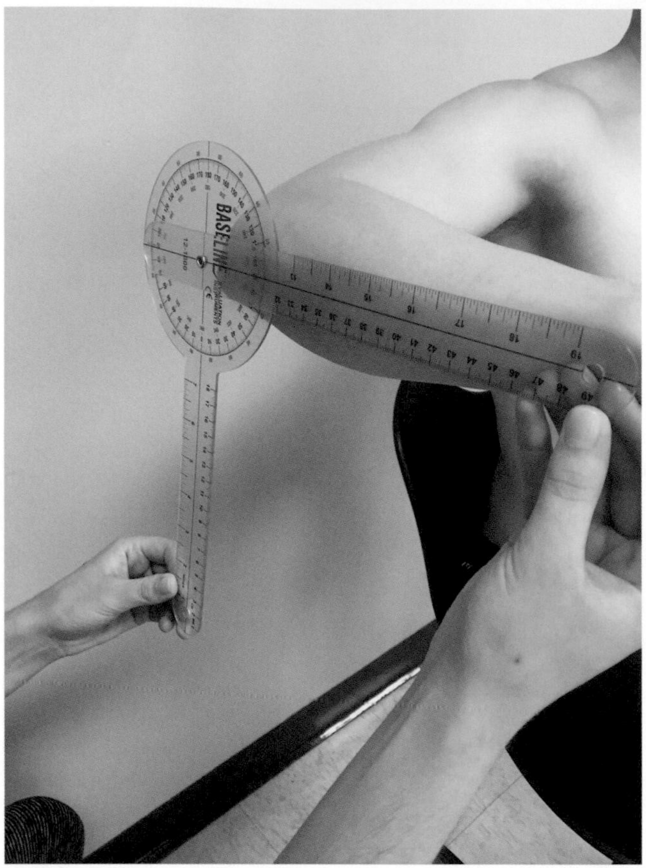

Figure 13-15. Shoulder external rotation, start position.

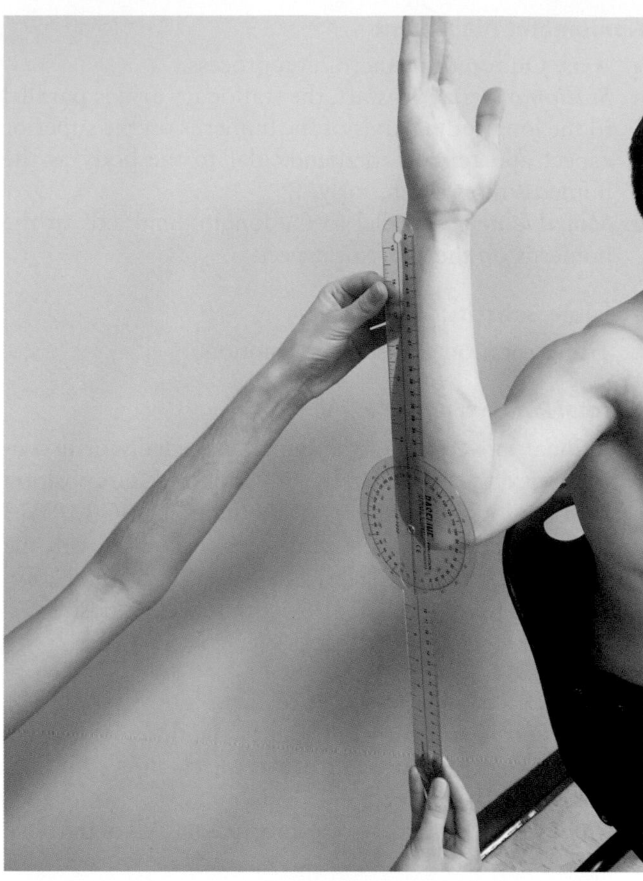

Figure 13-16. Shoulder external rotation, end position.

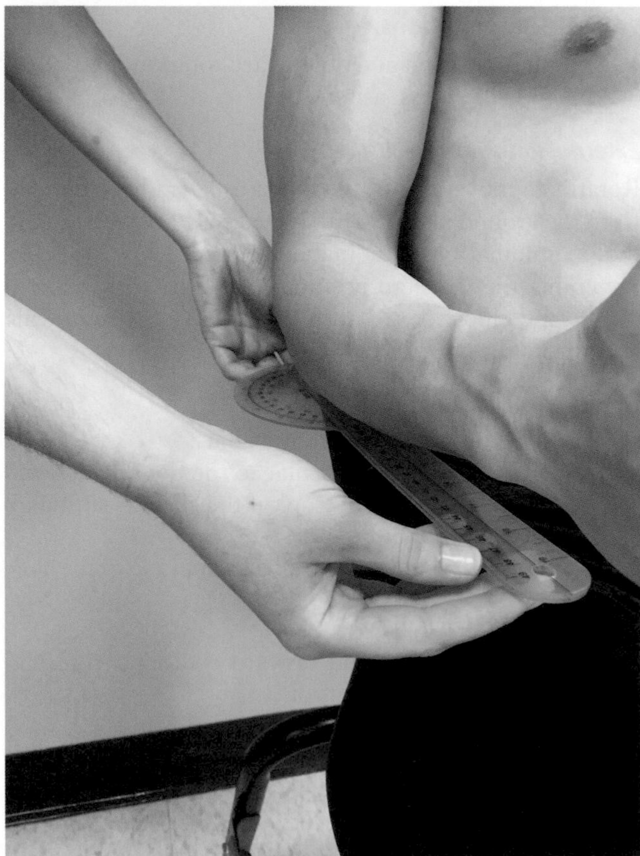

Figure 13-17. Shoulder internal and external rotation, alternative method, start position.

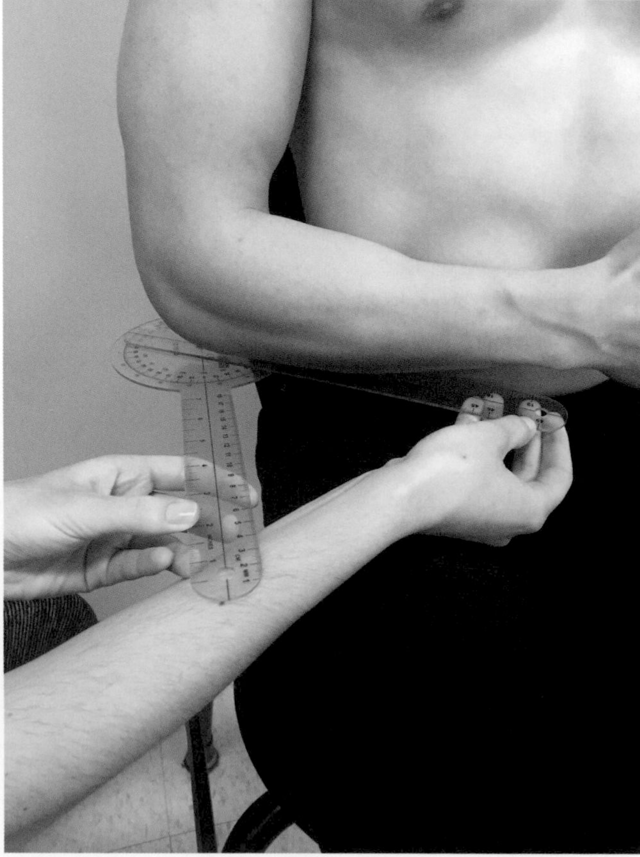

Figure 13-18. Shoulder internal rotation, alternative method, end position.

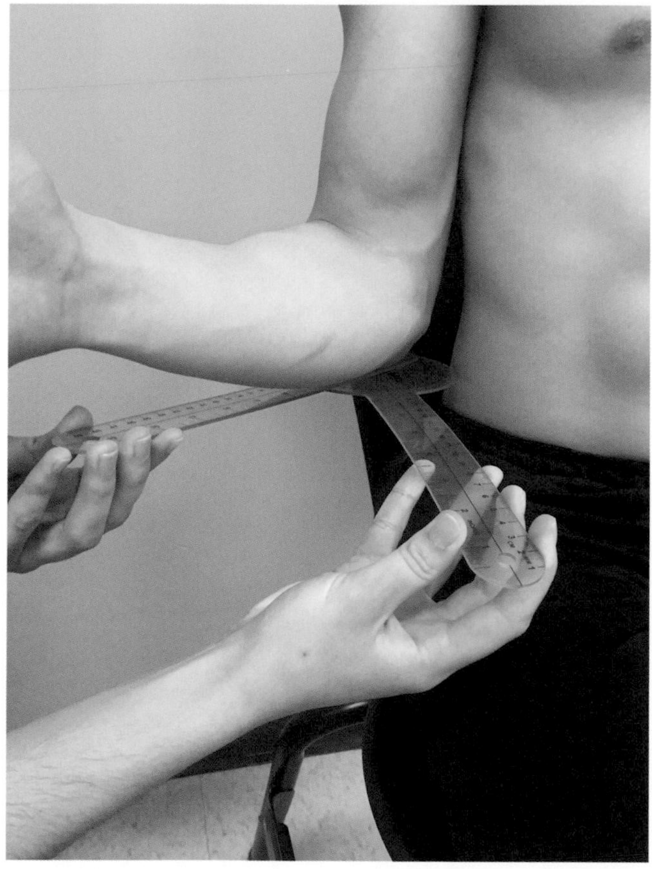

Figure 13-19. Shoulder external rotation, alternative method, end position.

Academy of Orthopedic Surgeons (AAOS)[19] and the American Medical Association (AMA)[20] do not provide norms for internal and external rotation in this position. Instead, the examiner measures the maximal possible ROM as available. Because there are no norms for this movement, the measurements are used to measure progress only.

This method is inaccurate for internal rotation if the UE is obstructed, such as if the client has a large abdomen.

Goniometer Placement

- *Axis:* Olecranon process of the ulna.
- *Stationary arm:* The stationary arm is along the longitudinal axis of the ulna on the inferior surface of the forearm and remains in that position, although the ulna moves away.
- *Movable arm:* Parallel to the longitudinal axis of the ulna and moves toward the abdomen during internal rotation and away from the abdomen during external rotation.

Possible Substitutions

- Trunk rotation, scapular retraction for external rotation, scapular protraction for internal rotation, and shoulder flexion.

Elbow Extension–Flexion (0°–150°)

Movement of the supinated forearm anteriorly in the sagittal plane (Figs. 13-20 and 13-21).

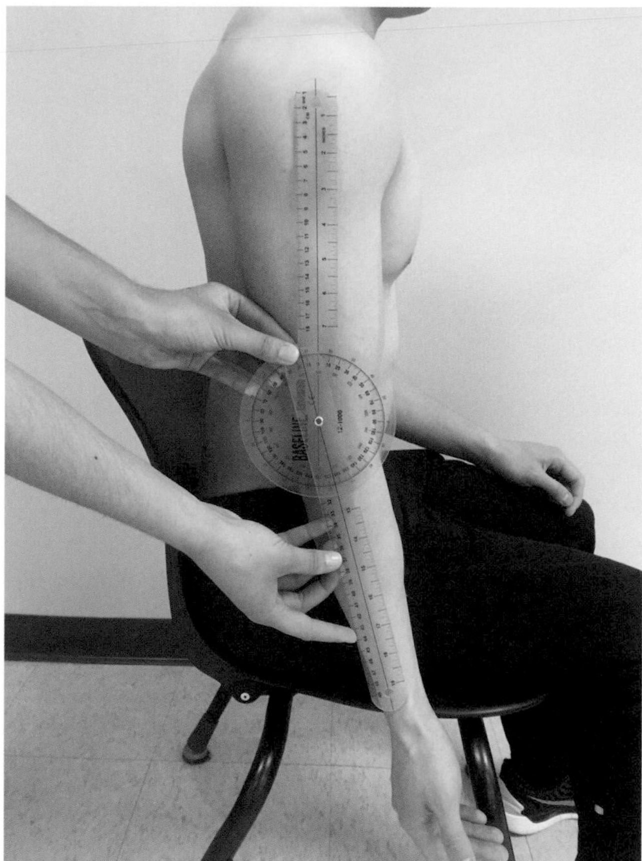

Figure 13-20. Elbow flexion, start position (elbow extension).

Goniometer Placement

- *Axis:* Lateral epicondyle of the humerus.
- *Stationary arm:* Parallel to the longitudinal axis of the humerus on the lateral aspect.
- *Movable arm:* Parallel to the longitudinal axis of the radius.

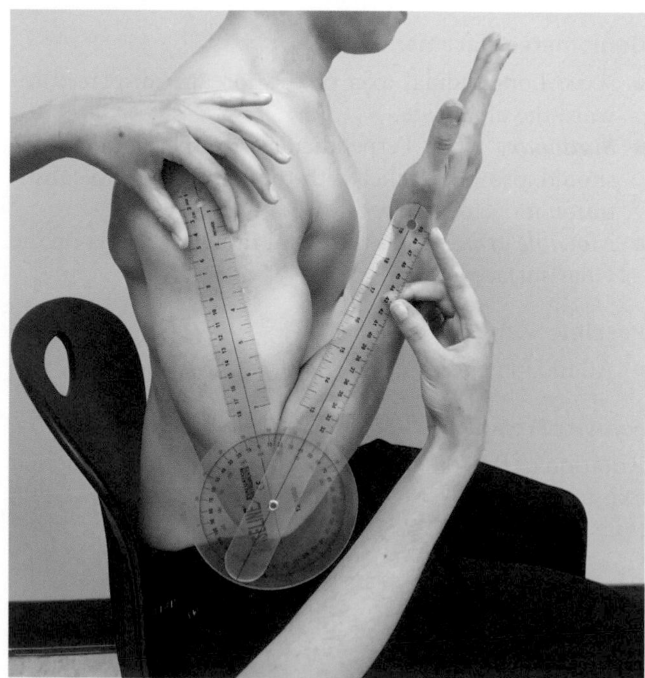

Figure 13-21. Elbow flexion, end position.

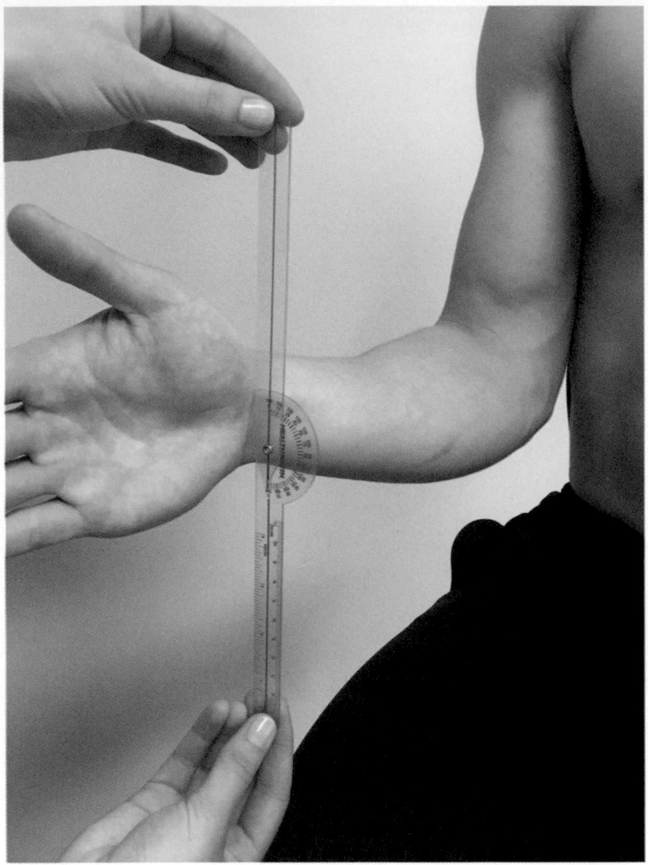

Figure 13-22. Supination, start position.

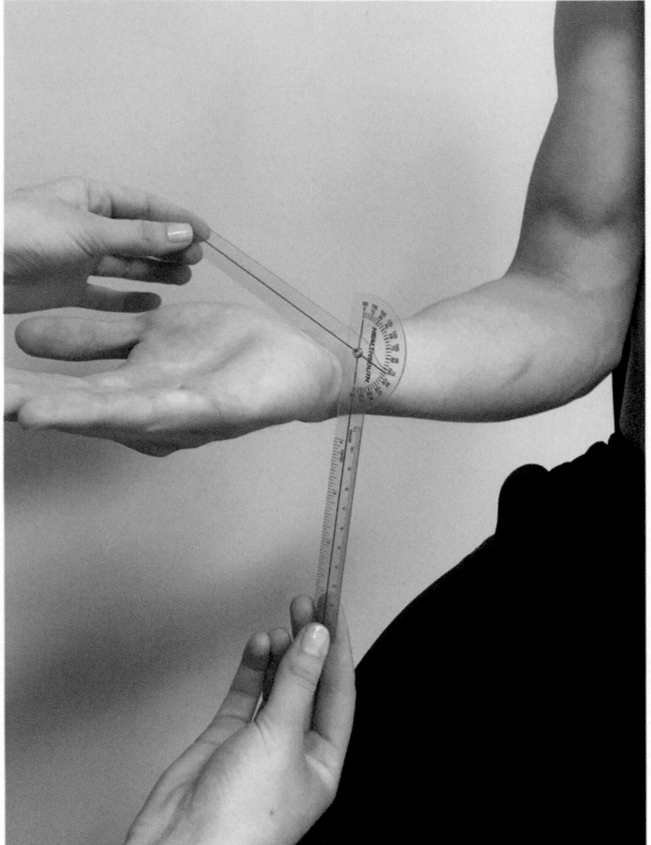

Figure 13-23. Supination, end position.

Forearm Supination (0°–80°)

Rotation of the forearm laterally around its longitudinal axis from midposition so that the palm of the hand faces up (Figs. 13-22 and 13-23). Starting position is with the humerus stabilized against the body, elbow flexed to 90°, and forearm in neutral.

Goniometer Placement

- *Axis:* Longitudinal axis of the forearm displaced toward the ulnar side.
- *Stationary arm:* Perpendicular to the floor, which should also be parallel with the humerus if no substitution movements are allowed.
- *Movable arm:* Across the distal radius and ulna on the volar surface.

Possible Substitutions

- Adduction and external rotation of the shoulder.

Forearm Pronation (0°–80°)

Rotation of the forearm medially around its longitudinal axis from neutral so that the palm of the hand faces down (Figs. 13-24 and 13-25).

Goniometer Placement

- *Axis:* Longitudinal axis of forearm displaced toward the ulnar side.

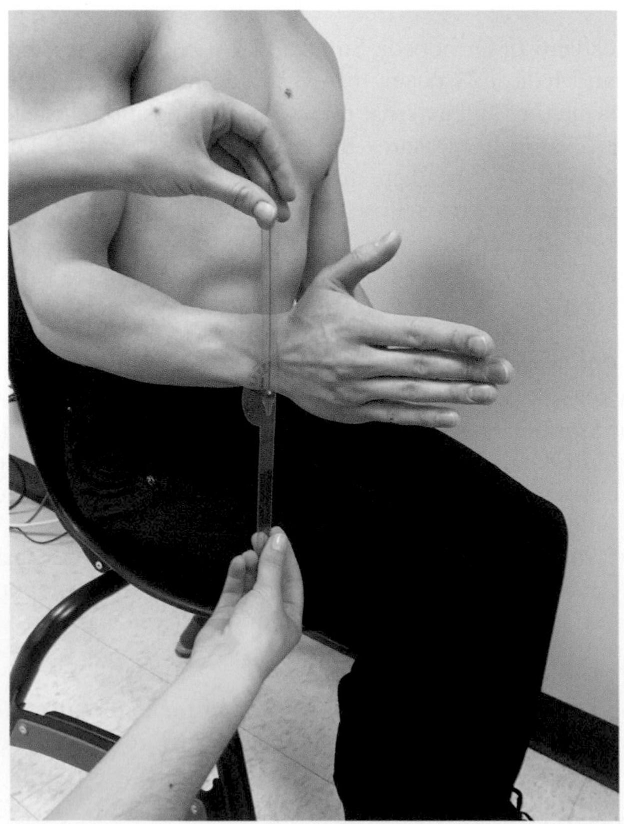

Figure 13-24. Pronation, start position.

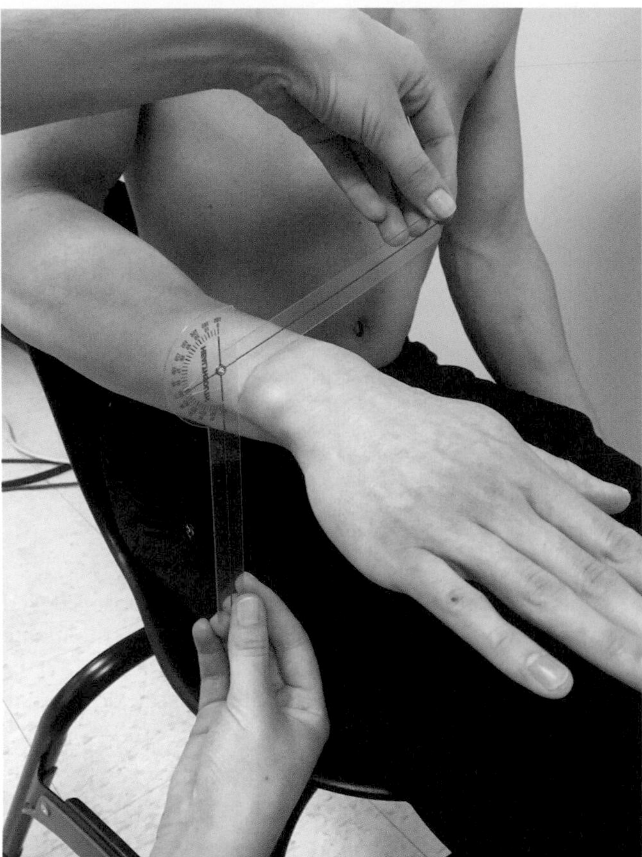

Figure 13-25. Pronation, end position.

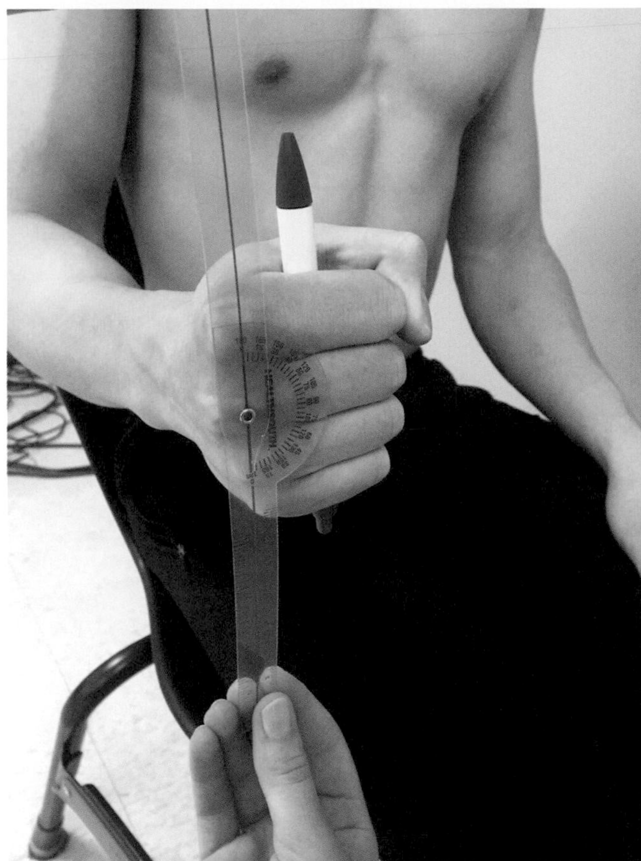

Figure 13-26. Forearm supination and pronation, alternative method, start position.

- *Stationary arm:* Perpendicular to the floor, which should also be parallel with the humerus if no substitution movements are allowed.
- *Movable arm:* Across the distal radius and ulna on the dorsal surface.

Possible Substitutions

- Abduction and internal rotation of the shoulder.

Supination and Pronation: Alternative Method

Although the distal forearm method described here for supination and pronation has been the gold standard, two additional methods (the handheld pencil and plumbline goniometer methods) have shown high interrater and intrarater reliability in a more functional measure of supination and pronation.[21] The handheld pencil method (Figs. 13-26 to 13-28) can be easily used in the clinic to determine functional forearm rotation. The standardized method is to have the client seated with hips and knees at 90°, feet flat on the ground, arms adducted to the sides with elbow flexed to 90°, and forearm unsupported in neutral. The client holds a standard 15-cm pencil in a tight fist, with the pencil extending from the radial aspect of the hand. The goniometer is aligned with the axis at the head of the third metacarpal, stationary arm perpendicular to the floor, and movable arm parallel to the pencil.

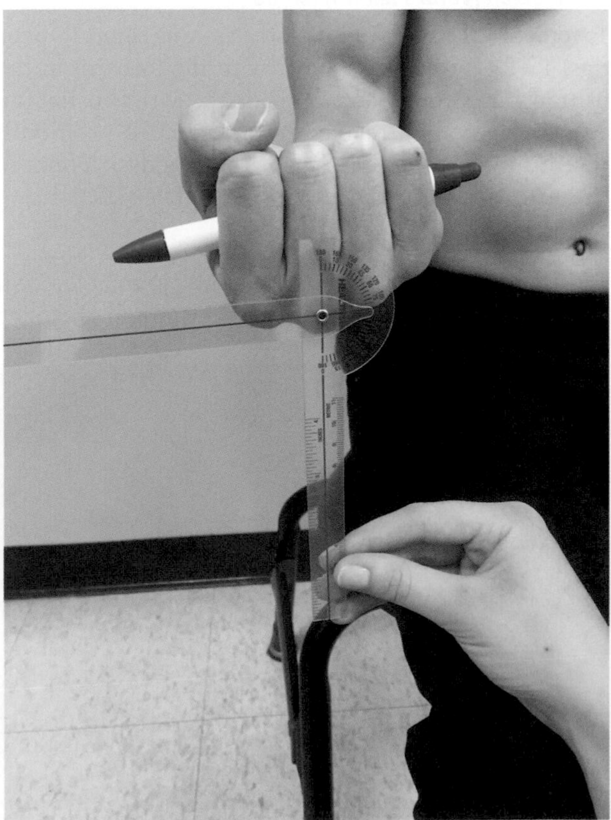

Figure 13-27. Forearm supination, alternative method, end position.

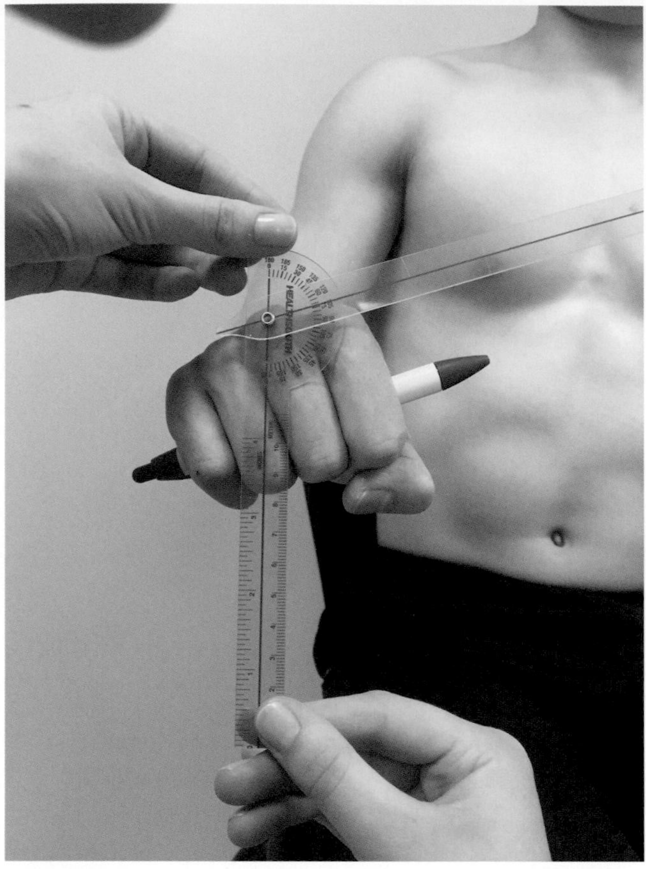

Figure 13-28. Forearm pronation, alternative method, end position.

Wrist Flexion (Volar Flexion) (0°–80°)

Movement of the hand volarly in the sagittal plane (Figs. 13-29 and 13-30). Start with the forearm in mid position on a table surface with the wrist in neutral. Keep the digits in a relaxed or an extended position to prevent any negative impact of the tenodesis effect on demonstrating the limits of motion.

Goniometer Placement

- *Axis:* On the dorsal aspect of the wrist joint in line with the base of the third metacarpal in the proximal capitate region. (*Note:* The lunate protrudes as the wrist is flexed forward, and the capitate is located distal to the lunate and proximal to the base of the third metacarpal.)
- *Stationary arm:* Along the midline of the dorsal surface of the forearm.
- *Movable arm:* Parallel to the longitudinal axis of the third metacarpal.

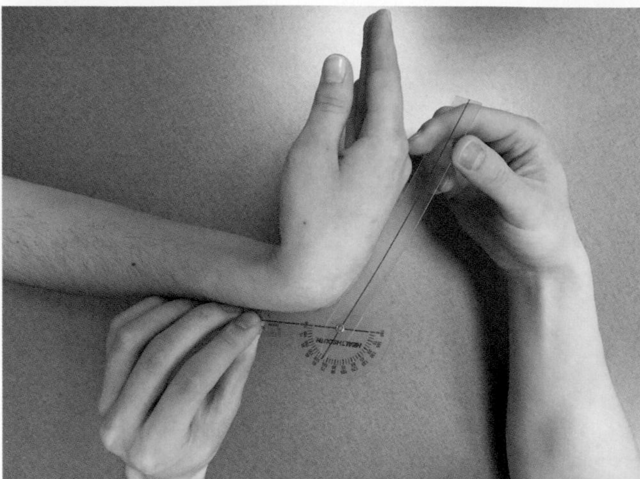

Figure 13-30. Wrist flexion, end position.

Wrist Extension (Dorsiflexion) (0°–70°)

Movement of the hand dorsally in the sagittal plane (Figs. 13-31 and 13-32). Again, prevent the tenodesis effect by reminding the client to relax or flex the fingers rather than trying to maintain them in full extension while measuring wrist motion.

Goniometer Placement

- *Axis:* On the volar surface of the wrist in line with the palmaris longus tendon in line with the third metacarpal at the level of the carpal bones.
- *Stationary arm:* Along the midline of the volar surface of the forearm.

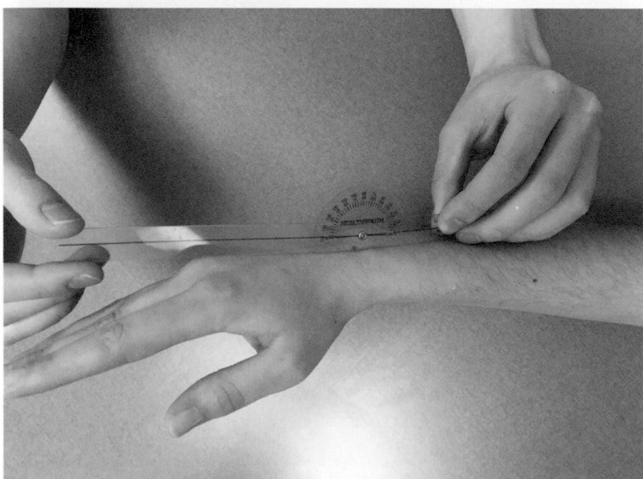

Figure 13-29. Wrist flexion, start position.

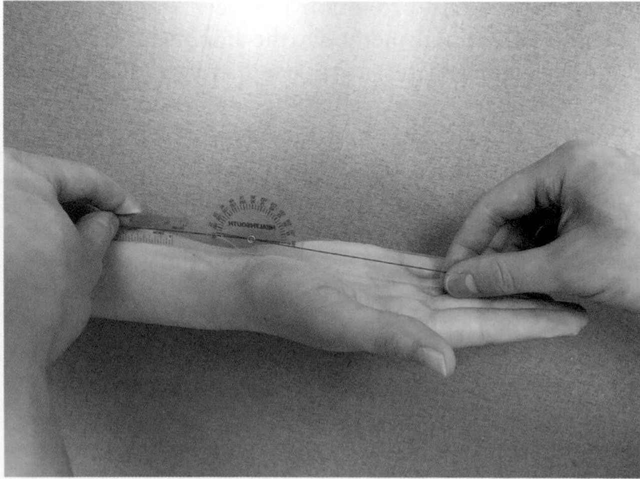

Figure 13-31. Wrist extension, start position.

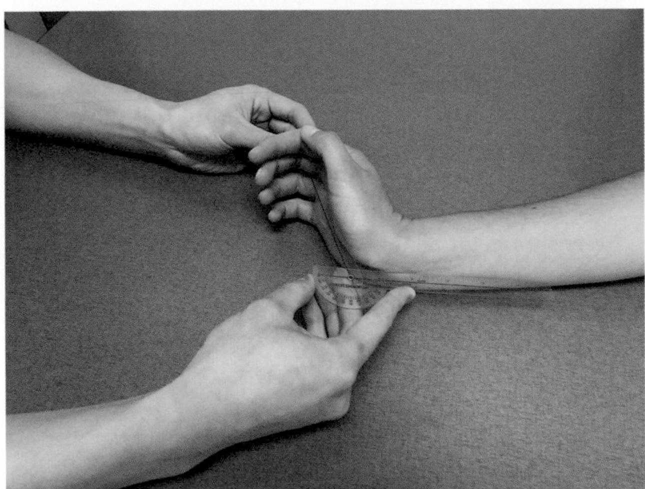

Figure 13-32. Wrist extension, end position.

- *Movable arm:* Parallel to the longitudinal axis of the third metacarpal. The movable arm may need to rest between the third and fourth digits if the digits prevent correct alignment.

Wrist Flexion and Extension: Alternative Method

Although the volar/dorsal method described here for wrist flexion and extension is the preferred method according to the American Society of Hand Therapists (ASHT), a lateral approach (Figs. 13-33 to 13-35) is acceptable if wounds or edema affect goniometer placement.[22] Start with the forearm and wrist resting on the table in neutral.

Goniometer Placement

- *Axis:* Over the styloid process of the radius, which is located on the lateral aspect of the wrist at the anatomical snuff box.
- *Stationary arm:* Parallel to the longitudinal axis of the radius.
- *Movable arm:* Parallel to the longitudinal axis of the second metacarpal.

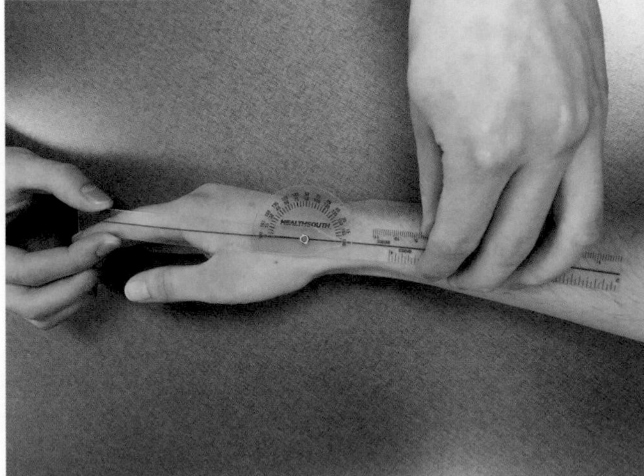

Figure 13-33. Wrist flexion and extension, alternative method, start position.

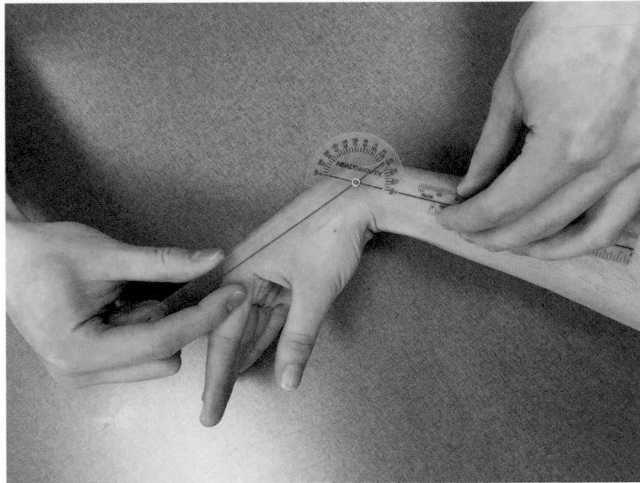

Figure 13-34. Wrist flexion, alternative method, end position.

Wrist Ulnar Deviation (0°–30°)

Movement of the hand toward the ulnar side in a frontal plane (Figs. 13-36 and 13-37). Starting position is with the forearm pronated on a table surface, wrist in neutral, and fingers extended.

Goniometer Placement

- *Axis:* On the dorsal aspect of the wrist joint in line with the base of the third metacarpal over the capitate bone where the motion is observed.

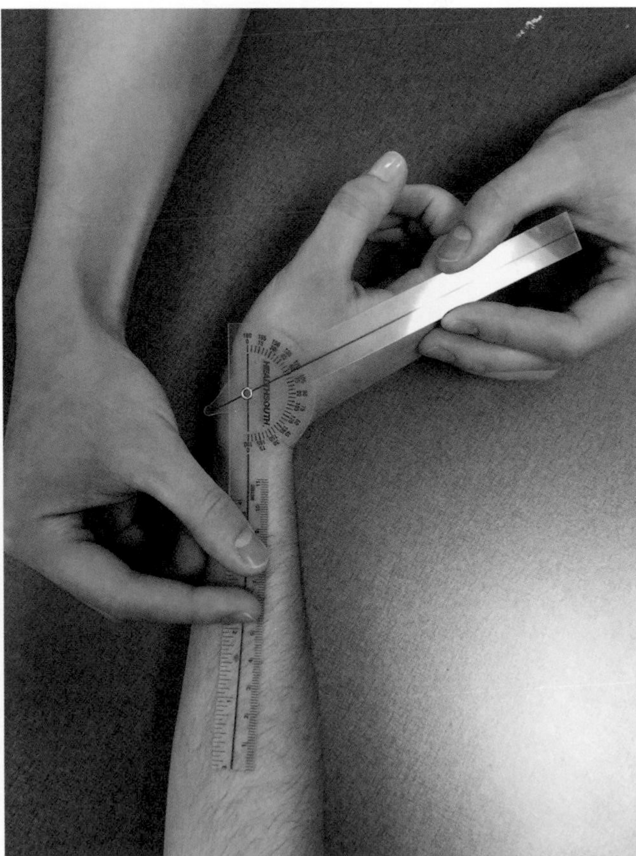

Figure 13-35. Wrist extension, alternative method, end position.

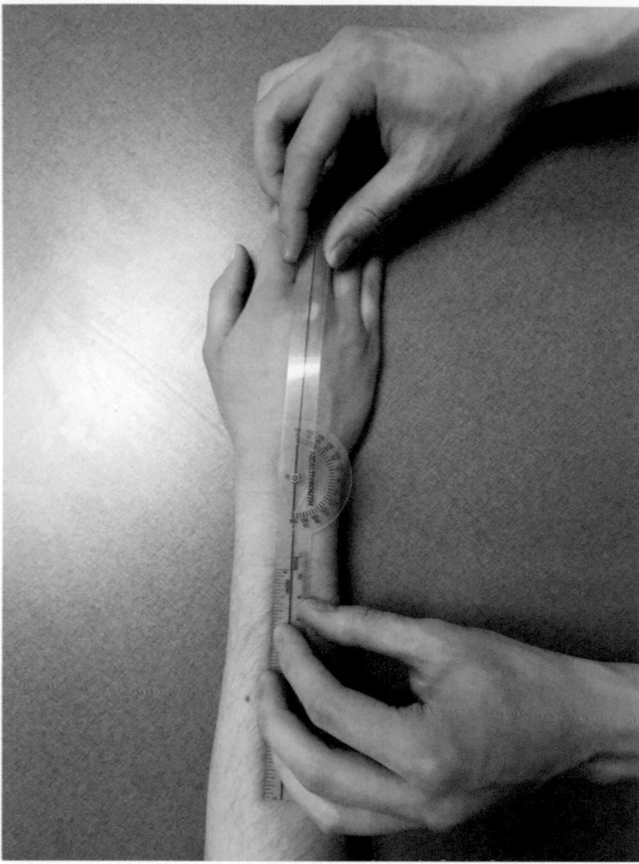

Figure 13-36. Wrist ulnar deviation, start position.

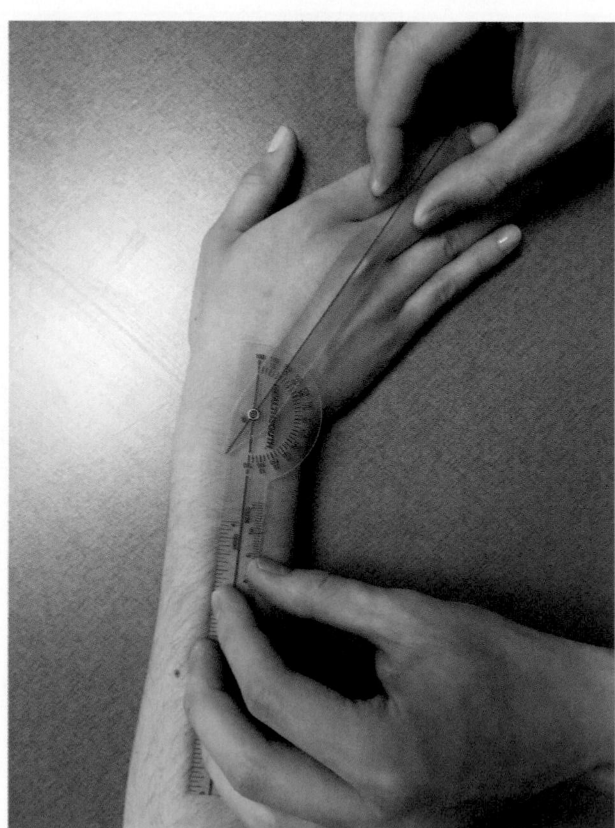

Figure 13-37. Wrist ulnar deviation, end position.

- *Stationary arm:* Along the midline of the forearm on the dorsal surface. After positioning the client, stabilizing the forearm can assist in isolating motion to the wrist.
- *Movable arm:* Along the midline of the third metacarpal. (*Note:* Do not be distracted by additional abduction of the third digit, and palpate the third metacarpal to ensure alignment.)

Possible Substitutions

- Wrist extension and wrist flexion.

Wrist Radial Deviation (0°–20°)

Movement of the hand toward the radial side in a frontal plane (Figs. 13-38 and 13-39).

Goniometer Placement

- *Axis:* On the dorsal aspect of the wrist joint in line with the base of the third metacarpal over the capitate.
- *Stationary arm:* Along the midline of the forearm on the dorsal surface. After positioning the client, stabilizing the forearm can assist in isolating motion to the wrist.
- *Movable arm:* Along the midline of the third metacarpal.

Possible Substitution

- Wrist extension.

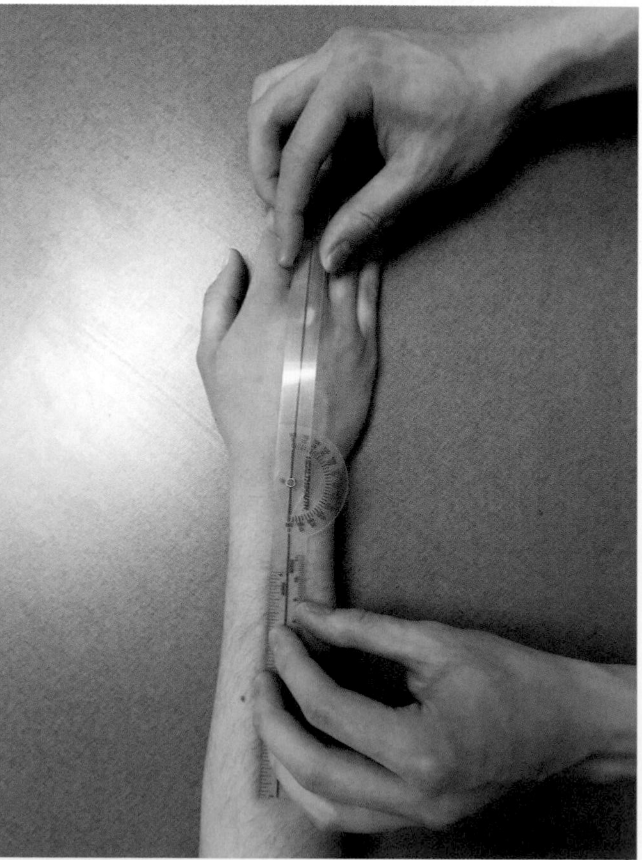

Figure 13-38. Wrist radial deviation, start position.

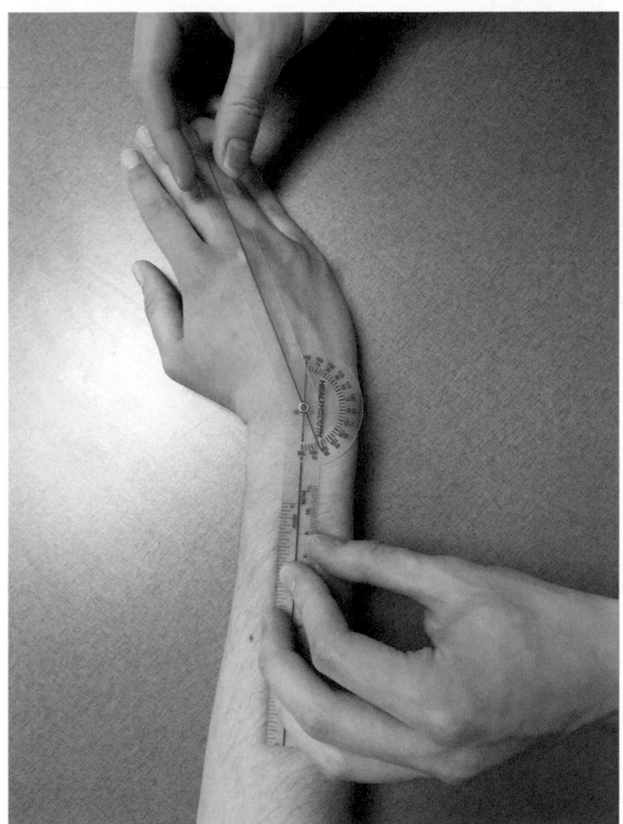

Figure 13-39. Wrist radial deviation, end position.

Thumb Carpometacarpal Flexion (0°–15°)

Movement of the thumb across the palm in the frontal plane (Figs. 13-40 and 13-41).

Goniometer Placement

- *Axis:* On the radial side of the wrist at the junction of the base of the first metacarpal and the trapezium.
- *Stationary arm:* To achieve proper alignment, place the shorter arm of the goniometer parallel to the longitudinal axis of the radius.

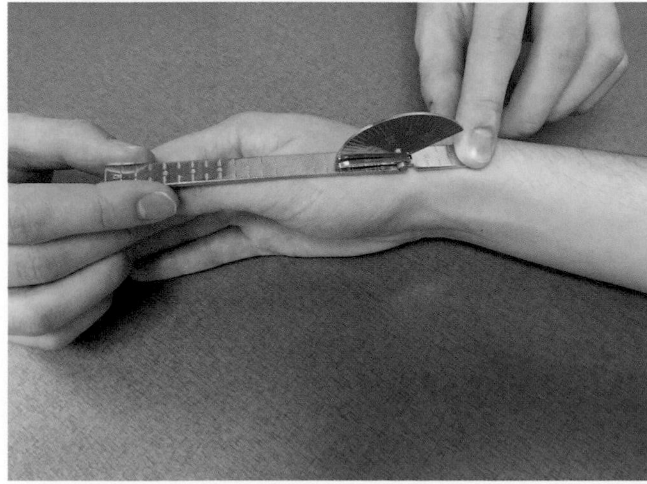

Figure 13-40. Thumb carpometacarpal flexion, start position.

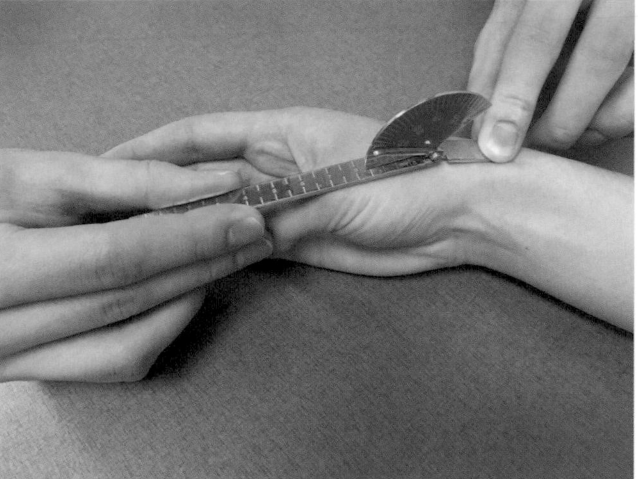

Figure 13-41. Thumb carpometacarpal flexion, end position.

- *Movable arm:* Place the longer arm of the goniometer parallel to the longitudinal axis of the first metacarpal. For accuracy, the arms of the goniometer must remain in full contact with the skin surface over the bones.

Thumb Carpometacarpal Extension/Radial Abduction (0°–50°)

Movement of the thumb away from the palm in the frontal plane (Figs. 13-42 and 13-43).

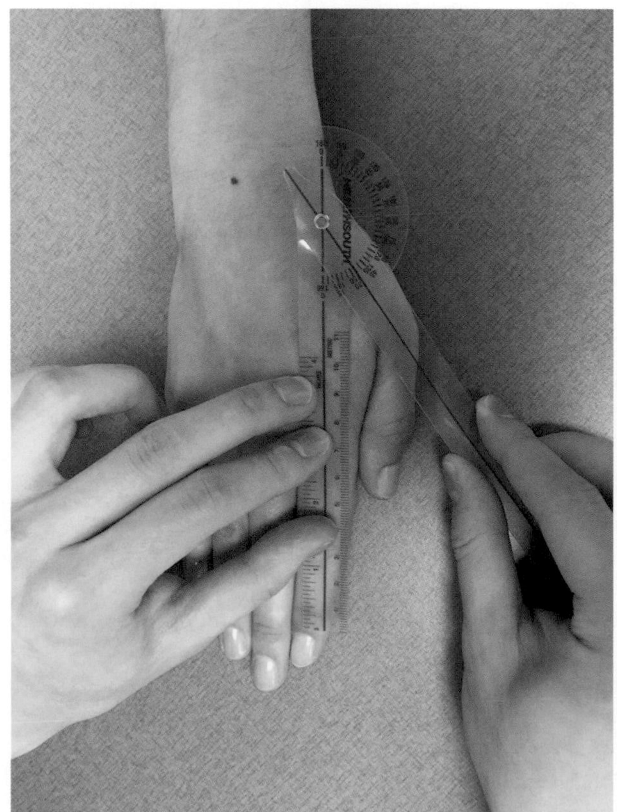

Figure 13-42. Thumb carpometacarpal extension/radial abduction, start position.

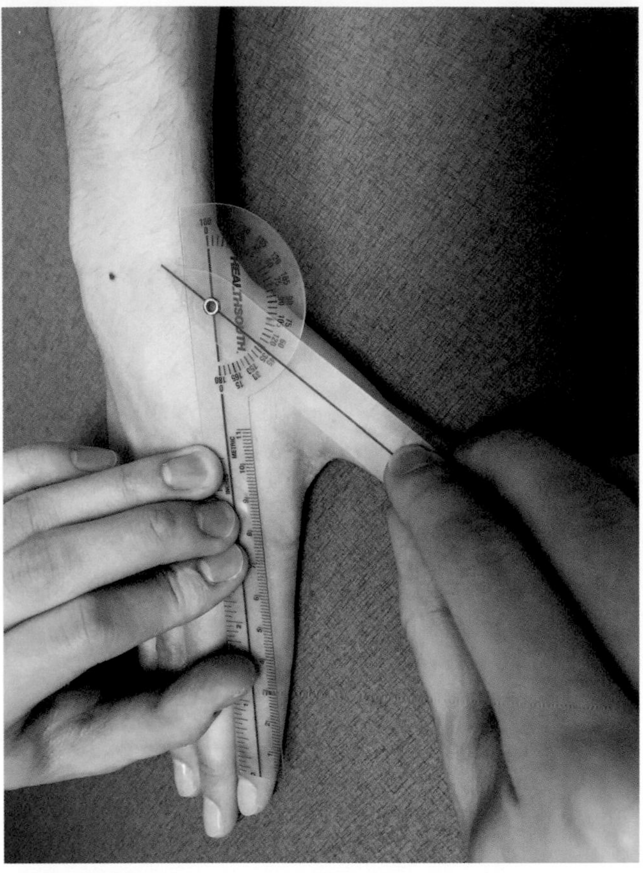

Figure 13-43. Thumb carpometacarpal extension/radial abduction, end position.

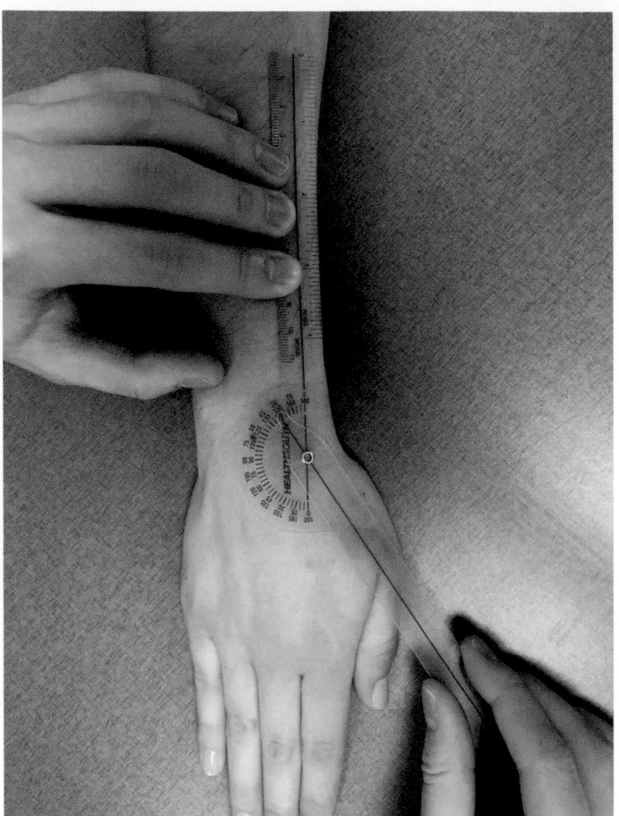

Figure 13-44. Thumb carpometacarpal extension/radial abduction, alternative method, start position.

Goniometer Placement

- *Axis:* On the dorsal side of the wrist at the junction of the base of the first metacarpal and the trapezium.
- *Stationary arm:* Parallel to the second metacarpal.
- *Movable arm:* Parallel to the first metacarpal.

Thumb Carpometacarpal Extension/Radial Abduction: Alternative Method

See Figures 13-44 and 13-45 for alternative methods.

Goniometer Placement

- *Axis:* On the dorsal side of the wrist at the junction of the base of the first metacarpal and the trapezium.
- *Stationary arm:* Parallel to the longitudinal axis of the radius.
- *Movable arm:* Parallel to the longitudinal axis of the first metacarpal.

Thumb Carpometacarpal Abduction/Palmar Abduction (0°–50°)

Movement of the thumb perpendicular to the palm in the sagittal plane (Figs. 13-46 and 13-47).

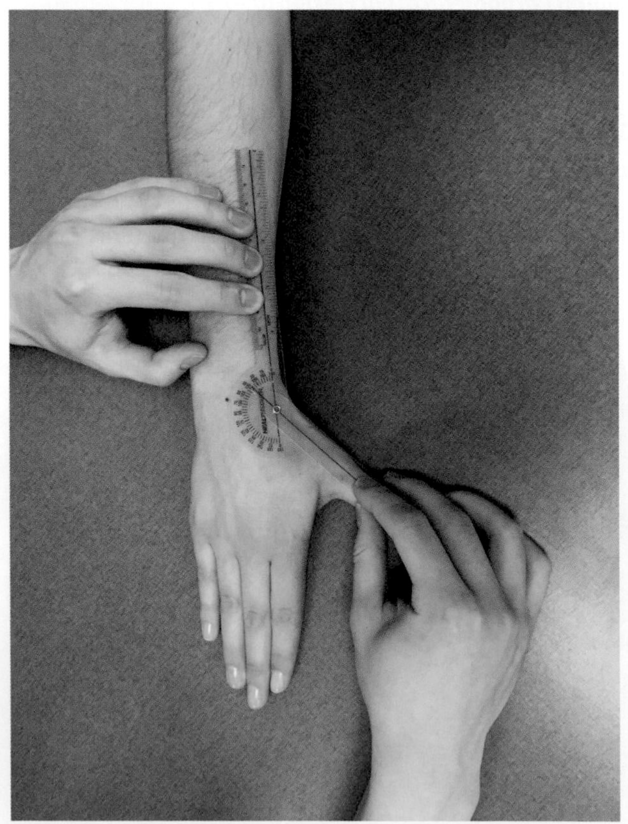

Figure 13-45. Thumb carpometacarpal extension/radial abduction, alternative method, end position.

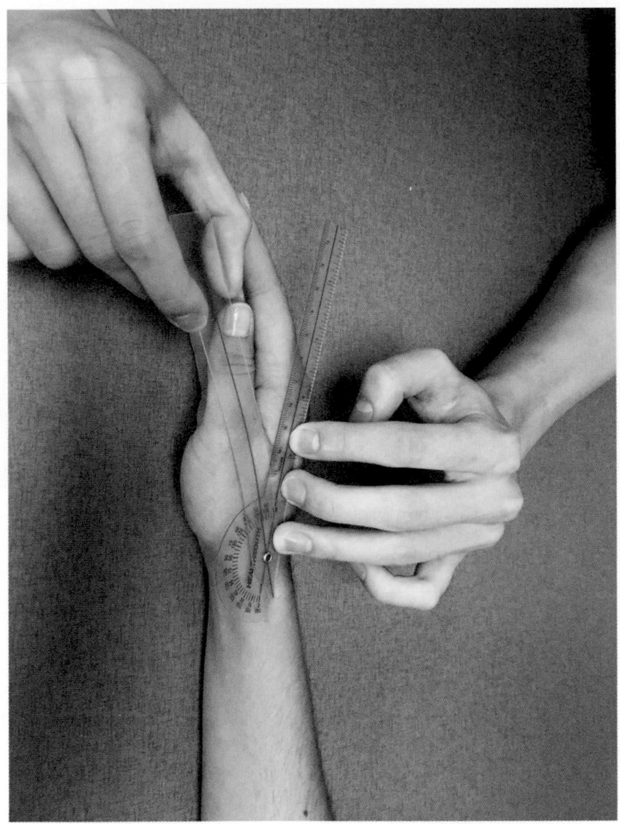

Figure 13-46. Thumb carpometacarpal abduction/palmar abduction, start position.

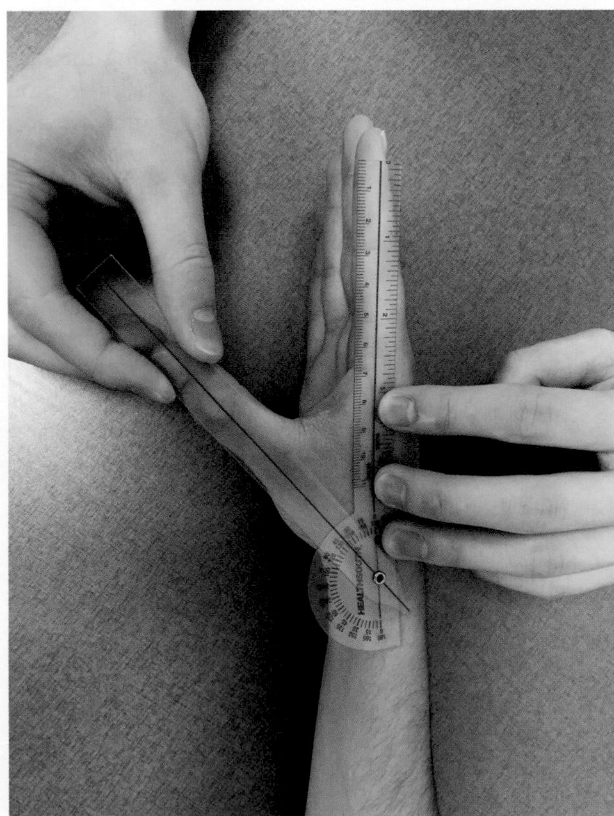

Figure 13-47. Thumb carpometacarpal abduction/palmar abduction, end position.

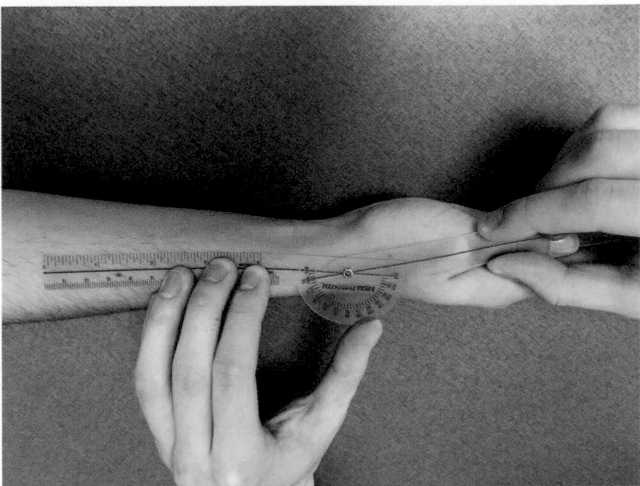

Figure 13-48. Thumb carpometacarpal abduction/palmar abduction, alternative method, start position.

Goniometer Placement

- *Axis:* On the radial side of the wrist at the junction of the base of the first metacarpal and the trapezium.
- *Stationary arm:* On the radial surface parallel to the second metacarpal.
- *Movable arm:* Parallel to the first metacarpal.

Thumb Carpometacarpal Abduction/Palmar Abduction: Alternative Method

See Figures 13-48 and 13-49 for alternative methods.

Goniometer Placement

- *Axis:* On the radial side of the wrist at the junction of the base of the first metacarpal and the trapezium.
- *Stationary arm:* Parallel to the longitudinal axis of the radius.

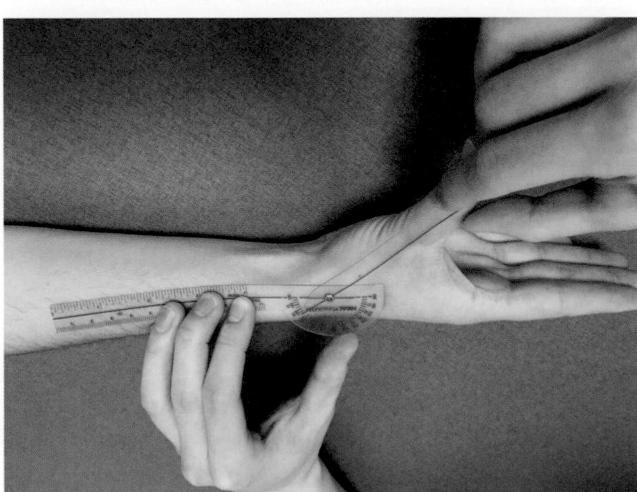

Figure 13-49. Thumb carpometacarpal abduction/palmar abduction, alternative method, end position.

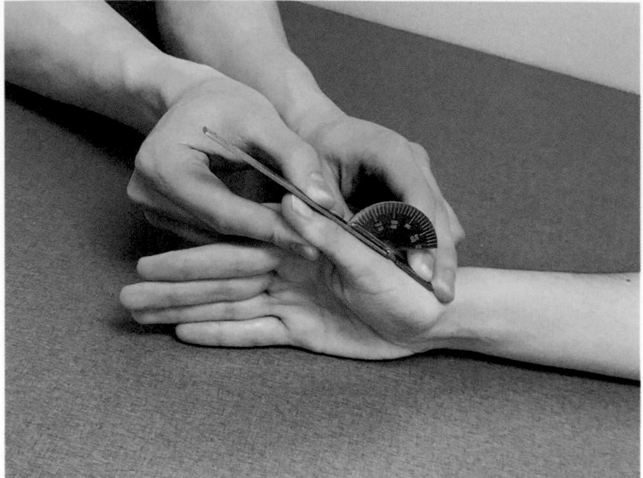

Figure 13-50. Thumb metacarpophalangeal flexion, start position (extension).

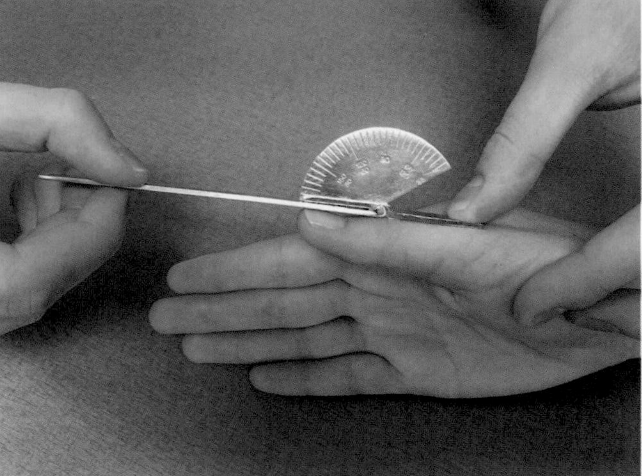

Figure 13-52. Thumb interphalangeal flexion, start position (extension).

- *Movable arm:* Parallel to the longitudinal axis of the first metacarpal.

Thumb Metacarpophalangeal Extension–Flexion (0°–50°)

Movement of the thumb across the palm in the frontal plane (Figs. 13-50 and 13-51).

Goniometer Placement

- *Axis:* On the dorsal aspect of the metacarpophalangeal (MP) joint.
- *Stationary arm:* On the dorsal surface along the midline of the first metacarpal.
- *Movable arm:* On the dorsal surface along the midline of the proximal phalanx of the thumb.

Thumb Interphalangeal Extension–Flexion (0°–80°)

Movement of the distal phalanx of the thumb toward the volar surface of the proximal phalanx of the thumb (Figs. 13-52 and 13-53).

Goniometer Placement

- *Axis:* On the dorsal aspect of the interphalangeal (IP) joint.
- *Stationary arm:* On the dorsal surface along the proximal phalanx.
- *Movable arm:* On the dorsal surface along the distal phalanx. (*Note:* If the thumbnail prevents full goniometer contact, shift the arms laterally to increase accuracy. Also, thumb MP and IP flexion and extension can be measured on the lateral aspect of the thumb using lateral aspects of the same landmarks.)

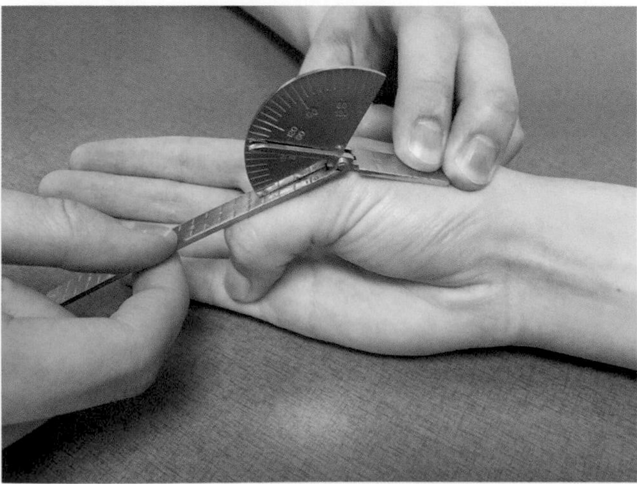

Figure 13-51. Thumb metacarpophalangeal flexion, end position.

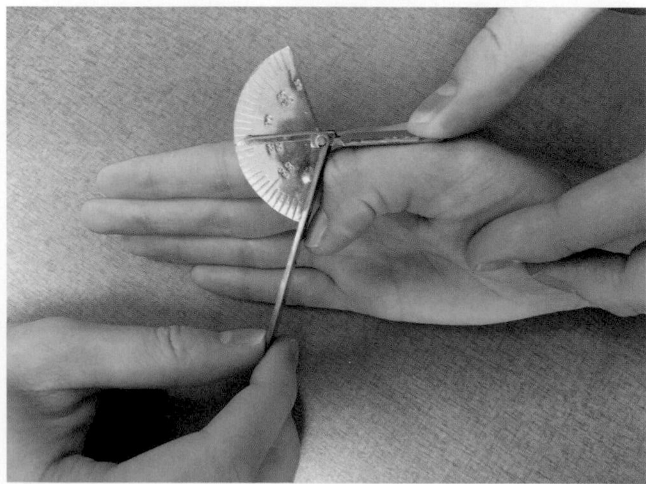

Figure 13-53. Thumb interphalangeal flexion, end position.

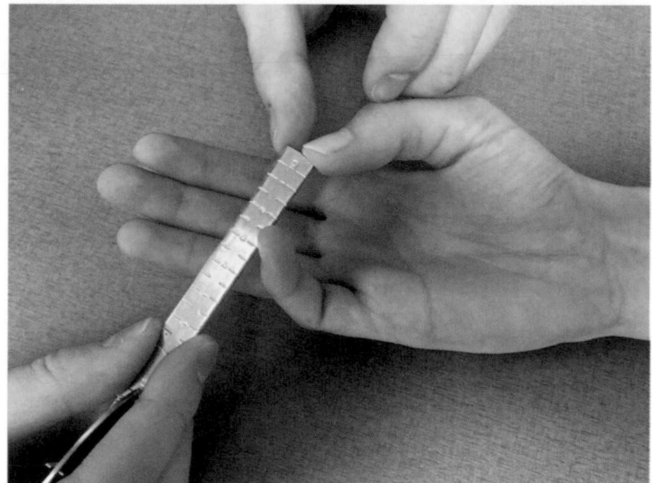

Figure 13-54. Measurement of opposition to the little finger using a centimeter ruler.

Opposition: Ruler Measurements

The pad of the thumb rotates to meet the pad of each finger. The little finger rotates to better meet the pad of the thumb. As a summary measure of opposition, record the distance from the tip of the thumb pad (not the thumbnail) to the tip end of the little finger (Fig. 13-54) or base of the little finger.

Finger Metacarpophalangeal Extension–Flexion

See Table 13-1 for ROM norms for fingers. Movement of the finger at the MP joint toward the palmar surface of the hand (Figs. 13-55 and 13-56 and Table 13-1). Hyperextension is normal at this joint.

Goniometer Placement

- *Axis:* On the dorsal aspect of the MP joint of the finger being measured.

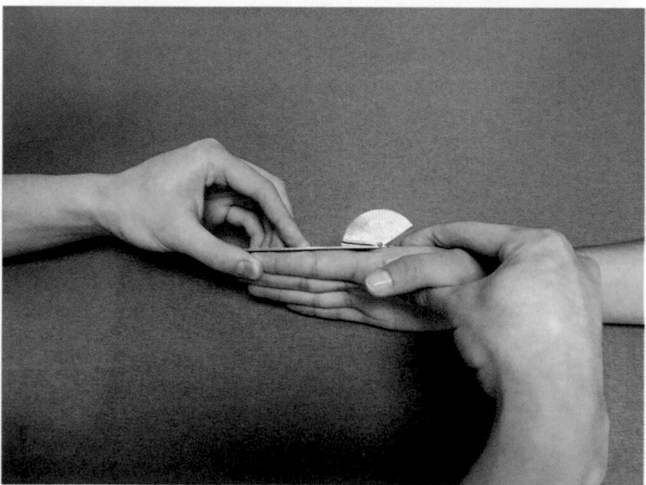

Figure 13-55. Finger metacarpophalangeal flexion, start position (extension).

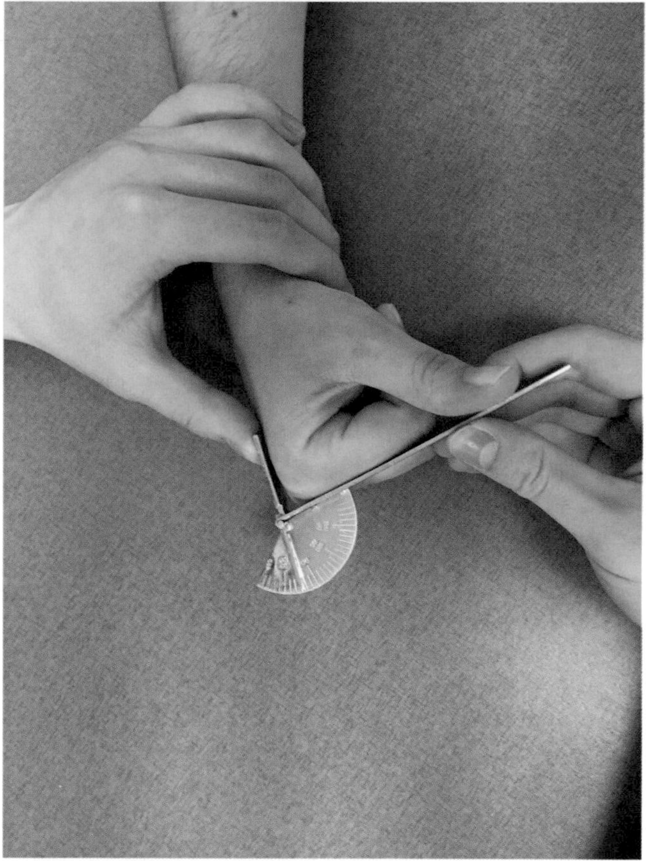

Figure 13-56. Finger metacarpophalangeal flexion, end position.

- *Stationary arm:* On the dorsal surface along the midline of the metacarpal of the finger being measured.
- *Movable arm:* On the dorsal surface along the midline of the proximal phalanx of the finger being measured.

Finger Metacarpophalangeal Hyperextension

Movement of the finger at the MP joint toward the dorsal surface of the hand (Figs. 13-57 and 13-58 and Table 13-1). The IP joints remain extended.[19,20]

Table 13-1. Range of Motion Norms for Fingers

	INDEX	LONG	RING	SMALL
Metacarpophalangeal flexion	0°–86°	0°–91°	0°–99°	0°–105°
Metacarpophalangeal hyperextension	0°–22°	0°–18°	0°–23°	0°–19°
Proximal interphalangeal flexion	0°–102°	0°–105°	0°–108°	0°–106°
Distal interphalangeal flexion	0°–72°	0°–71°	0°–63°	0°–65°

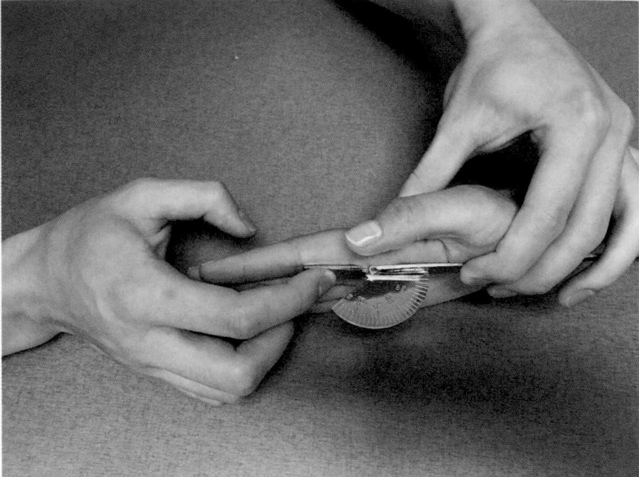

Figure 13-57. Finger metacarpophalangeal hyperextension, start position.

Goniometer Placement

- *Axis:* On the volar aspect of the MP joint of the finger being measured.
- *Stationary arm:* On the volar surface along the midline of the metacarpal of the finger being measured.
- *Movable arm:* On the volar surface along the midline of the proximal phalanx of the finger being measured.

Finger Proximal Interphalangeal Extension–Flexion

Movement of the middle phalanx toward the palmar surface of the proximal phalanx (Figs. 13-59 and 13-60 and Table 13-1).

Goniometer Placement

- *Axis:* On the dorsal aspect of the proximal interphalangeal (PIP) joint of the finger being measured.

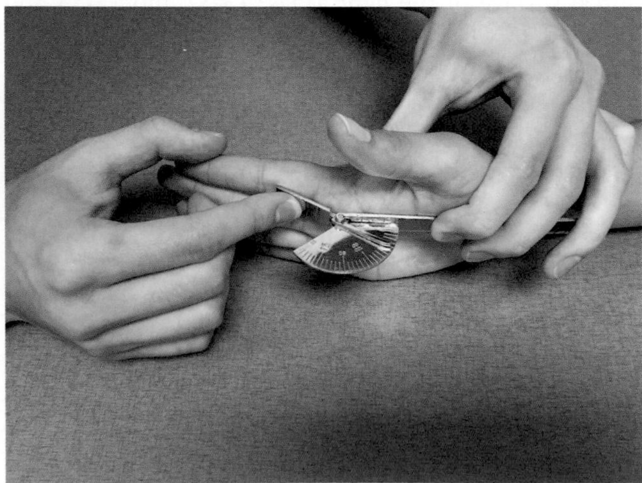

Figure 13-58. Finger metacarpophalangeal hyperextension, end position.

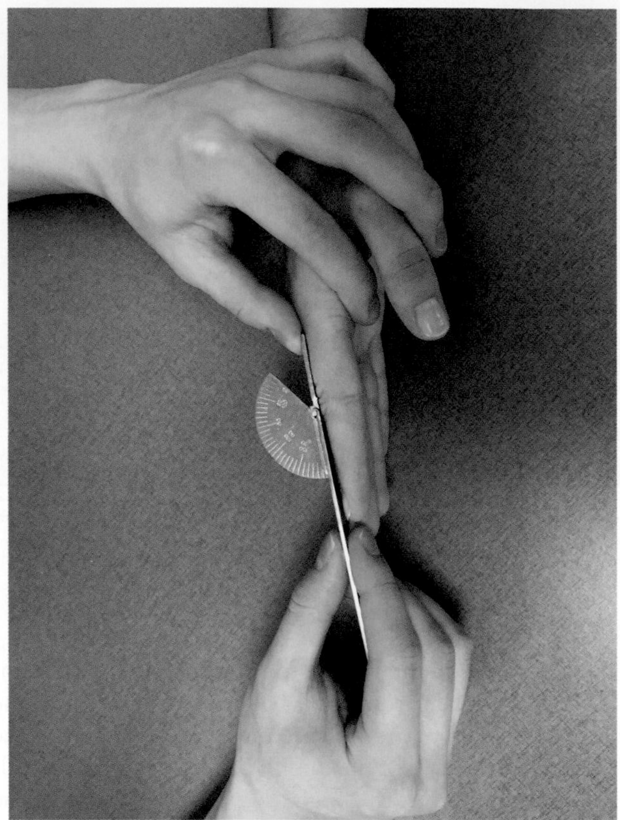

Figure 13-59. Proximal interphalangeal flexion, start position (extension).

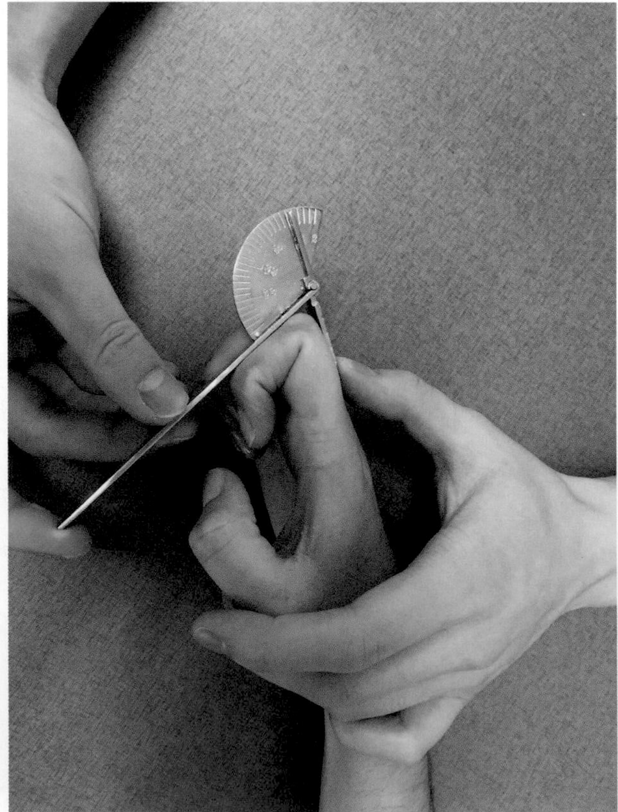

Figure 13-60. Proximal interphalangeal flexion, end position.

- *Stationary arm:* On the dorsal surface along the midline of the proximal phalanx of the finger being measured.
- *Movable arm:* On the dorsal surface along the midline of the middle phalanx of the finger being measured.

Finger Distal Interphalangeal Extension–Flexion

Movement of the distal phalanx toward the palmar surface of the middle phalanx (Figs. 13-61 and 13-62 and Table 13-1).

Goniometer Placement

- *Axis:* On the dorsal aspect of the distal interphalangeal (DIP) joint of the finger being measured.
- *Stationary arm:* On the dorsal surface along the midline of the middle phalanx of the finger being measured.
- *Movable arm:* On the dorsal surface along the midline of the distal phalanx of the finger being measured. (*Note:* If the fingernail prevents full goniometer contact, shift the arms laterally to increase accuracy. Finger PIP and DIP flexion and extension can be measured from the lateral aspect of each finger using the lateral aspect of the same landmarks. This method may be more accurate when joints are enlarged or when there is diffuse edema noted along the digit.)

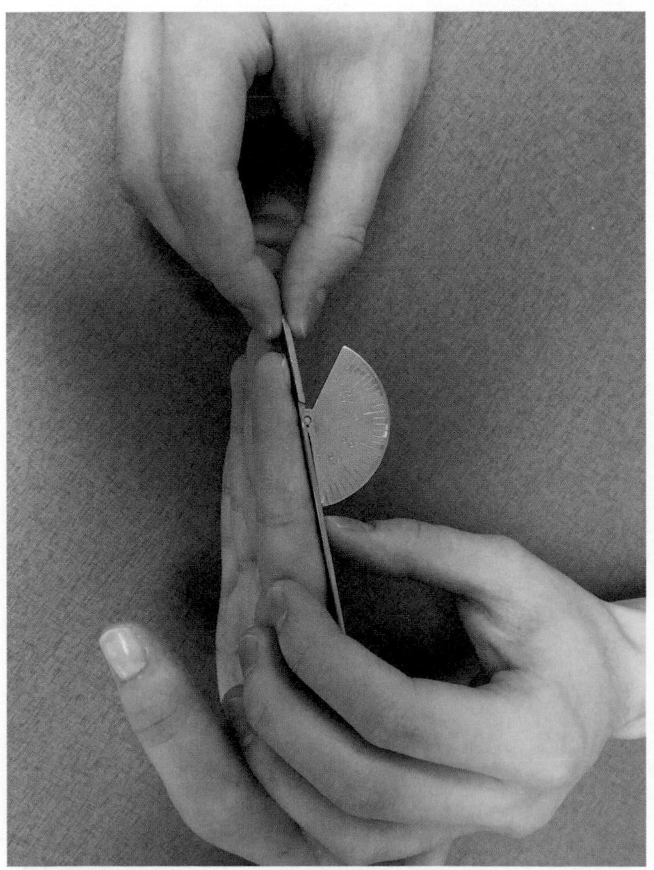

Figure 13-61. Distal interphalangeal flexion, start position (extension).

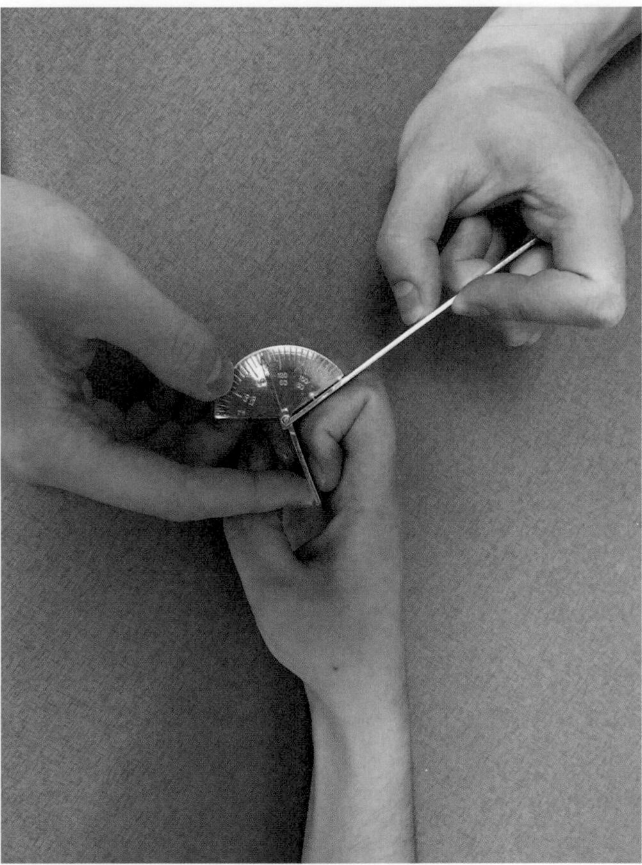

Figure 13-62. Distal interphalangeal flexion, end position.

Composite Measurement and Recording of Total Finger Flexion

A method of recording composite digital motion used by hand therapists is to sum the values for the degrees of flexion motion of the MP, PIP, and DIP joints, taking into consideration extension deficits.[23] Total active motion (TAM) or total passive motion (TPM) can then be expressed by a single number. The formula for calculating these values is as follows: (MP + PIP + DIP flexion) − (MP + PIP + DIP extension deficits) = TAM or TPM.

Another method for measuring combined flexion of the PIP and DIP joints or combined flexion of the MP, PIP, and DIP joints using a centimeter ruler is illustrated in Figures 13-63 and 13-64.

Finger Abduction and Adduction

Movement of the index, ring, and little fingers away from (abduction) (Fig. 13-65) or toward (adduction) the midline of the hand in a frontal plane. The middle finger, which is the midline of the hand, abducts in both radial and ulnar directions.

The AAOS[19] does not provide norms for this movement. Instead, the examiner measures the distance from the tip of the index finger to the tip of the little finger.

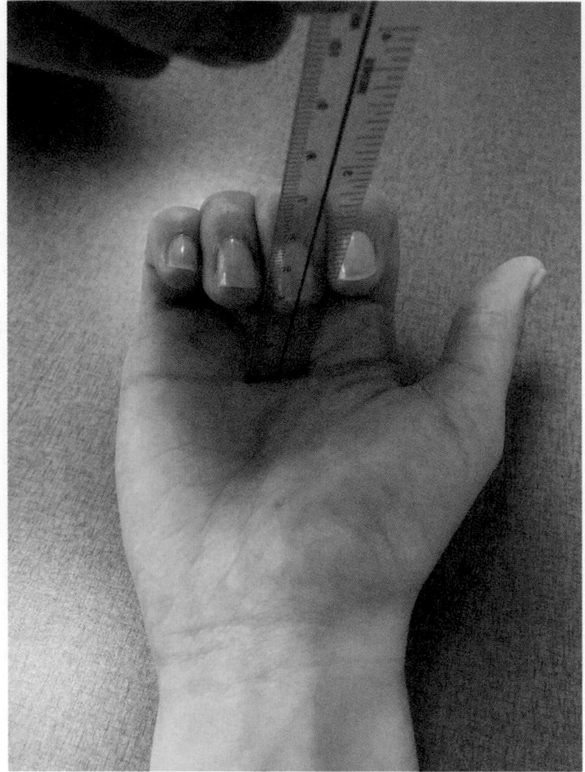

Figure 13-63. Proximal and distal interphalangeal combined finger flexion; ruler measurement placed at the distal palmar crease.

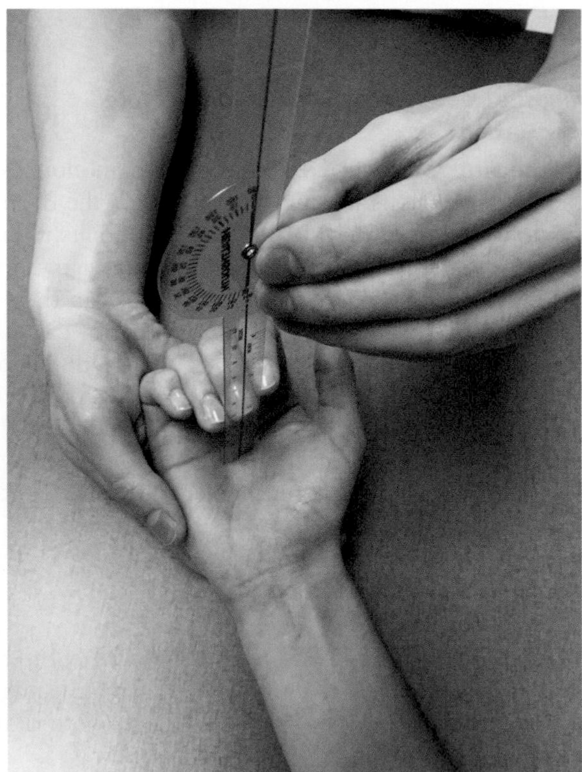

Figure 13-64. Metacarpophalangeal and proximal and distal interphalangeal combined finger flexion; ruler measurement placed at the proximal palmar crease.

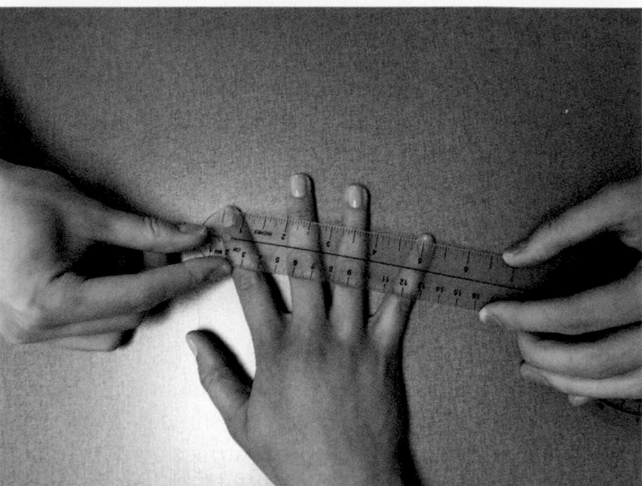

Figure 13-65. Finger abduction and adduction, ruler measurement.

The distance between individual fingers can be measured from tip to tip also. Because there are no norms for this movement, the measurements are used to measure progress only.

Metacarpophalangeal Deviation Correction Measurement

When there is ulnar deviation deformity of the MP joints, often seen in rheumatoid arthritis, this additional measurement is taken (Figs. 13-66 and 13-67).

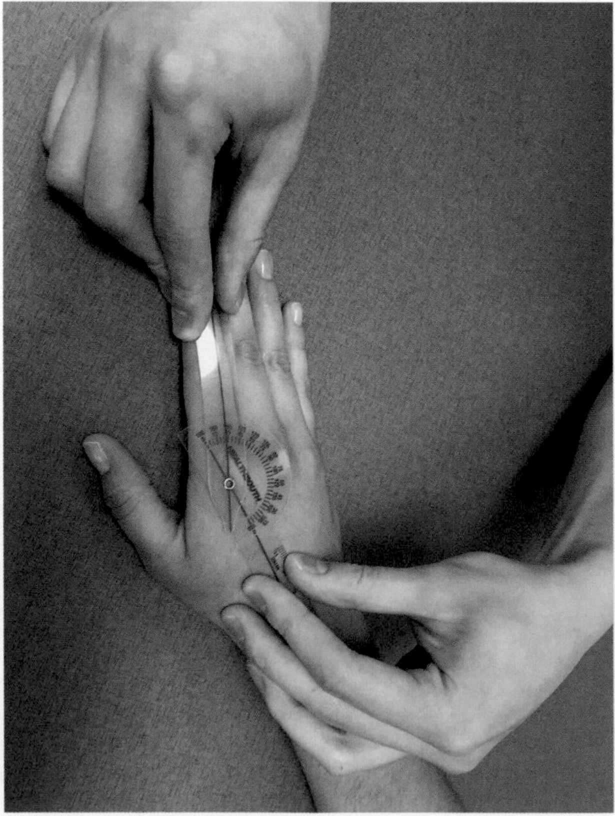

Figure 13-66. Metacarpophalangeal deviation correction, start position.

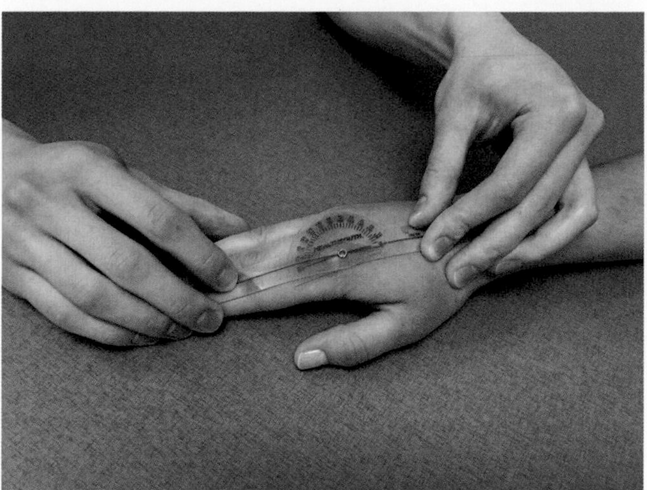

Figure 13-67. Metacarpophalangeal deviation correction, end position.

The AROM is compared with the PROM to determine whether muscle weakness is present. PROM is compared with the norm of 0° deviation to determine whether a fixed deformity exists.

Goniometer Placement

- *Axis:* Over the MP joint of the finger being measured.
- *Stationary arm:* Placed along the dorsal midline of the metacarpal.
- *Movable arm:* Placed along the dorsal midline of the proximal phalanx.

Accuracy

The therapist must place the axis and arms appropriately to ensure accuracy and reliability. The specific placement of the goniometer for each joint is described and demonstrated in this chapter. In addition to goniometer placement, multiple client-related and environmental factors can affect accuracy and reliability of ROM measurements. Client-related factors include pain, fear of pain, fatigue, and feelings of stress or tension. For the most accurate and reliable results, every effort should be taken to make the client physically and emotionally comfortable, including talking to the client and describing the procedure that is to follow. Environmental factors include time of day, temperature of the room, type of goniometer used, and training and experience of the tester. However, owing to the effect of various factors influencing ROM measurements, clinicians should adopt standardized methods of testing and should interpret and report goniometric results as ROM measurements only, not as measurements of factors that may affect ROM.[24]

Intrarater reliability is consistently higher than is interrater reliability for ROM testing using a universal goniometer. Intrarater reliability refers to *one* therapist consistently measuring the same joint angle over multiple trials, whereas interrater reliability concerns *multiple* therapists consistently measuring the same joint angle. It is advantageous to have the same therapist measuring a client's ROM repeatedly over time, rather than have multiple therapists, whenever possible.

AROM measurements are more reliable than are PROM ones. PROM measurements have the potential to be less reliable because of variability of the applied force.[24] This may be due to the position of the client affecting ROM. Therefore, therapists should record the testing position, and the same position should be used each time the client is retested.[25]

There are innovative instruments for measuring ROM. Clinicians must evaluate the efficacy and clinical utility of each as they arise. For example, the digital goniometer has adequate concurrent criterion-related validity as a tool for assessment of joint ROM and equivalent interrater and intrarater reliability to the universal goniometer. User surveys indicated that several of the novel features of the digital goniometer contributed to a higher likelihood that the device would be used by clinicians.[26] In addition, applications installed on smartphones are becoming more of a viable substitute for using a universal goniometer or an inclinometer. Research has shown that smartphone-based goniometers can yield the same accurate results of angular changes when compared to multiple examiners.[27] In another study, smartphone applications and visual inspection measurements of the finger joints with the radiographic measurements determined interrater reliability for these measurement tools agree and correlate well.[28] These studies suggest that new smartphone applications hold promise for providing accurate and reliable measures of ROM.

It is commonly believed that experience plays a major role in the reliability of ROM measurements. Increasing amounts of practice is an effective strategy for improving the accuracy of ROM measurements.[29] Thus, interrater reliability may be most dependent on practice.

Recording Range of Motion

Depending on the facility, ROM may be documented electronically or on paper, making it a part of the medical record and a legal document. This form should include the date that the measurements were taken, whether the measurements represent AROM or PROM, the starting and ending position for each movement, whether the right versus the left side was tested, and the physical or electronic signature of the therapist performing the measurements. A sample form is provided in Figure 13-68. When reading the goniometer, always state your results as a range using two numbers. The first number is the

Patient's Name ____________________

Type of motion: AROM ______

PROM ______

LEFT | RIGHT

Date	Date	Joint To Be Measured		Date	Date
		Shoulder			
		Flexion	0–180		
		Extension	0–60		
		Abduction	0–180		
		Horizontal abduction	0–45		
		Horizontal adduction	0–140		
		Internal rotation	0–70		
		External rotation	0–90		
		Internal rotation (alt)	0–90		
		External rotation (alt)	0–60		
		Elbow and Forearm			
		Flexion–extension	0–150		
		Supination	0–80		
		Pronation	0–80		
		Wrist			
		Flexion	0–80		
		Extension	0–70		
		Ulnar deviation	0–30		
		Radial deviation	0–20		
		Thumb			
		CM flexion	0–15		
		CM extension	0–20		
		MP flexion–extension	0–50		
		IP flexion–extension	0–80		
		Palmar Abduction	0–70		
		Radial Abduction	0–80		
		Opposition cm.			
		Index Finger			
		MP flexion	0–90		
		PIP flexion–extension	0–100		
		DIP flexion–extension	0–90		
		Abduction	no norm		
		Adduction	no norm		
		Middle Finger			
		MP flexion	0–90		
		PIP flexion–extension	0–100		
		DIP flexion–extension	0–90		
		Abduction	no norm		
		Adduction	no norm		
		Ring Finger			
		MP flexion	0–90		
		PIP flexion–extension	0–100		
		DIP flexion–extension	0–90		
		Abduction	no norm		
		Adduction	no norm		
		Little Finger			
		MP flexion	0–90		
		PIP flexion–extension	0–100		
		DIP flexion–extension	0–90		
		Abduction	no norm		
		Adduction	no norm		

Therapist's signature: ____________________

Figure 13-68. Sample range of motion recording form.

starting position of the extremity, and the second number is the limit of motion at end range. At reevaluation, compare the initial evaluation measurements to evaluate progress.

The most common method of determining ROM is the neutral zero method recommended by the Committee on Joint Motion of the AAOS.[19] The ROM normative data presented in this chapter is from the AAOS, as well as the AMA.[20] It is important to note that other sources have documented these averages differently, and these sources may be seen in practice as well. In the neutral zero method, the anatomical position is considered to be "0°" (zero start), or if a given starting position is different from anatomical position, it is defined as "0°." Measurement is taken from the stated starting position to the stated end position. If the client cannot achieve the stated starting and end positions, the actual starting and end positions are recorded to indicate limitations in movement. An example using elbow flexion is as follows:

0° to 150°: No limitation
20° to 150°: A limitation in extension (problem with the start position)
0° to 120°: A limitation in flexion (problem with the end position)
20° to 120°: Limitations in flexion and extension (problems with start and end positions)

To record hyperextension of a joint, which may be occasionally seen in MP and elbow joints, the AAOS recommends a separate measurement to describe the available ROM without confusion. For example, if 20° of elbow hyperextension (an unnatural movement) is noted, it should be recorded as follows:

0° to 150° of flexion
0° of extension
0° to 20° of hyperextension

If a joint is fused, the starting and end positions are the same, with no ROM. This is recorded as "fused at X°." If a joint that normally moves in two directions cannot move in one direction, the ROM-limited motion is recorded. For example, if wrist flexion is 15° to 80° with a 15° flexion contracture, the wrist cannot be positioned at zero or be moved into extension; therefore, wrist extension is −15° or a 15° extension lag.

Because there are various systems of notations, each having its own meaning, it is important to clarify the intended meaning to ensure consistency among therapists and physicians within the same facility.

Interpreting the Results

The initial evaluation is interpreted by reviewing the recording form to identify which joints have significant limitation. A significant limitation is one that decreases occupational functioning or may lead to deformity. Limits of motion scores can be used in several ways. The therapist can compare the scores of the involved to the uninvolved extremity. Some ranges of motion are different between dominant and nondominant sides; however, when these differences exist, they are minimal and may not be clinically significant. These results support the practice of using the opposite side of the body as an indicator of movement experienced preinjury or normal extremity ROM.[30] Another way in which to assess limitations of motion is to compare the client's scores with the average limits (norms) expected for each motion. The average limits stated by the Committee on Joint Motion of the AAOS[19] are commonly used and are included in this chapter with the directions for ROM of each joint.

The emphasis in occupational therapy is to enable occupational functioning. It is important to note that clients may be functional with less ROM than is noted in the norms for particular joints. A recent study quantified the motion requirements for the full upper limb and trunk during ADLs in healthy adults.[31] ROMs found in Gates et al. for the shoulder, elbow, and wrist were similar to those published previously.[32] The results of these studies justify clinicians' comparison of their clients' ROM with functional norms to evaluate impairments or assess the effects of interventions.

Comparing initial evaluation scores to mid- and posttreatment scores is important to assess the outcome and redirect treatment, if necessary. Interpretation of a reevaluation that shows improvement following treatment must be tempered with the realization that changes may occur because of instrumentation and procedures, differences among joint actions and body regions, passive versus active measurements, intrarater versus interrater measurements, and different client types.[24] For example, for ROM measurements to reflect actual change, the amount of change must exceed measurement error, which was found to be 5° for both the UEs and LEs.[33] Thus, an increase of 10° in shoulder flexion is considered an improvement, but 5° may be accounted for by measurement error.

Edema

Volumetric Measurement

Edema is one cause of limited ROM that can be quantified. Volumetric measures document changes in the mass of a body part by use of water displacement and is most often used to measure arm and hand edema. A water vessel that is large enough to allow submersion of the whole hand is used, as shown in Figure 13-69, and one that can be used to assess the whole arm is shown in Figure 13-70. When the limb is placed in the vessel, water is displaced and spills out into a collection beaker via the spout near the top and is then measured with a graduated cylinder. An edematous limb displaces more water

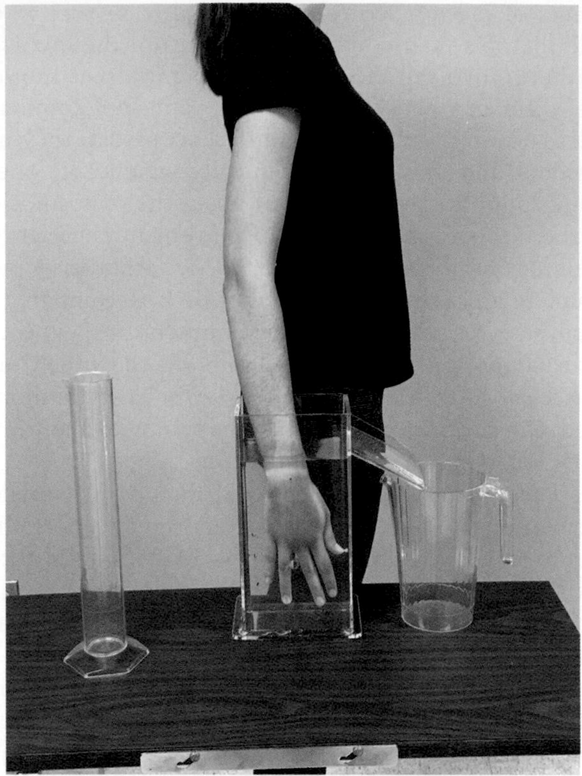

Figure 13-69. Measuring edema of the hand using a volumeter. Note the water being displaced into the graduated beaker as the hand is submerged.

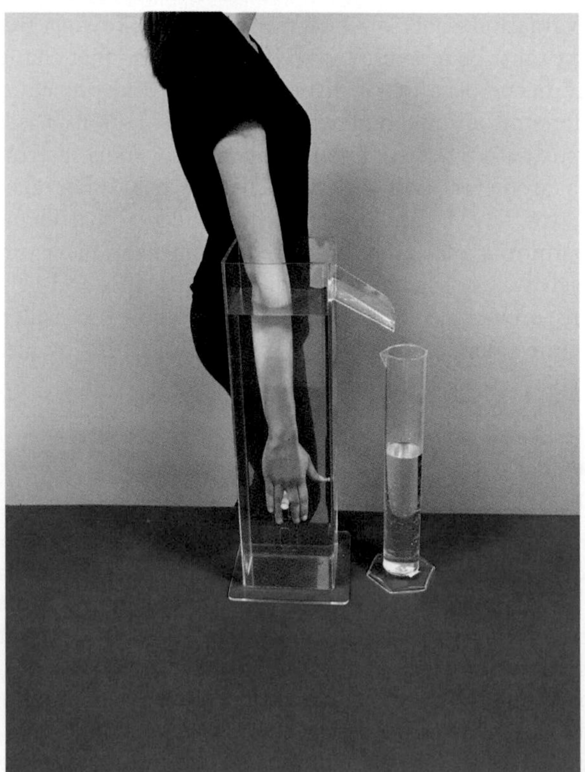

Figure 13-70. Measuring edema of the hand and arm using a volumeter. Note the water being displaced into the graduated beaker as the hand and are submerged.

than does a limb without swelling, so a lower reading is considered an improvement.

Precaution should be used with volumetry measurements. Immersing the hand in water is sometimes contraindicated, such as with open wounds or skin conditions, immediately postoperatively, with percutaneous pinning and external fixation devices, healing skin grafts, and suspicion of infection. It is also inappropriate if having the extremity in the dependent position during testing significantly increases pain and edema or if spasticity or paralysis impacts the measurement.[34]

Dodds et al.[34] examined therapists' ability to orient the extremity consistently within the volumeter and to measure the displaced water accurately. Following this protocol in the clinic setting, the therapist should follow the steps outlined in Box 13-3.

Box 13-3

Steps for Volumetry Measurements

1. An adjustable table should be set at a height that allows the client to keep the shoulder in neutral position when placing the hand in the volumeter on the tabletop. The therapist should ensure that the volumeter is stable, and the table is level.
2. The volumeter should be filled with room-temperature water to the point of overflow. Any excess water should be wiped out of the collection beaker.
3. The client should be positioned parallel to the volumeter with the volar forearm and palm of the hand facing his or her body. The client should stand to the side of the table that will allow his or her thumb to face the spout of the volumeter.
4. The client should be instructed to note the dowel in the volumeter and slowly lower his or her hand into the volumeter at a rate that allows the water to collect in the beaker below the spout until the web space between the third and fourth digits rests on the dowel and the water stops dripping. Tell the client to avoid touching the sides of the volumeter during the test.
5. The therapist should stand behind the client to support the trunk and prevent any rotation or leaning and can provide verbal cues to the client to prevent excess motion and ensure the hand is properly positioned. Instruct the client to remain silent until the test is complete to avoid motion from talking.
6. After the client removes his or her hand from the volumeter and dries it (provide a towel), the therapist uses the graduated cylinder to measure the amount of displaced water to the nearest 5 mL. The use of a 10-mL micropipette allows the therapist to measure the displaced water to the nearest 1 mL, thereby increasing accuracy. Occasionally, if more water is displaced than the cylinder will hold, multiple graduated cylinders will be needed, or the graduated cylinder must be dried out, and the remaining water measured and added.

To improve the reliability of volumetric measurement, modifications to the abovementioned instructions can include measurement of displaced water volume by means of a digital scale, utilization of a 3D anatomical marking system, and repositioning of the overflow spout and addition of a flow gate to a standard volumetric tank.[35]

If edema is found to be present, the short-term goal of treatment may be to decrease edema more than 10 mL, which is more than the standard error of measurement of less than 3 mL. However, it is important to remember the reasoning behind wanting the decrease in edema. The entire short-term goal may be written as, "The client will demonstrate a 10-mL decrease in volumeter measurement of edema of the right hand in order to increase hand function with dressing tasks."

Circumferential Measurement

Another method of measuring edema is the circumferential assessment. Volumetric and circumferential measurements have been found to be positively correlated.[36] A millimeter tape is used to measure the circumference of a body part not easily submerged (as required by volumetric measurement) or when the edema is very localized (such as to a single digit, making measurement of the entire hand unnecessary). With circumferential measurements (see Fig. 13-71 for an example of circumferential measurement), it is essential to measure at exactly the same place from test to test. Using anatomical landmarks can assist in the placement, such as over the third digit PIP joint or 5 cm proximal to the ulnar styloid.

Another method of measuring edema circumferentially is the figure-of-eight technique[37] (see Fig. 13-72). This method is typically used to measure the whole hand and is based on the understanding that edema of the hand tends to collect more dorsally. Using a 1/4-inch-wide tape measure with the wrist in neutral and fingers adducted, the tape is started at the medial aspect of the wrist just distal to the ulnar styloid. The tape is then run across the volar surface of the wrist to the most distal point of the radial styloid and then run diagonally across the dorsum of the hand to the fifth MP joint. The tape is then run across the heads of the metacarpals to the second MP joint and then back across the dorsum of the hand to the starting point. The measurement recorded is the distance measured by the tape in centimeters.

The figure-of-eight measurement technique may be especially appropriate when volumetry is contraindicated. Volumetry has been correlated with the figure-of-eight method[38]; however, the figure-of-eight method is easier to use, more time efficient, and cost-effective, particularly in the intensive care unit setting.

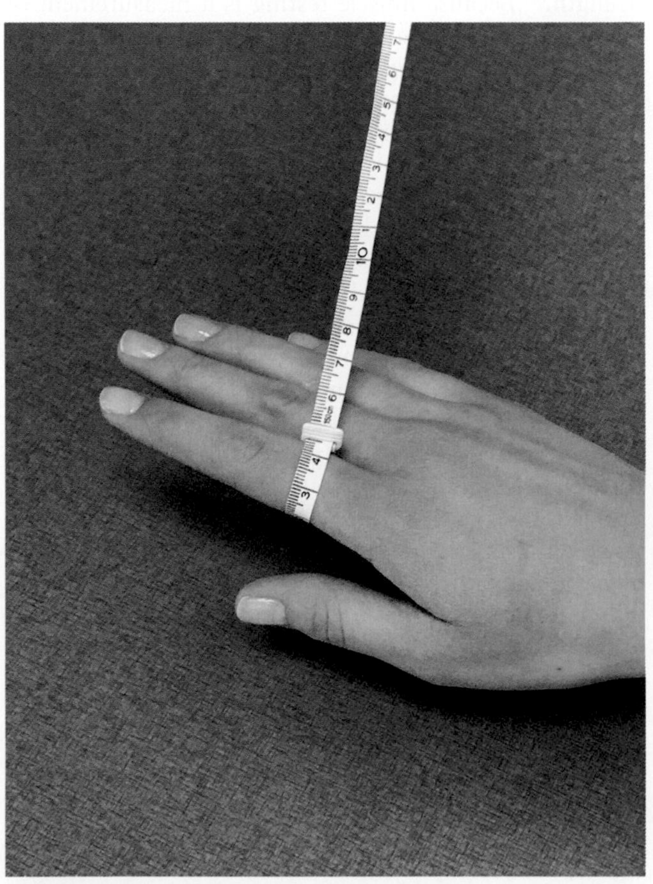

Figure 13-71. Measuring edema using circumferential method.

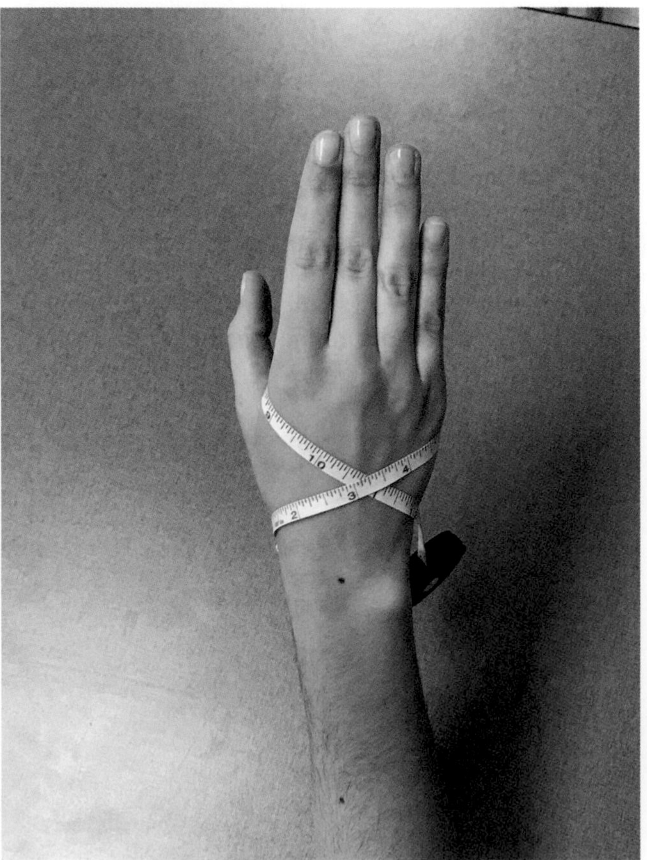

Figure 13-72. Measuring edema of the hand using the figure-of-eight method.

The perometer (see Fig. 13-73) is an optoelectronic automated method of measuring UE edema and has been shown to be a quick, hygienic, and a less operator-dependent method of limb volume assessment.[39,40] It is similar to computer-assisted tomography, but uses infrared beams to rapidly and automatically estimate limb volume. The volume of any part of the limb can be measured, the shape of the limb or limb segment can be displayed, and accurate calculations of change in volume can be made in seconds.[40] This automated method of measuring limb volume is a useful alternative in suitable clients in clinical and research applications.[39]

Typically, to interpret edema measurements, comparisons are made between the assessments of right and left limbs. It has been an accepted practice to assume that limbs are symmetrical or at least identical in volume. In fact, for the specific diagnosis of lymphedema, only a 2-cm circumferential difference or 200-mL limb volume difference must be noted.[41] When this assumption is challenged and the potential of asymmetry is considered, the next assumption is that the dominant limb is larger than the nondominant limb—with limb volume difference sometimes estimated to be up to 200 mL due to dominance.[40] Continued bilateral measurements over time are necessary to properly assess a limb volume change during follow-up evaluations, because it is important for documenting therapeutic progress.

Scar Tissue

Scar tissue, particularly scars that cross joints or run along tendons, can significantly impact motion. All wounds will heal with scar tissue, but not all scar tissue will impact motion. The size, color, and pliability of any wounds or scars should be described[42] with regard to how they affect joint motion during initial and subsequent evaluations. Typically, by manipulating the scar tissue with the fingers and pinching the skin around the scar, a therapist can determine whether any significant scar adhesions exist. Skin puckering around the scar with motion can also be a sign of adhesions. Adhesions will contribute to decreased ROM around a joint.

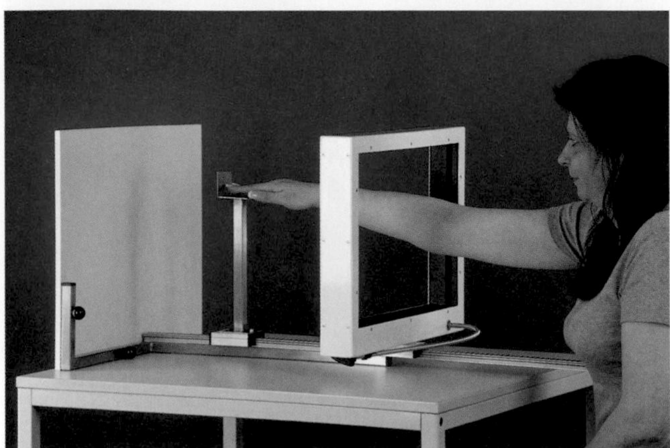

Figure 13-73. Perometer. (Picture courtesy of Pero-System Messgeraete.)

Muscle Strength Measurement

Muscular strength is the ability to perform activities that require high levels of muscular force—a key component of muscular fitness.[43] Weakness is a lack or reduction of the power in a muscle or muscle group. When weakness limits or impairs the individual's occupational functioning, determining the degree and distribution of weakness to establish an appropriate intervention plan is necessary. Treatment can be focused on remediating the weakness, or it can focus on alternative ways of accomplishing the task (compensation). Weakness can manifest in several forms. It can be general, such as being deconditioned after an illness, or it can be local, such as with a peripheral nerve lesion. In the former case, muscles throughout the body are assessed; in the latter case, just the muscles innervated by the involved nerve are tested. In both cases, the muscles to be tested are the ones contributing to the functional limitations on which treatment will focus.

A **maximum voluntary contraction** (MVC), the maximum amount of tension that can be produced under voluntary control, is commonly used to measure strength.[44] Because muscle testing is a measurement of voluntary contraction of an isolated muscle or a muscle group, strength testing is inappropriate for clients who lack the ability to contract a single muscle or a muscle group in isolation such as clients who exhibit patterned movement. For example, clients who have a difference in muscle strength due to a central nervous system event such as a stroke may exhibit patterned movement from hypertonicity. This results in a change in muscle tone that should not be tested with traditional MMT. That is, an increase in involuntary muscle tone cannot be equated with voluntary muscle contraction.

In this chapter, a technique called the "break test" is used. In the break test, the muscle to be tested is positioned at its greatest mechanical advantage and then an external force is applied. Once the extremity is positioned, the client is asked to hold the position as the tester imparts external force (i.e., his or her hand and own strength) to overcome the contractile force of the muscle or muscle group. Resistance applied at the end of the tested range is termed a *break test*. Resistance applied throughout the range is termed a *make test*.[45] The results of the strength testing differ depending on the method used. The isometric hold (break test) shows the muscle to have a higher test grade than does the resistance given throughout the range (make test). The make/break tests are both useful for assessing muscle strength and of being relatively comparable to the routine clinical strength examination.[46]

The therapist must ensure that providing resistance is not contraindicated by the diagnosis or the surgeon's orders for therapy. For example, putting resistance against a client with a healing fracture, following various surgeries such as tendon or nerve repairs, after chest/heart/lung surgery, initially after myocardial infarction, where there is a history of bone metastasis, or after recent back/neck surgery is contraindicated. Precautions should also be taken with various neurodegenerative disorders so as not to stress fatigued or weakened muscles.

The term *mechanical advantage* refers to the length–tension relationship of a muscle. The passive tension exerted by the elastic components in the lengthened muscle and surrounding tissue and the active tension generated by the contractile elements of the contracting muscle contribute to the total tension of a muscle.[47] A muscle is able to generate its greatest total tension or sustain the heaviest load when positioned at a length that gives it optimal mechanical advantage. This is usually slightly (10%) longer than resting length. Developed (active) tension, which is the total tension minus the elastic contribution, is greatest at resting length but decreases as the muscle shortens or lengthens. The length–tension principle is used to elicit the best response from prime movers, or muscles that have the sole or principle responsibility of the action, during muscle testing. Furthermore, this principle is used to reduce the contribution of synergist muscles (i.e., muscles that contribute to similar movements) when testing the prime mover (i.e., a muscle that contributes the most to a specific movement). Synergist muscles are placed at a mechanical disadvantage (either lengthened or shortened), whereas the prime mover is asked to resist the applied force.[47] For muscles or muscle groups too weak to resist an external force, muscle strength is evaluated by isotonic contraction, in which the muscle is required to move the mass of the body part against gravity without applied resistance or with the effect of gravity decreased.[48,49]

Gravity as resistance is considered an important variable and is used to test all motions when practical. Standard procedures for evaluation against gravity and with gravity eliminated are described in this chapter. Tests of the UE described here, for the most part, are motion tests for the purpose of evaluating strength in terms of functional ability. Tests of individual muscles in the wrist and hand are included because of the often increased responsibility of the occupational therapist in the rehabilitation of hand injuries. The specific movements of the face, head, neck, and trunk are important in the assessment of some clients; however, these movements are usually assessed as a whole for functional activities in many clients. Information on details of measuring these movements can be found in references listed at the end of this chapter.

Before the start of MMT, a ROM screen should be done to determine what ROM is available at each joint. Although the available range is considered to be full ROM for the purposes of muscle testing, notation should be made of any limitation. The muscle or muscle group is assigned a grade according to the amount of resistance it can take. Two grading systems are presented here: Table 13-2 equates the Medical Research Council[50] Oxford system with a descriptive grading system.[51]

Table 13-2. Muscle Testing Grading System

NUMERICAL GRADE	DESCRIPTIVE GRADE	DEFINITION
5	Normal	The part moves through full ROM against gravity and takes maximal resistance.
4	Good	The part moves through full ROM against gravity and takes moderate resistance.
4−	Good minus	The part moves through full ROM against gravity and takes less than moderate resistance.
3+	Fair plus	The part moves through full ROM against gravity and takes minimal resistance before it breaks.
3	Fair	The part moves through full ROM against gravity and is unable to take any added resistance.
3−	Fair minus	The part moves less than full range of motion against gravity.
2+	Poor plus	The part moves through full ROM in a gravity-eliminated plane, takes minimal resistance, and then breaks.
2	Poor	The part moves through full ROM in a gravity-eliminated plane with no added resistance.
2−	Poor minus	The part moves less than full ROM in a gravity-eliminated plane, no resistance.
1	Trace	Tension is palpated in the muscle or tendon, but no motion occurs at the joint.
0	Zero	No tension is palpated in the muscle or tendon, and no motion occurs.

ROM, range of motion.

The sequence of steps for testing every muscle or muscle group to ensure reliability and accuracy is outlined in Box 13-4.

There are additional considerations when performing an MMT. First, although fatigue differs for each person and each muscle, a rest of 2 minutes between maximum effort contractions of the same muscle is considered adequate.[52] Second, for the comfort and convenience of the client, all testing in one position is done before the client changes to another position.

To clarify among other systems, the scale proposed by the Medical Research Council (MRC) uses the numeral grades 0 to 5,[50] Kendall and McCreary use percentages,[49] and Daniels and Worthingham use differentiation between Normal, Good, Fair, Poor, Trace, and Zero.[48] In modified versions of the MRC scale, ROM is defined because it can be quantified more easily than resistance, even in clinical routine.[53] Another method to reflect muscle strength in general is to add together multiple measures from the MRC-sumscore which has excellent interrater reliability and is more easily assessed and sensitive when clients are bedridden or have significantly limited potential for movement.[54]

Box 13-4

Steps for Testing Every Muscle or Muscle Group

1. Explain the procedure and demonstrate the desired movement.
2. Position the client so that the direction of movement will be against gravity.
3. Stabilize proximal to the joint that will move to prevent substitutions.
4. Instruct the client to move actively to the end position. If the client cannot move actively against gravity, place the client in a gravity-eliminated position, and ask him or her to move actively in this position.
5. If the client can move actively against gravity, tell the client to hold the contraction at the desired position.
6. Apply resistance:
   a. to the distal end of the segment into which the muscle inserts
   b. in the direction the movement came from
   c. by starting with light resistance and increasing to maximal resistance over a 2- to 3-second period
7. Palpate over the prime mover to determine whether the muscle is contracting or whether gravity and/or synergistic muscles are substituting.
8. Record the appropriate grade according to the resistance tolerated before the muscle broke or by the amount of movement achieved without resistance in an against-gravity or gravity-eliminated position.

Manual Muscle Testing of the Upper Extremity

On the pages that follow, the reader will find narrative and pictorial descriptions to help in understanding and practicing measurement of UE strength.

Scapular Elevation

Prime Movers

Upper trapezius and levator scapulae.

Against-Gravity Position

- *Start position:* Client sitting erect with arms relaxed at side.
- *Stabilize:* Trunk is stabilized against the chair back.
- *Instruction:* "Lift your shoulders toward your ears like you are shrugging. Do not let me push them down."
- *Resistance:* The therapist places his or her hands over each acromion and pushes down toward scapular depression.
- *Substitution:* It could appear that the client's shoulders are elevated if he or she places hands on legs to push the shoulders into elevation (Fig. 13-74).

Gravity-Eliminated Position

- *Start position:* Prone with arms at side and therapist supporting under the shoulder.
- *Stabilize:* The trunk is stabilized against the mat or plinth.

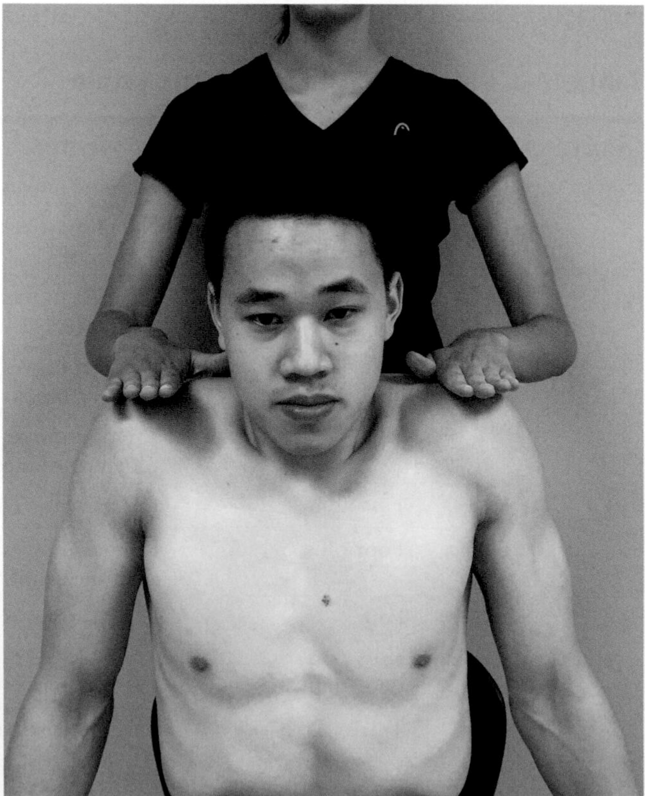

Figure 13-74. Scapular elevation against gravity.

- *Instruction:* "Lift your shoulder toward your ear."
- *Palpation:* The upper trapezius is palpated on the shoulder at the curve of the neck (Fig. 13-75). The levator scapula is palpated posterior to the sternocleidomastoid on the lateral side of the neck.

Scapular Depression

Prime Movers

Lower trapezius and latissimus dorsi.

Resistance Test

- *Start position:* This movement is tested in a gravity-eliminated position because the client cannot be positioned to move against gravity. The client lies prone with arms by the sides.
- *Stabilize:* The trunk is stabilized by the mat or plinth.
- *Instruction:* "Reach your hand down toward your feet."
- *Resistance:* The therapist's hand cups the inferior angle of the scapula; the therapist pushes up toward scapular elevation. When the inferior angle is not easily accessible because of tissue bulk, apply resistance at the distal humerus if the shoulder joint is stable and pain free.
- *Palpation:* Palpate the lower trapezius lateral to the vertebral column as it passes diagonally from the lower thoracic vertebrae to the spine of the scapula (Fig. 13-76). Palpate the latissimus dorsi along the posterior rib cage or in the posterior axilla as it attaches to the humerus.

Scapular Adduction/Retraction

Prime Movers

Middle trapezius and rhomboids.

Against-Gravity Position for the Middle Trapezius

- *Start position:* Prone with the shoulder abducted to 90° and externally rotated with the elbow flexed to 90°. Head is turned to contralateral side.

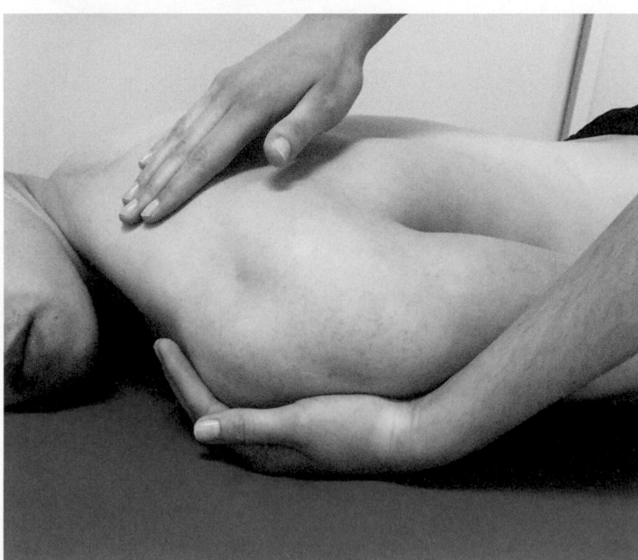

Figure 13-75. Scapular elevation, gravity eliminated.

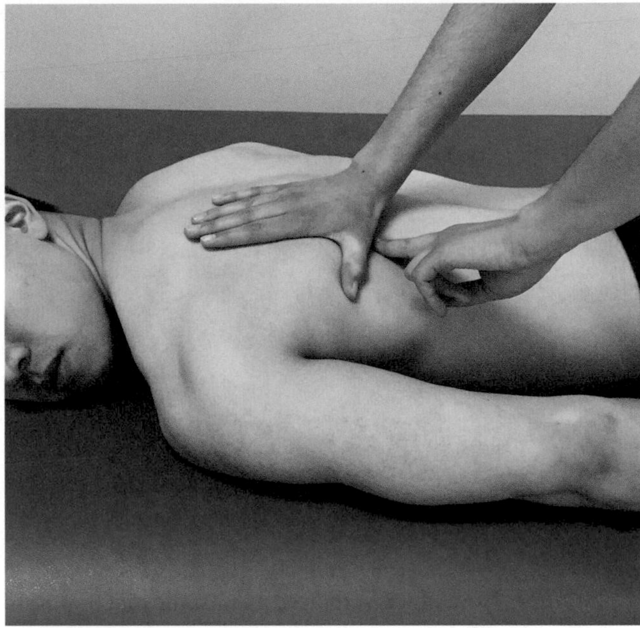

Figure 13-76. Scapular depression.

- *Stabilize:* The trunk is stabilized against the mat or plinth.
- *Instruction:* "Raise your elbow toward the ceiling. Do not let me push it down."
- *Resistance:* Apply resistance laterally at the vertebral border of the scapula or, if the shoulder is stable and pain free, apply resistance downward at the distal humerus (Fig. 13-77).

Against-Gravity Position for the Rhomboids

- *Start position:* Prone on the mat with the shoulder internally rotated and with the back of the hand resting on the lumbar region.

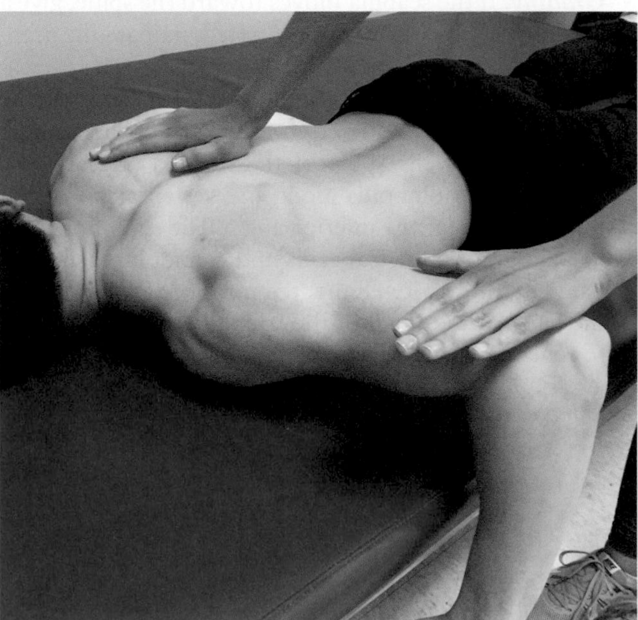

Figure 13-77. Scapular adduction against gravity, test for middle trapezius.

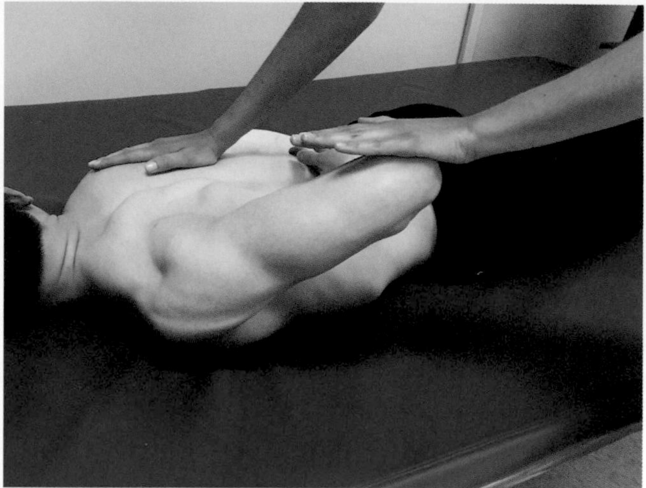

Figure 13-78. Scapular adduction against gravity, test for rhomboids.

- *Stabilize:* The trunk is stabilized against the mat or plinth.
- *Instruction:* "Lift your hand off of your back. Do not let me push it down."
- *Resistance:* Apply downward resistance against the distal humerus or, if the shoulder is unstable or painful, against the vertebral border of the scapula in the direction of scapular abduction (Fig. 13-78).

Gravity-Eliminated Position for the Middle Trapezius and Rhomboids

- *Start position:* Sitting erect with the humerus abducted to 90° and supported.
- *Stabilize:* The trunk is stabilized by the chair. Note a table or the therapist's arm can be used to support the arm of the individual being tested.
- *Instruction:* "Try to move your arm backward."
- *Grading:* If the scapula moves toward the spine, give a grade of 2. If no movement is noted, palpate the scapular adductors.
- *Palpation:* Palpate the middle trapezius between the vertebral column and vertebral border of the scapula at the level of the spine of the scapula (Fig. 13-79). Palpate the rhomboids along the vertebral border of the scapula near the inferior angle. The rhomboids are located deep to the trapezius and cannot be easily palpated in the gravity-eliminated position. Positioning of the hand in the small of the back allows the trapezius to remain relaxed so the rhomboids can be palpated.

Scapular Abduction/Protraction

Prime Mover

Serratus anterior.

Against-Gravity Position

- *Start position:* Supine with the humerus flexed to 90°. The elbow may be flexed or extended.
- *Stabilize:* The trunk is stabilized on the mat or plinth.
- *Instruction:* "Reach your arm toward the ceiling."

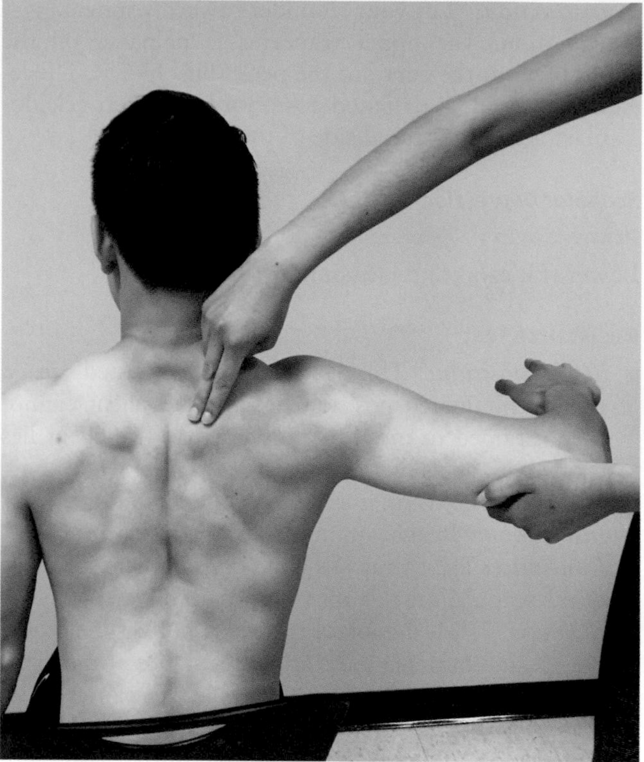

Figure 13-79. Scapular adduction, gravity eliminated. The therapist is pointing to the middle trapezius.

- *Resistance:* Resist this motion by grasping the distal humerus or by cupping the hand over the client's elbow and pushing down toward scapular adduction. If the glenohumeral joint is unstable or painful, resistance should be applied along the axillary border of the scapula (Fig. 13-80).

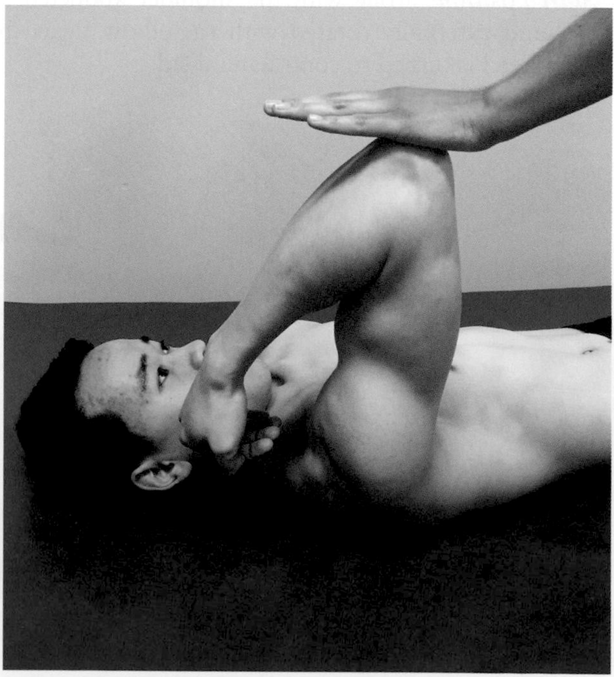

Figure 13-80. Scapular abduction against gravity.

Gravity-Eliminated Position

- *Start position:* Sitting erect with the humerus flexed to 90° and supported.
- *Stabilize:* The trunk is stabilized against the chair.
- *Instruction:* "Try to reach your arm forward."
- *Grading:* Movement of the scapula into abduction receives a grade of 2. If no movement occurs, palpate the serratus anterior.
- *Palpation:* Palpate the serratus anterior on the lateral ribs just lateral to the inferior angle of the scapula.
- *Substitution:* In the gravity-eliminated position, this motion can be achieved by inching the arm forward on a supportive surface using the fingers (Fig. 13-81).

Shoulder Flexion

Prime Movers

Anterior deltoid, coracobrachialis, pectoralis major (clavicular head), and biceps brachii.

Against-Gravity Position

- *Start position:* Sitting in a chair with the arm down at the side. Forearm in pronation to prevent substitution of the biceps brachii.
- *Stabilize:* Over the clavicle and the scapula.
- *Instruction:* "Lift your arm in front of you to shoulder height. Do not let me push it down."
- *Resistance:* The therapist's hand, placed over the distal end of the humerus, pushes down toward extension. Movement above 90° involves scapular rotation; these motions are separated for muscle testing, although they are not separated for ROM measurement.

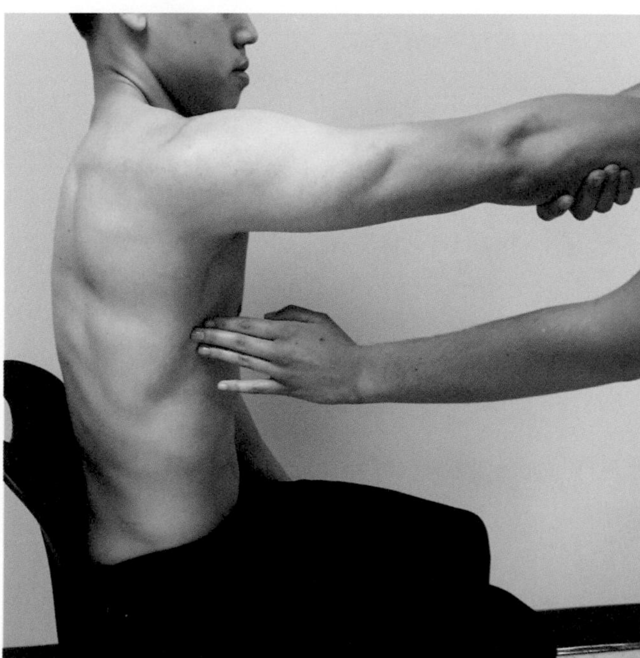

Figure 13-81. Scapular abduction, gravity eliminated.

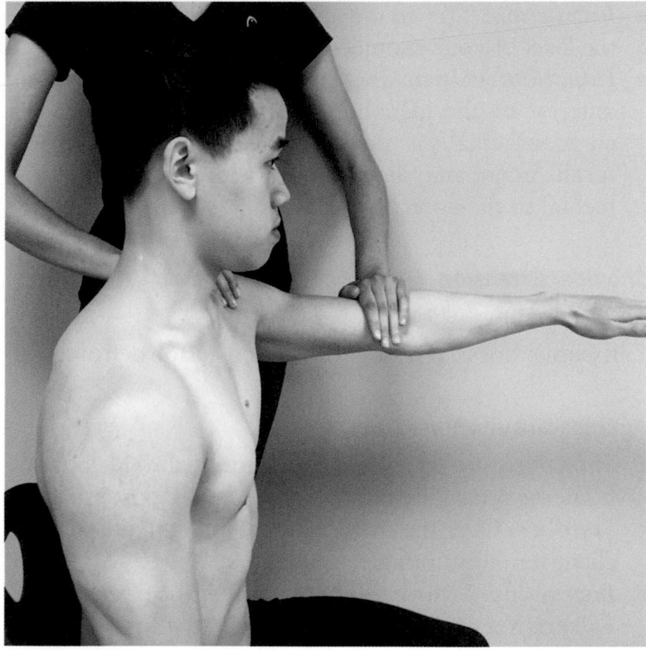

Figure 13-82. Shoulder flexion against gravity.

- *Substitutions:* Shoulder abductors, scapular elevation, or trunk extension (Fig. 13-82).

Gravity-Eliminated Position (Fig. 13-83)

- *Start position:* Lying on the side with the arm along the side of the body in neutral position; therapist supports the arm under the elbow.

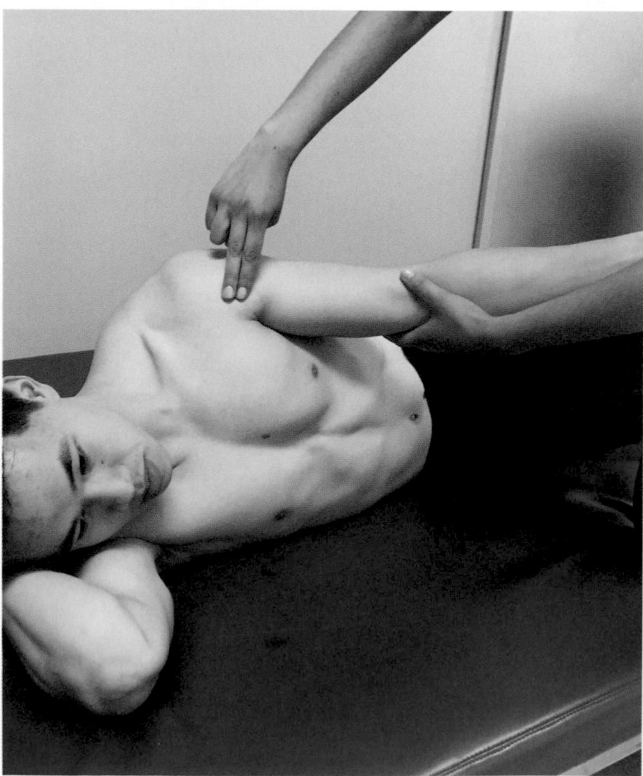

Figure 13-83. Shoulder flexion, gravity eliminated.

- *Instruction:* "Try to move your arm so your hand is at the level of your shoulder."
- *Palpation:* Palpate the anterior deltoid immediately anterior to the glenohumeral joint (Fig. 13-83). The coracobrachialis is too deep to easily palpate. The pectoralis major may be palpated below the clavicle, just medial to the anterior deltoid.

Shoulder Extension

Prime Movers

Latissimus dorsi, teres major, and posterior deltoid.

Against-Gravity Position

- *Start position:* Sitting with the arm by the side and the humerus internally rotated (palm facing posteriorly).
- *Stabilize:* Over the clavicle and scapula; make sure the client remains upright.
- *Instruction:* "Move your arm straight back as far as it will go. Keep your palm facing behind you."
- *Resistance:* The therapist's hand, placed over the distal end of the humerus, pushes forward toward flexion.
- *Substitutions:* Shoulder abductors, anterior tilting of the shoulder, and trunk flexion (Fig. 13-84).

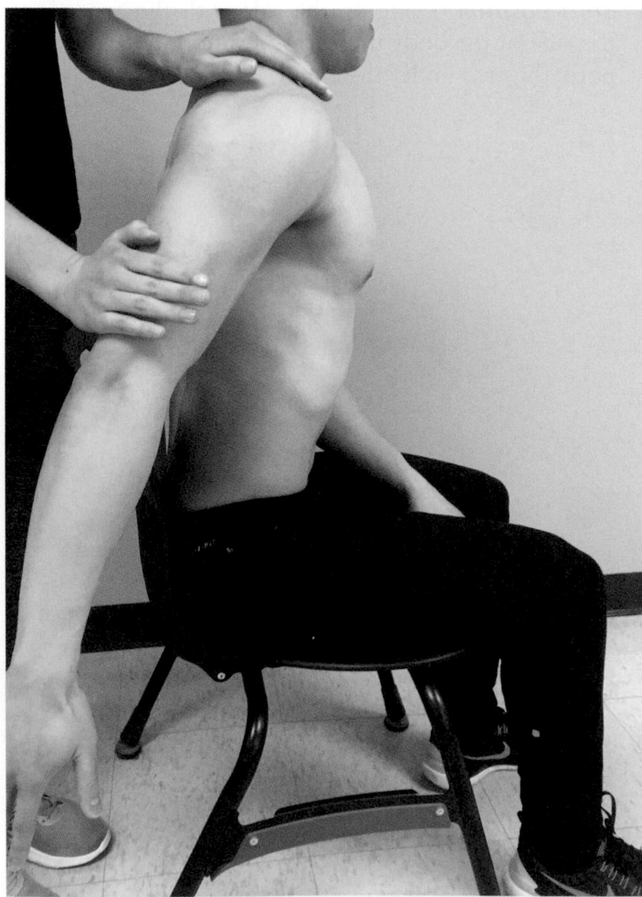

Figure 13-84. Shoulder extension against gravity.

Gravity-Eliminated Position (Fig. 13-85)

- *Start position:* Lying on the side with the arm along the side of the body and in internal rotation. Therapist supports the elbow during the motion.
- *Instruction:* "Try to move your arm backward."
- *Palpation:* The latissimus dorsi and teres major form the posterior border of the axilla (Fig. 13-85). The latissimus dorsi is inferior to the teres major. The posterior deltoid is immediately posterior to the glenohumeral joint.

Shoulder Abduction

Prime Movers

Supraspinatus and middle deltoid.

Against-Gravity Position

- *Start position:* Sitting erect with the arm down at the side and in neutral position.
- *Stabilize:* Over the clavicle and the scapula.
- *Instruction:* "Raise your arm out to the side to shoulder level. Do not let me push it down."
- *Resistance:* The therapist's hand, placed over the distal end of the humerus, pushes the humerus down toward the body. Movement above 90° involves scapular rotation and is not measured.
- *Substitutions:* The long head of the biceps can substitute if the humerus is allowed to move into external rotation; trunk lateral flexion (Fig. 13-86).

Gravity-Eliminated Position

- *Start position:* Supine with the arm supported at the side in neutral position. The therapist supports the elbow during the motion.

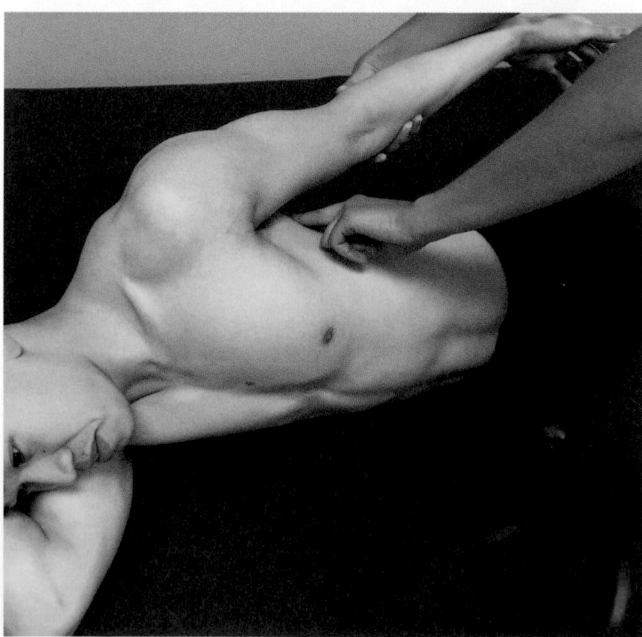

Figure 13-85. Shoulder extension, gravity eliminated.

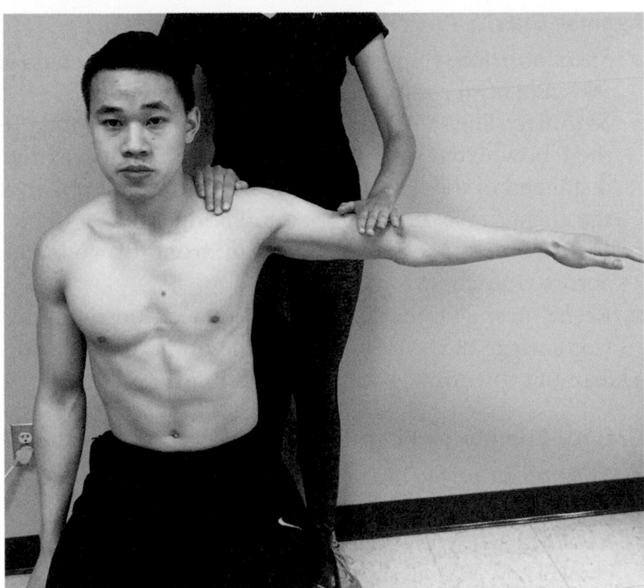

Figure 13-86. Shoulder abduction against gravity.

- *Instruction:* "Try to move your arm out to the side."
- *Palpation:* The supraspinatus lies too deep for easy palpation. Palpate the middle deltoid below the acromion and lateral to the glenohumeral joint (Fig. 13-87).

Shoulder Adduction

Prime Movers

Pectoralis major, teres major, and latissimus dorsi.

Gravity-Eliminated Position

The client cannot be positioned for this motion against gravity.

- *Start position:* Supine with the humerus abducted to 90° and the forearm in midposition.

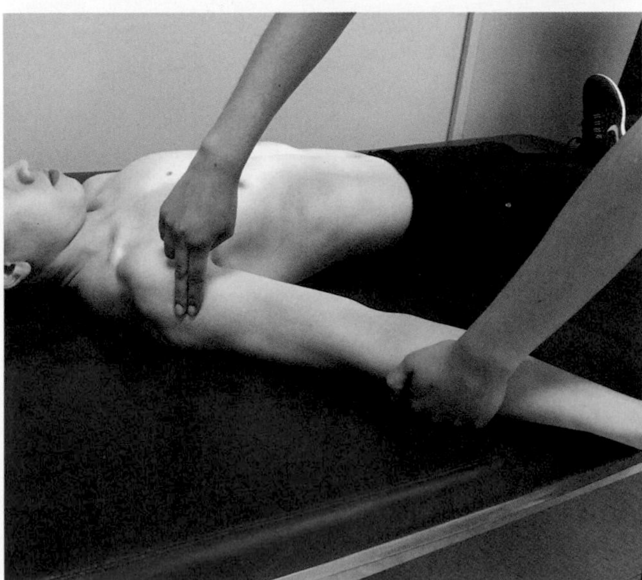

Figure 13-87. Shoulder abduction, gravity eliminated.

- *Stabilize:* The trunk is stabilized by the mat.
- *Instruction:* "Bring your arm down to your side, and do not let me pull it away."
- *Resistance:* The therapist's hand, placed on the medial side of the distal end of the humerus, attempts to pull the humerus away from the client's body.
- *Palpation:* The pectoralis major forms the anterior border of the axilla, where it may be easily palpated (Fig. 13-88). The latissimus dorsi and teres major form the posterior border of the axilla. The latissimus dorsi is inferior to the teres major.
- *Grading:* Antigravity grades can only be estimated; a question mark should be indicated in documentation. With experience, the therapist develops the skill to estimate reliably.
- *Substitutions:* On a supporting surface, the arm can be adducted with the use of the fingers.

Shoulder Horizontal Abduction

Prime Movers

Posterior deltoid, teres minor, and infraspinatus.

Against-Gravity Position

- *Start position:* Prone with the humerus abducted to 90° and supported by the mat. The elbow is flexed to 90° and is hanging over the edge of the table.
- *Stabilize:* The scapula and trunk are stabilized by the mat. Counterpressure over the contralateral scapula is helpful during action and resistance.
- *Instruction:* "Raise your elbow toward the ceiling."
- *Resistance:* The therapist's hand, placed on the posterior surface of the distal end of the humerus, pushes the arm down toward horizontal adduction (Fig. 13-89).

Gravity-Eliminated Position

- *Start position:* Sitting in a chair with the humerus supported in 90° of flexion and the elbow straight. The therapist supports the elbow.

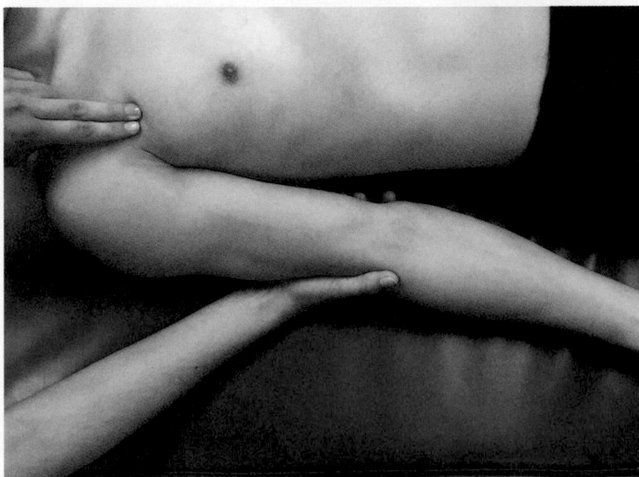

Figure 13-88. Shoulder adduction.

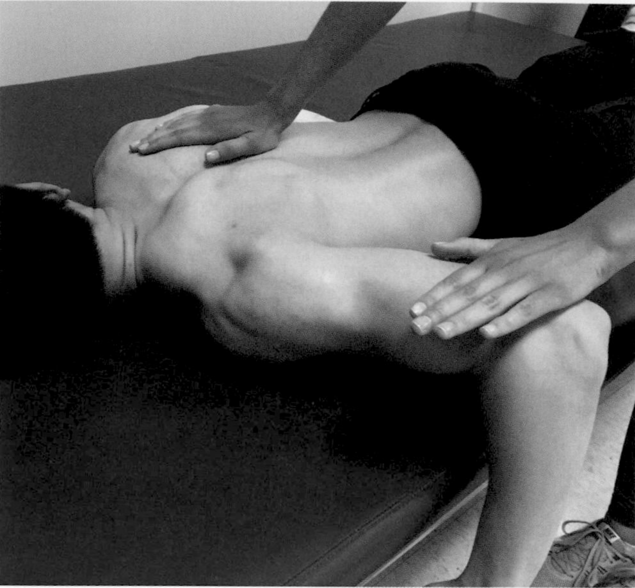

Figure 13-89. Shoulder horizontal abduction against gravity.

- *Stabilize:* The trunk is stabilized against the back of the chair.
- *Instruction:* "Try to move your arm out to the side."
- *Palpation:* Palpate the posterior deltoid immediately posterior to the glenohumeral joint.
- *Substitution:* Trunk rotation (Fig. 13-90).

Shoulder Horizontal Adduction

Prime Movers

Pectoralis major and anterior deltoid.

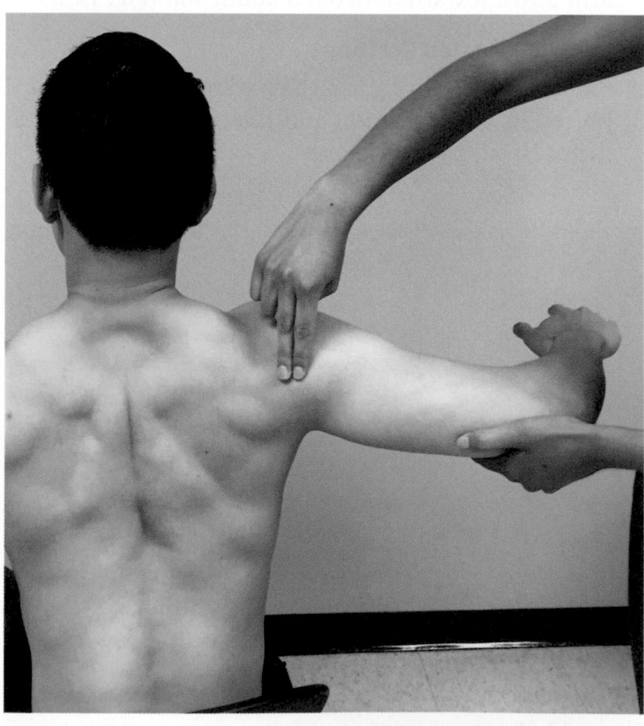

Figure 13-90. Shoulder horizontal abduction, gravity eliminated.

Against-Gravity Position

- *Start position:* Supine with the humerus abducted to 90° in neutral rotation and the elbow extended.
- *Stabilize:* The table stabilizes the scapula and trunk. If the elbow extensors are weak, be sure to support the distal end of the forearm so the hand does not fall into the client's face during horizontal adduction.
- *Instruction:* "Move your arm in front of you and across your chest."
- *Resistance:* The therapist's hand, placed on the anterior surface of the distal end of the humerus, pulls the arm out toward horizontal abduction (Fig. 13-91).

Gravity-Eliminated Position

- *Start position:* Sitting in a chair with the arm abducted to 90°.
- *Stabilize:* The trunk is stabilized against the back of the chair. The therapist supports the arm under the elbow.
- *Instruction:* "Try to bring your arm across your chest."
- *Palpation:* Palpate the pectoralis major along the anterior border of the axilla. The anterior deltoid is

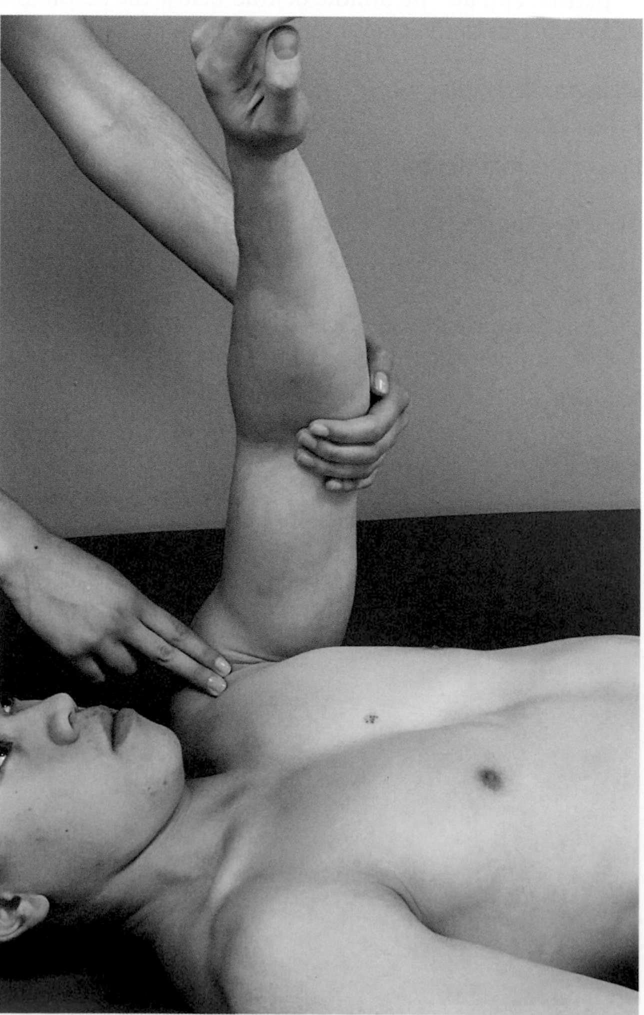

Figure 13-91. Shoulder horizontal adduction against gravity.

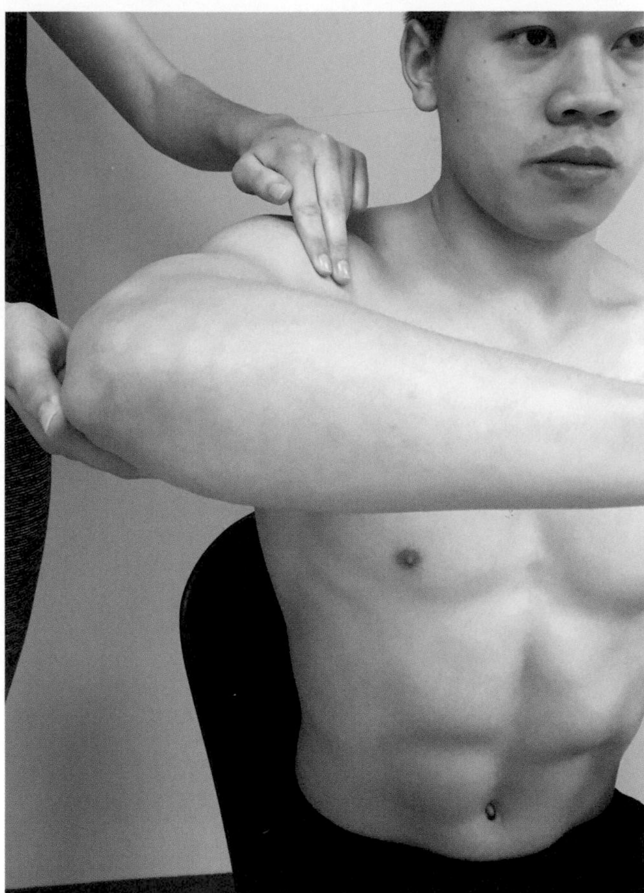

Figure 13-92. Shoulder horizontal adduction, gravity eliminated.

immediately anterior to the glenohumeral joint below the acromion process and superior to the pectoralis major (Fig 13-92).
- *Substitution:* Trunk rotation.

Shoulder External Rotation

Prime Movers

Infraspinatus, teres minor, and posterior deltoid.

Against-Gravity Position

- *Start position:* Prone with the humerus abducted to 90° and supported by the mat. A towel roll may be placed at the distal humerus for support to increase comfort. The elbow is flexed to 90° and is hanging over the edge of the table.
- *Stabilize:* The humerus is held just proximal to the elbow to allow only rotation.
- *Instruction:* "Lift the back of your hand toward the ceiling."
- *Resistance:* The therapist's hand, placed on the dorsal surface of the distal end of the forearm, pushes toward the floor. The therapist's other hand keeps the client's elbow supported and flexed to 90° to prevent supination.
- *Substitutions:* Scapula adduction combined with downward rotation can substitute. The triceps may substitute when resistance is applied (Fig. 13-93).

Gravity-Eliminated Position

- *Start position:* Prone with the entire arm hanging over the edge of the mat. The arm is in internal rotation.
- *Stabilize:* The trunk and scapula are stabilized on the mat.
- *Instruction:* "Try to turn your palm outward."
- *Palpation:* Palpate the infraspinatus inferior to the spine of the scapula (Fig. 13-94). The posterior deltoid can be palpated immediately posterior to the glenohumeral joint, as previously described. Palpate the teres minor between the posterior deltoid and the axillary border of the scapula; it is superior to the teres major.
- *Substitution:* Supination may be mistaken for external rotation in a gravity-eliminated position.

Alternative Gravity-Eliminated Position

- *Start position:* Sitting in a chair with the humerus adducted to the side and the elbow flexed to 90°.
- *Stabilize:* The distal end of the humerus is held against the body to allow only rotation.
- *Instruction:* "Try to move the back of your hand out to the side."
- *Palpation:* Same as previously described.
- *Substitutions:* Trunk rotation, scapular adduction, and elbow extension (Fig. 13-95).

Shoulder Internal Rotation

Prime Movers

Subscapularis, teres major, latissimus dorsi, pectoralis major, and anterior deltoid.

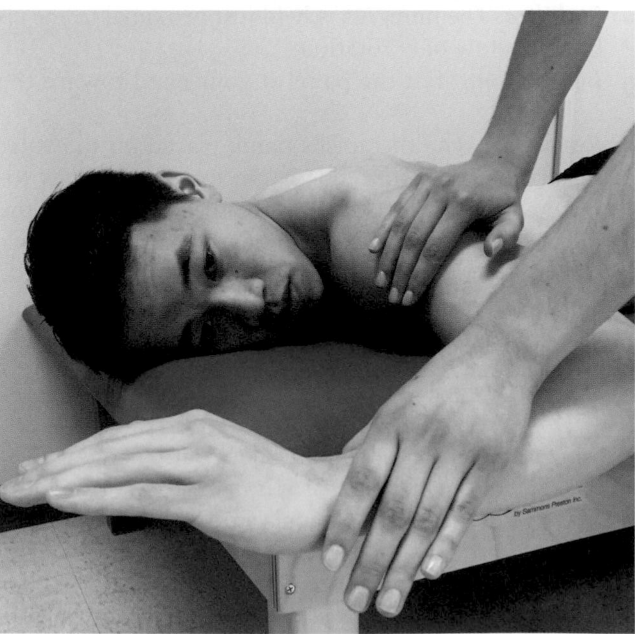

Figure 13-93. Shoulder external rotation against gravity.

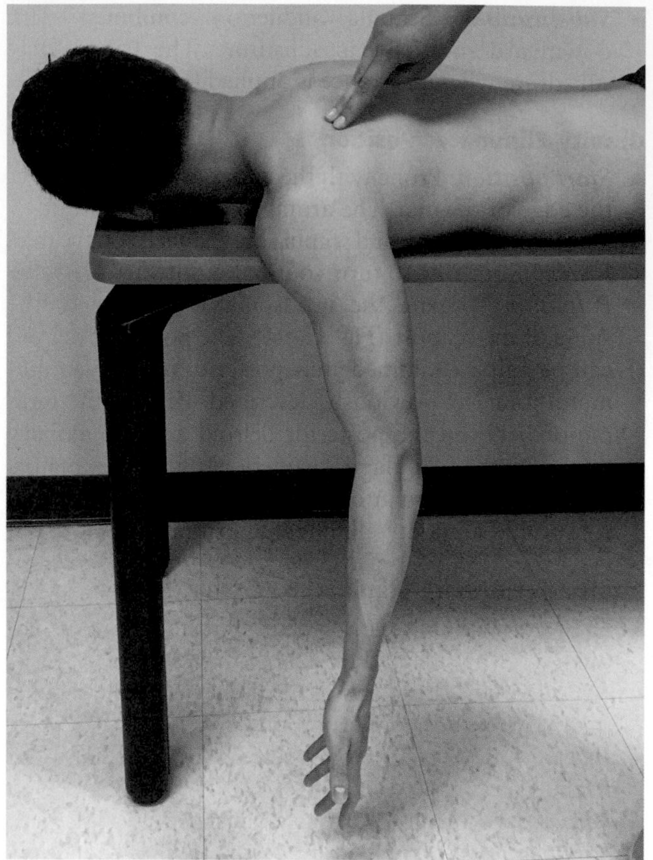

Figure 13-94. Shoulder external rotation, gravity eliminated.

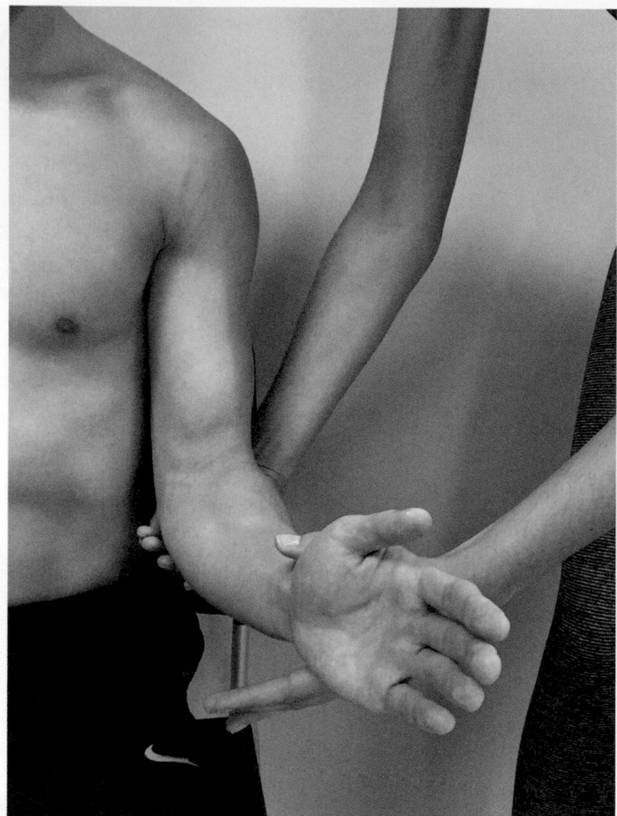

Figure 13-95. Shoulder external rotation, alternative position (shoulder adducted) with gravity eliminated.

Against-Gravity Position

- *Start position:* Prone with the humerus abducted to 90° and supported by the mat. A towel roll may be placed at the distal humerus for support to increase comfort. The elbow is flexed to 90° and hangs over the edge of the mat.
- *Stabilize:* The humerus is held just proximal to the elbow to allow only rotation.
- *Instruction:* "Lift the palm of your hand toward the ceiling."
- *Resistance:* The therapist's hand, placed on the volar surface of the distal end of the forearm, pushes toward the floor. The therapist's other hand keeps the client's elbow supported and flexed to 90° to prevent supination.
- *Substitutions:* Scapular abduction combined with upward rotation can substitute. The triceps can substitute as in external rotation (Fig. 13-96).

Gravity-Eliminated Position

- *Start position:* Prone with the entire arm hanging over the edge of the mat. The arm is in external rotation.
- *Stabilize:* The trunk and scapula are stabilized by the mat.
- *Instruction:* "Try to turn your palm inward."
- *Palpation:* The subscapularis is not easily palpated but may be found in the posterior axilla; otherwise, palpate the pectoralis major at the anterior border of the axilla.

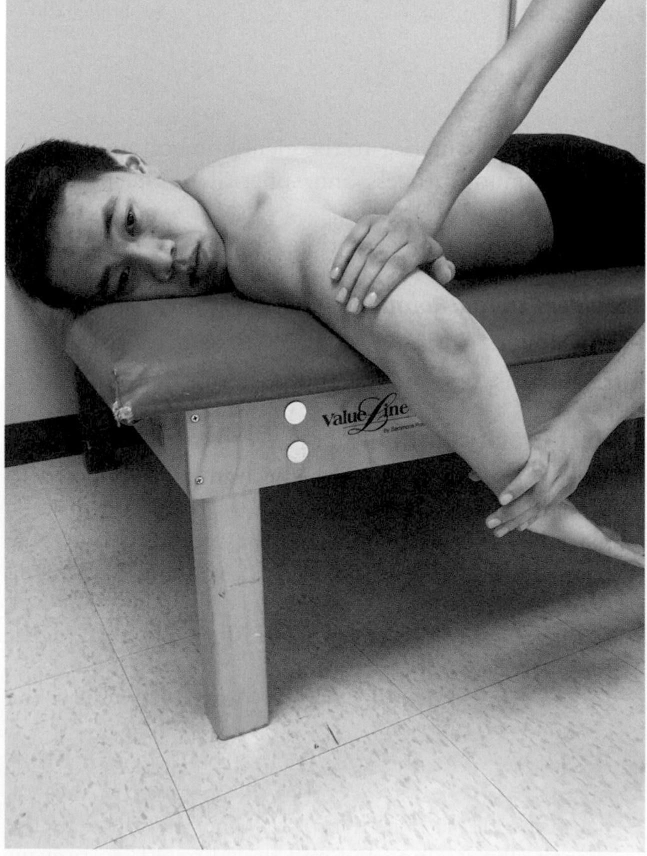

Figure 13-96. Shoulder internal rotation against gravity.

- ***Substitutions:*** Scapular abduction combined with upward rotation can substitute. Pronation may be mistaken for internal rotation in a gravity-eliminated position (Fig. 13-97).

Alternative Gravity-Eliminated Position

- ***Start position:*** Sitting in a chair with the humerus adducted to the side and the elbow flexed to 90°.
- ***Stabilize:*** The distal end of the humerus is held against the body to allow only rotation.
- ***Instruction:*** "Try to move the palm of your hand in toward your stomach."
- ***Palpation:*** Same as previously described.
- ***Substitutions:*** Scapular protraction, trunk rotation (Fig. 13-98).

Elbow Flexion

Prime Movers

Biceps brachii, brachialis, and brachioradialis.

Against-Gravity Position

- ***Start position:*** Sitting in a chair with the arm at the side. The position of the forearm determines which muscle is working primarily: (1) forearm in supination, biceps; (2) forearm in pronation, brachialis; and (3) forearm in neutral, brachioradialis.
- ***Stabilize:*** Stabilize the distal end of the humerus during the action. While applying resistance, provide counterpressure at the front of the shoulder.

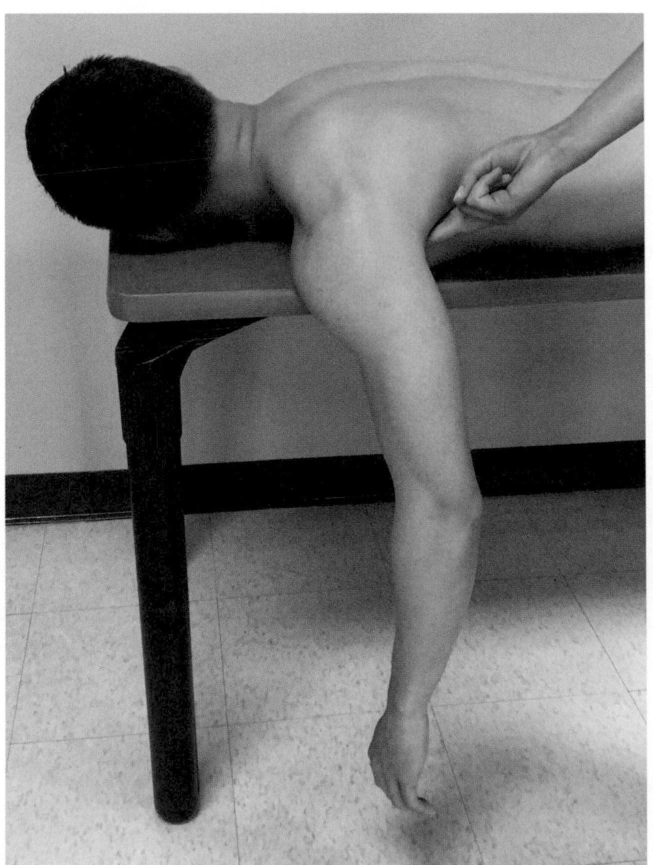

Figure 13-97. Shoulder internal rotation, gravity eliminated.

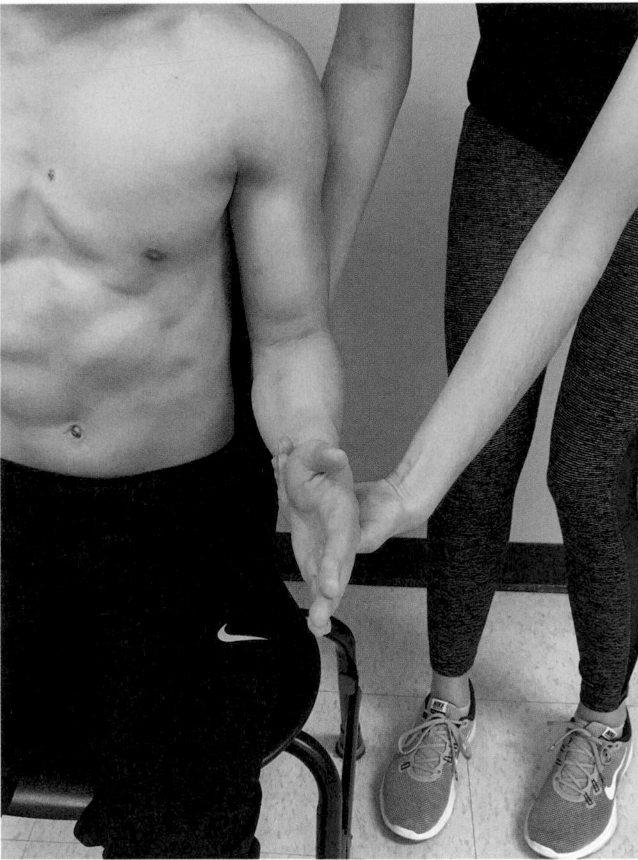

Figure 13-98. Shoulder internal rotation, alternative position (shoulder adducted) with gravity eliminated.

- ***Instruction:*** While the client is in each of the three forearm positions, say, "Bend your elbow, and do not let me pull it back down."
- ***Resistance:*** For each of the three positions, the therapist's hand is placed on the distal end of the forearm and pulls out toward extension (Fig. 13-99).

Gravity-Eliminated Position

- ***Start position:*** Sitting with the arm supported by the therapist in 90° of abduction and elbow extension. The position of the forearm determines which muscle is working, as described earlier.
- ***Stabilize:*** Distal humerus.
- ***Instruction:*** "Try to bend your elbow."
- ***Palpation:*** The biceps is easily palpated on the anterior surface of the humerus (Fig. 13-100). With the forearm pronated, palpate the brachialis just medial to the distal biceps brachii tendon. With the forearm in neutral, palpate the brachioradialis along the radial side of the proximal forearm.
- ***Substitution:*** In a gravity-eliminated plane, the wrist flexors may substitute.

Elbow Extension

Prime Mover

Triceps brachii.

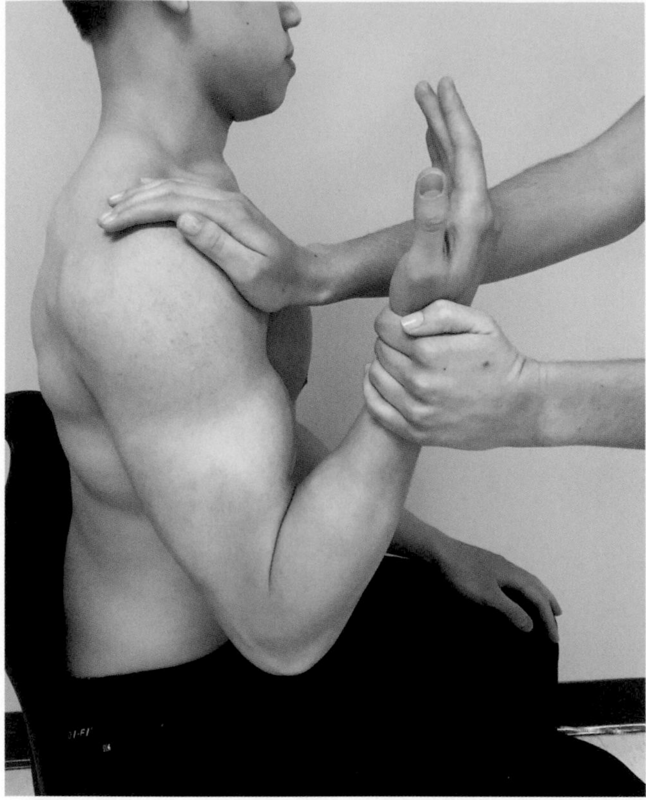

Figure 13-99. Elbow flexion against gravity.

Against-Gravity Position

- *Start position:* Prone with humerus abducted to 90° and supported on the table. The elbow is flexed, and the forearm is hanging over the edge of the table.
- *Stabilize:* Support the arm under the anterior surface of the distal humerus.
- *Instruction:* "Straighten your arm, and do not let me push it back down."
- *Resistance:* Apply resistance with the elbow at 10° to 15° less than full extension so that the elbow does not lock into position. The therapist's hand, placed on the dorsal surface of the client's forearm, pushes toward flexion (Fig. 13-101).

Gravity-Eliminated Position

- *Start position:* Sitting with the humerus supported by the therapist in 90° of abduction. The elbow is fully flexed.
- *Stabilize:* The humerus is supported and stabilized.
- *Instruction:* "Try to straighten your elbow."
- *Palpation:* The triceps is easily palpated on the posterior surface of the humerus.
- *Substitutions:* In the gravity-eliminated position, no external rotation of the shoulder is permitted, so as to avoid letting the assistance of gravity produce extension (Fig. 13-102).

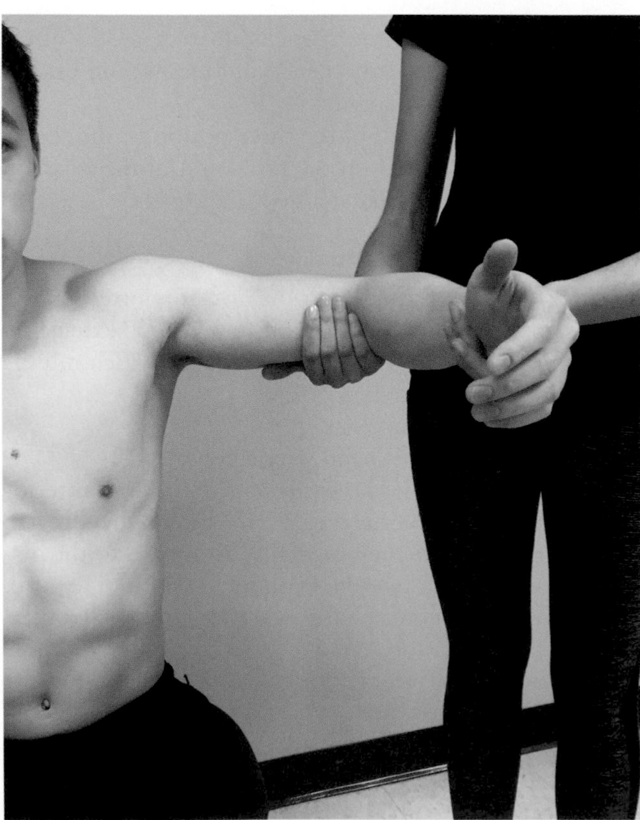

Figure 13-100. Elbow flexion, gravity eliminated.

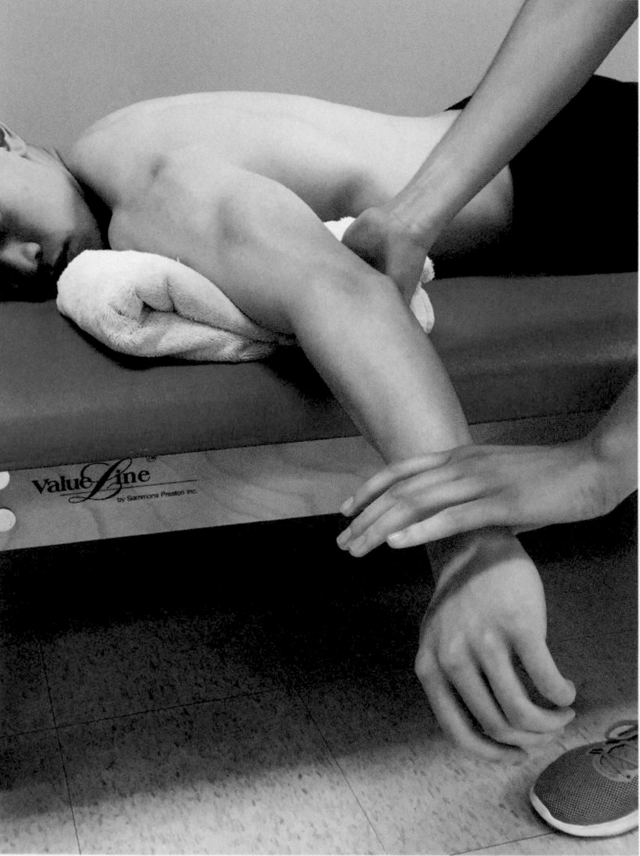

Figure 13-101. Elbow extension against gravity.

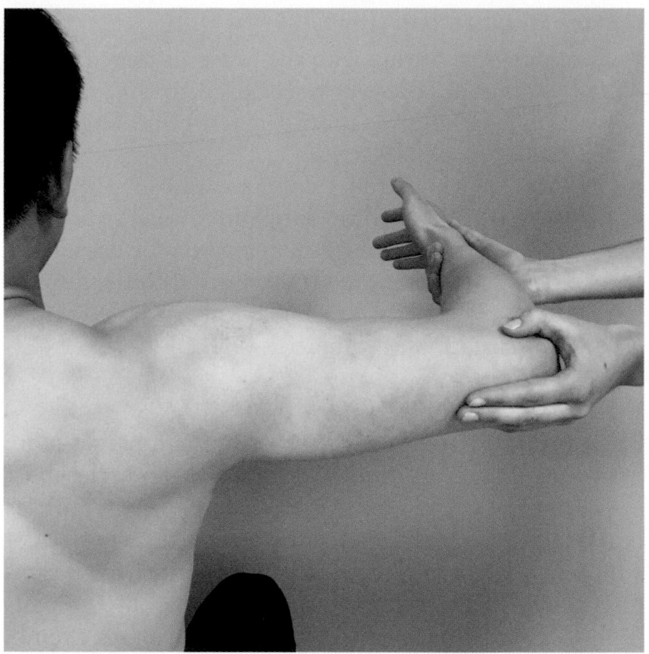

Figure 13-102. Elbow extension, gravity eliminated.

Pronation

Prime Movers

Pronator teres and pronator quadratus.

Against-Gravity Position

- *Start position:* Sitting with the humerus adducted, elbow flexed to 90°, and forearm supinated. The wrist and fingers are relaxed.
- *Stabilize:* The distal humerus is stabilized to keep it adducted to the body.
- *Instruction:* "Turn your palm to the floor, and do not let me turn it back over."
- *Resistance:* The therapist's hand encircles the client's volar wrist, with the therapist's index finger extended along the forearm. The therapist applies resistance in the direction of supination. An alternate method of applying resistance is to position the distal forearm between the therapist's opposing palms. The therapist applies resistance in the direction of supination.
- *Substitutions:* Shoulder abduction or internal rotation; wrist and finger flexors may substitute (Fig. 13-103).

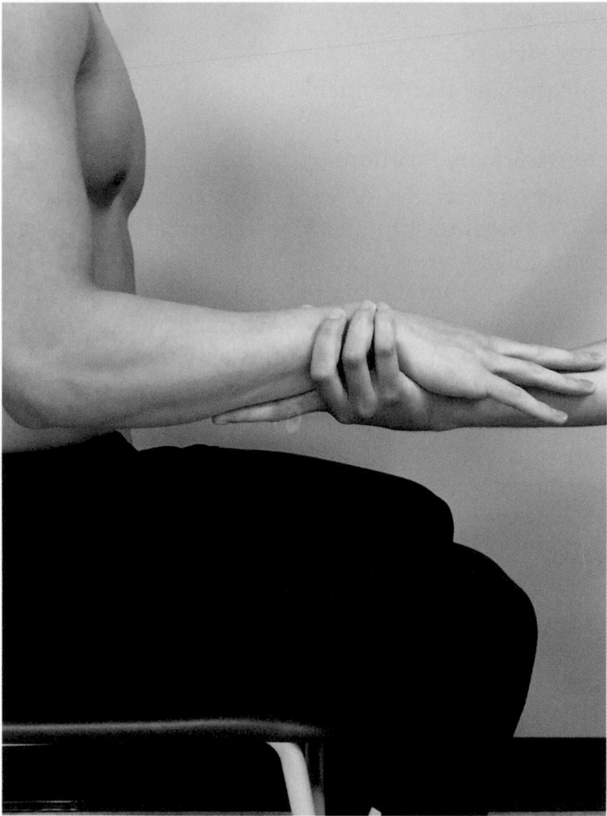

Figure 13-103. Pronation against gravity.

Gravity-Eliminated Position

- *Start position:* Sitting with the humerus flexed to 90° and supported. The elbow is flexed to 90°, and the forearm is in full supination. The wrist and fingers are relaxed.
- *Stabilize:* The humerus is stabilized.
- *Instruction:* "Try to turn your palm away from your face."
- *Palpation:* The pronator teres is palpated medial to the distal attachment of the biceps tendon on the volar surface of the proximal forearm. The pronator quadratus is too deep to palpate (Fig. 13-104).

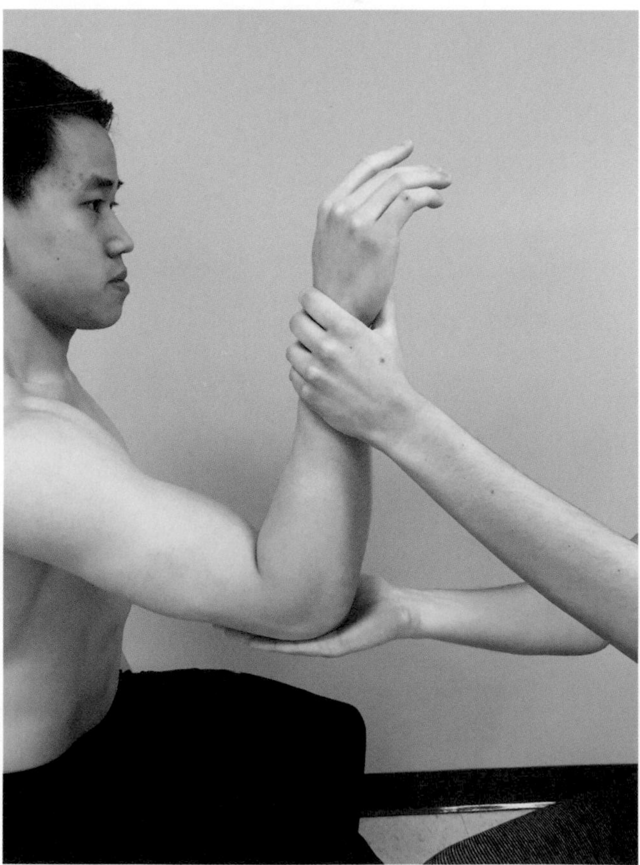

Figure 13-104. Pronation, gravity eliminated.

Supination

Prime Movers

Supinator and biceps brachii.

Against-Gravity Position

- *Start position:* Sitting with the humerus adducted, elbow flexed to 90°, and forearm pronated. The wrist and fingers are relaxed. (*Note*: To differentiate the supinator from the supination function of the biceps, isolate the supinator by extending the elbow. The biceps does not supinate the extended arm unless resisted.)[49]
- *Stabilize:* The distal humerus is stabilized.
- *Instruction:* "Turn your palm up toward the ceiling, and do not let me turn it back over."
- *Resistance:* The therapist's hand encircles the client's volar wrist, with the therapist's index finger extended along the forearm. The therapist applies resistance in the direction of pronation. An alternate method of applying resistance is to position the distal forearm between the therapist's opposing palms. The therapist applies resistance in the direction of pronation.
- *Substitutions:* Shoulder adduction or external rotation; wrist and finger extensors may substitute (Fig. 13-105).

Gravity-Eliminated Position

- *Start position:* Sitting with the humerus flexed to 90° and supported. The elbow is flexed to 90°, and the forearm is in full pronation. The wrist and fingers are relaxed.
- *Stabilize:* The humerus is stabilized and supported.
- *Instruction:* "Try to turn your palm toward your face."
- *Palpation:* The supinator is palpated on the dorsal surface of the proximal forearm just distal to the head of the radius. The biceps brachii is easily palpated on the anterior surface of the humerus (Fig. 13-106).

Wrist and Hand Measurement

Because many tendons of the wrist and hand cross more than one joint, test positions for individual muscles must include ways to minimize the effect of other muscles crossing the joint. In general, to minimize the effect of a muscle, place it opposite the prime action. For example, to minimize the effect of the extensor pollicis longus (EPL) on extension of the proximal joint of the thumb, flex the distal joint.

Wrist Extension

Prime Movers

Extensor carpi radialis longus (ECRL), extensor carpi radialis brevis (ECRB), and extensor carpi ulnaris (ECU).

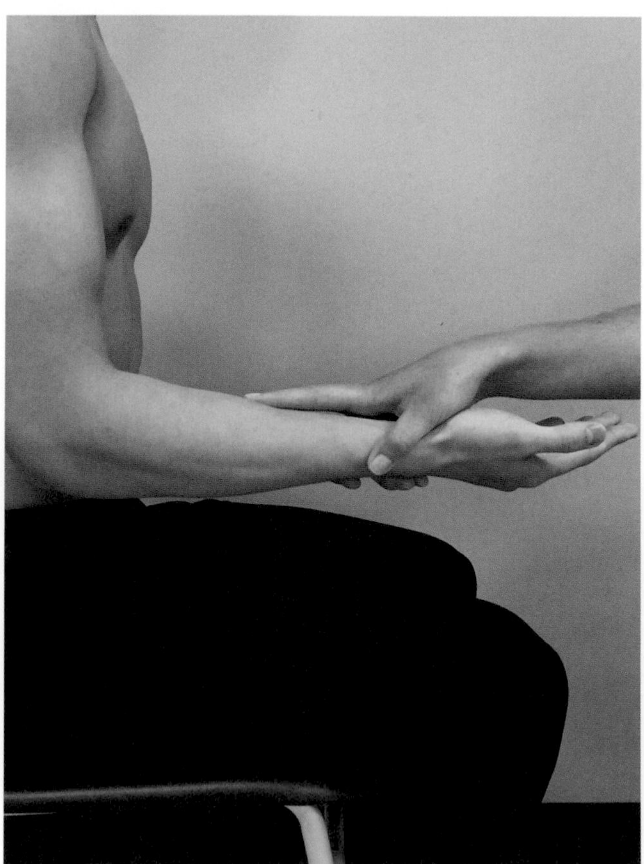

Figure 13-105. Supination, against gravity.

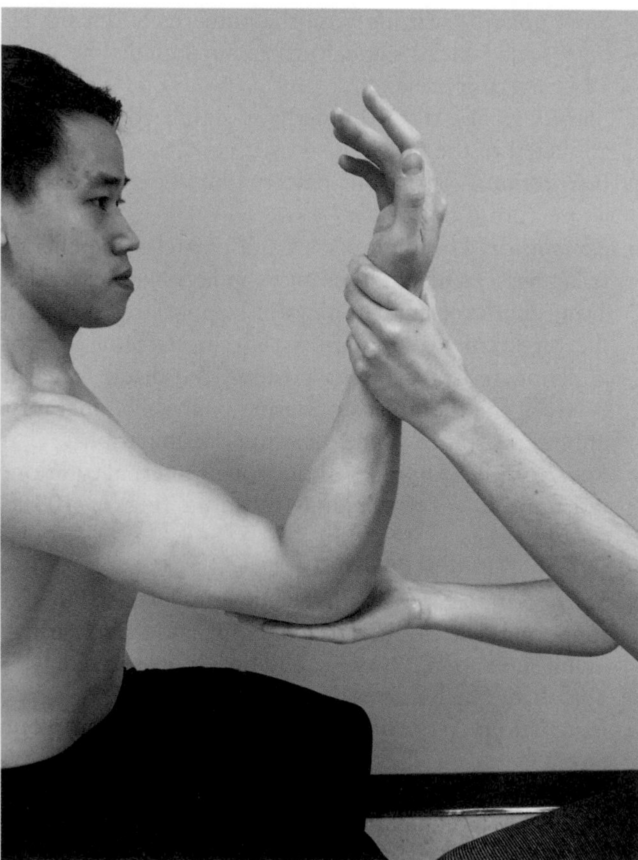

Figure 13-106. Supination, gravity eliminated.

Against-Gravity Position

- *Start position:* The forearm is supported on a table in full pronation with fingers and thumb relaxed or slightly flexed. The hand may hang over the edge of the table.
- *Stabilize:* The forearm is stabilized on the table.
- *Instruction:* "Lift your wrist as far as you can, and keep your fingers relaxed. Do not let me push it down."
- *Resistance:* Apply resistance to the distal metacarpals of the fingers toward flexion. Muscles individually as follows: To test the ECRL and ECRB, which extend and radially deviate, apply resistance to the dorsum of the hand on the radial side in the direction of flexion and ulnar deviation. To test the ECU, which extends and ulnarly deviates, apply resistance to the dorsum of the hand on the ulnar side and push in the direction of flexion and radial deviation.
- *Substitutions:* Extensor pollicis longus (EPL) and extensor digitorum communis (EDC) (Fig. 13-107).

Gravity-Eliminated Position

- *Start position:* The forearm is supported on the table in neutral with the wrist in a slightly flexed position.
- *Instruction:* "Try to bend your wrist backward."
- *Palpation:* Palpate the tendons at the dorsal wrist and the muscle bellies at the proximal dorsal forearm. Specifically, the tendon of the ECRL can be palpated at the base of the second metacarpal and the tendon of the ECRB at the base of the third metacarpal adjacent to the ECRL. The muscle belly of the ECRL is adjacent to the brachioradialis. The muscle belly of the ECRB is distal to the belly of the ECRL. Palpate the ECU tendon between the head of the ulna and the base of the fifth metacarpal. The muscle belly is approximately 2 inches distal to the lateral epicondyle of the humerus (Fig. 13-108).

Wrist Flexion

Prime Movers

Flexor carpi radialis (FCR), palmaris longus, and flexor carpi ulnaris (FCU).

Against-Gravity Position

- *Start position:* The forearm is supinated, the wrist is extended, and the fingers and thumb are relaxed.
- *Stabilize:* The forearm is stabilized on the table with the back of the hand hanging off the table to allow the wrist to go into slight extension.
- *Instruction:* "Bend your wrist all the way forward, and keep your fingers relaxed. Do not let me push it back."
- *Resistance:* Apply resistance to the distal metacarpals of the fingers toward extension. To test the FCR and palmaris longus, the therapist applies resistance over the heads of the metacarpals on the volar surface of

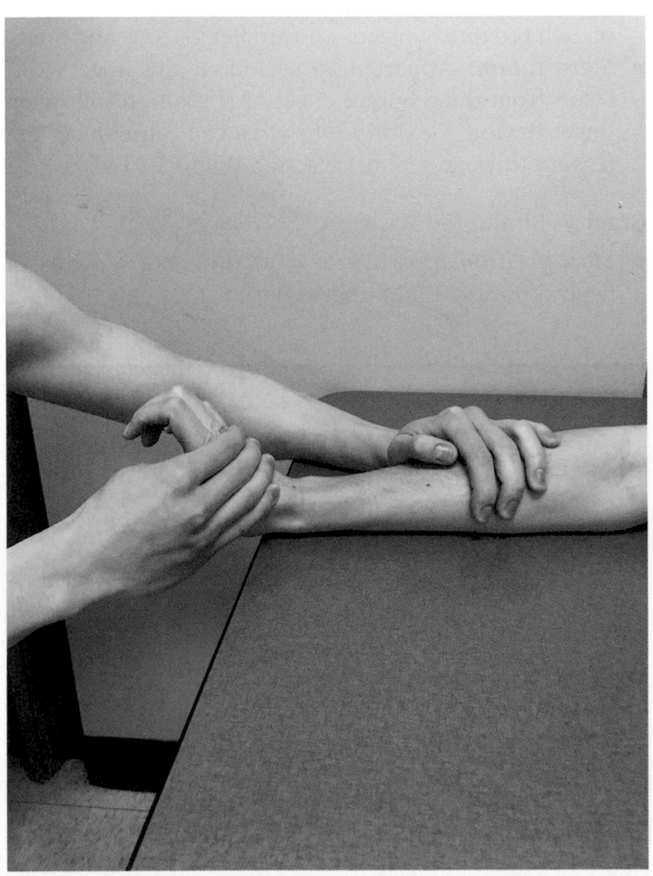

Figure 13-107. Wrist extension, against gravity.

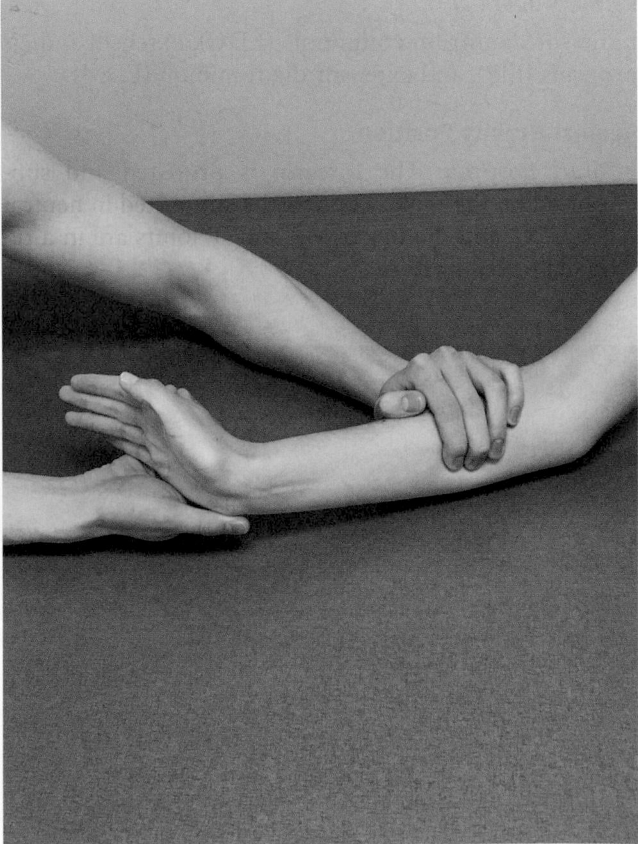

Figure 13-108. Wrist extension, gravity eliminated.

the hand toward extension. To test for the FCU, the therapist applies resistance over the head of the fifth metacarpal on the volar surface of the hand toward wrist extension and radial deviation.

- ***Substitutions:*** Abductor pollicis longus (APL), flexor pollicis longus (FPL), flexor digitorum superficialis (FDS), and flexor digitorum profundus (FDP) (Fig. 13-109).

Gravity-Eliminated Position

- ***Start position:*** Forearm in neutral, wrist extended, and fingers and thumb relaxed.
- ***Stabilize:*** The forearm rests on the table.
- ***Instruction:*** "Try to bend your wrist forward."
- ***Palpation:*** Palpate the tendons at the volar wrist. Specifically, the tendon of the FCR can be palpated at the base of the second metacarpal, radial to the palmaris longus (if present) and the tendon of the FCU just proximal to the pisiform bone on the ulnar aspect of the volar wrist. The palmaris longus is a weak wrist flexor. The tendon crosses the center of the volar surface of the wrist. It is not tested for strength and may not even be present; if it is present, it will stand out prominently in the middle of the wrist when wrist flexion is resisted or the palm is positioned with the thumb and fifth digit opposed to one another ((Figs. 13-110 and 13-111).

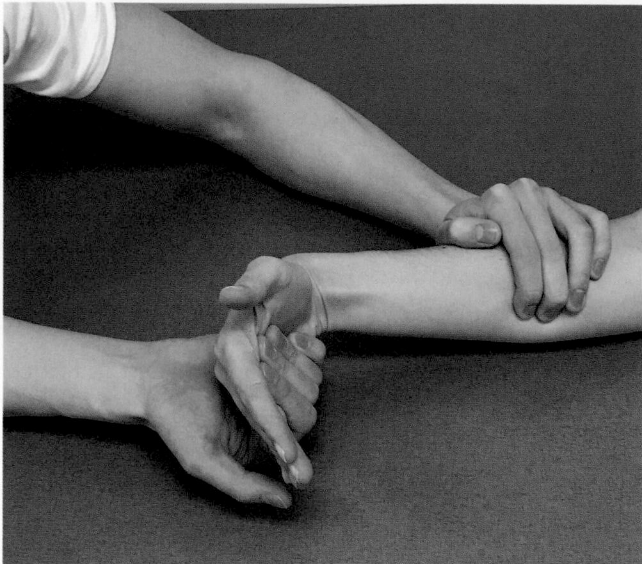

Figure 13-110. Wrist flexion, gravity eliminated.

Finger Metacarpophalangeal Extension

Prime Movers

Extensor digitorum communis (EDC), extensor indicis proprius (EIP), and extensor digiti minimi (EDM).

Against-Gravity Position

- ***Start position:*** The forearm is pronated and supported on the table. The wrist is supported in neutral position, and the finger MP and IP joints are in a relaxed flexed posture.
- ***Stabilize:*** Wrist and metacarpals.
- ***Instruction:*** "Lift this knuckle up as far as it will go (touch the finger that is to be tested). Keep the rest of your fingers bent. Do not let me push your knuckle down." (*Note:* Be sure to demonstrate this action.)
- ***Resistance:*** Using one finger, the therapist pushes the head of each proximal phalanx toward flexion, one at a time.
- ***Substitution:*** Apparent extension of the fingers can result from the rebound effect of relaxation following finger flexion. Flexion of the wrist can cause finger extension through tenodesis action (Fig. 13-112).

Gravity-Eliminated Position

- ***Start position:*** Forearm supported in neutral, wrist in neutral position, and fingers flexed.

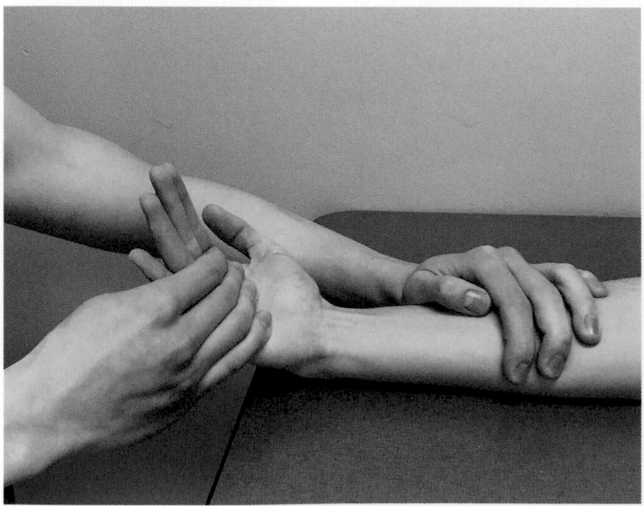

Figure 13-109. Wrist flexion, against gravity.

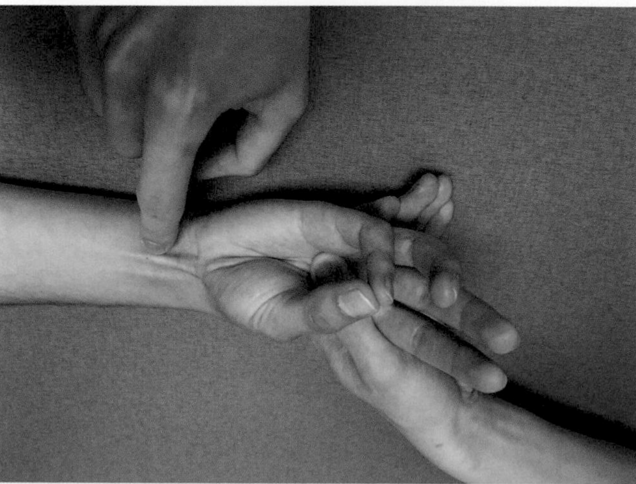

Figure 13-111. The therapist is pointing to the tendon of the palmaris longus as the client cups her hand to make this tendon stand out.

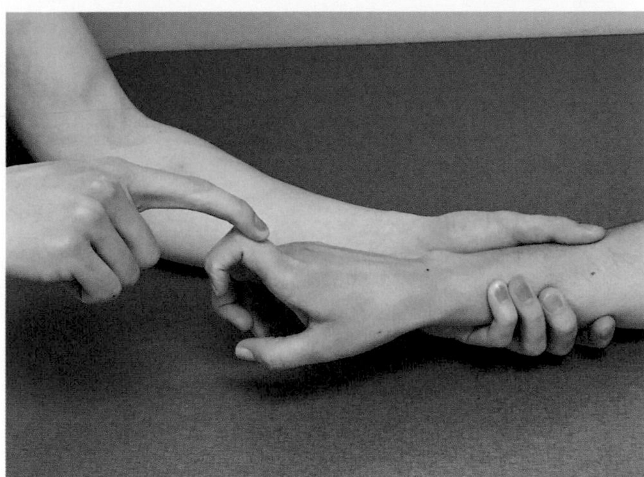

Figure 13-112. Finger metacarpophalangeal extension, against gravity.

- *Stabilize:* Wrist and metacarpals.
- *Instruction:* "Try to move your knuckles back as far as they will go, one at a time. Keep the rest of your fingers bent."
- *Palpation:* The tendons of the EDC are readily seen and palpated on the dorsum of the hand (Fig. 13-113). Both the EIP tendon and the EDM tendon are ulnar to the EDC tendon of their respective digits. Palpate the muscle belly of the EDC on the dorsal–ulnar surface of the proximal forearm. Often, the separate muscle bellies are discernible. Palpate the belly of the EIP muscle on the mid- to distal dorsal forearm between the radius and ulna (Fig. 13-113).

Finger Metacarpophalangeal Flexion

Prime Movers

Flexor digitorum profundus (FDP), flexor digitorum superficialis (FDS), dorsal interossei, palmar interossei, and flexor digiti minimi. The tests for the first four muscles are discussed under their alternative actions. The flexor of the little finger has no other action and is described here.

Against-Gravity Position for the Flexor Digiti Minimi

- *Start position:* Forearm supported in supination.
- *Stabilize:* Other fingers in extension.
- *Instruction:* "Bend the knuckle of your little finger toward your palm while you keep the rest of the finger straight."
- *Resistance:* Using one finger, the therapist pushes the head of the proximal phalanx toward extension. The therapist must be sure the IP joints remain extended.
- *Substitutions:* The FDP, FDS, or third palmar interosseus may substitute (Fig. 13-114).

Gravity-Eliminated Position

- *Start position:* Forearm supported in neutral.
- *Stabilize:* Other fingers in extension.
- *Instruction:* "Try to bend the knuckle of your little finger toward your palm while you keep the rest of the finger straight."
- *Palpation:* The flexor digiti minimi is found on the volar surface of the hypothenar eminence (Fig. 13-115).

Finger Proximal Interphalangeal Flexion

Prime Movers

Flexor digitorum superficialis (FDS) and flexor digitorum profundus (FDP).

Against-Gravity Position for the Flexor Digitorum Superficialis

- *Start position:* Forearm supinated and supported on the table; wrist and MP joints relaxed. To rule out the influence of the FDP when testing the FDS, hold all IP joints of the fingers not being tested in full extension

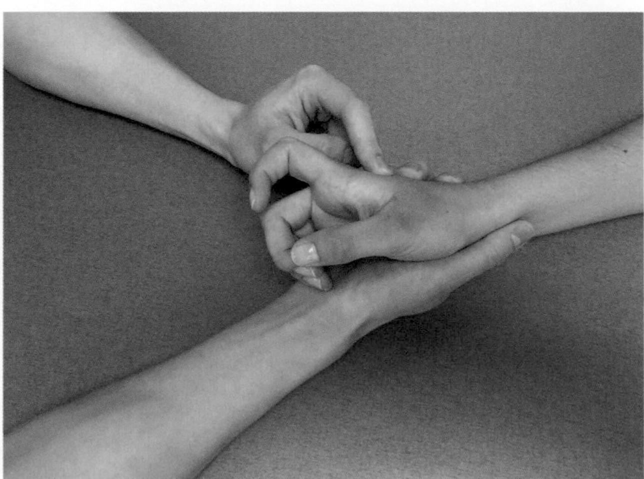

Figure 13-113. Finger metacarpophalangeal extension, gravity eliminated.

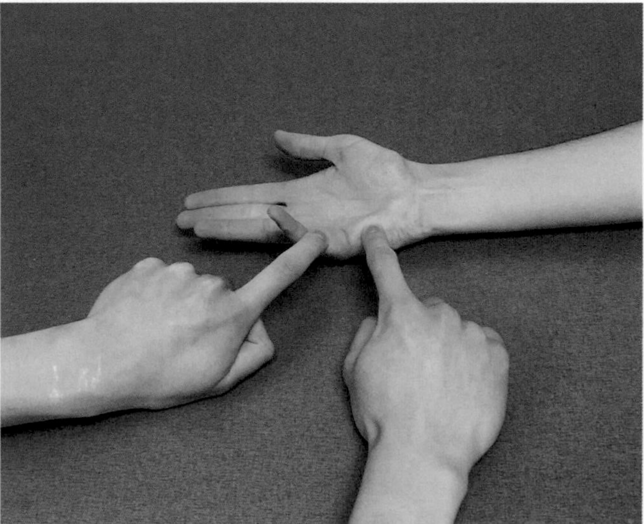

Figure 13-114. Finger metacarpophalangeal flexion, against gravity for the flexor digiti minimi.

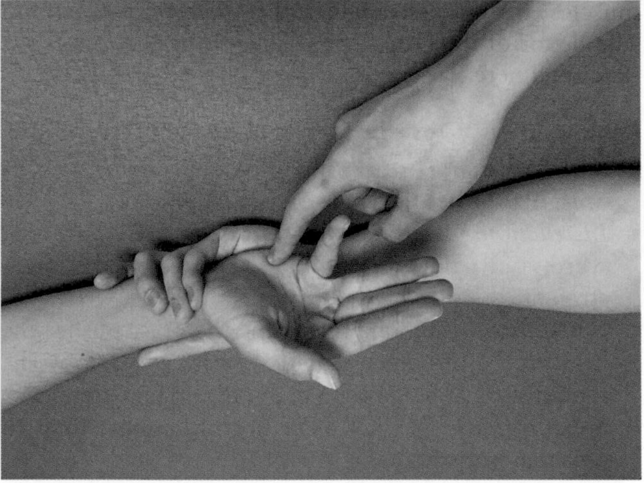

Figure 13-115. Finger metacarpophalangeal flexion, gravity eliminated.

to slight hyperextension. Because the FDP is essentially one muscle with four tendons, preventing its action in three of the four fingers prevents it from working in the tested finger. In fact, the client cannot flex the distal joint of the tested finger at all. In some people, the FDP slip to the index finger is such that this method cannot rule out its influence on the PIP joint of the index finger. This should be documented.

- *Stabilize:* All IP joints of the other digits of the hand.
- *Instruction:* Point to the PIP joint and say, "Bend just this joint."
- *Resistance:* Using one finger, the therapist applies resistance to the head of the middle phalanx toward extension.
- *Substitutions:* FDP. Wrist extension causes tenodesis action (Fig. 13-116).

Gravity-Eliminated Position

- *Start position:* Forearm supported in neutral with the wrist and MP joints relaxed in neutral position. Again, rule out the influence of the FDP by holding all the joints of the untested fingers in extension.
- *Stabilize:* Proximal phalanx of the finger being tested as well as all IP joints of the other digits of the hand.
- *Instruction:* Point to the PIP joint and say, "Try to bend just this joint."
- *Palpation:* Palpate the FDS on the volar surface of the proximal forearm toward the ulnar side (Fig. 13-117) and the tendons at the wrist between the palmaris longus and the FCU.

Finger Distal Interphalangeal Flexion

Prime Mover

Flexor digitorum profundus (FDP).

Against-Gravity Position

- *Start position:* Forearm supinated and supported on a table; wrist and IP joints relaxed.
- *Stabilize:* Firmly support the middle phalanx of each finger as it is tested to prevent flexion of the proximal IP joint; the wrist should remain in neutral position.
- *Instruction:* "Bend the last joint on your finger as far as you can."
- *Resistance:* The therapist places one finger on the pad of the client's finger and applies resistance toward extension.
- *Substitutions:* Rebound effect of apparent flexion following contraction of extensors. Wrist extension causes tenodesis action (Fig. 13-118).

Gravity-Eliminated Position

- *Start position:* The forearm is in neutral, resting on the ulnar border on a table. The wrist and IP joints are relaxed in neutral position.
- *Stabilize:* Firmly support the middle phalanx of each finger as it is tested to prevent flexion of the proximal IP joint; the wrist should remain in neutral position.

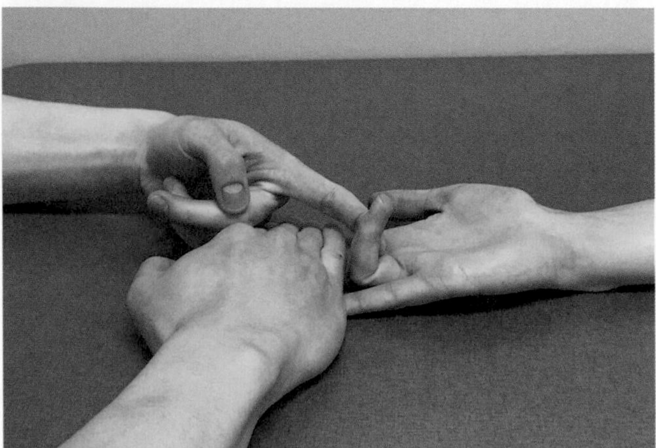

Figure 13-116. Finger proximal interphalangeal flexion, against gravity. The flexor profundus is prevented from substituting because the therapist is holding in extension all fingers not being tested.

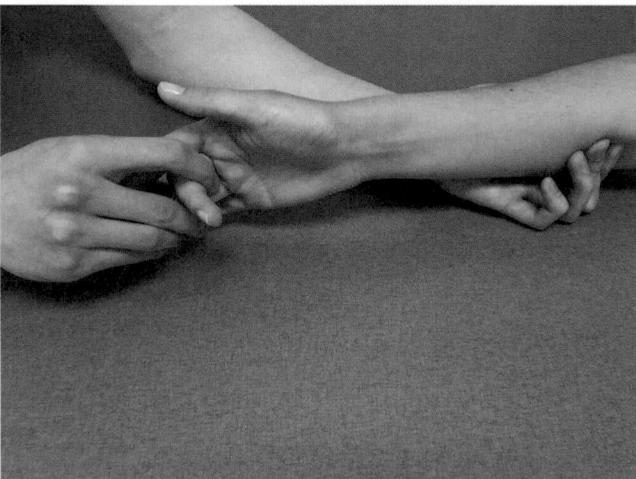

Figure 13-117. Finger proximal interphalangeal flexion, gravity eliminated.

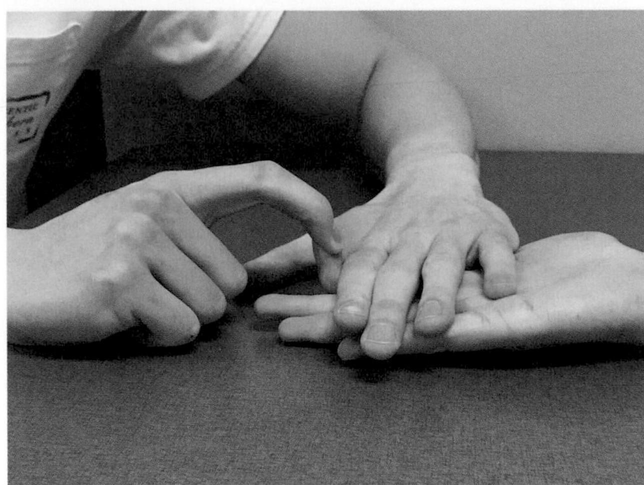

Figure 13-118. Finger distal interphalangeal flexion, against gravity. The other joints of the finger are prevented from flexing.

- *Instruction:* "Bend the last joint on your finger as far as you can."
- *Palpation:* Palpate the belly of the FDP just volar to the ulna in the proximal third of the forearm. The tendons are sometimes palpable on the volar surface of the middle phalanges (Fig. 13-119).

Finger Abduction

Prime Movers

Dorsal interossei (4) and abductor digiti minimi (ADM).

Gravity-Eliminated Position

These muscles are tested for all grades in the gravity-eliminated position.

- *Start position:* The pronated forearm is supported with the wrist neutral. The fingers are extended and adducted. Be sure the MP joints are in neutral or slight flexion.
- *Stabilize:* The wrist and metacarpals are gently supported.
- *Instruction:* "Spread your fingers apart, and do not let me push them back together."
- *Action:* The action of each finger is different because the midline of the hand is the third finger and abduction is movement away from midline. It is important to know which dorsal interosseus you are testing. The first dorsal interosseus abducts the index finger toward the thumb. The second dorsal interosseus abducts the middle finger toward the thumb. The third dorsal interosseus abducts the middle finger toward the little finger. The fourth dorsal interosseus abducts the ring finger toward the little finger. The ADM abducts the little finger ulnarly.
- *Resistance:* The therapist applies resistance at the radial or ulnar side of the head of the proximal phalanx in an attempt to push the finger toward midline. Applying resistance to the radial side of the heads of the index and middle fingers tests the first and second dorsal interossei. Applying resistance to the ulnar side of the middle, ring, and little fingers tests the third and fourth dorsal interossei and the ADM.
- *Substitutions:* Extensor digitorum communis (EDC).
- *Grading:* Normal finger abductors do not tolerate much resistance. If the fingers give way to resistance but spring back when the resistance is removed, the grade is 5. The grade is 4 if the muscle takes some resistance. The grade is 3 when there is full AROM. The grade is 2 if there is partial AROM. The grade is 1 when contraction is felt with palpation. The grade is 0 when no contractile activity is palpable.
- *Palpation:* Palpate the first dorsal interosseus on the dorsal web space and the ADM on the ulnar border of the fifth metacarpal. The other interossei lie between the metacarpals on the dorsal aspect of the hand, where they may be palpated; on some people, the tendons can be palpated as they enter the dorsal expansion near the heads of the metacarpals. When the dorsal interossei are atrophied, the spaces between the metacarpals on the dorsal surface appear sunken (Fig. 13-120).

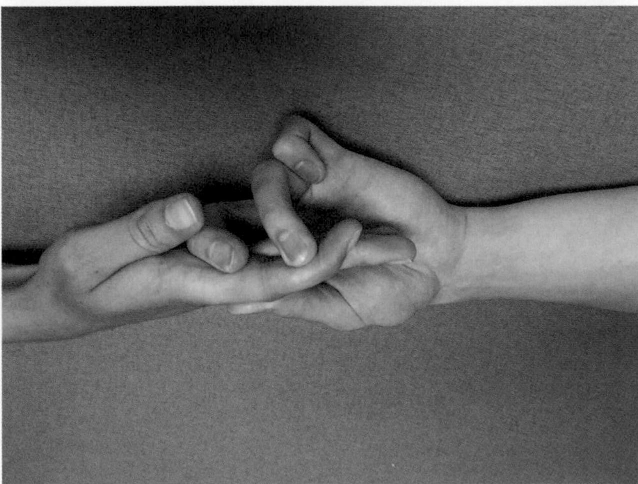

Figure 13-119. Finger distal interphalangeal flexion, gravity eliminated.

Finger Adduction

Prime Movers

Palmar interossei (3).

Gravity-Eliminated Position

These muscles are tested for all grades in the gravity-eliminated position.

- *Start position:* The forearm is pronated, and the MPs are abducted and in extension.
- *Stabilize:* Both of the therapist's hands are needed for resistance. The forearm and wrist can be supported on a table.

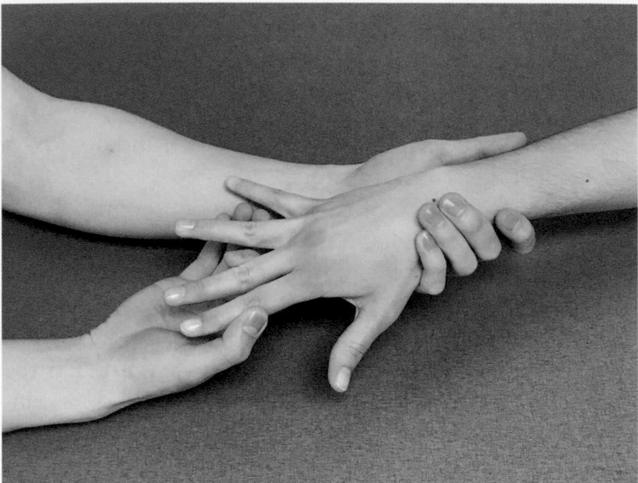

Figure 13-120. Finger abduction.

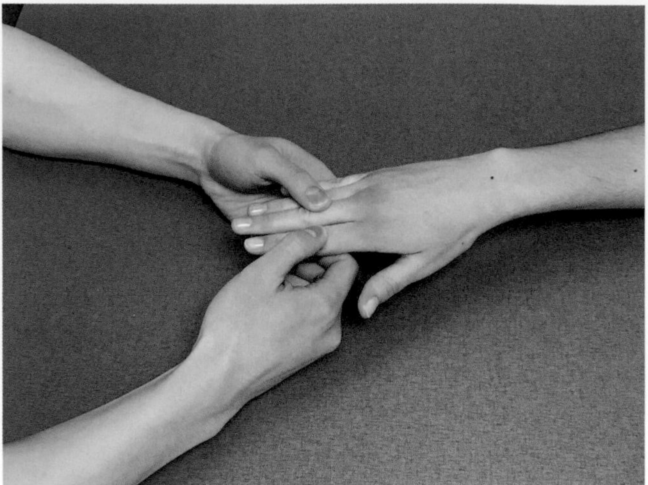

Figure 13-121. Finger adduction.

- *Instruction:* "Bring your fingers together and hold them. Do not let me pull them apart."
- *Action:* The action of each finger is different because the midline of the hand is the third finger and adduction is movement toward midline. The first palmar interosseus adducts the index finger toward the middle finger. The second adducts the ring finger toward the middle finger, and the third adducts the little finger toward the middle finger.
- *Resistance:* The therapist holds the heads of the proximal phalanx of two adjoining fingers and applies resistance in the direction of abduction to pull the fingers apart. For the index and middle finger pair, the first palmar interosseus is tested. For the middle and ring finger pair, the second palmar interosseus is tested. For the ring and little finger pair, the third palmar interosseus is tested.
- *Substitutions:* Extrinsic finger flexors.
- *Grading:* Normal finger adductors do not tolerate much resistance. If the fingers give way to resistance but spring back when the resistance is removed, the grade is 5. The grade is 4 if the muscle takes some resistance. The grade is 3 when there is full AROM. The grade is 2 if there is partial AROM. The grade is 1 when contraction is felt with palpation. The grade is 0 when no contractile activity is palpable.
- *Palpation:* The palmar interossei are usually too deep to palpate with certainty. When these muscles are atrophied, the areas between the metacarpals on the volar surface appear sunken (Fig. 13-121).

Thumb Metacarpophalangeal Extension

Prime Movers

Extensor pollicis brevis and extensor pollicis longus (EPL).

Against-Gravity Position

- *Start position:* Forearm supported in neutral, MP and IP joints flexed.
- *Stabilize:* Firmly support the first metacarpal in abduction.
- *Instruction:* "Straighten your thumb."

  To isolate the extensor pollicis brevis, instruct the client: "Straighten the knuckle of your thumb while keeping the end joint bent." (*Note:* You may have to move the thumb passively a few times for the client to get the kinesthetic input regarding this movement.)
- *Resistance:* The therapist's index finger, placed on the dorsal surface of the head of the proximal phalanx, pushes toward flexion.
- *Substitution:* EPL for the extensor pollicis brevis (Fig. 13-122).

Gravity-Eliminated Position

- *Start position:* Forearm pronated or supinated, MP and IP joints flexed.

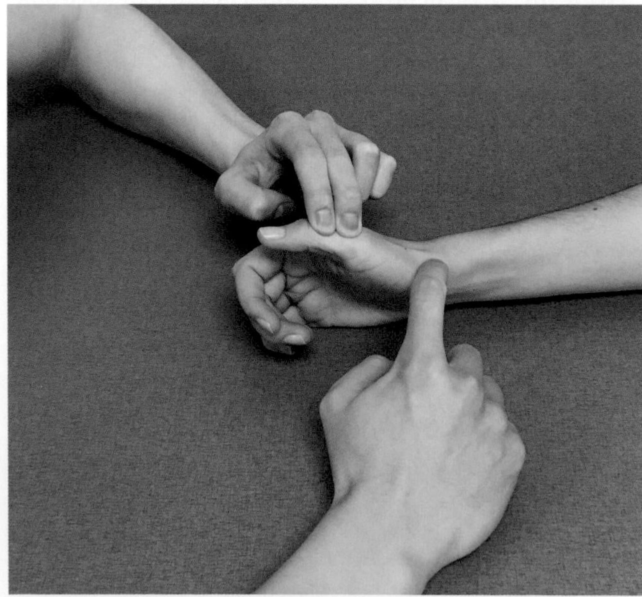

Figure 13-122. Thumb metacarpophalangeal extension, against gravity. The therapist is pointing at the extensor pollicis longus.

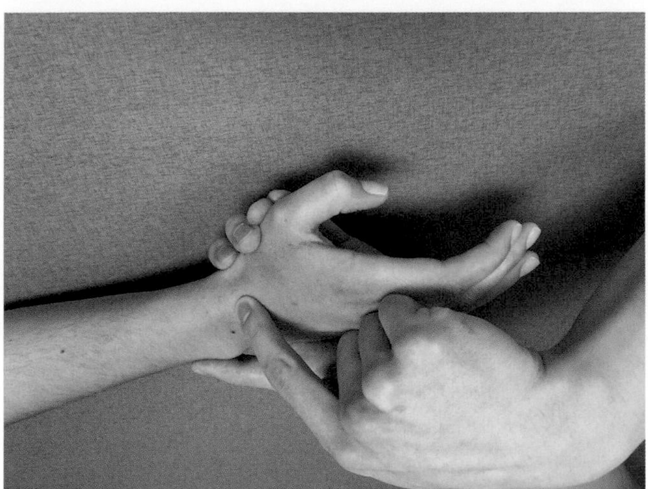

Figure 13-123. Thumb metacarpophalangeal extension, gravity eliminated.

- *Stabilize:* First metacarpal in abduction.
- *Instruction:*
  - EPL—"Try to straighten your thumb."
  - Extensor pollicis brevis—"Try to straighten the knuckle of your thumb while keeping the end joint bent."
- *Palpation:* Palpate the tendon of the EPL on the medial border of the anatomical snuffbox (Fig. 13-123). The tendon of the extensor pollicis brevis can be palpated on the lateral border of the anatomical snuffbox just medial to the tendon of the APL (Fig. 13-123).

Thumb Metacarpophalangeal Flexion

Prime Movers

Flexor pollicis brevis (FPB) and FPL.

Against-Gravity Position for the Flexor Pollicis Brevis

- *Start position:* Elbow flexed and supported on the table. Shoulder externally rotated and forearm supinated so that the palmar surface of the thumb faces the ceiling; thumb is extended at both the MP and IP joints.
- *Stabilize:* Firmly support the first metacarpal.
- *Instruction:* "Bend your thumb across your palm, keeping the end joint of your thumb straight. Do not let me pull it back out."
- *Resistance:* The therapist's finger pushes the head of the proximal phalanx toward extension.
- *Substitutions:* FPL; the abductor pollicis brevis (APB) and the adductor pollicis through insertion into the extensor hood (Fig. 13-124).

Gravity-Eliminated Position

- *Start position:* Forearm supinated to 90° so that the thumb can flex across the palm.
- *Stabilize:* First metacarpal.
- *Instruction:* "Try to bend your thumb into your palm, keeping the end joint of your thumb straight."
- *Palpation:* Palpate the FPB on the thenar eminence just proximal to the MP joint and medial to the APB (Fig. 13-125).

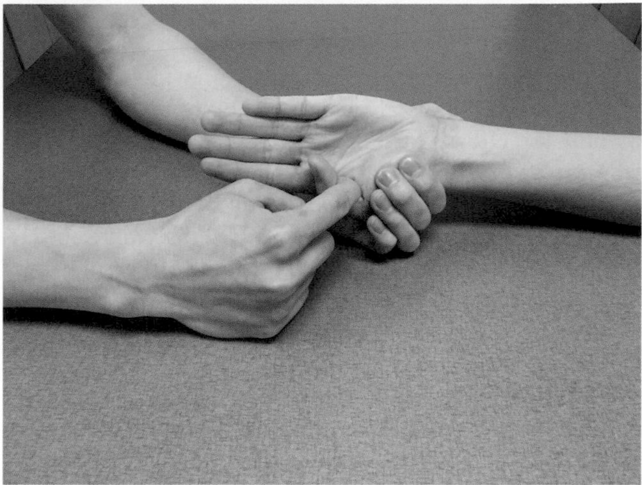

Figure 13-124. Thumb metacarpophalangeal flexion, against gravity.

Thumb Interphalangeal Extension

Prime Mover

Extensor pollicis longus (EPL).

Against-Gravity Position

- *Start position:* Forearm supported in neutral, wrist flexion of 10° to 20°, and thumb MP and IP flexion.

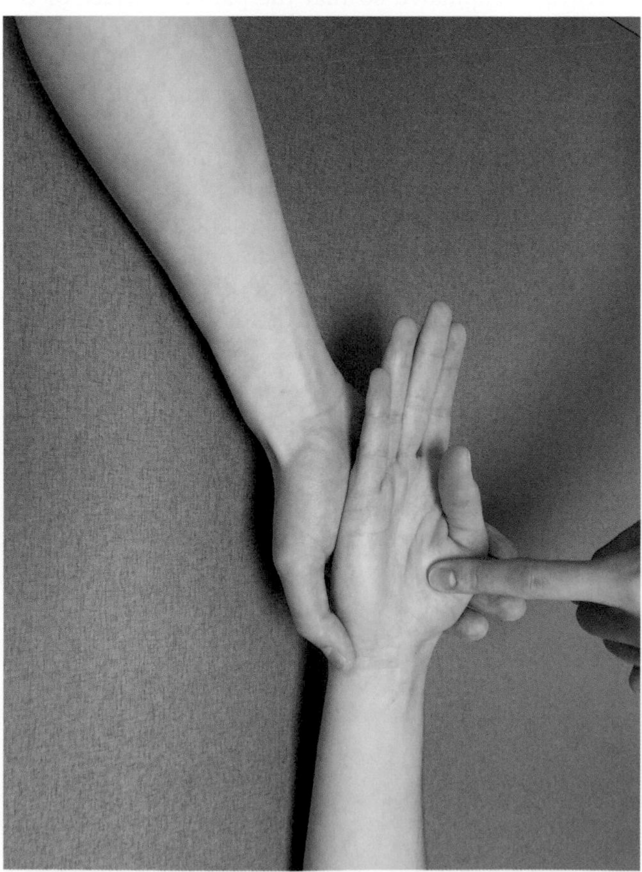

Figure 13-125. Thumb metacarpophalangeal flexion, gravity eliminated.

- *Stabilize:* Proximal phalanx into MP flexion.
- *Instruction:* "Straighten the end of your thumb."
- *Resistance:* The therapist places one finger over the dorsum of the distal phalanx (thumbnail) and pushes only the DIP toward flexion.
- *Substitutions:* Relaxation of the FPL produces apparent extensor movement as a result of a rebound effect. The APB, adductor pollicis, and FPB insert into the lateral aspects of the dorsal expansion, so they may produce thumb IP extension when the EPL is paralyzed (Fig. 13-126).

Gravity-Eliminated Position

- *Start position:* Forearm pronated or supinated, thumb flexed.
- *Instruction:* "Try to straighten the end of your thumb."
- *Palpation:* The tendon of the EPL may be palpated on the ulnar border of the anatomical snuffbox and on the dorsal surface of the proximal phalanx of the thumb (Fig. 13-127).

Thumb Interphalangeal Flexion

Prime Mover

Flexor pollicis longus (FPL).

Against-Gravity Position

- *Start position:* Elbow flexed and supported on a table. Forearm supinated so that the palmar surface of the thumb faces the ceiling; thumb extended at the MP and IP joints.
- *Stabilize:* Proximal phalanx, holding MP joint in extension.
- *Instruction:* "Bend the tip of your thumb as far as you can, and do not let me straighten it."
- *Resistance:* The therapist's finger pushes the head of the distal phalanx toward extension.
- *Substitution:* Relaxation of the EPL causes apparent rebound movement (Fig. 13-128).

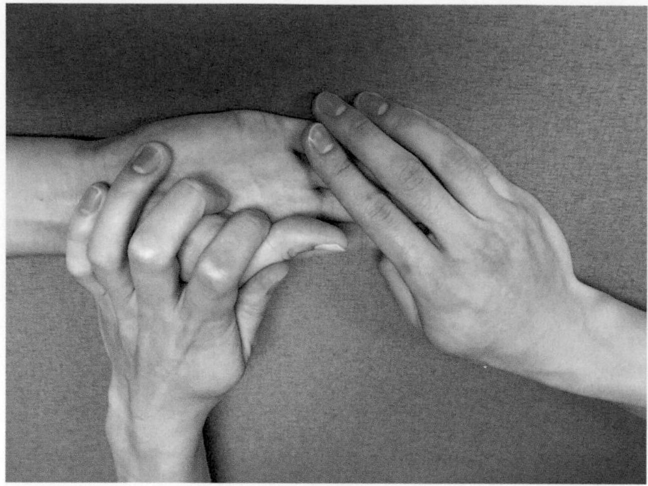

Figure 13-127. Thumb interphalangeal extension, gravity eliminated.

Gravity-Eliminated Position

- *Start position:* Forearm supinated to 90° so that the thumb can flex across the palm.
- *Stabilize:* Proximal phalanx, holding MP joint in extension.
- *Instruction:* "Try to bend the tip of your thumb as far as you can."
- *Palpation:* Palpate the FPL on the palmar surface of the proximal phalanx (Fig. 13-129).

Thumb (Palmar) Abduction

Prime Movers

Abductor pollicis longus (APL) and abductor pollicis brevis (APB).

Against-Gravity Position

- *Start position:* Forearm is supported in supination, wrist in neutral position, and thumb adducted.
- *Stabilize:* Support the wrist in neutral position by holding it on the dorsal and ulnar side.

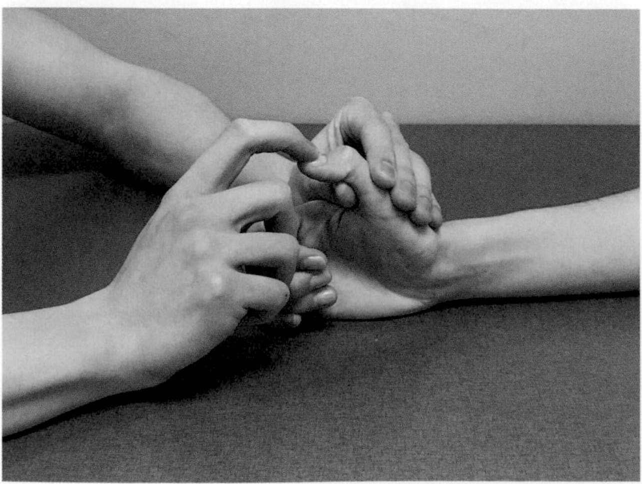

Figure 13-126. Thumb interphalangeal extension, against gravity.

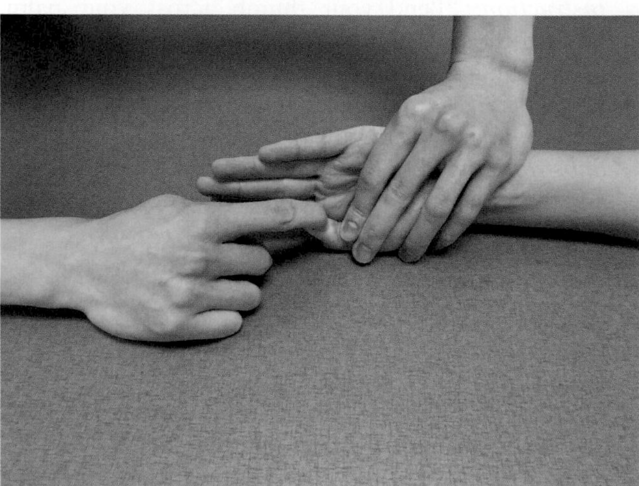

Figure 13-128. Thumb interphalangeal flexion, against gravity.

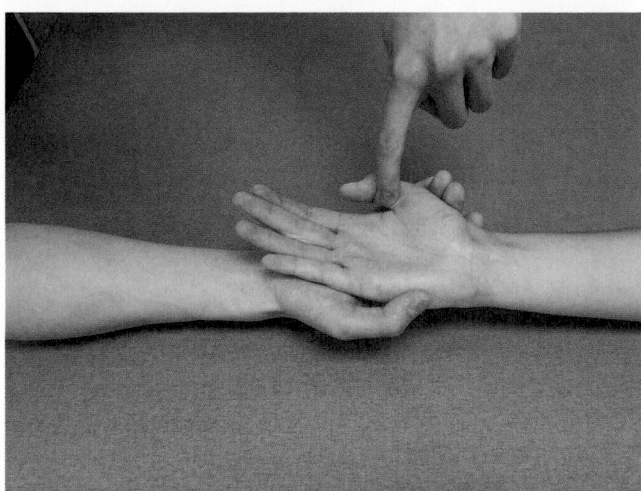

Figure 13-129. Thumb interphalangeal flexion, gravity eliminated.

- *Instruction:* "Lift your thumb directly out of the palm of the hand. Do not let me push it back in."
- *Resistance:* The therapist's finger presses the head of the first metacarpal toward adduction.
- *Substitutions:* APL may substitute for a weak APB, and APB may substitute for a weak APL; however, it is difficult to assess these muscles separately. The extensor pollicis brevis may also substitute (Fig. 13-130).

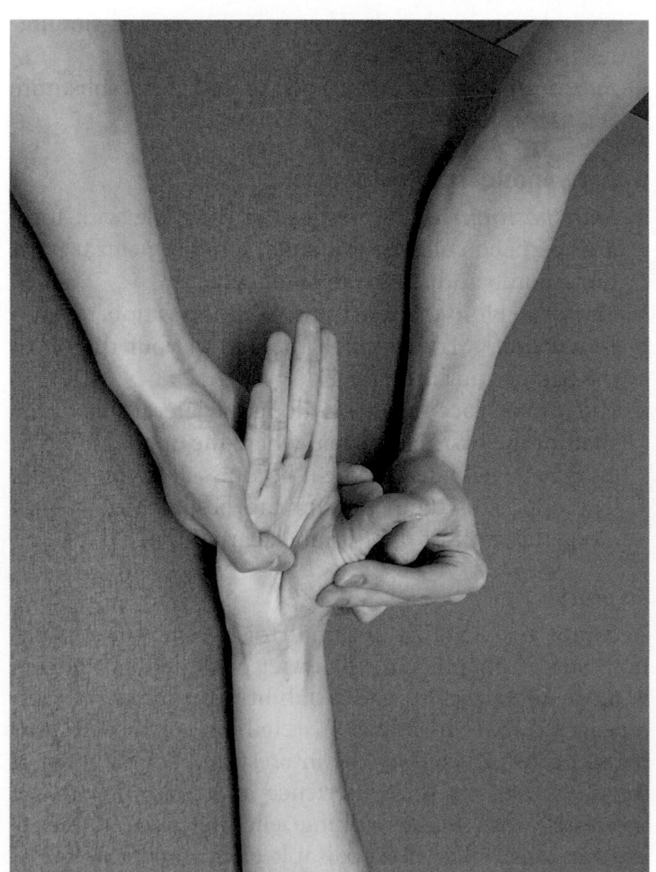

Figure 13-130. Thumb (palmar) abduction, against gravity.

Gravity-Eliminated Position

- *Start position:* Forearm and wrist are supported in neutral, thumb adducted.
- *Stabilize:* Support the wrist in neutral position by holding it on the dorsal and ulnar side.
- *Instruction:* "Try to move your thumb away from the palm of your hand."
- *Palpation:* Palpate the APL at the most lateral border of the anatomical snuffbox (Fig. 13-131) and the APB over the center of the thenar eminence.

Thumb Adduction

Prime Mover

Adductor pollicis.

Against-Gravity Position

- *Start position:* Forearm pronated, wrist and fingers in neutral position, thumb abducted, and MP and IP joints of the thumb in extension.
- *Stabilize:* Metacarpals of fingers, keeping the MP joints in neutral.
- *Instruction:* "Lift your thumb into the palm of your hand, and do not let me pull it out."
- *Resistance:* The therapist grasps the head of the proximal phalanx and tries to pull it away from the palm toward abduction.
- *Substitutions:* The EPL, FPL, or FPB may substitute (Fig. 13-132).

Gravity-Eliminated Position

- *Start position:* Forearm in midposition, wrist and fingers in neutral position, thumb abducted, and MP and IP joints of the thumb in extension.
- *Stabilization:* Metacarpals of fingers, keeping the MP joints in neutral.
- *Instruction:* "Try to bring your thumb into the palm of your hand."
- *Palpation:* Palpate the adductor pollicis on the palmar surface of the thumb web space (Fig. 13-133).

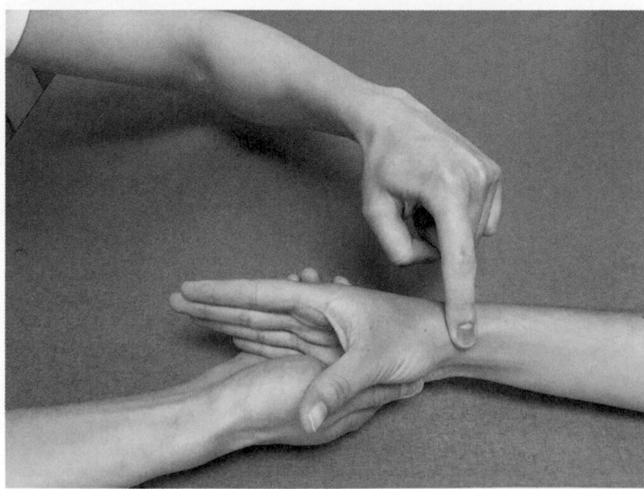

Figure 13-131. Thumb (palmar) abduction, gravity eliminated.

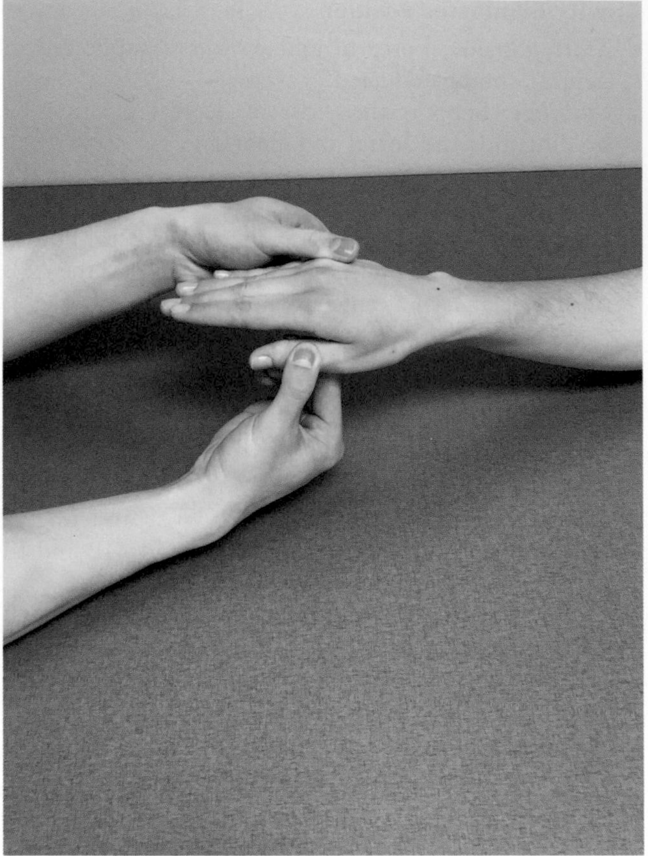

Figure 13-132. Thumb adduction, against gravity.

Opposition

Prime Movers

Opponens pollicis and opponens digiti minimi.

Against-Gravity Position

- *Start position:* Forearm supinated and supported, wrist in neutral position, thumb adducted and extended.
- *Stabilize:* Hold the wrist in a neutral position.

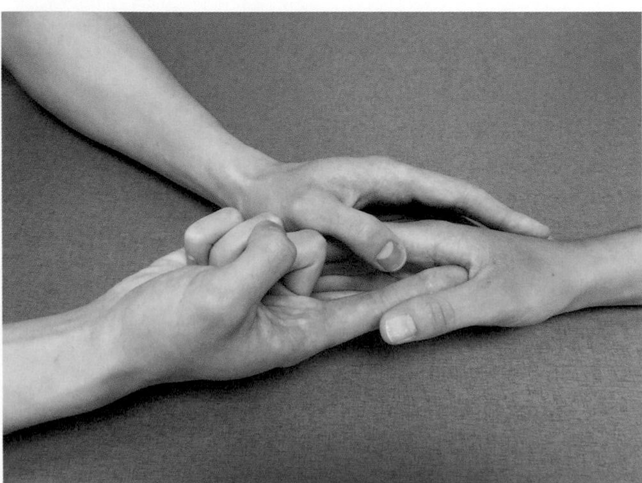

Figure 13-133. Thumb adduction, gravity eliminated.

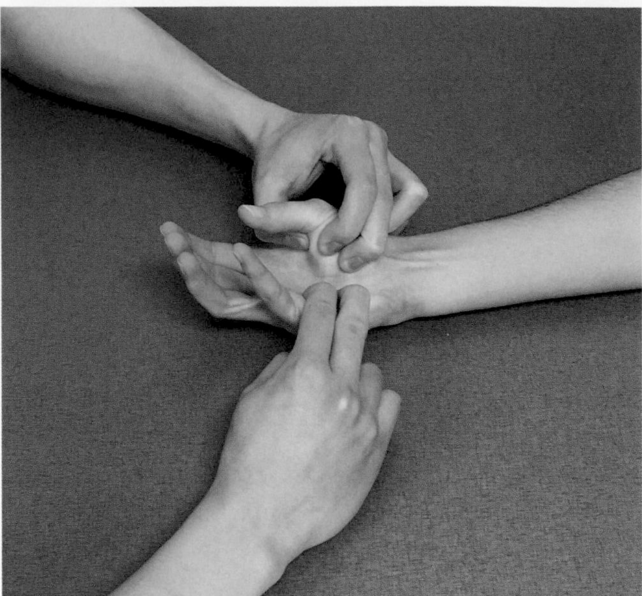

Figure 13-134. Opposition, against gravity.

- *Instruction:* "Touch the pad of your thumb to the pad of your little finger. Do not let me pull them apart."
- *Resistance:* To test the opponens pollicis, the therapist holds along the first metacarpal and attempts to pull the thumb away from the little finger. To test the opponens digiti minimi, the therapist holds along the fifth metacarpal and attempts to pull the little finger away from the thumb. These can be resisted simultaneously using both hands.
- *Substitutions:* The APB, FPB, or FPL may substitute (Fig. 13-134).

Gravity-Eliminated Position

- *Start position:* Elbow resting on the table with forearm perpendicular to the table, wrist in neutral position, thumb adducted and extended.
- *Stabilize:* Hold the wrist in a neutral position.
- *Instruction:* "Try to touch the pad of your thumb to the pad of your little finger."
- *Palpation:* Place fingertips along the lateral side of the shaft of the first metacarpal where the opponens pollicis may be palpated before it becomes deep to the APB. The opponens digiti minimi can be palpated volarly along the shaft of the fifth metacarpal (Fig. 13-135).

Accuracy

Accuracy of MMT is essential for meaningful evaluation. Strict adherence to the exact procedures of testing is most important to the reliability of the scores with repeated tests.[48] In addition, reliability of muscle testing scores is affected by the interest and cooperation of the client and by the experience and tone of voice of the tester, with higher volume eliciting greater muscle contractions.[55] The most suitable environment is free of distractions, is at a comfortable temperature, and has

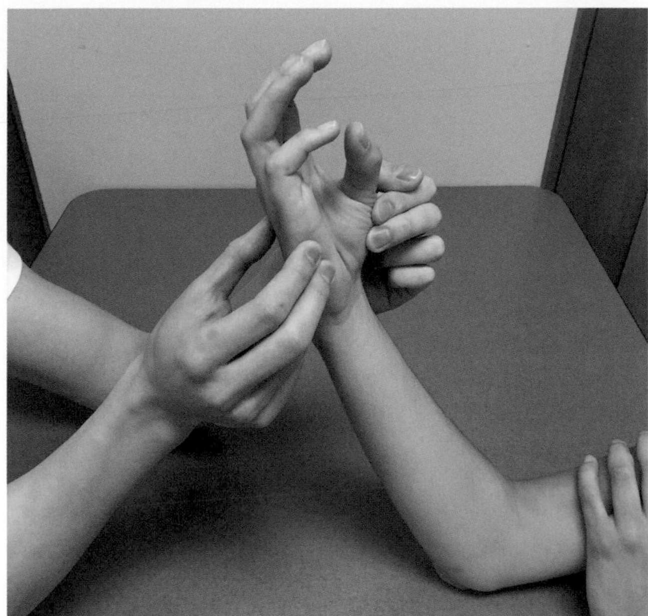

Figure 13-135. Opposition, gravity eliminated.

proper lighting. Other factors known to affect outcome are posture, fatigue, the client's ability to understand directions, the therapist's operational definitions of various grades, and test positions.[49] For reliability, these variables must be controlled from test to test and among therapists at the same facility. It is necessary for the inexperienced therapist to develop a kinesthetic sense of minimal, moderate, and maximal resistances by working with experienced therapists, each testing the same client and discussing the grade to be assigned.[51]

Recording Muscle Strength Scores

Muscle strength must be accurately documented in the medical record, identifying muscle or muscle group tested, grades assigned to the right and left sides, date of testing, and electronic or physical signature of the therapist performing the evaluation. A sample form is presented in Figure 13-136. On that form, the peripheral nerve and spinal segmental levels are listed beside each muscle to assist the therapist in interpreting the results of the muscle test.

Interpreting the Results

After recording all muscle test scores, the therapist reviews the scores and looks for the weak muscles and the distribution and significance of the weakness. Any muscle that grades "good minus" (4−) or below is considered weak. "Good plus" (4+) muscles are functional and usually require no therapy. "Good" (4) muscles may or may not be functionally adequate for the client, depending on his or her occupational task requirements.[48,50,51] The pattern of muscle weakness is important. The pattern may indicate general weakness caused by disuse secondary to immobilization, or it may reflect the level of spinal innervation in a client after spinal cord injury or the distribution of a peripheral nerve in the case of peripheral nerve injury. A pattern of imbalance of forces in agonist muscles (i.e., muscles that contract to make a movement) and antagonist muscles (i.e., muscles that relax to allow a movement) may be deforming; therefore, counter positioning or splinting should be considered along with strengthening of the weak muscles.

The pattern of significant strength is also important. For example, a muscle test of a client with an injured spinal cord that indicates some strength in a muscle innervated by a segment below the diagnosed level of injury is hopeful for more recovery. For muscles that are reinnervated proximally to distally after peripheral nerve injury, recording the pattern of return of strength in particular muscles helps track the progress of nerve regeneration.

Short-term goals move the client from the level of strength determined by testing to the next higher level. For example, if a muscle grades 3, the short-term goal is to improve strength to 3+; if it grades 3+, the goal is to increase strength to 4−, and so on. However, the goal should not purely reflect the numerical increase in the muscle strength. Improved strength should instead be reflected in some sort of functional task. For example, the short-term goal may state that the client will demonstrate an increase in left elbow muscle strength to 3+, as needed for independent hygiene tasks of brushing the teeth and washing the face. The required strength for occupational functioning must always be kept in mind when establishing goals.

If the muscle is being reevaluated, the scores are compared with those of the previous test. The frequency of reevaluation depends on the nature of expected recovery. Expected rapid recovery requires frequent reevaluation. For example, in a young, healthy individual recovering from a fracture that has been cleared by the surgeon to begin strengthening, it may be appropriate to reevaluate every 2 weeks until full strength is returned. However, in an individual recovering from a peripheral nerve injury when nerve healing is slow and expected to only heal 1 inch every month, it may be more appropriate to wait 4 weeks between reevaluations. If significant gains are noted in therapy and the client would benefit from a change in the treatment plan, then a reevaluation should be completed to document these gains and the change in treatment plan. If the repeated muscle test shows that the client is making gains, the program is considered beneficial, and its demands are upgraded. If repeated muscle tests show no gains despite program adaptations, the client is considered to have reached a plateau and to no longer benefit from remedial therapy. In that case, the focus of treatment shifts to teaching the client compensatory strategies and the use of adaptive equipment to enable participation in desired tasks and activities, as addressed in the rehabilitative frame of reference.[56]

There are, of course, exceptions to these standards. Clients with degenerative diseases are expected to get weaker; therefore, therapy is aimed at maintaining their

Patient's Name: ______________________________ Age: ________

LEFT Date	LEFT Date		RIGHT Date	RIGHT Date
		Scapula		
		ELEVATION		
		Upper trapezius (accessory) CN XI, C3-4		
		Levator scapulae (dorsal scapular) C5, C3-4		
		DEPRESSION		
		Lower trapezius (accessory) CN XI, C3-4		
		Latissimus dorsi (thoracodorsal) C6-8		
		ADDUCTION		
		Middle trapezius (accessory) CN XI, C3-4		
		Rhomboids (dorsal scapular) C5		
		ABDUCTION		
		Serratus anterior (long thoracic) C5-7		
		Shoulder		
		FLEXION		
		Anterior deltoid (axillary) C5-6		
		Coracobrachialis (musculocutaneous) C5-6		
		Pectoralis major-clavicular (pectoral) C5-6		
		Biceps (musculocutaneous) C5-6		
		EXTENSION		
		Latissimus dorsi (thoracodorsal) C6-8		
		Teres major (lower subscapular) C5-6		
		Posterior deltoid (axillary) C5-6		
		Triceps-long head (radial) C7-8		
		ABDUCTION		
		Supraspinatus (suprascapular) C5-6		
		Middle deltoid (axillary) C5-6		
		ADDUCTION		
		Latissimus dorsi (thoracodorsal) C6-8		
		Teres major (lower subscapular) C5-6		
		Pectoralis major (pectoral) C5-T1		
		HORIZONTAL ABDUCTION		
		Posterior deltoid (axillary) C5-6		
		HORIZONTAL ADDUCTION		
		Pectoralis major (pectoral) C5-T1		
		Anterior deltoid (axillary) C5-6		
		EXTERNAL ROTATION		
		Infraspinatus (suprascapular) C5-6		
		Teres minor (axillary) C5-6		
		Posterior deltoid (axillary) C5-6		
		INTERNAL ROTATION		
		Subscapularis (upper, lower subscapular) C5-7		
		Teres major (lower subscapular) C6-7		
		Latissimus dorsi (thoracodorsal) C6-8		
		Pectoralis major (pectoral) C5-T1		
		Anterior deltoid (axillary) C5-6		
		Elbow		
		FLEXION		
		Biceps (musculocutaneous) C5-6		
		Brachioradialis (radial) C5-7		
		Brachialis (musculocutaneous) C5-6 (radial) C7-8		
		EXTENSION		
		Triceps (radial) C6-8		

Figure 13-136. Sample form for recording manual muscle strength. (Reprinted with permission from Pansky B. *Review of Gross Anatomy*. 6th ed. New York, NY: McGraw-Hill; 1996.)

Patient's Name: ______________________ Age: ______________

LEFT RIGHT

Date	Date		Date	Date
		Forearm		
		PRONATION		
		Pronator teres (median) C6-7		
		Pronator quadratus (median) C8-T1		
		SUPINATION		
		Supinator (radial) C5-6		
		Biceps (musculocutaneous) C5-6		
		Wrist		
		EXTENSION		
		Ext. carpi radialis longus (radial) C6-7		
		Ext. carpi radialis brevis (radial) C7-8		
		Ext. carpi ulnaris (radial) C7-8		
		FLEXION		
		Flexor carpi radialis (median) C6-7		
		Palmaris longus (median) C7-8		
		Flexor carpi ulnaris (ulnar) C8-T1		
		Fingers		
		DIP FLEXION		
		1st flexor profundus (median) C8-T1		
		2nd flexor profundus (median) C8-T1		
		3rd flexor profundus (ulnar) C8-T1		
		4th flexor profundus (ulnar) C8-T1		
		5TH MP FLEXION		
		Flexor digiti minimi (ulnar) C8-T1		
		PIP FLEXION		
		1st flexor superficialis (median) C7-T1		
		2nd flexor superficialis (median) C7-T1		
		3rd flexor superficialis (median) C7-T1		
		4th flexor superficialis (median) C7-T1		
		ADDUCTION		
		1st palmar interosseus (ulnar) C8-T1		
		2nd palmar interosseus (ulnar) C8-T1		
		3rd palmar interosseus (ulnar) C8-T1		
		ABDUCTION		
		1st dorsal interosseus (ulnar) C8-T1		
		2nd dorsal interosseus (ulnar) C8-T1		
		3rd dorsal interosseus (ulnar) C8-T1		
		4th dorsal interosseus (ulnar) C8-T1		
		MP EXTENSION		
		1st extensor digitorum (radial) C7-8		
		2nd extensor digitorum (radial) C7-8		
		3rd extensor digitorum (radial) C7-8		
		4th extensor digitorum (radial) C7-8		
		Extensor digiti minimi (radial) C7-8		
		IP EXTENSION		
		1st lumbrical (median) C8-T1		
		2nd lumbrical (median) C8-T1		
		3rd lumbrical (ulnar) C8-T1		
		4th lumbrical (ulnar) C8-T1		

Figure 13-136. *(continued)*

Patient's Name: ______________________ Age: __________

LEFT Date	LEFT Date		RIGHT Date	RIGHT Date
		Thumb		
		EXTENSION		
		Extensor pollicis longus (radial) C7-8		
		Extensor pollicis brevis (radial) C7-8		
		FLEXION		
		Flexor pollicis longus (median) C8-T1		
		Flexor pollicis brevis (median) C8-T1		
		ABDUCTION		
		Abductor pollicis longus (radial) C7-8		
		Abductor pollicis brevis (median) C8-T1		
		ADDUCTOR		
		Adductor pollicis (ulnar) C8-T1		
		OPPOSITION		
		Opponens pollicis (median) C8-T1		
		Opponens digiti minimi (ulnar) C8-T1		
		Hip		
		FLEXION		
		Iliopsoas (femoral) L2-3		
		EXTENSION		
		Gluteus maximus (inf. gluteal) L5-S2		
		Knee		
		FLEXION		
		Hamstrings (tibial) L5-S2		
		EXTENSION		
		Quadriceps (femoral) L2-4		
		Ankle		
		DORSIFLEXION		
		Tibialis anterior (deep peroneal) L4-S1		
		Extensor digitorum longus (deep peroneal) L4-S1		
		Extensor hallucis longus (deep peroneal) L4-S1		
		PLANTARFLEXION		
		Gastrocnemius (tibial) S1-2		
		Soleus (tibial) S1-2		

Therapist's signature: ______________________ Date: __________

Figure 13-136. *(continued)*

strength and function for as long as possible, and efficacy is confirmed with repeat tests. A plateau for these clients is desirable; it indicates that the therapy is effective for maintaining strength and should be continued. Documentation of how this maintenance of strength impacts independence in ADL and IADL tasks should also be used to justify continued services. These clients often benefit from rehabilitation to maintain their current level of independence as well as learn compensatory techniques to conserve energy and maintain independence.[56]

Dynamometry

Other methods of muscle testing can provide more specific data regarding strength, such as isokinetic testing with Cybex and Biodex machines.[57] In addition, a strain gauge device or handheld dynamometer has been used for isometric strength testing. This type of dynamometer is placed directly against the body part being tested to register specific muscle strength when resistance is applied.[58,59] This is a different type of device from the dynamometer frequently used to measure grip strength (see Fig. 13-137).

Use of the handheld dynamometer includes placing it perpendicular to the limb segment with the joint in a gravity-eliminated position. The client is asked to build a maximum contraction against the dynamometer for a 1- to 2-second period and then to hold that contraction against the dynamometer for 4 to 5 seconds. The recorded measure is the maximum isometric value that was achieved by the client. This type of measurement is particularly helpful for quantifying antigravity strength, grades 3+ to 5.[60]

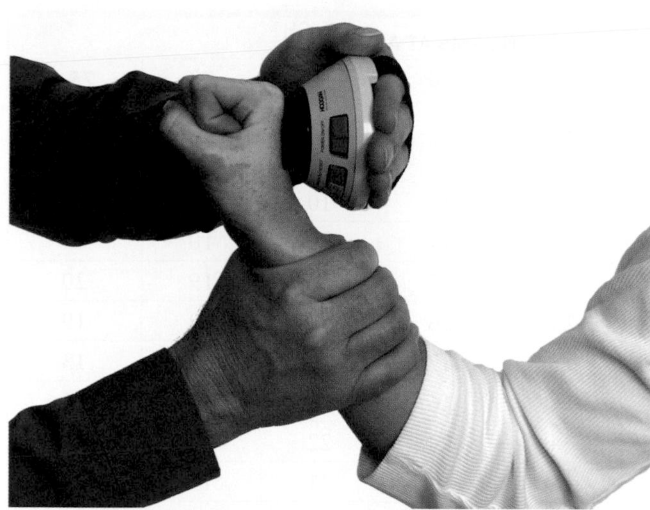

Figure 13-137. Example of handheld dynamometer for isometric strength testing. (Picture courtesy of Hoggan Scientific.)

The standardized positions and handheld dynamometer placement for each muscle group tested are described in detail by Hébert et al.[61] Owing to the expense, time required, and lack of correlation with MMT, all of these alternative methods of evaluating proximal muscle strength (Cybex, Biodex, and handheld dynamometry) are generally limited to research protocols.[62]

Grip and Pinch Strength Measurement

More specific measurements beyond MMT grading can demonstrate more discrete changes in grip and pinch strength. The ASHT recommends procedures for hand-grip strength, pinch strength, methods, and equipment.[22] Grip- and pinch-strength assessments can be compared to established norms or with measurements from the client's opposite hand (if the client does not fit the norms criteria) to ascertain whether there is a significant limitation. Normative data for both grip and pinch strength has long been established and frequently used as a reference for adults.[63] Other studies of normative values from heterogeneous populations are also available for reference.[64–70] Tables 13-3 and 13-4 list means and standard deviations (SD) for grip and pinch (tip, lateral, and palmar) measures from 628 adults, aged 20 to 75+.[63]

When individual scores are outside of these established norms, an individual with unilateral injury may also be compared to himself or herself using the 10% rule. In right-handed individuals, the dominant side is typically 10% stronger than is the nondominant side, although left-handed individuals typically demonstrate equal strength bilaterally.[71] For example, imagine a client recovering from a metacarpal fracture that can now demonstrate a full composite fist. He has an average score of 50 lb on the right dominant hand, and an average of 100 lb on the left nondominant hand. Using the 10% rule, the therapist would anticipate that 110 lb was the client's right-hand strength before injury. The therapist's assessment could be written as, "Client is 7 weeks post–metacarpal fracture with good return of motion. He demonstrates 45.5% of right-hand strength compared to the left and 42.7% compared to established norms for his age and gender. The client would benefit from continued occupational therapy services to increase strength needed for work and daily tasks." Grip and pinch measurements can be quickly and easily reevaluated over time to monitor the progress of the client and the effectiveness of the treatment plan.

Instruments

Grip-strength norms were originally established using the Jamar **dynamometer.**[63] This type of dynamometer is the most commonly used device for measuring grip strength in research,[64,70,72–75] and is recommended for clinical use by the ASHT.[22] However, interinstrument reliability, or the

Table 13-3. Grip Strength Norms in Pounds for Adults

		NORMS BY AGE											
		20	25	30	35	40	45	50	55	60	65	70	75+
Men	Right	121	121	122	120	117	110	114	101	90	91	75	66
	SD	21	23	22	24	21	23	18	27	20	21	21	21
	Left	104	110	110	113	113	101	102	83	77	77	65	55
	SD	22	16	22	22	19	23	17	23	20	20	18	17
Women	Right	70	74	79	74	70	62	66	57	55	50	50	43
	SD	14	14	19	11	13	15	12	12	10	10	12	11
	Left	61	63	68	66	62	56	57	47	46	41	41	38
	SD	13	12	18	12	14	13	11	12	10	8	10	9

N = 628; age range = 20 to 94.
SD, standard deviation.
Reprinted with permission from Mathiowetz V, Kashman N, Volland G, Weber K, Dowe M, Rogers S. Grip and pinch strength: normative data for adults. *Arch Phys Med Rehabil.* 1985;66:69–74.

Table 13-4. Pinch-Strength Norms in Pounds for Adults

			NORMS AT AGE						
			20	30	40	50	60	70	75+
Tip	Men	Right	18	18	18	18	16	14	14
		Left	17	18	18	18	15	13	14
	Women	Right	11	13	11	12	10	10	10
		Left	10	12	11	11	10	10	9
Lateral	Men	Right	26	26	26	27	23	19	20
		Left	25	26	25	26	22	19	19
	Women	Right	18	19	17	17	15	14	13
		Left	16	18	16	16	14	14	11
Palmar	Men	Right	27	25	24	24	22	18	19
		Left	26	25	25	24	21	19	18
	Women	Right	17	19	17	17	15	14	12
		Left	16	18	17	16	14	14	12

Tip pinch average standard deviation (SD): men, 4.0; women, 2.5. Lateral pinch average SD: men, 4.6; women, 3.0. Palmar pinch average SD: men, 5.1; women, 3.7. $N = 628$; age range = 20 to 94.

Reprinted with permission from Mathiowetz V, Kashman N, Volland G, Weber K, Dowe M, Rogers S. Grip and pinch strength: normative data for adults. *Arch Phys Med Rehabil.* 1985;66:69–74.

ability of multiple instruments to be used interchangeably, has been established between devices with various levels of confidence (see Table 13-5 for a listing of instruments used to measure grip strength).[71,76] There is a difference between electronic and hydraulic dynamometers with grip-strength measurements being approximately 10% higher when using hydraulic dynamometers.[77] Therefore, the same instrument should be used throughout each client's therapy. Although these instruments can be used with various levels of confidence against the norms, the selected instrument still must be calibrated every 4 to 12 months.[78] It is recommended to use the same instrument[79] at the same time of day using a standard protocol and instructions for body and instrument position when evaluating and reevaluating individual clients.[22,80] In the use of the Jamar dynamometer, there are five grooves along the handle used to select the grip position. The second grip position from the gauge is the standard position used for previous normative data and is recommended to increase reliability.[76,80] The assessment of grip strength with the Jamar Plus+ dynamometer is easier and faster if a single, standard handle position is used rather than multiple different positions. As well as providing accurate results, a single, standard handle position also reduces fatigue and increases the comparability of results to norms.[81] However, hand size[82] and nail length[83] may impact which position allows for maximum grip strength, so Boadella et al.[84] suggested that it may be more advantageous to allow the client to self-select their hand-grip position. It was also recommended that a change in score of at least 6 kg or 13 lb is needed to be clinically significant.[85]

In the past, it was thought that the vigorimeter could not be used interchangeably with a dynamometer.[71] However, it has always been an acceptable

Table 13-5. Dynamometer Equipment Interinstrument Reliability Compared to the Jamar Dynamometer

EXCELLENT	MODERATE TO EXCELLENT	LOW	UNCLEAR
■ Dexter ■ Baseline ■ Rolyan Hydraulic ■ Martin Vigorimeter	■ Baltimore Therapeutic Equipment (BTE) work simulator ■ BTE Primus ■ MicroFET 4 ■ DynEx	■ Sphygmomanometer ■ Vigorimeter ■ Smedley Dynamometer ■ Takei Dynamometer	■ Grippit dynamometer

Roberts HC, Denison HJ, Martin HJ, et al. A review of the measurement of grip strength in clinical and epidemiological studies: towards a standardised approach. *Age Ageing*. 2011;40(4):423–429. doi:10.1093/ageing/afr051; Sousa-Santos AR, Amaral TF. Differences in handgrip strength protocols to identify sarcopenia and frailty—a systematic review. *BMC Geriatr*. 2017;17(1):238. doi:10.1186/s12877-017-0625-y.

alternative hand strength–measuring device for clients whose diagnoses contraindicate stress on joints and/or skin, because it requires the client to squeeze a rubber bulb rather than a steel handle. More recently, the Jamar dynamometer and the vigorimeter have been found to have aspects of comparable validity, reliability, and responsiveness.[86] In fact, the vigorimeter has been found to be just as reliable as the dynamometer and more practical for populations that have difficulty adhering to the administrative constraints of the dynamometer.[87] The vigorimeter is a commercially available instrument for which norms have been published.[88]

The pinch norms can be used with the B & L, JTech, and NK pinch meters because they have been found to be interchangeably reliable.[89] However, there is a significant difference between the use of the commonly available mechanical pinch gauges and the newer electronic pinch gauges, with lateral pinch-strength measurements measuring approximately 18% higher with mechanical pinch gauges.[77] Therefore, it is recommended to always use the same instrument for each client for best reliability.

Calibration

As with any tool of measurement, the instrument must be calibrated and set at zero to start. Dynamometers and pinch meters can be calibrated by placing known weights on or suspending them from the compression part of the meter.[78] With this procedure, the Jamar dynamometer was found to be accurate to within 7%,[90] and the B & L pinch meter was found to be accurate within 1%.[91] Clinically this means that, if a client registered 50 lb for grip strength, the actual strength may range from 46.5 to 53.5 lb. Grip and pinch scores are considered abnormal if they are associated with a functional limitation and/or if they are three SD from the mean. For example, suppose a 40-year-old man had a mean average grip score of 50 lb after three trials for his dominant right hand. Table 13-3 shows that the mean average score for his age group is 117 lb, so the client's grip score was 67 lb less than is the mean normal score on the table. When the difference in his score is divided by the SD given in the table (21), he is 3.2 SD below the mean. He would be considered to have a significant limitation because his grip score is more than 3 SD below the mean.

Assessment of Grip Strength

There is significant clinical importance to following the standardized testing procedures for grip- and pinch-strength measurement as recommended by the ASHT.[22] Great attention should be paid to specific placement of the UE during testing, such as wrist,[92] forearm,[93] elbow,[94–96] and shoulder[97] positions. In addition, verbal instructions and encouragement can also alter outcomes.[55] To obtain the maximal hand-grip strength, at least three attempts or trials should be recorded.[98]

The specific protocol for testing grip strength according to the ASHT[22] is as follows:

1. The dynamometer should be calibrated and set on the second rung (if a different rung is used, such as for large hands, it should be noted and justified).
2. The dynamometer's dial should be turned away from the client and the examiner should gently support the base of the dynamometer.
3. The client should be seated in a chair without armrests, with feet fully resting on the floor, hips as far back in the chair as possible, and the hips and knees positioned at approximately 90°.
4. Shoulders should be adducted and neutrally rotated with the elbow flexed at 90° and the forearm in neutral position.
5. The wrist should be between 15° and 30° of extension (dorsiflexion) and 0° to 15° of ulnar deviation.
6. The task is demonstrated to the client.
7. After the dynamometer is positioned in the client's hand, the therapist says, "This test will tell me your maximum grip strength. When I say go, grip as hard as you can until I say stop. Before each trial, I will ask you, 'Are you ready?' and then tell you 'Go.' Stop immediately if you experience any unusual pain or discomfort at any point during testing. Do you have any questions? Are you ready? Go!" "Harder...harder...harder...Relax."
8. The client squeezes the dynamometer with as much force as he or she can three times, with each trial acquisition time being at least 3 seconds.
9. A rest break of at least 15 seconds is given between trials.
10. The score is the mean average of the three successive trials.

An alternative procedure that can be used is the Southampton protocol.[71] The main differences of the Southampton protocol are that the client's forearms are rested on the armrests of the chair, three trials on each side are elicited alternating sides (starting with the right hand), and the results are maximal grip score from all six trials. Note that research has suggested that a single trial is as reliable as multiple trials,[99] which may be appropriate for cases in which multiple trials would cause undue pain or stress; however, to assess maximal hand-grip strength, at least three attempts are needed.[98] See Figure 13-138 for standardized position for grip-strength testing, and Table 13-3 for grip-strength normative data.

Assessment of Pinch Strength

Three types of pinch are typically evaluated because they are involved in accomplishing occupational tasks and activities efficiently: the tip pinch, the lateral pinch, and the palmar pinch. The seating and positioning of the arm should be the same as with grip testing, with the addition that the fingers should be allowed to flex. With

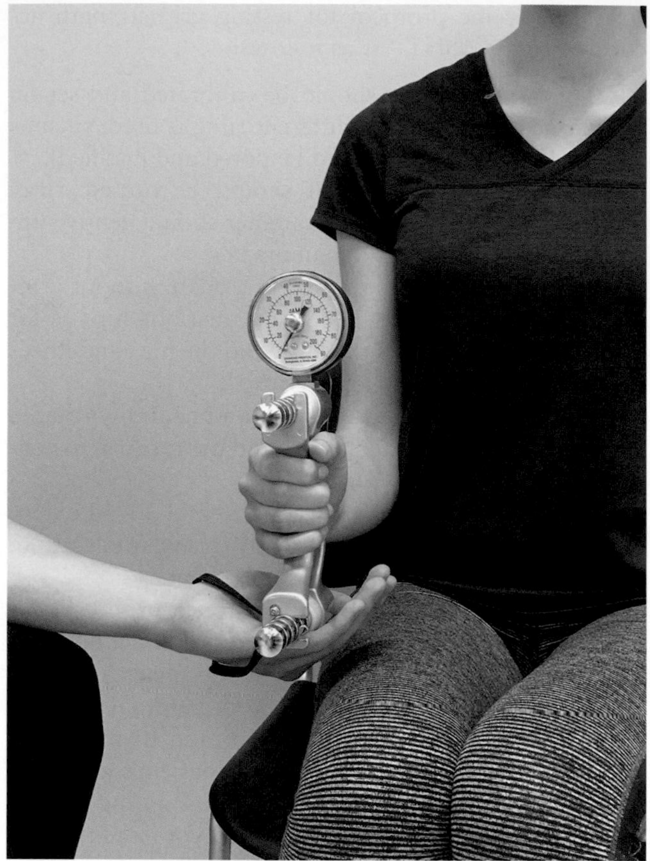

Figure 13-138. Measuring grip using a dynamometer. The client's upper arm is close to his body, and the elbow is flexed to 90°.

both tip and palmar pinch, it is important to note that to keep the forearm in a neutral position, the pinch gauge must be held vertically, and the wrist will naturally extend to assume the best testing position.[89] The following instructions are based on the ASHT[22] recommendations.

Tip Pinch

The pinch gauge is presented on its side at an angle of approximately 45°. The client pinches the ends of the pinch gauge between the tips of the thumb and index finger. The index finger is on the dial side and the fingertips must stop at the finger groove (as if the client is making an "O"). The thumb and index IP joints must be flexed. The middle, ring, and little fingers are flexed in the palm. The test is administered by first giving the client instructions and a demonstration. Next, the therapist says, "Are you ready? Pinch as hard as you can." The client is urged on as he or she attempts to pinch. Three trials, with a rest between each trial, are completed. The mean average of three trials is recorded. It is important to observe for any compensation techniques because some clients will naturally try to use the middle finger to assist without recognizing their deviance from the instructed test position. See Figure 13-139 for standardized position for tip pinch-strength testing, and Table 13-4 for tip pinch-strength normative data.

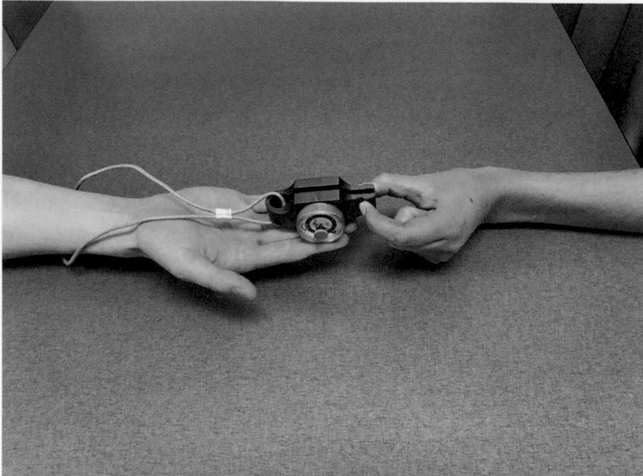

Figure 13-139. Measuring tip pinch strength with a pinch gauge.

Lateral Pinch: Key Pinch

The pinch gauge is presented in line with the forearm with the dial facing up. The client pinches the gauge between the pad of the thumb and the radial side of the middle phalanx of the index finger. The thumb is on the dial side and must stop at the finger groove. The IP joint of the thumb must be flexed. The fingers are flexed in the palm. The instructions and procedure are the same as for tip pinch, but the pinch gauge is held horizontally, as if holding a key. Interestingly, in a study of key pinch in children aged 5 to 12 years, differences were found according to age, but no significant differences were found by hand or gender in this age range. On the basis of these findings, comparing the right to left side in this age range should be possible as long as the injury or condition is not bilateral.[100] See Figure 13-140 for standardized position for lateral pinch-strength testing, and Table 13-4 for key pinch-strength normative data.

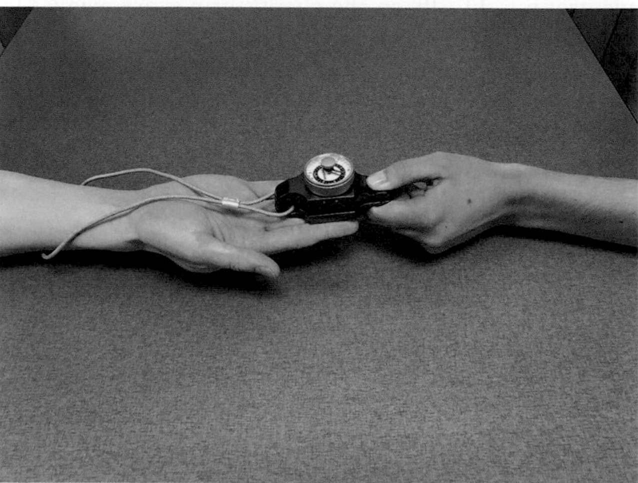

Figure 13-140. Measuring lateral pinch strength with a pinch gauge.

Palmar Pinch: Three-Jaw Chuck

The pinch gauge is presented on its side at an angle of approximately 45°. It is held between the pulp of the thumb and the pulp of the index and middle fingers. The index and middle fingers are on the dial side and the fingertips must stop at the finger groove. The thumb and fingers IP joints must be slightly flexed. The ring and little fingers are flexed in the palm. The client pinches the meter between the pad of the thumb and the pads of the index and middle fingers. The instructions and procedure are the same as for tip pinch. See Figure 13-141 for standardized position for palmar pinch-strength testing, and Table 13-4 for palmar pinch-strength normative data.

Endurance Measurement

Occupational therapists treat clients with a variety of conditions that can impact an individual's endurance, including cardiac or pulmonary impairments, a major trauma or illness requiring bed rest, loss of significant muscle function, or the need to use a prosthesis or adaptive equipment. There are two components of endurance. The first is **cardiorespiratory (CR) endurance**, which is the ability of the circulatory and respiratory system to supply oxygen during a task.[101] The second is muscular endurance, in which muscles continue to perform without fatigue.[101] Both of these aspects of endurance are vital to engage in ADL and IADL tasks, which is why occupational therapists refer to it as activity tolerance. Focusing on activity tolerance distinguishes the goal of occupational therapy from the goals of other professions that also address endurance. The therapist may evaluate one aspect or both depending on the client's symptoms.

Cardiorespiratory Aspects

The role of the occupational therapist here is most clearly seen in the role of therapists in cardiac rehabilitation programs, although these same principles may apply to an individual receiving therapy after prolonged bed rest or to an individual in home health with decreased endurance. Once an individual is cleared to begin a cardiac rehabilitation program from his or her physician following a cardiac event, activities that test CR fitness should progress slowly in terms of frequency, intensity, and time (duration) or FIT of exercise.[101] Activities to test CR fitness can begin with very light or light self-care tasks, progressing to moderately difficult IADLs, such as household management tasks, and then assessing vigorous activities such as return to work. The occupational therapist should assess the client's environment in which he or she performs tasks, such as the home and the workplace. This allows the occupational therapist to gain a better understanding of the activity demands and use task analysis to develop a program to return the client to the endurance level needed to complete tasks.

Another way to assess endurance is to ascertain the individual's perception of how hard he or she is working. Scales of perceived exertion, such as the rating of perceived exertion,[102] are based on psychophysics or the relating of a physical property to a subjective property via scaling procedures.[103] The Borg (15-point) scale of perceived exertion ranges from 6 (no exertion at all) to 20 (maximal exertion). This scale allows the person to assign one of a consecutive set of numbers with a corresponding descriptor of amount of exertion to the ongoing activity (e.g., 11, fairly light; or 17, very hard). Although subjective, multiplying the rating of exertion by 10 can provide a rough estimate of heart rate.[104] Therapists should be aware that perceived exertion for a given level of oxygen uptake is higher for arm work than for leg work.[103] The therapist should orient the client to the scale using the standardized instructions published by Borg[104] before the start of the activity. The scale should be enlarged and posted so that it can be seen easily from where the person is engaging in activity. At appropriate intervals depending on the task, the therapist prompts the client to rate exertion at that moment. The decision to continue depends on the goal and precautions for the particular client.

Another measure easily used when engaging in functional tasks is the talk test.[105] The client should be able to continue talking in full sentences during engagement in therapeutic tasks. This is correlated with the ventilator threshold, and when the client can no longer talk comfortably he or she has passed this threshold.[105]

These scales provide a good estimate when used repeatedly for the same client and therefore may be used clinically during ongoing continuous activity, such as walking, bicycling, scrubbing floors, painting a wall, mowing the lawn, raking leaves, and calisthenic exercises. Scales of perceived exertion do not apply to

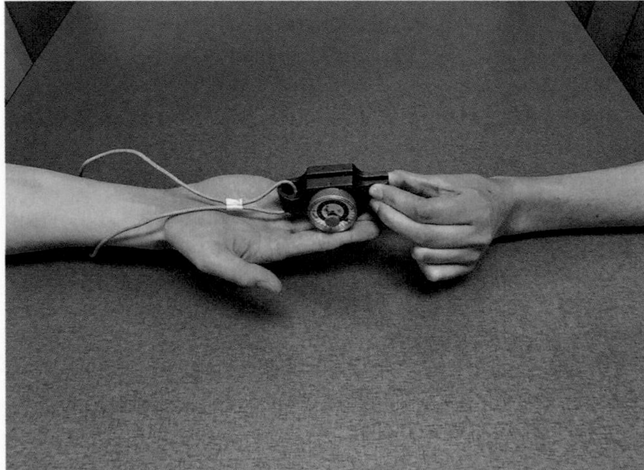

Figure 13-141. Measuring palmar pinch (or three-jaw chuck pinch) strength with a pinch gauge.

activities composed of sporadic variable movements, such as those that have frequent changes in intensity.

Muscular Aspects

Muscular fitness is a combination of muscular strength and muscular endurance.[101] This chapter has already explored the evaluation of muscular strength with MMT, grip, and pinch-strength testing. Muscular endurance is the ability of the muscle to perform multiple repetitions of a contraction without fatigue.[101] Endurance may be decreased because of local trauma or reduction of nerve innervation. In normal muscle contraction against low resistance, only a few of the available motor units are needed at any one time. The active and resting units take turns. If the person sustains a contraction that exceeds 15% to 20% MVC for the muscle group involved, blood flow to the working muscle decreases, causing a shift to anaerobic metabolism, which limits duration of contraction. The limitation is signaled by symptoms of muscle fatigue (cramping, burning, and tremor, which are secondary to the accumulation of lactic acid) and slowed nerve conduction velocity to the muscle fibers, which reduce tension and eventually result in an inability to hold the contraction.[101] Strength and endurance are closely related. As muscle gains strength, its endurance for a given level of work also increases. It is important to note that for neurologically disadvantaged muscles, such as after a stroke, fewer motor units or muscle fibers may be available than are required for daily activity. Such muscles work at as much as 50% to 75% MVC to do otherwise low-intensity work.[106]

Muscle endurance can be measured dynamically or statically. Dynamic assessments include the number of repetitions per unit of time. Static assessment is the amount of time a contraction can be held.[101,107] Frequency, intensity, and time (duration) of the activity are considerations when evaluating endurance. Intensity is related to both resistance and speed. The heavier the resistance or the faster the pace (speed), the higher the intensity. The intensity of the test activity must be kept constant from test to test to gauge improvement.

The decision to measure dynamically or statically depends on the functional goal of the client and his or her cardiopulmonary status. If the client's self-advancement and self-enhancement roles require mostly isotonic activity, endurance should be evaluated dynamically. To measure endurance in terms of number of repetitions, use a light repetitive activity such as sitting to fold washcloths. An activity like this can be adapted to measure UE endurance for light work by counting the number of washcloths the client can fold before becoming fatigued.

For some individuals, decreased endurance might need to be assessed with heavier repetitive tasks such as those that simulate their ability to return to work. In these cases, a functional capacity evaluation (FCE) may be appropriate. FCEs measure a client's occupational performance to participate in work or in the worker role. As a whole, it assesses the client's impairment (such as endurance), occupational performance overall, and the role performance of the work to which the client wants to return.[108] There are multiple components that are assessed in an FCE, including the record review, interview (of the client and employer), physical measures/musculoskeletal assessment, physiological measures, functional measures, and comparisons of testing with job requirements. Each feature of an FCE should be considered with care.[109]

A commonly used piece of equipment that may be used in an FCE is the Baltimore Therapeutic Equipment (BTE) work simulator. This equipment can be set up to simulate a variety of work and daily tasks, such as digging with a shovel, turning a knob, climbing a ladder or rope, and using a steering wheel (among other things). It is a helpful device to use when it is not feasible to perform the actual work task, or if the client needs to work on a specific component of the work task. A static trial can be completed to gain a numeric value for the individual's MVC for that task. Then, to test endurance, the therapist can set the resistance level at 20% to 30% of that maximum. The therapist can see on the equipment if the client is decreasing in speed and showing fatigue. The time, repetitions, and weight can be documented for later comparison to show progress in the area of endurance. Although these numbers can be used clinically to demonstrate progress, the therapist should use caution when relating them to work capacity.

If the client expects to return to a job or hobby that requires isometric contractions, such as maintaining grasp or holding loads, static endurance should be tested. To measure statically, the amount of time a person can hold an object or position requiring a certain level MVC is noted. Normally, a person can hold 25% MVC for 5 to 6 minutes, 50% MVC for 1 to 2 minutes, and 100% MVC only momentarily.[101]

Isometric holding increases blood pressure and stresses the cardiopulmonary system.[110] This is true especially if the person holds his or her breath (Valsalva maneuver) while holding the contraction. Therefore, clients being tested should talk (e.g., count or sing) while doing an isometric contraction to preclude breath holding. Isometric testing can produce arrhythmias and, therefore, electrocardiogram and blood pressure should be monitored during isometric testing of clients with heart disease or abnormalities. The results of isometric testing cannot be extrapolated to gauge isotonic aerobic exercise capacity.[110] However, blood pressure measurements performed during isometric hand-grip exercises may be a useful screening tool in evaluating prehypertensive individuals.[111]

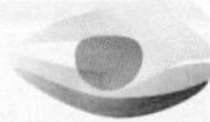

CASE STUDY

Client Information

Pat is a 42-year-old, right-handed person, who is 8 weeks status post open reduction internal fixation of a right humerus fracture following a gunshot wound during an assault in a parking lot in the city (about 45 minutes away). Pat's radial nerve (which is frequently injured during humerus fractures) was not lacerated, but Pat did have wrist drop for a week following the injury and surgery that has slowly been improving (neuropraxia). Pat complains of UE weakness, stiffness, and decreased motion. Pat also complains of pain and fatigue that are increasingly limiting ADLs, IADLs, and participation in meaningful activities.

Pat is a dental hygienist, who has a life partner who frequently travels for work. They live in a one-story house. Pat has two grown children and enjoys gardening, working out at the gym, and shopping. Pat was previously seen at another facility recommended by the injury lawyer but has decided to transfer to a new facility because it is closer to Pat's home. Pat recently had a follow-up with the surgeon, who referred Pat to occupational therapy for evaluation and to begin strength training.

Assessment Process

To determine Pat's perception of occupational dysfunction and Pat's priorities, the therapist administered the Canadian Occupational Performance Measure (COPM). To determine the extent that motion, strength, and endurance problems affected Pat's occupational functioning, AROM assessment, a manual muscle test on selected muscle groups, grip- and pinch-strength assessments, and engagement in 1 minute of wrist activity on the BTE for endurance during work tasks were administered.

Assessment Results

The results of the COPM are as follows:

- Difficulty holding dental hygienist tools for prolonged periods (performance 3, satisfaction 2).
- Difficulty with morning ADL, including showering and dressing. Pat has problems squeezing bottles, bathing the left side of the body such as the armpit and back, and putting on jewelry (performance 6, satisfaction 5).
- Difficulty engaging in shopping tasks because of the fear associated with it. Pat was on a shopping trip when the trauma occurred (performance 5, satisfaction 4).
- Inability to do heavy meal preparation activities, including cutting vegetables and carrying dishes (performance 6, satisfaction 4).
- Unable to garden as desired, specifically planting, digging with a trowel, and weeding (performance 3, satisfaction 2).

Grip and Pinch Strength

	Right	Left
Grip	18	58
Tip pinch	3	12
Lateral pinch	5	14
Palmar pinch	4	13

Active Range of Motion

Shoulder, wrist, and hand AROM within normal limits
Elbow extension–flexion right: 30°–120°
Elbow flexion left: 0°–150°
Elbow hyperextension left: 0°–5°
Supination right: 0°–60°
Supination left: 0°–90°
Pronation right: 0°–80°
Pronation left: 0°–90°

Pat has a 22-cm scar along the dorsal aspect of the arm that is red in appearance and flat. There is mild adhesion noted along the scar, and the scar does pucker with elbow motion.

Select Manual Muscle Strength

	Right	Left
Shoulder flexion	5	5
Shoulder abduction	4−	5
Elbow flexion	4	5
Elbow extension	4	5
Forearm supination	4	5
Forearm pronation	4	5
Wrist flexion	5	5
Wrist extension	3+	5
Digital extension	3+	5

Using the BTE, Pat demonstrated only five repetitions of wrist motion during 1 minute when set at 70% of Pat's MVC, which was 3 lb.

Occupational Therapy Problem List

- Decreased ability to perform morning ADL, including bathing and dressing, because of decreased motion, weakness, and low endurance.
- Decreased ability to perform meal preparation tasks because of weak grasp and pinch on the dominant side.
- Decreased ability to perform work-related tasks, including manipulating tools for prolonged periods of time because of weakness and decreased endurance of the muscles innervated by the radial nerve.
- Decreased ability to garden because of weakness and pain.
- Decreased engagement in shopping tasks depending on psychosocial factors.

Most Commonly Used Standardized Assessments for Motor Function

Instrument and Reference	Intended Purpose	Administration Time	Validity	Reliability	Sensitivity	Strengths and Weaknesses
Range of motion[19,20]	Measurement of joint range of motion	Full evaluation of all joints in the UE, 45 minutes to an hour	The concurrent validity between goniometry and digital inclinometry (for shoulder mobility) is good (intraclass correlation coefficient [ICC] ≥ 0.85) [112]	Interrater reliability for the measurement of passive movements of upper extremity joints varies with the method of measurement[4]	In the upper and lower extremities, measurement error is estimated at 5°[33]	*Strengths:* Relatively fast and inexpensive measure. Measurements are consistently more accurate when done by the same therapist with the client in the same position from test to test *Weaknesses:* Interrater reliability is consistently lower than is intrarater reliability. Accuracy of measurement is dependent on the consistent placement of the goniometer
Hand volumetry[34]	Edema measurement through the displacement of water	10–20 minutes	Water displacement correlated with geometric measurements in the arm ($r = 0.97$–0.98) and in the hand ($r = 0.81$–0.91)[36]	Test–retest reliability ($r = 0.999$)[35]	Variation of measurement 3–5 mL[34]	*Strength:* Easily accessible way of obtaining accurate measurement of edema *Weakness:* Hand must be immersed in water, so therapist must be aware of any contraindications. Takes considerable time
Figure-of-eight technique[37]	Edema measurement of the hand with circumferential tape assessment	1–4 minutes	Correlation coefficient between figure-of-eight technique and hand volumetry ICC = 0.83–0.95[37,38]	Intratester ICC for figure-of-eight ICC = 0.96–0.99; intertester reliability ICC = 0.94–0.99[37,113]	Recommend change of 1.16 cm to be clinically significant in clients with burns to the hands[114]	*Strengths:* Fast measurement. Can be used with individuals with open wounds or skin conditions *Weakness:* Larger studies of various client populations needed

Manual muscle testing[48,53,115]	Strength test of individual muscles and muscle groups	Depending on the number of muscles being tested, up to 1 hour	Spearman's correlation coefficients of the maximal relative force measurements with the median Medical Research Council and modified Medical Research Council score were both 0.78[53]	In a reliability test for intrinsic hand muscles, intrarater ($r = 0.71–0.96$) and interrater ($r = 0.72–0.93$) reliability.[116] In an evaluation of reliability for the deltoid muscles, Pollard et al.[117] found that two testers agreed exactly 82% of the time, ($\kappa = 0.62$)	Not established	*Strength:* No equipment needed *Weakness:* Dependent on training and experience of the tester
Handheld dynamometry[61]	Interval scale; measurement is in kilograms	Depending on the number of muscles being tested, up to 1 hour	Mean concurrent validity (ICC) varied from 0.78 to 0.93[118]	Interrater reliability ICC = 0.79–0.96, and intrarater reliability ICC = 0.87–0.98[119]	Norms established[59]	*Strength:* Reliable testing device *Weakness:* Expense of device
Grip strength test[22,80]	Measurement of grip strength by resistance in pounds or kilograms	5 minutes	Recommended by American Society of Hand Therapists as a valid measure of hand strength[22]	Test–retest reliability Jamar dynamometer $r > 0.8$,[80,120] and interrater reliability $r = 0.9$[71,76]	Norms established with gold standard Jamar dynamometer[63,65]; recommend 13-lb change for clinical significance[71]	*Strengths:* Quick and easy measure. Norms available *Weakness:* Dynamometers need to be calibrated regularly in order to be accurate
Pinch strength tests[22,80]	Measurement of pinch strength (tip, lateral, and palmar) by resistance in pounds or kilograms	5 minutes	Recommended by American Society of Hand Therapists as a valid measure of pinch strength[22]	Interrater reliability $r = 0.98$; test–retest reliability was $r = 0.81$[80]	Norms established[63,65]	*Strengths:* Quick and easy measure. Norms available *Weakness:* Pinch meters need to be calibrated regularly in order to be accurate
Borg rating of perceived exertion scale[103]	Measurement of perceived cardiorespiratory and muscular exertion	1 minute	Valid measure of exercise intensity.[121] Correlates with heart rate and oxygen uptake[122,123]	Reliable at high levels of exercise intensity[122]	More applicable at lower exercise levels with practice[122]	*Strength:* Good measure for individuals *Weakness:* Not consistent between individuals

References

1. Cyriax J. *Textbook of Orthopaedic Medicine: Diagnosis of Soft Tissue Lesions*. 8th ed. London, England: Bailliere Tindall; 1982.
2. Kaltenborn FM. *Manual Mobilization of the Extremity Joints*. 5th ed. Oslo, Norway: Olaf Norlis; 1999.
3. Paris SV. *Extremity Dysfunction and Mobilization*. Atlanta, GA: Institute Press; 1980.
4. Van de Pol RJ, Van Trijffel E, Lucas C. Inter-rater reliability for measurement of passive physiological range of motion of upper extremity joints is better if instruments are used: a systematic review. *J Physiother*. 2010;56(1):7–17. doi:10.1016/S1836-9553(10)70049-7.
5. Manning DM, Dedrick GS, Sizer PS, Brismée J. Reliability of a seated three-dimensional passive intervertebral motion test for mobility, end-feel, and pain provocation in patients with cervicalgia. *J Man Manip Ther*. 2012;20(3):135–141. doi:10.1179/2042618611Y.0000000023.
6. Barrett E, McCreesh K, Lewis J. Intrarater and interrater reliability of the flexicurve index, flexicurve angle, and manual inclinometer for the measurement of thoracic kyphosis. *Rehabil Res Pract*. 2013;2013:475870.
7. Barrett E, Lenehan B, O'Sullivan K, Lewis J, McCreesh K. Validation of the manual inclinometer and flexicurve for the measurement of thoracic kyphosis. *Physiother Theory Pract*. 2018;34:301–308. doi:10.1080/09593985.2017.1394411.
8. Van Blommestein AS, Lewis JS, Morrissey MC, MaCrae S. Reliability of measuring thoracic kyphosis angle, lumbar lordosis angle and straight leg raise with an inclinometer. *Open Spine J*. 2012;4(1):10–15. doi:10.2174/1876532701204010010.
9. Vohralik SL, Bowen AR, Burns J, Hiller CE, Nightingale EJ. Reliability and validity of a smartphone app to measure joint range. *Am J Phys Med Rehabil*. 2015;94(4):325–330. doi:10.1097/PHM.0000000000000221.
10. Milani P, Coccetta CA, Rabini A, Sciarra T, Massazza G, Ferriero G. Mobile smartphone applications for body position measurement in rehabilitation: a review of goniometric tools. *PM R*. 2014;6(11):1038–1043. doi:10.1016/j.pmrj.2014.05.003.
11. Legnani G, Zappa B, Casolo F, Adamini R, Magnani PL. A model of an electro-goniometer and its calibration for biomechanical applications. *Med Eng Phys*. 2000;22(10):711–722. doi:10.1016/s1350-4533(01)00009-1.
12. Wang PT, King CE, Do AH, Nenadic Z. A durable, low-cost electrogoniometer for dynamic measurement of joint trajectories. *Med Eng Phys*. 2011;33(5):546–552. doi:10.1016/j.medengphy.2010.12.008.
13. Yen TY, Radwin RG. Comparison between using spectral analysis of electrogoniometer data and observational analysis to quantify repetitive motion and ergonomic changes in cyclical industrial work. *Ergonomics*. 2000;43(1):106–132. doi:10.1080/001401300184684.
14. Blonna D, Zarkadas PC, Fitzsimmons JS, O'Driscoll SW. Validation of a photography-based goniometry method for measuring joint range of motion. *J Shoulder Elbow Surg*. 2012;21(1):29–35. doi:10.1016/j.jse.2011.06.018.
15. O'Neill BJ, O'Briain DM, Hirpara KM, Shaughnesy M, Yeatman EA, Kaar TK. Digital photography for assessment of shoulder range of motion: a novel clinical and research tool. *Int J Shoulder Surg*. 2013;7(1):23–27. doi:10.4103/0973-6042.109888.
16. Naylor JM, Ko V, Adie S, et al. Validity and reliability of using photography for measuring knee range of motion: a methodological study. *BMC Musculoskelet Disord*. 2011;12:77. doi:10.1186/1471-2474-12-77.
17. Fernández-Baena A, Susín A, Lligadas X. Biomechanical validation of upper-body and lower-body joint movements of kinect motion capture data for rehabilitation treatments. Presented at: Fourth International Conference on Intelligent Networking and Collaborative Systems; 2012:656–661; Bucharest, Romania. doi:10.1109/iNCoS.2012.66.
18. Zhou H, Hu H. Human motion tracking for rehabilitation—a survey. *Biomed Signal Process Control*. 2008;3(1):1–18. doi:10.1016/j.bspc.2007.09.001.
19. Greene WB, Heckman JD. *The Clinical Measurement of Joint Motion*. Rosemont, IL: American Academy of Orthopaedic Surgeons; 1994.
20. Gerhardt J, Cocchiarella L, Lea R. *The Practical Guide to Range of Motion Assessment*. Chicago, IL: American Medical Association; 2002.
21. Karagiannopoulos C, Sitler M, Michlovitz S. Reliability of 2 functional goniometric methods for measuring forearm pronation and supination active range of motion. *J Orthop Sports Phys Ther*. 2003;33(9):523–531. doi:10.2519/jospt.2003.33.9.523.
22. American Society of Hand Therapists. *American Society of Hand Therapists Clinical Assessment Recommendations: Impairment-Based Conditions*. 3rd ed. Mt. Laurel, NJ: American Society of Hand Therapists; 2015.
23. Ellis B, Bruton A. A study to compare the reliability of composite finger flexion with goniometry for measurement of range of motion in the hand. *Clin Rehabil*. 2002;16(5):562–570. doi:10.1191/0269215502cr513oa.
24. Norkin C, White DJ. *Measurement of Joint Motion: A Guide to Goniometry*. Philadelphia, PA: FA Davis; 2016.
25. Sabari JS, Maltzev I, Lubarsky D, Liszkay E, Homel P. Goniometric assessment of shoulder range of motion: comparison of testing in supine and sitting positions. *Arch Phys Med Rehabil*. 1998;79(6):647–651. doi:10.1016/S0003-9993(98)90038-7.
26. Carey MA, Laird DE, Murray KA, Stevenson JR. Reliability, validity, and clinical usability of a digital goniometer. *Work*. 2010;36(1):55–66. doi:10.3233/WOR-2010-1007.
27. Wellmon RH, Gulick DT, Paterson ML, Gulick CN. Validity and reliability of 2 goniometric mobile apps: device, application, and examiner factors. *J Sport Rehabil*. 2016;25(4):371–379. doi:10.1123/jsr.2015-0041.
28. Lee HH, St. Louis K, Fowler JR. Accuracy and reliability of visual inspection and smartphone applications for measuring finger range of motion. *Orthopedics*. 2018;42:e217–e221.
29. Akizuki K, Yamaguchi K, Morita Y, Ohashi Y. The effect of proficiency level on measurement error of range of motion. *J Phys Ther Sci*. 2016;28(9):2644–2651. doi:10.1589/jpts.28.2644.
30. Macedo LG, Magee DJ. Differences in range of motion between dominant and nondominant sides of upper and lower extremities. *J Manip Physiol Ther*. 2008;31(8):577–582. doi:10.1016/j.jmpt.2008.09.003.
31. Gates DH, Walters LS, Cowley J, Wilken JM, Resnik L. Range of motion requirements for upper-limb activities of daily living. *Am J Occup Ther*. 2016;70(1):7001350010p1–7001350010p10. doi:10.5014/ajot.2016.015487.

32. Aizawa J, Masuda T, Koyama T, et al. Three-dimensional motion of the upper extremity joints during various activities of daily living. *J Biomech*. 2010;43(15):2915–2922. doi:10.1016/j.jbiomech.2010.07.006.
33. Groth GN, VanDeven KM, Phillips EC, Ehretsman RL. Goniometry of the proximal and distal interphalangeal joints, part II: placement preferences, interrater reliability, and concurrent validity. *J Hand Ther*. 2001;14(1):23–29. doi:10.1016/S0894-1130(01)80021-1.
34. Dodds RL, Nielsen KA, Shirley AG, Stefaniak HA, Falconio MJ, Moyers PA. Test-retest reliability of the commercial volumeter. *Work*. 2004;22(2):107–110.
35. Tsang KKW, Norte GE, Hand JW. The assessment of hand volume using a modified volumetric technique. *J Test Eval*. 2012;40(2):329–333. doi:10.1520/JTE103841.
36. Sander AP, Hajer NM, Hemenway K, Miller AC. Upper-extremity volume measurements in women with lymphedema: a comparison of measurements obtained via water displacement with geometrically determined volume. *Phys Ther*. 2002;82(12):1201–1212.
37. Borthwick Y, Paul L, Sneddon M, McAlpine L, Miller C. Reliability and validity of the figure-of-eight method of measuring hand size in patients with breast cancer-related lymphoedema. *Eur J Cancer Care*. 2013;22(2):196–201. doi:10.1111/ecc.12024.
38. Maihafer GC, Llewellyn MA, Pillar WJ Jr, Scott KL, Marino DM, Bond RM. A comparison of the figure-of-eight method and water volumetry in measurement of hand and wrist size. *J Hand Ther*. 2003;16(4):305–310. doi:10.1197/S0894-1130(03)00155-8.
39. Mayrovitz HN, Sims N, Macdonald J. Assessment of limb volume by manual and automated methods in patients with limb edema or lymphedema. *Adv Skin Wound Care*. 2000;13(6):272–276.
40. Armer JM. The problem of post-breast cancer lymphedema: impact and measurement issues. *Cancer Invest*. 2005;23(1):76–83. doi:10.1081/CNV-200048707.
41. Casley-Smith JR, Casley-Smith JR. Modern treatment of lymphoedema. II. The benzopyrones. *Australas J Dermatol*. 1992;33(2):69–74. doi:10.1111/j.1440-0960.1992.tb00082.x.
42. McOwan CG, MacDermid JC, Wilton J. Outcome measures for evaluation of scar: a literature review. *J Hand Ther*. 2001;14(2):77–85. doi:10.1016/S0894-1130(01)80037-5.
43. American College of Sports Medicine. *Health-Related Physical Fitness Assessment Manual*. 4th ed. Philadelphia, PA: Wolters Kluwer Health/Lippincott Williams & Wilkins; 2014.
44. Maffiuletti NA, Aagaard P, Blazevich AJ, Folland J, Tillin N, Duchateau J. Rate of force development: physiological and methodological considerations. *Eur J Appl Physiol*. 2016;116(6):1091–1116. doi:10.1007/s00421-016-3346-6.
45. Palmer ML, Epler M. Principles of examination techniques. In: Palmer ML, Epler M, eds. *Clinical Assessment Procedures in Physical Therapy*. Philadelphia, PA: Lippincott Williams & Wilkins; 1990:8–36.
46. Van Der Ploeg RJO, Oosterhuis HJGH. The 'make/break test' as a diagnostic tool in functional weakness. *J Neurol Neurosurg Psychiatry*. 1991;54(3):248–251. doi:10.1136/jnnp.54.3.248.
47. Brody LT, Hall CM. *Therapeutic Exercise: Moving Toward Function*. 4th ed. Philadelphia, PA: Wolters Kluwer; 2018:1–779.
48. Hislop H, Avers D, Brown M. *Daniel's and Orthingham's Muscle Testing: Techniques of Manual Examination and Performance Testing*. 9th ed. St. Louis, MO: Elsevier Saunders; 2013.
49. Kendall FP, McCreary EK, Provance PG, Rodgers MM, Romani WA. *Muscles: Testing and Function with Posture and Pain*. 5th ed. Baltimore: Lippincott Williams & Wilkins; 2005.
50. Medical Research Council. *Aids to the Investigation of the Peripheral Nervous System*. London, England: Her Majesty's Stationary Office; 1976.
51. Clarkson HM. *Musculoskeletal Assessment: Joint Motion and Muscle Testing*. 3rd ed. Philadelphia, PA: Lippincott Williams & Wilkins; 2013.
52. Milner-Brown HS, Mellenthin M, Miller RG. Quantifying human muscle strength, endurance and fatigue. *Arch Phys Med Rehabil*. 1986;67(8):530–535.
53. Paternostro-Sluga T, Grim-Stieger M, Posch M, et al. Reliability and validity of the medical research council (MRC) scale and a modified scale for testing muscle strength in patients with radial palsy. *J Rehabil Med*. 2008;40(8):665–671. doi:10.2340/16501977-0235.
54. Escolar DM, Henricson EK, Mayhew J, et al. Clinical evaluator reliability for quantitative and manual muscle testing measures of strength in children. *Muscle Nerve*. 2001;24(6):787–793. doi:10.1002/mus.1070.
55. Johansson CA, Kent BE, Shepard KF. Relationship between verbal command volume and magnitude of muscle contraction. *Phys Ther*. 1983;63(8):1260–1265. doi:10.1093/ptj/63.8.1260.
56. Cole M, Tufano R. Biomechanical and rehabilitative frames. In: *Applied Theories in Occupational Therapy*. Thorofare, NJ: Slack Incorporated; 2008:165.
57. de Araujo Ribeiro Alvares JB, Rodrigues R, de Azevedo Franke R, et al. Inter-machine reliability of the biodex and cybex isokinetic dynamometers for knee flexor/extensor isometric, concentric and eccentric tests. *Phys Ther Sport*. 2015;16(1):59–65. doi:10.1016/j.ptsp.2014.04.004.
58. Bohannon RW. Hand-held dynamometry: a practicable alternative for obtaining objective measures of muscle strength. *Isokinet Exerc Sci*. 2012;20(4):301–315. doi:10.3233/IES-2012-0476.
59. Bohannon RW. Literature reporting normative data for muscle strength measured by hand-held dynamometry: a systematic review. *Isokinet Exerc Sci*. 2011;19(3):143–147. doi:10.3233/IES-2011-0415.
60. Hayes K, Walton JR, Szomor ZL, Murrell GAC. Reliability of 3 methods for assessing shoulder strength. *J Shoulder Elbow Surg*. 2002;11(1):33–39. doi:10.1067/mse.2002.119852.
61. Hébert LJ, Maltais DB, Lepage C, Saulnier J, Crête M. Hand-held dynamometry isometric torque reference values for children and adolescents. *Pediatr Phys Ther*. 2015;27(4):414–423. doi:10.1097/PEP.0000000000000179.
62. Watkins MP, Harris BA. Evaluation of skeletal muscle performance. In: Harms-Ringdahl K, ed. *Muscle Strength*. Edinburgh, Scotland: Churchill Livingstone; 1993:19–36.
63. Mathiowetz V, Kashman N, Volland G, Weber K, Dowe M, Rogers S. Grip and pinch strength: normative data for adults. *Arch Phys Med Rehabil*. 1985;66(2):69–74.
64. Peters MJH, Van Nes SI, Vanhoutte EK, et al. Revised normative values for grip strength with the jamar dynamometer. *J Peripher Nerv Syst*. 2011;16(1):47–50. doi:10.1111/j.1529-8027.2011.00318.x.

65. Werle S, Goldhahn J, Drerup S, Simmen BR, Sprott H, Herren DB. Age- and gender-specific normative data of grip and pinch strength in a healthy adult Swiss population. *J Hand Surg Eur Vol.* 2009;34(1):76–84. doi:10.1177/1753193408096763.
66. Lee-Valkov PM, Aaron DH, Eladoumikdachi F, Thornby J, Netscher DT. Measuring normal hand dexterity values in normal 3-, 4-, and 5-year-old children and their relationship with grip and pinch strength. *J Hand Ther.* 2003;16(1):22–28. doi:10.1016/S0894-1130(03)80020-0.
67. Angst F, Drerup S, Werle S, Herren DB, Simmen BR, Goldhahn J. Prediction of grip and key pinch strength in 978 healthy subjects. *BMC Musculoskelet Disord.* 2010;11:94. doi:10.1186/1471-2474-11-94.
68. Puh U. Age-related and sex-related differences in hand and pinch grip strength in adults. *Int J Rehabil Res.* 2010;33(1):4–11. doi:10.1097/MRR.0b013e328325a8ba.
69. Stegink Jansen CW, Niebuhr BR, Coussirat DJ, Hawthorne D, Moreno L, Phillip M. Hand force of men and women over 65 years of age as measured by maximum pinch and grip force. *J Aging Phys Act.* 2008;16(1):24–41.
70. Bohannon RW, Bear-Lehman J, Desrosiers J, Massy-Westropp N, Mathiowetz V. Average grip strength: a meta-analysis of data obtained with a jamar dynamometer from individuals 75 years or more of age. *J Geriatr Phys Ther.* 2007;30(1):28–30. doi:10.1519/00139143-200704000-00006.
71. Roberts HC, Denison HJ, Martin HJ, et al. A review of the measurement of grip strength in clinical and epidemiological studies: towards a standardised approach. *Age Ageing.* 2011;40(4):423–429. doi:10.1093/ageing/afr051.
72. Ashford RF, Nagelburg S, Adkins R. Sensitivity of the jamar dynamometer in detecting submaximal grip effort. *J Hand Surg.* 1996;21(3):402–405. doi:10.1016/S0363-5023(96)80352-2.
73. Cuesta-Vargas A, Hilgenkamp T. Reference values of grip strength measured with a jamar dynamometer in 1526 adults with intellectual disabilities and compared to adults without intellectual disability. *PLoS One.* 2015;10(6):e0129585. doi:10.1371/journal.pone.0129585.
74. Härkönen R, Harju R, Alaranta H. Accuracy of the jamar dynamometer. *J Hand Ther.* 1993;6(4):259–262. doi:10.1016/S0894-1130(12)80326-7.
75. Van Den Beld WA, Van Der Sanden GAC, Sengers RCA, Verbeek ALM, Gabreëls FJM. Validity and reproducibility of the jamar dynamometer in children aged 4–11 years. *Disabil Rehabil.* 2006;28(21):1303–1309. doi:10.1080/09638280600631047.
76. Sousa-Santos AR, Amaral TF. Differences in handgrip strength protocols to identify sarcopenia and frailty—a systematic review. *BMC Geriatr.* 2017;17(1):238. doi:10.1186/s12877-017-0625-y.
77. King TI. Interinstrument reliability of the jamar electronic dynamometer and pinch gauge compared with the jamar hydraulic dynamometer and B&L engineering mechanical pinch gauge. *Am J Occup Ther.* 2013;67(4):480–483. doi:10.5014/ajot.2013.007351.
78. Fess EE. A method for checking jamar dynamometer calibration. *J Hand Ther.* 1987;1(1):28–32. doi:10.1016/S0894-1130(87)80009-1.
79. Cadenas-Sanchez C, Sanchez-Delgado G, Martinez-Tellez B, et al. Reliability and validity of different models of TKK hand dynamometers. *Am J Occup Ther.* 2016;70(4):7004300010. doi:10.5014/ajot.2016.019117.
80. Mathiowetz V, Weber K, Volland G, Kashman N. Reliability and validity of grip and pinch strength evaluations. *J Hand Surg Am.* 1984;9(2):222–226. doi:10.1016/S0363-5023(84)80146-X.
81. Trampisch US, Franke J, Jedamzik N, Hinrichs T, Platen P. Optimal jamar dynamometer handle position to assess maximal isometric hand grip strength in epidemiological studies. *J Hand Surg Am.* 2012;37(11):2368–2373. doi:10.1016/j.jhsa.2012.08.014.
82. Ruiz-Ruiz J, Mesa JLM, Gutiérrez A, Castillo MJ. Hand size influences optimal grip span in women but not in men. *J Hand Surg Am.* 2002;27(5):897–901. doi:10.1053/jhsu.2002.34315.
83. Jansen CWS, Patterson R, Viegas SF. Effects of fingernail length on finger and hand performance. *J Hand Ther.* 2000;13(3):211–217. doi:10.1016/S0894-1130(00)80004-6.
84. Boadella JM, Kuijer PP, Sluiter JK, Frings-Dresen MH. Effect of self-selected handgrip position on maximal handgrip strength. *Arch Phys Med Rehabil.* 2005;86(2):328–331. doi:10.1016/j.apmr.2004.05.003.
85. Nitschke JE, McMeeken JM, Burry HC, Matyas TA. When is a change a genuine change?: a clinically meaningful interpretation of grip strength measurements in healthy and disabled women. *J Hand Ther.* 1999;12(1):25–30. doi:10.1016/S0894-1130(99)80030-1.
86. Draak THP, Pruppers MHJ, Van Nes SI, et al. Grip strength comparison in immune-mediated neuropathies: vigorimeter vs. jamar. *J Peripher Nerv Syst.* 2015;20(3):269–276. doi:10.1111/jns.12126.
87. Sipers WMWH, Verdijk LB, Sipers SJE, Schols JMGA, Van Loon LJC. The Martin vigorimeter represents a reliable and more practical tool than the jamar dynamometer to assess handgrip strength in the geriatric patient. *J Am Med Dir Assoc.* 2016;17(5):466.e1–466.e7. doi:10.1016/j.jamda.2016.02.026.
88. Fike ML, Rousseau F. Measurement of adult hand strength: a comparison of two instruments. *Occup Ther J Res.* 1982;2(1):43–49. doi:10.1177/153944928200200105.
89. MacDermid J, Evenhuis W, Louzon M. Inter-instrument reliability of pinch strength scores. *J Hand Ther.* 2001;14(1):36–42. doi:10.1016/S0894-1130(01)80023-5.
90. Shechtman O, Gestewitz L, Kimble C. Reliability and validity of the DynEx dynamometer. *J Hand Ther.* 2005;18(3):339–347. doi:10.1197/j.jht.2005.04.002.
91. Mathiowetz V, Vizenor L, Melander D. Comparison of baseline instruments to the jamar dynamometer and the B and L engineering pinch gauge. *Occup Ther J Res.* 2000;20(3):147–162. doi:10.1177/153944920002000301.
92. Yuvaraj Babu K, Saraswathi P. A study on influence of wrist joint position on grip strength in normal adult male individuals. *Int J Drug Dev Res.* 2014;6(3):161–164.
93. Richards LG, Olson B, Palmiter-Thomas P. How forearm position affects grip strength. *Am J Occup Ther.* 1996;50(2):133–138. doi:10.5014/ajot.50.2.133.
94. Dorf ER, Chhabra AB, Golish SR, McGinty JL, Pannunzio ME. Effect of elbow position on grip strength in the evaluation of lateral epicondylitis. *J Hand Surg Am.* 2007;32(6):882–886. doi:10.1016/j.jhsa.2007.04.010.
95. Kuzala EA, Vargo MC. The relationship between elbow position and grip strength. *Am J Occup Ther.* 1992;46(6):509–512. doi:10.5014/ajot.46.6.509.

96. Mathiowetz V, Rennells C, Donahoe L. Effect of elbow position on grip and key pinch strength. *J Hand Surg Am*. 1985;10(5):694–697. doi:10.1016/S0363-5023(85)80210-0.
97. Su C, Lin J, Chien T, Cheng K, Sung Y. Grip strength in different positions of elbow and shoulder. *Arch Phys Med Rehabil*. 1994;75(7):812–815.
98. Reijnierse EM, de Jong N, Trappenburg MC, et al. Assessment of maximal handgrip strength: how many attempts are needed? *J Cachexia Sarcopenia Muscle*. 2017;8(3):466–474. doi:10.1002/jcsm.12181.
99. Coldham F, Lewis J, Lee H. The reliability of one vs. three grip trials in symptomatic and asymptomatic subjects. *J Hand Ther*. 2006;19(3):318–327. doi:10.1197/j.jht.2006.04.002.
100. De Smet L, Decramer A. Key pinch force in children. *J Pediatr Orthop B*. 2006;15(6):426–427. doi:10.1097/01.bpb.0000218022.43277.f1.
101. American College of Sports Medicine. *ACSM's Guidelines for Exercise Testing and Prescription*. 10th ed. Philadelphia, PA: Wolters Kluwer; 2018.
102. Borg G. Psychophysical bases of perceived exertion. *Med Sci Sports Exerc*. 1982;14(5):377–381.
103. Russell WD. On the current status of rated perceived exertion. *Percept Mot Skills*. 1997;84(3, pt I):799–808. doi:10.2466/pms.1997.84.3.799.
104. Borg G. *Borg's Perceived Exertion and Pain Scales*. Champaign, IL: Human Kinetics; 1998.
105. Foster C, Porcari JP, Anderson J, et al. The talk test as a marker of exercise training intensity. *J Cardiopulm Rehabil Prev*. 2008;28(1):24–30. doi:10.1097/01.HCR.0000311504.41775.78.
106. Trombly CA, Quintana LA. Differences in responses to exercise by post-CVA and normal subjects. *Occup Ther J Res*. 1985;5(1):39–58. doi:10.1177/153944928500500103.
107. Fletcher GF, Ades PA, Kligfield P, et al. Exercise standards for testing and training: a scientific statement from the American Heart Association. *Circulation*. 2013;128(8):873–934. doi:10.1161/CIR.0b013e31829b5b44.
108. Gibson L, Strong J. A conceptual framework of functional capacity evaluation for occupational therapy in work rehabilitation. *Aust Occup Ther J*. 2003;50(2):64–71. doi:10.1046/j.1440-1630.2003.00323.x.
109. King PM, Tuckwell N, Barrett TE. A critical review of functional capacity evaluations. *Phys Ther*. 1998;78(8):852–866. doi:10.1093/ptj/78.8.852.
110. Williams MA, Haskell WL, Ades PA, et al. Resistance exercise in individuals with and without cardiovascular disease: 2007 update: a scientific statement from the American Heart Association Council on clinical cardiology and council on nutrition, physical activity, and metabolism. *Circulation*. 2007;116(5):572–584. doi:10.1161/CIRCULATIONAHA.107.185214.
111. Bond V, Adams RG, Obisesan T, et al. Cardiovascular responses to an isometric handgrip exercise in females with prehypertension. *North Am J Med Sci*. 2016;8(6):243–249. doi:10.4103/1947-2714.185032.
112. Kolber MJ, Hanney WJ. The reliability and concurrent validity of shoulder mobility measurements using a digital inclinometer and goniometer: a technical report. *Int J Sports Phys Ther*. 2012;7(3):306–13.
113. Leard JS, Breglio L, Fraga L, et al. Reliability and concurrent validity of the figure-of-eight method of measuring hand size in patients with hand pathology. *J Orthop Sports Phys Ther*. 2004;34(6):335–340. doi:10.2519/jospt.2004.1367.
114. Dewey WS, Hedman TL, Chapman TT, Wolf SE, Holcomb JB. The reliability and concurrent validity of the figure-of-eight method of measuring hand edema in patients with burns. *J Burn Care Res*. 2007;28(1):157–162. doi:10.1097/BCR.0b013e31802c9eb9.
115. Jepsen JR, Laursen LH, Larsen AI, Hagert CG. Manual strength testing in 14 upper limb muscles: a study of inter-rater reliability. *Acta Orthop Scand*. 2004;75(4):442–448. doi:10.1080/00016470410001222.
116. Brandsma JW, Schreuders TAR, Birke JA, Piefer A, Oostendorp R. Manual muscle strength testing: intraobserver and interobserver reliabilities for the intrinsic muscles of the hand. *J Hand Ther*. 1995;8(3):185–190. doi:10.1016/S0894-1130(12)80014-7.
117. Pollard H, Lakay B, Tucker F, Watson B, Bablis P. Interexaminer reliability of the deltoid and psoas muscle test. *J Manip Physiol Ther*. 2005;28(1):52–56. doi:10.1016/j.jmpt.2004.12.008.
118. Hébert LJ, Maltais DB, Lepage C, Saulnier J, Crête M, Perron M. Isometric muscle strength in youth assessed by hand-held dynamometry: a feasibility, reliability, and validity study. *Pediatr Phys Ther*. 2011;23(3):289–299. doi:10.1097/PEP.0b013e318227ccff.
119. Ottenbacher KJ, Branch LG, Ray L, Gonzales VA, Peek MK, Hinman MR. The reliability of upper- and lower-extremity strength testing in a community survey of older adults. *Arch Phys Med Rehabil*. 2002;83(10):1423–1427. doi:10.1053/apmr.2002.34619.
120. Bohannon RW, Schaubert KL. Test-retest reliability of grip-strength measures obtained over a 12-week interval from community-dwelling elders. *J Hand Ther*. 2005;18(4):426–428. doi:10.1197/j.jht.2005.07.003.
121. Chen MJ, Fan X, Moe ST. Criterion-related validity of the Borg ratings of perceived exertion scale in healthy individuals: a meta-analysis. *J Sports Sci*. 2002;20(11):873–899. doi:10.1080/026404102320761787.
122. Eston RG, Faulkner JA, Mason EA, Parfitt G. The validity of predicting maximal oxygen uptake from perceptually regulated graded exercise tests of different durations. *Eur J Appl Physiol*. 2006;97(5):535–541. doi:10.1007/s00421-006-0213-x.
123. Finucane L, Fiddler H, Lindfield H. Assessment of the RPE as a measure of cardiovascular fitness in patients with low back pain. *Int J Ther Rehabil*. 2005;12(3):106–111. doi:10.12968/ijtr.2005.12.3.19554.

Acknowledgments

Thank you to Ciara Fleer, OTS, Francis Phan, OTS, Emily Millard, OTS, and Jordan Sutton, OTS, students of the University of Central Arkansas, Occupational Therapy Department for contributing to the photography and for assisting in reviewing drafts of this chapter. Thank you to Margaret Standridge, CHT, OTR, and Marc Ellis, CHT, OTR for their assistance and consultation regarding many aspects of this chapter.

Chapter 14

Motor Function Intervention

Michael J. Borst

LEARNING OBJECTIVES

This chapter will allow the reader to:

1. Explain the biomechanical and physiological mechanisms that underlie occupational performance and therapeutic exercise.
2. Apply the conceptual framework for therapeutic occupation to conceptualize frames of reference, intervention approaches, and occupational performance.
3. Use methods to decrease edema and minimize contracture to prevent range of motion loss.
4. Apply principles from the biomechanical and motor learning frames of reference to occupation synthesis in order to improve range of motion, strength, and/or endurance.
5. Design interventions for clients who have impairments in edema, range of motion, strength, and/or endurance as needed to improve occupational performance.

CHAPTER OUTLINE

TERMINOLOGY

Client factors: basic structures and functions of a person that are used for occupational performance; edema, range of motion, strength, and endurance are all client factors[1]

Mechanical advantage (MA): ratio that describes how easily a force can move a resistance using a lever

Moment arm: the perpendicular distance from the axis of rotation to the line of force (force vector)[2] on a lever

Muscle endurance: the ability of a muscle to contract repeatedly or over time without a decrease in force produced[3]

Muscle strength: the maximum amount of force that is produced by a muscle in a single contraction[3]

Range of motion (ROM): the arc of rotational motion through which a bone moves around a joint; usually measured in degrees

Strain: the change in shape of an object that results from the stress placed on it[6]

Stress: the force acting on an object, divided by the cross-sectional area of that object[6]

Torque: the extent to which a force causes an object to rotate around an axis[2]

Occupational performance is influenced by **client factors** such as edema, **range of motion (ROM)**, **muscle strength**, and **muscle endurance.**[1] Occupational therapists sometimes help clients restore or establish these factors by synthesizing occupations, activities, or preparatory tasks designed to create change within the client.[1,4]

Musculoskeletal System

Occupational therapists need to understand the biomechanical and physiological principles behind musculoskeletal system function. This understanding allows occupational therapists to analyze and synthesize occupations to promote successful occupational performance.

Biomechanical Aspects

Biomechanics applies the principles of physics (such as motion and force) to the human body. Kinematics is the study of the motion of an object without regard to the forces that produced the motion.[2] In the human body, we see two types of motion, translation and rotation. Translation occurs when an object or body part moves in a straight line. Rotation occurs when an object or body part moves in a circular motion around an axis. For example, when you walk down a hallway, your head is moving down the hall in a translational manner. In contrast, rotational motion is occurring at your hip joints, knee joints, and ankle joints as each flexes and extends around an axis.[2] Translation and rotation often occur at the same time in the human body.

Kinetics is the study of forces on an object and how those forces change the motion of the object.[2] With regard to the human body, these forces might include muscle contraction, gravity, friction, and any external push or pull on a body part.

Most occupations involve motions and forces. For example, when a person places a glass on a cupboard shelf, muscles in the trunk (internal forces) coactivate to create stability before any arm motion is initiated. Muscles in the shoulder girdle activate synergistically to create force couples (two or more muscles pulling in different linear directions to create rotation in the same direction) that move the sternoclavicular, acromioclavicular, and glenohumeral joints. To raise the glass, the elbow flexor muscles activate concentrically causing elbow joint flexion (rotary motion). To cause this rotation, the elbow flexors must generate enough force to create sufficient internal **torque** to overcome the external torque created by the force of gravity acting on the glass's mass. The movement of the glass upward to the cupboard is an example of translational motion, in which the glass moves in a more or less linear manner, rather than rotating around an axis.

Torque

Any analysis of rotary motion requires an understanding of torque. There are two factors of torque: force and distance. Torque is created when a linear force acts on an object at a certain distance from that object's axis of rotation; this distance is measured perpendicular to the direction of the force. This perpendicular distance between the axis of rotation and a force's line of action (vector) is called the **moment arm.** Torque is calculated by multiplying the linear force by the distance from the line of force to the axis of rotation. Thus, in mathematical terms:

$$\text{torque} = \text{force times the moment arm}$$

In the metric system, force is measured in newtons, and the moment arm is often measured in meters. In the English system, force is measured in pounds, and the moment arm is often measured in feet. Torque is therefore often expressed in newton·meters or foot·pounds.

It is critical to understand the difference between force and torque. A force acts in a linear direction and tends to cause translation motion when directed at the center of an object's mass. In contrast, torque involves rotation around an axis, and the moment arm is just as important as the force in determining how much torque is produced. Returning to our example of lifting a glass up to a shelf, there are two torques involved at the elbow joint: an internal torque and an external torque. The internal torque is the product of the internal (biceps brachii) force acting on the radius bone times the internal moment arm (of the biceps) in relation to the elbow joint (Fig. 14-1A; we are considering only one elbow flexor muscle for the

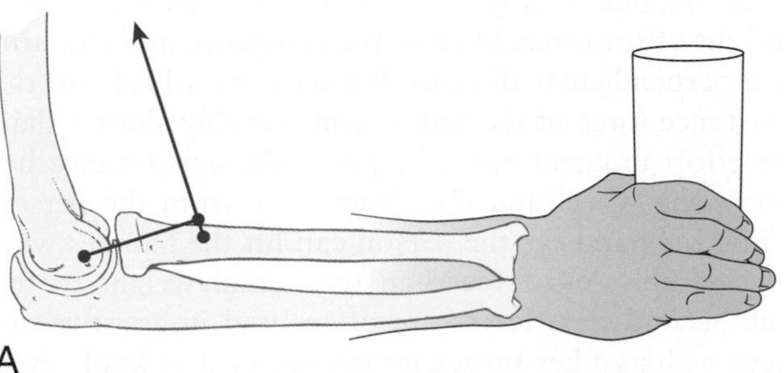

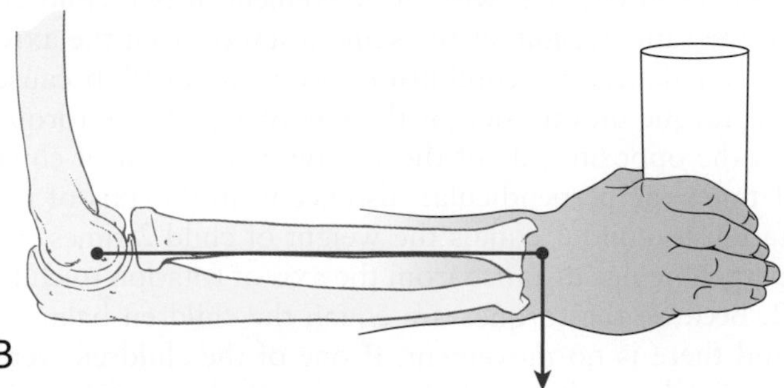

Figure 14-1. Internal and external torque. **A.** Internal (effort) torque. IF, internal force—Line of pull of biceps brachii. IMA, internal moment arm—Perpendicular distance between the IF of the biceps brachii and the axis of rotation. **B.** External (resistance) torque. EF, external force—Line of pull of combined weight of glass, hand, and forearm. EMA, external moment arm—Perpendicular distance between the EF and the axis of rotation.

sake of simplicity). The external torque is the product of the external force (the combined weight of the glass, forearm, and hand) times the external moment arm (of gravity) in relation to the elbow joint (Fig. 14-1B). If the internal torque is greater than the external torque, the muscle will activate concentrically (shorten) and the glass will go up. If the internal torque is less than the external torque, the muscle will activate eccentrically (lengthen while "trying" to shorten) and the glass will go down. If the internal torque is equal to the external torque, the muscle will activate isometrically (stay the same length), and the glass will be held still in midair.

To make an object easier to lift, we can reduce the external torque. This can be done in either of two ways: reduce the weight (force) of the object or reduce the distance (moment arm) between the object and the joint(s) responsible for the lifting. This is why therapists will teach clients to lift heavy objects closer to the body. Reducing the external moment arm will reduce the external torque and therefore also the internal torques required of the client's body. Similarly, when a therapist assists a client during a stand and pivot transfer, the therapist will stand as close to the client as is practicable in order to reduce the external moment arm and thus reduce the external torque, which in turn reduces the internal torques required of the therapist's body.

Levers

Another way to analyze torque production in rotary movement is through the description of levers. A lever consists of a rigid bar (such as a bone), an axis of rotation (such as a joint), and two opposing forces: effort and resistance. Effort is the force that causes movement, and resistance is the force that tends to keep an object from moving.[7] Sometimes, the effort force is simply termed force, and the resistance force is simply termed resistance. When analyzing human occupation, the force generated by muscles is termed internal force, and the force generated by objects outside of the body is termed external force. There are three classes of levers.

A first-class lever has the axis of rotation between the effort and resistance forces.[2] A common example of a first-class lever is the seesaw (Fig. 14-2A). A seesaw remains in balance, with no movement, if two children of the same weight sit the same distance from the axis. This balance, or equilibrium, is maintained because the torque on one side of the seesaw equals the torque on the opposite side of the seesaw. The weight of child 1 times the perpendicular distance from the axis of rotation to child 1 equals the weight of child 2 times the perpendicular distance from the axis of rotation to child 2. Because the torques are equal, the children balance, and there is no movement. If one of the children were heavier, he or she would have to move closer to the axis (shorten his or her moment arm) to decrease his or her torque and maintain equilibrium (Fig. 14-2B).

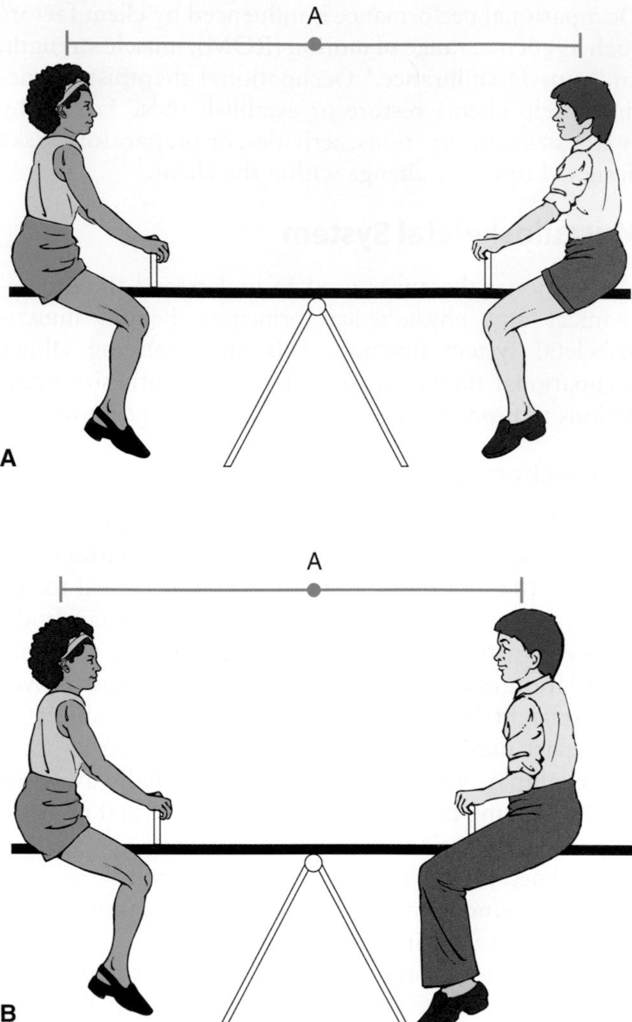

Figure 14-2. First-class lever. **A.** A seesaw as a first-class lever. Balanced equilibrium depicted by children on a seesaw. Both children weigh 60 lb, and they are equidistant from the axis. **B.** A seesaw as a first-class lever. The heavier child must be closer to the axis of the seesaw (shorten his moment arm) to maintain the equilibrium. A, Axis.

A second-class lever has the resistance force between the axis of rotation and the effort force.[2] A classic example of a second-class lever is a wheelbarrow used to move soil when gardening (Fig. 14-3). The resistance force (the pull of gravity on the soil) is between the axis and the effort force. Because the resistance moment arm (the perpendicular distance between the wheel and the resistance force of the soil) is considerably shorter than the effort moment arm (the perpendicular distance between the wheel and the effort force from the person lifting the handles), the person can lift the handles with considerably less force than the actual weight of the soil. Second-class levers are often used in assistive devices such as a key turner, jar opener, or doorknob lever. One disadvantage of second-class levers is that the arc of movement where the effort force is applied is always greater than the arc of movement where the resistance is

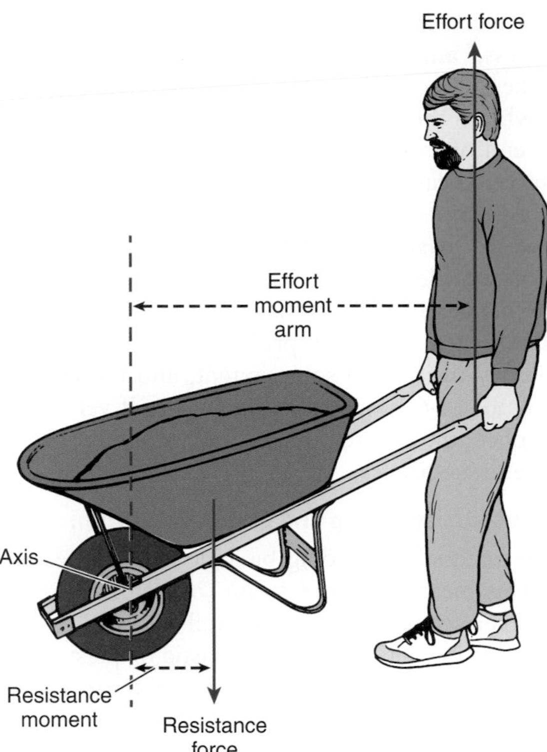

Figure 14-3. Second-class lever. A wheelbarrow as a second-class lever. The resistance force (from the soil) is between the axis (at the wheel) and the effort force (at the handles). Because the effort moment arm is longer than the resistance moment arm in a second-class lever, MA > 1, and less effort force is required to lift the resistance provided by the soil.

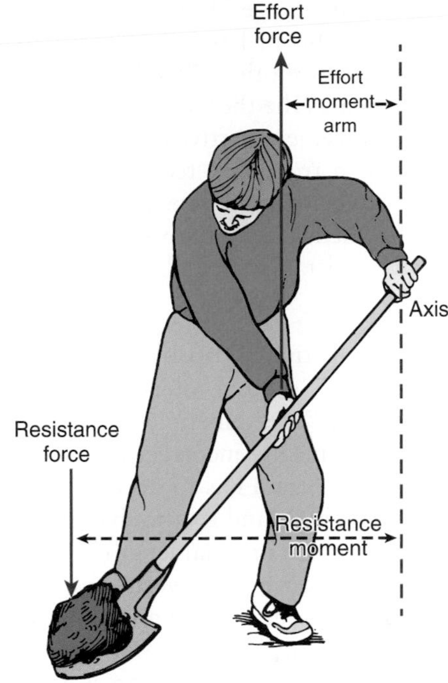

Figure 14-4. Third-class lever. A shovel can be a third-class lever, if the back hand is used to stabilize the shovel and the front hand to do the lifting.

applied. Thus, the end of a handheld jar opener must be moved several inches in order to move the jar lid itself only an inch.

A third-class lever has the effort force between the axis of rotation and the resistance force.[2] A shovel can be a third-class lever, if the person uses his or her back hand to stabilize the shovel and the front hand to do the lifting (Fig. 14-4). Because the resistance moment arm is longer than the effort moment arm, more effort force is required to lift the soil in the shovel; however, the soil will also move a greater distance than the hand that is doing the lifting moves. Third-class levers are often used in situations where the physical constraints of the lever require the effort moment arm to be shorter than the resistance moment arm. Most muscles in the human body are attached to bones in such a way as to create third-class levers, because the muscles need to be inside the body. Because the effort moment arm of a third-class lever is always shorter than the resistance moment arm, third-class levers always require the effort force to be greater than the resistance force in order to create an effort torque that is greater than the resistance torque. One advantage of third-class levers is that the arc of movement where the resistance is applied is always greater than the arc of movement where the effort force is applied. Thus the elbow flexor muscles can move the hand through an arc of about 2 feet with a muscle contraction of only a few inches.

Mechanical Advantage

Mechanical advantage (MA) is a ratio that describes how easily a force can move a resistance using a lever. MA can be expressed in terms of the length of the moment arms (MA = effort moment arm/resistance moment arm) or in terms of the force produced by the lever (MA = force out of the lever/force applied to the lever).[2]

A key turner extends the effort moment arm of the key (the distance between where effort force is applied to the key and the longitudinal axis of the key as it is turned), thus increasing the MA of the key (Fig. 14-5).

Physiological Aspects

A muscle–tendon unit consists of two components: elastic connective tissue that runs throughout the muscle belly and forms the tendons at the ends of the muscle–tendon unit, and muscle fibers that contract when stimulated by an alpha (lower) motor neuron. Both of these components are important in overall muscle–tendon unit functioning.

Elastic Connective Tissue Lengthening

In order to understand and evaluate interventions designed to increase ROM, it is essential to first review some basic definitions and principles of tissue biomechanics.[8] Active range of motion (AROM) occurs when the client uses his or her own muscles to actively move. Passive range of motion (PROM) occurs when an external force (such as the therapist or the client's other arm) causes the movement. Active assistive range of motion (AAROM) is a treatment technique used when a client does not have adequate strength to complete full AROM, and the client attempts to move actively while receiving passive assistance as well.

Stress and Strain

Stress is "the force acting on an object, divided by the cross sectional area" of that object.[6(p116)] The terms stress, force, and load are sometimes used interchangeably, but that is technically incorrect because force is a component of stress. **Strain** has to do with the resulting deformation of the object and is "the change in length of the object divided by the original length."[6(p116)]

The typical relationship between stress and strain in elastic connective tissue is shown in the stress–strain curve (Fig. 14-6). The *neutral zone* (NZ) represents the unfolding of the collagen fibers as stress is applied.[9] The NZ is also called the "toe" region of the curve.[2,10] As stress increases, the collagen fibers align along the line of stress,[9] and the tissue enters the "elastic zone" (EZ). The beginning of the EZ is where tissue resistance is first felt when a therapist performs PROM on a client's joint. The end of the EZ is the end of joint PROM. Application of increased stress after the end of the client's joint PROM can result in tissue microfailure (trauma)[9]; this is called the plastic zone (PZ). Because the tissue tears at a microscopic level in the PZ, the tissue elongation (strain) is permanent; however, that strain comes at the cost of inflammation and scar proliferation. The EZ and PZ probably overlap to some extent, and the clear border in Figure 14-6 is only for illustration. If yet more stress is applied, the failure point is reached, and gross rupture of the tissue occurs.

Viscoelasticity: Creep and Stress Relaxation

Some materials, including biologic tissues, are viscoelastic. This means that the strain (or deformation) of the tissue is a function of time as well as stress.[11] Viscoelastic tissues do not release their elastic or plastic strain all at once; instead, these changes occur more slowly over time. Viscoelasticity can be demonstrated in two ways

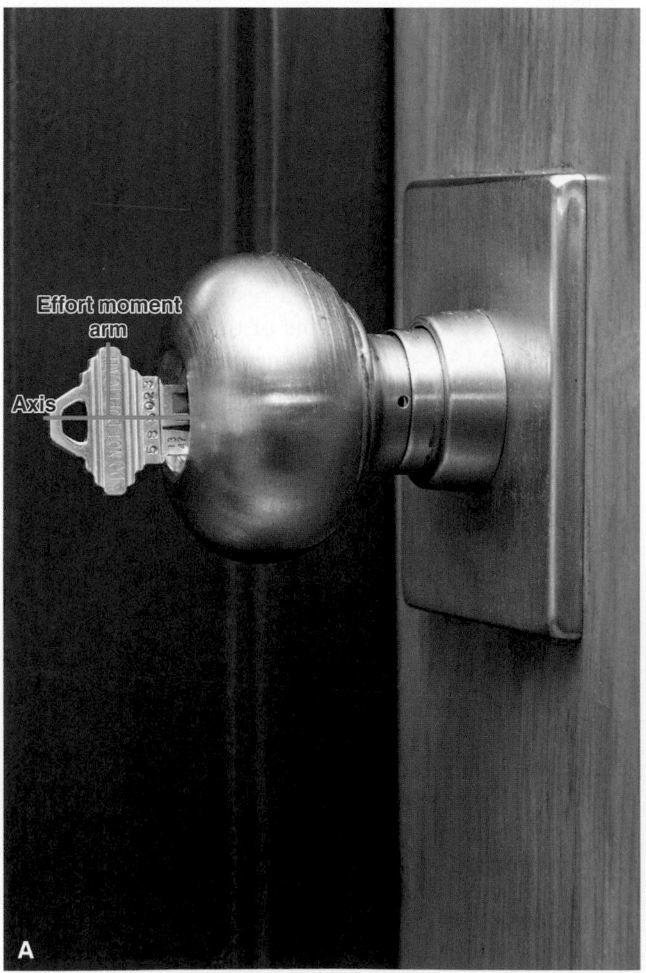

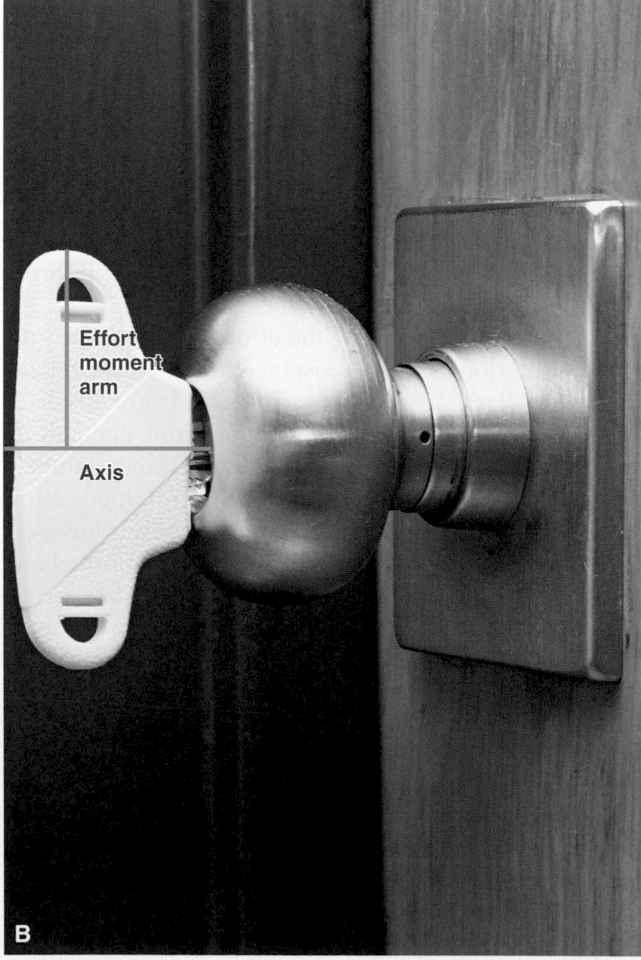

Figure 14-5. Mechanical advantage (MA). **A.** Opening a door with a key. The effort moment arm is half the width of the head of the key. **B.** Adding a key turner. The key turner doubles the effort moment arm, doubling the MA and cutting the effort force required by half.

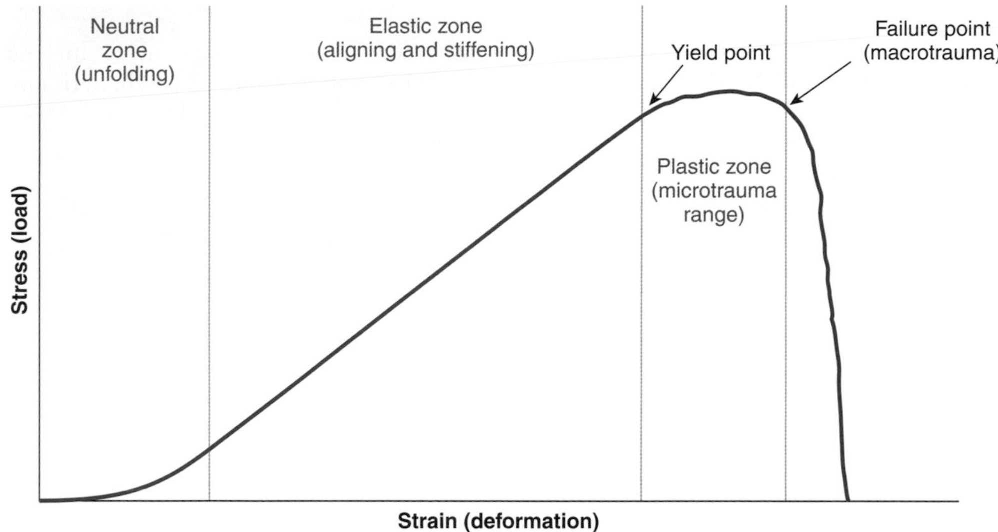

Figure 14-6. Stress–strain curve.

with the example of a tree branch (Fig. 14-7). If an object were hung on the branch (providing a constant stress), the weight of the object would result in some immediate deformation (strain), and additional deformation would occur over time as the object continued to hang on the branch. The additional deformation that occurs over time is due to viscoelasticity. This method of using viscoelasticity by applying a constant stress is called creep.[9–11]

Alternatively, if the tree branch were placed in the position that would result initially if the object were attached (but without the weight of the object) and held there by an external structure (thus maintaining a constant strain or deformation), the branch would adapt to that positioning and would not instantly return to its original position when the object constraining its movement were removed. This method of using viscoelasticity by maintaining a constant strain is called stress relaxation, because the stress decreases over time while the positioning (strain) is held constant.[9–11] Both stress relaxation and creep result from the viscoelastic nature of biologic materials.[11]

Some scholars have advocated creep as a method of permanently elongating biologic viscoelastic materials with stress[10]; however, others equate creep with plastic deformation caused by tissue microfailure and strongly caution against creep as a method of tissue elongation.[9] Still others define creep in biologic tissues as reversible elongation of a viscoelastic material over time in response to a continuous load.[2] It is critical to remember that when creep is used to elongate tissues, the point at which the tissue starts in the stress–strain curve is not stable; rather, it shifts to the right over time, moving closer to or into the PZ, as the tissue continues to deform in response to a constant load.[9–11] Thus, the use of creep to elongate tissue carries with it significant risk of tissue trauma, inflammation, and scarring or adhesion.

When stress relaxation is used to elongate tissues, the point at which the tissue starts in the stress–strain curve shifts downward over time, staying in the EZ as the tissue adapts to a held position (a constant amount of strain).[9–11] Thus, the use of stress relaxation to elongate tissue carries much less risk of tissue trauma.

Stimulating Tissue Growth

When adaptive shortening of elastic connective tissue creates a PROM deficit (as in a joint contracture), it is critical to understand that the preferred mechanism of elongation is tissue growth, instead of plastic or elastic changes caused by either creep or stress relaxation.[9,12,13] In order to promote tissue growth, Dr. Paul Brand advocated holding the tissue in "only a slightly lengthened position (within its elastic limit) for a period of hours or days" (using a constant strain, similar to stress relaxation, instead of a constant stress, as in creep).[9] An example of this method of stimulating tissue growth is the wearing of plugs of gradually increasing size (gauges) in the earlobes over time in order to create a large hole in intact earlobes (Fig. 14-8).

Prolonged Strain in the EZ

"Low-load prolonged stress"[13–17] is commonly advocated for remodeling elastic connective tissue. Although the concept is sound, the term is redundant and unclear, as load is a component of stress, and "low" is undefined, leaving it unclear whether the stress places the tissue in the elastic or PZs. Sometimes, the term low-load prolonged stretch is used, but this term should be avoided, as it is unclear whether stretch refers to the force on the object (stress) or the resulting change in length (strain). A more helpful term for the mechanism of stimulating tissue growth would be prolonged strain in the elastic zone.

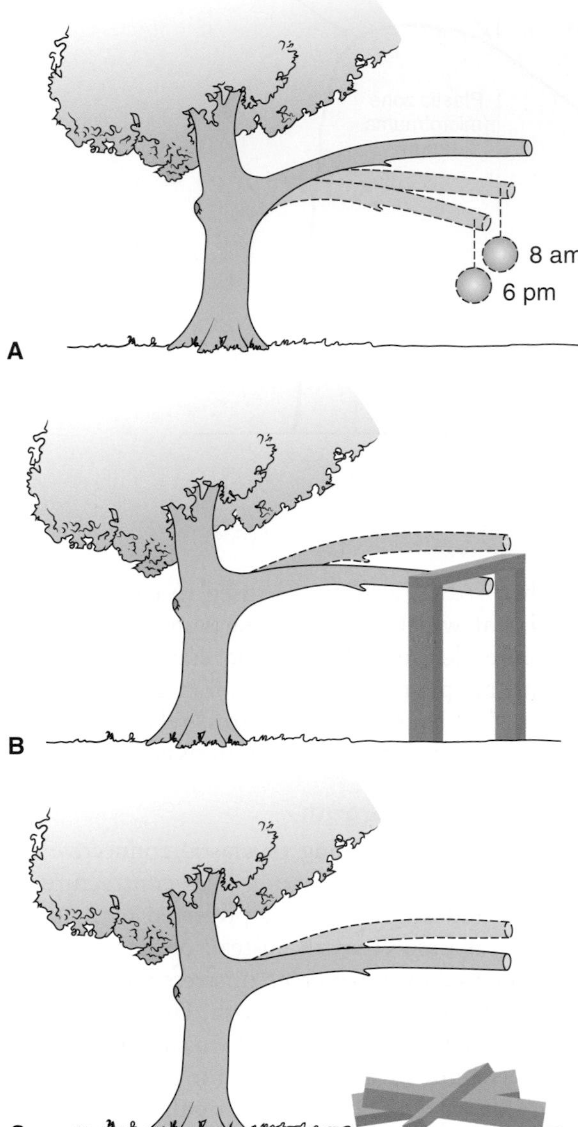

Figure 14-7. Viscoelasticity through creep and stress relaxation. **A.** Creep (constant stress). **B.** Stress relaxation (strain is held constant). **C.** Result of stress relaxation after the "hold" is removed.

Contractile (Muscle) Tissue

Skeletal muscle provides the force to produce movement of a bony lever around its joint axis. A muscle's strength and endurance depend on multiple factors, such as the size and type of muscle fibers, the number and frequency of motor units firing, and the length–tension relationship of the muscle. It is important to understand the basic contractile elements within muscle tissue.

The sarcomere (made up of actin and myosin filaments) is the basic contractile element of skeletal muscle and is located within the myofibril (Fig. 14-9). A motor unit consists of a single alpha motor neuron and the muscle fibers innervated by that neuron. When the alpha motor neuron is depolarized and causes the muscle fiber membrane to depolarize, calcium ions are released throughout the muscle fiber, causing the myosin heads to "grab" and "pull" on the actin filaments, shortening the sarcomere.[18]

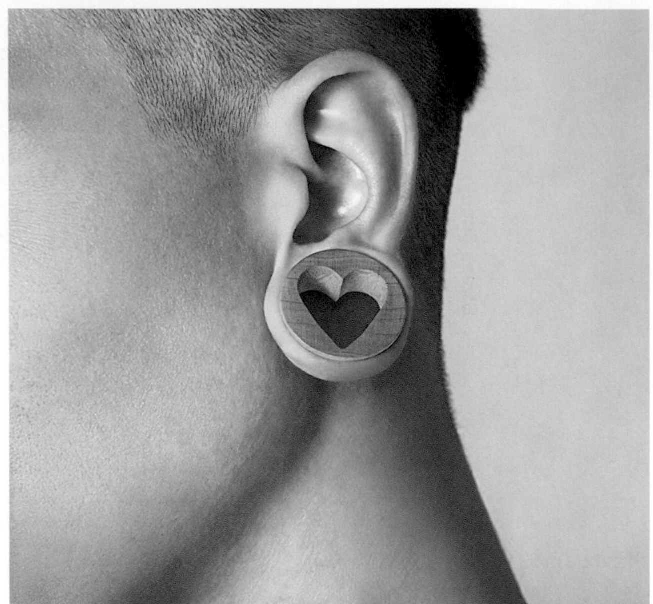

Figure 14-8. Tissue growth stimulated by the use of sequentially larger earlobe gauges to hold the tissue in an elongated position. (Shutterstock/Oleksii Fedorenko.)

Considerations for Lengthening Contractile (Muscle) Tissue

When stretching muscle tissue, the actin–myosin cross-bridges release and the sarcomeres lengthen temporarily.[19] The amount of lengthening available through this mechanism is proportional to the number of sarcomeres lined up end to end (in series) in an individual muscle. Thus, a fusiform muscle that has relatively many sarcomeres lined up end to end will have more range of muscle length than a pennate muscle.[20] For example, biceps brachii is a fusiform muscle that has a great range of muscle length as it activates across both the shoulder and the elbow joints simultaneously. The number of sarcomeres in series can decrease if a muscle is immobilized in a shortened position,[19] and prolonged strain in the EZ can increase the number of sarcomeres in series.[21]

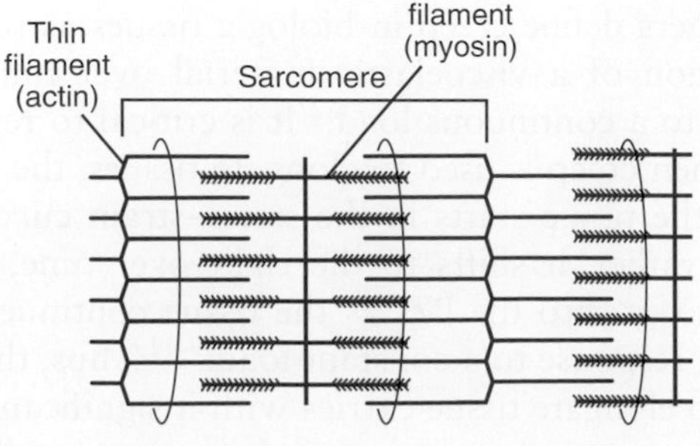

Figure 14-9. Sarcomere structure.

Considerations for Strengthening Muscle Tissue

The nature of a muscle's performance is influenced by the number and type of muscle fibers found in a single motor unit. Large muscles that typically contract with great force (such as gluteus maximus) have a greater proportion of motor units that have large neurons and up to 2,000 muscle fibers per motor unit.[22] These fibers are also typically fast-twitch fibers, which are capable of producing more force more quickly and also fatigue faster.[22] On the other hand, smaller muscles that typically contract with less force but produce more finely controlled movements (such as some facial muscles) have a greater proportion of motor units that have small neurons and as few as five muscle fibers per motor unit.[22] These fibers are typically slow-twitch fibers, which provide smaller, more controlled forces and do not fatigue as rapidly.[22]

The amount of force produced by a muscle activation is controlled through recruitment (the number of motor units that are activated) and rate coding (how frequently each motor unit is activated).[22] If more force is required, the brain can activate more motor units and/or activate each motor unit more frequently. Small motor units that produce less tension and thus require less energy are usually recruited first, but if they cannot produce adequate force, larger motor units are recruited to complete the action.

The force production of an individual muscle is proportional to the cross-sectional area of its muscle fibers. Because pennate muscles (in which the fibers attach to a tendon at an angle) can pack more muscle fibers in a given area, they tend to produce more force than fusiform muscles.[22] For example, the palmar and dorsal interosseous muscles are pennate muscles that pack a lot of fibers into a small space in the hand.

Finally, a muscle's ability to produce force depends on the length of its sarcomeres when it is activated. This phenomenon is illustrated using the active length–tension curve (Fig. 14-10). If a muscle is already fully shortened, its sarcomeres do not have room to shorten any further and thus cannot produce any additional force or tension (see the left side of the active length–tension curve). This phenomenon is called active insufficiency, and will result in apparent weakness in a multijoint muscle–tendon unit that has been shortened over all its joints simultaneously, even though the muscle's ability to produce force in a more neutral position is normal.[20] Muscles that cross only one joint tend not to have active insufficiency. If a muscle is fully passively lengthened, it will not be able to produce much force because most of the myosin heads are not in contact with the actin filaments and therefore cannot "pull" on the actin filaments to produce contractile force (see the right side of the active length–tension curve). If a muscle is in the middle of its length range, it has the greatest potential for force production, with enough actin–myosin cross-bridges to generate a lot of force and plenty of potential to shorten (see the middle of the active length–tension curve).

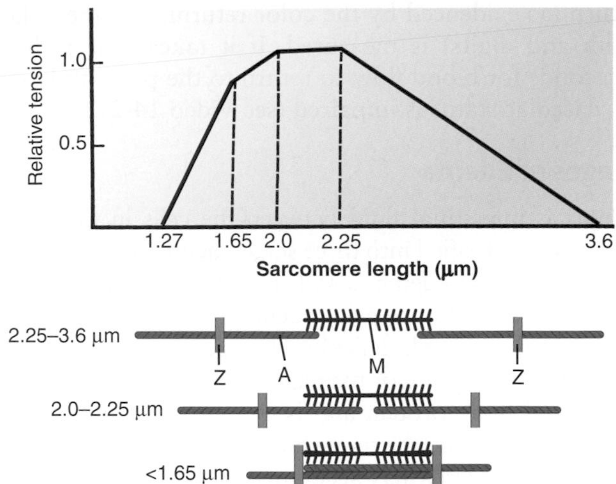

Figure 14-10. Active length–tension curve. The position of the myosin heads in relation to the actin filament determines the potential for force generation at a given muscle length.

Therapeutic Intervention for Edema

According to the biomechanical FOR, edema reduction is always a priority once structural stability has been addressed. Prompt edema management will result in improvements in ROM and pain, whereas unmanaged edema will worsen these issues and eventually result in contractures and adhesions between structures in the limb.[27] Edema management varies depending on the stage of the edema and the vascular status of the body part.

Vascular Status

Vascular flow may be impaired if there was damage to vascular structures or if a client has peripheral vascular disease. If vascular flow is impaired, interventions that involve limb compression, elevation, cold, or heat may be contraindicated.[27] Vascular status of a finger can be assessed using the capillary refill test, in which the client's fingertip is compressed so that it turns pale and then the time it takes for blood flow to return (as evidenced by the color returning in the fingertip pulp or under the fingernail) is measured. If it takes longer than 2 seconds for blood flow to return to the fingertip, vascular status is impaired (see Video 14-1).[28] Vascular status of the entire hand can be assessed by the Modified Allen's Test, in which firm pressure is placed over the client's radial and ulnar arteries just proximal to the volar wrist creases, the client flexes the digits into a fist and extends them again several times until the volar hand is pale, the pressure is released from one of the two arteries (radial or ulnar), and the time it takes for blood flow to

return (as evidenced by the color returning in the volar palm and digits) is measured. If it takes longer than 5 seconds for blood flow to return to the palm and digits, vascular status is impaired (see Video 14-2).[28]

Stages of Edema

Edema is interstitial fluid between the cells in the body and can be classified into three stages: acute, subacute, and chronic.[29] Acute edema is still quite fluid and mobile. In acute edema, the tissue pits (indents readily when pressed) deeply and rebounds quickly. The edema can be moved around with pressure or massage. Subacute edema has accumulated more protein and is more viscous as a result. In subacute edema, the tissue pits but is slow to rebound.

Chronic edema has accumulated even more protein, to the point that fibrotic adhesions start to form. In chronic edema, the tissue pits minimally, and the tissues may feel hard or leather-like. Measurement of edema is covered in Chapter 13; however, interstitial fluid can increase by 30% before being detected,[27] so edema measurement is not a valid method of ruling out the presence of edema.

Interventions for Acute Edema

For acute edema, the limb is elevated above the heart in order to use gravity to improve venous and lymphatic flow and reuptake of interstitial fluid.[27] Sometimes allied health professionals will consider a sling to be a form of elevation, but a sling often worsens arm edema because it holds most of the arm below the heart and also prevents active motion. Light compression with form-fitting garments can be helpful, such as gloves (Fig. 14-11) or hosiery, tubular sleeves such as Tubigrip (Mark One Health Care Products, Philadelphia, PA), or elastic wraps such as Coban (3M, St. Paul, MN). The therapist must be careful to keep the compression light, as compression above 60 mmHg will collapse the lymphatic pathways, inhibiting the body's natural pathways for resorbing edema, and compression above 75 mmHg can damage the lymphatic capillaries.[30] The garment or sleeve should be easily pulled away from the skin slightly, yet provide some compression.[29] Edema gloves often do not compress adequately in the webspaces between the fingers, and gauze 2 × 2s can be placed in the webspaces before donning the glove to improve the compression in this area, or the therapist can apply small (about 1 × 4 inches) hourglass-shaped strips of Kinesio Tape (Kinesio Holding Corporation, Albuquerque, NM) under light (10%) tension to the webspaces before donning the glove (Fig. 14-11). Sometimes, the proximal edge of Tubigrip or a compression glove will roll over, and this should be avoided by cutting a longitudinal slit in the sleeve or glove so the proximal edge can splay instead of rolling over. A rolled proximal edge will create a high-pressure area that will hinder the flow of edema through the lymphatic system. When using a self-adhesive elastic bandage such as Coban, start at the distal end of the limb or digit and wrap proximally with no tension, because self-adhesive bandages tend to tighten up on their own (see Video 14-3). When wrapping a digit, leave the tip open to observe skin color and circulation. In the inflammatory stage of wound healing (typically lasting 3–5 days after injury or surgery), cryotherapy can be used to prevent edema accumulation (see Chapter 24). AROM (especially overhead) and PROM can also decrease acute edema, but during the inflammatory stage of healing, immobilization is more appropriate to preserve structural stability and avoid increasing inflammation.

Interventions for Subacute Edema

Subacute edema contains more protein, which cannot be resorbed by the venous system, and thus requires techniques that utilize the lymphatic system. The lymphatic system consists of tiny initial lymphatic capillaries in the interstitium that are connected to surrounding tissues by anchor filaments. When tension is put on the surrounding tissues (usually by limb movement and muscle contraction), these anchor filaments open the initial lymphatic capillaries so they can extract the protein-laden

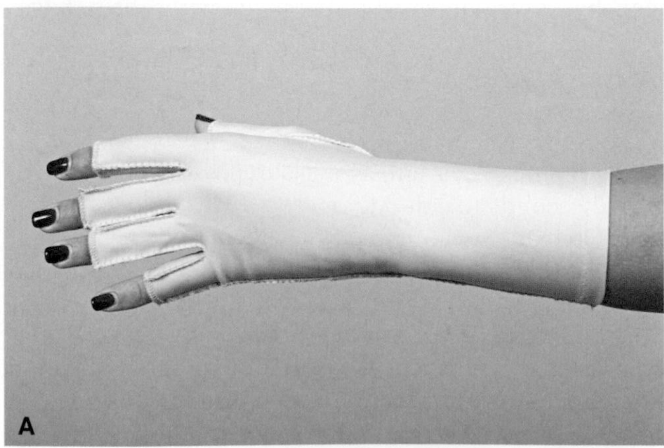

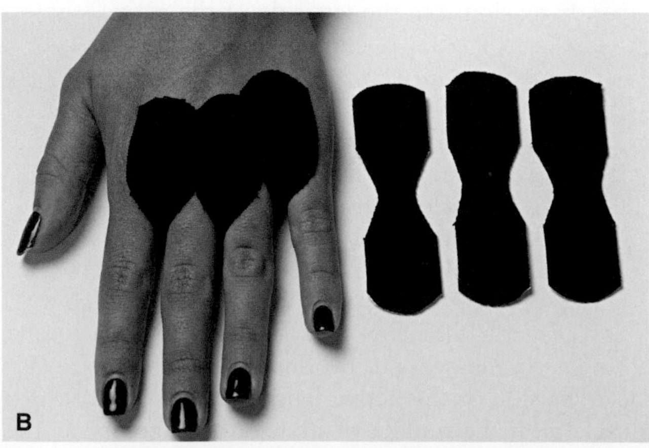

Figure 14-11. Edema glove compression. **A.** Edema glove. **B.** Kinesio Tape application for use under an eglove.

interstitial fluid.[29] Thus, most of our interventions for subacute edema involve some method of putting tension on these anchoring filaments so they can open the initial lymphatics, without applying so much compression that the lymphatic capillaries collapse.

AROM, PROM, and even light isometric exercise are methods the client can use to open the lymphatic capillaries. Kinesio Tape can also be used to provide light tension on the skin that may help open the initial lymphatics. Apply the Kinesio Tape with no stretch to skin that is stretched (i.e., with joints bent away from the surface you are taping) so that the tape wrinkles after application (Fig. 14-12). This method will provide light tension and light pressure with movement of the limb. Compression (as described under section Interventions for Acute Edema) can also be used in the same way for subacute edema. A "chip bag" or pad containing varying densities of foam chips can be used under a compressive glove or sleeve to help soften edema that has become more viscous. Chip bags can be fabricated easily by cutting scrap foam into small pieces and placing them in stockinette or between two layers of light tape such as Kinesio Tape (Fig. 14-13). After the tissues are well past the inflammatory stage of healing, mild heat (96°F–100°F) can be used to soften edema before exercise[29]; even the "neutral warmth" reflected by a pressure garment or very thin neoprene sleeve can help soften viscous edema.

Manual Edema Mobilization

Manual edema mobilization (MEM) is a set of techniques designed to promote normal functioning of the lymphatic system (see Video 14-4). MEM can move large amounts of interstitial fluid into the cardiovascular system in a short period, so it is contraindicated if the client has congestive heart failure or other severe cardiac problems, renal failure or other severe kidney problems, liver disease, or severe pulmonary problems; if the client has active cancer; if an infection is present; if a hematoma or blood clot is present; or over areas of inflammation (MEM proximal to areas of inflammation

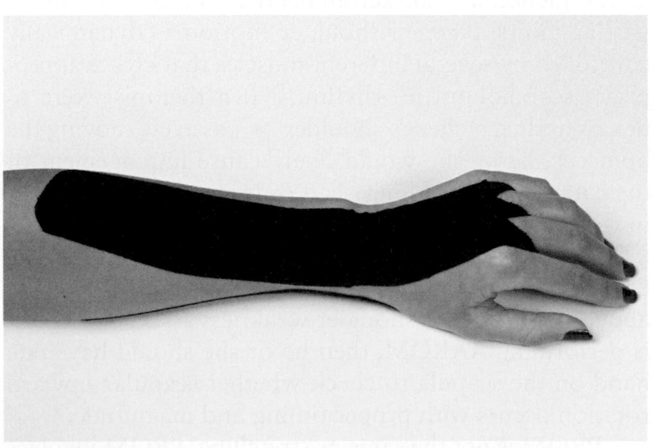

Figure 14-12. Kinesio Tape application for hand edema.

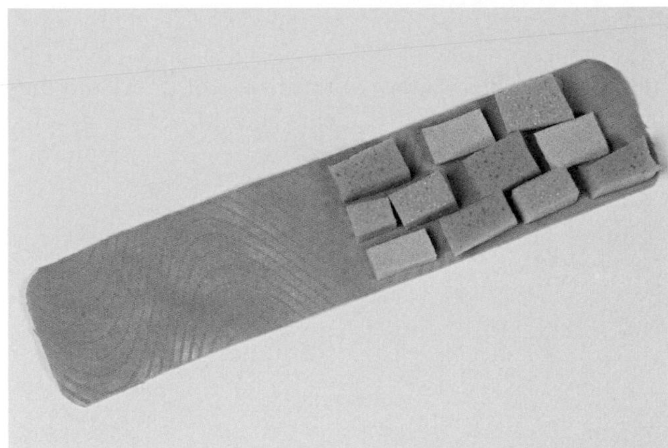

Figure 14-13. Construction of a chip bag using various densities of foam. The tape would be folded over to seal the foam chips in.

may be helpful).[30] MEM should be used with caution if the client has diabetes, because it may cause alterations in blood sugar; if the client has low blood pressure, because it may decrease blood pressure further; and if the client is pregnant, because it may increase feelings of morning sickness.[30]

MEM Principles

In contrast to the cardiovascular system, which uses the heart to push blood through the blood vessels, the lymphatic system uses pressure gradients to pull or draw the lymph proximally to areas of lower pressure. Thus, the techniques used in MEM are designed to create small pressure differentials to promote proximal lymphatic flow and to put light tension on the anchor filaments to open the superficial initial lymphatic capillaries. Furthermore, proximal areas must be cleared of lymph (creating lower proximal pressure) before lymph can flow out of distal areas. Finally, extra attention is paid to areas where lymph tends to accumulate, such as lymph nodes.

MEM Techniques

MEM techniques are used roughly in the following order, although they can be modified to fit each client's unique situation, as long as the basic principles listed previously are followed. First, deep diaphragmatic breathing is done for a couple of minutes to try to clear the proximal deep lymphatic structures. Second, shoulder AROM or PROM exercises are performed to further assist the proximal clearing.

Third, light skin-tractioning massage and ROM exercise is used to apply tension to the anchor filaments and open the lymphatic capillaries. The skin-tractioning massage should be applied directly to the skin (not through clothing) if at all possible. The pressure should be just enough to move the skin (rather than slide over the skin) and no more than that. More contact area between the massaging hand and the area being treated will result in more lymphatic capillaries being opened, so it is important for the therapist to use the entire surface of his or her relaxed palm and fingers to apply the light skin-tractioning massage. The massage is applied in a circular or U-shaped pattern with the top of the U pointing proximally. Each body segment (chest, upper arm, forearm, hand, digit) is divided into three sections, and five light skin-tractioning U's are applied in each section. Each body segment is first cleared by massaging the proximal section, then the middle section, and then the distal section. After clearing each segment, AROM or PROM of the adjacent joints is performed to further clear that segment. Once one segment is cleared with massage and exercise, then flow massage is performed. Flow massage involves the same light skin-tractioning U's to the same sections, but they are applied starting at the most distal section just cleared and then the next proximal section, and so on all the way to the contralateral chest. When performing the flow massage, one repetition is used in each section (instead of five), but the entire flow sequence is performed five times. Once a segment has been both cleared and flowed using this procedure, the next distal segment is cleared and flowed (e.g., after the upper arm is cleared and flowed, then the forearm is cleared and flowed).

Fourth, lymph nodes and other areas of potential lymph congestion (called pump points in MEM) are massaged using both hands simultaneously for a total of 20 to 30 U's. This massage can be done with slightly more pressure, but it is still important to keep the pressure light, remembering that you are not trying to push or force fluid proximally, but pull or draw it from more distal areas by creating lower pressures at the pump points. Pump points are located at the anterior shoulder and axilla, the medial elbow, the wrist, and the dorsal hand. Pump point massage can be incorporated into the light skin-tractioning massage between the clearing and flowing U's. More detailed information about MEM is available from other sources.[29,30]

MEM can and should be taught to outpatient clients as part of a home program as well. Although clients might not perform MEM exactly "by the book," in my experience, self-MEM can be very effective as long as the principles of clearing before flowing, light skin-tractioning massage, and AROM or PROM exercise are followed.

Interventions for Chronic Edema

Chronic edema has accumulated a substantial amount of protein that is becoming fibrotic. As a result, it can be very difficult to reduce. Hopefully, very few patients will reach this stage, but edema management does not always happen promptly. All of the interventions for subacute edema noted earlier are also appropriate for chronic edema. Additionally, low stretch or short stretch bandaging techniques can be used to treat chronic edema.[30]

Lymphedema

Lymphedema is edema that results from a lymphatic system that is not functioning properly because of damage from trauma, surgery, radiation therapy, and the like. Sometimes, the lymphatic system is congenitally inadequate. Whatever the cause, lymphedema requires the therapist to train the client in self-management techniques that work around the lymphatic system rather than with the lymphatic system, and therefore this area of practice requires specialized training.[29]

Therapeutic Intervention for ROM

Therapeutic Intervention to Prevent Loss of PROM

A client may be at risk for loss of PROM because of a variety of factors related to immobility, including coma, being on complete bed rest, paralysis, and trauma or surgical repair.[31] In these situations, elastic and contractile connective tissue can shorten, causing contracture, or lose elasticity, causing stiffness. Cartilage can thin, soften, and lose its ability to absorb the loads placed on it.[32] In some (but not all) situations, PROM intervention to prevent these impairments may be appropriate.

First, contraindications and precautions related to PROM must be considered. Remembering the first consideration of the biomechanical FOR (structural stability), the occupational therapist must be certain that the tissues involved can withstand any forces placed on them. If one is unsure what the movement and positioning restrictions are after surgery, it is the therapist's responsibility to contact the surgeon and find out. If, for example, a therapist were to move a client's fingers and/or wrist into full extension within a few weeks after a flexor tendon repair, he or she would likely rupture the repair. By breaking what the surgeon fixed, the therapist has created the need for a tendon reconstruction, involving multiple additional surgeries and several additional months of therapy. On the other hand, if the fingers and wrist are not ranged in a controlled fashion within safe limits, the repaired tendon will adhere to the surrounding tissues, and the outcome will be poor.

Shoulder PROM and AROM is another area where precautions need to be carefully considered. Shoulder motion is a complex phenomenon consisting of movements at the glenohumeral, acromioclavicular, and sternoclavicular joints. Normal shoulder motion is dynamically controlled by several different muscles that create appropriate scapulohumeral rhythm.[33] If a therapist were to flex or abduct a client's shoulder by passively moving the humerus, he or she would likely cause impingement of the rotator cuff and long head of biceps brachii tendons in the subacromial space. If the client's shoulder musculature is paralyzed (e.g., after stroke, spinal cord injury, or while comatose), the shoulder should not be ranged above 90°. If there is shoulder weakness and the therapist is performing AAROM, then he or she should have one hand on the scapula to check whether scapular upward rotation occurs with proper timing and magnitude.

PROM is not the same as stretching. PROM involves taking a joint through its available ROM without overpressure at the end of the range. This is accomplished with an external force: usually the therapist, a caregiver, or the client's other arm. Stretching, on the other hand, uses a prolonged hold in the EZ (near the end of the PROM).[19]

In order to maintain cartilage health, tissue length, and tissue elasticity, 5 to 10 repetitions of PROM in each available direction at each joint is recommended.[31] PROM should never be forced or cause pain. The total number of repetitions per day or week will depend on the client's situation. For example, a client with burns will need considerably more intensive intervention to prevent loss of ROM, and orthoses are often used to hold tissues in an elongated position for long periods.

Therapeutic Intervention for Limited ROM

Limited AROM or PROM at a joint can occur for a variety of reasons and become a concern when it causes a limitation in occupational performance. Full AROM is sometimes not required in order for a person to successfully complete his or her occupations and fulfill necessary roles. Functional ROM refers to the amount of AROM at a particular joint that is required to complete most activities of daily living (ADLs); however, what constitutes functional ROM depends on the occupations a client desires to perform. For example, a recent study indicated that elbow AROM of −27°/149° (give or take 5°–7°) was functionally adequate for basic ADLs (tying shoes, drinking, eating, and using a mobile phone).[34] However, some people may desire to perform occupations that require more elbow extension or flexion than that. When ROM impairments result in occupational performance limitations, those impairments become a concern for the occupational therapist and the client.

Differential Diagnosis of AROM Limitations

It is important to differentiate joint contracture from extensor lag, passive insufficiency, or tendon adhesion. Each of these causes is described next in more detail, and a differential flowchart for AROM loss is shown in Figure 14-14.

A lag exists when there is a loss of joint AROM in the direction of the active muscle (the agonist) but there is full passive motion.[35] A lag may be caused by agonist tendon adhesion, agonist muscle weakness, or some other factor that decreases the agonist force to the joint. A joint friction problem may exist when PROM is nearly normal but AROM is difficult and muscle weakness does not seem to be the problem.

Passive insufficiency occurs when an antagonist multijoint muscle–tendon unit that has become too short prevents full PROM in the direction of the agonist.[20] Passive insufficiency is easily diagnosed by changing the positioning of the other joints that are crossed by the antagonist multijoint muscle–tendon unit. If changing the position of one of these other joints changes the PROM available at the joint in question, then passive insufficiency is the cause. Tendon adhesion of the antagonist may appear similar to passive insufficiency, depending on the location of the adhesion.

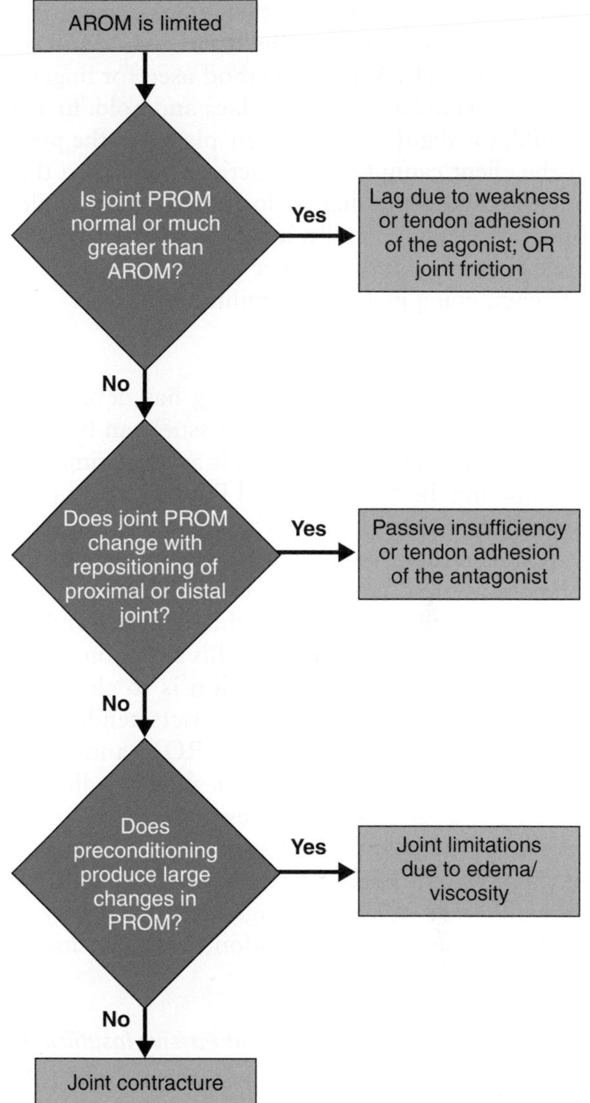

Figure 14-14. Differential diagnosis of limited AROM. AROM, active range of motion; PROM, passive range of motion.

A viscosity problem resulting from edema can sometimes look like a contracture. If PROM is limited and does not change with repositioning of other joints, preconditioning with 20 minutes of mild heat and AROM followed by about 10 minutes of stress applied in the EZ (e.g., a mild weighted stretch) can help differentiate between viscosity issues and joint contracture. If this preconditioning results in PROM gains of 20° or more, then the problem is likely increased viscosity from edema rather than a fixed contracture.[9,12]

If none of the preceding factors explain the limited AROM, it is likely that a joint contracture exists because of shortened elastic connective tissue such as ligaments, joint capsule, fascia, skin, or other connective tissues.

Intervention for a Lag

If a client has a lag that appears to result from muscle weakness (typically 2−/5 on the muscle strength grading scale in Chapter 13), then AAROM is appropriate (see Video 14-5). In AAROM, the client moves the joint as far as possible

on his or her own (actively), then gently assists it with the other hand to complete the ROM, while still trying to move it actively. Another method used for finger flexion or extension lag is called a place and hold. In a place and hold, the digit(s) are passively placed in the position that the client cannot achieve actively, and then the client tries to hold the digit(s) in that position while the support is released. Finally, if the client has 2/5 to 3−/5 muscle strength, light resistance can be used as tolerated for strengthening in a gravity-minimized plane.

Intervention for Tendon Adhesion

Tendon adhesion (in which scarring has developed between a tendon and surrounding tissue) can be difficult to treat and becomes more difficult as more time passes. Remembering the biomechanical FOR, our first priority is structural stability, so the therapist makes sure that any healing structures can withstand the stresses in the interventions described next. Therapy after a tendon repair is beyond the scope of this chapter, and other resources should be consulted in this situation.[36,37]

The goal with tendon adhesion is to elongate the adhesion so that it no longer restricts tendon excursion. Methods to do this include AROM and strengthening of the muscle–tendon unit that is adherent in order to put tension on the adhesion itself. Heat before exercise can help improve tissue extensibility as well (see Chapter 24). Finally, the tissues to which the tendon is adherent can be massaged in such a way as to pull them away from the tendon, putting tension on the adhesion.

Intervention for Muscle Shortness or Passive Insufficiency

A short or stiff muscle–tendon unit can limit AROM during occupational performance, particularly when it crosses multiple joints. Stretching is the initial option for lengthen a muscle–tendon unit. When stretching, the therapist or client uses a prolonged hold in the EZ (near the end of the PROM) in order to lengthen the muscle–tendon unit. To stretch, the joint(s) that the muscle–tendon unit crosses are held in a position opposite the action of that muscle–tendon unit. For example, if flexor digitorum profundus (which flexes the wrist and the finger metacarpophalangeal, proximal interphalangeal, and distal interphalangeal joints) is too short, those four joints would simultaneously be placed in extension and held there for a while to stretch the muscle–tendon unit (Fig. 14-15). If intrinsic musculature (which taken together flexes the finger metacarpophalangeal joints and extends the proximal interphalangeal and distal interphalangeal joints) is too short, those joints would simultaneously be placed in a position opposite the combined action of the intrinsics to stretch those muscle–tendon units (Fig. 14-16). *Active stretching* refers to stretching a muscle by performing and holding the opposite movement actively. *Passive stretching* refers to using an external force (such as the other hand) to hold the position

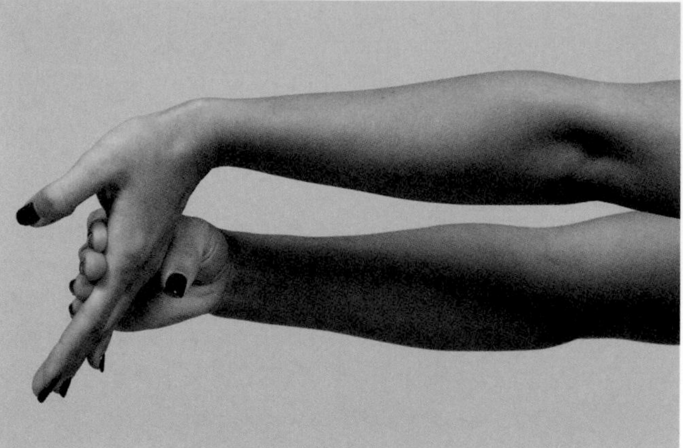

Figure 14-15. Passive stretch of flexor digitorum profundus.

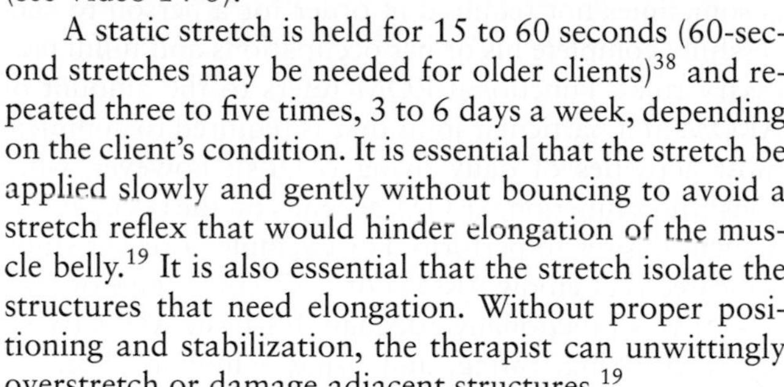

and tends to involve greater forces than active stretching (see Video 14-6).

A static stretch is held for 15 to 60 seconds (60-second stretches may be needed for older clients)[38] and repeated three to five times, 3 to 6 days a week, depending on the client's condition. It is essential that the stretch be applied slowly and gently without bouncing to avoid a stretch reflex that would hinder elongation of the muscle belly.[19] It is also essential that the stretch isolate the structures that need elongation. Without proper positioning and stabilization, the therapist can unwittingly overstretch or damage adjacent structures.[19]

Additional techniques that increase the range of shortened muscle are the proprioceptive neuromuscular facilitation techniques called contract relax (CR) and hold relax (HR) (see Video 14-7).[39,40] CR involves a maximal concentric contraction of the short muscle, usually performed at the point of limitation. The muscle is contracted concentrically and maximally for 5 to 8 seconds against resistance provided by the therapist and then relaxed. During the relaxation phase, the therapist gently moves the part in the direction opposite to the contraction and holds it there to stretch the muscle–tendon unit. For example, if there is a contracture of the elbow flexors, the elbow is passively extended as far as

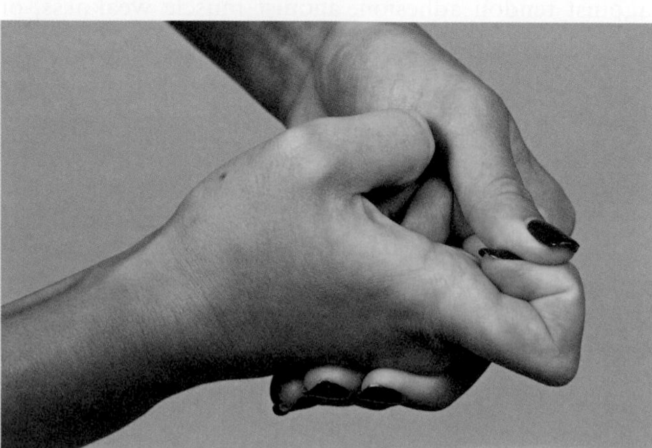

Figure 14-16. Passive stretch of the intrinsic muscles.

possible. The patient is instructed to contract the flexors maximally while the therapist provides resistance and then relax, at which point the therapist smoothly extends the elbow into a greater range. The CR technique can be repeated multiple times. HR is an essentially identical technique, except that it is done with a maximal isometric contraction against resistance provided by the therapist, rather than a concentric contraction. HR is used when the joint is painful or damaged in some way.

Joint Mobilization

Sometimes, altered arthrokinematics (the roll, slide, and spin of joint surfaces as a person moves) is the cause of limitations in joint ROM, especially after trauma such as a fracture. Arthrokinematic movements cannot be performed voluntarily, and therefore active movement or stretching cannot remediate arthrokinematic problems. Joint mobilization techniques are required to address altered arthrokinematics, and although these techniques are beyond the scope of this chapter, they are well addressed elsewhere.[41]

Intervention for Joint Contracture

When tissues have shortened to the point that they create a contracture at a joint, intermittent stretching is not likely to result in satisfactory improvement, and orthotic intervention is indicated. In order to improve the contracture, the tissues need prolonged strain in the EZ so that the body can grow new tissue in response to the strain (refer to section "Physiological Aspects"). This is most effectively done with either a static progressive orthosis or a serial static orthosis. Dynamic orthoses apply creep to the contracted tissues, which over time will move the tissues into the PZ, resulting in inflammation and scar proliferation.[9,42]

Therapeutic Intervention for Impaired Muscle Performance

Parameters for Therapeutic Exercise

When an occupational therapist designs an exercise program for a client, a number of interacting parameters need to be considered. Resistance or intensity refers to the external torque the client must overcome when doing the exercise and includes the force of gravity acting on a weight that might be held or strapped to a client's arm along with the weight of the arm itself, the tension in a TheraBand (The Hygenic Corporation, Akron, OH), or, in the case of an isometric exercise, an immovable object such as a desk or wall against which the client pushes. It is important to remember that external torque is the product of the external force and the external moment arm. The perpendicular distance between the joint axis of rotation and the external force's line of action is just as important as the external force itself. This is especially important to remember when using a cuff weight wrapped around an arm or a leg. If the cuff weight moves proximally on the extremity, the external moment arm will decrease and thus the external torque will decrease as well. Additionally, therapists sometimes instruct a client to hold a dumbbell in his or her hand with the arm at his or her side and the elbow positioned in 90° of flexion and then to rotate the forearm between pronation and supination to strengthen the pronator and supinator musculature. However, in this position, the weight will provide no resistance torque to pronation or supination because the center of gravity of the weight is in the middle of the hand, roughly in the same place as the forearm's axis of rotation, and thus the external moment arm is essentially zero.

Repetitions refers to the number of times an exercise is completed before a break, and that number is considered one set. Additional sets of repetitions may be completed after a rest break. Taken together, repetitions times sets times resistance = exercise volume. Frequency refers to the number of times a day or week the exercise routing is completed. The amount of rest between sets or exercise sessions is also an important consideration, especially in clients whose health is compromised or older clients. All of these parameters will vary depending on intervention goals (strength vs. endurance) as well as the health of the client.[3]

Two additional concepts need to be considered when designing intervention for impaired muscle performance. The overload principle states that in order to increase muscle performance, the demands on the muscle must be greater than the normal everyday demands to which the muscle is accustomed. Muscle demands may be increased by increasing resistance, repetitions, sets, or frequency. The Specific Adaptation to Imposed Demands (SAID) principle states that improvements in muscle performance will match (be specific to) the type of muscle activation, speed of muscle contraction, the joint positioning, the client's body position, and so on. Generalization of improvements to activities with different muscle demands will be limited. This principle provides a compelling argument for using occupational performance as a means to improve muscle performance.[3]

Types of Exercise

Static (Isometric) exercise is used when joint motion is painful or contraindicated because of joint instability. Isometric exercise can also remediate weakness at a particular point in the ROM. Isometric exercise is more effective with deconditioned individuals than with conditioned individuals. When designing an isometric exercise program to improve muscle performance, keep the following guidelines in mind[43]:

- Maximal isometric contractions against an immobile object will result in the quickest strength gains.
- Hold each contraction for 6 seconds, and no longer than 10 seconds.[3]
- Perform isometric holds every 15° to 20° throughout ROM, if possible.
- Repeat frequently throughout the day.

- Contraindication for isometric exercise: Clients with a history of cardiac or vascular disorders should avoid high-resistance isometric exercise.[3]
- Precaution for isometric exercise: Clients should not hold their breath, but instead count out loud and exhale while performing the exercise to avoid a Valsalva response, which increases blood pressure.[3]

Dynamic (Concentric and Eccentric) exercises are commonly used to promote strength gains throughout the arc of motion. In a concentric activation, the internal torque produced by the muscle is greater than the external torque produced by the resistance, so the muscle "wins." In an eccentric activation, the internal torque produced by the muscle is less than the external torque produced by the resistance, so the muscle "loses." Many exercises consist of a concentric phase immediately followed by an eccentric phase. During the eccentric phase, the therapist should instruct the client to slowly allow the resistance to "win" in order to ensure good eccentric muscle activation. If free weights are used to provide the resistance, the weight moves up when the muscle wins and moves down when the muscle loses (Fig. 14-17A). This, however, is not always the case with other methods of providing resistance. Elastic exercise bands can be anchored anywhere and will pull toward their anchor point (Fig. 14-17B). Thus with elastic bands, when the band is being lengthened by the client, the muscle is winning (concentric). When the band is shortening even though the muscles are trying to lengthen it, the muscle is losing (eccentric) (Fig. 14-17 B).

- Contraindications for dynamic exercise: Severe or acute joint or muscle pain during exercise; inflammation of joints and muscles; or severe cardiopulmonary disease[3]
- Precautions for dynamic exercise: Clients should not hold their breath, but instead count out loud and exhale while performing the exercise; avoid high resistance for clients with osteoporosis, children, and older adults; initiate exercise with low- to moderate resistance; correct substitutions; do not apply resistance to an unstable joint or healing fracture; avoid exercise volumes that excessively fatigue the client; and discontinue exercise if dizziness, pain, or unusual shortness of breath occurs.[3]

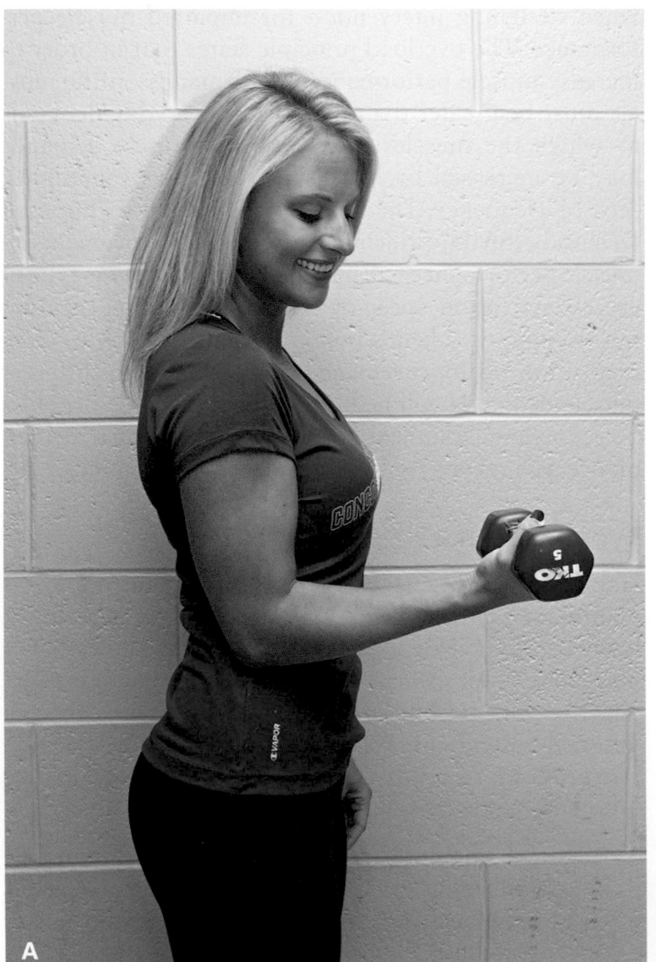

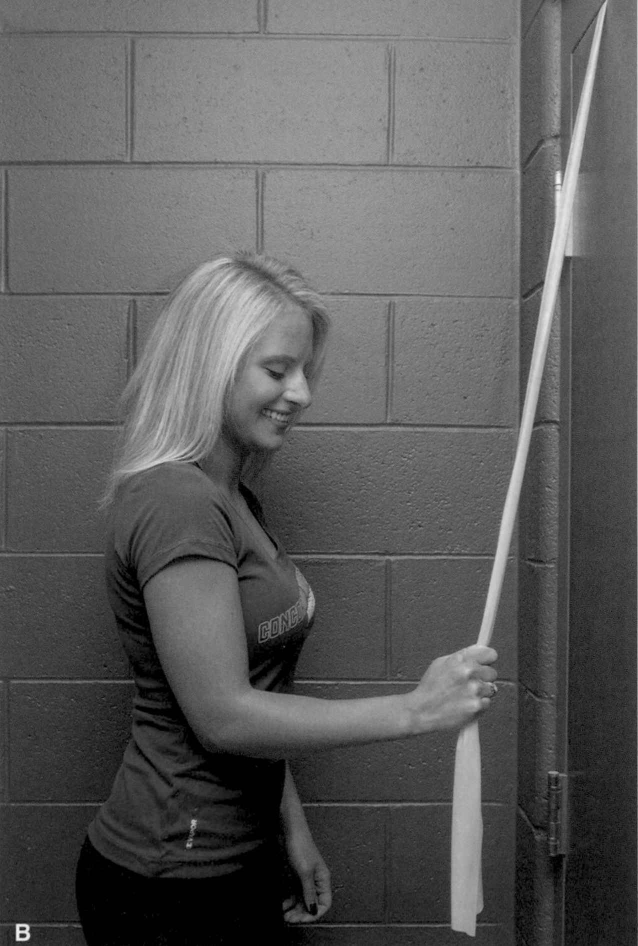

Figure 14-17. Methods of resistance. **A.** A dumbbell always exerts a downward force. **B.** An elastic resistance band pulls toward the place where it is anchored.

Methods of Resistance

In rote exercise, free weights and elastic bands such as TheraBand are often used because they are inexpensive and reasonably portable. Free weights also have the advantages of providing consistent resistance force and requiring dynamic stabilization similar to that which the client will need for occupational performance. Elastic bands are more portable and can be anchored anywhere (often between a closed door and its doorframe), allowing options for directions of resistance not easily achieved with free weights. On the other hand, elastic bands are quite variable in the amount of resistance they provide—when elongated to twice their resting length, they provide two to three times more resistance force than they provided initially when the slack was taken up.[43]

Occupation-Based Exercise

These same parameters and concepts will be considered when the occupational therapist synthesizes an occupational form in order to elicit a certain occupational performance from a client, although in a less formal way. Consider the occupation of making a simple meal in a kitchen. The therapist will take into account the weight of the utensils, any pots or pans that will be required, and the ingredients (that is, resistance); the number of times the client will likely have to lift or move these items in order to perform the occupation (that is, repetitions); the naturally built-in rest breaks, and so on. These parameters are probably not explicitly communicated to the client during occupational performance; however, the therapist carefully considers them when developing a treatment plan for the client.

Strength Training versus Endurance Training

Strengthening and endurance training are done at similar exercise volumes; however, strengthening is done with higher resistance and fewer repetitions, while endurance training is done with lower resistance and more repetitions.[3]

The concept of a repetition maximum (RM) is used when determining the appropriate resistance for a client. A RM is the most weight a client can lift (or resistance a client can move) with good form for a certain number of repetitions before fatigue begins to set in and the quality of the movement degrades. For example, a 1 RM would be the most weight a client can lift once with good form, with performance degrading on the second repetition. A 10 RM would be the most weight a client can lift 10 times with good form, with performance degrading on the 11th repetition. A client's 1 RM can be estimated by giving them a weight you think he or she will be able to lift 5 to 10 times and counting the actual number of repetitions completed before performance degrades. Use the Holten curve[44] to correlate the number of repetitions performed with a percentage of 1 RM (Table 14-1) and then divide the weight lifted by that percentage to estimate the client's 1 RM. For example, if a client could lift a 6 lb weight (at a particular joint in a particular direction) just 12 times, then 6 lb would be about 80% of the 1 RM. Dividing 6 lb by 0.8 would equal 7.5 lb, which is the estimated 1 RM.

Intervention to Prevent Loss of Muscle Strength

To prevent loss of muscle strength, the client must perform some type of muscle activation. When illness or injury results in immobilization or disuse, type I muscle fibers (which specialize in endurance and posture) atrophy before type IIA and B fibers (which specialize in power and strength).[3,19] Thus, exercises focusing on endurance with 30% to 40% of the client's 1 RM, 25 to 50 repetitions, and one to two sets may be most appropriate initially.[3] If the exercises are for maintenance of the client's current performance, the frequency of exercise can be as little as two to three times per week.[3] Clients that have recently been critically ill may require almost all of their available energy for healing and may thus not tolerate this exercise. The occupational therapist must consider the health, age, preillness conditioning level, and the client's response to exercise (including monitoring vital signs).

Sometimes during postoperative immobilization, a client is permitted to do "setting" (nonresisted isometric coactivation) exercises in order to prevent disuse atrophy. In this situation, just a few repetitions performed several times a day with no resistance may be appropriate,[3] but the therapist must check with the surgeon first to make sure these exercises will not compromise structural stability.

Intervention to Increase Muscle Endurance

For unconditioned and deconditioned clients, children, or the elderly, exercise that focuses on endurance with resistance that is 30% to 40% of 1 RM is most appropriate and may result in significant strength gains as well.[3] As the client gains endurance and strength, the therapist should first increase repetitions or sets before increasing resistance.[3] Three to five sets of up to 50 repetitions can be used before increasing resistance. When resistance is

Table 14-1. Holten Curve

PERCENTAGE OF 1 RM (%)	NUMBER OF REPETITIONS
100	1
95	2
90	4
85	7
80	11
75	16
70	22
65	25

increased, repetitions are initially decreased and then gradually increased again as the client improves.

Occupational performance is ideal for increasing endurance. Many everyday occupations involve repeated motions against light resistance, so it is easy to develop a treatment plan that will elicit this type of performance in the clinic or as a home program. When clients perform occupations that have many meaningful past associations, they will generally have a greater sense of purpose related to the impact of the occupation and will therefore perform it longer than they might perform a rote exercise.

Cardiovascular endurance is a related but different concept from muscle endurance. Increasing cardiovascular endurance is not addressed in this chapter.

Intervention to Increase Muscle Strength

As mentioned earlier, for deconditioned individuals, strengthening starts with increasing muscle endurance. When the client is ready for a strengthening regime, Progressive Resistive Exercises (PREs) provide one method of determining appropriate parameters.[43] The "DeLorme" PRE program involves three sets of 10 repetitions each: the first set is performed at 50% of the 10 RM, the second set at 75% of the 10 RM, and the third set at 100% of the 10 RM. This PRE program has the advantage of a built-in warm-up in the first two sets, but the client may be too fatigued to complete a third set at 100% of the 10 RM. The "Oxford" PRE program also involves three sets of 10 repetitions each, but the first set is performed at 100% of the 10 RM, the second set at 75% of the 10 RM, and the third set at 50% of the 10 RM. This PRE program accommodates client fatigue nicely, but would require a warm-up exercise beforehand to increase circulation and ready the muscles for work. Resistance should be increased gradually in increments of 5% to 10% of the client's 1 RM,[3,43] although somewhat larger increases might be acceptable when clients are just beginning resistive exercises and are using small (1–2#) weights.

Occupational performance can also be used to increase muscle strength and is often done when preparing clients to return to a job or sport. Throwing or hitting a ball, stacking boxes of various weights, and shoveling gravel are some examples. For clients with lower strength demands in their daily activities, making a meal in the kitchen may provide the appropriate resistance to increase muscle strength.

Considerations for Client Training Handouts

Anytime a client is trained in an exercise or other home program, materials must be provided for the client to keep. Verbal instruction is never enough, no matter how well the client appears to understand the instructions during the therapy session. If these instructions are provided in written form, they should be written at or below a fifth grade reading level. In a Microsoft Word document, you can check the Flesch–Kincaid Grade Level by enabling "Show Readability Statistics" in Word "Options" and performing a spelling and grammar check. Strategies for lowering the reading level include using only one- and two-syllable words and shortening sentence length.[45]

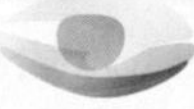

CASE STUDY

Patient Information

Bernard is an 89-year-old right-handed married man who fell in front of his house while watering some plants, sustaining a left distal radius fracture with multiple bone fragments and damage to the articular cartilage. He was hospitalized and had surgery to stabilize the fracture fragments with a plate and screws on the volar side of the radius. A temporary plaster splint was placed after surgery. After the surgery, he was discharged to a subacute rehabilitation facility for occupational therapy and physical therapy in order to improve his balance, general conditioning, and safe independence in self-care activities before returning home. At the subacute facility, his left arm was placed in a sling, and he was encouraged not to move it.

Assessment

The subacute occupational therapist observed Bernard performing basic ADLs and determined that he required total assistance with dressing his upper and lower body, putting on and taking off shoes and socks, and showering with his left arm bagged to keep water off the healing incisions. He required moderate assistance for shaving, brushing teeth, combing hair, eating, and toileting. He required minimal assistance for ambulation with a cane, but could walk only about 10 feet before requiring a rest break. Transfers to and from the bed required moderate assistance. Bernard spent most of the day in bed or in a wheelchair.

On the 10th day after surgery, an occupational therapist specializing in hand therapy was consulted. Bernard's left hand was swollen and discolored (see Fig. 14-18A), and his left fingers, wrist, elbow, and shoulder were all stiff. His left wrist had 30° of flexion and 10° of extension AROM, while his right wrist had 70° of flexion and 60° of extension AROM. He could wiggle his left fingers and thumb, but could not perform any functional grasp or pinch because of stiffness. Strength was not assessed in view of postoperative restrictions. Bernard was unable to use his left arm to perform any ADLs.

Short-Term Goals

Initial short-term goals set by the subacute occupational therapist included the following:

- Client will perform shaving, brushing teeth, and combing hair while standing at bathroom sink with minimal assistance within 2 weeks.

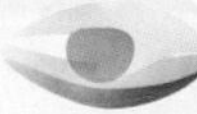

CASE STUDY *(continued)*

- In order to perform self-care occupations, client will ambulate from bedside to bathroom (about 20 feet) with minimal assistance within 2 weeks.

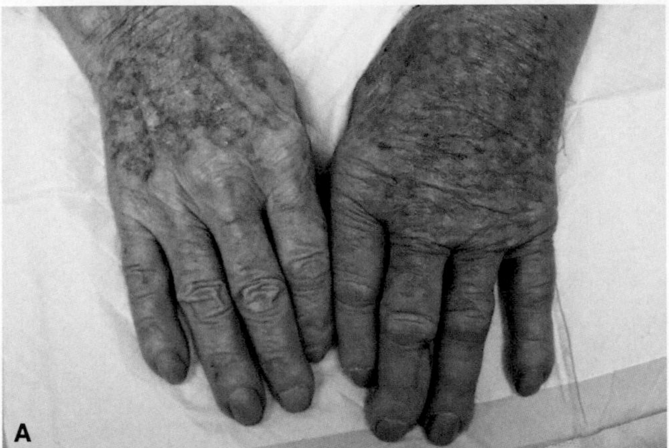

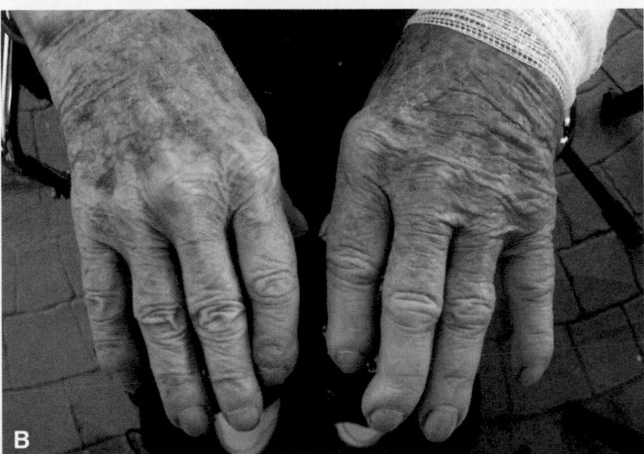

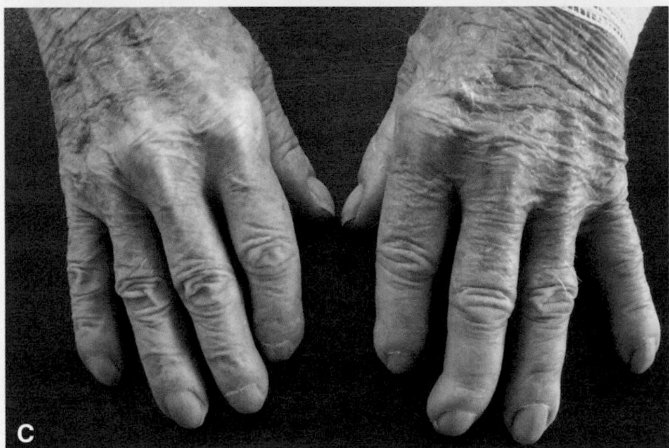

Figure 14-18. Edema intervention. **A.** Untreated edema in the left hand 10 days after surgery for a distal radius fracture. Note the discoloration, loss of wrinkles over the joints, and the loss of definition around the extensor digitorum (ED) tendons. **B.** Edema 1 day later, after one brief MEM treatment and discontinuing the sling. Note the increase in skin wrinkles, definition of the ED tendons, and more normal color. **C.** Continued reduction of edema 2 days later, after one additional brief MEM treatment.

- In order to perform ADLs, client will participate in 20 minutes of light aerobic exercise a day.

The following goals were added after the occupational therapist specializing in hand therapy was consulted:

- In order to dress and feed self independently, client will perform AROM of all left arm joints and self-PROM of left fingers and thumb daily with supervision within 2 days.
- In order to dress and feed self independently, client will don and doff custom thermoplastic volar wrist orthosis with supervision within 1 week.

Intervention

In addition to initial interventions aimed at general conditioning (recumbent bicycle), functional mobility, and self-care, the consulting occupational therapist recommended the following at 10 days after surgery (all with written approval from the hand surgeon):

- Replacing the temporary plaster splint with a custom thermoplastic volar wrist orthosis that would be easier to maintain and allow more finger motion
- Discontinuing the sling because it worsened the edema and joint stiffness in Bernard's left arm, as well as unnecessarily restricted his occupational performance
- Initiating MEM performed by the occupational therapist once daily
- Adding AROM for all joints of the left arm, from shoulder to fingers, with shoulder and elbow AROM performed overhead
- Adding self-PROM exercises for fingers and thumb

Progress

Twenty-four hours after discontinuing the sling and initiating a very brief MEM and AROM session, the edema in the left hand was considerably reduced (see Fig. 14-18B). Forty-eight hours after discontinuing the sling, and after two brief MEM and AROM sessions, the edema was reduced even more, and the color in the hand was returning to normal (see Fig. 14-18C). The stiffness in the shoulder and elbow was resolved within 2 weeks. Blocking exercises that isolated thumb interphalangeal joint AROM were initiated because of adherence of the flexor pollicis longus (FPL) tendon to the surgically placed volar plate. (FPL is the deepest tendon in the carpal tunnel and thus rests directly on the volar plate that was placed to stabilize the distal radius fracture.) Six weeks after surgery, hand strengthening with yellow (soft) Therapy Putty and passive wrist stretches were initiated. As Bernard's client factors improved, he was encouraged to perform his ADLs independently with less reliance on caregivers. After 2 months in subacute rehabilitation, the client performed shaving, brushing teeth, combing hair, dressing upper and lower body, and feeding self with supervision, and was discharged home.

Best Evidence for Motor Function Intervention

Intervention	Description	Participants	Dosage	Research Design and Evidence Level	Benefit	Statistical Significance and Effect Size
Occupation-Based Intervention[46]	Varied in the included studies: typing, handwriting, simulated ADLs, occupation as means/purposeful activity, playing games, modified constraint-induced movement therapy with occupation, and origami	Clients with upper extremity musculoskeletal disorders	Varied in the included studies; randomized controlled trials ranged from 3 to 6 weeks of occupation-based intervention	Systematic review of studies ranging from randomized controlled trials to case studies. Level I	Four of five randomized controlled trials found a significant benefit of occupation-based intervention (usually in addition to therapeutic exercise) versus therapeutic exercise alone.	Meta-analysis was not completed because of heterogeneity of studies.
Manual Edema Mobilization[47]	MEM + conventional therapy vs. conventional therapy	Clients with distal radius fracture and surgical intervention	Three times/week for 4 weeks, then 2 times/week for 2 weeks, then per therapist assessment	Randomized controlled trial. Level I	Clients treated with MEM + conventional therapy required 20% fewer visits and improved their ADL performance more quickly than those treated with conventional therapy alone.	Statistically significant difference in favor of the MEM group for number of edema treatments required ($p = 0.03$, effect size 5.1 edema treatments), and inability to perform ADLs at 3 weeks (but not 6 or 9 weeks) after inclusion in the study ($P = 0.03$, effect size NR). No statistically significant difference was found between groups in total number of therapy sessions ($P = 0.13$).
ROM, Stretching, Strengthening, and Joint Mobilization[48]	Varied in the included studies	Adults with musculoskeletal disorders of the shoulder	Varied in the 76 included studies	Systematic review of level I, II, and III studies. Level I	ROM, stretching, joint mobilization, and physical agents were beneficial for clients with adhesive capsulitis. Stretching, strengthening, and joint mobilization were beneficial for clients with general shoulder pain. ROM, stretching, strengthening, and joint mobilization were beneficial for clients with subacromial impingement syndrome.	Meta-analysis was not completed because of heterogeneity of studies.
DeLorme and Oxford PRE Programs[49]	DeLorme and Oxford PRE programs for knee extension with 2.75 kg increases each week (as tolerated)	Healthy adults (both male and female)	3 days a week for 9 weeks	Randomized controlled trial. Level I	Both PRE programs increased strength by 66.5%–96%. No difference was found between the two programs.	Difference between PRE programs in 10 RM increase after 9 weeks ($P < 0.65$). The study was underpowered to find such differences.

NR, not reported.

References

1. American Occupational Therapy Association. Occupational therapy practice framework: domain and process (3rd ed.). *Am J Occup Ther.* 2014;68(suppl 1):S1–S51. doi:10.5014/ajot.2014.682006.
2. Neumann DA. Getting started. In: Neumann DA, ed. *Kinesiology of the Musculoskeletal System: Foundations for Rehabilitation.* 3rd ed. St. Louis, MO: Elsevier; 2017:3–27.
3. Colby L, Borstad J. Resistance exercise for impaired muscle performance. In: Kisner C, Colby L, Borstad J, eds. *Therapeutic Exercise: Foundations and Techniques.* 7th ed. Philadelphia, PA: F. A. Davis; 2018:166–245.
4. Nelson DL, Jepson-Thomas J. Occupational form, occupational performance, and a conceptual framework for therapeutic occupation. In: Kramer P, Hinojosa J, Royeen CB, eds. *Perspectives in Human Occupation: Participation in Life.* Baltimore, MD: Lippincott Williams & Wilkins; 2003:87–155.
5. Nelson DL, Chapman LM. Occupational analysis and synthesis. *Ergoterapeuten (Norwegian Journal of Occupational Therapy).* 2015;58(3):46–53. https://www.ergoterapeuten.no/arkiv
6. Karduna AR. Understanding the biomechanical nature of musculoskeletal tissue. *J Hand Ther.* 2012;25(2):116–122. doi:10.1016/j.jht.2011.12.006.
7. Hamill J, Knutzen KM, Derrick TR. *Biomechanical Basis of Human Movement.* 4th ed. Philadelphia, PA: Lippincott Williams & Wilkins; 2015.
8. Flowers KR. Reflections on mobilizing the stiff hand. *J Hand Ther.* 2010;23(4):402–403. doi:10.1016/j.jht.2010.08.004.
9. Brand PW, Hollister AM, Thompson DE. Mechanical resistance. In: Brand PW, Hollister AM, eds. *Clinical Mechanics of the Hand.* 3rd ed. St. Louis, MO: Mosby; 1999:184–214.
10. Lis A, de Castro C, Nordin M. Biomechanics of tendons and ligaments. In: Nordin M, Frankel VH, eds. *Basic Biomechanics of the Musculoskeletal System.* 4th ed. Philadelphia, PA: Lippincott Williams & Wilkins; 2012:102–127.
11. Panjabi MM, White AA. *Biomechanics in the Musculoskeletal System.* New York, NY: Churchill Livingstone; 2001.
12. Flowers KR. A proposed decision hierarchy for splinting the stiff joint, with an emphasis on force application parameters. *J Hand Ther.* 2002;15(2):158–162.
13. Flowers KR, LaStayo PC. Effect of total end range time on improving passive range of motion. *J Hand Ther.* 1994;7(3):150–157. doi:10.1016/S0894-1130(12)80056-1.
14. McClure PW, Blackburn LG, Dusold C. The use of splints in the treatment of joint stiffness: biologic rationale and an algorithm for making clinical decisions. *Phys Ther.* 1994;74(12):1101–1107.
15. Glasgow C, Wilton J, Tooth L. Optimal daily total end range time for contracture: resolution in hand splinting. *J Hand Ther.* 2003;16(3):207–218. doi:10.1016/S0894-1130(03)00036-X.
16. McKee P, Hannah S, Priganc VW. Orthotic considerations for dense connective tissue and articular cartilage—the need for optimal movement and stress. *J Hand Ther.* 2012;25(2):233–243. doi:10.1016/j.jht.2011.12.002.
17. Schultz-Johnson K. Static progressive splinting. *J Hand Ther.* 2002;15(2):163–178.
18. Lorenz T, Campello M. Biomechanics of skeletal muscle. In: Nordin M, Frankel VH, eds. *Basic Biomechanics of the Musculoskeletal System.* 4th ed. Philadelphia, PA: Lippincott Williams & Wilkins; 2012:150–178.
19. Colby L, Borstad J, Kisner C. Stretching for improved mobility. In: Kisner C, Colby L, Borstad J, eds. *Therapeutic Exercise: Foundations and Techniques.* 7th ed. Philadelphia, PA: F. A. Davis; 2018:82–126.
20. Kendall FP, McCreary EK, Provance PG, Rodgers MM, Romani WA. *Muscles, Testing and Function.* 5th ed. Baltimore, MD: Lippincott Williams & Wilkins; 2005.
21. Boakes JL, Foran J, Ward SR, Lieber RL. Muscle adaptation by serial sarcomere addition 1 year after femoral lengthening. *Clin Orthop Relat Res.* 2007;456:250–253. doi:10.1097/01.blo.0000246563.58091.af.
22. Hunter SK, Senefeld JW, Neumann DA. Muscle: the primary stabilizer and mover of the skeletal system. In: Neumann DA, ed. *Kinesiology of the Musculoskeletal System: Foundations for Rehabilitation.* 3rd ed. St. Louis, MO: Elsevier; 2017:47–76.
23. Nelson DL. Occupation: form and performance. *Am J Occup Ther.* 1988;42(10):633–641. doi:10.5014/ajot.42.10.633.
24. Nelson DL. Therapeutic occupation: a definition. *Am J Occup Ther.* 1996;50(10):775–782. doi:10.5014/ajot.50.10.775.
25. Nelson DL. Why the profession of occupational therapy will flourish in the 21st century. *Am J Occup Ther.* 1997;51(1):11–24. doi:10.5014/ajot.51.1.11.
26. Lin K, Wu C, Tickle-Degnen L, Coster W. Enhancing occupational performance through occupationally embedded exercise: a meta-analytic review. *Occup Ther J Res.* 1997;17(1):25–47.
27. Villeco JP. Edema: therapist's management. In: Skirven TM, Osterman AL, Fedorczyk JM, Amadio PC, eds. *Rehabilitation of the Hand and Upper Extremity.* Philadelphia, PA: Elsevier Mosby; 2011:845–857.
28. Klein LJ. Evaluation of the hand and upper extremity. In: Cooper C, ed. *Fundamentals of Hand Therapy.* 2nd ed. St. Louis, MO: Elsevier Mosby; 2014:67–86.
29. Artzberger SM. Edema reduction techniques: a biologic rationale for selection. In: Cooper C, ed. *Fundamentals of Hand Therapy.* 2nd ed. St. Louis, MO: Elsevier Mosby; 2014:35–50.
30. Artzberger SM, Priganc VW. Manual edema mobilization: an edema reduction technique for the orthopedic patient. In: Skirven TM, Osterman AL, Fedorczyk JM, Amadio PC, eds. *Rehabilitation of the Hand and Upper Extremity.* Philadelphia, PA: Elsevier Mosby; 2011:868–881.
31. Kisner C. Range of motion. In: Kisner C, Colby L, Borstad J, eds. *Therapeutic Exercise: Foundations and Techniques.* 7th ed. Philadelphia, PA: F. A. Davis; 2018:61–81.
32. Falkel L. Tissue-specific exercises for the upper extremity. In: Cooper C, ed. *Fundamentals of Hand Therapy.* 2nd ed. St. Louis, MO: Elsevier Mosby; 2014:51–66.
33. Neumann DA. Shoulder complex. In: Neumann DA, ed. *Kinesiology of the Musculoskeletal System: Foundations for Rehabilitation.* 3rd ed. St. Louis, MO: Elsevier; 2017:119–174.

34. Sardelli M, Tashjian RZ, MacWilliams BA. Functional elbow range of motion for contemporary tasks. *J Bone Joint Surg Am.* 2011;93(5):471–477. doi:10.2106/jbjs.I.01633.
35. Cooper C. Hand impairments. In: Radomski MV, Latham CAT, eds. *Occupational Therapy for Physical Dysfunction.* 6th ed. Baltimore, MD: Lippincott Williams & Wilkins; 2008:1131–1170.
36. Pettengill K, Van Strien G. Postoperative management of flexor tendon injuries. In: Skirven TM, Osterman AL, Fedorczyk JM, Amadio PC, eds. *Rehabilitation of the Hand and Upper Extremity.* Philadelphia, PA: Elsevier Mosby; 2011:457–478.
37. Evans RB. Clinical management of extensor tendon injuries: the therapist's perspective. In: Skirven TM, Osterman AL, Fedorczyk JM, Amadio PC, eds. *Rehabilitation of the Hand and Upper Extremity.* Philadelphia, PA: Elsevier Mosby; 2011:521–554.
38. Brody LT. Impaired range of motion and joint mobility. In: Brody LT, Hall CM, eds. *Therapeutic Exercise: Moving Towards Function.* 4th ed. Philadelphia, PA: Wolters Kluwer; 2018:140–186.
39. Rust KL. Managing deficit of first-level motor control capacities using Rood and proprioceptive neuromuscular facilitation techniques. In: Radomski MV, Latham CAT, eds. *Occupational Therapy for Physical Dysfunction.* 6th ed. Baltimore, MD: Lippincott Williams & Wilkins; 2008:690–713.
40. O'Sullivan SB. Strategies to improve motor function. In: O'Sullivan SB, Schmitz TJ, eds. *Physical Rehabilitation.* 5th ed. Philadelphia, PA: F.A. Davis; 2007:471–522.
41. Kisner C. Peripheral joint mobilization/manipulation. In: Kisner C, Colby L, Borstad J, eds. *Therapeutic Exercise: Foundations and Techniques.* 7th ed. Philadelphia, PA: F. A. Davis; 2018:127–165.
42. Schultz K, Jacobs MA. Stiffness. In: Jacobs MA, Austin NM, eds. *Orthotic Intervention for the Hand and Upper Extremity: Splinting Principles and Process.* Philadelphia, PA: Wolters Kluwer; 2014:391–422.
43. Brody LT, Hall CM. Impaired muscle performance. In: Brody LT, Hall CM, eds. *Therapeutic Exercise: Moving Towards Function.* 4th ed. Philadelphia, PA: Wolters Kluwer; 2018:70–115.
44. Lorenz DS, Reiman MP, Walker JC. Periodization: current review and suggested implementation for athletic rehabilitation. *Sports Health.* 2010;2(6):509–518. doi:10.1177/1941738110375910.
45. Billek-Sawhney B, Reicherter EA. Literacy and the older adult. *Top Geriatr Rehabil.* 2005;21(4):275–281. doi:10.1097/00013614-200510000-00004.
46. Weinstock-Zlotnick G, Mehta SP. A systematic review of the benefits of occupation-based intervention for patients with upper extremity musculoskeletal disorders. *J Hand Ther.* 2018. doi:10.1016/j.jht.2018.04.001.
47. Knygsand-Roenhoej K, Maribo T. A randomized clinical controlled study comparing the effect of modified manual edema mobilization treatment with traditional edema technique in patients with a fracture of the distal radius. *J Hand Ther.* 2011;24(3):184–194. doi:10.1016/j.jht.2010.10.009.
48. Marik TL, Roll SC. Effectiveness of occupational therapy interventions for musculoskeletal shoulder conditions: a systematic review. *Am J Occup Ther.* 2017;71(1):7101180020p1–7101180020p11. doi:10.5014/ajot.2017.023127.
49. Fish DE, Krabak BJ, Johnson-Greene D, DeLateur BJ. Optimal resistance training: comparison of DeLorme with Oxford techniques. *Am J Phys Med Rehabil.* 2003;82(12):903–909. doi:10.1097/01.Phm.0000098505.57264.Db.

Chapter 15

Motor Control Assessment

Dawn M. Nilsen and Glen Gillen

LEARNING OBJECTIVES

This chapter will allow the reader to:

1. Understand how motor control supports occupational performance.
2. Understand the neurological and physiological basis of motor control.
3. Describe the classic signs associated with upper and lower motor neuron lesions.
4. Describe the various types of motor dysfunction seen in patients with central nervous system lesions.
5. Describe evaluation procedures used to assess motor control impairments.
6. Correctly interpret the results of motor control assessments.

CHAPTER OUTLINE

TERMINOLOGY

Apraxia: the inability to perform purposeful actions despite having normal muscle and sensory functions.

Ataxia: unsteadiness, incoordination, or clumsiness of movement.

Bradykinesia: slowness of movement.

Chorea: characterized by brief, abrupt, irregular, unpredictable, purposeless movements, primarily in the extremities and face.

Dysmetria: an improper measuring of distance during motor acts; results in overshooting (hypermetria) or undershooting (hypometria) a specific target.

Flaccidity: a state characterized by a complete absence of muscle tone.

Paresis/plegia: weakness or paralysis.

Rigidity: sustained muscle tension, causing the affected body part to become stiff and inflexible.

Spasticity: a velocity-dependent increase in tonic stretch reflexes; also denotes a form of muscular hypertonicity with exaggeration of tendon reflexes.

Tremor: involuntary rhythmic, oscillatory movements of the body or limbs; tremors that occur during precise intentional movements are known as intention tremors; tremors that occur at rest and stop upon the initiation of voluntary movements are called resting tremors.

Introduction

In all of our daily activities, we interact with the environment by sensing information and then acting on this information through the appropriate activation of the motor system. Sometimes, the relationship between what we sense in the environment and how we respond to it is very simple and direct. For example, when we inadvertently touch a hot stove while preparing breakfast, we will, without thought, quickly pull our hands away from the danger. Likewise, if we stand while riding a bus or train, our postural control system will respond to the train perturbations, allowing us to maintain an upright posture or protect ourselves should a sudden loss of balance occur. These movements are examples of reflexive movements. Reflexive movements are involuntary (performed without conscious control), stereotyped movements that are made in direct response to a sensory stimulus. They represent the simplest form of interaction with the world around us.

Although reflexive movements clearly serve a purpose during daily activities, most of our interactions with the environment are performed consciously and in very complex ways. For example, if we see or feel raindrops, we might respond to this sensory information by opening an umbrella, putting on our coat hood, or running to seek shelter. Each of the above actions represents a different response to the same sensory stimuli (raindrops), and each of these actions requires a unique set of voluntary movements. Unlike reflexive movements, voluntary movements are performed under conscious control. They are purposeful, goal-directed movements that are flexible and modifiable depending on the person and context. Voluntary movements allow us to interact with the environment we sense in a multitude of ways.

Most of our time is spent engaging in occupations that require an interplay between voluntary and reflexive movements to support performance. For example, this evening, we may have taken the train home, walked from the train station to our apartment, and rode the elevator to our apartment on the fourth floor. Once inside, we may have taken off our coat, slipped out of our shoes, and began preparing dinner by gathering necessary items from the refrigerator and cabinets. Activation of our postural control system combined with voluntary skilled limb movements were needed to support our functional mobility and engagement in these activities. As we can see from the previous example, any change in motor control can have tremendous impact on our ability to engage in daily occupations. Because occupational therapists treat various conditions that result in lost motor control (e.g., stroke, neurodegenerative diseases, spinal cord injuries), we must become proficient in the ability to identify, assess, and treat motor control impairments. This chapter provides an overview of (1) the neurological and physiological basis of motor control, (2) impact of motor control dysfunction on daily occupation, and (3) evidence-based assessment of motor control impairments. Interventions that address motor control impairments that interfere with daily occupational engagement are the focus of Chapter 16.

Neurological and Physiological Basis of Motor Control

According to Shumway-Cook and Woollacott, motor control is "the ability to regulate or direct the mechanisms essential to movement."[1] These researchers further stipulate that movement emerges from the interaction of multiple systems, including sensory/perceptual, cognitive, and motor/action systems.[1] These systems involve multiple brain regions working together in a cooperative manner, as illustrated in Figure 15-1. Central nervous system (CNS) regions important to the control of movement include the[1]:

- Spinal cord
- Brainstem
- Cerebellum
- Basal ganglia
- Sensorimotor areas of the cerebral cortex, including, but not limited to, the primary motor cortex, premotor cortex, supplementary motor area, and parietal cortex.

The interaction between the above regions involves both hierarchical and parallel processing.[1] In hierarchical processing, a signal is processed in a serial manner between higher and lower level brain regions. Higher levels of the motor hierarchy include cerebral cortex areas, such as the premotor cortex and supplementary motor area. These areas play important roles in the planning and programming of actions. Signals from these structures are conveyed to the primary motor cortex, which is thought to specify important execution commands (e.g., movement extent, direction, force, speed). Commands from higher centers are conveyed to lower levels of the motor hierarchy: the spinal cord via the corticospinal tract and the brainstem via multiple tracts (i.e., corticobulbar, corticoreticular, corticopontine, and corticorubro).[1] Ultimately, signals from the spinal cord and brainstem are sent to muscles for the generation of head, face, trunk, and limb movement (see Fig. 15-1).

Motor neurons that convey signals from higher to lower centers are called upper motor neurons (UMNs), whereas motor neurons that convey the final output signal to muscles are called lower motor neurons (LMNs).[2,3] Generally speaking, UMN cell bodies are contained in the gray matter of cerebral cortex motor areas and specific brainstem nuclei. The axons of these neurons are contained in the white matter and traverse the neuroaxis as descending motor tracts (i.e., corticospinal, corticobulbar, vestibulospinal, reticulospinal, and rubrospinal tracts).[3] LMN cell bodies are contained in

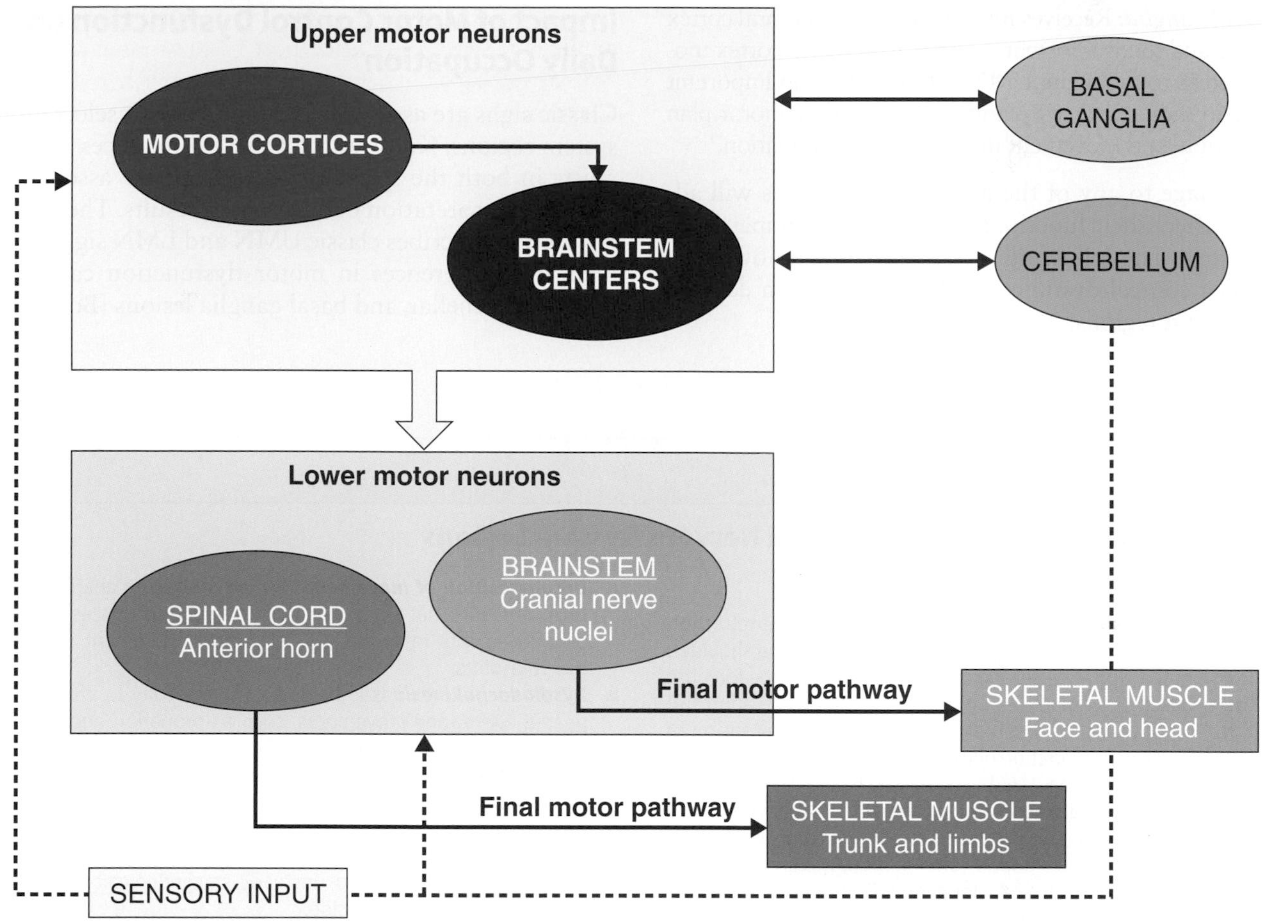

Figure 15-1. Regions of the central nervous system that are important to the control of movement. (Adapted from Purves D, Augustine GJ, Fitzpatrick D, Hall WC, LaMantia AS, White LE. *Neuroscience*. 5th ed. Sunderland, MA: Sinauer Associates; 2012.)

the gray matter of the spinal cord (anterior horn) and brainstem motor nuclei of select cranial nerves (see Chapter 20). The axons of these neurons are contained in spinal nerves and select cranial nerves.[2]

In contrast to hierarchical processing, parallel processing involves multiple brain regions that simultaneously process the same signal.[1] For example, both the cerebellum and the basal ganglia process information from cerebral cortical regions, and both send signals that modulate higher brain region activity, thereby regulating different aspects of motor control.[1] Both hierarchical and parallel processing in the motor system allow us to produce effective and efficient movements that underlie occupational performance. The following summarizes primary functions associated with key motor system regions:

- *Cerebral cortex:* Considered the highest level of the motor hierarchy. Includes (1) sensorimotor areas (e.g., premotor cortex, parietal cortex, supplementary motor area) that are involved in identifying the location of targets in space, choosing a course of action, and programming movements; and (2) the primary motor cortex that contains UMNs that convey signals that modulate lower level brain region activity.[1,3]
- *Spinal cord:* Considered the lowest level of the motor hierarchy. Contains LMNs that send final commands to muscles for reflexive and voluntary control of posture and limb movements. Receives and begins to integrate somatosensory input from the muscles, joints, and skin (via sensory neurons).[1,2]
- *Brainstem:* Contains important nuclei involved in the regulation of posture and movement (i.e., vestibular nuclei, reticular nuclei, pontine nuclei, red nucleus, and substantia nigra). Also contains cranial nerve nuclei (1) that receive somatosensory information from the head and face and that (2) control motor output to the neck, head, and face muscles.[1–3]
- *Cerebellum:* Receives information from the cerebral cortex about intended motor plans and compares that information with sensory information received from the spinal cord and brainstem. Sends information to cerebral cortex motor areas and the brainstem to modulate UMN activity. Plays an important role in modulating motor responses, updating motor plans, and motor learning.[1,4]

- *Basal ganglia:* Receives input from many cerebral cortex areas and sends information back to cerebral cortex motor areas to modulate UMN activity. Plays an important role in motor strategy planning, appropriate motor plan selection, and movement initiation and termination.[1,5]

Damage to any of the above brain regions will adversely affect their functions and negatively impact motor control. The following section provides an overview of motor control dysfunction that results from damage to key brain regions.

Impact of Motor Control Dysfunction on Daily Occupation

Classic signs are associated with damage to select motor system regions. Knowledge of these differences aid therapists in both the selection of appropriate assessments and the interpretation of assessment results. The following section describes classic UMN and LMN signs; highlights the differences in motor dysfunction caused by cortical, cerebellar, and basal ganglia lesions (Box 15-1);

Box 15-1

Motor Dysfunction Caused by Central Nervous System Lesions

Cortical Lesions

- ***Hemiplegic posture or pattern of spasticity*** includes retraction and depression of the scapula; internal rotation of the shoulder; flexion of the elbow, wrist, and fingers; pronation of the forearm; lateral flexion of the trunk toward the involved side; elevation and retraction of the pelvis; internal rotation of the hip; extension of the hip and knee; supination of the foot; and plantar flexion of the ankle and toes (Bobath, 1990).
- ***Hypotonia*** (decreased muscle tone) is less-than-normal resistance to passive elongation; the affected limb feels limp and heavy.
- ***Hypertonia*** (increased muscle tone) is more-than-normal resistance of a muscle to passive elongation. Both neural (spasticity) and mechanical (soft-tissue stiffness) factors contribute to this.
- ***Spasticity***, the neural component of hypertonus, is characterized by a velocity-dependent increase in tonic stretch reflexes and exaggerated tendon reflexes (Nagaoka & Kakuda, 2008). It is commonly accompanied by muscle clonus and clasp-knife reflex.
- ***Clonus*** is the oscillating contraction and relaxation of a limb segment caused by the alternating pattern of stretch reflex and inverse stretch reflex of a spastic muscle.
- ***Clasp-knife phenomenon or reflex*** is resistance to passive stretch of a spastic muscle that suddenly gives way, like the blade of a jackknife.
- ***Weakness*** is the inability to generate the necessary force for effective motor action.
- ***Loss of fractionation*** is the inability to move a single joint without producing unnecessary movements in other joints, resulting in stereotyped movement patterns instead of selective, flexible movement patterns.
- ***Apraxia*** is the inability to perform goal-directed motor activity in the absence of paresis, ataxia, sensory loss, or abnormal muscle tone. Apraxia is characterized by omissions, disturbed order of submovements within a sequence, clumsiness, perseveration, and inability to gesture or use common tools or utensils.
- ***Lead pipe rigidity*** is characterized by hypertonus in both agonist and antagonist muscles, with resistance to movement that is not velocity dependent and that is felt throughout the range of motion.

Cerebellar Lesions

- ***Intention tremor*** is the rhythmic oscillating movement that develops during precise intentional movements caused by involuntary alternating contractions of opposing muscles.
- ***Dysmetria*** is the inability to judge distances accurately; it results in overshooting or undershooting a specific target.
- ***Decomposition of movement***, or ***dyssynergia***, is characterized by movements that are broken up into a series of successive simple movements rather than one smooth movement involving multiple joints.
- ***Dysdiadochokinesia*** is impairment in the ability to perform repeated alternating movements, such as pronation and supination, rapidly and smoothly.
- ***Adiadochokinesia*** is the loss of ability to perform rapid alternating movements.
- ***Ataxia*** is unsteadiness, incoordination, or clumsiness of movement.
- ***Ataxic gait*** is a wide-based, unsteady, staggering gait with a tendency to veer from side to side.

Lesions of the Basal Ganglia

- ***Tremors at rest*** or ***nonintentional tremors*** stop at the initiation of voluntary movement but resume during the holding phase of a motor task when attention wanes or is diverted to another task. Tremors at rest are fatiguing.
- ***Cogwheel rigidity*** is characterized by rhythmic interrupted resistance of the muscles being stretched when the wrist or elbow is flexed quickly.
- ***Hypokinesia*** is slowness or poverty of movement. It includes *akinesia*, difficulty initiating voluntary movements, and ***bradykinesia***, slowness in carrying out movements. These symptoms are reflected in lack of facial expression, monotone speech, reduced eye movements, diminished arm swing during walking, and decreased balance and equilibrium responses seen in Parkinson disease.
- ***Festinating gait*** is characterized by small, fast, shuffling steps that propel the body forward at an increasing rate and by difficulty stopping or changing directions.
- ***Athetosis*** is characterized by slow, writhing involuntary movements, particularly in the neck, face, and extremities. Muscle tone may be increased or decreased. Athetosis ceases during sleep.
- ***Dystonia*** is characterized by powerful, sustained contractions of muscles that cause twisting and writhing of a limb or of the whole body, often resulting in distorted postures of the trunk and proximal extremities.
- ***Chorea*** is characterized by sudden involuntary purposeless, rapid, jerky movements and/or grimacing, primarily in the distal extremities and face (e.g., Huntington chorea).
- ***Hemiballismus*** is unilateral chorea in which there are violent, forceful, flinging movements of the extremities on one side of the body, particularly involving the proximal musculature.

From Fredericks CM Saladin LK, eds. *Pathophysiology of the Motor Systems: Principles and Clinical Presentations*. Philadelphia, PA: Davis; 1996.

and provides examples of how motor dysfunction impacts daily occupational engagement (Table 15-1).

UMN versus LMN Signs

As indicated earlier, UMN cell bodies are located in the gray matter of the cerebral cortex and the brainstem; the axons of these neurons make up the descending motor tracts (e.g., corticospinal tract, corticobulbar tract, vestibulospinal tract).[3] Damage to either the cell bodies or axons of these neurons, proximal to the anterior horn cells in the spinal cord, produces UMN signs.[3] Typical UMN signs include[3] (1) weakness (**paresis**) or paralysis (**plegia**) and disuse atrophy (muscle wasting), (2) **spasticity**, (3) hypertonicity, (4) hyperreflexia (exaggerated reflexes), and (5) a positive Babinski's sign (i.e., dorsiflexion of the great toe and outward fanning of the rest of the toes in response to firm stroking along the lateral aspect of the foot's sole). UMN signs are commonly seen after traumatic injuries (e.g., stroke, traumatic brain injury, spinal cord injury) that damage the motor cortex or corticospinal tract in the brain or spinal cord,[3] or as the result of diseases that damage UMNs (e.g., multiple sclerosis, primary lateral sclerosis).

Conversely, damage to LMN cell bodies (e.g., anterior horn cells located in the spinal cord) or axons (spinal, cranial, or peripheral nerves) results in LMN signs.[3] Typical LMN signs include[3] (1) flaccid paralysis followed by atrophy, (2) fibrillations or fasciculations (involuntary muscle contractions involving one or multiple groups of motor units, respectively), (3) hypotonia, and (4) hyporeflexia (diminished reflexes) or areflexia (absence of reflexes). LMN signs are associated with peripheral nerve injuries (e.g., median or radial nerve injury) or disease processes that damage LMNs (e.g., Guillain-Barré, spinal muscular atrophy).

Combinations of the abovementioned signs may present under certain circumstances. For example, disease processes that damage both types of motor neurons (e.g., amyotrophic lateral sclerosis) produce a combination of UMN and LMN signs. Likewise, a combination of signs is seen in spinal cord injuries that cause damage to descending motor tracts and anterior horn cells.

Dysfunction Caused by Cortical Lesions

Damage to cerebral cortex motor regions or the corticospinal tract most often results in UMN signs that are seen contralateral to the injury side.[3] In addition to these signs, the inability to fractionate movements,

Table 15-1. Impact of Common Motor Control Impairments on Daily Occupational Engagement

MOTOR CONTROL IMPAIRMENT	EXAMPLES OF IMPACT OF IMPAIRMENT ON FUNCTION
Apraxia	• Using awkward grasp and pinch patterns when retrieving objects for self-feeding • Difficulty maintaining the orientation of grooming objects toward the body • Difficulty with in-hand manipulation, such as handling coins and playing cards
Ataxia	• Presents with a wide-based, unsteady gait • Not able to coordinate reach patterns during bathing or leisure activities • Nystagmus may interfere with reading, bill paying, etc.
Bradykinesia	• Increased time needed to perform daily activities • Difficulty getting up and down from a chair • Difficulty throwing and catching a ball
Chorea, Athetosis, and Ballismus	• Interference with sleep/rest patterns due to flailing limbs • Impaired feeding and swallowing ability • Inability to participate in written communication (e.g., writing, keyboarding, texting)
Dysmetria	• Overshooting or undershooting items when attempting to retrieve them from cabinets during meal preparation • Overshooting or undershooting curbs and difficulty climbing steps during functional mobility
Hypotonicity	• Decreased ability to maintain an upright posture while seated in a chair • Decreased ability to maintain a standing position while preparing meals
Intention tremor	• Spillage of food from a spoon during feeding • Difficulty putting toothpaste on a toothbrush • Difficulty typing on a computer key board
Paresis	• Decreased ability to stabilize or manipulate grooming objects • Decreased ability to retrieve items from the refrigerator during meal preparation • Difficulty standing and weight shifting while manipulating clothing during toileting
Spasticity and rigidity	• Difficulty opening the hand or positioning the arm to wash and dry the affected upper extremity during bathing • Difficulty placing the affected limbs into clothing during dressing • Difficulty turning in bed

the development of stereotypical postures and movement patterns, and **apraxia** are common cortical lesion consequences.[1]

Cortical lesion deficits result in an inability to plan and produce effective and efficient movements, limiting daily occupational engagement. For example, paresis and tonal changes on one side of the body often negatively impact a person's ability to transfer, walk, and use his or her involved arm and hand to perform activities of daily living (ADLs).

Dysfunction Caused by Cerebellar Lesions

Damage to the cerebellum produces a variety of motor control impairments that generally impact coordination (ability to produce accurate, smooth, and controlled movements) and postural control, limiting occupational engagement.[4] For example, intention **tremor**, **dysmetria**, dysdiadochokinesia, movement decomposition, limb and truncal **ataxia**, and nystagmus are common after cerebellar damage. In addition, hypotonia and decreased deep tendon reflexes may be present.[1,4]

These coordination deficits can interfere with engagement in a wide range of activities. For example, intention tremors can cause spillage of food during feeding, and dysmetria can result in overshooting or undershooting target objects during ADL performance. Ataxic gait is common after cerebellar damage and is characterized by a wide base of support and unsteady gait pattern that increase fall risk. Nystagmus (rapid involuntary eye movements) may also be present and adversely impact vision, making tasks such as reading or computer use difficult.

Dysfunction Caused by Basal Ganglia Lesions

Basal ganglia damage can occur as a consequence of stroke, traumatic brain injury, or neurodegenerative disorders such as Parkinson or Huntington disease.[5] Basal ganglia lesions produce movement disorders that are generally described as hypokinetic (decreased motor activity) or hyperkinetic (increased motor activity) in nature.[5] Hypokinetic movement disorders are characterized by reduced voluntary movements and diminished or slowed automatic movements.[5] Conversely, hyperkinetic movement disorders are characterized by excessive involuntary movements. Clinical signs associated with basal ganglia lesions vary depending on lesion location and include resting or nonintentional tremors, **rigidity**, **bradykinesia**, athetosis, **chorea**, dystonia (sustained muscle contractions causing limb/body twisting and writhing), ballismus (flailing/flinging limb movement), and festinating gait (small, fast, shuffling steps).[1,5]

Like dysfunction caused by cortical or cerebellar damage, hypokinesia and hyperkinesia can negatively impact engagement in daily occupations. For example, bradykinesia can increase the time needed to complete daily activities, resulting in fatigue, whereas excessive involuntary movements can make performing tasks such as feeding, bathing, and dressing difficult or even impossible.

Motor Control Assessment

Because motor control impairments can deleteriously effect occupational performance, it is essential to assess patients' motor control. To develop effective intervention plans, therapists must determine which specific aspects of motor control are impaired—for example, poor coordination, impaired postural control, inability to motor plan, impaired upper and lower limb function, and spasticity. The following sections describe specific assessment procedures and review standardized assessments related to motor control.

Assessment of Motor Control Skills in Daily Living

It is critical for therapists to understand various body systems as they relate to occupational performance. Several standardized, valid, and reliable motor assessments allow therapists to assess patients during natural or simulated ADL performance.

The Assessment of Motor and Process Skills (AMPS)[6] is an example of an assessment that measures motor skills in a naturalistic setting using client-chosen occupations. Therapists evaluate motor and process skills within the context of basic and instrumental activities of daily living (IADL). The quality of patient ADL performance is assessed by rating the effort, efficiency, safety, and independence of 16 ADL motor (and 20 ADL process) skill items while performing chosen, familiar, and life-relevant ADL tasks. There are more than 100 tasks to choose from, ensuring a client-centered assessment approach. Evaluated motor skills include skills related to body position (stabilizes, aligns, positions), obtaining and holding objects (reaches, bends, grips, manipulates, coordinates), moving self and objects (moves, lifts, walks, transports, calibrates, flows), and sustaining performance (endures, paces).[6]

The Motor Assessment Scale (MAS)[7] is also a performance-based measure that evaluates motor function as it relates to everyday life (Box 15-2). It evaluates eight different areas of motor function[7]:

- Supine to side lying
- Supine to sitting over the edge of a bed
- Balanced sitting
- Sitting to standing
- Walking
- Upper arm function
- Hand movements
- Advanced hand activities.

Each task is performed three times, and best performance is recorded. All eight items are assessed using a 7-point scale, ranging from 0 to 6. A score of 6 indicates optimal motor behavior[7] (see the Assessment table at the end of this chapter).

Box 15-2

Abridged Criteria for Scoring Motor Assessment Scale

The score assigned on each item is the highest criterion met on the best performance of three. A 0 score is assigned if the patient is unable to meet the criteria for a score of 1.

0 1 2 3 4 5 6

Supine to Side Lying to Intact Side

1. Pulls self into side lying with intact arm, moving affected leg with intact leg.
2. Moves leg across actively and lower half of body follows. Arm is left behind.
3. Lifts arm across body with other arm. Moves leg actively; body follows in a block.
4. Actively moves arm across body; rest of body follows in a block.
5. Rolls to side, moving arm and leg; overbalances. Shoulder protracts and arm flexes.
6. Rolls to side in 3 seconds. Must not use hands.

Supine to Sitting on Edge of Bed

1. After being assisted to side lying, lifts head sideways; cannot sit up.
2. Side lying to sitting on edge of bed with therapist assisting movement.
3. Side lying to sitting on edge of bed with standby help assisting legs over side of bed.
4. Side lying to sitting on edge of bed with no standby help.
5. Supine to sitting on edge of bed with no standby help.
6. Supine to sitting on edge of bed within 10 seconds with no standby help.

Balanced Sitting

1. Sits only with support after therapist assists.
2. Sits unsupported for 10 seconds.
3. Sits unsupported with weight well forward and evenly distributed.
4. Sits unsupported with hands resting on thighs; turns head and trunk to look behind.
5. Reaches forward to touch floor 4 inches in front of feet and returns to starting position.
6. Sitting on stool, reaches sideways to touch floor and returns to starting position.

Sitting to Standing

1. Gets to standing with help (any method).
2. Gets to standing with standby help.
3. Gets to standing with weight evenly distributed and with no help from hands.
4. Gets to standing; stands for 5 seconds, weight evenly distributed, hips and knees extended.
5. Stands up and sits down with no help; even weight distribution; full hip and knee extension.
6. Stands up and sits down with no help three times in 10 seconds; even weight distribution.

Walking

1. Stands on affected leg with hip extended; steps forward with other leg (standby help).
2. Walks with standby help from one person.
3. Walks 10 feet alone. Uses any walking aid, but no standby help.
4. Walks 16 feet with no aid in 15 seconds.
5. Walks 33 feet, picks up small sandbag from floor, turns around, walks back in 25 seconds.
6. Walks up and down four steps with or without an aid three times in 35 seconds. May not hold rail.

Upper Arm Function

1. Supine, protracts shoulder girdle. Tester places arm in 90° flexion and supports elbow.
2. Supine, holds shoulder in 90° flexion for 2 seconds. (Maintains 45° external rotation and 20° elbow extension.)
3. From position in level 2, flexes and extends elbow to move palm to forehead and back.
4. Sitting, holds arm in 90° shoulder flexion with elbow extended, thumb pointing up, for 2 seconds. No excess shoulder elevation.
5. Achieves position in level 4; holds for 10 seconds; lowers arm. No pronation allowed.
6. Standing, arm abducted 90°, with palm flat against wall. Maintains hand position while turning body toward wall.

Hand Movements

1. Sitting, lifts cylindrical object off table by extending wrist. No elbow flexion allowed.
2. Sitting, forearm in midposition. Lifts hand off table by radially deviating wrist. No elbow flexion or forearm pronation allowed.
3. Sitting, elbow into side, pronates and supinates forearm through three-quarters of range.
4. Sitting, reaches forward to pick up 5-inch ball with both hands and puts ball down. Ball placement requires elbow extension. Palms stay in contact with ball.
5. Sitting, picks up plastic foam cup from table and puts it on table across other side of body.
6. Sitting, continuous opposition of thumb and each finger more than 14 times in 10 seconds.

Advanced Hand Activities

1. Reaches forward arm's length; picks up pen top; releases it on table close to body.
2. Picks up a jellybean from teacup with eight jellybeans and places it in another cup. Cups are at arm's length.
3. Draws horizontal lines to stop at a vertical line 10 times in 20 seconds.
4. Makes rapid consecutive dots with a pen on a sheet of paper. (Picks up and holds pen without assistance; at least two dots per second for 5 seconds; dots, not dashes).
5. Takes a dessert spoon of liquid to the mouth, without spilling. (Head cannot lower toward spoon).
6. Holds a comb and combs hair at the back of head. (Shoulder is externally rotated, abducted at least 90°; head is erect.)

The Action Research Arm Test (ARAT)[8] is a quick and easily administered assessment that uses simulated everyday activities to evaluate upper limb motor function. The ARAT consists of 19 items grouped in four categories: grasp, grip, pinch, and gross movement that generate 4 subscale scores. Test items include reaching, grasping, and transporting various size objects (i.e., blocks, marbles, cup with water). Items are timed (maximum allowable time is 60 seconds) and graded on a 4-point scale, ranging from 0 (unable to perform) to 3 (performs normally). Subscale scores range from 0 (unable to perform any item) to 18 (performs all items normally) for the grasp and pinch subscales, 0 to 12 for the grip subscale, and 0 to 9 for the gross movement subscale. Total scores range from 0 to 57, with higher scores indicating greater functional upper limb capacity.[8] The test is most useful for patients with some distal function (see the Assessment table).

Similarly, the Wolf Motor Function Test (WMFT)[9] has been used to document outcomes related to upper limb interventions and includes a variety of tasks such as basic reaching tasks (e.g., lifting arm from lap to table, extending elbow with and without a weight attached) and more functional activities involving fine motor control (e.g., picking up a pencil, turning a key in a lock). All tasks, excluding one, are unilateral and appropriate for both the dominant and nondominant arm. Because many tasks do not require distal control, it is appropriate for patients with a more involved upper extremity (UE). The therapist times task performance (maximum allowable time is 120 seconds) and qualitatively grades movement using a 6-point ordinal scale, ranging from 1 (doesn't attempt to use the UE for the task) to 6 (does attempt, movement appears normal)[9] (see the Assessment table).

It is also important to document clients' perception of their upper limb function. The Motor Activity Log (MAL)[10] is a self-report questionnaire (report by patient or family) related to actual use of the involved UE outside structured therapy time. The MAL uses a semi-structured interview format. Quality of movement ("How well" or quality of use scale) and amount of use ("How much" or amount of use scale) are graded on a 6-point ordinal scale. At present, there are 14-, 28-, and 30-item versions of the instrument.[10–12] Sample items include hold book, pick up a phone, use a towel, pick up a glass, write/type, steady myself, and use a television remote.[10]

Muscle Tone and Deep Tendon Reflexes

Muscle tone is defined as the involuntary resistance of a muscle to passive stretch. This resistance is felt when a body part is passively moved by an examiner. Normal muscle tone relies on the functioning of multiple motor system regions and is dependent on both neural factors (motor unit activity and the stretch reflex) and mechanical factors (muscle viscoelastic properties).[1]

Characteristics of normal muscle tone include the feeling of slight resistance to passive joint movement, and the ability to maintain body part position against gravity if support is removed. When muscle tone is normal, therapists will feel slight resistance when a muscle is passively stretched. Abnormalities in muscle tone often accompany damage to the motor system.[1,3] An increase in muscle tone (more than normal resistance to passive stretch) is called hypertonia. A decrease in muscle tone (less than normal resistance to passive stretch) is called hypotonia. Spasticity may accompany hypertonia. Spasticity is a velocity-dependent increase in the stretch reflex coupled with an exaggeration of deep tendon reflexes.[1,3]

Deep tendon reflexes involve direct activation of the stretch reflex, also known as the monosynaptic stretch reflex.[2,13] The stretch reflex is mediated by a two-neuron reflex arch involving the spinal or brainstem segment innervating the muscle. The sensory neuron innervates the muscle spindle, which is a complex sensory receptor found in skeletal muscle. The muscle spindle continuously provides the CNS with information about changes in muscle length. When the muscle spindle is lengthened (as occurs when a muscle tendon is tapped briskly with a reflex hammer), the sensory receptor discharges and excites the alpha motor neuron (located in either the anterior horn of the spinal cord or brainstem nuclei depending on the muscle involved), causing the muscle to contract.[2] Motor areas of the cerebral cortex and brainstem modulate stretch reflex activity, and this modulation plays an important role in the regulation of reflexive and voluntary movements.[3]

When deep tendon reflexes are normal, a brisk tap of a muscle's tendon will result in contraction of that muscle.[13] However, damage to the motor system may disrupt modulation of the stretch reflex, causing abnormalities in muscle tone and deep tendon reflexes. An increase in deep tendon reflexes (as occurs with spasticity) is called hyperreflexia. A decrease in deep tendon reflexes is called hyporeflexia, and an absence of deep tendon reflexes is termed areflexia.[13]

A severe form of hypertonicity is rigidity.[1] Common forms of rigidity include lead pipe rigidity, cogwheel rigidity, decorticate rigidity, and decerebrate rigidity.[2,3] In lead pipe rigidity, hypertonus is present in both the agonist and antagonist muscles (e.g., flexors and extensors of the elbow joint), and resistance is felt throughout the entire range of motion (ROM). In cogwheel rigidity, passive movement of the limb elicits ratchet-like, start-and-stop movements as tension in the muscle gives way and then increases again. These ratchet-like start-and-stop movements can be felt throughout the ROM.[3] Decorticate rigidity is characterized by abnormal flexor tone and abnormal flexor posturing of the upper limbs, and increased extensor tone and extensor posturing of the lower limbs.[2] This type of rigidity is associated with brain lesions that occur above the midbrain level, resulting in the removal of cortical influence on brainstem nuclei. Decerebrate rigidity is characterized by abnormal extensor tone and posturing of the upper and lower limbs in extension. This type of rigidity is associated with lesions impacting the brainstem.[2]

Muscle tone is assessed clinically by observing a muscle's response to passive stretch.[1] For example, when testing tone of the biceps muscle, therapists should place patients in a supine or seated position, place the elbow joint in a maximally flexed position, and then passively move the joint to a position of maximal extension over a period of ~1 second with repetition as needed to make an accurate determination; repetition should be kept to a minimum[14] (see Video 15-1).

The Modified Ashworth Spasticity Scale (MASS)[14] is a subjective rating scale that is often used to describe muscle tone and spasticity. As illustrated earlier, therapists attempt to move the part through its full ROM and the amount of resistance felt during passive movement is scored using a 6-point ordinal scale, ranging from 0 (no increase in muscle tone) to 4 (affected part is rigid in flexion or extension) (Box 15-3).[14] Evidence suggests the MASS is a reliable instrument for assessing tonal changes in patients with stroke[15] and those with profound intellectual and multiple disabilities[16]; however, its clinical utility with respect to other patient populations may be limited[17] (see the Assessment table).

Deep tendon reflexes are assessed by properly positioning the patient, palpating a muscle tendon, and tapping the muscle tendon briskly with a reflex hammer.[13] Figure 15-2 shows common testing positions for assessing the four common UE deep tendon reflexes. Box 15-4 highlights deep tendon reflexes commonly assessed in the upper and lower limbs, along with the grading scale used for reflex rating.

In addition to testing deep tendon reflexes, tests administered to determine the presence of pathological reflexes, such as a Hoffman's[18] or Babinski's sign,[18] can be useful to screen for UMN signs in the upper and lower limbs, respectively. The Hoffman's test is conducted by placing the patient in a comfortable standing or seated position. The therapist stabilizes the proximal interphalangeal joint of the third digit (middle finger) and applies a stimulus to the finger by "flicking" the fingernail between the therapists thumb and index finger[18] (Fig. 15-3). If the pathological reflex is present, adduction of the thumb and flexion of the index finger (positive Hoffman's sign) will occur in response to the stimulation (see Video 15-2). No movement of the thumb or index finger is considered normal (negative Hoffman's sign).[18] The Babinski's test is conducted with the patient in a supine or long sitting position. The therapist supports the patient's foot in neutral and applies stimulation to the plantar aspect of the foot, typically moving lateral to medial from the heel to the metatarsals, with the blunt end of a reflex hammer[18] (Fig. 15-4). If the pathological reflex is present, the great toe will extend along with fanning of the second through fifth toes (positive Babinski's sign).[18] A normal response is flexion of the toes (plantar reflex and negative Babinski's sign)[13] (see Video 15-3).

Box 15-3

Modified Ashworth Scale for Grading Spasticity

Grade	Description
0	No increase in muscle tone
1	Slight increase in muscle tone manifested by a catch and release or by minimal resistance at the end of the range of motion (ROM) when the affected part or parts are moved in flexion or extension
1+	Slight increase in muscle tone manifested by a catch, followed by minimal resistance throughout the remainder (less than half) of the ROM
2	Marked increase in muscle tone through most of the ROM, but affected parts are easily moved
3	Considerable increase in muscle tone; passive movement difficult
4	Affected part or parts rigid in flexion or extension

Reprinted with permission from Bohannon RW, Smith MB. Interrater reliability of a Modified Ashworth Scale of muscle spasticity. *Phys Ther.* 1987;67:207. Copyright 1987 by American Physical Therapy Association.

Postural Control

According to Shumway-Cook and Woollacott, postural control "involves controlling the body's position in space for the dual purposes of stability and orientation."[1] Normal postural control involves multiple body systems and senses working together to allow one to maintain a steady state in sitting and standing, react to perturbations to balance, and, most importantly, prevent falls. During development, major milestones such as lifting the head, crawling, and walking all contribute to postural control development. During this time, righting, equilibrium, and protective responses also develop. Righting reactions support positioning of the head vertically in space, alignment of head and trunk, and alignment of trunk and limbs. Equilibrium responses occur when posture is perturbed. Lastly, protective reactions occur to protect the face and head when equilibrium reactions fail.[1] Examples of standardized assessments

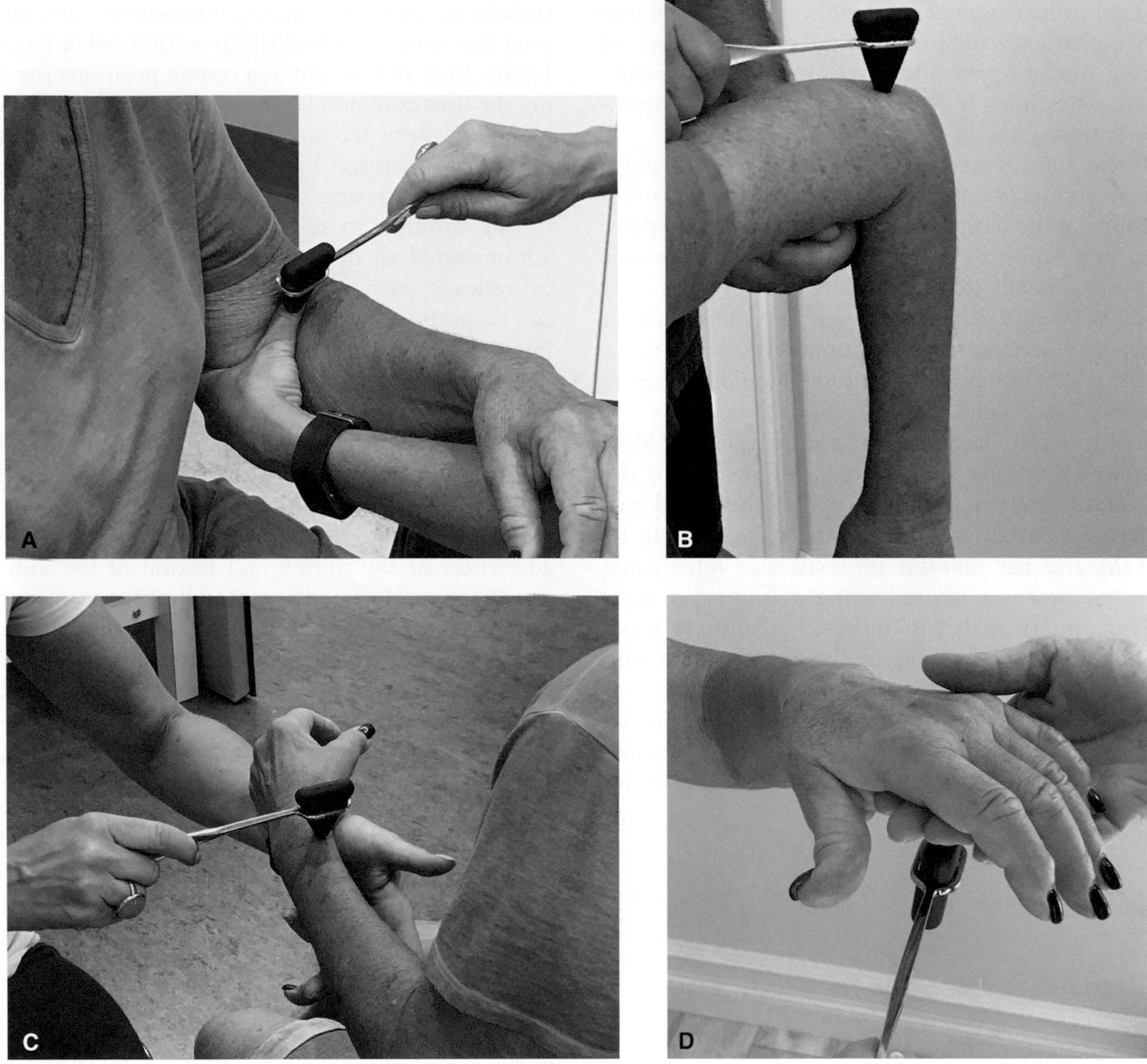

Figure 15-2. Testing positions for assessing the deep tendon reflexes in the upper extremity. **A.** Biceps. **B.** Triceps. **C.** Brachioradialis. **D.** Finger flexors.

for assessing postural control include the Berg Balance Scale[19] and the Functional Reach Test[20] (see the Assessment table and Fig. 15-5). Readers should see Chapter 17 for details on balance assessment.

Paresis and Selective Motor Control

As indicated earlier, weakness and the inability to fractionate or selectively control joint movement are common after damage to the descending motor system. These impairments are typically assessed by observing the resting posture of the limbs and trunk and by assessing patients' ability to produce voluntary movements during ADL performance.

For example, therapists may observe patients during activity engagement, such as feeding or grooming, while noting whether there is evidence of the following: (1) abnormal posturing of the limbs (see Box 15-1) or deviations in trunk alignment; (2) compensatory motor strategies (e.g., forward flexion of the trunk or hiking of the shoulder while reaching for objects); (3) weakness in specific muscle groups (e.g., inability to stabilize or hold objects in the hand because of weak finger flexors); (4) inability to selectively control certain joints (e.g., inability to grasp objects without flexing the elbow); (5) incorrect timing of movement components (e.g., finger closure prior to making appropriate contact with an object); and (6) inability to appropriately

Box 15-4

Assessment of Deep Tendon Reflexes

Deep Tendon Reflex with Spinal Segment[13]	Grading of Deep Tendon Reflexes
Biceps (C5, C6)	4+ = very brisk, hyperactive, clonus may be present
Triceps (C7–C8)	3+ = brisker than average (hyperreflexia)
Brachioradialis (C5–C6)	2+ = average, normal
Finger flexors (C7–C8)	1+ = diminished, low normal (hyporeflexia)
Quadriceps (patella) (L2–L4)	0 = no response
Gastrocnemius (Achilles) (S1)	

coordinate movement at adjacent joints (e.g., inability to hold objects in the hand while simultaneously extending the elbow and flexing the shoulder). If these deficits interfere with task performance, therapists may wish to perform additional testing. For example, manual muscle testing can be used to determine muscle strength (see Chapter 13), and standardized assessments, such as the Fugl-Meyer Assessment,[21] can be used to objectively measure the extent to which patients can isolate and coordinate individual joint movements.

The Fugl-Meyer Assessment (FMA) is a widely used instrument designed to evaluate motor recovery after stroke.[21] The test is based on earlier research describing the natural course of motor recovery following stroke and Brunnstrom motor recovery stages.[22] The FMA assesses UE motor function, lower extremity (LE) motor function, balance, sensation, and joint function. Maximum points are 66 for the UE, 34 for LE, 14 for balance, 24 for sensation, 24 for position sense, 44 for ROM, and 44 for joint pain (total possible score = 250). Each section can be scored separately.[22] The motor subtests have established reliability[23] and validity,[24] and they are responsive to changes overtime for stroke patients at various recovery stages[25–27] (see the Assessment table).

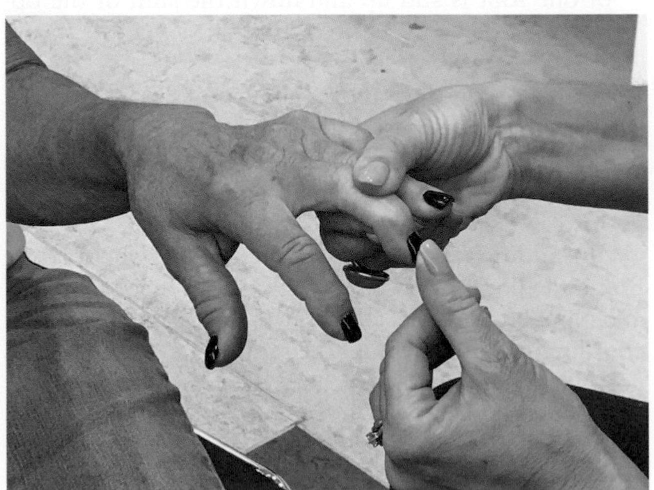

Figure 15-3. Testing position for administering the Hoffman's test.

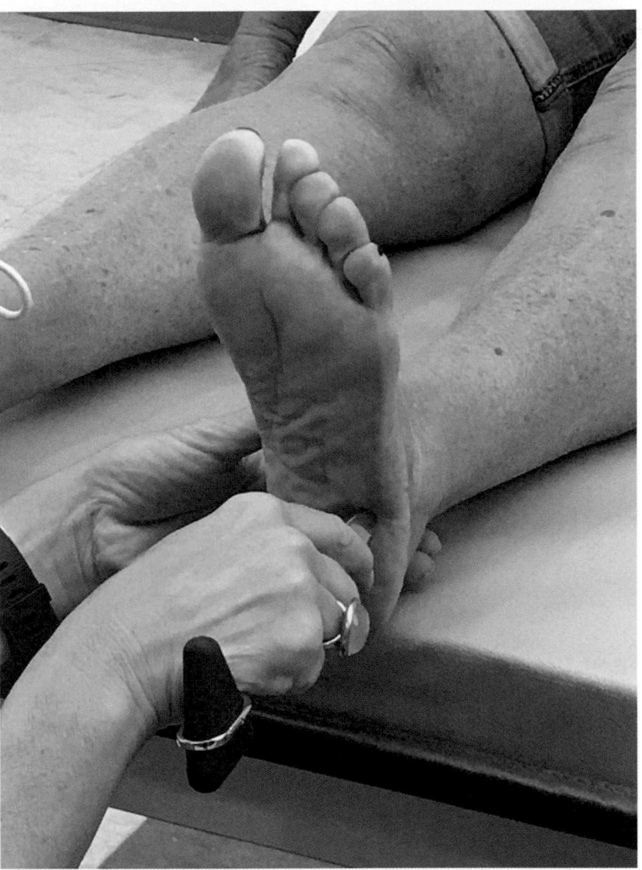

Figure 15-4. Testing position for administering the Babinski's test.

Coordination

As discussed earlier, coordination is the ability to produce accurate, smooth, and controlled movements. Like paresis, and the ability to fractionate movement, coordination is assessed by observing patients engaged in ADLs while noting movement quality or characteristics. For example, therapists may observe patients during activity participation (e.g., simple meal preparation or dressing) and note whether the patients have difficulty initiating or terminating movements, and whether movements appear slow or jerky. If coordination deficits interfere with function, therapists may further examine the extent of deficits. Examples of more formal clinical tests of coordination include the following[1]:

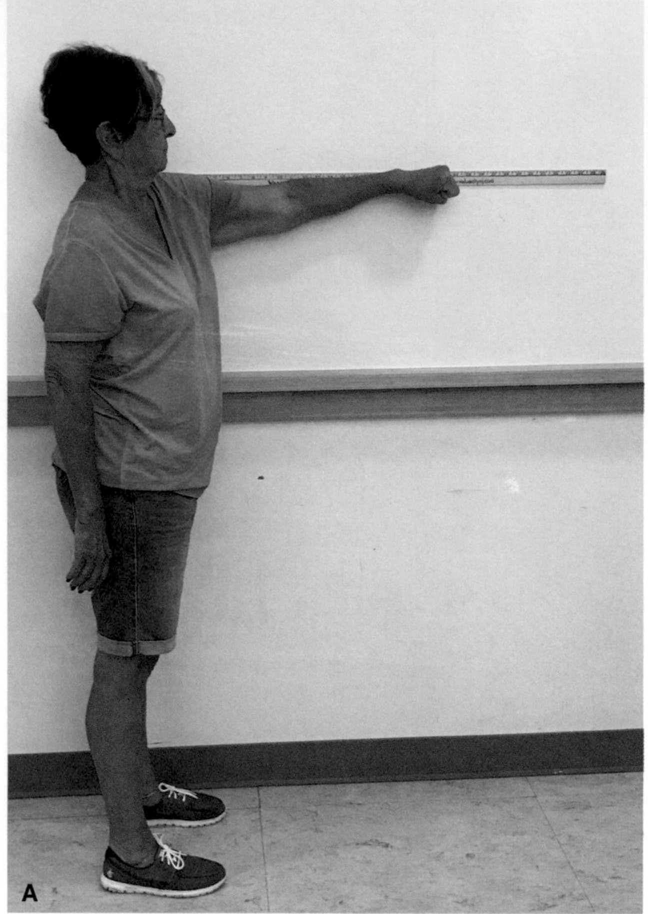

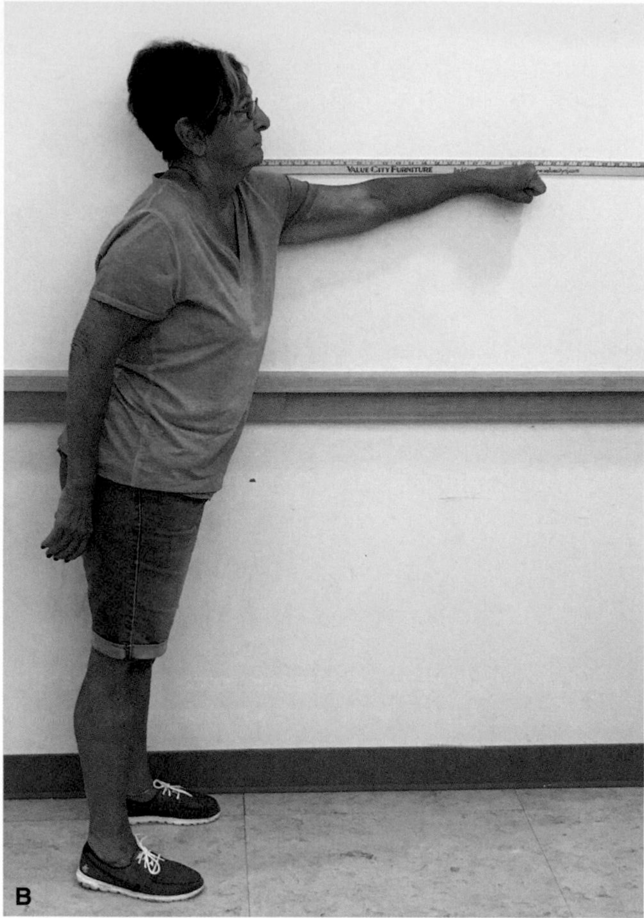

Figure 15-5. Functional Reach Test. **A.** Starting position: The assessor records the starting position at the third metacarpal head on the yardstick (or meter stick) and instructs the patient to "Reach forward as far as you can without taking a step." **B.** Ending position: The assessor records the location of the third metacarpal head on the yardstick (or meter stick). Scores are determined by assessing the difference between the start and end position in the reach distance.

- *Finger-to-Nose:* The shoulder is abducted to 90° with the elbow in extension. Patients are asked to bring the tip of their index finger to the tip of their nose. Alterations in the initial start position can be made to assess coordination in different movement plans.
- *Finger-Nose-Finger:* With patients in a seated position and therapists seated in front, patients are asked to move their index finger from their nose to the therapists' finger (Fig. 15-6). Position of the therapist's finger can be altered to change the distance and direction of the movement.
- *Pronation/Supination:* With the elbows flexed to approximately 90° and held close to the body, the patient alternately turns the palms up and down (see Video 15-4). Speed can be gradually increased.

- *Mass Grasp:* The patient alternates between opening and closing the hand. Speed can be gradually increased.
- *Finger Opposition:* The patient touches the tip of the thumb to the tips of the fingers in sequence. Speed can be gradually increased.
- *Tapping (Hand or Foot):* Patients are asked to tap their hand on their knee or the ball of their foot on the floor while maintaining the heel in contact with the floor.
- *Heel-Shin:* With the patient in supine, the heel of one foot is slid up and down the shin of the opposite LE.

Performance on the above clinical tests is typically graded subjectively using the following ordinal scale[1]: 5 = normal, 4 = minimal impairment, 3 = moderate impairment, 2 = severe impairment, and 1 = cannot perform.

In addition, standardized assessments such as the Box and Blocks Test (BBT),[28] Purdue Pegboard Test,[29] and Nine-Hole Peg Test[28] can be used to assess eye–hand coordination and manual dexterity. The BBT requires patients to move, one by one, the maximum number of wooden blocks from one compartment of a box to another of equal size, within 60 seconds. Patients are scored based on the number of blocks they transfer

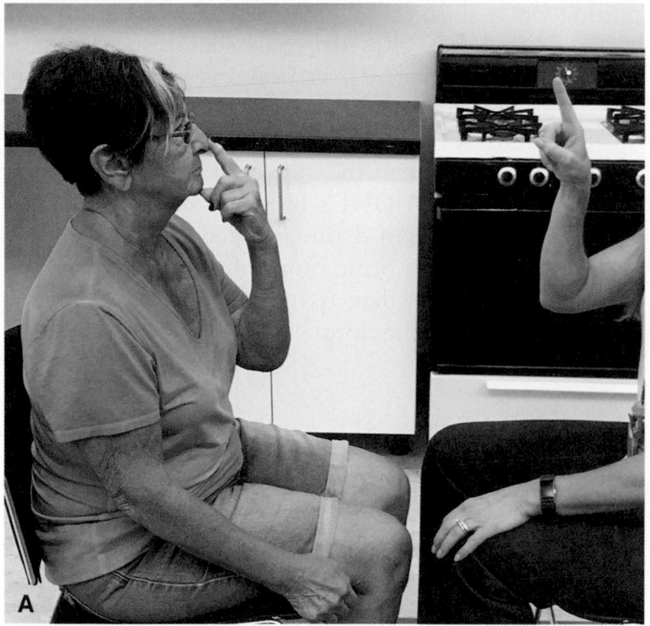

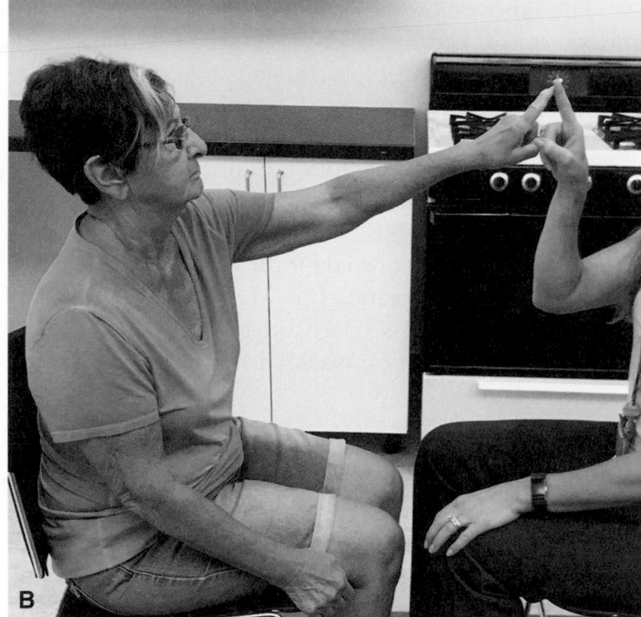

Figure 15-6. Finger-Nose-Finger test. Illustrates movement from patient's nose **(A)** to the therapist's finger **(B)**.

from one compartment to the other in the allotted time. Higher scores indicate better manual dexterity.[28] The BBT has established reliability, validity, and normative data and is responsive to change overtime as a measure of manual dexterity[28] (see the Assessment table).

The Purdue Pegboard consists of a board with 4 cups across the top and 2 vertical rows of 25 small holes centrally located on the board. The outside cups each contain 25 pins, the cup to the immediate left contains 40 washers, and the cup to the immediate right of center contains 20 collars. Patients are required to move as many pins as possible from the cups into the holes within 30 seconds. The test is performed with the right hand, left hand, and then both hands simultaneously. In the final subtest, patients use both hands to assemble as many pins, washers, and collars as possible within 60 seconds.[29]

The Nine-Hole Peg Test consists of a plastic board with a shallow round dish that contains pegs and nine holes oriented in three rows positioned below the cup. Patients are instructed to move the pegs into the holes, one by one, as quickly as possible; and then to move the pegs, one by one, back into the cup. The time required to complete the task is recorded.[28]

Motor Planning

The ability to motor plan and store motor plans allows one to effectively and efficiently interact with the environment. The saying "Once you learn how to ride a bicycle, you never forget" provides insight into motor plan function. When we repetitively practice a motor task, the plan to perform it, the sequence of one's movements, and the organization of movements all become stored as procedural memory. We develop motor plans throughout our life course. These motor plans, or praxicons, are thought to be stored in the left inferior parietal lobe. Destruction of praxicons or loss of the ability to access them can result from multiple brain trauma types. When this occurs, patients present with motor apraxia (or ideomotor apraxia).[30] During occupational performance, motor apraxia presents as clumsy and slower movements, simplified prehension patterns, inability to coordinate oral musculature (oral apraxia), inability to coordinate total body patterns such as rolling and supine-to-sit, poor gesture production, inability to coordinate joints and body parts, and poor task performance initiation.[31]

Several standardized evaluations relate to motor planning assessment. Although they differ in the number and order of items, they use similar procedures to detect motor apraxia. Procedures include imitation of gestures, performing transitive (with an object such as teeth brushing) and nontransitive (without an object such as saluting) movements on command, or via demonstration. Specific instruments include:

- Cambridge Apraxia Battery[32]
- Limb Apraxia Test[33]
- Kaufman Hand Movement Test[34]
- Ideomotor Apraxia Test[35]
- Florida Apraxia Screening Test[36]

The above-noted instruments screen for motor apraxia out of context. As occupational therapists, it is important that we adopt instruments that directly examine the impact of motor apraxia during ADL and IADL performance. Two such instruments are the ADL Observations to Measure Disabilities in those with Apraxia,[37] and the ADL-focused Occupation-based Neurobehavioral Evaluation (A-ONE, formerly known as the Árnadóttir OT-ADL Neurobehavioral Evaluation).[31]

The ADL Observations to Measure Disabilities in those with Apraxia is based on the structured observation of four activities: washing face and upper body, putting on a shirt or blouse, preparing food, and an individualized task chosen by the therapist. Scoring is based on independence, initiation, execution, and control. Items are scored from 0 to 3, with higher scores indicating more severe impairment.[37] The A-ONE is able to detect and document the impact of motor apraxia on basic ADLs.[31] The A-ONE's Independence Scale ranges from 0 (dependent) to 4 (independent). The Neurobehavioral Impairment Scale ranges from 0 (no neurobehavioral impairment detected) to 4 (unable to perform because of neurobehavioral impairment; needs maximum assistance).[31]

CASE STUDY

Patient Information

Nakai is a 34-year-old Native American male who was diagnosed with multiple sclerosis 2 years prior to this inpatient rehabilitation admission. His initial symptoms began approximately 3 years prior to this admission and consisted of diplopia, gait impairments, and problems with upper limb coordination. Nakai was admitted to the hospital because of worsening symptoms and an inability to complete basic self-care tasks such as feeding, grooming, dressing, and toileting.

Assessment Process and Results

The therapist began the assessment process by observing Nakai engaging in his morning self-care routine. She scored his performance using the Functional Independence Measure (FIM), because this is the standardized assessment typically used on the rehabilitation unit. Nakai's FIM scores were as follows:

- Feeding: 3 (moderate assistance)
- Grooming: 3 (moderate assistance)
- Bathing: 3 (moderate assistance)
- Upper body dressing: 4 (minimal assistance)
- Lower body dressing: 3 (moderate assistance)
- Toileting: 3 (moderate assistance)

Impairments in upper limb coordination appeared to be the significant limiting factor for the majority of activities observed. For example, while observing Nakai eating breakfast, she noted that he overshot items on his food tray when reaching with either his right or left hand. Attempts at hand-to-mouth patterns resulted in utensil stabbing around the mouth, and food and drink spillage. In an apparent attempt to control these jerky movements, Nakai often leaned on his forearms and brought his head toward his cup and spoon when attempting to eat or drink, rather than bringing the cup or spoon to his mouth. Because attempts to eat and drink continued to fail, Nakai became very frustrated and refused to continue eating. When observing Nakai attempt to toilet himself, she noted that he assumed a wide base of support and needed to use the grab bar to stabilize himself. Nakai was unable to manipulate his clothing or effectively perform toilet hygiene. Based on her observations, she decided to perform a formal assessment of Nakai's upper limb coordination to determine the extent of his deficits. The following clinical and standardized tests were performed:

- Finger-Nose-Finger
- Pronation/Supination (rapid alternating movements)
- BBT

Nakai was observed to have intention tremors and dysmetria, characterized by oscillating movements and overshooting of targets during Finger-Nose-Finger testing. Both his tremors and dysmetria increased as movement speed and distance requirements increased, or as movement direction changed. These deficits were present bilaterally and were only slightly more pronounced in the left UE. Nakai also had difficulty performing rapid alternating movements, particularly as movement speed increased, indicating the presence of dysdiadochokinesia. Again, these deficits were present bilaterally. Based on these tests, the therapist graded Nakai has having moderate impairments in bilateral upper limb coordination. BBT results revealed that Nakai was only able to transfer 50 blocks with his right hand and 46 with his left hand. Both of these scores are well below the norms for a 34-year old man, indicating manual dexterity impairment.

Occupational Therapy Problem List

- Decreased independence in the performance of basic self-care activities
- Bilateral impairment in upper limb coordination
- Bilateral impairment in manual dexterity

Occupational therapy (OT) interventions to address the above problem list are described in the case study presented in Chapter 16.

Examples of Commonly Used Standardized Motor Control Assessments

Instrument	Intended Purpose	Administration Time	Validity	Reliability	Sensitivity	Strengths and Weaknesses
ADL Observations to Measure Disabilities in those with Apraxia[38]	Structured observation of four activities: washing face and upper body, putting on a shirt or blouse, preparing food, and an individualized task chosen by the OT; each task is scored based on independence, initiation, execution, and control	Approximately 30–45 minutes based on impairment severity	Discriminant: Able to differentiate between those with and without apraxia. Construct: Highly associated with impairment tests of apraxia and the Barthel Index[38]	High internal consistency ($\alpha = 0.94$).[38] High inter-rater reliability for total score ($ICC = 0.98$).[38]	Sensitive for detecting disabilities in those with cognitive impairment compared to the Barthel Index and Motricity Index[39]	Strengths: Provides information related to how apraxia impacts everyday living. Weaknesses: Warrants further investigation
Action Research Arm Test (ARAT)[8]	Performance-based measure of UE capacity consisting of 19 items that are timed and rated on a 4-point ordinal scale: 0 = unable to perform any part of the task to 3 = performs normally	An average of 7–10 minutes. If all 19 items are tested, it takes ~20 minutes.	Adequate-to-high concurrent ($\rho = -0.55$ to -0.80) and convergent ($r = -0.38$ to -0.96) validity reported among stroke patients[40–42]	High internal consistency ($\alpha = 0.98$),[43] high test–retest reliability for both total score ($ICC = 0.98$–0.99)[23,41,42] and subscale scores ($ICC = 0.95$–0.99),[41,42] and high inter-rater reliability for both total score ($ICC = 0.92$–0.99)[41–43] and subscale scores ($ICC = 0.93$–0.99)[41,42]	Sensitive for detecting change in hand dexterity (standardized response mean [SRM] = 0.79),[44] and UE motor function ($SRM = 0.68$)[23] after stroke. Established MCID for acute (12–17 points)[40] and chronic (5.7 points)[45] stroke patients	Strengths: Established validity, reliability, and MCID across various stages of stroke recovery; administration of the ARAT is quick and easy. Weaknesses: Items are simulated ADLs and require the use of standardized equipment that can be costly.
Box and Block Test (BBT)[28]	Performance-based measure of manual dexterity that requires patients to transfer as many blocks from one compartment of a wooden box to another within 60 seconds	2–5 minutes	Predictive: The BBT, when performed at 1-week poststroke, is the best predictor of upper limb function at 5-months poststroke compared to grip strength, 9-Hole Peg Test, and the Stroke Rehabilitation Assessment of Movement.[46] High convergent validity between BBT and Minnesota Rate of Manipulation Test ($r = 0.91$)[47]	High test–retest reliability ($ICC = 0.97$; $ICC = 0.96$) for the right and left hand, respectively.[48] High inter-rater reliability ($r = 1.0$ and 0.99, right and left hands, respectively)[28]	Sensitive for detecting change in hand dexterity poststroke. ($SRM = 0.74$)[44]	Strengths: Quick and reliable administration. Weaknesses: Contrived task

(continued)

Examples of Commonly Used Standardized Motor Control Assessments (*continued*)

Instrument	Intended Purpose	Administration Time	Validity	Reliability	Sensitivity	Strengths and Weaknesses
Berg Balance Scale (BBS)[19]	Performance-based measure of balance consisting of 14 items graded on a 5-point ordinal scale with descriptors that vary based on item being scored	10–15 minutes	High concurrent ($r = 0.65–0.92$) and convergent ($r = 0.62–0.94$) validity reported among stroke patients.[19,49,50] Predictive validity for risk of falling in elderly,[19] adequately predictive of length of stay in rehabilitation unit,[51] and high predictive validity for motor ability 180 days after stroke[49]	High internal consistency ($\alpha > 0.83, 0.97$) for elderly long-term care residents and patients with stroke, respectively,[52] and high test–retest reliability ($ICC = 0.88$)[50] and inter-rater reliability ($ICC = 0.92$) among patients poststroke[53] and patients with PD ($ICC = 0.95$)[54]	Several studies have demonstrated that BBS is responsive to change over time in patients poststroke.[50] Established minimal detectable change (MDC) in acute (6.9 points)[53] and chronic (4.13 points)[50] stroke patients	Strengths: Established validity, reliability, and MDC; utilizes functional mobility task; quick, easy, and low cost to administer. Weaknesses: Significant ceiling effects noted for community-dwelling older adults and patients poststroke. Not suitable for severely affected patients because it assesses only one item related to balance while sitting .
Fugl-Meyer Assessment (FMA)[21]	Performance-based measure of motor impairment after stroke that consists of 50 (33 UE and 17 LE) items; the majority of items are scored on a 3-point ordinal scale: 0 = cannot perform to 2 = performs fully	30–45 minutes for the UE and LE subtests	Actual motor recovery poststroke parallels test items.[21] Adequate-to-high concurrent validity with MAS FMA-UE ($r = -0.50$) and FMA-LE ($r = -0.60$).[24] High convergent validity between the FMA-UE and the ARAT($r = 0.77–0.87$) and adequate($r = 0.54$) convergent validity between the FMA-UE and ADL subscores of the Functional Independence Measure (FIM)[23]	High inter-rater FMA-UE ($ICC = 0.97$) and FMA-LE ($ICC = 0.92$). High intra-rater reliability: UE ($r = 0.99$) and LE ($r = 0.96$) subtests[55]	Responsiveness of FMA has been reported for evaluating UE recovery in acute ($SRM = 0.74$)[23] and chronic ($SRM = 0.87$)[27] stroke patients. MCID has been established for acute (10 points)[26] and chronic (UE: 4.25–7.25 points[25] and LE: 6 points)[56] stroke patients	Strengths: Established reliability and validity and MCID across various stroke recovery stages. Administration times for UE and LE subtests are acceptable and low cost. Weaknesses: Test items are impairment focused and have little relevance to everyday activities.

Functional Reach Test[20]	Measures maximal forward reach distance while in standing position	~5 minutes	High concurrent validity with mobility skills ($r = 0.65$) and IADL ($r = 0.66$) and adequate concurrent validity with physical ADLs ($r = 0.48$).[57] Discriminant validity: significant difference between persons with high and low risk of falls. Predictive validity: score of 6 inches predictive of falls in the elderly[20]	High test–retest reliability: ($ICC = 0.92$)[20] and high inter-rater reliability ($r = 0.98$)[20] and intra-rater reliability ($r = 0.90$)[58]	Marginal significant change ($p = 0.07$) after physical rehabilitation, responsiveness index = 0.97[59]	Strengths: Established reliability and validity; quick, easy, and low cost to administer; a modified version exists for patients who cannot stand.[60] Weaknesses: Sensitivity is borderline
Modified Ashworth Spasticity Scale[14]	Assess muscle tone using a 6-point ordinal scale: 0 = normal muscle tone to 4 = rigid in flexion or extension	1–2 minutes per motion tested	High convergent validity with the FMA ($r = 0.94$); electromyography ($r = -0.79$); Box-Block Test ($r = -0.83$).[61] MASS was also negatively correlated with the FMA-UE ($r = -0.72$, $p < 0.05$) and the ARAT ($r = -0.41$, $p < 0.05$)[62]	Moderate test–retest reliability ($K = 0.47$–0.62). in adults with severe brain injury.[63] High inter-rater ($K_w = 0.84$) and intra-rater reliability ($K_w = 0.83$) for patients poststroke.[15] Adequate test–retest and inter-rater reliability ($K = 0.53$–0.77) for assessing spasticity in LE of patients with spinal cord injuries.[64] High inter-rater and intra-rater reliability $K_w = 0.8$ and $ICC = 0.8$ for persons with profound intellectual disabilities.[16] Reliability appears to be inadequate for children with cerebral palsy[17]	Sensitivity of the MASS is unclear as findings are mixed with respect to its ability to measure change overtime[65,66].	Strengths: Established validity and reliability for several patient populations; easy, quick, and low cost to administer. Weaknesses: Data on sensitivity is mixed

(*continued*)

Examples of Commonly Used Standardized Motor Control Assessments (*continued*)

Instrument	Intended Purpose	Administration Time	Validity	Reliability	SENSITIVITY	Strengths and Weaknesses
Motor Assessment Scale[7]	Performance-based measure of motor function consisting of eight items rated on a 7-point hierarchical scale: 0 = easiest task, 6 = hardest task	15–60 minutes for total MAS	High concurrent validity with FMA total scores ($r = 0.96$); adequate-to-high item-level validity between MAS and similar FMA items ($r = 0.65$–0.93); poor validity ($r = -0.10$) with FMA sitting balance[24]	High test–retest reliability ($r = 0.87$–1.00) and inter-rater reliability ($r = 0.89$–0.99)[7]	Medium-to-large effect sizes ($d = 0.50$–1.03) for six items and small effect sizes ($d = 0.36$–0.43) noted for two items[67]	Strengths: Established validity, reliability, and sensitivity; test items are functionally relevant; and easy and low cost to administer. Weaknesses: Sequence of scoring hierarchy of hand function and advanced hand activities scales are questioned; although a new hierarchical scoring system based on Rasch analysis has been developed.[68]
Motor Activity Log (MAL)[10]	Self-report measure of UE function that consists of 13 daily tasks rated using two 6-point ordinal scales that measure amount of UE use (AOU) and quality of UE movement (QOM)	20–30 minutes	High concurrent validity of the QOM scale with an objective accelerometer-based measure of arm movement: ($r = 0.91$)[11]	High internal consistency for AOU ($\alpha = 0.88$) and QOM ($\alpha = 0.91$).[69] Adequate-to-high test–retest reliability for the MAL-AOU ($r = 0.70$–0.85) and MAL-QOM ($r = 0.61$–0.71) subscales[69]	MAL is responsive to changes overtime *SRM*, and $RR > 1$ at postintervention and *ES*, *SRM*, and $RR > 1$ at 3-months follow-up.[70] MCID for QOM = 1.0–1.1 in acute stroke patients[71]	Strengths: Established validity, reliability, and sensitivity; measures patient's perception of actual use of post-stroke affected UE in real-life situations; quick, easy and low cost to administer. Weaknesses: Subjective measure
Wolf Motor Function Test (WMFT)[9]	Performance-based measure of UE capacity that consists of 2 strength items and 17 items that are timed and rated on 6-point ordinal scale, yielding a functional ability score (FAS) and a time score	30–45 minutes	Discriminates between healthy persons and those poststroke ($p \leq 0.05$).[9] Construct validity is supported by sensorimotor and kinematic measures of reach and grasp.[72] Moderate-to-high concurrent validity between ARAT total score and total WMFT FAS ($r_s = 0.86$, $p < 0.01$) and between ARAT score and WMFT medi an time score ($r_s = 0.89$, $p < 0.01$)[43]	High internal consistency ($\alpha = 0.96$–0.98).[72] High Inter-rater reliability: ($r = 0.95$–0.99)[9]	WMFT is responsive to changes overtime FAS ($d = 1.09$–1.63) and time ($d = 0.61$–0.85). MCID = 1.0–1.2[71]	Strengths: Established validity, reliability, and sensitivity; easy to administer, but requires standardized table template for item placement. Weaknesses: Several items assess at the impairment level and have little to do with function.

References

1. Shumway-Cook A, Woollacott M. *Motor Control: Translating Research into Clinical Practice*. 5th ed. Baltimore, MD: Lippincott Williams & Wilkins; 2017.
2. Mihailoff G, Haine DE. Motor system I: peripheral sensory, brainstem, and spinal influences on anterior horn cells. In: Haines D, ed. *Fundamental Neuroscience for Basic and Clinical Applications*. 5th ed. Philadelphia PA: Elsevier; 2018:346–354.
3. Mihailoff G, Haine DE. Motor system II: corticofugual systems and the control of movement. In: Haines D, ed. *Fundamental Neuroscience for Basic and Clinical Applications*. 5th ed. Philadelphia, PA: Elsevier; 2018:360–375.
4. Haines D, Mihailoff, GA. The cerebellum. In: Haines D, ed. *Fundamental Neuroscience for Basic and Clinical Applications*. 5th ed. Philadelphia, PA: Elsevier; 2018:394–412.
5. Ma T, Geyer, HL. The basal nuclei. In: Haines D, ed. *Fundamental Neuroscience for Basic and Clinical Applications*. 5th ed. Philadelphia, PA: Elsevier; 2018:377–389.
6. Fisher A. *Assessment of Motor and Process Skills*. 4th ed. Fort Collins, CO: Three Star Press; 2001.
7. Carr JH, Shepherd RB, Nordholm L, Lynne D. Investigation of a new motor assessment scale for stroke patients. *Phys Ther*. 1985;65(2):175–180.
8. Lyle RC. A performance test for assessment of upper limb function in physical rehabilitation treatment and research. *Int J Rehabil Res*. 1981;4(4):483–492.
9. Wolf SL, Catlin PA, Ellis M, Archer AL, Morgan B, Piacentino A. Assessing Wolf motor function test as outcome measure for research in patients after stroke. *Stroke*. 2001;32(7):1635–1639.
10. Uswatte G, Taub E. Constraint-induced movement therapy: new approaches to outcome measurement in rehabilitation. In: Struss D, Winocur G, Robertson IH, eds. *Cognitive Neurorehabilitation: A Comprehensive Approach*. Cambridge, England: Cambridge University Press; 1999.
11. Uswatte G, Taub E, Morris D, Vignolo M, McCulloch K. Reliability and validity of the upper extremity Motor Activity Log-14 for measuring real world arm use. *Stroke*. 2005;36:2493–2496.
12. Uswatte G, Taub E, Morris D, Light K, Thompson P. The Motor Activity Log-28 assessing daily use of the hemiparetic arm after stroke. *Neurology*. 2006;67(7):1189–1194.
13. Corbett J, Chen J. The neurologic examination. In: Haines D, ed. *Fundamental Neuroscience for Basic and Clinical Applications*. 5th ed. Philadelphia, PA: Elsevier; 2108:480–490.
14. Bohannon RW, Smith MB. Interrater reliability of a modified Ashworth scale of muscle spasticity. *Phys Ther*. 1987;67(2):206–207.
15. Gregson JL, Leathley M, Moore P, Sharma AK, Smith TI, Watkins CL. Reliability of the Tone Assessment Scale and the Modified Ashworth Scale as clinical tools for assessing poststroke spasticity. *Arch Phys Med Rehabil*. 1999;80:1013–1016.
16. Waninge A, Rook RA, Dijkhuizen A, Gielen E, van der Shans CP. Feasibility, test–retest reliability, and interrater reliability of the Modified Ashworth Scale and Modified Tardieu Scale in persons with profound intellectual and multiple disabilities. *Res Dev Disabil*. 2011;32:613–620.
17. Fosang A, Galea M, McCoy AT, Reddihough DS, Story I. Measures of muscle and joint performance in the lower limb of children with cerebral palsy. *Dev Med Child Neurol*. 2033;45(10):664–670.
18. Cook C, Roman M, Stewart KM, Leithe L, Isaacs R. Reliability and diagnostic accuracy of clinical special tests for myelopathy in patients seen for cervical dysfunction. *J Orthop Sports Phys Ther*. 2009;39(3):172–178.
19. Berg KO, Maki BE, Williams JI, Holliday PJ, Wood-Dauphinee SL. Clinical and laboratory measures of postural balance in an elderly population. *Arch Phys Med Rehabil*. 1992;73(11):1073–1080.
20. Duncan PW, Weiner DK, Chandler J, Studenski S. Functional reach: a new clinical measure of balance. *J Gerontol*. 1990;45(6):M192–M197.
21. Fugl-Meyer A, Jaasko L, Leyman I, Olsson S, Steglind S. The post stroke hemiplegic patient: a method for evaluation of physical performance. *Scand J Rehabil Med*. 1975;7(1):13–31.
22. Gladstone D, Danells CJ, Black SE. The Fugl-Meyer assessment of motor recovery after stroke: a critical review of tts measurement properties. *Neurorehabil Neural Repair*. 2002;16(3):232–240.
23. Rabadi M, Rabadi FM. Comparison of the action research arm test and the Fugl-Meyer assessment as measures of upper-extremity motor weakness after stroke. *Arch Phys Med Rehabil*. 2006;87:962–966.
24. Malouin FP, Pichard L, Bonneau C, Durand A, Corriveau D. Evaluating motor recover early after stroke: comparison of the Fugl-Meyer assessment and the motor assessment scale. *Arch Phys Med Rehabil*. 1994;74:796–800.
25. Page S, Fulk GD, Boyne P. Clinically important differences for the upper-extremity Fugl-Meyer scale in people with minimal to moderate impairment due to chronic stroke. *Phys Ther*. 2012;92:791–798.
26. Shelton F, Volpe BT, Reding M. Motor impairment as a predictor of functional recovery and guide to rehabilitation treatment after stroke. *Neurorehabil Neural Repair*. 2001;15(3):229–237.
27. Wei X, Tong K, Hu X. The responsiveness and correlation between Fugl-Meyer assessment, Motor Status Scale and the Action Research Arm Test in chronic stroke with upper extremity rehabilitation robotic training. *Int J Rehabil Res*. 2011;34(4):349–356.
28. Mathiowetz V, Volland G, Kashman N, Weber K. Adult norms for the Box and Blocks Test of manual dexterity. *Am J Occup Ther*. 1985;39(6):386–391.
29. Buddenberg L, Davis C. Test-retest reliability of the Purde Pegboard test. *Am J Occup Ther*. 1999;54(5):555–558.
30. Heilman K, Gonzalez RLJ. Apraxia. In: Heilman KM, Valenstein E, eds. *Clinical Neuropsychology* 5th ed. New York, NY: Oxford University Press; 2012.
31. Árnadóttir G. Impact of neurobehavioral deficits on activities of daily living. In: Gillen G, ed. *Stroke Rehabilitation: A Function-Based Approach*. 4th ed. St. Louis, MO: Elsevier; 2016.
32. Fraser C, Turton A. The development of the Cambridge apraxia battery. *Br J Occup Ther*. 1986;8:248–251.
33. Duffy RJ, Watt JH, Duffy JR. The construct validity of the Limb Apraxia Test (LAT): implications for the distinction between types of limb apraxia. *Clin Aphasiol*. 1994;22:181–190.
34. Neiman M, Duffy RJ, Belanger S, Coelho C. Concurrent validity of the Kaufman Hand Movement test as a measure of limb apraxia. *Percept Mot Skills*. 1994;79:1279–1282.
35. Dobigny-Roman N, Dieudonne-Moinet B, Tortrat D, Verny M, Forette B. Ideomotor apraxia test: a new test of imitation of gestures for elderly people. *Eur J Neurol*. 1998;5:571–578.
36. Rothi L, Raymer A, Heilman K. Limb praxis assessment. In: Gonzalez Rothi L, Heilman K, eds. *Apraxia: The Neuropsychology of Action*. London, England: Psychology Press; 1997:61–73.

37. van Heugten C, Dekker J, Deelman B, van Dijk A, Stehmann-Saris F, Kinebanian A. Measuring disabilities in stroke patients with apraxia: a validity study of an observational method. *Neuropsychol Rehabil.* 2000;10(4):401–414.
38. van Heugten CM, Dekker J, Deelman BG, Stehmann-Saris JC, Kinebanian A. Assessment of disabilities in stroke patients with apraxia: internal consistency and inter-observer reliability. *Occup Ther J Res.* 1999;19(1):55–70.
39. DonkerVoort M, Dekkler J, Deelman BG. Sensitivity of different ADL measures to apraxia and motor impairments. *Clin Rehabil.* 2000;16:299–305.
40. Lang C, Wagner JM, Dromerick AW, Edwards DF. Measurement of upper-extremity function early after stroke: properties of the Action Research Arm test. *Arch Phys Med Rehabil.* 2006;87:1605–1610.
41. Yozbatiran N, Der-Yeghiaian L, Cramer SC. A standardized approach to performing the Action Research Arm test. *Neurorehabil Neural Repair.* 2008;22:78–90.
42. Hsieh C, Hsueh I, Chiang F, Lin P. Inter-rater reliability and validity of the Action Research Arm test in stroke patients. *Age Ageing.* 1998;27:107–113.
43. Nijland R, van Wegne E, Verbunt J, van Wijk R, van Kordelaar J, Kwakkel G. A comparison of two validated tests for upper limb function after stroke: the Wolf Motor Function test and the Action Research Arm test. *J Rehabil Med.* 2010;42:694–696.
44. Lin KC, Chuang L, Wu C, Hsieh Y, Chang W. Responsiveness and validity of three dexterous function measures in stroke rehabilitation. *J Rehabil Res Dev.* 2010;47:563–572.
45. van der Lee J, Roords LD, Beckerman H, Lankhorst G, Bouter LM. Improving the Action Research Arm test: a unidimensional hierarchical scale. *Clin Rehabil.* 2002;16:646–653.
46. Higgins J, Mayo NE, Desrosiers J, Salbach NM, Ahmed S. Upper-limb function and recovery in the acute phase post-stroke. *J Rehabil Res Dev.* 2055;41(1):65–76.
47. Cromwell FS. *Occupational Therapists Manual for Basic Skills Assessment: Primary Prevocational Evaluation.* Pasadena, CA: Fair Oaks Printing; 1965.
48. Desrosiers J, Bravo G, Hébert R, Dutil É, Mercier L. Validation of the box and block test as a measure of dexterity of elderly people: reliability, validity and norms studies. *Arch Phys Med Rehabil.* 1994;75:751–755.
49. Mao H, Hsueh I, Tang P, Sheu C, Hsieh C. Analysis and comparison of the psychometric properties of three balance measures for stroke patients. *Stroke.* 2002;33:1022–1027.
50. Flansbjer U, Blom J, Brogardh C. The reproducibility of the Berg Balance Scale and the Single-leg Scale in chronic stroke and the relationship between the two tests. *P MR.* 2012;4:165–170.
51. Juneja J, Czyrny JJ, Linn RT. Admission balance and outcomes of patients admitted for acute inpatient rehabilitation *Am J Phys Med Rehabil.* 1998;77:388–393.
52. Berg K, Wood-Dauphinee S, Williams J. The Balance scale: reliability assessment with elderly residents and patients with an acute stroke. *Scand J Rehabil Med.* 1995;27(1):27–36.
53. Stevenson T. Detecting change in patients with stroke using the Berg Balance Scale. *Aust J Physiother.* 2001;47:29–38.
54. Leddy A, Crowner BE, Earhart GM. Functional gait assessment and balance evaluation system test reliability, validity, sensitivity, and specificity for identifying individuals with Parkinson disease who fall. *Phys Ther.* 2011;91(1):102–113.
55. Sandford J, Moreland J, Swanson LR, Stratford PW, Gowland C. Reliability of the Fugl-Meyer assessment for testing motor performance in patients following stroke. *Phys Ther.* 1993;73(7):447–454.
56. Pandian S, Arya K, Kumar D. Minimal clinically important difference of the lower-extremity Fugl–Meyer Assessment in chronic-stroke. *Top Stroke Rehabil.* 2016;23(4):233–239.
57. Weiner DK, Duncan P, Chandler J, Studenski SA. Functional reach: a marker of physical frailty. *J Am Geriatr Soc.* 1992;40(3):203–207.
58. Bennie S, Bruner K, Dizon A, Fritz H, Goodman B, Peterson S. Measurements of balance: comparison of the Timed Up and Go Test and Functional Reach Test with the Berg Balance Scale. *J Phys Ther Sci.* 2003;15:93–97.
59. Weiner DK, Bongiorni DR, Studenski SA, Duncan PW, Kochersberg GG. Does functional reach improve with rehabilitation? *Arch Phys Med Rehabil.* 1993;74:796–800.
60. Katz-Leurer M, Fisher I, Neeb M, Schwartz I, Carmelli E. Reliability and validity of the modified Functional Reach test at the sub-acute stage post-stroke. *Disabil Rehabil.* 2009;31(3):243–248.
61. Lin F, Sabbahi M. Correlation of spasticity with hyperactive stretch reflexes. *Arch Phys Med Rehabil.* 1999;80:526–530.
62. Lee G, An S, Lee Y, Lee D, Park D. Predictive factors of hypertonia in the upper extremity of chronic stroke survivors. *J Phys Ther Sci.* 2015;27:2545–2549.
63. Mehrholz J, Wagner K, Meibner D, et al. Reliability of the Modified Tardieu Scale and the Modified Ashworth Scale in adult patients with severe brain injury: a comparison study. *Clin Rehabil.* 2005;19:751–759.
64. Akpinar P, Atici A, Ozkan FU, et al. Reliability of the Modified Ashworth Scale and Modified Tardieu Scale in patients with spinal cord injuries. *Spinal Cord.* 2017;55:944–949.
65. Bakheit AM, Pittock S, Moore AP, et al. A randomized, double-blind, placebo-controlled study of the efficacy and safety of botulinum toxin type A (Dysport) in upper limb spasticity in patient with stroke. *Eur J Neurol.* 2001;8:559–565.
66. Pandyan AD, Vuadens P, van Wijck F, Stark S, Johnson GR, Barnes M. Are we underestimating the clinical efficacy of botulinum toxin (type A)? Quantifying changes in spasticity, strength and upper limb function after injections of Botox® to the elbow flexors in a unilateral stroke population. *Clin Rehabil.* 2002;16:654–660.
67. English C, Hillier SL, Stiller AK, Warden-Flood A. The sensitivity of three commonly used outcome measures to detect change amongst patients receiving inpatient rehabilitation following stroke. *Clin Rehabil.* 2006;20:52–55.
68. Sabari J, Woodbury M, Velozo CA. Rasch analysis of a new hierarchical scoring system for evaluating hand function on the motor assessment scale for stroke. *Stroke Res Treat.* 2014:730298.
69. van der Lee J, Beckerman H, Knol DL, de Vet HCW, Bouter LM. Clinimetric properties of the Motor Activity Log for the assessment of arm use in hemiparetic patients. *Stroke.* 2004;35:1410–1414.
70. Hammer A, Lindmark B. Responsiveness and validity of the Motor Activity Log in patients during the subacute phase after stroke. *Disabil Rehabil.* 2010;32(14):1184–1193.
71. Simpson L, Eng JJ. Functional recovery following stroke: capturing changes in upper-extremity function. *Neurorehabil Neural Repair.* 2013;27(3):240–250.
72. Edwards D, Lang CE, Wagner JM, Birkenmeier R, Dromerick AW. An evaluation of the Wolf Motor Function test in motor trials early after stroke. *Arch Phys Med Rehabil.* 2012(93):660–668.

Chapter 16

Motor Control Intervention

Dawn M. Nilsen and Glen Gillen

LEARNING OBJECTIVES

This chapter will allow the reader to:

1. Describe interventions that are commonly used to treat patients with motor control deficits.
2. Describe the characteristics of task-oriented training approaches used to remediate motor skill performance.
3. Describe how specific cognitive strategies can be implemented to supplement task-oriented training.
4. Describe how technology can be used to enhance task-oriented training approaches.
5. Describe interventions that target specific underlying neurological impairments.
6. Develop targeted intervention plans to improve motor skill performance in patients with neurological dysfunction.

CHAPTER OUTLINE

TERMINOLOGY

Action observation (AO): a multisensory approach thought to promote neural reorganization via activation of the mirror neuron system; involves a patient watching another person engage in task performance with the intention of imitating the task performance. Observation is typically followed by the patient physically performing the task.

Cognitive strategy training (CST): an intervention that consists of teaching internal and external compensatory approaches to execute activities of daily living (ADLs).

Constraint-induced movement therapy (CIMT): an intervention designed to overcome learned nonuse of an impaired limb; involves restraint of the less impaired limb and massed practice of the impaired limb via shaping and standard task practice.

Experience-dependent neuroplasticity: the brain's ability to change in response to environmental stimuli, experience, and learning.

Gesture training (GT): a behavioral training program consisting of gesture-production exercises (i.e., transitive, intransitive-symbolic, intransitive-nonsymbolic gestures).

High-amplitude movement training: a training approach that targets production of large amplitude movements, sensory recalibration to recognize these movements as normal, and self-cueing to maintain gains.

Mental practice (MP): an intervention that uses the cognitive rehearsal of an action in the absence of physical movements to improve task performance.

Mirror therapy (MT): an intervention that uses mirror visual feedback to create the illusion that an impaired limb is moving normally; involves placement of the impaired limb behind a mirror and the patient concentrating on the mirrored reflection of movements made by the less impaired limb in front of the mirror.

Motor apraxia: a disorder of the production praxis system; loss of access to praxicons (motor plans) so that purposeful movement cannot be produced or achieved because of defective planning and sequencing of movements, even though idea and task purpose are understood.

Task-oriented training (TOT): involves practicing common daily-life tasks with the intention of acquiring or reacquiring a skill.

Introduction

As indicated in Chapter 15, deficits that result from damage to the motor system (e.g., paresis, changes in muscle tone, incoordination, apraxia) can have a tremendous impact on our ability to engage in daily occupations. Thus, addressing motor skill performance and these underlying deficits is an important component of occupational therapy (OT) interventions for patients with motor control impairments.

It should be pointed out that various intervention approaches may be used when working with patients with motor control impairment. Often, these approaches are combined or the therapist may switch from one to another based on the patient's response or preference (see Section 5: Frames of Reference for Physical Disability Rehabilitation). For example, a combination of remediation and compensatory approaches may be used to improve occupational performance of patients with hemiparesis poststroke or those with bradykinesia and rigidity secondary to Parkinson disease (PD).

This chapter provides an overview of interventions that are commonly used to treat patients with deficits in motor control, including (1) task-oriented training (TOT) approaches; (2) approaches that combine TOT with cognitive strategies or that utilize technology to augment TOT; and (3) interventions targeting specific neurological impairments, specifically paresis and the inability to fractionate movement, changes in muscle tone, deficits associated with hyperkinetic and hypokinetic movement disorders (e.g., incoordination, bradykinesia), and apraxia.

Task-Oriented Training Approaches

Task-oriented training approaches are considered to be the most current approach related to the remediation of motor skill impairments.[1] Various terms have been used to describe TOT approaches in the literature. Examples include[1–3] task-specific training, repetitive task practice, repetitive task training, and functional task practice. A common thread in these approaches is the assumption that movement emerges as an interaction between many systems in the brain, is organized around a specific goal, and is constrained by the environment.[4] These approaches stress the importance of high-intensity repetitive practice of functional tasks that are chosen to address the motor deficits and goals of the patient.[3] The tasks are designed to challenge patients' current motor capabilities without overwhelming them; often referred to as the "just-right challenge."[5] In addition, training is structured to promote variability in practice, and feedback and coaching are strategically used to motivate the patient and provide useful performance-related information (see Chapter 34). This type of training is thought to promote **experience-dependent neuroplasticity** that remodels the brain after damage and results in recovery of lost function. Kleim and Jones[6] identified 10 key principles of experience-dependent neural plasticity (Table 16-1). Many of these principles are incorporated into TOT approaches.

Table 16-1. Principles of Experience-Dependent Plasticity

PRINCIPLE	DESCRIPTION
Use it or lose it	• Failure to drive brain functions can lead to functional degradation—over time, neural circuits not engaged in the performance of an activity will begin to degrade (e.g., failure to use the impaired limb after stroke may reduce the size of the cortical representation of that limb in the sensorimotor cortices)
Use it to improve it	• Training that drives a specific brain function can lead to an enhancement of that function—stresses the importance of practice to strengthen neural connections (e.g., playing the piano with the right hand may increase the size of the cortical representation of the right hand in the sensorimotor cortices and improve accuracy of playing the piano).
Specificity	• The nature of the training experience dictates the nature of the plasticity—learning, as opposed to rote use, is required to change neural connectivity; changes are dependent on the specific kinds of experience (e.g., learning to perform sit-to-stand transfers is needed to improve performance of transfers, as opposed to simply performing hip and knee flexion/extension exercises).
Repetition matters	• Induction of neural plasticity requires repetition—simple engagement of a neural circuit is insufficient to drive plasticity—stresses the importance of repeating a newly acquired skill for a period of time, so that the level of performance and brain reorganization is sufficient for the patient to continue to use the affected function outside therapy and to maintain gains.
Intensity matters	• Induction of plasticity requires sufficient training intensity—stresses the importance of high-intensity training and progression to continually challenge the patient.
Time matters	• Different forms of plasticity occur during different times during training—stresses the importance of recognizing that recovery of function after brain injury is a process and that there may be time windows during which certain types of training might be most beneficial.

Table 16-1. Principles of Experience-Dependent Plasticity (*continued*)

PRINCIPLE	DESCRIPTION
Salience matters	• The training experience must be sufficiently salient to induce plasticity—stresses the importance of selecting tasks that are motivating, stimulating, and important to the patient.
Age matters	• Training-induced plasticity occurs more readily in younger brains—important to keep in mind that change may occur more slowly as the brain ages.
Transference	• Plasticity in response to one training experience can enhance the acquisition of similar behaviors—stresses the importance of previous behavioral experiences and their ability to influence performance of related tasks.
Interference	• Plasticity in response to one experience can interfere with the acquisition of other behaviors—important to be aware of the fact that therapy that benefits one skill may interfere with performance of another skill.

Adapted from Kleim JA, Jones TA. Principles of experience-dependent neural plasticity: implications for rehabilitation after brain damage. *J Speech Lang Hear Res*. 2008;51:S225–S239.

TOT approaches have been used to improve upper extremity (UE) function, balance and mobility, and performance of activities of daily living (ADLs).[2,3] Components of TOT, as described in the literature, are contained in Box 16-1,[7] and Figure 16-1 provides examples of repetitive practice of a functional task (for an overview of the OT task-oriented approach, see Chapter 34). The subsequent section provides an example of a specific TOT approach designed to remediate UE function.

Constraint-Induced Movement Therapy

Constraint-induced movement therapy (CIMT) is an example of a TOT approach designed to address arm and hand motor impairments. CIMT was originally developed for patients with hemiparesis poststroke to counteract learned nonuse, a term coined by Taub et al.[8] in the early 1990s. This phenomenon was originally identified in animal studies and later applied to humans. Taub et al. hypothesized that the nonuse or limited use of an affected UE in individuals after a neurologic event results from a phenomenon of behavioral suppression.[8] Hypothesized causes of learned nonuse include therapeutic interventions implemented during the acute period of neurologic suppression, an early focus on adaptations to meet functional goals, negative reinforcement experienced by a patient as he or she unsuccessfully attempts to use the affected limb, and positive

Box 16-1

Task-Oriented Training Components

- ***Functional movements:*** A movement involving task execution that is not directed toward a clear ADL goal (e.g., moving blocks from one location to another).
- ***Clear functional goal:*** A goal that is set during everyday life activities and/or hobbies (e.g., washing dishes, grooming activity, dressing oneself, playing golf).
- ***Client-centered patient goal:*** Therapy goals that are set through the involvement of the patient himself or herself in the therapy goal decision process. The goals respect patients' values, preferences, and expressed needs and recognize the clients' experience and knowledge.
- ***Overload:*** Determined by the total time spent on therapeutic activity, the number of repetitions, the difficulty of the activity in terms of coordination, muscle activity type and resistance load, and the intensity, that is, the number of repetitions per time unit.
- ***Real-life object manipulation:*** Manipulation that makes use of objects that are handled in normal everyday life activities (e.g., cutlery, hairbrush).
- ***Context-specific environment:*** A training environment (supporting surface, objects, people, room, etc.) that equals or mimics the natural environment for a specific task execution in order to include task characteristic sensory/perceptual information, task-specific context characteristics, and cognitive processes involved.
- ***Exercise progression:*** Exercises with an increasing difficulty level that is in line with the increasing abilities of the patient in order to keep the demands of the exercises and challenges optimal for motor learning.
- ***Exercise variety:*** Various exercises are offered to support motor skill learning of a certain task because of the person experiencing different movement and context characteristics (within task variety) and problem-solving strategies.
- ***Feedback:*** Specific information on the patient's motor performance that enhances motor learning and positively influences patient motivation.
- ***Multiple movement planes:*** Movement that uses more than one degree of freedom of a joint, therefore occurring around multiple joint axes.
- ***Patient-customized training load:*** A training load that suits the individualized treatment targets (e.g., endurance, coordination, or strength training) as well as the patient's capabilities.
- ***Total skill practice:*** The skill is practiced in total, with or without preceding skill component training (e.g., via chaining).
- ***Random practice:*** In each practice session, the tasks are randomly order.
- ***Distributed practice:*** A practice schedule with relatively long rest periods.
- ***Bimanual practice:*** Tasks where both arms and hands are involved.

Adapted from Timmermans AA, Spooren AI, Kingma H, Seelen HA. Influence of task-oriented training content on skilled arm-hand performance in stroke: a systematic review. *Neurorehabil Neural Repair.* 2010;24(9):858–870.

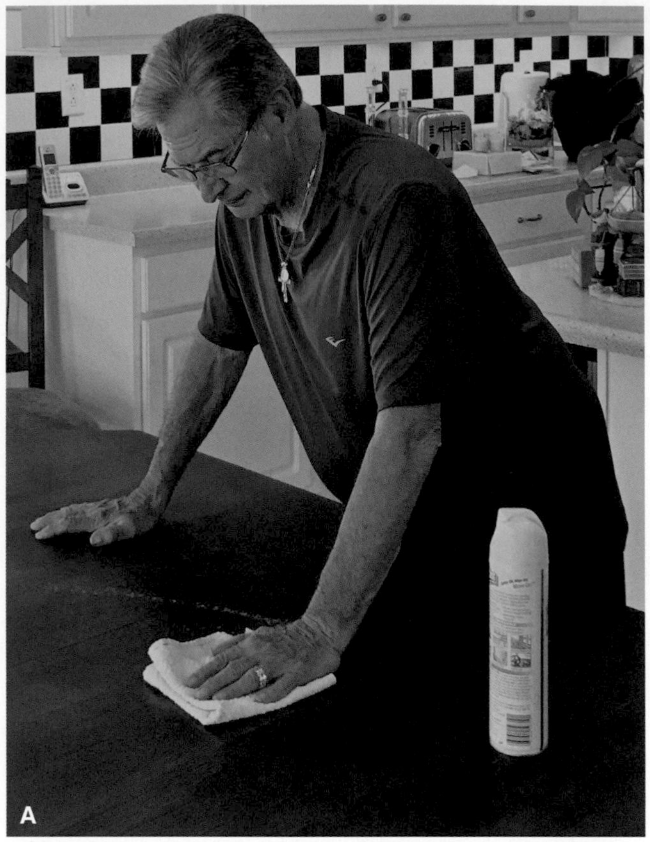

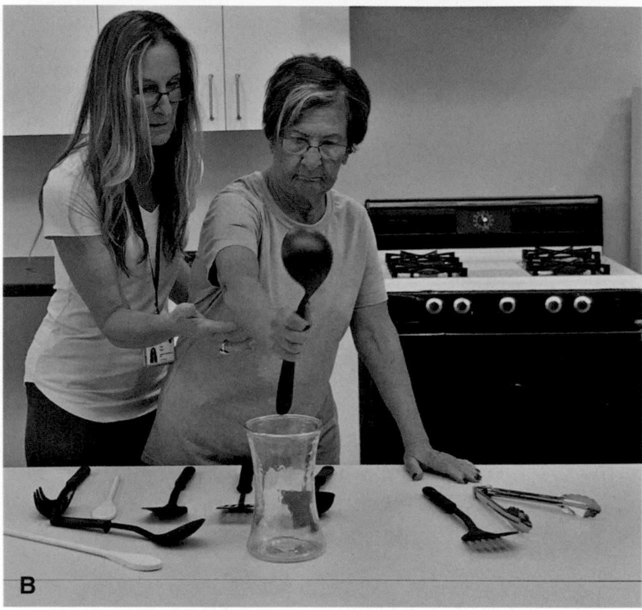

Figure 16-1. Examples of task-oriented training targeting remediation of upper extremity function and postural control. **A.** Dusting a table surface. **B.** Organizing a utensil caddy.

reinforcement experienced by the less involved hand and/or use of successful adaptations.[1]

CIMT is an intervention developed to reverse this acquired behavioral suppression. It consists of two main principles: (1) forced use of the impaired UE by restraining the less impaired UE in a sling or hand mitt for approximately 90% of waking hours and (2) massed practice (6–8 hours/day) of the impaired UE through shaping; a method of training in which a behavioral objective is approached in small successive steps that progressively increase in difficulty and standard (whole) task practice.[8–10] In the original protocol, the training was carried out over a period of 2 weeks. Since its original development and application, several modified CIMT (mCIMT) protocols have been introduced.[9] In mCIMT, the restraint time of the less impaired limb, the intensive training time of the impaired limb, or both the restraint and training times are reduced and/or distributed over a longer period of time.[9] Box 16-2 provides an example of the key features of the original protocol and examples of modified protocols. Figure 16-2 illustrates the main features of the task training: shaping and standard task practice.

CIMT has been found to induce changes in the cortical representation of the affected UE, and the majority of evidence accumulated to date suggests that both CIMT and mCIMT reduce UE motor impairments and improve UE motor skill performance in poststroke patients with some residual motor function in the wrist and hand. These improvements, however, may not readily translate to improved performance in ADL (see the Evidence table at the end of this chapter).[9]

More recently, mCIMT has been successfully used to improve arm and hand functioning of the more involved UE in patients with multiple sclerosis (MS)[11,12] and to improve fine and gross motor performance in patients with PD.[13]

Augmenting Task-Oriented Approaches

Approaches that combine TOT with cognitive strategies or that utilize technology to augment task training have been found to be feasible and effective for improving motor function after brain injury. In addition, several of these interventions may provide opportunities for self-directed practice outside traditional therapy sessions, or may be used with patients who have significant impairments in voluntary motor function. The following sections highlight the use of mental practice (MP), mirror therapy (MT), action observation (AO), virtual reality (VR), and robotics.

Use of Cognitive Strategies

Mental Practice

During **MP** (also called motor imagery [MI]), a patient cognitively rehearses an action in the absence of

Box 16-2

Constraint-Induced Movement Therapy

Original Protocol Based on the EXCITE Trail[10]	Modified Protocols
• Intervention length: 2 weeks. • Patients encouraged to wear a protective safety mitt on their less impaired UE for a goal of 90% of waking hours each day for a total of 14 days. • Training of the impaired limb for up to 6 hours on each week day consisting of two distinct types of task training: (1) shaping (adaptive or part-task practice—task objective is trained in small successive steps that progress in difficulty; each task is practiced in sets of individual trials of discrete movements); (2) standard task practice (functional activities [e.g., eating, writing] performed continuously for 15–20 minutes). • Behavioral techniques to enhance compliance with the program (i.e., behavioral contracts, mitt compliance device, daily practice schedule to encourage practice of two to three tasks daily at home and home diary to record task practice).	Dettmers and colleagues described the following protocol[63]: • Intervention length: 20 days. • Patients wore a resting hand splint on the less-affected hand on average for 9.3 hours/day, including the training sessions. • Intensive motor training of the affected UE for 3 hours/day for 20 consecutive weekdays training involved repetitive performance of daily activities (e.g., using clothes pins, picking up peas or dry berries out of a cup, opening and closing bottles). • Behavioral contract. Lin and colleagues described the following protocol[64]: • Intervention length: 3 weeks. • Unaffected hand restrained in a mitt for 6 hours/day. • Intensive training of the affected arm for 2 hours/weekday; typical practice activities included: picking up marbles, flipping over cards, stacking blocks, combing hair, and writing. • Log to record the hours of mitten wearing. Page and colleagues described the following protocol[65]: • Intervention length: 10 weeks. • Unaffected hand/wrist restrained in a mitt every weekday for 5 hours/day during an identified time of frequent arm use. • Individualized, ½-hour therapy sessions, 3 times/week: approximately 25 minutes of therapy focused on affected limb use during three agreed-upon daily activities (e.g., writing, brushing hair, drinking from a cup) using shaping techniques and 5 minutes of therapy was spent on more affected limb range of motion as needed. • Use of a home log to document device use and activities performed during restraint hours.

physical movements. Evidence suggests that MP activates many of the same brain regions that are activated by physical practice (PP).[14,15] It has been proposed that MP may prime the motor system and potentiate the effects of PP. MP is typically combined with TOT and is often facilitated via audio-taped scripts that the patient either listens to before or after task training.[16] MP may also be facilitated by visual prompts or verbal cues embedded into task training sessions.[16] Results of several systematic reviews suggest that MP combined with task

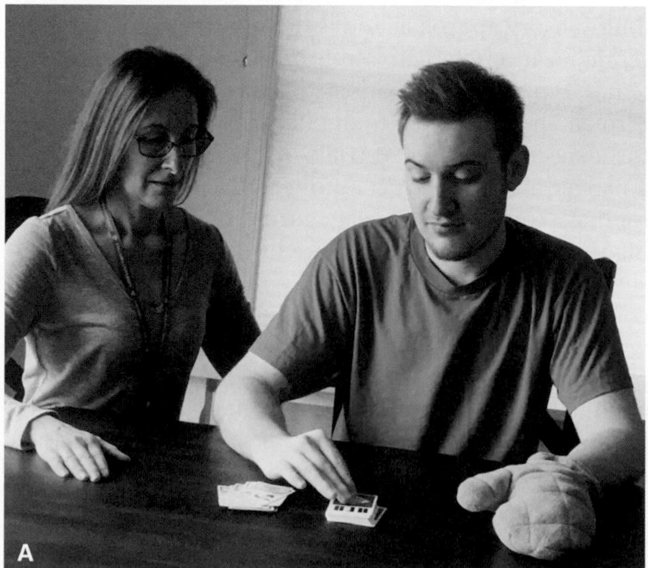

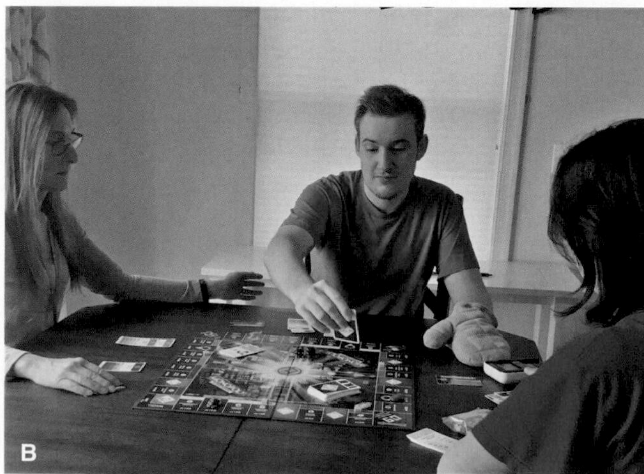

Figure 16-2. Constraint-induced movement therapy (CIMT). Examples of task training using the impaired hand while the unimpaired hand is restrained in a mitt. **A.** Shaping activity: multiple repetitions of flipping over cards. **B.** Standard (whole) task practice: playing a board game.

training improves motor function and ADL performance in patients after stroke.[14,15,17]

Research investigating whether MP benefits those with other neurological diseases, such as MS or PD, is sparse. Seebachher et al.[18] investigated the effect of a 4-week rhythmic-cued (metronome or music-based) MI program on walking, fatigue, and quality of life (QoL) in patients with MS. They found that compared to control participants, both forms of rhythmic-cued MI resulted in significant improvements in walking speed, distance and perception of ability, cognitive fatigue, and QoL (see the Evidence table).[18]

With respect to patients with PD, Tamir and colleagues[19] studied the effect of a 12-week intervention that combined MP and PP of callisthenic exercises (e.g., throwing and catching a ball while in broad tandem stance, reaching in different directions) and functional activities (sit-to-stand transitions, walking) administered for 1 hour per day, 2 days per week compared to a control group that received the same PP combined with relaxation exercise. They found that the intervention group had significantly faster performance of movement sequences, greater gains on the mental and motor subsets of the Unified Parkinson's Disease Rating Scale (UPDRS), and improved performance on cognitive tests (i.e., Clock drawing and Stroop test). Both groups improved on the ADL scale of the UPDRS.[19]

Conversely, Braun et al.[20] investigated the effect of a 6-week program that embedded MP in standard therapy on mobility tasks in patients with PD. They found no effect in favor of the MP intervention on any outcome measure (i.e., Timed Up and Go, 10-Meter Walk Test, Visual Analogue Scale to measure patient/therapist perception of effect on walking performance).[20] Further research with these patient populations is warranted.

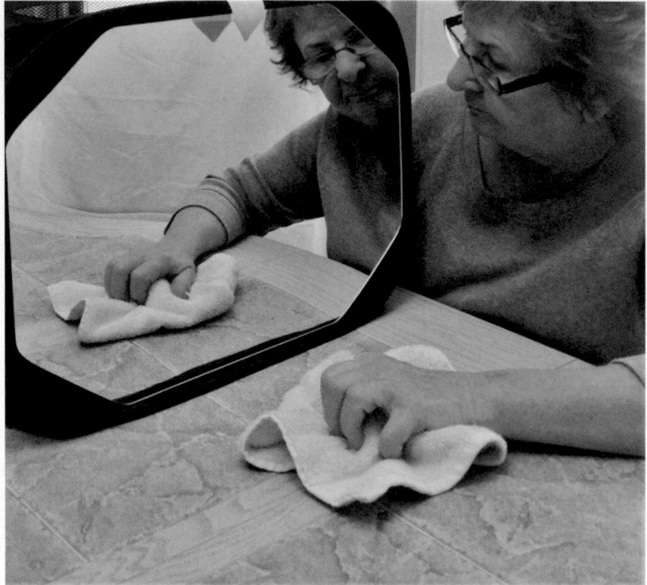

Figure 16-3. Example of mirror therapy. The impaired hand is placed inside the mirror box (hidden out of view), and the patient is asked to concentrate on the mirror reflection of the unimpaired hand grasping and releasing a washcloth.

Mirror Therapy

Mirror therapy (**MT**) is an intervention based on visual stimulation, specifically the use of mirror visual feedback.[21] During MT, a mirror is placed in approximately the midsagittal plane with the impaired limb position behind the mirror (hidden out of view). The unimpaired limb is positioned in front of the mirror, and the patient is asked to perform simple movements (e.g., opening and closing the hand, ankle dorsiflexion, plantar flexion) or simple functional tasks (e.g., grasping and releasing a washcloth, lifting a cup, stepping) while concentrating on the mirror reflection of the unimpaired limb (Fig. 16-3). This setup creates a visual illusion that the impaired limb is moving normally. During MT, patients are instructed to either keep the impaired limb in a resting position, or they are encouraged to attempt to move the impaired limb (as best as they are able) simultaneously with the unimpaired limb.[21]

Although the precise neural mechanisms underlying the beneficial effects attributed to MT remain unclear, evidence suggests that this type of training can improve motor function when combined with standard care. For example, a recent systematic review and meta-analysis found that MT reduces motor impairments, improves motor function, and improves ADL performance in patients with stroke.[21] MT has also been shown to improve movement speed of the more affected hand in patients with PD.[22]

Action Observation

Action observation (**AO**) is an intervention during which a patient observes a healthy person performing a task, either in a video or real demonstration, with the intention of imitating the task performance. AO is considered a multisensory approach and is thought to promote neural reorganization via activation of the mirror neuron system.[23] Typically, after patients watch an action being performed, they are asked to duplicate the action repeatedly for a specific number of trials or minutes. For example, a patient may be instructed to watch a video of a person folding a towel and then engage in the task of towel folding (Fig. 16-4). Often, tasks are broken down into small successive steps that are strung together with increasing complexity. For example, a patient may be instructed to watch a video of a person (1) reaching her hand out to pick up a cup; (2) reaching her hand out to pick up a cup and then lifting the cup to drink from it; and (3) reaching her hand out to pick up a cup, lifting the cup to drink from it, and then returning the cup to the table.[23]

Results of a recent systematic review and meta-analysis suggest that AO is beneficial for improving UE motor function, hand function, and independence in ADL in patients after stroke.[23] There is also some emerging evidence

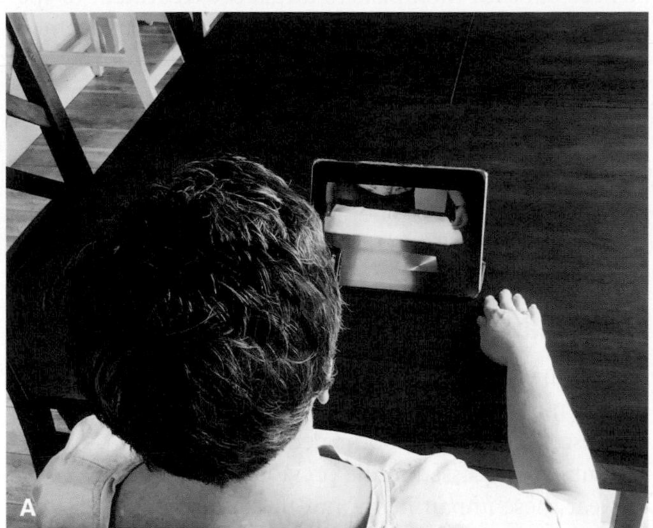

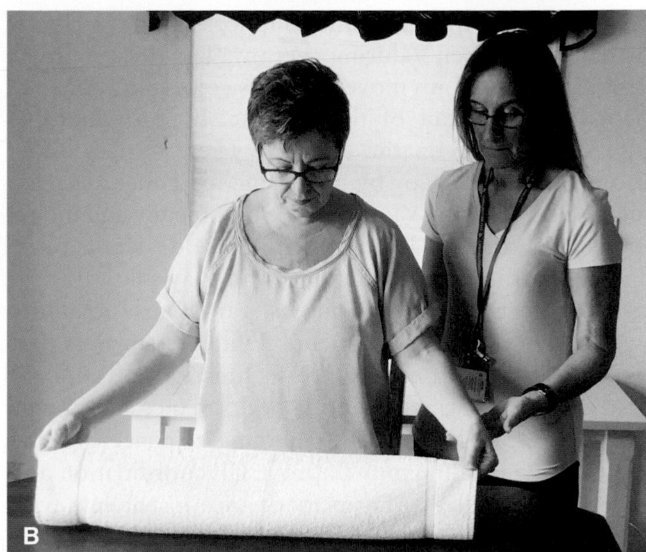

Figure 16-4. Example of action observation. **A.** Patient watches a prerecorded video of a model folding a towel. **B.** Following the viewing of the video, the patient performs the task of folding a towel.

that this intervention may improve functional mobility,[24] QoL,[24,25] and ADL performance[25] in patients with PD (see the Evidence table).

Use of Technology

Virtual Reality

VR is a treatment approach that allows for simulated practice of functional activities in a computer-based, interactive, simulated environment designed to replicate the real-world environment.[26] VR systems can vary in their degree of immersion of the user from high immersion (systems in which the user is represented within the virtual environment) to low immersion (single screen projection or desktop display).[26] Many commercially available gaming consoles (e.g., Nintendo Wii) are considered low immersion VR systems. Researchers suggest that VR training may be advantageous for the following reasons[26–28]: (1) it offers the patient an opportunity to engage in goal-directed tasks in an enriched environment; this may increase saliency, feedback, and motivation, thereby promoting a greater number of repetitions and adherence to training; (2) it may allow for unsupervised practice; and (3) it may offer patients with limited motor capabilities an opportunity to engage in trial tasks that might be unsafe to practice in the real world (e.g., crossing the street or pouring a hot cup of coffee).

VR training has been used as an intervention to improve motor function in patients with stroke,[26] PD,[27] and MS.[28] Laver et al.[26] conducted a systematic review and meta-analysis to determine the efficacy of VR on UE function and activity in patients after stroke. They found that VR was not superior to conventional therapy for improving UE function. However, when it was added to usual care (providing a higher dose of therapy), there was a statistically significant difference between the groups, favoring the addition of VR. They also reported that VR had a statistically significant effect for improving ADL.[26] These results suggest that VR may be beneficial when added to usual care. However, the effect of VR on participation restrictions or QoL could not be determined by the study.[26]

Dockx et al.[27] conducted a systematic review and meta-analysis to determine the effectiveness of VR for improving gait and balance, global motor function, ADL, QoL, cognitive function, and exercise adherence in patients with PD. The results of the review found that VR may have similar effects on gait, balance, QoL, and exercise adherence as compared to standard physiotherapy. Only one study included outcome measures related to ADL as defined in the review. No significant differences were noted between the VR group and standard care. Authors indicated that given the small number of studies conducted to date (eight studies were included in the review), generalization regarding VR effectiveness for patients with PD could not be determined.[27]

Finally, Massetti et al.[28] conducted a systematic review to investigate the results shown in previous studies investigating MS and VR. Ten studies were included in the review, and results from selected studies suggest that VR may improve arm movement and control, balance, and walking abilities in patients with MS. The authors suggest that VR might serve as an alternative intervention that motivates patients above traditional motor rehabilitation. However, no attempts were made to pool data contained in the studies, and the authors cautioned that further research is needed.[28]

Robotics

Overtime, advances in technology have led to the development of robotic training interventions for improving UE function after neurological injury. Robotic devices are specialized machines that support shoulder, elbow, or hand movements during therapy. The devices either provide passive limb movement, resist joint movements, or assist movement of the limb at single or multiple joints depending on the device.[29] These devices allow progression of therapy by increasing resistance, decreasing resistance, or by varying force parameters and movement amplitudes.[29] Training with these devices is often coupled with VR environments and may allow for increased repetition of movements, particularly for those with severe motor impairments. Evidence suggests that this type of arm training improves function and strength of the affected arm, and ADL performance in patients after stroke.[29] Additionally, emerging evidence suggests that robotic training may improve UE coordination and function, as well as ADL performance in patients with MS.[30,31] The use of robotic training devices is also being explored as a possible means for improving walking ability in patients with spinal cord injuries. Although some improvements in lower extremity motor function and activities have been reported, further studies are required to evaluate its effectiveness.[32]

Figure 16-5 provides an example of a robotic device, the ReoGo™, that allows controlled movements of the elbow and wrist and a small degree of shoulder motion.

Management of Specific Neurological Impairments

Although TOT should be considered foundational when attempting to improve motor skill performance, it may be necessary for therapists to target the treatment of specific neurological impairments to improve engagement in occupation. The following sections highlight the clinical management of common neurological impairments: paresis and inability to fractionate movement, changes in muscle tone, deficits associated with hypokinetic (e.g., bradykinesia) and hyperkinetic (e.g., ataxia) movement disorders, and apraxia.

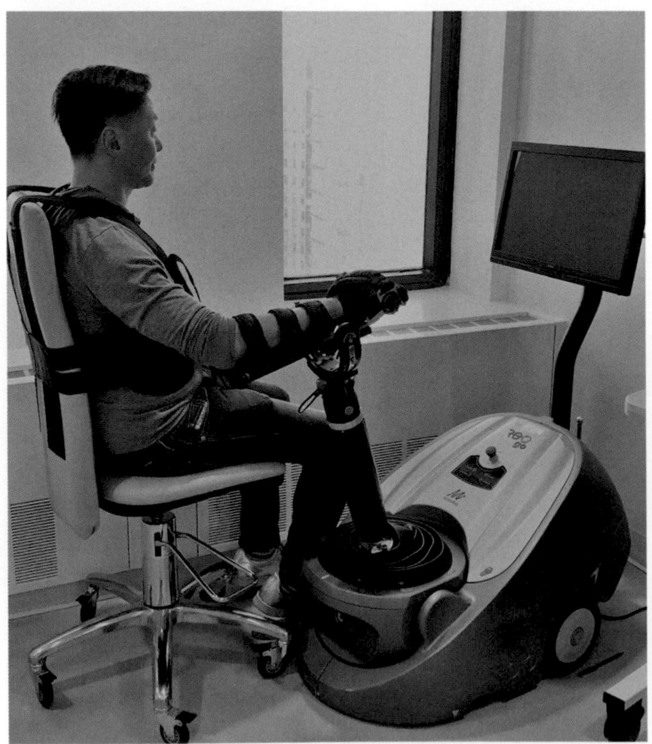

Figure 16-5. Example of a robotic device.

Intervention for Paresis and Inability to Fractionate Movement

As indicated in Chapter 15, paresis and the inability to fractionate movement are common consequences of lesions of the descending upper motor neuron system. All of the interventions discussed in the previous sections can be used to treat these impairments, but there are some additional clinical strategies that can be employed to specifically target recruitment of paretic muscles. Electromyogram biofeedback (EMG-BFB)[33] and electrostimulation (ES)[34] (also called neuromuscular electrical stimulation [NMES]) are technologies that can be used to assist patients with recruiting weak muscle groups or selectively controlling certain muscles groups during TOT (also see Chapter 24). EMG-BFB is a technique that amplifies and transduces an electrical signal generated from an electromyogram into a signal that is displayed in a simplified form to the patient, for example, by hearing a change in an auditory tone or by seeing a response on an oscilloscope display (device that is used to graph an electrical signal as it varies over time).[33] EMG-BFB may help patients learn how to recruit appropriate muscles groups during task training.

ES or NMES is a technique used to elicit a muscle contraction using electrical impulses. Electrodes, controlled by a specialized unit, are placed on the skin over predetermined areas related to the muscles targeted for recruitment. An electrical current is delivered from the unit through the electrodes and delivered to the muscle, causing the muscle to contract.[34] Figure 16-6 shows an example of the use of ES during task training. In this case, the muscles being targeted are weak wrist and finger extensors that are needed to open the hand in preparation for grasping a piece of fruit.

Strengthening programs may also be utilized to address paresis. Evidence suggests that exercise and strengthening interventions improve muscle strength and function after neurological injury without causing adverse effects (e.g., increasing muscle tone)[35] (for details on muscle strengthening, see Chapter 14).

Intervention for Flaccidity, Spasticity, and Rigidity

Changes in muscle tone are often seen as a consequence of damage to the motor system. Thus, managing changes in muscle tone is an important component of motor

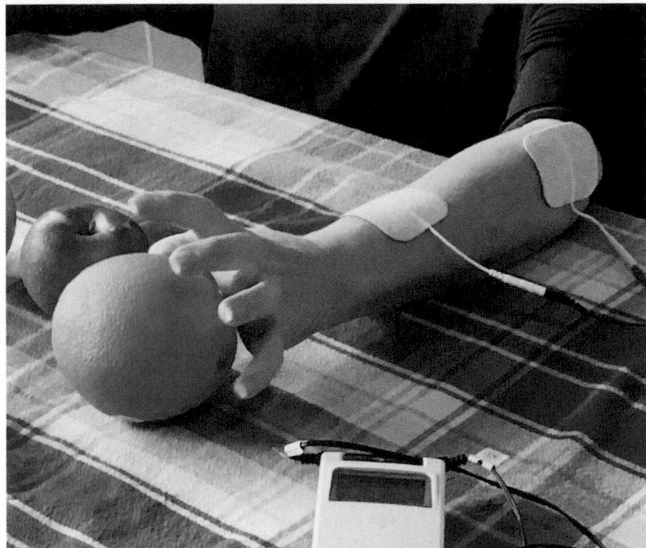

Figure 16-6. Example of the use of functional electrical stimulation to recruit paretic muscles. Stimulation is placed over the wrist and finger extensors to aid in opening the hand as the patient reaches to pick up a piece of fruit.

control intervention. Traditionally, neurophysiological approaches, including the application of various types of sensory stimuli (e.g., tactile, thermal, vibratory), have been used to either "facilitate" (in the case of flaccidity or low muscle tone) or "inhibit" (in the case of spasticity or rigidity) muscle tone, depending on the sensory modality used and how it is applied (e.g., duration, speed, intensity) (see Chapter 35). The following list provides examples of how practitioners have used sensory stimuli to either increase or decrease muscle tone; although it should be noted that evidence regarding their effectiveness to change muscle tone is lacking[4]:

- *Icing:*
  - Brief, rapid icing of the skin overlying a muscle belly has been used to increase muscle tone
  - Prolonged icing has been used to decrease muscle tone
- *Vibration:*
  - High-frequency vibration has been used to increase muscle tone
  - Low-frequency vibration had been used to decrease muscle tone
- *Tactile stimuli:*
  - Slow stroking over the skin has been used to inhibit muscle tone
  - Fast stroking over the skin has been used to facilitate muscle tone
- *Proprioceptive stimuli:*
  - Joint approximation and traction have been used to facilitate muscle tone

The techniques associated with the biomechanical approach (see Chapters 14 and 32), such as muscle stretching (including casting) and passive range of motion (ROM), are frequently used to manage hypertonicity and prevent the development of contractures. However, the effectiveness of these interventions for managing increased tone is unclear.[36,37] For example, results of a recent systematic review found that muscle stretch did not have a clinically important short-term effect on joint mobility, and it was uncertain whether stretch had clinically important short-term effects on pain or activity limitations in those with contractures.[37] Likewise, orthotic devices are frequently used to manage spasticity (see Chapter 22), although evidence supporting the effectiveness is lacking.[36,38]

Changing a patient's position has also been used to modulate tone. This is based on the assumption that placement of a patient in certain positions will activate primitive reflexes that may have reemerged as a consequence of brain injury. For example, placing a patient in prone may increase flexor muscle tone, whereas placing a patient in the supine position may increase extensor tone, secondary to activation of the tonic labyrinthine reflex. Appropriate positioning is also thought to maintain muscle length, thereby preventing the development of contractures.[4]

Finally, it should also be mentioned that physicians may utilize pharmacological treatments, such as baclofen or botulinum toxin, or utilize surgical procedures (e.g., dorsal root rhizotomy, motor point blocks, placement of spinal stimulators) to manage spasticity and rigidity. Although beyond the scope of OT practice, these treatments may reduce spasticity to a sufficient level, allowing patients to engage in other motor control interventions.

Intervention for Deficits Associated with Hyperkinetic and Hypokinetic Movement Disorders

Coordination disorders can be characterized as hyperkinetic (ataxia, hemiballismus, chorea, tremor, tics) or hypokinetic (bradykinesia, Parkinsonian disorders). Both types of disorders can have a serious negative impact on occupational performance (see Chapter 15).

There is limited evidence in terms of interventions for hyperkinetic disorders, such as ataxia. Llg et al.[39] described an intensive coordination training program for those living with ataxia due to cerebellar degeneration. The program lasted for 4 weeks (three 1-hour sessions per week). Exercises included the following categories:

1. static balance (e.g., standing on one leg)
2. dynamic balance (e.g., sidesteps, climbing stairs)
3. whole-body movements to train trunk–limb coordination

4. steps to prevent falling and falling strategies
5. movements to treat or prevent contracture

Training improved motor performance and reduced ataxia symptoms on both impairment measures and functional outcomes. In addition, subjects achieved personally meaningful goals in everyday life as measured by goal attainment scaling.

Miyai et al.[40] randomly assigned 42 patients with pure cerebellar degeneration to an immediate or delayed-entry control group in an inpatient rehabilitation setting. Physical therapy consisted of general conditioning; ROM exercise for trunk and limbs; muscle strengthening; static and dynamic balance exercise with standing, kneeling, sitting, and quadruped; mobilizing the spine while prone and supine; walking indoors and outdoors; and climbing up and down stairs. OT consisted of improving ADLs (e.g., hygiene, dressing, writing, eating), relaxation, balance exercises, reaching, coordinative tasks of the upper limbs and trunk, and dual motor tasks such as handling objects while standing and walking. The authors' findings include[40]:

- The immediate group showed significantly greater functional gains in ataxia, gait speed, and ADL than the control group.
- Improvement of truncal ataxia was more prominent than limb ataxia.
- The gains in ataxia and gait were sustained at 12 and 24 weeks, respectively.

It should be noted that many individuals living with hyperkinetic disorders have progressive diseases such as MS. Therefore, adaptive approaches are most likely to be a substantial component of intervention plans and have been recommended by various authors.[41] It has been hypothesized that many of the ineffective movement patterns observed in patients can be attributed to attempts to control the degrees of freedom (see Chapter 34). Therapists need to consider this during treatment planning when choosing activities. The degrees of freedom must be controlled carefully by stabilizing or eliminating use of some of the joints to decrease the number of joints involved (e.g., supporting the distal extremity on a table or substituting flat-hand stabilization for a hand grasp). Gillen has demonstrated a variety of methods to improve task performance in clients with ataxia by manipulating the degrees of freedom via positioning, splinting, movement retraining, and equipment.[42,43] Examples follow. See the case study of Nakai at the end of this chapter.[42]

- *Orthotics:* The goal is to provide joint stability in order to decrease control requirements.
  - Philadelphia collar
  - Opponens orthosis
  - Wrist supports
  - Task-specific orthoses (e.g., typing, writing)
- *Environmental modifications:* Utilizing the environment for stability. Focus on stabilizing the upper/lower trunk, stabilize arms, and decrease the degrees of freedom.
  - High back chairs
  - Forearm weight bearing on work surface or wall
  - Stabilize head on wall
  - Sit at a table against wall (anterior/lateral stability)
  - Use corner of wall (anterior/lateral stability)
  - Pillows and foam for support
  - Stabilize with one arm holding a chair
- *Retrain movements:*
  - Maintain arm contact with work surface or body (slide, don't reach)
  - Move upper limbs in flexion and adduction
  - Co-contract trunk
  - Push head into back of chair
  - Break down movement pattern to change target (for a feeding example, see Case Study)
  - Experiment with slow versus quick movements
  - Slide objects/tools on counter
  - Avoid reach into space
- *Adaptive devices:*
  - Soap on a rope
  - Electric toothbrush/razor
  - Coated utensils
  - Cup covers
  - Long straws
  - Weights
  - Dycem
  - Basket for transport
  - Adapted cutting boards
  - Suction brushes (nail, meal preparation, dish washing)
- *Assistive technology:*
  - Tilt-in-space power base
  - Tremor-dampening electronics
  - Contoured seating
  - High back chairs with head support
  - Speaker phone/headsets, bluetooth
  - Speech-to-text technology
- *Positioning:*
  - Semi-Fowler in bed
  - Tilt-in-space wheelchair for mobility
  - High back chairs
  - Avoid unsupported sitting
  - Lean against wall for sitting/standing
  - Platform walkers for gait
- *Therapeutic exercise to increase core stability:*
  - Closed chain strengthening
  - Proximal stability (core/scapula)

- Body weight as resistance
- Postural alignment
- Bridges, prone on elbow, quadruped, wall squats, kneeling, wheelchair pushups

Interventions to improve motor function for those with hypokinetic movement disorders such as PD have received more attention in the literature recently. A recent systematic review concluded the following[44]:

- The majority of relevant research addresses physical performance skills.
- There is a short-term benefit of physical activity for improving or maintaining physical performance skills.
- Task-specific training (particularly in enriched environments or contexts that utilize external supports, such as rhythmic cues) may benefit the development of new performance skills.
- Improvements appear to be specific to trained skills; lack of transfer to untrained skills or generalization of performance skill improvements to improvements in ADL or broader occupational performance outcomes.

The authors suggested that occupational therapists should encourage their clients with PD to engage in regular physical activity and help them find appropriate and meaningful forms of physical activity to ensure continued engagement.[44] There is anecdotal and emerging empirical evidence that engagement in specifically structured occupations can improve function and may in fact have a neuroprotective component. These include yoga (decreased limb bradykinesia and rigidity, increased strength and power, and improved QoL were seen after 12 weeks of training)[45]; boxing (improved mobility and endurance)[46]; and dance (improved balance and mobility).[47]

If one analyzes occupations such as boxing and dance (specifically Tango), it is clear that they require the use of high-amplitude movements. The Lee Silverman Voice Treatment Big (LSVT Big) is a protocol-driven **high-amplitude movement training** program. The program is 1 month, including four 1-hour sessions per week. The key aspects of this program include the combination of (1) an exclusive target on increasing amplitude (bigger movements in the limb motor system), (2) a focus on sensory recalibration to help patients recognize that movements with increased amplitude are within normal limits, even if they feel "too loud" or "too big", and (3) training self-cueing and attention to action to facilitate long-term maintenance of treatment outcomes.[48]

Intervention for Apraxia

Motor apraxia is a disorder of the production praxis system and may be defined as the loss of access to praxicons (motor plans) so that purposeful movement cannot be produced or achieved because of defective planning and sequencing of movements, even though idea and the purpose of task are understood.[49]

The person knows what to do related to the task at hand and has the overall concept of what to do. If language is intact and the person is questioned, he or she can explain the purpose of the task at hand. Instead, he or she cannot program, plan, or produce the movements necessary to accomplish the task, despite having the sensory and motor skills to execute the task. Clinical observations related to errors during task performance may include the following[49–52]:

- Difficulties related to motor planning in general, resulting in awkward or clumsy movements.
- Difficulties when planning movements to cross the body's midline (e.g., difficulty adjusting the grasp on a hairbrush when moving it from one side of head to the other).
- Difficulty orienting the UE or hand to conform to objects (e.g., picking up a juice bottle with the radial side of the hand down instead of a typical cylindrical grip).
- Inflexible and static hand patterns (e.g., not being able to manipulate coins out of the palm of the hand to insert them into a vending machine).
- Difficulty sequencing movements such as the sequence to get out of bed, or sequencing complex upper limb movements such as picking up the phone and lifting it to the ear.
- Spatial orientation and spatial movement errors (e.g., moving scissors laterally instead of forward).
- Difficulty coordinating two or more joints (e.g., coupling the shoulder and elbow movements for cutting). In general, the more joints involved in the tasks, the more degraded the motor planning.
- Difficulty timing movement (e.g., delay in initiation of movement, pauses, or difficulty related to movement speed).
- Poor gesture-production ability, particularly when gesturing the use of an object (transitive gestures).
- Using a body part as an object when asked to pantomime use of an object—common diagnostic screen for motor apraxia.
- Movements are imprecise.

Recent reviews have examined the available evidence to determine the most appropriate evidence-based interventions for those living with apraxia. A systematic review by West et al.[53] determined that two studies that documented changes in ADL status using the Barthel Index (BI) showed a small and short-lived therapeutic effect. They determined that this change was not clinically significant and did not persist. They recommended that higher quality research be conducted.

In 2011, Cicerone et al.[54] updated their clinical recommendations for cognitive rehabilitation of people with traumatic brain injury (TBI) and stroke, based on a systematic review of the literature from 2003 through 2008.[55] Their practice standard related to apraxia is stated as "specific gestural or strategy training is recommended for apraxia during acute rehabilitation for left hemisphere stroke."

Similar to Cicerone et al.,[54] Gillen et al.[56] identified two potential interventions: cognitive strategy training (CST) and gesture training (GT). Both of these are described further in the sections that follow.

Cognitive Strategy Training

CST consists of teaching internal and external compensatory approaches to execute ADLs. Techniques include internal rehearsal, verbalizing actions during ADL execution, and external cueing. Building on the research of Donkervoort et al.,[57] Geusgens et al.[58] examined their data to see whether CST had a greater transfer effect to nontrained tasks than usual OT alone. Although analysis showed both treatment groups improved on trained and nontrained tasks, the CST group showed greater improvement on nontrained tasks. These data indicate a greater transfer effect in the CST condition (see the Evidence table).

van Heugten and colleagues[59] described an intervention study designed for use by occupational therapists based on teaching clients strategies to compensate for the presence of apraxia. The treatment was focused on training activities that were relevant to the individual client. The therapist and client decided on which activities to focus. Interest checklists were also used to choose activities in addition to focusing on activities that were important to carry out in the future. Every 2 weeks, other activities were chosen.

The focus of the intervention was error specific and determined by the specific problems observed during standardized ADL observations. Specifically, interventions focused on errors related to the following:

- *Initiation:* inclusive of developing a plan of action and selection of necessary and correct objects
- *Execution:* performance of the plan
- *Control:* inclusive of controlling and correcting the activity to ensure an adequate end result

Difficulties related to *initiation* were treated via specific *instructions*. Instructions were hierarchical in nature and could include verbal instructions, alerting the client with tactile or auditory cues, gesturing, pointing, handing objects, or starting the activity together. *Assistance* was the intervention provided when problems related to *execution* of the activity occurred. Also hierarchical, assistance could range from various types of verbal assist, stimulating verbalization of steps, naming the steps of the activity, to physical assistance such as guiding movements (Fig. 16-7). When having difficulty with *control* (i.e., clients do not detect or correct the errors they make during the activity), *feedback* was provided. Feedback ranged from verbal feedback related to knowledge of results to taking control of the task and controlling for errors. The specific strategy training intervention protocol is included in Box 16-3. van Heugten and Geusgens[60] have more recently described the process of CST (Box 16-4).

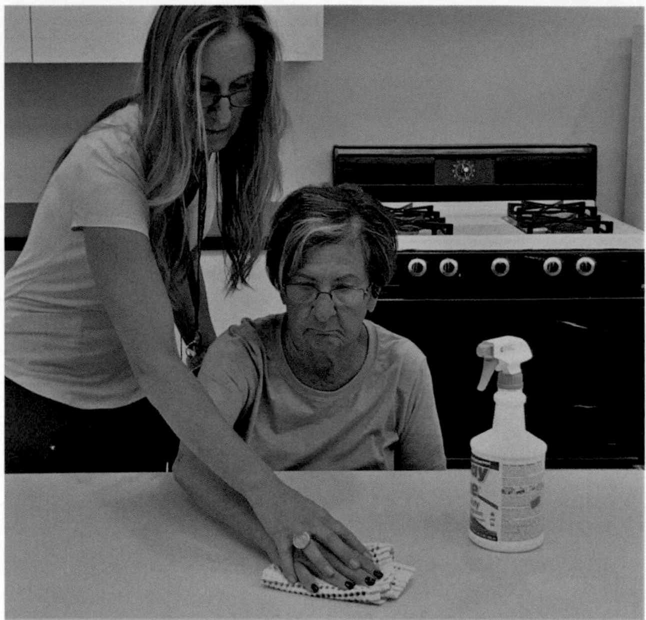

Figure 16-7. Example of intervention for apraxia when errors in task execution are noted. Therapist is providing physical assistance by guiding the patient's movements during the task of washing down a table surface.

Gesture Training

Smania et al.[61] first described **GT** for apraxia. The authors described GT as a behavioral training program consisting of gesture-production exercises. The rehabilitation program is made up of three sections[61]:

1. *Transitive gestures:* (1) patient is asked to show the use of common tools (e.g., spoon), (2) patient is shown a picture illustrating a transitive gesture (e.g., using a spoon), (3) patient is required to produce the corresponding gestural pantomime, and (4) patient is then presented with a picture of a common tool (e.g., a spoon) and required to pantomime the use of that object.
2. *Intransitive-symbolic gestures:* (1) patient is shown two pictures, one illustrating a given context (e.g., a man eating a sandwich) and the other showing a symbolic gesture related to that context (e.g., the gesture of eating), after presentation; (2) patient is asked to reproduce the symbolic gesture; (3) patient is asked to produce the correct gesture (e.g., the gesture of eating) after presentation of the context picture alone (e.g., a man eating a sandwich); and (4) patient is asked to produce the correct gesture

Box 16-3

Cognitive Strategy Training

The specific interventions are built up in a hierarchic order, depending on the patient's level of functioning. The therapist can use instructions, assistance, and feedback.

Instructions (for those not able to *initiate* task performance)

The occupational therapist can give the following instructions:

- Start with a verbal instruction.
- Shift to a relevant environment for the task at hand.
- Alert the patient by:
  - Touching
  - Using the patient's name
  - Asking questions about the instruction
- Use gestures, point to the objects.
- Demonstrate (part of) the task.
- Show pictures of the activity.
- Write down the instruction.
- Place the objects near the patient, point to the objects, put the objects in the proper sequence.
- Hand the objects one at a time to the patient.
- Start the activity together with the patient one or more times.
- Adjust the task to make it easier for the patient.
- Finally, take over the task because all efforts did not lead to the desired result.

Assistance (for those with difficulties *executing* the task)

The following forms of assistance can be given by the therapist:

- There is no need to assist the patient during the execution of the activity.
- Verbal assistance is needed:
  - By offering rhythm and not interrupting performance.
  - To stimulate verbalization of the steps in the activity.
  - To name the steps in the activity or name the objects.
  - To direct the attention to the task at hand.
- Use gestures, mimics, and vary intonation in your speech.
- Show pictures of the proper sequence of steps in the activity.
- Physical assistance is needed:
  - By guiding the limbs.
  - In positioning the limbs.
  - To use aids to support the activity.
  - To take over until the patient starts performing.
  - To provoke movements.
- Finally, take over the task.

Feedback (for those with difficulty *controlling* or correcting errors)

Feedback can be offered in the following ways:

- No feedback is necessary because the result is adequate.
- Verbal feedback is needed in terms of the result (knowledge of results).
- Verbal feedback by telling the patient to consciously use the senses to evaluate the result tell the patient to see, hear, feel, smell, or taste.
- Physical feedback is needed in terms of the result (knowledge of results):
  - To evaluate the posture of the patient.
  - To evaluate the position of the limbs.
  - To support the limbs.
- Physical feedback is given by pointing or handing the objects to the patient.
- Verbal feedback is needed in terms of performance (knowledge of performance).
- Physical feedback is needed in terms of performance (knowledge of performance).
- Place the patient in front of a mirror.
- Make video recordings of the patient's performance and show the recordings.
- Take over the control of the task and correct possible errors.

Adapted from van Heugten CM, Dekker J, Deelman BG, van Dijk AJ, Stehmann-Saris JC, Kinebanian A. Outcome of strategy training in stroke patients with apraxia: a phase II study. *Clin Rehabil.* 1998;12:294–303.

Box 16-4

Cognitive Strategy Training

Strategies for instructions to support the preparation of the performance when the client's performances deficits occur in the ***orientation*** phase:

- Give instructions more than once and use extra attention.
- Ask questions about the performance.
- Demonstrate the performance or its parts.
- Give a written description of the performance.
- Show pictures of the task performance.
- Show objects needed for the task.
- Hand objects to the client one by one.
- Take over performance or its parts.

Strategies for instructions to support the preparation for the performance when the client's performance deficits occur in the ***execution*** phase are guidance strategies:

- Show pictures.
- Guide with verbal support.
- Guide with physical support.
- Start with a slow tempo.
- Start with only one object.
- Show objects needed for the task.
- Hand objects to the client (one by one).
- Take over the performance or its parts.

Strategies for instructions to support the preparation for the performance when the client's performance deficits occur in the ***control*** phase are feedback strategies:

- Give verbal feedback.
- Show the result in a mirror.
- Make video recordings to show to the client.
- Ask questions about the result ("Did you put on your socks?").
- Make pictures to show to the client.

Adapted from van Heugten CM, Geusgens C. Strategies to compensate for apraxia among stroke clients. In: Söderback I, ed. *International Handbook of Occupational Therapy Interventions.* New York, NY: Springer; 2009.

(e.g., the gesture of eating) following the presentation of a picture showing a new, but similar contextual situation (e.g., a man eating canned food with a fork).
3. ***Intransitive-nonsymbolic gestures:*** (1) patient is asked to imitate meaningless intransitive gestures (six proximal and six distal joint movements, half are static and half dynamic) previously shown by the examiner.

Smania et al.[62] assessed how GT affects functional independence in ADL. The researchers completed a study with 41 left hemisphere patients after stroke. In addition to the neuropsychological test battery, they included a caregiver questionnaire regarding patient ADL independence. An additional 2-month post-training follow-up assessment was included. Results showed that the GT group's performance improved significantly on ideational, ideomotor, and gesture comprehension tests. Performance on these tests and measures of ADL independence was correlated.

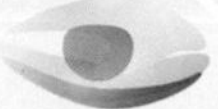

CASE STUDY

Nakai is a 34-year-old Native American male who was diagnosed with MS 2 years prior to this inpatient rehabilitation admission. His initial symptoms began approximately 3 years prior to this admission and consisted of diplopia, gait impairments, and problems with upper limb coordination. Nakai was admitted to the hospital because of worsening symptoms and an inability to complete basic self-care tasks such as feeding, grooming, dressing, and toileting. See Chapter 15 for assessment results. Based on the assessment results, two control parameters guided the development of Nakai's intervention plan[42]:

- As the degrees of freedom (number of joints involved in the task) increased, tremors increased and functional control decreased. When the degrees of freedom were controlled (decreased) during treatment sessions, UE trajectories were smoother and resulted in an improved ability to interact with the environment and perform functional activities.
- When engaged in activities that challenged his postural stability, his tremors worsened. Observations to support this hypothesis included progressive worsening of tremors as he moved from supine to sitting to standing; improvement of tremors while seated in high back chairs and semi-reclined postures where his trunk was supported (i.e., semi-sitting position with knees flexed and supported by pillows on the bed); and worsening of tremors when Nakai became increasing posturally insecure or when he was required to control his trunk against gravity (i.e., reaching beyond his arm span, weight shifting during ADL).

Nakai confided that he felt humiliated when staff had to assist him with feeding and oral care, thus improving independence in feeding and oral care became primary goals. To meet these goals, orthotic devices were provided in an effort to decrease motor control requirements and to stabilize the cervical spine as well as the distal UEs. A semirigid cervical collar was prescribed as well as off-the-shelf wrist supports. In addition, an electric toothbrush was provided to reduce the need for rapid alternating movements, and Dycem was used to stabilize his plate during eating. Nakai's feeding position promoted postural security and was characterized by leaning into the table in a position of forearm weight bearing to stabilize his upper trunk. In addition, his hand-to-mouth movement pattern was modified from a continuous trajectory from plate to mouth to a three-step pattern as follows:

1. Slide hand and utensil across the table and manipulate food onto the utensil.
2. Bring the hand to a point approximately 2 inches from the mouth (to decrease the effects of intention and smaller target size on worsening tremors).
3. Relax and place food in the mouth.

Likewise, Nakai's movement patterns and positioning during oral care were adapted to use the environment for UE stabilization and to minimize reaching into space. His positioning during oral care was modified to one of standing in front of a wall in a position of forearm weight bearing while simultaneously co-contracting his trunk to promote postural stability. With the electric toothbrush stabilized, Nakai was taught to systematically move his mouth around the toothbrush.

In addition, Nakai was provided with two MP CDs. One CD verbally prompted Nakai to imagine performing the task of eating using the new three-step pattern and modified positioning. The other CD verbally prompted him to imagine performing the task of brushing his teeth using the new positioning and movement pattern of moving his mouth around the stabilized toothbrush. Nakai was encouraged to use the tapes outside therapy sessions prior to task performance.

Breaking tasks down, decreasing the degrees of freedom with orthotics, increasing postural stability via positioning, the use of adaptive equipment, and supplementing the training with MP resulted in increased control of the desired movement patterns and improved task performance. Nakai was able to eat independently with utensils and perform oral care with the aid of an electric toothbrush, albeit with effort and increased time. Continued practice eventually decreased the time required to eat and perform oral care to performance levels acceptable to Nakai.

Best Evidence for Motor Control Intervention

Intervention	Intervention Description	Participants	Dosage	Research Design and Evidence Level	Benefit	Statistical Significance and Effect Size
Action Observation[25]	Both groups received conventional therapy. In addition, patients in the case group were asked to observe and subsequently execute different daily actions presented via video clips. Controls observed video clips without motor content and subsequently performed the same actions as the case participant.	$N = 15$ patients with PD, ages 18–75, normal or corrected vision, normal auditory acuity, relatively cognitively intact, and the absence of depression. Case group: $n = 7$; Control group: $n = 8$. Groups did not differ statistically on any of the baseline characteristic, except for disease severity—cases were worse than controls.	Dosage information not provided in the study	Case–Control Level 2	Findings suggest AO may improve autonomy in daily living activities	Both groups improved after treatment, but change scores were higher in the cases as compared to the controls on both the UPDRS ($p = 0.004$) and the Functional Independence Measure ($p = 0.002$).
Cognitive Strategy Training[58]	Strategy training integrated into OT. The focus of training is determined by problems noted during ADL performance as they relate to initiation, execution, and control. Instruction, assistance, and feedback are used depending on the problems identified as compared to standard OT.	$N = 113$ patients with left hemispheric stroke and apraxia. Strategy training group: $n = 56$; Usual treatment group: $n = 57$. Groups did not differ statistically on any of the baseline characteristics with the exception of age: strategy training group was older.	Eight weeks of treatment according to group randomization. Experimental group had on average 25 (standard deviation [SD] = 9.8) sessions, resulting in 15 (SD = 7.7) hours of OT. Control group had on average 27 (SD = 15.6) sessions, resulting in 19 (SD = 15.0) hours of OT	Single-blind, randomized controlled trial (RCT) Level 1	Transfer effects from trained to nontrained tasks were noted for both groups, suggesting both forms of treatment resulted in transfer of training; although, the effect was larger in the group that received the strategy training intervention.	ADL change scores of nontrained task improved in both groups over time ($p = 0.00$). Change score on the ADL observations of nontrained tasks (week 8–week 0) was larger in the strategy training group than in the usual treatment group ($t = 1.78$, $p = 0.040$). No significant differences between the groups on trained tasks or on trained and untrained tasks at 5-month follow-up.
Constraint-induced movement therapy (CIMT) and modified CIMT (mCIMT)[9]	Forced use of the affected UE by restraining the unaffected UE with a sling or hand splint/mitt and massed practice of the affected limb via shaping and standard task practice	Forty-two RCTs were included, involving 1,453 participants who had a stroke and had some residual motor power of the paretic arm with limited pain or spasticity; more men (64%) than women; mean age range and time after stroke varied	CIMT: $n = 9$ studies mCIMT: $n = 29$ studies Restraint time of unimpaired limb, training intensity of impaired limb, and treatment duration varied across studies accordingly	Systematic review and meta-analysis Level 1	Reduces UE motor impairments and improves UE function in stroke survivors with some residual motor function in the affected UE. However, these improvements may not readily translate to improved performance of ADLs. No differences in adverse effects between CIMT and control conditions	Nonsignificant effects for disability (SMD 0.24, 95% confidence interval [CI] −0.05 to 0.52) and QoL (mean difference [MD] 6.54, 95% CI −1.2 to 14.28). Significant effects for (1) upper limb function (SMD 0.34, 95% CI 0.12–0.55); (2) perceived upper limb function (quality of use: MD 0.68, 95% CI 0.47–0.88) and amount of use (MD 0.79, 95% CI 0.50–1.08); (3) arm motor impairment (SMD 0.82, 95% CI 0.31–1.34); (4) dexterity (SMD 0.42, 95% CI 0.04–0.79)

(*continued*)

Best Evidence for Motor Control Intervention (*continued*)

Intervention	Intervention Description	Participants	Dosage	Research Design and Evidence Level	Benefit	Statistical Significance and Effect Size
MI with rhythmic cueing[18]	Participants in experimental group were engaged in a 30–40-minute group (two to three people) session to get familiar with use of MI. Then, they were provided with study CDs containing verbal prompts to facilitate kinesthetic imagery of walking combined with either music or metronome and rhythmic cues used to carry out home-based MI program. Control group received standard care.	$N = 101$ patients diagnosed with mild-to-moderate MS without overt signs of cognitive impairment or depression. 85 females and 16 males; mean age was 44.1 ± 12.0 years. Groups did not differ statistically on any of the baseline characteristics.	Seventeen minute sessions per day, for 6 days/week for a total of 4 weeks. Participants recorded their practice sessions in a diary; participants practiced a median 5 (4–6) times per week	RCT Level 1	Home-based rhythmic-cued MI improves walking, fatigue, and QoL in people with mild-to-moderate MS. It appears music-cued MI may be more effective. The intervention was reported to be safe, convenient, and without adverse events.	Rhythmic-cued MI significantly improved walking speed as compared to controls ($p < 0.0001$, with a large effect size (ES) of $\eta^2 = 0.581$) and walking distance compared to controls ($p < 0.0001$, with a large ES of $\eta^2 = 0.596$). Participants walking perception improved significantly in the MI groups, and improvements were clinically meaningful in the metronome group compared to controls. Cognitive and total fatigue significantly improved in the MI groups, whereas physical fatigue improved only after music-cued MI. Psychosocial fatigue did not improve. Health-related QoL (HRQoL) significantly improved in the MI groups as compared to the control group, with greater improvements noted with music-cued MI.
Power Yoga Program[45]	Yoga practice using Vinyasa style that incorporates vigorous, fitness-based positions. The program used fast transitions from one posture to another. Strength, power, flexibility, and balance were addressed by stabilizing body extremities and strengthening core muscles. Control group received usual care and three nonexercise health education classes.	$N = 27$ elderly (60–90) patients with PD (Hoehn & Yahr stages I–III), ambulatory (at least 50 feet); able to get up and down from floor with minimal assistance and relatively cognitively intact. Yoga group: $n = 15$; Control group: $n = 12$. Groups did not differ statistically on any of the baseline characteristics.	The yoga program was given as group class for 1 hour per session, 2 sessions per week for 12 weeks.	RCT Level 1	Yoga program reduced bradykinesia and rigidity, increased muscle strength and power, and improved QoL in older patients with PD.	Significant effects in favor of the yoga group for: (1) bradykinesia: decrease in the upper limb (UL) (4.5 points) and lower limb (LL) (2.5 points) scores, with large ES (UL: $g = -1.75$; LL: $g = -1.11$, $p < 0.001$); (2) rigidity: (decrease in 2.6 points) with a large ES ($g = -0.64$, $p = 0.001$); (3) improved muscle strength and power ($p < 0.05$) with small ($g = 0.16$, $p = 0.023$) to large ($g = 0.80$, $p < 0.001$), ES seen across various tests; (4) improved mobility ($g = -0.82$, $p = 0.025$), ADL ($g = -0.46$, $p = 0.035$) domains and the sum score ($g = -0.70$, $p = 0.016$) of Parkinson's Disease Questionnaire

References

1. Gillen G, Nilsen DM. Motor function and occupational performance. In: Schnell B, Gillen G, eds. *Willard and Spackman's Occupational Therapy, Centennial Edition*. 13th ed. Philadelphia, PA: Wolters Kluwer; 2019.
2. French B, Thomas LH, Coupe J, et al. Repetitive task training for improving functional ability after stroke. *Cochrane Database Syst Rev.* 2016;(11):CD006073.
3. Nilsen DM, Gillen G, Geller D, Hreha K, Osei E, Saleem GT. Effectiveness of interventions to improve occupational performance of people with motor impairments after stroke: an evidence-based review. *Am J Occup Ther.* 2015;69(1):6901180030p6901180031–6901180030p6901180039.
4. Shumway-Cook A, Woollacott M. *Motor Control: Translating Research into Clinical Practice*. Baltimore, MD: Lippincott Williams & Wilkins; 2017.
5. Page SJ, Boe S, Levine P. What are the "ingredients" of modified constraint-induced therapy? An evidence-based review, recipe, and recommendations. *Restor Neurol Neurosci.* 2013;31(3):299–309.
6. Kleim JA, Jones TA. Principles of experience-dependent neural plasticity: implications for rehabilitation after brain damage. *J Speech Lang Hear Res.* 2008;51:S225–S239.
7. Timmermans AA, Spooren AI, Kingma H, Seelen HA. Influence of task-oriented training content on skilled arm-hand performance in stroke: a systematic review. *Neurorehabil Neural Repair.* 2010;24(9):858–870.
8. Taub E, Miller N, Novack TA, et al. Technique to improve chronic motor deficit after stroke. *Arch Phys Med Rehabil.* 1993;74:347–354.
9. Corbetta D, Sirtori V, Castellini G, Moja L, Gatti R. Constraint-induced movement therapy for upper extremities in people with stroke. *Cochrane Database Syst Rev.* 2015;(10):CD004433.
10. Wolf SI, Winstein C, Miller JP, et al. Effect of constraint-induced movement therapy on upper extremity function 3 to 9 months after stroke: the EXCITE randomized clinical trial. *JAMA.* 2006;296:2095–2104.
11. Mark VW, Taub E, Uswatte G, et al. Phase II randomized controlled trial of constraint-induced movement therapy in multiple sclerosis. Part 1: effects on real-world function. *Neurorehabil Neural Repair.* 2018;32(3):223–232.
12. Barghi A, Allendorfer JB, Taub E, et al. Phase II randomized controlled trial of constraint-induced movement therapy in multiple sclerosis. Part 2: effect on white matter integrity. *Neurorehabil Neural Repair.* 2018;32(3):233–241.
13. Lee KS, Lee WH, Hwang S. Modified constraint-induced movement therapy improves fine and gross motor performance of the upper limb in Parkinson disease. *Am J Phys Med Rehabil.* 2011;90(5):380–386.
14. Braun S, Kleynen M, van Heel T, Kruithof N, Wade D, Beurskens A. The effects of mental practice in neurological rehabilitation; a systematic review and meta-analysis. *Front Hum Neurosci.* 2013;7:390.
15. Nilsen DM, Gillen G, Gordon AM. Use of mental practice to improve upper-limb recovery after stroke: a systematic review. *Am J Occup Ther.* 2010;64(5):695–708.
16. Malouin F, Jackson PL, Richards CL. Towards the integration of mental practice in rehabilitation programs. A critical review. *Front Hum Neurosci.* 2013;7:576.
17. Barclay-Goddard RE, Stevenson T, Poluha W, Thalman, L. Mental practice for treating upper extremity deficits in individuals with hemiparesis after stroke. *Cochrane Database Syst Rev.* 2011;(5):CD005950.
18. Seebacher B, Kuisma R, Glynn A, Berger T. The effect of rhythmic-cued motor imagery on walking, fatigue and quality of life in people with multiple sclerosis: a randomised controlled trial. *Mult Scler.* 2017;23(2):286–296.
19. Tamir R, Dickstein R, Huberman M. Integration of motor imagery and physical practice in group treatment applied to subjects with Parkinson's disease. *Neurorehabil Neural Repair.* 2007;21(1):68–75.
20. Braun S, Beurskens A, Kleynen M, Schols J, Wade D. Rehabilitation with mental practice has similar effects on mobility as rehabilitation with relaxation in people with Parkinson's disease: a multicentre randomised trial. *J Physiother.* 2011;57(1):27–34.
21. Thieme H, Morkisch N, Mehrholz J, et al. Mirror therapy for improving motor function after stroke. *Cochrane Database Syst Rev.* 2018;(7):CD008449.
22. Bonassi G, Pelosin E, Ogliastro C, Cerulli C, Abbruzzese G, Avanzino L. Mirror visual feedback to improve bradykinesia in Parkinson's disease. *Neural Plast.* 2016;2016:8764238.
23. Borges LR, Fernandes AB, Melo LP, Guerra RO, Campos TF. Action observation for upper limb rehabilitation after stroke. *Cochrane Database Syst Rev.* 2018;(10):CD011887.
24. Di Iorio W, Ciarimboli A, Ferriero G, et al. Action observation in people with Parkinson's disease. A motor–cognitive combined approach for motor rehabilitation. A preliminary report. *Diseases.* 2018;6(3), 58.
25. Buccino G, Gatti R, Giusti MC, et al. Action observation treatment improves autonomy in daily activities in Parkinson's disease patients: results of a pilot study. *Mov Disord.* 2011;26(10):1963–1964.
26. Laver KE, Lange B, George S, Deutsch JE, Saposnik G, Crotty M. Virtual reality for stroke rehabilitation. *Cochrane Database Syst Rev.* 2017;(11):CD008349.
27. Dockx K, Bekkers EM, Van den Bergh V, et al. Virtual reality for rehabilitation in Parkinson's disease. *Cochrane Database Syst Rev.* 2016;(12):CD010760.
28. Massetti T, Trevizan IL, Arab C, Favero FM, Ribeiro-Papa DC, de Mello Monteiro CB. Virtual reality in multiple sclerosis—A systematic review. *Mult Scler Relat Disord.* 2016;8:107–112.
29. Mehrholz J, Pohl M, Platz T, Kugler J, Elsner B. Electromechanical and robot-assisted arm training for improving activities of daily living, arm function, and arm muscle strength after stroke. *Cochrane Database Syst Rev.* 2018;(9):CD006876.
30. Carpinella I, Cattaneo D, Abuarqub S, Ferrarin M. Robot-based rehabilitation of the upper limbs in multiple sclerosis: feasibility and preliminary results. *J Rehabil Med.* 2009;41(12):966–970.
31. Gijbels D, Lamers I, Kerhofs L, Alders G, Knippenberg E, Feys P. The Armeo Spring as training tool to improve upper limb functionality in multiple sclerosis: a pilot study. *J Neuroeng Rehabil.* 2011;8:5.
32. Swinnen E, Duerinck S, Baeyens JP, Meeusen R, Kerckhofs E. Effectiveness of robot-assisted gait training in persons with spinal cord injury: a systematic review. *J Rehabil Med.* 2010;42(6):520–526.

33. Woodford H, Price C. EMG biofeedback for the recovery of motor function after stroke. *Cochrane Database Syst Rev.* 2007;(2):CD004585.
34. Pomeroy VM, King L, Pollock A, Baily-Hallam A, Langhorne P. Electrostimulation for promoting recovery of movement or functional ability after stroke. *Cochrane Database Syst Rev.* 2006;(2):CD003241.
35. Harris JE, Eng JJ. Strength training improves upper-limb function in individuals with stroke: a meta-analysis. *Stroke.* 2010;41(1):136–140.
36. Katalinic OM, Harvey L, Herbert RD, Moseley AM, Lannin NA, Schurr K. Stretch for the treatment and prevention of contractures. *Cochrane Database Syst Rev.* 2010;(9):CD007455.
37. Harvey LA, Katalinic OM, Herbert RD, Moseley AM, Lannin NA, Schurr K. Stretch for the treatment and prevention of contractures. *Cochrane Database Syst Rev.* 2017;(1):CD007455.
38. de Jong LD, Nieuwboer A, Aufdemkampe G. Contracture preventive positioning of the hemiplegic arm in subacute stroke patients: a pilot randomized controlled trial. *Clin Rehabil.* 2006;20(8):656–667.
39. Llg W, Synofzik M, Brotz D, Giese A, Schols L. Intensive coordinative training improves motor performance in degenerative cerebellar disease. *Neurology.* 2009;73:1823–1830.
40. Miyai I, Ito M, Hattori N, et al. Cerebellar ataxia rehabilitation trial in degenerative cerebellar diseases. *Neurorehabil Neural Repair.* 2012;26(5):515–522.
41. Marsden J, Harris C. Cerebellar ataxia: pathophysiology and rehabilitation. *Clin Rehabil.* 2011;25:195–216.
42. Gillen G. Improving activities of daily living performance in an adult with ataxia. *Am J Occup Ther.* 2000;54:89–96.
43. Gillen G. Improving mobility and community access in an adult with ataxia: a case study. *Am J Occup Ther.* 2002;56:462–466.
44. Foster ER, Bedekar M, Tickle-Degnen L. Systematic review of the effectiveness of occupational therapy-related interventions for people with Parkinson's disease. *Am J Occup Ther.* 2014;68(1):39–49.
45. Ni M, Mooney K, Signorile JF. Controlled pilot study of the effects of power yoga in Parkinson's disease. *Complement Ther Med.* 2016;25:126–131.
46. Combs SA, Diehl M, Chrzastowski C, et al. Community-based group exercise for persons with Parkinson disease: a randomized controlled trial. *NeuroRehabiltiation.* 2013;32(1):117–124.
47. Rios RS, Anang J, Fereshtehnejad S, Pelletier A, Postuma R. Tango for treatment of motor and non-motor manifestations in Parkinson's disease: a randomized control study. *Complement Ther Med.* 2015;23(2):175–184.
48. Fox C, Ebersbach G, Ramig L, Sapir S. LSVT LOUD and LSVT BIG: behavioral treatment programs for speech and body movement in Parkinson disease. *Parkinsons Dis.* 2012;2012:391946.
49. Arnadoittir G. *The Brain and Behavior: Assessing Cortical Dysfunction Through Activities of Daily Living.* St. Louis, MO: Mosby; 1990.
50. Árnadóttir G. Impact of neurobehavioral deficits on activities of daily living. In: Gillen G, ed. *Stroke Rehabilitation: A Function-Based Approach.* 4th ed. St. Louis, MO: Elsevier; 2016.
51. Gillen G. *Cognitive and Perceptual Rehabilitation: Optimizing Function.* St. Louis, MO: Elsevier/Mosby; 2009.
52. Heilman KM, Gonzalez R. Apraxia. In: Heilman KM, Valenstein E, eds. *Clinical Neuropsychology* 5th ed. New York, NY: Oxford University Press; 2012.
53. West C, Bowen A, Hesketh A, Vail A. Interventions for motor apraxia following stroke. *Cochrane Database Syst Rev.* 2008;(1):CD004132.
54. Cicerone KD, Langenbahn DM, Braden C, et al. Evidence-based cognitive rehabilitation: updated review of the literature from 2003 through 2008. *Arch Phys Med Rehabil.* 2011;92(4):519–530.
55. Cicerone KD, Dahlberg C, Malec JF, et al. Evidence-based cognitive rehabilitation: updated review of the literature from 1998 through 2002. *Arch Phys Med Rehabil.* 2005;86(8):1681–1692.
56. Gillen G, Nilsen DM, Attridge J, et al. Effectiveness of interventions to improve occupational performance of people with cognitive impairments after stroke: an evidence-based review. *Am J Occup Ther.* 2015;69(1):6901180040p6901180041–6901180040p6901180049.
57. Donkervoort M, Dekker J, Stehmann-Saris FC, Deelman BG. Efficacy of strategy training in left hemisphere stroke patients with apraxia: a randomised clinical trial. *Neuropsychol Rehabil.* 2010;11(5):549–566.
58. Geusgens C, van Heugten C, Donkervoort M, van den Ende E, Jolles J, van den Heuvel W. Transfer of training effects in stroke patients with apraxia: an exploratory study. *Neuropsychol Rehabil.* 2006;16(2):213–229.
59. van Heugten CM, Dekker J, Deelman BG, van Dijk AJ, Stehmann-Saris JC, Kinebanian A. Outcome of strategy training in stroke patients with apraxia: a phase II study. *Clin Rehabil.* 1998;12:294–303.
60. van Heugten CM, Geusgens C. Strategies to compensate for apraxia among stroke clients. In: Söderback I, ed. *International Handbook of Occupational Therapy Interventions.* New York, NY: Springer; 2009.
61. Smania N, Girardi F, Domenicali C, Lora E, Aglioti S. The rehabilitation of limb apraxia: a study in left-brain-damaged patients. *Arch Phys Med Rehabil.* 2000;81(4):379–388.
62. Smania N, Aglioti SM, Girardi F, et al. Rehabilitation of limb apraxia improves daily life activities in patients with stroke. *Neurology.* 2006;67:2050–2052.
63. Dettmers C, Teske U, Hamzei F, Uswatte G, Taub E, Weiller C. Distributed form of constraint-induced movement therapy improves functional outcome and quality of life after stroke. *Arch Phys Med Rehabil.* 2005;86(2):204–209.
64. Lin KC, Wu C, Wei TH, Lee CY. Effects of modified constraint-induced movement therapy on reach-to-grasp movements and functional performance after chronic stroke: a randomized controlled study. *Clin Rehabil.* 2007;21:1075–1086.
65. Page SJ, Levine P, Leonard AC. Modified constraint-induced therapy in acute stroke: a randomized controlled pilot study. *Neurorehabil Neural Repair.* 2005;19(1):27–32.

Chapter 17

Balance Assessment and Intervention

Allison Chamberlain Miller

LEARNING OBJECTIVES

This chapter will allow the reader to:

1. Recognize how balance contributes to daily occupational participation and performance.
2. Describe how impaired balance contributes to occupational dysfunction.
3. Understand the neurological and physiological basis of balance.
4. Describe screening skills for balance, sit-to-stand transfers, and functional ambulation.
5. Differentiate between static and dynamic balance.
6. List standardized assessments designed to evaluate balance and fall risk.
7. Describe appropriate intervention approaches in daily occupation for balance, sit-to-stand transfers, functional ambulation, and fall prevention.
8. List evidence-based interventions for the treatment of balance.

CHAPTER OUTLINE

TERMINOLOGY

Balance: an even distribution of weight enabling someone to remain upright and steady.

Base of Support (BoS): area of contact between body and support surface.

Center of Mass (CoM): anatomical point representing the mean position of total body weight; also known as *center of gravity*.

Dynamic: body positioning during active motion.

Ipsilateral: belonging to or occurring on the same side of the body.

Postural adjustments: strategic changes in body alignment that minimize changes in CoM during weight shifting in a variety of planes and directions.

Postural control: the motor act of maintaining, achieving, or restoring a state of balance during any activity.

Static: body positioning without motion.

Weight shift: transfer of body mass from one supporting limb or body part to another.

Balance and Impairment in Daily Occupation

Balance is a critical skill for participation in many daily occupations. It is required for activities performed in sitting or standing, including the ability to transition between sitting and standing and to perform functional ambulation. The *Occupational Therapy Practice Framework: Domain and Process* (3rd ed.)[1] refers to balance as both a client factor and a performance skill necessary for participation in a person's chosen occupations. Many studies have supported a correlation between sitting balance scores and occupational independence, length of stay in inpatient settings, and occupational performance after stroke.[2] Impaired balance not only impacts an individual's ability to perform an occupation, it is also a leading cause of falling. Falls are a major health concern in the United States because they lead to high medical costs, a decline in quality of life, and can even be fatal. Balance deficits and falls can cause decreased levels of occupational participation and independence.[3]

Neurological and Physiological Basis of Balance

Achieving and maintaining balance is a complex skill that requires the coordination of musculoskeletal systems and sensorimotor neural systems.[4,5] An individual may experience reduced sensation or motor weakness that impairs balance, and other body systems such as vision are often used to compensate for those deficits.[6] Neurologically, balance is regulated by the sensory and motor systems, including processing of vestibular (righting and equilibrium reactions), visual, and tactile, and proprioceptive information.[7] Cranial nerve 8, known as the vestibulocochlear nerve, is responsible for sense of balance and spatial orientation.[8] Proprioception senses body position and movement[8] and is one factor associated with fall risk in older adults because it declines with age and has been linked to gait disorders.[9]

This processing plays an important role in trunk or **postural control** mechanisms. Each time a person moves, his or her body's **center of mass (CoM)** changes its relationship to the **base of support (BoS)**.[7] Postural control skills allow us to stay in balance by maintaining our body's CoM within the BoS.[7] Individuals with asymmetric postural alignment and impaired postural control tend to be fearful of falling during **static** sitting or standing without support, and this fear increases with **dynamic** movement attempts.[7] Control during **postural adjustments** is required for all reaching from a sitting or standing position.[10] Additionally, if an individual is unable to bear or **weight shift** to one side of his or her body, caused by orthopedic or neurological deficits, balance may be impaired because of asymmetrical postural alignment and control.[11]

Decreased trunk strength and weakness in one or both of the lower extremities can also contribute to impaired balance. Lower extremity weakness is common in older adults, as strength begins to decrease annually around the age of 50, and this weakness can increase the risk of falling.[12,13] This is particularly true for the hip flexors, knee extensors and flexors, and ankle plantar flexors and dorsiflexors.[4,13] Individuals with lower extremity weakness have a decreased ability to recover from balance loss, related to an increased risk of falling.[13] There is a relationship between reduced physical activity, muscle weakness, and balance deficits in clients with chronic obstructive pulmonary disease (COPD), for example.[4]

At times, some individuals experience impaired balance because of multiple factors, such as after a stroke. For example, individuals who have experience a stroke often exhibit balance deficits related to reduced weight bearing on the affected lower extremity, increased postural sway during standing, reduced sensation, unilateral inattention, delayed equilibrium reactions, impaired postural adjustments on the affected side, and uneven weight distribution during functional movements.[11]

Neurologically based balance disorders are those for which an individual feels unsteady or dizzy even while still or laying down and require different evaluation and treatment than those discussed in this chapter, as prescribed by a physician. Certain medications have side effects that can negatively affect balance, as well as high or low blood pressure, viral or bacterial infection in the ear, or specific change of position of the head that displaces the vestibular structures of the inner ear. There are over a dozen different balance disorders, each with different causes and treatments that should be diagnosed and prescribed by a physician. For example, benign paroxysmal positional vertigo (BPPV) can be treated by physical or occupational therapists who are trained in the Epley maneuver, a series of simple movements to help dislodge displaced vestibular structures of the inner ear that are likely causing the balance impairment.[14,15]

Screening of Balance Skills

Balance is impaired when an individual is unable to maintain a sitting or standing position without support or assistance, whether while remaining static or during dynamic movement. Impaired balance can create skill impairment for reaching from a sitting or standing position, transferring from sitting to standing, and performing functional ambulation. This can result in a higher risk of falling as well as decreased independence in meaningful occupations.

Signs Indicating Dysfunction in Balance

Occupational therapists often work with clients who require physical assistance to maintain an upright sitting or standing posture.[6] Signs indicating dysfunction in daily occupation can be observed by analyzing the individual's postural alignment, such as whether or not the shoulders are even, if he or she is leaning more to one side than the other, or if he or she is simply unable to maintain sitting while unsupported. This is best observed on a firm surface that requires unsupported sitting, such as on the edge of a client's bed or on a therapy mat.[7] The ability to flex and extend the trunk can be observed to recognize signs of decreased core strength. Observation of an individual's ability to perform postural adjustments and maintain control while reaching away from the body or across midline during functional tasks can also reveal signs indicating dysfunction in daily occupation.[10] Other signs or precautions include impaired righting reactions, decreased depth perception in reaching for an item, or self-report that the individual is feeling dizzy or lightheaded.

To maintain standing balance, the goal is to maintain one's CoM over the BoS during weight shifting in a variety of directions, from one leg to the other.[7] The quality of alignment of a weight-bearing leg can be assessed by observation of the following optimal characteristics: at least 90° of ankle dorsiflexion (foot flat on an even surface), active extension at the knee (not locked), active hip extension, and neutral position of the pelvis.[7]

Possible Causes of Impairment

As discussed, there are several possible causes of impaired balance, which may occur singularly or in combination. It is important to start by understanding the client's medical history because certain diagnosis may be at a higher risk of balance impairment based on the neurological or physiological basis of the condition. It is also important to be aware that anxiety regarding falling, especially if the individual has a history of falling, can affect safety during unsupported sitting and standing tasks. Because there are several possible causes of impaired balance, multifactorial screening and assessment is recommended to determine the individualized needs of the client.

Screening Instructions

Currently, there are no studies regarding how occupational therapists assess and document sitting balance, suggesting that there is a not a commonly accepted method.[2] Objective, skilled documentation is of increasing importance because other health care professionals refer clients to occupational therapists for discharge recommendations[2] and third-party reimbursement often requires standardized, measureable data to justify intervention. It is important to record the baseline balance performance of the client at initial evaluation to measure progress throughout intervention and plan for discharge.[6] This section offers instructions for screening for sitting and standing balance using a grading system in order to provide measurable documentation and outcome measurements. Screening for balance offers a quick option for therapists to detect and measure potential balance impairments before completing a standardized assessment of balance, which only exists for standing balance.[2]

Before screening an individual for balance, sit-to-stand transfers, or functional ambulation, the therapist should review the client's history and create an occupational profile. It is important to note the client's diagnoses, medications and possible side effects, any history of falling, and prior level of function. The therapist should also assess the client's blood pressure because abnormal levels can create dizziness and increase the risk of falling or injury. Ensure the client's safety at all times, starting by assessing balance in sitting (see Fig. 17-1). This means another therapist's assistance may be required to stand by the client while assessing reaching ability.

Balance can be measured by grading it to detect the severity of any balance impairments and provide objective data. Grading includes static and dynamic balance for both sitting and standing. All grades must be qualified with the assistive device being used by the client. If no device is being used, that must be stated. Balance is graded on a scale from *Normal*, to *Good*, *Fair*, and *Poor* (see Table 17-1).[16] The therapist should screen static balance before dynamic balance for both sitting and standing.

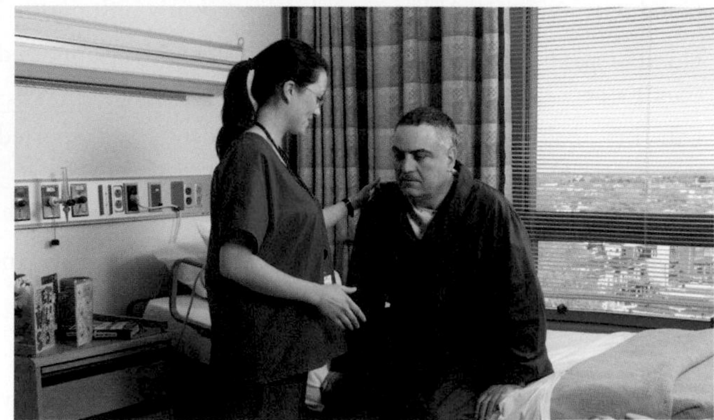

Figure 17-1. Standing in front of patient and assessing for balance deficits or complaints of dizziness before standing, for safety.

Table 17-1. Balance Grades

STATIC SITTING BALANCE	
Normal (N)	Able to maintain unsupported sitting balance against maximal resistance
Good (G)	Able to maintain unsupported sitting balance against moderate resistance
Good−/Fair+ (G−/F+)	Able to maintain unsupported sitting balance against minimal resistance
Fair (F)	Able to sit unsupported without balance loss and without UE support
Fair− (F−)	Able to maintain sitting balance with UE support
Poor+ (P+)	Able to maintain sitting balance with minimum assistance from individual or chair
Poor (P)	Unable to maintain sitting balance. Requires moderate/maximum support from another individual or chair
DYNAMIC SITTING BALANCE	
Normal (N)	Able to sit unsupported, able to weight shift and cross midline maximally
Good (G)	Able to sit unsupported, able to weight shift and cross midline moderately
Good−/Fair+ (G−/F+)	Able to sit unsupported, able to weight shift and cross midline minimally
Fair (F)	Able to sit unsupported, minimal weight shift to front/ipsilateral side, difficulty crossing midline
Fair− (F−)	Able to sit unsupported, able to reach to ipsilateral side, unable to weight shift
Poor+ (P+)	Able to sit unsupported with minimal assistance and reach to ipsilateral side, unable to weight shift
Poor (P)	Able to sit supported with moderate assistance and reach to front/ipsilateral side, cannot cross midline or weight shift
STATIC STANDING BALANCE	
Normal (N)	Able to maintain unsupported standing balance against maximal resistance
Good (G)	Able to maintain unsupported standing balance against moderate resistance
Good−/Fair+ (G−/F+)	Able to maintain unsupported standing balance against minimal resistance
Fair (F)	Able to stand unsupported without UE support and without balance loss for 1–2 minutes
Fair− (F−)	Requires minimal assistance or UE support to maintain standing without balance loss
Poor+ (P+)	Requires moderate assistance and UE support to maintain standing without balance loss
Poor (P)	Requires maximum assistance and UE support to maintain standing without balance loss
DYNAMIC STANDING BALANCE	
Normal (N)	Able to stand independently unsupported, able to weight shift and cross midline maximally
Good (G)	Able to stand independently unsupported, able to weight shift and cross midline moderately
Good−/Fair+ (G−/F+)	Able to stand independently unsupported, able to weight shift and cross midline minimally
Fair (F)	Able to stand independently unsupported, weight shift, and reach ipsilateral side; difficulty crossing midline without balance loss
Fair− (F−)	Able to stand with supervision and reach ipsilateral side; unable to weight shift
Poor+ (P+)	Able to stand with minimal assistance and reach ipsilateral side; unable to weight shift
Poor (P)	Able to stand with moderate assistance and minimally reach ipsilateral side; unable to cross midline

UE, upper extremity.
Adapted from: *Grading for Balance: Graded Posture Movement Ability of Individual* by Stanbridge College.

Static Sitting Balance Screening

- Determine whether the client is able to sit unsupported without balance loss and without upper extremity (UE) support.
  - If so, apply pressure with your hands to the client's trunk in the anterior, posterior, and lateral directions.
    - Determine whether the client is able to maintain balance against minimal, moderate, or maximal resistance; gradually increasing the amount of resistance to the extent that the client is able to tolerate safely and comfortably.
  - If not, determine whether the client can maintain balance with UE support or if the client requires minimum or moderate/maximum support from another individual or chair.

Dynamic Sitting Balance Screening

- If the client is able to sit unsupported, determine whether and how far he or she is able to weight shift and cross midline by asking the client to reach for an item in multiple planes including crossing midline and reaching to the contralateral, or opposite, side of the body. Make sure that the client is not using the other UE for support. Classify this as weight shifting and crossing midline minimally, moderately, or maximally.
- If the client is able to sit unsupported but has difficulty crossing midline, determine whether he or she can complete any amount of weight shifting or reaching to the **ipsilateral** side of the body (see Fig. 17-2).
- If the client is unable to sit unsupported, determine whether he or she needs minimal or moderate assistance to maintain sitting. This will indicate that the client is unable to reach to the ipsilateral side, weight shift, or cross midline.
- If a client requires maximum assistance to maintain sitting, you do not need to screen for dynamic balance because this indicates an absence of, or *Poor*, dynamic sitting balance.

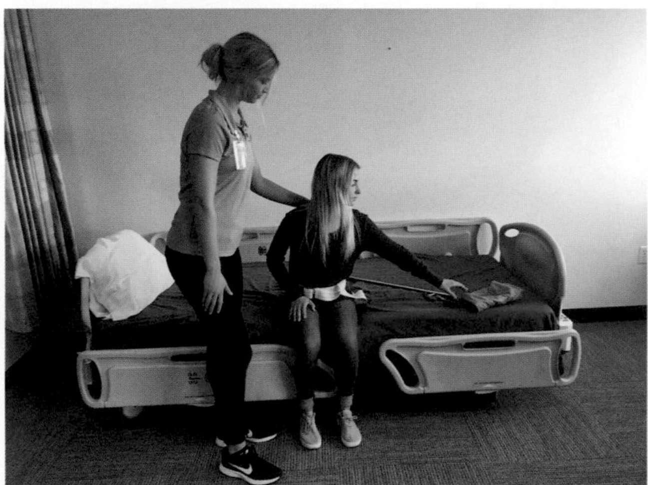

Figure 17-2. Dynamic sitting balance screening.

Static Standing Balance Screening

- Determine whether the client can stand supported without UE support and without balance loss for 1 to 2 minutes.
  - If so, apply pressure with your hands to the client's trunk in the anterior, posterior, and lateral directions (see Fig. 17-3).
    - Determine whether the client is able to maintain balance against minimal, moderate, or maximal resistance; gradually increasing the amount of resistance to the extent the client is able to tolerate safely and comfortably.
  - If not, determine whether the client can maintain standing without loss of balance with UE support and minimum, or moderate, or maximum support from another individual or assistive device.

Dynamic Standing Balance Screening (see Videos 17-1 and 17-2)

- If the client is able to stand independently unsupported, determine whether he or she is able to weight shift and reach across midline to the contralateral side minimally, moderately, or maximally. This can be accomplished by again asking the client to reach for an item and gradually increasing the distance as tolerated.

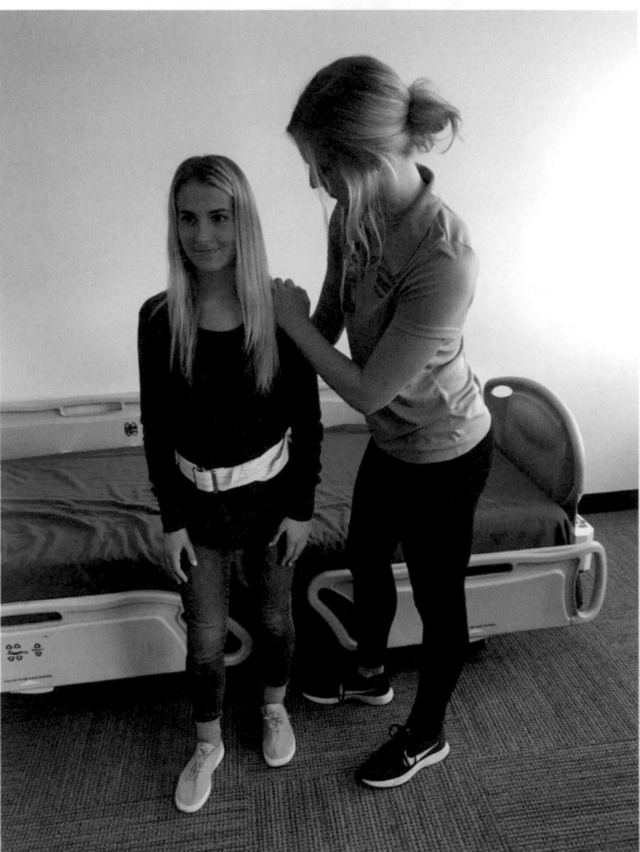

Figure 17-3. Static standing balance screening.

- If the client is able to stand independently unsupported, but cannot reach to the contralateral side, screen his or her ability to weight shift and reach to the ipsilateral side as well as cross midline.
- If the client is able to stand with supervision and reach to the ipsilateral side, determine whether he or she is able to weight shift.
- If the client is able to stand with minimal or moderate assistance, determine whether he or she is able to weight shift, reach to the ipsilateral side, or cross midline.
- If a client requires maximum assistance to maintain standing, you do not need to screen for dynamic balance because this indicates an absence of, or *Poor*, dynamic standing balance.

See Figures 17-4 and 17-5 for examples of a dynamic standing balance screening.

Another option for screening balance using a grading scale is a tool offered by Kansas University titled the *Kansas University Sitting and Standing Balance Scale* (KUSSBS).[17] This sitting balance and standing balance scale measures balance on a numerical grading scale, ranging from 0 (i.e., client performs 25% or less of sitting activity; maximum assist) to 5 (i.e., client independently moves and returns to center of gravity in all planes >2 inches). The standing balance portion has been shown to be reliable and valid in the inpatient rehabilitation setting with a small sample in one study.[6]

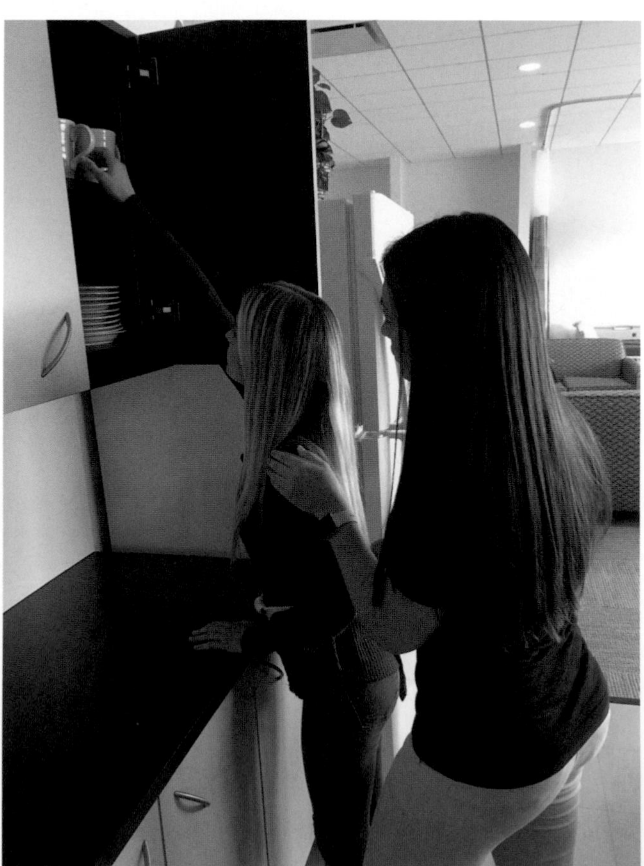

Figure 17-4. Dynamic standing balance screening.

Assessing Impact on Daily Occupational Function

In addition to measuring the client's balance grade, it is also very important to determine the impact of balance impairments on his or her daily occupational performance. The best way to accomplish this is through skilled observation and measurement of the amount of assistance required by the client during occupational performance because there are currently no existing standardized assessments of balance that are occupation based.[2] Additionally, it is essential to examine the client's context and environment, including both the physical and social environment. It is also necessary to determine the client's risk for falling as well as any impact a balance deficit has on his or her occupational participation and performance. Observe the client for signs indicating dysfunction in daily occupations, as discussed earlier.

If a problem is identified through screening, an in-depth assessment should be used to better evaluate the severity of the impairment. Balance is assessed while observing the client during movement in sitting and standing, including looking in a variety of directions, reaching for items in different directions, and walking in various conditions.[10] These movements require anterior movement of the pelvis, flexion of the trunk at the hips, using the lower extremities to create a BoS, and shifting body weight and CoM toward the direction of the object during reaching.[10] See the Assessment table at the end of this chapter for standardized assessments that can be used to assess standing balance deficits, including fall risk.

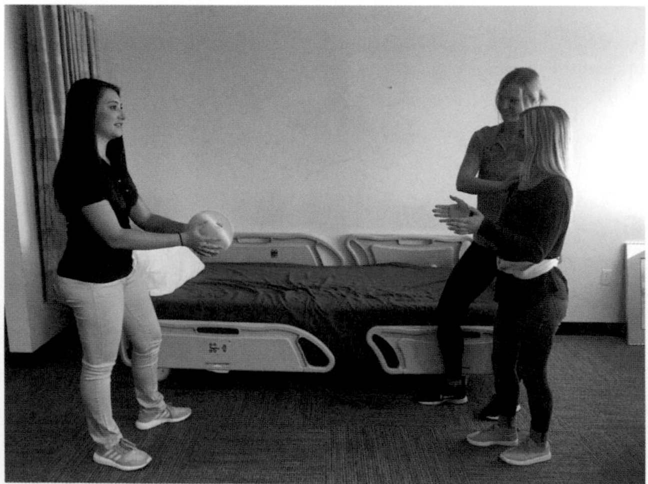

Figure 17-5. Dynamic standing balance screening.

Overview of Interventions for Balance Impairment

The therapist should create an individualized, multifactorial treatment plan that combines approaches as needed to address the cause(s) of the balance deficit(s). The approach or approaches used to address balance impairment can be determined by the underlying cause of the deficit and if there is potential to improve the deficit through remediation or if compensation and adaptation would be more appropriate. At times, it is necessary to begin with a compensatory and/or adaptive approach to increase safety and independence during the process of remediation. Remedial techniques include increasing range of motion, strength, and/or endurance where motor dysfunction has an effect on balance and fall prevention.[18] Improving these motor skills may lead to an increased ability to maintain static or dynamic sitting and standing postures. Compensatory techniques introduce clients to techniques for using their UE(s) or weight shifting techniques to offset deficits that cannot be remediated or that are in the process of remediation. Adaptation techniques include several environmental options, such as adding adaptive equipment or devices to the client's environment to increase safety and independence. Some clients may benefit from a combination of all three approaches. Specific interventions are discussed next.

Specific Interventions for Balance Impairment

Remediation of Balance Impairments

If screening and assessment indicate that client factors can be improved, a remediation, or biomechanical, approach is appropriate. Exercises and occupation-based activities can be incorporated into treatment to improve core, UE, and lower extremity strength or activity tolerance, if indicated, by gradually increasing the weight and/or repetition of the activity. Preparatory methods should be used to treat edema and/or pain, such as modalities, manual techniques, and splinting or positioning, if applicable. If a client demonstrates soft-tissue stiffness causing impaired postural control or alignment, the therapist should begin with passive stretching before engaging in active balance activities.[7] However, if the cause of impaired postural control is because of postural insecurity, the therapist can provide additional external support via physical "handling" to allow the client to safely and fully participate in the planned activity.[7]

There is a history of evidence to support the use of therapeutic exercise to increase strength and balance and reduce the risk of falling.[19,20–22] The occupational therapist should select exercises to target any muscles that have been identified as debilitated during the assessment of strength with the use of manual muscle testing. As mentioned previously, this may include core, UE, or lower extremity muscles. Core and lower extremity muscles have a direct influence on remediating balance, whereas UE muscle strengthening may be needed for the use of compensatory and adaptive techniques for mobility and other occupations, listed in the subsequent section. Resistive exercises to increase strength for improved balance should be incorporated with the use of functional activities to provide contextual, dynamic challenges while ensuring client safety. Other forms of exercise that have been shown to improve balance through greater strength, endurance, flexibility, and postural control include yoga,[9,23] tai chi (see Fig. 17-6),[24] and repetitive task training.[21] See the Evidence table at the end of this chapter for evidence of remediation intervention studies.

Reaching can be improved by gradually increasing activity demands for reaching during daily occupation training or with rote exercises (see Fig. 17-7), while seated unsupported as long as safely tolerated. Balance can be improved by increasing activity demands for tasks completed in sitting or standing with the least amount of support or assistance as required to reach a higher balance grade as measured during the initial screening.

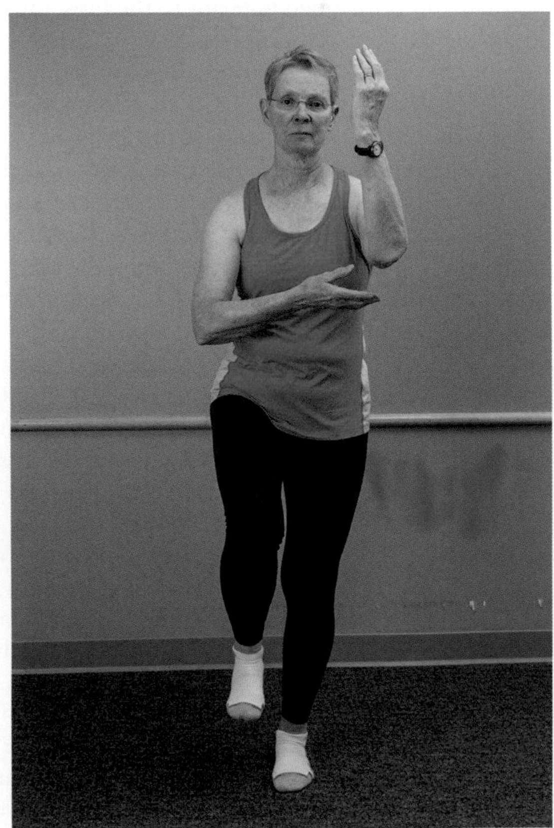

Figure 17-6. Tai chi is an exercise strategy to help restore control and balance to movement patterns.

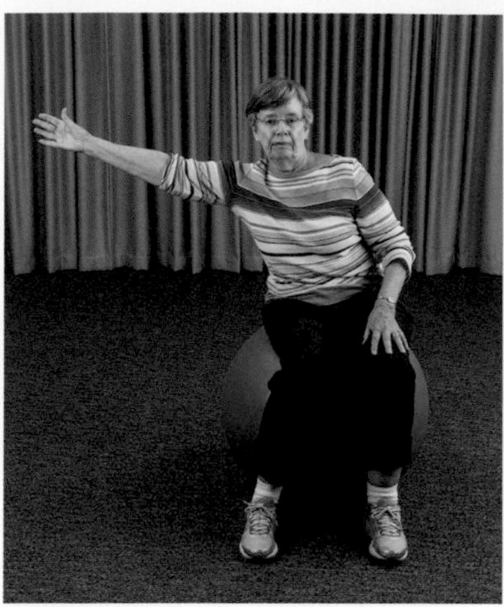
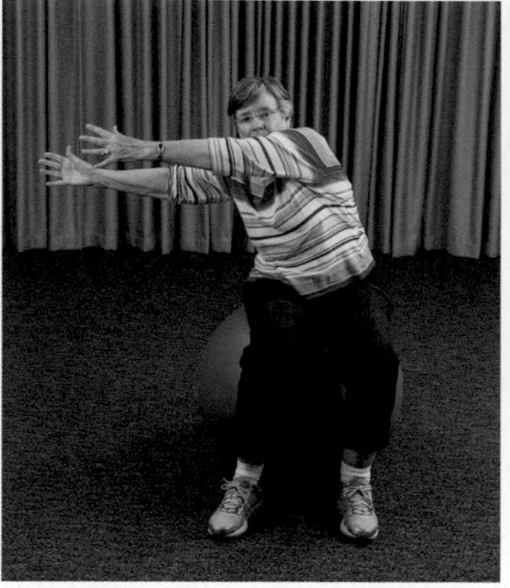
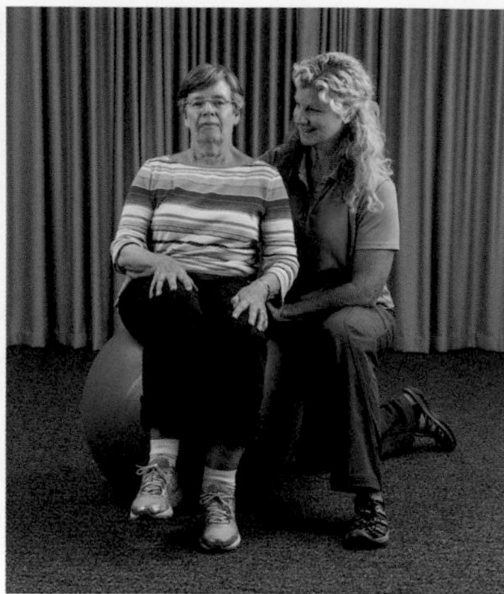

Figure 17-7. A variety of balance activities can be performed on a therapeutic ball, such as bilateral reaching.

In treating sitting balance deficits, the therapist should work to develop the client's understanding of this alignment, awareness of postural adjustments, and learning through occupation-based challenges that require active weight shifting.[7] The therapist starts by ensuring that the client achieves optimal postural alignment for performing daily tasks in sitting. This position can be described as having the pelvis in neutral to anterior tilt with equal weight bearing on the ischial tuberosities, the trunk extended in a midline orientation, the shoulders symmetrical and positioned anterior to the hips, the hips and knees flexed and neutrally rotated, and both feet securely on the floor and ready to accept weight (see Fig. 17-8).[7] To help a client develop awareness of alignment and adjustments, the therapist can provide verbal and/or visual cues through the use of questions, such as "are you sitting up straight?," and of a mirror or video recording to recognize errors and challenge the client to correct his or her posture before continuing the activity.[7]

Occupation-based challenges that require active weight shifting include incorporating tasks that demand the client to move in a variety of planes, such as backward and forward, to the left and to the right, rotating the trunk to the left or right, and any combination of those movements plus upward or downward directions (see Fig. 17-9).[7] In each direction, weight shifting is accompanied by postural adjustments. By requiring the client to shift weight in a variety of planes, he or she can improve his or her ability to look and reach for moving objects to improve balance for self-care tasks such bathing, dressing, and grooming and household tasks such as meal preparation, laundry, and cleaning.[7] Throughout these tasks consisting of weight shifting and reaching, core muscle strengthening occurs, further improving balance for daily occupations.[7] Similar to sitting balance exercises, standing balance can be challenged by exercising lower extremity muscles during tasks performance that requires weight shifting by reaching for objects in a variety of planes while in standing.[7]

Compensating for Balance Impairments

If balance skills cannot be remediated or if compensation for balance is necessary during the remediation of underlying skills, there are several options. The client can participate in education for the following:

- Safe weight shifting techniques
- Bracing with the contralateral UE
- Getting dressed lying in bed

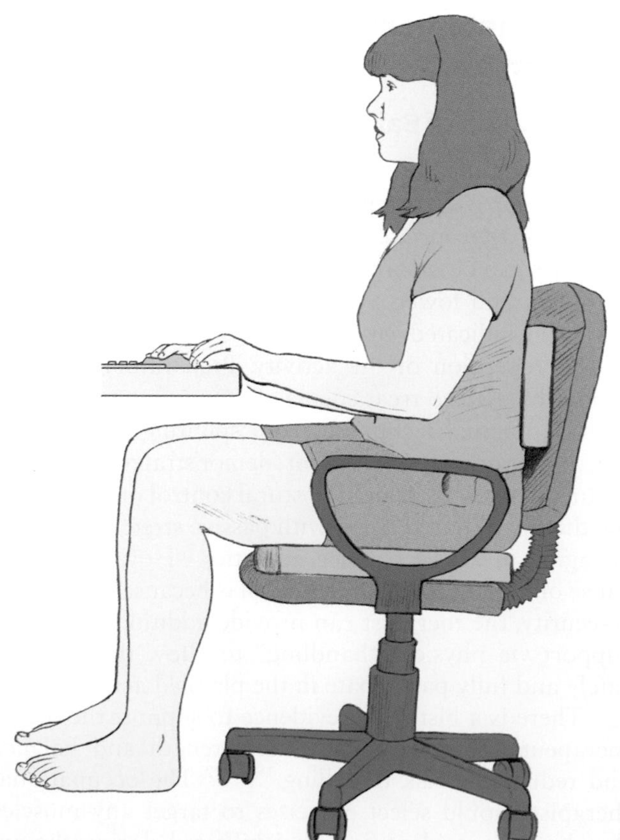

Figure 17-8. Optimal postural alignment in sitting.

- Learning to complete all pieces of lower body dressing in sitting and standing only one time to pull pants up around hips
- Using alternate methods of lower body dressing to decrease the need to bend toward the floor
- Performing toileting hygiene in sitting when possible
- Pulling pants up over the knees before standing from toilet to prevent pants from falling to the floor while standing
- Performing standing activities in front of a chair in case of loss of balance or the need to take a seated rest break
- Learning to position self directly in front of a workspace to avoid reaching outside the BoS during housekeeping tasks, such as cooking, unloading the dishwasher, transferring laundry, and cleaning
- Making the bed while still lying in it
- Wearing a terry cloth bathrobe to dry off after the shower instead of towel drying.

Adapting for Balance Impairments

There are several environmental adaptations that can be made to increase safety and independence for a balance impairment that cannot be improved or while the client is in the process of remediation. Many supports can be added to the home environment such as:

- Grab bars
- Stair railings
- Electronic lift chairs
- Stair lifts
- Toilet safety frames/handles
- Shower chair/bench
- Nonslip adhesive surfaces for the bathtub/shower or stairs
- Use of adaptive devices such as canes, walkers, and wheelchairs
- Use of a reacher and other long-handled items
- A pant clip for toileting clothing management
- Positioning equipment that can be added to wheelchair seating systems for postural support/alignment
- Bed rails for transfers or sitting balance
- transfer boards for lateral (seated) transfers.

Additionally, the environment can be arranged to increase safety and independence, such as:

- Setting up the environment to decrease reaching distance required to complete a task
- Setting up the environment to allow for tasks to be completed in sitting, such as a table in the kitchen for food prep
- Placing hygiene/grooming tools on the bathroom counter within reach from a chair.

The therapist should work with the client to design adaptations specific to that client's performance skills and environment.

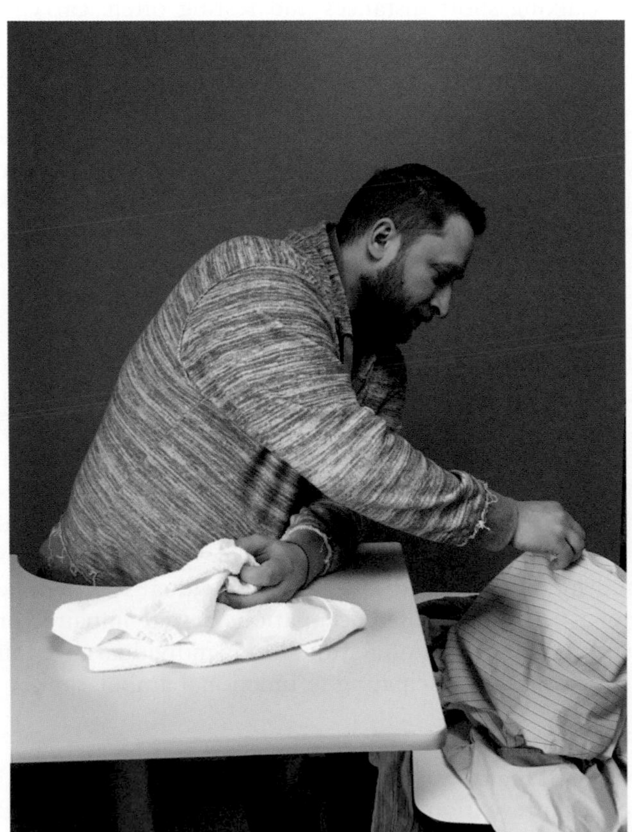

Figure 17-9. Laundry is placed to the left of a right-handed person to encourage reaching and development of dynamic standing balance.

Functional Mobility

Functional mobility training includes interventions aimed at improving a client's ability to perform bed mobility, transition between standing and sitting, and to perform daily activities while standing and walking. Balance is essential for safe, independent functional mobility. Treatment for functional mobility is similar to balance interventions, in that it provides for remediation of strength and postural adjustments to improve safety and performance of daily occupations.[7]

Standing Up and Sitting Down

Safely transitioning between standing and sitting is essential for the performance of daily occupations. Optimal performance of sit-to-stand transfer requires intact balance with the integration of adequate mobility at the pelvis and hips, postural alignment, postural adjustments, weight shifting, and strength in the core and lower extremities (see Fig. 17-10).[7] After screening and assessment, remediation training should address any of these components that are impaired, as discussed earlier. If the limitation is suspected to be related to impaired motor planning, rather than balance, refer to Chapters 15 and 16.

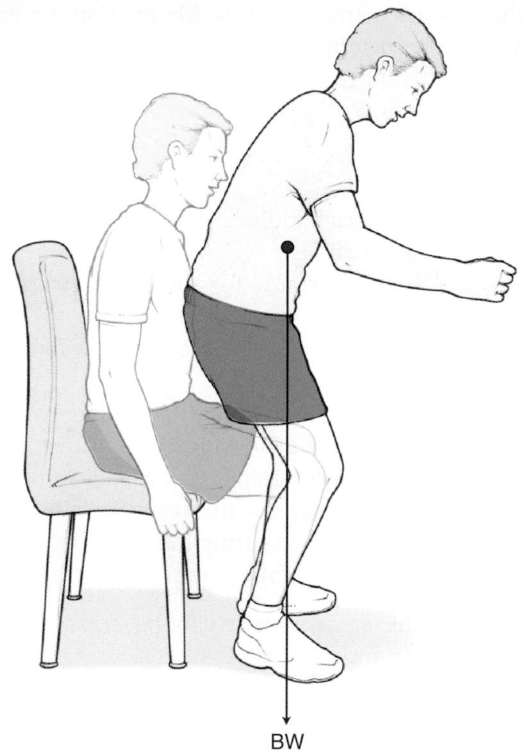

Figure 17-10. Initial phase of the sit-to-stand movement involves trunk lean and horizontal weight shift to position the center of gravity over the new base of support (feet). The movement of the center of gravity in several directions is often used to study balance. BW, body weight.

When remediation of sit-to-stand transfer is not possible or safe, training should include transition to adaptation approaches. Using arm rests or grab bars to push down, reach back, pull, or steady oneself with the UE(s) is a commonly helpful and safe technique when transitioning between sitting and standing. It should be noted that this technique is not ideal for clients recovering from stroke or brain injury because these body mechanics contradict essential motor strategies.[7] When a client is unable to achieve sit-to-stand transfer, another compensatory strategy for transferring from one surface to another is known as a squat pivot. With this approach, the client is not required to shift weight between the lower extremities. These alternative approaches are intended for clients who will not progress to walking.[7]

There are several environmental adaptations that can assist an individual with achieving sit-to-stand transfer, including raising the height of seating surface, grab bars, and using chairs with armrests. Further examples were provided in the section on Adapting for Balance Impairments.

Functional Ambulation

Walking is another essential skill for the performance of many daily occupations. Occupational therapists address walking with clients who wish to improve their performance in many functional activities that involve walking, such as bathroom, kitchen, vocational, leisure, and educational occupations. The most common risk factors for impaired functional ambulation are older age, decreased physical activity, obesity, strength or balance impairment, and chronic diseases such as diabetes or arthritis.[23] Functional ambulation training in occupational therapy often centers around safety and fall prevention while enabling a client to increase participation and independence in valued occupations. Physical therapists provide specific evaluation and treatment to prevent and reduce gait deviations. Occupational therapists work with physical therapists to maximize efficient gait patterns during occupation-based intervention for activities that require the use of the UEs while walking.[7] Many of the occupation-based interventions for balance remediation previously described in this chapter contribute to improved functional ambulation. This includes improving stability and facilitating proper postural adjustments during activities in sitting and standing that require weight shifting and reaching in a variety of directions[7] and exercises to increase strength and balance. Interventions for functional ambulation should be determined based on the client's identification of valued occupations.[7]

Compensatory techniques for functional ambulation include the use of energy conservation techniques, such as walking short distances and resting often, carrying less/lighter objects while walking, walking at a slower pace, as well as holding onto furniture or other sturdy objects for balance. Many clients will independently incorporate the use of atypical body mechanics to compensate for weakness or other deficits affecting functional ambulation. The occupational therapist should work with the client to ensure compensatory strategies are safe and should not cause additional structural damage that may further impair functional ambulation.

Primary adaptive techniques for functional ambulation include the use of adaptive devices, such as canes, crutches, walkers, and wheelchairs (see Fig. 17-11). Other adaptive techniques include the use of a shopping or utility cart for balance and/or object transportation. The environment will likely need to be modified to create accessibility with adaptive devices. The occupational therapist should work with the client to devise strategies and modifications to allow the individual to continue to participate in valued occupations despite impaired or absent functional ambulation. Many individuals live full lives without participating in functional ambulation.

Fall Prevention

Much of the research on balance interventions is related to fall prevention. Treatment of balance, sit-to-stand transfer, and functional ambulation are important components of fall prevention. However, they are only part of the picture in preventing falls because there are other

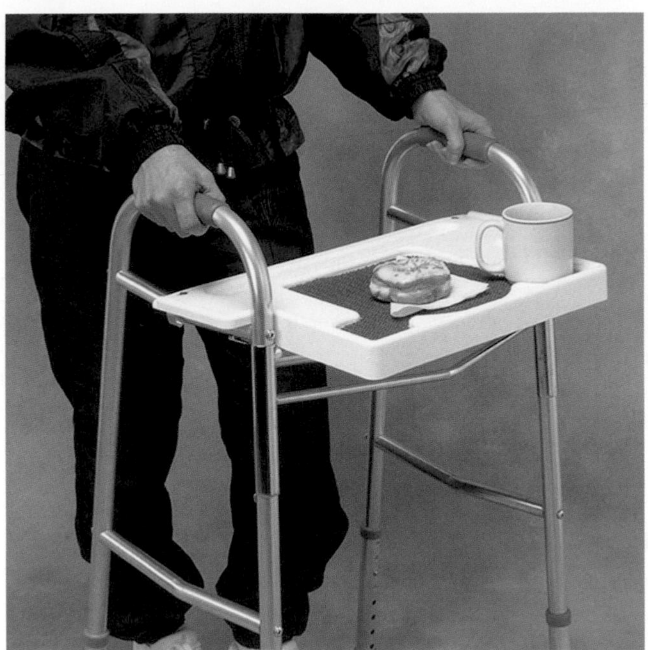

Figure 17-11. Walker with tray to adapt functional mobility.

risk factors. Evidence suggests that individuals with an identified risk of falling benefit from an individualized, multifactorial approach that may include a combination of the following: functional ambulation training and advice on the use of appropriate adaptive device(s), medication review and modification if necessary (especially psychotropic medications), exercise programs (with balance training as a component), treatment of postural hypotension, modification of environmental hazards, and treatment of cardiovascular disorders. For individuals living in institutional settings (i.e., assisted living and long-term care), staff education is also recommended.[25–27] The therapist's role in an interdisciplinary approach to the treatment of balance and fall prevention may include functional ambulation and adaptive device training, exercise programs (including balance training), environmental assessment and modification, and staff education. There are proven benefits of exercise and balance training in preventing falls, though there is no conclusive agreement on the type, duration, or intensity of exercise. There is also emerging evidence to support the use of virtual reality in therapy to improve balance for individuals who have had a stroke.

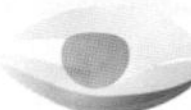

CASE STUDY

Patient Information

Anna is a 76-year-old woman who presented to her primary care physician with complaints of common cold symptoms and shortness of breath at rest. Her physician found that her oxygen saturation was below 90% and recommended that she be admitted to an acute care hospital. She was diagnosed with left lower lobe pneumonia and treated with intravenous antibiotics, steroids, and supplemental oxygen. Anna has a past medical history of COPD. She was discharged from the hospital to a skilled nursing facility for rehabilitation and medication management. Anna is retired, widowed, and lives alone in a single-story home. She often sleeps in the recliner because it is easier for her breathe with her head elevated. Prior to admission, Anna was functioning at the modified independent level with activities of daily living (ADLs), requiring extra time and some compensatory strategies or adaptive equipment to complete tasks. She is inactive most of the day, outside minimal ADL and instrumental activities of daily living (IADLs) participation. Anna reports relying more on her daughter in the past few months for shopping for groceries, getting the mail, and taking out the trash. Her son-in-law mows her lawn and removes snow as needed. She does not spend much time out of the house or socializing because she reports it takes a lot of energy, she is afraid of falling in the community, and her finances are limited. She admits that she does not keep up well with housekeeping tasks and prepares simple meals. She reports falling once or twice in the past 6 months while in the bathroom and kitchen and is afraid of showering, which she reports doing about 1 to 2 times a week.

Assessment Process and Results

The occupational therapist interviewed Anna to complete an occupational profile. The evaluation was completed through observation of functional tasks and motor assessments. Her oxygen saturation was assessed at 97% oxygen at rest and 89% with activity. Anna does not appear to have any cognitive, sensory, or visual perceptual deficits. Her UE range of motion and strength are within functional limits (4/5 during manual muscle testing), however, she demonstrates weakness in her lower extremity muscles because of inactivity (3+/5 during manual muscle testing). During screening, she demonstrates Good−/Fair+ (G−/F+) static and dynamic sitting balance and Fair—(F−) static and dynamic standing balance, requiring a front-wheeled walker and standby assistance for functional ambulation resulting from impaired balance related to fatigue and lower extremity weakness. Anna participated in the Functional Reach Test, demonstrating an ability to reach 6 inches, indicating a moderate risk for falls. Anna tolerates standing

(continued)

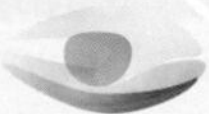

CASE STUDY *(continued)*

1 to 2 minutes and needs to rest after 2 to 3 minutes of total functional activity. She is able to perform upper body dressing and grooming tasks while seated with setup and standby assistance. She displays shortness of breath, and increased time is required for task completion. She requires minimal assistance for upper body bathing while seated. Anna requires moderate assistance with lower body dressing, bathing, and hygiene tasks secondary to increased shortness of breath when bending over and fatigue and impaired balance while performing tasks in standing, such as pulling pants over her hips. Anna is fearful of falling and requires minimal assistance for functional transfers and moderate assistance for tub transfers. She requires minimal assistance for toileting, clothing management, and hygiene because of fatigue and balance deficits. Anna requires minimal verbal cues to safely manage oxygen tubing for fall prevention because she is not used to performing functional tasks while on oxygen.

Occupational Therapy Problem List

- Sitting and standing balance
- General and standing activity tolerance
- Lower extremity weakness
- Setup and standby assistance needed for upper body dressing
- Moderate assistance needed for lower body dressing, bathing, and hygiene
- Setup and standby assistance needed for upper body hygiene and grooming while seated
- Minimal assistance needed for toileting
- Minimal assistance needed for functional transfers
- Moderate assistance needed for tub transfers
- Standby assistance needed for functional ambulation with a front-wheeled walker
- At risk of falling because of fatigue, balance, and oxygen tubing management
- Reduced IADL participation and performance

Occupational Therapy Goal List

Anna's goal is to return home with modified independence in ADLs and perform IADLs at her prior level of function without the use of oxygen.

- Increase safety and independence with all ADLs
- Decrease risk of falling
- Increase IADL participation and independence
- Establish a routine with increased activity as tolerated to prevent deconditioning
- Return home at highest functional level with home health therapy and support from her daughter and son-in-law as needed

Intervention

- Remediation of sitting and standing balance, activity tolerance, and lower extremity strength through exercises and occupation-based treatment activities.
- Education and incorporation of compensatory and adaptive strategies as needed to increase independence and safety with ADLs and IADLs, including energy conservation techniques, setting up the home environment to make commonly used items easy to reach, a bath bench and grab bars in the tub, compensatory strategy for tub transfers, a raised toilet safety frame with handles, a chair in her bathroom and kitchen, emergency call system in case of falls, adaptive equipment for lower body dressing and bathing, and a walker if still needed upon discharge from skilled nursing facility.
- Increased independence and decreased risk of falling with home environment assessment to incorporate identified compensatory and adaptive techniques.
- Referral to home health occupational therapist after discharge to further address performance in home environment, IADLs performance, creation of a more active routine to prevent deconditioning, such as home exercise program, and methods to increase social participation and leisure occupational participation.

Psychometric Properties of Assessments of Balance

Instrument and Reference	Intended Purpose	Administration Time	Validity	Reliability	Sensitivity	Strengths And Weaknesses
Berg Balance Scale[28]	Measuring balance across 14 tasks	15–20 minutes	Concurrent validity: $r = 0.91$ with the Tinetti Balance Subscale[29]; $r = -0.81$ with Timed Up-and-Go Test (TUG)[30] or $r = -0.74$ with the TUG.[31] Discriminant validity: discriminates among persons using various types of walking aids[28]	Inter-rater reliability: Intra-class correlation coefficient (ICC) = 0.98 for total scale; ICC = 0.71–0.99 for individual items.[28] For total scale: ICC = 0.97[32] and 0.95.[33] Test–retest reliability: ICC = 0.99 for total scale.[28] ICC for tests 1 week apart = 0.98[32] and 0.96.[34] Internal consistency: Cronbach's $\alpha = 0.96$[35] and 0.92–0.98[32]	Significant changes in scores at 6 and 12 weeks poststroke.[36] Minimal detectable change value = 7 points[34]	*Strengths:* Measures many aspects of balance; consistent reports of excellent reliability; evidence of validity.[10] *Weaknesses:* Long administration time. Has floor and ceiling effects.[32] Not predictive of falls.[32,33]
Functional Reach Test[37]	To assess the functional standing balance performance of older adults[38]	1–2 minutes	Concurrent validity: $r = 0.71$ with center of pressure excursion.[37] Discriminant validity: Significant difference between persons with high and low risk of falls. Predictive validity: score ≤6 inches predictive of falls in elderly[39]	Inter-rater reliability: $r = 0.98$ Test–retest reliability: ICC = 0.92[37]	Marginal significant change ($p = 0.07$) after physical rehabilitation, responsiveness index = 0.97[40]	*Strengths*: Brief, functional test; excellent reliability; evidence of validity.[10] *Weakness*: Sensitivity is borderline.[10]
Tinetti Performance Oriented Mobility Assessment (POMA)[29]	To measure balance and gait[41] of older adults to determine mobility status and changes over time and determine risk of fall. Individual scores	10–15 minutes	Concurrent validity with TUG −0.56 to −0.68 (all three subtests); Discriminant validity: discriminates among persons using various types of walking aids[43]	Inter-rater reliability $r = 0.87$[41]; 0.80–0.93 (all three subtests)[43] Test–retest reliability: Spearman $R = 0.72–0.86$ (all three subtests)[43]	Sensitive (0.70 with 0.52 specificity) to 1 or more falls in 225 community-dwelling elders. With a high cutoff score, 125 tested positive, but sensitivity decreased rapidly with other cutoff values.[44]	*Strengths*: Brief administration time; reliable and valid tool for assessing mobility status.[41] *Weaknesses:* The gait subtest has lower reliability and validity, limiting the ability of the POMA scale for predicting falls.[42,43]

(continued)

Psychometric Properties of Assessments of Balance (*continued*)

Instrument and Reference	Intended Purpose	Administration Time	Validity	Reliability	Sensitivity	Strengths And Weaknesses
	are combined to [illegible] measures: overall [illegible] assessment score (POMA-[illegible]), overall balance assessment score (POMA-B), and a combined score (POMA-T).[42]					
Timed Up-and-Go Test (TUG)[30]	An objective clinical measure for assessing functional mobility, balance, and the risk of falling[45]	1–2 minutes (86 second average time including instructions)[46]	Convergent validity: Moderately or strongly correlated with Tinetti balance scores ($r = -0.55$), Tinetti gait scores ($r = -0.53$), and Tinetti walking speed ($r = 0.66$).[46] Discriminant validity: Excellent—older adults who had experienced a fall in the previous year, used a walking aid, and suffered greater ADL disabilities required a longer time to complete the TUG.[46]	Inter-rater reliability: ICC ≥ 0.87[47] Test–retest reliability: Pearson correlation coefficients (r) = 0.73–0.99[47]	Higher pooled specificity (0.73, 95% CI, 0.51–0.88) than sensitivity (0.32, 95% CI, 0.14–0.57)[48]	*Strengths*: Brief administration time; reliable and valid measure of functional mobility[30]; good test–retest reliability and discriminant validity; Clients may be more willing to participate in TUG than other measures.[46] *Weaknesses*: May not be accurate in predicting fall risk[46,48]; may be more appropriate for older persons who are frail or use mobility aids[46]; does not address performance while performing a simultaneous motor task.[45]

Evidence Table of Remediation Intervention Studies

Intervention	Description	Participants	Dosage	Research Design and Evidence Level	Benefit	Statistical Significance And Effect Size
Therapeutic exercise[22]	Progressive resistance and balance exercises combined with motivational group discussions (see study for details)	Community-dwelling individuals with a stroke 1–3 years prior	Twice weekly × 12 weeks	Randomized controlled trial—Level I	Significant improvement in balance	Berg Balance Scale—MD 2.5 vs. 0 points; effect size (ES), 0.72; $p < 0.01$
Yoga[23]	A yoga-based rehabilitation intervention on balance, balance self-efficacy, fear of falling (FoF), and quality of life	People with chronic stroke	Twice per week × 8 weeks. Seated, standing, and floor postures with relaxation and meditation	Prospective, randomized pilot study—Level I	Significant improvement in balance. Potential in improving multiple poststroke variables as a complement to rehabilitation in medical- and community-based settings. May be cost-effective	Balance (Berg Balance Scale)—41.3 ± 11.7 vs. 46.3 ± 9.1; $p = 0.001$ FoF—51% vs. 46% with FoF; $p < 0.001$
Tai chi[24]	A tailored tai chi program to improve postural control	People with idiopathic Parkinson disease	Sixty minutes, twice per week × 24 weeks	Randomized, controlled trial—Level I	Reduced balance impairments in patients with mild-to-moderate Parkinson disease. Additional benefits of improved functional capacity and reduced falls	The tai chi group performed consistently better than resistance training and stretching groups (between-group difference in the change from baseline, 5.55 percentage points; 95% confidence interval [CI], 1.12–9.97; and 11.98 percentage points; 95% CI, 7.21–16.74, respectively) and in directional control (10.45 percentage points; 95% CI, 3.89–17.00; and 11.38 percentage points; 95% CI, 5.50–17.27, respectively).
Repetitive task training[21]	Training approaches that include performance of goal-directed, individualized tasks with frequent repetitions of task-related or task-specific movements	People with motor impairments after stroke	Nine studies included outcome measures addressing balance and mobility.	Systematic review—Level I	Seven of the nine studies reported positive effects for improving balance and mobility.	None reported

References

1. American Occupational Therapy Association. Occupational therapy practice framework: domain and process (3rd ed.). *Am J Occup Ther.* 2014;68(suppl 1):S1–S48. doi:10.5014/ajot.2014.682006.
2. Franc IA. Balancing act: documenting sitting balance in acute care. *OT Practice.* 2018;23(3):8–11. doi:10.7138/otp.2018.2303.f1.
3. Cercone ML, Grulke-Kidd KM, Haskin AS, Medearis KM, Wegner CJ, Herlache-Pretzer E. Establishing normative values for the Barnett Balance Assessment tool: a preliminary study. *Open J Occup Ther.* 2014;2(2). doi:10.15453/2168-6408.1081.
4. Beauchamp MK, Sibley KM, Lakhani B, et al. Impairments in systems underlying control of balance in COPD. *Chest.* 2012;141(61):1496–1503. doi:10.1378/chest.11-1708.
5. Maki BE, McIlroy WE. Control of rapid limb movements for balance recovery: age-related changes and implications for fall prevention. *Age Ageing. 2006;35(suppl 2):*ii12–ii18. doi:10.1093/ageing/afl078.
6. Kluding P, Swafford BB, Cagle P, Gajewski BJ. Reliability, responsiveness, and validity of the Kansas University Standing Balance Scale. *J Geriatr Phys Ther.* 2006;29(3):93–99. doi:10.1519/00139143-200612000-00003.
7. Sabari JS, Capasso N, Feld-Glazman R. Optimizing motor planning and performance in clients with neurological disorders. In: Radomski MV, Trombly Latham CA, eds. *Occupational Therapy for Physical Dysfunction.* 7th ed. Baltimore, MD: Lippincott, Williams, and Wilkins. 2014:614–674.
8. Herron DG. The ups and downs of motion sickness. *Am J Nurs.* 2010;110(12):49–51. doi:10.1097/01.NAJ.0000391242.75887.17.
9. Wooten SV, Signorile JF, Desai SS, Paine AK, Mooney K. Yoga meditation (YoMed) and its effect on proprioception and balance function in elders who have fallen: a randomized control study. *Complement Ther Med.* 2018;36:129–136. doi:10.1016/j.ctim.2017.12.010.
10. Almhdawi K, Mathiowetz V, Bass JD. Assessing abilities and capacities: motor planning and performance. In: Radomski MV, Trombly Latham CA, eds. *Occupational Therapy for Physical Dysfunction.* 7th ed. Baltimore, MD: Lippincott, Williams, and Wilkins. 2014:242–275.
11. Pollock SP, Durward BR, Rowe, PJ. What is balance? *Clin Rehabil.* 2000;14:402–406. doi:10.1191/0269215500cr342oa.
12. Goodpaster BH, Park SW, Harris TB, et al. The loss of skeletal muscle strength, mass, and quality in older adults: the health, aging and body composition study. *J Gerontol A Biol Sci Med Sci.* 2006;10(1):1059–1064. doi:10.1093/gerona/61.10.1059.
13. Carty CP, Barrett RS, Cronin NJ, Lichtward GA, Mills PM. Lower limb muscle weakness predicts use of a multiple- versus single-step strategy to recover from forward loss of balance in older adults. *J Gerontol A Biol Sci Med Sci.* 2012;67(11):1246–1252. doi:10.1093/gerona/gls149.
14. Balance Disorders. MedicineNet.com. https://www.medicinenet.com/vestibular_balance_disorders/article.htm#how_is_a_balance_disorder_diagnosed. Accessed March 28, 2018.
15. NIDCD Fact Sheet: Balance Disorders. U.S. Department of Health and Human Services: National Institutes of Health. https://www.nidcd.nih.gov/health/balance-disorders. NIH Pub. No. 00-4374. Published December, 2017. Updated March 6, 2018. Accessed March 29, 2018.
16. Grading for Balance: Graded Posture Movement Ability of Individual. Stanbridge College. http://mystudyfocussheet.weebly.com/uploads/1/2/6/2/12621943/grading_for_balance-graded_posture_movement_ability_of_individual-v3.pdf. Accessed March 28, 2018.
17. Prost E. Kansas University Balance Scale. Geriatric Examination Tool Kit. University of Missouri, School of Health Professions, Department of Physical Therapy. http://geriatrictoolkit.missouri.edu/balance/ku-balance-scale/index.htm. Updated February 15, 2018. Accessed March 28, 2018.
18. Chang P-FJ, Kuo Y-F. Functional improvement in older adults after a falls prevention pilot study. *Open J Occup Ther.* 2013;1(2). doi:10.15453/2168-6408.1029.
19. Brown CJ, Flood KL. Mobility limitation in the older patient: a clinical review. *JAMA.* 2013;310(11):1168–1177. doi:10.1001/jama.2013.276566.
20. Peterson MD, Gordon PM. Resistance exercise for the aging adult: clinical implications and prescription guidelines. *Am J Med.* 2011;124:194–198. doi:10.1016/j.amjmed.2010.08.020.
21. Nilsen DM, Gillen G, Geller D, Hreha K, Osei E, Saleem GT. Effectiveness of interventions to improve occupational performance of people with motor impairments after stroke: an evidence-based review. *Am J Occup Ther.* 2015;69(1):6901180030p1–6901180030p9. doi:10.5014/ajot.2015.011965.
22. Vahlberg B, Cederhom T, Lindmark B, Zetterberg L, Hellström K. Short-term and long-term effects of a progressive resistance and balance exercise program in individuals with chronic stroke: a randomized controlled trial. *Disabil Rehabil.* 2017;39 (16):1615–1622. doi:10.1080/09638288.2016.1206631.
23. Schmid AA, Van Puymbroeck M, Altenburger PA, et al. Poststroke balance improved with yoga: a pilot study. *Stroke.* 2012;43(9):2402–2047. doi:10.1161/STROKEAHA.112.658211.
24. Fuzhong L, Harmer P, Fitzgerald K, et al. Tai chi and postural stability in patients with Parkinson's disease. *N Engl J Med.* 2012;366(6):511–519. doi.org/10.1056/NEJMoa1107911.
25. Gillespie LD, Robertson MC, Gillespie WJ, et al. Interventions for preventing falls in older people living in the community. *Cochrane Database Syst Rev.* 2009;(2). doi:10.1002/14651858.CD007146.pub2.
26. Gillespie LD, Roberston MC, Gillespie WJ, et al. Interventions for preventing falls in older people living in the community. *Cochrane Database Syst Rev.* 2012;(9). doi:10.1002/14651858.CD007146.pub3.
27. American Geriatrics Society, British Geriatrics Society, and American Academy of Orthopaedic Surgeons Panel on Fall Prevention. Guideline for the prevention of falls in older persons. *J Am Geriatr Soc.* 2001;49:664–672. doi:10.1046/j.1532-5415.2001.49115.x.
28. Berg K, Maki B, Williams JI, Holliday PJ, Wood-Dauphinee S. Clinical and laboratory measures of postural

balance in an elderly population. *Arch Phys Med Rehabil.* 1992;73:1073–1080.
29. Tinetti ME. Performance-oriented assessment of mobility problems in elderly patients. *J Am Geriatr Soc.* 1986;34:119–126. doi:10.1111/j.1532-5415.1986.tb05480.x.
30. Podsiadlo D, Richardson S. The timed "up and go": a test of basic mobility for frail elderly persons. *J Am Geriatr Soc.* 1991;39:42–148. doi:10.1111/j.1532-5415.1991.tb01616.x.
31. Salavati M, Negahban H, Mazaheri M, et al. The Persian version of the Berg Balance Scale: inter and intra-rater reliability and construct validity in elderly adults. *Disabil Rehabil.* 2012;34(20):1695–1698. doi:10.3109/09638288.2012.660604.
32. Blum L, Korner-Bitensky N. Usefulness of the Berg Balance Scale in stroke rehabilitation: a systematic review. *Phys Ther.* 2008;88:559–566. doi:10.2522/ptj.20070205.
33. Wirz M, Müller R, Bastiaenen C. Falls in persons with spinal cord injury: validity and reliability of the Berg Balance Scale. *Neurorehabil Neural Repair.* 2010;24:70–77. doi:10.1177/1545968309341059.
34. Learmonth YC, Paul L, McFadyen AK, Mattison P, Miller L. Reliability and clinical significance of mobility and balance assessments in multiple sclerosis. *Int J Rehabil Res.* 2012;35:69–74. doi:10.1097/MRR.0b013e328350b65f.
35. Berg K, Wood-Dauphinee S, Williams JI, Gayton D. Measuring balance in the elderly: preliminary development of an instrument. *Physiother Can.* 1989;41:301–311. doi:10.3138/ptc.41.6.304.
36. Wood-Dauphinee S, Berg K, Bravo G, Williams I. The Balance Scale: responsiveness to clinically meaningful changes. *Can J Rehabil.* 1997;10:35–50.
37. Duncan PW, Weiner DK, Chandler J, Studenski S. Functional reach: a new clinical measure of balance. *J Gerontol.* 1990;45:M192–M195. doi:10.1093/geronj/45.6.M192.
38. Lin Y-H, Chen T-R, Shan C, Tang Y-W. A reliability study for standing Functional Reach Test using modified and traditional rulers. *Percept Mot Skills.* 2012;115(2):512–520. doi:10.2466/15.03.10.PMS.115.5.512-520.
39. Duncan PW, Studenski S, Chandler J, Prescott B. Functional reach: predictive validity in a sample of elderly male veterans. *J Gerontol.* 1992;47:M93–M98. doi:10.1093/geronj/47.3.M93.
40. Weiner DK, Bongiorni DR, Studenski S, Duncan PW, Kochersberger GG. Does functional reach improve with rehabilitation? *Arch Phys Med Rehabil.* 1993;74:796–800. doi:10.1016/0003-9993(93)90003-S.
41. Kegelmeyer DA, Kloos AD, Thomas KM, Kostyk SK. Reliability and validity of the Tinetti Mobility Test for individuals with Parkinson disease. *Phys Ther.* 2007;87:1369–1378. doi:10.2522/ptj.20070007.
42. Amini DA. Motor assessments. In: Asher IE, ed. *Occupational Therapy Assessment Tools: An Annotated Index*. 3rd ed. Bethesda, MD: AOTA Press; 2007.
43. Faber MJ, Bosscher RU, van Wieringen PCW. Clinimetric properties of the performance-oriented mobility assessment. *Phys Ther.* 2006;86(7):944–954.
44. Panzer VP, Wakefield DB, Hall CB, Wolfson LI. Mobility assessment: sensitivity and specificity of measurement sets in older adults. *Arch Phys Med Rehabil.* 2011;92:905–912. doi:10.1016/j.apmr.2011.01.004.
45. Chan PP, Si Tou JI, Tse MM, Ng SS. Reliability and validity of the Timed Up and Go test with a motor task in people with chronic stroke. *Arch Phys Med Rehabil.* 2017;98:2213–2230. doi:10.1016/j.apmr.2017.03.008.
46. Lin M-R, Hwang H-F, Hu M-H, Isaac H-D, Wang Y-W, Huang F-C. Psychometric comparisons of the Timed Up and Go, One-Leg Stand, Functional Reach, and Tinetti balance measure in community-dwelling older people. *J Am Geriatr Soc.* 2004;52:1343–1348. doi:10.1111/j.1532-5415.2004.52366.x.
47. Morris S, Morris ME, Iansek R. Reliability of measurements obtained with the Timed "Up & GO" test in people with Parkinson disease. *Phys Ther.* 2001;81(2):810–818. doi:10.1093/ptj/81.2.810.
48. Barry E, Galvin R, Keogh C, Horgan F, Fahey T. Is the Timed UP and Go test a useful predictor of risk of falls in community dwelling older adults: a systematic review and meta-analysis. *BMC Geriatr.* 2014;14(14):1–14. doi:10.1186/1471-2318-14-14.

Chapter 18

Communication Assessment and Intervention

Anne Escher, Sue Berger, and Anne Carney

LEARNING OBJECTIVES

This chapter will allow the reader to:

1. Describe the impact of communication impairment on occupational performance.
2. Identify conditions in adults that lead to communication impairment.
3. Understand communication impairment patterns based on diagnosis or described lesion.
4. Discuss the role of the occupational therapist in screening and evaluating occupational performance for people with communication impairment.
5. Select occupational performance assessment methods and instruments based on individual characteristics, including communication abilities.
6. Discuss strategies to adapt self-report assessments to support individuals with communication impairments to participate in collaborative goal setting, complete outcome measures, and engage in research.
7. Describe specific interventions to support communication performance.
8. Use interventions to support occupational performance for people with communication impairments.
9. Understand the role of speech language pathologists and the importance of collaboration.

CHAPTER OUTLINE

TERMINOLOGY

Acalculia: acquired impairment of the ability to perform basic mathematical operations.

Agraphia: acquired writing impairment that frequently co-occurs with aphasia.

Alexia: acquired reading impairment that frequently co-occurs with aphasia.

Anomia: condition that refers to difficulty with word retrieval.

Aphasia: language disorder resulting from damage to certain areas of the brain and is characterized by difficulty with speaking, understanding, reading, or writing.

Apraxia of speech (AoS): motor speech disorder that limits the ability to plan and program the production of speech.

Dysarthria: motor speech disorder caused by weakness or difficulty controlling the muscles for speech, which may result in slurred or mumbled sounding speech.

Communication Function and Impairment in Daily Occupation

Communication imbues most daily occupations. Many activities in which people engage throughout the day involve communication, including instrumental activities of daily living (IADL), education, work, play, leisure, and social participation. Whereas some activities of daily living (ADL) may be performed independently without communication, many basic ADLs require communication when individuals need to direct caregivers for assistance.

Given that communication is such an important part of occupational performance, occupational therapists must understand and respond to clients' communication challenges. The *Occupational Therapy Practice Framework: Domain and Process*[1] categorizes communication management as an IADL, defined as:

> Sending, receiving, and interpreting information using a variety of systems and equipment, including writing tools, telephones (cell phones or smartphones), keyboards, audiovisual recorders, computers or tablets, communication boards, call lights, emergency systems, Braille writers, telecommunication devices for deaf people, augmentative communication systems, and personal digital assistants.

This definition focuses primarily on technology use, but communication also includes verbal and nonverbal information exchange. The American Speech-Language-Hearing Association describes functional communication skills as "forms of behavior that express needs, wants, feelings, and preferences that others can understand."[2] This chapter uses a broad conceptualization of communication that includes both communication management (sending, receiving, and interpreting information from systems including other people) and functional communication (being able to express needs and wants in ways that others can understand) to address how communication influences occupational performance.

Communication influences occupational performance in multiple and complex ways. People's quality of life and rates of psychosocial health indicators (frustration, hopelessness, depression) can all be impacted by the onset of communication challenges.[3,4] Additionally, researchers have found that people with communication impairments have lower rates of participation in meaningful activities.[3]

Worrall and colleagues[4] found that because communication impairments significantly impact relationships, people with **aphasia** (a language disorder characterized by difficulty with speaking, understanding, reading, or writing) identified social, leisure, and work participation as key rehabilitation goals. People with aphasia post-stroke desire to contribute to society in meaningful ways and to practice altruism.[4] Such meaningful goals, however, are often overlooked in rehabilitation settings. Practitioners may not recognize how best to engage clients and inadvertently fail to address clients' self-identified occupational performance goals. Despite the fact that collaborative goal setting has been shown to increase both motivation and the likelihood of achieving goals,[5] people with communication impairments are rarely included in the goal-setting process.[6] Along with occupational performance impairments, limited involvement in collaborative goal setting, and difficulty participating in the rehabilitation process, clients with communication impairments are often excluded from research, unless studies specifically address communication impairment.[7]

Neurological and Physiological Basis of Communication

In 1861, Paul Broca—French anatomist, anthropologist, and neurologist—encountered a patient who lost the ability to produce meaningful speech but retained his ability to comprehend language. During autopsy of the patient, Broca observed a lesion located in the left posterior inferior frontal gyrus. Broca subsequently observed lesions in the same frontal lobe area in other patients with similar losses of spoken language. This area, which became known as Broca's area, continues to be a region critical for speech production. More than a decade later, Carl Wernicke—a German anatomist, neurologist, and psychiatrist—observed a loss of language comprehension that he linked to lesions located in the left posterior temporal lobe. This area became known as Wernicke's area and remains a key region for language comprehension (Fig. 18-1). Although Broca and Wernicke's areas remain critical for the production and comprehension of language, there is an increasing body of research using neuroimaging techniques that has clarified our understanding of how the brain processes language. This rapidly evolving body of research has implicated the involvement of widespread brain networks for language processing in both the left and right hemispheres.[8,9]

Neuroanatomical Structures and Functions

An overview of central and peripheral nervous system areas that possess large roles in the support of speech and language is explained in the subsequent sections (for further reading, refer to Bhatnagar,[10] Duffy,[11] Helm-Estabrooks et al.,[12] and Seikel et al.[13]).

The Central Nervous System: Brain

The lips, tongue, and teeth are among the articulators that help us make speech sounds. The brain, however, is responsible for the planning, initiation, and coordination of the motor movements of those articulators, as well as for selecting the words, grammatical structures, and tone with which we choose to convey our needs, wants, thoughts, and feelings.

Although recent evidence indicates that language functions are supported by widespread neural networks

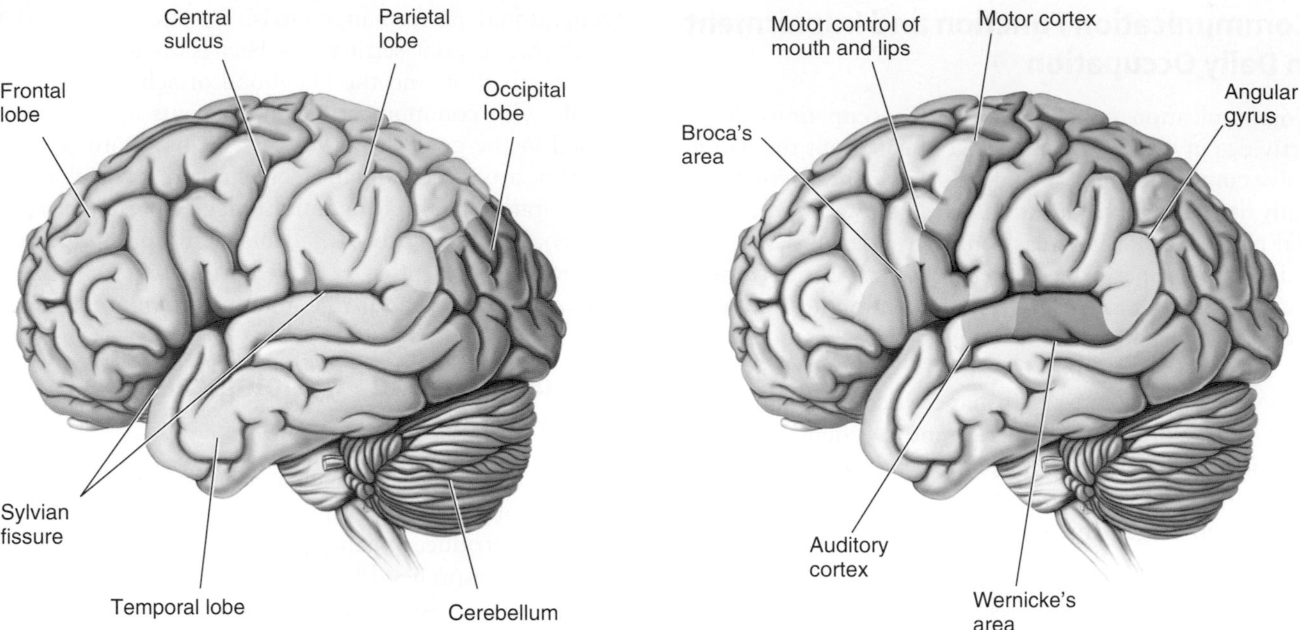

Figure 18-1. Two lateral views of the left hemisphere of the brain, which for the majority of people is the language-dominant hemisphere. Broca's area is located in the left frontal lobe and Wernicke's area in the left temporal lobe.

across both hemispheres, cerebral dominance for language remains a firmly established principle.[14] For most of the population—upward of 95% of right handers and 70% of left handers—the left hemisphere is dominant for language. The remaining 30% of left handers may have either bilateral dominance or right hemisphere language dominance.[15] This is evidenced clinically: individuals who sustain strokes in the left hemisphere may experience the language disorder known as aphasia; whereas strokes sustained in the right hemisphere are characterized by impairments related to attention, perception, problem-solving, memory, and/or social communication (e.g., difficulty following the turn-taking rules of conversation or interpreting nonverbal communication such as facial expression or tone).

In addition to lateralization of brain functions, another key principle related to the understanding of communication is neuroplasticity, or the brain's ability to change and reorganize in response to experiences. Although the brain's plasticity is greatest during childhood, the capacity for reorganization continues throughout the life span. Adults who sustain traumatic brain injury (TBI) or stroke provide evidence for the brain's ongoing ability to reorganize itself, as observed when uninjured regions of the brain assume language functions previously associated with injured areas.[16]

Frontal Lobe

The frontal lobe contains the primary motor cortex or "motor strip," which is involved in the control of voluntary motor movements on the opposite side of the body. A motor homunculus, or "little human," serves as a neurological map, representing the region where motor processing occurs for each body part (Fig. 18-2). The homunculus is distorted because the amount of cortical space designated for each body part does not correspond

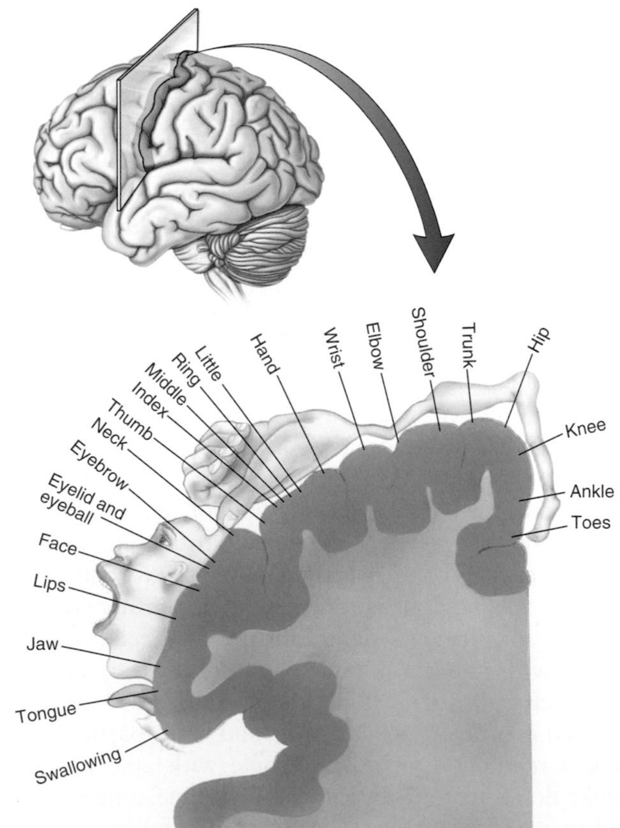

Figure 18-2. A motor homunculus acts as a neurological map that indicates the location in the frontal lobe where motor activity is processed for different parts of the body.

to body part size, but rather to processing complexity. For example, the lips and tongue are oversized in the homunculus because the small and precise movements required to form speech sounds take up more cortical space than the less nuanced movements of the hip or knee.

The premotor and supplementary motor cortices of the frontal lobe are linked to the initiation and planning of motor activity. The frontal lobe of the language-dominant hemisphere also contains Broca's area, known to be important for speech production. Another critical area of the frontal lobe is the prefrontal cortex, which is linked to executive functions such as planning, problem-solving, and judgment, as well as mood, personality, and emotion. Lesions in the prefrontal region, such as those resulting from TBI, can lead to impairment in inhibition, impulse control, flexibility, and self-monitoring, which can negatively impact social communication or pragmatics.

Temporal Lobe

The temporal lobe is responsible for hearing and analyzing auditory information. Areas within the temporal lobe in the language-dominant hemisphere that transform auditory stimuli into meaning include the auditory cortex, auditory association area, and Wernicke's area. The temporal lobe is also home to the hippocampus, which is critical for memory.

Parietal Lobe

The main function of the parietal lobe is related to processing somesthetic sensations (e.g., tactile sensation and proprioception). Damage to the left (or language-dominant) parietal lobe can also result in reading impairments (**alexia**), writing impairments (**agraphia**), calculation impairments (**acalculia**), and aphasia.

The Peripheral Nervous System: Cranial Nerves

There are 12 paired cranial nerves (CNs) that relay motor and sensory information to and from the brain to parts of the head and neck, as well as to certain sensory organs and glands. CNs serve a critical role in the production of speech as well as in nonverbal communication. The CNs are numbered I through XII based on the location from which they enter and/or exit the brain or brainstem (Fig. 18-3).

The CN pairs that are most important for communication are CN V, CN VII, CN IX, CN X, CN XI, and CN XII. CN V, the trigeminal nerve, supports jaw movement, which is important for articulation. CN VII, the facial nerve, is responsible for facial expression and movement of the lips, which is critical for the production of labial and labiodental sounds (i.e., sounds involving the lips such as "m" and "p," and sounds involving the lips and teeth such as "f" and "v"). CN IX, the glossopharyngeal nerve, is a smaller CN that is closely linked to CN X, the vagus nerve. CN X supports movement of the vocal folds or vocal cords, which allows for phonation or the production of sound. CN X is also responsible for movement of the soft palate, which is involved in resonance. CN XI, the spinal accessory nerve, supports gestures involving the head and shoulders that are important for nonverbal communication (e.g., shrugging shoulders and shaking head). Lastly, CN XII, the hypoglossal nerve, is responsible for tongue movement, which is a key articulator for speech production.

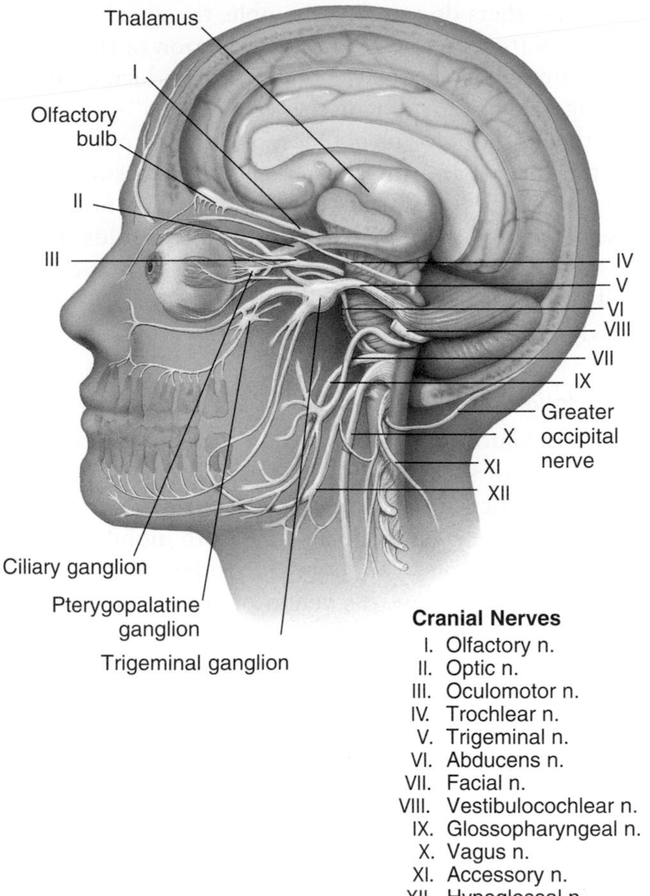

Figure 18-3. A lateral view of the 12 cranial nerves.

Anatomy and Physiology of Speech

The systems involved in speech production include respiration, phonation, articulation, and resonance. An overview of each system follows.

Respiration

Air from the lungs provides the energy source for speaking. During speech production, inhalations become shorter in duration, whereas exhalations become longer. Weaknesses or changes to the musculature in the respiratory system may contribute to hypophonia or reduced loudness.

Phonation

During speech production, the air from the lungs travels through the larynx and passes between the vocal folds (or vocal cords). Some speech sounds involve voicing, whereas others do not. For example, the vocal folds are adducted (together) during the production of the voiced "z" sound, whereas the vocal folds are abducted (apart) during the production of the voiceless "s" sound. To feel the vibration or its absence, one can place the hand on the throat, and produce and hold both sounds for several seconds. Trauma, stroke, and other neurological diseases can weaken or paralyze the vocal folds. Paralysis of one vocal fold will still allow for phonation, but will result in a breathy quality. If both vocal folds are paralyzed, phonation can be absent.

Articulation and Resonance

The articulatory and resonance systems shape air into the sounds of speech. Once air passes between the vocal folds, the articulators interact to create the speech sounds known as phonemes. Humans have both mobile and immobile articulators. The mobile articulators include the tongue, the lower jaw, the velum or soft palate, and the lips. The immobile articulators are the alveolar ridge of the upper jaw (the ridge located just behind the upper front teeth and in front of the hard palate), the hard palate, and the teeth. Consider the action required to produce the "t" sound versus the "v" sound: the tongue makes contact with the alveolar ridge to make the "t" sound, whereas the teeth make contact with the lower lip to make the "v" sound.

Resonance is the way that airflow is modified as it passes through the oral and nasal cavities. The velum or soft palate, which is located just behind the hard palate along the roof of the mouth away from the alveolar ridge, differentiates nasal sounds from non-nasal sounds. In English, the nasal sounds are "n," "m," and the "ng", the latter of which is the sound at the end of the word "sing." To form these sounds, the velum lowers, allowing air to travel through the nasal cavity. Resonance disorders include hyponasality and hypernasality. Hyponasality occurs when inadequate air travels through the nasal cavity for the production of nasal sounds, similar to how people sound when they have a cold or congestion. Hypernasality, or nasal speech, occurs when too much air is allowed to flow through the nasal cavity during speech, such as in individuals with cleft palate. Resonance disorders can result from trauma, stroke, or neurological disease, such as amyotrophic lateral sclerosis (ALS) and multiple sclerosis.[13]

Conceptual Foundation Underlying the Role of Occupational Therapy for Communication Impairment

The *International Classification of Functioning, Disability, and Health*[17] (ICF) is a framework used by health care professionals to describe, organize, and guide assessment and intervention for individuals of all ages and health conditions. The classification system provides a common language for health care professionals when discussing clients, groups, and populations. The ICF includes a section labeled *voice and speech functions* under body functions and *structures involved in voice and speech* under body structures. Within *activities and participation,* there is an entire chapter on communication with sections on *communicating-receiving, communicating-producing,* and *conversation and use of communication devices and techniques.* This section is separate from chapters on *domestic life, interpersonal interactions and relationships, education, work and employment,* and *community, social and civic life,* all activities that involve communication. The ICF section about environmental factors addresses the physical, social, and societal environments that influence one's ability to communicate. Even personal factors, not elaborated upon in the ICF, influence communication.[18] For example, people who are assertive might request others to repeat comments or slow down to facilitate understanding, whereas others may not verbalize such requests and struggle to engage in conversation. Each of these major ICF groupings (e.g., body function and environments) can be a facilitator or barrier to communication. Understanding the interaction between them can guide occupational therapy assessment and intervention.

The Participation, Environment, Occupation (PEO) model[19] is another way to conceptualize communication that overlaps with the ICF. The focus of occupational therapy is to enable participation, for this chapter, focusing on communication participation. The PEO model contends that the interaction of person factors, environmental factors, and occupations—considered together—supports or limits participation. Assessing and addressing the occupational and environmental factors related to communication are within the scope of occupational therapy practice, whereas assessing and providing intervention at the body function/body structure level of the person factors related to communication are not. Rather, occupational therapists refer to speech language pathologists (SLPs) to address speech and language impairments. SLPs understand the underlying mechanisms of speech and language, and thus, much of their assessment and intervention focuses on remediating impairments, identifying compensatory strategies, and supporting goals that are meaningful to clients. Occupational therapists focus on participation and supporting clients to engage in the occupations of choice, despite communication impairments. Therefore, occupational therapists use compensatory and adaptive strategies to support occupational performance in people with communication impairments.

Most importantly, occupational therapists use an ecological approach—focusing on participation within an individual's natural environment—when assessing how communication influences occupational performance and providing intervention to support communication

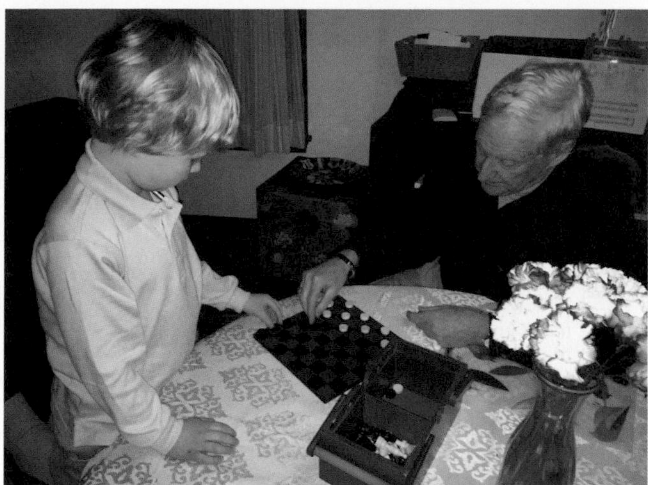

Figure 18-4. Playing checkers with grandchild in the home environment.

participation (Fig. 18-4). For example, although an individual may perform well communicating in a private treatment room during occupational therapy, the same individual may struggle to communicate at home when the television is on in the background, or at a party while many people are talking at once. Occupational therapists consider communication in both ideal and naturalistic settings to determine supports and barriers to participation. Therapy goals focus on supporting individuals to communicate where they live, work, and play.

Communication: Disorders, Signs and Symptoms, and Causes

Communication disorders in adults may start in childhood or can arise due to an acquired illness or injury. The following section describes some acquired speech and language disorders seen in the adult population, including apraxia of speech (AoS), dysarthria, and aphasia.

Speech Disorders

AoS and dysarthria are considered motor speech disorders. They result from neurological injury or illness and affect an individual's ability to plan, program, control, or execute speech production.

Apraxia of Speech

Apraxia of speech (AoS) is predominantly characterized by a reduced overall speech rate and distortions in articulation and prosody, or the rhythm of speech. In the area of articulation, sounds may be imprecise, distorted, substituted, added, or deleted. In the area of prosody, disruptions include segregating words into individual syllables and equalizing stress across syllables.[11] AoS is caused by illness or injury to the left or language-dominant hemisphere, most commonly after stroke. AoS frequently co-occurs with aphasia and dysarthria. TBI and neurodegenerative disease can also result in AoS.

Dysarthria

Dysarthria is a motor speech disorder resulting from muscle weakness or difficulty controlling the muscles that are used for speech and is typically caused by stroke, brain injury, tumors, or neurodegenerative disease. Dysarthria is characterized by "abnormalities in the strength, speed, range, steadiness, tone, or accuracy of movements required for the breathing, phonatory, resonatory, articulatory, or prosodic aspects of speech production."[11] Individuals who have dysarthria may slur or mumble speech sounds, or may speak too slowly, quickly, softly, or loudly. There are several different types of dysarthrias that can often be associated with underlying neuropathophysiology. Parkinson disease, for example, is associated with hypokinetic dysarthria, which is characterized by variable speech rate, monopitch, monoloudness, and imprecise articulation. Individuals with ALS typically develop a mixed flaccid–spastic dysarthria, which is characterized by reduced speech rate, imprecise articulation, hypernasality, strained or strangled vocal quality, monopitch, and monoloudness.[20]

Language Disorders

Aphasia: Definitions and Subtypes

Aphasia is a disorder resulting from damage to the brain's language areas. Because most of the population possess language centers in the left cerebral hemisphere, strokes, brain tumors, TBIs, infections, and neurodegenerative diseases that damage the left hemisphere may result in aphasia. The hallmark of aphasia is the presence of **anomia**, or difficulty with word retrieval (i.e., problems finding desired words). Additionally, varying degrees of impairment may exist in comprehension, reading (alexia), writing (agraphia), and math skills (acalculia), depending on the aphasia type and severity of damage.

One of the most common methods for differentiating aphasia subtypes is referred to as the "Boston Classification System."[12] Because all aphasias cannot be classified according to this system, and given that aphasia subtypes may evolve over time with both spontaneous recovery and treatment, a comprehensive speech and language evaluation is important to gain a complete understanding of client strengths and weaknesses with regard to speaking, listening, reading, writing, and functional communication skills. A brief description of three aphasia subtypes is provided that follows.

Broca Aphasia

Broca aphasia, also known as expressive aphasia, is the most common subtype of nonfluent aphasia. In Broca aphasia, spoken utterances can range from single words to short agrammatic phrases that contain mostly nouns and verbs, but are limited in the use of function words, such as articles, auxiliary verbs, and prepositions.

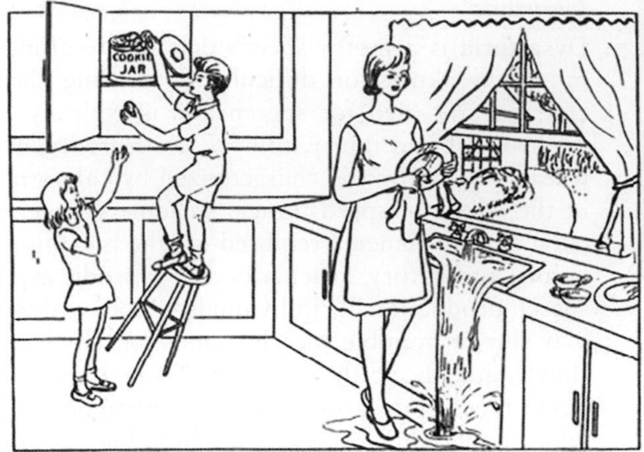

Transcription of an Individual with Broca Aphasia in Response to Cooking Theft Picture:
"Water dripping. Boy" (point to girl) "Girl" (pointing to boy) Okay. Okay... Mother... Mother.".. (What's going on?) "No."

Partial Transcription of an Individual with Wernicke Aphasia in Response to Cooking Theft Picture:
"Oh, this one? Yeah, He's looking at this...Uh this. I know it's a w..wife, and the thing, right at the thing you know the...And it looka...It's a speed...speela...they...she didn't. as it she's so closing it. She didn't close it, so it's open, see? It's up, looka this...it's right down fallin' off.

Figure 18-5. The "Cookie Theft" picture stimulus and transcriptions. (From Goodglass H, Kaplan E, Barresi B, et al. *The Boston Diagnostic Aphasia Examination: BDAE-3 Long Form Kit.* Austin, TX: Pro Ed; 2001. Used with permission from Pro-Ed.)

Spoken communication may seem halting and effortful, which can, in turn, lead to abandoned communication attempts. Although comprehension is commonly described as good or even "intact," clients with Broca aphasia may struggle to understand complex syntax such as passive sentence structures (e.g., "the dog was chased by the bicyclist," as opposed to the active version, "the bicyclist chased the dog"). See Figure 18-5 for an example of a person with Broca aphasia, describing the "Cookie Theft" picture stimulus.

Wernicke Aphasia

Wernicke aphasia is a type of fluent and receptive aphasia in which auditory comprehension is impaired. Although individuals with Wernicke aphasia speak in full sentences that retain intonation and melody, they struggle to convey meaning and their spoken utterances are marked by semantic paraphasias or word substitution errors (e.g., "wife" for "son"), as well as jargon in the form of made-up words and phrases. Clients with Wernicke aphasia have variable awareness of both their expressive and receptive errors, which often results in communication breakdowns. Reading and writing are also typically impaired. See Figure 18-5 for an example of a person with Wernicke aphasia, describing the "Cookie Theft" picture stimulus.

Global Aphasia

Global aphasia is a severe form of nonfluent aphasia in which spoken output and auditory comprehension are both significantly impaired. In global aphasia, individuals have severe anomia and may produce stereotypic utterances or repeated phrases (e.g., "Yeah, right") during attempts to verbalize.

Primary Progressive Aphasia

Primary progressive aphasia (PPA) is a gradual worsening of language skills caused by progressive degeneration of nerve cells in the brain's language areas. PPA differs from aphasia in that it is a degenerative disease. PPA is typically caused by either frontotemporal lobar degeneration or Alzheimer disease.[12]

Communication: Assessing Impact on Occupational Performance

The following section focuses on assessment of occupational performance as it is impacted by communication challenges. The strategies described in the subsequent sections also support collaborative goal setting.

Screening

Occupational therapists always observe and consider client's communication abilities as they influence occupational performance; however, occupational therapists do not screen for communication impairment. Rather, they screen for occupational performance difficulties related to communication challenges. Occupational therapists should perform chart reviews and ask family members or other health care team members about clients' communication abilities. Occupational therapists use clinical observation skills to note whether clients appear to understand what is being said (e.g., whether client responses fit posed questions). At times, it can appear that clients understand everything while they make eye contact, nod, and smile; however, some clients are skilled at masking their communication impairment. When questioning a client's comprehension, it is advisable to screen by providing instructions for the client to follow (such as "pick up the pen") or posing yes/no questions to confirm marital status or living situation. If the client demonstrates communication difficulties, referral to an SLP should be made. Having both an SLP and occupational therapist involved in a client's care will increase the client's potential to improve both communication skills and occupational performance.

Assessing Impact on Daily Occupational Function

For clients with impaired language or speech, occupational therapists should use strategies such as adaptations and modifications to support participation in the evaluation and collaborative goal-setting process. See Table 18-1 for approaches to goal setting and assessment modification based on a review of empirical evidence, universal design principles for learning, and health literacy. For example, adapting questionnaires by placing one question per page, bolding key words, and using sans serif font can make reading easier for some people (Fig. 18-6). In addition, using photographs with simple captions may support comprehension (Fig. 18-7). When administering Likert scales, therapists should use large print and emoticon or smiley faces to denote positive and negative sides. The use of slash marks instead of scale numbers can be considered, depending on the client's level of numeric understanding (Fig. 18-8). There is initial evidence that assessments that have been modified to support communication can still be valid and reliable.[21]

Some assessments have been developed specifically for adults with impaired communication. For example, the Life Interests and Values Cards (LIV),[22] developed by an SLP and occupational therapist team, incorporates many of the strategies in Table 18-1. This measure provides visual cues and uses line drawings depicting different activities in which clients may participate. Visual cues are provided by a large green check mark and red X to facilitate client understanding of the two-pile sort system, in which clients sort activity cards into the categories of "want to do" and "don't want to do."

When assessing clients with communication impairments, it is imperative to assess not only their physical functioning and ADL/IADL performance but also other ways in which their communication impairment impacts their daily lives. For instance, clients with communication impairments may find themselves isolated because

Table 18-1. Key Principles for Modifying Outcome Measures

PRINCIPLE	DESCRIPTION	EXAMPLE
1. Modify the presentation	Use large sans serif font; font that has extra flare is harder to read. Place one item per page to allow clients to focus on one item at a time (see Fig. 18-6).	Modify the Stroke Impact Scale[47] to present one question per page, with larger font.
2. Use simple vocabulary and syntax	Short and clear sentences with commonly used words are best.	When asking clients to rate performance on the Canadian Occupational Performance Measure,[48] use "How good are you at cooking?" instead of "How would you rate your performance in cooking?"
3. Use pictures	Photographs and line drawings are effective if the picture is clear without extra unnecessary details.	Use pictures, the LIV,[22] or Activity Card Sort (ACS)[49] to support both client comprehension and expression of interest in activities (see Fig. 18-6).
4. Provide choices and simplify options	Ask close-ended or yes/no questions. Reduce number of options.	When administering the ACS, ask clients to sort into two piles instead of four to five. Ask them to first sort activity cards into "want to do/do not want to do," then to sort cards from the "want to do" pile into "hard to do" vs. "easy to do."
5. Provide support	Allow clients time to process questions and formulate responses. Provide scaled levels of support.	Repeat questions, restate questions, and verify responses. For example, "How good are you at cooking?" Restate as "How well are you able to make meals?" Verify as "So, you don't cook well?"
6. Adapt the testing environment	Ensure quiet environments with few distractions and provide additional materials.	Provide paper, pen, and visuals (such as maps or letter boards) as needed. Ensure clients are comfortable (doesn't need to use bathroom).

From Haley K, Womack J, Helm-Estabrooks N, Caignon D, McCulloch K. *The Life Interest and Values Cards*. Chapel Hill: University of North Carolina Department of Allied Health Sciences; 2010; Berger S, Escher A, Hildebrand M, Tabor Connor L. Modifying outcome measures to support participation for people with aphasia. *OT Pract*. 2017;22:10–13; Herbert R, Haw C, Brown C, Gregory E, Brumfitt S. Accessible information guidelines: making information accessible for people with aphasia. 2012. https://www.stroke.org.uk/sites/default/files/accessible_information_guidelines.pdf1_.pdf.

How much help do you need for each of the following?

	A lot of help	Some help	A little help	No help
Putting on shirt	1	2	3	4
Putting on pants	1	2	3	4
Putting on socks	1	2	3	4
Putting on shoes	1	2	3	4

How much help do you need to **put on your shirt?**

A lot of help	**Some help**	**A little help**	**No help**
1	2	3	4

Figure 18-6. The top image shows a section of a sample questionnaire regarding self-care. The bottom image shows a modified version of the sample self-care questionnaire, with the following changes made to presentation to support comprehension: one question per page, font changed to sans serif, keywords bolded, shaded row to differentiate numerical choice from word choice, and emoticons.

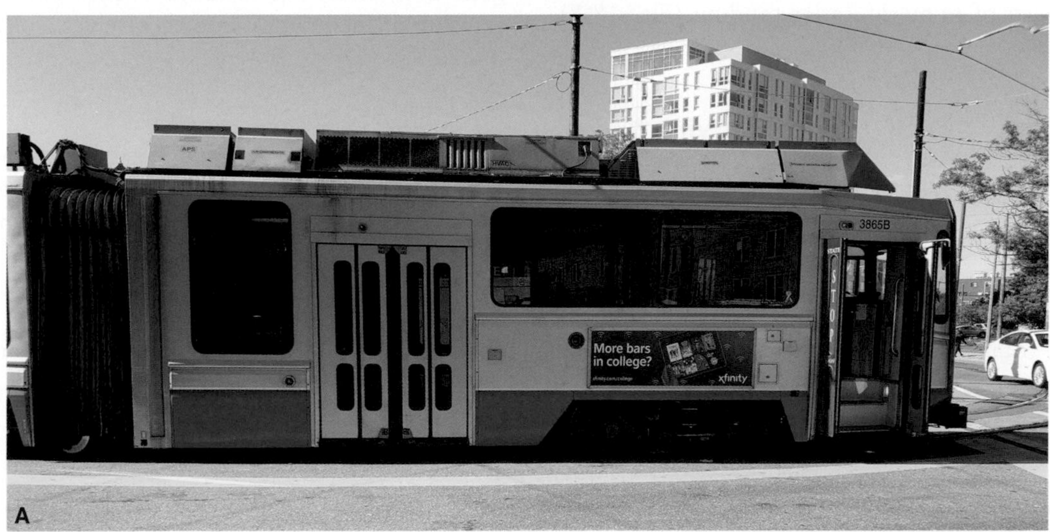

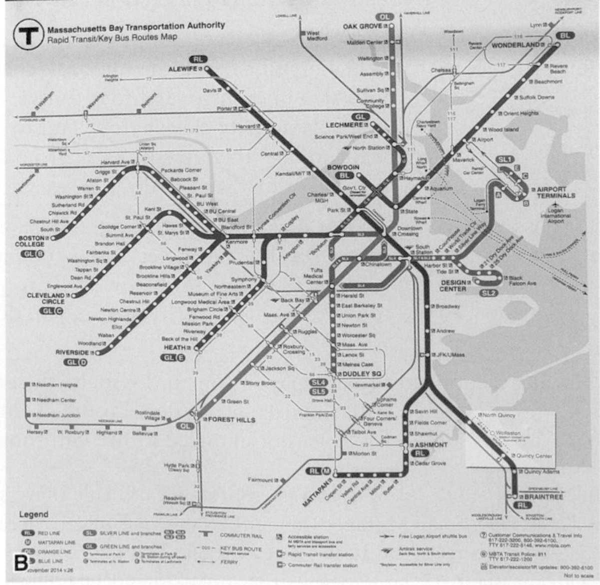

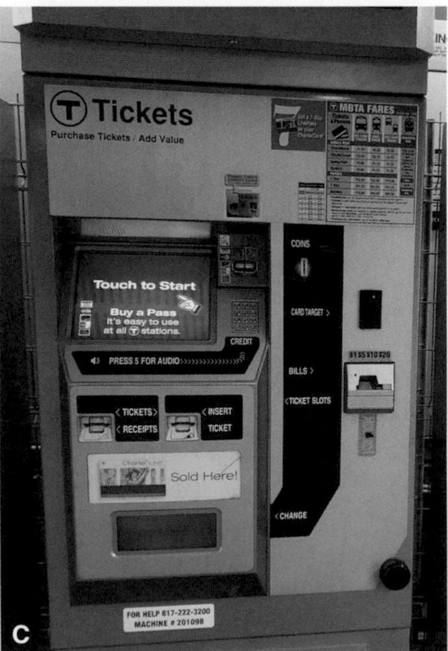

Figure 18-7. A to C. Examples of additional photos to use during evaluation to support collaborative goal setting.

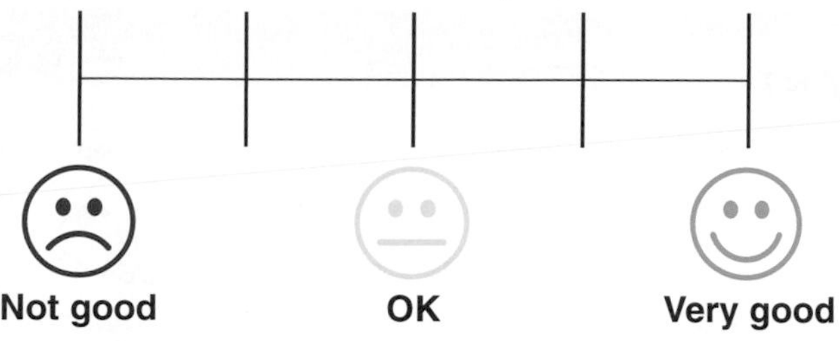

Figure 18-8. Example of a simplified Likert scale using only slash marks, emoticons, and simple words in large font.

of their inability to converse easily with friends and family. Therapists should consider administering an assessment to understand clients' psychosocial status, such as the Geriatric Depression Scale.[23] When administering assessments, it is important to ensure that instruments are accessible to clients by making appropriate modifications as noted earlier and using strategies listed in Table 18-1.

Instruments in the Assessment table at the end of this chapter focus on occupational performance, occupational participation, and communication participation. The Assessment table includes a sampling of instruments developed specifically for people with impaired communication, as well as other evaluations that were developed for a generic population and are user friendly or easily modified for people with communication difficulties. Many additional assessments exist that are administered by SLPs and which provide information related to the impact of communication impairment on participation and quality of life. For example, occupational therapists may encounter results from the following assessments in client charts and research studies: the ASHA Functional Assessment of Communication Skills for Adults[24] (a measure completed by an individual familiar with the client's communication who rates communication independence across functional tasks), ASHA Quality of Communication Life Scale[25] (a self-rating scale that assesses the impact of communication impairment on relationships, communication, and participation), and the Assessment for living with aphasia[26] (a pictographic, self-report assessment of quality of life for individuals with aphasia).

Specific Interventions for Communication Dysfunction

The following are a sampling of evidence-based interventions that occupational therapists can use to maximize participation of clients with communication difficulties. Occupational therapists collaborate with both SLPs and clients in the selection and use of the most appropriate interventions to support participation when communication is impaired (see the Evidence table at the end of this chapter for a selection of evidence related to interventions for communication dysfunction).

Augmentative and Alternative Communication

Augmentative and alternative communication (AAC) includes low- and high-tech solutions and strategies that support communication. Augmentative strategies are used to supplement speech, whereas alternative strategies are used when speech is nonfunctional or absent. The most appropriate AAC for a client varies based on the condition, the client's abilities and challenges, and the context. The type of AAC also depends on the client's recovery stage and continuum.[27] For example, in acute care environments, focusing on communicating basic needs such as expressions of pain or thirst through picture boards may be appropriate. In later recovery stages, when functional status is more stable, the selection of high-tech solutions may be a better option.

AAC includes unaided and aided systems. Unaided systems are strategies that require only the individual and include gesturing, making facial expressions, and using body and sign language. Although some strategies may come naturally, learning to intentionally gesture and exaggerate body language can support communication when speech is limited. Slowing the rate of speech or over articulating are strategies to improve speech intelligibility.

Aided systems require the use of a tool or device and can be as simple as pen and paper or as high tech as a computer. There is strong evidence that low- and high-tech AAC are effective to support communication in functional situations based on multiple systematic reviews.[28,29] Using letter, word, or picture boards or books are options for many (Fig. 18-9). Personalizing these boards by including family member names or favorite foods can make communicating easier and quicker by simply pointing to words instead of spelling them out. It is important to note that word or alphabet boards may not be helpful for those with aphasia. Often clients who struggle to speak due to aphasia will also have difficulty writing and spelling. Sometimes people who struggle to speak or read, however, can point to a first letter or picture, helping the recipient of the information to make educated guesses.

The number and variety of high-tech options to support communication has significantly increased over the past 20 years with the development of many types of computers, tablets, and cell phones, all with accessibility features (Fig. 18-10). However, while many speech generating devices allow users to designate gender, age, and language, digitized speech, although improving, does not sound like human voice.[30]

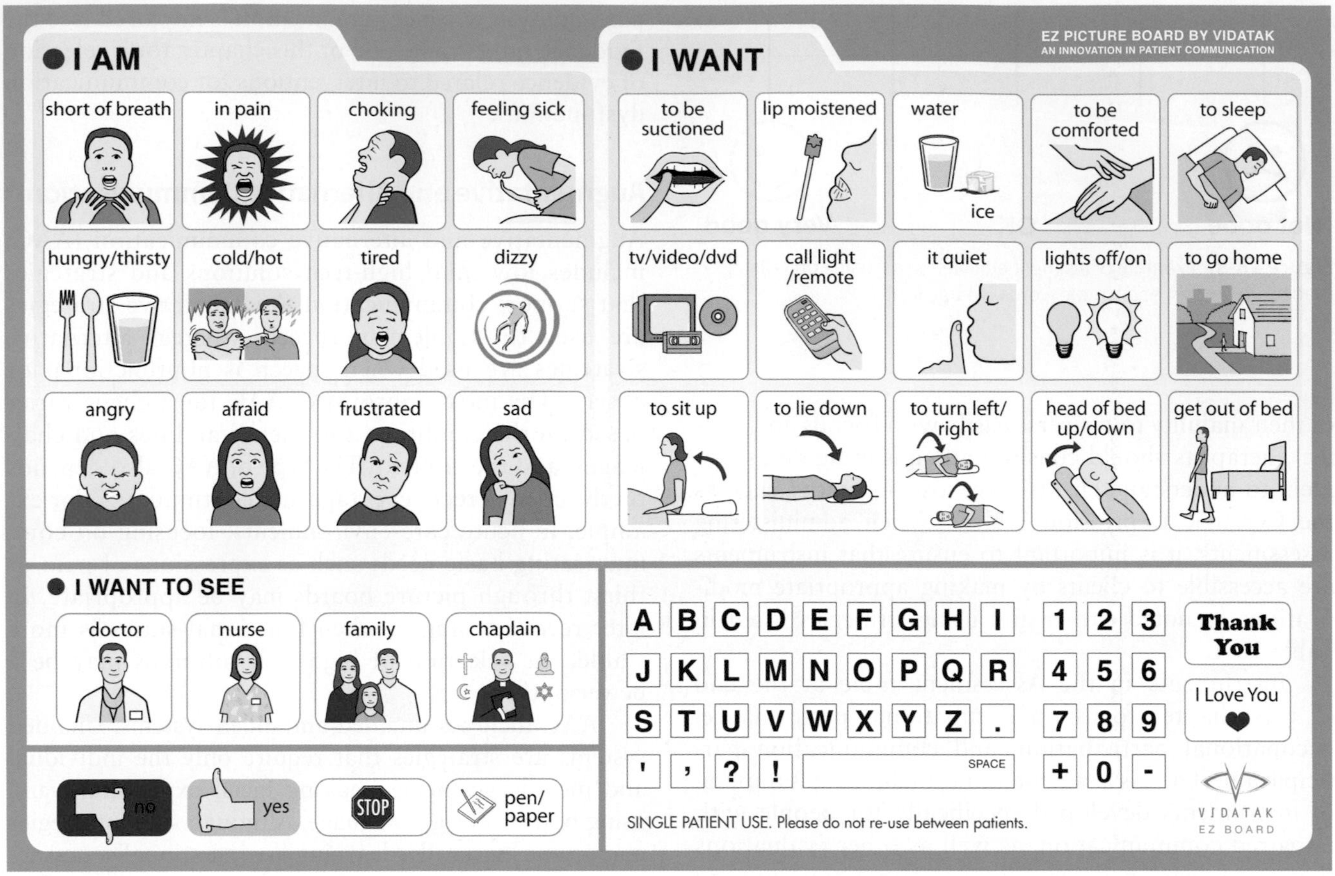

EZ PICTURE BOARD BY VIDATAK
AN INNOVATION IN PATIENT COMMUNICATION
I AM
short of breath
in pain
choking
feeling sick
hungry/thirsty
cold/hot
tired
dizzy
angry
afraid
frustrated
sad
I WANT
to be suctioned
lip moistened
water
ice
to be comforted
to sleep
tv/video/dvd
call light /remote
it quiet
lights off/on
to go home
to sit up
to lie down
to turn left/ right
head of bed up/down
get out of bed
I WANT TO SEE
doctor
nurse
family
chaplain
no
yes
STOP
pen/ paper
A B C D E F G H I
J K L M N O P Q R
S T U V W X Y Z .
' , ? !
SPACE
1 2 3
4 5 6
7 8 9
+ 0 -
Thank You
I Love You
SINGLE PATIENT USE. Please do not re-use between patients.
VIDATAK
EZ BOARD

Figure 18-9. Example of a picture board.

9:06 AM Tue Mar 5
31%
Settings
General
Accessibility
Apple ID, iCloud, iTunes & App Store
Update Apple ID Settings
Airplane Mode
Wi-Fi
Bluetooth On
Cellular Data Off
Notifications
Sounds
Do Not Disturb
Screen Time
General 1
Control Center
Display & Brightness
VISION
VoiceOver Off
Zoom Off
Magnifier On
Display Accommodations On
Speech
Larger Text On
Bold Text
Button Shapes
Reduce Transparency Off
Increase Contrast Off
Reduce Motion Off
On/Off Labels
INTERACTION
Switch Control Off
AssistiveTouch Off
Touch Accommodations On
Speech features include the option of "Speak Selection" that allows the user to hear selected text.
AssistiveTouch features support users who have difficulty using the touch screen (e.g., options such as single tap, double tap, long press, or customized gestures).

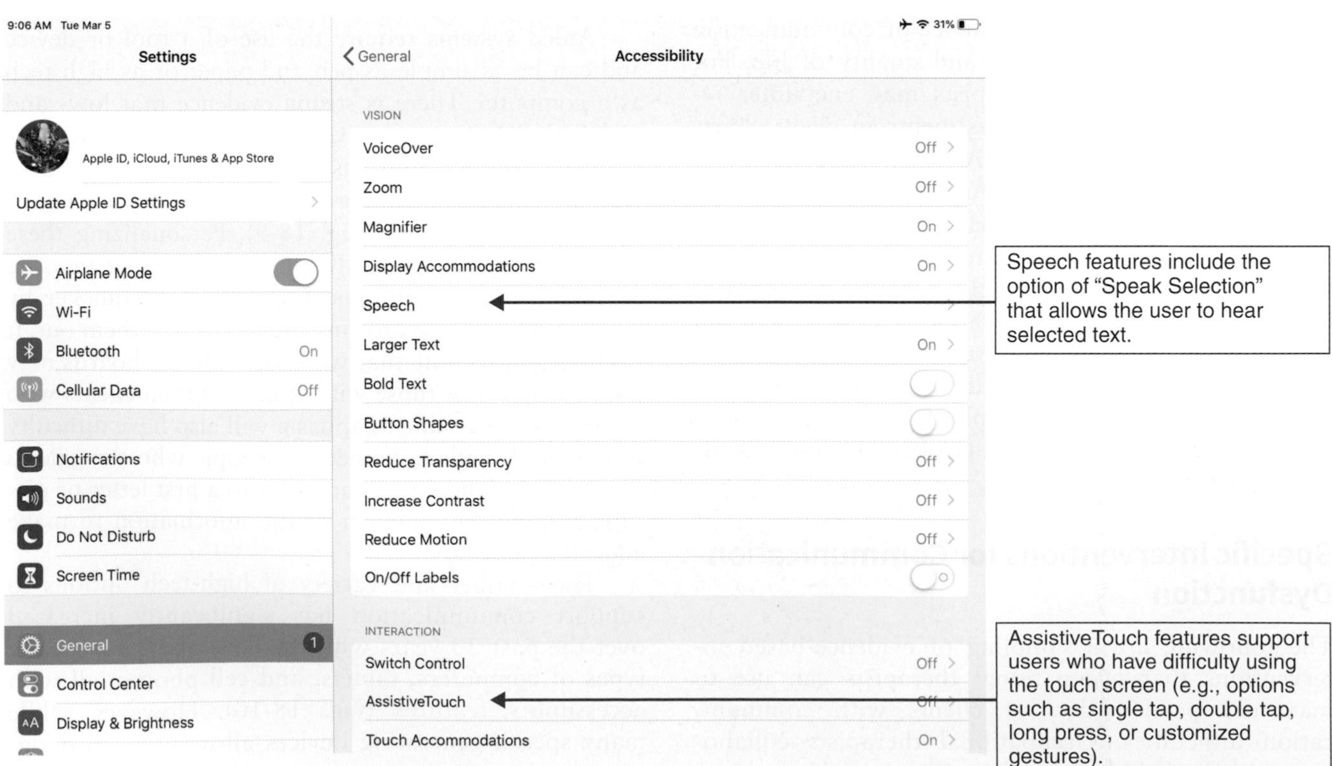

Figure 18-10. Screenshot of the general accessibility page on an iPad with two features highlighted.

To address this challenge, some people who anticipate the future loss of their voice, for example those with ALS, can choose to record and store their own voice through message banking.[31]

Computers, tablets, and cell phones can be operated through touch technology or adapted for use with eye gaze, optical head pointers, joy sticks, or through visual or oral scanning. Because technology changes often, it can be helpful to refer clients to an AAC specialist, typically an occupational therapist or SLP who specializes in this practice area. Some have questioned whether AAC decreases client motivation to improve natural speech skills or limits language development, but research has demonstrated otherwise.[32] AAC, when used in conjunction with natural speech, can actually improve speech.

Many people abandon or stop using their AAC device even when still needed, despite possessing well-designed and appropriately chosen systems.[33] Clients abandon devices for a variety of reasons, including stigma, slow speed, equipment failure, cultural differences, inadequate training, and lack of support from family members or caregivers.[33] Therapists can help prevent AAC abandonment by assuring a good match of the device to the user's physical, cognitive, and communication abilities; providing adequate training for users, family, and caregivers; and offering realistic expectations.[34] Providing opportunity to practice AAC use in the client's natural environment offers meaning and motivation, is key to successful AAC use, and improves social participation.

It is critical to remember that technology is a tool. The end goal of AAC is not the use of technology, but rather increased communication participation. Focusing on this goal will help the therapist collaborate with the client to select the most appropriate technology.

Partner Training

Communication is reciprocal, and clients' ability to express themselves also involves the people who are attempting to understand what is being said. Most of the literature regarding the effectiveness of care partner training addresses the care partners of people with aphasia.[35,36] Evidence exists, however, regarding the effectiveness of training care partners of people with social communication challenges resulting from TBI,[37] intellectual disability,[38] dementia,[39] and other conditions.

There are several standardized partner training protocols,[37,40] which include a combination of the following features: education, personalized goal setting, modeling, role-play, feedback, practice, and homework. Whereas SLPs are typically the professionals who administer partner training interventions, occupational therapists can provide suggestions, strategies, and encouragement

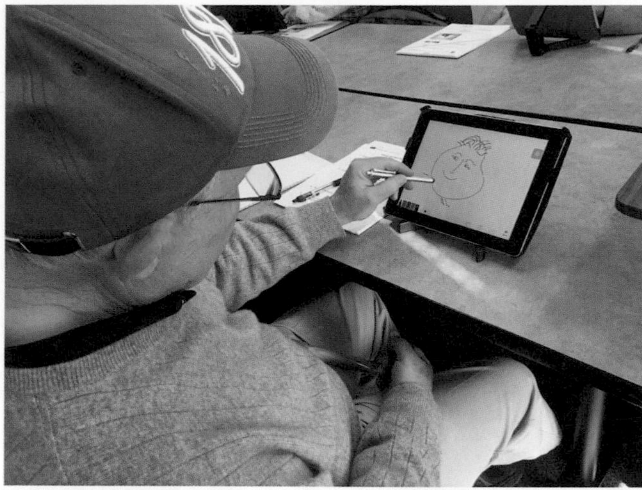

Figure 18-11. Use of technology (iPad and stylus) to support expression of ideas.

to care partners and should incorporate partner training strategies when working with clients who struggle to communicate. Strategies that care partners can use to support the expression of persons with communication difficulties include[27]:

- Providing written choices
- Asking closed-ended (yes/no) questions
- Making available writing/drawing utensils, paper, maps, photos, objects, and technology, as appropriate (Fig. 18-11)
- Listening actively without interrupting
- Allowing extended response time
- Encouraging

Strategies that partners can use to support the comprehension of persons with communication difficulties include:

- Using multiple modalities such as pictures, calendars, maps, and gestures along with spoken words (Fig. 18-12)
- Emphasizing keywords through tone or vocal volume
- Using short, simple sentences and familiar words
- Repeating or paraphrasing
- Using age-appropriate language and intonation
- Speaking slowly
- Limiting number of questions posed
- Keeping volume at a normal tone

Some common partner communication challenges to be aware of include (1) overcompensating by speaking very slowly or with a childish voice, (2) providing little time for the person to communicate and respond, (3) speaking for the person, (4) asking about information that is obvious or already known, and (5) preventing the influence of natural consequences (e.g., failing to demonstrate interest in topics when they are initiated).[37]

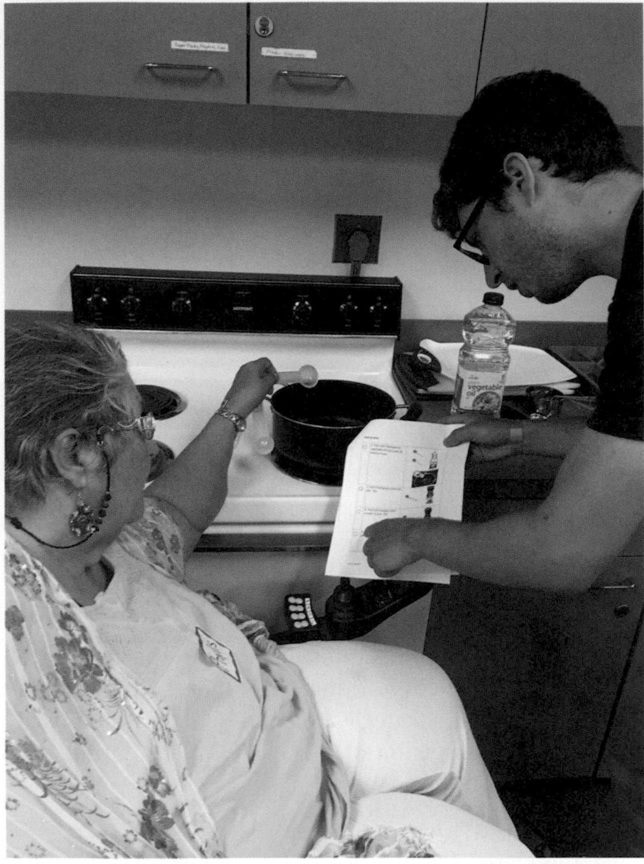

Figure 18-12. Example of partner using strategy to support comprehension.

Script Training

Script training involves teaching someone to use scripts to communicate, and evidence supports this approach for people with aphasia[41] and AoS.[42] Script training is based on both the importance of stories in everyday life and on whole task training. All people use stories, or scripts, throughout daily conversation. For example, many therapists have a set response to the question, "What is occupational therapy?" When students first enter occupational therapy school, this script may not yet have been practiced and is often said slowly, with limited confidence, and unclearly. Practice of this script takes place with peers and family members, focusing on both keywords and phrases (part task training), and explaining occupational therapy in full. With whole task training, this important "story" becomes perfected.

Script training is typically performed by SLPs, but occupational therapists can support both SLPs and clients to develop scripts in a variety of ways including:

- Collaborating with clients to determine situations in which scripts would support participation.
- Increasing technology accessibility by heightening keyboard contrast using stickers, practicing typing techniques, and exploring computer and tablet accessibility features (for clients using computers to develop scripts).
- Providing clients opportunity to practice using scripts in simulated and authentic environments.

Participation as Intervention

Improving communication skills can lead to increased participation, but as importantly, participation in meaningful occupations can improve communication. In a qualitative study of adults with aphasia, participants reported numerous benefits of volunteer activity participation including improved communication.[43] Volunteer experiences provided these individuals with opportunity and motivation to communicate, and increased overall confidence and self-esteem (Fig. 18-13). Dalemans and colleagues[44] discuss the importance of social participation for people with aphasia, emphasizing that social engagement provides people with voice and respect. Social participation also affords individuals who struggle to communicate the opportunity to be a part of society and to feel ordinary.

Although therapy groups often focus on improving specific skills, participants in aphasia groups reported joining groups primarily to meet other people and develop friendships.[45] Group members reported placing greater value on interactions and relationships developed during groups than on any specific skill or activity (Fig. 18-14). Although therapy groups are valuable to facilitate communication and social engagement, there is strong evidence to support the importance and positive benefits of social participation in naturally occurring environments. Engaging in motivating and authentic conversations can improve communication skills, self-confidence, and overall participation.[30]

Adaptive Strategies

The role of occupational therapy is unlimited when working with clients with communication challenges, and supporting communication and participation are key foci. Some strategies to support participation in both therapy and the home for people with decreased communication by adapting activities and/or the environment include the following:

- ***Ask clients to use tablets or cell phones to photograph their home environments for therapists.*** This involves clients in the assessment of and interventions for home adaptations.

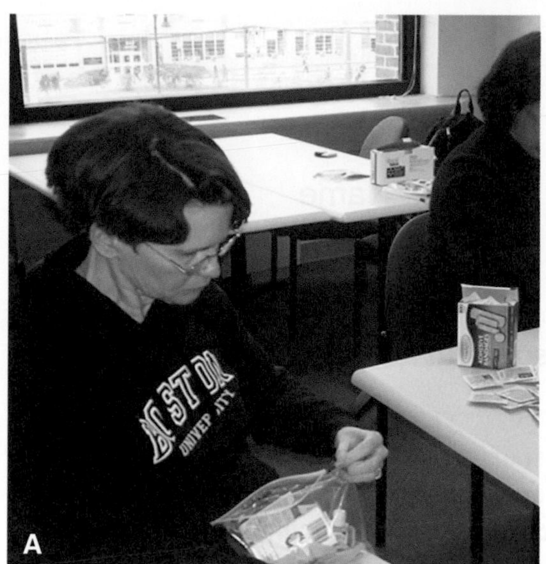

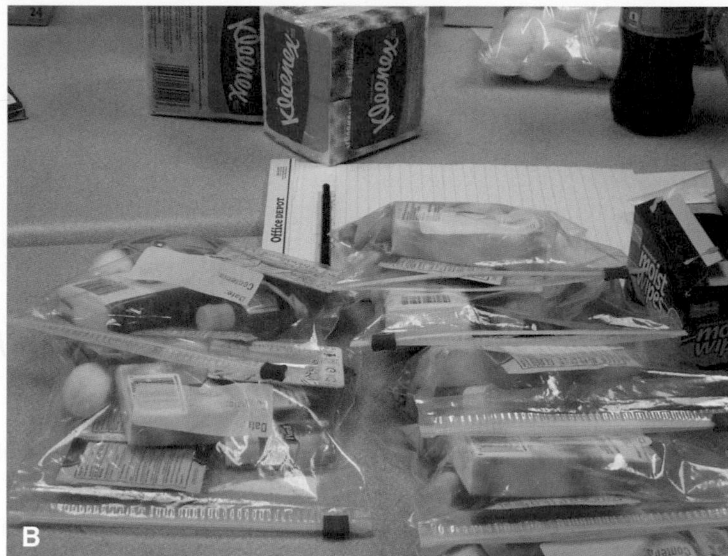

Figure 18-13. A, B. Volunteering to make first aid kits for a homeless shelter provides opportunity for communication along with increased confidence and a chance to give back to the community.

- ***Choose quiet environments with few distractions.*** For example, when possible, therapists should communicate in private rooms instead of large clinic settings. Ask clients for permission to turn off the radio before engaging in conversation. Encourage clients to find quiet environments when socializing. Dining with one friend instead of a large group may make communicating easier.
- ***Plan for emergency situations with clients.*** It is important to determine whether clients have medical

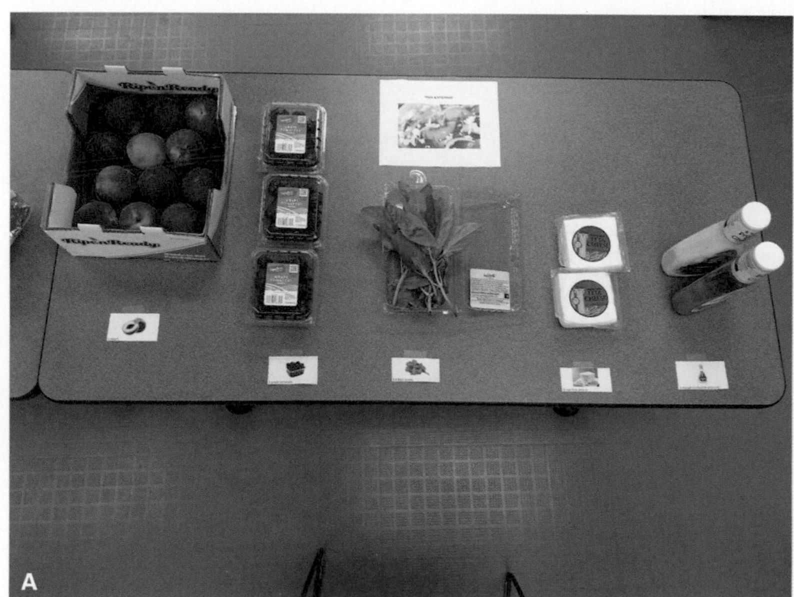

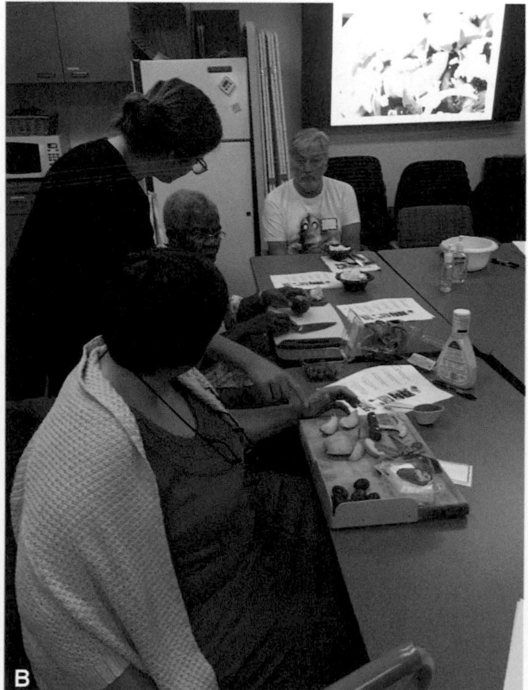

Figure 18-14. A, B. Collaborating with others with communication impairment to make a peach salad, using adapted recipes and visual cues.

alert buttons or can use a phone to call 911. If clients cannot use a cell phone to verbally communicate with others, they can still obtain help by calling the 911 system, which will send help without the need for clients to speak.

- *Discourage multitasking.* Singularly focusing on the task of talking is easier than talking combined with another activity such as eating or watching television. During therapy, provide directions, ensure that clients understand all directions, and then allow clients to perform therapy activities. The avoidance of multitasking while talking is particularly important for clients with communication difficulties resulting from Parkinson disease.[46]
- *Contact telephone company representatives to explore available options for clients.* For example, Speech-to-Speech (STS) services employ people who are trained in understanding a variety of speech disorders. STS communication assistants relay information to the person on the other end of the phone.[27]
- *Support clients to advocate for themselves.* For example, develop an information card (Fig. 18-15) with clients which explains their communication difficulty. Clients can then share this card with people in stores or social environments.

Finally, contextual factors are critical to consider when providing intervention for clients with impaired communication. For example, virtual contexts, such as talking on the phone, can be challenging for some people with impaired communication. Temporal contexts, such as time of day, can also influence communication due to fatigue or medication schedule. Personal contexts, such as socioeconomic status, may influence clients' ability to access AAC. Cultural contexts, as well, may support or hinder communication. For example, religious dress may limit some observable facial expressions. These are only several of the many contextual factors to consider when working with clients with communication challenges.

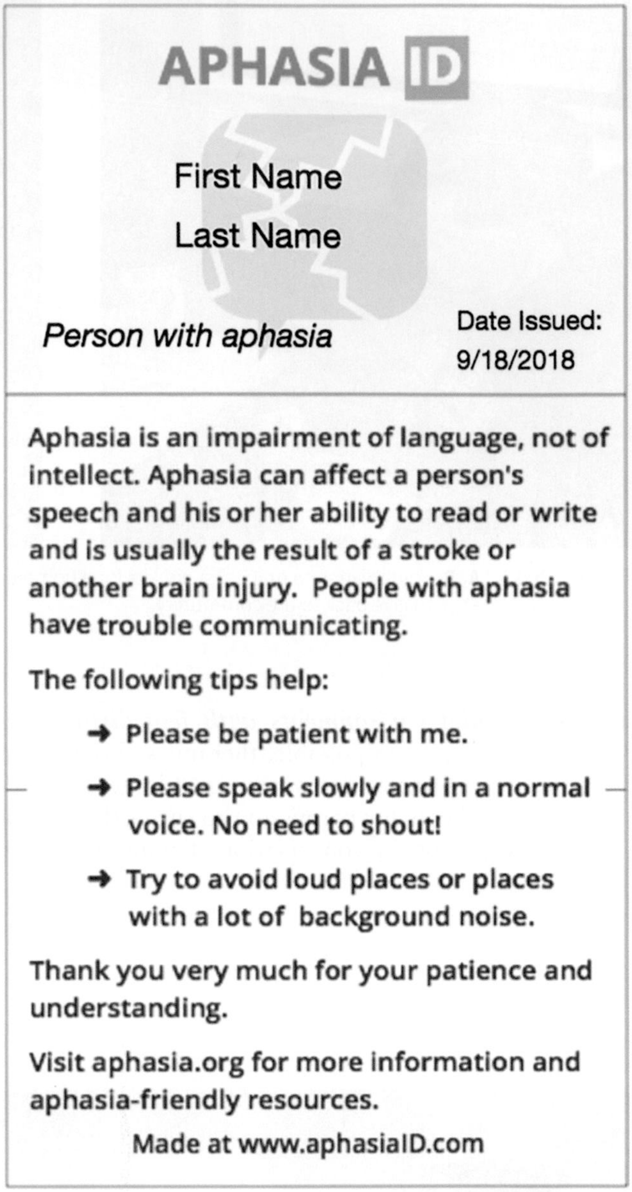

APHASIA ID

First Name
Last Name

Person with aphasia

Date Issued:
9/18/2018

Aphasia is an impairment of language, not of intellect. Aphasia can affect a person's speech and his or her ability to read or write and is usually the result of a stroke or another brain injury. People with aphasia have trouble communicating.

The following tips help:

- **Please be patient with me.**
- **Please speak slowly and in a normal voice. No need to shout!**
- **Try to avoid loud places or places with a lot of background noise.**

Thank you very much for your patience and understanding.

Visit aphasia.org for more information and aphasia-friendly resources.

Made at www.aphasiaID.com

Figure 18-15. Example of information card. Printed with permission from http://aphasiaid.com.

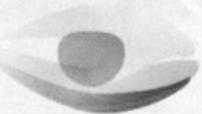

CASE STUDY

Patient Information

Sheng is a 69-year-old Asian American male who lives with his wife, Tuyen, in a small single-family house, 15 minutes from the city. He worked as a mail carrier until retiring at age 66. Tuyen worked as a part-time nurse but was able to leave her job to care for her husband after he experienced a stroke 1 month ago. Sheng and Tuyen have two grown children and three grandchildren. Their daughter and two grandsons live approximately 25 minutes away; their other adult children live several hours away.

Sheng reported being a quiet, hard-working man who enjoys his family, home, and hobbies. Aside from going out to eat once or twice a week and visiting family, he stated that he keeps to himself. Tuyen, however, described herself as very social and active. They have been married for 45 years and consider themselves to be decidedly fortunate.

Prior to his stroke, Sheng and Tuyen shared very traditional roles. Tuyen completed all household tasks, including cooking, cleaning, and shopping, whereas Sheng's home responsibilities included yard work, car maintenance, and financial management. Both reported contentment with this arrangement.

CASE STUDY *(continued)*

Assessment Process and Results

Sheng was seen, with his wife, in an outpatient setting 4-weeks poststroke. Initial information was obtained through review of Sheng's chart. Medical notes stated that Sheng experienced a left middle cerebral artery stroke; SLP documentation reported Broca nonfluent aphasia and that Sheng had strong auditory comprehension skills and utterances of two to three words in length. The occupational therapist observed Sheng walk into the clinic (using a straight cane and ankle-foot-orthosis), take off his coat (slowly but independently), and open his water bottle by stabilizing it between his legs. From observation, it was noted that Sheng had right-sided upper extremity paresis and lower extremity weakness. Tuyen was very anxious about leaving Sheng to participate in activities alone because of his communication struggles; she expressed concern that he may become lost and unable to communicate his need for help.

After an initial informal interview with Sheng and Tuyen to gather background information, the Canadian Occupational Performance Measure (COPM) was administered to identify Sheng's self-reported, most important daily activities that had become challenging poststroke. Photo cards from the Activity Card Sort (ACS) and Life Interests and Values (LIV) were used to support Sheng's ability to share his priorities. The occupational therapist asked Sheng to perform multiple photo card sorts, each time using just two categories per sort: (1) "want to do" and "don't want to do"; and (2) "want to do" pile sorted into "do same" or "do less."

Then, using cards from the "do less" pile, the therapist asked Sheng to prioritize his most important activities and rate the performance (P) and satisfaction (S) of each activity using a Likert scale ranging from 1 to 10 (where 1 = poor performance and low satisfaction). Using an adapted scale with large font, visual icons, simplified language, and positioning the photo of each identified activity next to the rating scale, Sheng listed the following four activities as high priority:

- Using the computer (P = 2, S = 5)
- Presenting a gift to Tuyen (P = 1, S = 1)
- Using transportation independently (P = 1, S = 6)
- Fishing independently (P = 1, S = 2)

Based on evaluation findings, the therapist learned that Sheng previously completed many errands independently but now sits in the car waiting as Tuyen completes errands. Sheng enjoyed reading but is unable to read easily now; used the computer to send and answer e-mail messages, but can no longer complete this activity independently; was the family driver but no longer drives; and loved to fish both alone and with family, but now has difficulty holding the fishing pole. He shared that he is independent in self-care activities (e.g., bathing, dressing, toileting, eating) and spends much of his day watching television. Tuyen expressed that she is anxious about Sheng's independent use of paratransit and that she is unsure about how to arrange this service for him.

Occupational Therapy Problem List

- Nonfluent aphasia
- Right-sided hemiparesis
- Limited participation in self-reported desired activities
- Dependent on Tuyen to go outside the home

Occupational Therapy Goal List

By the end of 2 months, Sheng will:

1. Report that he went fishing with son and was able to independently use adapted fishing pole
2. Independently use cell phone for emergencies, and to call and answer family members
3. Use paratransit to attend therapy sessions, once arranged by wife
4. Make or purchase a surprise gift for wife

Intervention

Tuyen attended Sheng's first three occupational therapy sessions, often answering for him when questions were posed. Sheng sat quietly, appearing content for Tuyen to respond, and gesturing to her to respond when he needed help communicating. When given time, however, Sheng was able to communicate with the therapist and answer questions using gestures, words, photos, and, at times, paper and pencil. For example, he drew a picture of a boat to explain that he preferred fishing from a boat in contrast to a dock.

During these first sessions, the occupational therapist provided Tuyen with strategies to support her ability to communicate with Sheng (e.g., asking close-ended questions, listening without interrupting, allowing time for Sheng to respond) and worked with him to adapt a fishing pole holder based on his requirements and suggestions. Sheng became excited and enthusiastic for more occupational therapy sessions. Unfortunately, Tuyen fractured her ankle after falling and was unable to transport Sheng to therapy. As a result, he missed the next session and reported that Tuyen could not drive for 6 weeks. The therapist took this opportunity to address the use of paratransit. While Sheng was eager to use paratransit independently, Tuyen expressed concern. Through several phone calls, the therapist instructed Tuyen in the process of scheduling paratransit services. Tuyen followed through and arranged for Sheng to be picked up for his next therapy session. Because Tuyen could not as yet travel with him, the therapist arranged for a hospital volunteer to drive to the house and accompany Sheng on the paratransit van, to and from therapy. The therapist called Tuyen when Sheng arrived to assure her of his safety. Sheng again took paratransit in the following week,

(continued)

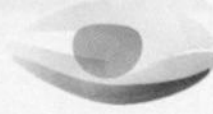

CASE STUDY *(continued)*

but this time alone. When he arrived at the clinic, Sheng called Tuyen, with support from the therapist, and using the cell phone that Tuyen gave him for emergencies. Sheng expressed elation to be able to attend therapy on his own and allow Tuyen time to herself. During these next sessions, the therapist worked with Sheng to practice two scripts that he developed with the SLP for telephone use: one to let his wife know that he arrived at a designated location safely, and one for emergencies (e.g., calling 911). Sheng also learned to use his phone's camera and photographed himself and his wife. In therapy, he made a collage frame, framed this photo, and wrapped it as a gift for Tuyen. To support Sheng's ability to write a card, the therapist found five possible sentences that might convey his thoughts (e.g., "Thank you for everything;" "I appreciate all you do."). Sheng chose one, copied the words onto the card in his writing, and signed his name.

In the final occupational therapy session, Tuyen joined him via paratransit. She was still unable to drive but enjoyed getting out of the house. During this session, the occupational therapist reinforced strategies that worked for communication and encouraged Sheng to advocate for himself (e.g., request people to speak more slowly). Because Tuyen was so impressed by Sheng's ability to call her using the phone, she planned to purchase a simple smartphone (e.g., the Jitterbug) so that he could call his children and grandchildren and gain assistance in case of emergencies. During the final session, COPM outcome measures were repeated, and Sheng's ratings improved significantly, as follows:

- Using the computer (P = 2, S = 5)
- Presenting a gift to Tuyen (P = 5, S = 8)
- Using transportation independently (P = 8, S = 6)
- Fishing independently (P = 5, S = 9)

Most Commonly Used Communication Standardized Assessments

Instrument and Reference	Intended Purpose	Administration Time	Validity	Reliability	Sensitivity	Strengths and Weaknesses
Activity Card Sort (ACS)[49]	Measures level of activity in instrumental, social, and leisure activities	~60 minutes	Concurrent validity adequate to strong; construct validity satisfactory to excellent[49]	Internal consistency generally considered strong; test–retest considered excellent[49]	Not available	Created for older adults; cards support communication; no ADL photos
Canadian Occupational Performance Measure (COPM)[48]	Measure of a client's perception of his or her performance and satisfaction of daily activities; identifies areas of difficulty in occupational performance	~15–30 minutes	Concurrent, criterion, convergent, divergent, construct, content validity all acceptable[48]	Test–retest: consistently acceptable[48]	Considered responsive to change[48]	Focus on occupational performance and challenges; encourages client-centered, occupation-based practice. Needs to be modified to be accessible to people with communication challenges.
Communicative Participation Item Bank[50]	Measures the extent to which communication impairment disrupts communicative participation	~10 minutes	Valid for use with people with aphasia[51]; content validity strong[50]	Not available	Not available	Self-report; can be used for community-dwelling adults with different communication disorders, including MS, ALS, and Parkinson disease
Goal Attainment Scaling (GAS)[52]	Evaluation of intervention effectiveness based on level of individualized goal achievement	Variable	Can have strong validity when GAS intervals are precisely developed[53]	Considered a reliable measure with precise GAS intervals[53]	Sensitive to change[53]	Individualized, criterion referenced; predicts expected outcomes. Can be time-consuming and challenging to create five ordinal levels of goal attainment. Reliability and validity highly dependent on abilities of the person writing the GAS goals.[53]
Life Interests and Values Cards (LIV)[22]	Developed for SLP, OT, PT to facilitate communication of client-centered interests and goal setting	~45 minutes	Considered valid instrument to elicit involvement in life activities for people with aphasia[54]	NA	NA	Facilitates communication with people with aphasia and explores their interests and goals. Not an outcome measure. Includes friends and family member questionnaire.
Stroke Impact Scale[47]	Outcome assessment for people poststroke, measuring ADL, IADL, mobility, communication, emotion, memory and thinking, and participation	~15–20 minutes	High-to-adequate concurrent validity[55]	High internal consistency; good test–retest reliability[55]	Not adequate evidence[55]	Diagnosis specific—just for use poststroke; communication items along with more global items

ADL, activities of daily living; ALS, amyotrophic lateral sclerosis; IADL, instrumental activities of daily living; MS, multiple sclerosis; NA, not applicable; OT, occupational therapy; PT, physical therapist; SLP, speech language pathologist.

Evidence Table of Communication Intervention Studies

Intervention	Description	Participants	Dosage	Research Design and Evidence Level	Benefit	Statistical Significance and Effect Size
Augmentative and Alternative Communication (AAC) for adults with decreased communication[28]	Use of AAC to support communication	Eighteen studies of adults aged 60+ with communication impairment (for any reason) and use AAC to support communication	Varied (and not reported in many studies)	Systematic review Level I	Technology was beneficial as an assistive communication tool. Older adults were receptive to technology. Simpler the technology, the better. Older adults, with or without disability, benefit from AAC to support communication.	No statistical analysis
AAC for people with aphasia[29]	Use of high-tech communication devices	Thirty articles focusing on AAC use by adults with aphasia (1989–2016)	Total of 13 different types of AAC systems were used in 30 interventions.	Systematic review Level I	People with aphasia demonstrated improvement in functional communication (communication during telephone conversations, everyday activities, written communication, and face-to-face interaction) using high-technology AAC.	No statistical analysis
Partner training for caregivers of people with dementia[39]	Communication skills training for professional or nonprofessional caregivers to improve communication or interaction with people with dementia	Twelve studies focusing on communication skills training for health care professionals and lay caregivers of people with dementia in nursing homes ($n = 8$) or home ($n = 4$)	Interventions were small groups or face-to-face trainings. Hands-on practice and feedback provided. Dosage varied from two sessions at 1 hour each to five sessions at 2.5 hours each.	Systematic review Level I	Many strategies found to be effective in improving caregivers' communication skills including: • Verbal skills including using one-step instructions, person's name, and biographical and positive statements • Nonverbal and emotional skills, including making eye contact, providing enough time, and actively listening • Attitudes toward people with dementia, including avoiding over-nurturing and increasing opportunities for pleasant events • Behavioral management skills, including using distraction and setting realistic goals • Usage of tools, including memory books and aids • Self-experiences, including reflecting on what works and what doesn't • Theoretical knowledge, including knowledge about dementia, culture, and communication	No statistical analysis

Partner training with people with aphasia and their care partners[35]	Teaching people who interact with individuals with aphasia to use strategies and resources to support communication	Twenty-five articles focusing on training partners of people with aphasia	Amount of training varied from 1.25 hours to as many as 100 hours (most common was 10–15 hours of training).	Systematic review Level I	Language impairment—less than half the studies that measured this demonstrated improvement. Communication activity/participation—more than half the studies that measured this demonstrated improvement. Psychosocial adjustment/QoL—all studies that measured this showed improvement Communication partners—improvement noted in strategy use and psychosocial adjustment.	No statistical analysis
Script training[41]	Script training for people with chronic, nonfluent aphasia	Six studies focusing on script training that explored outcomes related to rate of speech and verbal output	All studies focused on personally meaningful scripts Intervention varied including: • Number of scripts practiced (from 1 to 20) • Length of intervention (from 2 to 16 weeks)	Critical review Level V	Improvement noted in all studies for increasing rate of speech and use of script-related words in other contexts; evidence also showed increased confidence in communication and increased social participation.	No statistical analysis
Community aphasia group participation[45]	Participation in community-based group programs for people with aphasia	Individuals with severe aphasia, $N = 7$, 49–79 years old, 1–10 years after aphasia	2 months to 9 years of group participation	Qualitative study—Phenomenological approach Level V	Three themes: • Initially perceive community group as high risk • Benefited from structure • Opportunity for authentic interaction and chance to highlight individual strengths	NA

NA, not applicable; QoL, quality of life.

References

1. Occupational therapy practice framework: domain and process (3rd edition). *Am J Occup Ther*. 2014;68(suppl 1):S1–S48. doi:10.5014/ajot.2014.682006.
2. American Speech-Language-Hearing Association. Definition of communication and appropriate targets. https://www.asha.org/NJC/Definition-of-Communication-and-Appropriate-Targets/. Accessed July 10, 2019.
3. Hilari K. The impact of stroke: are people with aphasia different to those without? *Disabil Rehabil*. 2011;33(3):211–218. doi:10.3109/09638288.2010.508829.
4. Worrall L, Sherratt S, Rogers P, et al. What people with aphasia want: their goals according to the ICF. *Aphasiology*. 2011;25(3):309–322. doi:10.1080/02687038.2010.508530.
5. Locke EA, Latham GP. Building a practically useful theory of goal setting and task motivation. A 35-year odyssey. *Am Psychol*. 2002;57(9):705–717.
6. Rosewilliam S, Roskell CA, Pandyan A. A systematic review and synthesis of the quantitative and qualitative evidence behind patient-centred goal setting in stroke rehabilitation. *Clin Rehabil*. 2011;25(6):501–514. doi:10.1177/0269215510394467.
7. Brady MC, Fredrick A, Williams B. People with aphasia: capacity to consent, research participation and intervention inequalities. *Int J Stroke*. 2013;8(3):193–196. doi:10.1111/j.1747-4949.2012.00900.x.
8. Friederici AD. The brain basis of language processing: from structure to function. *Physiol Rev*. 2011;91(4):1357–1392. doi:10.1152/physrev.00006.2011.
9. Price C. A review and synthesis of the first 20 years of PET and fMRI studies of heard speech, spoken language and reading. *Neuroimage*. 2012;62(2):816–847. doi:10.1016/j.neuroimage.2012.04.062.
10. Bhatnagar S. *Neuroscience for the Study of Communicative Disorders*. 5th ed. Philadelphia, PA: Lippincott Williams & Wilkins; 2018.
11. Duffy JR. *Motor Speech Disorders: Substrates, Differential Diagnosis, and Management*. 3rd ed. St. Louis, MO: Elsevier Mosby; 2013. https://www.elsevier.com/books/motor-speech-disorders/duffy/978-0-323-11267-3. Accessed August 12, 2018.
12. Helm-Estabrooks N, Albert ML, Nicholas M. *Manual of Aphasia and Aphasia Therapy*. 3rd ed. Austin, TX: Pro Ed; 2014.
13. Seikel J, Drumright D, King D. *Anatomy & Physiology for Speech, Language, and Hearing*. 5th ed. Clifton Park, NY: Cengage Learning; 2016.
14. Wada J, Rasmussen T. Intracarotid injection of sodium amytal for the lateralization of cerebral speech dominance 1960. *J Neurosurg*. 2007;106(6):1117–1133. doi:10.3171/jns.2007.106.6.1117.
15. Knecht S, Dräger B, Deppe M, et al. Handedness and hemispheric language dominance in healthy humans. *Brain*. 2000;123(12):2512–2518. doi:10.1093/brain/123.12.2512.
16. Kiran S. What is the nature of poststroke language recovery and reorganization? *ISRN Neurol*. 2012;2012:1–13. doi:10.5402/2012/786872.
17. World Health Organization. *International Classification of Functioning, Disability and Health (ICF)*. Geneva, Switzerland: World Health Organization. http://www.who.int/classifications/icf/en/. Accessed June 27, 2018.
18. Threats T. Access for persons with neurogenic communication disorders: influences of personal and environmental factors of the ICF. *Aphasiology*. 2007;21(1):67–80. doi:10.1080/02687030600798303.
19. Law M, Cooper B, Strong S, Stewart D, Rigby P, Letts L. The person-environment-occupation model: a transactive approach to occupational performance. *Can J Occup Ther*. 1996;63(1):9–23.
20. Hanson EK, Yorkston KM, Britton D. Dysarthria in amyotrophic lateral sclerosis: a systematic review of characteristics, speech treatment, and augmentative and alternative communication options. *J Med Speech Lang Pathol*. 2011;19:12–30. http://link.galegroup.com/apps/doc/A266957325/AONE?sid=googlescholar. Published September 1, 2011. Accessed August 21, 2018.
21. Tucker FM, Edwards DF, Mathews LK, Baum CM, Connor LT. Modifying health outcome measures for people with aphasia. *Am J Occup Ther*. 2012;66(1):42–50. doi:10.5014/ajot.2012.001255.
22. Haley K, Womack J, Helm-Estabrooks N, Caignon D, McCulloch K. *The Life Interest and Values Cards*. Chapel Hill: University of North Carolina Department of Allied Health Sciences; 2010.
23. Yesavage JA, Brink TL, Rose TL, et al. Development and validation of a geriatric depression screening scale: a preliminary report. *J Psychiatr Res*. 1982;17(1):37–49.
24. Frattali CM, Thompson CK, Holland AL, et al. *American Speech-Language-Hearing Association Functional Assessment of Communication Skills for Adults (ASHA FACS)*. Rockville, MD: American Speech-Language-Hearing Association; 2018.
25. Paul DR, Frattali C, Holland AL, Thompson CK, Caperton CJ, Slater SC. *The American Speech-Language-Hearing Association Quality of Communication Life (QCL) Scale Manual*. Rockville, MD: American Speech-Language-Hearing Association; 2004.
26. Kagan A, Simmons-Mackie N, Victor J, Carling-Rowland A, Hoch J, Huijbregts M. *for Living with Aphasia (ALA)*. 2nd ed. Toronto, Canada: Aphasia Institute; 2014.
27. Wallace T, Bradshaw A. Technologies and strategies for people with communication problems following brain injury or stroke. *NeuroRehabilitation*. 2011;28(3):199–209. doi:10.3233/NRE-2011-0649.
28. Antunes TPC, Oliveira ASB de, Hudec R, et al. Assistive technology for communication of older adults: a systematic review. *Aging Ment Health*. 2019;23(4):417–427. doi:10.1080/13607863.2018.1426718.
29. Russo MJ, Prodan V, Meda NN, et al. High-technology augmentative communication for adults with post-stroke aphasia: a systematic review. *Expert Rev Med Devices*. 2017;14(5):355–370. doi:10.1080/17434440.2017.1324291.
30. Beukelman DR, Mirenda P. *Augmentative and Alternative Communication; Supporting Children and Adults with Complex Communication Needs*. 4th ed. Baltimore, MD: Brookes Publishing; 2013.

31. ALS Worldwide. Message banking: preserve your voice. http://alsworldwide.org/whats-new/article/messagebanking.com-preserve-your-voice. Accessed June 27, 2018.
32. Millar DC, Light JC, Schlosser RW. The impact of augmentative and alternative communication intervention on the speech production of individuals with developmental disabilities: a research review. *J Speech Lang Hear Res.* 2006;49(2):248–264.
33. Johnson JM, Inglebret E, Jones C, Ray J. Perspectives of speech language pathologists regarding success versus abandonment of AAC. *Augment Altern Commun.* 2006;22(2):85–99. doi:10.1080/07434610500483588.
34. Baxter SEP, Evans PJS. Barriers and facilitators to the use of high-technology augmentative and alternative communication devices: a systematic review and qualitative synthesis. *Int J Lang Commun Disord.* 2012;47(2):115–129.
35. Simmons-Mackie N, Raymer A, Cherney LR. Communication partner training in aphasia: an updated systematic review. *Arch Phys Med Rehabil.* 2016;97(12):2202–2221.e8. doi:10.1016/j.apmr.2016.03.023.
36. Sorin-Peters R, Patterson R. The implementation of a learner-centred conversation training programme for spouses of adults with aphasia in a community setting. *Aphasiology.* 2014;28(6):731–749. doi:10.1080/02687038.2014.891094.
37. Togher L, McDonald S, Tate R, Rietdijk R, Power E. The effectiveness of social communication partner training for adults with severe chronic TBI and their families using a measure of perceived communication ability. *NeuroRehabilitation.* 2016;38(3):243–255. doi:10.3233/NRE-151316.
38. Ogletree BT, Bartholomew P, Kirksey ML, et al. Communication training supporting an AAC user with severe intellectual disability: application of the communication partner instruction model. *J Dev Phys Disabil.* 2016;28(1):135–152. doi:10.1007/s10882-015-9444-2.
39. Eggenberger E, Heimerl K, Bennett MI. Communication skills training in dementia care: a systematic review of effectiveness, training content, and didactic methods in different care settings. *Int Psychogeriatr.* 2013;25(3):345–358. doi:10.1017/S1041610212001664.
40. Kagan A, Black SE, Duchan JF, Simmons-Mackie N, Square P. Training volunteers as conversation partners using supported conversation for adults with aphasia (SCA): a controlled trial. *J Speech Lang Hear Res.* 2001;44(3):624–638. doi:10.1044/1092-4388(2001/051).
41. Anderson J. The effectiveness of script training intervention on the rate of speech and percentage content use in the speech of persons with chronic, non-fluent aphasia. 2013. https://www.uwo.ca/fhs/lwm/teaching/EBP/2012_13/Anderson_J.pdf.
42. Youmans G, Youmans SR, Hancock AB. Script training treatment for adults with apraxia of speech. *Am J Speech Lang Pathol.* 2011;20(1):23–37. doi:10.1044/1058-0360(2010/09-0085).
43. Pearl G, Sage K, Young A. Involvement in volunteering: an exploration of the personal experience of people with aphasia. *Disabil Rehabil.* 2011;33(19–20):1805–1821. doi:10.3109/09638288.2010.549285.
44. 50. Dalemans R, Wade DT, van den Heuvel WJ, de Witte LP. Facilitating the participation of people with aphasia in research: a description of strategies. *Clin Rehabil.* 2009;23(10):948–959. doi:10.1177/0269215509337197.
45. Lanyon L, Worrall L, Rose M. Combating social isolation for people with severe chronic aphasia through community aphasia groups: consumer views on getting it right and wrong. *Aphasiology.* 2018;32(5):493–517. doi:10.1080/02687038.2018.1431830.
46. LaPointe LL, Stierwalt JAG, Maitland CG. Talking while walking: cognitive loading and injurious falls in Parkinson's disease. *Int J Speech Lang Pathol.* 2010;12(5):455–459. doi:10.3109/17549507.2010.486446.
47. Duncan PW, Wallace D, Lai SM, Johnson D, Embretson S, Laster LJ. The stroke impact scale version 2.0. Evaluation of reliability, validity, and sensitivity to change. *Stroke.* 1999;30(10):2131–2140.
48. Law M, Baptiste S, Carswell A, McColl M, Polatajko H, Pollock N. *Canadian Occupational Performance Measure.* 5th ed. Toronto, Canada: CAOT Publications ACE; 2008. http://www.thecopm.ca/.
49. Baum C, Edwards D. *Activity Card Sort.* 2nd ed. Bethesda, MD: AOTA Press; 2008. https://myaota.aota.org/shop_aota/prodview.aspx?TYPE=D&PID=763&SKU=1247.
50. Baylor C, Yorkston K, Eadie T, Kim J, Chung H, Amtmann D. The communicative participation item bank (CPIB): item bank calibration and development of a disorder-generic short form. *J Speech Lang Hear Res.* 2013;56(4):1190–1208. doi:10.1044/1092-4388(2012/12-0140).
51. Baylor C, Oelke M, Bamer A, et al. Validating the communicative participation item bank (CPIB) for use with people with aphasia: an analysis of differential item function (DIF). *Aphasiology.* 2017;31(8):861–878. doi:10.1080/02687038.2016.1225274.
52. Kiresuk TJ, Sherman RE. Goal attainment scaling: a general method for evaluating comprehensive community mental health programs. *Community Ment Health J.* 1968;4(6):443–453. doi:10.1007/BF01530764.
53. Krasny-Pacini A, Evans J, Sohlberg MM, Chevignard M. Proposed criteria for appraising goal attainment scales used as outcome measures in rehabilitation research. *Arch Phys Med Rehabil.* 2016;97(1):157–170. doi:10.1016/j.apmr.2015.08.424.
54. Haley KL, Womack J, Helm-Estabrooks N, Lovette B, Goff R. Supporting autonomy for people with aphasia: use of the life interests and values (LIV) cards. *Top Stroke Rehabil.* 2013;20(1):22–35. doi:10.1310/tsr2001-22.
55. Mulder M, Nijland R. Stroke impact scale. *J Physiother.* 2016;62(2):117. doi:10.1016/j.jphys.2016.02.002.

Chapter 19

Swallowing and Eating Assessment and Intervention

Wendy Avery

LEARNING OBJECTIVES

This chapter will allow the reader to:

1. Discuss normal swallowing.
2. Define basic terminology related to dysphagia care.
3. Identify types of dysphagia and their presentation.
4. Identify diagnoses in which dysphagia is commonly seen.
5. Describe how to perform a clinical dysphagia assessment.
6. Employ basic compensatory and rehabilitative strategies to treat dysphagia.
7. Name and describe the execution of commonly used compensatory swallowing maneuvers.
8. Discuss precautions for the occupational therapist and the patient during dysphagia evaluation and intervention.
9. Describe instrumental evaluation procedures for dysphagia.
10. Describe instrumental interventions for dysphagia.

CHAPTER OUTLINE

TERMINOLOGY

Aspiration: the entrance of food or secretions into the larynx below the level of the vocal cords.

Bolus: any food or liquid in the mouth.

Deglutition: the act of swallowing.

Direct therapy: any therapeutic technique or intervention involving ingestion of food or liquids.

Dysphagia: difficulty with any stage of swallowing.

Eating: the ingestion of food and liquid, including the preoral, oral preparatory, oral, pharyngeal, and esophageal stages.

Feeding: taking or giving nourishment.

Fiberoptic endoscopic evaluation of swallowing (FEES): the direct visualization of the swallow using a small illuminated camera at the end of a flexible tube (endoscope), which is introduced into the pharynx through the nose.

Indirect therapy: any therapeutic technique that addresses the prerequisite capacities associated with swallowing without the ingestion of food or liquid.

Instrumental evaluation: imaging and diagnostic studies to provide critical information about the unseen parts of the oral, pharyngeal, and esophageal stages of swallowing.

Mechanical dysphagia: a swallowing and eating impairment caused by the loss of oral, pharyngeal, or esophageal structures; weakness; and/or sensory deficits caused by trauma or surgery.

Modified barium swallow (MBS): moving radiographic images of swallowing structure and physiology, as recorded on DVD. It was formerly referred to and still seen in the literature as "videofluoroscopy."

Paralytic dysphagia: lower motor neuron involvement that causes weakness and sensory impairment of oral and pharyngeal structures, including weakness or absence of the swallowing reflex.

Pseudobulbar dysphagia: upper motor neuron involvement, causing hypotonicity or hypertonicity of oral and pharyngeal structures and a slow or poorly coordinated swallowing reflex.

Swallowing: the ingestion of nourishment, beginning with introduction of food into the mouth and ending with reception of food into the stomach; it includes the preoral, oral preparatory, oral, pharyngeal, and esophageal stages.

Swallowing and Eating Function and Impairment in Daily Occupation

Normal **swallowing** and **eating** functions encompass a wide range of skills, including the sensory and motor skills related to swallowing and eating, as well as cognition and perception. Swallowing and eating are critical functions that "fuel" all other occupations and activities of daily living (ADLs). **Dysphagia,** or difficulty with any stage of swallowing, can interfere with functional independence for many recipients of occupational therapy services in multiple settings. The incidence of dysphagia is increasing as the US population is aging.[1] Dysphagia has been shown to be correlated with ADL dependence, including loss of dependent eating in rehabilitation[2] and nursing home populations.[3] Dysphagia can lead to dehydration,[4] pressure ulcers,[5] and malnutrition.[6] Malnutrition, in particular, is common in all health care settings.[7]

Dysphagia frequently causes pulmonary complications caused by **aspiration**. These complications include aspiration pneumonia,[8] airway obstruction,[9] and death.[8] Impairment in eating and swallowing can lead to reduction in the ability to participate in rehabilitation as well as basic and instrumental ADLs. For most people, eating is a pleasurable daily experience and the challenges posed by dysphagia can greatly limit the enjoyment of this activity. The reduced ability to participate in social and cultural activities that include food can profoundly affect an individual.[10]

Neurological and Physiological Bases of Swallowing and Eating

Deglutition (the act of swallowing) is a complex process involving both volitional and nonvolitional behaviors. The cranial nerves execute the sensory and motor processes that constitute swallowing. Cortically mediated factors, including appetite, attitude, attention span, appreciation of food, and body position, influence swallowing and must be considered in evaluation and treatment. The oral, pharyngeal, and esophageal structures involved in swallowing are illustrated in Figure 19-1.

The stages of swallowing include the preoral, oral preparatory, oral, pharyngeal, and esophageal stages.

Preoral Stage

In the preoral stage, food is visually and olfactorily appreciated. This stimulates salivation, and there are preparatory movements of the mouth to ready the oral cavity to receive and mobilize foods and liquids. Spontaneous upper extremity movements occur as the person reaches for and grasps utensils, cups, or finger foods and brings them into the mouth.

Oral Preparatory Stage

In the oral preparatory stage, food is received and contained by the mouth. It is then formed into a **bolus** of food and mixed with saliva. Pureed or liquid boluses require little mastication and may briefly be held centrally in the mouth by the tongue and cheek musculature. Solid food may need to be bitten off in order to be contained in the mouth. The bolus is chewed in a rotary motion and moved between the left and right molars. The buccal muscles contract to prevent food from pocketing between the cheeks and the teeth. Once masticated or formed, the bolus is brought to the center of the tongue.

Oral Stage

In the oral stage, the cheek and tongue muscles retain the bolus centrally in the mouth. The tongue squeezes the bolus against the hard palate, moving it posteriorly to the level of the faucial arches.

Pharyngeal Stage

In the pharyngeal stage, the soft palate elevates to close off the nasopharynx. The larynx and hyoid elevate and protract, minimizing the size of the laryngeal vestibule (its opening) as the epiglottis tips to cover the vestibule. Breathing stops (termed swallowing apnea), reducing the possibility of aspiration or laryngeal penetration of

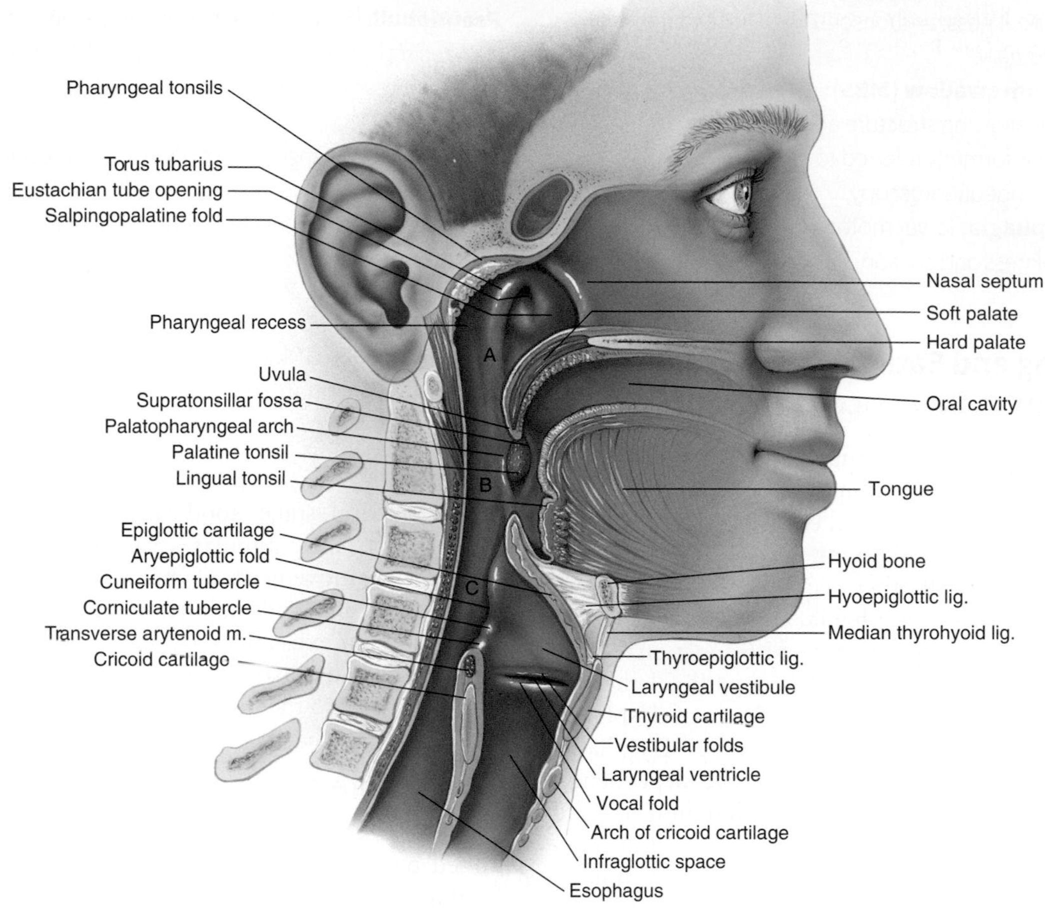

Figure 19-1. Oral, pharyngeal, and esophageal structures involved in swallowing.

food or liquid. The vocal cords close. Simultaneously, the pharyngeal constrictor muscles sequentially contract to propel the bolus through the pharynx. The elevation of the larynx causes the upper esophageal sphincter (UES) to relax, allowing the bolus to pass through it.

Esophageal Stage

In the esophageal stage, the UES returns to its normal tonic state, and the bolus is transported through the esophagus via esophageal peristalsis and gravity. The lower esophageal sphincter relaxes, allowing the bolus to pass through into the stomach.

The preoral, oral preparatory, and oral stages are voluntary. The length of the oral preparatory, oral, and pharyngeal stages vary with bolus type.[11] Oral transit time, the length of time to accomplish the oral stage, has been assumed to be 1 to 1.5 seconds[12]; however, recent research indicates no present consensus.[13] The pharyngeal stage is involuntary, although volitional movements can alter it. The pharyngeal stage is most effective in an upright position.[14] Normal pharyngeal transit time is less than 1 second.[11] The esophageal stage takes 8 to 10 seconds.[15] Although the patient's position may affect the esophageal stage because of the effects of gravity, this stage is involuntary.[15]

Impaired Swallowing

Many disease processes and trauma cause dysphagia, including those that affect the central and peripheral nervous systems, motor end plates, muscles, and other anatomical structures.

Types of Dysphagia

Dysphagia may be named by the location of its source: paralytic, pseudobulbar, and mechanical. **Paralytic dysphagia** results from lower motor neuron involvement that causes weakness and sensory impairment of oral and pharyngeal structures, including weakness or absence of the swallowing reflex. **Pseudobulbar dysphagia** results from upper motor neuron involvement, causing hypotonicity or hypertonicity of oral and pharyngeal structures and a slow or poorly coordinated swallowing reflex. **Mechanical dysphagia** is caused by loss of oral, pharyngeal, or esophageal structures; weakness; and/or sensory deficits caused by trauma or surgery, including tracheostomy. Pulmonary complications may worsen the presentation (see Boxes 19-1 and 19-2).

Evaluation of Swallowing and Eating Skills

Clinical dysphagia assessment involves two components: a clinical assessment and an **instrumental evaluation**.

Clinical Assessment

Clinical assessment of dysphagia must be thorough, with examination of all areas relevant to swallowing. It is best done using a reliable and valid tool.[34] A reliable and valid tool allows for accurate assessment and reassessment by different test administrators and ensures that each test item provides accurate assessment of performance components.

History, Nutrition, and Respiratory Considerations

The clinician reviews the patient's medical and surgical history, with special attention to any diagnoses and procedures that are relevant to dysphagia. The patient and caregiver also provide information about any history of swallowing disorders. Specific signs and symptoms, and modifications in behaviors relevant to mealtime are noted, as are changes in food intake and weight loss. The

Box 19-1

Respiratory Considerations Contributing to Dysphagia

Pulmonary Concerns

Respiratory problems may contribute to dysphagia and vice versa because the respiratory and swallowing mechanisms share anatomy and physiology.

Secretion Management

The patient's airway must be clear of excessive secretions. Intermittent suctioning through the nose or tracheostomy may be needed to clear the airway. The occupational therapist should work closely with nursing and respiratory staff to assess whether airway protection and the ability to maintain oxygenation are adequate. Personnel should be available to suction the airway as necessary.

Tracheostomy

A tracheostomy tube reroutes breathing through a stoma in the neck. Tracheostomy tubes may be temporary or permanent and are used to keep the airway open (Fig. 19-2). Tracheostomies provide easy access for suctioning or ventilator use but can cause or exacerbate dysphagia. They cause reduced smell and taste sensation because the patient is not breathing through the nose. Tracheostomy reduces the ability to clear the upper airway if laryngeal penetration occurs. It increases the risk of aspiration caused by pooling in the pharynx, delays trigger of the swallow reflex, decreases duration of vocal cord closure, and reduces laryngeal movement. An inflated tracheostomy cuff further reduces laryngeal elevation and increases the risk of silent aspiration.[16] An "open" tracheostomy, in which the tube is not covered or "capped," eliminates the subglottic pressure, reducing the force of the swallow response.[17]

Mechanical Ventilators

Ventilators are machines that assist patients to breathe if they cannot do so on their own. Positive-pressure ventilators may be used temporarily, to assist a patient through an acute illness, or chronically, for a patient with a long-term respiratory challenge. Positive-pressure ventilators deliver breaths to patients through a tube in the nose or mouth, or through a tracheostomy. Patients who use a ventilator to breathe via a tracheostomy may be able to eat by mouth. As breathing ceases during the swallow, a well-coordinated swallow is needed to interpose the swallow between inhalation and exhalation. Patients who have had mechanical ventilation for more than a week have been shown to have multiple swallowing deficits once the ventilator is removed.[18] Patients who are ventilator dependent via tracheostomy are prone to aspiration during eating.[18]

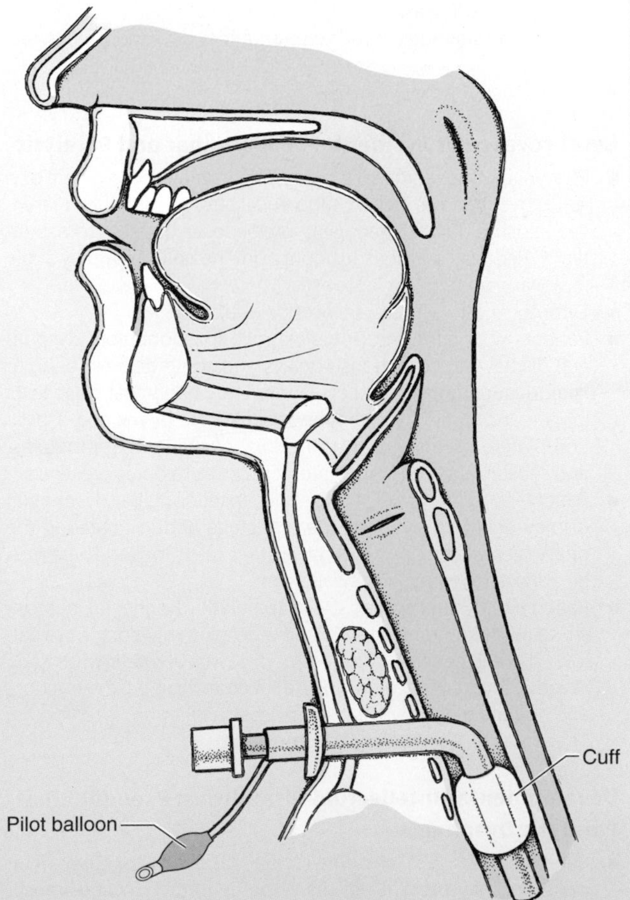

Figure 19-2. Tracheostomy tube. Tubes are available in different sizes and may come with or without the cuff as pictured. The pilot balloon is used to inflate the cuff with a syringe and indicates relative inflation of the cuff. The inflated cuff prevents food or secretions from falling further into the airway.

Box 19-2

Clinical Dysphagia Presentation for Various Diagnostic Groups

This is not an exhaustive list of diagnoses prone to dysphagia; however, it includes those most often encountered.

Alzheimer Disease: Pseudobulbar Dysphagia

- Decreased attention span and apraxia for swallowing and self-feeding may be seen.
- Oral and pharyngeal responses are slow, and a need for physical and verbal cues to self-feed are needed.
- Difficulty with self-feeding is common, and challenges with initiating the meal may be present.[19]
- Agitation and behavioral challenges can hamper the eating process.[19]
- Clients prefer sweet-flavored and pureed foods.
- Clients are prone to aspiration[20] and more difficulty with self-feeding in later stages of the disease.[19]

Brain Injury: Pseudobulbar, Paralytic Dysphagia

- Type and severity of dysphagia in brain injury depends on the injury cause, neural location, and size of brain lesion.
- Behavioral and cognitive problems affect self-feeding and swallowing.
- There may be motor difficulty with the oral and pharyngeal phases, including aspiration.[21]
- Abnormal pathological reflexes can affect oral and pharyngeal control.
- Overall mealtime may be slow.

Cerebrovascular Accident: Pseudobulbar and Paralytic

- Pharyngeal and laryngeal sensory deficits may occur in right and left hemispheric as well as subcortical strokes.[22] Reduced laryngeal closure during swallowing predisposes patients to aspiration.[23] Reduced oral sensory input from the bolus may play a role in slowing pharyngeal responses.[24]
- Symptoms vary with lesion location and size.
- Patients with right hemispheric stroke (pseudobulbar dysphagia) display mild oral transit delays and some delay in pharyngeal trigger and laryngeal elevation. The pharyngeal stage lasts longer, and there may be penetration of the larynx and aspiration.[8] There may be neglect or denial of swallowing problems, and sensory loss can slow motor responses to bolus presence.
- Patients with left hemispheric stroke (pseudobulbar dysphagia) display delays in initiating the oral stage and in triggering the pharyngeal stage. The pharyngeal stage takes longer. There may be apraxia for eating and swallowing.
- Patients with subcortical stroke (paralytic dysphagia) demonstrate mild oral transit delays and a delay in triggering the swallow. There is general weakness of pharyngeal swallow, as seen in reduced laryngeal elevation, reduced tongue base retraction, and unilateral pharyngeal weakness. Aspiration is common. There may also be reduced UES opening.

Developmental/Intellectual Disabilities: Pseudobulbar, Paralytic Dysphagia

- Cerebral palsy (CP) and intellectual disability, together or in isolation, may present deficits of bolus formation and transit, delayed swallow reflex, pharyngeal dysmotility, esophageal disease, and aspiration.[25]
- Abnormal oral reflexes, and oral hyposensitivity or hypersensitivity may be observed.
- Poor postural, head, neck, and limb control can affect swallowing.
- Behaviors such as eating too quickly and putting too much food in the mouth can affect efficiency and safety of swallowing.[26]

Head and Neck Cancer: Mechanical Dysphagia

- Swallowing problems with head and neck cancer vary with tumor type, size, and location.[27]
- Bolus control and containment problems result from surgery to the lip.
- Resection of tumor from the floor of the mouth causes difficulty with bolus control, reduced laryngeal elevation, and its accompanying reduction in UES opening.
- Glossectomy, or removal of some or all of the tongue, causes difficult or absent bolus mobilization; a resection of the tongue base limits the elevation needed to initiate the pharyngeal swallow.
- Unilateral laryngeal cancer may require a vertical laryngectomy or hemilaryngectomy; this may cause reduced vocal cord closure, reduced posterior tongue movement, and reduced UES opening.
- Supraglottic laryngectomy reduces glottic closure, laryngeal elevation, and opening of the UES.
- Extensive cancer of the larynx necessitates a total laryngectomy, which separates the foodway and airway tracts and creates a permanent anatomical tracheostomy. Although aspiration is no longer a threat, there is reduced movement through the pharynx, remaining laryngeal tissue, and esophagus.
- Adjunctive radiation therapy causes edema in areas adjacent to the radiation field, fibrosis, and reduced salivary flow, causing dry mouth or xerostomia.
- Radiation therapy combined with chemotherapy without surgery can reduce tongue base movement, laryngeal elevation, and pharyngeal range of motion and speed.
- Radiation therapy combined with surgery can cause longer oral transit time, increased pharyngeal residue, and reduced UES opening.

Multiple Sclerosis: Pseudobulbar, Paralytic Dysphagia

- Dysphagia symptoms vary with location of plaques in the central and peripheral nervous systems. Dysphagia worsens with disease progression.[28]
- Weakness of the oral structures and the neck muscles may be seen.[28]
- Delayed pharyngeal swallow and weakness of pharyngeal contractions may be seen.[28]

Neoplasms of the Brain: Pseudobulbar, Paralytic Dysphagia

- Dysphagia may be due either to a tumor or to metastasis in the brain or to medical or surgical interventions.
- Symptoms vary with the location and extent of the client's neoplasm and interventions, and symptoms may be similar to those found in clients with stroke.[29]

Parkinson Disease: Pseudobulbar Dysphagia

- Impulsiveness and poor judgment can affect swallowing.
- Jaw rigidity, abnormal head and neck posture, impaired coordination of tongue movements and mastication. Mastication and orofacial motions are affected[30] along with tongue control.[31] Alterations in the pharyngeal aspect of the swallow occur,[32] including pharyngeal residue and delayed pharyngeal elevation. Abnormal head, neck, and trunk posture along with difficulty coordinating upper extremity movements for self-feeding are seen.
- Feeding and swallowing may be too slow and laborious to allow sufficient nutritional intake.
- Orofacial fatigue may make eating and swallowing more difficult as a meal progresses.[33]

current nutritional sources are recorded, including the length of time the patient has been NPO (from the Latin term, *nil per os*), or not eating by mouth, if applicable. The therapist also documents any cultural and religious dietary preferences and practices. Information regarding respiratory status is gathered from the hospital chart and staff, including the presence of a tracheostomy and/or mechanical ventilation, and the level of independence with secretion management.

Assessment of Cognitive, Perceptual, and Physical Abilities

Important cognitive and perceptual considerations include the level of alertness and arousal, orientation, ability to attend to a **feeding** session or meal, ability to follow multistep commands, and any visual deficits or unilateral neglect. The clinician notes the patient's insight into his or her dysphagia and observes head, neck, trunk, and limb control and endurance for being out of bed at mealtimes. The ability to self-position and self-feed, and the need for or use of adaptive eating equipment are assessed.

Assessment of Oral and Pharyngeal Abilities

Once direct physical assessment begins, the clinician must observe universal precautions to prevent exposure to pathogens for both the clinician and the patient. The occupational therapist then assesses aspects of oral and pharyngeal control, as noted in the subsequent section. A stethoscope may be used to listen for pooling of fluid above the level of the vocal cords because pooled liquids resonate during breathing.[35] The therapist rates the patient's hunger and level of enthusiasm for a snack or meal.

Lip Closure

- The function of lip closure is to contain solid and liquid boluses in the mouth and to help collect the food into a bolus for swallowing.
- Signs of dysfunction include food loss through the mouth, possibly only on one side.
- Causes of impairment include oral motor weakness or muscle tone impairment.
- The impact on eating function includes the inability to keep the bolus in the mouth and initiate a swallow because pressure cannot be generated in the oral pharynx to initiate posterior bolus movement or a swallow.
- Lip closure is assessed by asking the patient to hold the lips closed over a tongue depressor. It is also assessed by observing bolus loss from the mouth during a food trial.

Bolus Containment within the Cheeks

- The cheeks function to hold the bolus within the oral cavity.
- Signs of dysfunction include food particles pocketing in the cheek or between the cheek and the teeth after the swallow.
- Causes of impairment include oral motor weakness or muscle tone impairment.
- The impact on eating function may include incomplete swallowing of the bolus, food remaining in mouth that could be aspirated later (food or secretions enter the larynx below the level of the vocal cords), and/or inability to form a cohesive bolus with more solid foods.
- To assess, observe lack of movement on the affected side or sides. Assess after the swallow by having the patient open the mouth and examine with a flashlight. Run your gloved finger inside the cheek to check for food pocketing.

Jaw Closure/Chewing

- The function of mastication (of solids) is to break down food to form a bolus.
- Signs of dysfunction include "chomping" (nonrotary chewing), or slowed or absent chewing.
- Causes of impairment include decreased muscle tone or jaw strength, neurological injury, or trauma.
- The impact of dysfunction includes the inability to break down food and form a bolus.
- To assess, have the patient open the mouth and examine with a flashlight. Large particle food remnants may be observed.

Tongue Motions

- The tongue moves food in the mouth to form a bolus and begins propulsion of the bolus to the pharynx.
- Signs of dysfunction include the inability to move the bolus side to side for chewing on either molar surface, lack of bolus formation, and/or the inability to form a bolus or propel the bolus posteriorly.
- Causes of impairment include decreased muscle tone or strength, neurological injury, or trauma.
- The impact of dysfunction is the inability to control a liquid bolus or move a bolus posteriorly.
- Assess by asking the patient to open the mouth and protrude or move the tongue from side to side.
- Dysfunction is indicated by tongue lateralization to only one side (which indicates weakness on the opposite side) and an inability to oppose the tip of the tongue outside the mouth to the left, right, superiorly, and inferiorly.

Soft Palate Function

- The function of the soft palate is to cover the nasopharynx during swallowing.
- Signs of dysfunction include nasal regurgitation (food enters the nasal cavity).
- Causes of dysfunction include decreased or altered muscle tone due to neurological injury.
- The impact of dysfunction is nasal regurgitation during swallowing, which may be associated with nasal vocal quality and aspiration.
- Assess by having the patient open the mouth, push the tongue down gently so that the uvula and soft palate are visualized, and examine uvula elevation

when the patient phonates "ah." The uvula may not elevate, or elevation may be asymmetrical. Soft palate function is most accurately visualized on **modified barium swallow** (MBS).

Gag Reflex

- The presence of the gag reflex indicates sensitivity in the pharynx, which helps to protect the airway if food is misdirected there.
- Signs of dysfunction may be laryngeal penetration or aspiration, detectible on MBS.
- Causes of dysfunction include neurological injury or trauma from surgery.
- The impact of dysfunction is difficulty protecting the airway and lack of coughing if airway protection is challenged.
- Assess by a tongue depressor. Carefully stroke the back of the soft palate or posterior pharynx and then watch for throat clearing or cough.

Vocal Quality

- Normal vocal quality suggests good vocal cord strength, which is important as the vocal cords close during the swallow for airway protection.
- Signs of dysfunction include wet or hoarse voice or absence of voice.
- Causes of dysfunction include neurological injury, trauma, or the presence of a tracheostomy.
- The impact of dysfunction can include decreased airway protection during or in between swallows, and increased risk of laryngeal penetration or aspiration.
- Assess by listening to the quality of the patient's voice. If wet or wet hoarse, there may be limited vocal cord ability to close during the swallow.

Volitional Cough

- Both volitional and reflexive cough help to protect the airway.
- Signs of dysfunction include lack of volitional cough. Causes of dysfunction include neurological injury, trauma from surgery, and the presence of a tracheostomy.
- The impact of dysfunction includes decreased airway protection, increased risk of laryngeal penetration, or aspiration.
- Assess by asking the patient to cough, or observe lack of cough when the airway appears challenged; may best be evaluated by MBS.

Laryngeal Elevation

- Elevation and slight anterior tipping of the larynx occurs during normal swallowing.
- Signs of dysfunction include lack of upward movement of the larynx during swallowing.
- Causes of dysfunction include neurological injury, trauma, surgery, or the presence of a tracheostomy.
- The impact of dysfunction includes the inability to effect a swallow.
- Laryngeal elevation may be palpated during bedside evaluation and assessed during MBS.

The Feeding Trial

Precautions for the therapist and patient are outlined in Box 19-3.

Interventions that maximize performance can be initiated before the feeding trial begins (see Figs. 19-3 to 19-5). Prior to the feeding trial portion of an evaluation (with snacks or meals), measures must be taken to optimize the patient's swallowing performance. Because these strategies do not involve ingestion of food, they are **indirect therapy** techniques.

- The patient should be evaluated in a quiet environment to encourage concentration.
- Position the patient upright in a chair to minimize the risk of aspiration. The patient's feet should be

Box 19-3

Precautions for the Therapist and Patient

The occupational therapist is physically close to the patient during eating and is exposed to oral secretions and respirations. Likewise, the patient is exposed to pathogens on the therapist's clothing and hands and in the therapist's respiratory tract. Universal (also called standard) precautions should be used. The use of gloves is mandatory anytime the therapist touches the face, neck, or oral cavity. Use of a gown and mask may be advised.

Dysphagia patients are prone to difficulty with airway obstruction and aspiration during eating. For the safety of the patient, the swallowing therapist should be trained in suctioning of the airway, the Heimlich maneuver, and cardiopulmonary resuscitation.

Signs and Symptoms of Potential or Actual Aspiration

Although laryngeal penetration or aspiration may be silent, occurring without overt warning signs and symptoms, the following indicates that it may occur or be occurring. If observed during a dysphagia evaluation, these signs or symptoms can indicate that a feeding trial should not be initiated or should be discontinued. Specific items of concern are as follows:

1. The patient cannot remain awake for the clinical evaluation.
2. The oral and/or pharyngeal sensation and motion assessment reveal poor ability to manipulate and contain the bolus.
3. The bolus remains in the mouth, and the patient cannot initiate or complete the oral preparatory stage within a reasonable time.
4. There is excessive coughing or choking before, during, or after swallowing.
5. There is no swallow response once the oral stage is completed.
6. There is a change in voice quality, often wet, or no voice after swallowing.
7. Severe pooling or wetness is heard on auscultation or by the naked ear; secretions are poorly managed.
8. Silent aspiration is suggested by a change in the patient's color and/or respiratory rate, increased congestion on auscultation of the chest, and/or a reduction in oxygen level in the blood as recorded by pulse oximetry.

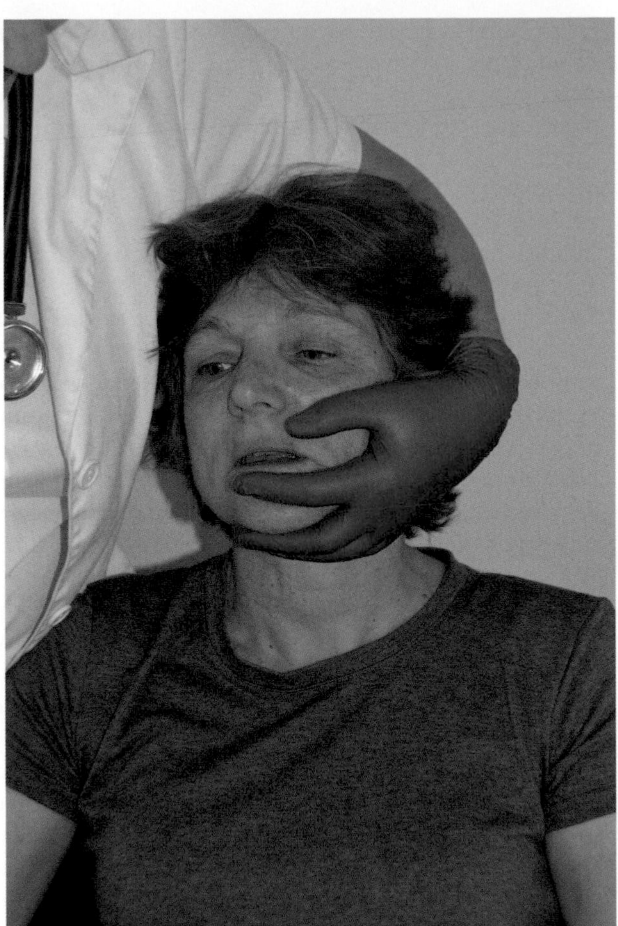

Figure 19-3. The therapist uses a half-Nelson position to assist with head and neck control. The therapist can also assist with jaw, cheek, and lip control at the same time.

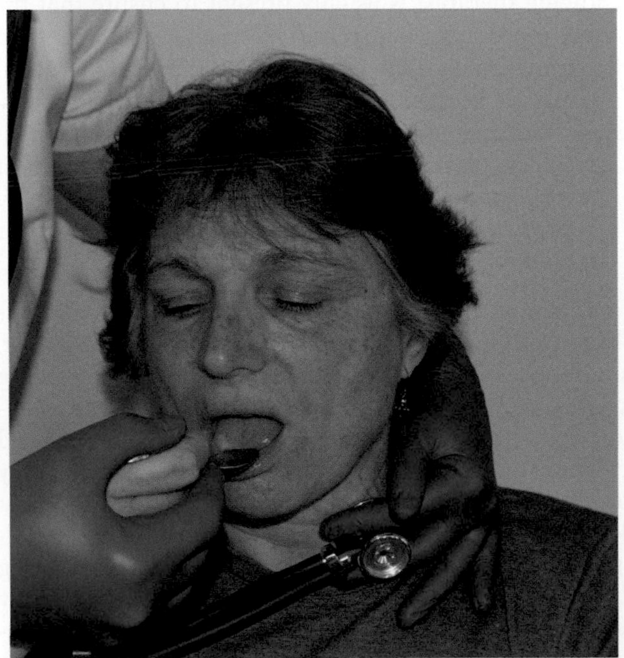

Figure 19-4. The therapist facilitates auscultation of the swallow using a stethoscope. The therapist may be able to facilitate head position and guide self-feeding while listening to the sounds of the swallow.

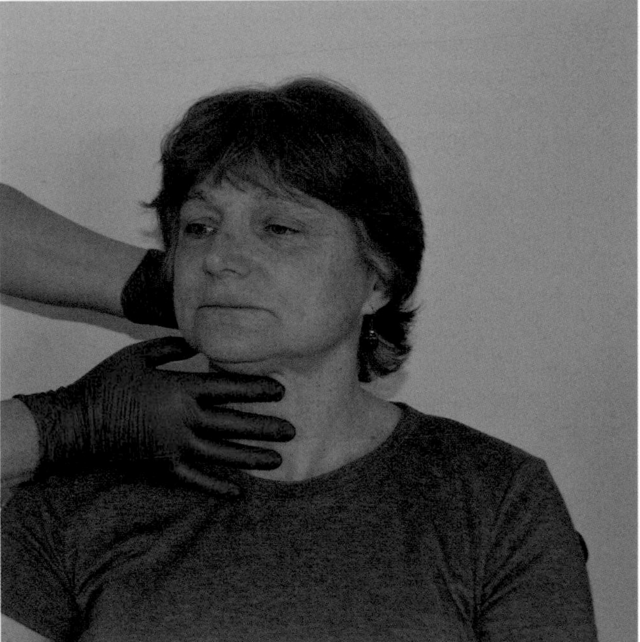

Figure 19-5. The therapist palpates the neck during swallowing. The first finger is under the chin, the second finger is at the base of the tongue, the third finger is over the thyroid cartilage, and the fourth finger is at the base of the throat. A very light touch should be used so as not to inhibit motion.

supported, and the arms should be free for self-feeding. Patients with pseudobulbar dysphagia may need special attention to seating and positioning before eating and special positioning devices; they may need assistance to maintain head and neck alignment and facilitation to stimulate oral and pharyngeal motions prior to and during eating (see Fig. 19-3).

- Oral hygiene activities should be completed before the trial because this stimulates sensation and range of motion of oral structures.
- Present a simplified visual array of food and utensils for the patient with visual neglect and/or other visual deficits. "Anchors," colorful cues to call attention to the side of the plate, are helpful for patients with neglect.
- Present appetizing, culture-specific foods, utensils, and tableware.
- Provide adaptive equipment and/or use hand-over-hand guidance to facilitate self-feeding.
- Provide simple explanations and one-step verbal directions if necessary.
- If the patient eats too quickly or is confused by multiple food choices, present one food at a time.
- Use small-bowled utensils and verbal or manual assistance to load just a teaspoon-sized bolus. Pinch the straw to limit the amount of liquid consumed or use a covered cup with a small opening.

The safest food textures are chosen for the trial. Easy-to-manage foods and thick fluids are attempted first, especially if the patient has been NPO and/or has a diagnosis or clinical picture that suggests a high risk of aspiration. During the oral stage, the clinician observes bolus containment, formation, propulsion, and mastication. During the pharyngeal stage, the clinician assesses laryngeal elevation, voice quality after swallow, repetitive swallows, and cough reflex. The therapist should observe for signs and symptoms of laryngeal penetration or aspiration, especially during the first feeding trial (see Fig. 19-3). The evaluation concludes with a summary, recommendations, and plan.[16]

Specific techniques are helpful during the feeding trial. Auscultation (listening) to the swallow with a stethoscope held lateral to the larynx (Fig. 19-4) can reveal the efficiency and safety of the oral and pharyngeal stages.[35] Gentle palpation of the neck (Fig. 19-5) during the swallow reveals symmetry, strength, and speed of oral pharyngeal movement and may be done simultaneously with auscultation. If the patient can self-feed, palpation and auscultation may be performed at the same time. If the patient needs help to self-feed, auscultation and guiding with hand-to-mouth efforts may be done together.

Recommendations and Plan

Once the clinical evaluation is complete, recommendations and a plan are formulated. Recommendations may include (1) whether eating by mouth is advisable, (2) whether an instrumental evaluation is advised, (3) whether a nutritional consultation with a dietitian is needed, (4) recommended diet type, (5) mealtime seating and positioning, (6) mealtime supervision, (7) adaptive equipment, and (8) type and amount of assistance. Evaluation of the patient is ongoing, and with additional information from clinical observations, instrumental evaluations, and input from other dysphagia team members, the treatment plan and goals change.

Instrumental Evaluation

Clinical assessment accompanies instrumental evaluation, which uses imaging and diagnostic studies to provide critical information about the unseen parts of the oral, pharyngeal, and esophageal stages of swallowing. Various types of instrumental evaluations for dysphagia include the following:

- *Electromyography.* Electrodes are placed either into the muscle via a small needle or on the skin over a muscle to record contractions of the muscle. Surface electrodes have been used to assess aspects of oral bolus management in neurological dysphagia patients and pharyngeal, laryngeal, and esophageal activity.[36]
- *Fiberoptic endoscopic evaluation of swallowing.* A fiberoptic laryngoscope, a narrow flexible tube with a small camera on its tip, is introduced through the nose into the nasopharynx, where structures including the palate, pharynx, and larynx are viewed for assessment of anatomy and movement. Food is administered in different consistencies to observe posterior oral and pharyngeal function and airway protection during eating.
- *Manometry.* A catheter with transducers to measure pressure is introduced into the esophagus. The force, timing, and sequence of the esophageal contractions are measured.
- *Scintigraphy.* A radioactive isotope is mixed with food. As the bolus is swallowed, a gamma camera tracks the radioactive particles. This test measures the speed of bolus transit and can accurately measure the amount of bolus that is aspirated.
- *Ultrasonography.* An ultrasound transducer held under the chin produces images of oral and pharyngeal stages of swallow, revealing the mobility of structures and boluses swallowed.
- ***Modified barium swallow.*** The patient is seated between a movable camera and a fluorescent screen. Radiographic images of oral, pharyngeal, and esophageal structures are delivered to a screen from the camera as barium or barium-impregnated fluids and foods are swallowed. The images are recorded on DVD. Figure 19-6 illustrates a videofluoroscopic image of the oral, pharyngeal, and upper esophageal structures. Swallowing pathology and the effectiveness of compensatory swallowing techniques and positions can be observed. The patient may be positioned in a lateral and/or anteroposterior position to view structure and function from both perspectives. MBSs are often repeated to assess progress. A swallowing therapist is usually present to ensure that the test reproduces compensatory maneuvers and food textures being used and to ensure that it mimics real eating as accurately as possible. In some instances, the therapist may perform the MBS. Occupational therapists assisting with or performing MBS must be expert swallowing clinicians; they must be fully trained in use of the equipment and procedures used in videofluoroscopy.

These evaluations are usually performed by a radiologist, often together with the occupational therapist. Aspiration of food or fluid may be silent.[37] Imaging studies, such as MBS (see Fig. 19-6) and **fiberoptic endoscopic evaluation of swallowing** (FEES), are needed to identify aspiration. These procedures, however, may not identify aspiration in all instances because client skills can change and the testing situation in the radiology suite may not reliably approximate an actual eating situation. Although not always able to reliably identify aspiration, these procedures do provide important information about the quality of the swallow and the efficacy of compensatory therapy techniques used during swallowing.

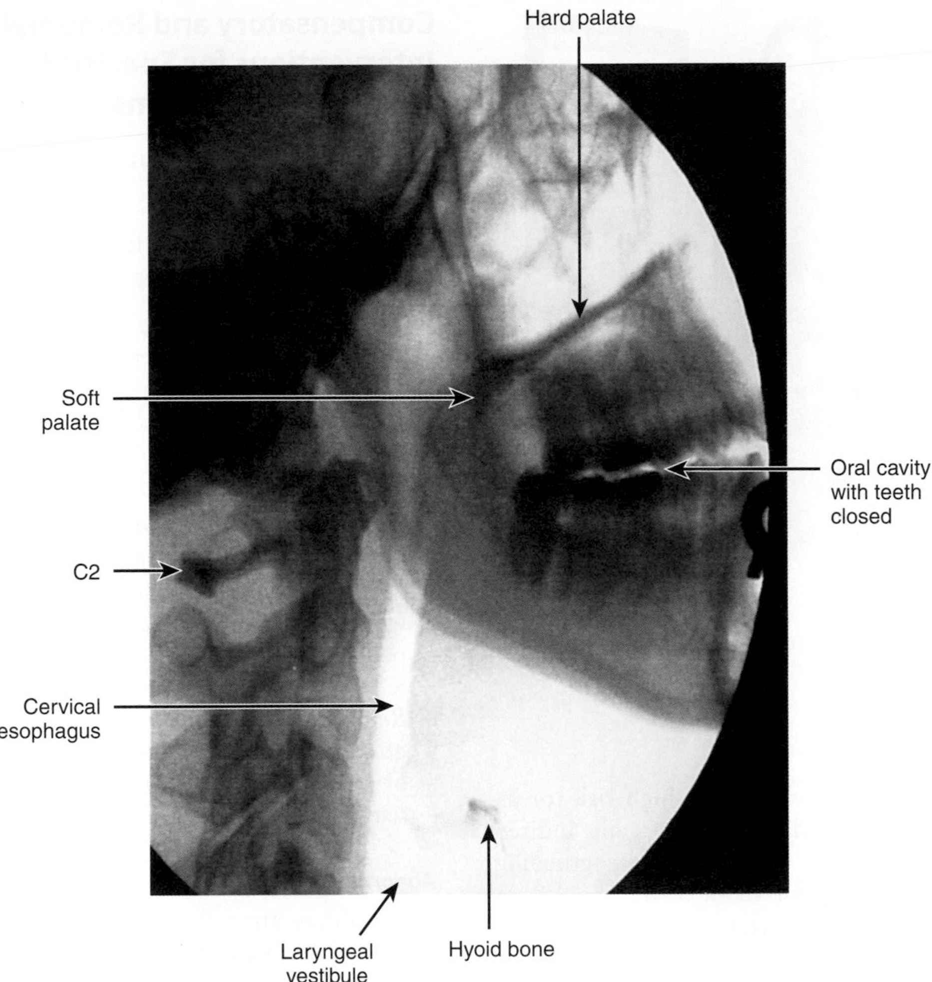

Figure 19-6. A videofluoroscopic image of the oral, pharyngeal, and esophageal structures. (Image courtesy of Bette Pomerleau, MS, SLP, and Ray Autiello, LPN, RT, of Universal Mobile Services, Haverhill, MA.)

Conceptual Foundations Underlying Interventions for Swallowing and Eating Impairment

The intervention approach for patients with dysphagia depends on the prognosis of their illness or condition.

Remedial and Compensatory Dysphagia Therapy

Remedial, also referred to as rehabilitative treatment, focuses on restoring a more normal level of swallowing function. Potential for partial or full recovery is anticipated when goals are strictly remedial. For example, a remedial approach may be used with an acute stroke patient for whom complete or near-complete recovery is anticipated. One example is surface electromyography that provides patients with improved awareness of swallowing function, providing for better swallowing. This intervention has been shown to be useful in populations with stroke[38] and nonstroke disorders.[39] VitalStim is a specially designed neuromuscular stimulation unit that facilitates contraction of the muscles used in swallowing, by placing surface electrodes on the neck (see Fig. 19-7).

Compensatory treatment circumvents impairments with the use of alternative strategies and techniques. These techniques are used when full recovery is not anticipated, for example, for a patient with advancing Parkinson disease. Compensatory techniques may also be used to enable a safe, functional swallow prior to recovery of normal swallowing, for example, with a patient with acute pneumonia. Thus, these approaches may be used in tandem. Goals may be remedial and then change to compensatory once a plateau in function or relatively normal function is reached.

Indirect and Direct Therapy

Another consideration is the type of therapeutic techniques used. Indirect therapy addresses the prerequisite abilities or the capacity to swallow without ingestion

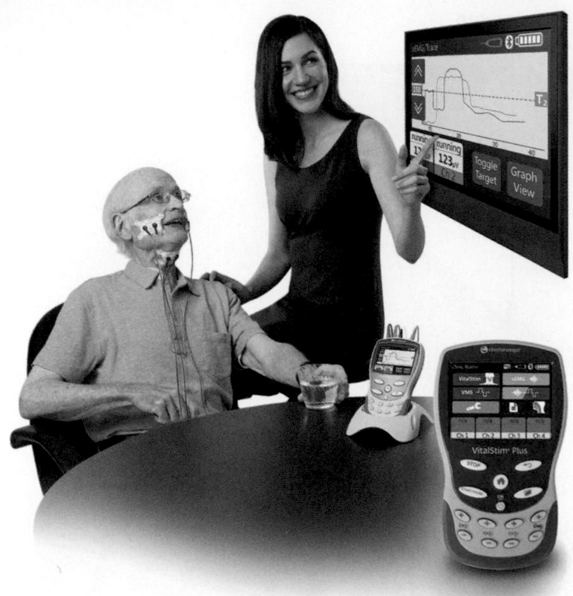

Figure 19-7. Instrumental intervention: VitalStim. (© 2018 DJO, LLC VitalStim is a registered trademark of DJO, LLC.)

of food or liquid. Patients who are at high risk for aspiration often begin with indirect therapy only. Indirect therapy can include range of motion, strengthening, and coordination exercises for weak or hypotonic oral and pharyngeal musculature; strengthening of pharyngeal and laryngeal structures; techniques to reduce or stimulate sensitivity of oral musculature; and techniques to improve the pharyngeal swallowing response. Indirect therapy also involves increasing the patient's level of arousal to implement treatment and manipulating the environment to optimize behaviors that affect swallowing.

Direct therapy rehabilitates prerequisite abilities or the capacity to swallow during therapeutic snacks or meals. This involves exercises and/or the use of compensatory swallowing maneuvers that include ingestion of food. Indirect therapy may continue once direct therapy has begun. An individualized treatment plan usually includes a selection of direct and indirect techniques. The complexity of interventions depends on the ability of the patient and/or caregiver to process complex information. Treatment techniques may be evaluated by MBS or FEES to assess their efficacy, especially in the pharyngeal stage where the effects of techniques are unseen. Although not discussed in depth here, optimizing self-feeding skills is an important goal to address together with swallowing goals. Although not yet supported in the literature, the sensory inputs and motor patterns used for self-feeding are likely related to those used in the partly voluntary swallow, and facilitating both skills enhances each.

Compensatory and Remedial Interventions for Specific Eating and Swallowing Problems

Specific Eating and Swallowing Problems

Swallowing Apraxia

Swallowing apraxia is difficulty or inability to swallow in the absence of motor or sensory deficits.

- *Remedial intervention:* Provide a natural mealtime setting, enhance self-feeding skills to facilitate oral skills, and provide a variety of boluses to stimulate oral movements.

Weakness of Cheeks and Lips

- *Compensatory intervention:* Provide soft solids and thick fluids for easy oral manipulation. Place food at the back and stronger side of the mouth. Tilt the head toward the stronger side. Massage the cheek to prevent pocketing. Hold the lips closed. Inspect the mouth after meals to check for residue.
- *Remedial intervention:* Use tapping, vibration, and quick stretches to stimulate movement. Provide range of motion and stretching exercises, progressing to resistive sucking and blowing exercises.

Abnormal Oral Reflexes

Oral reflexes are reflexive motions that are seen in infants and extinguished with development. They may reappear in adults with neurological injury. Rooting, biting, tongue thrust, sucking, and a hyperactive gag response are all reflexes that may be observed.

- *Compensatory intervention:* Avoid stimuli that provoke rooting, biting, tongue thrusting, sucking, or hyperactive gag reflexes. Elicit movements that are antagonistic to the undesirable reflex (e.g., encourage mouth opening to weaken the bite reflex). Seat the patient with the body well supported to minimize proximal extensor tone, which can provoke abnormal distal movements and reflexes.

Facial and Intraoral Hypersensitivity

Hypersensitivity to normal touch on the face and in the mouth can occur following neurological injury.

- *Remedial intervention:* Provide systematic desensitization to the face and intraoral area. If sensory defensiveness affects the whole body, a program of graded sensory stimulation to the body should precede stimulation to the oral area, followed by careful introduction of food. Use systematic desensitization with guided imagery to reduce muscle tone and anxiety regarding eating and mouth sensitivity.

Oral Hyposensitivity

Oral hyposensitivity can occur following neurological injury and involves reduced sensation of the oral cavity to contact from a bolus or liquid.

- *Compensatory intervention:* Place the bolus on areas of the mouth that are more sensitive. Use warmer or colder boluses, flavorful food, and heavy or viscous boluses to stimulate sensation.[36,40]
- *Remedial and compensatory intervention:* Use a sensory diet that provides heightened tactile and proprioceptive input to the intraoral structures to stimulate sensation and movement before and during a meal or snack.

Reduced Lingual Control

Reduced lingual (tongue) control occurs when neurological injury has affected coordinated tongue motions required for speech and swallowing.

- *Compensatory intervention:* Introduce a diet requiring little oral manipulation, including soft solids and thick fluids. Use a posterior and/or lateral placement of food on the stronger side. Inspect the mouth for residue after meals.
- *Remedial intervention:* Introduce active and passive tongue range of motion exercises and activities. Provide quick stretches to the tongue with a tongue depressor or gloved fingers. Provide articulation and tongue strengthening exercises.

Slow Oral Transit Time

Slow oral transit time is slowed oral propulsion and manipulation of the bolus due to weakness or neurological injury.

- *Compensatory intervention:* Use cold boluses to hasten oral transit time (be cautious that they do not melt into a difficult-to-manage liquid). Sour boluses, such as those infused with lemon juice, can speed oral manipulation.

Delayed Swallow

A delayed swallow occurs when the oral and pharyngeal stages of the swallow do not occur in a timely way. As noted earlier in the chapter, the normal oral phase takes 1 to 1.5 seconds and the pharyngeal phase takes less than 1 second.

- *Compensatory intervention:* Use highly flavored boluses to reduce swallowing delays.[36] Use chin tuck to enhance airway protection.[41] Increase bolus volume and viscosity to reduce pharyngeal delay time.
- *Remedial intervention:* Try thermal-tactile stimulation: stroke the anterior faucial arches with an iced laryngeal mirror (Fig. 19-8), which hastens initiation and overall speed of swallowing immediately after application.[42]

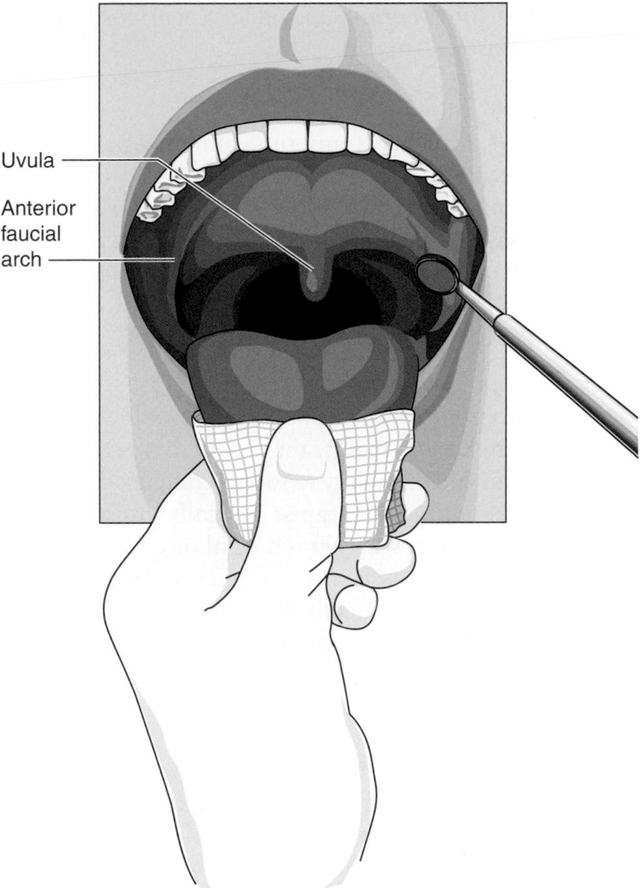

Figure 19-8. Thermal-tactile stimulation of swallow. An iced laryngeal mirror is used to stroke the faucial arches to elicit or improve strength of the swallowing reflex.

Reduced Laryngeal Elevation

Laryngeal elevation is the (normal) elevation of the larynx that occurs during the swallow; it accompanies a slight forward tipping of the larynx.

- *Compensatory intervention:* Use the Mendelsohn maneuver to prolong elevation of the larynx[43] or a chin tuck to elevate the larynx.[41] Use a supraglottic or super-supraglottic swallow to clear or minimize any material in airway. These swallow procedures are used by patients to close the larynx during the swallow to prevent food and liquids from entering the lungs.
- *Remedial intervention:* Use Shaker exercises (a program of neck flexion exercises) to strengthen suprahyoid musculature and prolong opening of the UES.[41]

Reduced Laryngeal Closure

During the swallow, the larynx (which includes the vocal cords) closes to protect the airway from penetration by food or liquid.

- *Compensatory intervention:* Use a supraglottic or super-supraglottic swallow to enhance airway protection, or use a chin tuck to elevate and close off the larynx.

- *Remedial intervention:* Introduce vocal cord adduction exercises.

Tracheostomy

Occlusion of a tracheostomy tube minimizes aspiration and improves swallow biomechanics.[44] Use of a one-way speaking valve, usually a Passy-Muir valve, can decrease frequency of aspiration.[45] Dysphagia often improves with decannulation (removal of tracheostomy).[46]

Compensatory Swallowing Maneuvers

Compensatory swallowing maneuvers use volitional movement to improve the quality of the swallow. Most of them are complex and require the patient to possess a good attention span and the ability to follow complex directions.

The occupational therapist typically must try different interventions, whether remedial or compensatory, preferably with the assistance of MBS, to assess which techniques work most effectively. Clinicians should work under the guidance of an experienced occupational therapist when using a technique that is new to them.

Chin Tuck

This maneuver moves the base of the tongue back and narrows the opening to the larynx, thus protecting the airway.[47] Have the patient tuck the chin down toward the chest while swallowing.

Effortful Swallow

An effortful swallow helps to elevate the base of the tongue during swallowing.[48] The patient squeezes hard with the throat muscles while swallowing.

Mendelsohn Maneuver

This technique prolongs opening of the UES.[43] The patient pushes the tongue into the roof of mouth and attempts to keep the Adam's apple up while swallowing.

Head/Neck Rotation

Head/neck rotation closes the weaker side of the pharynx and uses the stronger intact musculature in cases of unilateral weakness of the pharynx and/or vocal folds. Head/neck rotation also improves the quality of the swallow.[49] The patient turns the head to the weaker side while swallowing.

Supraglottic Swallow

Named for use with supraglottic laryngectomy patients, the supraglottic swallow compensates for weak vocal cord closure and reduces penetration of food into the larynx during swallowing by closing the vocal cords.[49] The patient swallows while holding the breath and then coughs. The volitional cough that is done after swallowing helps to ensure that anything in the airway returns to the pharynx to be reswallowed.

Super-Supraglottic Swallow

This technique reduces penetration of food into the larynx during swallowing by narrowing the opening to the airway.[49] The patient holds the breath and bears down. The patient should be instructed to maintain the breath-hold and bearing down while swallowing. Afterward, the patient volitionally coughs.

Progression of Diet with Swallowing Therapy

The occupational therapist typically must try different interventions, whether remedial or compensatory, preferably with the assistance of MBS, to assess which techniques work most effectively. Clinicians should work under the guidance of an experienced occupational therapist when using a technique that is new to them.

As indirect therapy begins, some patients may receive all nutrition, hydration, and medication via a nonoral source, such as intravenous or gastrostomy tube feedings. As the patient recovers the ability to swallow without laryngeal penetration or aspiration, direct therapy with the therapist present begins during snacks and progresses to meals. As improvement continues and the patient learns compensatory techniques, he or she may progress to eating under the supervision of nursing personnel and trained significant others and then progress to eating independently. Calorie counts are initiated by the dietitian to assess the adequacy of oral intake. Once food intake improves and calories are consistently sufficient, nonoral feeding sources may be used only for hydration and/or medication. Finally, as the patient improves and fluids and medications are safely ingested by mouth, the use of nonoral feeding sources can be discontinued. Diet textures are upgraded as skills develop. Depending on the diagnosis and potential for recovery, patients may level off at any point in the described progression.

Dysphagia Diets

Dysphagia diets are designed to provide stepwise gradation of food and fluid textures that are matched to the patient's improving oral and pharyngeal skills. A diet of mechanical soft foods (foods that have been chopped or ground) that form a moist, cohesive bolus, and thickened fluids may reduce the incidence of aspiration compared with pureed foods and thin fluids.[36] Specific textures and stronger flavors can stimulate optimal oral and pharyngeal motion; for example, stronger and spicy flavors may stimulate swallowing responses.[36,40] Patients may have strong preferences; those with dementias may prefer sweet flavors and reject foods that require chewing. Dysphagia diets for most patients follow this general progression:

1. Thick purees, such as pudding and applesauce
2. Very soft moist chewables, such as soft cooked vegetables, fruits, and soft pastas

3. Drier chewables, such as cookies and breads
4. Foods requiring biting, firmer chewables such as meats, and mixed textures like cereals and milk or pills and water.

The progression of fluids advances as follows:

1. No fluids at all
2. Honey-thick fluids
3. Nectar-thick fluids
4. Thin, flavored fluids
5. Water

Fluids are easily thickened with commercial thickeners, which can be mixed with hot or cold beverages. Unthickened or "free" water is sometimes provided to dysphagia clients on the assumption that consuming small amounts of water creates little risk of pneumonia and can improve hydration.[50] This may best be assessed by FEES as opposed to MBS because the latter uses barium or barium-infused food or liquid that may change the swallowing ability.

Because bacterial pathogens in the mouth may be aspirated into the lungs, meticulous oral hygiene before and after meals is needed with any oral intake to reduce the risk of pneumonia.[51] It is important that all caregivers know and understand an individual patient's diet so that no foods or fluids are provided that are contraindicated.

Patient and Caregiver Training

Although the occupational therapist alone may carry out treatment, the plan for intervention also includes education of the patient, nursing staff, and caregivers. The patient and family should understand the cause and prognosis of the patient's dysphagia and the importance of strategies to be carried out at home. It may be helpful to have the patient view the MBS or FEES to fully comprehend his or her condition and the benefits of compensatory techniques. Mealtime seating, adaptive equipment, and the type and amount of assistance must be taught to caregivers. Meal preparation practice and community outings can reinforce diet modifications, enhance patient and family education in various settings, and motivate the patient.

As the emphasis on evidence-based practice and rehabilitation advances, clinicians must keep abreast of new knowledge. The author encourages the reader to explore further learning and expertise in dysphagia care. Early discharge from acute care and rehabilitation hospitals, and minimized staffing in health care facilities, create situations in which competence in dysphagia intervention has become a mandatory skill for occupational therapists. Occupational therapists, with their background in the many abilities and capacities that influence eating and swallowing, make logical primary swallowing therapists.

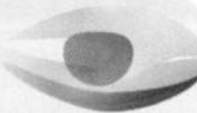

CASE STUDY

Patient Information

Dominick is a 73-year-old Italian American male with a left hemispheric cerebrovascular accident (CVA). He was admitted to an acute care hospital with aphasia and right upper extremity weakness, with a prior history of hypertension, transient ischemic attacks (TIAs) with aphasia, and chronic heart failure.

Assessment Process and Results

A dysphagia evaluation was performed using a standardized dysphagia assessment. The evaluation revealed that Dominick had hypotonicity and reduced control of his lips, cheek, and tongue on the right side. Decreased airway protection skills were evidenced by his inability to phonate because of vocal cord weakness, inability to cough volitionally, and reduced laryngeal elevation as palpated during swallowing. He was not aphasic. Dominick was able to swallow foods from a beginning level dysphagia diet, including foods with soft, moist textures, such as pudding and applesauce, with mild food spillage out of the right side of his mouth because of poor lip control, delayed formation and propulsion of the bolus, and delayed initiation of the swallow. He had difficulty grasping utensils and cups because of hypotonicity of his dominant right hand.

Occupational Therapy Problem List

- Dominick showed hypotonicity of oral, pharyngeal, and laryngeal structures, resulting in a delay in and reduced coordination of bolus control both in the mouth and in propelling the bolus posteriorly to initiate a swallow.
- He also demonstrated a delay in initiation of the swallow.
- His reduced upper extremity control resulted in awkward use of his dominant arm to self-feed.

Occupational Therapy Goal List

- Dominick will tolerate a more advanced dysphagia diet, adding soft chewables such as cooked fruit and soft pasta.
- Dominick will tolerate these textures without clinical signs of aspiration.
- Dominick will be independent in vocal cord adduction exercises.
- Dominick will support the right side of his lower lip and massage the right cheek during the oral preparatory stage to prevent food spillage and pocketing in his right cheek.
- Dominick will feed himself with his right hand with built-up utensils and an adapted cup while weight bearing on his right elbow.

Intervention

Dominick was seen daily for occupational therapy during 1 week as a hospital inpatient. Constant supervision at mealtime was accomplished, and all meals and snacks took place with him seated upright in a chair. Occupational therapy intervention addressed exercises and positioning to enhance tone and control of oral motor skills, laryngeal exercises to strengthen his vocal cords and improve laryngeal elevation, and facilitation of tone and movement in his hypotonic right upper extremity to improve self-feeding skills. Dominick and his caregiver were educated and given handouts on the nature of his dysphagia, exercises, and mealtime procedures and precautions.

Dominick was discharged from the hospital to home in the company of his wife. He and his wife were taught to thicken fluids with commercial thickeners at home. As his vocal cord strength returned, his volitional cough became stronger, and he gradually became able to speak in a loud whisper; vocal cord strengthening exercises continued. Dominick was able to discontinue use of external lip control strategies as oral motor control returned. He continued use of built-up utensils and weight bearing at the elbow while self-feeding. He continued with outpatient occupational therapy and speech-language pathology to address voice issues for 4 more weeks.

Most Commonly Used Standardized Assessments for Dysphagia

Instrument and Reference	Intended Purpose	Administration Time	Validity	Reliability	Sensitivity	Strengths and Weaknesses
Mann Assessment of Swallowing Ability[52]	Evaluation of swallowing function	15–20 minutes	Validity was tested to determine 71% sensitivity.	Inter-rater reliability testing determined 82% for agreement on the presence of dysphagia; 75% for the presence of aspiration.	Accuracy of diagnosing dysphagia 72%	Standardized in hospital and inpatient rehabilitation setting, standardized for CVA patients
Dysphagia Outcome and Severity Scale[53]	Rating of dysphagia severity	5–10 minutes	Not tested	Inter-rater 90% and intra-rater 93%	Not tested	Parameters are not defined; thus, clinician's expertise is needed; it can be completed regardless of patient's cognition and language status; an MBS must be completed for scoring.
Dysphagia Evaluation Protocol[54]	Evaluation for dysphagia in acute and rehabilitation patients with acute and chronic dysphagia	30–45 minutes including feeding trial	Determined by experts to possess face validity	Inter-rater 89%; overall agreement on test items; Intra-rater 93%	Accuracy of predicting aspiration, penetration, or pooling, 60%	Comprehensive evaluation that helps to development a comprehensive eating and swallowing treatment plan
McGill Ingestive Skills Assessment[55]	Evaluation of feeding and swallowing skills in the elderly with various conditions, not including trauma or head and neck cancer	The length of a meal: 20–30 minutes	Construct validity determined in comparison with two ADL scales (The Functional Independence Measure and the Modified Mini-Mental State Exam) at 0.45 and 0.25, respectively, $p < 0.05$	Inter-rater reliability > 0.80 for most subscales	Known groups validity determined for those with dentures at 0.01 with $p < 0.05$	For use in tertiary care nursing facilities in those with neurogenic dysphagia

Best Evidence for Dysphagia Interventions Used in Occupational Therapy

Intervention	Description	Participants	Dosage	Research Design and Evidence Level	Benefit	Statistical Significance and Effect Size
Immediate effects of thermal-tactile stimulation on timing of swallow in idiopathic Parkinson disease[56]	Effect of thermal-tactile stimulation as assessed prestimulation and poststimulation by videofluoroscopy	Thirteen patients with Parkinson disease and dysphagia	Thermal-tactile stimulation applied to faucial pillars in pharynx	Pre–post nonexperimental design Level III	Median pharyngeal transit time for swallowing both fluid and paste textures was improved. Oral transit time was unaffected with both textures.	Pharyngeal transit time for fluids: $p < 0.004$; for paste: $p < 0.01$
A randomized study of three interventions for aspiration of thin liquids in patients with dementia or Parkinson disease[57]	Comparison of three interventions for aspiration in patients with dementia and/or Parkinson disease: chin-down posture, nectar-thickened liquids, and honey-thickened liquids	711 patients who aspirated on thin liquids assessed with videofluoroscopy	1. Chin-down posture 2. Nectar-thickened liquids 3. Honey-thickened liquids	Randomized controlled study Level I	Honey-thickened fluids were more effective than nectar-thickened fluids to eliminate aspiration, and both were more effective than chin-down position with thin fluids.	1. Chin down vs. nectar thickened, $p < 0.001$ 2. Chin down vs. honey thickened, $p < 0.0001$ 3. Nectar thickened vs. honey thickened, $p < 0.0001$

References

1. Leder SB, Suiter DM, Agogo GO, Coonery LM. An epidemiologic study on ageing and dysphagia in the acute care geriatric hospitalized population: a replication and continuation study. *Dysphagia*. 2016;31(5):619–625.
2. Nakayama E, Tohara H, Hino T, et al. The effects of ADL on recovery of swallowing function in stroke patients after acute phase. *J Oral Rehabil*. 2014;41(12):904–911.
3. Melgaard D, Baandrup U, Bogsted M, Bendtsen MD, Hansen T. The prevalence of oropharyngeal dysphagia in Danish patients hospitalized with community-acquired pneumonia. *Dysphagia*. 2017;32(3):383–392.
4. Leibovitz A, Baumoehl Y, Lubart E, Yaina A, Platinovitz N, Segal R. Dehydration among long-term care elderly patients with oropharyngeal dysphagia. *Gerontology*. 2007;53(4):179–183.
5. Sura L, Madhavan A, Carnaby G, Crary MA. Dysphagia in the elderly: management and nutritional considerations. *Clin Interv Aging*. 2012;7:287–298.
6. Namasivayam AM, Steele CM. Malnutrition and dysphagia in long-term care: a systematic review. *J Nutr Gerontol Geriatr*. 2015;34(1):1–21.
7. Cereda E, Pedrolli C, Klersy C, et al. Nutritional status in older person according to healthcare setting: a systematic review and meta-analysis of prevalence data using MNA®. *Clin Nutr*. 2016;35(6):1282–1290.
8. Bock JM, Varadarajan V, Brawley MC, Blumin JJ. Evaluation of the natural history of patients who aspirate. *Laryngoscope*. 2017;127(suppl 8):S1–S10.
9. De Lima Alvarenga EH, Dall'Oglio GP, Murano EZ, Abrahao M. Continuum theory: presbyphagia to dysphagia? Functional assessment of swallowing in the elderly. *Eur Arch Otorhinolaryngol*. 2018;275(2):443–449.
10. Higgs S, Thomas J. Social influences on eating. *Curr Opin Behav Sci*.2016;9:1–6.doi:10.1016/j.cobeha.2015.10.005.
11. Cassiani RA, Santos CM, Parreira LC, Dantas RO. The relationship between the oral and pharyngeal phases of swallowing. *Clinics (Sao Paulo)*. 2011;66(8):1385–1388.
12. Mendell DA, Logemann JA. Temporal sequence of swallow events during the oropharyngeal swallow. *J Speech Lang Hear Res*. 2007;50(5):1256–1271.
13. Soares TJ, Moraes DP, de Medeiros GC, Sassi FC, Zilberstein B, de Andrade CRF. Oral transit time: a critical review of the literature [in English, Portuguese]. *Arq Bras de Cir Dig*. 2015;28(2):144–147.
14. Rosen SP, Abdelhalim SM, Jones CA, McCullouch TM. Effect of body position on pharyngeal swallowing pressures using high-resolution manometry. *Dysphagia*. 2017;33:389–398. doi:10.1007/s00455-017-9866-3.
15. Mashimo H, Goyal RK. Physiology of esophageal motility. *GI Motility Online*. 2006. doi:10.1038/gimo3.
16. Latella D, Meriano C. Clinical evaluation of dysphagia. In: Avery W, ed. *Dysphagia Care and Related Feeding Concerns for Adults*. 2nd ed. Bethesda, MD: AOTA Press; 2010:83–120.
17. Ding R, Logemann JA. Swallow physiology in patients with trach cuff inflated or deflated: a retrospective study. *Head Neck*. 2005;27(9):809–813.
18. Gross RD, Mahlmann J, Grayhack JP. Physiologic effects of open and closed tracheostomy tubes on the pharyngeal swallow. *Ann Otol Rhinol Laryngol*. 2003;112(2):143–152.
19. Macht M, Wimbish T, Clark BJ, et al. Postextubation dysphagia is persistent and associated with poor outcomes in survivors of critical illness. *Crit Care*. 2011;15(5):R231.
20. Edahiro A, Hirano H, Yamada R, et al. Factors affecting independence in eating among elderly with Alzheimer's disease. *Geriatr Gerontol Int*. 2012;12(3):481–490.
21. Van der Maarel-Wierink CD, Vanobberben JN, Bronkhorst EM, Schols JM, de Baat C. Risk factors for aspiration pneumonia in frail older people: a systematic literature review. *J Am Med Dir Assoc*. 2011;12(5):344–354.
22. Terre R, Mearin F. Prospective evaluation of oro-pharyngeal dysphagia after severe traumatic brain injury. *Brain Inj*. 2007;(13–14):1411–1417.
23. Alvarez-Berdugo D, Rofes L, Casamitjana JF, Padron A, Quer M, Clave P. Oropharyngeal and laryngeal sensory innervation in the pathophysiology of swallowing disorders and sensory stimulation treatments. *Ann N Y Acad Sci*. 2016;1380(1):104–120.
24. Power ML, Hamdy S, Singh S, Tyrrell PJ, Turnbull I, Thompson DG. Deglutitive laryngeal closure in stroke patients. *J Neurol Neurosurg Psychiatry*. 2007;78(2):141–146.
25. Warabi T, Ito T, Kato M, Takai H, Kobayashi N, Chiba S. Effects of stroke-induced damage to swallow-related areas in the brain on swallowing mechanics of elderly patients. *Geriatr Gerontol Int*. 2008;8(4):234–242.
26. Sullivan PB. Gastrointestinal disorders in children with neurodevelopmental disabilities. *Dev Disabil Res Rev*. 2008;14(2):128–136.
27. Samuels R, Chadwick DD. Predictors of asphyxiation risk in adults with intellectual disabilities and dysphagia. *J Intellect Disabil Res*. 2006;50(pt 5):522–527.
28. Ward EC, van As-Brooks C. *Head and Neck Treatment, Rehabilitation, Outcomes*. 2nd ed. San Diego, CA: Plural Publishing; 2014.
29. Poorjavad M, Derakhshandeh F, Etemadifar M, Soleymani B, Minagar A, Maghi AH. Oropharyngeal dysphagia in multiple sclerosis. *Mult Scler*. 2010;16(3):362–365.
30. Wesling M, Brady S, Jensen M, Nickell M, Statkus D, Escobar N. Dysphagia outcomes in patients with brain tumors undergoing inpatient rehabilitation. *Dysphagia*. 2003;18(3):203–210.
31. Bakke M, Larsen SL, Lautrup C, Karlsborg M. Orofacial function and oral health in patients with Parkinson's disease. *Eur J Oral Sci*. 2011;119(1):27–32.
32. van Lieshout PH, Steele CM, Lang AE. Tongue control for swallowing in Parkinson's disease: effects of age, rate, and stimulus consistency. *Mov Disord*. 2011;26(9):1725–1729.
33. Noyce AJ, Silveira-Moriyama L, Gilpin P, Ling H, Howard R, Lees AJ. Severe dysphagia as a presentation of Parkinson's disease. *Mov Disord*. 2012;27(3):457–458.
34. Solomon NP. What is orofacial fatigue and how does it affect function for swallowing and speech? *Semin Speech Lang*. 2006;27(4):268–282.
35. Borr C, Hielscher-Fastabend M, Lücking A. Reliability and validity of cervical auscultation. *Dysphagia*. 2007; 22(3):225–234.

36. Stepp CE. Surface electromyography for speech and swallowing systems: measurement, analysis, and interpretation. *J Speech Lang Hear Res*. 2012;55(4):1232–1246.
37. Leder SB, Suiter DM, Green, BG. Silent aspiration risk is volume-dependent. *Dysphagia*. 2011;26(3):310.
38. Chen YW, Chang KH, Chen HC, Liang WM, Wang YH, Lin YN. The effects of surface neuromuscular electrical stimulation on post-stroke dysphagia: a systematic review and meta-analysis. *Clin Rehabil*. 2016;30(1):24–35.
39. Tan C, Liu Y, Li W, Liu J, Chen L. Transcutaneous neuromuscular electrical stimulation can improve swallowing function in patients with dysphagia caused by non-stroke diseases: a meta-analysis. *J Oral Rehabil*. 2013;40(6):472–480.
40. Rofes L, Arreola V, Martin A, Clave P. Natural capsaicinoids improve swallow response in older patients with oropharyngeal dysphagia. *Gut*. 2013;62(9):1280–1287.
41. Sze WP, Yoon WL, Escoffier N, Rickard Liow SJ. Evaluating the training effects of two swallowing rehabilitation therapist using surface electromyography—Chin tuck again resistance (CTAR) exercise and the Shaker exercise. *Dysphagia*. 2016;31(2):195–205.
42. Nakamura T, Fujishima I. Usefulness of ice massage in triggering the swallow reflex. *J Stroke Cerebrovasc Dis*. 2013;22(4):378–382.
43. Inamoto Y, Saitoh E, Ito Y, et al. The Mendelsohn maneuver and its effects on swallowing: kinematic analysis in three dimensions using dynamic area detector CT. *Dysphagia*. 2018;33:419–430. doi:10.1007/s0045-017-9870-7.
44. Kim YK, Lee SH, Lee JW. Effects of capping the tracheostomy tube in stroke patients with dysphagia. *Ann Rehabil Med*. 2017;41(3):426–433.
45. Elpern EH, Borkgren Okonek M, Bacon M, Gerstung C, Skrzynski M. Effect of the Passy-Muir tracheostomy speaking valve on pulmonary aspiration in adults. *Heart Lung*. 2000;29(4):287–293.
46. Kim YK, Choi JH, Yoon JG, Lee JW, Cho SS. Improved dysphagia after decannulation of tracheostomy in patients with brain injuries. *Ann Rehabil Med*. 2015;39(5):778–785.
47. Saconato M, Chiari BM, Lederman HM, Goncalves, MI. Effectiveness of chin-tuck maneuver to facilitate swallowing in neurologic dysphagia. *Int Arch Otorhinolaryngol*. 2016;20(1):13–17.
48. Clark HM, Shelton N. Training effects of the effortful swallow under three exercise conditions. *Dysphagia*. 2014; 29(5):553–563.
49. McCabe D, Ashford J, Wheeler-Hegland K, et al. Evidence-based systematic review: oropharyngeal dysphagia behavioral treatments. Part IV—Impact of dysphagia treatment on individuals' postcancer treatments. *J Rehabil Res Dev*. 2009; 46(2):205–214.
50. Gillman A, Winkler R, Taylor NE. Implementing the free water protocol does not result in aspiration pneumonia in carefully selected patients with dysphagia: a systematic review. *Dysphagia*. 2017;32(3):345–361.
51. Terpenning M. Geriatric oral health and pneumonia risk. *Clin Infect Dis*. 2005;40(12):1807–1810.
52. Antonios N, Carnaby-Mann G, Crary M, et al. Analysis of a physician tool for evaluating dysphagia on an inpatient stroke unit: the modified Mann assessment of swallowing ability. *J Stroke Cerebrovasc Dis*. 2010;19(1):49–57. doi:10.1016/j.jstrokecerebrovasdis.2009.03.007.
53. O'Neil KH, Purdy M, Falk J, Gallo L. The dysphagia outcome and severity scale. *Dysphagia*. 1999;14(3):139–145. https://link.springer.com/article/10.1007/PL00009595.
54. Avery-Smith W, Dellarosa DM, Rosen AB. *Dysphagia Evaluation Protocol*. San Antonio, TX: Therapy Skill Builders; 1997.
55. Lambert HC, Gisel EG, Groher ME, Wood–Dauphinee S. McGill Ingestive Skills Assessment (MISA): development and first field test of an evaluation of functional ingestive skills of elderly persons. *Dysphagia*. 2003;18(2):101–113. https://link.springer.com/article/10.1007/s00455-002-0091-2.
56. Regan J, Walshe M, Tobin WO. Immediate effects of thermal-tactile stimulation on timing of swallow in idiopathic Parkinson's disease. *Dysphagia*. 2010;25(3):207–215.
57. Logemann JA, Gensler G, Robbins J, et al. A randomized study of three interventions for aspiration of thin liquids in patients with dementia or Parkinson's disease. *J Speech Lang Hear Res*. 2008;51(1):173–183..

Acknowledgments

The author thanks Janice P. Alden and Cheryl A. McCarthy for their assistance with photographs used in this chapter. Thanks also to Bette Pomerleau, MS, SLP, and Ray Autiello, LPN, RT, formerly of Universal Mobile Services in Haverhill, Massachusetts, for their assistance with the modified barium swallow image reproduced in this chapter.

Chapter 20

Cranial Nerve Assessment

Sharon A. Gutman and Dawn M. Nilsen

LEARNING OBJECTIVES

This chapter will allow the reader to:

1. Describe the 12 paired cranial nerves with regard to function, neuroanatomical location, and motor/sensory transmission.
2. Demonstrate appropriate screening procedures to assess the function of all 12 cranial nerves.
3. Predict distinct lesion symptoms based on specific cranial nerve damage.
4. Describe how specific cranial nerve damage will likely impair patient function in daily life activities.
5. Correctly interpret the results of a cranial nerve screening examination.

CHAPTER OUTLINE

TERMINOLOGY

Ageusia: a sensory disorder involving loss of taste; may result from olfactory, facial, or glossopharyngeal nerve damage.

Anesthesia: a sensory disorder involving insensitivity to all sensation; may result from trigeminal nerve damage.

Anosmia: a sensory disorder involving loss of smell; may result from olfactory nerve damage.

Bitemporal hemianopia: an ocular condition in which vision has been lost in the temporal field halves of both eyes; results from optic chiasm damage.

Contralateral homonymous hemianopia: an ocular condition in which vision has been lost in the same field halves of both eyes; results from optic tract lesions.

Dysarthria: a speech disorder in which words are slurred; may result from glossopharyngeal, vagus, and hypoglossal nerve impairment.

Dysphagia: an eating disorder involving difficulty manipulating and transporting solids/liquids from the oral cavity to the pharynx; can result from damage to the following cranial nerves: trigeminal, facial, glossopharyngeal, vagus, accessory, and hypoglossal nerves.

Dysphonia: a speech disorder involving decreased vocal volume or hoarseness; may result from glossopharyngeal and vagus nerve impairment.

Dyspnea: a respiratory disorder involving difficulty breathing; may result from glossopharyngeal and vagus nerve impairment (in this case, dyspnea results from rapid heartbeat causing shortness of breath).

Hemianopia: an ocular condition in which vision has been lost in one-half of a visual field; results from damage to the optic tract.

Homonymous quadrantanopia: an ocular condition in which vision has been lost in a specific visual field quadrant; results from optic pathway lesions.

Near triad: an extraocular response in which three ocular changes occur that allow a visual target to be brought into focus: convergence, lens accommodation, and pupillary constriction.

Nystagmus: an ocular condition in which both eyeballs involuntarily oscillate when moved to a visual field extreme; may result from impairment of the vestibulocochlear nerve.

Strabismus: an ocular condition involving deviation of one eyeball as it sits in the orbital socket; may result from extraocular cranial nerve impairment.

Cranial Nerve Function and Impairment in Daily Occupation

The cranial nerves (CNs) are 12 pairs of peripheral nerves located in or near the brainstem and carry sensory and motor information to and from the structures of the head, face, and neck. Five CNs (olfactory, optic, facial, vestibulocochlear, and glossopharyngeal nerves) are responsible for the special sense functions of vision, audition (hearing), olfaction (smell), and gustation (taste).[1–4] Damage to these CNs can cause impairment of the special senses associated with them. Unilateral blindness, or loss of vision in one eye, can result in a failure to attend to objects in that lost visual field, creating significant safety risks. For example, patients may bump into furniture or walls, trip over items on the floor, fail to identify oncoming traffic while crossing the street, or miss needed items in a handbag such as one's keys. Hearing loss can impair one's ability to identify safety signals in the environment, such as smoke alarms, ambulance sirens, or automobile horns. When smell is lost, patients may fail to identify food burning on a stove or the presence of gas or mold in the home environment. Because of the neuroanatomical organization of the pathways connecting olfaction and gustation, lost smell is commonly accompanied by suppressed taste.[5] When both smell and taste are compromised, patients may experience decreased appetite (critical in the frail elderly) and are at risk for food poisoning if left to prepare meals independently.[1–4]

The extraocular CNs (oculomotor, trochlear, and abducens nerves) are responsible for eyeball movements up, down, medially, and laterally. When one or more of these nerves are damaged, vision remains but is impacted by **strabismus** (deviation of one eyeball as it sits in the orbital socket), diplopia (double vision), or lost pupillary reflex (pupil constriction in response to light).[1–4] These conditions can severely impair a patient's safe negotiation of the environment. The presence of a strabismus can impact one's ability to safely traverse steps, curb cuts, and uneven surfaces (sand, gravel, dirt), placing the patient at risk for falls. Patients with diplopia, whose vision is doubled, may become unsafe drivers, unable to determine the true location of other cars and pedestrians. Such patients, who may also fail to correctly grasp objects such as pot handles and drinking glasses, often drop items of daily living, resulting in possible safety incidents. When patients are engaged in hot meal preparation, they are at increased risk for scalds if hot food and drinks are spilled.

The vestibulocochlear nerve mediates equilibrium, or balance. When this CN is damaged, a patient's balance and protective responses become impaired, placing the patient at risk for falls and injury.[1–4] Environments in which transitional movements are required (negotiating steps, ramps, and curb cuts; getting in and out of a car; getting on and off of a toilet; rising from bed) can pose a fall risk.

Six CNs have roles in swallowing (trigeminal, facial, glossopharyngeal, vagus, accessory, and hypoglossal nerves) and, if impaired, can result in **dysphagia**, choking, and food aspiration. Aspiration of oropharyngeal contents into the lungs can result in lower respiratory tract infections. In the frail elderly with compromised immunity, such infections can fatally lead to aspiration pneumonia.[1–4]

Neurological and Physiological Basis of Cranial Nerve Function

The 12 paired CNs predominantly originate from the brainstem and exit the brain between the midbrain and the medulla (see Fig. 20-1). Each CN is named and numbered from rostral (toward the head) to caudal (toward the tail or posterior body), and collectively, the CNs are considered to be part of the peripheral nervous system. This means that damage to a CN has the potential to resolve similarly to other peripheral nerve structures. It should be noted, however, that CN cell bodies, or nuclei, are located directly within the brainstem, or within the central nervous system. When CN cell bodies are destroyed as a result of disease or injury, resolution is not possible and the lost CNs function will not be recovered.[1–4]

When CN impairment occurs, ipsilateral (same side as the lesion) symptoms commonly result because most nerves do not cross midline. As noted earlier, several CNs carry sensory information that mediate the special sense functions of olfaction, vision, audition, and gustation. Several CNs carry somatic motor components that innervate the skeletal muscles of the head and neck. Other CNs carry somatic sensory components that transmit sensory messages between the

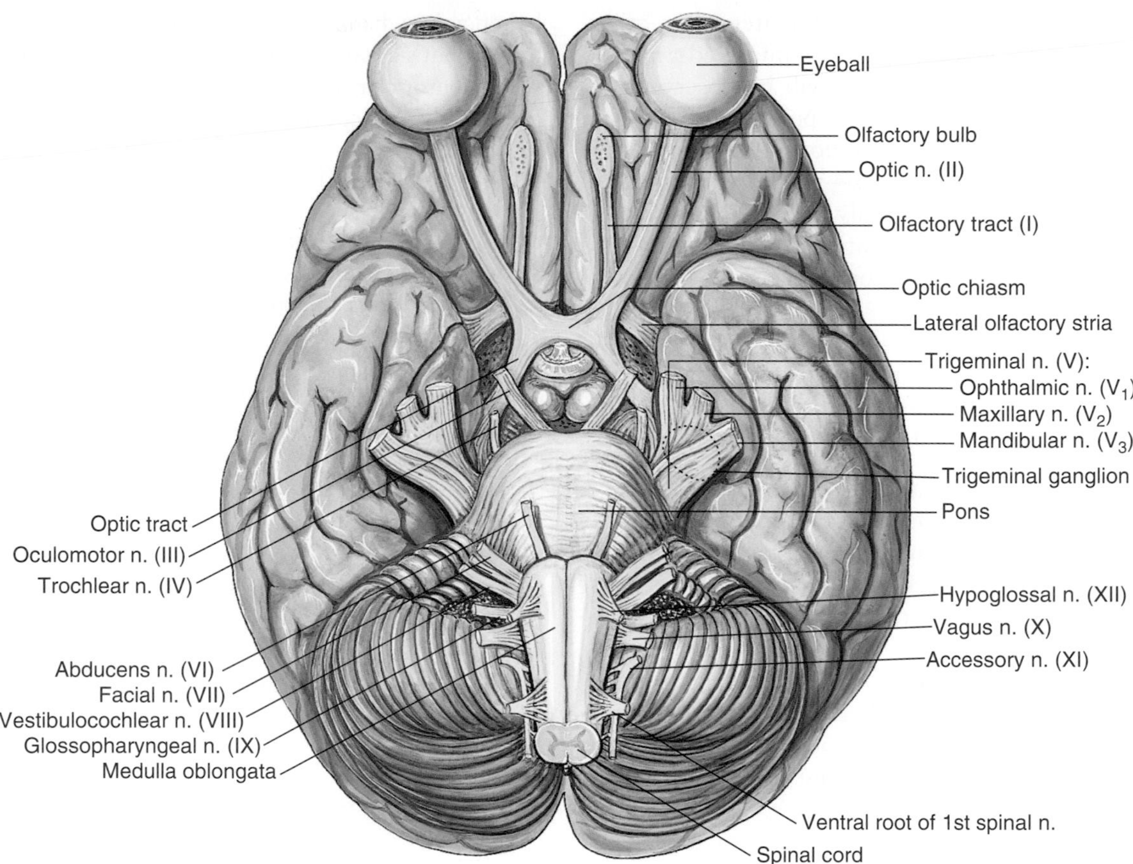

Figure 20-1. The 12 paired cranial nerves.

brain and the skin of the face and head. Some CNs transmit visceral motor and sensory signals (responsible for innervation of cardiac muscle, smooth muscle, and glands located throughout the body) and are considered to be part of the parasympathetic division of the autonomic nervous system (ANS). The ANS is responsible for our vegetative or critical life functions, such as respiration, heart rate, temperature, and blood pressure. The parasympathetic nervous system is the division of the ANS responsible for slowing heart rate, respiration, and metabolism and promoting digestion. Several CNs are mixed nerves that carry combinations of the abovementioned components, allowing them to serve multiple functions.[1–4]

This chapter describes each CN with regard to (1) function, (2) neuroanatomical location, (3) type of sensory and/or motor information transmitted, (4) screening procedures, and (5) signs indicating dysfunction in daily occupation. The intervention of specific CN impairments is not described in this section but can be found in Chapters 8, 12, 14, 17, and 19, addressing the intervention of visual, sensory, motor, balance, and swallowing disorders.

Cranial Nerve Screening Procedures

Cranial Nerve I: Olfactory Nerve

CN I is a special sensory nerve that mediates olfaction, or smell. The olfactory nerve's sensory receptors are chemoreceptors located in the olfactory epithelium in close proximity to the nasal mucosa. Chemoreceptors in the nose convey olfactory signal to the olfactory bulb located in the inferior frontal lobes. Olfactory messages then travel to the areas of the brain concerned with the processing, interpretation, integration, and storage of olfactory information. For example, olfactory messages travel to the hippocampal formation in the temporal lobes, a structure responsible for long-term memory storage, including memories associated with scent and odor. The storage of odor memories in the hippocampus accounts for why specific scents can elicit long-term memories more efficiently than any other sense. Olfactory messages are then sent to the hypothalamus, thalamus, and, finally, to the orbitofrontal cortex, where they are interpreted and integrated with gustatory information. This is why lesions of the olfactory nerve can impact taste sensation in addition to smell.[5–7]

If an olfactory nerve lesion is unilateral—in other words, if only one olfactory nerve is impaired and the other is preserved—no symptoms will be observed because the preserved nerve will compensate for the one that is lost. Bilateral lesions—lesions that oblate the function of both olfactory nerves—result in **anosmia**, or loss of smell. Anosmia commonly occurs as a result of traumatic brain injury. When patients present with loss of smell, **ageusia** (loss of taste) occurs as well.[5–8]

Screening Procedures

Olfactory nerve function is assessed by testing the patient's sense of smell using the screening procedures outlined as follows (see Fig. 20-2 and Video 20-1)[6,7,9]:

- The patient should be seated with vision occluded.
- Each olfactory nerve should be screened separately by presenting scents to one nostril at a time.
- Ask the patient to block one nostril; the therapist should screen the opposite nostril by presenting one odor stimulus at a time.
- Use four scents that are familiar to the patient (peppermint, cinnamon, coffee, and vanilla). Avoid pungent odors (ammonia and acetic acid) that can stimulate nerve endings in the mucosal lining, which is innervated by the trigeminal nerve. Stimulation of the trigeminal nerve may cause patients to believe that they can smell the odor stimulus, thus giving a false-positive result.
- Ask whether the patient smells the odor stimulus. The ability to smell the odor is more important than the actual identification of the specific stimulus.
- Provide the patient with a verbal choice of specific odors if he or she has word-finding difficulties or cannot identify each specific odor, but can smell them.

Assessing Impact on Daily Function

To determine how olfactory nerve impairment may impact daily function, ask the following questions. It is beneficial to have a close family member corroborate the patient's answers, particularly if the patient is elderly with memory problems or has a head injury. If possible, observe the patient in the home environment.

- Do you have difficulty smelling foods cooking on the stove?
- Have you ever burned food (on the stove, in the oven, or in the toaster) because you didn't smell it?
- Have you ever mistakenly eaten spoiled food because you didn't notice through smell or taste that it had perished?
- Do you have any problems tasting your food? Have you experienced a decrease in appetite because food doesn't seem to have a taste anymore?

If possible, the therapist should prepare toast or coffee while the patient is seated nearby but with body turned to prevent visual cues. Ask whether and when the patient can identify the smell of the selected stimulus. Patients who cannot identify the stimulus scent may be at risk for the abovementioned safety incidents and should receive an in-depth evaluation.

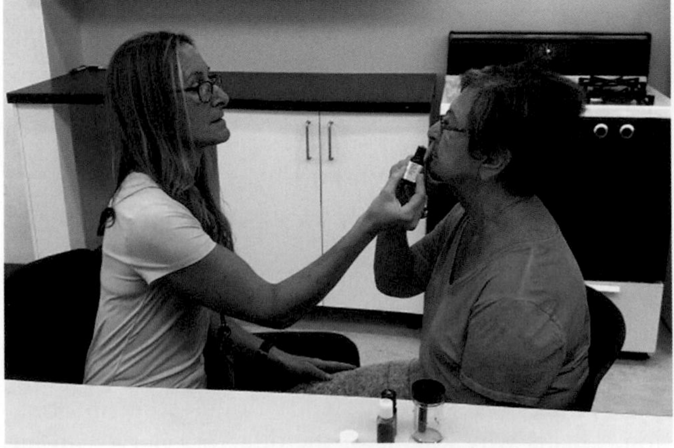

Figure 20-2. Olfactory nerve screening.

Cranial Nerve II: Optic Nerve

CN II is a special sensory nerve responsible for visual acuity, or the accuracy of sight rather than the interpretation of a visual stimulus. The optic nerve mediates the afferent limb of the pupillary light reflex, in which the pupil constricts when exposed to direct light. When photoreceptors (rods and cones) of the retina are stimulated by light, they send visual information through the optic nerves to the optic chiasm. The optic chiasm is the point at which some optic fibers cross over to the opposite side, whereas others remain uncrossed. These crossed and uncrossed fibers then exit the chiasm, forming the optic tracts. Visual messages travel from the optic tracts to several locations, including the thalamus (a primary relay center for visual information), hypothalamus (involved in circadian rhythm regulation), and midbrain (responsible for visual reflexes and the unconscious detection of visual information). Visual messages then travel to the occipital lobes for visual detection and interpretation.[1–4,10,11]

Screening Procedures

Optic nerve function is assessed by screening the patient's visual acuity and visual fields. It should be noted that while therapists perform visual acuity and visual field tests, ophthalmologists perform funduscopic examinations in which the retina and optic head are inspected. Visual acuity and visual field function are assessed using the screening procedures outlined in the subsequent section.[9–11]

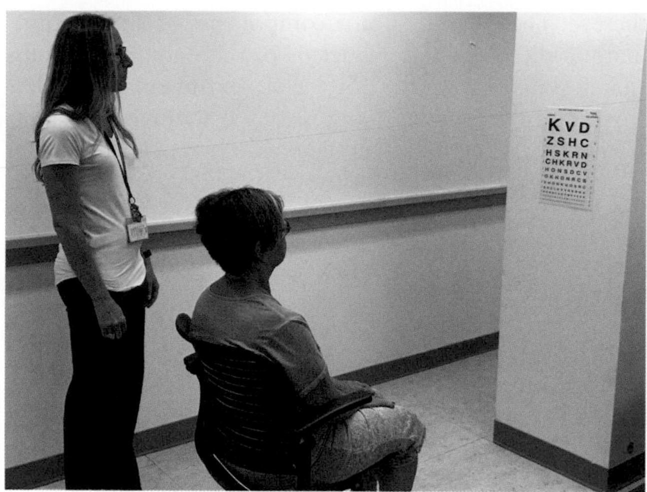

Figure 20-3. Screening visual acuity: Optic nerve screening.

Visual Acuity Test (Snellen Eye Chart)

- The patient should be seated at a distance of 20 feet from the chart (see Fig. 20-3 and Video 20-2).
- First, screen each eye separately (monocular vision). If the patient wears corrective lenses, test the patient with lenses on.
- Then, screen both eyes together (binocular vision). Patients should wear their prescribed corrective lenses.
- Ask the patient to read the top line from left to right.
- Then, instruct the patient to read each successive line below the top line, if possible.
- The number listed beside each letter line indicates the number of feet at which that line can be read by an individual with normal vision. Note the last line for which the patient correctly identified more than 50% of letters.
- Document the patient's score for the tested eye as the distance at which the patient could read the letters (20 feet), over the number listed on the chart next to the last line read (in which the patient could correctly identify more than 50% of letters).
- Record the number of letters missed by the patient in the last line read. For example, a score of 20/40−1 indicates that the patient could read at a distance of 20 feet all but one of the letters in the line that a normally functioning eye can read at 40 feet.
- If the patient scored 20/40 or lower, an ophthalmology referral should be made.

Visual Field Test (Confrontation Testing)

An examination of visual fields provides important information about the functioning of the visual pathway from the optic nerve to the visual cortex; the most common method of visual field testing is called confrontation testing. The eye's visual field encompasses the area of central to peripheral vision when the eye focuses straight ahead. Visual fields are assessed by identifying the point at which patients are first able to detect a visual stimulus along each peripheral perimeter. Visual fields are screened in the vertical and horizontal planes in four quadrants: (1) superior (upper) and (2) inferior (lower) nasal fields, and (3) upper and (4) lower temporal quadrants. When a patient gazes straight ahead, a stimulus positioned directly in front of him or her is considered to be at 0°. A stimulus positioned directly over the patient's head is considered to be at 90°. A stimulus positioned directly in line with the ears and held about 1.5 feet away from the head is also said to be at 90°.[9–11]

- The therapist should be positioned in front of the seated patient (see Fig. 20-4 and Video 20-3).
- Screen one eye at a time.
- Occlude the opposite eye by asking the patient to cover that eye with the palm of the hand or by holding an occluder over the eye.

- Ask the patient to gaze directly ahead at the therapist's nose. Move the visual stimulus in the horizontal plane from the 90° position to the 0° position. Instruct the patient to verbally indicate when he or she first sees the visual stimulus (finger or pen cap).
- Document the horizontal plane position at which the patient first identified vision of the stimulus.
- Repeat these procedures in the vertical plane.

Normal horizontal peripheral vision is 85°; normal peripheral vertical vision is 45°. Therapists should suspect the presence of a visual field deficit if a patient scores more than 5° below these norms. A field deficit may also be indicated if one of the peripheral fields is abnormally small; referral to a specialist for further testing should be made. Visual pathway lesions cause specific types of visual deficits. For example, if a patient reports the presence of a blind spot within a visual field, retinal damage is indicated. Unilateral blindness (loss of vision in one eye, but not the other) suggests an optic nerve lesion. **Hemianopia** is a condition in which vision has been lost in half of a field of one eye. A **contralateral homonymous hemianopia** occurs when vision has been lost in the same field halves of both eyes, indicating a lesion

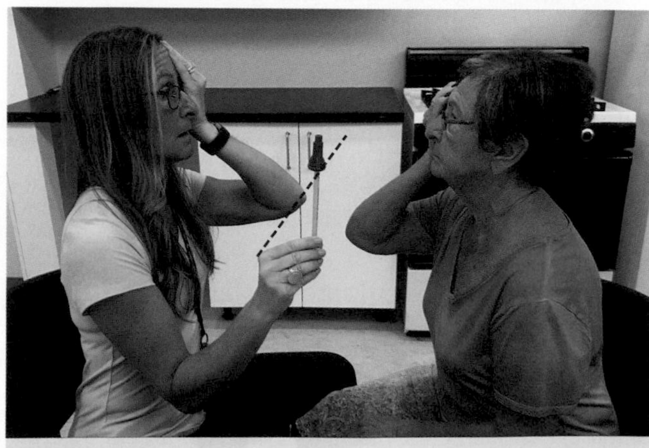

Figure 20-4. Screening visual fields (confrontation): Optic nerve screening.

of the optic tract. **Bitemporal hemianopia** is a condition in which vision is lost in the temporal field halves of both eyes and usually results from damage to the optic chiasm. Loss of a specific visual field quadrant is called a **homonymous quadrantanopia** and commonly results from lesions of the optic pathways as they project from the lateral geniculate bodies to the primary visual cortex.[9–11]

Assessing Impact on Daily Function

To determine whether visual acuity problems have impacted daily function, provide reading materials (book or magazine) and observe the patient while reading. If the patient squints while reading or attempts to move the reading material closer to or further from the eyes (normal reading material should be held at a distance of ~1.5 feet), visual acuity may be impaired.

- Ask whether the patient can easily identify coins held at arm's length.
- Ask the patient if reading fine print (such as a magazine or phone book) is difficult.
- Ask the patient to demonstrate a fine motor activity (such as threading a needle, tying a fishing pole hook, or texting on a smartphone) to determine whether squinting occurs or if the patient attempts to reposition the object closer to or further from the eyes.

To determine whether and how a visual field deficit has impacted daily function, again observe the patient while reading. If the patient moves the reading material horizontally to maintain its view within his or her visual field, instead of fluidly scanning the lines, a visual field deficit may be indicated.

Allow the patient to participate in a simple cold meal preparation activity, such as making a sandwich. Place all items on a table in a 3-foot span. Observe whether the patient ignores items falling within the range of one particular visual field, or moves the head or body unusually in order to see objects in all visual field ranges. When patients ignore items falling within a visual field, or move the head/body unusually in order to see all objects, a possible field deficit may be indicated.

Ask whether the patient has recently tripped or fallen because he or she didn't see steps or objects on the ground. Ask whether the patient has bumped into furniture or walls while ambulating. Such experiences may indicate possible field deficits.

Cranial Nerve III: Oculomotor Nerve

Three CNs are collectively referred to as the extraoculomotor nerves: CN III, CN IV, and CN VI. CN III consists of both somatic and visceral motor components and mediates eye movements, pupillary constriction, and lens accommodation—all important for the coordination of eye and head movements. The oculomotor nerve originates in the midbrain and exits the superior orbital fissure to reach both somatic and visceral motor targets located in the eye. The somatic motor components of CN III originate in the oculomotor nucleus of the midbrain and ipsilaterally innervate four of the six extraocular muscles: superior rectus (upward and medial eye movements), inferior rectus (downward and medial eye movements), medial rectus (medial eye movements), and inferior oblique (upward and lateral eye movements), as well as the levator palpebrae muscle that lifts the upper eyelid.[1–4,12]

The visceral motor components of the oculomotor nerve originate in the Edinger-Westphal preganglionic nucleus of the midbrain. Axons of these neurons ipsilaterally innervate the sphincter pupillae and ciliary muscles, which are responsible for pupillary constriction and lens accommodation. respectively.[1–4,12]

As noted earlier, CN II mediates the afferent limb of the pupillary light reflex, whereas CN III mediates the efferent limb. The pupillary reflex occurs when light is shined into the eye and the pupil receiving the light constricts (referred to as the direct response). At the same time, the pupil of the opposite eye constricts (referred to as the consensual response).[9,12]

CN III is also involved in the **near triad** or near response. This response involves activation of both somatic and visceral motor components. When gazing from a distant target to a closer one, three ocular changes occur that allow the visual target to be brought into focus. In the first change, referred to as convergence, both eyes move medially (through the somatic motor activation of the medial rectus muscles) to align the eyes with the closer target. Simultaneously, lens curvature increases. This visceral motor response is referred to as lens accommodation and increases the lens' refractive power. Pupillary constriction is the third change (visceral motor) and increases the eyes' field depth.[9,12]

Screening Procedures

CN III is assessed conjointly with the other extraoculomotor nerves (CN IV and CN VI) by examining ocular alignment and range of motion, pupillary light reflex, and convergence.[9,12]

Ocular Alignment

- The patient should be seated and instructed to gaze straight ahead. Note any abnormalities in ocular alignment:
  - *Esotropia:* Medial or internal strabismus; one eye is inwardly misaligned.[13]
  - *Exotropia:* Lateral or external strabismus; one eye is outwardly misaligned.[13]
  - *Hypertropia:* Vertical strabismus; one eye sits higher than the other.[13]
  - *Hypotropia:* Vertical strabismus; one eye sits lower than the other.[13]
- Dim the lighting and shine a pen light at the bridge of the patient's nose. Note symmetrical corneal reflection. If corneal reflection appears asymmetrical, strabismus is indicated.

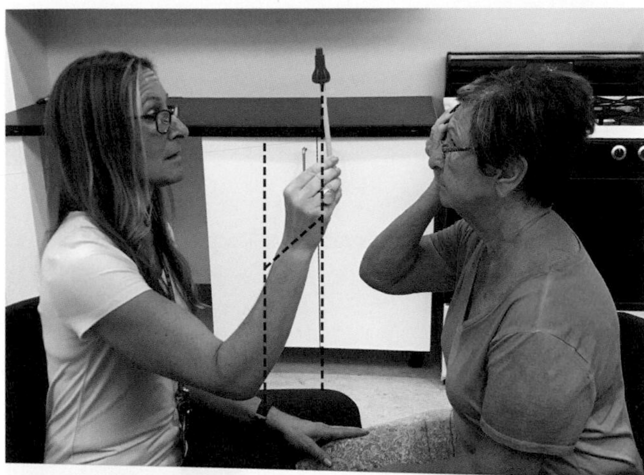

Figure 20-5. Screening ocular range of motion: Oculomotor nerve screening.

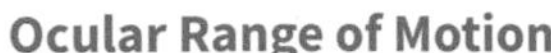

Ocular Range of Motion

- The patient should be seated with the therapist positioned in front (see Fig. 20-5 and Video 20-4).
- Test one eye at a time.
- Occlude vision of the eye not being tested by asking the patient to cover the eye with the palm or using an occluder.
- Instruct the patient to maintain the head in a fixed position and visually scan a moving stimulus (finger or pen cap) presented by the therapist.
- Move the visual stimulus slowly in the shape of an H. Note any impairment in ocular range of motion (inability to move the eye up, down, medially, or laterally).

Pupillary Light Reflex: Direct Response

- The patient should be seated and instructed to gaze straight ahead. Note any asymmetry of pupil size.
- Dim the room lighting to increase the patient's pupil size.
- Shine a penlight into one eye for ~2 seconds. Note whether the pupil constricts quickly or sluggishly. Impairment is indicated if pupil constriction is sluggish or fails to occur.
- Repeat the procedure for the opposite eye.
- Using a penlight, shine light into both eyes at the same time allowing equal amounts of light to fall on both eyes. Turn the penlight on and off, and observe whether both pupils dilate and constrict at the same time and to the same degree. Impairment is indicated if both pupils do not dilate and constrict simultaneously and to the same degree.

Pupillary Light Reflex: Consensual Response

- In a dimly lit room, place one hand on the patient's nose between the eyes to limit light exposure to the eye being tested.
- Shine a penlight into one eye and observe the pupillary reflex in the opposite eye (both eyes should constrict).
- Document whether the pupil of the unstimulated eye fails to constrict simultaneously with the pupil of the illuminated eye. Impairment is indicated if the pupil of the unstimulated eye does not constrict at the same time and to the same degree as the pupil of the opposite eye.

Convergence

- The patient should be seated with the therapist positioned in front (see Fig. 20-6 and Video 20-5).
- Hold a pencil (or similar visual stimulus) in front of the patient (~18 inches away from the nose), and instruct the patient to visually fixate on the pencil.

- Slowly move the pencil toward the patient's nose in a straight line. Instruct the patient to maintain gaze fixated on the pencil as it is moved closer to the nose.
- Observe for simultaneous medial movement of both eyes. Record the distance at which convergence was broken (when the patient could no longer medially invert both eyes). Convergence is normally broken at ~3 to 4 inches from the nose.
- Note any asymmetry in eye movements or pupillary constriction. Impairment is indicated if asymmetrical eye movements occur or if the pupils fail to constrict as the eyes converge.

CN III lesions (oculomotor nerve palsy) will result in paralysis of the ipsilateral extraocular muscles (superior rectus, inferior rectus, medial rectus, and inferior oblique). The patient will be unable to move the eye upward, downward, or inward; the eye will assume a downward lateral strabismus in the orbit because of the unopposed actions of the lateral rectus and superior oblique muscles (see Fig. 20-7). Partial or complete ptosis (drooping of the upper eyelid) may also occur. The affected eye's pupil will be dilated with impairment of the pupillary light reflex. Convergence will also be impaired because of weakness of the medial rectus muscle,

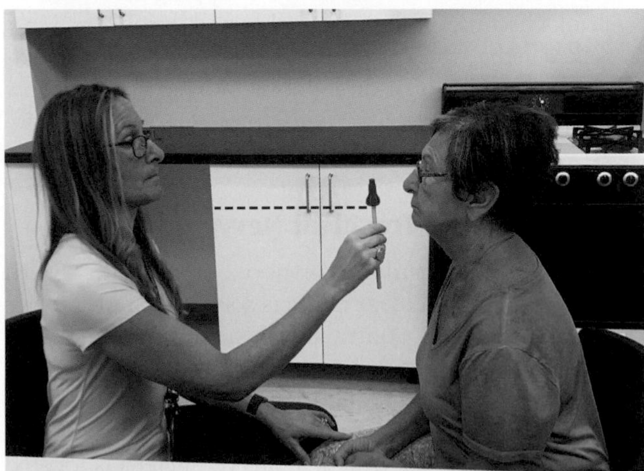

Figure 20-6. Screening convergence: Oculomotor nerve screening.

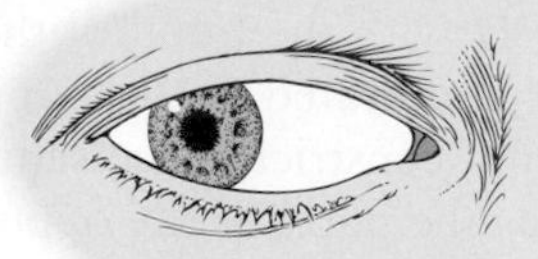
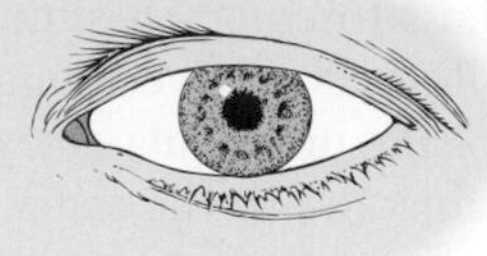

Figure 20-7. Downward lateral strabismus: Oculomotor nerve dysfunction.

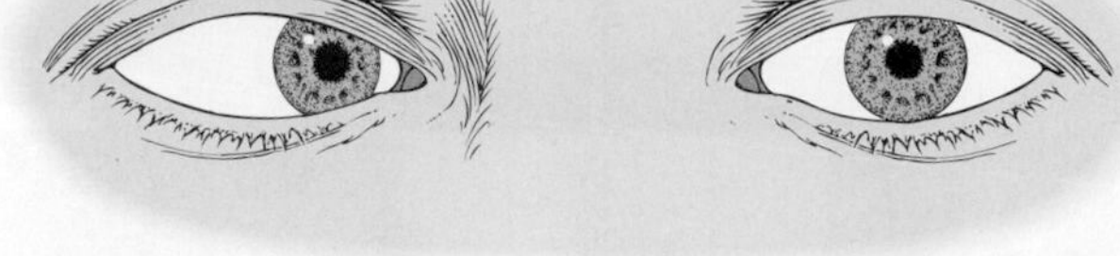

Figure 20-8. Vertical medial strabismus: Trochlear nerve dysfunction.

and as a result, the patient may complain of diplopia or blurred vision, particularly when viewing objects at close range.[9,12]

Assessing Impact on Daily Function

To determine whether extraoculomotor nerve impairment has impacted daily function, therapists should observe for the presence of strabismus, diplopia, or blurred vision because these conditions can severely affect one's ability to negotiate the physical environment.

- Ask whether the patient has tripped or experienced any recent falls at home or in the community.
- Ask whether the patient has difficulty safely traversing steps, curb cuts, and uneven surfaces such as gravel driveways and uneven sidewalks.

The presence of diplopia and blurred vision can severely affect driving, meal preparation, and any activity involving reading such as phone use.

- Ask whether the patient has difficulty driving as a result of diplopia or blurred vision, and ever experiences difficulty determining the true location of cars and pedestrians.
- Ask whether the patient has recently experienced any safety incidents in the kitchen as a result of diplopia or blurred vision, such as misperceiving the location of and failing to accurately grasp pot handles, drinking glasses, stove knobs, and plates. Has the patient scalded himself or herself by dropping hot food or drinks because of diplopia or blurred vision?
- Ask whether the patient has difficulty using a smartphone as a result of diplopia or blurred vision. Allow the patient to demonstrate use of a smartphone to observe possible deficits.

Cranial Nerve IV: Trochlear Nerve

CN IV is an extraoculomotor nerve, along with CN III and CN VI. The trochlear nerve is a somatic motor nerve that innervates the contralateral superior oblique eye muscle, which is responsible for depression (downward eyeball movement), abduction (lateral eyeball movement), and intorsion (inward eyeball rotation) movements of the eye. The trochlear nerve nucleus is located in the caudal midbrain and yields axons that decussate before exiting the midbrain, making it the only motor CN that crosses midline. CN IV exits the skull through the superior orbital fissure, where it enters the orbit to reach its target.[1–4]

The function of CN IV is assessed conjointly with the other two extraoculomotor nerves (CN III and CN VI) through examination of ocular alignment and range of motion. A trochlear nerve lesion will result in paralysis of the contralateral superior oblique muscle, causing the patient to experience difficulty moving the contralateral eyeball downward and laterally. This occurs because of the unopposed action of the medial and superior rectus muscles, which pull the eyeball upward and inward. As a result, a vertical medial strabismus may be apparent (see Fig. 20-8), and the patient may complain of diplopia at both far and near distances.[1–4,14,15]

For screening procedures and assessment of daily functional impact, see CN III.

Cranial Nerve V: Trigeminal Nerve

CN V is a mixed nerve with both somatic motor and sensory components. The nerve originates in the pons and divides into three branches (ophthalmic, maxillary, mandibular) before exiting the skull. The ophthalmic and maxillary branches only carry sensory information; the mandibular branch carries both motor and sensory information. Along with CN III, CN IV, and CN VI, the ophthalmic branch exits the skull through the superior orbital fissure. The maxillary and mandibular branches exit the skull through the foramen rotundum and foramen ovale, respectively.[1–4]

The motor nucleus of CN V is located at the mid-pontine brainstem and yields axons that ipsilaterally innervate the muscles of mastication, the anterior belly of the digastric muscle, the tensor veli palatini, and the tensor tympani. This branch of the trigeminal nerve also mediates the efferent limb of the masseter reflex.[1–4]

The somatic sensory components of the trigeminal nerve ipsilaterally innervate the face, head, cornea, and conjunctiva of the eye; the mucosa of the nasal cavity and sinuses; and the inner oral cavity, including the teeth and anterior two-thirds of the tongue. The ophthalmic branch of the trigeminal nerve mediates the afferent limb of the corneal reflex.[1–4]

Screening Procedures

CN V is assessed by examining motor function of the jaw, testing facial sensation, and eliciting the corneal and masseter reflexes.[9,16]

Motor Function

Assess the muscles of mastication for strength and symmetry.

- The patient should be in a seated position with the therapist positioned in front.
- Instruct the patient to open the mouth. Note any jaw deviation to one side or asymmetry of the opened mouth (see Video 20-6).
- Instruct the patient to move the jaw from side to side. Note any asymmetry of jaw movement.
- Instruct the patient to bite down on a tongue depressor. Gently attempt to pull the tongue depressor, and ask the patient to resist your attempts to remove it. Note any asymmetry between right and left jaw strength.

Sensory Function

Assess sensation on the patient's face, head, and inner oral cavity. Evaluate the intact side prior to the suspected involved side.

- The patient should be seated with vision occluded.
- Use a cotton swab applicator to stroke the inner oral cavity.
- Use a cotton swab to stroke the patient's forehead, cheek, jaw, and chin (see Fig. 20-9 and Video 20-7).
- Ask the patient to verbally identify the facial area being touched. Note any areas of **anesthesia** (insensitivity to sensation). If areas of anesthesia are detected, repeat the procedure using the bare wooden end of a cotton swab applicator to assess sensation of sharp items. If sensory deficits are found for sharp items, repeat the procedure using test tubes of hot and cold water to assess temperature detection.

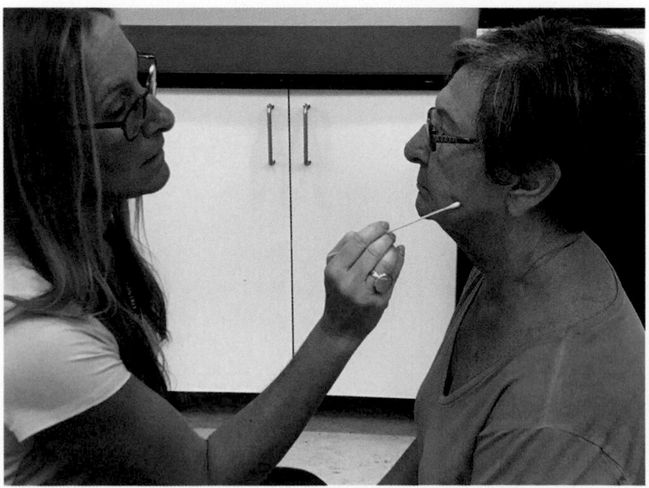

Figure 20-9. Screening sensory function of the trigeminal nerve.

Reflexes

Example: Corneal Reflex (Blink Reflex)

- Gently touch the patient's cornea using a sterile cotton swab.
- The stimulated eye should close (direct response) along with simultaneous closure of the opposite eye (consensual response).

Masseter Reflex

- Using a reflex hammer, gently tap the chin (see Video 20-8).
- The masseter muscle should contract.

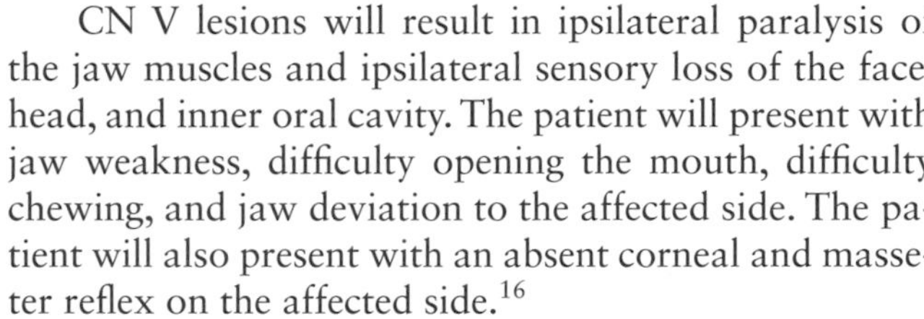

CN V lesions will result in ipsilateral paralysis of the jaw muscles and ipsilateral sensory loss of the face, head, and inner oral cavity. The patient will present with jaw weakness, difficulty opening the mouth, difficulty chewing, and jaw deviation to the affected side. The patient will also present with an absent corneal and masseter reflex on the affected side.[16]

Assessing Impact on Daily Function

When CN V is damaged, patients will have difficulty chewing food, may unknowingly pocket food in the inner oral cavity, and may drool or allow food and liquids to escape from the mouth area on the affected side. Therapists should ask patients if they have difficulty chewing food and should check for the above conditions by observing the patient during eating and drinking.

Male patients may be at risk for razor cuts during shaving on the affected side of the face; all patients may be at risk for undetected abrasions to the affected side of the head resulting from minor accidents and falls. Therapists should ask patients and their family members if such events have recently occurred.

An absent corneal reflex may increase the risk of eye irritation, infection, or injury, and therapists should ask patients and family members if such ocular problems have recently occurred.

Cranial Nerve VI: Abducens Nerve

CN VI is one of the extraoculomotor nerves, along with CN III and CN IV. Like the trochlear nerve (CN IV), CN VI is a somatic motor nerve that innervates the ipsilateral lateral rectus eye muscle (responsible for lateral eye movements). The nucleus of CN VI is located in the caudal pons and yields axons that exit the brainstem at the pons–medullary junction. Along with CN III and CN IV, CN VI exits the skull through the superior orbital fissure, where it enters the orbit to reach its target.[1–4]

CN VI is assessed conjointly with the other two extraoculomotor nerves by examining ocular alignment and range of motion. When CN VI is damaged, paralysis of the ipsilateral lateral rectus muscle occurs, and the patient will have difficulty moving the affected eyeball laterally. This condition occurs because the medial rectus muscle, which pulls the eyeball medially, is working unopposed and a medial strabismus may be apparent. Such patients will be unable to move the eye past midline and may experience diplopia and blurred vision.[9,17]

For screening procedures and assessment of daily functional impact, see CN III.

Cranial Nerve VII: Facial Nerve

CN VII is a mixed nerve that contains both somatic and visceral sensory and motor components. The sensory portion of the nerve innervates the taste receptors on the anterior tongue, whereas the motor portion innervates the muscles of facial expression, the stapedius muscle (located in the middle ear), posterior belly of the digastric muscle, and the efferent limb of the corneal reflex. Axons of the visceral motor neurons are responsible for ipsilateral innervation of the lacrimal gland (for tear production) and the submandibular and sublingual salivary glands (for saliva production).[1–4]

CN VII originates at the pons–medullary junction, enters the temporal bone through the internal acoustic meatus, and exits the temporal bone through the stylomastoid foramen. Although CN VII is referred to as one nerve, it actually consists of two comingled nerves: the nerve proper and the intermediate nerve.[1–4]

Screening Procedures

CN VII is assessed through an examination of the motor function of the muscles of facial expression, taste sensation on the anterior tongue, and the corneal reflex.[9,18,19]

Motor Function

The muscles of facial expression should be evaluated for strength and symmetry.

- The patient should be seated with the therapist positioned in front.
- Instruct the patient to smile, frown, and pucker the lips. Note any asymmetry between both sides of the face during these facial movements.
- Ask the patient to blow the cheeks up with air. Gently push on the patient's cheeks while instructing him or her to resist your manual pressure. Note any asymmetry between cheek strength (see Fig. 20-10 and Video 20-9).

- Instruct the patient to elevate the eyebrows and forehead. Preserved ability to wrinkle the forehead with lower facial muscle weakness indicates an upper motor neuron lesion (commonly resulting from stroke). Ipsilateral paralysis of both the forehead and facial expression muscles indicates a lower motor neuron lesion (commonly resulting from CN damage).

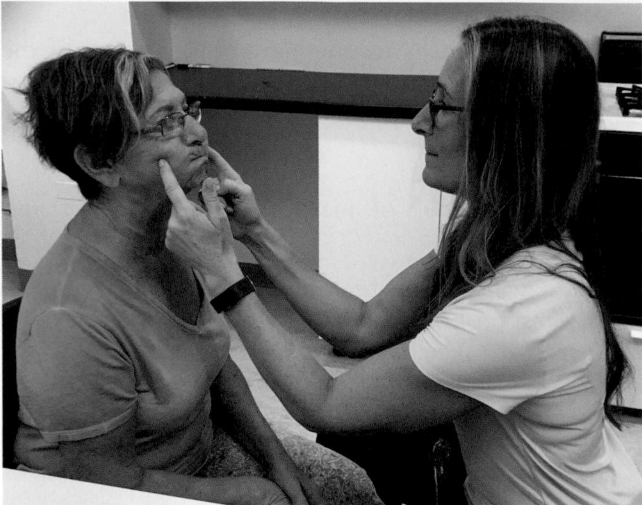

Figure 20-10. Screening motor function of the facial nerve.

Sensory Function

Taste sensation on the anterior aspect of the tongue should be evaluated. Always assess the intact side prior to the suspected involved side.

- The patient should be seated with vision occluded.
- One at a time, present sweet, salty, and sour solutions to the anterior tongue (senses sweet) and middle and lateral tongue (senses sour and salty). Ask whether the patient can taste and identify each substance type.

Corneal Reflex

See section on Screening Procedures for CN V.

A lesion to CN VII will result in ipsilateral paralysis of the muscles of facial expression, lost taste sensation on the anterior two-thirds of the tongue, changes in tear and saliva production, and an absent corneal reflex. Because the facial nerve gives off branches that innervate the stapedius muscle, patients with CN VII lesions may complain of ipsilateral hyperacusis, or increased sound sensitivity.[9,18,19]

Assessing Impact on Daily Function

To assess whether and to what extent a CN VII lesion has impacted a patient's daily function, determine the following. Corroborate patient responses with close family members.

- Ask whether the patient has experienced changes in appetite because food no longer tastes appealing or the same. Determine whether weight loss has occurred and if nutritional intake has been impacted.
- Because patients may pocket food in the mouth as a result of oral muscular weakness, observe patients while eating and drinking.
- Ask whether the patient has withdrawn from social participation because of asymmetrical facial control and movement.

- Ask the patient if increased or decreased tear and saliva production have interfered with daily life activities such as reading, eating/drinking, and driving. Over production may cause blurred vision and an inability to control drooling. Underproduction may cause dry eye and mouth.
- If the corneal reflex is absent, the patient may be more susceptible to eye irritations, infection, and injury. Ask if any of these have recently occurred.
- Ask whether the patient has been bothered by loud noises and, as a result, has changed routines relating to social participation, entertainment, and phone use.

Cranial Nerve VIII: Vestibulocochlear Nerve

CN VIII is a special sensory nerve responsible for audition and balance. The nerve originates in the pons–medullary junction and exits the skull to enter the inner ear through the internal acoustic meatus. CN VIII consists of two branches: cochlear and vestibular. The cochlear branch mediates the function of audition by transmitting sensory signals (sound waves) originating from fluid movement in the cochlea to the brain. The vestibular branch mediates balance/equilibrium by transmitting sensory signals about body and head position that originated from fluid movement in the vestibular apparatus (semicircular canals and otolith organs) to the cortex and cerebellum.[1–4]

The vestibulocochlear nerve is assessed by examining the special sensory functions of hearing and balance and by screening for the presence of **nystagmus** (rapid eye movements that result from activation of the vestibulo-ocular reflex).

Auditory Branch of the Vestibulocochlear Nerve

Assessing the auditory branch involves screening the function of hearing. Auditory screens are usually performed by an audiologist to distinguish between conductive and sensorineural hearing[9,20–22]:

- Conductive hearing loss results from impairment of the outer and middle ear structures.[20,21]
- Sensorineural hearing loss results from impairment to the inner ear structures, vestibulocochlear nerve, and/or temporal lobe.[20,21]

Two tests are commonly used to distinguish between conductive and sensorineural hearing loss: Weber Test and Rinne Test.[22] Both ears are tested.

- *Weber Test:* Strike a tuning fork and place it against the middle of the patient's forehead. Sound is heard through bone conduction and should be heard equally in both ears. If sound is heard louder in one ear, a conductive hearing loss in that ear is indicated (see Fig. 20-11 and Video 20-10).

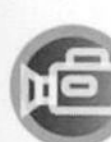

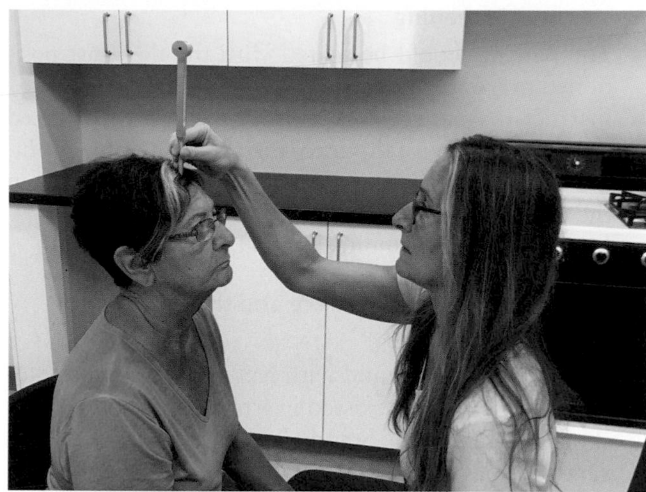

Figure 20-11. Weber test: Vestibulocochlear nerve.

- *Rinne Test:* Strike a tuning fork and place it against the mastoid bone. When the patient indicates no longer being able to hear the sound, move the tuning fork next to the auditory canal (see Fig. 20-12 and Video 20-11). Sound heard through air conduction is usually twice as long as bone conduction. If the patient no longer hears the sound when the tuning fork is moved to the auditory canal, conductive hearing loss is indicated. If sensorineural hearing loss has occurred, both bone conduction and air conduction will be impaired, and sound will be heard louder in the opposite ear.

Vestibular Branch of the Vestibulocochlear Nerve

Assessing the vestibular branch involves screening for the presence of nystagmus and evaluating balance and equilibrium responses.[9,20]

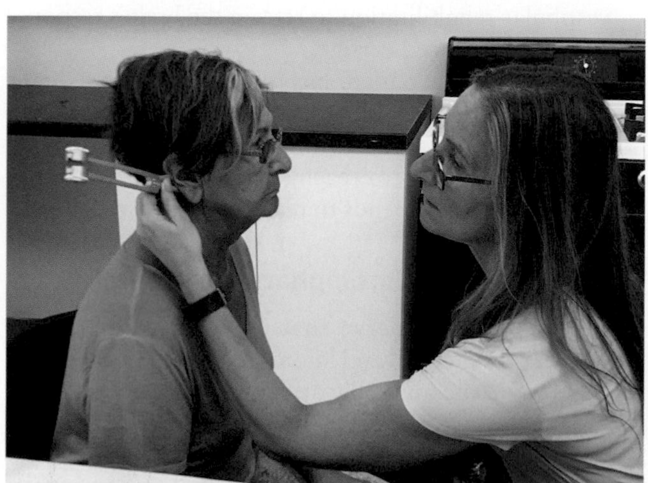

Figure 20-12. Rinne test: Vestibulocochlear nerve.

Nystagmus Screening

- The patient should be seated with the therapist positioned in front.
- Instruct the patient to maintain the head in a fixed position while visually tracking a moving object (finger or pen cap) held at a distance of ~15 inches from the patient's nose.
- Move the visual stimulus in an H and X pattern.

Romberg Test (To Test Balance and the Presence of Protective Responses)

- Ask the patient to stand with feet together while holding arms next to or crossed in front of the body (shoes should be removed). Stand close to the patient to prevent possible falls (see Video 20-12).
- Instruct the patient to first stand with eyes open and then with eyes closed. Observe for increased sway or loss of balance.
- Gently displace the patient's balance and check for protective responses.

CN VIII lesions can result in ipsilateral sensorineural hearing loss and/or tinnitus (ringing in the ears), vertigo (dizziness), nystagmus, and impaired balance and equilibrium responses.[20–22]

Assessing Impact on Daily Function

To assess whether and to what extent a CN VIII lesion has impacted a patient's daily function, determine the following. Corroborate patient responses with close family members.

- Ask whether the patient has problems with hearing during conversation (in-person or via phone use), television viewing, or driving; misses information as a result; or has withdrawn from social participation.
- Ask whether the patient has recently experienced dizziness (with or without nausea) for periods of time that has impacted the ability to participate in daily activities. Patients with vestibular neuritis may require vestibular rehabilitation to retrain the brain's response to motion-induced vertigo.
- Ask whether the patient has recently experienced falls or feels unsteady on his or her feet in daily activities such as bathing and dressing. Observe the patient as he or she attempts to reach above to retrieve items in high cabinets and bends to reach items in low cabinets.

Cranial Nerve IX: Glossopharyngeal Nerve

CN IX is a mixed nerve that contains both somatic and visceral sensory and motor components. CN IX originates in the medulla at the level of the postolivary sulcus and exits the skull through the jugular foramen. The nerve's motor components mediate swallowing (along with CN X, vagus nerve) and secretion of the parotid gland. The sensory components of CN IX are responsible for (a) taste sensation on the posterior tongue region; (b) sensation (pain, temperature, touch) of the external auditory meatus and posterior tongue region; and (c) visceral sensation of the pharynx, parotid gland, and carotid body and sinus. CN IX and CN X conjointly play primary roles in the gag and swallowing reflexes.[1–4]

Screening Procedures

CN IX and CN X functions are screened together.[9,23]

Sensory Function

See section on Screening Procedures for evaluating taste sensation for CN VII, facial nerve. Use the same procedures, but instead apply bitter substances to the posterior region of the tongue.

Motor Function

The gag and swallow reflexes are assessed.

Gag Reflex. Swipe a tongue depressor or cotton swab applicator at the back of the patient's throat and observe for immediate contraction of the pharyngeal muscles and elevation of the palate.

Swallow Reflex. Present the patient with different foods of varying textures and viscosities (solids, pureed, thick and thin liquids) one at a time. Observe the patient's ability to swallow, noting signs of food aspiration, coughing, throat clearing, or wet vocal quality (indicating food pocketing in the larynx).

Assessing Impact on Daily Function

To assess whether and to what extent CN IX impairment has impacted the patient's daily activities, determine the following. Corroborate patient responses with close family members.

- Ask whether the patient has recently experienced difficulty swallowing solid food and/or liquids, including coughing and choking.
- If the patient indicates the presence of swallowing difficulties, determine which types of foods/liquids are most problematic.
- Ask whether swallowing difficulties have altered the patient's food intake (has the patient begun to eat less or lost weight), nutritional intake (is the patient eating a sufficient amount and array of food for adequate nutrition), and social eating with others (does the patient avoid eating with others).

Cranial Nerve X: Vagus Nerve

Similar to CN IX, CN X is a mixed nerve that contains both (a) somatic and visceral motor components and (b) somatic and visceral sensory components. Along with CN IX, CN X originates in the medulla at the level of the postolivary sulcus (caudal to CN IX) and exits the skull through the jugular foramen.[1–4]

CN X's motor components mediate swallowing, speaking, digestion, and cardiorespiratory processes. The nerve's sensory components are responsible for (a) sensation of the skin at the external auditory meatus, the external ear, and the dura of the posterior cranial fossa; (b) taste at the epiglottis and base of the tongue; and (c) visceral sensation from the larynx, pharynx, heart, aortic arch, lungs, and gastrointestinal tract. As mentioned previously, both CN IX and CN X conjointly mediate the gag and swallowing reflexes.[1–4]

Screening Procedures

When evaluating the gag and swallowing reflexes, CN IX and CN X are assessed together (see section on Screening Procedures for CN IX). The vagus nerve is additionally assessed by evaluating the function of the palatal muscles, voice quality, and breathing using the following screening procedures.[9,24,25]

- The patient should be seated with the therapist positioned in front.
- Instruct the patient to say "ah" while observing the soft palate and uvula to detect whether the uvula is maintained in midline. Weakened palatal muscles on one side will cause the uvula to be pulled toward the opposite side.
- Observe the patient's articulation of speech. Check for the presence of dysarthria (slurred speech) and **dysphonia** (decreased vocal volume or hoarseness).
- Observe the patient's respiratory status and check for the presence of **dyspnea** (difficulty breathing).

In addition to swallowing and speaking difficulties, impairment of the vagus nerve may also result in dyspnea and changes in heart rate, such as tachycardia (rapid heart rate at resting).[9]

Assessing Impact on Daily Function

To assess whether and to what extent CN X impairment has impacted the patient's daily activities, determine the following. Corroborate patient responses with close family members.

- Ask whether the patient experiences difficulty clearly and audibly articulating speech in conversation, has difficulty communicating through speech in-person or by phone, and/or has withdrawn from social participation because of speech difficulties.
- Ask whether the patient experiences rapid heart rate at rest and if this interferes with any daily life activities, such as eating, sleeping, reading, or television viewing.

Cranial Nerve XI: Accessory Nerve

CN XI is considered to be a somatic motor nerve that ipsilaterally innervates two muscles: the sternocleidomastoid (SCM) and trapezius muscles. The SCM is responsible for (a) head lateral flexion to the same side and (b) head rotation to the opposite side. The trapezius muscle mediates the scapular movements of elevation, depression, rotation, and retraction.[1–4]

CN XI has two nerve roots: spinal and cranial. The spinal nerve root originates from motor neurons in the cervical segments of the spinal cord (C1–C6). These motor neurons yield axons that ascend the cervical segments and enter the cranial cavity through the foramen magnum. The spinal root, along with CN IX and CN X, exits the skull via the jugular foramen to reach its motor targets. The CN root originates in the caudal medulla from motor neurons located in the nucleus ambiguus and dorsal motor vagal nucleus. The cranial root exits the skull via the jugular foramen and immediately combines with CN X.[26,27]

Screening Procedures

CN XI is primarily assessed by evaluating the function of the spinal nerve root as it innervates the SCM and trapezius muscles.[9,27]

Sternocleidomastoid Muscle

- The patient should be seated with the therapist positioned in front.
- Assess the uninvolved side first, followed by the involved side.
- Instruct the patient to flex the head laterally (toward the same side) and rotate the head to the opposite side (see Video 20-13).

- Ask the patient to resist your attempts to gently return the head toward a neutral midline position.
- Note asymmetry of movement and strength, and check for atrophy of the affected SCM muscle.

Trapezius Muscle

- Instruct the patient to shrug both shoulders toward the ears and maintain that position.
- Ask the patient to resist your attempts to gently depress the shoulders (see Fig. 20-13 and Video 20-14).

- Note asymmetry of movement and strength, and check for atrophy of the affected upper trapezius muscle.

A CN XI lesion will result in paralysis or weakness of the SCM and trapezius muscles. As a result, the patient will have difficultly rotating the head to the opposite side (of the lesion) and will present with drooping of the affected shoulder. The patient may also experience swallowing difficulties (dysphagia) resulting from weakened laryngeal muscles innervated by the CN root.[9,27]

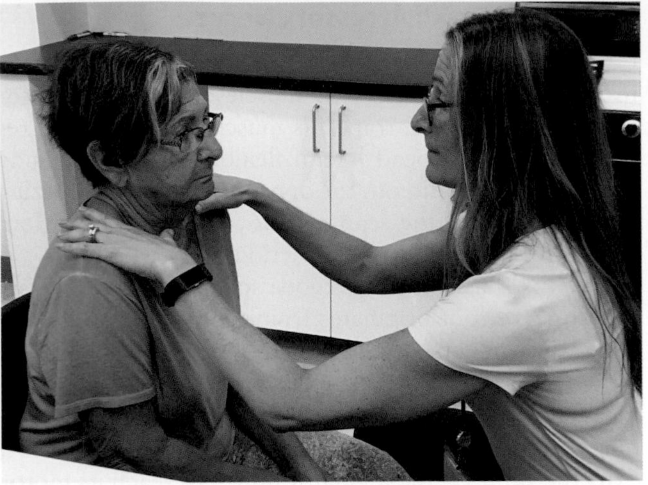

Figure 20-13. Screening trapezius muscle function: Accessory nerve.

Assessing Impact on Daily Function

To assess whether and to what extent CN XI impairment has impacted the patient's daily activities, determine the following. Corroborate patient responses with close family members.

- Ask whether the patient has difficulty turning his or her head while driving, bathing, grooming, dressing, and in response to noise or someone's voice. Observe the patient's ability to rotate the head directly within these activities.
- Ask whether the patient has difficulty reaching above his or her head to retrieve items from overhead cabinets, putting on a coat or over-the-head sweater, or brushing one's hair. Observe the patient during these activities.
- If swallowing difficulties are noted, use the screening procedures outlined in the sections addressing CN V, CN VII, CN IX, and CN X to determine how such impairment has impacted daily life function.

Cranial Nerve XII: Hypoglossal Nerve

CN XII is a somatic motor nerve that innervates ipsilateral tongue muscles and is responsible for tongue movements required in swallowing (oral stage) and speaking. The nerve originates in the hypoglossal nucleus located within the caudal medulla, yields motor axons that exit the medulla at the preolivary sulcus, and exits the skull through the hypoglossal canal.[1–4]

Screening Procedures

CN XII function is assessed by examining tongue movement.[9,28,29]

- The patient should be seated with the therapist positioned in front.
- Instruct the patient to protrude the tongue. Observe whether the tongue deviates toward the ipsilateral side. Also note the presence of unilateral or bilateral fasciculations (muscle twitches or fast, involuntary muscle contractions) and/or atrophy of the tongue muscles.
- Instruct the patient to move the tongue from side to side. Observe any asymmetry in tongue movement.
- Instruct the patient to push the tongue against the right cheek, then the left.
- Ask the patient to resist your attempts to depress each cheek as he or she pushes the cheek outward. Note any asymmetry in tongue strength.

CN XII lesions result in ipsilateral tongue muscle paralysis. Such patients present with ipsilateral weakness and atrophy of tongue muscles, deviation of the protruded tongue to the affected side, and possible fasciculations in the ipsilateral tongue muscles. Patients commonly experience dysphagia resulting from an inability to use tongue muscles to manipulate food into a bolus that can be transported to the pharynx. **Dysarthria** (slurred speech) may also occur secondary to an inability to use the tongue to produce sound and enunciate words.[9,25,28,29]

Assessing Impact on Daily Function

To assess whether and to what extent CN XII impairment has impacted the patient's daily activities, determine the following. Corroborate patient responses with close family members.

- Ask whether the patient has recently experienced difficulty swallowing solid food, including coughing and choking.
- Ask whether swallowing difficulties have altered the patient's food intake (has the patient begun to eat less or lost weight), nutritional intake (is the patient eating a sufficient amount and array of food for adequate nutrition), and social eating with others (does the patient avoid eating with others).
- Ask whether the patient experiences difficulty clearly articulating speech in conversation, has difficulty communicating through speech in-person or by phone, and/or has withdrawn from social participation because of speech difficulties.

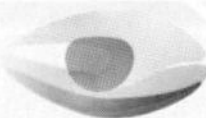

CASE STUDY

Patient Information

Mateo is a 63-year-old retired Hispanic man who reports facial weakness, diminished taste, persistent tearing, and increased aural sensitivity, all present on the right side only. He reports that symptoms occurred suddenly 2 weeks ago and were noticeable upon waking. No other unusual health events were reported other than a viral infection that fully cleared 2 weeks prior to the reported symptoms.

Assessment Process

Because the therapist suspected CN VII, facial nerve damage, Mateo was screened for the following: (1) bilateral strength and symmetry of the muscles of facial expression, (2) taste sensation on the anterior aspect of the tongue, and (3) corneal reflex function.

Assessment Results

Mateo was observed to have asymmetry and weakness of the facial muscles on the right side including his forehead muscles, indicating lower motor neuron impairment (found in CN damage) as opposed to upper motor neuron involvement (found in stroke). Taste sensation, particularly sweet and salty, were absent on the anterior two-thirds of the tongue. In response to stimulation of the right cornea, it was noted that the corneal reflex was absent on that side. During evaluation, it was observed that Mateo's right eye teared continuously and he repeatedly wiped saliva from the right corner of his mouth. He stated that eye tearing often caused blurred vision, which interfered with reading and television viewing. He reported using cotton balls in his right ear to reduce sound sensitivity that had recently developed and was aggravated by television viewing, phone use, and street sounds such as police sirens. Although Mateo reported no change in eating and dietary habits, his daughter, who was present at the evaluation, mentioned that her father was eating less and now preferred to eat alone in his room rather than with family. In response, Mateo stated that he was experiencing difficulty containing food and fluid in his mouth and that foods didn't taste as good as they used to. Bell's palsy,[30] impairment of CN VII, was suspected, and referral made for a full neurological evaluation.

Occupational Therapy Problem List

- Weakness and asymmetry of right-sided facial muscles with apparent difficulty handling foods and liquids. The patient appears to be withdrawing from social participation as a result. An in-depth dysphagia evaluation is warranted.
- Increased right-sided tear and saliva production causing blurred vision in daily occupations such as reading and phone use.
- Increased right-sided sound sensitivity that appears to be interfering with daily occupations, such as phone use, television viewing, and community participation.
- Reduced taste sensation on the anterior two-thirds of the tongue, causing decreased appetite. An in-depth nutritional evaluation should be made.

Commonly Used Standardized Assessments in Cranial Nerve Evaluation

Instrument and Reference	Intended Purpose	Administration Time	Validity	Reliability	Sensitivity	Strengths and Weaknesses
Berg Balance Scale (BBS)[31]	Performance-based assessment of balance in the elderly	15 minutes	Concurrent validity was established with Barthel Index ($r = 0.67$), Timed Up-and-Go ($r = 0.76$), and Tinnetti Balance Test ($r = 0.91$).	Inter-rater reliability = 0.98. Internal consistency = 0.96	BBS was able to identify fallers with 100% accuracy.	Strengths: Short administration time, high reliability and moderate-to-high validity, and high sensitivity. Weaknesses: Test activities are not based in daily occupational activities.
Dysphagia Evaluation Protocol[32]	Observation-based assessment of swallowing difficulties for adults	30 minutes	Face and content validity reported to be high based on a panel of experts.	Inter-rater reliability ranged from 0.85 to 1.00. Test–retest reliability ranged from 0.83 to 1.00.	Not established	Strengths: Developed for use by occupational therapists, high validity and reliability, and short administration time. Weaknesses: Sensitivity not established.
Full Range Test of Visual-Motor Integration[33]	Paper-and-pencil test of visual motor skills for children and adults	10–30 minutes	Content validity reported to be high based on a panel of experts. Concurrent validity with Developmental Test of Visual-Motor Integration ($r = 0.85$).	Internal consistency = 0.91. Test–retest reliability = 0.85. Inter-rater reliability = 0.96	Not established	Strengths: High reliability and validity, short administration time Weaknesses: Paper-and-pencil test that is not ecologically valid (based in daily occupation), instrument is expensive.

References

1. Nowinski WL, Thaung TSL, Chua BC, et al. Three-dimensional stereotactic atlas of the adult human skull correlated with the brain, cranial nerves, and intracranial vasculature. *J Neurosci Methods*. 2015;246:65–74. doi:10.1016/j.jneumeth.2015.02.012.
2. Wilson-Pauwels L, Stewart PA, Akesson EJ, Spcaey S. *Cranial Nerves: Function and Dysfunction*. 3rd ed. Shelton, CT: People's Medical; 2010.
3. Damodaran O, Rizk E, Rodriguez J, Lee, G. Cranial nerve assessment: a concise guide to clinical examination. *Clin Anat*. 2014;27(1):25–30. doi:10.1002/ca.22336.
4. Binder DK, Sonne C, Fischbein NJ. *Cranial Nerves: Anatomy, Pathology, Imaging*. New York, NY: Thieme Medical; 2010.
5. Cecchini MP, Cardobi N, Sbarbati A, et al. Post-traumatic taste disorders: presentation of three meaningful cases. *Ital J Anat Embryol*. 2017;122(1):57. doi:10.13128/IJAE-21449.
6. Abolmaali N, Gudziol V, Hummel T. Pathology of the olfactory nerve. *Neuroimaging Clin N Am*. 2008;18(2): 233–242. doi:10.1016/j.nic.2007.10.002.
7. Nordin S, Brämerson A. Complaints of olfactory disorders: epidemiology, assessment and clinical implications. *Curr Opin Allergy Clin Immunol*. 2008;8(1):10–15. doi:10.1097/ACI.0b013e3282f3f473.
8. Coello AF, Canals AG, Gonzalez JM, Martín JJA. Cranial nerve injury after minor head trauma: clinical article. *J Neurosurg*. 2010;113(3):547–555. doi:10.3171/2010.6.JNS091620.
9. Corbett JJ, Santiago ME. The neurologic examination. In: Haines DE, ed. *Fundamental Neuroscience for Basic and Clinical Applications*. 4th ed. Philadelphia, PA: Elsevier Saunders; 2014:454–467.
10. Allen KF, Gaier ED, Wiggs JL. Genetics of primary inherited disorders of the optic nerve: clinical applications. *Cold Spring Harb Perspect Med*. 2015;5(7): a017277. doi:10.1101/cshperspect.a017277.
11. May PJ, Corbett JJ. Visual motor systems. In: Haines DE, ed. *Fundamental Neuroscience for Basic and Clinical Applications*. 4th ed. Philadelphia, PA: Elsevier Saunders; 2014:389–404.
12. Sadagopan KA, Wasserman BN. Managing the patient with oculomotor nerve palsy. *Curr Opin Ophthalmol*. 2013;24(5):438–447. doi:10.10097/ICU .0b013e3283645a9b.
13. Quoc EB, Milleret C. Origins of strabismus and loss of binocular vision. *Front Integr Neurosci*. 2014;8:71. doi:10.3389/fnint.2014.00071.
14. Engel JM. Treatment and diagnosis off congenital fourth nerve palsies: an update. *Curr Opin Ophthalmol*. 2015;26(5): 353–356. doi:10.1097/ICU.0000000000000179.
15. Robles L. Central trochlear nerve palsy due to stroke: report and clinical correlation of two cases. *Can J Neurol Sci*. 2016;43:417–419. doi:10.1017/cjn.2015.344.
16. Heir GM, Nasri-Heir C, Thomas D, et al. Complex regional pain syndrome following trigeminal nerve injury: report of 2 cases. *Oral Surg Oral Med Oral Pathol Oral Radiol*. 2012;114(6):733–739. doi:10.1016/j.oooo.2012.06.001.
17. Azarmina M, Azarmina H. The six syndromes of the sixth cranial nerve. *J Ophthalmic Vis Res*. 2013;8(2):160–171.
18. Hohman MH, Hadlock TA. Etiology, diagnosis, and management of facial palsy: 2000 patients at a facial nerve center. *Laryngoscope*. 2014;124(7):E283–E293. doi:10.1002/lary.24542.
19. Baricich A, Cabrio C, Paggio R, Cisari C, Aluffi P. Peripheral facial nerve palsy: how effective is rehabilitation? *Otol Neurotol*. 2012;33(7):1118–1126. doi:10.1097/MAO.0b013e318264270e.
20. De Foer B, Kenis C, Van Melkebeke D, et al. Pathology of the vestibulocochlear nerve. *Eur J Radiol*. 2010;74(2): 349–358. doi:10.1016/j.ejrad.2009.06.033.
21. Chin CJ, Dorman K. Sudden sensorineural hearing loss. *CMAJ*. 2017;189(11):E437–E438. doi:10.1503/cmaj.161191.
22. Butskiy O, Ng D, Hodgson M, Nunez DA. Rinne test: does the tuning fork position affect the sound amplitude at the ear? *J Otolaryngol Head Neck Surg*. 2016;45(1):21. doi:10.1186/s40463-016-0133-7.
23. Steele CM, Miller AJ. Sensory input pathways and mechanisms in swallowing: a review. *Dysphagia*. 2010; 25(4):323–333. doi:10.1007/s00455-010-9301-5.
24. Cohen SM, Kim J, Roy N, Asche C, Courey M. Prevalence and causes of dysphonia in a large treatment-seeking population. *Laryngoscope*. 2012;122(2):343–348. doi:10.1002/lary.22426.
25. Jordan LC, Hillis AE. Disorders of speech and language: aphasia, apraxia, and dysarthria. *Curr Opin Neurol*. 2006;19(6):580–585. doi:10.1097/WCO.0b013e3280109260.
26. Liu H, Wo H, Chung I, Kim IB, Han SH. Morphological characteristics of the cranial root of the accessory nerve. *Clin Anat*. 2014;27:1167–1173. doi:10.1002/ca.22451.
27. Restrepo CE, Tubbs RS, Spinner RJ. Expanding what is known of the anatomy of the spinal accessory nerve. *Clin Anat*. 2015;28(4):467–471. doi:10.1002/ca.22492.
28. Fletcher A. Persistent isolated unilateral hypoglossal nerve palsy. *Med Case Rep*. 2017;3:1. doi:10.21767/2471-8041.100004.
29. Stino A, Smith B, Temkit M, Reddy SN. Hypoglossal nerve palsy: 245 cases. *Muscle Nerve*. 2016;54:1050–1054. doi:10.1002/mus.25197.
30. Eviston TJ, Croxson GR, Kennedy PGE, Hadlock T, Krishnan AV. Bell's palsy: aetiology, clinical features and multidisciplinary care. *J Neurol Neurosurg Psychiatry*. 2015;86:1356–1361. doi:10.1136/jnnp-2014-309563.
31. Berg K, Wood-Dauphinee S, Williams J, Gayton, D. Measuring balance in the elderly: preliminary development of an instrument. *Physiother Can*. 1989;41:304–311. doi:10.3138/ptc.41.6.304.
32. Avery-Smith W, Rosen AB, Dellarosa DM. *Dysphagia Evaluation Protocol*. San Antonio, TX: NCS Pearson; 1997.
33. Hammill DD, Pearson NA, Voress JK, Reynolds CR. *Full Range Test of Visual–Motor Integration: Examiner's Manual*. Austin, TX: Pro-Ed; 2006.

Chapter 21

Environmental Assessment and Modification: Home, Work, and Community

Tracy Van Oss, Martha J. Sanders, and Pamela Hewitt

LEARNING OBJECTIVES

This chapter will allow the reader to:

1. Identify common environmental modification assessments used in the home, workplace, and community.
2. Understand the purpose and processes of conducting home, workplace, and community environmental assessments.
3. Determine how to ensure that individuals and populations fit living spaces.
4. Incorporate universal design principles into the planning of living spaces.
5. Understand common modifications to enhance safety and functional performance of clients with disabilities in the home, workplace, and community.

CHAPTER OUTLINE

TERMINOLOGY

Accessibility: the ease with which the physical environment may be reached, entered, and used by all individuals.

Aging in place: the idea that environments can be modified to support changes in functional performance as a result of aging, thus ensuring continued residence in one's own home.

Anthropometrics: the science of measuring body size and proportions and applying measurements to the design of equipment and spaces.

Environmental modification: alteration of physical environments to improve safety and occupational performance.

Ergonomics: a set of principles to improve worker efficiency and comfort and to decrease injury risk by designing workplaces, equipment, and work processes that fit workers.

Physical environment: the features of a person's surroundings that are built or exist in nature.

Universal design: a set of principles for the built environment that enhance optimal function and convenience for all individuals, regardless of ability.

Visitability: the concept that homes can be accessible for persons in wheelchairs to visit.

Environmental Assessment and Modification

The environment influences human behavior and provides the context within which all occupational roles are performed. Numerous stakeholders including clients, family, contractors, designers, physicians, and employers are interested in promoting healthy and safe environments for clients. Occupational therapists uniquely focus on clients' occupations within the location in which they are performed. Therapists consider how the environment supports and optimizes clients' safe engagement in chosen occupations in the present and future. Thus, therapists are well suited to perform environmental assessments and modifications in the home, workplace, and community. **Environmental modifications** are defined as adaptations applied to the **physical environment** to promote safety and full participation. The American Occupational Therapy Association (AOTA) has developed evidence-based practice guidelines for home modification interventions.[1] Federal, state, and local regulations impact environmental modifications relative to building codes, accessibility, and safety.

History and Legislative Standards

Occupational therapists' role in environmental modifications at home, work, and in the community has been shaped by legislation that supports the rights of individuals with disabilities to full societal participation. **Accessibility** to public buildings, employment settings, and housing choices is fundamental to individuals' safety and meaningful community participation. The following section outlines key legislation impacting environmental modifications.

American National Standards Institute

Founded in 1918, the American National Standards Institute (ANSI) develops standards to ensure the safety and health of US consumers as well as the protection of the environment.[2] ANSI develops building and design standards to allow for accessibility in conjunction with the Americans with Disability Act (ADA), the US Department of Housing and Urban Development (HUD), and Fair Housing Accessibility Guidelines. For example, ANSI determined specifications for the turning radius needed for a standard wheelchair to enter and exit a room. These specifications are used as a guide for both public spaces and private remodelers designing bathroom modifications for wheelchair users.

Fair Housing

The Fair Housing Act Accessibility Guidelines (FHAAG), established in 1968, mandated accessibility in multifamily housing and ensured rights for people with disabilities for equal access to housing options. According to this law, individuals cannot be denied the opportunity to modify a rented home to meet their needs for accessibility; however, renters endure modification costs.[3] Specific accessibility requirements have been established to ensure that the design and construction of public residential buildings comply with the Fair Housing Act (e.g., buildings must have accessible entrances or routes).

Americans with Disabilities Act

The Americans with Disabilities Act (ADA)[4] extended equal rights protection to individuals with disabilities. The ADA outlined three areas in which state and local government became responsible for providing reasonable accommodations that ensured access to employment, public services, facilities, transportation, accommodations, and telecommunications. Title I mandated that employers accommodate individuals in hiring and employment who are qualified and who meet disability criteria. Titles II and III mandated accessibility to private and public facilities, recreational facilities, state and local government buildings including businesses and schools, and public transportation. Many buildings and spaces constructed prior to 1990 may still contain accessibility barriers.

The ADA was revised in 2008 (Amendments Act 2008) to expand its application to a larger group.[5] The definition of "disability" was revised to include impairments that substantially limit participation in major life activities, such as work. The 2010 ADA Standards for Accessible Design outline how both public-sector and private-sector services, programs, and facilities should comply with and implement accessibility requirements.[6]

Building Standards

Building standards support accessibility by providing specific architectural dimensions and building guidelines for applicable private and public facilities. In 2004, the US Access Board released the updated ADA-ABA (Architectural Board Act) Accessibility Guidelines for new or altered buildings, which provide accessibility requirements for public and private facilities.[7] The specifications in these guidelines are based on adult and child dimensions and anthropometrics, and are applied during the design, construction, or alteration of buildings and facilities covered by ADA titles II and III. Specifications are provided for most aspects of the built environment, including the space required for maneuvering wheelchairs in corridors and rooms, washrooms, building entrances, and parking lots.

Standards for Specific Environments

Building accessibility standards apply to public and private businesses with public access; however, additional standards are often developed for specific environments, such as workplaces, playgrounds, and daycare centers. Occupational Safety and Health Administration (OSHA) standards are aimed at creating safe environments for workers. Although these legislative acts do not mandate involvement by health care professionals, occupational therapists are well suited to ensure that legislative requirements are met, clients are aware of available services, and planned environmental modifications meet clients' identified current and future needs.

Universal Design

In 1997, a group of American advocates developed the principles of **universal design** that have been commonly adopted in a variety of nations. Universal design principles highlight strategies to promote accessibility, inclusive design, and safety in activities available to a wide range of people. Universal design is based on the idea that all environments, products, and communication systems—not only those serving people with disabilities—should be developed to facilitate ease of use, safety, and optimal function. Because most existing environments have not been built using universal design principles, environmental modifications are commonly needed to increase accessibility. The following principles summarize key universal design principles.[8]

Equitable Use

Equitable use refers to design that is useful and marketable for all users. For example, automatically opening doors decrease the need for strength, and motor and cognitive skills. In addition to being useful for people with functional limitations, automatic doors are helpful to any worker carrying packages through doorways. Automatically opening doors and curb cuts are useful for people using scooters and wheelchairs, as well as parents with strollers. Furniture with adjustable chair and table heights are similarly useful for all people.

Flexibility in Use

Flexibility in use refers to design that accommodates a wide range of individual preferences and abilities. Seats or benches placed in public places, such as parks or malls, allow people of all ages to rest and those with pulmonary issues to conserve energy. A no-step entrance and a curbless shower are also examples of universal design features in the home.

Simple and Intuitive Use

Simple and intuitive use addresses multiple ways to present information. Products that are designed for use by everyone should use simple language and universally recognized symbols, such as red faucet labeling for hot water and blue for cold. Other examples include product assembly instructions that use diagrams instead of language. Similarly, international retailers use diagram labeling for products having an international audience.

Perceptible Information

Perceptible information refers to design that communicates necessary information effectively to users, regardless of environmental conditions or users' sensory abilities. An example includes interior automobile gas cap labels displaying the location of the car side on which the gas cap is located. Another example includes home fire alarms that have visual and auditory signals and large dial displays. Also in this category are products or devices that provide verbal, written, and tactile information regarding use.

Tolerance for Error

Tolerance for error refers to design that minimizes hazards and the possibility of adverse consequences from accidental or unintended actions. Examples are red light indicators on stoves to alert users that surfaces are still hot, and refrigerator signals that alert users when doors are left ajar. Staircases that have two railing levels at differing heights to accommodate shorter and taller individuals to enhance safety is another example.

Low Physical Effort

Low physical effort refers to design that can be used effectively, comfortably, and with minimal fatigue. When traveling, moving sidewalks allow passengers to reduce energy expenditure, especially with luggage in tow. Useful products may include lever door handles and rocker switches for people with poor hand strength or loss of fine motor abilities. Groceries can become heavy at any life stage, and the installation of a package shelf can be beneficial when entering the home. Long-handled equipment such as reachers can reduce bending to retrieve items from the floor and aid in lower body dressing. The use of built-up utensils can reduce fatigue when preparing meals requiring repetitive movements such as stirring, peeling, and cutting. Also included in this category are devices and products that are touch-activated, such as can openers and faucets.

Size and Space for Approach and Use

This refers to design that promotes approach, reach, manipulation, and use, regardless of the user's body size, posture, or mobility. Examples include raised kitchen appliances such as dishwashers to reduce bending, microwaves located in pullout drawers to reduce reaching, and sink faucets positioned in counter fronts for easier access. Additional examples include push-button door openers located at appropriate heights for all users, and entryways that accommodate wheelchair maneuverability.

Measuring for Fit: Understanding Anthropometrics

Anthropometrics is the study of human body dimensions such as height, weight, leg length, and body segment length as applied to living and working spaces, furniture, and equipment. Anthropometrics is the basis for designing spaces that "fit" an individual or group in the home, workplace, or community. Because human dimensions vary with population, age, ethnicity, and clinical conditions, it is important to understand how anthropometric measurements are applied to space planning. For general space planning, occupational therapists, designers, and architects depend on tables of body sizes in order to design spaces that "fit" the majority of individuals (i.e., 95% of the largest and 5% of the smallest users). Individuals, however, who are unique, at the extremes of size, who are pregnant, or who have disabilities, may require individual measurement to ensure a proper "fit" for their space.[9] The following steps for measuring a person or population to ensure "fit" applies to home, work, and community settings.

Steps to Use Anthropometric Measurements to Design Space

1. Identify the target user population.
2. Identify the criteria that are important to the user (e.g., comfort, use, clearance through an area).
3. Identify important body dimensions (e.g., thigh length for a chair seat).
4. Determine whether the space is being designed for one person or for a population (consider averages and extremes).
5. Measure body parts or find data from anthropometric data tables. Measure length of body segments between joints using a measuring tape or calipers.
6. Consider other factors impacting use of space (e.g., wearing heavy clothing in cold temperatures may impact fit, and use of walkers or wheelchairs).
7. Create a mock-up or virtual model that can be tested with a user.

Purposes for Environmental Assessments

Occupational therapists perform home, work, and/or community assessments to improve clients' or populations' occupational performance. Therapists need to clearly identify the purposes of such assessments in order to select evaluation instruments that can gather the most appropriate information.

Overall Independence

Occupational therapists are consulted to promote independence for individuals with disabilities that limit engagement and mobility as a result of chronic or short-term (e.g., postoperative) conditions. Each condition may require a slightly different evaluation focus. For example, clients in wheelchairs will need identification of environmental modifications to accommodate wheelchair use; clients with visual impairment may need modifications to enhance visual function (e.g., increased lighting, color contrast, and low-tech aids); and clients with dementia may need modifications to compensate for memory and wayfinding problems. Each client's medical history and daily life needs should be clearly identified at the onset of the evaluation.

Home Safety and Fall Prevention

Fall prevention refers to strategies and modifications designed to minimize fall risk in the home and other environments. For older adults, falls can have devastating consequences, including long-term disability, the potential need for extended care, loss of confidence, depression, social isolation, and even premature death. Research on the effectiveness of home interventions provided by occupational therapists indicates that environmental modifications can effectively reduce falls in older adults.[10] Fall prevention interventions address such environmental features as physical structure, furniture, rugs, lighting, and stairs. Home safety evaluations address additional hazards such as overloaded electrical outlets and tangled cords placed in walking paths, unsafe use of appliances and stoves leaking gas, and chemical (radon, carbon monoxide detectors) and biological hazards (mold, dust mites). Whereas therapists may detect such hazards during home safety evaluations, other consultants will perform chemical and biological testing.

Aging in Place

According to the American Association of Retired Persons (AARP), 89% of people aged 50 years and older who are considering options for housing express preferences for remaining at home, within familiar settings and communities, and with family and friends.[11] Adults 50+ define successful aging as taking care of oneself, independently making choices, participating in community activities, and pursuing desired hobbies and interests.[12] Additional considerations that promote **aging in place** are the high cost of nursing homes and assisted living facilities, which lead older adults to remain in their homes with supportive services, environmental modifications, and/or renovations. Occupational therapists identify clients' current needs and anticipate potential future needs to promote safe aging in place, such as relocating a master bedroom and bath downstairs (to avoid stair use), and building an accessible house entrance.

Community Livability

Livability addresses the structure, accessibility, services, and enhancements that promote quality of life for all community inhabitants. **Visitability** is the incorporation of basic features into the homes of persons using mobility devices to facilitate ease of entrance, exit, visit, or stay, for any length of time.[13] The advocacy group, Concrete Change, developed by Eleanor Smith, asserts that all home environments should be designed to improve livability and visitability for home inhabitants and visitors.[14] For example, basic home features that should be incorporated into all homes and that enhance accessibility of visitors using wheelchairs include no-step entrances, wide doorways of 32 inches, and access to first-floor bathrooms.

Injury Prevention and Productivity

Workplaces must meet ADA standards to promote equal access to job opportunities and public spaces for individuals with disabilities. A workplace evaluation may have the additional foci of preventing injuries and improving productivity. Although injury prevention programs include analyses of job tasks and worker body mechanics, work environments are evaluated to examine conditions that promote safety and health, while reducing injury risk. Environmental conditions, such as workstation design, noise, and lighting, impact productivity by affecting ease-of-task completion.

Home Environment Assessment and Modification

Understanding the Client: The Occupational Profile

Occupational therapists seek to understand how people interact with their environments to engage in desired occupations. Using occupational profiles, the client–therapist interaction begins by determining the client's previous roles and occupations, and present desires and expectations for activity participation. Therapists obtain important client characteristics, including age, height, weight, medical conditions, hospitalizations, and past medical history. Therapists also obtain information about client performance patterns, activity demands, ambulation modes, and current or anticipated future use of assistive devices and adaptive equipment. Additional questions and use of standardized assessments and observation allow therapists to assess visual impairment, balance and coordination, cognition, and safety awareness.

Evidence suggests that home environment interventions are most effective when they consider the specific needs of individual clients rather than generically addressing a checklist of common home safety concerns.[15,16] The need for home modifications will vary among individuals occupying similar spaces, depending on factors such as health status, cognitive and visual-perceptual function, physical mobility, financial resources, and whether clients live alone or with others. For example, a home evaluation for a client with dementia may focus on the need for memory cues, wayfinding strategies, and safety systems, whereas a home evaluation for a client with spinal cord injury (SCI) may focus on the home's physical structural characteristics that require modification to promote occupational participation. Therapists identify barriers to participation and make personalized recommendations for environmental modifications that ensure optimal independence and safety for each client.

Team Approach: Including a Variety of Stakeholders

Throughout the assessment process, occupational therapists collaborate with caregivers to ensure that recommendations for adaptations support caregiving activities. Therapists also work collaboratively with other professionals to plan and complete modifications. Building professionals—such as contractors, designers, architects, and building code officials—are not part of typical health care teams, but provide important structural, zoning, and financial information related to environmental interventions. To effectively achieve desired outcomes, interprofessional team members must similarly perceive client goals and engage in collaborative problem-solving.

Funding Options

Funding options vary greatly by region, health insurer, and needed environmental modifications. Possible funding and resources for assistance with modifications may include Rebuilding Together, Area Agencies on Aging, Centers for Independent Living, and the Bureau of Rehabilitation Services. Many individuals without sufficient financial resources or assistance, however, will often need to "pay out of pocket." Employers may fund workplace accommodations for employees with disabilities and are required to accommodate ADA-specific issues that are financially feasible. Some insurers may subsidize home and/or workplace accommodations. Community organizations with grant funds may also financially sponsor services that improve community and home accessibility.

Creating the Problem List

Once assessments have been completed, occupational therapists should compile a list of areas in which client occupational roles cannot be met because of environmental conditions. This list should be specific and co-created by clients, therapists, and community stakeholders. The problem list should include criteria to promote the desired goal, which may, in turn, yield a number of solutions. Each client problem list is unique to the individual, and therapists create personalized intervention plans that address all identified needs. Examples of problems may include cognitive challenges effecting safe meal preparation, balance impairments limiting safe tub transfers, and visual-perceptual deficits impacting reading medication labels.

The Process of Home Assessment and Modification

Once a home assessment referral is made, therapists should plan to bring writing instruments (e.g., laptop or pad), tape measures, and cameras. The reason for a home safety evaluation should be clear regarding the client's safety needs and desires for role resumption. For example, some clients will require a home modification evaluation because they have begun permanently using a wheelchair, whereas others may desire to age in place. Most referrals will require evaluation of both the exterior and interior home environments. The following provides guidelines for assessment and modification of home environments.

Entryways, Ramps, and Home Exteriors

Therapists begin home assessments by examining the home's entryway. Pathways leading to front or back doors should be well lit with gentle slopes and textured surfaces that are even throughout all walkways. Trees or shrubs should be well maintained to prevent fallen berries or leaves from creating slippery conditions. Access to stairs should be clutter free with slip-resistant surfaces and adequate handrails. Universal design features such as a package shelf outside the door, or an overhang above the door, can mitigate unnecessary struggling and risk. Thresholds into the home should be flush with the floor or no higher than 0.5 inches to prevent tripping. A 5 × 5 foot space (1.5 × 1.5 meters) both outside and inside the doorway should be present to provide an adequate turning radius for wheelchair users. Use of appropriate lighting is one of the most important features, as well as a doorbell that is lit or has a vibrating device/alarm or amplification. Finally, use of a keyless entry system can be installed for ease of access into the home. If entering via the garage, a garage door remote control and inside light are needed to minimize safety hazards. Box 21-1

Box 21-1

Recommended Minimal Lighting Levels

Location or Workplace	Activity	Illuminance Range (Lux)
Home		
Exterior lights	Safety, orienting	50–100
Interior entry		1,000
Bedroom/living room	Reading, dressing, watching TV, telephone calling	200 (reading 750)
Bathroom	Grooming, hygiene, reading	200, sink area 500
Dining room	Eating, socializing	200 ambient (500 on table)
Kitchen	Reading, preparing, cooking	200, 500 prep area (combination of ambient and local or task lighting)
Work		
Hallways, stairwells	Safety, general mobility	60
Warehouses	Tasks with large size and high contrast	200–400
Office work (data entry)	Reading, computer work, writing, laboratories	300, 500 on desk surface
Industrial drawing	Gross assembly, machine work, buffing	750–1,500
Industry detailed drawing, small scale, cognitive visual tasks	Fine assembly, inspection, detailed drawing blueprints	2,000–4,000
Industry or health care, extremely small, prolonged, and exacting tasks	Visual performance of the highest order	3,000–6,000
Industry or health care precise, very special or life-sustaining task	Surgery, industrial fine sewing	10,000–20,000
Community		
Hallways, stairwells, bathrooms, maintenance rooms, stairways, interiors	Orienting, occasional visual tasks	200 (1,000 for older adults)
Conference rooms	Reading, conversing	300
Retail stores	Read, select, handle	750

Compiled from Illuminating Engineering Society of North America. *The Lighting Handbook*. 10th ed. New York, NY: Illuminating Engineering Society of North America; 2011.

provides minimum illuminance levels for both exterior and interior spaces based on recommendations from the Illuminating Engineering Society of North America.[17,18]

After assessing the home entrance and analyzing the information gained from the client's evaluation, therapists apply skilled judgment to select appropriate ramp types. Portable ramps offer flexibility in time and installation and are often used for temporary health conditions (Fig. 21-1). Permanent ramps are recommended for clients who have health conditions that will not improve or will worsen over time resulting in the necessity of a wheelchair for functional mobility. In this case, it is recommended that the therapist work with a Certified Aging in Place Specialist (CAPS) builder to accurately measure slope, run, and direction changes based on the topography of the entrance's approach. If a ramp is present or needed, it should comply with ADA standards. Each landing must be at least 60 × 60 inches (1.5 × 1.5 meters), and the slope of the ramp should be a maximum of 1 feet (30.48 cm) of rise for each 12 feet (3.65 meters) of run.[2] Ramps should also possess handrails on each side and can be located inside the garage if warranted.

Exterior Stairs, Elevators, and Lifts

Whereas ramps are one option for creating a step-free entrance, lifts may be another alternative. An aesthetically pleasing option is the use of soil and ground covering to create a gradual sloping feature called an earth berm (Fig. 21-2). Elevators also allow accessibility to all home levels (see Fig. 21-3). Stair lifts are another alternative for persons to safely move from one home level to another. Cognition should be assessed for safety when navigating stair lifts as part of the clinical reasoning process. If clients have short-term memory deficits, display inability to process new directions, or have dementia or Alzheimer disease, an alternative to a stair lift may be necessary because neurocognitive deficits will impact client safety, especially when exiting the chair at the top of the stairs (Fig. 21-4).

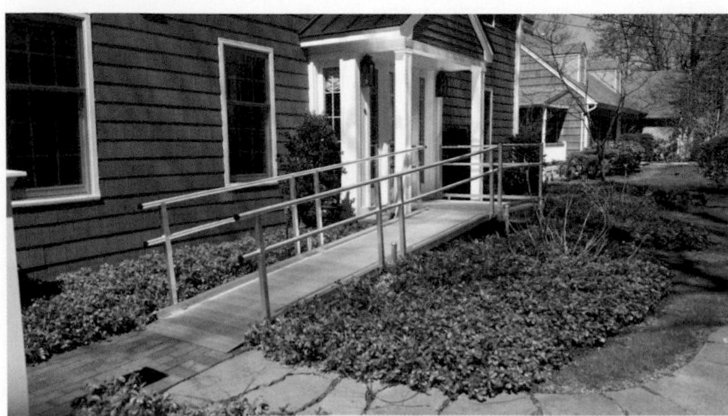

Figure 21-1. Portable ramp. (Reprinted with permission from Gregg Frank.)

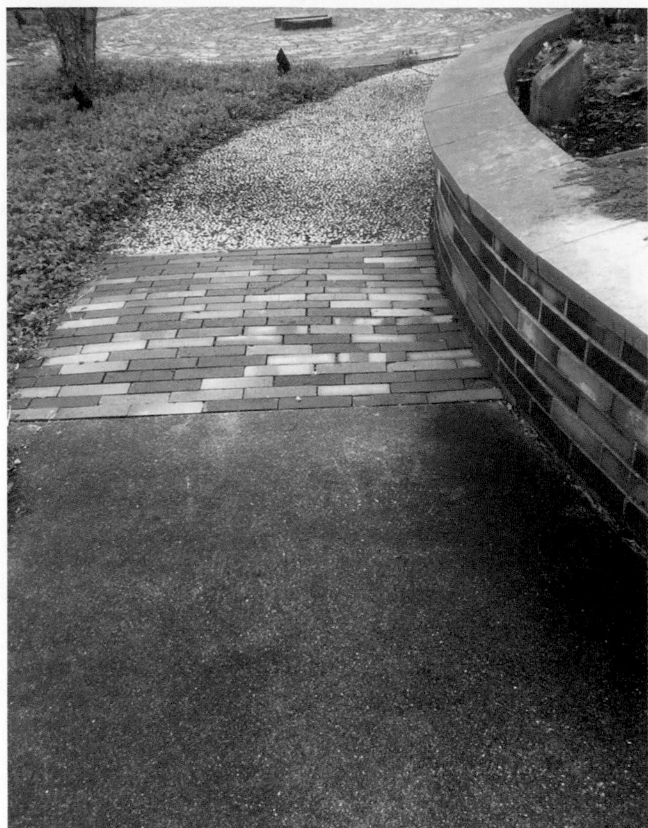

Figure 21-2. Universally designed entryway. (Reprinted with permission from Amy Wagenfeld.)

Stairs: Exterior and Interior

Stairs throughout the home must be well lit with a light switch at the top and bottom of each staircase. The flat part of the steps, or the treads, should be 11 to 12 feet (~28 to 30 cm) deep and 36 inches (~91 cm) wide.

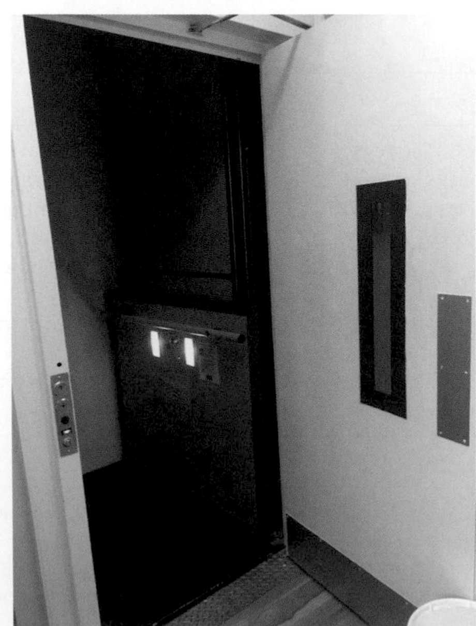

Figure 21-3. Vertical platform elevator for wheelchair users.

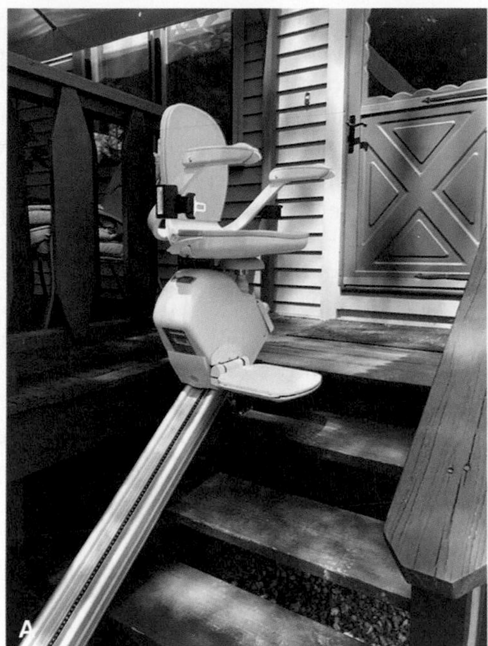

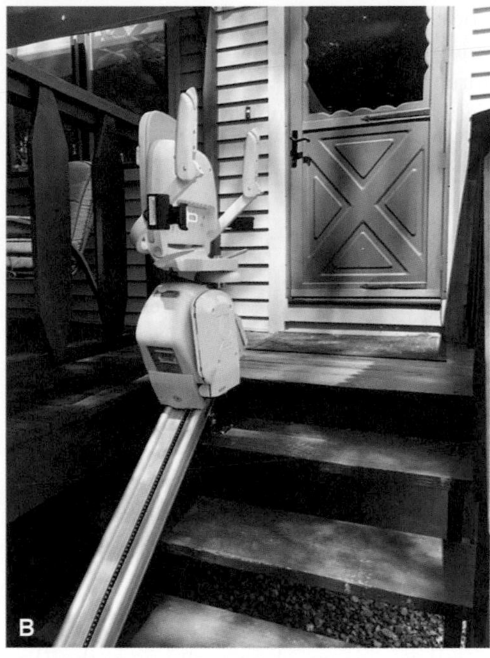

Figure 21-4. Outdoor stair lift. (Reprinted with permission from Justin Oakley.)

Treads should have a nonslip surface, have color contrast between risers and steps for clients with low vision, and be clutter free. A landing at every 10 steps is helpful for older adults who need to stop and rest because of limited endurance.

Use of a bilateral, sturdy handrail is another important component to keep clients safe while climbing or descending stairs. Handrails should be about 34 inches (~86 cm) from the floor, 1.5 inches (~4 cm) from the wall, and extend 1 to 2 inches (~2 to 5 cm) beyond the top and bottom steps. Handrails should be tightly secured to wall studs and support the appropriate weight of all users.[2]

Doors

There are many door styles, including sliding doors, barn doors, bifold doors, and pocket doors, and clients may choose one for multiple purposes, including wheelchair accessibility. The client and therapist will consider the door style as well as hardware (e.g., hinges and doorknobs), the width of the open door clearance, the threshold height, and the door weight. Ideally, to prevent injury to hands propelling a wheelchair, an opening of 36 inches (~91 cm) is recommended. Standard doors can be adapted by removing the door hardware to gain additional open space. Replacing standard hinges with swing-clear offset hinges allows doors to swing open and out of the way of the door frame. This action provides an additional 2 inches (~5 cm) clearance (on the door side of the frame) for people using wheelchairs and walkers. Door knobs should be replaced with lever-style handles to enhance ease of use, particularly for clients with limited hand mobility secondary to injury or disease. A keyless entry and peephole can be considered, as well as their ideal height for users.[2]

When assessing doorway thresholds for potential trip hazards or for wheelchair propulsion, a zero threshold is ideal. In the home interior, the threshold can be removed and filled with a replacement surface that is level with the floor. If the occupational therapist is assessing the entire home for functional mobility safety, recommendations can be made to install the same flooring throughout the house so that zero thresholds exist between doorways and rooms.

When assessing exterior doors, it is important to note that although exterior door thresholds cannot be removed, they can be replaced with lower height thresholds to allow easier wheelchair mobility and reduce fall risk. Also, note that exterior doors are heavier and can be difficult to open. In this case, therapists may recommend power door openers similar to those used in public dwellings.

As with all home modification recommendations, collaboration with the client and caregiver is most important in determining a list of priorities for safety, functional mobility, and cost. Although standards are set by ANSI 117.1 for accessible doorways and entrances in public dwellings, occupational therapists can customize doorways for individual clients in private homes.

Lighting and Outlets

Utilization of natural light by opening curtains or shades is a simple suggestion for improving lighting. Care must be taken, however, to avoid glare or even overlighting at midday (a problem for those with macular degeneration or aging eyes). Repositioning furniture near clean windows might offset the need for electrical lights, particularly during the day. Use of automatically lighting nightlights in bedrooms, bathrooms, and hallways is important for older adults and persons with low vision to prevent unintentional injuries in the evening and in darkly lit home areas. A seemingly simple act such as requesting family members or friends to occasionally change light bulbs can eliminate unnecessary climbing that may precipitate a fall.

A light switch should be located at each room's entrance and connected to a light source for that specific room. Touch control table lamps, remote controls, and multiple light switch styles are available, including motion activated and sound- or voice-sensor switches, depending on the client's individual preference and needs. Light-up rocker and slider switches can be installed to help clients easily detect light switch location in the dark to reduce fall risk. The color of furniture, appliances, and walls should contrast with floors and countertops to enhance visual detection. Electrical outlets are often low to the floor, making them difficult to reach; however, extension cords should be used sparingly and should be tacked to the wall to ensure clear walking paths (for recommended minimal lighting levels in the home, see Box 21-1).[17,18]

Interior Floors, Hallways, Doorways, and Windows

Interior floor surfaces should be smooth and slip resistant and can include low pile carpeting or nonglare, nonslip surfaces such as sand-finished tile or hardwood floors with a satin, low-shine finish. Area rugs, throw rugs, and runners without nonslip rubber backing should be discouraged because of their potential to cause tripping and falls. Therapists, however, must acknowledge clients' desire to keep rugs, and in this case, rugs can be made less hazardous by placing nonslip rubber mats underneath or using double-sided tape to secure them in place.

Doorways and hallways throughout the home should be well lit and clutter free to prevent falls. Use of neutral color paint that contrasts with the floor is optimal to promote visual performance and safety. Hallways should be at least 36 inches (~91 cm) wide to accommodate wheelchairs, and thresholds between rooms should be eliminated or maintained at 0.5 inches (~1 cm) or lower. A clear space in front of and behind doorways with at least 60 inches (~1.5 meters) of space is optimal for all users. If doorways to rooms along the hallway are narrow, adjustments can be made to remove some of the mechanisms within the door to increase the doorframe width for wheelchair clearance. Additionally, by adding swing-clear offset hinges to interior doors, a 34-inch (~86 cm) opening can be achieved with minimal reconstruction by the builder. Also, lever handles set no higher than 44 inches (~1 meter) from the floor create easy-to-open doors and can facilitate improved use of the home for all. It is important to remove or repair flooring that is warped, worn, or buckled for safety purposes. Additionally, electrical outlets should be within reach and not overloaded.[2]

Finally, recommendations for windows and window treatments should consider the client's ability. Some windows are electronically operated and open and close with ease; other windows rely on remote controls to open and close blinds for safety and privacy; and others are simply manual. Windows should not be overlooked because they may be the only exit in home fires. Therapists should assess the client's ability to both open and close windows, as well as access to windows. Furniture and clutter preventing window access should be removed.

Bathrooms

There are several features that can be modified in the bathroom to make activities of daily living (ADLs) more manageable, comfortable, and safe. Bathroom recommendations may include a door that is at least 32 inches (~81 cm) wide, one that swings out, or a pocket door that slides within the wall. There should be sufficient floor space in the bathroom for safe transfers from a wheelchair for toileting or bathing. The use of grounded fault circuit indicator (GFCI) outlets (i.e., grounded outlet to minimize short circuit and fire risk), rubber-backed bathmats to reduce slipping, anti-scald detectors to maintain water temperature below 120°, and the provision of bathroom phone access are preventive recommendations to promote bathroom safety.

Numerous toilet options exist relative to height, color, and capabilities. A typical toilet can be purchased with a 17 to 19 inch-height (~43 to 48 cm) height with varying types of seating options. Toilet heights can be increased or lifts added to make sitting and standing easier. Other options include light-up toilet seats for night use or bidet toilet seats to wash, dry, and keep perineal areas clean (Fig. 21-5). Automatic options with remotes or flush sensors exist. There should be at least 18 inches

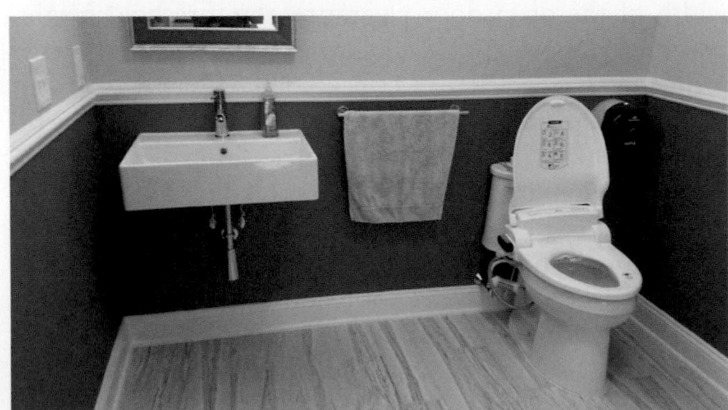

Figure 21-5. Bidet toilet seat and suspended sink. (Reprinted with permission from Gregg Frank.)

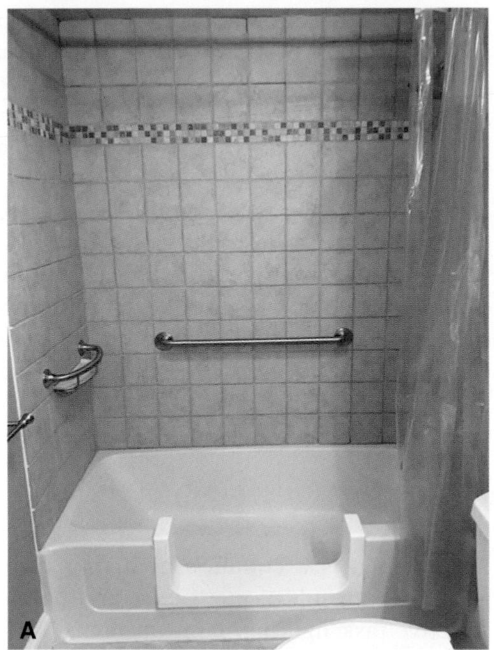

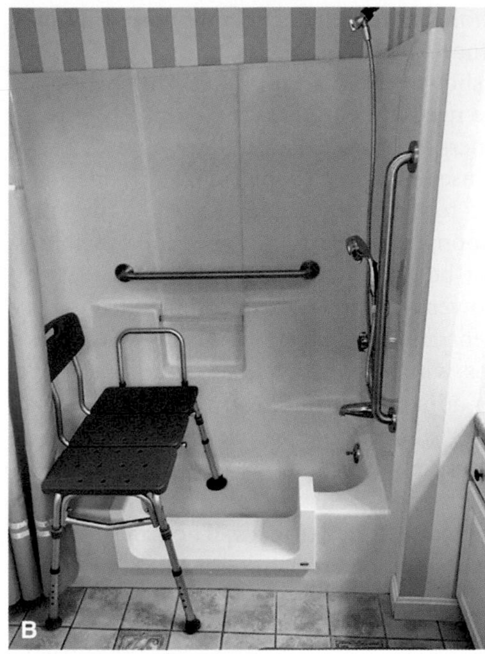

Figure 21-6. A and **B,** Cut-out bathtub. (Reprinted with permission from Justin Oakley.)

(~46 cm) of free space in front of the toilet and 42 inches (~1 meter) of space on one side for adequate transfers from another seated position if needed. Open-ended toilet paper holders should be within easy reach. An added toilet paper/grab bar option may also be considered.[2]

The sink and counter should be 34 inches (~86 cm) from the floor, with knee space beneath for persons needing to sit to perform self-care activities. Counters should be rounded and clutter free, with daily used items placed within easy reach. There should also be one lever handle located in the sink front to control hot and cold water temperature. A mirror that is adjustable or tilts downward will benefit persons who are seated.

The bathtub–shower combination should have a nonslip surface and temperature water controls that can be easily reached from outside the tub. Positioning soaps and towels nearby can eliminate reaching and possible balance loss. Bottled soaps are less likely to drop to tub floors and cause potential falls compared to handheld soaps. Use of handheld showers and tub seats or benches are frequent recommendations, particularly for clients with balance problems, low endurance, and lower extremity mobility limitations. There are, however, cut-out tubs that allow clients to use a small opening to walk in and out of the bathtub (Fig. 21-6). Finally, for clients who bathe in tubs but may have difficulty rising, there are hydraulic bathtub lifts.

One needed modification may be to replace bathtubs with curbless showers to facilitate bathing from a wheelchair (Fig. 21-7). Curbless or roll-in showers can be uniquely created through collaboration between occupational therapists, clients, and contractors. Use of smaller floor tiles that are mildew resistant may reduce slipping and potential mold exposure. Placement of seating options, faucets, and shower heads should be aligned with user and/or caregiver needs in mind. Rolling shower chairs should be able to easily glide over shower dams if necessary. Another consideration may be a shower bay, which is a portable shower system with a shower chair that attaches to a sink.

Walk-in shower stalls should also have nonslip surfaces and easy-to-reach soaps, towels, and water controls. The use of fold down seats with handheld shower heads offers the option of sitting in the shower for persons with limited endurance or balance. Grab bars in the shower provide extra security for persons requiring stability or assistance with transfers. Walk-in showers

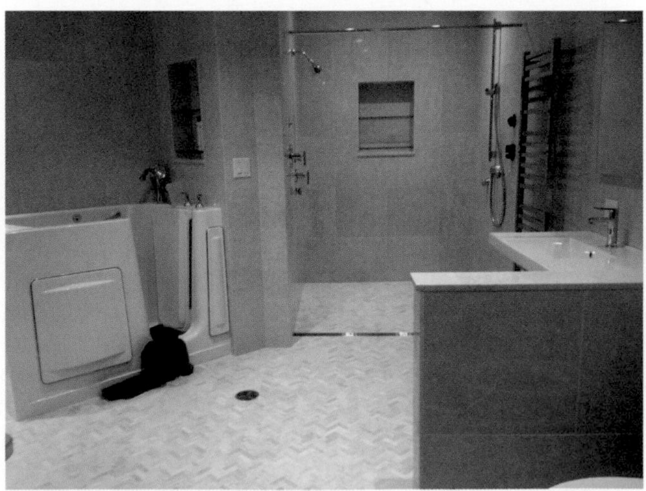

Figure 21-7. Shower and walk-in soaking tub. (Reprinted with permission from Gregg Frank.)

without thresholds can be beneficial for persons with decreased balance or who use roll-in shower chairs.

Inside the shower itself, adaptations can be installed that can fit the needs for all. Shower pumps for shampoos, conditioners, and body soaps allow for easy use of these regularly used items. Therapists may provide adaptive equipment for shower use, including bath mitts, long-handled sponges, or suction-cupped foot scrubbers. Shower seats or benches with backs/rails (some swivel) or tub slide shower chairs may be recommended to promote safe tub entrance and exit. Handheld showers and shower combos with on/off switches to control water while seated, or adjustable height showerheads, allow all persons to sit or stand while bathing. If bathmats are troublesome for some to use on a daily basis, therapists can replace mats with nonskid mildew-resistant bath strips that adhere to floor surfaces. The safest shower doors are made of tempered, laminate safety glass and should be recommended if clients have needed financial resources. Otherwise, shower curtains with bottom weights should be recommended. If there is no light source in the shower area, the shower curtain should be made of clear mildew-resistant plastic to allow light from the main bathroom light fixture (usually at the ceiling or sink). Finally, there may be need for a visual display to identify water temperature to prevent scalding.

Pedestal sinks or vanities with under-cabinet leg room can be used with clients using a wheelchair or seat for self-care activities. Lever faucets, touch control faucets, or auto turn-off faucets can be useful depending on client needs. Sinks can have faucet handles offset to the side or front for ease of use. Mirrors with tilt options are helpful for those who sit at the sink. Therapists should be certain that all necessary items are positioned on the countertop within easy reach and that cabinets have C- or D-shaped handles if hand function is limited.

Grab bars can be obtained in a variety of lengths, circumferences, and textures and can be purchased from the local pharmacy, home center store, or online. The type and style of grab bar can be chosen by the homeowner and therapist for appropriate weight capacity and functional use. Therapists will also make recommendations for grab bar location based on a user's current and predicted future abilities. It is important to make sure that clients never use towel racks, soap dishes, or sinks from which to push or pull, because these items will not withstand excessive pressure. Installers should collaborate with clients and therapists to meet recommended requirements for specific users. Grab bars must be installed by licensed contractors for optimal safety and sealed with silicone on shower walls to prevent leaks. Use of grab bars next to toilets, and in and around shower stalls and tubs, can support clients needing assistance or stability with transfers.

When renovating bathrooms, nonglare bathroom surfaces and lighting should be selected, with color contrast between floor and wall tiles. Task lighting positioned at the top and sides of sink mirrors, and on shower ceilings, best promote safe function. Nightlights are useful for safe entry in the dark, and heat lamps should be considered to control temperature variation and increase drying time (thereby decreasing rushing and potential accidents).

Bathroom storage should be considered for catheter, oxygen tank, and colostomy equipment and supplies. When working with bariatric clients, special equipment should be considered to accommodate weight for tub benches, roll-in shower commode chairs, and toilet commodes placed over existing toilets (to increase height and provide safety rails). When clients use caregiver assistance, therapists must consider how the environment will be used by a dyad.

Kitchen

The kitchen is a common area that can become dangerous as a result of utensil use and hot surfaces. Using effective task lighting, light-up utensil drawers, or natural light for mealtime prep and eating can eliminate potential kitchen injuries. Phones and fire extinguishers should be easily accessible in case of emergencies. Doorways should be wide enough with low thresholds to allow easy and safe access to kitchens.

Several styles of refrigerators with adjustable shelves, a variety of door arrangements, and options including water and ice dispensers exist. Refrigerator door openings vary and include side by side, freezer on bottom or top, and combinations and can be selected based on client preference and function. Dishwashers at least 8 inches off the ground reduce reaching demands; it is also important to make sure that sufficient space exists to allow wheelchair users to be positioned next to the dishwasher. Many dishwashers are now designed with waist height drawers for convenience and safety.[2]

Wall-mounted ovens with pull-down or side-swinging doors at convenient heights can make cooking easier. Use of push-button controls at the stove front instead of back limits excessive reaching and reduces burn risk. Use of tilted or angled mirrors above stoves allows seated users to view inside pots. Cooktops also have a variety of options available to meet client needs and preferences. Burners should be staggered and sit below smooth, glass tops for easy cleaning and safety. Stove knobs should be located at stove fronts to prevent potential burns when reaching over hot burners. Cooktops should also sit atop counters that allow sufficient knee space for seated users. Stovetops should have indicator lights to alert homeowners that burners may still be hot. Clutter-free, nonglare, heat-resistant counters with rounded edges and smooth surfaces promote safe and efficient use of this potentially dangerous area.

Microwaves are used frequently by older persons who receive "Meals on Wheels" or who heat leftover food provided by family, friends, or neighbors. Microwaves should have a shelf nearby, touchpad controls with tactile cues as needed, and be located at an adequate height from the floor appropriate for the user. Microwaves can also be installed as drawer options. There should be a clear path and safe method to transfer hot items to and from the stove, microwave, or cooktop. This may include utility cart use or sliding items on the counter rather than lifting them.

Multiple or adjustable counter heights can be suitable for many users. Storing frequently used items on the counter can also reduce reaching or bending. There are multiple storage options with pullout drawers, electronic adjustable counters and shelving, rollout shelves, and mixer lifts for those who use this heavy appliance. Use of D- or C-shaped handles on shelves or cabinets are useful for all users. Dishes, glassware, and utensils should be within reach for easy access, whereas heavy pots and pans can be stored below counters in slide-out drawers. Upper cabinets can be easily reached at 48 inches from the floor and lower cabinets at 6 inches for seated users. Use of Lazy-Susans on deep shelves or in corner cabinets can improve access and limit unnecessary reaching. It is important for therapists to assess clients' ability to access upper and lower cabinets, and reposition supplies to enhance safe meal preparation.

Kitchen sinks are easily accessible from seated positions at 34 inches (~86 cm) from the floor with no more than 6.5-inch ((16.5 cm) deep basins.[2] Use of single lever handle faucets, instead of individual knobs, allows control of hot and cold water with one handle. Retractable spray hoses, anti-scald devices, and lever handles located near the counter front best support kitchen safety. Knee space beneath counters and sink benefits wheelchair users or persons needing to sit. Insulation or panels placed in front of pipes should be added to protect legs from potential burns. Placement of garbage disposal switches, if present, should be within easy reach. Finally, placement of trash cans, compactors, and/or recycling bins should be assessed and positioned for easy and frequent use (Fig. 21-8).

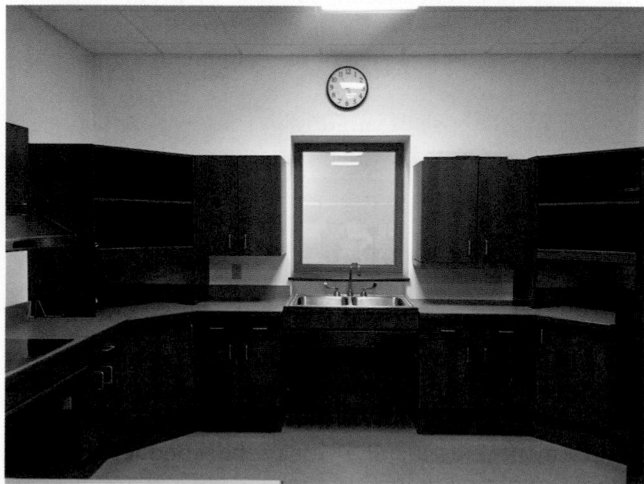

Figure 21-8. Kitchen with raised dishwasher and adjustable stove, oven, and cabinets.

Living and Dining Rooms

Living and dining room areas are common spaces in which people spend considerable time each day. The placement of cordless phones in these areas is important should emergencies arise requiring calls for assistance. Central vacuum system use can eliminate the need to lift and carry a vacuum cleaner. It is important to assess how well clients are able to sit down onto and rise from furniture, particularly low and armless chairs. Recommendations for persons having difficulty with sit-to-stand transfers may include use of firm cushions for increased support, chairs with bilateral arms, adding risers or leg extenders to furniture to increase seat height, or power lift chair use. It is additionally important to make sure that clear walking paths exist to reduce fall risk. Recommendations may be made to reduce obstacles, clutter, and glare and enhance mobility with the rearrangement of furniture and strategic lighting placement. This may include painting walls light colors that provide contrast to furniture; using touch control table lamps, task lighting, and motion-, sound-, or voice-sensor switches; and using remote controlled, rocker, slider light, or light-up light switches that can be easily located in the dark. Windows should be easy to open, and shear curtains that cover entire windows should be used to allow natural light without glare or shadows commonly occurring from vertical and horizontal blinds (which can increase fall risk). Easy-to-read or preprogrammed thermostats are also needed in this space.

Bedrooms

Bedrooms can be individualized for the person(s) occupying this space. Beds should be specific to client height, weight, and health condition. It is important to assess how well clients are able to sit down onto and rise from their beds. Recommendations to increase bed mobility may include risers up to 4 inches (~10 cm) to increase bed height or adjustable beds that raise and lower electronically. Programmed vibrating beds can also be recommended to serve as morning alarms and alert clients of ringing doorbells or the presence of smoke or fire (such beds can be connected to smoke alarms). When clients require assistance to get out of bed, simple bed rails, floor-to-ceiling poles, trapeze bars, or ceiling lifts may be necessary. Clients should be instructed to keep flashlights and phones near the bed, use automatically lighting nightlights, and remove clutter to enhance safety and reduce fall risk. Recommendations for bedroom furniture should consider client mobility needs and wheelchair use relative to furniture height and layout. Chairs with armrests are useful to assist with transfers and dressing, and bedside commodes with absorption pads in the basin can limit nighttime ambulation (further reducing fall risk).

Closets

Closets should be assessed for ease of access and item retrieval relative to client mobility limitations. There are many closet space configurations. Sliding doors may limit a client's ability to perceive and access all closet items at once, whereas bifold doors may impede a seated user's access when attempting to reach inside. Some clients may prefer to remove closet doors completely to increase easier access to items inside. Shelving and double-hung rods should be adjusted to a client's height and reaching limitations; pull-down closet rods that lower clothing within a client's reach may be beneficial. Hanging shoe bags and racks maintain these items' accessibility and reduce clutter. For persons with visual impairments, stick-on wall lights and tagging clothes to identify colors may be helpful. Closet lighting should be of sufficient intensity to allow searching for and matching clothing colors.

Home Safety Technologies

Assistive technology can greatly improve clients' quality of life and should be considered when making recommendations for modification of the home or daily routine. Some technologies are appropriate for caregiving, whereas others are designed for client use to enhance occupational participation. Therapists must determine the need for technology based on clients' objectives and wishes, nature of their health condition (e.g., progressive and worsening or temporary such as postsurgical recovery), and cognitive functional level. Therapists will additionally need to collaborate with caregivers and family to determine budgets for technology because financial status will influence decision-making.

Choices for home modification technology are dependent on training needs as well as device complexity. According to Georgia's Assistive Technology Act Program, assistive technology can be categorized into three main categories based on use and needed training.[19]

Low Technology

Low-technology items are devices or equipment that require minimal training by the occupational therapist, may be less expensive, and do not have complex or mechanical features.[19] Examples for the home include under-cabinet jar openers, lever-style handles for doors and faucets, C-shaped cabinet handles, rocker light switches, and double-sided carpet tape. Examples of low-technology items used in daily activities include reachers, long-handled shoe horns, dressing sticks, and built-up handled utensils.

Medium Technology

Medium-technology items are devices or equipment that require moderate training by the therapist, may have some complex features, and may be electronic or battery operated. Medium-technology items are more expensive than low-technology devices and are primarily adaptations to the home.[19] Some examples include hot water regulators to prevent scalding, tub benches and seats, grab bars, handheld shower heads, raised toilet seats, versa frames, and large button telephones.

High Technology

High technology refers to the most complex devices or equipment that likely require maximal training by the therapist, have digital or electronic components, and may be computerized. As a result of these factors, such items can be costly.[19] It is imperative that therapists determine the need and potential successful use of these technologies prior to obtaining them for clients. Examples of such technology include stair lifts; walk-in tubs; tub hydraulic lift seating systems; electronic transfer ceiling track systems; power door openers; wheelchair elevator systems; adjustable height kitchen counters, cabinets, and appliances; power stand assist chairs; electronic adjustable beds; life alert systems; and electronic medication management devices.

Home Safety Technologies

These can be categorized separately as advanced systems that can be installed directly in the home to enhance client safety. Many of these technologies would be recommended by the therapist when working with clients with low vision or hearing loss. Examples of smart home technology command centers for phone and alarm systems include vibrating beds that awaken clients when smoke or fire is detected and flashing lights or audible alarms that alert clients to emergencies and ringing phones.

Safety in the kitchen is of particular concern for clients with dementia. To prevent burns and fires resulting from short-term memory loss, electronic home technologies that sense motion can be installed in the kitchen. Such systems can provide audio cues to remind clients to return to the stove if the system detects lack of motion after a set time. The system can also be programmed to automatically turn off the stove in this situation. Sensor systems and webcams are additionally recommended to monitor client whereabouts within and exiting the home, as in the case of sun downing and nighttime wandering seen in late-stage dementia.

Workplace Environmental Assessment

Purpose of Conducting a Workplace Assessment

The purpose of workplace environmental assessments is to prevent injuries and promote comfort, safety, and productivity for employees and workgroups. Workplace environmental assessments may be conducted along with **ergonomic** job analyses that identify the sequences of job tasks, body motions and postures, time spent in specific postures, and risk factors for musculoskeletal disorders. Workplace environmental assessments may be requested by (1) the worker's physician or insurance company to promote safe return to work, (2) the company safety department to promote injury prevention, or (3) human resources for ADA issues. In all cases, input from workers, supervisors, and employers are critical to understand worker challenges, personal and organizational resources, company expectations, and productivity standards. If a worksite assessment is for an individual worker, therapists will collect information through the occupational profile about the worker's medical history, pattern of discomfort, and current functional limitations.

Preparing for the Worksite Visit

Prior to assessing a worksite environment, therapists should contact the company to clearly identify the reason for the visit, request a job description, and set a visit date. A job description identifies the primary job function and duties that are considered essential to the job. The job description will typically include qualifications such as education, needed experience, skills, and work conditions (hours, location). Therapists can verify this information with the company contact person and client. This will help therapists identify worker priorities for the assessment. Therapists will then identify the specific tasks, task sequences, physical and cognitive demands, and worker positions needed to accomplish the job.

Therapists should consult relevant workplace standards, guidelines, and resources from OSHA, National Institute for Occupational Safety and Health (NIOSH), and professional organizations for a particular workplace. For example, lighting guidelines from the Illuminating Engineering Society (IES) provide recommendations for various job tasks (see Box 21-1).[17] Assessment supplies will be determined by the nature of the worksite visit. Typical supplies for office and industry visits may include personal protective equipment (PPE) as required by the workplace (e.g., steel-toed footwear and protective glasses), assessment recording tools (e.g., forms, computer), measuring tape, force strain gauges (e.g., Chatillon gauges, handheld force gauges), stopwatches, light meters and thermometers, and cameras (with video recording capacity).

Components of an Environmental Assessment

Similar to the home assessment, therapists should observe a worker or representative perform required job tasks in order to understand how the workstation supports the job. Features of the work environment that impact job task performance are addressed here. All workstations address reach and clearance, which are two important considerations in a worker's ability to access the task being performed and "fit" into the workspace provided. The size of the worker (see section on Measuring for Fit: Understanding Anthropometrics, p. 407) is critical for determining the appropriate reach, clearance, heights, and workstation design.

- *Clearance* refers to sufficient headroom, legroom, and elbowroom in the work area. Clearances should always be designed for the largest user (95th percentile). The therapist will observe, measure, and determine whether clients have adequate legroom, armroom, and headroom (if in cramped spaces).
- *Reach* refers to the location of controls and materials accessed to perform a task. Usual manual work should be conducted close to one's body (14 inches [~35 cm]). The tools, staplers, phones, and calculators may be located within about 24 inches (~61 cm) of the individual to minimize awkward postures. Reach should be designed for the smallest user (5th percentile) to minimize awkward postures[9] (Fig. 21-9).

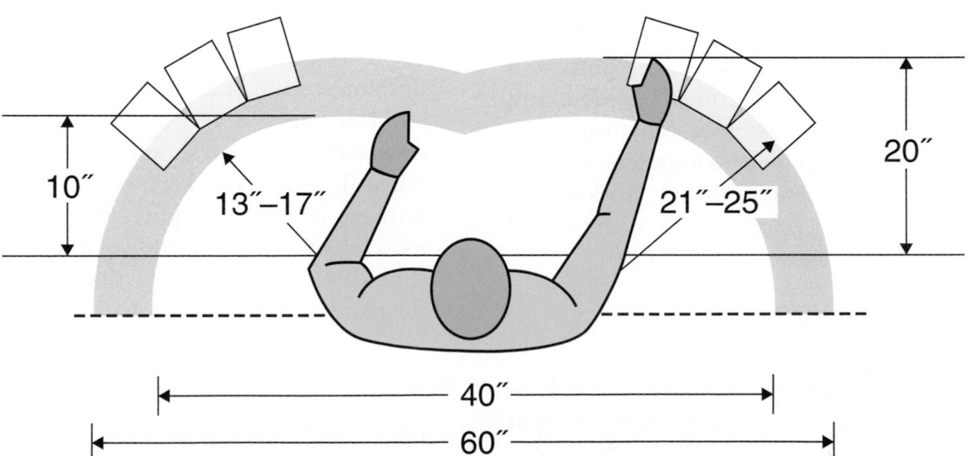

Figure 21-9. Reach envelope. The primary work zone for table top work is within about 10 to 14 inches (~25 to 35 cm) of the elbow. This zone should include frequently used work equipment such as the keyboard and primary equipment. The secondary work zone, within about 20 inches (~21 cm) of the elbow, includes items such as phones, calculators, and less frequently used tools.[34] Document in the public domain and may be freely copied.

Therapists should consult normative data for anthropometric information related to sitting, standing, and reaching relative to hand tool and equipment design. These are measured when workers are sitting and then again standing depending on the workstation.

Task Requirements and Workstation Design

The task requirements of the job dictate worker posture and body motions. Therapists should note the visual requirements of the job (e.g., location of visual cues, objects to manipulate, or information) because these will determine worker head position. Visual information that is positioned directly in a worker's line of sight will promote an upright head/neck posture. Visual information that is placed lower (such as a laptop monitor) will require workers to flex their neck and trunk to view images. Computer screens placed far from the body (beyond arm's length) and low (below head height) will cause workers to flex the neck and trunk forward to view the screen.

Similarly, worker posture also results from placement of workstation equipment. If work surfaces and equipment are placed too high, workers must reach for objects, prompting shoulder flexion and fatigue. If work surfaces are too low, workers must bend their trunks, contributing to low back discomfort. The working areas of desks or benches should be close to the body and unobstructed.[20,21]

Seated Workstations

Seated work is common in offices, call centers, laboratories, dental offices, and seated assembly workstations. Well-designed seated workstations can minimize discomfort from prolonged sitting. Discomfort arising from low back, neck, or shoulder pain reduces work efficiency and may contribute to musculoskeletal disorders over time if awkward postures are sustained.

Computer workstations are examples of seated stations that include a chair, computer (desktop or laptop) with keyboard and monitor, desk (traditional or standing), input device (mouse, trackball), lights, and other office equipment such as document holders and calculators. In laboratories or assembly environments, task-specific equipment will replace computers, such as microscopes or micrometers. The following workstation components should be assessed for workers using seated or standing computer workstations (Fig. 21-10).

Computer Workstation Components

Ergonomic Chair

Well-fitting ergonomic chairs can minimize the risk of long-term neck, back, and even leg problems when fit properly.

- *Height adjustment:* Elbows should be aligned with the desk, keyboard, or working surface. Feet should be flat on the floor or on a footrest.

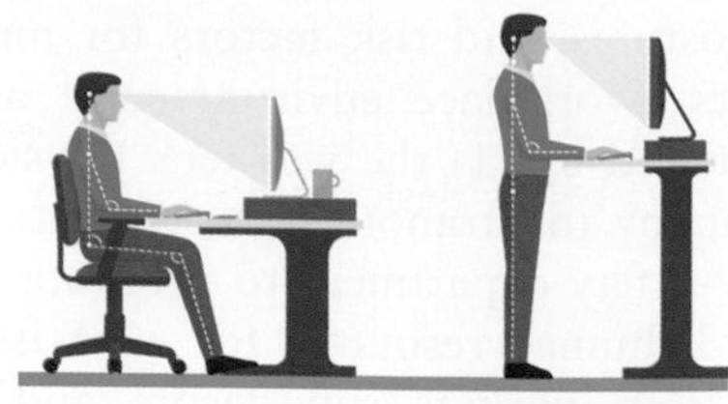

Proper Posture

Head/neck upright, facing forward	☐	Hips perpendicular to floor	☐
Shoulders at one's side	☐	Low and mid back supported back	☐
Elbows bent to about 90°	☐	Knees bent to 90°	☐
Wrists straight	☐	Feet flat on floor or footrest	☐

Adjust Your Workstation

Monitor		Chair	
Top of screen slightly below eye level	☐	Elbows at height of keyboard	☐
Monitor about arm's length from body	☐	Backrest fits in small of back	☐
Good screen contrast	☐	Seat pans supports leg, knees bend	☐
Monitor directly in front of you	☐	Able to lean back to rest back	☐

Careful Keyboarding		Lighting	
Keyboard flat or negative tilt	☐	Position desk to avoid reflections	☐
Mouse close to keyboard	☐	Place monitor perpendicular to window	☐
Use as little force as necessary	☐	Focus task light on document	☐
Wrists straight	☐	Task light on non dominant side	☐

Figure 21-10. Seated and standing computer workstation checklist. (Developed by Martha Sanders, 2018.)

- *Lumbar and thoracic support:* The worker's back should be in contact with the backrest and comfortably fit the lumbar curve.
- *Seat pan length:* Seat pan length should support the thighs yet allow workers to fully bend the knees to 90° (chair seat should extend to about 2 inches (~5 cm) behind the knees). Seat edges should be rounded and upholstered.
- *Seat angle:* Seat angle should be 100° to 110° and allow the worker to access the desk, as well as allow movement backward by 5° to relax the spine.
- *Footrest:* Footrests should support the feet if workers are unable to reach the floor. Footrests also promote upright posture in chairs and relieve pressure on thighs and low back.
- *Armrest:* Armrests should barely reach the elbows when flexed at 90°. Perspectives differ with regard to armrest use when typing. Armrests are customarily used when relaxing; however, if used while typing, care should be taken to ensure that posture is upright and the trunk is not flexed forward.

Desk or Surface

- Desk height should be about same as elbow height when flexed to 90° to access keyboards. Chairs must be height adjusted if desks are not adjustable.
- Desk surfaces should have rounded edges or wrist rests.

Keyboard

- Keyboards may be placed close to desk edges or on keyboard trays below desk surfaces.
- Keyboards should be flat or positioned at a negative tilt.
- Keyboard width should be approximately shoulder width to minimize internal rotation of the arms.

Computer Monitor

- Workers should face the monitor directly (and should not rotate the trunk or neck).
- Monitors should be positioned at about arm's length away from the body.
- Monitors should be positioned perpendicular to the window to avoid sun glare.
- Screen tops should be at eye level or slightly lower.
- Laptop stands are needed to attain the correct height of laptop monitors.

Input Device Mouse or Input Device

- Mouses should be positioned close to the keyboard.
- Traditional mouses should fit the transverse arch of hand.
- Various mouse and input device options include vertical mouses (forearm positioned in neutral), handshoe mouses (contours to fingers and thumb), trackballs, touchpads, and styluses.

Laptop computers are heavily used for personal and workplace use but present challenges for optimal setup. When laptop computers are used on desk surfaces, monitors are too low; when laptops are placed on raised surfaces to improve monitor placement, keyboards are too high, causing excessive reach.

Standing Workstations

Standing workstations are common in industrial settings for assembly tasks, warehousing, and manual materials handlings. Standing for long periods without breaks, particularly on hard surfaces, can be associated with leg, low back, and foot pain (such as plantar fasciitis). Work surfaces that are low create the need for excessive neck flexion, as shown in Figure 21-11. Standing workstations must be evaluated to determine the optimal work surface height, reach, clearance, and posture needed for essential tasks. Additional considerations are flooring, the presence of ergonomic mats, rest areas (chairs), and the duration of time spent in standing, walking, and carrying tasks.

Lifting Workstations

Frequent lifting of heavy loads in awkward positions contributes to the development of low back pain. Therapists should determine the safe lifting limits for workers and the workstation factors that promote safe lifting and decrease low back pain risk. The NIOSH Lifting Equation is based on the assumption that a healthy person can lift 51 lb (~23 kg) when an object is located at the ideal height for the person, lifted close to the body, carried a reasonable distance, and possesses good handholds. When workstation design conditions change requiring greater bending and reaching, the load that a worker can safely carry decreases.

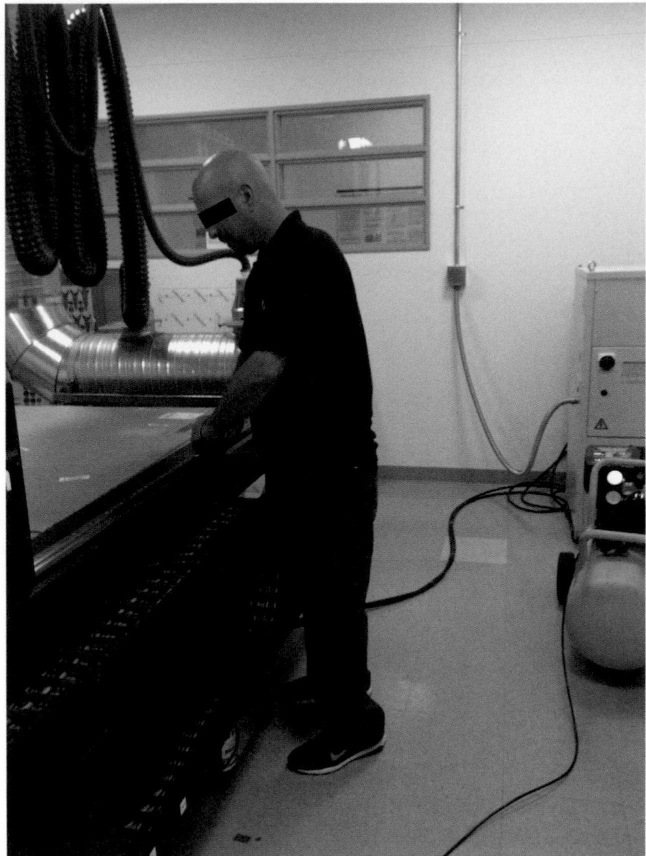

Figure 21-11. Standing workstation. Worker standing at a laser machine. Note flexion of neck and extension of elbows resulting from low height of working surface. Worker would benefit from an ergonomic mat for prolonged standing.

Standardized tests such as the NIOSH Lifting Equation and the Liberty Mutual Tables can be consulted to guide therapists in (a) identifying key variables that impact workers' ability to lift and (b) providing the level or risk in the current workstation.

Lighting

Lighting is most commonly assessed at the location where the task is performed using a light meter. This measure of light, *illuminance*, refers to the light intensity on the surface where work is performed. Additionally, therapists can use a lighting checklist to gather information about the worker's perceived ease in completing tasks based on current lighting conditions.[22]

Noise

Noise-induced hearing loss can occur when workers are exposed to high intensities of noise over 85 to 90 dB. Companies in which workers are exposed to continuous noise are required to determine noise level, provide audiometric testing for workers, and institute a hearing conservation program for workers exposed to 85 dB per day. Noise-related testing is typically performed by occupational safety and health personal according to OSHA standards.[20]

Temperature

Most indoor environments are temperature controlled at 70 to 73 (~21 to 23 Celsius). Extreme considerations such as workers' regular exposure to high heat, humidity, or cold, for example, should be reported. Such temperature extremes may be particularly detrimental for individuals with arthritis or Raynaud phenomenon.[22,23]

Flooring

Floor surfaces are important considerations in workplace fall prevention, ease of moving equipment, and standing workstation comfort. Although therapists may not be involved in the initial floor selection, they can make recommendations for individual workstation safety and comfort. In general, slip-resistance surfaces are recommended, particularly where moisture or wet floors may occur. This type of coating, however, creates increased friction for pushing carts or equipment. Companies must determine flooring based on safety and tasks performed. In general, ergonomic mats are recommended for standing workstations to reduce leg and foot fatigue. All mats and rugs should be secured to the floor to prevent tripping hazards.[21]

Interventions for Work Environments

Workstation design influences a worker's postures, work patterns, workflow, and, ultimately, comfort and productivity throughout the day. Therapists should ensure that workstation layout—including the location of objects, surface heights, and visual displays—is well organized.[21] Therapists must keep in mind that workstation equipment recommendations alone do not ensure clients' appropriate equipment use and adjustment. Therapists must educate workers about proper postures and body mechanics, train them in workstation adjustments, and follow up to ensure that recommended practices are carried out.[23,24]

Workplace Layout

Workspaces should be organized in a logical manner to minimize wasted effort. The location of frequently used items, task sequences, and workflow should all be considered. Personalized items (e.g., family and pet photos) should be placed away from the direct working area. Several key principles, also emphasized in universal design principles, help determine optimal item placement[21]:

- *Importance principle:* Place the most important items in the most easily accessible location.
- *Frequency-of-use principle:* Place the most frequently used items in convenient, close-to-reach locations.
- *Function principle:* Place items with similar functions together (staples, paper clips, scissors).
- *Sequence-of-use principle:* Lay out items in the same sequence in which they are used.

Because workspace is at a premium, only frequently used items should be placed in the worker's reachable distance (Fig. 21-9).

Workstation Design

Workstations should be designed specific to the tasks performed and promote a worker's neutral posture. A neutral posture is a biomechanically advantageous position that allows the body to efficiently use its muscles. A neutral posture is achieved when the head is upright and the neck is slightly flexed, the shoulders are at the sides and flexed less than 20° to 25°, the elbows are flexed to about 90°, and the wrists are in 0° of flexion. Positions that deviate from a neutral posture require more energy to sustain. Workstations should incorporate adjustability to accommodate changes in the tasks performed and other workers occupying the workspace.

In general, work equipment or controls that are regularly used should be located within a worker's "reach envelope." This refers to a semicircular shell in front of workers that allows them to easily access work tasks when the elbows are flexed to 90° and objects are within 14 inches of the body. Items located outside the primary zone should be accessed less frequently. Figure 21-9 illustrates the reach envelope. The worker should not reach above shoulder height or behind the back on a frequent basis.

Seated Workstation Adjustments

Seated work requires little physiological effort and provides stability for precise work. Prolonged sitting, however, increases spinal compression forces and the potential for static loading on the neck and shoulders; careful readjustment is critical for employees assuming seated positions for much of the day.[21] Although some offices or seated workstations have adjustable furniture and equipment, workers may not be familiar with proper computer workstation setup and sometimes use equipment "right out of the box" (e.g., on the lowest chair setting). Many valuable online resources and videos demonstrate proper computer setup.[25] The following are steps to examine worker posture and adjust equipment to promote a neutral posture (Fig. 21-12).

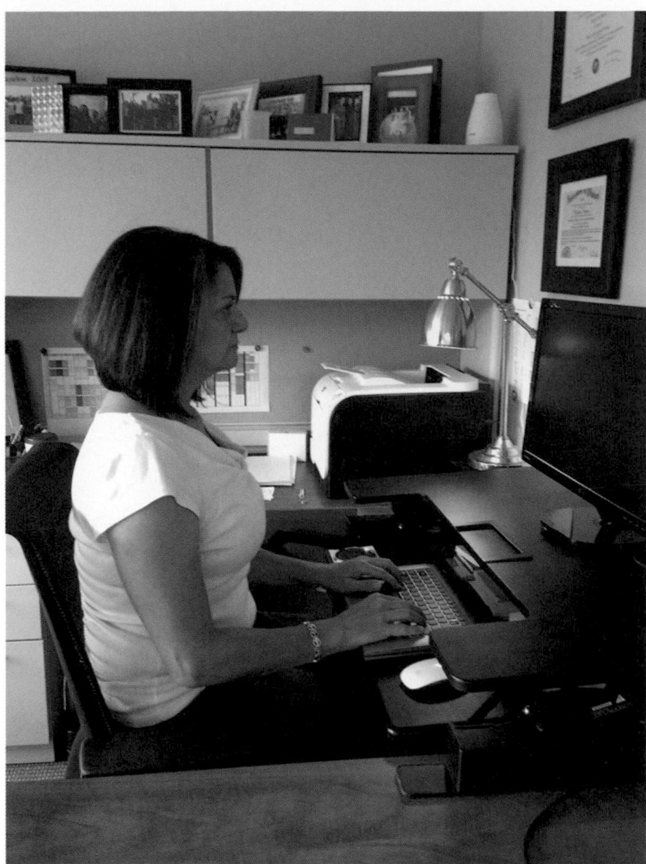

Figure 21-12. Seated workstation.

Computer Workstation Adjustment Process

1. Observe the worker regularly performing work tasks and record each body part's posture in the evaluation process.
2. Position clients in a neutral sitting posture. Align the elbows and wrists with the keyboard so that the fingers can access the middle row with the wrists straight.
3. Move the keyboard to the location for best access.
4. Move the mouse close to the keyboard to minimize reach.
5. Check that the palms are not resting on the hard edges of the computer or desk.
6. Adjust chair height (up if shoulders are flexed when reaching for the keyboard; down if elbows are extended when reaching for the keyboard). Ensure that elbows, wrists, and keyboard are aligned in a neutral wrist position (straight).
7. Adjust chair features. Seat pans should fully support the thighs. Seat pans that are too deep (long) cause users to sit forward and lose contact with the backrest. Seat pans that are too short create increased pressure under the thighs and potential instability. Lower the chair arms if they touch the desk directly. Adjust the lumbar support up or down.
8. Determine the need for a footrest (if person's feet do not touch ground).
9. Ensure that clients face the monitor. Identify head/neck position in relation to the monitor. Adjust the monitor height or determine the need for a laptop stand.

Laptop computers should make use of a laptop stand to raise the monitor height and a peripheral keyboard placed on the desk to ensure that workers are keying without excessive reaching. Therapists should demonstrate several optimal positions that workers should assume throughout the day to promote movement and position change.

Standing Workstation Adjustments

Standing workstations are common in assembly, warehousing, and machining tasks. The same principles exist relative to working in a neutral position of the upper extremity; however, hip and lower extremity posture need to be addressed along with concerns for prolonged standing.

Workers should stand with hips midway between an anterior and posterior pelvic tilt. Foot rails or a low stool can be used for intermittent foot placement both to relieve stress on the low back (as it promotes a neutral pelvis) and to change leg position. Anti-fatigue mats promote small postural changes to stimulate venous pump to the legs and should be placed on hard floor surfaces to minimize leg, feet, and low back discomfort. The following guidelines consider the position of the body during a task to leverage stability or force.[21]

- Precise work requires a higher work surface to provide proximal stabilization (2 to 4 inches [~5-10 cm] above the elbow for drafting work or precise assembly).
- For light assembly work, the work surface can be 2 to 4 inches (~5-10 cm) below the elbow to best utilize upper extremity musculature forces.
- Heavy work requires a lower work surface (about 4-5 inches [~10-25 cm] below the elbow) to leverage body and trunk strength. Heavier work requires a lower work surface to increase available muscle forces.

All work surface edges should be rounded or padded to avoid compression of soft-tissue structures.

Lifting Workstation Adjustments

Modification of lifting workstations can minimize injury risk. Principles rely on the use of mechanical assists and proper heights relative to the worker.[20] Adjustability is key for multiple individuals using the same workstation (Fig. 21-13).

- Use mechanical assists to transfer loads between surfaces.
- Use adjustable surfaces to lift loads at waist height.
- Reduce the size of containers lifted to minimize awkward reaches.
- Design handles, hooks, or handholds to promote firm object grasp.
- Change jobs from pulling to pushing.

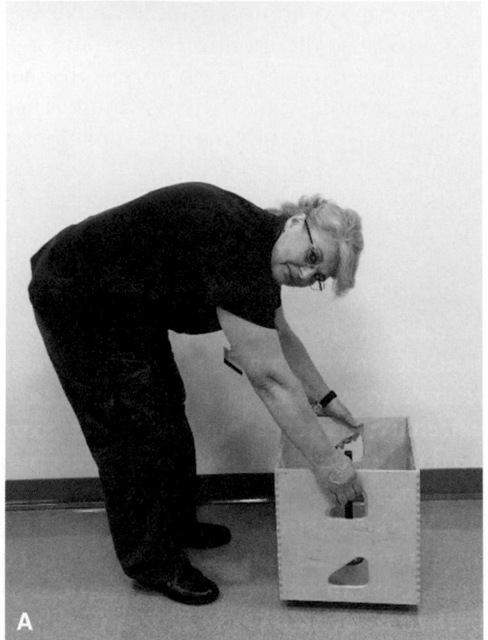

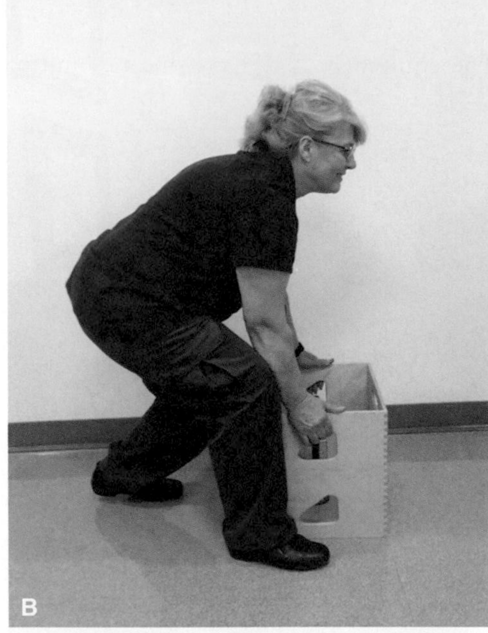

Figure 21-13. Lifting workstation. **A.** Improper lifting with a flexed trunk and load far from body. **B.** Proper straight back and load.

Sit–Stand Workstations and Physical Activity

Sit–stand workstations are increasingly recognized as beneficial in promoting changes in body position for sedentary workers.[26] Sedentary or seated work has been associated with the development of chronic disease, cancers, obesity, and increased mortality.[27] Much effort has been undertaken to promote movement and overall increased activity in the workplace.

Hedge[25,28] promotes a combination of sit–stand–move routines for office workers (sit 20 minutes, stand 8 minutes, move 2 minutes), noting that simply moving from a prolonged sitting to a prolonged standing position is not beneficial. Sit–stand workstations are one way to promote postural changes that may decrease musculoskeletal strain from either position alone (Fig. 21-14). Although training is required for all ergonomic modifications, the use of sit–stand workstations in particular requires education regarding the duration of time for each posture, proper workstation height, and continued importance of movement. Research suggests that sit–stand stations can decrease musculoskeletal discomfort and fatigue and improve mood without jeopardizing productivity. Such gains, however, were not realized in research studies unless ergonomic training accompanied equipment use.[24]

Sit–Stand Options

Numerous options now exist for sit–stand workstations. Decisions about which sit–stand equipment to adopt depend on factors such as space allotment, cost, ease of surface adjustment up or down, and the amount of workspace needed around the keyboard. Ideas for creating sit-and-stand areas or buying dedicated sit–stand equipment are provided as follows:

- Different work areas can be designated for sitting and standing work. Create a separate work area at a desk; then move to another location for standing work.

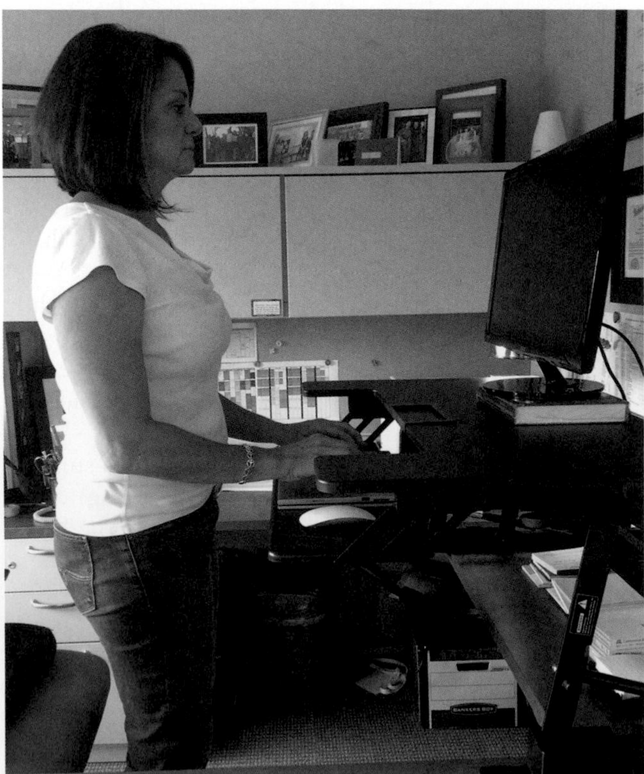

Figure 21-14. Sit–stand workstation.

- Desktop sit–stand equipment. An adjustable surface is placed on top of a desk and manually raised and lowered. The equipment may have one or multiple levels for placement of a monitor and keyboard. Limited work area exists around the keyboard (Fig. 21-14).
- Adjustable desks (crank or electric) allow the entire desk surface to raise to standing or lower to sitting. Ample workspace around the keyboard is available.

Community Environmental Assessment and Modification

Occupational therapists promote environments that enable clients to participate in community roles with the same opportunities and dignity as that of individuals without disabilities. For example, it is not acceptable for wheelchair users to be forced to use freight elevators at the back of buildings, endure safety risks to maneuver sidewalk curbs, or require others to lift them over even a few steps to enter buildings. In order for persons with physical disabilities to fully engage in and feel included in community life, they should experience easy, convenient, and safe access to desired places, services, and programs. ADA legislations and universal design principles are now applied in mainstream design approaches to promote access across most community settings.[29]

Community Environmental Assessment

A number of instruments are available to assess community environments. Some assessments target the person–environment fit and enable clients to identify aspects of the home and community environments that hinder desired occupational participation (e.g., physical characteristics and social attitudes) (see Boxes 21-2 and 21-3). Other community assessments, such as online livability indices, rank environmental areas, services, and amenities that most impact life: housing affordability and access; safe and convenient transportation; neighborhoods that provide access to life, work, and play; environments with clean air and water; access to health services; civic and social involvement opportunities; and inclusiveness and diversity (Box 21-3). Therapists can work with clients to examine communities that best fit their needs as they transition from one life stage to another. Other instruments measure built environmental features associated with physical activity and walking, including architectural, traffic, transportation, and aesthetic features as well as proximity to services and retailers. These features can have a positive impact on the ability of persons with disabilities to access their neighborhood community.

Box 21-2

Descriptions of Home Environmental Assessments

Assessment and Description

Cougar Home Safety Assessment[35]**:** Identifies potential safety issues in residences.

I-HOPE[15]**:** Home assessment for older adults (https://starklab.wustl.edu/i-hope-kit/).

Home Environment Lighting Assessment (HELA)[36]**:** Near-task home lighting assessment for older adults with low vision.

Home Environmental Assessment Protocol (HEAP)[37]**:** Environmental hazards specific to individuals with dementia.

Home Falls and Accidents Screening Tool (HOMEFAST)[38]**:** Preventive health assessment to determine fall risk of older persons in the home.

Home for Life Design, Home Assessment App, and Solution: Mobile platform to conduct home assessments efficiently (www.homeforlifedesign.com).

Housing Enabler[39]**:** Predicts problems arising as a consequence of a client's functional limitations and barriers in the home.

Safety Assessment of Function and the Environment for Rehabilitation Health Outcome Measurement and Evaluation (SAFER-HOME), Version 3[40]**:** Used to evaluate change over time of clients' functional abilities and task completion in the home.

TVO Bathroom Assessment[41]**:** A bathroom assessment of both environmental and functional aspects to promote safety, reduce falls, and encourage aging in place.

Westmead Home Safety Assessment (WeHSA)[42]**:** Identifies and prioritizes home hazards with client input specific to falls in older adults.

Community Environmental Modification

Client-Specific Modifications

The impetus for community environmental modifications can be generated from a specific client's needs or those of an entire community. When therapists serve clients for whom occupational participation is impeded because of community environmental barriers, therapists should work with community stakeholders (e.g., city officials and planners, and business owners) to present a client's case and strategize feasible solutions that benefit not only the

Box 21-3

Descriptions of Community Environmental Assessments

Assessment and Description

Livability Index[43]**:** Ranks seven areas of environment, services, amenities that are important to community life.

Senior Walking Environmental Assessment Tool–Revised (SWEAT-R)[44]**:** Addresses built environment features related to physical activity for older adults.

Neighborhood Walkability Scale (NEWS)[45]**:** Used to assess the perception of neighbor design features by area residents.

Irvine Minnesota Inventory (IMI): Focuses on the built environment related to physical activity, specifically walking, in the community.

client but all community members. Examples may include the incorporation of benches in public areas (e.g., public gardens, malls, museums) for clients who fatigue easily as a result of disease or injury; the availability of ATM machine screen magnification for clients with visual deficits; the provision of simple pictorial instructions for clients with cognitive deficits who use kiosk machines to purchase subway and bus transportation cards; the addition of grocery store aisle signage using food photos for clients with visual or literacy deficits; and the installation of appropriately timed pedestrian walk signals displaying timed, street crossing countdowns for clients with mobility or cognitive impairment. In these instances, therapists can present possible solutions and work with community planners and business owners to strategize implementation.

Population-Based Modifications

Occupational therapists can also serve as consultants for populations or groups desiring community modifications that benefit all members. When considering population-based modifications for communities, therapists will work as a member of a collaborative team with municipal officials, city planners, ADA specialists, business owners, and community members. For example, when working to build a new accessible recreational center and park for a school or town, it is imperative to work with city officials to determine and comply with zoning requirements and budgets. Therapists should seek community residents' input when evaluating how well a community promotes walking, socializing, safety, and intellectual stimulation; identification of barriers, such as inaccessible transportation, should also be made. Once identified, therapists can generate recommendations, based on client and community priorities, to create spaces and plans with local municipalities. Ideally, solutions should benefit all community members through inclusive and universal design concepts. Funding for projects may be secured through grants, fundraising, or other community sources.

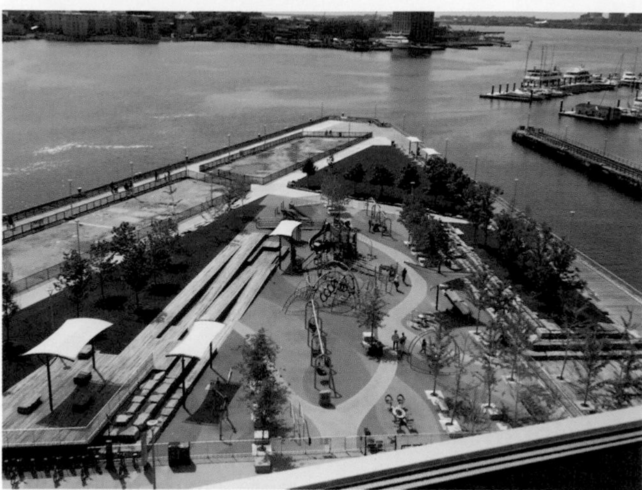

Figure 21-15. Accessible community space with playground. (Reprinted with permission from Amy Wagenfeld.)

In general, paths and surfaces should accommodate a wide range of people, including users of scooters and wheeled mobility devices, parents with strollers, and two people in wheelchairs strolling together or in tandem.[30] Surfaces should be level, and transitions from one level to another should be achieved with ramps, earth berms, and lifts. Options for handrails and seating benefit persons with limited endurance and balance problems. Indoor seating areas should be strategically placed in large walking areas, such as shopping malls, home center stores, supermarkets, schools, and parks. Signage should be simple, contain symbols or illustrations, and have limited printed text to accommodate persons with visual or cognitive impairment, or poor literacy. Lighting should enhance safety, provide clear vision of paths and walkways, be evenly distributed across a space but also minimize glare, and should highlight task-specific activities such as kiosk use (Fig. 21-15).

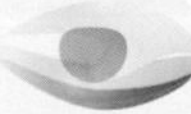

CASE STUDY

Patient Information

Dyani is a 19-year-old Native American female with a recent C-7 complete SCI resulting from a motor vehicle collision. After a short acute care hospitalization and rehabilitation center stay, Dyani was discharged home. The occupational therapist at the rehab center made recommendations for a custom wheelchair; there are plans for a portable ramp to enter the family home and a drop-arm bedside commode. Dyani received training for and is now independent in transfers and ADLs. She plans to continue therapy in the home.

Reason for Occupational Therapy Referral

The family has requested a home assessment for additional recommendations regarding bathroom modifications to increase self-care independence. Dyani's insurance company has agreed to provide homecare assessment and services.

Assessment Process and Results

The therapist met with Dyani and her family to learn about the existing bathroom environment, concerns regarding bathroom use, and plans for ADL routines. Dyani prefers to shower each evening and perform bowel and bladder routines in the morning. The current bathroom has a standard toilet, bath/shower combination, sink, and large closet. The therapist observed Dyani's current bathroom area use and used the TVO Bathroom assessment to document environmental enablers and hindrances in this space (Box 21-4). Although Dyani was taught to safely use a tub bench with supervision while in rehab, she

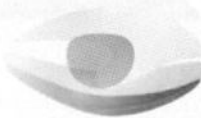

CASE STUDY (continued)

is elated to learn that the bathroom can be modified to allow her to complete ADLs independently and alone.

Occupational Therapy Problem List

- Decreased independence in self-care and basic ADLs
- Difficulty with sink and shower water controls
- Difficulty transferring to the tub bench without assistance from caregivers
- Unable to reach the toilet paper located behind the toilet
- Unable to see herself in the mirror for grooming

Occupational Therapy Goal List

(All within 2 weeks after modifications)

- Dyani will perform toilet hygiene with modified independence and adaptive toilet seat controls.
- Dyani will use a rolling shower seat for transfers in and out of the roll-in shower with modified independence.
- Dyani will perform grooming tasks independently.
- Dyani will independently control water temperature with one-touch lever handles.

Intervention

The family was willing and able to make modifications to the bathroom to allow Dyani to perform self-care and ADLs as independently as possible. The use of a toilet seat bidet with remote facilitated hygiene while seated allowed Dyani the dignity to perform this task without assistance. Partial closet space was used to build a roll-in shower, and with the use of a roll-in shower chair, Dyani was able to bathe on her own. Additional modifications that increased independent bathing were a handheld shower with control, touchless soap/shampoo dispensers, and lever handles to control water temperature at the sink and the shower. Additionally, a roll-under sink, mirror at sink height, and adequate lighting assisted Dyani to perform grooming tasks. A closet portion was maintained for medical supplies and storage.

Once the above modifications were completed, Dyani was seen again by the occupational therapist. The results of the post-TVO assessment showed no further areas to modify. Dyani was able to use the bathroom without assistance to perform self-care and ADLs safety and independently.

Box 21-4

Sample from TVO Bathroom Assessment

Primary Bathroom

ADEQUATE LIGHTING

# of Lights ____________________ Accessibility of Switches: _______Yes _______No

- # of Lights: Identify the number of light fixtures in the bathroom, *not* the number of bulbs
- Accessibility of Switches: Can all users use switch appropriately? Can all users reach light switch?

COMMENTS: If users cannot reach switch, identify the reason why (i.e., height, location of switch). Also note the type of switch (i.e., rocker, flip, knob, motion sensor, dimmer)

SINK/VANITY

Height of Sink: ___________

Height: Measurement should be taken from top surface of sink to floor (~34 inches or 86 cm)

Water Control

Type/Style _________________ Able to manipulate: _______Yes _______No

Water Control: Identify if it is a handle, knob, motion activated

Accessible Mirror: _______ Yes _______No

Accessible Mirror: Is the mirror located at an eye level for all users?

Storage Access ____________________________

Storage: Identify location (i.e., above or below sink).

COMMENTS:

TOILET

**When assessing this area of the bathroom: Ask client to demonstrate ability to properly get on and off toilet. Also ask for client to reach for toilet paper when sitting on the toilet and toilet handle.*

Height ___________

Height: Measure from floor to top of seat (standard height: 17 inches or 43 cm).

Toilet Handle

Able to Manipulate: _______Yes _______No

Toilet Paper Dispenser:

Location ___________ Distance from Toilet ___________

Able to Use: _______Yes _______No

Distance of toilet paper dispenser: Measure from edge of toilet to dispenser.

COMMENTS: Identify client's functional capabilities.

Selected Assessments for Home Environments

Instrument and Reference	Intended Purpose	Administration Time	Validity	Reliability	Sensitivity	Strengths and Weaknesses
The Housing Enabler[39]	Questionnaire to assess the congruence or fit between an individual with a functional impairment and the home environment. Measures functional limitations (15 items) and physical environmental barriers (188 items).	Up to 2 hours depending of functional limitations and physical environment	Content item selection based on literature review and expert option; adjusted after pilot studies	Inter-rater: Studies report excellent results ranging from 81% to 100% agreement; test–retest: interclass correlation (ICC) range—0.92–0.98.	Person–environment fit scores captured significant differences between baseline and follow-up by means of signs and McNemars's tests.	Strengths: Meticulous development and testing. Up-to-date website. Widely used in Europe. Useful for both clinical and research purposes. Weaknesses: Rating training more difficult to arrange outside Europe. Time-consuming to administer.
Home Falls and Accident Screening Tool (HOME FAST)[38]	Health care provider completed questionnaire; designed to identify risk of falls as a result of home hazards; may be used as an outcome measure to evaluate interventions for improving function in the home environment.	20–30 minutes	Content: Based on the literature; field testing with 83 older adults; review of content and field testing data by an expert panel; reduced number of items; content further examined in a cross national validation (Australia, Canada, the United Kingdom) where occupational therapists, physiotherapists, and nurses responded to a survey regarding the content and weighting of items.	Inter-rater: Evaluated ($n = 40$) using k for individual items and weighted k for the total number of hazards; overall weighted k was 0.56 (considered fair-to-good agreement); k values for individual items indicated 4 items had excellent reliability, 20 items had fair-to-good reliability, and 1 item (hazardous outside paths) had poor reliability.	Sensitivity shown by comparison of expert ratings and second ratings of home hazards; 68.6% agreement (95% confidence interval [CI] 63.4-73.6) ($n = 844$ sample ratings)	Strengths: Can be quickly administered as a screening assessment. Research has been conducted in various countries. Initial psychometric research is positive. Initial evidence suggests may be useful as an outcome measure. Weaknesses: Further examination of the predictive validity, responsiveness, and test–retest reliability would strengthen our understanding of the measure.

Safety Assessment of Function and the Environment for Rehabilitation Health Outcome Measurement (SAFER-HOME) Version 3[40]	SAFER-HOME based on SAFER tool: Designed to measure intervention effectiveness and changes in safety intervention over time (12 domains: living situation, mobility, environmental hazards, kitchen, household, eating, personal care, bathroom and toilet, medication, addiction and abuse, leisure, communication and scheduling, and wandering)	45–90 minutes	Content: For both the SAFER and the SAFER-HOME established through review by experts and clinicians as well as statistical analysis of completed measures	Internal consistency: Cronbach's for total scores = 0.8593; subscales ranged from 0.539 to 0.789	No formal studies have directly examined sensitivity to detect change; preliminary investigations show promising results; occupational therapists (n = 95) administered the SAFER-HOME V1 twice; 76% indicated the assessment measured changes in the client.	Strengths: Comprehensive coverage of home safety. Developed and tested rigorously. Comprehensive training manual provided. Weaknesses: Length of administration may be problematic in some clinical situations. Further research on responsiveness to change needed.
Westmead Home Safety Assessment (WeHSA)[42]	Assessment to identify fall hazards in the home environments of older adults	One home visit	Content: Established through content analysis of the literature and a rigorous expert review process	Inter-rater: Tested in a sample of 21 clients' homes; c values of >0.75 for 34 items and between 0.4 and 0.75 for 31 items; k could not be calculated for some items.	Not established	Strengths: Comprehensive and systematic assessment of home hazards specific to falls in older adults. Manual is helpful and provides operational definitions for key hazards. Weaknesses: Does not address home hazards besides falls. Further psychometric testing required.
Work Environment Impact Scale (WEIS)[46]	Worker capacities and perceptions A worker's perception of impact of work environment on performance, satisfaction, and physical, social, and emotional well-being	30 minutes	Content validity good to moderately good; internal consistency satisfactory (0.72)	Test–retest good-to-moderate at 0.35–0.78 (median 0.61)	Discriminates levels of work environment among subjects; targets impact of environment on users	Strengths: Short administration time, moderate-to-good validity, and reliability Weaknesses: Scores based on observation; not norm-referenced; costs to purchase

Evidence Table of Intervention Studies for Home Environmental Modifications

Intervention	Description	Participants	Dosage	Research Design and Evidence Level	Benefit	Statistical Significance and Effect Size
Home modification by an occupational therapist[31]	Steps to living environment modifications: (1) comprehensive assessment (interRAI HC instrument), (2) identify the needs and wishes of clients, (3) home visits to provide counseling and plan the modifications, (4) after modifications occupational therapist teach clients how to correctly use the new materials	All participants were at least 65 years old and frail. Frailty was assessed by the Edmonton Frailty Scale.	From four to five visits	Quasi-experimental design Comparison between three groups of intervention (home modifications by occupational therapist; home modifications by occupational therapist with a case management component; other interventions without home modifications) and a control group Level II	Home modifications by an occupational therapist showed a significant reduction of falls at 6 months combined or not with a case management component (the sample consisted of 1,565 people).	Clients receiving home modifications by an occupational therapist had a lower chance of falling in the next 6 months (odds ratio [OR] = 0.46). Similar results for interventions combining case management and home modifications (OR = 0.39). No impact from projects providing other types of interventions than home modification (OR = 1.20).
Comparison of environmental assessment and modification provided by an occupational therapist vs. an unqualified trained assessor[32]	Westmead Home Safety Assessment and strategies to address hazards	Community-dwelling adults aged 70 years and older with a recent history of falls (controls $n = 78$; occupational therapist assessor, $n = 87$; trained assessor $n = 73$)	1.5- to 2-hour home assessment and two follow-up phone calls	Randomized controlled trial Level I	Participants in the group had significantly fewer falls at 12-month follow-up; no change in fall rate for those in trained assessor group (controls).	Occupational therapist group: Incident rate ratio (IRR) = 0.54; confidence interval (CI) = 0.36–0.83, $p = 0.005$ Trained assessor group: IRR = 0.78; CI = 0.51–1.12; $p = 0.34$

Ergonomic prevention programs to improve positioning and workstation design for microscope workers[23]	Two intervention groups: One group education-only (handouts, information); second group education + training (slide presentation, handouts, discussion), and onsite adjustment of workstation	Fifty-one laboratory workers randomized into three groups: education-only = 16; education and training = 24; control group = 11.	Education + training delivered as a 1-hour slideshow presentation and handouts followed by onsite workstation adjustment for 15 minutes	Three groups, randomized, control group Level I	Workers showed improved position, workstation design, and work behaviors following intervention as measured by the Laboratory Assessment Checklist.	Education-only ($p = 0.002$) and education + training ($p = 0.000$) showed significantly improved scores as compared to control group. Education + training showed stronger gain than education-only group. Within-group effect size: Control group—0.71; Education-only group—1.02; education-training group—2.09.
Computer ergonomics program to improve postural comfort in university workers using computers[33]	Ergonomics interview, group ergonomics educational session, and individual consult in workers' offices	Healthy university employees (25); females = 22, males = 3	Intervention delivered in one session: 15 minutes intake, 45 minutes educational session, 15 minutes onsite consult; postural discomfort scale (1–10) completed each week for 6 weeks.	Single subject Level 4	Improvements in workstation adjustment and decreased discomfort	Highest discomfort levels reported in the neck (14/25 reported pain above 5); 21 (84%) of 25 participants reported less discomfort on discomfort rating scale. Most common area of adjustment was the chair.

References

1. Siebert C, Smallfield S, Stark S. *Occupational Therapy Practice Guidelines: Home Modification*. Bethesda, MD: AOTA Press; 2014.
2. American National Standards Institute. *ICC A117.1-2009, Standard and Commentary: Accessible and Usable Building and Facilities: Code and Commentary*. Washington, DC: International Code Council; 2009.
3. United States Department of Housing and Urban Development. History of fair housing. https://www.hud.gov/program_offices/fair_housing_equal_opp/aboutfheo/history.
4. Americans with Disabilities Act of 1990. Pub. L. No. 101-336, 42 U.S.C. § 12101. 1990.
5. ADA Amendments Act of 2008. Pub. L. No. 110-325. 2008. http://www.ada.gov/pubs/ada.htm. Accessed June 14, 2018.
6. United Stated Department of Justice Civil Rights Division. Information and Technical Assistance on the Americans with Disability Act. ADA standards for accessible design. https://www.ada.gov/2010ADAstandards_index.htm. Published 2004. Accessed June 15, 2018.
7. United States Access Board. ADA and ABA accessibility guidelines. https://www.access-board.gov/guidelines-and-standards/buildings-and-sites/about-the-ada-standards/.
8. North Carolina State University Center for Universal Design. Definitions: accessible, adaptable, and universal design. https://projects.ncsu.edu/design/cud/pubs_p/docs/Fact%20Sheet%206.pdf.
9. Pheasant S, Haselgrave C. *Bodyspace: Anthropometry, Ergonomics and the Design of Work*. 3rd ed. London, England: Taylor & Francis; 2007.
10. Pighills AC, Ballinger C, Pickering R, Chari S. A critical review of the effectiveness of environmental assessment and modification in the prevention of falls amongst community dwelling older people. *Br J Occup Ther*. 2015;79(3):133–143.
11. American Association of Retired Persons. These four walls...Americans 45+ talk about home and community. https://assets.aarp.org/rgcenter/il/four_walls.pdf. Published 2003. Accessed June 14, 2018.
12. Kochera A, Straight A, Guterbock T. Beyond 50.05. A report to the nation on livable communities: creating environments for successful aging. http://assets.aarp.org/rgcenter/il/beyond_50_communities.pdf. Published 2006. Accessed June 17, 2018.
13. Young D, Van Oss T, Wagenfeld A. Universal design for a lifetime: interprofessional collaboration and the role of occupational therapy in environmental modifications. *OT Pract*. 2014;19(13):CE1–CE8.
14. Maisel J, Smith E, Steinfeld E. *Increasing Home Access: Designing for Visitability*. Washington, DC: AARP Public Policy Institute; 2008.
15. Stark SL, Somerville EK, Morris JC. In home occupational performance evaluation (I-HOPE). *Am J Occup Ther*. 2010;64(4):580–589.
16. Velligan DI, Diamond P, Mueller J, et al. The short-term impact of generic versus individualized environmental supports on functional outcome sand target behaviors in schizophrenia. *Psychiatry Res*. 2009;168:94–101.
17. Illuminating Engineering Society of North America. *The Lighting Handbook*. 10th ed. New York, NY: Illuminating Engineering Society of North America; 2011.
18. Illuminating Engineering Society. *Lighting the Visual Environment for Seniors and the Low Vision Population. ANSI/IES RP-28-16*. New York, NY: Illuminating Engineering Society of North America; 2016.
19. Georgia Institute of Technology. What is assistive technology. http://www.gatfl.org/assistive.php. Accessed June 15, 2018.
20. Bridger RS. *Introduction to Ergonomics*. 3rd ed. Boca Raton, FL: CRC Press; 2009.
21. Kroemer KHE, Grandjean E. *Fitting the Task to the Human: A Textbook of Occupational Ergonomics*. 6th ed. Boca Raton, FL: CRC Press; 2009.
22. Canadian Centre for Occupational Health and Safety. Lighting ergonomics—Checklist. https://www.ccohs.ca/oshanswers/ergonomics/lighting_checklist.html. Published 2018. Accessed June 15, 2018.
23. Darragh AR, Harrison H, Kenny S. Effect of an ergonomics intervention on workstations of microscope workers. *Am J Occup Ther*. 2008;62:61–69.
24. Robertson M, Ciriello V, Garabet A. Office ergonomics training and a sit-stand workstation: effects on musculoskeletal and visual symptoms and performance of office workers. *Appl Ergon*. 2013;44:73–85.
25. Hedge A. Sit-stand working programs. http://ergo.human.cornell.edu/CUESitStandPrograms.html. Published 2016. Accessed June 14, 2018.
26. Karol S, Robertson M. Implications of sit-stand and active workstations to counteract the adverse effects of sedentary work: a comprehensive review. *Work*. 2015;52:255–267.
27. Biwas A, Oh PI, Faulkner GE, et al. Sedentary time and its association with risk for disease incidence, mortality, and hospitalization in adults: a systematic review and meta-analysis. *Ann Intern Med*. 2015;162(2):123–132.
28. Hedge A. *Ergonomic Workplace Design for Health, Wellness and Productivity*. Boca Raton, FL: CRC Press; 2016.
29. Ostroff E. Universal design: the new paradigm. In: Preiser WFE, Ostroff E, eds. *Universal Design Handbook*. New York, NY: McGraw-Hill; 2001.
30. Witterbottom D, Wagenfeld A. *Design for Healing Spaces Therapeutic Gardens*. Portland, WA: Timber Press; 2015.
31. Maggi P, de Almeida Mello J, Delye S, et al. Fall determinants and home modifications by occupational therapists to prevent falls. *Can J Occup Ther*. 2018;85(1):79–87. doi:10.1177/0008417417714284.
32. Pighills AC, Torgerson DJ, Sheldon TA, Drummond AE, Bland JM. Environmental assessment and modifications to prevent falls in older people. *J Am Geriatr Soc*. 2011;59:26–33.
33. Lindstrom-Hazel D. A single-subject design of ergonomic intervention effectiveness for university employees in a new facility. *Work*. 2008;31:83–93.
34. Center for Disease Control, National Institute of Occupational Safety and Health. *Elements of ergonomic programs: A Primer Based on Workplace Evaluations of Musculoskeletal Disorders*. Cincinnati, OH: NIOSH; 1997:102. Publication No. 97-117.
35. Fisher GS, Ewonishon K. *Cougar Home Safety Assessment. Version 4.0*. Dallas, PA: Misericordia University; 2006. http://www.misericordia.edu/uploaded/documents/academics/ot/ot_research/home_safety/ot_finalcougar07.pdf. Accessed June 14, 2018.
36. Perlmutter MS, Bhorade A, Gordon M, Hollingsworth H, Engsberg JE, Baum MC. Home lighting assessment for

clients with low vision. *Am J Occup Ther*. 2013;67:674–682. doi:10.5014/ajot.2013.006692.

37. Gitlin LN, Schinfeld S, Winter L, Corcoran M, Boyce AA, Hauck W. Evaluating home environments of persons with dementia: interrater reliability and validity of the Home Environmental Assessment Protocol (HEAP). *Disabil Rehabil*. 2002;24(1–3):59–71.
38. Mackenzie L, Byles J, Higginbotham N. Reliability of the home falls and accidents screening tool (HOME FAST) for identifying older people at increased risk of falls. *Disabil Rehabil*. 2002;24(5):266–274.
39. Iwarsson S, Slaug B. *The Housing Enabler: An Instrument for Assessing and Analysing Accessibility Problems in Housing*. Nävlinge, Sweden: Veten & Skapen HB and Slaug Data Management; 2001.
40. Chiu T, Oliver R, Ascott P, et al. *Safety Assessment of Function and the Environment for Rehabilitation Health Outcome Measurement and Evaluation (SAFER–HOME). Version 3*. Toronto, Ontario, Canada: COTA Health; 2006.
41. Van Oss T, Rivers M, Heighton B, Macri C, Reid B. Bathroom safety: environmental modifications to enhance bathing and aging in place in the elderly. *OT Pract*. 2012;17(16):14–16, 19.
42. Clemson L, Fitzgerald MH, Heard R. Content validity of an assessment tool to identify home fall hazards: the Westmead Home Safety Assessment. *Br J Occup Ther*. 1999;62(4):171–179.
43. AARP. AARP livability index. https://livabilityindex.aarp.org/. Published 2015. Accessed June 15, 2018.
44. Michael Y, Keast E, Chaudhury H, Day K, Mahmood A, Sarte AF. Revising the senior walking environmental assessment tool. *Prev Med*. 2009;48:247–249.
45. Saelens BE, Sallis JF, Black JB, Chen D. Neighborhood-based differences in physical activity: an environment scale evaluation. *Am J Public Health*. 2003;93(9):1552–1558.
46. Wastberg BA, Haglund B, Eklunda M. The work environment impact scale—self-rating (WEIS-SR) evaluated in primary health care in Sweden. *Work*. 2012;42:447–457. doi:10.3233/WOR-2012-1418.

Chapter 22

Upper Extremity Orthoses

Nancy S. Hock and Lori DeMott

LEARNING OBJECTIVES

This chapter will allow the reader to:

1. Define and discuss key concepts and terms related to orthoses.
2. Identify major purposes for using orthoses.
3. Explain general precautions relative to the use of orthoses.
4. Identify key factors to consider when selecting the most appropriate orthosis.
5. Given a photograph or illustration, identify the orthosis and a clinical problem for which it may be used.
6. Select an appropriate orthosis for a given diagnosis based on a specific clinical need.
7. Identify additional methods of support for the upper extremity.

CHAPTER OUTLINE

TERMINOLOGY

Arm sling: a fabric orthosis that supports the proximal upper extremity to restrict motion, reduce pain, or prevent or reduce shoulder subluxation.

Arm trough: an upper extremity positioning device that supports the lower arm and is attached to a wheelchair armrest.

Dynamic orthosis: a device that applies a mobile force using rubber bands or springs; primarily used to regain joint mobility or facilitate function.

Lapboard: a portable tabletop that is applied to a wheelchair to provide a working surface or support one or both upper extremities; also known as a lap tray.

Mobile arm support (MAS): a device that supports and facilitates arm movement by compensating for gravitational forces and may be used for remediation in clinical intervention or compensation during occupations such as self-feeding; also known as a dynamic arm support.

Orthosis: any externally applied device added to a person's body to support, align, position, immobilize, prevent or correct deformities, assist weak muscles, allow tissue proliferation and remodeling, or improve function.

Serial casting: applying casts at routine intervals as range of motion improves, with the goal of restoring joint mobility or increasing soft-tissue length.

Serial static orthosis: remolding or fabricating new static orthoses as range of motion improves, with the goal of restoring joint mobility or increasing soft-tissue length.

Static orthosis: a device that has no moving parts; primarily used to support, stabilize, protect, or immobilize.

Static progressive orthosis: orthosis that uses nondynamic forces to elongate soft tissue to decrease contractures through the application of incrementally adjusted static force to promote lengthening of contracted tissues.

Introduction

Orthoses are often an integral component of occupational therapy for patients with physical dysfunction. Orthotics entails prescription, selection, design, fabrication, testing, and training in the use of these special devices.

Successful use of an orthosis is made possible only through an integrated team approach including the patient, his or her significant others, and health care providers. Several rehabilitation professionals may bring their expertise to different aspects of the orthotic process. The physician typically prescribes the device. The certified orthotist is an expert in the design and fabrication of high-temperature thermoplastic orthoses, especially complicated spinal, lower extremity, and upper extremity orthoses used to restore function. The rehabilitation engineer is an expert in technical problem-solving involving mechanical and/or electrical solutions to unique needs of patients.

The occupational therapist, as an expert in adapting the upper extremities for use in occupational performance tasks, has the major responsibility for the recommendation of appropriate orthoses, the design and fabrication of custom thermoplastic orthoses, and the testing and training in the use of orthoses. Occupational therapists often collaborate with orthotists and rehabilitation engineers to solve problems encountered by patients in performing their occupations and activities of daily life. The therapist presents the parameters of the problem to these professionals in terms of the patient's abilities and limitations and the functional and psychological goals that the prescribed device should meet or allow. The orthotist or engineer then proposes technical solutions, and together they apply them to the patient and evaluate the outcome.

Finally, and possibly most importantly, the patient and caregivers bring key physical, psychological, social, and functional characteristics to the orthotic process and should be considered the primary members of the team. For the orthosis to be successful, all team members must work in close collaboration.

Classification of Orthoses

The numerous kinds of upper extremity orthoses vary according to the body parts they include, their mechanical properties, and whether they are custom-made, custom-fit, or prefabricated.

According to the Centers for Medicare and Medicaid, an **orthosis** is an externally applied device used to support a weak upper extremity, or to restrict or eliminate motion. The term splint refers to casts or strapping for reduction of fractures or dislocations.[1] Historically, the term splint has been used to describe what we now call an orthosis. This can be confusing for students and novice therapists, as well as referral sources and payers. The term splint should not be used by therapists when describing or documenting the fabrication or recommendation of an orthosis. A therapist can incorporate an orthosis into a patient's treatment plan without a prescription, but in order to obtain reimbursement, a prescription from a physician is required, or a certificate of medical necessity must be signed by a physician.

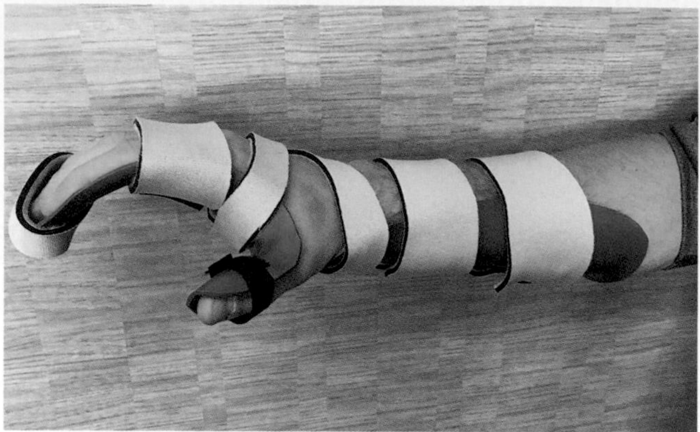

Figure 22-1. Custom-fabricated static forearm-based resting hand orthosis with wrist in slight extension, thumb palmarly abducted, and metacarpal and interphalangeal joints in slight flexion.

Basic Types of Orthoses

Orthosis fall into four categories: static, serial static, static progressive, and dynamic. The **static orthosis** (Fig. 22-1), which has no moving parts, is used primarily to provide support, stabilization, protection, or immobilization. Static orthoses can either be prefabricated (Fig. 22-2) or custom fabricated. **Serial static orthoses** can be used to lengthen tissues and regain passive range of motion (ROM) by placing tissues in an elongated position for prolonged periods.[2,3] With this process, orthoses are remolded as tissue remodeling occurs,

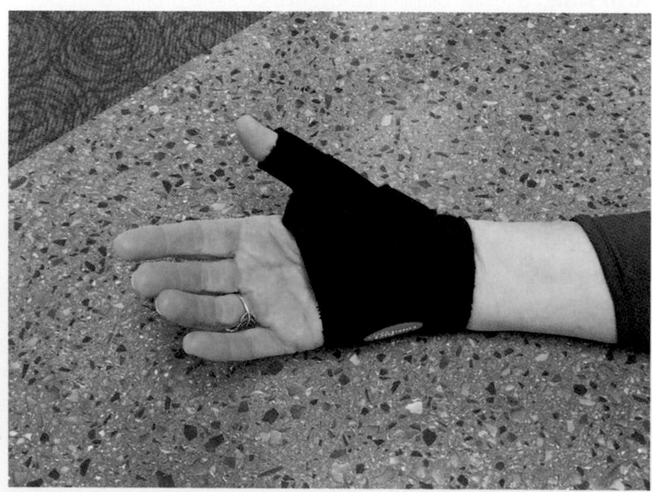

Figure 22-2. Prefabricated neoprene hand-based thumb support.

and ROM increases. Serial static orthoses are typically custom fabricated. Because immobilization causes such unwanted effects as atrophy and stiffness, a static orthosis should never be used longer than physiologically required and should never unnecessarily include joints other than those being treated. The benefits of orthosis use must outweigh the problems associated with its use.

Static progressive orthoses use nondynamic components, such as Velcro, hinges, screws, or turnbuckles, to create a mobilizing force to regain motion. This type of orthosis, termed inelastic mobilization, offers benefits not available with serial static or dynamic orthosis use, because the same orthosis can be used without remolding, and adjustments can be made more easily as motion improves.[4] Static progressive orthoses can either be custom fabricated or prefabricated.

Dynamic orthoses use moving parts to permit, control, or restore movement. They are primarily used to apply an intermittent, gentle force with the goal of lengthening tissues to restore passive motion. Forces may be generated by springs, rubber bands, or elastic cords. This type of orthosis use is termed elastic mobilization.[4] Dynamic orthoses can be either custom fabricated or prefabricated.

When using a dynamic, serial static, or static progressive orthosis to increase ROM to address soft-tissue contracture, two concepts are critical. The first is that the force must be gentle and applied over a long time.[4,5] Safe force must be determined based on tissue tolerances, which will vary between patients. Providing excessive force can result in an undesirable inflammatory response, which could lead to tissue damage or microtrauma.[6]

The second concept is that, to be effective and prevent skin problems, the line of pull must be at a 90° angle to the segment being mobilized.[7] To ensure this, forces are directed by an outrigger, a structure extending outward from the orthosis. Violating this principle could result in either distal or proximal migration of components of the orthosis, which would limit gains in passive ROM.

Outriggers may be high profile or low profile (Fig. 22-3). Each design has distinct advantages and disadvantages. Selection of outrigger design must be based on the specific patient's needs and abilities. High-profile outriggers are inherently more stable and mechanically efficient, require fewer adjustments to maintain a 90° angle of pull, and require less effort for the patient to move against the dynamic force. Low-profile outriggers are less bulky but require more frequent adjustments and greater strength to move against the dynamic force.[4,7]

When deciding between using a serial static, dynamic, or static progressive orthosis to improve passive joint motion or to increase tissue length through tissue remodeling, therapists must consider the current stage of healing to provide the appropriate amount of tension. Figure 22-4 demonstrates the appropriate type of orthosis recommended across the continuum of healing.[4,8]

In addition to functioning as a mobilization orthosis, dynamic orthoses can also be used to assist weak or paralyzed muscles. These dynamic orthoses may be intrinsically powered by another body part or by electrical stimulation of the patient's muscles and typically support the patient's return to functional use of the upper quadrant.

Orthosis Terminology

One challenge when discussing orthoses is the lack of uniform terminology in the medical literature, which makes it difficult to compare and contrast features and outcomes when a single orthosis may be known by many names. There are names of orthoses that are sometimes misunderstood by referring physicians and therapists, such as wrist cock-up, resting hand, and finger gutter. There is an international coding system (ICS) that is currently used for reimbursement.[9] Descriptions are based on body parts that the orthosis crosses. For example, a forearm-based resting hand orthosis would instead be called a Wrist Hand Finger Orthosis (WHFO). A Healthcare Common Procedural Coding System (HCPCS) is used to code orthoses using L codes. For example, a Hand Finger Orthosis (HFO) would be coded using L3913 for reimbursement.[9] These codes identify the correct reimbursement, but do not inform the payer the purpose of the custom orthosis.

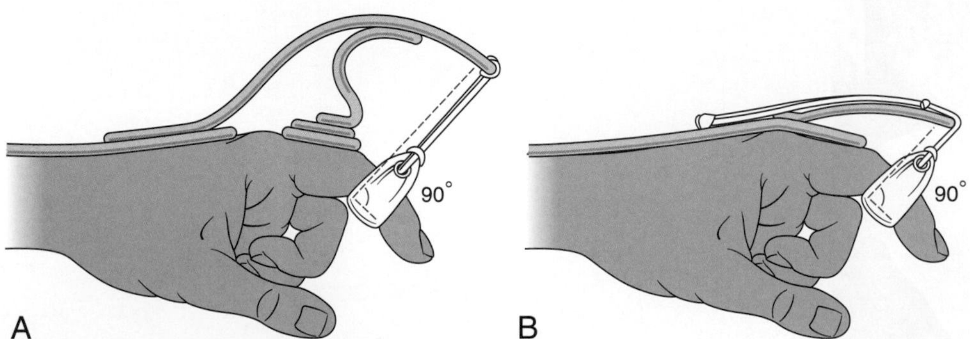

Figure 22-3. Outriggers directing proper 90° line of pull. **A.** High profile. **B.** Low profile. (Adapted with permission from Hunter JM, Mackin EJ, & Callahan AD, eds. *Rehabilitation of the Hand: Surgery and Therapy*. 4th ed. St Louis, MO: Mosby; 1995.)

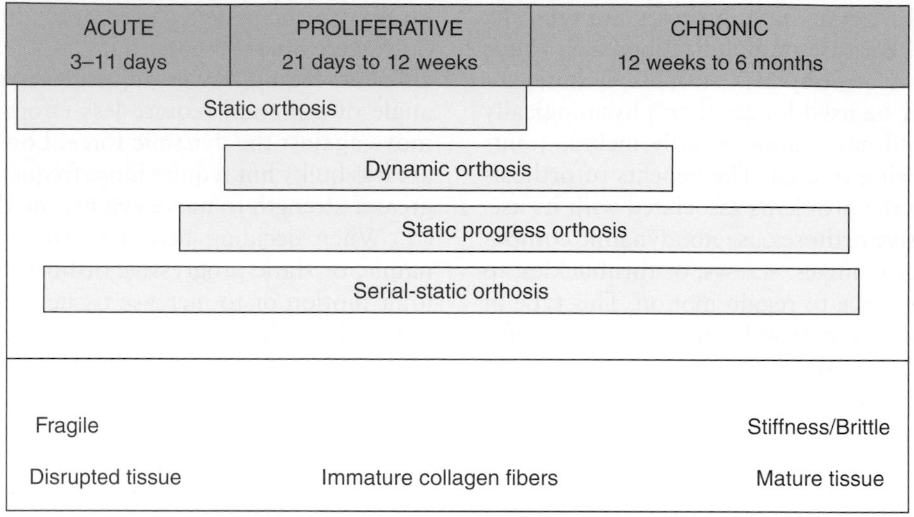

Figure 22-4. Mobilization orthosis based on the stage of healing.(From Fess EE, Gettle KS, Phillips CA, Janson JR. *Hand and Upper Extremity Splinting: Principles and Methods*. 3rd ed. St Louis, MO: Mosby; 2005; Glasgow C, Tooth LR, Fleming J, Peters S. Dynamic splinting for the stiff hand after trauma: predictors of contracture resolution. *J Hand Ther*. 2011;24(3):195–206. doi:10.1016/j.jht.2011.03.001.)

To simplify, organize, and describe a standardized professional nomenclature, the American Society of Hand Therapists (ASHT) developed the Expanded Splint/Orthosis Classification System (ESCS). It classifies orthoses based on the following six criteria:

1. Articular/nonarticular
2. Anatomic focus
3. Kinematic direction
4. Purpose
5. Number of secondary joints included
6. Number of joints included.[7]

According to this system, a wrist cock-up orthosis is a wrist extension immobilization, type 0, because no other joints are affected. Although the intent was to serve as a universal language for referral, reimbursement, communication, and research, the system has not been widely used outside the hand therapy community. Table 22-1 provides descriptions of the common term for orthoses used in clinical discussions, the ICS, and also the ESCS.

Orthosis Selection

Orthosis provision is a beneficial intervention strategy available to therapists when used correctly and appropriately. The end goal of orthosis use should always relate

Table 22-1 Orthoses Terminology

COMMON CLINICAL TERMINOLOGY	INTERNATIONAL CODING SYSTEM[10]	ASHT SCIENTIFIC CLASSIFICATION ECSC[4]
Wrist control orthosis	(WHO) Wrist hand immobilization orthosis (wrist 20° extension)	Wrist extension mobilization; type 0 [1]

Table 22-1 Orthoses Terminology (*continued*)

COMMON CLINICAL TERMINOLOGY	INTERNATIONAL CODING SYSTEM[10]	ASHT SCIENTIFIC CLASSIFICATION ECSC[4]
Ulnar gutter orthosis 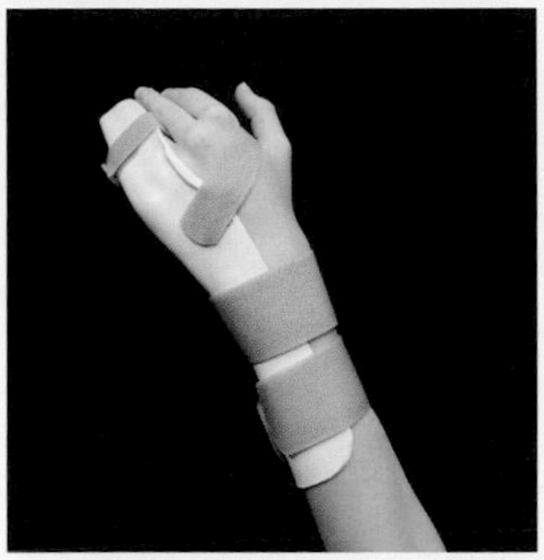	(WHFO) Wrist hand finger immobilization orthosis (wrist 30° extension, RF-SF MP joint 60° flexion, RF-SF IP joint full extension)	Wrist extension immobilization; type 1 [5]
Dorsal blocking orthosis 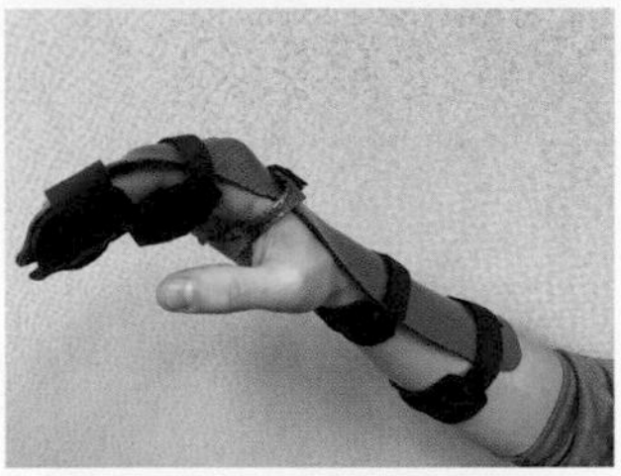	(WHFO) Wrist hand finger dorsal blocking orthosis (wrist 30° flexion, MP joint 70° flexion, IF-SF IP joint full extension)	IF-SF extension restriction orthosis, type 1 [13]
Long opponens orthosis 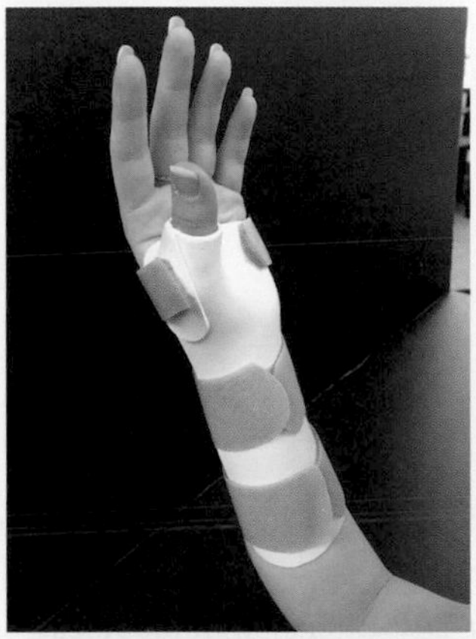	(WHFO) Wrist hand finger orthosis: thumb immobilization (wrist 30° extension, thumb CMC joint palmar ABD, MP joint 20° flexion, IP joint free)	Wrist radial deviation immobilization; type 2 [3]
Short opponens 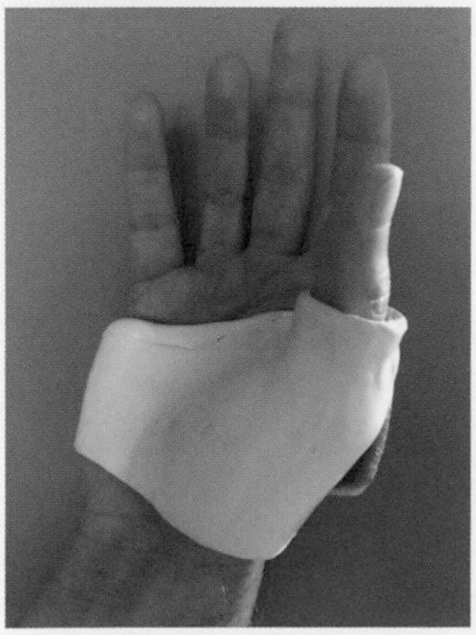	(HFO) Hand finger orthosis (thumb CMC joint 30° flexion and palmar ABD, MP joint 10° flexion)	Thumb CMC joint abduction immobilization; type 1 [2]

(*continued*)

Table 22-1 Orthoses Terminology (*continued*)

COMMON CLINICAL TERMINOLOGY	INTERNATIONAL CODING SYSTEM[10]	ASHT SCIENTIFIC CLASSIFICATION ECSC[4]
Clam shell 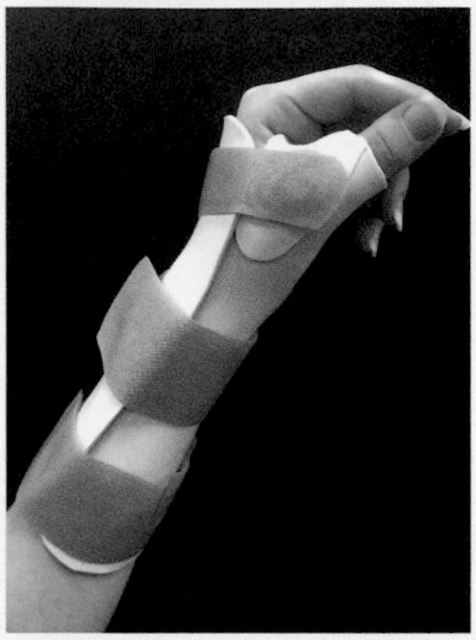	(WHFO) Wrist hand finger orthosis: circumferential (wrist 30° extension, thumb palmarly abducted)	Wrist extension mobilization; type 0 [1]
Yoke orthosis 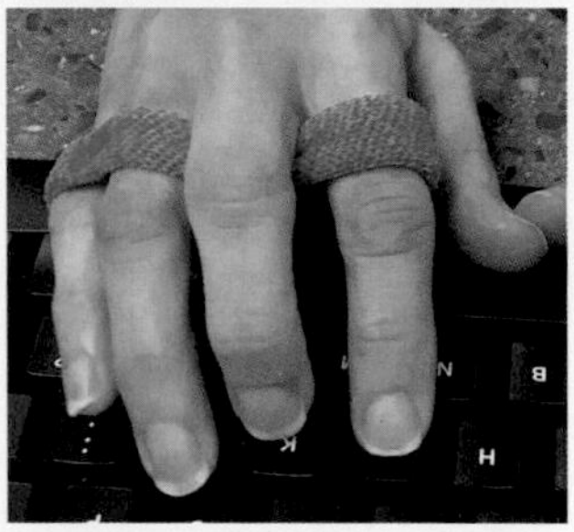	(FO) Finger orthosis: limits MF flexion	MF metacarpal joint extension transmission; type 1 [3]
Sugar tong 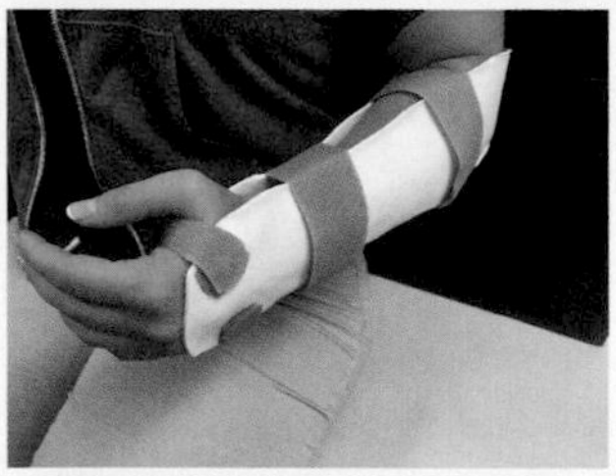	(EWHO) Elbow wrist hand orthosis: distal radioulnar joint immobilization orthosis (forearm neutral and wrist 30° extension)	Wrist neutral immobilization; type 1 [2]
Mallet finger orthosis 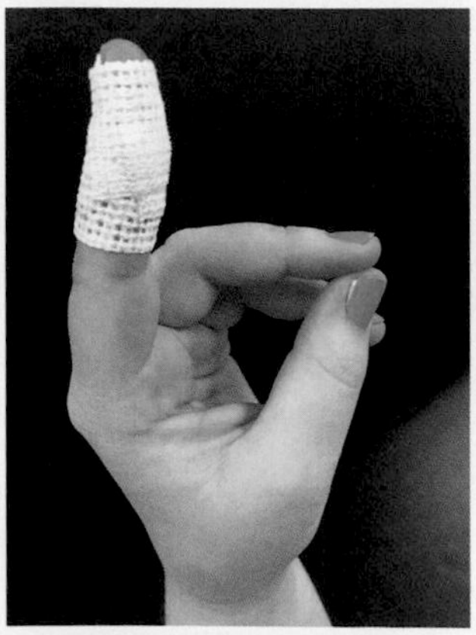	(FO) Finger orthosis: DIP joint immobilization	Index finger DIP extension immobilization; type 0 [1]

Table 22-1 Orthoses Terminology (*continued*)

COMMON CLINICAL TERMINOLOGY	INTERNATIONAL CODING SYSTEM[10]	ASHT SCIENTIFIC CLASSIFICATION ECSC[4]
Long arm orthosis	(EO) Elbow orthosis (elbow −60° extension)	Elbow flexion immobilization; type 0 [1]
Finger gutter orthosis	PIP/DIP joint extension immobilization (FO) Finger orthosis (0° extension)	Middle finger pip joint extension immobilization; type 1 [0]

Examples are inclusive, not exclusive.
ABD, abduction; CMC, carpal metacarpal; DIP, distal interphalangeal; IF, index finger; IP, interphalangeal joint; MF, middle finger; MP, metacarpal; PIP, proximal interphalangeal; RF, ring finger; SF, small finger.

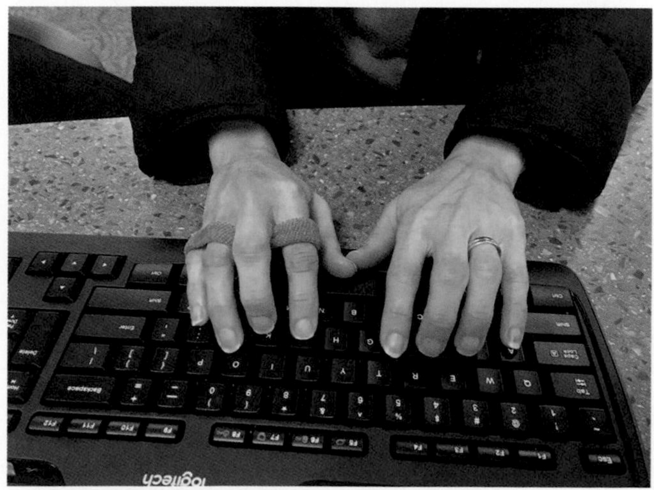

Figure 22-5. Yoke orthosis to limit middle finger metacarpal flexion to allow return to computer use.

to the patient's return to function (Figs. 22-5 to 22-7). The diagnosis of the patient directs the purpose of the orthosis—whether to immobilize, lengthen soft tissue, or substitute for nerve loss. The therapists must consider not only the anatomic and physiological needs for proper orthosis design but also a holistic approach when determining the correct orthosis to also promote function.[11] Additionally, the orthosis must also provide aesthetic appeal and comfort.[12] Otherwise, the orthosis may be recommended and fabricated, but the patient may choose to not use it. Therefore, the therapist must think critically and often creatively with careful consideration of each patient's unique physical and psychosocial needs, as well as personal factors and contexts.[11,13]

The therapist's multifaceted role is to evaluate the need for an orthosis clinically and functionally; to select the most appropriate orthosis (custom fabricated

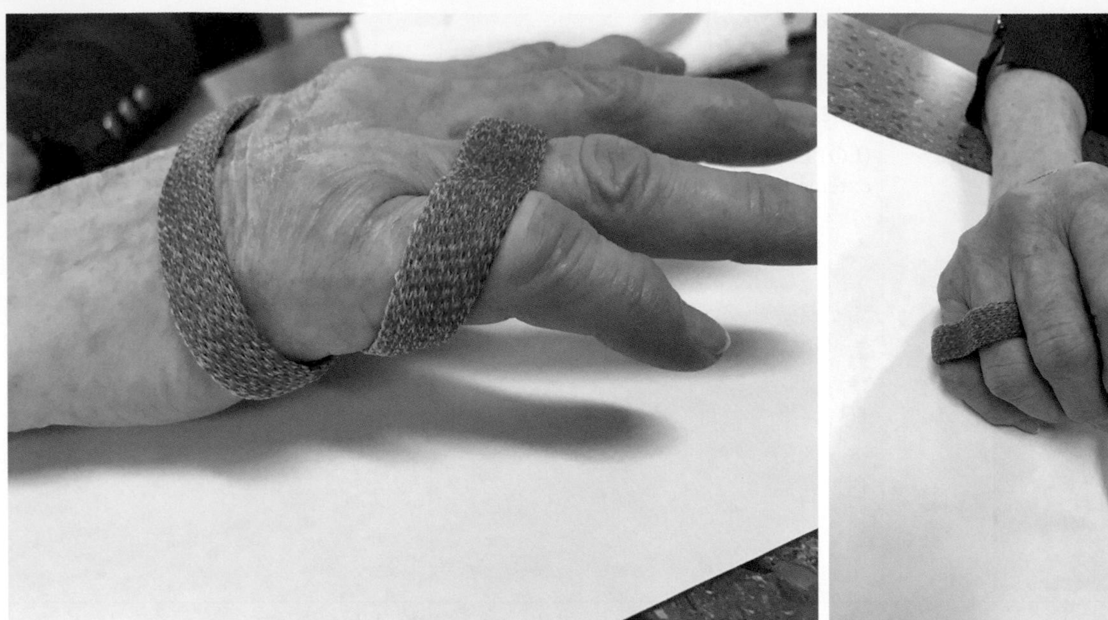

Figure 22-6. Anticlaw orthosis to allow return to writing.

or prefabricated); to provide or fabricate the orthosis; to assess the fit of the orthosis; to teach the patient and caregivers the purpose, care, and use of the orthosis; and to provide related training as needed. The therapist must take a leadership role to ensure that the treatment team, including the patient and caregivers, work collaboratively in every phase of the orthotic process. A patient-centered, occupation-based approach empowers the patient and caregivers to participate actively. This also positions them as the experts in the patient's occupations, lifestyle, values, image, and activity contexts, which complements the expertise that the health care professionals bring. The therapist should clearly explain rationales, make clinically sound recommendations, and offer choices to the patient whenever possible. This helps establish each team member's accountability and increases the likelihood that the patient will actually use the orthosis as instructed.

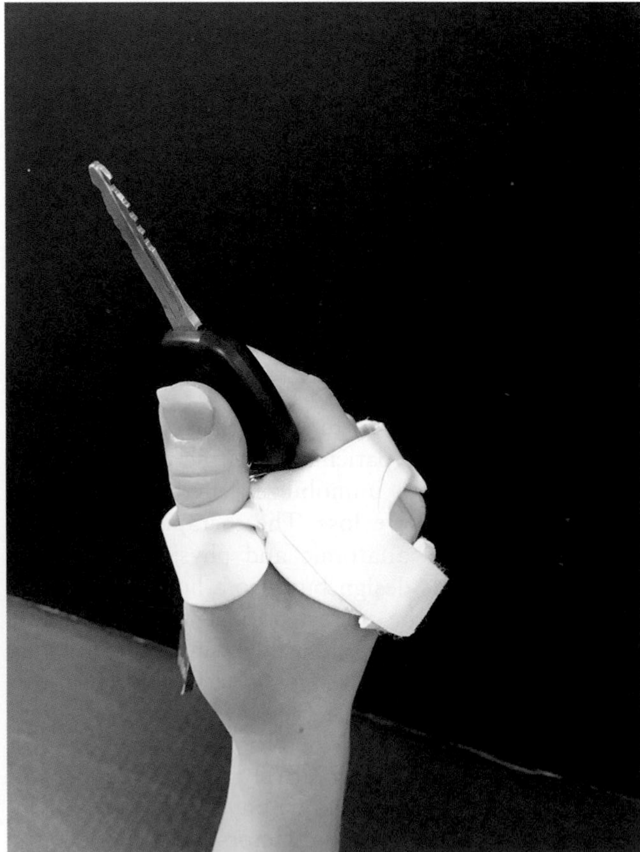

Figure 22-7. Orthosis for combined ulnar and median nerve pathology. Orthosis prevents clawing and supports thumb in a position of opposition for use with pinch tasks.

When deciding to incorporate an orthosis into a treatment plan, the following key questions should be considered:

- What is the primary clinical or functional problem?
- What are the indications for and goals of orthosis use?
- How will the orthosis affect the problem and the patient's overall function?
- What benefits will the orthosis provide?
- What limitations will the orthosis impose?
- What evidence is available related to the orthosis use?

Based on these considerations, the therapist must select or design the most appropriate orthosis. In some cases, the best choice is no orthosis at all.

The growing array of commercial products has led to a greater number of choices. The first choice to be made is whether the orthosis should be custom fabricated or prefabricated. Materials must also be considered. The therapist must be familiar with properties, benefits, and drawbacks of each. Options abound, with rigid, semi-rigid, and soft materials available (see Chapter 23).

When making an orthosis selection, several key factors must be carefully weighed:

- Among the orthosis-related factors are type, design, purpose, fit, comfort, cosmetic appearance, cost to purchase or fabricate, weight, ease of care, durability, ease of donning and doffing, effect on uninvolved joints, and impact on function.
- Patient-related factors include clinical and functional status, attitude, lifestyle, preference, occupational roles, living and working environments, social support, issues related to safety and precautions, ability to understand and follow through, and financial or insurance status.

Orthosis Adherence

Previous literature suggested that patient education on orthosis use and a wearing schedule, the comfort of the orthosis, and involving the patient in the preference of orthosis and family support all improve compliance with use of an orthosis. However, a more recent systematic review of adherence to orthosis wear in adults with acute upper limb injuries found little published scientific evidence and concluded that existing studies were of varied quality. Authors suggested future research is needed to examine the relationship between orthosis adherence and socioeconomic status as well as other patient characteristics.[14] Additional review of the literature concluded there is limited evidence to correlate orthosis material selection with adherence, but indicated some evidence to support the use of behavioral approaches with orthosis adherence.[15] With the relatively small base of literature on orthoses, therapists must continue to put their clinical judgments and experience to the test and strive to develop evidence-based practice related to observed outcomes and factors that influence successful use of orthoses as an intervention.

The therapist must consider, carefully monitor, and teach both the patient and caregiver to report any of these problems that may be related to orthotic use:

- Impaired skin integrity (pressure areas, blisters, maceration, dermatological reactions)
- Pain
- Swelling
- Stiffness
- Sensory disturbances/numbness
- Increased stress on uninvolved joints
- Functional limitations

Should problems with orthosis wear arise, the therapist should examine both the orthosis and the wearing schedule. The orthosis itself may not fit properly or comfortably. The patient's functional demands may outweigh the benefits of orthosis wearing, or the wearing schedule may be too complex. Actively engaging the patient in the problem-solving process is likely to improve the outcome. Although it is important to strive for the ideal, therapists must remain realistic in the scope of the patient's daily life.

Theoretical Foundations for the Use of Orthoses as a Therapeutic Intervention

There are remedial, compensatory, and adaptive approaches when incorporating an orthosis as part of an intervention plan. Using the Biomechanical Frame of Reference, remediation integrates an orthosis to improve ROM, strength, or endurance.[16] For example, following a distal radius fracture, patients may demonstrate extreme digit stiffness preventing them from holding small objects such as coins and medication, or even grasping a fork or toothbrush. Use of a mobilization orthosis to increase digit flexion allows the patient to be able to make a fist and to increase their functional performance. Remediation involves regaining a skill that was present prior to the onset of an injury or disease.[17] Return to grasping coins, medication, and a toothbrush are all examples of skills regained through remedial use of an orthosis as an intervention.

In contrast, the Rehabilitative Frame of Reference promotes the use of compensatory strategies and adaptations to increase functional performance.[16] For example, patients with C4–C5 spinal cord injuries with tetraplegia can use **mobile arm support** (**MAS**) to perform activities they otherwise could not. These patients will exhibit weak deltoid and biceps muscles, limiting their functional performance. The use of MAS can allow these patients to participate in self-feeding, driving a power wheelchair, playing games, writing, using electronic devices, and performing grooming tasks.[18]

Compensatory strategies may be recommended along with adaptive techniques. Thermoplastic material used for custom orthoses fabrication can be molded to create adaptive handles to promote participation in activities of daily living. When working with patients following C4–C5 spinal cord injury, the MAS may allow the patients to bring their hand to their face for self-feeding, and adaptations to eating utensils and cups may allow the patients to use their distal extremities for functional use.

Purposes of Orthoses

Orthoses are categorized according to several purposes, including:

- Support a painful joint
- Immobilize for healing
- Protect tissues

- Provide stability
- Restrict unwanted motion
- Restore mobility
- Substitute for weak or absent muscles
- Prevent contractures
- Modify tone

Although a specific orthosis is discussed under the category for which it is most commonly used, that purpose may not be its only one. Also, a single orthosis may fulfill several functions simultaneously. The orthoses presented here are by no means an exhaustive list but a representative sampling of commonly used or historically significant orthoses. Inclusion of specific orthoses should not be interpreted as an endorsement of one type over another. Whenever possible, published evidence-based data have been included. Because the intent of this chapter is to provide an overview of orthoses, the reader is encouraged to explore the references and resources for more detailed information.

Immobilization to Support a Painful Joint

Pain in a joint or soft tissues can result from a wide variety of causes, including acute trauma (such as sprains and strains), nerve irritation (such as carpal tunnel syndrome and cubital tunnel), inflammatory conditions (such as tendonitis and rheumatoid arthritis [RA]), and joint instability (such as degenerative arthritis, ligamentous laxity, and shoulder subluxation). When resting a joint is indicated to relieve pain, protect joint integrity, and/or decrease inflammation, supportive orthoses can be used. These orthoses are often worn all day or all night or both to provide the maximum benefit, or they may be worn only during selected activities. Unless contraindicated, the orthosis should be removed at least once a day for skin hygiene and gentle ROM exercises to prevent loss of joint mobility. The following are common examples of orthoses used for pain relief.

Supporting a Painful Shoulder

Subluxation occurs secondary to weakness of the rotator cuff muscles and the weight of the dependent arm, resulting in inferior displacement of the humeral head from the glenoid fossa.[19] There are many factors that contribute to glenohumeral joint subluxation. These may include improper positioning, a lack of support when in the upright position, as well as pulling on the hemiplegic arm during transfers.[20] **Arm slings** have been developed to prevent or correct shoulder subluxation or reduce pain in patients who have subluxation caused by brachial plexus injuries, hemiplegia, or central cord syndrome injuries. Sling designs are numerous, with some commercially available and others fabricated by the therapist.

Certain slings support and immobilize the whole arm. These slings, such as the standard pouch and the double arm cuff sling, restrict motion by keeping the humerus in adduction and internal rotation and the elbow in flexion. Although these slings may take some of the weight off of the affected shoulder, these supports typically facilitate an increase in flexor tone in the synergy pattern, decrease arm swing during ambulation, impact body image, and restrain function that could limit recovery (Fig. 22-8).[20] Other sling designs support the shoulder but leave the rest of the arm free for function,

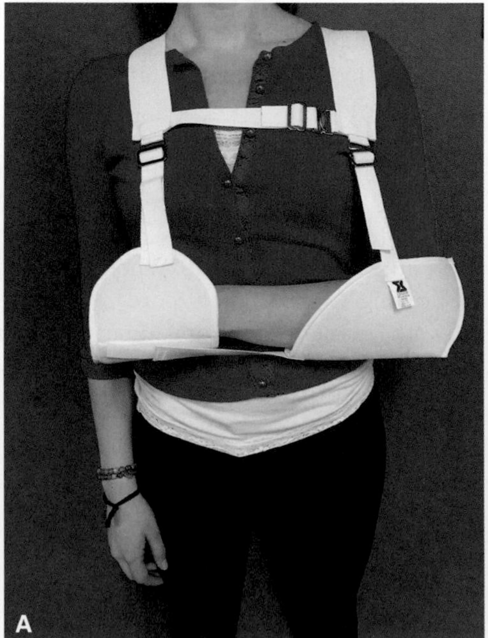

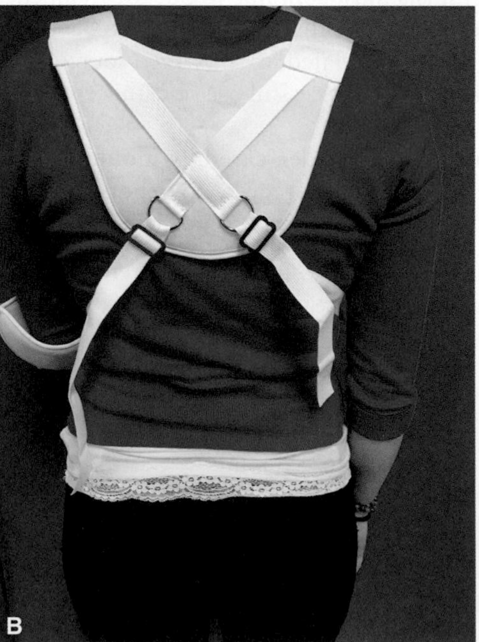

Figure 22-8. Sling that facilitates increased flexor tone in a synergy pattern and does not promote functional use of upper quadrant. **A,** Front View; **B,** Rear View.

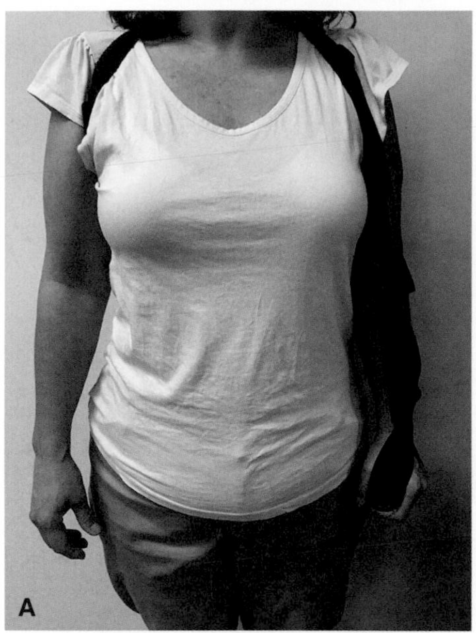

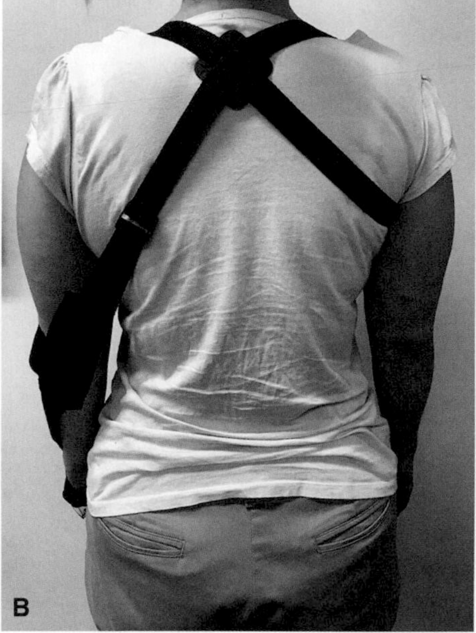

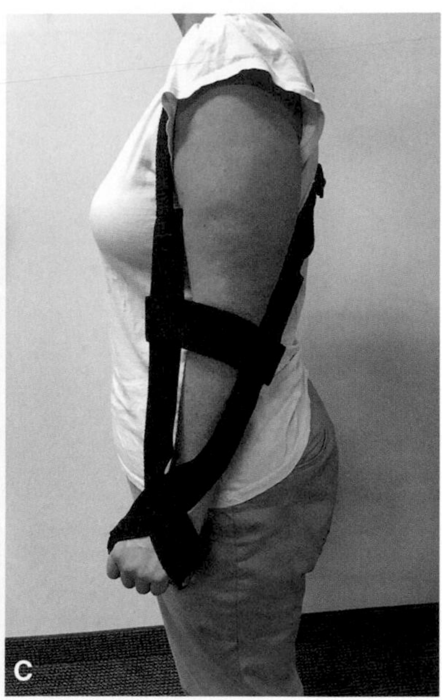

Figure 22-9. GivMohr sling that provides distal support, but holds upper quadrant to the side of the body instead of a flexor synergy pattern. **A,** Front view; **B,** Rear view; **C,** Side view.

such as a humeral cuff sling, GivMohr and OmoNeurexa sling (Figs. 22-9 and 22-10).

The use of supports in reducing shoulder subluxation remains controversial and lacks empirical evidence. A systematic review by Ada et al. found no evidence to conclude that supportive devices are effective in preventing or reducing subluxation or in decreasing pain after stroke.[21] A systematic review by Nadler and Pauls concluded that application of slings to an already subluxed shoulder resulted in a decrease in vertical subluxation during use, but these changes were not maintained when the orthosis was removed.[19] Authors also concluded that slings with support to the proximal humerus were less effective than those that supported the upper extremity with a distal attachment. Previous literature suggest the benefits of supporting the forearm and elbow in flexion using slings such as the Hemi sling, Harris sling, or Triangular sling to decrease subluxation. More recent evaluation of the GivMohr and OmoNeurexa identified these slings as effective in decreasing subluxation during use, but the benefit to these products is that they allow elbow motion and also hold the upper extremity in a more neutral extended position at the side of the body.[19] This review also provided some support for the use of a sling for 4 weeks to decrease pain at the glenohumeral joint following stroke.[19]

The patient's acceptance of the sling also must be considered. Relative ease of donning and doffing the sling is imperative so the limb is not damaged further from improper wearing. More definitive research on the effectiveness of slings and orthoses in the management

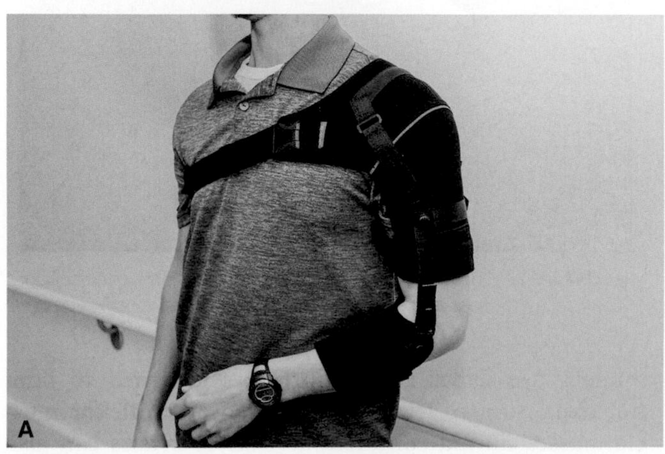

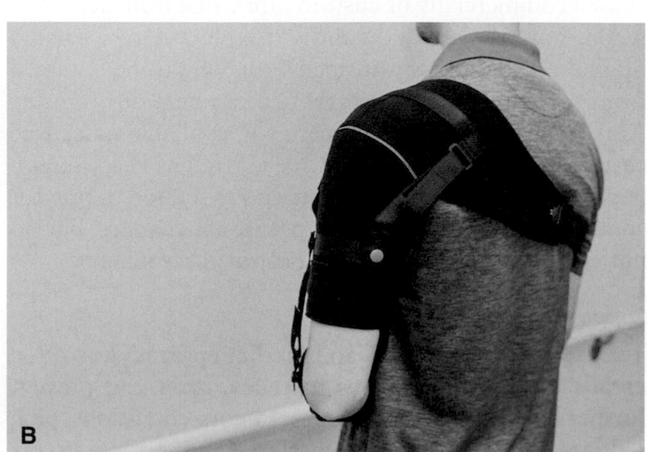

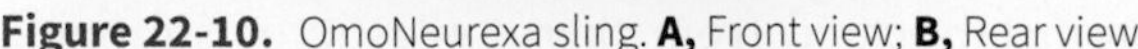

Figure 22-10. OmoNeurexa sling. **A,** Front view; **B,** Rear view.

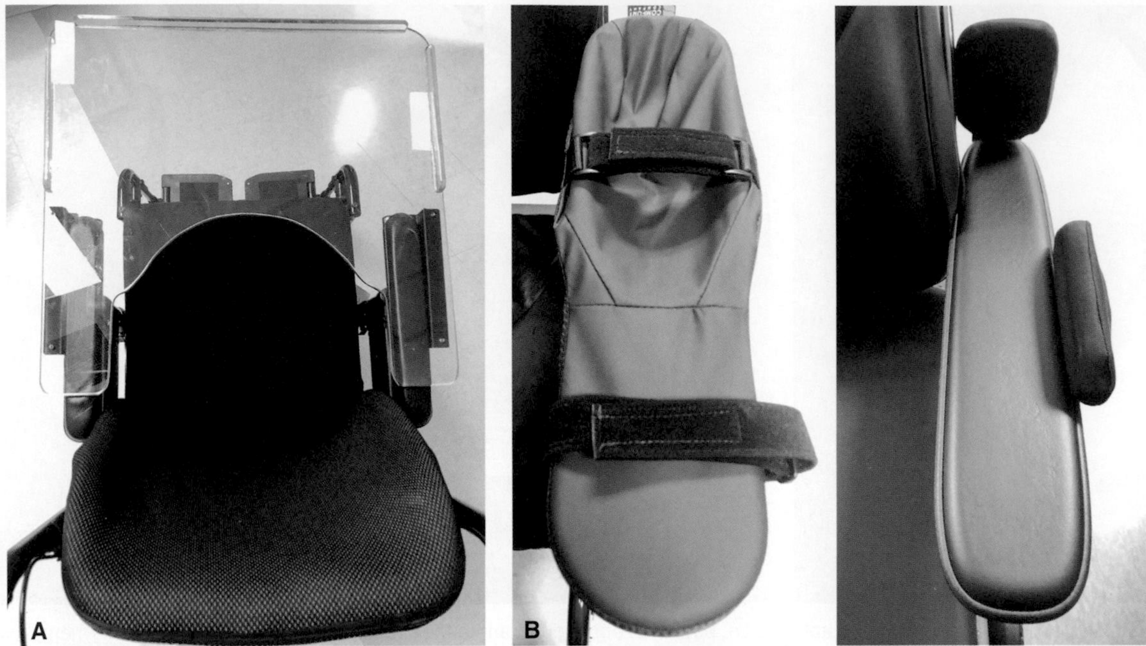
Figure 22-11. Lap board (A) and arm troughs (B) to support the upper extremity.

of the flaccid or subluxed shoulder is needed, and therapists should carefully consider all options before recommending slings.

Arm troughs, lapboards, and half-lapboards are also used to support the painful shoulder when the patient is seated in a wheelchair and also have been demonstrated to decrease glenohumeral joint subluxation during use.[20] It is important to remember that these supports lack the constant relationship between the patient and the support as exists with slings.

Lapboards are generally indicated for patients with poor trunk control or visual field deficits and for those who require greater variability of upper extremity positioning or a work surface. Arm troughs and half-lapboards are used for patients who need a device that does not interfere with wheelchair propulsion or transfer activities (Fig. 22-11). Full and half-lapboards can be purchased commercially or custom fabricated from acrylic or wood. Some designs allow the half-lapboard to be rotated up and out of the way, instead of having to be removed from the wheelchair when the patient needs to transfer. Arm troughs are also commercially available or can be custom-made. Lap boards and arm troughs keep the upper extremity abducted and externally rotated to prevent contractures. These allow for positional changes, but do not always provide consistent proper positioning.[22]

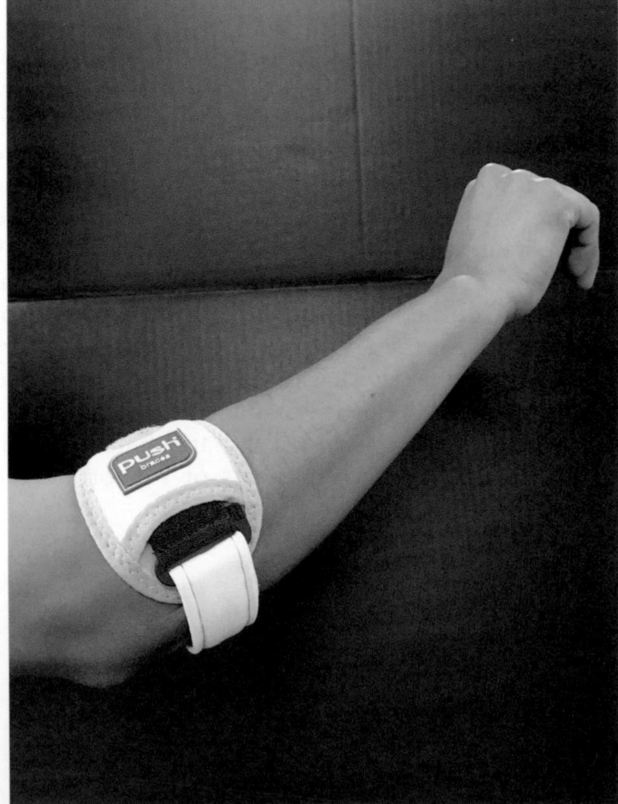

Figure 22-12. Counterforce strap used to limit muscle contraction of the wrist extensors and decrease pain in the lateral elbow region.

Supporting a Painful Elbow

The treatment of lateral and medial epicondylitis often entails the use of orthoses to relieve pain and prevent further stress to affected tissues. In both conditions, pain reduces grip strength and function. Counterforce braces (Fig. 22-12), of which there are several commercial models, are wide, nonelastic bands designed to limit full expansion of the forearm extensor or flexor muscle masses during contraction.[23] These braces can also be custom fabricated from thermoplastic or strapping materials. The literature reports wide variation in the success of braces.[24] Instruct the patient that complications can result from the brace being applied too tightly, including nerve compression syndromes. The patient must be carefully taught accordingly.

A wrist orthosis placing the wrist in 35° to 40° of extension and worn alone or in conjunction with a counterforce brace is often prescribed to rest the forearm musculature.[23] A study by Jafarian et al. found that use of a counterforce brace resulted in immediate increase in pain-free grip strength, whereas a wrist orthosis did not.[25] Conversely, Garg et al. found that pain relief was significantly better with a wrist orthosis than with a counterforce brace.[26] However, Sadeghi-Demneh and Jafarian found a greater reduction in pain with the use of a counterforce strap as compared to a wrist orthosis.[27] The prescription of orthoses must be based on the patient's symptoms. It is vital that the cause of the problem and the biomechanics of loading forearm musculature are also addressed in relation to all activity demands.

Supporting a Painful Wrist or Hand

Resting hand orthoses are used to support the wrist, fingers, and thumb. The normal resting position of the hand is determined anatomically by the bony architecture, capsular length, and resting tone of the wrist and hand muscles. This is typically 0° to 20° of wrist extension, 20° to 30° of metacarpophalangeal (MCP) joint flexion, 10° to 30° of proximal interphalangeal (PIP) joint flexion, and slight distal interphalangeal (DIP) joint flexion, the thumb carpometacarpal (CMC) in slight extension and abduction, and the thumb MP and IP in slight flexion (see Fig. 22-1).[4]

A resting hand orthosis is commonly prescribed for patients with RA. A randomized controlled trial found that in addition to pain relief, nighttime use of resting hand orthoses improved hand strength and functional status.[28] With RA, the orthosis should be in a position of comfort, regardless of whether this is the ideal anatomical position.[4] During an acute exacerbation of the disease, orthoses are generally worn at night and during most of the day and removed at least once for hygiene and gentle ROM exercises. It is recommended that orthosis use continue for at least several weeks after the pain and swelling have subsided.[4]

Wrist extension, or cock-up, orthoses are probably the most commonly prescribed type of orthosis for the upper extremity. Indications for use include sprains, strains, tendonitis, arthritis, carpal tunnel syndrome, following cast removal of wrist fractures, and other conditions that cause pain. A wrist orthosis typically positions the wrist in 10° to 30° of extension, which is thought to be the best position for hand function.[4] A well-fitting orthosis is one that clears the distal palmar and thenar creases to allow for unrestricted mobility of the fingers and thumb and that conforms to the palm to support the arches of the hand. Wrist orthoses may be volar (Fig. 22-13), dorsal, or circumferential and can be custom fabricated or prefabricated. Because these orthoses are intended to provide wrist support while allowing functional use of the hand, fit and comfort are crucial.

A growing variety of prefabricated orthoses are available, with designs and materials offering a range of soft to rigid support. Elasticized wrist orthoses with an adjustable metal stay that slides into a volar pocket (Fig. 22-14) are commonly used because they are cost-effective and readily available. The drawbacks of these orthoses are that they do not fully support the palmar arches, they do not completely clear the palmar and thenar creases, and the metal stay is often prepositioned at a 35° to 45° angle of extension. Therefore, it is critical to fit and adjust the stay to the desired angle before issuing the orthosis. Other commercial products are made of wire-foam, neoprene, leather, canvas, and other fabric blends, all of which offer features having distinct advantages and disadvantages.

Orthoses vary in the amount of motion they allow or restrict. Collier and Thomas compared ROM at the wrist with three commercial supports and a custom-made volar thermoplastic orthosis.[29] The prefabricated orthoses allowed the same amount of motion (wrist flexion to about neutral and wrist extension to

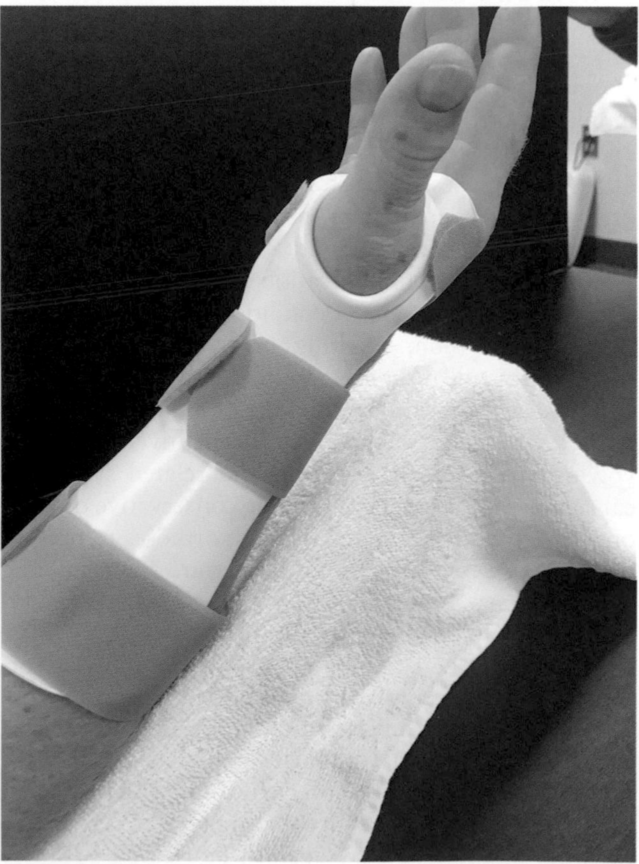

Figure 22-13. Volar wrist immobilization orthosis.

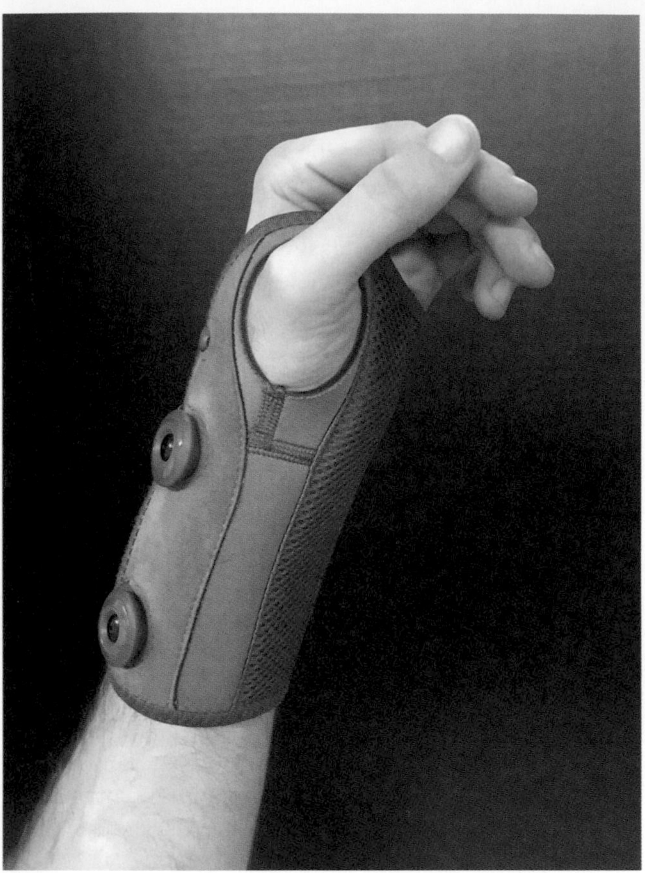

Figure 22-14. Prefabricated wrist support.

about 26°–31°). In contrast, the custom-fabricated thermoplastic orthosis allowed less wrist flexion (not past 14° of wrist extension) and more wrist extension (about 40°). This suggests a custom-fabricated thermoplastic orthosis may be more appropriate for conditions where limited wrist flexion is desired.

Another common indication for a wrist orthosis is carpal tunnel syndrome, a condition caused by median nerve compression, resulting in symptoms including pain, sensory disturbances, muscle weakness, swelling, stiffness, and frequent dropping of items. Symptoms often are worse at night or with repetitive activity involving wrist flexion. For pain and related symptoms caused by carpal tunnel syndrome, conservative or postoperative treatment often uses wrist orthoses to prevent the elevation of carpal tunnel pressure by restricting wrist motion.[30] A neutral position (Fig. 22-13) is recommended, avoiding wrist extension.[31]

There is a consensus that prefabricated wrist orthoses, which often place the wrist in excessive extension, may not be of any benefit unless they are modified to a less extended position. A systematic review of orthosis use for carpal tunnel syndrome showed benefits from various orthosis types and wrist angles, with evidence suggesting that custom-fabricated orthoses and full-time orthosis wear promote better results.[32] Orthosis use is most effective when initiated early after symptom onset. Control of wrist position alone may be insufficient, and blocking the MPs in slight flexion may also be needed to decrease intratunnel pressure.[30]

A long opponens orthosis (Fig. 22-15), also known as a long thumb spica, can relieve pain from wrist and thumb arthritis or from de Quervain tenosynovitis of the abductor pollicis longus and extensor pollicis brevis. This orthosis is typically based on the volar or radial aspect of the forearm and extends distally to immobilize the thumb CMC and MP joints. The wrist is generally positioned in slight extension, with the thumb in slight flexion and palmar abduction to enable opposition to the index and middle fingers.[33] If the thumb IP joint or the extensor pollicis longus tendon is involved, the IP joint can be included in the orthosis as well. Prefabricated orthoses often provide a softer support and are easier to use for function, whereas custom-made thermoplastic orthoses give more rigid immobilization.

A thumb CMC stabilization orthosis, or a hand-based thumb orthosis, is a static orthosis that encompasses the first metacarpal to provide stability, reduce pain, and increase hand function. It restricts motion

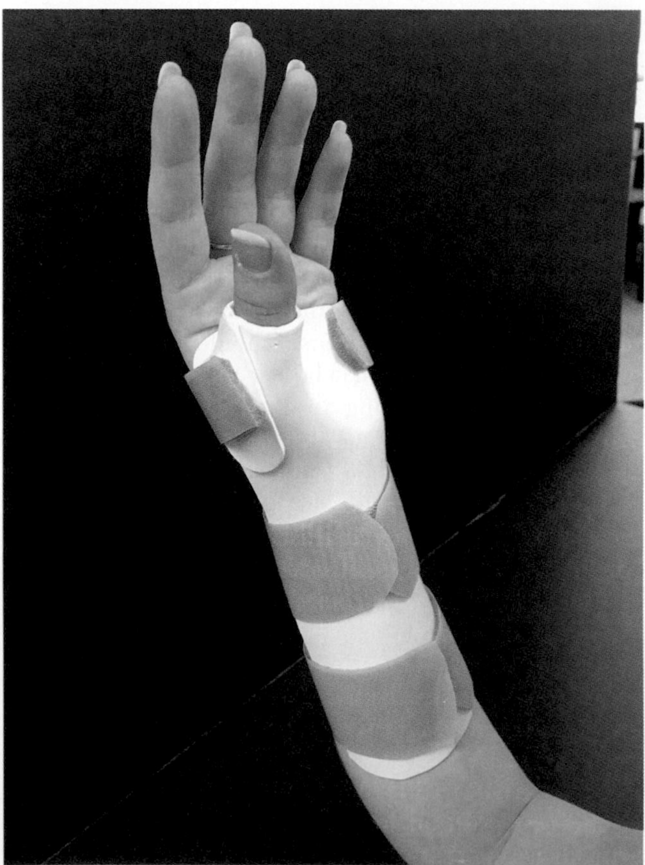

Figure 22-15. Long opponens orthosis/forearm-based wrist and thumb orthosis.

of the CMC and MP joints but leaves the wrist relatively mobile and the thumb IP free. A static thumb MP orthosis allows for CMC and IP motion and can be used when the disorder is localized to the MP joint alone.

Indications for hand-based thumb spica include RA or osteoarthritis (OA) of the thumb CMC or MP joints or trauma to soft tissues, such as the ulnar collateral ligament of the MP. The thumb is generally positioned to enable opposition to the fingers for function while in the orthosis. When used with arthritis, the orthosis is worn during functional activities and at night. If ligament damage is suspected, the orthosis is worn at all times.

For a precise fit and rigid support, orthoses can be custom fabricated from thermoplastic materials (Fig. 22-16). Newer commercial products made of soft, breathable elastic material have moldable thermoplastic stays to enable a custom-fit, combining comfort and ease of fabrication with the required individualized rigid support. Rigid support may not always be needed. In comparing a custom-made thermoplastic orthosis and a soft neoprene support for OA of the thumb CMC joint, Weiss et al. found that the prefabricated neoprene orthosis (Fig. 22-2) provided greater pain relief and function and was preferred over the custom thermoplastic orthosis by 72% of the subjects.[34] Sillem et al. similarly found that patients preferred a soft prefabricated orthosis even though a more rigid custom orthosis provided greater pain reductions.[35] Bani et al. found a greater reduction in pain with a custom thermoplastic orthosis than with a neoprene-prefabricated orthosis.[36] Systematic reviews found evidence for the effectiveness of orthosis use to relieve pain and improve function in CMC OA, found evidence of varying patient orthosis preferences, but found no evidence of orthosis design superiority.[37,38]

If the thumb or finger IP joints are painful from trauma or arthritis, lateral, dorsal, or volar gutter orthoses may be used for pain relief. Silicone-lined sleeves (Fig. 22-17) or pads can protect painful joint nodules from external trauma.

Pain, volar subluxation, and ulnar deviation of the MCPs are common sequelae of RA. MCP ulnar deviation supports may be used to provide stability, realign joints, reduce joint stress, and relieve pain. They may delay the progression of deformity, but do not correct or prevent it.[39] These supports may be worn alone or incorporated into a resting hand orthosis.

Prefabricated and custom-designed orthoses with dividers or straps to align the digits include dynamic and static and soft and rigid. However, rigid static orthoses

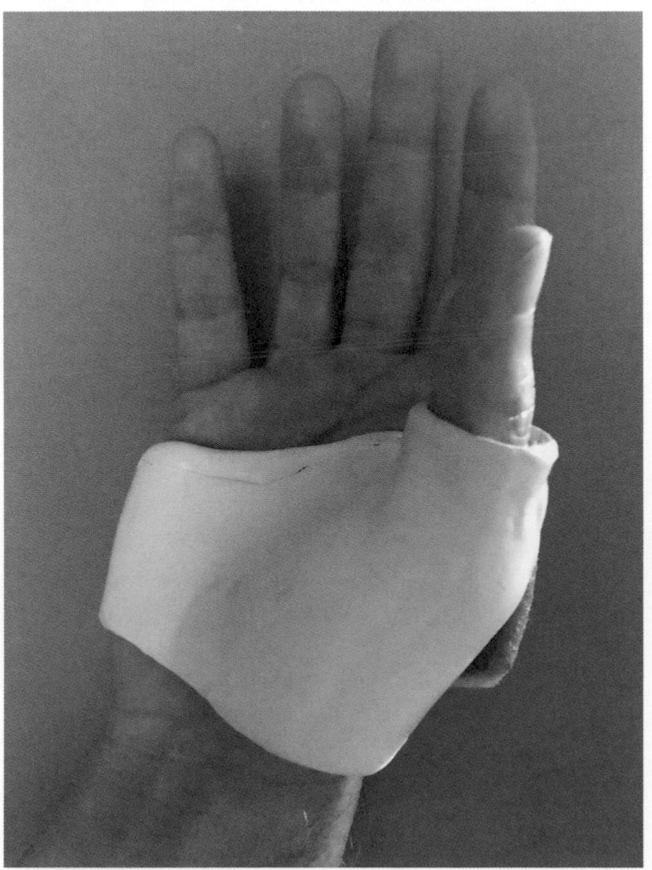

Figure 22-16. Custom-fabricated hand-based thumb carpal metacarpal orthosis or short opponens orthosis.

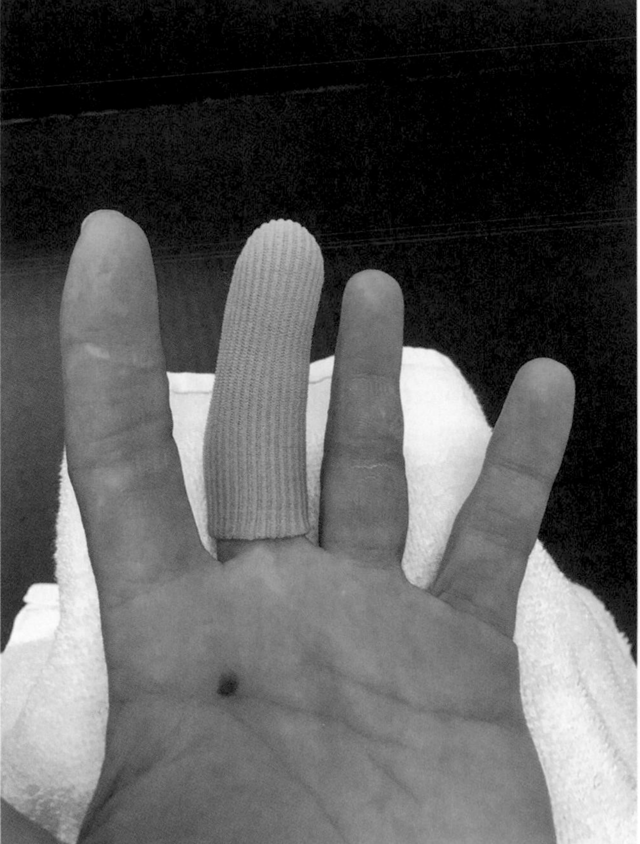

Figure 22-17. Digit sleeve.

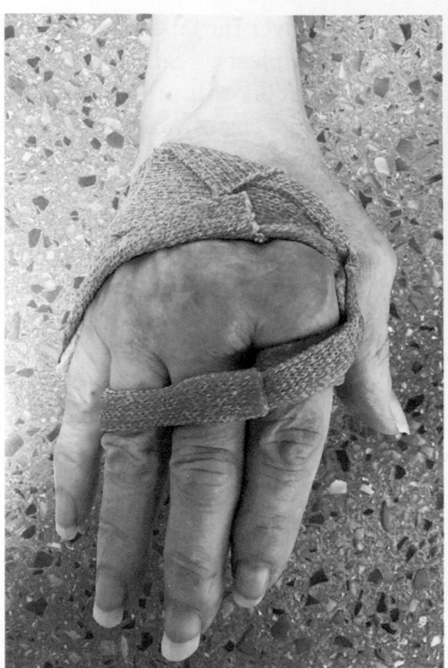

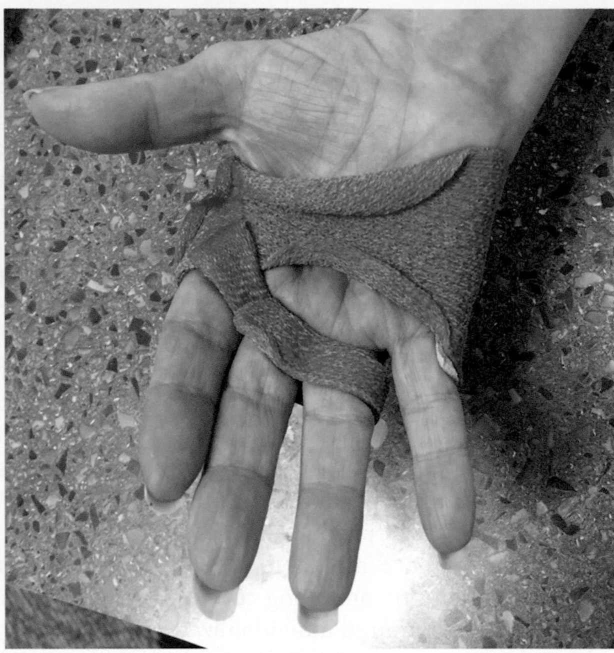

Figure 22-18. Custom-fabricated ulnar drift orthosis used to reduce ulnar drift of the digits, which is seen with individuals with rheumatoid arthritis.

(Fig. 22-18) used to achieve passive correction of deformity can create focal pressure points on the digits. The prime indicator for use and selection of an MCP ulnar deviation support should be the patient's preference.[40]

Immobilize for Healing or to Protect Tissues

Many of the orthoses previously discussed for pain relief can also be used to immobilize for healing or protection following injury or surgery. For example, a type of sling used to relieve traction pain associated with a brachial plexus injury can also protect the nerve structures from overstretching during the healing phase. A thumb MP orthosis that relieves pain from arthritis may also be used while an acutely injured collateral ligament heals.

Immobilize or Protect the Shoulder, Upper Arm, or Elbow

The sling is the simplest and most commonly used device for the upper extremity when there is a need to limit motion of the shoulder yet allow for some motion of the arm on the thorax. The basic arm sling (Fig. 22-19) consists of a forearm pouch or cuffs, a strap, and a mechanism for adjusting and securing the strap. To adjust a sling for patient use:

- Place the patient upright.
- Ensure the elbow is flexed to 90° and is seated properly in the sling, with the hand and wrist also supported as the design allows.
- Adjust the strap or straps so the arm is comfortably supported.
- Check for comfort.
- Teach both the patient and caregiver how to properly don and doff the sling.
- Monitor the axilla and areas where sling straps cross the body for signs of moisture and skin breakdown.
- Monitor for signs of edema and joint stiffness.

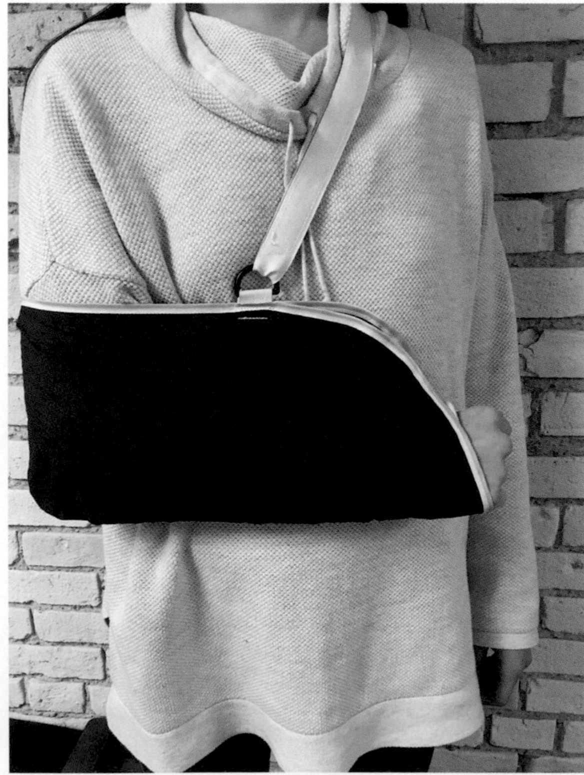

Figure 22-19. Basic sling for immobilization.

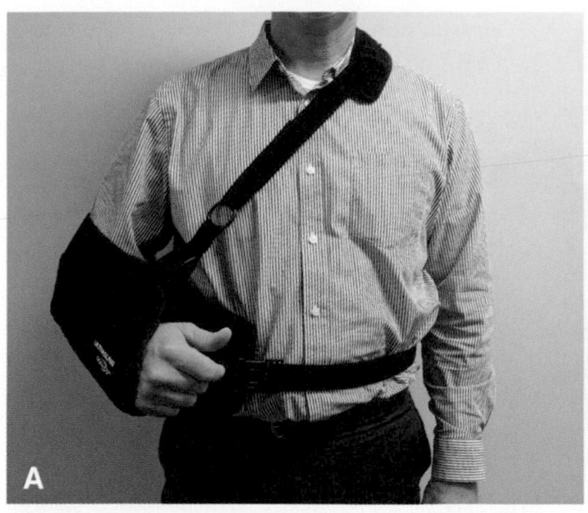
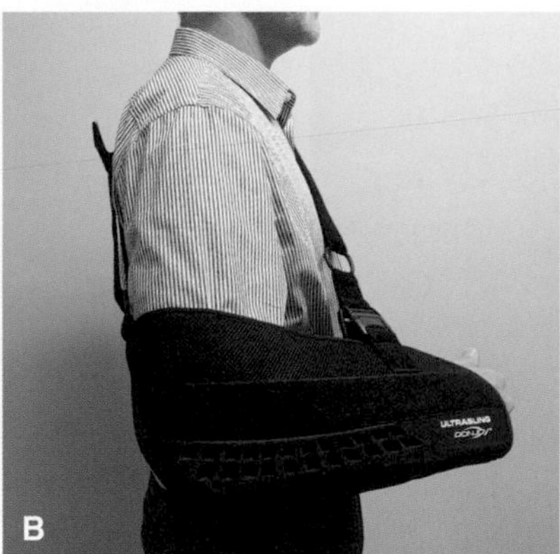
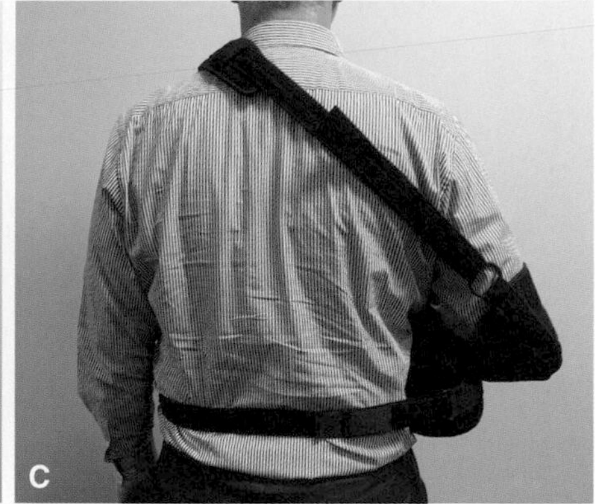

Figure 22-20. Shoulder immobilizers commonly used following to protect a rotator cuff repair. **A,** Front view; **B,** Side view; **C,** Rear view.

To further limit mobility, shoulder immobilizers (Fig. 22-20) can be used. These devices, which relatively immobilize the shoulder and elbow, are typically used following shoulder surgical reconstructions, arthroplasty, and rotator cuff repair. Immobilizers are more complex than slings, involving strapping that wraps the body to stabilize the arm against the trunk. Several commercial designs are available.

Foam abduction pillows or wedges may be used to maintain the arm at a certain elevation from the body. Abduction braces, sometimes called airplane orthoses, are commercially available or custom fabricated from thermoplastics. These devices are based on the trunk and can position the shoulder in varying degrees of abduction or rotation and the elbow in varying degrees of flexion or extension. Commercial braces offer ease of adjustability with the use of wrenches but may need extra padding to prevent skin breakdown. Indications for use include postoperative shoulder rotator cuff repairs, burns, and skin grafts to the axillary region.

The treatment of humeral shaft fractures often involves functional fracture bracing. A humeral fracture brace provides external stabilization and alignment of the fracture by compressing surrounding soft tissues while allowing for early mobilization of the shoulder and elbow. These braces may be prefabricated or custom fabricated by the therapist from low-temperature thermoplastics. They are circumferential in design, with D-ring or Velcro straps to allow for a secure closure and size adjustments as edema subsides. They should be lightweight and made of a perforated material for ventilation. Excellent results with the use of functional fracture bracing of the humerus have been reported.[41] A Sarmiento brace (Fig. 22-21) is the typical prefabricated choice for conservative treatment of humeral shaft fractures.[42] Whether the brace is prefabricated or custom fabricated, the therapist should ensure that its distal end does not block elbow flexion motion and that its proximal end does not unnecessarily limit shoulder motion.

Casts, orthoses, and hinged braces can be used to immobilize and protect the elbow following fractures, burns, ligamentous injuries, or other surgical procedures. Casts offer rigid immobilization and may be made according to a circumferential, posterior, or anteroposterior bivalve design that allows the cast to be removed for wound care or ROM. Hinged braces are frequently used to protect healing ligaments by limiting certain amounts of motion of the elbow. Thermoplastic orthoses may be anterior or posterior and may be secured by Velcro straps or an elastic wrap. Anterior elbow extension orthoses (Fig. 22-22) are most commonly used to immobilize and position the elbow following skin grafting.

Immobilize or Protect the Wrist or Hand

The maintenance of normal hand function requires strong tissue repair with free gliding between adjacent

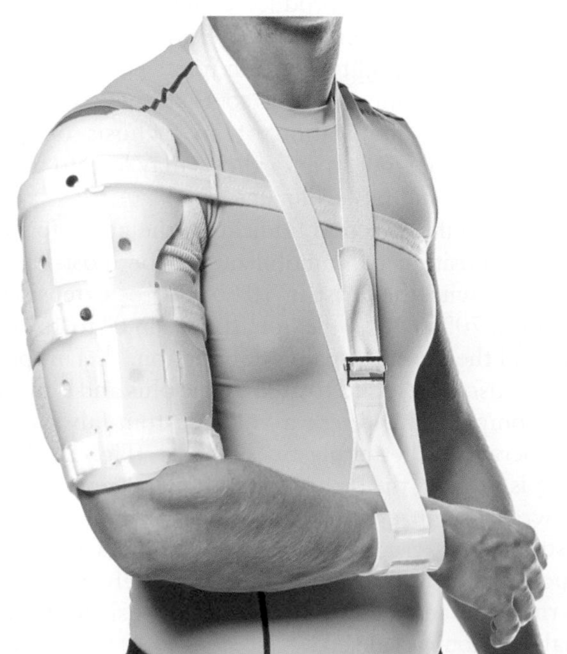

Figure 22-21. Sarmiento brace—humeral fracture brace to immobilize humeral shaft fracture. (Courtesy of BraceAbility.)

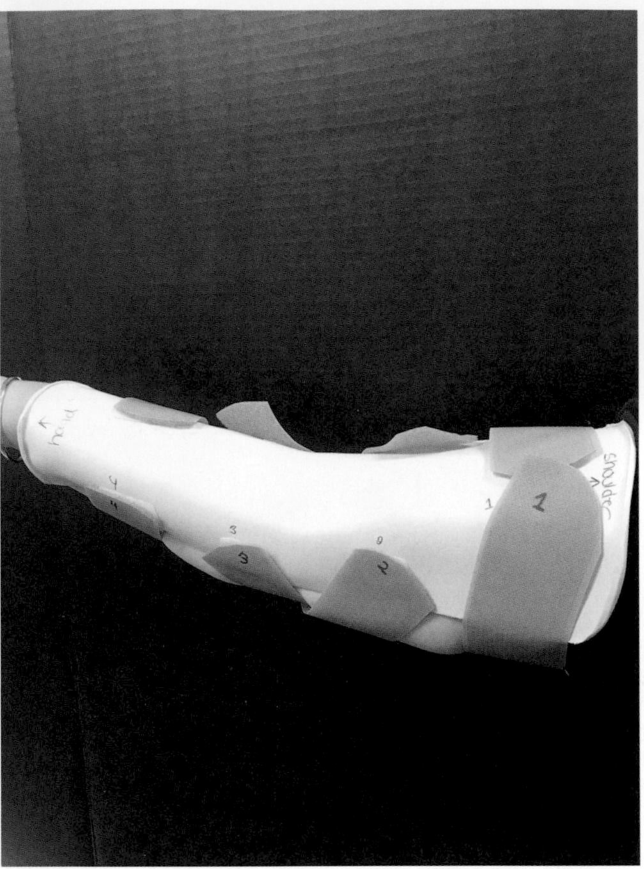

Figure 22-22. Elbow extension orthosis.

structures. Proper positioning of the wrist and hand is critical to prevent complications due to injury, edema, and tissue healing. Orthosis use in the early stages of healing can counteract the typical joint contractures of the injured hand that produce common deformities of wrist flexion, MCP extension, IP flexion, and thumb adduction. It is essential to position joints correctly and keep uninvolved joints moving so that they will not stiffen.[43] Incorrect application of an orthosis or improper positioning while in an orthosis may lead to both joint limitations and tissue damage.

Unless specifically contraindicated, the antideformity, or safe, position of immobilization for most hand conditions is with the wrist in 10° to 30° of extension, the MCPs in 70° to 90° of flexion, the IPs in 0° to 15° of flexion, and the thumb in palmar abduction.[4,43] This position may also be referred to as intrinsic plus and is most often accomplished through a volar custom-fabricated low-temperature thermoplastic orthosis (Fig. 22-23). If edema is present, the orthosis should be secured by an elastic wrap or gauze wrap to avoid a tourniquet effect from straps. It is crucial never to force joints into the ideal position but to position joints as closely as possible to the ideal and serially revise the orthosis until the optimal position is realized.

Antideformity orthoses are integral to the treatment of acute dorsal hand burns because even a small burn can

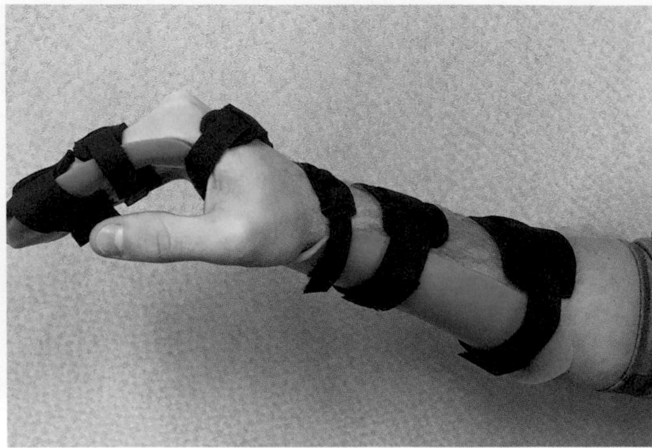

Figure 22-23. Forearm-based immobilization orthosis in an intrinsic plus position.

lead to significant deformity or contracture.[44] The most commonly recommended positions for joints is with the wrist in 15° to 30° of extension, the MCPs in 50° to 70° of flexion, the IPs in full extension, (Fig. 22-23), and the thumb in palmar abduction or midway between palmar and radial abduction with the MP and IP in slight flexion to full extension to prevent common burn-related contractures.[45] Custom-fabricated orthoses, preferably of a perforated material, ensure the best fit. Orthoses may have to be adjusted daily for optimal fit and maintenance of proper joint positioning. For the grafting and rehabilitation phases of burn treatment, orthosis design varies with the positions necessary to counteract the contractile forces of the scars.

Wrist orthoses, as discussed in the previous section, may be used for protection or immobilization of wrists following cast removal or to treat soft-tissue injuries. Athletic injuries to the wrist and hand, such as contusions, sprains, strains, fractures, and joint dislocations, often require the use of protective orthoses to enable the patient to continue participation in sports. As with other orthoses, selection of material and design should be carefully tailored to the patient's needs. Materials may be thermoplastic, fiberglass, or neoprene. Selection should be based on the degree of immobilization required, material durability and breathability, the player's sport position, governing rules of the sport, and the safety of other players.

Treatment of tendon injuries and repairs may involve static positioning to immobilize the tendon for healing using a dynamic orthosis to protect the tendon while allowing controlled motion to increase tendon repair strength and gliding. Flexor tendon repair protocols vary, but a protective dorsal blocking orthosis (Fig. 22-24) positioning the wrist and MCPs in flexion and blocking the IP joints at 0° of extension is typically used. Rubber band traction may be added to hold the digits in a flexed position or to enable resistive extension

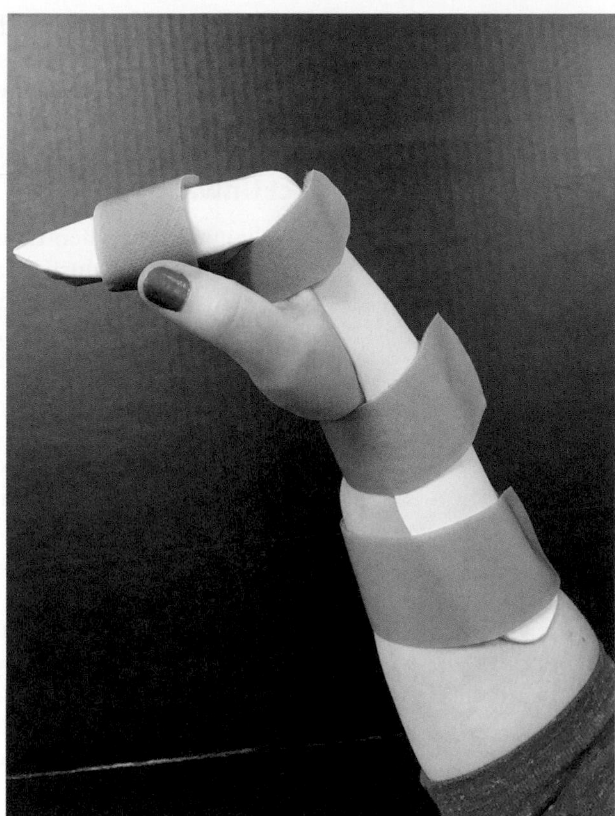

Figure 22-24. Dorsal blocking orthosis used to protect a repair of a digit flexor tendon.

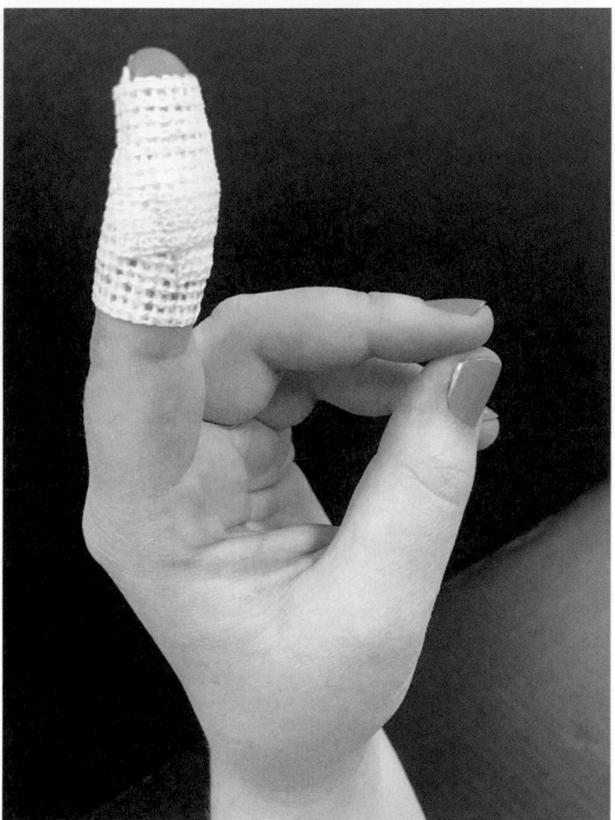

Figure 22-25. Use of Quick Cast to protect terminal extensor tendon (Mallet finger).

and passive flexion exercises. The orthosis is custom fabricated from low-temperature thermoplastic and is often worn for as long as 6 weeks.[46]

Treatment and orthoses for extensor tendon injuries are based on the level of injury. For injuries at the DIP level that may result in a mallet finger deformity, the DIP is immobilized for 6–8 continuous weeks in a slightly hyperextended position.[47] The PIP joint is left free. The orthosis used may be volar, dorsal, or circumferential and is typically custom fabricated for the best results. Thermoplastics, Quick Cast, or Orficast may be used for fabrication. Excellent results for the treatment of mallet finger (Fig. 22-25) have been reported with various orthoses.[48] For injuries at the PIP level, treatment includes Quick Cast (Fig. 22-26) or thermoplastic immobilization with the PIP in absolute 0° of extension for 6 to 8 continuous weeks to prevent boutonniere deformity. For more proximal tendon injuries, orthoses may involve static positioning, dynamic assists, or both.[47]

Relative motion orthoses are sometimes used following a more proximal extensor tendon laceration to limit MCP flexion. This is sometimes referred to as a yoke orthosis (Fig. 22-6). The position of the bar fabricated out of thermoplastics or Orficast material limits MCP flexion, therefore minimizing the extensor tendon glide.[49]

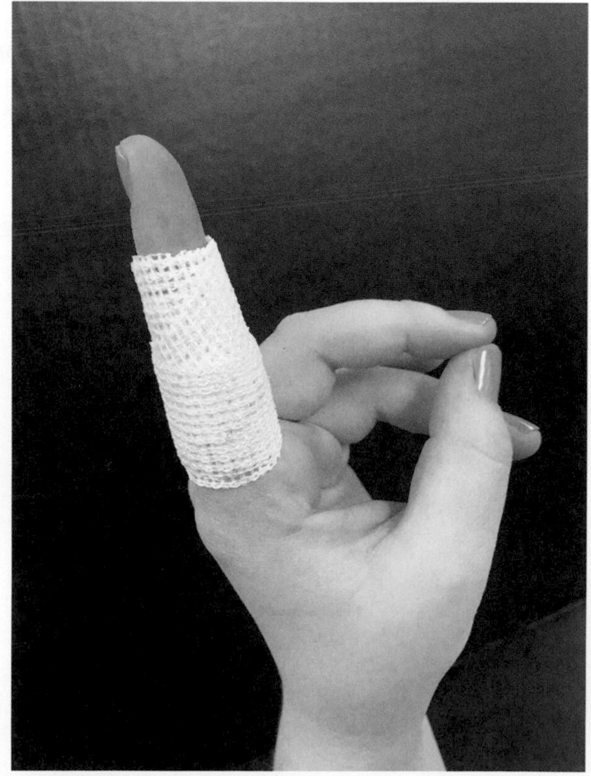

Figure 22-26. Use of Quick Cast to hold proximal interphalangeal joint in extension following central slip injury.

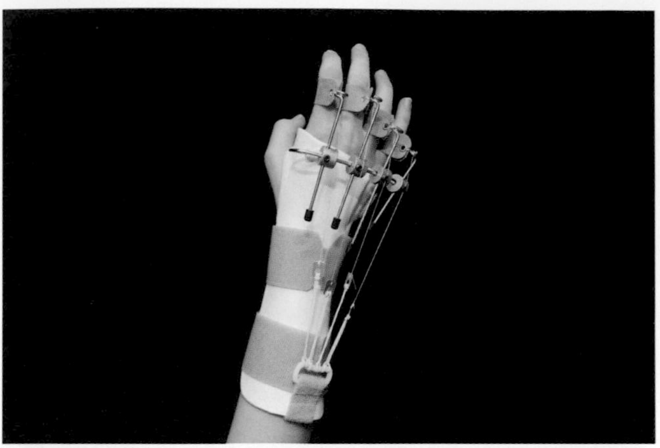

Figure 22-27. Forearm-based dynamic metacarpophalangeal extension orthosis.

Orthosis fabrication is an integral part of postoperative MCP arthroplasty treatment. Early positioning and motion following arthroplasty often uses a dynamic MCP extension assist (Fig. 22-27) to support the wrist, control MCP position and alignment, allow guided motion, and assist with extensor power. This controlled stress allows for joint capsule remodeling over time.[50] Dynamic MCP extension assists may use high-profile or low-profile outrigger designs. They have slings to support the MCPs in neutral extension and deviation and to provide rotatory alignment. Outrigger kits are commercially available, or the outrigger may be hand fabricated. The dynamic extension orthosis may be supplemented by a static positioning orthosis at night.[4,50]

To protect digits but allow for stabilization or controlled motion of the MCP, PIP, or DIP joints following injury or surgery, buddy straps (Fig. 22-28) that connect an injured finger to an adjacent finger, can be used. Common indications for these include stable fractures, PIP joint dislocations, collateral ligament injuries, and staged flexor tendon reconstructions.[4,39]

Provide Stability or Restrict Unwanted Motion

Orthoses can be helpful in stabilizing joints when their integrity has been compromised by an acute injury or a chronic disease such as arthritis. Stabilization or restriction of motion can often greatly facilitate functional use of a limb.

Stabilize or Restrict Motion of the Shoulder or Elbow

In addition to the purposes previously described, slings, and hinged elbow orthoses can also be used to provide proximal stability that may enable improved distal function.

Stabilize or Restrict Motion of the Wrist or Hand

It is essential to determine the position in which a joint needs to be supported relative to hand dominance and task requirements because specific functional demands vary greatly among individual patients. The wrist is considered by many to be the key to ultimate hand function, and therefore wrist orthoses are commonly prescribed to provide stability. Dorsal wrist orthoses allow for the greatest palmar sensation but are least supportive, volar wrist orthoses are most commonly prescribed and provide a moderate amount of stability, and circumferential wrist orthoses provide the greatest amount of stability.[51] For optimum mechanical advantage to support the weight of the hand, the forearm portion of the orthosis should be two-thirds the length of the forearm.[4,51]

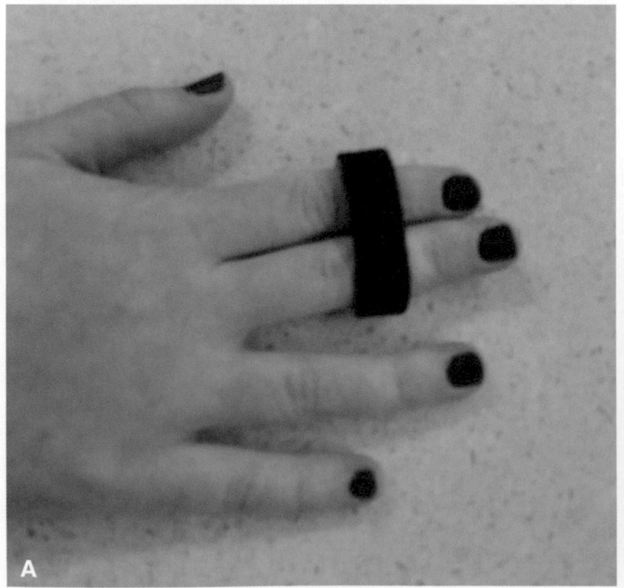

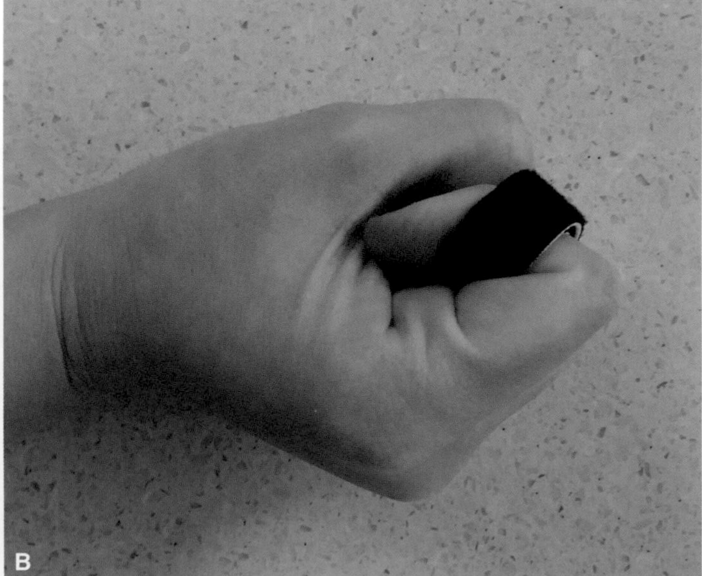

Figure 22-28. **A,** Buddy straps using an adjacent digit to support an injured digit. **B,** Can also be used to encourage movement of an injured finger by strapping it to the adjacent digit.

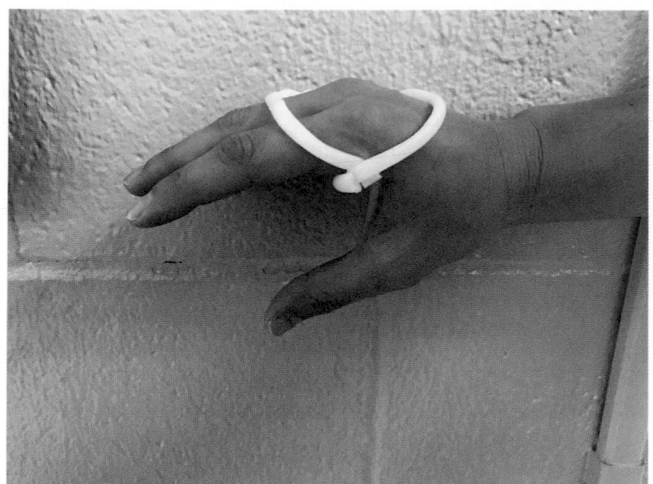

Figure 22-29. Lumbrical bar orthosis for anticlaw.

A lumbrical bar is a hand-based orthosis that extends over the dorsal aspect of the proximal phalanges to restrict unwanted hyperextension of the MCPs that can result from an ulnar nerve or combined median and ulnar nerve injury. By blocking this motion, IP flexion contractures can be prevented and functional hand opening can be improved as the power of the long finger extensors is transferred to the IPs for extension. Custom-fabricated thermoplastic orthoses (Fig. 22-29) provide for an intimate and streamlined fit.[52]

This same principle of restricting undesired motion is used in a PIP hyperextension block, also known as a swan-neck orthosis. Swan-neck deformities are common sequelae of RA and a possible complication following an extensor tendon injury or repair. These deformities often cause difficulty with hand closure, as PIP tendons and ligaments can catch during motion, and the finger flexors have less of a mechanical advantage to initiate flexion when the PIP is hyperextended. By blocking the PIP in a slightly flexed position, the patient can flex the PIP more quickly and easily.[39,40]

For short-term use or for trial purposes, custom-fabricated thermoplastic swan-neck orthoses (Fig. 22-30) may suffice. For long-term use or for use on adjacent digits, commercial swan-neck orthoses are often recommended because they are more durable, less bulky, more easily cleaned, and more cosmetically appealing. Custom-ordered ring splints made of silver or gold are attractive, durable, streamlined, and adjustable for variations in joint swelling, but they are more costly. Silver splints have also been shown to improve dexterity.[53] Prefabricated splints made of polypropylene (Fig. 22-31), also available commercially, offer some of the benefits of silver splints with less cost. In a study comparing commercial silver and polypropylene splints, both were equally

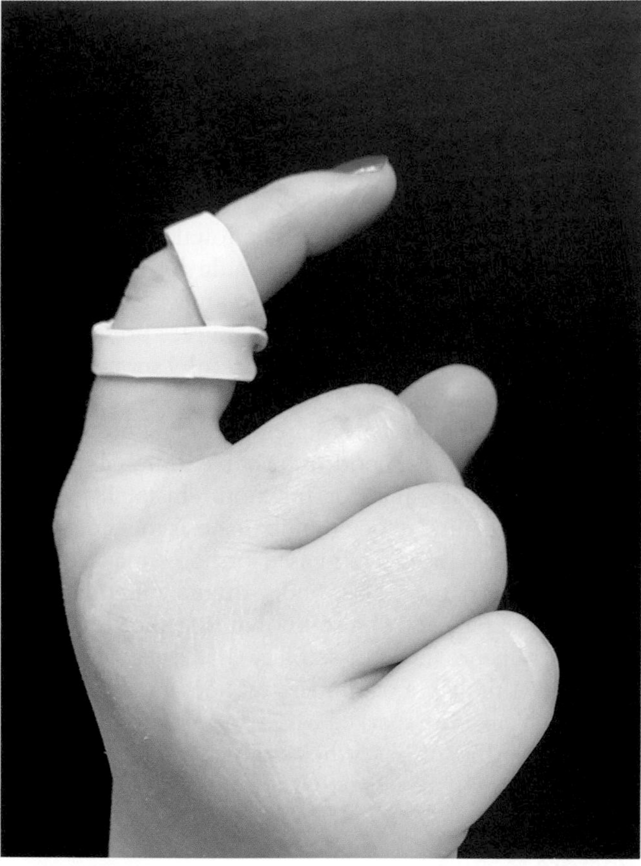

Figure 22-30. Custom-fabricated orthosis to block proximal interphalangeal joint hyperextension and to prevent swan-neck deformity.

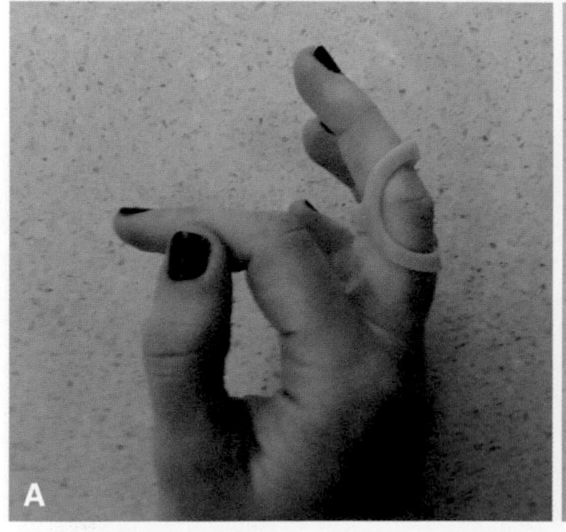

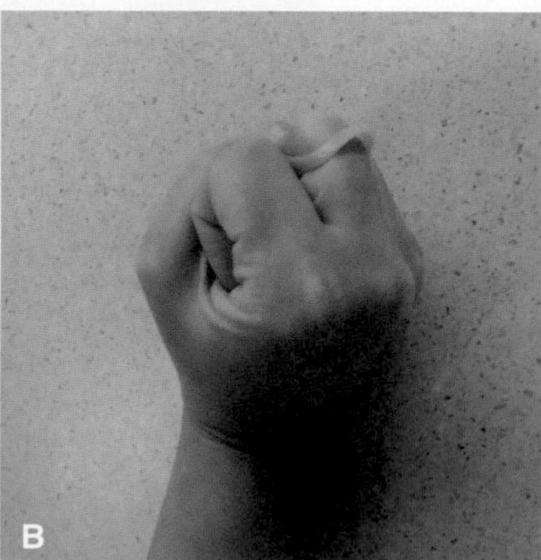

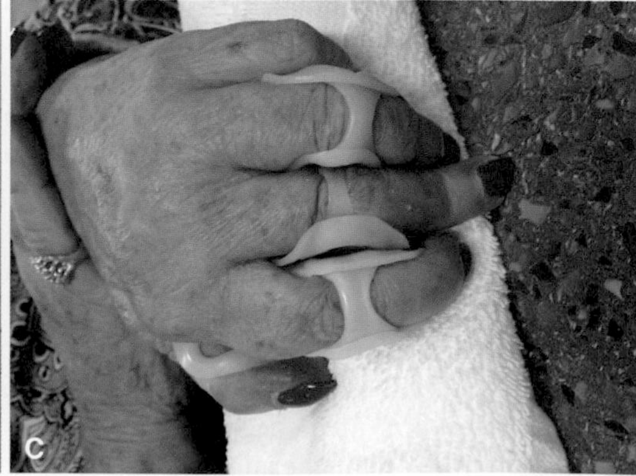

Figure 22-31. 3 Point Products Oval 8 orthosis to prevent swan-neck or boutonniere deformity. **A,** Support and stability; **B,** Mobility; **C,** Alignment.

effective and acceptable to patients.[54] Heavy-duty metal splints, such as Murphy ring splints, may benefit patients who use their hands in highly demanding tasks. Swan-neck splints can also be used to provide lateral stability to unstable IP joints of the fingers or thumb.

Flexible boutonniere deformities may benefit from immobilization to block the PIP in a more extended position to allow for greater functional hand opening. These orthoses may be custom-made by the therapist or custom ordered from the companies that fabricate swan-neck splints. Because there is direct pressure over the PIP, the dorsal skin must be carefully monitored for signs of breakdown.

Thumb stability is a requirement for almost all prehensile activities, so support of unstable thumb joints may have a particular value for function.[4] Instability of the CMC often requires a long thumb orthosis that crosses the wrist because shorter hand-based orthoses may not adequately support the CMC. Short thumb immobilization orthosis (see Fig. 22-16) also known as a short opponens orthosis, can provide MP stability and a stable post for pinching. Although a circumferential design is commonly used, problems with marked MP deformity can make donning and doffing of the orthosis difficult, and direct pressure over the MP may lead to a breakdown of fragile skin.

Restore Mobility

Orthoses play an integral role in the restoration of mobility by lengthening soft tissue or impacting joint contractures that can occur as a result of poor positioning, trauma, scarring, or increased muscle tone.[55] As described earlier in this chapter, custom-fabricated serial static, dynamic, or static progressive orthoses may be used to provide a low load of pressure over a prolonged period of time to impact contracture management. This can also be used in the management of tone following neurological pathology.

A therapist implementing an orthosis program to regain motion must understand how orthoses work to affect positive change. ROM is gained not by tissue stretching but by actual tissue elongation from new cell growth.[4,5] Inelastic mobilization applies constant forces needed to remodel tissues and is the most effective means for gaining motion in chronically stiff joints. Elastic mobilization is most indicated for acute joint stiffness or more supple joints because forces can be more easily controlled and fine adjustments made.[4] The forces used must be gentle and carefully applied, and the tissue must be closely monitored for signs of excessive stress, such as redness and inflammation, which are indicators of tissue damage or microtrauma.[6]

Fixed contractures and chronically stiff joints often respond best to inelastic mobilization from serial casting. Casting material is ideal because it conforms intimately and is more rigid than thermoplastics. Casts are changed as motion gains are achieved. In a systematic review of upper extremity casting in central nervous system disorders, however, there was insufficient high-quality evidence on the long-term benefits from casting, and there was high variability in casting protocols.[56] Therefore, it is not possible to make specific recommendations for practice.

Dynamic mobilization orthoses are more effective when used for early contractures.[8] Orthoses can be removed for hygiene and function and are worn at night so as not to interfere with use of the extremity. This decrease in wearing time, however, means that tissues are not kept under constant tension, which may result in less rapid gains. The amount and direction of force must be carefully monitored and adjusted as joint angles change. Static progressive mobilization orthosis use is often indicated for fixed or chronic contractures. However, static progressive force should more commonly be used with extension mobilization programs as patients may not tolerate a prolonged position in maximum flexion.[3]

Restore Mobility of the Shoulder, Elbow, or Forearm

A serial static abduction orthosis can be used to apply pressure to and elongate burn scars in the axilla. The benefits of wearing this type of orthosis must be carefully weighed against the complete lack of function that it imposes. For flexion contractures of the elbow, thermoplastic anterior elbow extension orthoses (see Fig. 22-22), serial casts or dropout casts, and dynamic elbow extension or static progressive elbow extension (Fig. 22-32) orthoses can be used.

Serial casting, which typically entails changing the cast weekly, can safely reposition joints without providing undue stress to tissues.[2,3] Contractures that develop as a result of increased tone, such as in the patient with a brain injury, casting is often used in conjunction with nerve blocks, Botox injections, or other surgical procedures. Great care must be taken with

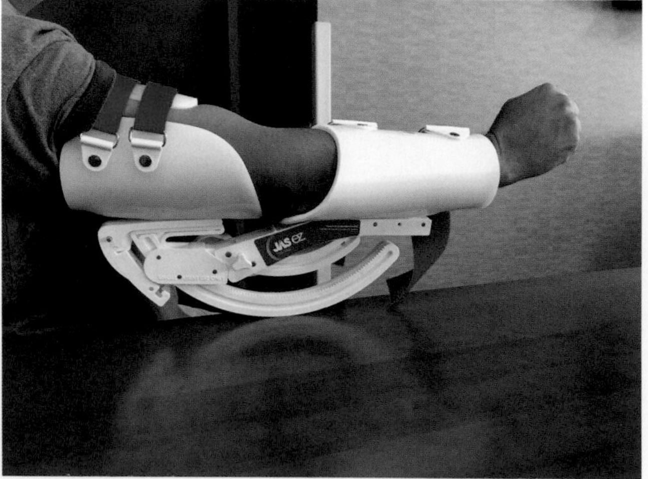

Figure 22-32. Static progressive elbow extension orthosis.

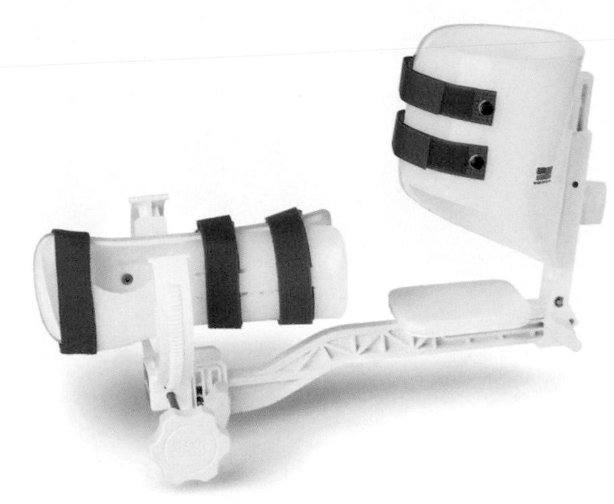

Figure 22-33. Static progressive forearm orthosis. (Courtesy of Joint Active Systems.)

casting in the presence of severe tone, because pressure areas may develop.

Loss of forearm rotation, often seen following spinal cord injury, peripheral nerve injury, or fracture, can be treated with a dynamic or static progressive forearm orthosis. Orthoses can be custom fabricated[4] or obtained commercially as a preformed product or kit (Fig. 22-33). Altering the direction of force when using these orthoses can produce supination or pronation.

Restore Mobility of the Wrist or Hand

Serial static thermoplastic wrist orthoses, dynamic wrist orthoses, and static progressive wrist orthoses can be used for limitations in wrist flexion or extension. These may be custom fabricated or preformed. Dynamic or static progressive component kits can also be purchased commercially. This allows the therapist to custom mold the orthosis base while more easily assembling force units.

Lack of MCP flexion can devastate hand function. Many dynamic orthosis designs to regain MCP motion are available. Custom-fabricated thermoplastic orthoses use individual finger loops over the proximal phalanx (Fig. 22-34). When using dynamic force, these loops are attached to rubber bands or springs that provide the needed force for sustained tension. When using static progressive force, the loops are attached to nylon cord or Velcro straps for tension. An outrigger is used to direct the line of pull at 90°. It is important to clear the distal palmar crease so as not to block full flexion ROM. These orthoses may be forearm based or hand based, depending on the mechanical advantage needed, degree of stiffness, and the patient's wrist strength and stability.[4]

Limited PIP flexion makes grasp difficult, and limited PIP extension interferes with the ability to open the hand in preparation for grasp or to release objects. PIP flexion contractures are a frequent complication of trauma or poor positioning and extension contractures can be seen following dorsal hand burns or prolonged immobilization for fracture management.

To address these contractures, forearm or hand-based dynamic thermoplastic orthoses similar to those designed for MCP flexion and extension can be used. A hand-based prefabricated dynamic PIP extension orthoses or prefabricated static progressive orthosis (Fig. 22-35) can be used to isolate PIP extension. Static progressive force can be applied for flexion to the MP or the IP joints (Fig. 22-36) using a custom-fabricated orthosis. Glasgow et al. also found the duration of dynamic orthotic is a key factor in PIP joint contracture resolution, with flexion motion obtained more quickly than extension.[57] Securing the MCP joint in flexion using a custom hand-based orthosis can also assist in promoting PIP extension (Fig. 22-37).

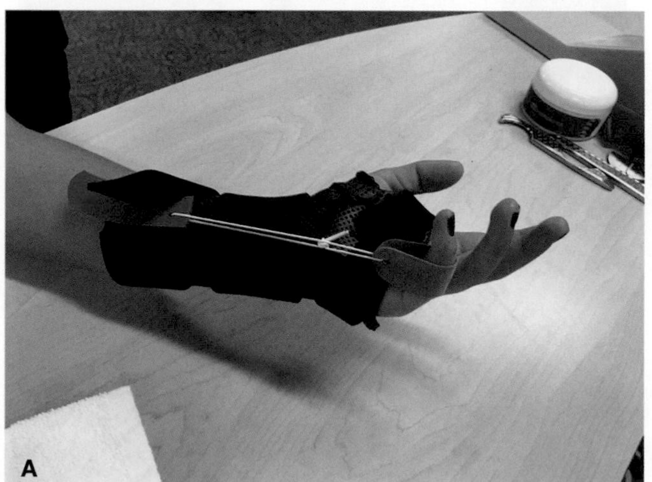

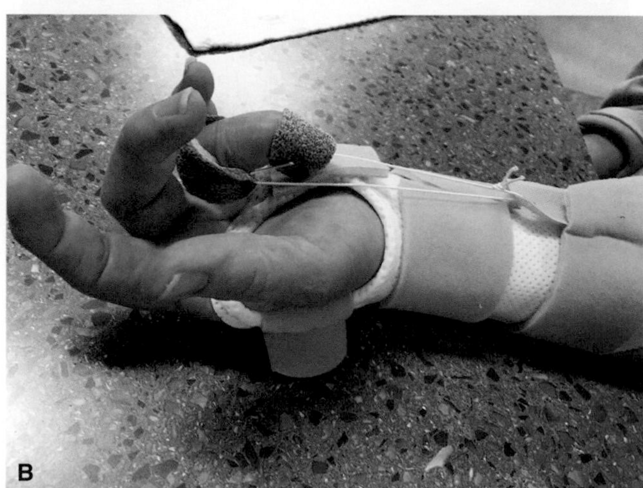

Figure 22-34. A. Forearm-based static progressive metacarpophalangeal flexion orthosis. **B.** Forearm-based static progressive orthosis for three joint flexion.

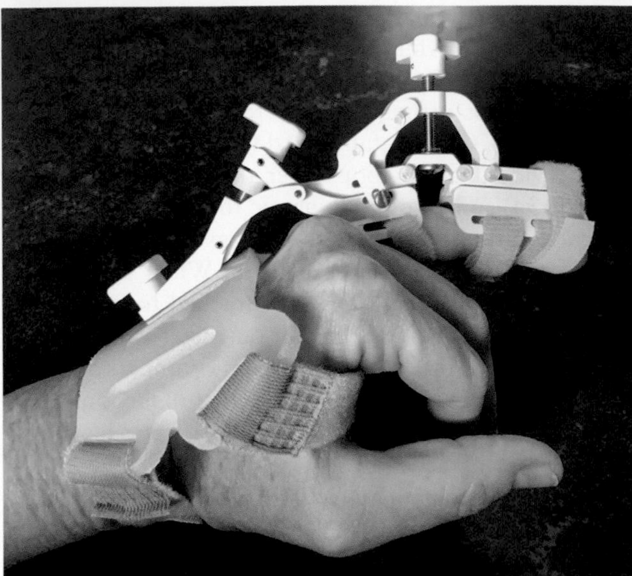

Figure 22-35. Prefabricated hand-based static progressive proximal interphalangeal extension orthosis.

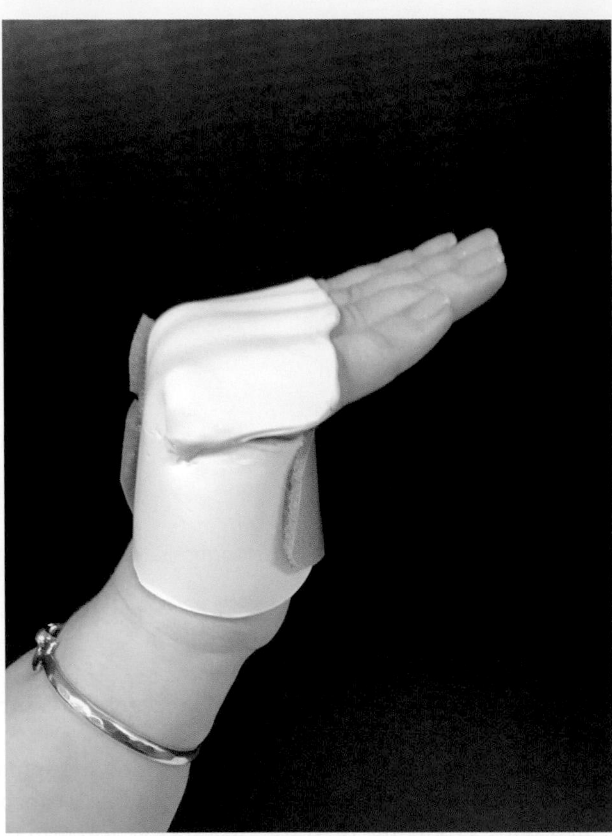

Figure 22-37. Hand-based dorsal metacarpophalangeal flexion orthosis to promote proximal interphalangeal extension.

Thermoplastic gutter (Fig. 22-38), circumferential orthoses, and dynamic mobilization orthoses are useful in the treatment of mild contractures, whereas serial digital casting (Fig. 22-39) has been advocated for moderate to severe contractures.[2] Casting offers the advantages of intimate conformity, rigidity, breathability, and uniform

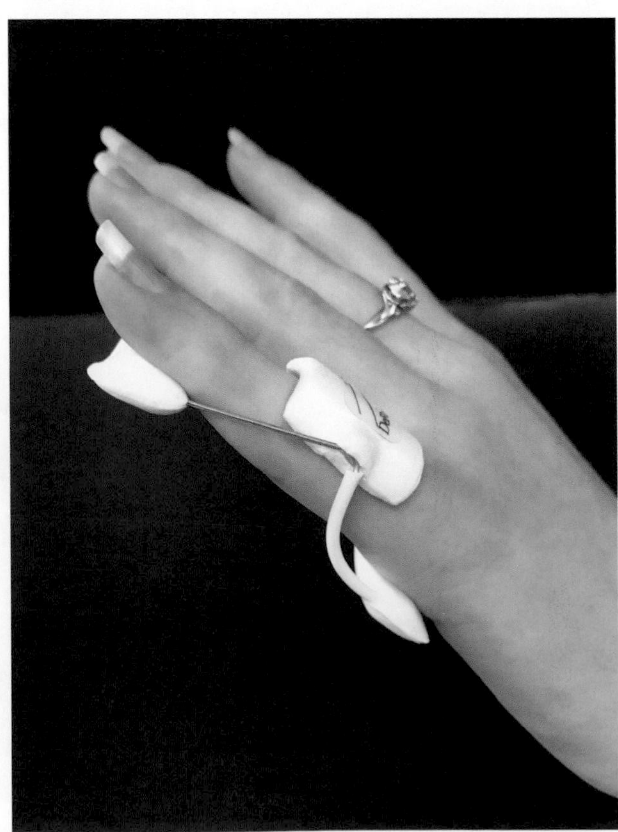

Figure 22-36. Dynamic PIP extension orthosis.

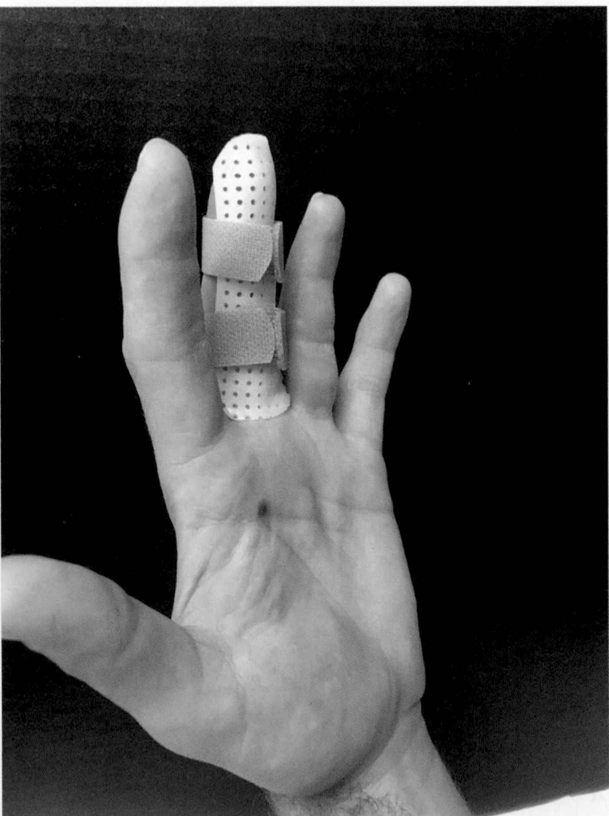

Figure 22-38. Custom-fabricated thermoplastic digit extension/gutter orthosis.

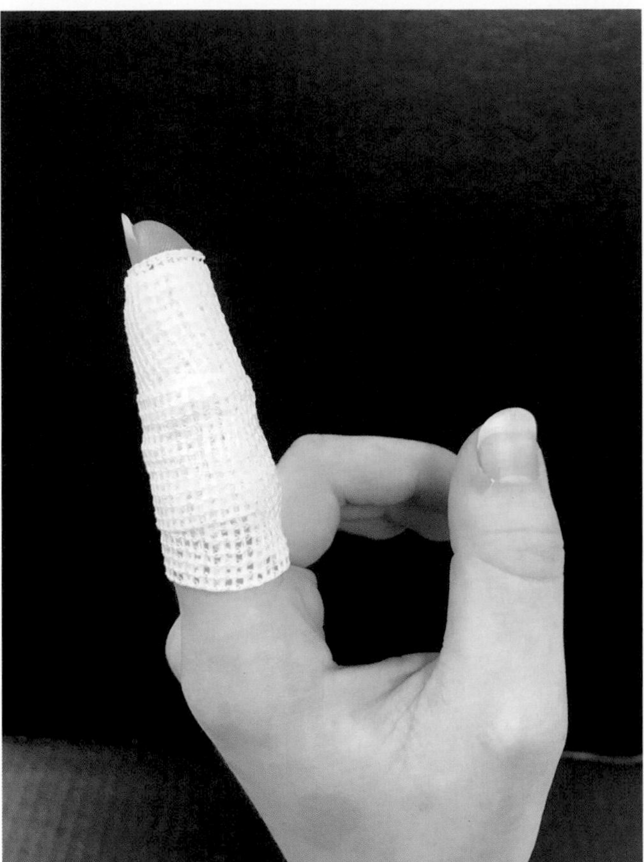

Figure 22-39. Quick Cast digit extension orthosis.

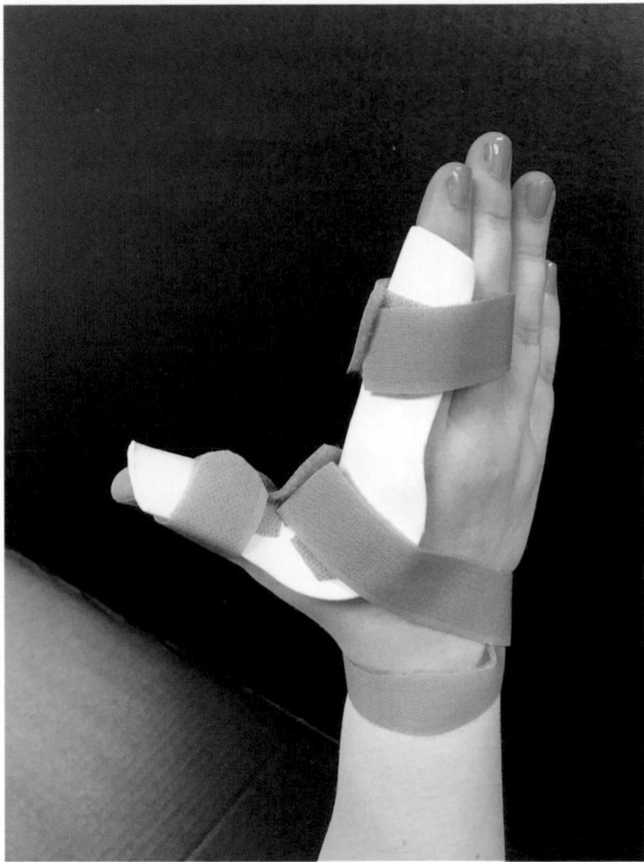

Figure 22-40. Web spacer orthosis.

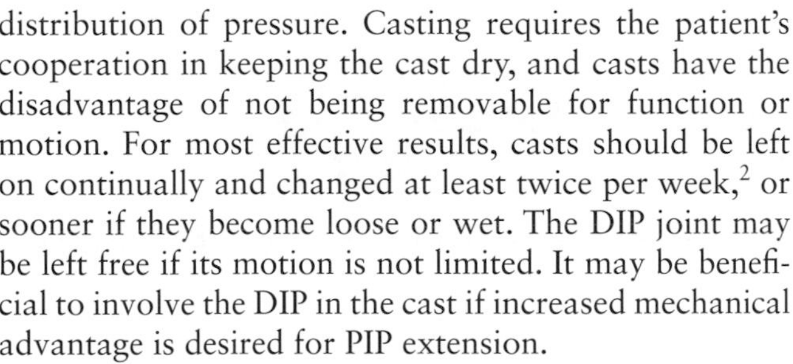

distribution of pressure. Casting requires the patient's cooperation in keeping the cast dry, and casts have the disadvantage of not being removable for function or motion. For most effective results, casts should be left on continually and changed at least twice per week,[2] or sooner if they become loose or wet. The DIP joint may be left free if its motion is not limited. It may be beneficial to involve the DIP in the cast if increased mechanical advantage is desired for PIP extension.

Adduction contractures of the thumb, which are commonly seen in burns and median nerve injuries, are most often treated with serial static thumb abduction orthoses, which conform to the first web space (Fig. 22-40). It is important to ensure that abduction forces are directed to the CMC joint by involving as much of the distal aspect of the first metacarpal as possible.[4] Strapping must be designed to apply pressure in the proper direction and to prevent distal migration of the orthosis. This often requires a strap that crosses the wrist.

Substitute for Weak or Absent Muscles

Orthoses are commonly used to assist patients in maximizing the functional use of an affected upper extremity. Orthoses may be used temporarily, as in the case of recovering nerve injuries or neurological diseases such as Guillain-Barré, or they may be prescribed for long-term use, such as in complete spinal cord injury or progressive neuromuscular conditions like amyotrophic lateral sclerosis. They are generally worn only during the day or for specific functional tasks. An orthosis that is successful in improving the ability to function is often much more accepted and appreciated by the patients than orthoses prescribed for other purposes.

Substitute for Weak or Absent Shoulder or Elbow Muscles

A MAS (Fig. 22-41) can support the shoulder and forearm to encourage motion of weak proximal musculature, allow for distal function against gravity, and enable occupational performance as well as prevent loss of motion and provide pain relief. Contraindications to use include glenohumeral joint instability, and care must be taken to ensure that the humeral head does not sublux or impinge on the supraspinatus when the arm is in the device.

A MAS is a mechanical device that supports the weight of the arm and provides assistance to shoulder and elbow motions through a linkage of ball-bearing joints.[58] The MAS is either powered or nonpowered and is typically mounted to a patient's wheelchair, but it can also be attached to a tabletop or even a floor stand for trial use. The mechanical principles are threefold: (1) use

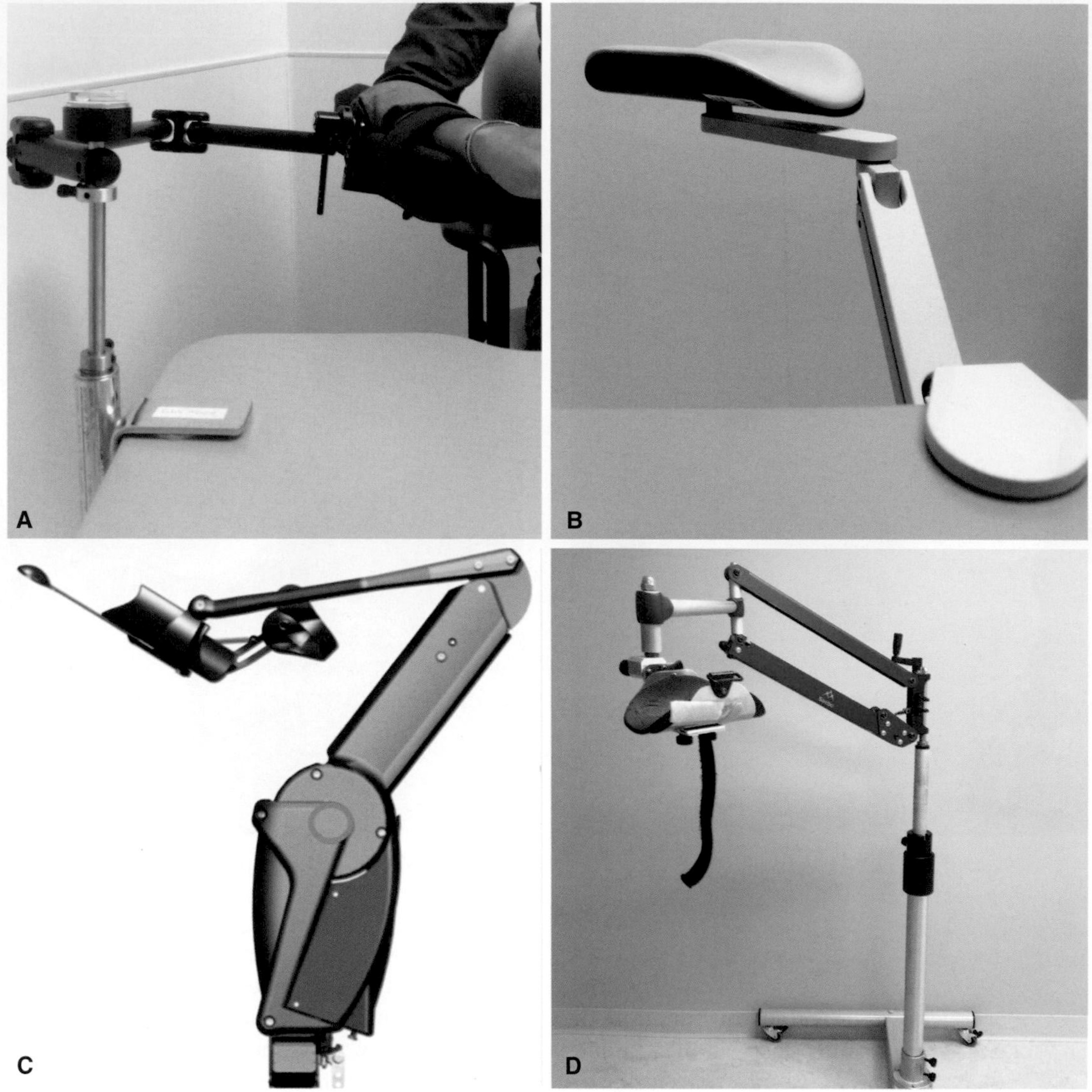

Figure 22-41. Mobile arm supports: In order of low to high complexity, the arm supports are listed left to right, top to bottom: **A.** Ergorest arm support. **B.** Jaeco nonelevating mobile arm support. **C.** SaeboMAS mobile arm support, typically used in clinical sessions for remediation. **D.** 0540 powered arm support, mounted on the person's power wheelchair in place of the armrest for consistent support. (Courtesy of Cara E. Masselink, MS, OTR/L, ATP.)

of gravity to assist weak muscles, (2) support of the arm to reduce the load on weak muscles, and (3) reduction of friction by ball-bearing joints. The MAS may be nonelevating or elevating and may be used in clinical intervention or compensation during occupations. Criteria for use include:

- A defined functional need
- An adequate source of power from the neck, trunk, shoulder girdle, or elbow muscles
- Adequate motor control such that the patient can contract and relax functioning muscles
- Sufficient passive joint ROM, with 0° to 90° of shoulder flexion and abduction, 0° to 30° of external rotation, full internal rotation and elbow flexion, and 0° to 80° of pronation preferred
- Stable trunk positioning
- A motivated patient
- A supportive environment that provides the patient with the opportunity and assistance to use the device

Patients who may benefit include those with cervical spinal cord injury,[18] muscular dystrophy, Guillain-Barré syndrome, amyotrophic lateral sclerosis, poliomyelitis, and polymyositis. The benefits of MASs include[18,59]:

- Opportunity for movement and decreased risk of joint contractures
- Supported use of upper quadrant to improve available strength
- Improved posture
- Decreased compensatory movements

- Increased independence in many activities of daily living
- Increased social participation
- Improved confidence

It is also important to note the psychological factors impacted by the use of a MAS. Patients report improved independence and confidence as a result of performing additional activities. Patients also report improved performance of intimate tasks such as hugging or shaking hands.[59]

Selection of MAS components, assembly of parts, and balance and adjustment of the MAS generally require additional training. Therefore, to fit and educate a patient on the use of a MAS, either additional training or consultation with an experienced therapist to ensure the best possible fit to provide the patient with the maximal mechanical advantage is needed.

Substitute for Weak or Absent Wrist or Hand Muscles

The combination of sensory loss and motor imbalance due to a peripheral nerve injury greatly impairs normal hand function. It is impossible to build an external device that can substitute for the intricately balanced muscles that an orthosis attempts to replace.[3] In supporting nerve palsies with an orthosis, the key concept is to understand the patient's condition and neuromuscular status so as to prescribe or design an appropriate orthosis to increase function. Orthoses should keep areas of intact sensibility free if possible, should be as simple as possible, and should not immobilize joints unnecessarily. The orthosis program must be closely monitored and altered in response to nerve recovery as the patient's muscle status changes. In a study to assess factors that influenced orthosis wear in peripheral nerve lesions, the only significant variable was a positive effect as perceived by the patient; 52% of patients reported terminating wear because the orthosis hindered their daily life and 23% reported terminating wear because the orthosis had not been of any use. Interestingly, the highest effectiveness score was for day orthoses for the dominant hand aimed at replacing function.[60]

Radial nerve palsy, commonly associated with humeral fractures, can result in the complete loss or partial weakness of wrist, finger, and thumb extensors and weakness of forearm supination and thumb abduction. The loss of wrist extensor strength devastates hand grasp. Not only is the patient unable to position the hand properly, but the inability to stabilize the wrist in extension impairs normal function of the long finger flexors. Loss of extrinsic finger extension is much less of a functional problem because the unaffected intrinsic muscles can actively extend the IPs. Supporting the wrist in extension is the primary goal of an orthosis for radial nerve palsy, and the use of a simple static wrist orthosis may suffice in improving hand function.[4]

There are many prefabricated radial nerve orthoses as well as custom orthosis designs available to dynamically extend the wrist, MCPs, and thumb (Fig. 22-27). It is usually preferable not to include the thumb because of the limitation in intrinsic motion it imposes and the danger of stressing the MP collateral ligament through poorly directed forces. Caution should be used when prescribing a dynamic orthosis because strong unopposed flexors may easily overcome the dynamic forces trying to hold the wrist and hand in extension, negating functional benefits.

A custom-fabricated radial nerve orthosis, also known as a Colditz orthosis, is designed to allow for partial wrist and full finger motion and a facsimile of a normal tenodesis effect. This orthosis consists of a low-profile outrigger attached to a dorsal forearm base. Nonelastic cords connect the orthosis base to finger loops. The cord length is adjusted so that, when the MCPs actively flex, the wrist is brought into extension. Conversely, when the wrist flexes, the cord tension causes the MCPs to extend. Minimal training is required for the patient to be able to use the orthosis functionally, and grasp and release of objects is greatly enhanced. Further advantages of this orthosis are the maintenance of normal hand arches, the absence of thermoplastic material covering the palm, the low-profile design, and the facilitation of wrist extensor strength as return of nerve function occurs.[3] Preformed orthoses and outrigger kits are commercially available.

Orthosis use following median nerve palsy is geared toward substituting for weak or absent thenar muscles that render the thumb unable to pull away from the palm and oppose to the fingers. This is most often accomplished through a custom-fabricated thermoplastic opponens orthosis that stabilizes the thumb in a position of abduction and opposition to enable pulp-to-pulp pinch (Fig. 22-16). Although such an orthosis often greatly improves fine motor prehension, this must be individually assessed because substitution patterns from unaffected thumb muscles may provide sufficient thumb function.[3,4] Patients may choose to wear an orthosis for opposition for selected activities only.

In the presence of ulnar nerve palsy, the hand assumes a claw position, or intrinsic-minus position, with ring and small finger hyperextension of the MCPs and flexion of the IPs. This is a result of weakness or loss of lumbrical and interossei muscles, which are responsible for MCP flexion and IP extension. The prime objective of an orthosis is to assist in grasp and release of objects by preventing the claw position. This is accomplished by an anticlaw orthosis, which blocks the MCPs in slight flexion, allowing the force of the unaffected long finger extensors to extend the IPs.

Dynamic orthoses, such as prefabricated spring wire orthoses, do not work well because the spring tension is usually not sufficient to hold the MCPs in flexion when the patient actively opens the hand. Thus, the MCPs hyperextend against the force, which actually strengthens the long extensors and encourages deformity.[3]

A static custom-fabricated thermoplastic orthosis is advocated as the best solution. It should be nonbulky, carefully molded to distribute pressure evenly over the dorsum of the proximal phalanges, and designed so as not to obstruct full flexion of all joints.[3,4] The orthosis may include just the affected ring and small fingers (Fig. 22-6) or may include all fingers to distribute pressure more effectively and comfortably. An orthosis is also used in the treatment of combined median and ulnar nerve injuries, resulting in the clawing of all four fingers and limitations in thumb abduction (Fig. 22-7).

Static orthoses, which allow passive holding of functional implements such as utensils or pens, may also be used in the presence of wrist or hand weakness. A hand-based universal cuff (Fig. 22-42), a wrist support with a universal cuff, and a short or long design Wanchik Writer orthosis are examples of these orthoses.

Orthoses may also be used to facilitate distal motion and motor reeducation in neurologically impaired upper extremities. The SaeboFlex (Fig. 22-43) dynamic orthosis uses a fixed wrist support and a finger/thumb spring system that assists with opening the hand during grasp-and-release activities. The Ness H200 Hand Rehabilitation System (Fig. 22-44) supports the wrist in a functional position and uses low-level electrical stimulation to assist finger and thumb motion. Specialty training in fitting and use of these devices is required, and evidence of their efficacy is limited, pending more independent studies.[61,62]

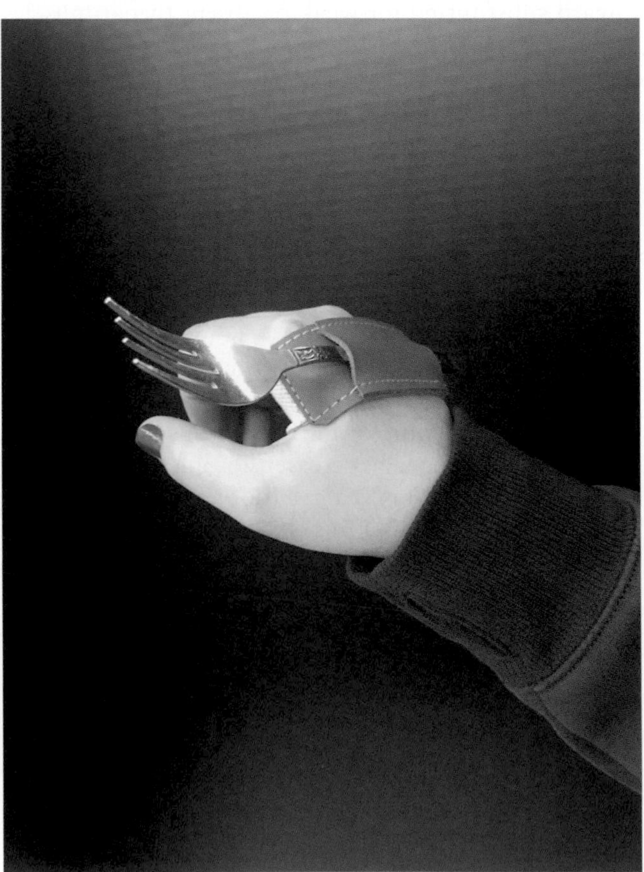

Figure 22-42. Hand-based universal cuff used to secure fork for self-feeding.

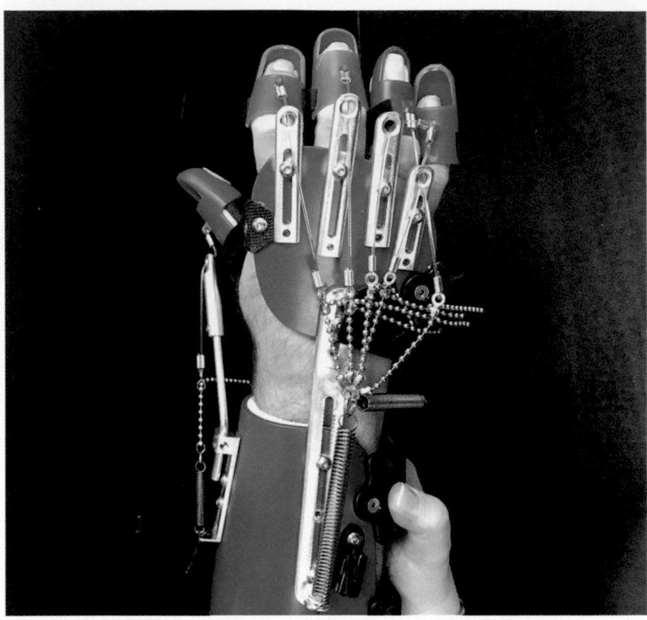

Figure 22-43. SaeboFlex orthosis—Uses dynamic forces to assist with release with allowing grasp to enable return to purposeful activities.

Prevent Contractures or Modify Tone

Careful attention to positioning in the presence of wound healing, muscle imbalance, abnormal muscle tone due to stroke or brain injury, or motor disorders such as cerebral palsy is critical in the prevention of loss of ROM, which can lead to functional or skin hygiene problems. Many of the static orthoses and casts previously mentioned for immobilization, stabilization, or substitution can be used for this purpose. Examples of these orthoses include acute burn immobilization orthosis to prevent wrist and digital contractures, wrist extension orthoses to

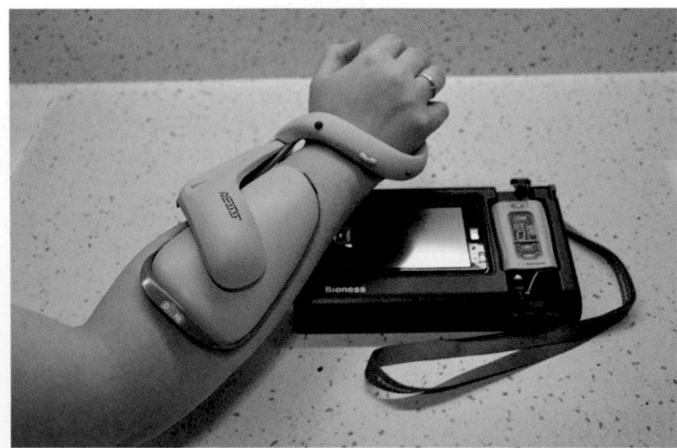

Figure 22-44. Ness H200—Device uses a low-level electrical stimulation to activate weak or paralyzed muscles within the forearm to improve hand function.

prevent contractures caused by wrist drop, thumb abduction orthoses to prevent thumb adduction contractures, and anticlaw orthoses to prevent MCP hyperextension and IP flexion contractures. Lapboards, arm troughs, and suspension arm slings can help to position the upper extremities properly. Bivalved plaster casts or anteroposterior orthoses can be used to maintain ROM, especially in the presence of increased tone. Care must be taken to avoid pressure problems by ensuring that casts are properly padded and that the skin is closely monitored.

Ideally, these orthoses should not limit function, exert excessive stress on soft tissues, or interfere with movement of uninvolved joints. If orthoses are not required for functional use, it is often possible for patients to wear static immobilization orthoses at night only. In addition to the prevention of contractures, orthoses may be used to prevent shortening of the muscle–tendon unit. For example, a volar thermoplastic orthosis worn at night to position the wrist and fingers in maximum composite extension can help to prevent extrinsic tightness of the long finger flexors.[2]

The use of orthoses in the modification of tone in the wrist and hand continues to be controversial in the literature and in practice. Opponents of orthosis use argue that an orthosis may lead to increased muscle tone, joint stiffness, and muscle atrophy and may interfere with treatment aimed at facilitation and functional use. Proponents of orthosis use contend that an orthosis can reduce tone and prevent joint contracture. In a systematic review of hand orthosis use to prevent contracture and reduce spasticity following stroke, Lannin and Herbert found insufficient evidence to either support or refute its effectiveness.[63] Tyson and Kent concluded from their systematic review that current evidence suggests orthosis use does not improve function, motion, or pain following stroke.[64] Garros et al. also studied a volar dorsal orthosis worn by patients with wrist and hand spasticity poststroke.[65] The results showed an increase in patient-rated occupational performance at 3 months, but no long-term follow-up was done.

Common static orthosis designs include resting pan orthoses, finger spreaders or abduction orthoses, and cone orthoses.[13] Several prefabricated orthoses are commercially available, but no clinical studies have been done to establish their fit and effectiveness.

Efficacy and Outcomes

Although the use of upper extremity orthoses is an accepted practice with much clinical and intuitive support, the state of best evidence about upper extremity orthoses is limited (see the Evidence table at the end of this chapter). Good, valid studies of current practice are needed to enhance our knowledge of orthosis use efficacy and variables that lead to optimum outcomes.

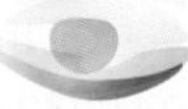

CASE STUDY

Patient Information

Tom, a 25-year-old full-time graduate student, has sustained a shaft fracture of his left dominant hand small finger metacarpal (MCP) following a fall on the ice when walking his dog. The fracture is 10 days old and stable. His performance patters include the roles of a full-time graduate student, a part-time employee as a server at a local restaurant, a son, and a brother. His leisure activities include bike riding, snowboarding, reading, and playing guitar. Tom lives with two other students in a small campus apartment. Tom was referred to occupational therapy for custom orthosis fabrication and treatment to address limits in active ROM and edema.

Initial Assessment

The Disabilities of Arm Shoulder and Hand Questionnaire (DASH) was administered to identify patient factors impacted by the injury. The DASH is a 30-item self-report questionnaire used to measure symptom and function in people with musculoskeletal disorders.[66] Tom's score indicated that he was 65% disabled for activity and participation. The DASH prompted discussion regarding several functional activities that are limited and are important to him. He complained of difficulty writing, using the keyboard for school tasks, grasping plates and cups for work tasks, preparing meal, and playing the guitar. At the time of the initial occupational therapy evaluation, the fracture healing is in the primary callus formation state of osteoblastic activity and that pain-free active ROM out of orthosis is allowed. Active ROM was assessed, and limitations were noted at the wrist in all planes, the MCP, PIP, and DIP joints of the long, ring, and small fingers. Total active motion (TAM) for the long finger was 210°, 195° for the ring finger and 185° for the small finger. The patient demonstrated 35° of wrist extension, 30° of wrist flexion, 15° of radial deviation, and 15° of ulnar deviation. Edema was noted at the dorsum of the hand and also in the digits. Measurements were taken with a tape measure to objectively assess edema. Fine motor coordination was assessed using the 9 Hole Peg test with limitations noted in speed—requiring 20.90 seconds for the left dominant involved hand and only 17.83 seconds for the right hand. The thumb, index finger, and middle finger can be used for nonresistive pinch activities. Resistive activities are restricted until there is evidence of bone healing. Therefore, hand strength was not assessed during the initial evaluation. Patient complains of a pain level of 6/10 at the fracture site.

Occupational Therapy Problem List

- Tom requires increased time to complete school-related tasks, such as typing and writing.

(continued)

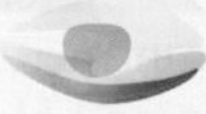

CASE STUDY *(continued)*

- Tom is unable to perform the required work tasks of a server and is currently working seating customers instead.
- Tom requires increased time to complete basic activities of daily living and is unable to squeeze a shampoo bottle and fasten his pants.
- Tom complains of difficulty sleeping secondary to hand pain.
- Tom is unable to play the guitar secondary to restrictions.
- Tom requires minimal assistance for meal preparation tasks to open jars, cut meat and vegetables, and lift pots and pans.

Occupational Therapy Goals

- Tom will be independent with donning and doffing orthosis in 1 week.
- Tom will demonstrate at least 240° TAM including three joint flexion of long, ring, and small fingers for use to hold small objects in his palm within 4 weeks.
- Tom will report a pain level of no greater than 2/10 to be able to sleep through the night within 2 weeks.
- Tom will perform meal preparation with modified independence within 6 weeks.
- Tom will return to work part time as a server within 8 weeks.
- With increased strength and ROM, Tom will independently squeeze shampoo bottle within 8 weeks.

Occupational Therapy Intervention

The occupational therapist fabricated a wrist hand finger immobilization orthosis (Fig. 22-45) to include the ring and small finger. This forearm-based orthosis protects the site of the fracture with support to both the palmar and dorsal aspects of the hand with the wrist in 20° to 30° of extension, the MCP joints in 70° of flexion, and the IP joints in full extension. Tom was educated in the care of the orthosis and how to don and doff the orthosis. At this time, Tom is required to wear the orthosis for all activities and while sleeping. Tom can remove the orthosis five times per day to perform recommended exercises. During treatment, the orthosis is monitored for correct fit because adjustments will be needed as dorsal hand edema subsides. Occupation-based interventions are directed to improve his performance to return to his activities of daily living, work, school, and leisure tasks.

Tom is provided a home exercise program that includes tendon gliding exercises and active ROM for his wrist. These exercises should assist in decreasing edema, but Tom is also educated in edema management techniques such as elevation and the use of a compression glove.

Owing to precautions related to fracture healing, Tom's performance of functional tasks is restricted. Most activities will be performed using his uninvolved, nondominant extremity. Tom is able to use his involved, dominant extremity for nonresistive tasks using his thumb, index, and long fingers. Adaptive occupation is addressed through the use of assisted devices or modifications.

Progress

Because there is physiological evidence of callus formation that usually occurs between 4 and 6 weeks, Tom's orthosis is modified from forearm based to hand based. Bone callus formation indicates bone maturation and strength, and with this information, there is a corresponding change in the expectation of use and the patient's occupational capacity is increased. Tom is able to remove the orthosis for light activities of daily living, including showering, keyboard use, cell phone use, and light dressing tasks.

Active ROM was assessed to monitor progress. TAM of digits increased to 230° of the long finger, 215° of the ring, and 208° of the small. Wrist flexion increased to 45°, extension increased to 42°, radial deviation increased to 22°, and ulnar deviation increased to 25°. Tom also demonstrates a decrease in edema, a decrease in reports of pain to 3/10, and improved fine motor coordination with a decrease in time required to complete the 9 Hole Peg test in 18.65 seconds.

Following evidence of clinical union confirmed by x-ray (usually 6–8 weeks following fracture), Tom's hand strength can be assessed, and he can begin to use his dominant hand for resistive tasks. The orthosis is typically discontinued at this time. Tom is able to return to work as a server and all other resistive functional tasks such as playing the guitar, riding his bike, and preparing meals.

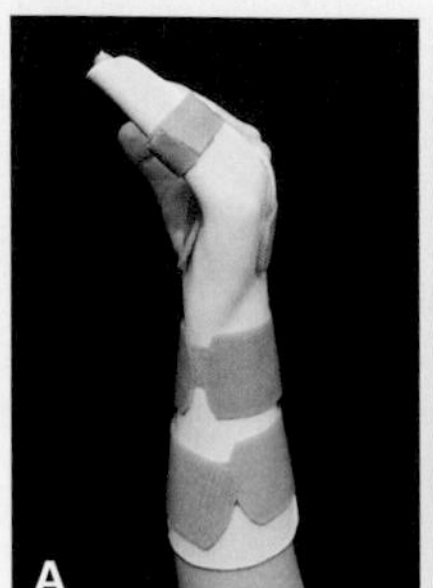

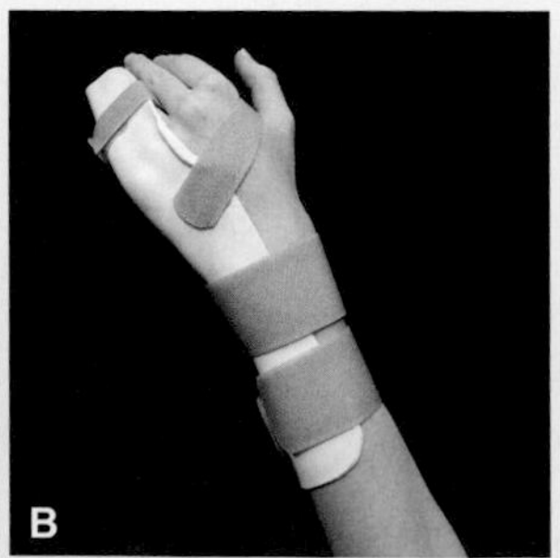

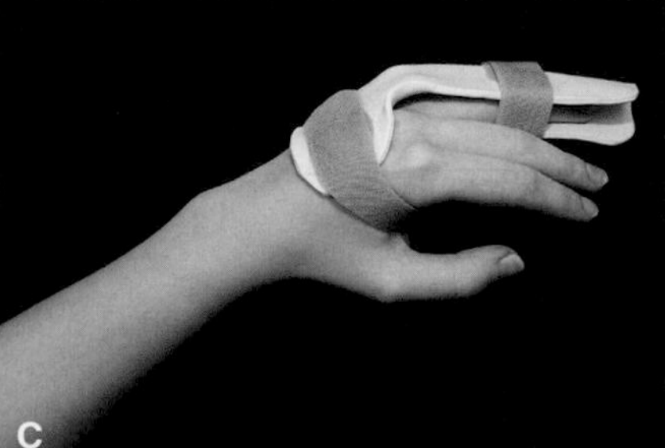

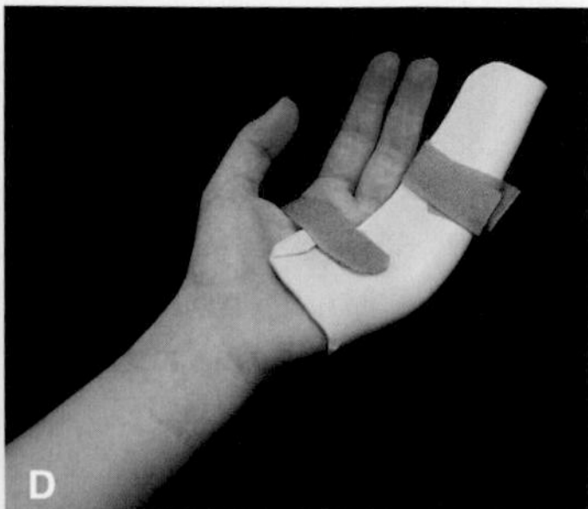

Figure 22-45. Forearm-based immobilization orthosis for metacarpal fracture. **A, B.** Wrist is in slight extension, and ring and small fingers are immobilized in metacarpophalangeal (MCP) flexion and interphalangeal (IP) full extension to protect fracture for approximately 4 weeks. **C, D.** Hand-based immobilization orthosis with MCP in flexion and IP joints to ring and small fingers in full extension to protect fracture for 4 to 8 weeks dependent on activity.

Best Evidence for Use of Orthotics as Intervention

Intervention	Description of Intervention	Participants	Dosage	Level of Evidence	Benefit	Statistical Probability and Effect Size
Immobilization orthosis for thumb OA[67]	Different types of orthosis and designs	Fourteen publications including a total of 580 subjects	At least 2 weeks of orthosis use was recommended.	Systematic review; Level I evidence	Immobilization of the CMC joint is effective regardless of design and reduces pain and improves function.	Impact of orthosis use on hand strength was inconclusive. Significant effect was noted with reduction in pain and improved hand function. Analysis of results was not reported secondary to variances in studies.
Treatment strategies for treatment of thumb OA[68]	OA treatment strategies: joint protection, CMC immobilization orthosis, thumb isometric exercises	Sixty subjects	6-Week treatment program, including orthosis use, exercises, assistive device education, and joint protection education	Pre–post design; Level II evidence	Statistical and clinical differences were noted in pain, ROM, and functional use.	80% power established with sample size. Significant improvements in pain ($p < 0.0001$), active motion (right $p = 0.003$, left $p = 0.0001$), and Canadian Occupational Performance Measure (COPM) ($p = 0.0001$).
Wrist orthosis and patient education as treatment for carpal tunnel syndrome[69]	Effects of wearing a wrist support orthosis and receiving education on activities, which increase pressure in the carpal tunnel	Random assignment: 30 in treatment and 24 in control group	Intervention group: 8 weeks orthosis use and patient education (150 minutes of treatment time)	Randomized controlled trial; Level I evidence	Benefits were noted with improved grip strength, decreased pain, improved sensation, and improved function.	Power and effect sizes were not reported. Significant differences found in post-test of intervention group with the Boston Carpal Tunnel Questionnaire ($p = 0.001$), visual analog scale (VAS) ($p = 0.001$), Phalen's test ($p = 0.031$), grip strength ($p = 0.020$), Purdue Pegboard ($p = 0.021$), and monofilament test ($p < 0.001$).

(continued)

Best Evidence for Use of Orthotics as Intervention (*continued*)

Intervention	Description of Intervention	Participants	Dosage	Level of Evidence	Benefit	Statistical Probability and Effect Size
Orthosis intervention for thumb OA thumb CMC[38]	Effectiveness of custom-fabricated orthosis and prefabricated orthoses to reduce pain	469 subjects in 12 studies	Orthotic wear for 2 weeks up to 7 years, various wearing schedules	Systematic review of 12 studies published in 2000 or later; Level I evidence	Significant decrease in pain at short term ($\leq$45 days) and long term ($\geq$3 months)	Significantly reduction in hand pain at short-term (<3 months) and long-term ($\geq$3 months) follow-up, with a standardized mean difference of 0.37 (95% confidence interval [95% CI] 0.03, 0.71) and 0.80 (95% CI 0.45, 1.15). Unable to determine effects size because of lack of homogeneity of study design, methods, and orthosis design.
Orthosis intervention and therapy for thumb CMC OA[70]	Hand orthosis and therapy benefits over time; baseline, 6 weeks, 3 months, and 12 months	122 subjects	Subjects were provided an orthosis for use and therapy to include a home exercise program and education in appropriate pinch patterns. Specific dosage varied between subjects. Subjects were treated for up to 12 weeks, 2 times per week.	Prospective observation cohort; longitudinal; Level II evidence	Improvement in pain and function. Fifteen percent of subjects eventually sought surgical intervention after 2.2 years.	Reports of pain in last week decreased from 49 to 36 over 12 months on a VAS, $p < 0.05$. Reports of pain with activity decreased from 60 to 21 over 12 months, $p < 0.05$. Michigan Hand Questionnaire (MHQ) scores decreased from 65 to 69 ($p < 0.05$), which was not clinically relevant.

References

1. Centers for Medicaid and Medicare. Durable medical equipment, prosthetics, orthotics, and supplies (DMEPOS) quality standards. https://www.cms.gov/Medicare/Provider-Enrollment-and-Certification/MedicareProviderSupEnroll/downloads/dmeposaccreditationstandards.pdf. Published 2008. Accessed August 22, 2018.
2. Bell-Krotoski J. Tissue remodeling and contracture correction using serial plaster casting and orthotic positioning. In: Skirven T, Osterman A, Fedorczyk J, Amadio P, eds. *Rehabilitation of the Hand and Upper Extremity*. 6th ed. Philadelphia, PA: Mosby; 2011:1599–1609.
3. Colditz JC. Therapist's management of the stiff hand. In: Skirven TM, Osterman AL, Fedorczyk JM, Amadio PC, eds. *Rehabilitation of the Hand and Upper Extremity*. 6th ed. Philadelphia, PA: Mosby; 2011:894–921.
4. Fess EE, Gettle KS, Phillips CA, Janson JR. *Hand and Upper Extremity Splinting: Principles and Methods*. 3rd ed. St Louis, MO: Mosby; 2005.
5. Bell-Krotoski J, Breger-Stanton D. The forces of dynamic orthotic position: ten questions to ask before applying a dynamic orthosis to the hand. In: Skirven T, Osterman A, Fedorczyk J, Amadio P, eds. *Rehabilitation of the Hand and Upper Extremity*. Philadelphia, PA: Elsevier Mosby; 2011. doi:10.1016/B978-0-323-05602-1.00123-9.
6. Flowers KR, Lastayo PC. Effect of total end range time on improving passive range of motion. *J Hand Ther*. 2012;25(1):48–55. doi:10.1016/j.jht.2011.12.003.
7. Fess EE. Orthoses for mobilization of joints: principles and methods. In: Skirven T, Osterman A, Fedorczyk J, Amadio P, eds. *Rehabilitation of the Hand and Upper Extremity*. 6th ed. Philadelphia, PA: Elsevier Mosby; 2011. doi:10.1016/B978-0-323-05602-1.00124-0.
8. Glasgow C, Tooth LR, Fleming J, Peters S. Dynamic splinting for the stiff hand after trauma: predictors of contracture resolution. *J Hand Ther*. 2011;24(3):195–206. doi:10.1016/j.jht.2011.03.001.
9. Healthcare Common Procedure Coding System. 2018 HCPCS L codes. https://www.hcpcsdata.com/Codes/L. Published 2018. Accessed November 6, 2018.
10. Webster JB, Murphy D. *Atlas of Orthoses and Assistive Devices*. 5th ed. Philadelphia, PA: Elsevier; 2018.
11. McKee PR, Rivard A. Biopsychosocial approach to orthotic intervention. *J Hand Ther*. 2011;24(2):155-163. doi:10.1016/j.jht.2010.08.001.
12. McKee PR, Rivard A. Foundations of orthotic intervention. In: Skirven T, Osterman A, Fedorczyk J, Amadiio P, eds. *Rehabilitation of the Hand and Upper Extremity*. Philadelphia, PA: Elsevier Mosby; 2011:1565–1580.
13. Amini D, Rider D. Occupation-based splinting. In: Coppard B, Lohman H, eds. *Introduction to Splinting: A Clinical Reasoning and Problem-Solving Approach*. 3rd ed. St Louis, MO: Mosby; 2008:15–28.
14. O'Brien L. Adherence to therapeutic splint wear in adults with acute upper limb injuries: a systematic review. *Hand Ther*. 2010;15(1):3–12. doi:10.1258/ht.2009.009025.
15. Cole T, Robinson L, Romero L, O'Brien L. Effectiveness of interventions to improve therapy adherence in people with upper limb conditions: a systematic review. *J Hand Ther*. 2017;32:175–183.
16. Kielhofner G. *Conceptual Foundations of Occupational Therapy Practice*. 4th ed. Philadelphia, PA: F.A. Davis; 2009.
17. Nelson D, Jepson-Thomas J. Occupational form, occupational performance, and a conceptual framework for therapeutic occupation. In: Kramer P, Hinojosa J, Brasic C, eds. *Perspectives on Human Occupation: Participation in Life*. Baltimore, MD: Lippincott Williams & Wilkins; 2003:87–155.
18. Atkins MS, Baumgarten JM, Yasuda YL, et al. Mobile arm supports: evidence-based benefits and criteria for use. *J Spinal Cord Med*. 2008;31(4):388–393.
19. Nadler M, Pauls MMH. Shoulder orthoses for the prevention and reduction of hemiplegic shoulder pain and subluxation: systematic review. *Clin Rehabil*. 2017;31(4):444–453. doi:10.1177/0269215516648753.
20. Paci M, Nannetti L, Rinaldi LA. Glenohumeral subluxation in hemiplegia: an overview. *J Rehabil Res Dev*. 2005;42(4):557. doi:10.1682/JRRD.2004.08.0112.
21. Ada L, Foongchomcheay A, Canning C. Supportive devices for preventing and treating subluxation of the shoulder after stroke. *Cochrane Database Syst Rev*. 2005;(1):CD003863. doi:10.1002/14651858.CD003863.pub2.
22. Stolzenberg D, Siu G, Cruz E. Current and future interventions for glenohumeral subluxation in hemiplegia secondary to stroke. *Top Stroke Rehabil*. 2012;19(5):444–456. doi:10.1310/tsr1905-444.
23. Fedorczyk J. Elbow tendinopathies: clinical presentation and therapist's management of tennis elbow. In: Skirven T, Osterman A, Fedorczyk J, Amadio P, eds. *Rehabilitation of the Hand and Upper Extremity*. 6th ed. Philadelphia, PA: Mosby; 2011:1098–1108.
24. Borkholder CD, Hill VA, Fess EE. The efficacy of splinting for lateral epicondylitis: a systematic review. *J Hand Ther*. 2004;17:181–199. doi:10.1197/j.jht.2004.02.007.
25. Jafarian FS, Demneh ES, Tyson SF. The immediate effect of orthotic management on grip strength of patients with lateral epicondylosis. *J Orthop Sports Phys Ther*. 2009;39(6):484–489. doi:10.2519/jospt.2009.2988.
26. Garg R, Adamson GJ, Dawson PA, Shankwiler JA, Pink MM. A prospective randomized study comparing a forearm strap brace versus a wrist splint for the treatment of lateral epicondylitis. *J Shoulder Elbow Surg*. 2010;19(4):508–512. doi:10.1016/j.jse.2009.12.015.
27. Sadeghi-Demneh E, Jafarian F. The immediate effects of orthoses on pain in people with lateral epicondylalgia. *Pain Res Treat*. 2013;2013:353597. doi:10.1155/2013/353597.
28. Silva AC, Jones A, Silva PG, Natour J. Effectiveness of a night-time hand positioning splint in rheumatoid arthritis: a randomized controlled trial. *J Rehabil Med*. 2008;40(9):749–754. doi:10.2340/16501977-0240.
29. Collier SE, Thomas JJ. Range of motion at the wrist: a comparison study of four wrist extension orthoses and the free hand. *Am J Occup Ther*. 2002;56:180–184. doi:10.5014/ajot.56.2.180.
30. Evans RB. Therapist's management of carpal tunnel syndrome: a practical approach. In: Skirven T, Osterman A, Fedorczyk J, Amadio P, eds. *Rehabilitation of the Hand and Upper Extremity*. 6th ed. Philadelphia, PA: Mosby; 2011:666–667. doi:10.1016/B978-0-323-05602-1.00107-0.

31. Cha YJ. Changements de la distribution de la pression selon les angles du poignet et la posture des mains dans une orthèse de poignet. *Hand Surg Rehabil.* 2018;37(1):38–42. doi:10.1016/j.hansur.2017.09.007.
32. Piazzini DB, Aprile I, Ferrara PE, et al. A systematic review of conservative treatment of carpal tunnel syndrome. *Clin Rehabil.* 2007;21(4):299–314. doi:10.1177/0269215507077294.
33. Lohman H. Thumb immobilization splints. In: Coppard B, Lohman H, eds. *Introduction to Splinting: A Clinical Reasoning and Problem-Solving Approach.* 3rd ed. St Louis, MO: Mosby; 2008:156–187.
34. Weiss S, Lastayo P, Mills A, Bramlet D. Splinting the degenerative basal joint: custom-made or prefabricated neoprene? *J hand Ther.* 2004;17(4):401–406.
35. Sillem H, Backman CL, Miller WC, Li LC. Comparison of two carpometacarpal stabilizing splints for individuals with thumb osteoarthritis. *J Hand Ther.* 2011;24(3):216–225; quiz 126; discussion 227-30. doi:10.1016/j.jht.2010.12.004.
36. Bani M, Arazpour M. Comparison of custom-made and prefabricated neoprene splinting in patients with the first carpometacarpal joint osteoarthritis. *Disabil Rehabil Assist Technol.* 2013;8(3):232–237. doi:10.3109/17483107.2012.699992.
37. Egan MY, Brousseau L. Splinting for osteoarthritis of the carpometacarpal joint: a review of the evidence. *Am J Occup Ther.* 2007;61(1):70–78. doi:10.5014/ajot.61.1.70.
38. Kjeken I, Smedslund G, Moe RH, Slatkowsky-Christensen B, Uhlig T, Hagen KB. Systematic review of design and effects of splints and exercise programs in hand osteoarthritis. *Arthritis Care Res.* 2011;63(6):834–848. doi:10.1002/acr.20427.
39. Beasley J. Therapist's examination and conservative management of arthritis of the upper extremity. In: Skirven T, Osterman A, Fedorczyk J, Amadio P, eds. *Rehabilitation of the Hand and Upper Extremity, 2-Volume Set.* 6th ed. Philadelphia, PA: Mosby; 2011:1330–1343.e2. doi:10.1016/B978-0-323-05602-1.00103-3.
40. Harrell P. Splinting of the hand. In: Bartlett S, ed. *Clinical Care in the Rheumatic Diseases.* 3rd ed. Atlanta, GA: Association of Rheumatology Health Professionals; 2006:261–266.
41. Ekholm R, Tidermark J, Törnkvist H, Adami J, Ponzer S. Outcome after closed functional treatment of humeral shaft fractures. *J Orthop Trauma.* 2006;20(9):591–596. doi:10.1097/01.bot.0000246466.01287.04.
42. Koch PP, Gross DFL, Gerber C. The results of functional (Sarmiento) bracing of humeral shaft fractures. *J Shoulder Elbow Surg.* 2002;11(2):143–150. doi:10.1067/mse.2002.121634.
43. Pettengill KM. Therapist's management of the complex injury. In: Skirven T, Osterman A, Fedorczyk J, Amadio P, eds. *Rehabilitation of the Hand and Upper Extremity.* 6th ed. Philadelphia, PA: Mosby; 2011:1238–1251.
44. Kamolz LP, Kitzinger HB, Karle B, Frey M. The treatment of hand burns. *Burns.* 2009;35(3):327–337. doi:10.1016/j.burns.2008.08.004.
45. Tufaro PA, Bondoc SL. Therapist's management of the burned hand. In: Skirven T, Osterman A, Fedorczyk J, Amadio P, eds. *Rehabilitation of the Hand and Upper Extremity.* 6th ed. Philadelphia, PA: Mosby; 2011. doi:10.1016/B978-0-323-05602-1.00026-X.
46. Pettengill KM, van Strien G. Postoperative management of flexor tendon injuries. In: Skirven TM, Osterman AL, Fedorczyk JM, Amadio PC, eds. *Rehabilitation of the Hand and Upper Extremity.* 6th ed. Philadelphia, PA: Mosby; 2011:457–478.
47. Evans RB. Clinical management of extensor tendon injuries: the therapist's perspective. In: Skirven T, Osterman A, Fedorczyk J, Amadio P, eds. *Rehabilitation of the Hand and Upper Extremity.* 6th ed. Philadelphia, PA: Mosby; 2011:521–554.
48. Pike J, Mulpuri K, Metzger M, Ng G, Wells N, Goetz T. Blinded, prospective, randomized clinical trial comparing volar, dorsal, and custom thermoplastic splinting in treatment of acute mallet finger. *J Hand Surg Am.* 2010;35(4):580–588. doi:10.1016/j.jhsa.2010.01.005.
49. Pitts DG, Fess EE. Orthoses: essential concepts. In: Cooper C, ed. *Fundamentals of Hand Therapy: Clinical Reasoning and Treatment Guidelines for Common Diagnoses of the Upper Extremity.* 2nd ed. St Louis, MO: Mosby; 2013:103.
50. Lubahn J, Wolfe T, Feldscher S. Joint replacement in the hand and wrist: surgery and therapy. In: Skirven T, Osterman A, Fedorczyk J, Amadio P, eds. *Rehabilitation of the Hand and Upper Extremity.* 6th ed. Philadelphia, PA: Mosby; 2011:1376–1407.
51. Lohman H. Splints acting on the wrist. In: Coppard B, Lohman H, eds. *Introduction to Splinting: A Clinical Reasoning and Problem-Solving Approach.* 3rd ed. St Louis, MO: Mosby; 2008:119–155.
52. Duff S V., Estilow T. Therapist's management of peripheral nerve injury. In: Skirven T, Osterman A, Fedorczyk J, Amadio P, eds. *Rehabilitation of the Hand and Upper Extremity, 2-Volume Set.* 6th ed. Philadelphia, PA: Mosby; 2011:619–633.e2. doi:10.1016/B978-0-323-05602-1.00045-3.
53. Zijlstra TR, Heijnsdijk-Rouwenhorst L, Rasker JJ. Silver ring splints improve dexterity in patients with rheumatoid arthritis. *Arthritis Care Res.* 2004;51(6):947–951. doi:10.1002/art.20816.
54. van der Giesen FJ, van Lankveld WJ, Kremers-Selten C, et al. Effectiveness of two finger splints for swan neck deformity in patients with rheumatoid arthritis: a randomized, crossover trial. *Arthritis Rheum.* 2009;61(8):1025–1031. doi:10.1002/art.24866.
55. Michlovitz SL, Harris BA, Watkins MP. Therapy interventions for improving joint range of motion: a systematic review. *J Hand Ther.* 2004;17(2):118–131. doi:10.1197/j.jht.2004.02.002.
56. Lannin NA, Novak I, Cusick A. A systematic review of upper extremity casting for children and adults with central nervous system motor disorders. *Clin Rehabil.* 2007;21(11):963–976. doi:10.1177/0269215507079141.
57. Glasgow C, Fleming J, Tooth LR, Hockey RL. The long-term relationship between duration of treatment and contracture resolution using dynamic orthotic devices for the stiff proximal interphalangeal joint: a prospective cohort study. *J Hand Ther.* 2012;25(1):38–47. doi:10.1016/j.jht.2011.09.006.
58. Mulcahey MJ. Upper limb orthoses for the person with spinal cord injury. In: Hsu JD, Michael JW, Fisk JR, eds. *AAOS Atlas of Orthoses and Assistive Devices.* 4th ed. Philadelphia, PA: Mosby; 2008:203–217.
59. Kumar A, Phillips MF. Use of powered mobile arm supports by people with neuromuscular conditions. *J Rehabil Res Dev.* 2013;50(1):61–70.

60. Paternostro-Sluga T, Keilani M, Posch M, Fialka-Moser V. Factors that influence the duration of splint wear in peripheral nerve lesions. *Am J Phys Med Rehabil*. 2003;82(2):86–95. doi:10.1097/01.PHM.0000046628.64857.59.
61. Alon G, Levitt AF, McCarthy PA. Functional electrical stimulation enhancement of upper extremity functional recovery during stroke rehabilitation: a pilot study. *Neurorehabil Neural Repair*. 2007;21(3):207–215. doi:10.1177/1545968306297871.
62. Farrell JF, Hoffman HB, Snyder JL, Giuliani CA, Bohannon RW. Orthotic aided training of the paretic upper limb in chronic stroke: results of a phase 1 trial. *NeuroRehabilitation*. 2007;22(2):99–103.
63. Lannin NA, Herbert RD. Is hand splinting effective for adults following stroke? A systematic review and methodological critique of published research. *Clin Rehabil*. 2003;17(8):807–816. doi:10.1191/0269215503cr682oa.
64. Tyson SF, Kent RM. The effect of upper limb orthotics after stroke: a systematic review. *NeuroRehabilitation*. 2011;28(1):29–36. doi:10.3233/NRE-2011-0629.
65. Garros D dos SC, Gagliardi RJ, Guzzo RAR. Evaluation of performance and personal satisfaction of the patient with spastic hand after using a volar dorsal orthosis. *Arq Neuropsiquiatr*. 2010;68(3):385–389.
66. Beaton DE, Davis A, Hudak PL, McConnell S. The DASH (Disabilities of the Arm, Shoulder and Hand) outcome measure: what do we know about it now? *Hand Ther*. 2001;6(4):109-118. doi:10.1177/175899830100600401.
67. de Almeida PHT, MacDermid J, Pontes TB, Dos Santos-Couto-Paz CC, Matheus JPC. Differences in orthotic design for thumb osteoarthritis and its impact on functional outcomes: a scoping review. *Prosthet Orthot Int*. 2017;41(4):323–335. doi:10.1177/0309364616661255.
68. Shankland B, Beaton D, Ahmed S, Nedelec B. Effects of client-centered multimodal treatment on impairment, function, and satisfaction of people with thumb carpometacarpal osteoarthritis. *J Hand Ther*. 2017;30(3):307–313. doi:10.1016/j.jht.2017.03.004.
69. Hall B, Lee HC, Fitzgerald H, Byrne B, Barton A, Lee AH. Investigating the effectiveness of full-time wrist splinting and education in the treatment of carpal tunnel syndrome: a randomized controlled trial. *Am J Occup Ther*. 2013;67(4):448–459. doi:10.5014/ajot.2013.006031.
70. Tsehaie J, Spekreijse KR, Wouters RM, et al. Outcome of a hand orthosis and hand therapy for carpometacarpal osteoarthritis in daily practice: a prospective cohort study. *J Hand Surg Am*. 2018;43(11):1000–1009.e1. doi:10.1016/j.jhsa.2018.04.014.

Acknowledgments

The authors acknowledge the following contributions:

- Cara Masselink: Figures 22-11 and 22-41
- Kristy McKamey: Figures 22-10 and 22-44
- Holly Greives: Figure 22-20
- Matt Oaks: Figures 22-28; 22-31
- BraceAbility: Figure 22-21
- Joint Active Systems: 22-33

The authors also thank the occupational therapy students at Western Michigan University in Grand Rapids for their assistance with several photos in this chapter.

Chapter 23

Upper Extremity Orthoses Fabrication

Nancy S. Hock

LEARNING OBJECTIVES

This chapter will allow the reader to:

1. Describe the anatomical, biomechanical, and mechanical principles applied to the construction of custom-fabricated orthoses.
2. List the primary reasons to use orthoses as a therapeutic intervention.
3. Recognize factors affecting compliance with orthoses.
4. Explain design, pattern-making, and construction for three custom-fabricated orthoses.
5. Describe the orthosis fabrication process.

CHAPTER OUTLINE

TERMINOLOGY

Custom-fabricated orthosis: an individually made device for a specific patient that is based on clinically determined measurements or tracings and involves the use of basic materials such as plastic, metal, leather, or cloth in uncut or unshaped sheets.

Custom-fit orthosis: a prefabricated device that is not manufactured for an individual and may need assembly, fitting, trimming, or molding.

Dynamic orthosis: a device that applies a mobile force with rubber bands or springs in one direction while allowing active motion in the opposite direction.

Fibroblastic phase: a stage of wound healing that follows the inflammatory phase, during which fibroblasts proliferate and initiate collagen production in the healing of tissues.

Inflammatory phase: a stage of wound healing immediately following injury or surgery, characterized by edema and infiltration of leukocytes and macrophages to begin healing tissue.

Maturation phase: a stage of wound healing that follows the fibroblastic phase, characterized by wound contraction, remodeling, and maturation of the healed tissues.

Orthosis: a device that is applied to the body to provide immobilization, avoid deformity, correct deformity, protect healing structures, limit motion, or to allow tissue proliferation and remodeling for the upper extremity.

Prefabricated orthosis: a device that is obtained off the shelf, but may require adjustment.

Splint: casts or strapping that are used to reduce fractures or dislocations; this term is used primarily by physicians or clinicians applying a cast.

Static progressive orthosis: a device designed to elongate soft tissue to decrease contractures through the application of incrementally adjusted static force to promote lengthening of contracted tissues.

Orthosis Fabrication Introduction

To effectively construct a hand **orthosis**, one must appreciate the significance, biomechanics, and anatomy of the human hand. Mary Reilly described the significance of hand function in her 1961 Eleanor Clarke Slagle lecture when she suggested, "That man, through the use of his hands as they are energized by mind and will, can influence the state of his own health."[1(p88)] Others have suggested that hands are among the features that distinguish human beings from other living creatures. Hands are most certainly important to occupational performance.

Pathology of the upper extremity can result in impairments of many client factors including limitations in joint mobility or muscle strength, swelling, sensory impairment, and pain. Occupational therapists often address these impairments by incorporating an orthosis into a patient's intervention plan to enhance performance skills and occupational performance.

In this chapter, we introduce the biomechanical and anatomical structures of the hand that occupational therapists consider when fabricating an orthosis. We then provide basic information about the construction of orthoses, appreciating that practice and further training are required to develop expertise in this area. A **splint** refers to casts or strapping used to reduce fractures or dislocations. The word splint/splinting should not be used when documenting orthosis fabrication.[2]

Anatomical and Biomechanical Considerations When Fabricating Custom Orthoses

A functional understanding of the human body requires the appreciation of three major areas of scientific study: musculoskeletal anatomy, neuromuscular physiology, and biomechanics.[3] Recovery of hand function following disease or injury may be optimized when the abovementioned scientific study are combined with an understanding of function in occupation and orthosis fabrication.

Anatomy

The anatomy of the hand informs the concept, design, and construction of custom-fabricated or custom-fit hand orthoses. Such consideration requires a basic review of the macrostructure of tissues and component structures that contribute to functional interaction with the environment.

Anatomic Principles Applied to Custom Orthosis Fabrication

- Bones create structural support and arches of the hand. Orthoses conform to structure and arches to create dual obliquity and support a functional position.
- Joints create levers for movement. The more stable a joint, the less motion; the more actual degrees or planes of motion, the less stable.
- Muscles create movement of joints. Orthosis design is intervention specific, encouraging motion, stability, or immobilization of tissue and joints.
- Neuromuscular physiology is the organ system that drives function. Orthosis design must allow neuron to muscle fiber communication in order to be a beneficial intervention.
- The integumentary system encapsulates the body. Understanding the relationship of skin creases to joints is important for orthosis design and construction.

The metacarpals vary in length and height. Metacarpals of the radial fingers are longer than the ulnar fingers of the hand. The metacarpal heads on the radial side of the hand are higher than those on the ulnar side of the hand, an effect more pronounced when the hand is closed. The therapist must apply this concept of dual obliquity to the construction of an orthosis. That is, the orthosis must be longer and higher on the radial side of the hand[4] (Fig. 23-1).

Bone

The specific functions of bone that must be considered for orthosis fabrication include structural support, levers for body movement, and protection of underlying

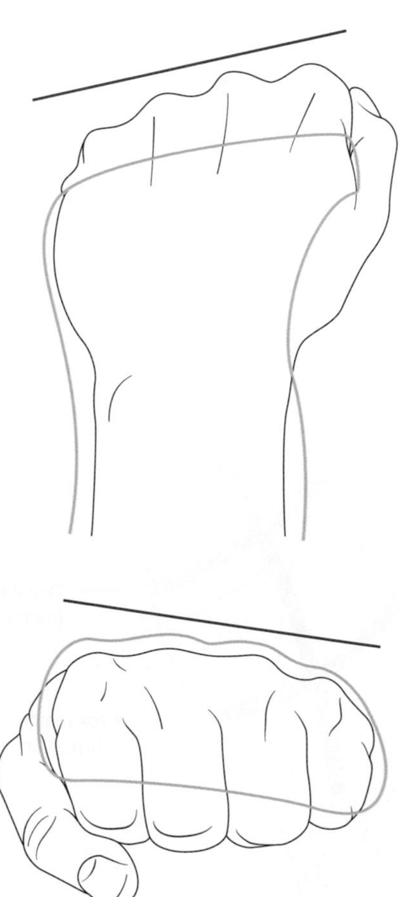

Figure 23-1. Concept of dual obliquity applied to orthosis fabrication.

structures. Bones are categorized according to shape and size. Long bones have a shaft that acts as a rigid tube; each end of the shaft is expanded, creating a basic component of a joint. Short bones are cube shaped, as long as they are wide. Flat bones are broad and thin with flat or curved surfaces, and sesamoid bones are round.[5] The three primary arches of the hand are assured by the structural anatomy of the bones. An orthosis must conform to these concave arches to support a functional position of the hand (see Fig. 23-2). The distal transverse arch is formed by the metacarpal heads of the index, long, ring, and small fingers. The longitudinal arch extends from the wrist to the long or index finger. The oblique arch is formed through opposition of the thumb and small finger.[6] It is important to maintain these arches throughout the fabrication process. Otherwise, collapse or flattening of these arches may result in decreased functional return of the hand.[7]

Joint

A joint can be defined according to structure or function. Structurally, it is a place where two or more bones are joined to one another by soft tissue. The major function of a joint is to allow movement. The hand consists of joints that have space between the articulating bones that allow for movement. Joints surfaces create bony prominences that should be considered during orthosis fabrication as they can be pressure areas. Adequate orthosis design requires conformity to bony prominences, assuring proper fit and reduced risk of pressure points from orthosis use (Fig. 23-3). Joints are constructed to allow for a balance between mobility and stability.[5]

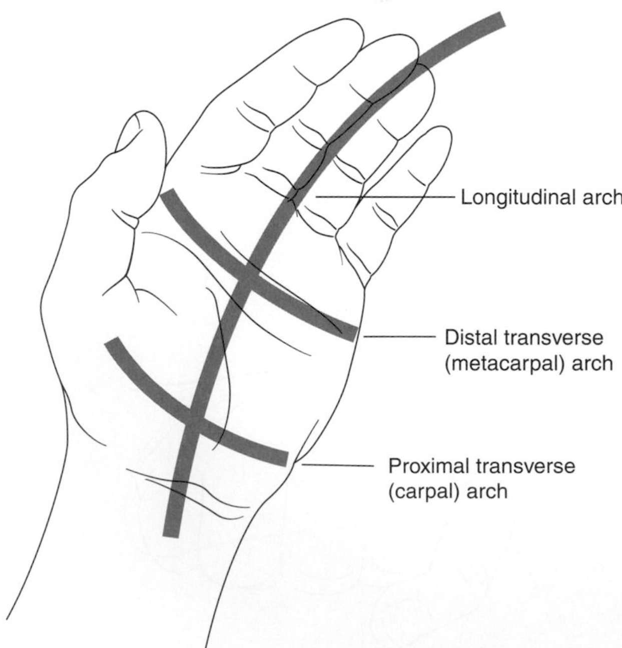

Figure 23-2. Arches of the hand must be supported in orthosis fabrication.

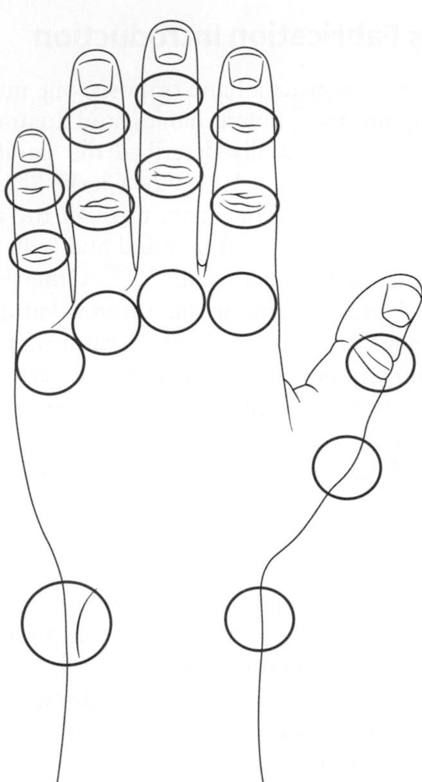

Figure 23-3. Bony prominences can lead to pressure points, especially over the back of the hand. Careful contouring of the thermoplastic material can minimize this problem.

The motion available at joints within the hand is variable. The more mobile a joint, the less stable it is. When a joint has inherently less stability, it is at higher risk for injury. It is important to note there is increased joint mobility on the ulnar side of the hand as compared to the radial side, and this should be considered during orthosis fabrication.[7] Additionally, there is basically no motion allowed at the carpometacarpal (CMC) joints of the index and long fingers and only a small amount of motion that occurs at the CMC joints of the ring and small.[8] The concepts of joint stability and mobility must be considered in custom orthosis design and construction to assure the orthosis is safe and performs as intended.

Muscle

Most skeletal muscles have attachments to two bones: the origin, where it begins, and the insertion, where it ends. Musculotendinous structure crosses a joint or joints located between the origin and insertion. When a muscle contracts, it shortens toward its center; when the contraction force is sufficient, one or both of the bones to which the muscle is attached will be pulled toward the center of the muscle.[5] The joint or joints between the muscle's origin and insertion function to allow movement. Understanding the action of a joint caused by the forces applied by muscle and other generated forces is critical to orthosis design.

Integumentary System

As the largest organ system of the human body, skin completely encapsulates the body and permits unrestricted mobility.[9] Dorsal hand skin is relatively thin with creases directly over articulations. Volar skin is fibrous and thick with more defined creases. As with dorsal digital creases, the volar digital creases directly correlate with joint location. The palmar creases are often used as landmarks for orthosis fabrication.[10] For example, the distal palmar crease is a landmark for the distal aspect of a volar-based orthosis to allow motion at the metacarpophalangeal (MCP) joints. The thenar crease should also be considered during orthosis fabrication to allow full movement of the thumb. The wrist crease should be clear for hand-based orthoses to allow full wrist flexion[10] (see Fig. 23-4).

Biomechanical Principles Applied to Custom Orthosis Fabrication

When wearing an orthosis, external forces are applied, thus requiring a basic knowledge of anatomy and biomechanics to ensure proper fit of the orthosis and appropriate outcomes. An orthosis with poor fit can result in skin breakdown and poor compliance.

Proper Position with Custom Orthosis Fabrication

Proper positioning of the extremity in an orthosis is vital to minimize the risk of joint contracture following injury to the hand.

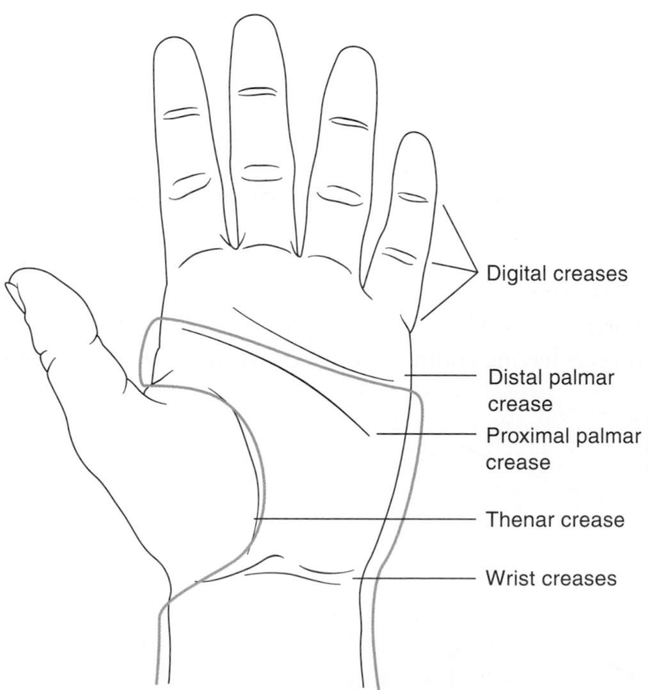

Figure 23-4. Creases of the hand provide landmarks for the distal ends of the orthosis. For a wrist support orthosis, the distal end of the orthosis should not block the thenar eminence or distal palmar crease.

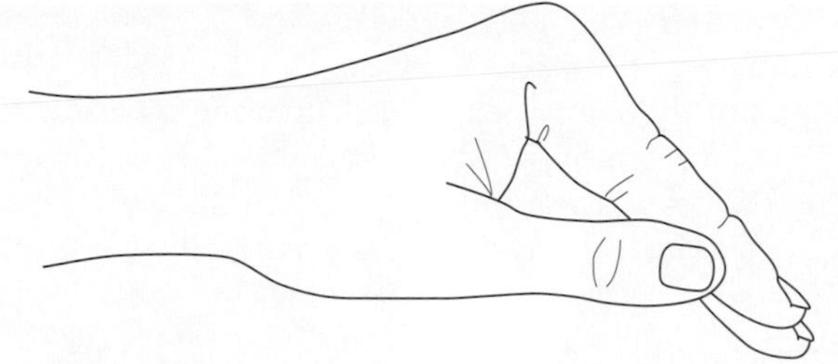

Figure 23-5. Position of safe immobilization or intrinsic plus position.

- The intrinsic plus position is the appropriate position for immobilization. Dobson et al. recommend the 0–30° of wrist extension, the MCP joints in 70–90° of flexion, and the interphalangeal (IP) joints in full extension. This position creates tension on the collateral ligaments, preventing the development of joint stiffness or contracture[11] (Fig. 23-5).
- Natural hand postures impact function. When the forearm is supinated, the wrist is in neutral to slight radial deviation, and when the forearm is pronated, the wrist has increased ulnar deviation. An orthosis fabricated in supination, for a patient whose occupations are primarily done in pronation, will likely result in poor fit and compliance.
- The normal biomechanics of digit flexion result in convergence toward the scaphoid bone. This must be taken into account when fabricating a dynamic or static progressive orthosis to address passive digit flexion and provide the appropriate direction of force (Fig. 23-6).

Mechanical Principles Applied to Orthosis Construction

90° Angle for Dynamic or Static Progressive Orthosis Fabrication

Orthoses using outriggers with springs, nylon lines, or elastic bands/cords should be fabricated by considering the line of the force as well as the degree of the pull.

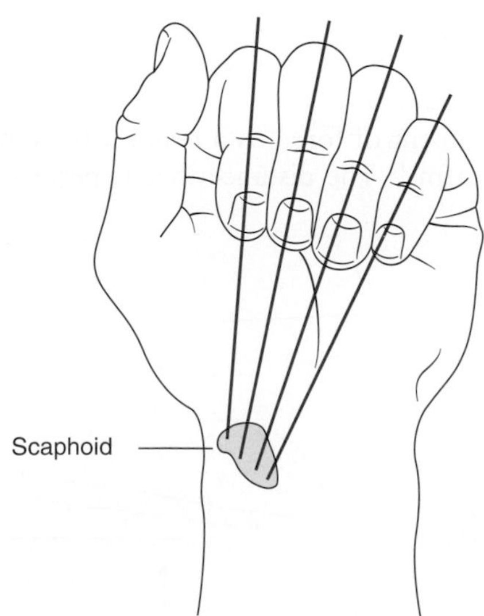

Figure 23-6. Digits flex toward the scaphoid.

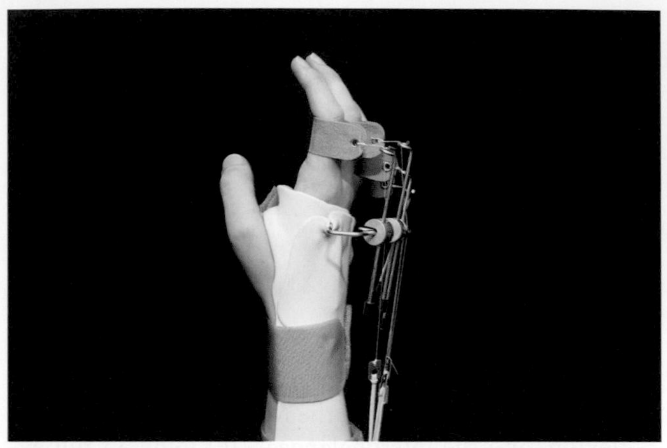

Figure 23-7. Demonstrating correct angle of pull from outrigger.

- In dynamic or **static progressive orthoses**, the line of pull (force) must be at a 90° angle to the joint at which motion is intended (see Fig. 23-7). Maintaining this angle allows the force to be correctly applied to the joint to improve passive motion. This also prevents compression or distraction of the articulating surfaces.[12]
- The magnitude of force applied through dynamic traction can be measured using a Haldex gauge.[13] However, it can also be determined through experience. The clinician should look not only at blanching of the skin but also at patient tolerance of the orthosis and outcomes. If the patient has tolerated an orthosis for a long period of time, but no gains were made, force could be increased. If the patient was only able to tolerate the orthosis for a short period of time and no gains were made, force should be decreased.

The therapist risks putting excessive pressure to the joints and soft tissues if the force delivered by either side of the joint axis is not in balance with the other side of the orthosis.[14] Unbalanced mechanical advantage can create problems such as skin breakdown or joint compression.

Torque

Torque (moment of force) is a result a force multiplied by a lever arm.[15] The distance that is perpendicular to the force is known to be the moment arm of that force.[16] The moment arm multiplied by the force produces the torque force.[7] A mechanical advantage is created by the ratio between the lever length from which the force is applied and the length of the lever arm where the force is delivered.[12] Clinicians must consider Newton's Third Law when determining forces to deliver with the use of an orthosis, as with every action, there is an equal and opposite reaction.[16] Excessive force, despite a satisfactory level arm, could result in migration of the orthosis, causing skin irritation or breakdown, pain, and poor compliance impacting desired outcomes.

Levers

Mechanical advantage occurs when a lever system is efficient.[7] The more efficient the lever system, the less force is needed to create a change. Upper extremity anatomy consists of several basic lever systems. The first-class lever system is the basis of mechanical principles for immobilizing the hand (Fig. 23-8). First-class levers provide forces on opposite sides of the axis, similar to a seesaw. Second-class levers have an axis at one end of a rigid lever, and the resistance is between the axis and the force, such as a wheelbarrow. Third-class levers are commonly found in the musculoskeletal system and have an axis at one end, while the force is provided through a long moment arm.[7] Second-class levers have greater efficiency than third-class levers. Most orthoses have a first-class lever system.[17]

With constant resistance, the force in the lever system can be decreased by increasing the length of the force arm. In the case of a wrist support orthosis, the forearm trough is the force arm, and the metacarpal bar serves as the resistance arm. The longer the forearm trough, the less pressure is transferred from the weight of the hand to any one part of the forearm in contact with the orthosis or strap. Using this principle, the forearm trough should be designed as long as possible without interfering with elbow motion, approximately two-thirds the length of the forearm.

Stress/Force

Force occurs when there is a push or pull created by two objects having contact. Compressive and sheer forces can

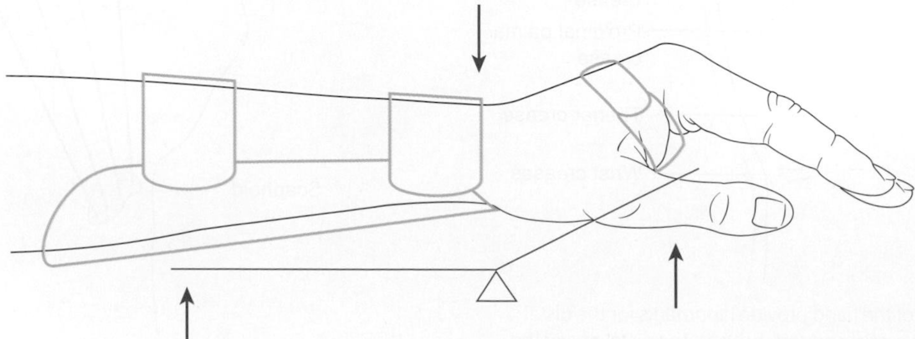

Figure 23-8. The orthosis as a class 1 lever system.

occur with orthosis use.[16] Compressive forces act in directions toward each other, and shear forces act parallel to one another, but in opposite directions.[7] Clinicians can control this force by increasing the area where force is applied, as pressure is created by the force divided by the area where it is created.[12] Otherwise, these forces can lead to tissue breakdown. When designing and constructing an orthosis, these principles must be considered for optimal outcomes. This means that a wide, long orthosis applies less pressure in any one area than a narrow, short orthosis. A forearm-based orthosis should cover at least two-thirds the length of the forearm to avoid sheering. A contoured orthosis requires more material and surface area contact than an uneven or point-pressured design over a prominence. Padding may actually increase pressure to the hand if the orthosis is not well molded.

Three Points of Pressure

To immobilize or mobilize a joint using an orthosis, three points of pressure are used. These forces guide orthosis design and direct strap placement to ensure proper force application. Three linear forces are created using a middle force that pulls in an opposite direction from the other two forces.[10]

Add Strength through Contouring Tensile Characteristics

The response a material has to stress and the degree of strain produced in an elastic body is described in Hooke's law of elasticity. This law suggests that if the same material is curved, the level of energy stored is greater, and the material can more effectively withstand force.[18] This means that contour mechanically increases a material's strength. Therefore, orthoses should be constructed with contour and extend midway around the part being immobilized to create increased strength and maximum comfort.[4] Curved and contoured edges are preferred over square edges.

Patient Considerations When Choosing to Incorporate Orthoses into the Treatment Plan

As with any intervention, the clinician considers many patient factors in determining the appropriateness of an orthosis.

- The clinician should evaluate the patient's neurovascular status (sensation and blood supply), mobility, motor function, edema, tone, and cognition prior to orthosis design and construction.
- Sensory deficits in the hand are concerning because the patient may be unable to feel pressure points or areas of irritation from the orthosis. This may lead to skin breakdown or injury.
- In the case of hypersensitivity, wearing an orthosis can protect the fingertip or hand from unpleasant stimuli.
- Edema may also indicate the need for close monitoring of orthosis fit and comfort. As edema diminishes, the orthosis will require modification or remolding to maintain proper fit.
- Changes in range of motion (ROM) and edema may occur during the course of dynamic or static progressive orthosis intervention, thus requiring frequent modifications to ensure proper biomechanics. Changes in tone may warrant modification to a serial static orthosis. Therefore, ongoing assessment is required when using an orthosis in a treatment plan to ensure fit, proper biomechanics, and comfort to ensure appropriate outcomes.

When designing an orthosis, it is important to maintain the thumb in a functional position to ensure prehension to the index and long fingers. Typically, the thumb is held in palmar abduction and opposition to these fingers for effective prehension, unless thumb movement is contraindicated following a postoperative protocol. While forming the orthosis, the clinician may have the patient grasp a pen or other object to test the thumb motion needed to achieve functional prehension. When designing a splint for the patient with carpal tunnel syndrome, the clinician should be aware of a wrist position that results in the lowest pressure in the carpal canal. Cha recommends a neutral position, avoiding wrist extension.[19] Fufa et al. recommend an intrinsic plus position for contracture prevention following hand burns with the wrist in 20–30° of extension, MCP joints in 70–90° of flexion, IP joints in full extension, and thumb palmarly abducted.[20]

Considerations for Designing an Orthosis

The following questions should be taken into account when determining the appropriate orthosis design:

- What is the patient's provisional diagnosis?
- Is there a good reason to fabricate an orthosis? If so, what does the orthosis need to accomplish?
- Does the benefit of using an orthosis outweigh the benefits of not using an orthosis?
- Does the clinical evaluation support the provisional diagnosis and orthosis intervention?
- What are the implications of an orthosis on various anatomical factors (e.g., affected structures, number of joints)?
- Biomechanically, should the orthosis be static, static progressive, or dynamic?
- What are the mechanical considerations? Forearm or hand based? Volar or dorsal design?
- Can the treatment goals be achieved with a **prefabricated orthosis**?
- Does the patient understand the purpose and benefits of the orthosis?
- Can the patient don and doff the orthosis as required?
- What can be done to support patient adherence to wearing the orthosis?

Theoretical Foundations for the Use of Orthoses as a Therapeutic Intervention

There are many reasons to introduce an orthosis into a patient's therapeutic program. An orthosis can be used as a method of remediation as well as compensation. Using the biomechanical frame of reference, remediation allows patients to restore ROM, strength, and endurance.[21] For example, a patient who has experienced radial nerve compression following a midshaft humeral fracture will demonstrate limitations in wrist, digit, and thumb extension, causing the extremity to have significant limitations in functional performance. Use of a forearm-based dynamic extension orthosis will significantly improve function of the upper extremity. This increase in functional use will improve ROM at the glenohumeral joint, improve the strength of digit flexors, and increase endurance for occupation. This is especially important, given the length of time required for nerve regeneration.

Using the rehabilitative frame of reference, compensation allows patients to return to function despite limitations.[21] An orthosis can be used as compensatory because it can substitute for motor loss or a lack of stability. For example, following prolonged median nerve compression at the carpal tunnel, patients may lose the ability to oppose the thumb to digits. This presents as a significant functional challenge when attempting to grasp items. Using a hand-based thumb orthosis that holds the thumb in palmar abduction will allow compensation for this limitation in motion. The use of this orthosis may also prevent contracture of the thumb in adduction because this is many times associated with distal median nerve pathology.

Adaptation is many times needed to alter or change how a task is completed to increase a patient's ability to complete meaningful tasks. Thermoplastic material can be used to improve occupational performance by softening scraps of the material to enlarge handles, alter grip-and-pinch patterns, and create loops to grasp items needed for function. For example, thermoplastic material can be twisted with loops to create an apparatus for a patient suffering from a C6 spinal cord injury to don pants, it can be added to a key to improve the ability for it to be grasped, and it can be added to eating utensils to improve use.

Phases of Tissue Healing

Fess reported that an orthosis can be used to limit motion following a sprain/strain, nerve or vessel repair, or fracture.[22] Therefore, clinicians must have at least basic knowledge of the several phases of wound healing when incorporating an orthosis in a treatment plan. The first phase of wound healing is the **inflammatory phase**, also called the exudative stage. During this stage, there is a clearing of debris to prepare for tissue repair.[23] During

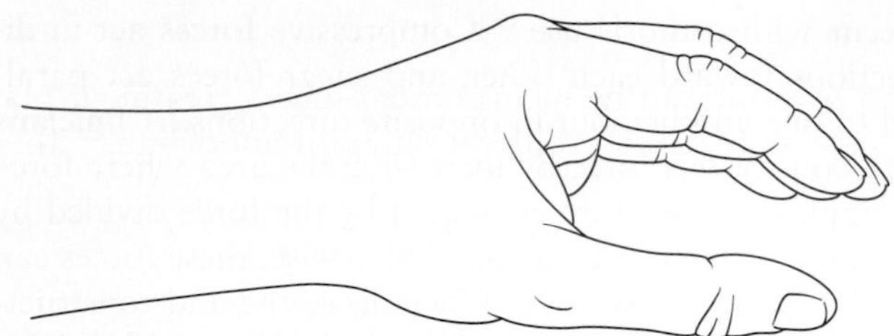

Figure 23-9. Functional position of the hand.

the inflammatory phase, the therapist may use a static orthosis to immobilize and protect the healing tissues in the hand and wrist. An orthosis in the position of safe immobilization is also known as the intrinsic plus position, with the wrist slightly extended, MCPs flexed, and IP joints fully extended (see Fig. 23-5). Incorporating an orthosis in the functional position may be considered in the latter two phases of tissue healing (Fig. 23-9). This places the wrist in slight extension as in the intrinsic plus orthosis, and MCP joints and IP joints in slight flexion while placing the thumb in palmar abduction.

The second phase of healing is the **fibroblastic phase**, also called the reparative stage. During this phase, an orthosis may be used to mobilize healing tissues while still protecting them. As the strength of the healing tissue increases, the third stage of healing, the **maturation phase** or remodeling phase, occurs.[23] Low-load force may be applied through use of a **static progressive orthosis** or a **dynamic orthosis**, designed to lengthen contracted tissues through application of incrementally adjusted static force. As maturation progresses, the tissues can tolerate an increased amount of stress.[24]

It is important to provide the appropriate amount of stress to tissue during the healing process. The speed at which tissue healing and maturation occurs varies among individuals.[25] Providing high levels of force through an orthosis at the incorrect time in the healing process may lead to tissue damage or microtrauma.[26] Understanding of the healing process allows therapists to better identify the orthosis needs of their patients. Initially, a dynamic orthosis will address limitations in joint stiffness, which are not resolved with passive mobilization. If the tissue matures and a hard end-feel is noted during passive range of motion (PROM), a serial static or static progressive orthosis will likely be required.[25]

Reasons to Use Orthoses

There are many reasons to include an orthosis as part of an intervention plan. These include[22]:

- Improve function
- Avoid deformity
- Correct deformity
- Protect healing structures
- Limit motion
- Allow tissue proliferation and remodeling

Influence of Orthosis Use on Tissue Remodeling

An orthosis can be incorporated into a treatment plan to promote tissue proliferation and remodeling.[22] Total end range time (TERT) is described as the total time a stiff joint is held at its passive end range with tension provided by an orthosis.[26] Flowers reported temporarily elongating tissue with a stretch technique is not effective because of the viscoelastic properties of soft tissue.[27] Instead, using an orthosis to hold a joint at its end range for a long period of time to promote a growth response, actually lengthens tissue. Ideal tissue remodeling occurs with gentle elongation of tissues.[28] There is a direct relationship between the length of time a dynamic orthosis is used to provide tension and improved passive motion.[29] Glasgow et al. recommend orthosis intervention to impact contracture resolution within 1–2 months postinjury.[30] A 6-hour daily wearing time is identified as optimal at TERT.[29,31]

Patient Adherence to Orthosis Use

Patient adherence profoundly influences the effectiveness of any intervention. Even the most expertly designed and constructed orthosis will not benefit the patient if it is not worn. Adherence to a therapeutic program is influenced by intrinsic and extrinsic factors. Intrinsic factors are derived from the patient's perception of hand function, the seriousness of the injury, and the perceived efficacy of the treatment or rehabilitation.[32] The clinician must understand that a patient's perception of the effectiveness of the orthosis in achieving the goals of rehabilitation can influence his or her willingness to wear an orthosis.[15,33] An informed patient takes ownership and adheres to orthosis use.

Extrinsic factors likely to influence adherence include time restriction, discomfort or pain, forgetting to perform the home program or orthosis application, interference with family or social activities, and a lack of positive feedback.[32] Cole et al. recommend applying behavioral approaches, such as providing feedback and encouragement, to promote self-efficacy and improve adherence to treatment plan.[34] In the interest of being client centered, it is helpful to collaborate with the patient to identify effective options that are also acceptable to the patient.

Strategies to Promote Orthosis Compliance

- Incorporate the patient's preferences (as able) in orthosis design.
- When possible, educate family members of the importance of orthosis use.
- Educate the patient on benefits of orthosis use and possible outcomes if it is not used.
- Instruct in proper orthosis wear and care, including orthosis hygiene.
- Make sure the orthosis fits properly and feels comfortable.
- Incorporate aesthetics into the orthosis design for improved cosmesis.
- If possible, offer options (custom-fabricated or prefabricated) to the patient.
- Provide for easy application and removal of the orthosis.
- If feasible, collaborate with the patient on a wearing schedule.

Considerations Regarding Thermoplastic Orthosis Construction

Material Properties

Low-temperature thermoplastic material is typically used with custom orthosis fabrication. This material becomes moldable at a low temperature of 140–170°, allowing molding of the orthosis directly on the patient's skin versus high-temperature thermoplastic, which requires a temperature of 210°.[35] There are several things to consider when selecting thermoplastic material. First is the resistance to stretch, which is how much resistance there is to pulling or stretching when the material is heated or softened. Material with a high resistance to stretch will tolerate firm handling and is typically used for larger orthoses and when working with patients with spasticity. Material with a low resistance to stretch is more appropriate for smaller orthoses, but can be challenging for the novice therapist. The drapability of the material should also be considered. Drapability impacts the material's ability to conform to the skin surface, providing good fit with minimal handling.[36] Some material has memory, allowing the material to return to its original shape when reheated. This material turns clear when heated, to indicate it is ready to be molded.[37] This feature is important when an orthosis requires frequent modifications, as with serial static orthoses.

It is important to base material selection on the type of orthosis you are fabricating, the experience level of the therapist, and characteristics of the patient. Properties of various thermoplastic materials are outlined in Table 23-1. For example, a novice therapist using a material with minimal resistance to stretch may have difficulty overstretching the material and should instead allow gravity to do much of the work instead of stroking or pulling on the material. Material with a low resistance to stretch may also show fingerprints and/or nail marks if held too firmly, impacting aesthetics of the orthosis and potentially patient wearing compliance.

There are several other considerations for selecting thermoplastic material. Material comes in various thicknesses, such as 1/16″, 1/12″, 3/32″, or 1/8″. A thicker material is suitable for orthoses that require firm support, when working with patients with spasticity or abnormal

Table 23-1 Properties of Various Thermoplastic Materials

THERMOPLASTIC MATERIAL	PROPERTIES	DISTRIBUTERS/MATERIALS
Minimum resistance to stretch	Comfortable Drapability Avoid heavy handling Not for the novice fabricator Hand-forearm-based orthoses	*Performance Health* • RolyanPolyform *North Coast Medical* • Clinic *Orfit* • OrfitFlex NS
Moderate resistance to stretch	Drapability (good balance) Tolerates greater handling For novice and experienced Various orthosis sizes	*Performance Health* • TailorSplint *North Coast Medical* • Preferred *Orfit* • Orfilight
Maximum resistance to stretch (with memory)	Translucent when heated Tolerates repeated heating Can use with spasticity Tolerates firm handling Larger orthoses	*Performance Health* • AquaplastResilient *North Coast Medical* • Encore *Orfit* • Tecnofit
Maximum resistance to stretch (without memory)	Resistant to stretching/fingerprints Rigidity Tolerates firm handling Larger orthoses	*Performance Health* • Synergy *North Coast Medical* • Solaris *Orfit* • Orfibrace NS

tone, or with fracture bracing. A thinner material is appropriate when fabricating finger- or hand-based orthoses or when working with children.[38] Material can also be purchased with various levels of perforation to provide greater ventilation and for fabricating circumferential orthoses.[38] These features are important when placing an orthosis over a wound dressing or when there is skin maceration.

A material's self-adherence or bonding ability must be considered when the orthosis design requires attaching two or more pieces of material together. An example is attaching an outrigger to an orthosis. Polyform (Performance Health) is one example of a material that has a coating, or laminate, on the surface that resists self-adherence until it is modified.[39] This coating must be removed before attaching straps or other permanent attachments using a solvent or scraping the surface. Uncoated material provides effective bonding if pressed together when heated.[38] This technique can be challenging for the novice therapist if the material is accidentally folded onto itself during handling.

Material is available in multiple colors. Purchasing several colors, however, may not be feasible or cost-effective if working in a small clinic environment. Many adult patients prefer a material that matches their skin tone to avoid drawing attention to their injury or limitation. It is important to note that darker colors show less wear and tear and look cleaner. However, when working with older adults and those with low vision, contrasting colors may aid with strap application and prevent the orthosis from getting lost or mixed into laundry.[40]

Technological advances have allowed incorporation of an antimicrobial agent into several thermoplastic materials. This is important because orthoses are often worn continuously against the skin, and a moist environment can lead to bacteria build-up and an unpleasant smell. Antimicrobial protection may make the orthosis easier to clean.

High-temperature thermoplastics are also available for rigid immobilization. They require use of a band saw for cutting and an oven for heating.[4] These high-temperature thermoplastics have high-impact strength, but do not contour well, making them unsuitable for orthosis fabrication.

Material can be purchased from various companies. An employer may have established contracts with certain suppliers, thus limiting thermoplastic material and supplies. To that end, it is important to be familiar with the basic properties of material to best select certain thermoplastics from each supplier.

Thermoplastic material can be purchased in individual sheets or in a case of 4. To prevent waste, these sheets need to be cut into smaller pieces with a utility knife. Material can also be purchased in precut patterns, thus eliminating cutting prior to heating, a time saver in orthosis fabrication (see Fig. 23-10).

Soft lightweight materials, such as neoprene or thickened closed cell foam, are also available to support the hand and wrist. These materials provide light restriction, which may be desirable for patients who do not tolerate hard thermoplastic orthoses. A prefabricated orthosis requires less time and effort to prepare on the part of the therapist; however, evidence suggests custom-fabricated orthoses are preferred over prefabricated for some diagnoses.[37] The clinician should consider the patient's tolerance to any material being used when recommending prefabricated orthoses or custom-made orthoses.

Necessary Basic Equipment for Orthosis Fabrication

Fabricating a custom orthosis requires many supplies beyond thermoplastic material. An electric fry pan, splint pan, or hydrocollator is required to soften thermoplastic material. A utility knife and extra blades are needed to cut sheets of material into smaller pieces to fit within the splint pan, and heavy-duty chrome-plated scissors are needed to cut material after it is softened. Many experienced therapists use Gingher scissors for this task. An all-purpose pair of scissors is needed to cut Velcro loop strapping and Velcro hook. A heat gun is needed for spot-heating areas of the orthosis. A pair of needle-nosed pliers is useful for removing Velcro hook. If more complicated orthoses, such as dynamic or static progressive, will be fabricated, additional equipment will be required, including a hole punch to insert a rubber band post. Outrigger wire, wire benders, wire cutters, and bonding solvent are necessary to attach an outrigger to the orthosis. Finger loops, nail hooks, elastic bands/cords, springs, nylon outrigger line, super glue, and D-ring attachments or safety pins are all needed to attach the outrigger to the hand. Moleskin or close cell foam can also be used to reduce friction or stress to the skin.

Custom Orthosis Construction

Orthosis Design

As previously discussed, the primary determination of orthosis design is identified by the provisional diagnosis. The design process is multifactorial, incorporating not only the clinical condition that led to the need for the orthosis, but also taking into account the client factors identified in a thorough assessment of the patient and his or her performance skills, occupations, and performance patterns. Design decisions are also informed through review of the evidence and knowledge of the biomechanical and physiological factors relevant to the orthosis design. It is also important to consider the cost of the orthosis because thermoplastic material is expensive and orthosis fabrication can be time-consuming, both of which impact potential cost to the patient. If a prefabricated orthosis that provides the same purpose is available, it may be a more cost-effective option than a **custom-fabricated orthosis**. Examples of orthoses are shown in Figure 23-11.

Thermoplastic Material Selection

To reiterate, in order to select the material that best meets the patient's needs and aligns with the purpose of the orthosis, the therapists should be familiar with the properties of various thermoplastics.

Steps in Custom Orthosis Fabrication

1. Design orthosis.
2. Select appropriate material.
3. Make a pattern/Check on patient.
4. Cut thermoplastic material using utility knife.
5. Heat thermoplastic material.

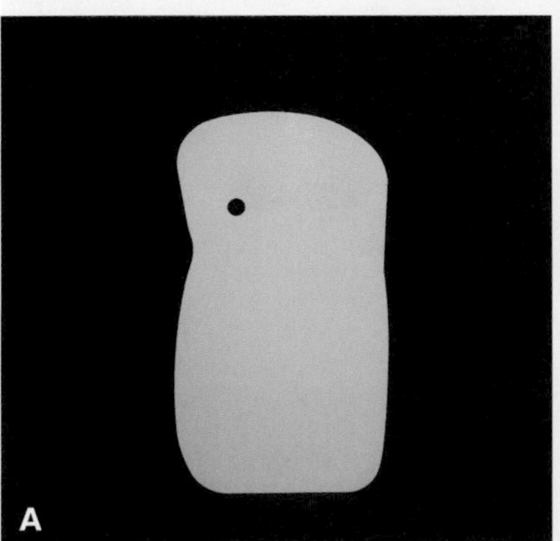

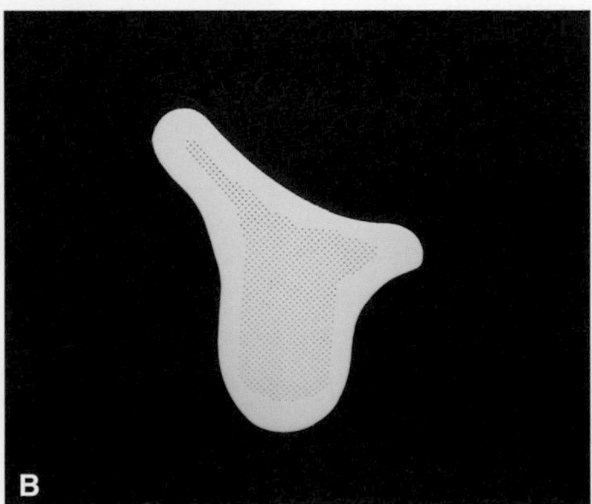

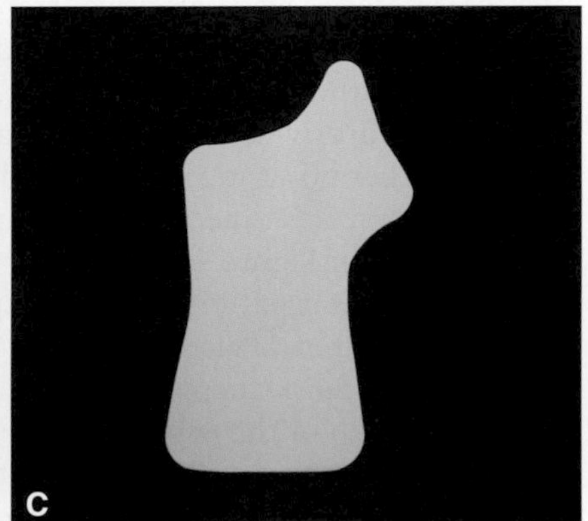

Figure 23-10. Precut thermoplastic material. **A,** Wrist immobilization orthosis; **B,** Hand-based thumb immobilization orthosis; **C,** Forearm-based wrist and thumb immobilization orthosis.

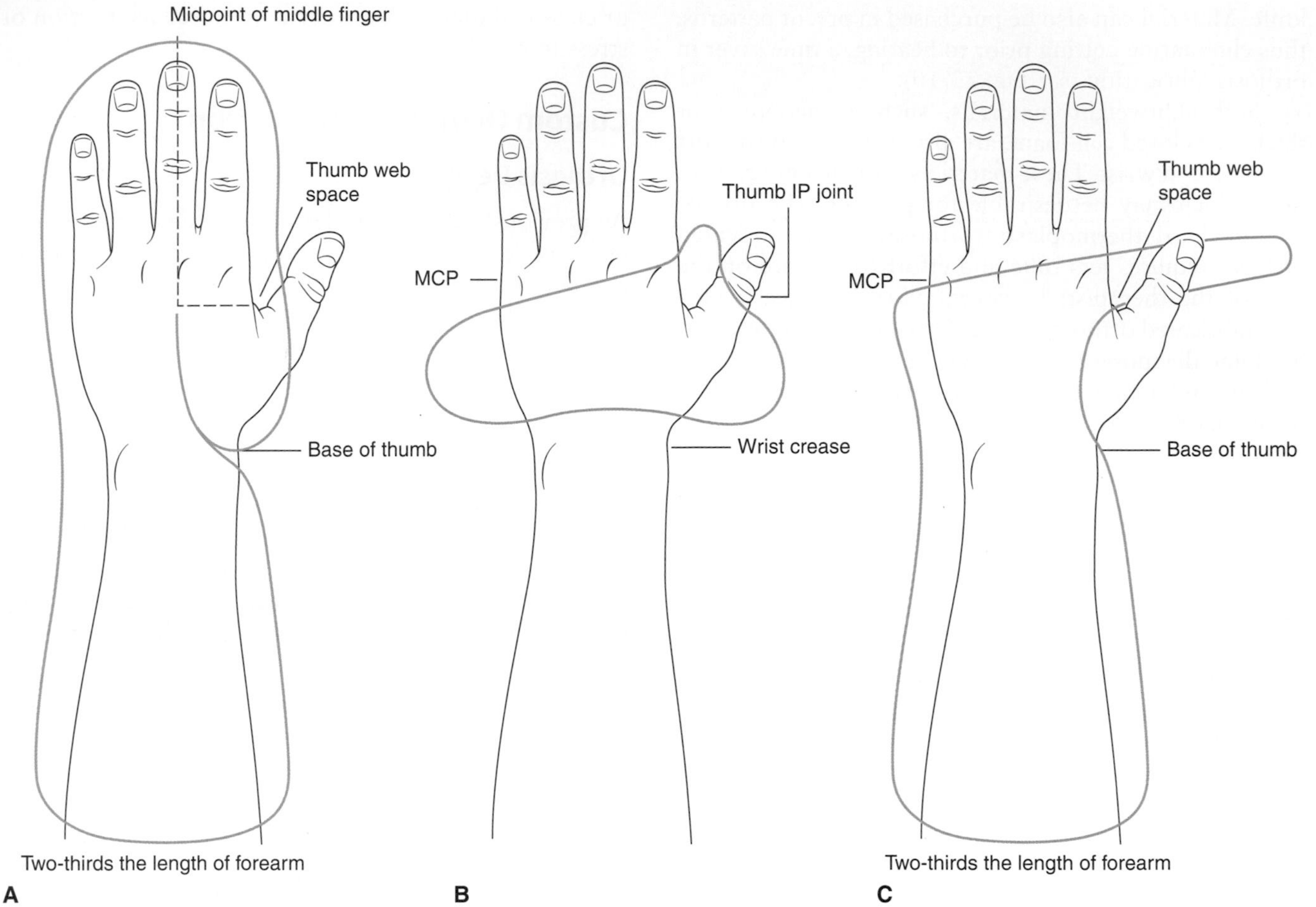

Figure 23-11. **A.** Resting orthosis. **B.** Hand-based thumb orthosis. **C.** Dorsal wrist orthosis. IP, interphalangeal; MCP, metacarpophalangeal.

6. Score material outlining pattern with scissors.
7. Cut outlined softened material with scissors.
8. Form orthosis.
9. Finish edges.
10. Apply straps, padding, and attachments.
11. Evaluate the orthosis for fit, function, and comfort.

Making a Proper Pattern

After establishing the orthosis design, a proper pattern must be created. This is a critical step in custom orthosis fabrication because a well-designed pattern results in an orthosis with appropriate support, function, and fit. Moving forward without a proper pattern could result in waste of thermoplastic material and a waste of the patient and therapist's time. Three common splint patterns are illustrated in Figure 23-11. Paper towels provide an excellent moldable pattern, but any type of paper can be used for the pattern. Place the patient's hand directly on the paper and mark the anatomical landmarks according to the design of the orthosis (see Fig. 23-12).

The pattern must extend beyond the lateral borders of the hand and forearm to allow the splint to form a trough, which will extend halfway around the surface being immobilized to provide adequate support. This is critical to prevent sheering or pressure from the orthosis. When creating a forearm-based orthosis that is either dorsal, volar, or lateral, extend the forearm trough two-thirds the length of the forearm. Once the pattern is drawn, cut it out and then place it on the patient to assure appropriate fit (see Fig. 23-13, and also look ahead at Figs. 23-23 and 23-26).

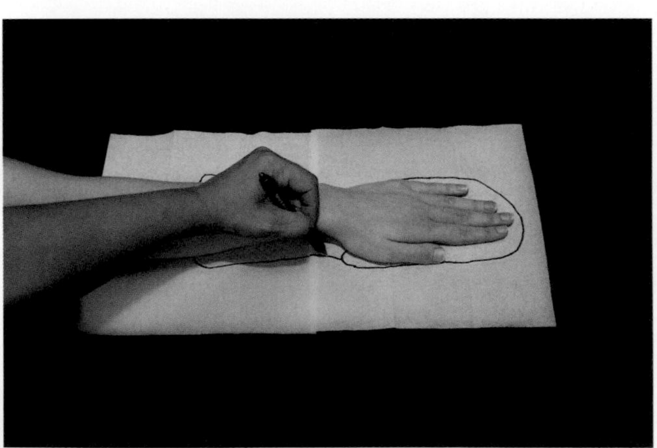

Figure 23-12. Drawing a pattern for a resting hand orthosis on a patient.

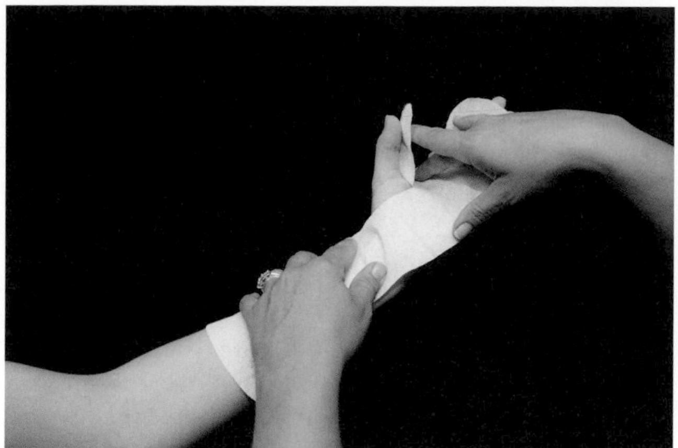

Figure 23-13. Fitting the pattern on the patient.

Modifications are easily achieved by reducing the pattern, adding paper for extra length or width, as needed. If the patient is unable to lay the hand flat for pattern drawing due to deformity or spasticity, use the uninvolved hand for pattern-making and flip the pattern over for the contralateral side. A pattern can be adjusted for edema or other variations before transferring the pattern to the thermoplastic material. When the pattern fits as designed, use scissors to score it onto heated thermoplastic material. The pattern can be cut out using heavy-duty scissors.

Cutting Thermoplastic Material

Thermoplastic material can be purchased in either 18 × 24 or 24 × 36 inches sheets. Cut the full sheet with a utility knife by scoring and bending it (Fig. 23-14); place the bent material over the edge of a firm table to cut the pieces completely apart (see Fig. 23-15). Doing so also results in a manageable sheet of thermoplastic that is likely to fit in a splint pan and reduces waste. Heat the thermoplastic and score the outline of the pattern using scissors (see Fig. 23-16). Do not use a pen or marker to trace the pattern on your material because it is difficult to completely remove and impacts the aesthetics of the orthosis. After ensuring the material is soft,

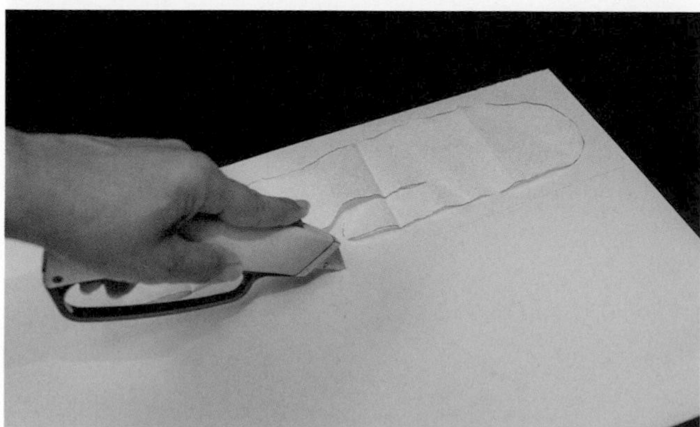

Figure 23-14. Scoring thermoplastic material with a utility knife.

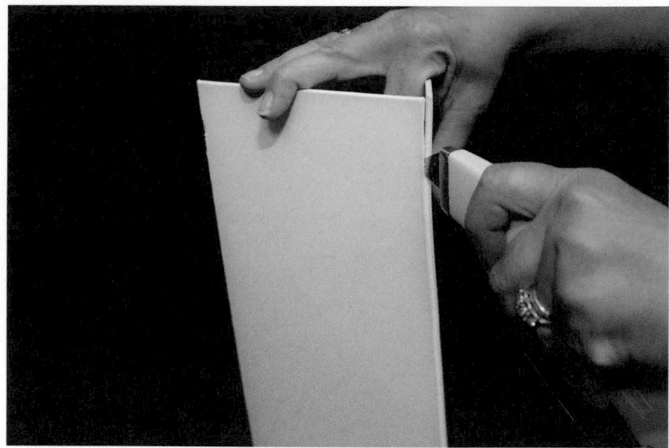

Figure 23-15. Cutting thermoplastic material with a utility knife.

and to avoid cut marks, cut out the pattern using long strokes with sharp, heavy-duty straight-edged scissors (see Fig. 23-17).

Cutting the material after heating eliminates rough edges, reduces stress to therapists' hands, and saves time in the finishing step. Minimize fingerprinting by maintaining the material on the work surface, not on a terry cloth towel, and handling it by sliding your flattened hand under the material, lifting as little as possible, and retaining the material horizontally while cutting to avoid stretching.

Heating Thermoplastic Material

Electric fry pans, splint pans, and hydrocollators are typically used to heat thermoplastic materials (Fig. 23-18). If using a hydrocollator, prevent material from stretching or dropping to the bottom using a heat pan liners to cradle the material. Water temperature is usually kept at 150°F to 160°F for most materials, but the recommended temperature varies between materials. Always consult the manufacturer's recommendations for specific materials. Keep a thermometer in the water to ensure consistent temperature. Typical heating time for most materials is about

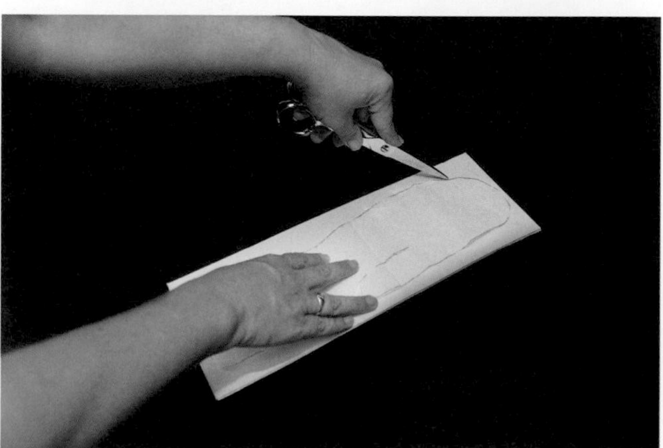

Figure 23-16. Scoring heated material with scissors to outline pattern.

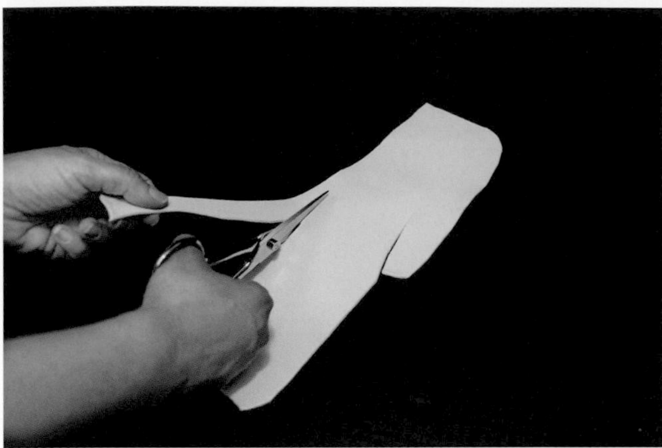

Figure 23-17. Cutting the thermoplastic material.

1 minute. Check the material to ensure that it is heated uniformly before forming the orthosis on the patient. The working time for thermoplastic material varies from 1 to 6 minutes, depending on the material properties. Thin materials cool more rapidly than thick. Heat guns do not uniformly soften thermoplastic material, hence are recommended only for spot heating when attachments are required, minor adjustment, and edge finishing.

Forming the Material into an Orthosis

Once the entire piece of material is heated, use tongs or a spatula to remove the material from the water by holding the edge, allowing you to grab the material with your fingers, taking caution not to stretch the pattern. Be mindful to not to put your fingers in the hot water. At this point, the entire piece of thermoplastic material should feel soft and easily moldable. Lay the material on a towel to briefly dry. If the material is too hot, let it cool slightly before placing it on the patient to assure tolerance and comfort. A rule of thumb is that if you cannot comfortably hold the material on your own arm, you should allow it to cool prior to placing it on your patient. As a reminder, when using a material with draping qualities, it is best to let gravity assist the positioning.

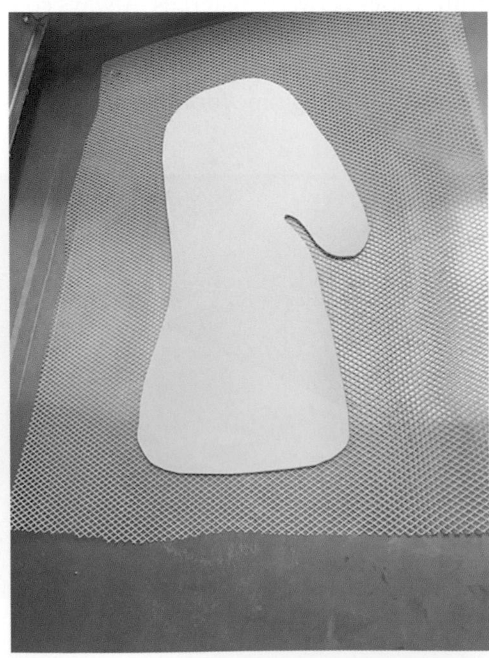

Figure 23-18. Heating cut-out thermoplastic material.

Proper Patient Positioning during Orthosis Fabrication

Ideally, your patient should be seated during orthosis fabrication. This enables the extremity to remain in a relaxed position. This positioning allows the therapist to respect the biomechanical principles of the hand, such as the palmar arch. To that end, the therapist must also find a position that the patient can comfortably maintain. This may require some creativity, such as using a plinth so that the patient can be in supine if he or she exhibits restricted shoulder or elbow motion.

Proper upper extremity positioning during orthosis construction can make the difference between use and noncompliance. For example, if the orthosis is formed with the patient's forearm in supination, the orthosis trough may impose undue forearm pressure when it is moved toward the more common functional pronation position. The problem is reduced when the orthosis is formed in neutral, creating enhanced comfort during functional use. To assist with fabrication, place the extremity in a position to allow gravity to assist with molding. This reduces the amount of handling required from the therapist. After placing the patient's hand and forearm in the desired position, apply the heated thermoplastic material. Avoid gripping or squeezing the material (Fig. 23-19).

Finishing Edges of the Orthosis

Smooth edges are important to prevent pressure points. Cutting the material at the required temperature allows the edges to seal smoothly without requiring additional work (Fig. 23-20).

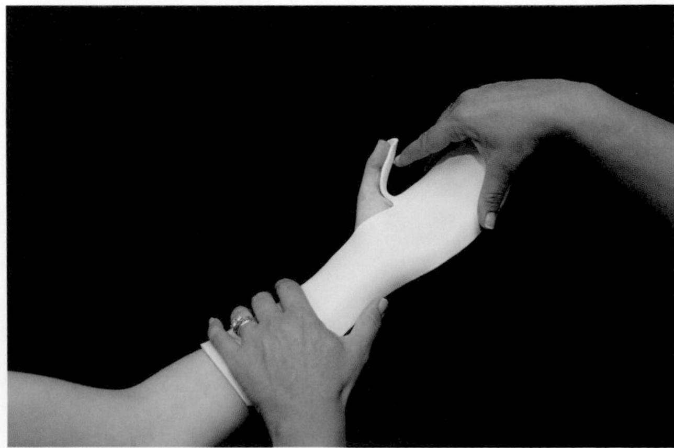

Figure 23-19. Forming the forearm-based resting hand orthosis on the patient.

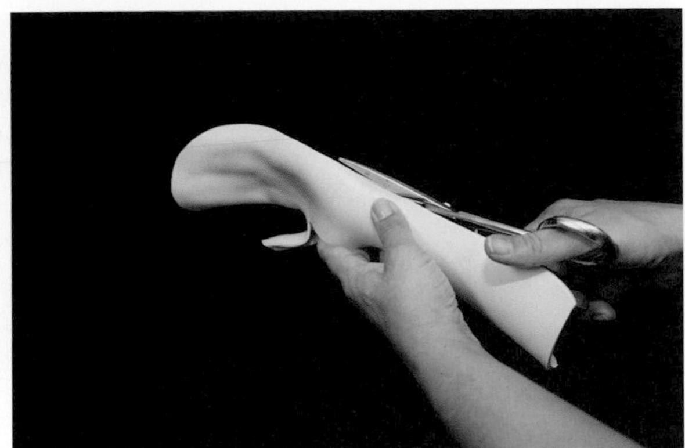

Figure 23-20. Trimming the orthosis to improve fit.

When using some perforated materials or rough-cut thermoplastics, it may be necessary to smooth the edges by dipping the edge of the orthosis into the hot water and cutting it to produce a smooth edge or alternatively, smooth it lightly with fingertip pressure. Flare the proximal portion of forearm-based orthoses to finish the edge to avoid pinching during full elbow flexion.

A heat gun produces a very hot stream of dry heat. It should never be directed toward the patient's skin. To avoid damage to the motor, set the heat gun on a cool setting before turning it off.

Applying the Straps

Straps attach the orthosis to the patient. Their location must be carefully planned to achieve optimal surface contact for pressure dispersion and positional stability. Apply adhesive-hook Velcro to the orthosis and use loop or foam strapping material to hold the orthosis securely on the patient. Hook Velcro adheres well to the orthosis if the surface is prepared for the bond. This is done by removing the nonstick finish on the thermoplastic. Use a heat gun to spot heat the part of the orthosis that will receive the Velcro hook and press a cotton towel into the material. Then spot heat the sticky side of the Velcro with a heat gun before applying it to the thermoplastic (Fig. 23-21).

Other preparation techniques include applying a solvent or scraping the plastic with the sharp edge of a scissor blade. There are also variations that may be used to apply Velcro hook. A full piece of sticky-back Velcro should be applied on the forearm portion of the orthosis to prevent it from falling off when the orthosis is donned or doffed. Two pieces on the edge of the orthosis can be applied on the hand portion of the orthosis.

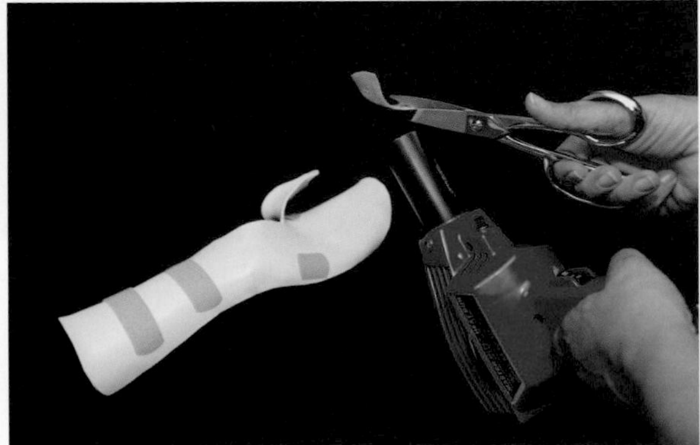

Figure 23-21. Heating Velcro hook to attach to orthosis.

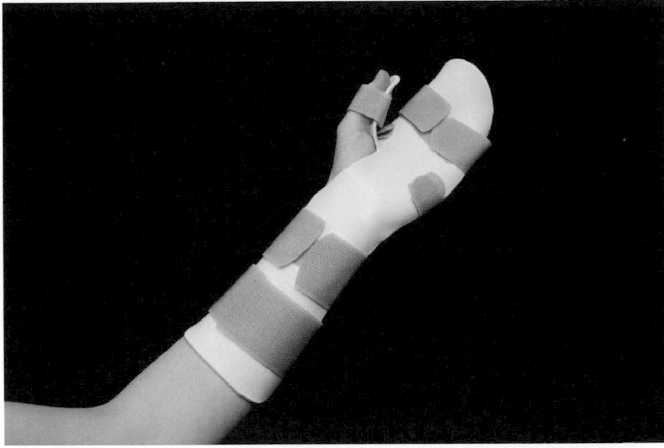

Figure 23-22. Finished forearm-based resting hand orthosis on the patient.

Beyond Velcro, other strapping options include durable foam, neoprene, and elastic strapping, which are all available in a variety of widths. Applying clinical reasoning to determine the proper strapping material is critical. Two-inch straps should always be used when securing an orthosis over the forearm. One-inch straps can be used in the hand. Foam strapping may be more appropriate when using an orthosis on fragile skin. Strap placement should also be considered when fabricating an orthosis over a nerve or vessel graph, skin graph, or when there is compromised skin integrity. It is best to round the corners of the strapping material to improve aesthetics and comfort. Straps should also be an hourglass shaped when crossing a web space.

The finished forearm-based resting hand orthosis constructed in Figures 23-12 through 23-21 is shown in Figure 23-22.

Figures 23-23 through 23-25 depict the process of making a hand-based thumb orthosis, and Figures 23-26 through 23-29 depict the process of making a dynamic extension orthosis.

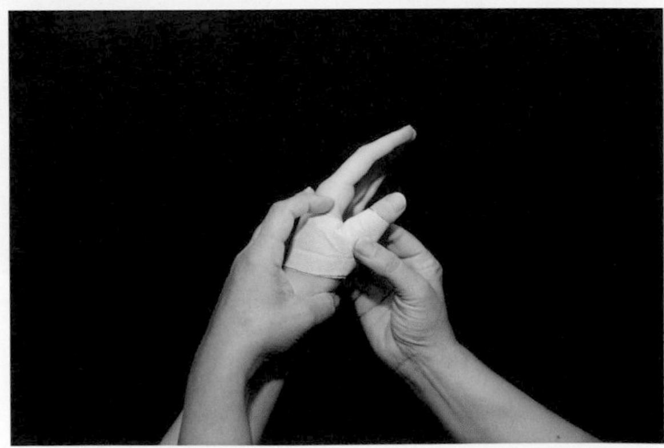

Figure 23-23. Fitting the pattern on the patient for a hand-based thumb orthosis with thumb in functional position.

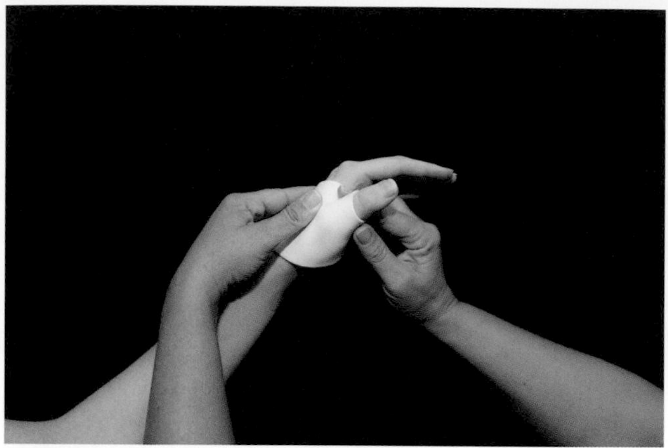

Figure 23-24. Forming the orthosis on the patient.

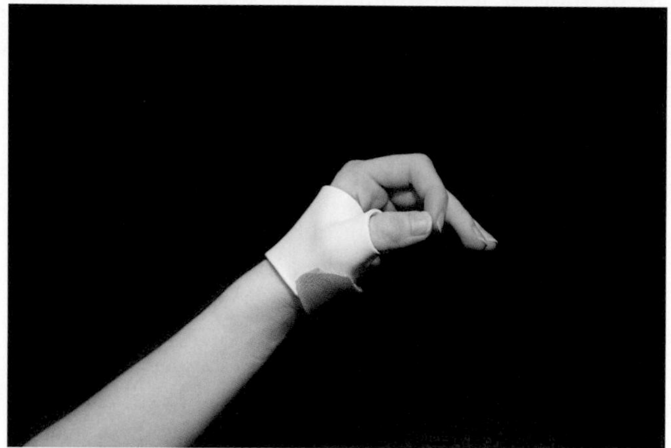

Figure 23-25. Finished hand-based thumb orthosis on patient.

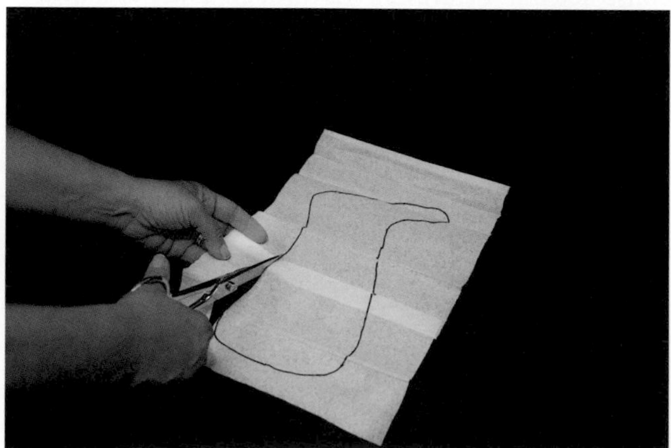

Figure 23-26. Cutting out pattern for base of dynamic metacarpophalangeal extension orthosis.

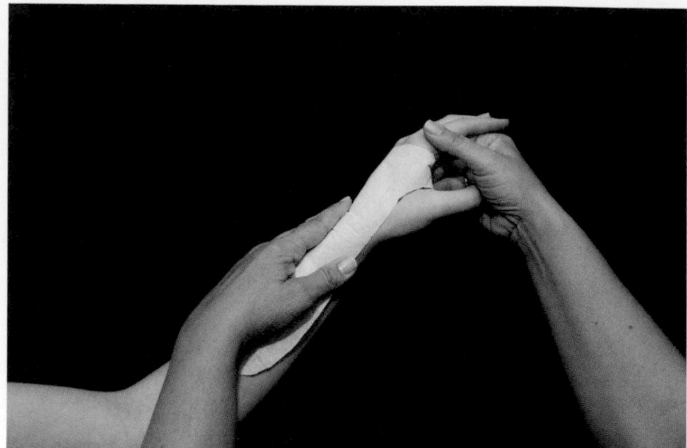

Figure 23-27. Fitting the pattern for the wrist orthosis base on the patient.

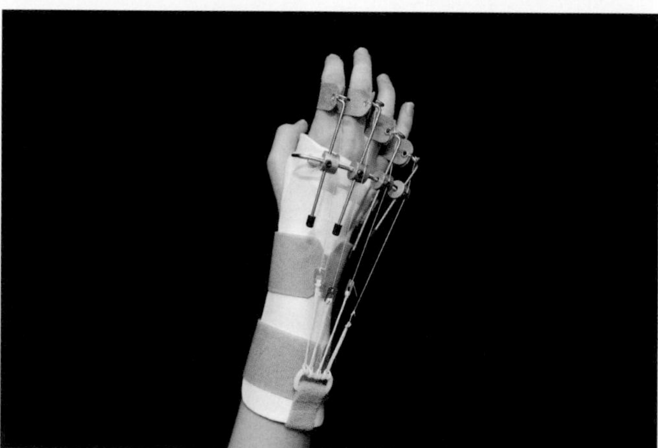

Figure 23-28. Finished forearm-based dynamic metacarpophalangeal extension orthosis.

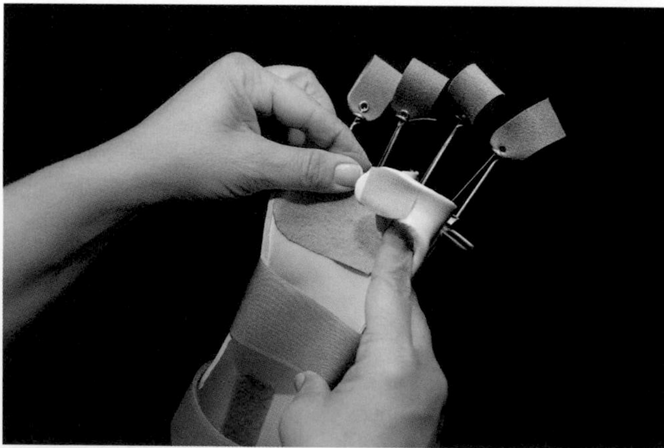

Figure 23-29. Applying moleskin to the distal aspect of the orthosis.

Outrigger Attachments

Outriggers and pulleys can be attached to a dynamic or static progressive orthosis after its base is complete. An outrigger is best considered as an extension to the orthosis base, providing the desired angle to direct a static progressive or dynamic force. Outriggers can be created by bending wire. Outriggers can also be made by rolling or pressing softened thermoplastic into shape.[41] Alternatively, commercial outriggers can be purchased (see Fig. 23-30 commercially available outriggers). The therapist should consider the requirements of the outrigger, determining whether it is to be high or low profile, single or multiple finger, static progressive, or dynamic.[42] If the outrigger requirements are of a very specific or complex application, it is best to purchase custom kits, which increases orthosis fabrication costs.

Process for Creating a Custom Outrigger

A technique to create a custom outrigger with thermoplastic material such as Polyform is described in the following. It is best to use the same material used for the splint base.

1. Heat a piece of material and place it on a cotton towel.
2. Cover the material on all surfaces with the towel and press the towel into the material.
3. The impression of the towel indicates the removal of laminate from the material.
4. Remove the material from the towel and press the warm material into the shape of a solid tube.
5. The material can be reheated in the splint pan as needed and rolled into a tube and then flattened.
6. Reheat the material to allow flexibility to conform it to the hand for precise construction.

If you elect to add any type of outrigger or pulley, prepare the orthosis surface for optimal bond. Use a heat gun to spot heat the material to receive the outrigger or pulley and press a cotton towel into the material to remove the laminate. Spot heat the post or area of the outrigger that will contact the base and attach it to the base while both pieces are heated.

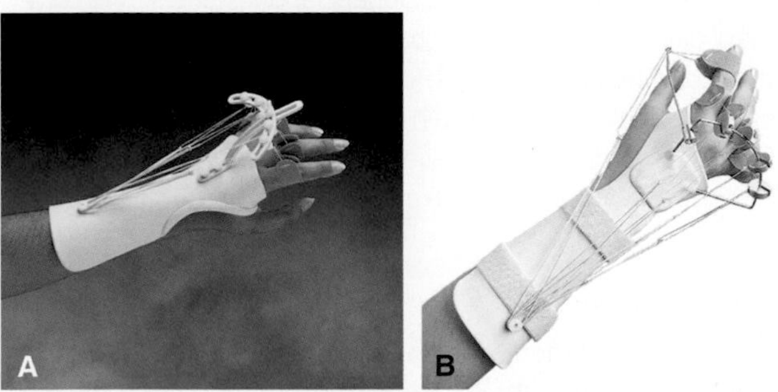

Figure 23-30. Commercially available outriggers. **A.** The Base 2 Multi-Digit MP Extension Kit through North Coast Medical. (Courtesy of North Coast Medical.) **B.** Phoenix Outrigger Kit. (Courtesy of Human Factors Engineering.).

Bonding solvent or scraping the surface of the base can also remove the laminate. The outrigger or pulley attachment points should be treated similarly. Use a heat gun as described earlier and press them together. To increase the material bond, gently pull and push the base and outrigger enough to stress the material, gradually forcing them tighter together, but not enough to separate or shift the position of attachment. As the material cools, hold the pieces together for adequate bonding. They can be cooled with cool water or a cold spray before starting the next attachment.

The described technique will omit the need for additional reinforcement. If an alternate technique is used, heat another piece of thermoplastic and apply it over the outrigger base attachment. Always prepare surfaces with dry heat for effective bonding. Dynamic splints may be prone to slide distally because of the force or pull on the orthosis base. You can control this migration with appropriate strap placement and a friction-enhanced material that is in contact with the skin. Silicone gel or Microfoam tape (available through Performance Health) provides light friction to keep the orthosis base in place. Rubber bands, coil springs, or elastic thread provide the tension to a dynamic orthosis. They can be attached to the orthosis base with a thermoplastic hook, Velcro tabs, or thumbscrews placed proximal to the outrigger on the orthosis base. Pulleys or line guides such as Velcro hook and loop can redirect the line of pull as needed for dynamic or static progressive flexion orthoses. Monofilament (fishing line) attached to the rubber band creates a smooth excursion for the rubber band tension as it pulls over the outrigger or under the pulley (see Fig. 23-28).

The monofilament attaches to a finger sling, fingernail hook, or tab to provide the appropriate tension and angle of pull. Dynamic orthoses may incorporate commercially available hinges, which provide a movable axis at a joint. Static progressive orthoses use locking hinges and various types of inelastic components such as Velcro strips, monofilament line, MERiT components, and Click Strips.[43] Hinges and turn screws may also be used for static progressive orthoses to provide adjustable positioning of stiff joints in the optimal position tolerated by the patient. These components allow for adjustments as the patient achieves increased mobility.[24]

The Use of Padding

When padding an orthosis, allow extra space in the design and molding phases to contour over a bony prominence, to avoid additional pressure in this area. Some padding can be applied before forming the orthosis. When applying the padding after orthosis construction, ensure that the material padding is measured to fit only the material enlarged to accept padding (see Fig. 23-29). To reduce scissor damage, cut the padding before removing the pad backing. Then, place padding over the thermoplastic area in need of padding, assuring proper placement. Remove the backing and apply padding to the orthosis (see Fig. 23-29).

If padding is applied to the thermoplastic before heating, the excess water should be squeezed out before applying the orthosis to the patient. Stockinette liners can be used instead of padding for light protection, and sticky-back moleskin is also available as a thin, soft padding material. Please note that padding should never substitute for a well-fitting orthosis.

Evaluating Fit and Comfort

Once orthosis fabrication is complete, the therapist performs a checkout to verify its fit and comfort and to ensure that the patient understands its use and care (see Figs. 23-22, 23-25, and 23-28).

Training and Education

Patients must understand the goal and purpose of orthosis use. It may also be helpful to inform them of the consequences of failing to comply with orthosis wear. This information should be provided in written and verbal form. If the patient has a cognitive deficit, provide instructions to a caregiver. Patients or caregivers also need to receive instructions to watch for pressure points, edema, and excessive dynamic tension, and on how to adjust the orthosis, if feasible. Ensure that patients know how to clean their orthosis and to keep thermoplastic orthoses away from heat so they do not lose their shape. Schedule a follow-up visit if you anticipate needing to modify the orthosis, and always provide a method for patients or caregivers to contact you with questions or concerns about their orthosis.

Orthosis Checkout

After fabrication is complete, ask the patient to wear the orthosis for about 20 minutes and then remove it. This can be done while providing the patient with instructions for orthosis use or when reviewing a home program. During this time, if redness or blanching is identified and does not readily resolve, it may be an indication of a pressure area.[13] Modify the orthosis if signs of excessive pressure are present and then reevaluate fit and comfort. This is critical to ensure proper use, prevent skin breakdown, and avoid unnecessary trips to return to the clinic for modifications.

Prior to sending the orthosis home with the patient, consider the following questions:

- Does the orthosis achieve the purpose?
- Does the orthosis maintain proper position at rest and perform as required with stress?
- Does the orthosis contour to and fit the hand considering arches and bony prominences?
- Does the orthosis extend beyond necessary structures causing undue restrictions?
- Is the orthosis long enough to support immobilized structures?
- Is the orthosis finished with smooth edges and resolved pressure points?
- Can the patient apply and remove the orthosis independently?
- Does the patient understand wear and care instructions?

In summary, orthotic intervention requires a client-centered approach by a skilled therapist. This requires practice and mentorship. Custom orthosis fabrication is an important component in a holistic rehabilitation process to meet the occupational performance goals of the patient and should not be considered as just the application of a device. By combining applicable knowledge, principles of orthosis fabrication, skill, and creativity with the patient's needs, the therapist can meet the challenges imposed on the patient to meet the goals of rehabilitation.

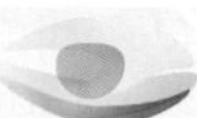

CASE STUDY

Patient Information

Sarah is a 62-year-old, right-hand–dominant female who has been diagnosed with osteoarthritis of the CMC joint of the thumb of her right hand. Sarah was referred to outpatient occupational therapy for conservative management to reduce hand pain and improve function.

Sarah reports she lives with her husband of 30 years in a one-story home. Her performance patterns include the roles of a part-time employee as a librarian, a wife, and a mother of three and grandmother of eight. Her leisure occupations include reading, baking, and gardening. Client factors that affected include independence in all functional mobility and modified independence for most basic activities of daily living (ADL) because of increased time for buttoning, tying shoes, zippers, and fasteners. She complains of difficulty with tasks, such as turning a key, grasping books, writing, opening jars and bottles, performing cooking tasks, and using gardening tools due to pain, limited strength, and decreased mobility. She complains of swelling and redness at the base of her right thumb after prolonged use and reports a pain level of 2/10 at rest and 7/10 with activity on the visual analog scale.

Assessment Results

During the assessment, Sarah demonstrated limitations in grip-and-pinch strength as compared to her contralateral hand. She also demonstrated decreased thumb palmar and radial abduction and localized edema at the CMC joint of

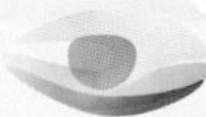

CASE STUDY (continued)

the thumb and the proximal phalanx. Sarah also demonstrated increased time when completing the 9 Hole Peg Test as compared to her nondominant hand, thus demonstrating decreased fine motor coordination. Ligament stress testing revealed slight joint instability and tenderness with palpation at her right thumb CMC joint. Sarah's sensation was intact, and no redness or inflammation present. Right-digit and wrist active range of motion (AROM) was within functional limits.[44]

Occupational Therapy Problem List

- Sarah requires increased time to complete ADL tasks, such as buttoning, tying shoes, and zippers secondary to poor fine motor coordination; decreased AROM in thumb abduction; and decreased pinch strength.
- Sarah demonstrates difficulty completing baking tasks, secondary to difficulty stirring and lifting pans.
- Sarah reports difficulty pulling weeds and digging with hand trowel.
- Sarah complains of difficulty sleeping, secondary to hand pain.
- Sarah is unable to open jars and bottles, secondary to decreased grip-and-pinch strength.

Occupational Therapy Goal List

- Sarah will demonstrate decreased time required to complete the 9 Hole Peg Test to be equal to nondominant hand to perform buttoning tasks independently.
- Sarah will demonstrate increased grip strength by 6 lb to lift baking pans with modified independence with use of a custom-fabricated hand-based orthosis.
- Sarah will sleep through the night with use of a custom-fabricated hand-based orthosis.
- Sarah will demonstrate increased pinch strength by 4 lb to independently open pop bottles.

Intervention

Sarah was fitted with a custom-fabricated hand-based thumb orthosis made from a 1/16-inch thermoplastic material with the thumb placed in palmar abduction and the IP joint free. She received instruction on her program of orthosis wear and care, pain-free strengthening to thumb extensors and abductors, wrist strengthening, and AROM exercises.[45] Sarah was also educated to perform strengthening exercises to her first dorsal interosseous muscles to reduce subluxation at the thumb CMC joint.[46] Joint protection, energy conservation, and the benefits of adaptive equipment use were introduced.[47] Sarah stated that her orthosis felt comfortable and that she was able to don and doff it without difficulty. A follow-up appointment was scheduled for an orthosis check, review of all instructions, and options for adaptive equipment.

Progress

At follow-up, Sarah reported tolerating the orthosis well and wearing it at night time and as needed during the day. She is able to work and garden with the orthosis on. Sarah reported speaking with her supervisor at work and that they agreed to have her spend a greater amount of her work shift at the checkout counter and less time shelving books to help lessen pain. She reported compliance with her home exercise program and has integrated joint protection strategies and adaptive equipment into her daily routine. Sarah purchased an electronic reading device to avoid the prolonged pinch required to hold open a book. She now uses a potato peeler with an enlarged grip, and has a pouring stand for pots and pans. Sarah also reported using home paraffin baths to help alleviate joint pain.

Best Evidence for Orthotic Interventions Used in Occupational Therapy

Intervention	Description	Participants	Dosage	Research Design and Evidence Level	Benefit	Statistical Significance and Effect Size
Dynamic orthosis to address proximal interphalangeal (PIP) joint contracture[29]	Determine the relationship between PIP joint contracture resolution and weeks of treatment using dynamic orthosis	Forty-one subjects with a total of 48 stiff PIP joints	Flexion deficits maximized gains after 12 weeks of orthosis use and extension deficits continued to demonstrate gains after 17 weeks of orthosis use.	Prospective cohort study; Level II evidence	Improvements in flexion noted on average 1.77° per week and improvements in extension noted on average 77° per week of orthosis use.	$p<0.001$ for both flexion and extension when examining the relationship between duration of orthosis use and gains in AROM. No effect size was described.
Orthosis intervention for hand osteoarthritis[45]	Effectiveness of custom-fabricated orthosis and prefabricated orthoses to reduce pain	Four hundred and sixty-nine subjects in 12 studies	Orthotic wear for 2 weeks up to 7 years, various wearing schedules	Systematic review of 12 studies published in 2000 or later; Level I evidence	Significant decrease in pain at short term (≤45 days) and long term (≥3 months)	Significantly reduction in hand pain at short-term (<3 months) and long-term (≥3 months) follow-up, with a standardized mean difference of 0.37 (95% confidence interval [95% CI] 0.03, 0.71) and 0.80 (95% CI 0.45, 1.15). Unable to determine effects size owing to lack of homogeneity of study design, methods, and orthosis design.
Mobilizing orthoses[31]	Assess the time of orthosis use in a 24-hour period using TERT and gain in PROM	Forty-three subjects randomly assigned to two groups. Thirty-two subjects completed the intervention for 4 weeks. Following exclusion, a final sample of 11 participants was obtained.	Use of a mobilizing orthosis either <6 hours per day or 6–12 hours per day	Prospective sequential clinical trial with random assignment; Level I evidence	Daily TERT of >6 hours resulted in faster contracture resolution as compared to daily TERT of <6 hours per day over a 4-week treatment period.	The only statistically significant predictor was group assignment ($p = 0.005$). Pretreatment joint stiffness ($p = 0.162$) and joint type ($p = 0.463$) were not significant.
Tested the validity of TERT theory[26]	Assessed the theory if an increase in PROM is directly related to the amount of time a stiff joint is held at its end range	Fifteen subjects with 20 PIP flexion contractures between 15° and 60°	Group A was casted for 6 days in end range extension and then casted 3 days in end range extension. Group B was casted for 3 days in end range extension and then 6 days in end range extension.	Experimental with random assignment; Level I evidence	Total gains in PROM following 3 days of continuous casting was 60° and total gains in PROM following 6 days of continuous casting was 106°.	$p < 0.005$ indicating TERT was a valid theory.

References

1. Reilly M. Occupational therapy can be one of the greatest ideas of 20th century medicine. *Am J Occup Ther.* 1962;16:87–105.
2. Centers for Medicaid and Medicare. Durable medical equipment, prosthetics, orthotics, and supplies (DMEPOS) quality standards. https://www.cms.gov/Medicare/Provider-Enrollment-and-Certification/MedicareProvider-SupEnroll/downloads/dmeposaccreditationstandards.pdf. Published 2008. Accessed August 22, 2018.
3. Hamilton N, Weimer W, Luttgens K, eds. *Kinesiology: Scientific Basis of Human Motion.* 12th ed. Boston, MA: McGraw-Hill; 2011.
4. Fess E, Gettle K, Phillips C, Janson J eds. *Hand and Upper Extremity Splinting: Principles and Methods.* 3rd ed. St Louis, MO: Elsevier Mosby; 2004.
5. Muscolino J. *Kinesiology: The Skeletal System and Muscle Function.* 2nd ed. St Louis, MO: Mosby; 2011.
6. Sangole AP, Levin MF. Arches of the hand in reach to grasp. *J Biomech.* 2008;41(4):829–837. doi:10.1016/j.jbiomech.2007.11.006.
7. Samuels V. *Foundation in Kinesiology and Biomechanics.* Philadelphia, PA: F.A. Davis; 2018.
8. Pratt N. Anatomy and kinesiology of the hand. In: Skirven T, Osterman A, Fedorczyk J, Amadio P, eds. *Rehabilitation of the Hand and Upper Extremity.* Philadelphia, PA: Elsevier Mosby; 2011:3–17.
9. Hedman T, Quick C, Richard R, et al. Rehabilitation of burn casualties. In: Pasquina P, Cooper R, eds. *Textbooks of Military Medicine: Care of the Combat Amputee.* Washington, DC: Office of The Surgeon General at TMM Publications Borden Institute Walter Reed Army Medical Center; 2009:277–379.
10. Coppard B. Anatomic and biomechanical principles related to orthotic revision. In: Coppard B, Lohman H, eds. *Introduction or Orthotics: A Clinical Reasoning & Problem-Solving Approach.* 4th ed. St Louis, MO: Elsevier Mosby; 2015:53–73.
11. Dobson P, Taylor R, Dunkin C. Safe splinting in hand surgery. *Ann R Coll Surg Engl.* 2011;93(1):94. doi:10.1308/003588411X12851639108033.
12. Fess E. Orthoses for mobilization of joints: principles and methods. In: Skirven T, Osterman A, Fedorczyk J, Amadio P, eds. *Rehabilitation of the Hand and Upper Extremity.* 6th ed. Philadelphia, PA: Elsevier Mosby; 2011.
13. Bell Krotoski J, Breger-Stanton D. The forces of dynamic orthotic position: ten questions to ask before applying a dynamic orthosis to the hand. In: Skirven T, Osterman A, Fedorczyk J, Amadio P, eds. *Rehabilitation of the Hand and Upper Extremity.* Philadelphia, PA: Elsevier Mosby; 2011.
14. Levangie P, Norkin C, eds. *Joint Structure and Function: A Comprehensive Analysis.* 4th ed. Philadelphia, PA: F.A. Davis; 2005.
15. Mckee P, Rivard A. Foundations of orthotic intervention. In: Skirven T, Osterman A, Fedorczyk J, Amadiio P, eds. *Rehabilitation of the Hand and Upper Extremity.* Philadelphia, PA: Elsevier Mosby; 2011:1565–1580.
16. Karduna AR. Understanding the biomechanical nature of musculoskeletal tissue. *J Hand Ther.* 2012;25(2):116–122. doi:10.1016/j.jht.2011.12.006.
17. Austin G, Jacobs M. Mechanical principles. In: Jacobs M, Austin N, eds. *Splinting the Hand and Upper Extremity: Principles and Process.* Baltimore, MD: Lippincott Williams & Wilkins; 2003.
18. Encyclopaedia Britannica. Hooke's law. In: *Encyclopaedia Britannica*; 2018.
19. Cha YJ. Changes in the pressure distribution by wrist angle and hand position in a wrist splint. *Hand Surg Rehabil.* 2018;37(1):38–42. doi:10.1016/j.hansur.2017.09.007.
20. Fufa DT, Chuang S-S, Yang J-Y. Postburn contractures of the hand. *J Hand Surg.* 2014;39(9):1869–1876. doi:10.1016/j.jhsa.2014.03.018.
21. Kielhofner G. *Conceptual Foundations of Occupational Therapy Practice.* 4th ed. Philadelphia, PA: F.A. Davis; 2009.
22. Fess E. A history of splinting: to understand the present, view the past. *J Hand Ther.* 2002;15:97–132. doi:10.1053/hanthe.2002.v15.0150091
23. von der Heyde, R., Evans R. In: Skirven T, Osterman A, Fedorczyk J, Amadio P, eds. *Wound Classification and Management.* 6th ed. Philadelphia, PA: Elsevier Mosby; 2011.
24. Schultz-Johnson K. Static progressive splinting. *J Hand Ther.* 2002;15(2):163–178. doi:10.1053/hanthe.2002.v15.015016.
25. Colditz J. Therapist's management of the stiff hand. In: Skirven T, Osterman A, Fedorczyk J, Amadio P, eds. *Rehabilitation of the Hand and Upper Extremity.* 6th ed. Philadelphia, PA: Elsevier Mosby; 2011.
26. Flowers KR, Lastayo P. Effect of total end range time on improving passive range of motion. *J Hand Ther.* 2012;25(1). doi:10.1016/j.jht.2011.12.003.
27. Flowers KR. Reflections on mobilizing the stiff hand. *J Hand Ther.* 2010;23(4):402–403. doi:10.1016/j.jht.2010.08.004.
28. Boccolari P, Tocco S. Alternative splinting approach for proximal interphalangeal joint flexion contractures: no-profile static-progressive splinting and cylinder splint combo. *J Hand Ther.* 2009;22(3):288–293. doi:10.1016/j.jht.2009.04.001.
29. Glasgow C, Fleming J, Tooth LR, Hockey RL. The long-term relationship between duration of treatment and contracture resolution using dynamic orthotic devices for the stiff proximal interphalangeal joint: a prospective cohort study. *J Hand Ther.* 2012;25(1). doi:10.1016/j.jht.2011.09.006.
30. Glasgow C, Tooth LR, Fleming J, Peters S. Dynamic splinting for the stiff hand after trauma: predictors of contracture resolution. *J Hand Ther.* 2011;24(3):195–206. doi:10.1016/j.jht.2011.03.001.
31. Glasgow C, Wilton J, Tooth L. Optimal daily total end range time for contracture: resolution in hand splinting. *J Hand Ther.* 2003;16(3):207–218. doi:10.1016/S0894-1130(03)00036-X.
32. Sandford F, Barlow N, Lewis J. A study to examine patient adherence to wearing 24-hour forearm thermoplastic splints after tendon repairs. *J Hand Ther.* 2008;21(1):44–53. doi:10.1197/j.jht.2007.07.004.
33. O'Brien L. Adherence to therapeutic splint wear in adults with acute upper limb injuries: a systematic review. *Hand Ther.* 2010;15(1):3-12. doi:10.1258/ht.2009.009025.

34. Cole T, Robinson L, Romero L, O'Brien L. Effectiveness of interventions to improve therapy adherence in people with upper limb conditions: a systematic review. *J Hand Ther.* 2017. doi:10.1016/j.jht.2017.11.040.
35. Orifit. What are Low Temperature Thermoplastic Materials (LTTPs)? https://www.orfit.com/faq/what-are-low-temperature-thermoplastic-materials-lttps/. Published 2018. Accessed August 23, 2018.
36. Orifit. Orifit Catalog. https://www.orfit.com/app/uploads/52000E-Physical-Rehabilitation-Products-Catalogue.pdf. Published 2018. Accessed August 23, 2018.
37. Coppard B, Blanchard S. Orthotic processes, tools, and techniques. In: Coppard B, Lohman H, eds. *Introduction or Orthotics: A Clinical Reasoning & Problem-Solving Approach.* 4th ed. St Louis, MO: Elsevier Mosby; 2015: 27–52.
38. North Coast Medical. Hand Therapy Catalog. https://www.ncmedical.com/item_2223.html. Published 2018. Accessed August 23, 2018.
39. Performance Health. Performance Health Catalog. http://online.flipbuilder.com/ffcx/jzqo/mobile/index.html. Published 2018. Accessed August 23, 2018.
40. Riley M, Lohman H. Orthotic intervention for older adults. In: Coppard B, Lohman H, eds. *Introduction or Orthotics: A Clinical Reasoning & Problem-Solving Approach.* 4th ed. St Louis, MO: Elsevier Mosby; 2015:346–365.
41. Flinn S, Bailey J. Mobilization orthoses: Serial-static, dynamic, and static-progressive orthoses. In: Coppard B, Lohman H, eds. *Introduction or Orthotics: A Clinical Reasoning & Problem-Solving Approach.* 4th ed. St Louis, MO: Elsevier Mosby; 2015.
42. Austin G, Slamet M, Cameron D, Austin N. A comparison of high-profile and low-profile dynamic mobilization splint designs. *J Hand Ther.* 2004;17:335–343. doi:10.1197/j.jht.2004.04.003.
43. Vazquez N. Introduction to a new method for inelastic mobilization. *J Hand Ther.* 2002;15(2):205–209. doi:10.1053/hanthe.2002.v15.0150201.
44. Biese J. Arthritis. In: Cooper C, ed. *Fundamentals of Hand Therapy: Clinical Reasoning and Treatment Guidelines for Common Diagnoses of the Upper Extremity.* St Louis, MO: Elsevier Mosby; 2007:348–375.
45. Kjeken I, Smedslund G, Moe RH, Slatkowsky-Christensen B, Uhlig T, Hagen K. Systematic review of design and effects of splints and exercise programs in hand osteoarthritis. *Arthritis Care Res.* 2011;63(6):834–848. doi:10.1002/acr.20427.
46. McGee C, O'Brien V, Van Nortwick S, Adams J, Van Heest A. First dorsal interosseous muscle contraction results in radiographic reduction of healthy thumb carpometacarpal joint. *J Hand Ther.* 2015;28(4):375–381. doi:10.1016/j.jht.2015.06.002.
47. Kurtz P. Conservative management of arthritis. In: Burke S, Higgins J, McClinton M, Saunders R, Valdata L, eds. *Hand and Upper Extremity Rehabilitation: A Practical Guide.* 3rd ed. St Louis, MO: Elsevier Churchill Livingstone; 2006:649–658.

Acknowledgments

The authors have no financial connections with the named products in this chapter.

Collectively, we would like to thank Charles Quick and Priscillia Bejarano for providing a strong foundation from the seventh edition of this text.—N.S.H.

I would like to thank Sommer Groendyke for assisting with photography. I would also like to thank my amazing family and friends who have offered support during the development of this chapter.—N.S.H.

Chapter 24

Physical Agent Modalities and Biofeedback

Alfred G. Bracciano

LEARNING OBJECTIVES

This chapter will allow the reader to:

1. Describe a theoretical framework for the use of physical agents within occupational therapy.
2. Describe types of physical agents, their classification, and mechanism of action.
3. Discuss professional, ethical, and regulatory issues related to physical agent use.
4. Discuss sources of evidence and the clinical use of physical agents.
5. Identify the phases of healing and the biophysiological impact of physical agent modalities (PAMs) on the process.
6. Define pain, pain theory, and the influence of PAMs on pain modulation.
7. Compare the primary classifications of PAMs: thermal agents, electrotherapeutic agents, and mechanical devices.
8. Describe the biophysiological effects of thermal agents (heat/cold) on the healing process.
9. Identify precautions, contraindications, and basic principles underlying PAMs commonly used in occupational therapy.
10. Demonstrate clinical reasoning in the therapeutic use of PAMs in occupational therapy treatment.

CHAPTER OUTLINE

TERMINOLOGY

Biofeedback: involves procedures or techniques used to provide individuals with auditory or visual cues, or feedback, to learn and gain volitional control over a physiological response.

Cryotherapy: the application of a superficial cold agent to decrease the tissue temperature of the body.

Deep thermal agents: therapeutic modalities used for the application of energy to soft-tissue structures that penetrate to a depth of 5 cm or more.

Low-level laser (light) therapy (LLLT): modalities that apply low-level (low-power) lasers or light-emitting diodes (LEDs) to the body to facilitate biostimulation.

Neuromuscular electrical stimulation (NMES): an electrotherapeutic modality that applies low levels of alternating current to selected muscle nerves to facilitate a sensory or motor response.

Phonophoresis: the use of therapeutic ultrasound to move a topical medication into the underlying tissue by increasing cell membrane permeability.

Physical agents: therapeutic interventions or technologies, which use force or energy to manipulate the healing process and biophysiology of the body.

Superficial thermal agents: modalities that apply energy to modify tissue temperature to a depth of 1 to 2 cm.

Thermotherapy: the therapeutic use or application of heat that is greater than body temperature, to conduct the heat from the device/modality to the body, thus elevating tissue temperature.

Thermal agents: physical agents that provide a change in tissue temperature, either through the application of heat or cold.

Transcutaneous electrical nerve stimulation (TENS): an electrotherapeutic modality that delivers low-level modulated alternating current to the body to stimulate sensory nerves or a physiological response to modulate the perception of pain.

Ultrasound: a therapeutic modality that applies sound energy to soft tissue, causing thermal and nonthermal effects to modify or produce a biophysiological response.

Introduction

Physical agent modalities (PAMs) are those procedures and interventions that are systematically applied and use various forms of force or energy to modify specific client factors when neurological, musculoskeletal, or skin conditions are present that may limit occupational performance. Physical agents are used in preparation for or concurrently with purposeful and occupation-based activities.[1,2] Understanding the biophysiological effects of physical agents on the anatomical systems (client factors) involved in injury or disability is requisite for safe and effective use.

Classifying types of physical agents provides a framework for determining the effect and energy applied to tissues. There are four primary classifications of physical agents:

1. **Thermal agents** provide a change in tissue temperature, heating or cooling tissue, and include hot packs, cold packs, and **ultrasound (US)**, which have a thermal and mechanical effect.
2. Electromagnetic agents use magnetic and electrical fields or spectrums and move through the air without need for a specific conductor or medium through which to focus the energy.
3. Electrotherapeutic modalities use electrical current.
4. Mechanical agents apply force (energy) or controlled stress to anatomical structures to manipulate tissue healing.

Physical agents are described by depth of penetration and mechanism of action. Superficial thermal agents, such as hot or cold packs, penetrate 1 to 2 cm, whereas deep thermal agents penetrate to 5 cm. US has either a deep or superficial effect depending on parameters set and has either a thermal (heating effect) or nonthermal, mechanical (healing) effect, leading to different biophysiological impact.

Superficial thermal agents include hydrotherapy/whirlpool, cryotherapy, Fluidotherapy, hot packs, paraffin, and infrared heating. **Deep thermal agents** include therapeutic US, phonophoresis (the use of US to deliver medication), and short wave and microwave diathermy. Electrotherapeutic agents include neuromuscular electrical stimulation (NMES), functional electrical stimulation (FES), **transcutaneous electrical nerve stimulation (TENS)**, high-voltage galvanic stimulation (HVGS), electrical stimulation for tissue repair (ESTR), and iontophoresis that is the use of electrical current to administer medication. Electromagnetic agents include low-level laser (light) therapy (LLLT) or cold lasers that have a therapeutic effect for tissue healing and pain modulation for both acute and chronic pain. Electromagnetic agents also include diathermy, which uses short wave or high-frequency microwaves to influence tissue healing, or higher frequencies that cause tissue heating.

Competency and Regulatory Issues

Changes in health care require clinicians with the ability to implement and articulate the science supporting our scope of practice.[3,4] Physical agents are tools therapists can leverage as a component of the therapeutic process to facilitate patient outcomes and engagement in occupation.[5] When applied judiciously within correct parameters, physical agents are safe and effective. Without a complete understanding of the biophysiological effects on the body, errors can lead to tissue damage, burns, and potentially life-threatening events with iontophoretic medications.

A therapist should always include occupation and performance as key components in the clinical reasoning process to effectively use physical agents. The American Occupational Therapy Association (AOTA) specifies that physical agents may only be applied by therapists with documented evidence of possessing the theoretical background and technical skills for safe and competent integration of the modality into occupational therapy intervention plans.[6] This statement should be of critical concern to clinicians practicing in states without specific regulatory language or licensing requirements regulating physical agents.

The intent of licensure and regulatory language is to protect the public health, safety, and welfare and to ensure that service providers have the minimal necessary competency. Clinical use of physical agents is associated with risk in terms of client safety and professional liability. There are three primary issues when deciding whether to use physical agents in clinical practice: (1) AOTA's position on the use of PAMs; (2) personal competency in the specific agent used; and (3) federal, state, and institutional rules and guidelines regarding physical agent use in occupational therapy practice.

It is beyond the scope of this chapter to present all information needed to use physical agents safely and effectively. The reader is encouraged to obtain additional training and education in safe and efficacious physical agent use and to meet all state regulatory requirements. Incorrect use can disrupt healing and cause injury. Therapists have an ethical and legal responsibility to ensure they possess the fundamental training and education to safely use physical agents. All therapists who anticipate using physical agents should contact their respective state regulatory board to obtain the most current information and should be able to document and defend their education and training in meeting regulatory requirements.

Theoretical Framework for Clinical Application

A frequent argument against physical agent use in clinical practice is the apparent "lack" of evidence-based research. Research is often contradictory, lacking in rigor, consistency in design, and with variability of therapeutic parameters or measures. This does not mean the research is insignificant or not applicable; the parameters or amount of energy applied may be inconsistent because of variability of the clinical diagnosis and research design inefficacy.[7]

Physical agents are often applied without appreciation of their biophysiological impact. Understanding the impact of force and energy on injured body systems is critical. The Occupational Therapy Practice Framework states that client factors are needed, either "in whole or in part," for an individual to successfully engage in an occupation.[8] Use of physical agents provides a means of applying force or energy to client factors to facilitate healing, decrease pain, and improve occupational performance.

The body's response to injury is a dynamic series of events at a micro and macro level.[9,10] Pain is a warning sign, indicating potential or actual tissue damage. Pain is associated with acute injury, becoming chronic when continuing beyond the stage where tissue healing has occurred. Pain is afferent and efferent with two primary theories: the gate control theory and the opioid theory.[11,12] Clinical conditions may involve damage to soft-tissue structures. Healing is the body's attempt to repair and replace injured or damaged tissue and return structures to homeostasis and function. The connection between the impact of disease or injury to body systems and structures requires understanding the biophysiological responses to therapeutic interventions, including physical agents that modify and facilitate healing.

Tissue healing is a complex series of events with physical and psychological components. A wound is a pathological state with disruption of the normal anatomical tissue structure and loss of function. Healing involves a variety of repair mechanisms as the body attempts to compartmentalize the injury and restore damaged tissue function. Comorbidities, advanced age, foreign object presence, infection, poor nutrition, and medications may slow the healing process.[13] The three phases of healing include inflammation, proliferation, and maturation. These processes are overlapping and occur in all injuries, including soft-tissue structures such as tendons, muscles, ligaments, nerves, articular capsules, and vascular structures.

Physical agents use force or energy, including heat, cold, light, water, sound, electricity, and the electromagnetic spectrum, to manipulate healing through impact on the unique client factors involved in the injury or condition. Physical agents modulate pain, facilitate or stabilize movement, decrease edema, increase circulation and tissue extensibility, improve strength and functional movement, and manipulate scar and skin conditions with the end goal of successful performance in occupational tasks. Physical agents are integrated within a comprehensive occupational therapy approach and are applied to the body for specific goals and objectives.

Phase I: Inflammatory Phase

The initial response to tissue injury is inflammation, consisting of vascular and cellular components lasting up to 72 hours. The initial response is vasodilation causing the wound to bleed, cleaning the area, and removing foreign bodies to prevent infection. Vasoconstriction then occurs, with aggregation of platelets, blood coagulation, and an encapsulation of the impacted area to compartmentalize and limit further damage. Fluid from the vascular system is released along with histochemicals such as histamine, prostaglandins, bradykinins, and growth factors, causing an increase in hydrostatic pressure and swelling. Inflammation is characterized with the classic signs of redness, heat, swelling, and associated pain, and changes in skin color (petechia) with red, blue, or purple tissue discoloration. Injury to soft tissues below the skin is dependent on the nature of the causative factor, location (superficial or deep), and the material properties of the tissue.

Inflammation prepares the wound for the proliferative phase of healing. Chronic inflammation indicates an abnormality in the healing response. Prolonged inflammation can lead to scar tissue development, decreased range of motion (ROM), and function loss. Too little inflammation can delay or slow healing. The primary goal during the inflammatory phase is to decrease or limit factors that prolong or prevent inflammation.

Treatment activities and interventions are focused on assisting the role of the macrophage activity through use of antibiotics; debridement; wound cleaning and dressings; position, rest, ice/cryotherapy, and compression; low-intensity pulsed ultrasound (LIPUS); and limiting active, forceful movements or activities that may disrupt the healing tissue. The main goal is to minimize all factors that can prevent or prolong inflammation.

Phase II: Proliferative Phase

Macrophage activity cleans the debris and wound in preparation for injured tissue to be repaired. The proliferative phase overlaps with inflammation, epithelialization, fibroplasia, and angiogenesis to resurface the area and strengthen the wound. Proliferation lasts approximately 3 weeks. Fibroblasts synthesize collagen molecules. Granulation tissue occurs when the body forms a matrix of connective tissue, including collagen, filling in the wound bed and closing the wound. Wound contraction pulls the outer edges of the wound together and from the bottom up. Collagen becomes cross-linked increasing tensile strength of the scar. Fibroblasts grow in the wound as inflammation decreases, with collagen synthesis affected by age, tension, pressure, and stress, and continuing for approximately 2 to 4 weeks.

Angiogenesis, cell budding with capillary development, occurs. Epithelialization provides a protective layer between the wound and the external environment. Proliferation can be facilitated through physical agent use such as LIPUS and electrical stimulation. As tissue heals and strengthens, controlled motion can be initiated. Care must be taken to avoid applying too much force or energy to the tissue. Infections, edema, or incorrect handling can cause the area to become enflamed, complicating and delaying healing.

Phase III: Maturation Phase

The maturation phase lasts from 21 days up to 2 years. During maturation, the new tissue is modified and gains strength and flexibility. Collagen fibers mature to assume the characteristics of the tissue they are replacing. When fully remodeled, new tissue has approximately 80% of the tissue's preinjured strength. During the maturation phase, new tissue is fragile, but slowly gains strength and flexibility. Healing can be delayed or interrupted owing to local or systemic factors, including moisture, infection, maceration, nutrition, and comorbidities such as diabetes and age.

Because the tissue has increased tensile strength, greater forces and energy can be systematically applied to the healing tissue to foster differentiation, tissue extensibility, and function. Physical agents that impact the maturation phase include heat, electrotherapy, thermal US, diathermy, superficial thermal agents, iontophoresis, dynamic splinting, and use of silicone and compressional wraps and dressings.

Pain

Pain is the body's response to potential or actual tissue damage and is a protective function. Pain negatively affects occupational performance because of decreased ROM, guarding of an extremity, muscle weakness, and a myriad of psychosocial and behavioral aspects including sleep disorder, irritability, anxiety, depression, and emotional distress. Pain is classified as acute or chronic and triggered by injury causing release of endogenous pain-producing substances, including bradykinin, histamine, and leukotrienes. Pain may be referred from the body structure to a different site or area. Acute pain has an identifiable cause and resolves during the course of normal healing. Chronic pain persists beyond the normal stage of healing, or past 3 months.

Pain perception is both afferent and efferent. There are two primary pathways involved in pain perception: the gate control theory and the opioid theory. The gate control theory involves both a peripheral and central mechanism consisting of small-diameter A-delta fibers that carry fast pain signals and C-fibers that carry chronic or continuous pain—both of which impact T cells in the spinal cord dorsal horn and which inhibit or transmit signals to higher brain centers. Stimulation of A-beta fibers overrides or shuts down pain transmitting nerve pathways and accounts for the effectiveness of heat, massage, and other thermal modalities.

The endogenous opiate theory involves the body's natural histochemicals, enkephalins, endorphins, serotonin, and dopamine in an efferent process that blocks pain neurotransmitters, effectively closing the gate. These neurotransmitters can be stimulated by muscle fatigue or intense exercise, intense pain, acupuncture, laughter or meditation, and TENS or electrotherapy.

Incorporating Physical Agents into Typical Occupational Therapy Treatment

Physical agents are a precursor or an adjunct to functional activity, movement, and engagement in occupational tasks and are a consideration after thorough examination and evaluation. Physical agents are used to address pain and to impact biophysiological client factors interfering with occupational engagement. Physical agents should be considered to facilitate tissue healing and improve occupational performance in patients presenting with pain, inflammation, edema, muscle spasm or guarding, decreased ROM, and muscle weakness.

Superficial Thermal Agents

Thermal therapy is the application of heat or cold to change the cutaneous, intra-articular, or core temperature of soft tissue. The application of heat is referred to as **thermotherapy**. The application of cold is referred to as **cryotherapy**. Thermal agents modify or change the cutaneous, intra-articular temperature of soft tissue to impact the symptoms of specific clinical conditions. Thermotherapy can be applied locally to produce a biophysiological change in tissue and is used with musculoskeletal or soft-tissue injuries. Most thermal applications are passive and place the extremity in a dependent position, contributing to edema.

Thermal conductivity refers to the ability of different tissues, such as the skin, muscle, bone, and blood, to conduct or absorb energy, resulting in temperature changes. Adipose tissue acts as a barrier or insulating layer, inhibiting energy transfer (heat/cold) to deeper tissues and minimizing tissue temperature change. Thermal agents are categorized as superficial, penetrating to a depth of 1 to 2 cm, or deep, penetrating to a depth of 5 cm. Deep thermal agents include diathermy and US. Hot packs, cold packs, paraffin, and Fluidotherapy are examples of superficial methods. Because of ease and convenience, thermal agents are often used as part of home programs. Patients and families are provided education in precautions, contraindications, and application instructions.

Thermotherapy or Heat Agents

Thermotherapy, or heat agents, increase biophysiological effects. Primary considerations for use involve determining whether the condition is acute or chronic, location and tissue depth involved, and whether to increase or decrease the biophysiological effects. Heat can be beneficial to tissue healing in chronic conditions, inflammation, and scar tissue; heat tends to worsen acute inflammation and edema. Physiological effects of heat include increased tissue temperature; metabolic activity; capillary permeability; lymphatic and venous drainage; axon reflex activity; elasticity of muscles, ligaments, and articular capsule fibers; formation of edema; decreased muscle tone; spasticity; and viscosity.

General dosage guidelines provide a starting point for agent selection and for application parameters. *Dosage* refers to the amount of heat or cold applied to tissue that then elevates tissue temperature. A positive physiological effect occurs when soft-tissue temperature is increased to the range of 104°F to 113°F (38°C–45°C). If soft tissue is heated to temperatures less than 104°F (38°C), cell metabolism may not be stimulated adequately enough to elicit a therapeutic response. If tissue is heated to a temperature greater than 113°F (45°C), tissue damage may occur.

Superficial thermal agents will heat or cool the surface tissue to a depth of 1-2 cm. The normal temperature range of the body varies between 36.3-37.3°C (97.3-99.1°F). The therapeutic range for the physiological effects of heat occur between 104-113 °F (40-45°C). Mild applications of heat ≤40°C (104°F) provide relaxation and pain relief. Many home remedies (dry heating pad, whirlpool) provide this dosage. An increase of 2-3°C in temperature (ranging from 42-43°C; 107-109 F) provides a moderate dose, increases blood flow and decrease pain and spasm. Vigorous doses, an increase 4-5°C, (43-45°C; 107-113 F) elevate tissue temperature with vascular, metabolic, and connective-tissue responses. With higher temperature increases beyond 45°C (113°F), burning of the tissue and discomfort will occur. Therapists should closely monitor the patients skin color and response during application.

Cryotherapy or Cold Agents

Cryotherapy or cold agents slow down or decrease biophysiological effects, including local tissue temperature, local metabolism, nerve conduction velocity, leukocyte and phagocyte delivery, lymphatic and venous drainage, muscle excitability, muscle spindle depolarization, and edema (Fig. 24-1). Cryotherapy also causes vasoconstriction of arterioles and capillaries, increases viscosity,

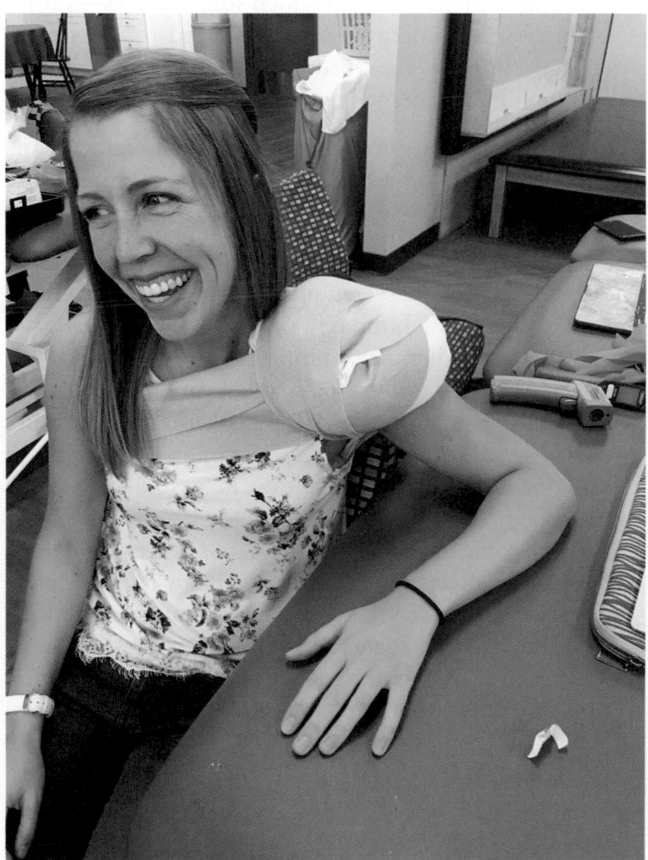

Figure 24-1. Application of ice pack for cooling of tissue. Note the use of wrapping to maintain the ice pack in place and to provide greater energy conduction.

and has an anesthetic effect. Physiological effects of cold occur at 80.6°F (27°C). Care must be taken when applying cryotherapy because frostbite can occur if left on too long. Contraindications include patients with cold sensitivities such as cold urticaria, cryoglobulinemia or Raynaud disease, or past history of frostbite.

Mechanisms Underlying Function/Action

The principle underlying thermal therapy is the application of heat or cold to change the cutaneous, intra-articular or core temperature of soft tissue. The mechanism for energy transfer (heat/cold loss or gain) is accomplished through the process of conduction, convection, or conversion.

- **Conduction** occurs when there is direct contact between the modality and tissue, each possessing different temperatures. Because body temperature is less than that of a hot pack, heat is transferred and absorbed by the body.
- **Convection** refers to thermal energy transfer to a body part as the energy (heat/cold) circulates around the extremity in the air, liquid, or other medium. An example of convection is Fluidotherapy or whirlpool.
- **Conversion** refers to tissue temperature change when energy is transformed from one form into another. An example is thermal US, in which sound waves—a form of mechanical energy—are transferred to kinetic energy as they are absorbed by the tissue that vibrates, turning kinetic energy into heat.

Four primary biophysiological effects of thermotherapy are analgesic, vascular, metabolic, and connective-tissue responses.

- **Analgesic effects** reduce pain symptoms. Heat acts selectively on free nerve endings, tissues, and peripheral nerve fibers, which directly or indirectly reduces pain, elevates pain tolerance, and promotes relaxation.
- **Vascular effects** aid in pain relief and in decreasing muscle spasm and spasticity. As tissue temperature elevates, substances such as histamines are released into the bloodstream, resulting in vasodilation. This increased blood flow reduces ischemia, muscle spindle activity, tonic muscle contractions, spasticity, and pain.
- **Metabolic effects** influence tissue repair and modulate pain. In addition to the vascular effect of increased circulation, thermal agents affect inflammation and healing because of chemical reactions. Increases in blood flow and oxygen within the tissues bring a greater number of antibodies, leukocytes, nutrients, and enzymes to injured tissues. Pain is reduced through removal of by-products of the inflammatory process. Nutrition is enhanced at the cellular level and repair occurs.
- **Connective-tissue response** to heat refers to the fact that biological tissues are more easily stretched after heating. Collagen is the primary component protein of the skin, tendon, bone cartilage, and connective tissue. Tissues containing collagen can become shortened because of immobilization or limited ROM as a result of weakness, injury, or pain. Improvement in the properties of collagen and extensibility of tissues occurs when heat is combined with passive or active mobilization and/or engagement in occupation. This ultimately results in reduced joint stiffness and increased ROM.

Clinical Conditions for Which Modality Can Be Used

Thermotherapy and cryotherapy are used when a change or variation in tissue temperature to impact tissue biophysiology is the intended effect. Cryotherapy is used with acute, inflammatory conditions; thermotherapy (heat), with subacute and chronic conditions. Common conditions, which may benefit from heat, include musculoskeletal disorders where there is movement limitation, muscle guarding or spasm, scar tissue, osteoarthritis, joint pain, and stiffness. Deeper tissues require longer applications to reach a therapeutic temperature and the associated biophysiological effects. Superficial structures, such as the hand or dorsal aspect of the forearm, require shorter time periods for superficial agents to reach a therapeutic effect. Adipose tissue acts as an insulator; heating tissues located below body fat may require longer time periods.

Injuries in the early inflammatory phase should be treated with cryotherapy, not heat, to avoid increased edema and to facilitate movement into the proliferative healing phase. Tissues in the remodeling recovery stage should be treated with heat to facilitate the remodeling processes of collagen alignment and differentiation. Following heat application, there is a 10-minute window of opportunity where the viscoelastic properties of collagen, tendon, and muscle are at optimal points. Patients with limited ROM secondary to scar tissue development, or adhesions such as adhesive capsulitis (frozen shoulder), benefit from heat agent use. Patients with joint stiffness, muscle guarding, or pain can use either heat or cold agents depending on their preference.

Precautions

Care must be used to avoid burning patient skin. In addition to determining tissue depth and the amount of adipose tissue, three primary factors to consider when applying thermal agents (hot/cold) are the rate at which the temperature is applied to targeted tissue, application duration, and tissue area or volume.

Elderly, obese, thin, and fragile patients should be monitored closely—including blood pressure and respiration—and observed for systemic reactions. Patients can be burned when tissue temperatures have been elevated beyond 113°F (45°C); however, individual sensitivity to heat varies from patient to patient. Heat should be avoided in patients with sensory loss, confusion or comatose, acute hemorrhage, cancer, peripheral vascular disease, acute inflammation, or inability to communicate with therapists. Patients' skin condition should be monitored during and 5 minutes after application. Therapeutic heating should always be discontinued if patients report pain or burning during application.

Thermotherapy: Hot Packs

Hot packs provide a moderate or vigorous dose of moist heat and are available in a variety of sizes and shapes that contour to extremities. Hot packs are stored in thermostatically controlled tanks in which the water is maintained at temperatures between 158°F and 168°F (70°C–76°C), high enough to kill bacteria.

Clinical Conditions for Which Modality Can Be Used

Hot packs are used for a variety of subacute and chronic musculoskeletal conditions, arthropathies, joint contractures, pain, and muscle spasm.

Effect

Biophysiological effects including analgesic, vascular, metabolic, and connective-tissue responses.

General Instructions for Hot Packs

The temperature of the hot pack can be maintained for approximately 30 to 45 minutes when removed from the tank. Dry padding should be used between hot packs and skin to avoid burns and maintain temperature between 104°F and 115°F (40°C–46°C).

- Skin should be protected with a minimum of six Turkish towels to avoid burns with the patient placed in a comfortable position.
- Commercial hot pack covers are comparable to two Turkish towels; the hot pack is placed inside the hot pack cover. When using commercial covers, a minimum of four additional towel layers are placed over the treated area.
- Owing to high temperatures, hot packs should never be placed directly on skin. Larger hot packs, which are heavier, may be uncomfortable, necessitating use of the correct size for the treated area. Extra padding and care should be used when hot packs are placed over or around bony prominences.
- If toweling and hot pack covers become damp from repeated use, more heat is transferred from the hot pack to the body. Therefore, padding should be rotated and allowed to dry, or more layers of padding will be needed to avoid tissue burns.
- To facilitate conduction, hot packs draped over an extremity can be positioned and secured with an elastic bandage. This will pull the hot pack tighter to the skin, increasing conduction. Care should be used because it may cause a more vigorous exchange of heat and burn the patient.
- The patient's skin should be checked after 5 minutes of application for redness, blistering, or potential burns, and the patient asked about his or her comfort level. Patients should be closely monitored for a systemic reaction, and hot packs should be removed if patients express discomfort or pain.
- Hot packs should be left on for 15 to 20 minutes to achieve a therapeutic effect. Patients often think that hot packs should be "hot" when ideally they should be warm, but not uncomfortable.
- Following application, hot packs should be removed and placed in the hydrocollator. Therapists should assess patient skin for redness, blistering, or burns. If there is evidence of overheating, cold packs can be applied to the area to stop the overheating response. Following application, it will take approximately 30 minutes for hot packs to return to a therapeutic temperature range.

Thermotherapy: Whirlpool

Whirlpool is the use of water that can be circulated or agitated to remove gross contaminants and toxic debris, including surface bacteria, increase local circulation, decrease wound pain, decrease suppuration, decrease fever, help soak and gently remove dressings, and, ultimately, accelerate healing.[14,15] Whirlpools or hydrotherapy can be used for mild, moderate, or vigorous heat dosages. Whirlpools consist of a stainless steel or fiberglass tank that vary in size and are mobile or stationary consisting of a turbine, drain, and thermostatically controlled water. The turbine mixes air and water that provides water aeration and can be adjusted to increase water agitation. Smaller "hand" whirlpools typically hold 25 gallons of water.

Effect

- Debridement or cleaning open wounds can be achieved by soaking or irrigating the area. Agitation can be used for wound care or removing macerated or dry skin following cast removal. When used with warm water, vasodilation occurs with the biophysiological effects, including increased blood flow, oxygen, nutrition, and metabolic activity.
- Increased blood flow facilitates movement of leukocytes and aids in phagocytosis.
- Water buoyancy allows for active movement of the extremity in a gravity-minimized environment.
- Patients may report decreased pain and increased ROM if actively moving the extremity in the whirlpool.

Clinical Conditions for Which Modality Can Be Used

- Whirlpool can be used for healing tissue and open wounds and for debridement of macerated or dry tissue following cast removal (Colles, wrist, or digital fractures).

- Limited ROM: Whirlpool baths are more effective than hot packs when used to increase ROM with patients after radial fracture.[15,16]
- Careful determination of patients with open wounds is necessary. Whirlpool facilitates the healing process when used judiciously and affects the inflammatory healing phase. Whirlpool loosens necrotic tissue and slough, cleansing the wound and stimulating granulation tissue. Water agitation must be controlled.

General Instructions for Whirlpool

- Review patient evaluation and diagnosis for consideration of the healing stage and integrity of the healing structures to determine whether whirlpool is an effective medium to use. If used too early in the healing process, viable granulation tissue may be disrupted, and the healing process impacted.
- Fill the whirlpool with the appropriate level of water to cover the agitator.
- Monitor water temperature to avoid burns; add hot/cold water as needed.
- If used for debridement, low agitation should be used with tepid or body temperature water (92°F; 33°C). Remove bandages or dressings. Adjust clothing to avoid getting wet.
- Position patient at a comfortable height and support the extremity for comfort.
- Turn on the turbine and adjust the agitation to the desired level.
- Treatment time is between 10 and 20 minutes. Monitor patient response.
- Thorough tank and turbine cleaning are necessary. Chemical agents can be added to avoid infection.

Precautions

- Patients with skin grafts, intravenous, active infection, or conditions, which would be exacerbated by the dependent position, are contraindicated for whirlpools.
- Clean and sanitize the tank to prevent contamination or infection. Appropriate additives such as chloramine-T (Chlorazine), a bactericidal, should be added to the water.
- Do not use with patients who lack sensation in the extremity.
- Determination of water temperature, turbine agitation, and time length in the water is based on the goals for whirlpool use and on the healing stage.
- Do not leave patient unattended.

Thermotherapy: Fluidotherapy

Fluidotherapy uses fine particles of organic cellulose circulated in a hot air stream inside a containment unit to heat an extremity through convection (Fig. 24-2). The force of the air and circulating particles can be graded via the blower speed.

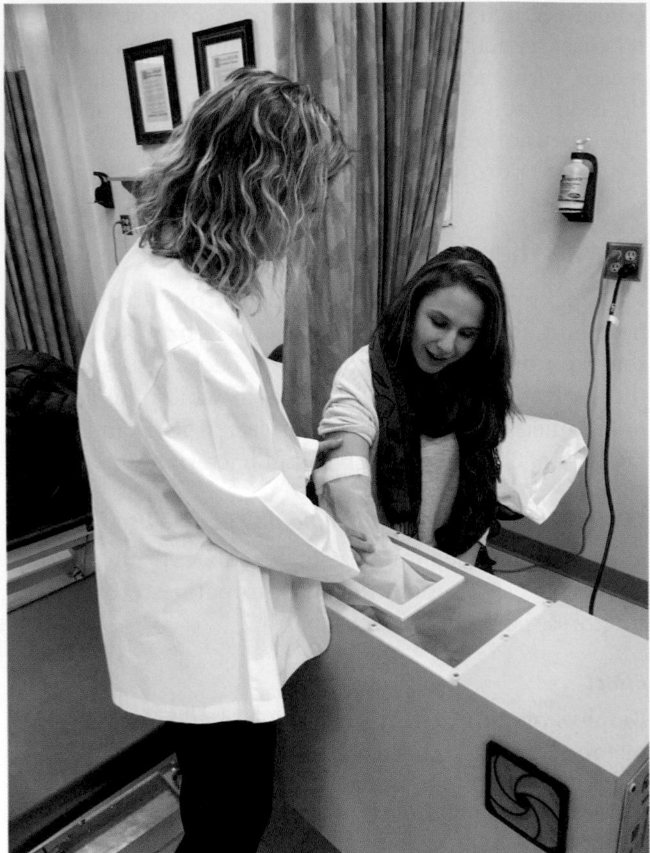

Figure 24-2. Fluidotherapy uses fine particles of organic cellulose circulated in a hot air stream inside a containment unit to heat an extremity through convection.

Effect

- Fluidotherapy simultaneously performs the functions of applied heat, massage, sensory stimulation, levitation, and pressure oscillations.
- Biophysiological effects of heat applications:
    - Relieves localized pain and increases localized blood circulation and ROM.
    - Decreases minor pain and stiffness associated with osteoarthritis.

Clinical Conditions for Which Modality Can Be Used

- Decreased ROM
- Hypersensitization
- Pain and stiffness
- Desensitization of digital amputations/painful neuromas
- Acute or subacute traumatic or nontraumatic musculoskeletal disorders of the extremities

Precautions

- Patients who may have difficulty regulating systemic temperature

Contraindications

- Cancerous lesions in treated area
- Open wounds, sutures, staples, or infections
- Systemic infectious diseases with fever or inability to suppress or modulate body temperature
- Severe circulatory obstruction disorders (arterial, venous, or lymphatic)

General Instructions for Fluidotherapy

- Review patient evaluation and diagnosis for consideration of the healing stage and integrity of the healing structures to determine whether Fluidotherapy is an effective medium to use.
- Patient should thoroughly wash the extremity and remove jewelry.
- Preheat the Fluidotherapy unit and set the temperature. Temperature is controlled by a thermostat and set between 105°F and 118°F (40.5°C–47.7°C).
- Place the extremity in the machine; ensure that the sleeve is fully closed around the extremity to avoid loss of the medium.
- Instruct patient if active movement is desired or if positional heat/stretch will be applied.
- Treatment time is approximately 20 minutes.
- Adjust the air flow for desired effect and sensory input.

An advantage of Fluidotherapy is the ease of implementation: the patient can actively exercise the extremity as the tissue heats up, the therapist has easy access to the extremity to provide active-assistive and passive mobilization, and the dry cellulose particles can provide desensitization therapy. Because of the medium, open lesions or wounds must be covered completely before use to avoid contamination or the cellulose medium from entering the wound.

Thermotherapy: Paraffin Baths

Paraffin baths involve application of a warmed melted mineral wax mixture that provides moist superficial heat that can be applied by dipping the extremity into the medium or brushed onto the skin surface (Fig. 24-3). Commercial units can be purchased for home use. Paraffin temperature should be checked regularly and monitored prior to use because there is no thermostat or way to modulate temperature.

Effect

Biophysiological effects of superficial heat:

- Increased blood flow
- Increased metabolic effects
- Pain modulation
- Decreased muscle spasm
- Increased tissue extensibility
- Softened skin; provides moisture

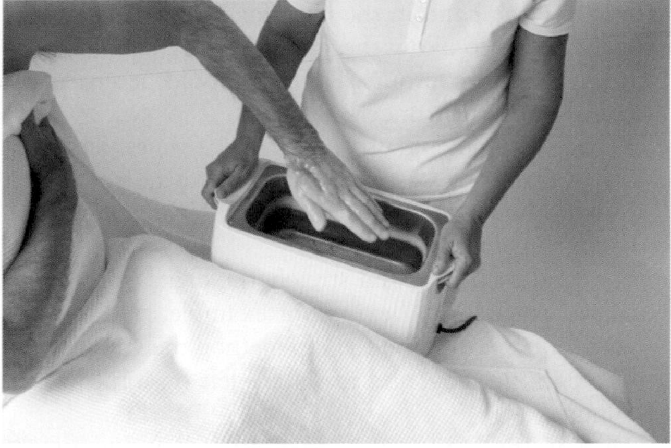

Figure 24-3. Paraffin baths involve application of a warmed melted mineral wax mixture that provides moist superficial heat that can be applied by dipping the extremity into the medium or brushed onto the skin surface.

Clinical Conditions for Which Modality Can Be Used

- Arthritis/osteoarthritis
- Joint stiffness
- Pain
- Acute or subacute traumatic or nontraumatic musculoskeletal disorders of the extremities
- Limited ROM
- Hand injuries, digital fractures

Contraindications

- Cancerous lesions in treated area
- Open wounds, suture, staples, cuts, lacerations, or abrasions
- Infections or systemic infectious diseases with fever or inability to suppress or modulate body temperature
- General physiological heat contraindications and precautions
- A disadvantage to paraffin treatment is that the hand needs to remain still during the heating process, limiting active and active-assistive mobilization.

General Instructions for Paraffin Bath

Therapeutic paraffin baths consist of a thermostatically controlled heating unit filled with a commercial mixture of paraffin wax and mineral oil. Mineral oil lowers paraffin melting point.

- Review patient evaluation and diagnosis for consideration of the healing stage and integrity of the healing structures to determine whether paraffin is an effective medium to use.
- Remove jewelry; avoid placing clothing in contact with the wax.
- Check paraffin temperature to ensure a therapeutic range between 125°F and 130°F (48.8°C–54.4°C).

- Immerse the hand in the bath for 1 to 2 seconds and withdraw it to allow the paraffin to harden and conform to hand contours. Patients should be instructed not to move their fingers or wrists.
- Repeat the gloving process 8 to 10 times. The first dip is always deepest to avoid hotter wax from being caught under the existing layers with the potential to burn the patient.
- For positional heat and stretch, the digits of the hand can be placed into flexion, for example, held in place with Coban tape, and the dip method then applied.
- The paraffin, bag, and towel are left on for 15 to 20 minutes.
- The paraffin is removed and discarded after treatment end.

Cryotherapy

Cryotherapy or cold therapy is the therapeutic application of physical agents to lower tissue temperature.

General Instructions for Cryotherapy

Cryotherapy applications, because of their colder temperatures than the body, conduct heat out of the body into the cooling agent. This can be achieved through conduction, such as the application of a cold pack on an extremity, or convection, placing the extremity in a cold-water bath. A less commonly used method involves topical cold sprays, which are liquid when applied, but absorb heat as the medium evaporates, effectively cooling the area. In addition to these application methods, heat can also be transmitted out of the body through evaporation.

Selection of the cooling agent used is based on the volume or area to be treated, the cooling agent rate or intensity, and the duration or time for which the modality is applied. Consideration of the anatomical structure depth (deep or superficial) and adipose tissue amount are also critical factors. Therapists should monitor patients' skin and response to the modality. Commonly used cooling agents include commercial and homemade ice packs, and ice massage. Cold packs can be made by combining three-parts water to one-part isopropyl alcohol in a plastic zip-seal bag and freezing. The alcohol will keep the mixture from fully freezing, resulting in a slushy soft cold pack similar in consistency to some commercial gel packs. Cold packs should always be covered with a material such as toweling or a pillow case. A dry covering will make the initial contact with the patient more comfortable and slow the cooling process.

Effect

- Primary biophysiological effects of cryotherapy are analgesic, vascular, metabolic, and neuromuscular. Cold therapy agents decrease tissue temperature to a depth of 2 cm.[17]
- The analgesic effect of cold decreases pain through counterirritation and by decreasing nerve conduction velocity in superficial sensory nerves.[18,19]
- Vascular effects include both vasoconstriction (when cold is applied for <15 minutes) and vasodilation (when cold is applied for longer than 15 minutes).[17] Decreased circulation.
- Short-term application of cold therapy can help reduce edema.
- Metabolic processes are slowed decreasing inflammation, edema, and tissue repair.
- Neuromuscular effects influence muscle tone. Cold therapy can temporarily reduce spasticity in patients with upper motor neuron lesions.[20]
- Decrease muscle spasm, nerve conduction velocity, and may break the cycle of pain-spasm-pain
- Decrease pain

Clinical Conditions for Which Modality Can Be Used

- Inflammatory phase, post surgical procedures, and combined with compression following acute injuries[21]
- Cold is used in the management of acute inflammation, trauma, and pain due in part to vasoconstriction and decreased metabolic rate, and can be more effective when combined with compression.[22]
- Edema
- Exercise-induced delayed muscle soreness
- Arthritic exacerbation, acute bursitis, or tendonitis
- Spasticity
- Acute or chronic pain secondary to muscle spasm

Contraindications

- Hypertension (due to secondary vasoconstriction)
- Raynaud disease
- Rheumatoid arthritis
- Local limb ischemia
- History of vascular impairment, such as frostbite or arteriosclerosis
- Cold allergy (cold urticaria)
- Paroxysmal cold hemoglobinuria

Precautions

- Changes in skin temperature occur quickly and tissue may be damaged before the desired biophysical effects are achieved.
- Monitor the skin for tissue damage.
- Caution is advised for patients with decreased sensation or mentation.
- Cold therapy normally turns skin pink or light red. It should be immediately discontinued if skin turns bright red, white, pale, or grayish yellow, or develops welts.

Cryotherapy: Ice Massage

General Instructions for Ice Massage

Ice massage is a localized application of cold directly onto the skin surface and is often used to treat relatively small areas or to break the pain cycle of a trigger point, muscle spasm, or spasticity (Fig. 24-4).

- Review patient evaluation and diagnosis for consideration of the healing stage and integrity of the healing structures to determine whether ice massage is an effective medium to use.
- A towel should be placed under the area to be treated to collect the water as the ice melts.
- Inform patients of the treatment process and the sensations they may experience.
- Ice cubes or water placed in a paper or Styrofoam cup and frozen can be used as the medium. Cups are easier for therapists to use, because of the insulating effect of the cup on their fingers.
- The ice cube or cup is rubbed in small, slow circles staying in direct contact with the skin.
- Patients will subjectively describe cooling stages as a "burning" feeling, "aching," and "numbness."
- Treatment times are relatively short, approximately 5 to 10 minutes because of the limited treatment area.

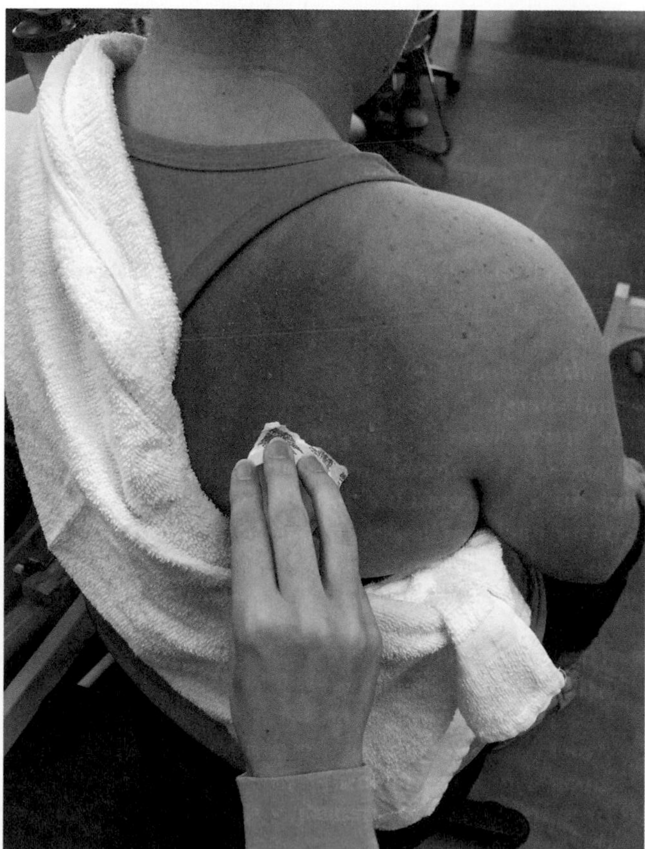

Figure 24-4. Ice massage. Note the towel used to drape the treatment area and the redness of the tissue secondary to cooling.

- Discontinue ice massage shortly after the patient reports "numbness," indicating analgesia.
- Monitor the patient for signs of cold intolerance or tissue damage.

Ice massage is an inexpensive, relatively convenient way to apply a localized application of cold, leading to analgesia. Some patients will not tolerate the intensity of the application and the sensory response of burning and aching that occur. Alternative methods for cooling should be considered for those individuals.

Cryotherapy: Cold Packs

General Instructions for Cold Packs

Cold packs are convenient, effective, and can easily be made at home using a simple bag of ice or frozen peas. Commercial units are stored in thermostatically controlled freezers, which maintain sealed gel packs at an effective temperature. Gel packs can be used over and recooled. Gel packs warm more quickly than ice packs made with ice cubes and have an effective application of approximately 10 minutes.

- Review patient evaluation and diagnosis for consideration of the healing stage and integrity of the healing structures to determine whether cryotherapy is an effective medium to use.
- Describe the treatment technique and process to patients. Inform patients of the sensations they may experience during cooling stages. Instruct patients to inform the therapist if they encounter discomfort, pain, or distress.
- Depending on the patient and treatment area, a dry thin towel or pillow case is placed over the treatment area; a moist thin towel or paper towel can be used if a more rapid energy transfer rate is needed.
- Ice packs are made by placing cubed or crushed ice into a plastic bag and sealing it. A thin towel can be placed over the treated tissue and the ice pack conformed to the treatment area.
- Ace wraps or elastic straps can be used to hold ice packs in place and conform more directly to treatment areas.
- Ice packs or cold packs are applied for approximately 10 to 15 minutes.

Ultrasound

US is a form of mechanical energy in which a piezoelectric crystal expands and contracts, creating sound waves that are propagated longitudinally in a frequency between 1.0 and 3.0 MHz. Therapeutic US has both a healing and heating effect (Fig. 24-5).

Four variables must be selected to safely apply therapeutic US:

1. **Frequency** (1 or 3 MHz), which determines sound wave penetration depth

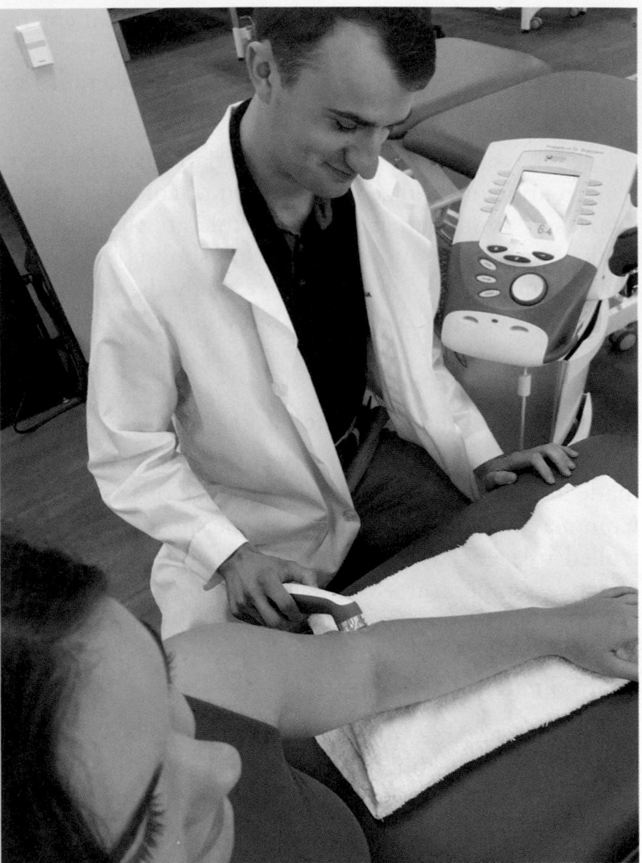

Figure 24-5. Application of therapeutic ultrasound. Effective treatment area is equal to twice the size of the soundhead.

2. **Duty cycle** (or pulsed or continuous) (20%, 50%, 100%), which is the on/off time of the US wave and determines the amount of energy transmitted to the underlying tissue
3. **Intensity** (0–2.5 W/cm^2), which determines sound wave strength
4. **Duration** (0–16 minutes), which determines treatment length and amount of energy applied

Effect

US uses acoustic energy or sound waves and is a deep or superficial modality. US has two primary effects: a thermal (heat) or nonthermal (mechanical) effect to facilitate tissue healing. *Thermal effects* refer to biophysiological changes produced by cellular heating, whereas *nonthermal*, mechanical effects refer to biophysiological changes produced by the cellular effects of cavitation, microstreaming, or acoustic streaming. Both thermal and nonthermal US can be used to facilitate healing and improve occupational function.

A lubricant gel is necessary to transmit the sound energy to a small area of tissue over the treatment area. Sound energy is transmitted longitudinally, causing the cells to compress and decompress. When sound energy encounters bone, it is deflected, causing a transverse or shear wave that is negligible in terms of tissue temperature elevation.[17] Sound energy has peaks and valleys that affect penetration depth and is referred to as beam nonuniformity ratio (BNR). These factors create hot spots and potential tissue overheating. To avoid tissue overheating, the transducer is moved in slow circles over the treatment area.

Body fluids such as blood and water have the lowest impedance and acoustic absorption coefficient. Bone, along with other protein-dense structures—such as scars, joint capsules, ligaments, and tendons—possess high impedance and absorption coefficients, absorbing the sound energy allowing for targeted application.[23,24]

Energy Distribution

Frequency

Frequency refers to the number of cycles or waves that are produced each second. Clinically, frequencies of 1 MHz travel further and penetrate to a depth between 3 and 5 cm. A frequency of 3 MHz penetrates superficially to 1.5 cm. Frequency selection is determined by the depth of the anatomical structure to be treated.

Intensity

Intensity describes the strength of the acoustic energy at the application site and is a significant factor in determining tissue response. Intensity is documented as Watts per square centimeter (W/cm^2). As US is absorbed into tissue, the molecules oscillate, converting sound energy into kinetic energy resulting in a heating effect.

Duty Cycle

Duty cycle determines the amount of acoustic energy transmitted, contributes to determining the tissue response, and reflects the ratio of on/off time. *Continuous ultrasound* (100%) refers to the constant flow of sound energy. *Pulsed ultrasound* refers to an interruption in the acoustic energy as the US machine cycles on-and-off. Commonly used duty cycles are 20% (healing), 50% (warming), and 100% (heat) or continuous acoustic energy. The determination of which duty cycle to use is based on pathology, healing stage, and treatment area.[17]

- Thermal effects can occur with frequencies of 1 or 3 MHz and use of continuous US (100% duty cycle).
- Less vigorous forms of heat may be applied (50%) for patients in the subacute, proliferative healing phase along with lower intensities (0.3–0.7 W/cm^2) resulting from the decreased strength, integrity, and viability of the healing structures.
- Acute injuries in the inflammatory healing phase can be treated with nonthermal US parameters of 0.2 W/cm^2.[23,25,26]

Types of Clinical Conditions: Heal (Nonthermal) or Heat (Thermal) Ultrasound

A thorough evaluation of a patient is necessary to confirm the clinical diagnosis, symptoms and functional deficits, healing stage, and tissue depth to be treated. Clinicians may use US to achieve thermal or nonthermal effects based on desired therapeutic effect.

- Clinical diagnoses that benefit from US to facilitate healing include tendinitis, bursitis, epicondylitis, trigger points, contusions, pain, acute or chronic inflammation, bone fractures, and tendon repairs (nonthermal).
- Thermal US is often used when patients present with scar tissue, joint contracture, adhesive capsulitis, movement limitation, or decreased ROM secondary to soft-tissue injury and pain.
- Therapeutic parameters and outcomes of thermal US vary in the research but demonstrate effectiveness (Table 24-1).[27–29]

Thermal doses of US are dependent on the treatment goal and presenting problem. It is important to respect the stretching window following high-intensity applications because tissue temperature will cool approximately 2°C (3.6°F) within 5 to 10 minutes.[30,31]

When treating subacute inflammation, thermal effects should be mild—that is, an increase in tissue temperature of approximately 1°C (1.8°F). Moderate thermal effects are used for pain modulation/altered nerve conduction velocity, muscle relaxation/stiffness, muscle spasm, and chronic inflammation.

Nonthermal US exerts mechanical effects at the cellular level to facilitate the healing process but does not elevate tissue temperature. US is applied using a 20% duty cycle. Nonthermal effects of pulsed US occur at the cell membrane because of stable cavitation, acoustic streaming, and micro massage.[32,33] Second-order effects of nonthermal US are caused by the destabilization of the cellular membrane. This contributes to the enhancement of the inflammatory response to accelerate tissue healing.[34,35]

Phonophoresis

Phonophoresis is the use of US to facilitate the delivery of topically applied drugs or medication to selected tissue. Anti-inflammatory medication, such as betamethasone, is administered using US to decrease the inflammatory process. Research related to its effectiveness is inconsistent because of variability in treatment parameters. Phonophoresis does not allow therapists to effectively dose or measure the amount of drug patients receive. Other methods such as iontophoresis may be a more appropriate choice.[36]

Table 24-1. Clinical Parameters for Ultrasound Based on Healing Stage

TISSUE STATE	INTENSITY REQUIRED AT THE LESION (W/cm^2)
Acute (inflammatory phase)	0.2
Subacute (proliferative phase)	0.3–0.7
Chronic (maturation phase)	0.8–2.0

Contraindications

Most contraindications and precautions for US use are because of thermal effects.

- Hemorrhagic regions, reproductive organs
- Impaired sensation
- Over electronic implants (pacemakers, neurostim systems)
- Directly over the spinal cord after laminectomy
- Over areas suspected to be cancerous or precancerous
- In front of the upper neck (carotid sinus)
- Over joints or tissues that have been injected with medication within the last 3 months
- Over plastic or cement implants
- Directly over the skull or bony prominences (bony part of elbow)

Precautions

- Acute inflammation
- Epiphyseal plates
- Fracture healing (high dose)
- Breast implants
- Application of cryotherapy
- Primary repair of tendon or ligament

General Instructions or Directions for Ultrasound Use

- Review patient evaluation to determine whether US is indicated for the clinical condition; review precautions and contraindications.
- Determine treatment tissue depth (superficial or deep) to establish frequency. Identify tissue healing phase to determine therapeutic parameters (heat or heal). Check skin condition.
- Clean the area and sound head; apply US gel to the targeted tissue.
- Explain the procedure to patients; they may feel a gentle warmth, but not intense heat or pain during application.
- Remove jewelry, position the patient, and drape area being treated.
- Set the therapeutic parameters of frequency (deep 1 MHz or superficial 3 MHz), duty cycle (20% heal, 50% warm, 100% heat), intensity (0.2 W/cm^2 heal; higher intensities to heat), and treatment time (10–15 minutes for large area and vigorous dose and 1 MHz; 2–7 minutes for small areas and 3 MHz).

Table 24-2. Thermal and Nonthermal Effects of Therapeutic Ultrasound

THERMAL EFFECTS	NONTHERMAL EFFECTS
Increases extensibility of collagen fibers	Increases phagocytic activity of macrophages/attracts immune cells to tissue
Decreases muscle stiffness	Increases protein synthesis
Reduces muscle spasm	Increases capillary density
Alters nerve conduction velocity/diminishes pain perception	Regenerates tissue
Increases metabolism and blood flow	Heals wounds and fractures
Provides all of the effects of nonthermal ultrasound	

- Move soundhead slowly, approximately 4 cm per second, keeping the soundhead in contact with the skin. Positional heat and stretch technique can be used to increase ROM.
- If patient reports pain or heat, add additional gel, decrease intensity and duty cycle, and move the sound head.
- When treatment is complete, wipe the gel off and clean the soundhead.
- Document the treatment, therapeutic parameters, and patient response.

The larger the treatment area, the greater the time required. The area that can be effectively treated is twice the size of the soundhead. The transducer should be kept flat during application with a gentle pressure and adequate amount of US gel. Preset intensities should be avoided because they will likely not be effective in generating desired treatment outcomes and benefits of therapeutic US.[29,37] Research has identified that higher doses of US energy and longer applications were found to have more positive outcomes (Table 24-2).

Precautions for Ultrasound Use

Patients should be monitored during US, and any pain or discomfort may indicate that the intensity is too high or that there is an inadequate amount of gel. When using US as a thermal agent, one must follow general contraindications and precautions for any thermal modality.

Electrotherapy

Advances in technology, a focus on pain control, clinical outcomes, and availability, have facilitated the increased interest and use of electrotherapy in clinical practice. Electricity is a form of energy consisting of charged particles (electrons) and which has magnetic, chemical, mechanical, and thermal properties. There are a variety of electrotherapeutic devices available, which use specific currents and modifications to impact tissue healing, muscle strength and endurance, pain modulation, inflammation, and muscle spasm. Surface electromyography biofeedback monitors the electrical activity level in muscles (helps determine how well someone is able to recruit muscle activity on their own) and is often paired with NMES.

Forms of Electrotherapy

- **Neuromuscular electrical stimulation (NMES)** uses pulsating, alternating current to activate muscles through stimulation of intact peripheral nerves to cause a motor response. Stimulation of the motor nerve is used to decrease muscle spasm, strengthen muscle, and for muscle pumping that can reduce edema. NMES to innervated muscle is used for muscle reeducation, atrophy prevention, and muscle spasm and edema reduction.
- **Functional electrical stimulation (FES)** is electrical stimulation used to activate targeted muscle groups for orthotic substitution or to facilitate performance of functional activities or movements. FES is often used with individuals who have shoulder subluxation, weak grasp/release, or foot drop after a stroke.
- **Transcutaneous electrical nerve stimulation (TENS)** uses pulsed alternating current for pain control. TENS uses surface electrodes placed strategically over the area of pain to stimulate afferent sensory nerve fibers to modulate pain perception. TENS is used for targeting smaller areas, trigger points, muscle spasm, and acupuncture points.
- **Electrical muscle stimulation (EMS)** is electrical stimulation of denervated muscle to facilitate viability and to prevent atrophy, degeneration, and fiber fibrosis. EMS facilitates nerve regeneration and muscle reinnervation.
- **Interferential current therapy (IFC)** utilizes two channels (four electrodes placed in a vector pattern) simultaneously with different frequencies. This allows deeper tissue penetration to facilitate pain reduction and physiological effects. IFC is used for treatment of large areas and deeper tissues.
- **Iontophoresis** is the use of low-voltage direct current to ionize topically applied medication into tissue. Iontophoresis is often used in the treatment of inflammatory conditions or for scar formation and management.
- **Electrical stimulation for tissue repair (ESTR)**, also known as high-voltage galvanic stimulation (HVGS), has been used for tissue healing. Because of its complexity, use requires highly advanced training, and therefore, it is not reviewed in this chapter.

Principles of Electricity

The clinical use of electrotherapy and integrating the concepts and parameters necessary for safe use require advanced training and knowledge. The reader is encouraged to pursue additional education and training to ensure service competency and safe, effective use of electrotherapy. It is beyond the scope of this textbook to discuss all aspects of electrotherapy, but the primary concepts will be highlighted.

There are two primary forms of electrical current, alternating current (AC) and direct current (DC), both of which can be modified or pulsed. DC is unidirectional, with the electrons moving continuously in one direction, and the electrodes maintaining their polarity. AC is characterized by periodic changes in the polarity of the current flow (positive-to-negative, sinus wave form). The current is uninterrupted and bidirectional, without any true positive or negative pole. Household electricity uses AC. Pulsed current is the term used when electron flow is periodically interrupted for very short periods of milliseconds or microseconds. *Modulation* refers to changes or modifications made in one or more aspects of the current.

Electric current is represented graphically by a waveform and provides a visual representation of the current flow. The amplitude (intensity/output) is the level or distance the impulse rises above or below a baseline (zero electric charge), whereas the pulse duration is the length of time that is required to complete the shape of the electrical flow. A pulsed waveform is classified as either monophasic (consisting of a single phase), biphasic (two phases with current flow in both directions), or polyphasic (multiple phases). Electrical stimulation at low current intensity evokes a sensory response. If the current intensity is high enough to exceed the motor threshold, a muscle contraction will occur.

The principles underlying all forms of electrotherapy include selection of the appropriate form of electrotherapy based on the therapeutic goals for the patient, and the concepts of amplitude, pulse duration, and pulse frequency. The peak amplitude is the most frequent level of intensity used in clinical settings and is measured in amperes, micro amperes, or for most electrotherapy equipment used clinically milliamperes (mA), which is one thousandth of an ampere, a measure for small electric currents. Pulse duration (pulse width) consists of the length of time the electric flow is "on" and is measured in microseconds or milliseconds (ms). As pulse width increases, more muscle fibers are stimulated. A narrow pulse width is typically better for pain control.[38] The pulse rate or pulse frequency is the number of pulses or wave forms per second and is measured in pulses per second (pps) or Hz. If pulse duration is too short, an action potential won't be reached. The higher the intensity and frequency of pulses, the stronger the muscle contraction.

Duty cycle is the ratio the time the current is on to the time the current is off. For example, a treatment protocol in which electrical stimuli are delivered for 10 seconds followed by a 50-second off period is expressed as a 1:5 duty cycle. Most common duty cycles/protocols used for NMES are 1:1, 1:3, and 1:5 to allow for greater volitional extremity movement.

Effects

Human tissue is either excitable or nonexcitable. Excitable tissues respond to intensity, pulse duration, and pulse frequency. Excitable tissues, such as nerves and muscles, can initiate and propagate an action potential.

The diameter of the nerve, depth of the nerve, and duration of the pulse affect a nerve's response to electrical stimulation (Fig. 24-6). Sensory nerves are stimulated first, followed by motor nerves, pain fibers, and finally muscle fibers. As the amplitude is increased, motor nerves reach threshold and with sufficient intensity, contraction of all muscle fibers attached to that nerve (motor unit) occurs.

In volitional movement, there is asynchronous recruitment of muscle. Electrodes act as the interface between the skin surface and the current flow from the stimulation device. Electrodes come in several sizes and should be selected based on muscle size and number of motor units stimulated. Electrodes are self-adhesive and should only be used with the same patient to avoid cross contamination.

Neuromuscular Electrical Stimulation

Neuromuscular electrical stimulation (NMES) refers to the use of electricity to elicit a muscle contraction of paralyzed or paretic muscles and is used for muscle reeducation, muscle strengthening, preventing disuse atrophy, and edema control, and requires an intact peripheral nerve (Fig. 24-7). FES is the use of NMES as

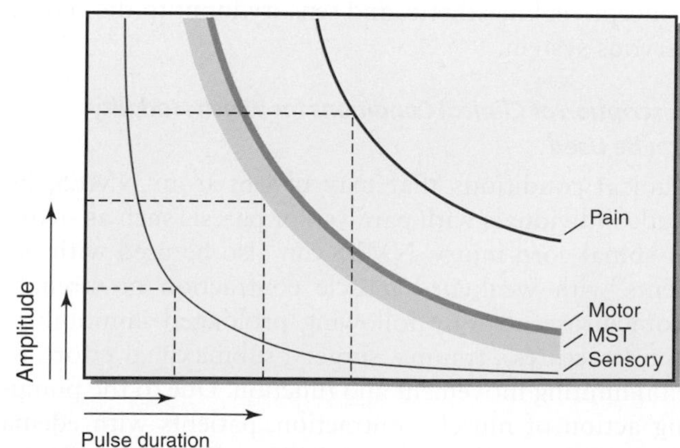

Figure 24-6. The strength–duration curve of an electrical stimulus describes the relationship between the amplitude and duration of the stimulus needed to depolarize a specific nerve to achieve a response. MST, maximum sensory threshold.

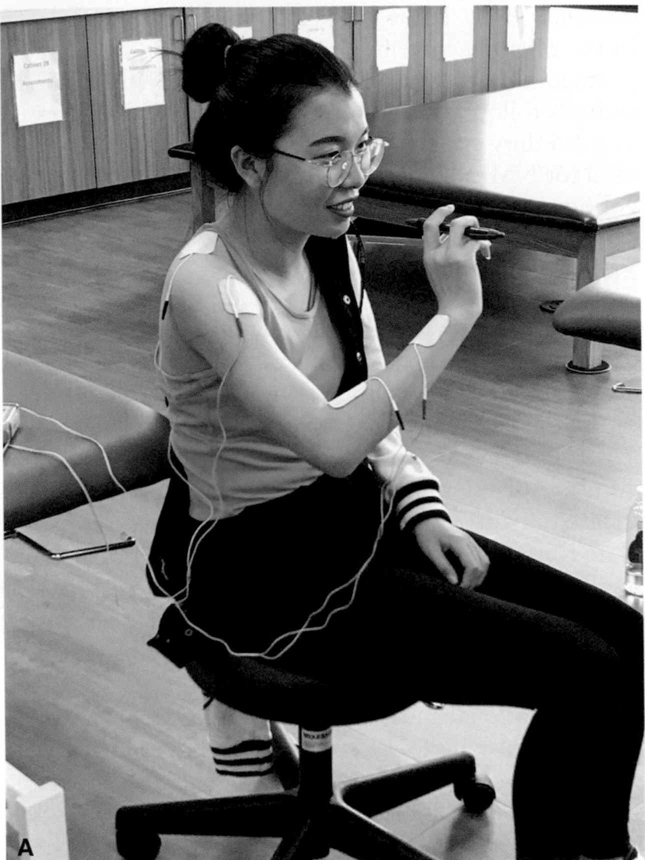

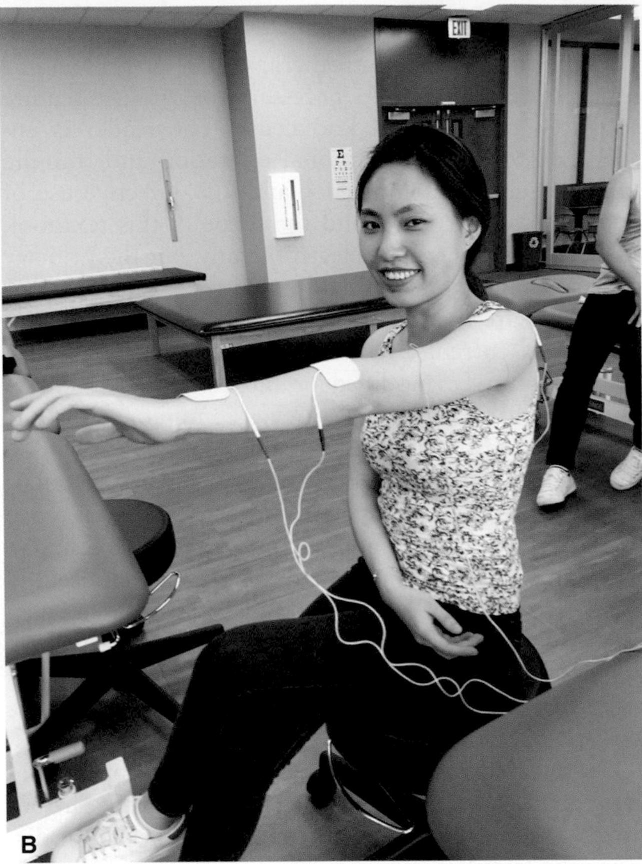

Figure 24-7. A and **B,** Multichannel reaching. Common electrode placements for reaching patterns using two channels of stimulation.

an orthotic substitute (neuroprosthesis) to assist with a functional activity and movement.[39,40]

Mechanisms Underlying Function/Effect

Stimulation of targeted peripheral or motor nerves with sufficient pulse width, frequency and amplitude to tetany, produces movement of an extremity to improve or restore motor function. Stimulation also provides proprioceptive, kinesthetic, and sensory input to the central nervous system.

Description of Clinical Conditions for Which Modality Can Be Used

Clinical conditions that may benefit from NMES, include individuals with paralysis or paresis such as stroke or spinal cord injury. NMES can also be used with patients with weakened muscle contraction or strength from disuse atrophy following prolonged immobilization (fractures), trauma, surgery, submaximal effort, or pain limiting movement and function. Due to the pumping action of muscle contraction, patients with edema may also be candidates for NMES or FES.[41–43]

Precautions

Review precautions listed in the equipment's operating manual before applying electrical stimulation. The lowest effective current should be applied to patients with impaired mentation or sensation. Level of motor response and skin condition should be closely monitored. Areas of skin irritation, damage, or skin lesions can cause decreased tissue impedance and increased current that may result in pain and should be avoided.

Contraindications

Electrical stimulation should not be applied to the craniofacial or cervical region of patients who have stroke or seizure histories; areas of phrenic nerves or bladder stimulators; over the carotid sinus; near diathermy devices; over or near superficial metal pins, plates, or hardware; and patients with cancer, infection, tuberculosis, active hemorrhage, and cardiac pacemakers.

General Instructions or Directions for Use

- The patient should be reevaluated to determine whether the injury or problem is appropriate for NMES use and to identify therapeutic goals.
- Review precautions, contraindications, and identify movement patterns to determine which muscles or muscle groups are active, inactive, or weak. Identify which muscles will be targeted for stimulation and what movement patterns are required. Check and

clean the area to be treated, do not place electrodes over cuts, abrasions, or lacerations.

- Review the specific characteristics of the equipment and select the parameters for the NMES unit that will be used.
- Explain the procedure to patients and describe the sensation they will experience (tingling/vibrating) followed by muscle twitching, fasciculations, and, finally, tetany with muscle contraction and joint movement.
- Place the primary electrode over the bulk of the muscle fibers consistent with the desired contraction and/or movement with the other electrode parallel to the muscle fibers and at the distal or proximal end of the muscle (near origin or insertion). Connect the leads to the electrodes and stimulator (Fig. 24-8).
- Pulse rate for muscle contraction should be 30 to 35 pps for healthy patients (ortho); higher frequencies (such as 50 pps) will fatigue spastic muscles. Phase durations between 200 and 400 μs will stimulate the motor nerve.
- Set the on/off time (duty cycle) for the intended amount of time with consideration of a 1:1, 1:3, or 1:5 ratio.
- Gradually increase the amplitude until sufficient to reach a tetanic contraction. Treatment time is between 10 and 30 minutes. For orthopedic patients or to increase muscle strength, the amplitude/intensity should be increased to the patient's maximum tolerance.
- Modify the electric current if the patient reports pain or discomfort. If the contraction is intolerable, a sensory response can be achieved by decreasing the amplitude or by modifying the pulse duration/width to 150 to 200 μs. As the patient can tolerate the stimulation, parameters can be changed.
- When treatment is over, remove electrodes and check patient skin. When the patient displays volitional movement patterns, stimulation can be set at a sensory level to cue the patient as to the desired movement pattern, or the duty cycle can be modified to a 1:3 or 1:1 ratio for strength and endurance.

Transcutaneous Electrical Nerve Stimulation

TENS uses surface electrodes and low-voltage pulsed electrical current to stimulate superficial nerves to modulate the patient's pain perception.

Mechanism Underlying Function/Effect

Treatment applications using electrical stimulation for pain control employ pulsed or AC in a variety of stimulation patterns. Stimulation type is based on the physiological response to the stimulation with the goal being pain relief and comfort. Four levels of stimulation used include subsensory, sensory, motor, and noxious levels. Two primary theories on which the modulation of pain

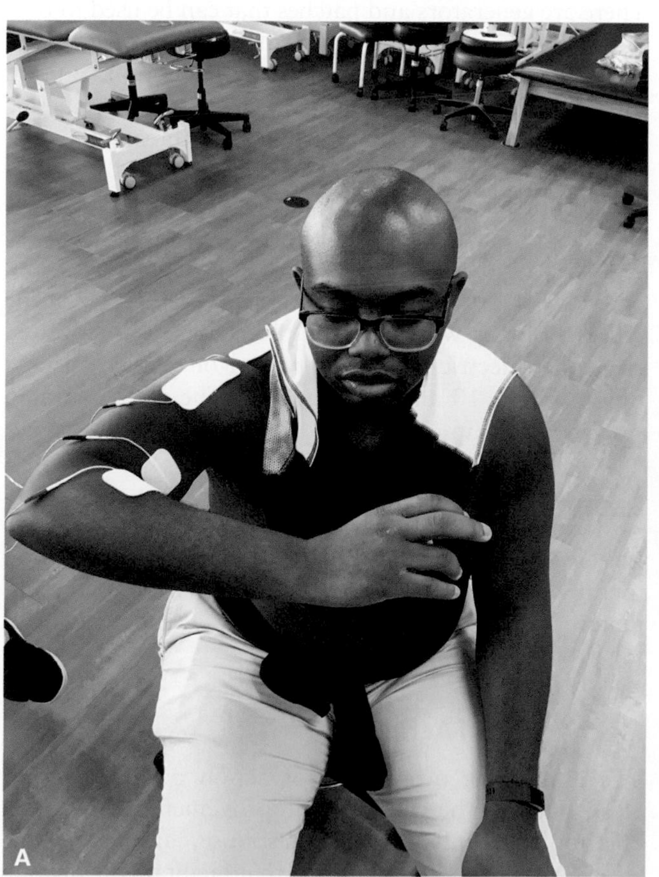

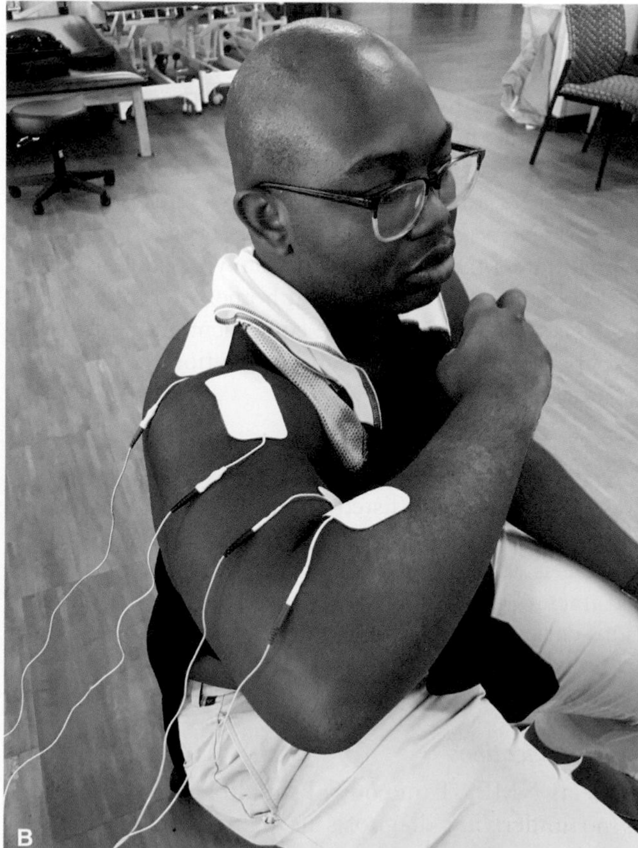

Figure 24-8. **A** and **B,** Multichannel reaching. Common electrode placements for reaching patterns using two channels of stimulation.

with TENS is based are the gate control theory and the opioid theory.[11,44] Gate theory involves stimulation of afferent nerves to block pain by closing the gate in the spinal column to pain signals. Opioid theory asserts that natural beta endorphins are released with the application of intense beat frequency of TENS that inhibits pain signal transmission and occurs with muscle fatigue or physiological stress.[45,46]

Clinical Conditions for Which Modality Can Be Used

Pain is one of the most common complaints that cause patients to seek medical care. Adequate pain management facilitates occupational function. TENS can be used to manage pain in musculoskeletal disorders, pre- and post-surgically, and for both acute and chronic pain.[46,47]

General Instructions

- Treatment employs pulsed or AC in a variety of stimulation patterns.
- Review the clinical diagnosis, presenting signs and symptoms, and determine appropriateness for TENS use.
- Explain the treatment to the patient; describe current sensation (tingling, buzzing).
- Clean the area where the electrodes will be placed. Remove jewelry and clothing over the treatment area. Ensure skin integrity.
- Optimal electrode placements correlate with pain structures and sources, and include dermatomes, motor, trigger, and acupuncture points.
- Position electrodes securely to maintain conductivity. Electrodes can be parallel, crossed, front/back, bracketed, or crisscrossed over the area of pain. If the patient doesn't achieve pain modulation, electrodes should be moved and a different wave form tried. Increase amplitude after 10 minutes to avoid accommodation to the stimulation.
- Treatment time varies between 30 and 60 minutes. Patient can use the TENS unit as needed for pain or maintain a three to four times daily schedule.
- TENS units are often used at home. Therapists should explain the purpose of the equipment and instruct the patient in its operations and precautions (verbally and in writing).

Precautions

Review precautions listed in the equipment's operating manual before applying electrical stimulation. Amplitude is increased to patient comfort and tolerance. Parameters can be changed to avoid nerve accommodation. Patients should be instructed to avoid overactivity to prevent tissue damage or further injury by engaging in activities without pain sensation.

Contraindications

Same as NMES. Pain control should be avoided if there is no underlying diagnosis as pain is a protective response to potential or actual tissue damage.

Iontophoresis

Iontophoresis is an active drug delivery system that uses direct current to deliver medication through the skin. Iontophoresis is easily applied, the amount of drug is consistent, and it is essentially painless.

Mechanism of Action

The most commonly used medication for musculoskeletal conditions is dexamethasone, which has a negative ion. Because direct current is used, the like (same) charge is applied to the medicated electrode, repelling the medicated ion into the tissue. The black, negative lead is placed over the medicated electrode with the red lead connected to the dispersive electrode 4 to 5 inches away. Like charges repel the ion into the tissue where it exerts a biophysiological effect; for dexamethasone, it decreases inflammation.

Clinical Conditions for Which Modality Can Be Used

Iontophoresis can be used for treatment of acute inflammatory conditions such as epicondylitis, carpal tunnel syndrome, glenohumeral bursitis, ulnar nerve inflammation, wrist tendinitis, and tenosynovitis. Therapists should thoroughly understand patient pathophysiology, medications, and potential drug interactions. Documented orders should be obtained from physicians prior to using iontophoresis.[48]

General Instructions

There are generators and patches that can be used to provide iontophoresis. Primary consideration is clinical diagnosis, area to be treated, and medication selection. Caution must be used because medications may cause an allergic or anaphylactic reaction, which is a life-threatening condition and medical emergency. Patients should be asked for a list of current medications, any known allergies, sensitivities, or reactions to foods or medications.

Medication is placed in the electrode reservoir and positioned over the treatment tissue. The polarity of the ion determines which lead is placed on the medicated electrode. Electric current is turned on with treatment time between 10 and 20 minutes.[49] The most common side effect is skin irritation.

Laser Therapy (Low-Level Laser Therapy)

Low-level laser therapy (LLLT), or photobiomodulation therapy, is the application of a monochromatic, collimated red and near-infrared light to facilitate the healing process and modulate pain.

Mechanism of Action

The underlying mechanism of action of LLLT is not clear, but may be caused by improvement in microcirculation, the inflammatory response, and adenosine triphosphate production (ATP) that facilitate the healing process. There are physiological and therapeutic effects at a cellular level causing a disruption in the histochemicals and cell membrane that modify the inflammatory response, facilitating healing and modulating pain.[50,51] LLLT lasers do not produce heat, sound, or vibration; have no thermal effect; and are called cold lasers.

Clinical Conditions for Which Modality Can Be Used

LLLT impacts the tissue at the cellular level. Research varies but supports its use for wound healing, inflammatory arthropathies, soft-tissue injuries, and pain modulation.[52]

General Instructions

LLLT appears to affect the three phases of healing, particularly the inflammatory process and fibroplasia. LLLT increases connective-tissue repair and modifies the cell membrane, allowing histochemical changes that occur with healing and decreasing the inflammatory process. There are different wavelengths that vary from 600 to 900 nm and are most commonly used to treat a variety of musculoskeletal conditions. Patients and therapists should wear appropriate safety goggles, and the laser should never be aimed into the eyes. LLLT should not be used with patients with active cancer or secondary metastasis unless used for pain control for palliative care. LLLT should not be applied over the abdomen of pregnant women or those with seizure history.

Surface Electromyographic Biofeedback

Biofeedback refers to those procedures or techniques that provide individuals with an auditory or visual cue, "feedback," to gain volitional control over a physiological response. Biofeedback provides an external mechanism for monitoring a specific physiological function and response, and through instant feedback, allows individuals to attempt to control or modify their behavior or response.

Clinical Conditions for Which Modality Can Be Used

Biofeedback is used to treat a variety of conditions, including migraine headaches, pain, anxiety, behavioral disorders, hyper/hypotension, paralysis, and movement disorders. In rehabilitation, surface electromyographic (sEMG) feedback is used for muscle reeducation and can be paired with electrical stimulation to provide movement and enhance motor control. It can also be used for women's health and pelvic floor disorders and incontinence. Clinical use of sEMG paired with electrical stimulation has been demonstrated to be effective for improving performance and functional movements in the hemiplegic upper extremity (UE); dysphagia, muscle dysfunction, and myoclonus following spinal cord injuries; focal hand dystonia; and movement dysfunction in children with cerebral palsy.[53–56]

Mechanism of Action

Biofeedback uses surface electrodes and instrumentation to measure and display the physiological response of the body, including respiratory, cardiovascular, and neuromuscular. Clinically, feedback measures activity in the neuromuscular system and is used for motor reeducation, retraining of functional movement, and to improve performance in activities of daily living (ADLs). Biofeedback provides immediate feedback (auditory or visual), allowing patients to objectively measure, determine, and quantify muscle activity and track motor performance changes.

Following a stroke, there is often a disruption of motor control and an impairment in sensation, kinesthesia, and proprioception in the affected extremities, limiting functional ability and movement. sEMG provides a mechanism for providing feedback to enhance motor return and movement patterns.

General Instructions

Use of sEMG biofeedback for muscle reeducation uses auditory and visual feedback, which measures muscle activation level. These parameters or threshold for activation can be adjusted, which also allows grading of the activity or movement depending on the goal and sensory and kinesthetic feedback.

- Surface electrodes are placed over the targeted muscles to detect the electrical impulse that is generated with muscle contraction.
- Dependent on the threshold parameter, with the onset of a muscle contraction, the biofeedback unit will alert the patient through auditory or visual stimulus or both.
- As the contraction strengthens and movement progresses, the auditory tone may become louder as additional muscle fibers are recruited.
- Feedback sensitivity can be adjusted to provide the patient with immediate feedback about the desired movement or unwanted muscle activity.
- sEMG can be paired with electrical stimulation to allow for completion of developing movement patterns, such as reach, grasp, or release.
- As motor function improves, more complex movement patterns can be added to the therapy program.
- For chronic pain or muscle spasm, sEMG provides feedback related to hyperactive muscle contraction (spasm), alerting the patient to consciously relax those muscles.

As with all physical modalities used in occupational therapy, biofeedback is a component of the occupational therapy process and is used in preparation for or concurrently with purposeful and occupation-based activities.

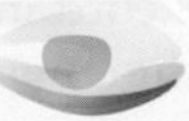

CASE STUDY

Patient Information

Marie is a 36-year-old African American female who experienced a stroke affecting her left side secondary to a prothrombotic disorder with no prior history. The stroke occurred while vacationing with her husband and two sons (age 9 and 12). She was initially stabilized at a small community hospital, then airlifted to a university hospital where she was treated and began inpatient rehabilitation. She made consistent progress at the facility and was independent for most basic level ADLs. Her discharge plans included recommendation for outpatient treatment. She was discharged home with orders to continue outpatient therapy. Marie lives in a small town in a rural community. Prior to the cerebrovascular accident (CVA), she was employed as a lead surgical nurse at an area hospital. She was actively involved in her community and the children's school and was responsible for most household activities including cooking, preparing her son's school lunches, laundry, and cleaning. Marie attended extracurricular school activities such as soccer and baseball, assisted with classroom and school activities when her schedule permitted, and was actively involved in her church. She was right-hand dominant and independent in ADLs and instrumental ADLs (IADLs) prior to the CVA.

Assessment Process and Results

Marie was accompanied by her husband for the initial evaluation, was alert and oriented, but appeared apprehensive and subdued. Speech was clear, though slow, and responses appropriate. Marie ambulated independently, demonstrating good dynamic balance using a standard cane and left ankle-foot orthosis (AFO). She displayed dynamic active movement in the left UE. Assessment results revealed fluctuating tone with volitional movement and difficulty combining left shoulder, elbow, and forearm/hand motions for performance of efficient forward, side, and overhead reaching; or when attempting to reach, combined with grasp/release patterns. She displayed fluctuating flexor tone in the biceps and finger flexors when attempting to grasp and move objects using the left UE, minimal left unilateral neglect, and diminished tactile sensation of the left arm and hand. She displayed increased flexor tone in the biceps, gross grasp, and beginning finger extension and release when attempting to grasp objects such as cups. She displayed active should flexion and abduction (0°–95°); elbow movement lacked 30° of active extension, but full passive extension was present. Active elbow flexion was 30° to 100° with flexor synergies noted when fatigued. Endurance was low. No confusion or cognitive impairment was noted.

Marie reports independence for feeding, drinking, and dressing, but requires additional time to complete tasks using compensatory techniques rather than consistent, active left UE use as an assist. She attempts to use the left UE for self-care and IADL tasks but mentions that she frequently becomes frustrated owing to lack of endurance and tonal changes. Marie is independent in gait and ambulation using a standard cane and AFO as an assist, and transfers independently with good static and dynamic balance. She requires minimal assistance for higher level IADL tasks, such as meal preparation, laundry, and bathing.

The significant limiting factor identified by Marie was the inability to use her left UE more functionally and fluidly with better reach, grasp, and release patterns to facilitate independence and completion rate. The Canadian Occupational Performance Measure (COPM) was administered to the client. Marie identified the following occupations as most important to her and in which she wants to engage: meal preparation, laundry, driving, and return to work.

Occupational Therapy Problem List

The following problems were identified during the assessment:

- Decreased initiation of IADL secondary to endurance and tonal changes
- Decreased functional use of the left UE to complete ADLs and IADLs
- Developing reach and grasp patterns with fluctuating tone with volitional movement
- Decreased strength and endurance for return to work and functional independence
- Dependent for community mobility on public transportation

Occupational Therapy Goal List

- Marie will be independent for ADLs and IADLs, demonstrating active arm reach and hand grasp/release patterns for object manipulation.
- Marie will display active grasp and release patterns of the UE to manipulate large objects as a component of meal preparation.
- Marie will independently complete a laundry load using her left UE to assist in loading laundry/dryer machines and folding laundry.
- Marie will return to work on a part-time basis, increasing to full-time employment as endurance improves.

Intervention

To facilitate and strengthen an active reach-and-release pattern overriding flexor synergies, NMES electrical stimulation was used to strengthen volitional movement patterns of mass extension/reach of the left UE. Participation in food preparation and laundry was incorporated into the stimulated movement patterns and was triggered using an external trigger to the stimulator. Active participation in movements and activities, combined with electrically stimulated movement, was used to strengthen and facilitate outcomes.[42,57]

Owing to increased flexor tone in the left biceps and wrist/finger flexors, targeted muscles for NMES to facilitate a mass reach-and-release pattern will involve a dual-channel stimulation, targeting the muscles of the left anterior deltoid and triceps/posterior deltoid (channel 1) and wrist/finger extensors (channel 2).

NMES Parameters

- **Rate:** 35 pps
- **Waveform:** Asymmetrical

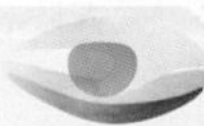

CASE STUDY (continued)

- **On:Off Cycle**:
  - 1:3
  - 1:3 to 1:1 for endurance
  - 1:5 for power
- **Ramp:** 2 seconds

Reeducation

- Proceed with 10 to 20 minutes of muscle stimulation as tolerated.
- May need to adjust for accommodation.
- Watch for signs of fatigue.
- To improve strength and endurance, treatment time should start at 30 minutes per session and increase to 60 minutes daily, 4 to 6 days per week. Research is variable in terms of length of treatment and frequency, but some studies indicate that longer treatment times, even at a sensory level without muscle contraction, and if treatment occurs more often (3–6 days/week), will improve function and hemiplegic UE use.[58–60]

Best Evidence for Physical Agent Modalities Used in Occupational Therapy

Intervention	Description	Participants	Dosage	Research Design and Evidence Level	Benefit	Statistical Significance and Effect Size
Neuromuscular Electrical Stimulation (NMES)[61]	The study used a specially designed NMES system to target shoulder flexion, elbow extension, and wrist-and-finger extension to improve motor control and functional use of the UE in chronic stroke patients.	15 participants with chronic (>1 year following CVA) upper limb hemiparesis	Upper limb training for 60 minutes/day, 6 days/week, for 2 weeks, using both a shoulder-and-elbow stimulation device and a wrist-and-finger stimulation device	Randomized controlled trial Level I	Multi-muscle stimulation approach and method appears to be a feasible approach and adjunctive method for chronic stroke patients. Participants demonstrated improved motor control and functional upper limb use.	Significant improvements in the UE component of the Fugl-Meyer (F-M) assessment and Action Research Arm Test (ARAT) scores ($p < 0.01$) were found. There were also significant reductions in Modified Ashworth Scale scores for the elbow and wrist flexors ($p < 0.01$).
NMES[62]	Systematic review of FES following CVA to determine effect of electrical stimulation (FES) in improving activity and to investigate whether FES is more effective than training alone	18 articles included in review; randomized and controlled trials Population: poststroke	Varied with each study	Systematic review and meta-analysis of 18 research articles Level I	FES moderately improved activity (specifically UE activity) when compared with no intervention or training alone.	FES had a moderate effect on activity (standardized mean difference [SMD], 0.40; 95% confidence interval [CI], .09 - .72) compared with no or placebo intervention. FES had moderate effect on activity (SMD, 0.56; 95% CI, .29 - .92) compared with training alone. When subgroup analyses were performed, FES had large effect on upper limb activity (SMD, 0.69; 95% CI, .33 - 1.05) and small effect on walking speed (mean difference, 0.08 m/s; 95% CI, .02 - .15) compared with control groups.
NMES[63]	Use of NMES to the hand muscles combined with repetitive task practice to determine effect on skilled hand performance in patients following CVA. All participants received repetitive task practice, but control group received sham electrical stimulation.	40 patients poststroke between the ages of 45 and 65 (first CVA)	NMES for 30 minutes, 3×/week for 8 weeks	Randomized controlled trial (pre/post-treatment measurements) Level I	Repetitive task practice therapy combined with electrical stimulation improved skilled hand performance in terms of hand motor function, skills, and ROM in stroke patients. Patients in experimental group showed significant improvement in fine motor control and hand function compared with those in control group.	Motor assessment scale score was 4.25 ± 0.63 for experimental group and 3.35 ± 0.74 for control group ($t = -3.50$ and $p = 0.0001$). Time to complete Jebsen Taylor Test was 180.90 ± 7.04 for experimental group and 192.80 ± 6.87 for control group ($t = 4.50$ and $p = 0.0001$).
Functional Electrical Stimulation (FES)[64]	FES and use of advanced iterative learning control (ILC) technology to improve functional control and UE use	Five CVA patients, aged >18 years and at least 6 months post-CVA	60 minutes/session for 18 treatment sessions	Randomized controlled trial Level I	Combining low-cost technology with advanced FES controllers ILC, strengthens upper limb movement and function and may decrease UE impairments poststroke.	A one-tailed, paired t test, with a significance level of $p < 0.05$, was used to compare pre- and postintervention F-M and ARAT outcome measures.

References

1. Bracciano A, McPhee S, Rose B. Physical agent modalities a position paper. *Am J Occup Ther*. 2012;66:S78–S80.
2. AOTA. Scope of practice. *Am J Occup Ther*. 2014;68(S04):S34–S40.
3. Richard L, Furler J, Densley K, et al. Equity of access to primary healthcare for vulnerable populations: the IMPACT international online survey of innovations. *Int J Equity Health*. 2016;15:64.
4. Ruano AL, Shadmi E, Furler J, et al. Looking forward to the next 15 years: innovation and new pathways for research in health equity. *Int J Equity Health*. 2017;16(1):35.
5. Hildenbrand W, Lamb A. Occupational therapy in prevention and wellness: retaining relevance in a new health care world. *Am J Occup Ther*. 2013;67(3):266.
6. Bracciano A, McPhee S, Rose B. Physical agent modalities. *Am J Occup Ther*. 2012;66(6):78–80. doi:10.5014/ajot.2012.66S78.
7. Tygiel PP. On "exposure to low amounts of ultrasound energy..." Alexander LD, Gilman DRD, Brown DR, et al. Phys Ther. 2010;90:14–25. *Phys Ther*. 2010;90(3):461; author reply 461–462.
8. American Occupational Therapy Association. Occupational therapy practice framework: domain and process (3rd edition). *Am J Occup Ther*. 2014;68(suppl 1): S1–S48.
9. Treede RD. The international association for the study of pain definition of pain: as valid in 2018 as in 1979, but in need of regularly updated footnotes. *Pain Rep*. 2018;3(2):e643.
10. Cohen M, Quintner J, van Rysewyk S. Reconsidering the international association for the study of pain definition of pain. *Pain Rep*. 2018;3(2):e634.
11. Melzack R. Evolution of the neuromatrix theory of pain. The Prithvi Raj lecture: Presented at the third world congress of world institute of pain, Barcelona 2004. *Pain Pract*. 2005;5(2):85–94.
12. Doleys DM. Chronic pain as a hypothetical construct: a practical and philosophical consideration. *Front Psychol*. 2017;8:664.
13. Gupta S, Andersen C, Black J, et al. Management of chronic wounds: diagnosis, preparation, treatment, and follow-up. *Wounds*. 2017;29(9):S19–S36.
14. Tao H, Butler JP, Luttrell T. The role of whirlpool in wound care. *J Am Coll Clin Wound Spec*. 2013;4(1):7–12.
15. Szekeres M, MacDermid JC, Grewal R, Birmingham T. The short-term effects of hot packs vs therapeutic whirlpool on active wrist range of motion for patients with distal radius fracture: a randomized controlled trial. *J Hand Ther*. 2018;31(3):276–281.
16. Szekeres M, MacDermid JC, Birmingham T, Grewal R, Lalone E. The effect of therapeutic whirlpool and hot packs on hand volume during rehabilitation after distal radius fracture: a blinded randomized controlled trial. *Hand (N Y)*. 2017;12(3):265–271.
17. Bracciano A. *Physical Agent Modalities: Theory and Application for the Occupational Therapist*. 3rd ed. Thorofare, NJ: Slack, Inc.; 2019.
18. Bleakley CM, Davison GW. Cryotherapy and inflammation: evidence beyond the cardinal signs. *Phys Ther Rev*. 2010;15(6):430–435.
19. Bongers CC, Hopman MT, Eijsvogels TM. Cooling interventions for athletes: an overview of effectiveness, physiological mechanisms, and practical considerations. *Temperature*. 2017;4(1):60–78.
20. Abd El-Maksoud GM, Sharaf MA, Rezk-Allah SS. Efficacy of cold therapy on spasticity and hand function in children with cerebral palsy. *J Adv Res*. 2011;2(4): 319–325. doi:10.1016/j.jare.2011.02.003.
21. Gillette CM, Merrick MA. The effect of ICE on intramuscular tissue temperature. *J Sport Rehabil*. 2017:1–15.
22. Dupuy O, Douzi W, Theurot D, Bosquet L, Dugue B. An evidence-based approach for choosing post-exercise recovery techniques to reduce markers of muscle damage, soreness, fatigue, and inflammation: a systematic review with meta-analysis. *Front Physiol*. 2018;9:403.
23. Harrison A, Lin S, Pounder N, Mikuni-Takagi Y. Mode & mechanism of low intensity pulsed ultrasound (LIPUS) in fracture repair. *Ultrasonics*. 2016;70:45–52.
24. Kimura IF, Gulick DT, Shelly J, Ziskin MC. Effects of two ultrasound devices and angles of application on the temperature of tissue phantom. *J Orthop Sports Phys Ther*. 1998;27(1):27–31.
25. ter Haar G. Basic physics of therapeutic ultrasound. *Physiotherapy*. 1978;64(4):100–103.
26. ter Haar G. Therapeutic ultrasound. *Eur J Ultrasound*. 1999;9(1):3–9.
27. Draper D, Prentice W. Therapeutic ultrasound. In: Prentice W, ed. *Therapeutic Modalities for Physical Therapists*. Chicago, IL: McGraw Hill; 2002:290–292.
28. Lioce EE, Novello M, Durando G, et al. Therapeutic ultrasound in physical medicine and rehabilitation: characterization and assessment of its physical effects on joint-mimicking phantoms. *Ultrasound Med Biol*. 2014;40(11):2743–2748.
29. Robertson VJ, Baker KG. A review of therapeutic ultrasound: effectiveness studies. *Phys Ther*. 2001;81(7):1339–1350.
30. Zhang N, Chow SK, Leung K, Cheung W. Ultrasound as a stimulus for musculoskeletal disorders. *J Orthop Translat*. 2017;9:52–59. doi:10.1016/j.jot.2017.03.004.
31. Draper DO, Schulthies S, Sorvisto P, Hautala AM. Temperature changes in deep muscles of humans during ice and ultrasound therapies: an in vivo study. *J Orthop Sports Phys Ther*. 1995;21(3):153–157.
32. Apfel R. Acoustic cavitation: a possible consequence of biomedical uses of ultrasound. *Br J Cancer*. 1989; 45:140.
33. Leighton R, Watson JT, Giannoudis P, Papakostidis C, Harrison A, Steen RG. Healing of fracture nonunions treated with low-intensity pulsed ultrasound (LIPUS): a systematic review and meta-analysis. *Injury*. 2017;48(7):1339–1347. doi:10.1016/j.injury.2017.05.016.
34. Coskun ME, Coskun KA, Tutar Y. Determination of optimum operation parameters for low-intensity pulsed ultrasound and low-level laser based treatment to induce proliferation of osteoblast and fibroblast cells. *Photomed Laser Surg*. 2018;36(5):246–252.
35. Beheshti A, Shafigh Y, Parsa H, Zangivand AA. Comparison of high-frequency and MIST ultrasound therapy for the healing of venous leg ulcers. *Adv Clin Exp Med*. 2014;23(6):969–975.

36. Kutlay S, Kars E, Oztuna D, Ergin S. Is steroid phonophoresis effective in the treatment of subacromial impingement syndrome? Randomized controlled study. *Ann Phys Rehabil Med.* 2018;61:e12. doi:10.1016/j.rehab.2018.05.027.
37. Bayat M, Virdi A, Jalalifirouzkouhi R, Rezaei F. Comparison of effects of LLLT and LIPUS on fracture healing in animal models and patients: a systematic review. *Prog Biophys Mol Biol.* 2018;132:3–22.
38. Bickel CS, Gregory CM, Dean JC. Motor unit recruitment during neuromuscular electrical stimulation: a critical appraisal. *Eur J Appl Physiol.* 2011;111(10):2399–2407.
39. Knutson JS, Fu MJ, Sheffler LR, Chae J. Neuromuscular electrical stimulation for motor restoration in hemiplegia. *Phys Med Rehabil Clin N Am.* 2015;26(4):729–745.
40. Bouton C. Cracking the neural code, treating paralysis and the future of bioelectronic medicine. *J Intern Med.* 2017;282(1):37–45.
41. Kim T, Kim S, Lee B. Effects of action observational training plus brain-computer interface-based functional electrical stimulation on paretic arm motor recovery in patient with stroke: a randomized controlled trial. *Occup Ther Int.* 2016;23:39–47.
42. Doucet BM, Lam A, Griffin L. Neuromuscular electrical stimulation for skeletal muscle function. *Yale J Biol Med.* 2012;85(2):201–215.
43. Bosques G, Martin R, McGee L, Sadowsky C. Does therapeutic electrical stimulation improve function in children with disabilities? A comprehensive literature review. *J Pediatr Rehabil Med.* 2016;9(2):83–99.
44. Zhou M, Li F, Lu W, Wu J, Pei S. Efficiency of neuromuscular electrical stimulation and transcutaneous nerve stimulation on hemiplegic shoulder pain: a prospective randomized controlled trial. *Arch Phys Med Rehabil.* 2018;99:1730–1739.
45. Goldberg JS. Revisiting the Cartesian model of pain. *Med Hypotheses.* 2008;70(5):1029–1033.
46. do Carmo Almeida TC, Dos Santos Figueiredo FW, Barbosa Filho VC, de Abreu LC, Fonseca FLA, Adami F. Effects of transcutaneous electrical nerve stimulation on proinflammatory cytokines: systematic review and meta-analysis. *Mediators Inflamm.* 2018;2018:1094352.
47. AminiSaman J, Mohammadi S, Karimpour H, Hemmatpour B, Sharifi H, Kawyannejad R. Transcutaneous electrical nerve stimulation at the acupuncture points on relieve pain of patients under mechanical ventilation: a randomized controlled study. *J Acupunct Meridian Stud.* 2018;11:290–295.
48. Bracciano A. *Physical Agent Modalities: Theory and Application for the Occupational Therapist.* 3rd ed. Thorofare, NJ: Slack, Inc.; 2018.
49. Rigby JH, Draper DO, Johnson AW, Myrer JW, Eggett DL, Mack GW. The time course of dexamethasone delivery using iontophoresis through human skin, measured via microdialysis. *J Orthop Sports Phys Ther.* 2015;45(3):190–197.
50. Awotidebe AW, Inglis-Jassiem G, Young T. Low-level laser therapy and exercise for patients with shoulder disorders in physiotherapy practice (a systematic review protocol). *Syst Rev.* 2015;4:60.
51. Bicknell B, Liebert A, Johnstone D, Kiat H. Photobiomodulation of the microbiome: implications for metabolic and inflammatory diseases. *Lasers Med Sci.* 2019;34:317–327.
52. Stanos S, Mogilevsky M, Vidakovic LR, McLean J, Baum A. Physical medicine approaches to pain management. In *Current Therapy in Pain, Smith, H.S. (ed.).* Philadelphia, PA: Elsevier, Inc.; 2009:527–540. doi:10.1016/B978-1-4160-4836-7.00073-0.
53. Garcia-Hernandez N, Garza-Martinez K, Parra-Vega V. Electromyography biofeedback exergames to enhance grip strength and motivation. *Games Health J.* 2018;7(1):75–82.
54. Amorim GO, Balata PMM, Vieira LG, Moura T, Silva HJD. Biofeedback in dysphonia—progress and challenges. *Braz J Otorhinolaryngol.* 2018;84(2):240–248.
55. Benfield JK, Everton LF, Bath PM, England TJ. Does therapy with biofeedback improve swallowing in adults with dysphagia? A systematic review and meta-analysis. *Arch Phys Med Rehabil.* 2019;100:551–561.
56. Elmelund M, Biering-Sorensen F, Due U, Klarskov N. The effect of pelvic floor muscle training and intravaginal electrical stimulation on urinary incontinence in women with incomplete spinal cord injury: an investigator-blinded parallel randomized clinical trial. *Int Urogynecol J.* 2018;29:1597–1606.
57. Wilson RD, Knutson JS, Bennett ME, Chae J. The effect of peripheral nerve stimulation on shoulder biomechanics: a randomized controlled trial in comparison to physical therapy. *Am J Phys Med Rehabil.* 2017;96(3):191–198.
58. Bickel CS, Yarar-Fisher C, Mahoney ET, McCully KK. Neuromuscular electrical stimulation-induced resistance training after SCI: a review of the Dudley protocol. *Top Spinal Cord Inj Rehabil.* 2015;21(4):294–302.
59. Auchstaetter N, Luc J, Lukye S, et al. Physical therapists' use of functional electrical stimulation for clients with stroke: frequency, barriers, and facilitators. *Phys Ther.* 2016;96:995–1005.
60. Carda S, Biasiucci A, Maesani A, et al. Electrically assisted movement therapy in chronic stroke patients with severe upper limb paresis: a pilot, single-blind, randomized crossover study. *Arch Phys Med Rehabil.* 2017;98(8):1628.e2–1635.e2.
61. Noma T, Matsumoto S, Shimodozono M, Iwase Y, Kawahira K. Novel neuromuscular electrical stimulation system for the upper limbs in chronic stroke patients: a feasibility study. *Am J Phys Med Rehabil.* 2014;93(6):503–510.
62. Howlett OA, Lannin NA, Ada L, McKinstry C. Functional electrical stimulation improves activity after stroke: a systematic review with meta-analysis. *Arch Phys Med Rehabil.* 2015;96(5):934–943.
63. Gharib NM. Efficacy of electrical stimulation as an adjunct to repetitive task practice therapy on skilled hand performance in hemiparetic stroke patients: a randomized controlled trial. *Clin Rehabil.* 2015;29(4):355.
64. Meadmore KL, Exell TA, Hallewell E, et al. The application of precisely controlled functional electrical stimulation to the shoulder, elbow and wrist for upper limb stroke rehabilitation: a feasibility study. *J Neuroeng Rehabil.* 2014;11:105.

Chapter 25

Wheelchair and Seating Selection

Michelle L. Lange

LEARNING OBJECTIVES

This chapter will allow the reader to:

1. Recognize when wheelchair seating is indicated for a client.
2. Recognize when current wheelchair seating is not appropriate and requires modification or replacement.
3. Describe general components of a wheelchair seating assessment.
4. Describe general seating system categories.
5. Recognize when client mobility is inefficient and intervention is indicated.
6. Describe general components of a wheelchair mobility assessment.
7. Describe major mobility device categories.
8. Describe impact of manual wheelchair configuration on self-propulsion.
9. List several proportional and nonproportional power wheelchair driving methods.
10. Describe strategies to develop further competence in the area of wheelchair seating and mobility.

CHAPTER OUTLINE

TERMINOLOGY

Manual wheelchair (MWC): a mobility base consisting of a frame, rear wheels, and front casters designed for self-propulsion or dependent mobility.

Power assist add-ons: additions to a manual wheel chair that are placed under and behind the wheelchair and can be activated to assist in propulsion as needed for longer distances.

Power assist wheels: alternative to standard wheels on a manual wheelchair to increase the force of the client's propulsion stroke for increased distance and speed.

Power-operated vehicle (POV): (aka scooters) mobility bases that have three or four wheels, a driving tiller, and a consumer-style seat.

Power wheelchair (PWC): a mobility base consisting of a frame, drive wheels, and casters designed for independent mobility through a driving method such as a joystick.

Pressure injury: a breakdown of the skin and sometimes underlying tissues owing to unrelieved pressure in conjunction with other contributing factors.

Primary support surfaces: the seat, back, footplates, and arm pads of the wheelchair and seating system.

Secondary supports: anterior (e.g., pelvic positioning belt or anterior trunk support), posterior (e.g., calf strap), or superior (e.g., foot straps) supports.

Secondary support surfaces: anterior (e.g., anterior lower leg support aka knee block), lateral (e.g., lateral trunk support), posterior (e.g., posterior head support), and medial (i.e., medial knee support) support surfaces designed to keep the client aligned with the primary support surfaces.

Shear: forces created when body tissues and seating surfaces move laterally in relation to each other.

Wheelchair Seating and Mobility in Daily Occupation

Wheelchair seating and mobility is an area of assistive technology (AT) that is broad and deep. This chapter is intended as an introduction to this area of practice. The entry-level occupational therapist should be able to screen a client to determine whether a formal seating and mobility evaluation is required. Referral can then be made to a qualified wheelchair seating and mobility team.

Think about how your body is positioned right now. Perhaps you are sitting at a desk, leaning forward over this book, highlighter in hand. We each position our bodies for specific tasks to optimize our functioning. If a person is seeking a position of rest while watching a football game, he or she may sink back into the couch cushions to minimize the effort required to sustain his or her position. Assuming the best position for a specific task provides stability to optimize function during occupation. For clients who have motor, visual, cognitive, and/or sensory impairments, assuming and sustaining the most appropriate position may only be possible through wheelchair seating.[1] The seating system may allow the client to participate in activities of daily living (ADLs), work tasks, school tasks, or use ATs such as a wheelchair or a speech-generating device (SGD).

We are mobile people. We are often on the move, whether to accomplish a specific task of daily occupation or just for the sake of movement itself. Our clients require movement, as well. If a person is nonambulatory or inefficient in his or her mobility, a variety of mobility devices are available. When augmented mobility devices, such as walkers, are inadequate to meet someone's needs, wheelchairs can provide dependent or independent mobility. Lack of efficient mobility is a significant barrier to participation and independence in occupation.

Motor, Visual, Cognitive and Sensory Impairments That Underlie the Need for Seating and Mobility Devices

Who can benefit from wheelchair seating and mobility interventions? Anyone who requires a mobility base also requires a seating system. In general, a mobility base is indicated if a client needs dependent or independent mobility that cannot be achieved through ambulation or use of augmented mobility devices. Seating systems not only provide a surface to sit on, but also can provide postural support and pressure relief.

Specific impairments may indicate a need for wheelchair seating.[1] Motor impairments may limit the client's ability to assume and sustain an upright sitting posture. Maintaining this posture relies on the body's ability to balance muscle groups (flexors and extensors). If the client has low or high muscle tone, the ability to balance these muscle groups is diminished. If a client has muscle weakness, he or she may be unable to assume or maintain a sitting posture as adequate muscle strength and endurance is not present. If paralysis is present, the brain is unable to communicate with the nerves controlling muscle groups. Visual impairments can also impact posture. We rely on vision to dictate an upright and midline posture. For example, people with impaired or lack of vision often display asymmetrical head positions. If a client has significant cognitive impairment, he or she may not shift his or her weight in response to discomfort, increasing risk for pressure injuries. This is common in people with advanced dementia. Finally, clients who lack sensation (often due to spinal cord injury) will not feel discomfort and so are less likely to shift their weight, again increasing risk for pressure injuries.

Specific impairments may also indicate a need for a wheelchair for mobility.[1] Motor impairments limit a person's ability to ambulate and may also limit ability to use mobility devices. Motor impairments impacting mobility include decreased motor skills, decreased coordination, abnormal muscle tone, muscle weakness, and paralysis. Impaired vision can certainly impact our ability to move throughout the environment, though many people with impaired or no vision are successfully mobile. Using a mobility device, particularly a power wheelchair (PWC), requires certain cognitive skills, though many toddlers are successful at this task. Finally, moving through space is a multisensory task, and clients with sensory issues may require time to accommodate to this activity.

These impairments may be seen in clients with a variety of diagnoses, across the age span and in multiple environments. Diagnosis, age, and environment may dictate more specific interventions.

Wheelchair Seating and Mobility Screening and Assessment

Wheelchair seating and mobility interventions may be recommended for a client who does not have any equipment, perhaps due to young age or an acquired injury. Current equipment may no longer be meeting a client's needs, and reassessment is required. Screening can help us determine whether a client is positioned adequately in his or her current seating system before a recommendation for a formal assessment (see Box 25-1).

Wheelchair Seating Screening

When screening a client in his or her current seating system, the following items are noted:

- Is the pelvis in a neutral position in the seating system, without tilt, obliquity, or rotation?
- If the pelvis is not in a neutral position, can you correct the pelvis, and is this corrected position maintained over time in the current seating system?

Box 25-1

How Do I Know if the Client Is Positioned Adequately in His or Her Mobility Base?

Positioning Checklist

This checklist is designed to screen the student to determine whether a formal seating evaluation is required. Please refer the student, as indicated, to a qualified wheelchair seating team in your area.

___ 1. Pelvis: is the pelvis in a neutral position within the seating system?
This includes neutral pelvic tilt, obliquity, and rotation.

___ 2. Pelvis: if the pelvis is not in a neutral position, can you correct the pelvis, and is this corrected position maintained over time in the current seating system?

___ 3. Trunk: is the trunk upright and midline?

___ 4. Head: is the head upright and midline, balanced over the trunk, without neck hyperextension?

___ 5. Lower extremities: are the lower extremities aligned with the pelvis?
Without adduction, abduction, or rotation?

___ 6. Back height: with the pelvis in a neutral orientation, is the back at the correct height?
For students who require full support or who use anterior trunk supports, this is at or just above the shoulders.

___ 7. Seat depth: with the pelvis in a neutral orientation, is there approximately 1 inch between the end of the cushion and the back of the knee?
If there is more than 1 inch, the seat depth is too short.
If the back of the knee is contacting the front of the seat or not allowing the pelvis to be placed in a neutral tilt, the seat depth is too long.

___ 8. Lower leg length: with the pelvis in a neutral orientation, is the distance between the top of the seat and the footplate correct?
If the distal thighs are unweighted, the distance may be too short.
If the feet are not making full contact with the footplates, the distance may be too long.
If you marked "No" for any of these items, further assessment is indicated.

- Is the trunk upright and midline?
- Is the head upright and midline, balanced over the trunk, without neck hyperextension?
- Are the lower extremities aligned with the pelvis, without adduction, abduction, or rotation?
- Back height: With the pelvis in a neutral orientation, is the back at the correct height? For clients who require full support or who use anterior trunk supports, this height should be at or just above the shoulders.
- Seat depth: With the pelvis in a neutral orientation, is there approximately 1 inch between the end of the cushion and the back of the knee? If there is more than 1 inch, the seat depth may be too short. If the back of the knee/calf is contacting the front of the seat or not allowing the pelvis to be placed in a neutral tilt, the seat depth is too long.
- Lower leg length: With the pelvis in a neutral orientation, is the distance between the top of the seat and the footplate correct? If the distal thighs are unweighted, the distance may be too short. If the feet are not making full contact with the footplates, the distance may be too long.

If the answer to any of these items is "no," then further seating assessment is indicated.

The Wheelchair Seating and Mobility Assessment Team

The wheelchair seating and mobility assessment team includes the client, caregivers, clinicians (occupational and/or physical therapists), and the equipment supplier. Wheelchair seating falls under the area of Complex Rehabilitation Technology (CRT). Occupational therapists need to understand the importance of appropriate positioning and recognize when a seating system is not meeting a client's needs. Occupational therapists who perform these assessments typically have additional training and experience and may be certified in this area by the Rehabilitation Engineering and Assistive Technology Society of North America (RESNA) as an assistive technology professional (ATP) and/or seating and mobility specialist (SMS). The equipment supplier working with CRT should also have specialized training, experience, and certification including the ATP and sometimes the CRTS (Certified Complex Rehabilitation Technology Supplier, available through the National Registry of Rehabilitation Technology Suppliers/NRRTS). See Most Commonly Used Standardized Assessments for Mobility table at the end of this chapter.

Wheelchair Seating Assessment

Wheelchair seating assessment includes gathering information/intake, assessment of current posture and equipment, the mat examination, simulation, equipment trials, fabrication and fitting, and follow-up. The intake is more than just gathering information and demographics. It provides critical information to develop client parameters that are then matched to appropriate equipment. The intake provides context and direction and should include client goals, home and vehicle accessibility, medical issues, independence in ADLs, and current equipment. Assessment of the client's posture in the current equipment includes noting the position of the pelvis, trunk, neck and extremities.

The mat examination is a key part of wheelchair seating assessment. The purpose of the mat examination is to determine available range of motion for a seated posture, where support surfaces are required and what seated angles will be used.[2] What we can support with our hands, the seating system can also support (see Figs. 25-1 and 25-2).

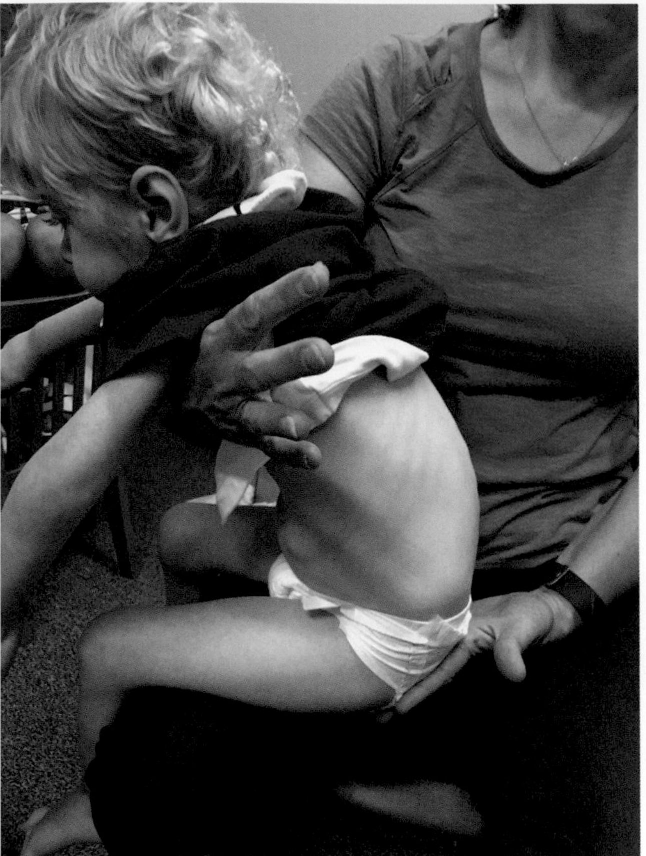

Figure 25-1. Client sitting on examiner's lap, uncorrected.

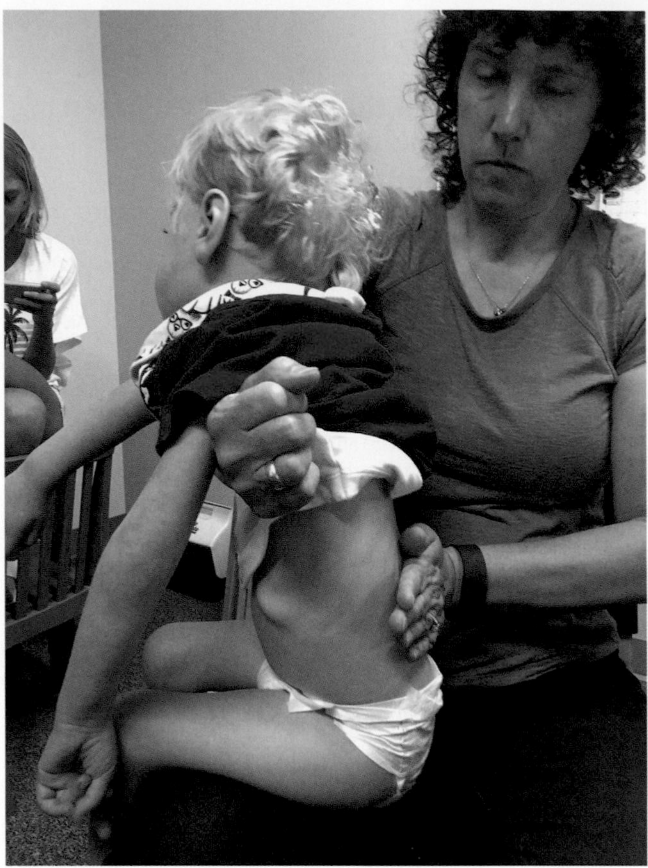

Figure 25-2. Client sitting on examiner's lap with hands-on support.

During the mat examination, describe reflexes and muscle tone and the influence of these on body movements and posture. Note any range of motion limitations. When noting postural challenges, look for the causes and not just the effect. The client is examined sitting on the edge of the mat table as well as in supine. On the edge of the mat table, note the position of the head, shoulders, upper extremities, trunk, pelvis, hips, and lower extremities (see Fig. 25-1). Determine what angles and support are required to achieve a neutral position (see Fig. 25-2). Supine allows examination without the influence of gravity. The evaluator places the pelvis in a neutral position and then begins to flex the hip. When the pelvis begins to rock posteriorly, this indicates the end of available hip flexion, which, in turn, determines the seat-to-back angle of the seating system. This is rechecked with the knees at 90° of extension or more to ensure the client can be placed at this amount of hip flexion with the feet on the footplates (see Fig. 25-3).

The mat examination determines the approximate available range, where support is required and at what angles. Simulation allows us to "test drive" our recommendations to fine-tune and assess effectiveness. This requires a seating simulator or equipment that can be trialed. Pressure mapping may occur at this stage of the assessment to determine whether pressure is well distributed. Pressure mapping can also be used with the client's current seat.

Wheelchair Mobility Screening

Wheelchair mobility is all about efficiency. Efficiency is a combination of time and effort. If the current method of mobility is taking too long or too much effort, then another method of mobility may be more appropriate. For example, if a high school student is using a **manual wheelchair** (**MWC**) to self-propel between classes and is often late to class and too fatigued to learn, this is not

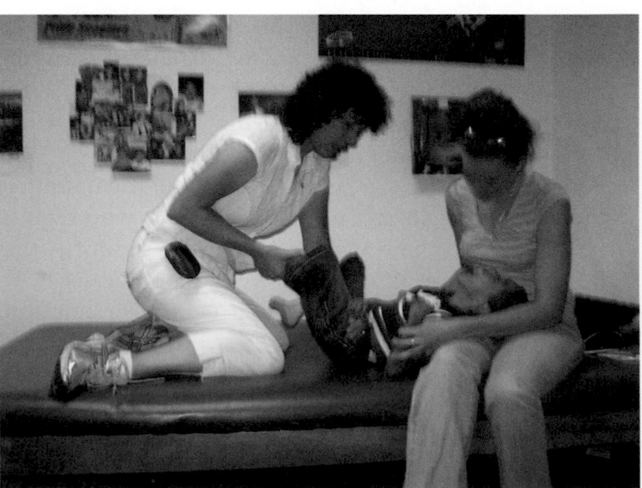

Figure 25-3. The mat examination in supine.

efficient. That same student may be able to use a PWC for these longer distances, arriving to class on time and ready to participate.

Safety is also a concern. If a client can ambulate, but is inefficient, he or she may be at risk of falling, in addition to taking too long and using too much energy. Energy expenditure is a significant medical concern. Energy conservation is required for clients with cardiopulmonary insufficiency. Fatigue can lead to an exacerbation of symptoms (e.g., clients with multiple sclerosis), lead to an increase in muscle tone (e.g., clients with cerebral palsy), or limit how long a person can use his or her mobility base. Some clients may not achieve independent mobility in any mobility base and will still require a base for dependent use, allowing a caregiver to push. To summarize, if a client is not currently mobile or is inefficient or unsafe in his or her mobility, further evaluation is required.

Wheelchair Mobility Assessment

Assessment is typically done with a wheelchair supplier. Many MWC and PWC are considered CRT, which is typically recommended by a professional who is a certified as an ATP or SMS. The assessment determines the most appropriate wheeled mobility category, which is addressed in more detail later in this chapter. If power mobility is being assessed, the evaluation determines the client's readiness for this task. If the client is an appropriate candidate for a PWC, the evaluation also determines the most appropriate seating system, driving method, power seating (e.g., power tilt), and other required features.

Conceptual Foundation Underlying Interventions for Seating and Mobility Impairment

What are the goals of providing wheelchair seating and mobility? First and foremost is function. The seating system should provide optimal and aligned postural support and stability to improve functional skills and compensate for motor, sensory, visual, and cognitive impairment. Function will vary by client. For one client, proper seating may result in increased independence in ADLs. For another client, the seating system may promote vision, breathing, and swallowing by aligning the trunk and head. The wheelchair provides mobility, whether independent or dependent, and that increases function.

Other goals of wheelchair seating and mobility include:

- **Postural alignment:** To the degree possible, to the evaluation team strives for the client to approach an upright and symmetrical alignment. Range of motion losses and orthopedic changes may limit the client's ability to fully achieve neutral alignment, sometimes referred to as a fixed or nonreducible asymmetry. In this case, the team corrects what is flexible or reducible and accommodates what is fixed or nonreducible. It is important not to place a joint or muscle on stretch because this leads to pain, possible damage, and may elicit a stretch reflex, leading to the muscle tightening further.
- **Postural support and stability:** Once the most aligned position is identified, primary and secondary support surfaces, as well as secondary supports, are identified to provide adequate postural support to maintain that position. The more force required to maintain a position, the larger the support may need to be to adequately distribute pressure. For example, it is not appropriate to use a lateral trunk support that is only a few inches wide along the side of the ribcage if significant force is required at this area to maintain trunk alignment. A larger lateral trunk support will provide increased support and pressure distribution.

Adequate postural support typically increases stability for the client. Stability is essential to allow the client to be functional and to disassociate the extremities or head from the trunk.[3] Proximal stability increases distal control.

- **Pressure distribution:** The more pressure is distributed over a surface, the less likely the client will develop focused areas of pressure, which can lead to injury. Sitting on a bean bag provides more pressure distribution/contact than sitting on a flat metal bleacher. Various materials have features that better distribute pressure and so are often used in wheelchair seating systems. Distributing pressure can reduce client risk of developing pressure injuries.
- **Pressure relief:** Pressure distribution itself is not adequate to prevent pressure injury development.[4] It is also essential that the pressure is relieved for periods of time. If you are sitting through a long movie, you relieve pressure by getting up out of your seat. Clients using wheelchair seating and mobility typically perform a weight shift, such as using a tilt system. Some cushions off-load or completely unweight the ischial tuberosities to prevent pressure from developing in this area.
- **Mobility:** The mobility base is designed to provide independent or dependent mobility for the client.

Wheelchair seating and mobility is *not* intended to meet therapy goals, such as stretching, strengthening, and balance. For example, if a client has tight hamstrings, the wheelchair should not intentionally place the hamstring on stretch (e.g., using a footrest hanger with a large angle). This only results in eliciting a stretch response and can actually lead to a loss of range in this muscle. Some therapists have advocated for less postural support in a wheelchair seating system in an effort to increase trunk and head control. It is unrealistic to work on trunk and head control all day, and this reduces the client's ability to be functional in his or her wheelchair. These goals are best addressed in therapy, rather than in the wheelchair itself.

Specific Interventions for Skill Dysfunction

Wheelchair Seating System Categories

Wheelchair seating systems fall into a hierarchy of categories. The decision-making process matches the client's needs and goals, which have been determined in the evaluation, to the simplest category possible. Many funding sources require that documentation address why a less costly seating system was not recommended. This isn't just about cost savings; our documentation must reflect that a hierarchy of options was considered.

Seating systems are comprised of primary support surfaces, secondary support surfaces, and secondary supports. **Primary support surfaces** include the seat, back, footplates, and arm pads of the wheelchair and seating system and are the minimal surfaces required to maintain a seating position.[5] **Secondary support surfaces** include anterior (e.g., anterior lower leg support aka knee block), lateral (e.g., lateral trunk support), posterior (e.g., posterior head support), and medial (e.g., medial knee support) support surfaces and are designed to keep the client aligned with the primary support surfaces. **Secondary supports** include anterior (e.g., pelvic positioning belt or anterior trunk support), posterior (e.g., calf strap), or superior (e.g., foot straps) supports, which are also referred to as soft goods.

Wheelchair seating systems fall into the following general categories:

- Sling upholstery
- Captain's seat (available only on power mobility bases)
- Linear seating
- Generic contoured seating
- Aggressively contoured seating
- Molded seating

Sling upholstery is commonly found on transport and fleet wheelchairs (these mobility base categories will be discussed further in this chapter). The seating and back surfaces consist of a vinyl sling. The seat depth and back height are not adjustable. Sling upholstery does not provide adequate postural support or pressure distribution for any client, so this option is used on bases where the client is only seated for short periods of time (e.g., from the car to the doctor's office). The "hammocking" of these slings tends to promote a pelvic posterior tilt, trunk kyphosis, and lower extremity adduction and internal rotation (see Fig. 25-4).

Captain's seats are similar to the seats found in many motor vehicles. These include generic contours that fit an "average" sized person. Captain's seats are used on many scooters or consumer-level PWCs. These are comprised of foam and vinyl and may include a separate head support. This category of seating is not designed for a client who sits in his or her mobility base for long periods of time, but rather for the client who transfers to other seating (e.g., a standard chair) once arriving at his or her destination. Pressure distribution and postural support are minimal (see Fig. 25-5).

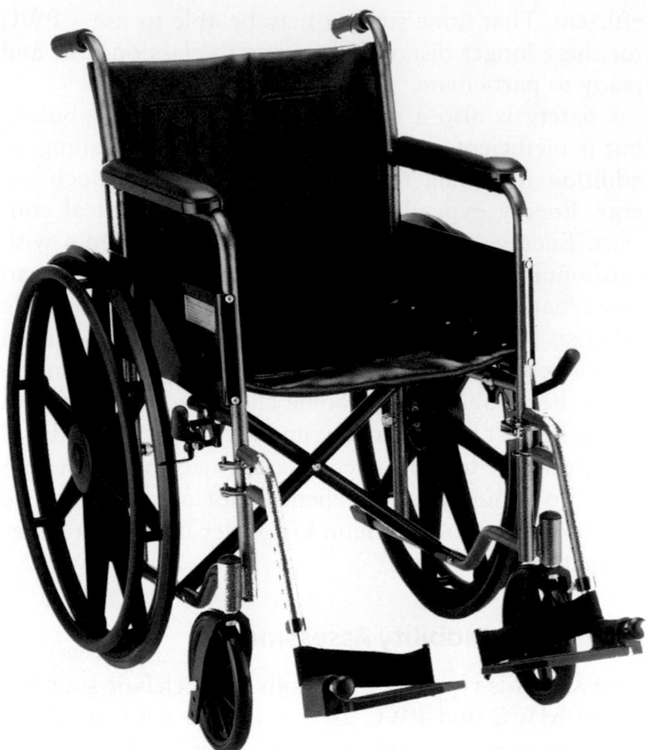

Figure 25-4. Sling seat and back. (Courtesy of pngimg.com.)

Linear seating is comprised of flat surfaces, both on the primary support surfaces and the secondary support surfaces. This category of wheelchair seating includes a wide variety of material and upholstery types. The exact dimensions of the seating system are specified to achieve the required seat width and depth, as well as back width and height. Linear seating is often used with the pediatric population because this can easily be grown. Generic contours are sometimes used to encourage the client to remain in position within the seating system. The seating system may be custom build for an individual or be comprised of "off-the-shelf" cushions and/or backs (see Fig. 25-6).

Aggressively contoured seating systems use a variety of strategies to provide more intimate contact with the client's body for increased postural support and pressure distribution. These contours can also impede transfers and movement within the seating system, so it is imperative to determine, through evaluation, if a lesser seating category will still meet the client's needs and goals.

Molded seating systems provide the most contact with the client. This category of seating is often selected for clients who have significant orthopedic asymmetries

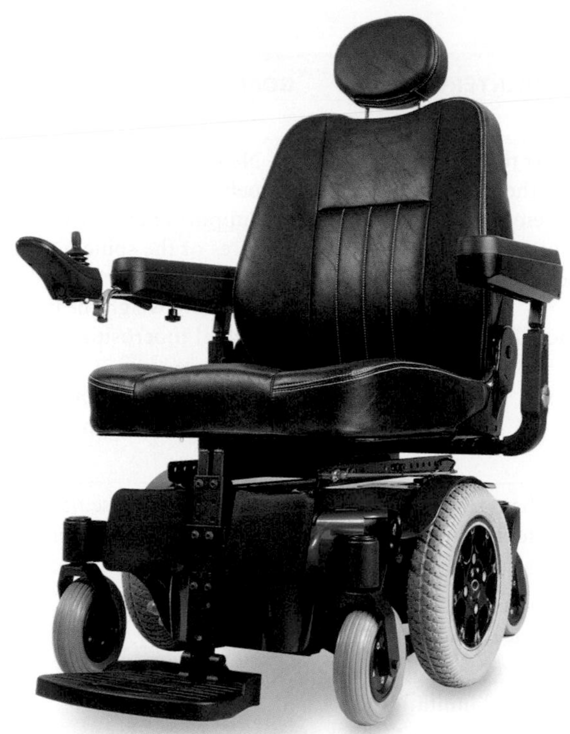

Figure 25-5. Captain's seat. (© Sunrise Medical.)

(e.g., significant scoliosis) and require very intimate contact for postural support and pressure distribution. Once the client is placed in the desired position, his or her "shape" is captured using a variety of techniques that are unique to each manufacturer. For example, the client may be placed on top of thin plastic bags filled with small beads. Air is gradually removed from the bag, and the bag is "shaped" to the client. Once the shape is captured, the seating system is manufactured based on this information. Molded seating systems are the most difficult to modify for growth or other changes (see Fig. 25-7).

Common Positioning Challenges and Strategies

In general, wheelchair seating interventions include mitigating pressure issues, determining angles of support, using specific strategies to address common positioning challenges, and then matching needs to specific product solutions. This can be quite complex and is addressed in-depth in other resources[1] (see Table 25-1).

Pressure

The National Pressure Ulcer Advisory Panel (NPUAP) defines a **pressure injury** (formerly referred to as pressure sores or pressure ulcers) as "localized injury to the skin and/or underlying tissue usually over a bony prominence, as a result of pressure, or pressure in combination with shear and/or friction."[6] Pressure injuries, just like the term suggests, are caused by pressure over an area of tissue, which leads to reduced or loss of blood flow

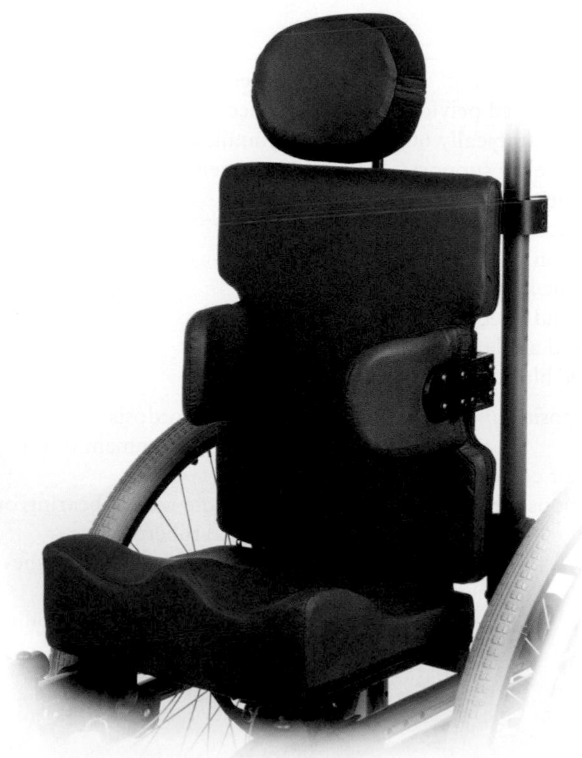

Figure 25-6. Off-the-shelf cushion. (© Sunrise Medical.)

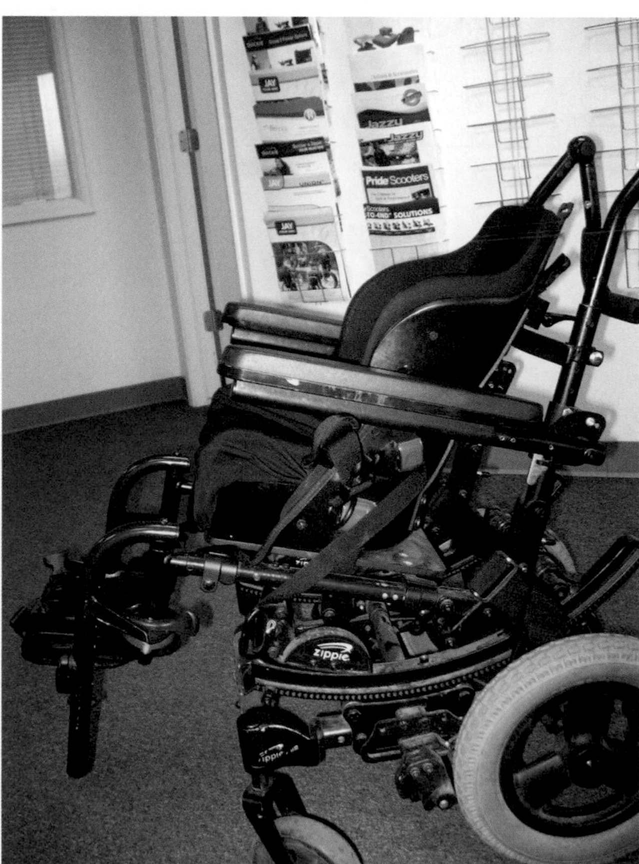

Figure 25-7. Molded seating system.

Table 25-1 Positioning Chart

PROBLEM	POSSIBLE CAUSE	SUGGESTIONS FOR INTERVENTION	GOALS
Pelvis			
Posterior Pelvic Tilt • Top of the pelvis is tipped backward.	• Low abdominal/trunk tone	• Provide support to posterior superior surface of the pelvis to block rearward movement • Anteriorly sloped seat • Drop the footrests to allow hip extension • Biangular back, PSIS pad	• Neutral alignment of the pelvis • Support anatomical curvatures of the spine (i.e., prevent kyphosis) • Promote weight bearing on ischial tuberosities, reduce pressure risks • Best alignment for biomechanical function
	• Tight hamstrings	• Open thigh-to-back angle and/or decrease thigh-to-calf angle	(e.g., of trunk musculature) Increase proximal stability for function
	• Depth of wheelchair seat cushion or platform is too long	• Provide appropriate seat depth to allow hip and knee flexion	
	• Limited ROM, particularly limited hip flexion	• Accommodate fixed limitation in hip flexion by opening seat-to-back angle >90° • Contoured or molded seating system	
	• Sliding forward on seat	• Provide antithrust or aggressively contoured seat • Stabilize pelvis using appropriately angled pelvic belt (typically 60°) or anterior pelvic stabilizer (e.g., subASIS bar) • Change upholstery type	
	• Extensor thrust	• Pelvic stabilization using appropriately angled pelvic positioning belt (typically 60°) or rigid anterior pelvic support • Antithrust seat or aggressively contoured seat • Change position in space if thrust is caused by tonic labyrinthine reflex • Increase hip and knee flexion, hip abduction, and ankle dorsiflexion • Anterior knee blocks	Conserve energy Reduce friction Maintain alignment with other components
Anterior Pelvic Tilt • Top of the pelvis is tipped forward.	• Low trunk tone • Muscle weakness • Lordosis	• Place pelvic positioning belt across ASIS • Belly binder or corset • See interventions for lordosis	• Reduce lordosis • Neutral alignment of the pelvis • Promote weight bearing on ischial tuberosities • Best alignment for biomechanical function • Increase proximal stability for function

Table 25-1 Positioning Chart (*continued*)

PROBLEM	POSSIBLE CAUSE	SUGGESTIONS FOR INTERVENTION	GOALS
Pelvic Elevation • Pelvis moves upward off seating surface	• Extensor tone • Discomfort	• Extensor thrust interventions • Four-point seatbelt • Dynamic footrest hangers or footplates	• Conserve energy • Reduce shear • Maintain alignment with other components • Provide consistent positioning for access
Pelvic Rotation • One side of the pelvis is forward	ROM limitation in the hip: • Abduction • Adduction • Hip flexion • Windswept posture	• Align pelvis in neutral and accommodate asymmetrical lower extremity posture	• Neutral alignment of pelvis • Support anatomical curvatures of the spine (i.e., prevent kyphosis) • Promote weight bearing on ischial tuberosities, reduce pressure risks
	• Fixed limitations in spine, pelvis, and/or femoral mobility (i.e., rotational scoliosis)	• Pelvis may need to assume asymmetrical posture in order to keep head and shoulders in neutral position.	• Best alignment for biomechanical function (e.g., of trunk musculature) • Prevent subsequent trunk rotation
	• Unequal thigh length • Hip dislocation	• Check measurement from the pelvis to the plane of the popliteal fossa with the pelvis in neutral position, if possible • Create an appropriate seat surface depth for each limb, if fixed	• Increase proximal stability for distal function • Increase pressure distribution over posterior trunk
	• Asymmetrical surface contract over posterior buttocks and trunk	• Create contour back surface to "fill-in," if fixed	
	• Discomfort	• Identify source and remediate, or refer to physician	
	• Tone and/or reflex activity • ATNR	• Use positioning such as lower extremity abduction with hip, knee flexion, and ankle dorsiflexion • Pull pelvic belt back on forward side of pelvis • Anterior knee block on forward side • Antithrust seat • Aggressively contoured, if fixed	
Pelvic Obliquity • One side of the pelvis is higher.	• Scoliosis • ATNR • Surgeries • Discomfort	• Change angle of pull of pelvic belt • Wedge: under low side to correct, under high side to accommodate	• Best alignment for biomechanical function (e.g., of trunk musculature) • Level pelvis • Equalize pressure under pelvis • Prevent subsequent trunk lateral flexion • Reduce fixing to increase function

(*continued*)

Table 25-1 Positioning Chart (*continued*)

PROBLEM	POSSIBLE CAUSE	SUGGESTIONS FOR INTERVENTION	GOALS
Painful or Dislocated Hip	• Increased muscle tone • Poorly formed socket because of lack of weight bearing • Surgeries	• Use softer materials under and/or around hip • Avoid lateral contact with hip • Provide lateral support along distal thigh • Determine what positions relieve discomfort	• Comfort
Pelvic Amputation A I IV S II A III	• Hemipelvectomy • Sacral agenesis	• Generally an orthotic is made • Cushion is straight forward as the orthotic is being positioned • If no orthotic, then molded seating system	• Neutral alignment of trunk over pelvis • Support anatomical curvatures of the spine • Pressure distribution • Best alignment for biomechanical function • Increase proximal stability
Trunk			
Lateral Trunk Flexion or Scoliosis • Scoliosis may be C curve, S curve, and/or rotational	• Increased tone on one side • Musculature imbalance, may have pelvic involvement • Decreased trunk strength or decreased tone, causing asymmetrical posture • Habitual posturing for functional activity or stability • Fixed scoliosis	If flexible: • Generic contoured back • Lateral trunk supports (may need to be asymmetrically placed, one lower at the apex of lateral convexity) • Anterior trunk supports to correct any rotation (see forward trunk flexion interventions) If fixed: • Refer to physician to explore medical or surgical procedures, x-rays • TLSO • Aggressively contoured or molded back to allow for fixed curvature of spine and/or rib cage • Horizontal tilt under seat to right head, if pressure distribution is good	• Neutral alignment of trunk over pelvis, if flexible • Minimize subsequent changes in pelvic and lower extremity posture • Level head over trunk for increased vision, social interaction • Pressure distribution
Forward Trunk Flexion or Kyphosis	• Flexion at hips • Flexion at thoracic area • Flexion at shoulder girdle with gravitational pull downward • May occur from increased or floppy tone, abdominal weakness, poor trunk control, weak back extensors • Increased tone (i.e., hamstrings) pulling pelvis back into posterior tilt • Posterior pelvic tilt • Habitual seating in an attempt to increase stability • Fixed kyphosis	If flexible: • Anterior trunk support • Chest strap • Shoulder straps • Shoulder retractors • TLSO • May be a rotational component • posterior trunk support • Correct posterior pelvic tilt • Increase trunk extension with biangular back, PSIS pad, and so on If fixed: • Open seat-to-back angle to match pelvis angle • Contoured back • Tilt seating system to allow upright head	• Prevent spinal changes and subsequent pelvic changes • Neutral alignment of trunk over pelvis • If flexible, anatomical alignment • Increase head control • Trunk extension • Pressure distribution • Maintain good visual field

Table 25-1 Positioning Chart (*continued*)

PROBLEM	POSSIBLE CAUSE	SUGGESTIONS FOR INTERVENTION	GOALS
Trunk Extension or Lordosis • Hyperextension of the lumbar area • Often combined with anterior pelvic tilt 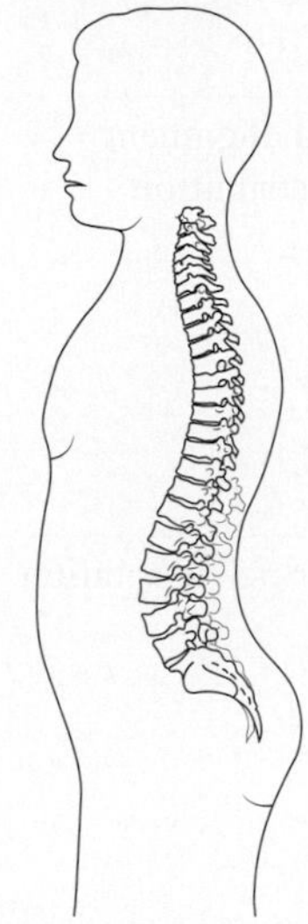	• Tight hip flexors or overcorrection of tight hip flexors • Increased tone pulling pelvis forward into an anterior tilt • Habitual posturing in an attempt to lean forward for functional activities • "Fixing" pattern to extend trunk against gravity (e.g., in conjunction with shoulder retraction.)	If flexible: • Provide lower back support as needed • Biangular back • May need to change seat-to-back angle • Do not overcorrect limited hip flexion • Anterior trunk support (vest or belly binder) If fixed: • Molded seating system	• Neutral alignment of trunk over pelvis • Pressure distribution • Reduce subsequent shoulder retraction and fixing to allow function • Reduce subsequent anterior pelvic tilt
Trunk Rotation • Often seen in combination with lateral trunk flexion and pelvic rotation 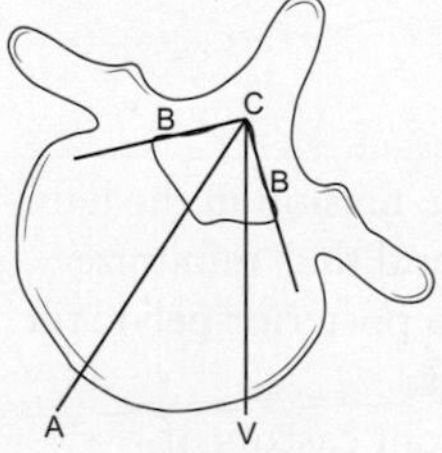 B C B A V	• Pelvic rotation • See lateral flexion causes	If flexible: • Use anterior supports on forward side If fixed: • Consider placing pelvis asymmetrically in seating system so that trunk and head face forward • Molded back to distribute pressure	If flexible: • Neutral alignment of trunk over pelvis • Correct pelvic rotation If fixed: • Pressure distribution • Forward facing posture
Lower Extremities			
Hip Flexion 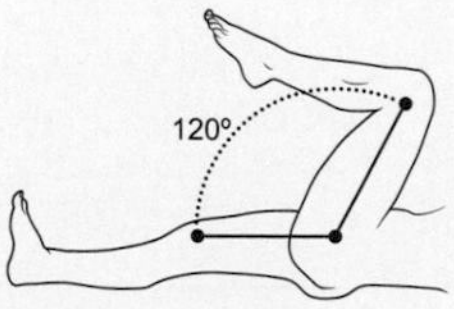 120°	• Decreased ROM of hip flexors • Fixing with hip flexors because of lack of hip extension or stability • Poor positioning • Poor ROM management	If flexible: • Superior thigh pads or strapping thighs or feet superiorly • Padded lap tray (underside) If fixed: • Do not overcorrect and cause anterior pelvic tilt	• Prevent anterior pelvic tilt • Prevent lordosis
Hip Extension 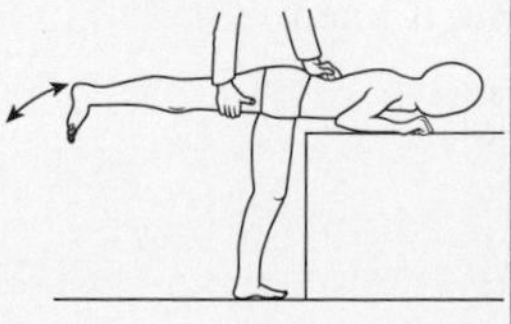	• Decreased ROM of hip extensors • Increased extensor tone • Poor positioning • Poor ROM management	If flexible: • Dynamic options If fixed: • Open seat-to-back angle • Increase knee flexion, if hamstrings are tight • Contoured seating system	• Prevent further loss of range leading to a more reclined, and less functional, position affecting vision, feeding, and respiratory • Avoid putting extensors on stretch

(*continued*)

Table 25-1 Positioning Chart (*continued*)

PROBLEM	POSSIBLE CAUSE	SUGGESTIONS FOR INTERVENTION	GOALS
Hip Adduction 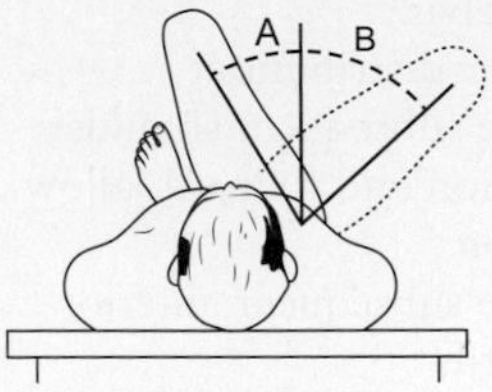 A B	• Extensor tone • Decreased ROM of hip adductors	• Medial knee blocks • Anterior knee blocks • Leg troughs • Contoured seat	• Pressure distribution • Anatomical alignment • Prevent stimulation of stretch reflex or initiation of extensor tone patterns • Prevent hip internal rotation • Ease ADLs
Hip Abduction 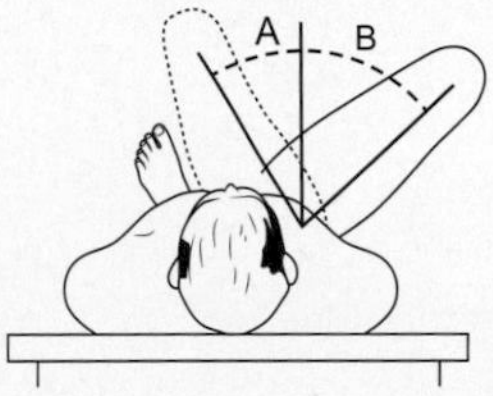 A B	• Decreased ROM of hip abductors • Initial low tone • Surgeries	• Lateral knee blocks • Lateral pelvic/thigh supports • Leg troughs • Contoured seat	• Anatomical alignment • Pressure distribution
Windswept Posture • One leg is abducted, the other is adducted. 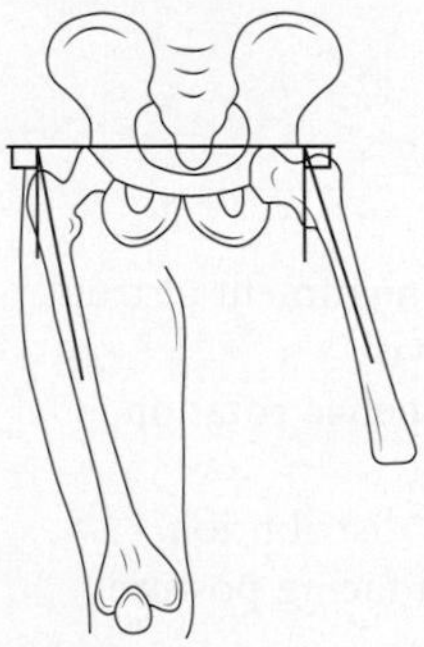	• Pelvic rotation • Range limitations	• Pelvic rotation interventions • Hip adduction and abduction interventions • Sleep positioning	• Same as for pelvic rotation
Knee Flexion 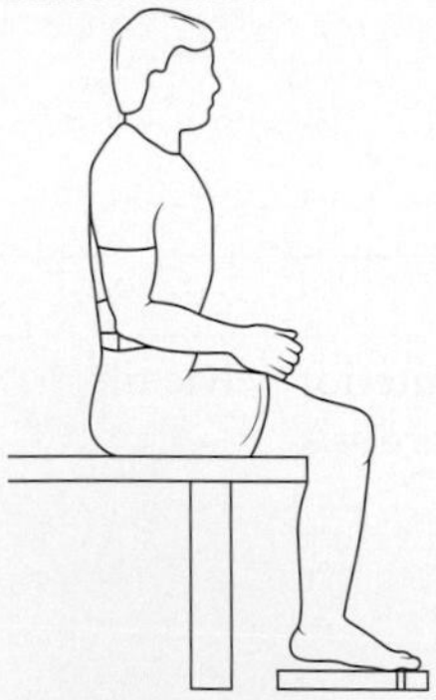	• Decreased ROM of hamstrings • Flexor tone • Structural knee issues	If flexible: • Refer to physician to explore medical or surgical procedures If fixed: • Open seat-to-back angle • Anteriorly sloped seat • Move footrests back • Bevel front edge of seat	• Decrease tension in the hamstrings and thus minimize pull into posterior pelvic tilt • Comfort • Clear front castors of wheelchair • Ease transfers
Knee Extension 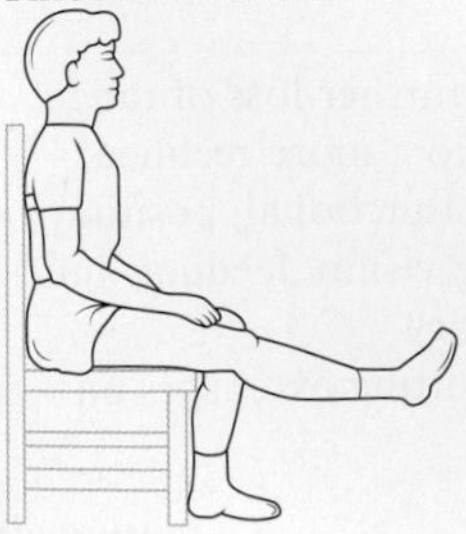	• Extensor tone • Decreased range in quadriceps • Over lengthening of the hamstrings • Structural knee changes	If flexible: • Dynamic options • Refer to physician to explore medical or surgical procedures • Provide alternative positioning to stretch quadriceps If fixed: • Elevating legrests	• Alleviate pull on pelvis and lower leg • Accommodate in extended position, if fixed

Table 25-1 Positioning Chart (*continued*)

PROBLEM	POSSIBLE CAUSE	SUGGESTIONS FOR INTERVENTION	GOALS
Leg Length Discrepancy	• Pelvic rotation • Hip dislocation • Surgeries • Unequal femur length	• Correct any pelvic rotation, if possible • Asymmetrical seat depth	• To provide adequate pressure distribution for each leg • To correct any pelvic rotation
Lower Extremity Extensor Tone	• Extensor tone • Total extensor patterns • Reflex activity (i.e., pressure under ball of foot) • Spasms • Using stable surface at feet to initiate movement	Minimize hip extension: • See extensor thrust strategies under pelvic posterior tilt • Dynamic options Minimize knee extension: • Shoeholders with ankle straps • Anterior lower leg blocks • Dynamic options	• Prevent initiation of total extensor pattern • Prevent pelvic elevation • Increase endurance • Reduce shear • Reduce wear and tear on equipment
Lower Extremity Edema • Fluid retention and/or swelling	• Feet consistently lower than knees • Constriction at knees • Medical issues (i.e., blood pressure, decreased circulatory function)	• Provide alternative positioning out of the chair to elevate the legs • Open the thigh-to-calf angle if ROM is possible and hamstrings are not put on stretch; must evaluate pull on pelvis • Check that feet are supported • Raise footrests to alleviate pressure on distal thigh • Check for pressure areas around proximal lower leg	• Minimize potential for constriction, pressure, or edema • Comfort
Ankle Limitations	• Tonal patterns • Lack of weight bearing • Surgery • Discomfort	• Angle adjustable foot plates (sagittal and frontal planes) • Padded foot boxes • Molded foot support	• Accommodate fixed distortions • Prevent pressure to foot • Protect feet from injury • Comfort
Foot Distortions	• Tonal patterns • Lack of weight bearing • Surgery	• Angle adjustable footplates (sagittal and frontal planes) • Padded foot boxes • Molded foot support • Adaptive footwear to pad feet	• Prevent pressure to foot • Protect feet from injury • Comfort
Lower Extremity Amputation	• Congenital • Acquired	Below knee • Increase pressure distribution along thigh as much as possible • Use calf pad or panel to support lower leg • Avoid weight bearing on distal end of leg • Above knee • Ensure pelvis is level	• Distribute pressure • Comfort • Not to interfere with transfers

(*continued*)

Table 25-1 Positioning Chart (*continued*)

PROBLEM	POSSIBLE CAUSE	SUGGESTIONS FOR INTERVENTION	GOALS
Upper Extremities			
Shoulder Retraction • Often in conjunction with elbow flexion	• Increased tone in scapular adductors or retractors • Weakness of muscles in shoulder girdle with decreased ability to protract shoulder • "Fixing" pattern to extend trunk against gravity, stabilize, or as a righting response • Anxiety, startle	• Build up posterior back support with wedges or increased foam behind scapular area • Adjust tilt-in space • Strap forearms (trunk must be anteriorly supported) • Provide stability elsewhere to breakup fixing pattern	• Neutral alignment for function • Reduce risk of injury (arms may get caught in doorways) • Breakup fixing patterns for function • Reduce neck hyperextension often seen in conjunction with scapular retraction • Protect integrity of shoulder girdle
Elbow Extension • Often in conjunction with shoulder horizontal abduction	• Muscle imbalance • Habitual pattern to laterally stabilize trunk • Habitual pattern to extend trunk • ATNR • Anxiety, startle • Effort or stress	• Pad attached to back cushion or tray to block upper extremity laterally and/or posteriorly • Strap forearms	• Neutral alignment for function • Reduce risk of injury (arms may get caught in doorways) • Minimize orthopedic risks to elbow joint • Breakup muscle tone patterns for function
Uncontrolled Movement of Upper Extremities	• Increased tone due to effort • Athetosis/dystonia • Anxiety	• Block or strapping to decrease movement • Forearm weights • Dynamic strapping to allow some movement but decreasing extraneous movement • Distal stabilizer for independent grasp	• Stabilization • Reduce anxiety • To allow dependent tasks, such as feeding, to proceed
Self-Abusive Behavior	• Self-abuse • Self-stimulation	• Same as uncontrolled movement interventions • Provide alternate sensory input, if appropriate	• To reduce risk of injury to user or others • To calm
Shoulder Subluxation or Dislocation • Usually in conjunction with upper extremity weakness	• Decreased shoulder or upper extremity strength • Paralysis • Decreased muscle control • Decreased tone • Increased tone • Postures that continually pull humerus	• Upper Extremity Support System (tray) • Widened armrests • Arm trough • Posterior or lateral elbow blocks • Forearm straps • Dual shoulder straps crossing the clavicle and acromion processes • Slings	• Comfort • Enhance functional use of arm • Prevent further loss of integrity of shoulder girdle
Head			
Decreased or No Head Control	• Decreased neck strength • Hyperextension of neck in compensation for poor trunk control • Forward tonal pull • Visual impairment, particularly a vertical midline shift	• Posterior head support • Providing only support at the neck may elicit increased neck extension and may not provide adequate surface area support, particularly in tilt • Change pull of gravity against head by reclining or tilting seating system Solutions for little or no head control: • Collars • Forehead strap or pad • Snug lateral supports • Chin support/orthosis • Superior head support (head pod) • Refer to behavioral optometrist, if appropriate	• Elongation of neck extensors (if shortened by neck hyperextension) • Capital flexion (e.g., "chin tuck") • Visual attention to the environment, peers, and so on • Increased function • Improved swallow, feeding, breathing • Prevent subsequent orthopedic changes to neck and shoulder girdle • Prevent overstretching of neck extensors and shortening of neck flexors (if head is usually hanging down)

Table 25-1 Positioning Chart (*continued*)

PROBLEM	POSSIBLE CAUSE	SUGGESTIONS FOR INTERVENTION	GOALS
Lateral Neck Flexion	• Decreased neck strength • Muscle imbalance/tone • ATNR • Scoliosis • Visual impairment, particularly a horizontal midline shift	• Address scoliosis • Headrest with lateral support • Posterior support with three-point lateral control; either side of head and along jawline that is deviated laterally • Custom molded headrest • Horizontal tilt, if severe and if pressure OK • Refer to behavioral optometrist, if appropriate	• Prevent subsequent orthopedic changes to neck and shoulder girdle • Right head for vision, feeding, and respiratory status

ADLs, activities of daily living; ASIS, anterior superior iliac spine; ATNR, asymmetrical tonic neck reflex; PSIS, posterior superior iliac spine; ROM, range of motion; TLSO, thoracolumbosacral orthosis.

and subsequent tissue death. Many factors place the client at a higher risk of pressure injury, including heat, moisture, poor pressure distribution, lack of sensation, incontinence, poor hygiene, poor nutrition, prior pressure injuries, immobility, friction, **shear** (forces created when body tissues and seating surfaces move laterally in relation to each other), inactivity, and decreased mental status. Pressure injuries are staged with stage 1 being the least amount of damage and stage 4 begin the most involved.

In general, wheelchair seating can reduce risk of pressure injury in several ways. First, seat shape and materials can be used to distribute pressure over as large an area as possible (see Table 25-2). A highly contoured shape can distribute pressure well, but can also impede independent transfers. Some cushion materials that distribute pressure well are less stable and so do not provide as much postural control. Risk of pressure injury must be weighed against function. Second, pressure relief unweights specific areas of the body for specific lengths of time. Tilt and recline can be used to relieve pressure under the buttocks while shifting weight to the posterior trunk for short periods of time (see Fig. 25-8). The client may also be able to shift his or her weight (e.g., a forward lean) within the seating system. Third,

Table 25-2 Cushion Types and Examples

CLASSIFICATION	ADVANTAGES	DISADVANTAGES	EXAMPLE
Foam	Lightweight	Uneven pressure relief	T-Foam by Alimed
	Easily sized, shaped	Poor durability	
	Low cost	Hard to clean	
Gel-filled	Self-contouring	Heavy to move	Jay Cushion by Jay Medical
	Posture control	Temperature sensitive	
	Sitting balance	Leaking, maintenance	
Air-filled	Lightweight	Reduced control/balance	High or Low Profile by Roho
	Even pressure relief	Requires attention to air-pressure tending	
	Little shear	Potentially requires repair of puncture/air leaking	
Honeycomb	Lightweight	Uneven pressure relief	Supracor Stimulite Contoured
	Easy to clean	Difficult to shape	
	Low maintenance	Excessive thickness	
Custom-contoured foam	Surface area coverage	Expense	Contour U Pindot by Invacare
	Reduced shearing	Longevity with change	
	Better postural control	Reduced weight shift	
Alternating pressure systems	Scheduled relief cycle	Cost and availability	Bellows Air Support Equipment by Talley Medical
	Reduces user effort	Uneven pressure relief	
	Self-contouring	Unsteady sitting balance	

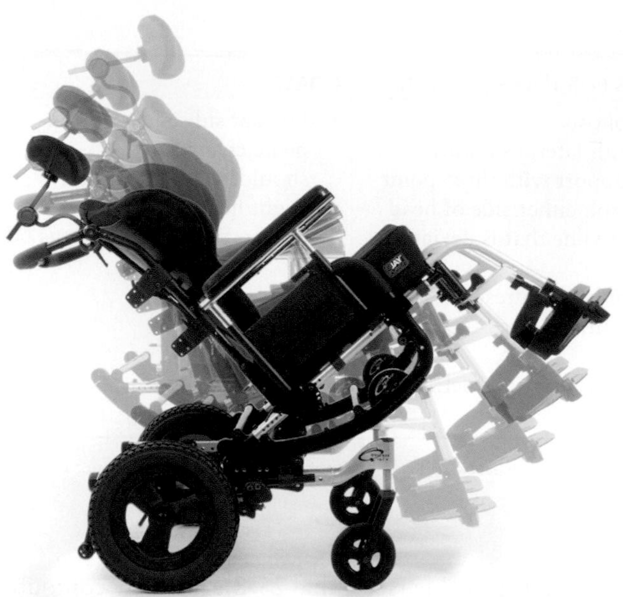

Figure 25-8. Tilt-in space wheelchair. (© Sunrise Medical.)

seating and upholstery materials that reduce both heat and moisture can be used.

Angles of Support

Seating systems are more than support surfaces and strapping. Angles are essential to optimize biomechanics and subsequent function. Stability allows for dissociation and control of movement. An appropriate wheelchair seating system matches the required seated angles identified during the mat examination to accommodate range limitations, optimize trunk and head control, and provide stability.

The primary seated angles that must be determined include the pelvis (trunk-to-upper leg angle), the knee (upper leg-to-lower leg angle), and the ankle (lower leg-to-foot angle). It is also important to determine the overall position in space, including tilt and recline.

The trunk-to-upper leg angle is often referred to as the seat-to-back angle, referring to the angle between the seat rails and back canes of the wheelchair frame. This angle will be different from the client's actual trunk-to-upper leg angle, so it is important to measure both and clearly communicate what is required to the team. A neutral seat-to-back angle is at 90°. Let's try this for a moment. Sit up nice and tall with your trunk-to-upper thigh angle at about 90°. Although this position may make your Grandma proud, it is difficult to maintain because of the muscle strength required. For a client with low muscle tone, particularly in the trunk; muscle weakness; or paralysis, this position often cannot be achieved or maintained. For clients with abnormal muscle tone, co-contraction of the flexors and extensors in the trunk are impaired, also impacting the ability to sit at this angle. The angle is often "opened" past 90° to provide a position of rest and to recruit gravity to assist the client in maintaining upright sitting. If this angle is too open, extensor tone may increase, and the client may not be in a functional position. Often, an angle of just 100° can be adequate—again, this is determined during the mat examination.

Occasionally, a client will be placed in a closed seat-to-back angle (<90°), sometimes referred to as a "task performance position." This position has been demonstrated to improve upper extremity control in some clients and may need to be combined with a posterior tilt to prevent the client from falling forward.

The upper leg-to-lower leg angle is primarily determined by hamstring length and the front castors of the wheelchair. If the hamstrings are tight, this angle must not be open enough to place the muscles on stretch. Pulling on the hamstrings will only lead to the client sliding forward into a posterior pelvic tilt to relieve this stretch. However, if angle is closed, the footplate may interfere with the front castors, getting in the way for turning. Various product design strategies are available to address this issue.

The lower leg-to-foot angle is primarily determined by ankle range. The footplate angle can be adjusted on many wheelchair frames to accommodate limitations in plantar or dorsiflexion, as well as inversion and eversion. If a client must be positioned in plantar flexion owing to range limitations, this can affect ground and castor clearance.

The client's position in space can be changed manually by a caregiver on some MWCs or independently by the client on a PWC. This includes recline and tilt. These technologies are used for a variety of reasons. Recline opens the seat-to-back angle (see Fig. 25-9), whereas tilt moves the entire seating system posteriorly without changing the seated angles (see Fig. 25-8). Anterior and lateral tilts are also available, but posterior tilt is by far the most common.

Advantages of recline and tilt include:

- Pressure redistribution
- Postural management
- Fatigue management
- Medical management

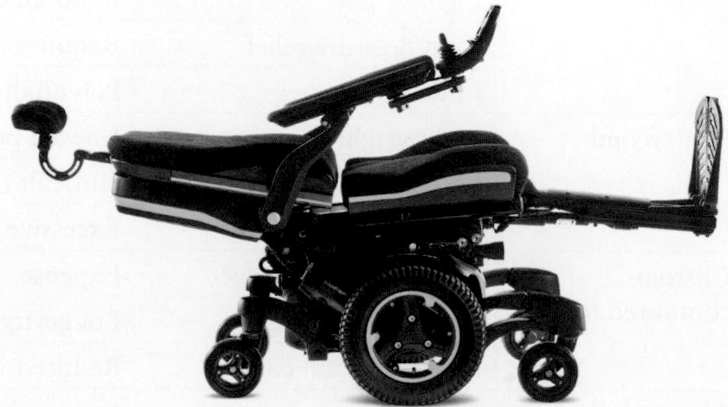

Figure 25-9. Recline with elevating legrests on a power wheelchair. (© Sunrise Medical.)

Recline also allows for easier catheterization in the wheelchair, provides passive range of motion at the hips and knees, may relieve orthostatic hypotension, and may ease transfers. However, opening the seat-to-back angle can lead to shear forces, which can disrupt alignment and increase pressure over the sacral area. Opening this angle can also set off spasms in some clients and will pull the client out of position if range is limited at the hips or knees.

Tilt maintains the seated angles that may inhibit muscle tone and help to maintain the client's posture. Any other AT devices remain in position in relation to the client (such as a mounted SGD). Range limitations are accommodated, and tilt systems can be used with contoured and molded seating systems because there is no shear during movement to disrupt alignment with these intimate shapes.

Common Positioning Challenges

It is beyond the scope of this chapter to address specific wheelchair seating strategies in depth. It is important, however, to understand common positioning challenges and recognize when intervention is required. Please refer to Appendix 2 for further information. These positioning challenges may be flexible or fixed and are often seen in combination with one another.

Common positioning challenges seen at the pelvis include tilt, rotation, and obliquity. A posterior pelvic tilt is a very common challenge and occurs when the pelvic tips posteriorly. Let's try it. Sit on your hands for a moment. You should be able to feel two bony prominences. These are your ischial tuberosities (ITs). Let your pelvis slide forward. The ITs have now moved forward and off your hands. What is your spine doing? A posterior pelvic tilt leads to a flexed trunk or kyphosis. Sit up straight again and then tip the top of your pelvis forward. This is an anterior pelvic tilt. The ITs have now moved posteriorly. What is your spine doing? Anterior pelvic tilt leads to a hyperextended lower spine or lordosis. Sit up straight again and place one knee further forward of the other. One IT is now off of your hand. Your pelvis is now rotated, with one side forward of the other. If you then attempt to face forward, your spine will be rotated, as well. Finally, return to a neutral position and then cross one leg over the other. This creates a mild obliquity, where one side of the pelvis is higher than the other. Both ITs are still over your hands; however, one side is creating more pressure. Think about what your spine is doing. Pelvic obliquity leads to a lateral trunk lean or scoliosis.

Common positioning challenges seen at the lower extremities include hip adduction and abduction, hip or knee flexion, hip or knee extension, and ankle and foot limitations. Any of these positions deviate from a neutral lower leg position and need to be addressed through the wheelchair seating system.

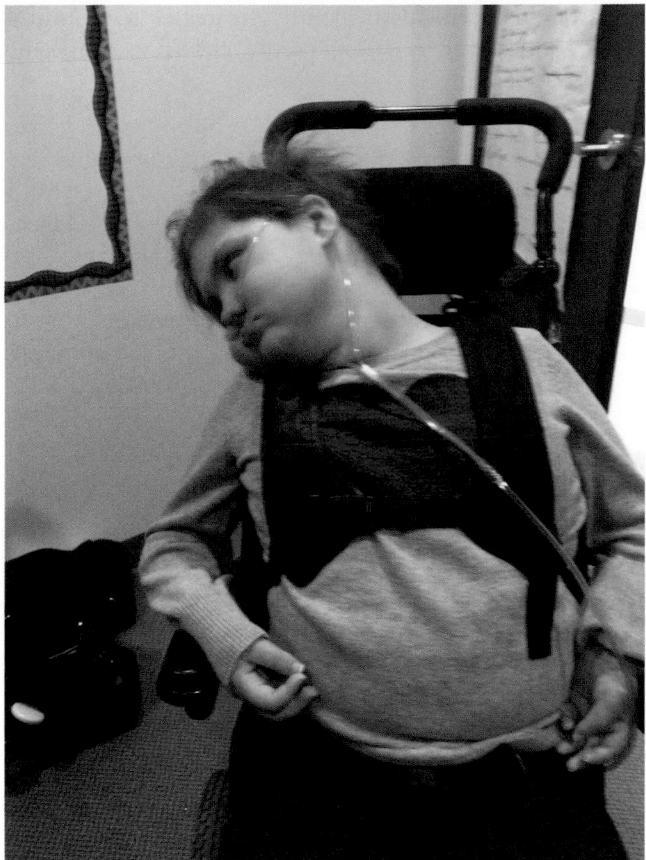

Figure 25-10. Poor head position.

Common positioning challenges seen at the head include decreased head control, lack of any head control, and lateral flexion and rotation. Although a wide variety of head supports are available (see Figs. 25-10 and 25-11), a thorough mat examination and seating

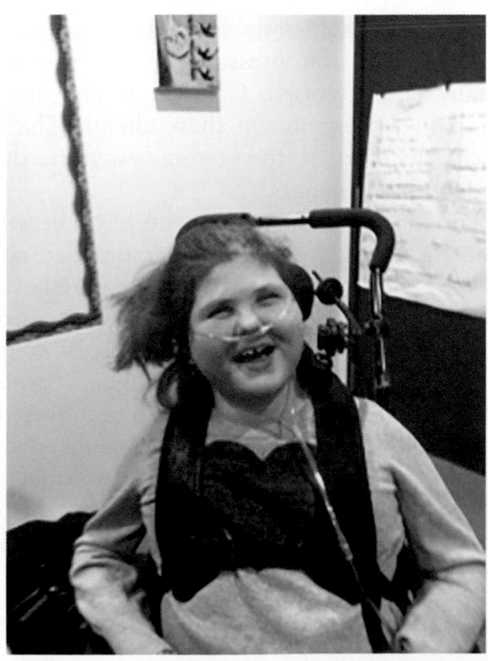

Figure 25-11. Corrected head position with appropriate head support.

assessment is critical to identify strategies to optimize head control and position before choosing a specific head support.

Seating assessment:

- Identifies pressure injury risks and makes related recommendations to mitigate this risk
- Determines the appropriate angle of support surfaces and components
- Identifies specific seating challenges
- Develops intervention strategies and matches this to appropriate products. These interventions can be applied to multiple seating system categories.

Specific Populations

Wheelchair seating recommendations will vary based on specific client populations. Common populations requiring wheelchair seating include pediatrics, bariatrics, and geriatrics as well as degenerative conditions. Geriatric clients may have limited funding because of their living situation (e.g., long-term care facility) and by Medicare funding regulations. These clients often have comorbidities that impact their seating needs, such as diabetes, osteoporosis, kyphosis, and dementia. Skin and underlying tissues also become more fragile as we age, increasing pressure injury risk. All too frequently, geriatric clients do not receive optimal equipment because of seating equipment being misconstrued as a restraint.[7] Services are often limited in this population, and competent wheelchair seating evaluation is critical.

Bariatric clients have larger body dimensions and require wheelchairs and seating systems that accommodate those dimensions as well as have higher weight limits. Seating goals are different with this population. Rather than focus on posture, the seating system primarily accommodates body size and shape, as well as protects the client from pressure injuries. Skin integrity is typically compromised. Comfort is also important because pain is common in these clients. The client's weight can fluctuate, so the seating system needs to accommodate these changes.

When working with a client who has a degenerative condition, the seating system must accommodate changing needs. Often, more postural support is required over time, and pressure risk may increase as movement decreases. The client's body shape may change because of weight loss, muscle atrophy, and/or orthopedic changes. Depending on the specific diagnosis, these changes can occur rapidly. It is important to anticipate needs, so the recommended equipment can meet those needs for as long as possible.

Wheelchair seating can be fairly straightforward for clients who are not at risk for pressure injuries and who do not require much postural support or stability for alignment and function. However, many clients have more complex needs. It is critical to screen clients who use or need wheelchair seating to ensure that their needs are being adequately met. Screening can direct the occupational therapist to make a referral to a wheeled seating and mobility team for comprehensive evaluation.

Wheeled Mobility Categories

Wheeled mobility products are categorized in a hierarchy from simple to complex and are matched to client need and ability through a mobility assessment. The assessment determines the simplest device that will meet a client's needs and goals, and documentation generally must include why a lesser category of mobility device would not meet those needs. Much of this determination centers on efficiency, which is a combination of effort and time to move between specific locations. As discussed in the section on Mobility Screening, even if a client can move a mobility device, use must be efficient, or a higher mobility category may be indicated.

Augmented Mobility Devices

Augmented mobility devices include walking aids (canes and crutches), walkers, and gait trainers. These are not considered wheeled mobility devices; however, many people use both. This is an important category to keep in mind because this is a simpler category than dependent mobility bases and so must be addressed in documentation.

Dependent Mobility Bases

Dependent mobility bases are not designed for self-propulsion and include adaptive strollers, transport chairs, and the following MWCs: tilt-in space, reclining, and standard. Adaptive strollers are most often used with very young children who require small dimensions and specific features including the ability to face the caregiver (for careful monitoring), tilt, recline, and ease of transport (folding and lightweight) (see Fig. 25-12).

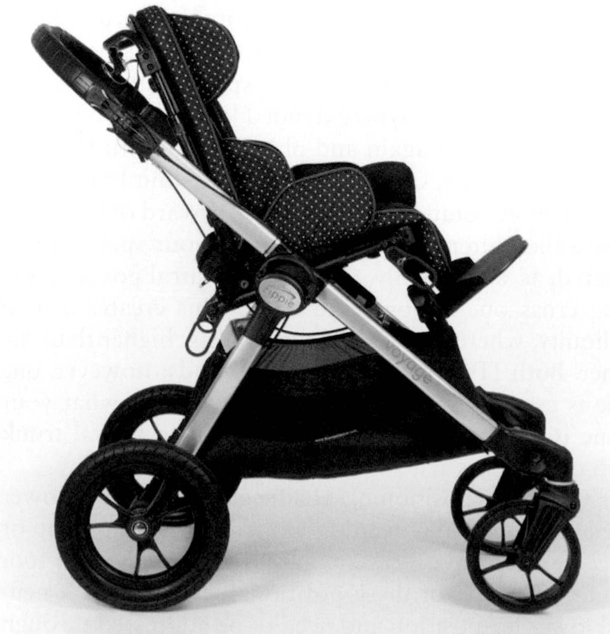

Figure 25-12. Adaptive stroller. (© Sunrise Medical.)

Caregivers are often more willing to accept an adaptive stroller than a pediatric MWC for very young children. Strollers are also used as a backup to an MWC at times, owing to ease of use and transport.

Transport chairs are designed just for that—transport. The client may take short trips in this dependent mobility base, for example, from the car to the doctor's office waiting room. The client would typically ride in a standard passenger seat in the vehicle and then transfer to a waiting room chair. Transport chairs are inexpensive but include minimal seating and offer no frame adjustments. The small wheels provide no opportunity for self-propulsion and are difficult to push over varied terrain. Standard wheelchairs (see Fig. 25-4) are similar to transport chairs and are designed for temporary use. These are commonly used in hospitals to transport a client from one location to another. These are inexpensive and fold for transport but are too heavy for self-propulsion and have very limited seating and frame adjustment options.

Tilt-in space MWCs (see Fig. 25-8) are not generally designed for self-propulsion. The few models that are designed for self-propulsion are quite heavy. Clinical indicators for use of tilt were addressed earlier in this chapter. Most tilt wheelchairs can support a wide variety of seating systems, grow, fold, and include a wide variety of frame adjustments to meet a specific client's needs. Reclining MWCs are also not designed for self-propulsion and are not intended for long-term use. Instead, reclining wheelchairs are typically used postsurgery to provide a more open seat-to-back angle. Seating options and frame adjustments are limited. The reclining mechanism creates a high degree of shear.

Manual Mobility Bases

MWCs fall into many categories, which are primarily dictated by Medicare. The categories are in a hierarchy, from simplest to most complex. Documentation generally must indicate why a "lesser" category of MWC will not meet a client's needs.

- **Standard wheelchair (K0001):** Dependent wheelchair (see earlier), weight over 35 lb, limited sizes, adjustments, modifications, and seating (see Fig. 25-4)
- **Standard hemi wheelchair (K0002):** Standard wheelchair with lower seat to floor height to allow for foot propulsion. *Hemi* refers to decreased control on one side of the body, such as clients who have had a stroke. This client may propel with one arm and one foot. This is not an ideal wheelchair for any form of self-propulsion owing to weight and lack of adjustment.
- **Lightweight wheelchair (K0003):** Weighs less than 36 lb, 28 lb average. More sizes available, but little or no frame adjustments. Limited options and accessories. Appropriate for a client who cannot propel a standard wheelchair but can propel a lightweight wheelchair. Not designed for long-term use or extensive self-propelling.

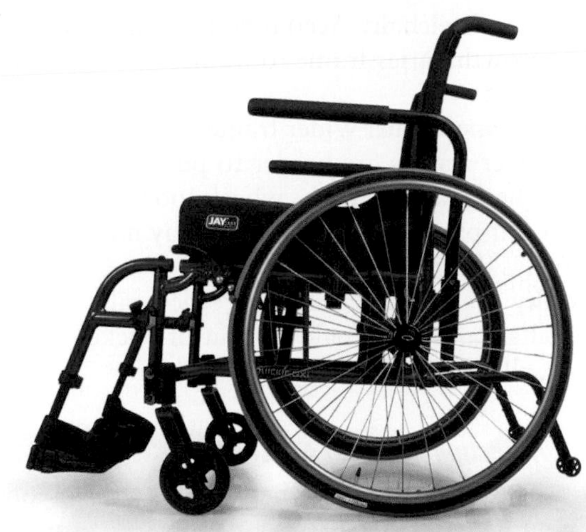

Figure 25-13. Lightweight wheelchair K0004. (© Sunrise Medical.)

- **Lightweight wheelchair (K0004):** Weighs less than 34 lb, average 26 lb. More sizes, options and accessories, minimal frame adjustments, and minimal adjustable axle plate. Appropriate for a client who cannot propel a lesser category of wheelchair owing to weight and setup and requires frame adjustments to optimize self-propulsion (see Fig. 25-13).
- **Custom lightweight and ultra lightweight wheelchair (K0005):** Weighs less than 30 lb, as low as 17 to 18 lb. Greatest degree of options: size, frame adjustments, suspension, and casters. Designed to maximize self-propulsion efficiency and reduce repetitive stress injury (RSI) risk. Appropriate for a client who is self-propelling using both arms for a significant time period. Rigid and folding frame options. Folding frames are easier to transport and often have more growth. Rigid frames are lighter, more durable,[8] and more energy efficient (see Fig. 25-14).

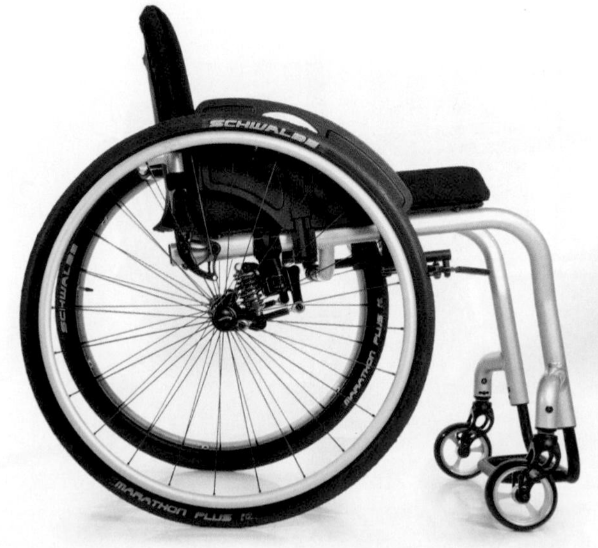

Figure 25-14. Ultra lightweight wheelchair. (© Sunrise Medical.)

- **Pediatric wheelchair:** Accommodates smaller dimensions, growth varies frame to frame, low seat to floor height.
- **Bariatric wheelchair:** Wider frames, higher weight limits. Heavier frames are harder to push, and the width of the wheelchair places the wheels too far from the client for self-propulsion. The frame may not fit through doorways if very wide.
- **Specialty wheelchairs:** These are generally a second wheelchair and often paid for out-of-pocket. Includes sports, all terrain, and beach wheelchairs.

Manual Wheelchairs—Power Assist

Power assist wheels replace the standard wheels on an MWC to increase the force of the client's propulsion stroke for increased distance and speed. Conversely, the power assist wheels can also help the client slow down the wheelchair when descending an incline. These are indicated for clients who do not have enough strength and endurance for longer distances or varied terrain, but do not require a PWC. Power assist wheels do add to the weight of the wheelchair and need to be charged. **Power assist add-ons** are placed under and behind the wheelchair and can be activated as needed for longer distances. The client pushes the wheels, and the power assist will continue movement of the wheelchair without additional wheel contact. The client can adjust his or her course by short pushes on either wheel as movement continues forward. Power assist can bridge the distance between MWC and PWC and minimize risk of RSI.

Power Mobility Bases

Power-operated vehicles (POVs), also known as scooters, are available in three- and four-wheel bases (see Fig. 25-15). Many clients prefer scooters because these do not look like a wheelchair. The three-wheel versions are more maneuverable, but also less stable and may tip during turns. The four-wheel versions are more stable, but have a larger turning radius. Seating options are limited. The client drives using a tiller, similar to controlling a bicycle. The seat sometimes swivels to the side to ease transfers. Scooters generally have less power, speed, and range than PWCs.

Power wheelchairs (PWCs) are available in consumer-level and complex rehab-level bases. Consumer-level PWCs include a standard captain's style seat, joystick access, and limited power seating. Complex rehab-level PWCs include a full range of seating, driving methods, and power seating options (see Fig. 25-16). Complex rehab-level PWCs also include advanced features, such as infrared (IR) transmission to control devices in the environment; mouse emulation to control computers, tablets, smartphones, and SGDs; and the ability to interface certain AT devices so that the PWC driving method can also be used to access these devices.

Manual Wheelchair Self-propulsion Considerations

If a client is able to self-propel an MWC, there are a number of factors to consider in order to maximize the client's efficiency and reduce RSI risk. Generally, the lighter the wheelchair, the more efficient it is to propel. This includes the weight of components and seating. Placement of the rear wheel is also important. If the rear wheel is placed behind the client, the wheelchair is more stable, but the propulsion stroke is less efficient. If the rear wheel is placed too far forward, the wheelchair will be tippy rearward. Configuration must achieve a balance of stability and maneuverability that fits an individual's needs. For example, if the client performs "wheelies" to manage certain obstacles, the

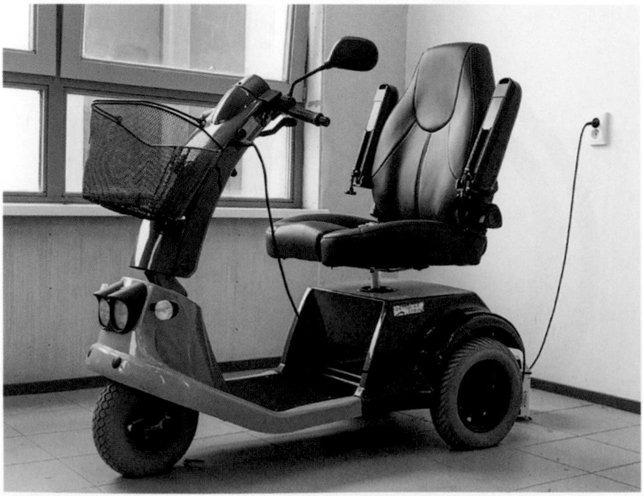

Figure 25-15. Scooter. (Courtesy of Pixabay.com.)

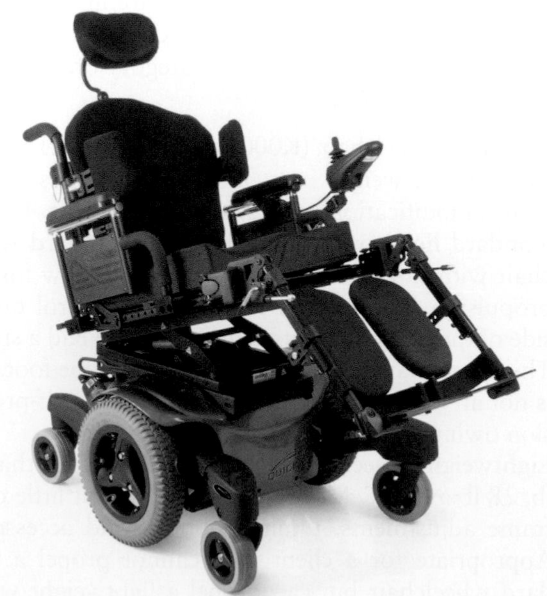

Figure 25-16. Complex rehab power wheelchair. (© Sunrise Medical.)

point of balance of the wheelchair must allow for this function. Another consideration for rear wheel placement is optimizing self-propulsion and reducing RSI risk. With an arm hanging down at the client's side, the axle should be in line with the shoulder and the tip of the middle finger.

Research has demonstrated that people using MWCs tend to use one of four propulsion patterns. This includes a semicircular, single-loop over, double-loop over, and arcing pattern. The propulsion patterns that are most efficient and less likely to lead to RSI are the semicircular or double loop.[9] It is important to train the client in the use of this pattern during self-propulsion. Camber changes the angle of the wheels in relation to the ground. Increasing camber increases stability and maneuverability in turning. This also increases the overall width of the wheelchair base.

The front caster also impacts propulsion. Smaller casters allow tight turns and result in less interference with the footplates. However, larger casters better manage varied terrains. The client should be positioned so that most of his or her weight is over the rear wheel. If client is positioned too far forward, the front casters are "loaded," which impedes turning and increases caster wear.

The most efficient means of self-propulsion is using both hands. If the client is unable to do so, a PWC may be indicated. If the client only needs to move short distances, time is not an issue, and surfaces are level and flat, other propulsion methods may be used including one hand, one hand and one foot, or both feet. One-handed propulsion requires a special wheelchair modification. These dual rims allow full directional control with one hand. When both rims are moved forward at the same time, the wheelchair moves forward. If only one rim is moved, the wheelchair will turn in one direction. The client must have large enough hands to grip both rims and have good grip strength. A combination of one hand and one foot may be used for short distances and is often used by clients who have had a stroke. The seat to floor height must be low enough for the feet to rest on the floor, and propulsion tends to be slow and takes a lot of energy. This movement pattern may pull the pelvis forward. Propelling with both feet also requires a low wheelchair and generally pulls the pelvis forward into posterior pelvic tilt.

MWC skills are often trained in therapy and include transfers, wheelies, getting back into the wheelchair from a fall, and even maintenance. The main goal of an MWC is independent mobility, if attainable. Mobility needs to be as efficient as possible and limit RSIs. If a client is not efficient in one category of MWC, consider the next category. If the client is not efficient in any category of MWC, consider power assist, a POV, or a PWC. A seating and mobility evaluation team will have access to the equipment required to make these determinations.

Power Wheelchair Considerations

Drive Wheel Configuration

Complex rehab PWCs are available in front wheel drive (FWD), mid or center wheel drive (MWD), and rear wheel drive (RWD) configurations. Each configuration has advantages and disadvantages, which much be matched to the client's specific needs, including driving method and environment. RWD was more commonly used in the past and is known to be quite stable on a variety of terrains. RWD has the largest turning radius, and the front casters may interfere with the footplates during turns. FWD allows the client to move up close to tables and has no caster interference because these are behind the client; however, these bases tend to "fishtail" at faster speeds. MWD has the smallest turning radius and is the most intuitive to drive (see Fig. 25-16). These MWD bases do not perform well on aggressive outdoor terrain.

Power Seating

Power seating has many clinical benefits for clients using a PWC.

- **Power tilt:** The advantages of tilt were explored earlier in this chapter under section on Angles of Support.
- **Power recline:** The advantages of recline were also explored earlier in this chapter under section on Angles of Support (see Fig. 25-9).
- **Power tilt/recline** are sometimes used in combination on a PWC. Using these technologies in combination helps to maintain the client's posture, particularly upon return to upright, while providing greater pressure relief through recline.
- **Power adjustable seat height** (see Fig. 25-17) increases seat to floor height that extends functional reach, allows the client to choose an optimal height for a specific transfer, provides access to a variety of work surface heights, expands visual field, and increases social interaction and participation.
- **Power elevating legrests (ELRs)** (see Fig. 25-9) are often used in combination with a power recline system. ELRs provide passive range of motion at the knees and may improve circulation and reduce edema if used in

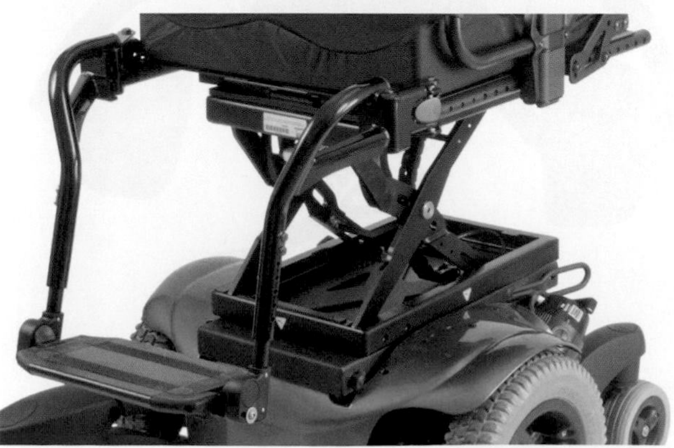

Figure 25-17. Power adjustable seat height. (© Sunrise Medical.)

combination with a power tilt to raise the legs above the level of the heart. ELRs can pull the pelvis forward if the client does not have adequate hamstring length.

- **Power stand** extends the hips and knees partially or fully and provides all the benefits of stationary standing. In addition, standing from a wheelchair extends functional reach, expands the client's visual field, increases social interaction and participation, and increases compliance with a standing program. The client must have adequate range of motion and have medical clearance to participate in a standing program.

Driving Methods

Most clients using a PWC drive with a joystick. However, a joystick may be too difficult for a client to use due to muscle weakness, paralysis, abnormal muscle tone, or lack of motor control. A wide variety of alternative driving methods are available to provide independent driving for these clients.

Joysticks are a proportional driving method. The driver has proportional directional control and speed control. The joystick handle can be moved in a 360° circle, resulting in 360° of wheelchair movement. The farther the joystick handle is deflected from center, the faster the wheelchair will move. If a client cannot use a standard joystick, a variety of other proportional driving methods are available, including mini proportional joysticks that require significantly less force and travel to drive the PWC. This driving method works well for clients with muscle weakness.

Digital driving methods are nonproportional and utilize switches. Each switch represents a discreet direction: forward, left, right, and reverse. Speed is not controlled through the driving switch, but rather through other strategies. Any switch type can be used in any location the client can activate the switch for driving. A common digital driving method is the head array (see Fig. 25-18 and

Videos 25-1 and 25-2). This head support contains proximity switches in the rear and side pads. Proximity switches are activated when the client's head approaches the pad. No force is required, as these are electrical switches. The materials and upholstery of the pad do not activate this switch type. If the client moves his or her head toward the rear pad, the PWC moves forward. If the client moves his or her head toward the left pad, the wheelchair turns to the left. Finally, if the client moves his or her head toward the right pad, the wheelchair turns to the right.

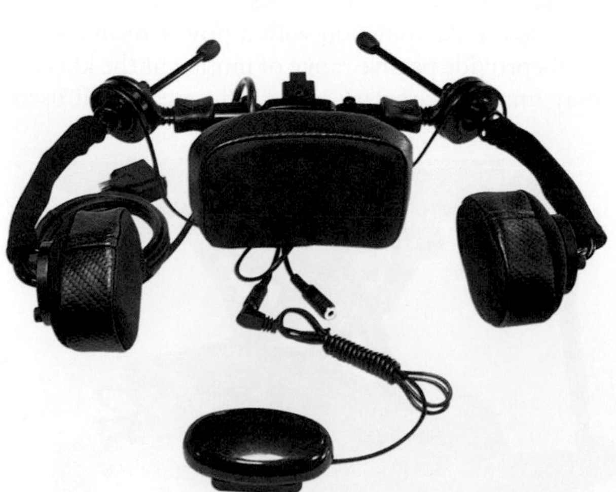

Figure 25-18. Head array driving method. (Permission to use from Stealth Products, iDrive Head Array.)

A wheeled seating and mobility assessment team can evaluate a client to determine the best driving method owing to level of experience as well as availability of driving methods to trial during the evaluation.

Programming

Programming optimizes drive performance and efficiency. This also enables control of other features such as speed, reverse, and power seating through the driving method. Programming is often performed by the equipment supplier, but can also be done by the clinician. An external programmer or computer is required. It is possible to program a PWC to be downright dangerous, so the programmer must be well qualified. The clinician, even if not actively programming, can observe the client's driving and direct needed changes that the supplier can then implement.

Other Features

Complex rehabilitation PWCs are just that ... complex! Each PWC manufacturer uses a unique electronics system with specific parameters. Besides driving and changing position in space through power seating, the client can take advantage of other features including:

- **Infrared (IR) transmission:** Many devices in the home environment receive IR signals, such as audiovisual equipment. The PWC can store or learn IR signals and then transmit these to the device. Another area of AT that provides this level of control is electronic aids to daily living (EADLs). IR transmission from the PWC poses a few challenges, however. The client must be in the wheelchair—if the client is in bed, he or she will not have this control without using an EADL. Many devices that traditionally have received IR signals now receive a combination of IR and radiofrequency (RF) signals (e.g., audiovisual equipment). The PWC is not able to learn and transmit RF signals. As IR is being replaced with other technologies, many clients are using the wireless network in their home to control devices in the environment using Apps or voice-based smart home assistants (e.g., Alexa).
- **Mouse emulation:** PWCs can "pair" through Bluetooth with devices such as a computer, tablet, smartphone, or SGD. Specific capabilities vary by PWC electronics system. The device must support mouse access. For example, Apple tablets and smartphones do not currently support mouse access.

- **Interfacing:** Many clients who use a PWC, particularly those requiring alternative driving methods, also require power seating and may use other AT devices, such as an SGD. Using a separate access method to control each device or feature is not typically realistic, because of lack of motor control. Interfacing allows the PWC driving method to be used as the access method for interfaced devices as well. Interfacing has many advantages and disadvantages and requires careful assessment.

Pediatric Power Mobility

Power mobility isn't just for adults. Research has clearly demonstrated that even very young children can use power mobility.[10] Furthermore, research has shown a clear link between the onset of independent mobility and overall motor, cognitive, visual, and psychosocial development. If a child cannot efficiently use any other mobility device, power mobility should be considered.

Mobility Training

The average teenager must spend 40 to 50 hours practicing how to drive over a period of a year before even taking a driver's test for a license. This teen typically has average motor, vision, and cognitive skills and has observed drivers his or her entire life. Many PWC candidates have impaired motor, vision, and/or cognitive skills; have never seen anyone drive a PWC before; and receive little training. Mobility training can be used to develop readiness to use a PWC as well as to optimize driving skills.

Power mobility can be complicated. Assessment is a team effort, including the CRT supplier. PWCs can provide independent mobility to clients who would otherwise be dependent or inefficient in their mobility. A variety of driving methods can provide access even to clients with complex needs.

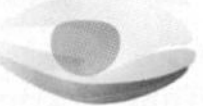

CASE STUDY

Patient Information

Taylor is a teenage boy with the diagnosis of cerebral palsy. He was first evaluated by an occupational therapist specializing in wheelchair seating and mobility at age 8 in conjunction with his private occupational therapist, the complex rehab equipment supplier, and his speech language pathologist. At that time, Taylor attended elementary school and lived at home with his mother in an apartment.

Occupational Therapy Goal List

The goals of this assessment were to evaluate his current positioning, determine a means of independent mobility, and determine a means for Taylor to access an SGD.

Assessment Process and Results

Taylor was positioned in a linear seating system in a tilt-in space MWC (see Fig. 25-19). Taylor was seen twice for seating assessment. A number of changes were recommended at the first appointment. At the second appointment, the team evaluated the effectiveness of these changes and made further recommendations.

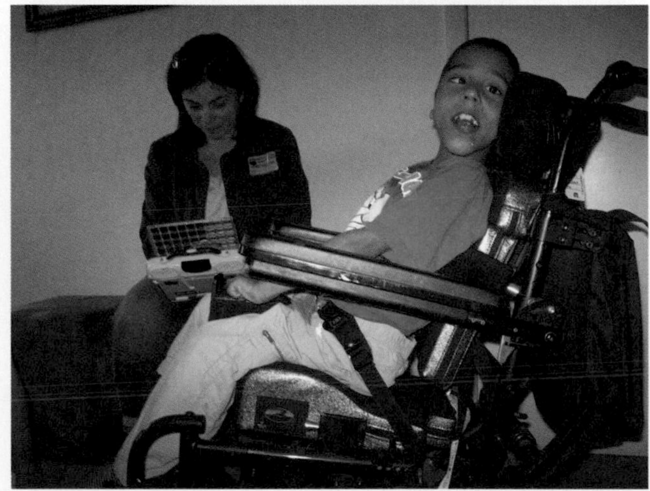

Figure 25-19. Taylor in manual tilt-in space wheelchair and linear seating system and anterior vest.

Wheelchair Seating

Taylor was seated in a linear seating system comprised of an antithrust seat, biangular back, lateral thoracic pads, shoulder straps, pelvic positioning belt, shoe holders, and a standard head support. The seat-to-back angle was approximately 90°. When Taylor was seen at the first appointment at his home, he was wearing an anterior vest for trunk support and this was replaced with shoulder straps to minimize risk of asphyxiation on the vest (as this tends to move up toward the throat when tightened) and to provide better support of the upper trunk (by providing more targeted support). Taylor tended to extend into a posterior pelvic tilt, and the antithrust well was thought to be too long. An antithrust seat employs a "curb" that is positioned immediately in front of the ITs to limit forward migration. Because the "well" posterior to this curb was too long, Taylor could slide forward. This was modified to the correct length; however, Taylor continued to move into a posterior pelvic tilt when reassessed at the second appointment. The angle of the pelvic positioning belt was also changed at the first appointment from a 45° to a 60° angle, which better controls the position of the pelvis, but did not prevent Taylor's posterior pelvic tilt. The back was too short and needed to be replaced owing

(continued)

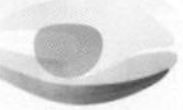

CASE STUDY *(continued)*

to growth. The medial knee support was no longer needed after recent hip surgery (adductor release) and was so removed. A different head support that provided better support was also recommended.

After these initial changes, Taylor continued to demonstrate strong extension and move into a posterior pelvic tilt. He had been unable to tolerate his AFOs and so was not wearing shoes or contacting the footrests consistently. As his feet were not kept in contact with the footplates using ankle straps or shoe holders, he could extend his legs, increasing overall extension and making a neutral pelvis very challenging to maintain. He was on oral Baclofen to reduce muscle tone, and his resting tone was not as much of a challenge as his dynamic tone. Options to control the position of pelvis included a four-point pelvic positioning belt, subASIS bar, and anterior knee blocks. The team did not believe that adding an additional angle of pull on the pelvic positioning belt would control his pelvis (a four-point belt has two straps on either side of the pelvic to provide two angles of pull). He was so short (only 23 lb) that the team was concerned that a subASIS bar (a rigid padded anterior pelvic support) or knee blocks (pads placed anterior to the lower leg, just under the knees) would be too large or could cause harm. Taylor was also at high risk for developing spinal asymmetries due to high muscle tone. The team recommended a molded seating system to control the position of the pelvis and reduce overall extension through intimate contact with a larger surface area of the body. This system would also reduce the risk or delay the onset of spinal asymmetries because of the intimate contact and support of the trunk. The seat could also be moved between the MWC and a future PWC.

Wheelchair Mobility

When Taylor was seen for his first appointment, he was screened for power mobility. Switches were placed on mounts behind and to either side of his head on his MWC. When Taylor activated a switch, the chair was pushed by this therapist in the corresponding direction. Taylor quickly demonstrated cause-and-effect, directional concepts, stop-and-go concepts and adequate vision to navigate a parking lot outside his home.

At the second appointment, Taylor's linear seating system was placed into a PWC base with a head array. This access method consists of a tripad head support with proximity switches embedded in each pad for directional control. At this point of the evaluation, Taylor was very frustrated and upset, but was able to drive the evaluation PWC outside the equipment supplier's office. Based on his performance, the team was confident that Taylor would be able to use a PWC with some basic mobility training.

The team decided to wait for Taylor to receive his molded seating system before recommending a PWC. The molded seating system was placed in an evaluation PWC (see Fig. 25-20), and Taylor once again drove outside the equipment supplier's office, but with better control positioned in this new seat (see Video 25-3).  A PWC was recommended with a head array, power tilt, and center mount footplate with shoe holders and padded straps. A reset switch would be needed to allow Taylor, as he developed competence, to access reverse, the power tilt, speeds, and use the right directional switch to send switch signals to the SGD through interfacing. Taylor was able to access an SGD using a switch by the right side of his head, and interfacing allowed him to use a switch in this location for both right turns (PWC) and communication (SGD).

The home was not accessible to a PWC, and the family did not have an accessible vehicle (they were able to transport the MWC). The PWC could be used at his school, providing Taylor independent mobility in an accessible environment. The PWC could also be transported on the accessible school bus so that Taylor could bring the chair home at times to drive outside. The family was pursuing an adaptive van.

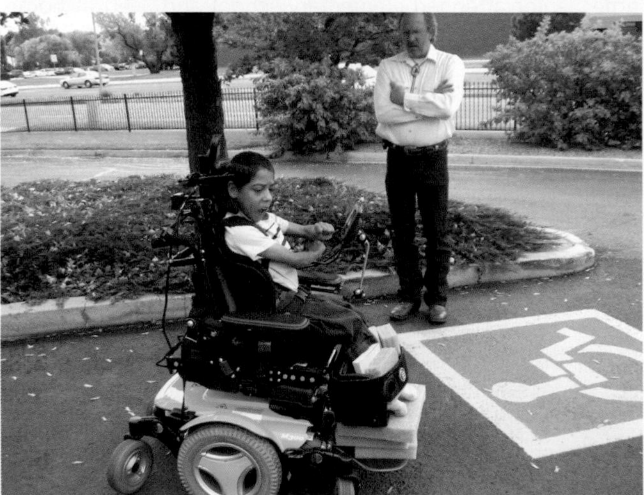

Figure 25-20. Taylor in his new seat and an evaluation power wheelchair.

Most Commonly Used Standardized Assessments for Mobility

Instrument and Reference	Intended Purpose	Administration Time	Validity	Reliability	Sensitivity	Strengths and Weaknesses
Functional Mobility Assessment (FMA)	To measure effectiveness of wheeled mobility and seating interventions	45–60 minutes	Content validity established	Test–retest reliability scores above acceptable level[11]	Measures change in function effectively[12]	Completed at evaluation and specific follow-up dates
Canadian Occupational Performance Measure	To capture a client's self-perception of performance over time	20–60 minutes	Content validity established[13]	Test–retest reliability scores above acceptable[13]	Successful in detecting changes over time	Broad focus on occupational performance in all areas, but not wheelchair focused
Power-Mobility Indoor Driving Assessment (PIDA)	To assess the indoor mobility of persons who use power chairs or scooters and who live in institutions	60–120 minutes	Content validity established[14]	Test–retest and inter-rater reliability confirmed[14]	Evaluates change over time	Measures mobility status, not the level of function in other self-care activities
Power-Mobility Community Driving Assessment (PCDA)	To assess the community mobility of persons who use power chairs or scooters	60–120 minutes	Content and concurrent validity results[15]	Moderate-to-good reliability[15]	Evaluates change over time	Useful tool to identify where clients are able to drive safely in community settings and identify specific learning needs
Wheelchair Skills Test	Documents a set of representative wheelchair skills	30 minutes	Valid[16]	Reliable[16]	Can measure change in function over time	Easy and inexpensive to measure. Accompanying training program
Functioning Every day with a Wheelchair (FEW)	To measure function while in wheelchair	45–60 minutes	Good test–retest validity Content validity[17]	Excellent inter-rater reliability[17]	Can measure change in function over time	Self-report tools are not always accurate, though two performance-based companion tools were developed, which validated the FEW.

References

1. Lange ML, Minkel J, eds. *Seating and Wheeled Mobility: A Clinical Resource Guide.* Thorofare, NJ: Slack Incorporated; 2018. https://www.healio.com/books/health-professions/occupational-therapy/%7B-0494f75e-c42b-4f30-96d8-175a3fd90747%7D/seating-and-wheeled-mobility-a-clinical-resource-guide
2. Minkel J. Seating and mobility evaluations for persons with long-term disabilities: focusing on the client assessment. In: Lange ML, Minkel J, eds. *Seating and Wheeled Mobility: A Clinical Resource Guide.* Thorofare, NJ: Slack Incorporated; 2018. https://www.healio.com/books/health-professions/occupational-therapy/%7B0494f75e-c42b-4f30-96d8-175a3fd90747%7D/seating-and-wheeled-mobility-a-clinical-resource-guide
3. Sparacio J. Postural support and pressure management considerations for prop sitters. In: Lange ML, Minkel J, eds. *Seating and Wheeled Mobility: A Clinical Resource Guide.* Thorofare, NJ: Slack Incorporated; 2018. https://www.healio.com/books/health-professions/occupational-therapy/%7B0494f75e-c42b-4f30-96d8-175a3fd90747%7D/seating-and-wheeled-mobility-a-clinical-resource-guide
4. Chisholm J, Yip J. Pressure management for the seated client. In: Lange ML, Minkel J, eds. *Seating and Wheeled Mobility: A Clinical Resource Guide.* Thorofare, NJ: Slack Incorporated; 2018. https://www.healio.com/books/health-professions/occupational-therapy/%7B0494f75e-c42b-4f30-96d8-175a3fd90747%7D/seating-and-wheeled-mobility-a-clinical-resource-guide
5. Waugh K, Crane B. Standardized measures of the person, seating system, and wheelchair. In: Lange ML, Minkel J, eds. *Seating and Wheeled Mobility: A Clinical Resource Guide.* Thorofare, NJ: Slack Incorporated; 2018. https://www.healio.com/books/health-professions/occupational-therapy/%7B0494f75e-c42b-4f30-96d8-175a3fd90747%7D/seating-and-wheeled-mobility-a-clinical-resource-guide
6. The National Pressure Ulcer Advisory Panel. Pressure injury stage. 2016. http://www.npuap.org/resources/educational-and-clinical-resources/npuap-pressure-injury-stages. Accessed June 15, 2018.
7. Babinec M, Cole E, Crane B, et al. The Rehabilitation Engineering and Assistive Technology Society of North America (RESNA) position on the application of wheelchairs, seating systems, and secondary supports for positioning versus restraint. *Assist Technol.* 2015;27(4):263–271. doi:10.1080/10400435.2015.1113802.
8. Liu HY, Hong EK, Wang H, Salatin B. Evaluation of aluminum ultralight rigid wheelchairs versus other ultralight wheelchairs using ANSI/RESNA standards. *J Rehabil Res Dev.* 2010;47(5):441. doi:10.1682/JRRD.2009.08.0137.
9. Slowik JS, Requejo PS, Mulroy SJ, Neptune RR. The influence of wheelchair propulsion hand pattern on upper extremity muscle power and stress. *J Biomech.* 2016;49(9):1554–1561. doi:10.1016/j.jbiomech.2016.03.031.
10. Rosen L, Plummer T, Sabet A, Lange M, Livingstone R. RESNA position on the application of power mobility devices for pediatric users. *Assist Technol.* 2017:1–9. doi:10.1080/10400435.2017.1415575.
11. Kumar A, Schmeler MR, Karmarkar AM, et al. Test-retest reliability of the functional mobility assessment (FMA): a pilot study. *Disabil Rehabil Assist Technol.* 2013;8(3):213–219. doi:10.3109/17483107.2012.688240.
12. Powers PJ, Fly V, Law M, et al. Functional mobility outcomes of individuals using wheelchairs. Platform Presentation at International Seating Symposium; 2013.
13. Tuntland H, Aaslund MK, Langeland E, Espehaug B, Kjeken I. Psychometric properties of the Canadian Occupational Performance Measure in home-dwelling older adults. *J Multidiscip Healthc.* 2016;9:411. doi:10.2147/JMDH.S113727.
14. Dawson D, Chan R, Kaiserman E. Development of the power-mobility indoor driving assessment for residents of long-term care facilities: a preliminary report. *Can J Occup Ther.* 1994;61(5):269–276. doi:10.1177/000841749406100507.
15. Letts L, Dawson D, Bretholz I, et al. Reliability and validity of the power-mobility community driving assessment. *Assist Technol.* 2007;19(3):154–163. doi:10.1080/10400435.2007.10131872.
16. Smith EM, Low K, Miller WC. Interrater and intrarater reliability of the wheelchair skills test version 4.2 for power wheelchair users. *Disabil Rehabil.* 2018;40(6):678–683. doi:10.1080/09638288.2016.1271464.
17. Kumar A, Schmeler MR, Karmarkar AM, et al. Test-retest reliability of the functional mobility assessment (FMA): a pilot study. *Disabil Rehabil Assist Technol.* 2012;8(3):213–219. doi:10.3109/17483107.2012.688240.

Chapter 26

Assistive Technology

Debra K. Lindstrom and Cara Masselink

LEARNING OBJECTIVES

This chapter will allow the reader to:

1. Explain how the model(s) of occupational therapy practice and assistive technology can be used to address occupational goals.
2. Describe the roles of other professionals on an interprofessional technology team.
3. Describe and give examples of direct and indirect access methods.
4. Explain the purpose of positioning and mounting platforms or accessories such as switches using technology for remediation.
5. Explain the purpose of positioning and mounting platforms or accessories such as switches using technology for compensation.
6. Identify the platform, hardware, software, transmission method (if applicable), and target in a clinical situation.
7. Explain questions to include in an occupational profile for device access and how that is similar/different for electronic aids to daily living (EADLs) access.
8. Identify simple through complex compensatory technology for navigation, selection, and text entry.
9. Describe barriers to successful use of commercially available smarthome technology.

CHAPTER OUTLINE

TERMINOLOGY

Access method: the process the person uses to activate a target. It can be either direct (any target can be spontaneously selected) or indirect (multiple steps needed to select and activate target).

Control method: the type of action a target requires to produce an effective response. It can be discrete (e.g., power off) or continuous (e.g., volume up).

Electronic aids to daily living (EADLs): commercial- or disability-specific products that enable a person with physical, cognitive, or psychosocial deficits to control electronics in his or her physical environment, including appliances, home theater systems, lights, doors, and more.

Latched switch activation: a switch action that requires one-switch press to turn on the target and one to turn off the target.

Macro: the programming of two or more infrared (IR) codes on one icon to activate multiple targets with one activation.

Momentary switch activation: a switch action that turns on a target for the length of time that the switch is pressed, and is most common in a 1:1 format.

Navigation: the process of browsing and isolating targets on device display.

Selection: the process of activating a target on a device display.

Switch: hardware that closes an electrical circuit when activated. It may be activated through touch, proximity, or other means.

Switch scanning: an indirect access method that groups customized selections on the device display using a scan box; the scan box is moved and a target is activated using programmed switches.

Timed switch activation: a switch action that turns a target on for a specified (often adjustable) amount of time, then turns it off automatically.

Word acceleration techniques: software-based strategies that increase typing speed and may assist with spelling, includes word completion and word prediction.

Technology as an Enabling Part of Occupational Performance

Occupational therapists use technology in two main ways. First, technology can enable the remediation of body function and performance skill deficits. Second, technology enables occupational performance, by helping the person compensate for deficits. In occupational therapy, assistive technology (AT) is often used. The formal definition of AT that is accepted by the American Occupational Therapy Association is taken from The Assistive Technology Act of 2004: "The term 'assistive technology device' means any item, piece of equipment, or product system, whether acquired commercially off the shelf, modified, or customized that is used to increase, maintain, or improve functional capabilities of individuals with disabilities."[1]

Technology is used to compensate for limitations in performance skills and body functions using AT or universally available technology to allow a person to complete an occupational task of his or her choice. The same technology can be used to remediate a performance skill or body function (occupation as a means) using a task requiring actions with technology positioned to strengthen or improve performance skills and body functions.

Theoretical Foundations for the Use of Technology in Occupational Therapy

In one way or another, technology (assistive or universal) has been used by occupational therapists for either occupation as an end (compensation) or occupation as a means (remediation). Technology can be included in most of the major models used in occupational therapy that incorporate the environment. The ecological models of practice that specifically address the environment lend themselves well to be guides for assessment and intervention that includes technology.[2] The Person-Environment-Occupation-Performance (PEOP) model[3] is specifically identified AT (as well as universal technology) as being part of the environmental component of the model and follows the World Health Organization's *International Classification of Functioning, Disability and Health* (ICF). This model specifically designates any technology needed as being part of the environmental factor of the framework.[4]

The theoretical frameworks for using technology for either remediation or compensation are the same frameworks used for other types of remediation interventions. Technology can be used to remediate

- Range of motion, strength, and endurance in the biomechanical framework
- Cognitive skills in the cognitive rehabilitation framework

Postural control, balance, gait, and coordination in the motor learning framework technology are used as compensation in the rehabilitation framework. Although technology applications can be guided through general occupational therapy practice models such as the PEOP, several models have been developed to specifically address guiding AT recommendations. Cook and Hussy[5] introduced the Human Activity Assistive Technology (HAAT) model, Anson[6] developed the Human Interface Assessment (HIA), and Scherer[7] developed the Matching Persons with Technology (MPT) model. Anson's HIA illustrates technology as the missing piece or interface between a people whose performance skills (human) are not sufficient to perform the demands of the desired occupational task. In these AT models, the technology provides the link that bridges the gap between what the person can do and what the person needs to do to complete the occupational task. Thinking about the technology as the bridge for the person can be helpful to understanding how the occupational therapist needs to conduct an assessment to determine what the person can do and then compare what the person is able to do with the demands of the task the person wants to complete.

Assessment and Clinical Considerations for Using Technology

Because an occupational therapist completes an assessment for the match between a person and technology, there is a significant amount of information that needs to be considered. The occupational therapist will use information gathered from the occupational profile (including contextual information) as well as physical, visual, cognitive, and perceptual assessments of the person's related abilities in order to determine the best technology and positioning needed (see Fig. 26-1). For remediation, intervention often occurs primarily in the clinical setting with the goal to improve physical, cognitive, and/or perceptual abilities. When addressing equipment that will enable occupation as an end goal, trials with equipment should occur over a period of time and be generalized to the context where the person will use them. Following the Occupational Therapy Practice Framework,[8] the role of the occupational therapist is to consider not only the physical demands of using a device but also the psychological, social, emotional, and mental demands of using the device within the specific contexts in which the person will use the device(s). Ideally, equipment trials should occur within the environments where the person plans to use them (i.e., home and community). It is always recommended that the occupational therapist create a situation where the person can try using several devices prior to deciding which actual device will be recommended.

Occupational therapists must consider potential equipment abandonment and the person's decision to stop using the device, when recommending equipment. Critically, assessing equipment abandonment requires taking a "devil's-advocate" approach and listing the reasons why the person may not use the device once he or she receives it. This list may include things such as:

- Usability: The device takes too long or is too difficult to set up or clean. It requires assist of another person to turn on or off. It is too heavy or too big to transport.
- Aesthetics: The person does not like the size, weight, color, or style of the device.
- Durability: The device is not sturdy enough for daily use. The warranty is too short and the device malfunctioned, or the tech support is poor.
- Prognosis: The person only needed a device for a short time. The recommended device did not consider improving or declining abilities.

Trialing equipment provides an opportunity for the person to get an idea of whether or not there are some predisposing factors that might contribute to him or her not wanting to use the device in the future, and to discuss these factors prior to ordering the device. If unable to trial equipment, check into the company's return policy. Whether the device is funded with public money, private money, or personal funds, it is not a good use of anyone's money to recommend the purchase of a device that will soon be discarded or no longer needed.

Interprofessional Team

Matching appropriate technology with the person requires a team approach for optimal outcomes.

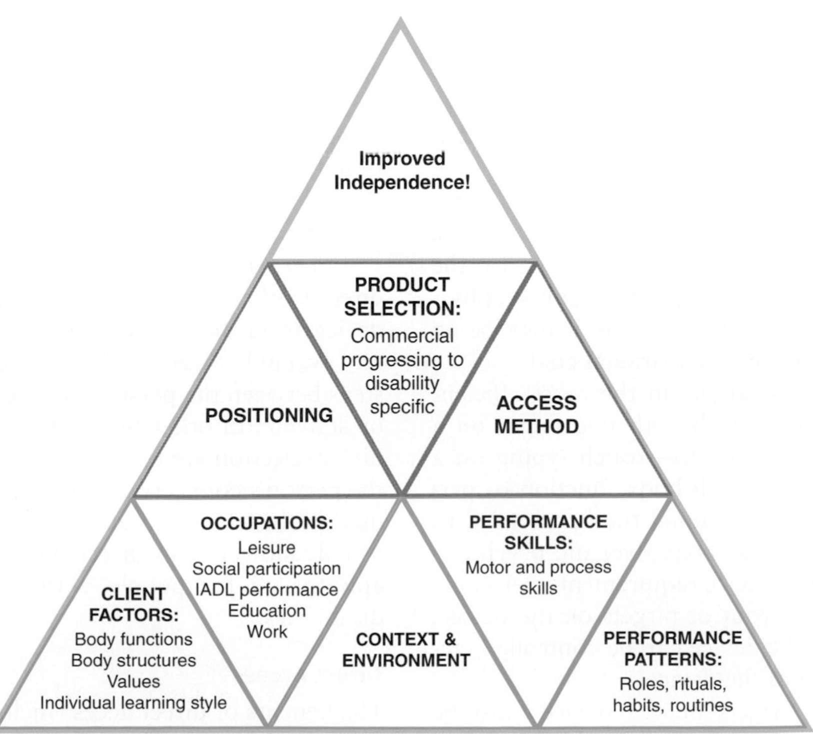

Figure 26-1. In the assistive technology hierarchy, technology services are based on the domain of occupational therapy.

The person arrives at an AT evaluation with preexisting community and health care teams. The home and community team includes the person and his or her family as well as other providers such as caregivers, teachers, and support coordinators. The health care team may consist of concurrent active therapy services that may include, but is not limited to, physical and speech therapy, physicians, and social workers. Introducing technology often requires additional professionals. The Rehabilitation and Engineering Society of North America names engineers and technologists, suppliers and manufacturers, and vocational rehabilitation personnel as crucial to the interprofessional team.[9] In addition, orthotists and prosthetics may add value when configuring custom equipment for people with significant physical disabilities. It is the responsibility of the occupational therapist to ensure that needed team members are included whenever possible in the process to cover the scope of the person's needs. Each included profession should focus on their scope of practice and collaborate on the spheres of shared influence.

Foundational Concepts for Access and Positioning

Whether a person calls his or her friend by touching the phone icon on him or her cell phone's display and pressing "Jim," or saying, "Hey Siri, call Jim," he or she is accessing his or her phone in order to meet the goal of talking to his or her friend. The position of the phone may hinder or enable access; the position may enable control of the phone by touch or, if the phone is far away, may hinder access by voice recognition. The method a person uses to control an object and the position of the object make a significant difference to the usability of the device. An **access method** is the way the person activates a target. A target may be a variety of objects, such as an individual icon on a phone, a key (or keys) on a keyboard, and icons on a computer monitor, toys, lights, or even a door. The target should be motivating for the person and appropriate for their age and cognitive, physical, and psychosocial needs. In addition, it may be an important part of meeting an occupational goal.

People tend to access targets in the most efficient way, whether that's using touch with one finger on a remote control, or 10 fingers when touch typing on a keyboard. To match people with body function or performance skill deficits, occupational therapists need to consider the person's physical, cognitive, and psychosocial abilities as well as the device requirements. This may include considering the layout of targets on the device, the different ways that the device can be controlled (accessed), and positioning of the device.

The layout of the targets on the device must be considered throughout trials of access and positioning, including:

- The targets displayed on the desktop and placed in folders
- The frequency of use, with more frequently used targets placed within easy access
- The spacing of targets
- The color of the background and of the targets
- The labels on the targets, with text and/or symbols

Visual perception and coordination are important considerations with layout because deficits may impair the person's ability to discriminate between icons and may impact the optimal spacing of the targets. The layout should match the person's abilities and goals. Changing the organization of the targets may improve the person's ability to accurately direct select to complete a task efficiently. However, if the goal is remediation of physical abilities, placing the targets at the periphery of the person's range of motion will facilitate reaching and coordination.

Access

The occupational therapy evaluation, especially the performance analysis of physical abilities, will provide the basis for the selection of appropriate access methods to try. When trialing access methods, the occupational therapist must concurrently consider the person's specific occupational goals. An appropriate access method must allow the person to do what he or she want to do, within an appropriate time period. For example, a person may make a phone call or text by voice, but when he or she needs to review an appointment in his or her calendar, he or she may need to don a stylus to open his or her calendar, scroll, and select (see Fig. 26-2). The occupational therapists must ensure that the person is able to place both phone calls and texts, as well as use his or her calendar, if this contributes to his or her occupational competence. The occupational therapist must use clinical reasoning and careful clinical observation when selecting an access method.

There are two main types of access: direct and indirect methods. A person is using direct access to use a device when he or she is able to spontaneously select any available target. Indirect access requires connecting steps between the person and the desired target to select or activate. In other literature, the terms direct and indirect selection are used; however, because access relates the person's connection with the occupational goal, it is used in this chapter. Indirect access is less strenuous but usually slower than direct, but often the only or most appropriate for people with more complex physical disabilities.

Direct Access

The benefits of direct access include efficiency and intuitiveness. For example, the most efficient typists usually use eight fingers and two thumbs to type, using direct

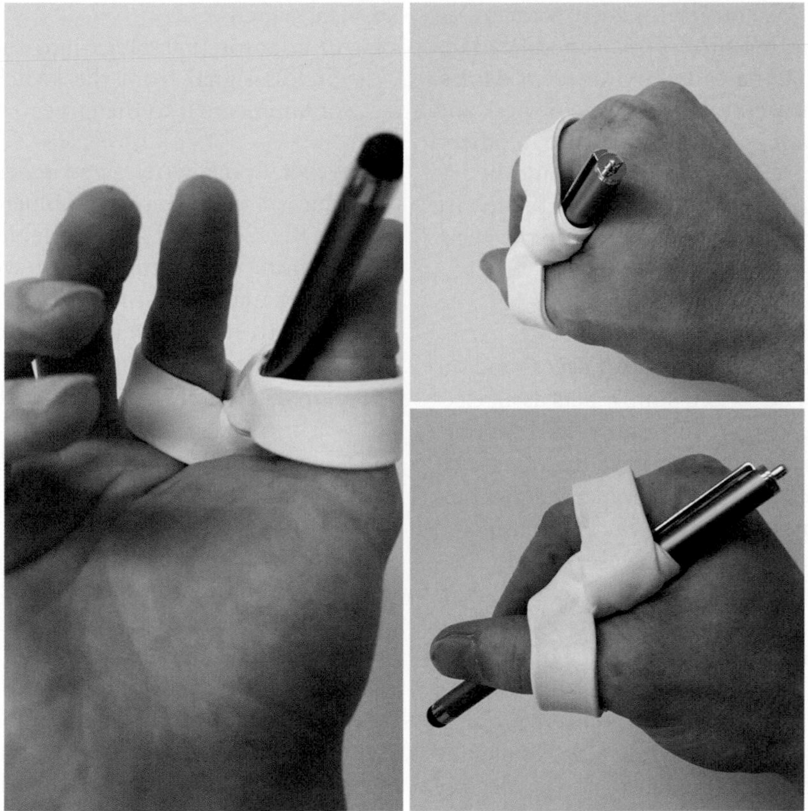

Figure 26-2. Example of a Figure 8 holder for a stylus made from splinting material..

access on a keyboard. Direct access requires lower cognitive demands than indirect access, but the person must possess the range of motion, endurance, dexterity, strength, and eye-hand coordination that allows for the accurate selection of various targets. Digits (fingers, toes), voice, or eye gaze may be utilized to directly activate a selected target. Direct access may require additional tools, such as a stylus or a keyguard (a raised grid that lies on top of the device's display), to improve accuracy. Using a combination of tools and body functions may be more complex, but may allow for greater occupational competence.

Voice recognition, or speech recognition, may be used for direct access. Key components that must be considered for the person to use voice recognition are:

- Does the person have a consistent, clear voice? If he or she is fraught with respiratory illnesses frequently his or her voice quality changes considerably throughout a day or week, voice recognition may not be the best access method.
- Is the person capable of learning new commands, or do he or she have a good support system that is able to devote significant time to training?
- Is the person able to problem solve? If the desired action does not occur, is the person able to identify why (after learning the software)?

More complex access is through eye gaze because it requires unique positioning of the device, minimal movement by the person, and often congruent eye movement. Also, the eye gaze device needs to be recalibrated every time the person moves away from the device and returns (as may occur during a pressure relief, if the device is not mounted correctly on the wheelchair frame). The increased complexity of this device requires more caregiver support and technological knowledge to use on a daily basis, but can be very effective for people with minimal physical movement. Voice and eye gaze can be efficient, but the person must demonstrate appropriate cognitive and physical abilities. Also, a backup method for times when the person is fatigued or has a cold may be needed to enable occupational performance and to avoid equipment abandonment.

Options within software (which directs device function and includes computer programs, apps, and operating systems) or device settings may enable a direct access method to be used with greater accuracy. Activating a "hold" setting will decrease the sensitivity of a touchscreen and require the user to linger on a selected target, within a specified area, for a period of time before it activates. Setting a "repeat" will ignore repeated touches within the same area. An "activate on release" setting will allow the person to drag his or her hand across the monitor, activating the last target touched prior to releasing contact with the monitor. Touch modifications are not universal and may be called by different names. Touch accommodations are built into some devices and operating systems, but are in add-on software in others. If touch modifications are required, they should be trialed within the specific operating system and software that the person will be using when completing the occupational goal.

Switch Use

A **switch** may be used in direct or indirect access and for a wide variety of tasks. The switch simply acts as an electricity conductor or interrupter. When at rest, or not activated, a space exists in the connection so that the target is turned off; when activated, the electrical circuit is completed and the target turns on. The switch is considered hardware because it is a physical object (see Fig. 26-3).

Each switch has different physical and sensory characteristics that must be matched with the user's physical and cognitive needs. Physical characteristics of a switch include the color, size (width, length, and depth), and the force and amount of movement required for activation and deactivation. Sensory characteristics include the auditory, tactile, or visual feedback it provides the user with activation. People with poor strength may need a switch that requires a low force for activation, such as the Micro Light (AbleNet) or Pal Pad (Abilitations) switches. When movement is very limited, the Candy Corn proximity switch (AbleNet) activates with close movement without direct contact.

Switches may be wired or wireless. Wireless switches do not necessarily connect through a wireless connection; they often connect via a Bluetooth connection. Most wireless switches consist of two pieces of hardware:

- The switch
- An adaptor that plugs into the target to receive the wireless signal from the switch when activated, and communicate it to the target

However, some wireless switches are "all-in-one" and capable of connecting via Bluetooth to devices (such as the Blue2 Switch from AbleNet). Wired switches are often more consistent, have fewer pieces to lose, and are lower maintenance; but the wires must be carefully managed to ensure the wires do not get tangled. Wireless switches require charging or batteries and often need to be paired (sometimes before each use) with the device to work.

The simplest type of switch use requires no software and can be thought of in a 1:1 format, which is when one switch activates one target. A 1:1 switch format may be used with battery operated toys that are modified with switch ports for switch control, or with simple electronic aids to daily living (EADLs) devices (see section on EADL). Although very basic, a 1:1 switch setup introduces the foundational concept of "cause" and "effect." The user learns that when he or she activates a switch (cause), something desirable happens (effect). When trialing the switch, the occupational therapist should practice (and keep data) for trial and error with various targets to determine the best switch the person is capable of using to motivate activation of the device. A 1:1 switch format represents direct access. Once the person demonstrates competency with the concept of cause and effect, the switch access can be expanded into a 1:many format. 1:many formats are considered indirect access, as the person uses one or two switches to access many targets, and may not spontaneously access any target at any time.

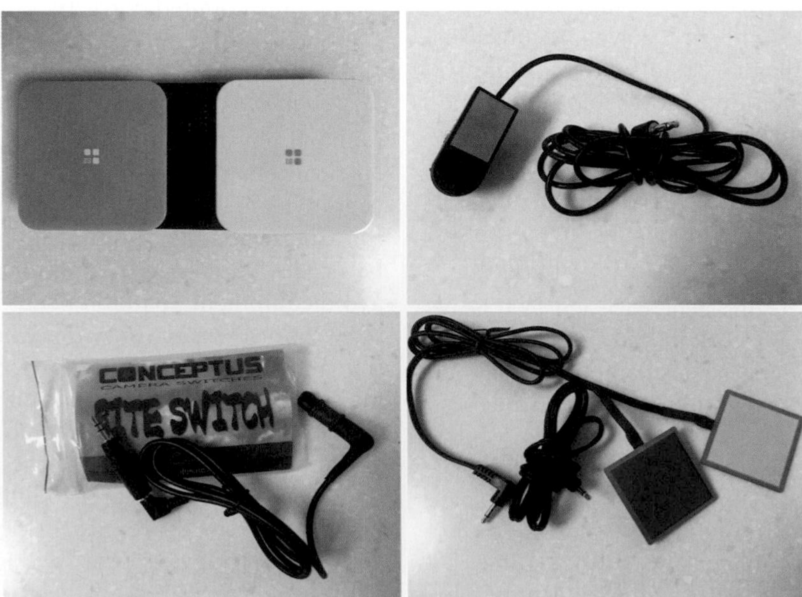

Figure 26-3. Switches with various characteristics. Examples of switches top to bottom, left to right (wireless) Blue2 (AbleNet Inc.); (wired) Micro Light (AbleNet Inc.), Bite Switch (Conceptus), Pal Pad (Adaptivation).

Indirect Access

The most common indirect access method commonly found on commercial- and disability-specific devices is switch scanning. **Switch scanning** uses software and hardware to provide a person with very limited physical movement access to multiple selections by only activating one target via a software or hardware interface (see Fig. 26-4). Software interfaces that allow switch scanning include some phones, tablets, most computer operating systems and some augmentative communication software. The software interface should display icons that, when activated, execute an action such as to speak a phrase, turn on or off the television, change a channel, open the internet, or open an app. Icons in the software can be programmed with different actions that can be configured for the person's unique needs.

To increase independence and participation, switch scanning can increase access to targets in a 1:many format. In a 1:many format, one-switch activation starts a scan pattern (highlighting boxes) that moves across available targets in specific, programmable, sequence. Common scan patterns include linear, row-column, column-row, and group or block scanning. A linear scan pattern moves across targets one target at a time. This is the slowest scan pattern, but appropriate for people with cognitive or visual deficits. Linear scan patterns allow for auditory scanning (when the software speaks a description of each target that the scan box highlights). Row-column scan patterns require the following three-switch presses:

- First switch press: To move the scan box down each row of icons.
- Second switch press: Select the desired row that the desired icon is in; this starts the scan box moving across each column in the selected row.
- Third switch press: Select the desired icon when the scan box highlights it, thereby selecting the icon.

Column-row and group or block scanning are variations of the row-column pattern. When considering an appropriate scan pattern, the type of scan initiation needs to be considered. Two main types of scan initiation exist:

- Automatic: The scan box starts moving with one-switch activation and scans the targets automatically.
- Manual: The user must activate the switch to advance the scan box.

An automatic scan initiation (method used to advance the highlighting box when scanning) is less physically exerting, but requires the person to respond to a set timing. A manual scan initiation requires two unique switch actions, usually programmed on two different switches. The manual scan initiation does not require the person to respond to set timing, but requires more switch activations to navigate to desired targets. It also requires greater cognition to differentiate between the unique actions of two switches.

Switch scanning can be complicated and overwhelming at times, but for people with complex needs, it may provide opportunities for occupational participation that would be otherwise out of reach. The Scanning Wizard website (www.scanningwizard.com) allows for trials of various settings and gathers objective data with printed reports of trials. In addition, each trial provides recommendations that may contribute to more efficient switch setup. Using the Scanning Wizard on a computer requires a Universal Serial Bus (USB) switch adaptor, such as the Swifty (Origin Instruments), to connect wired or wireless switches to the computer. Scanning Wizard documents may be used as a tool to introduce people to switch scanning, to educate users on the benefits of different switches or switch setups, and to contribute to improved clinical decision-making.

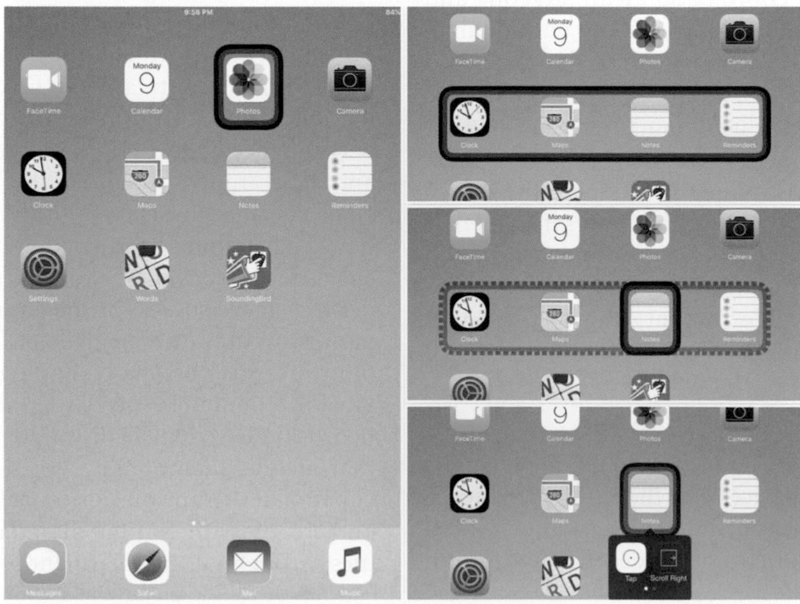

Figure 26-4. Row-column 1-switch scanning on an iPad platform.

Positioning and Mounts

When occupational therapists consider positioning of a device, the person's available active range of motion, strength, endurance, dexterity, coordinated movement, and most consistent voluntary isolated movement (fingers when possible) need to be considered. Additionally, the person's environment(s) and contexts, the number of caregivers, and whether or not the caregivers are consistent, make a difference. To find the ideal placement for a device or switch for the person, different angles, depths, and heights should be trialed. The person's specific accuracy and endurance (length of continuous use) with access should be measured during these trials, to be documented to justify the final equipment selection.

When evaluating for access, the position of the person and the device (which may be an augmentative communication device, tablet, keyboard, or switch) may make a significant difference in accuracy and endurance during active use. The person's vision and physical abilities need to be considered from the onset. Small changes may make a big difference for access. Ensuring that the person's trunk is securely supported may provide a solid base of support that facilitates upper extremity movement. Providing a solid surface as reference for a forearm or elbow may improve accuracy of direct access. The size of the display and the distance between the display and the person should also be considered. When using a smartphone, the person may anchor their thenar eminence on the side of the device and access all quadrants with their thumb or part of a digit. This "hold" allows people with tone or tenodesis to effectively use a touchscreen when the device is stabilized. However, for 7 inches tablets and larger, the user must hover their isolated digit over the display. If the display is on an angle perpendicular to the table (approximately 60°), the user may improve their coordination with targeting and activating icons by stabilizing their elbow on the tabletop while reaching toward the device with an isolated digit. Trials with various positions and access methods are necessary to decide which configuration will meet the person's needs best.

The end goal of positioning is to secure the device in a position that is consistent, stable, and safe, whether the person is in a bed or wheelchair. Mounts may roll (*Tobii Dynavox* ConnectIT Floorstand, or *Daedalus* Technologies' Daessy Rolling mount) or prop the device into an upright position for tabletop use. There are two main categories of mounts that exist:

- **Flexible:** Adjustable, and allows for movement of the device into various positions without tools. This is best for lightweight devices and those that need to be used in a portrait (vertical) and landscape (horizontal) position. These are often not funded through health insurance. Examples are tabX Tablet Holder from *Modular Hose* and Hover from *AbleNet*.
- **Fixed:** Remain in a static position, requiring tool adjustment to change position. Often heavy duty and able to support heavy devices. May be funded through health insurance when recommended for a speech-generating device. An example is the Rigid and Positioner Mounts, available from *Daessy*.

Flexible mounts (adjustable cradle, arm, and clamp that allow for movement of the device into various positions without tools) are often one piece, whereas a fixed mount (a cradle or mounting plate, arm(s), and clamp that remain in a static position, unless adjusted using tools to change position) is ordered specifically for one main configuration and has multiple parts. A mounting cradle attaches to the person's seating device or bed, allowing for removal of the device and mount for transfers. The stem of the mount fits into the mounting cradle and may have more than one joint and stem to improve specific positioning. A mounting plate specific for the device allows for secure positioning of the device onto the mount. With fixed mounts, careful consideration of the person's use of the device and mount should be considered. It is important to remember that the person will be involved with multiple occupational tasks that need to be taken into account when considering a fixed mount.

Technology Used for Remediation: Occupational-as-a-Means

An occupational therapist uses technology for remediation within an intervention session, or across intervention sessions, to remediate the specific performance skills and person factors that are limiting them in completing their occupational goals. Prior to using technology for remediation, the occupational therapist must gather the same kind of assessment information as he or she would prior to any other treatment. Occupational profile information regarding the person's occupational goals and performance analysis data regarding performance skills and body functions allow the therapist to creatively challenge the physical, cognitive, or perceptual limitations. When done appropriately, the *just-right-challenge* engages the person in exerting maximum effort in order to achieve success at the game, while really addressing restoration of their deficits. The feeling of "flow"[10] motivates the person. Technology for remediation may include computer software, tablet-based apps, lightboards, and virtual reality (VR), as well as accessories that include intentionally positioned switches. The occupational therapist needs to use their clinical reasoning and creativity to continually adapt and grade the activities throughout the treatment session (see Fig. 26-5).[11]

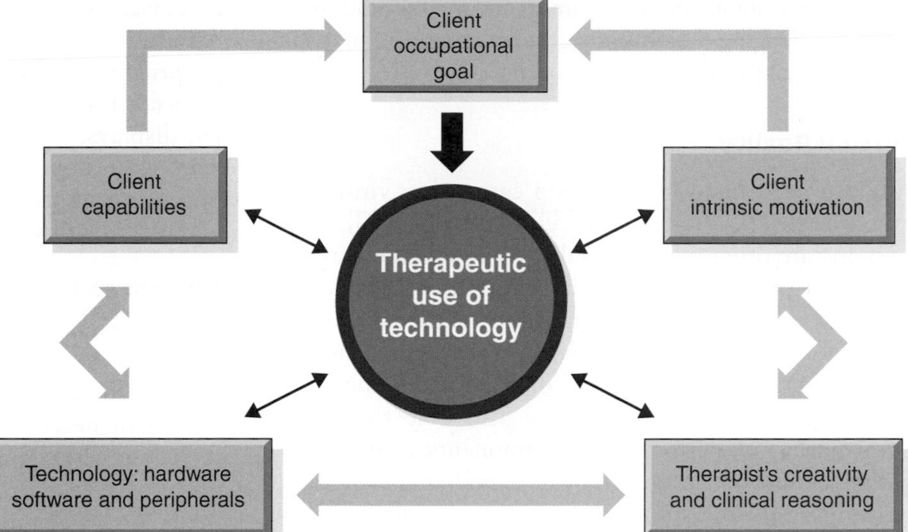

Figure 26-5. Rakoski's therapeutic use of technology model. (From Rakoski DR, Ferguson RC. The virtual context of occupation: integrating everyday technology into everyday practice. OT Practice. 2013;18:CE.1–CE.8.)

General Guidelines for Therapeutic Use of Technology

Occupational therapists should consider the following when using technology in a clinical session (see Fig. 26-6):

- Remediation activity should always be connected to body function or performance deficit(s) that hinder occupational competence.
- The software program (games, activities, and apps) should relate to the person's intrinsic motivation, encouraging the person to engage in the software to achieve a feeling of "flow"[10] and providing a *just-right-challenge* that balances vigilance, anxiety, and boredom.
- The occupational therapist should engage in the activity for the duration to gauge difficulty and engagement, adjusting the software or hardware maintain the "just right" challenge. The intention is not to "set someone up" to work independently.
- The occupational therapist should determine, prior to use, what objective data from the person's interaction with the technology will be gathered for documentation. The data gathered and documented should relate to the person's deficits, not engagement in technology (e.g., accuracy with movement, distance reached and repetitions, length of engagement with sustained attention, number of items recalled using short-term memory).
- When addressing cognitive, visual, or perceptual deficits, initial setup for physical access to the controls should not be challenged; the person's focus needs to be on the therapeutic part of the treatment, not the access or activation.
- When the person's deficits are physical in nature, the occupational therapist should consider:
  - Writing goals should focus on the strength, range, coordination, or endurance needed to complete the person's targeted occupational goal. The intervention techniques used would include technology for remediation; the focus of occupational therapy intervention is not the technology itself.
  - Computer program/game/app choice should reflect the person's interests (obtained in the occupational profile) in order to enable the person's intrinsic motivation. Activity choice should facilitate use of the person's hindering physical deficits when accessing the controls on the computer/device.

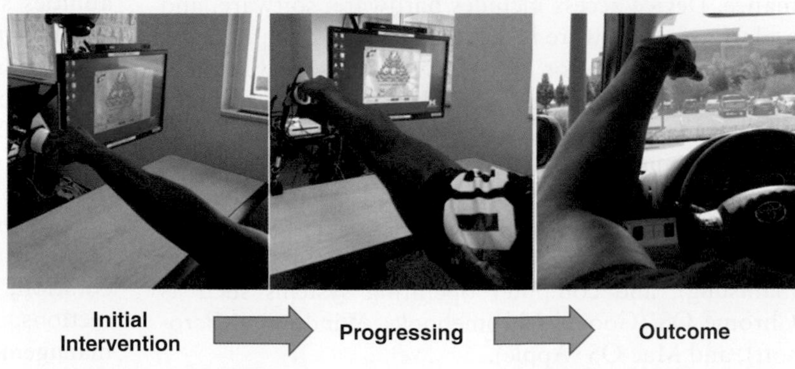

Figure 26-6. Person with an end goal to activate garage door opener on visor in car strengthens their upper extremity by activating raised switch in computer game, an example of therapeutic use of technology.

- Controlling the program/game/app should be a challenging action that requires repetition of a specific physical ability that needs to be restored.[11]

Virtual Reality

VR can be defined in two main categories: virtual environment (VE) and commercial gaming (CG).[12] VE systems are often more specialized and created with the intention of using for remediation and are considered immersive VR. CG systems may be adapted for use in occupational therapy interventions and may also be called exergaming.[13] CG are considered nonimmersive VR. Occupational therapists are also able to address remediation of performance components using VR to influence subcortical reactions to remediate balance and postural stability following the motor control theory. Any VR system used in occupational therapy should have the capability of being personalized and customized so that the occupational therapist can grade the task to create the *just-right-challenge* as the person is engaged with the technology.[14] See the Evidence table at the end of this chapter for descriptions of systematic reviews reporting on the evidence of VR interventions used for remediation.

Assistive Technology for Occupational Performance

When people experience physical, psychosocial, or cognitive limitations due to a significant congenital or acquired injury or disease, they may need adaptations or devices to allow them to fully participate in the occupations of their choice. This section focuses on adaptations that can be made to electronics, including appliances, home theater systems, lights and doors, phones, tablets, and computers. Adapted seating and augmentative communication devices are discussed in other chapters.

Device Access

Device access is the use of a device, including phones, tablets, and computers, to enable occupational performance. Device access includes hardware, software, and a platform. Hardware is the actual, physical equipment. A keyboard, monitor, hard drive, mouse, tablet, and phone are all examples of hardware. Software directs device function and includes computer programs, apps, and operating systems. A device (hardware) and operating system (software) make up a platform. Examples of commonly used platforms include smartphone and tablet operating systems include iOS (Apple), Android (Samsung), and computer operating systems such as Chrome OS (Google Chromebook), Windows (Microsoft), and Mac OS (Apple).

Another consideration in device access is the type and number of ports that the device contains. Examples of device ports include USB, high-definition multimedia interface (HDMI), and Ethernet. Some devices have proprietary ports, for example, Apple's Thunderbolt. In order for the Thunderbolt port to work with external displays, an adapter dongle is needed. These small details are important to consider and should be noted during device trials, to ensure that the recommended equipment will work for the person as intended.

Evaluating for Device Access

Many occupations are enabled by device use, such as online banking, connecting with friends and families on social media, researching a diagnosis, and shopping for clothes or necessities; however, people vary in the way they complete these tasks. For example, online banking may be accessed through an app on a smartphone or tablet, or a website using an Internet web browser. Paying bills, a similar, connected, task may be completed through automatic withdrawal from a bank account, using bill pay services through the bank, or using standard mail. None of these options are wrong, but they all take different paths to meet the same goal.

When occupational therapists work with persons, the person's occupational goal(s) direct the device setup and targets that must be accessed. When matching a person with hardware and software, the occupational therapist should first consider the person's medical condition, including whether it is acute or chronic, temporary or permanent, or static or progressive. Interview the person or his or her caregiver about:

- *Environments:* Home, work, and other community environments
- *Previous device setup:* Determine what has worked and what has not.
- *Current device setup (if one exists):* Document the hardware, software, and platform(s) available.
- *Internet:* Wireless or wired, whether data are capped or unlimited, and if it is a public or private connection. Internet carrier and type is important to know because many software packages are direct downloads from the Internet or require Internet access to work.

The person's physical, cognitive, and psychosocial abilities should be assessed just as they are in a typical occupational therapy evaluation (see Fig. 26-1). Hand dominance, range of motion, muscle strength, fine motor and gross motor coordination, sensation, visual acuity, and visual perception should all be documented. The person's balance both seated and standing (if applicable) should be measured, as well as his or her ability to transport items safely. The person's cognitive abilities, including (but not limited to) orientation, attention, and memory, ability to follow directions, safety, sequencing, organization, and time management, should be assessed. This information will be used in the documentation to support the person's need for and ability to use recommended equipment.

The assessment process for these abilities is available in other chapters of this textbook.

Evaluating for Navigation and Selection

After the occupational profile and performance analysis, occupational performance should be assessed in device trials on the person's preferred platform. Device trials need to consider two main concepts:

- *Navigation:* The way a person moves around their computer display. This is often completed through use of mouse control or touchscreen access.
- *Selection:* The primary mouse actions (left single clicks, left double clicks, right clicks, and click and drag mouse actions) and primary touchscreen actions (quick tap, double tap, and tap and hold to activate software or files) that are necessary to open and close programs, files, and select items after navigation.

The person's ability to use his or her current mouse setup or device setup (for touchscreen devices) should be observed and documented. If the person does not use a mouse, start with a standard USB wired, touchpad mouse, or touchscreen device setup at a 60° angle on a table. The goal of navigation is to match the person with the least restrictive (or most standard) equipment that enables occupational performance. This will allow the person to generalize the setup to other devices, if needed.

During the trial, the person should be asked to identify icons in all quadrants of the device screen. Vision and light reading skills can also be observed during this task. If assessing mouse use, the person should be asked to perform:

- *Primary mouse actions:* Left single clicks, left double clicks, right clicks, and click and drag mouse actions
- *Primary touchscreen actions:* Quick tap (single click), double tap (double click, not all touchscreens use this action), and tap and hold to activate software or files
- *Gestures (programmed touch or mouse sequences that execute specific actions):* Available on some mice and touchscreens. May include swipe, pinch, or Apple's 3-D Touch

Efficiency (length of time for navigation), accuracy (number of inaccurate activations), and usability (if the mouse, touchscreen, or gestures support or hinder performance) should be documented.

There are two main movements that a mouse will control. A proportional control enables mouse movement in all directions from one piece of hardware. For example, a standard USB mouse moves the around the monitor in response to physical movement of the mouse. Switched control mouse pointer movement can be identified by one defined activation that produces one defined result. An activation can be made through a sip or a puff, separate switches, or various keys on the keyboard. For example, Mouse Keys (built into the major operating systems) enables four to eight keys (typically select keys on a number pad, keyboard, or the arrow keys) to control the mouse pointer in specific directions; up, down, left, and right. Mouse clicks when using Mouse Keys depend on the platform used. Proportional control is more common and intuitive than switched, but switched may provide more flexibility for physical conditions such as tone or when teaching cause and effect.

Few formal assessments for navigation and selection exist. For computers, the Compass Software for Access Assessment, available from *Koester Performance Research*, assesses different mouse skills including aiming, dragging, and selecting items from a menu. Quantitative results from the software can be gathered at evaluation (baseline) and with each trial. This information contributes to improved decision-making about final equipment and greater justification in the documentation supporting the recommended equipment.

Hardware and Software Associated with Navigation

Hardware, the physical equipment associated with navigation, includes various types of mice, styli, and touchscreens. Each piece of navigation hardware trialed should be evaluated for advantages and disadvantages in relationship to the person's physical, cognitive, and psychosocial strengths and weaknesses. Hardware will be explored starting with simple and moving to complex.

Touchscreens, wired USB mice, and touchpad mice on laptops are simple hardware that offer proportional control for navigation. Wired USB mice and touchpad mice are often included in the price of the laptop, as touchscreens are on tablets. However, people with physical disabilities may not be able to use this equipment successfully. Wired USB mice and touchpad mice require the user to connect the hardware movement to mouse pointer movement. The user must effectively initiate and terminate digit flexion and distinguish between single and double mouse clicks. To execute a click and drag action, the user must exert downward force while moving the hardware horizontally and vertically. Impaired upper extremity strength, fine motor coordination (including the ability to stabilize forearm, wrist, and digit movements), and decreased sensation are a few of the physical deficits that may impede mouse use.

Although touchscreens are more intuitive, they require a greater combination of gross motor skills, fine motor skills, and dexterity than a mouse. A stylus is hardware that may be trialed when the person is unable to isolate a digit; commercial options and patterns for self-fabrication exist (see Figure 8 holder in Fig. 26-2). Touchscreens for commercial devices are often capacitive touchscreens, meaning that they require flow of an electrical current to recognize an activation. This can be tested; if the device responds to the gentle touch of a pencil eraser, it is not a capacitive touchscreen, and virtually anything can be used as a stylus (although sharp objects are not recommended). Many disability-specific devices are not capacitive touchscreens. Conducting an Internet search for "disability, stylus" will bring up options, including those with large grips, telescoping models, and for different body parts including mouth- and head-controlled styli.

Wired USB mice and touchpad mice are considered "simple," low complexity hardware, but more complex options exist. Medium complexity mice include commercial options such as trackballs or trackpads. Medium complexity mice require less gross motor movement than a wired mouse. Also, the wired or wireless nature of the mouse allows for increased distance between the person and the device display. This may allow the user to stabilize their forearm on the tabletop, which may improve accuracy. In all navigation trials, the same mouse actions should be assessed, and data on the person's performance should be documented.

Hardware-only navigation methods are often described as "plug-and-play" equipment, meaning that they work when plugged into the appropriate port. Software may provide additional adjustment to facilitate competence. Simple software such as the device's mouse or display options may enhance performance. Available mouse and display options are unique to each platform. Mouse pointer options often include pointer speed, size, and color. The size of the icon and text can be changed, and display modifications can increase the contrast of content. *Koester Performance Research* produces the Pointing Wizard, a downloadable software onto a Windows computer. This wizard assesses the person's navigation and selection in relationship to the computer's *Ease-of-Access* settings, recommending changes for greater efficiency and accuracy after performing simple tasks. Use of the Pointing Wizard may improve outcomes for people using a mouse with a Window's platform.

Many medium complexity mice may pair with add-on software as well for increased functionality. For example, the TrackballWorks software, Kensington, enables the programming of trackball mouse clicks for the typical single click, double click, click and drag, and right click. Or, for increased function, the buttons may be programmed to page up and page down; scroll up and scroll down; cut, copy, or paste; and more. Pairing a Kensington trackball with TrackballWorks software may increase the efficiency of navigation for a person with disabilities.

Hardware and software options are available for smartphones, tablets, and computers that improve the accessibility of navigation using switched control. As previously stated, the operating system function Mouse Keys provides switched control. Similarly, a disability-specific product, the Hitch 2.0, *AbleNet*, enables five switches, each that execute a defined mouse pointer movement such as up, down, left, or right. For device access, switches offer access through a 1:many format, where one or two switches may enable access to an entire device display through accompanying software. The software may be built-in to the device (e.g., the iOS accessibility option "Switch Control") or may be an add-on (e.g., E Z Keys from *Words+*). For iOS devices, the Hitch+, *AbleNet*, serves as an interface between an iOS platform and switch(es). Customizing the scanning options for the person is necessary to enable performance; these options are described comprehensively in the previous sections.

Switch Use and Indirect Access

Disability-specific navigation options offering proportional control range from joysticks to eye gaze. Ranging from simple to complex, there are joysticks, trackballs, head-controlled mice, mouth-controlled mice, and eye gaze (see Fig. 26-7) as follows:

- ***Disability-specific joysticks and trackballs:*** Often exist as plug-and-play hardware or may be programmed through the person's power wheelchair joystick using a Bluetooth transmission method. Examples are the n-Abler Pro Joystick and the Optima Joystick, both from *Infogrip*.
- ***Head-controlled mouse:*** Uses infrared (IR) sensors in a camera-like device to track reflective dots placed on the person's head, nose, or hat brim. Examples are TrackerPro *AbleNet* and Headmouse Extreme *Origin Instruments*, both plug-and-play options.
  - Mouse pointer speed is influenced by the placement of the camera-like device, with closer positioning translating to faster pointer movement.
- ***Mouth-controlled mice:*** Mounted joystick moved by a person's mouth or chin. Examples are the Jouse 3, *Compusult Limited*, QuadJoy 3 from *Ergoguys*, and the Quadstick FPS from *Quadstick*.
- ***Eye gaze:*** Camera-like device mounted in front of computer monitor that tracks eye movement. Requires calibration prior to use. Examples are PCEye Mini from *TobiiDynavox* and the mGaze Eye Tracker from *School Health*.

Remember that the abovementioned disability-specific products discuss controlling mouse pointer movement. The person will need access to mouse clicks using hardware or software as well!

Hardware and Software Associated with Selection

In order for navigation to be meaningful to the user, the user must also have a method to select an item. **Selection** is often completed using the primary mouse actions and primary touchscreen actions discussed during device navigation trials, which are actions that are necessary to open and close programs, files, and select items after navigation. Efficient device access will enable the person to navigate to an intended icon, and select accurately after one attempt. Double clicks, differentiating between right and left clicks and performing click

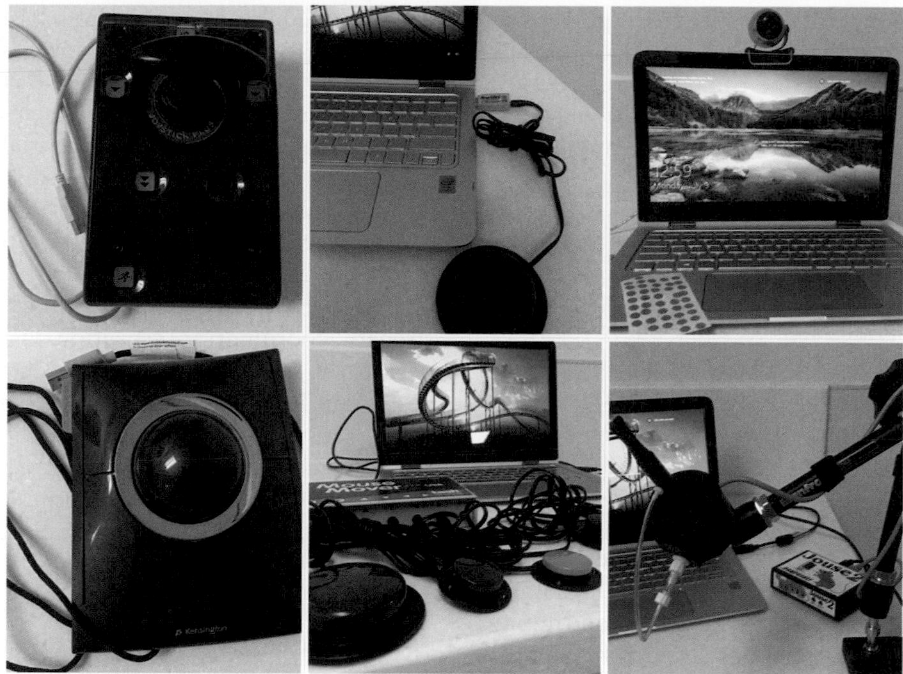

Figure 26-7. Examples of common navigation and selection methods, from left to right and top to bottom—Roller Joystick from Traxys, Swifty USB switch adapter, Orin Instruments and Jelly Bean switch, AbleNet Inc., TrackerPro head-controlled mouse from AbleNet Inc., SlimBlade trackball, Kensington, Mouse Mover/Hitch Computer Switch Interface from Able26Net Inc., Jelly Bean and Specs Switches from AbleNet Inc., and Jouse 3 from Compusult Limited.

and drag actions, can all be difficult for a person with physical and cognitive deficits. However, performing all of these actions are often necessary for complete device access. Traditional USB or wireless mouse clicks can be modified using a range of complexity of hardware and software:

- *Switch selection for proportional mouse pointer movement:* Enables mouse clicks through an external switch to separate mouse pointer movement from mouse clicks. The mouse pointer movement is proportional through the mouse (whether hand, mouth, or eye controlled), but an external switch is plugged into an adaptor for mouse clicks. Examples of adaptors are the Swifty (*Orin Instruments*) for the computer or Tapio (*Orin Instruments*) for iOS devices. Some disability-specific devices may have built-in switch ports. A person will also need a switch and mouse for mouse pointer movement.
- *Dwell software:* A nonphysical method for selection. Dwell software is available in some operating systems, free, or may be built-in the software of a head-controlled, mouth-controlled, or eye gaze navigation system. The software often "sits" on top of the device display, offering options in icon format for left click, double click, click and drag, or right click. Dwell software requires sequencing multiple steps for effective use:
    - First, the mouse pointer or gaze must stabilize on the selected icon for a specified amount of time. The amount of time that stabilization is required is customizable.
    - The software will select the icon after the dwell time and apply the action to the next area (the size of which is also customizable) that the mouse pointer or gaze "dwells" on.
    - The timing and area must be customized to the user for effective use. Too slow or too fast, and the person will likely grow frustrated. If the selection area is too large, the action may select more than one item; however, too small and the person may not be able to stabilize the pointer or their gaze.
- *Eye blink:* Available in many eye gaze systems. Length of blink is customizable.

Selection methods should be intentionally explored because selecting icons can cause frustration if difficulties and inaccurate activations persist.

Considerations with Navigation and Selection

Hardware and software for navigation often need various trials, over a period of time, to determine the optimal setup. For people with inconsistent presentation, such as tone, difficulty maintaining optimal positioning, or cognition that changes over the period of a day or week, the recommended equipment must provide access at their best and worst times of function. People with degenerative diagnoses may need equipment that will continue to provide access as their condition progresses. With trials, change one thing at a time. Often, a "mix-and-match" approach is optimal for hardware and software. Some people may require one method for navigation and another for selection.

Text Entry

Navigating and selecting icons to move between and within software programs are necessary, but to really utilize the full capabilities of a device, the person needs a method to enter text. Text entry (entering text on a device, generally in the form of phrases and sentences) consists of entering text on a device, generally in the form of phrases and sentences. Consider navigating social media. Scrolling through newsfeeds and seeing friends and family's faces may be fun, but without the ability to comment and socially participate by entering text, the inherent meaning in this occupation (keeping in touch with friends and family) is lost. There are many skills that are needed for successful spontaneous text entry, including composing the text (figuring out what needs to be said), grammar, and spelling (how to say it). After the text is entered, proofreading skills are necessary to ensure that the intended message is conveyed. For responsive text entry, when returning pleasantries through email, for example, reading fluency is an important secondary skill.

Evaluating for Text Entry

When assessing text entry, it is important to ask questions regarding the various components that contribute to successful text entry during the occupational profile:

- Does the person read, and how proficiently?
- How is his or her spelling ability?
- When the person uses a device now, does he or she type out his or her own content? Or, does he or she speak it to the device or another person?
- Is the content appropriate (in context, spelling, and grammar)? Does he or she identify and fix mistakes?
- Most importantly, what occupations does he or she perform that require successful text entry? The answer to this question is important to keep in mind during the evaluation and throughout the hardware and software trials.

If the person only wants to do text entry for recreation such as researching his or her diagnosis online and keeping in touch with his or her son who lives three states away, text entry demands may be minimal. In addition, an informal message with minimal-to-moderate spelling or grammar mistakes will be understood. However, if the person uses text entry for more formal purposes, such as work as an attorney, he or she may be expected to compose pages of text in professional language with good organization and accurate spelling and grammar. Similarly, a financial advisor will likely need to enter many numbers into spreadsheets and proprietary software or websites. Each of these examples requires different skills. If the intricacies of text entry were not considered during the device trial, the occupational therapy intervention may not actually enable the needed occupational performance.

The performance analysis for text entry remains similar to navigation and selection. Each person's available body functions, including range of motion, muscle strength, coordination, sensation, vision, and cognition, need to be assessed. The person's strengths and weaknesses can be paired with the access methods discussed in previous text because text entry methods are available that accommodate each access method. The occupational therapist should perform specific observation of current text entry, preferably using the person's preferred platform, including:

- *Positioning:* An effective seated position, with supported trunk if needed, will facilitate effective bilateral upper extremity movement. Owing to the many items (keys) that the person needs to access with text entry, positioning is a greater factor to successful direct access (any available target can be spontaneously selected) than with navigation and selection.
- *Text composition:* Spontaneous and responsive text entry, including the person's proofreading or ability to identify and fix mistakes.
- *Typing method:* Typing using a hunt-and-peck method refers to using one or two digits, on one or both hands, to activate keys. A touch typist places his or her hands on the home row, using all 10 digits to activate keys.

Consider the body functions that are needed for each type of typist. Hunt-and-peck typists require visual attention to the keyboard because they do not have consistent hand placement and often do not have the keyboard memorized. Touch typists are generally able to type without visual attention to the keyboard. Requiring visual attention to the keyboard to enter text decreases text entry speed and corrections. Some research is available regarding text entry rates (TER) for different types of access interfaces that have been used by people with physical disabilities to help the occupational therapist in the selection process.[15]

There are more formal assessments for text entry than for navigation and selection. Typing speed, measured in words per minute (wpm), is important to document. The Compass Software for Access Assessment from *Koester Performance Research* assesses various word and sentence text entry. Furthermore, the software will assess performance with alternative hardware and software. This allows the clinician to gather information at baseline (with the person's own setup or a standard setup used for evaluation) and then with the various recommended equipment during trials. Wpm or data from the Compass Software gathered at evaluation (baseline) and with each configuration of hardware and software during trials (after appropriate trial period) will provide important information that can be used when making final equipment recommendations.

As with navigation, the goal of text entry is to match the person with the least restrictive (or most standard) equipment that enables occupational performance. This increases the generalizability of their setup to other devices, allowing for successful text entry in various contexts and settings.

Hardware for Text Entry

The physical and sensory characteristics that apply to switches also apply to hardware for text entry. Physical characteristics of hardware for text entry include the color (and contrast), size (width, length, and depth of each key and the keyboard), and the force and movement required for activation and deactivation of a key (see Fig. 26-8). Sensory characteristics of hardware for text entry include the auditory, tactile, and/or visual aspects of the keys and keyboard, both when stationary and when in use. Assessing these characteristics of the hardware apart from the person, then observing how the different characteristics interact with the person's body function strengths and deficits during use of the hardware, will contribute to greater clinical reasoning skills as well as support the occupational therapist when justifying the selected hardware in documentation.

Devices come standard with their own text entry method. The devices that most often come with hardware keyboards are Chromebooks, laptop, and desktop computers. Software keyboards that "pop up" on displays, called on-screen keyboards, exist also. Smartphones and tablets come with on-screen software keyboards, although an external physical keyboard may be a very useful accessory for some people. Both commercial- and disability-specific keyboards exist. Keyboards may be large, standard, or compact in size; may or may not have a number pad; and may connect to the device through a wired or wireless connection (with wireless often connecting to the device through Bluetooth).

Basic Trials for Text Entry

Trials for text entry should start with positioning. As with navigation and selection, the distance between the keyboard and the person may make a significant difference. Laptop keyboards may be too close to the person and encourage a kyphotic position; if this occurs, there are two options:

1. Trial an external keyboard (wired or wireless) to increase the distance between the display and the keyboard. The display then can be raised into a more appropriate position.
2. Trial a second monitor. The second display may be extended (so the person has two displays) or duplicated (the content on the primary display is copied onto the secondary display). The laptop keyboard can continue to be used for text entry, whereas the monitor can be placed at a height that encourages an upright trunk position.

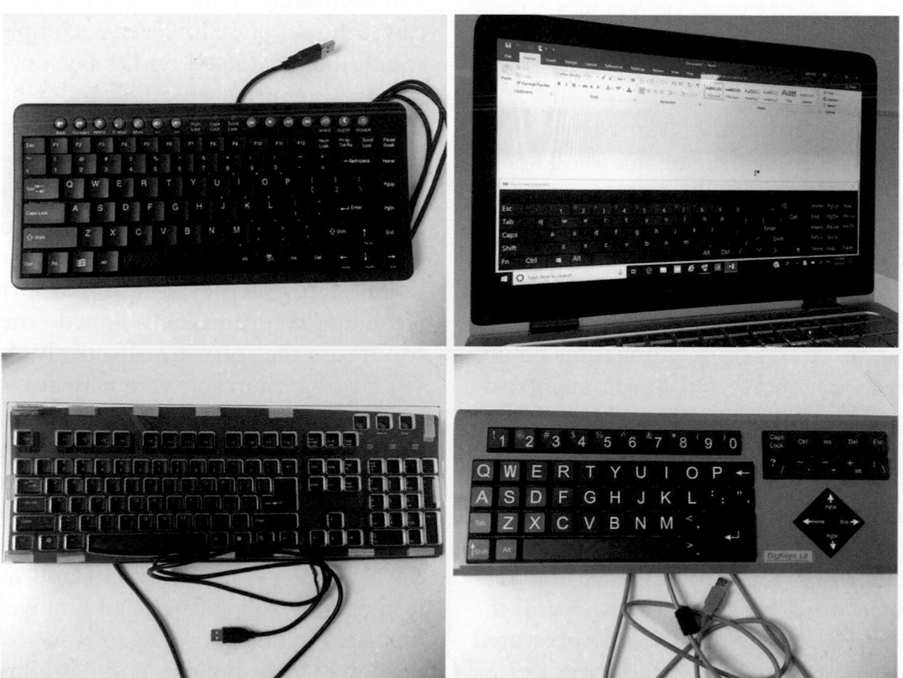

Figure 26-8. Common equipment for text entry including (left to right, top to bottom) compact keyboard (multiple manufacturers), on-screen keyboard (built-in to OS), Keyboard with Keyguard from Infogrip, Inc., and BigKeys keyboard, Greystone Digital.

When making a recommendation, consider the person's environments and what will increase efficiency and independence. Does the person transport his or her laptop often? If so, a keyboard will likely be easier to carry and set up than a second monitor.

Devices contain accessibility settings that may change how the keyboard (physical or on-screen) accepts touch. Using built-in accessibility settings is less complex than changing hardware or adding on software and is generalizable between devices with the same platform. The accessibility options on a device are located in the device's settings, often under an "Accessibility" or "Ease-of-Access" label. Accessibility settings for text entry that apply to physical or on-screen keyboards often include:

- *Slow Keys:* Controls the amount of time a person must press down a key before the key is activated; allows people with ataxic movements to move around various keys before they settle on the intended key.
- *Bounce Keys:* Ignores multiple (same) key presses for a set period of time after that key is pressed; is helpful for people with tremors, when the person has difficulty gauging the force of a movement or difficulty terminating fine motor movement.
- *Repeat Keys:* Ignores any key presses for a specified amount of time after the first key is pressed; may help a person who has poor coordination and difficulty controlling extraneous movements.
- *Sticky Keys:* Enables keyboard access to two-key actions for one-handed typists. Holds down the Shift, Control, Command, Alt, or Windows key with one key press and then applies that action to the next key pressed. For example, if a one-handed typist wished to type a capital "S," he would press the "Shift," release the "Shift," and press "S," which would result in typing a capital "S."

Commonly, people will turn on the "Caps Lock" Key, press the "S," and press "Caps Lock" again; using Sticky Keys reduces one key press. Keyboard shortcuts (such as "Control-C" for copying highlighted content) are efficient with Sticky Keys. These built-in operating systems should be trialed prior to trialing other hardware keyboards.

Another option to trial before purchasing equipment is the on-screen keyboard. On-screen keyboards are prevalent on touchscreen devices, but Chromebooks and Windows and Mac computers also have on-screen keyboards built-in to the operating system. Features of the keyboards vary between manufacturers. Some of the keyboards use **word acceleration techniques** such as word prediction and word completion. When the keyboard presents choices to complete a started word, the keyboard is using word completion. Words presented that predict the next word the person will type, before the person starts typing, is called word prediction. Many on-screen keyboards learn the person's typing style and form the word prediction list around common words and phrases typed. When the person clicks on a presented word, the word will be inserted on the display where the cursor lies. This may increase text entry speed for the person in that fewer letters are typed, and a decreased chance of spelling error exists. However, the person must visually scan the word list while typing and be able to select the appropriate word. On-screen keyboards also maintain the person's vision on the display. If the person must have visual attention to the keyboard when typing and has physical deficits, an on-screen keyboard is good text entry software to try. Trialing built-in software options that guide keyboard access is less complex than physical hardware or add-on keyboard software and should be explored prior to progressing to more complex equipment.

Voice recognition (also called speech recognition or voice-to-text) software enables access to text entry when people are performing other tasks, or when people need to make a quick note. Some device voice recognition software programs are more like systems. They may also manage reminders, set alarms, and make phone calls. Most all devices have a type of voice recognition software built-in to the operating system; however, they vary widely. Components of voice recognition include dictation and transcription (process of translating the person's speech into text, completed by the software program used; may or may not need internet access, depending on the voice recognition program). The person dictates, or speaks, into a microphone. The software transcribes the entry, attempting to translate the person's speech into text accurately. Built-in voice recognition software is perceived as simple. However, a complete activity analysis should be conducted on the person, including the physical and cognitive strengths and deficit areas, goals, and the voice recognition software. Each platform's voice recognition software requires knowledge of unique commands to work at the highest potential, and therapists should research the capabilities of the software on the platform prior to recommending the equipment. Additional steps, such as pressing a button to activate and terminate dictation, may impede the ability of the person to use the software effectively. Additionally, built-in voice recognition software may not work without access to the Internet. If the person has a data-capped Internet service, inconsistent access to Internet, or a public hook-up, built-in voice recognition may not be the best access method for consistent text entry.

Built-in software will work most effectively within the operating system software and should be specifically tested in add-on software and on web pages. The manufacturers of add-on software and web designers may, or may not, have built-in compatibility with accessibility options.

More Complex Trials for Text Entry

A wide variety of commercial keyboards exist, and the inventory changes daily. If specific physical or sensory characteristics of a commercial keyboard appear as though it may improve function, through the in-depth analysis of the person and the hardware, the new keyboard should be trialed. The addition of typing splints (such as the Wanchik Slip-on Typing Aid from Patterson Medical) may be trialed on keyboards for text entry also, although the need to put the splint on and store it should also be considered.

Although changing the keyboard hardware may improve direct access, hardware may be difficult to generalize from one computer system to another. Hardware also requires transportation and setup for effective use. Common disability-specific keyboards include:

- ***Large key keyboards:*** Keyboard with large keys, may accommodate for vision deficits or ataxic movements because of tone. However, the large size limits the stabilization of the palm or forearm, which often improves accuracy of movement. An example is BigKeys LX from BigKeys.
- ***Keyboard with Keyguard:*** Keyguards are made from solid material that lies on top of a keyboard, with a hole for each key, which allows the person to stabilize his or her hand on top of the keyguard and facilitates digit isolation to press the desired key. Keyguards exist for standard and large keyboards, and on-screen tablet keyboards. Keyguards for on-screen keyboards should be recommended cautiously because the orientation of the display (and sometimes the software or app) changes the keyboard location and size.

  An example is the Keyboard with Keyguard/USB, available from *Infogrip*.

  If built-in options and hardware do not work, add-on software may improve text entry.

Add-on software may be local (installed on the person's own computer only) or networked (accessible through any computer on a network, most often in a vocational environment). Add-on software may also need permission from an information technology (IT) department to install and may or may not work with proprietary software (such as that for accounting, or data entry). Add-on software is available to assist with text entry and pretext entry skills, such as reading, spelling, and text composition. Common add-on software that specifically addresses text entry includes simple on-screen keyboards to more complex options such as voice recognition software. In the past 5 years, add-on onscreen keyboards that support text entry using various access methods have faded out as built-in on-screen keyboards have improved. Currently, most add-on on-screen keyboards are a combination of text entry, navigation, and selection software. E Z Keys (*Words+*) is an example of a software system that provides control of text entry, navigation, and selection for access methods including single and two-switch scanning and eye gaze. The PCEye Mini *TobiiDynavox* software package includes an on-screen keyboard as well.

The Jouse 3 (*Compusult Solutions for AT*) takes another approach. Although the Jouse 3 may be used with an on-screen keyboard, the hardware has built-in Morse code. Morse code, an indirect access method, matches each letter of the alphabet with a combination of dots and dashes. The code for each letter itself takes time to learn, but enables text entry of the full alphabet using one or two switches (in this case, the Jouse 3 acts as the switch). Other hardware and software is available to use Morse code as a text entry method as well. Although it is rarely used, it can be quite efficient for people with significant physical limitations.

Add-on voice recognition software also exists, most notably the commercial products within the Dragon series (*Nuance Communications, Inc.*). Voice recognition software does two things: enables text entry by voice and assists with spelling. Dragon will not spell a word wrong, but may transcribe the wrong word. This has produced some amusing (although often not professional) entries that either will need outside proofreading assist before publication, or a tolerant audience. Add-on voice recognition has evolved into a powerful product. Whereas the early editions, like Dragon Dictate, required stilted and supremely clear speech on a Windows-only platform, the newer products span various platforms and thrive on natural speech patterns. The Dragon products on laptops and computers do not require Internet access to work. However, the person's voice profile is local to one machine. This means that any custom words, commands, or training that the person has done will remain on the computer that he or she trained them on.

If voice recognition is not appropriate, other add-on software programs exist that assist with spelling, grammar, and proofreading. WordQ (*ST4 Learning*) provides options for spelling with a word list that provides word prediction and word completion options. These options may be read aloud and may also be read in context of their definition to aid comprehension and word choice. The software also facilitates proofreading using options that speak aloud each letter, word, or sentence as typed. Finally, the software may act as a text-to-speech software and will read aloud highlighted words anywhere on the computer. WordQ is easy to use because it floats above other software programs and is customizable. *Grammarly* (available from company by the same name) is another software program that assists with syntax in writing. It can be configured for use online or off-line. As with any software though, it is necessary to customize these programs to the person's needs to reduce risk of equipment abandonment.

There are other robust programs that aid with reading digital content, called text-to-speech programs. Text-to-speech programs range greatly from simple (such as Google Chrome extension SpeakIt! and text-to-speech shortcuts built into MacOS and Adobe Reader), to moderate (Read & Write Gold, *TextHelp*), to complex (WYNN Wizard from *Access Ingenuity* and *Kurzweil Education*). These software programs should not be confused with screen readers (such as JAWS from *Freedom Scientific*), which read aloud the content on a computer screen to aid navigation for people with visual impairments. Text-to-speech readers may be used to provide a multisensory reading environment to aid reading fluency, comprehension, and attention to task, or to accommodate for physical deficits and the inability to manage a physical book. When choosing text-to-speech software, it is important to first look at the file format of the content. File formats dictate the way that digital information is stored and displayed, with common formats being .doc (Microsoft Office Word document), .pdf (Portable Document Format, which preserves the document's format), and .jpg (images). Check to ensure that the text-to-speech software can read aloud the content in that file format. Components to consider in text-to-speech software include the quality and customizability of the voices, the ability to highlight and extract text, text masking properties, and bookmarking (the ability to return to specific place in the text). The person's needs should be considered as well. Consider if the person is using the software for leisurely reading or for vocational purposes.

Electronic Aids to Daily Living

Electronic aids to daily living (EADLs) enable a person with physical, cognitive, or psychosocial deficits to control electronics in his or her physical environment, including appliances, home theater systems, lights, doors, and more. EADLs encompass a wide category of commercial- and disability-specific products, with the commercial products advancing in capability and accessibility over the past few years. EADLs are exciting and captivating, and they appear deceptively simply. However, advancing technology has contributed to this being an increasingly complex category that now extends to smarthome technology, smart televisions, DVD players and smart DVD players, home theater systems, and smarthome theater systems, as well as smart speakers, smart hubs, and more. The addition of wireless features into today's technology requires that occupational therapists must examine each person's own technology carefully and conduct in-depth research before cautiously recommending additional technology for accessibility. Although no-tech options exist that support the performance of occupations in the person's own environment, this section is focused on the occupations that involve technology. Several research studies have focused on people's perceptions and subjective meanings of how EADL have affected people's lives with limited mobility.[16,17]

Evaluating for EADL Equipment

The basic technology and routines of the person are essential to evaluate when conducting the occupational profile.

1. Identify the person's main occupation-based goals and priorities.
2. Document routines for the occupation-based goals. Include the frequency of engagement, the process used, and the specific equipment. For example, if a person mentions watching television. Ask if the person likes to watch shows or movies and ask if he or she uses a television, Netflix, Amazon Prime, or another method. If the person uses a television, ask about cable or satellite services and ask if he or she uses a digital video recorder (DVR). Ask about smartspeakers such as Amazon Alexa, and smarthubs such as the Samsung SmartThings Smart home Hub. When exploring the person's equipment, take note of the brand and product name, whether or not it has smart features, why and when the person uses it (e.g., at night to watch evening shows, during the day watching Netflix), and how the person accesses it (e.g., pushes buttons on an IR remote control).

Performance analysis for EADLs begins with an assessment of the person's available body functions, including range of motion, muscle strength, coordination, sensation, vision, and cognition. The person's physical, cognitive, and psychosocial strengths and weaknesses should be considered alongside the previously discussed access methods, with potential access methods noted. During observation of occupational performance, the occupational therapist should observe the person using his or her current equipment.

A few important concepts are necessary to understand when describing EADLs (see Fig. 26-9). First, appliances and electronics may use discrete or continuous **control methods**:

- *Discrete control method:* Executes two actions, for example, power on and off an appliance or open and close blinds; or selects one target, such as a channel for the television or a prestored radio station
- *Continuous control method:* Allows for increasing flexibility in the outcome. This is necessary for adjusting volume on a television or radio or when raising and lowering the head of a bed.

Transmission methods are also important. Transmission methods are the ways that an EADL device communicates with a target (in this example, the television). There are four main transmission methods:

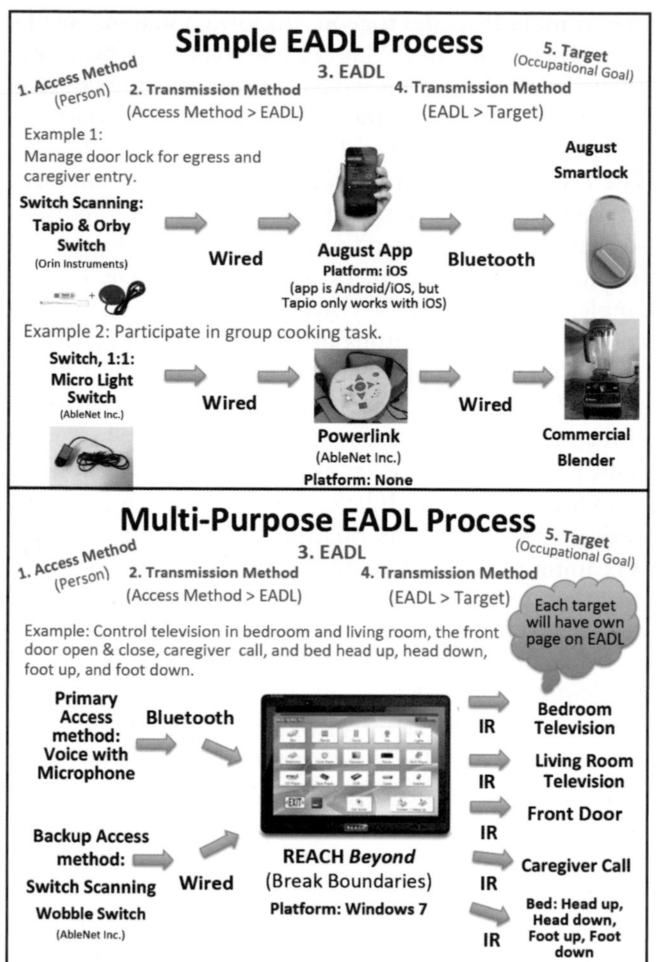

Figure 26-9. Simple and Complex EADL including the access method and transmission method to the device; transmission method from device to target for both. EADL, electronic aids to daily living.

- *Direct connection:* A wired connection exists between the EADL device and the target. Direct connections may increase the consistency of the equipment working, but they require that the person to remain in a limited area while the device is in use (e.g., landline phone, a bed control, some external speakers).[18]
- *House wiring:* Enables signals to be carried from one room to another within the wiring built into houses. Modules that plug into the wall receive information from a remote control and activate or deactivate simple appliances such as radios, fans, or lamps. An example is an X10 device, seen in many older devices.
- *Infrared (IR):* Uses invisible light to transmit unique codes to the target. IR requires an open "line of sight" between the remote control and the target in order for the target to receive the light, which limits IR to a single room. IR allows for discrete or continuous control through unique IR commands that exist for each brand, product, and action. Most televisions controlled by a remote control use an IR transmission.
- *Radio frequency (RF):* Uses RF waves to communicate with the target object (e.g., most garage doors). The receiver for the garage door is inside of the garage, out of the "line of sight." However, when activated, the RF waves pass through the closed garage door to activate the opener, which opens the door. RF has expanded with advancing technology and now contains subcategories as follows:
  - **Bluetooth** uses low-power radio waves to connect items within close proximity, often a maximum of 30 feet, or shorter depending on building infrastructure and interference. EADL devices may use Bluetooth, but Bluetooth can be a less reliable transmission method than wireless. However, devices such as smart door locks and light bulbs may use Bluetooth.
  - **Wi-Fi** uses the existing wireless Internet network to connect objects. Apps on smartphones that control a smart television, cable, or satellite box often use Wi-Fi.
  - **Wireless** is similar to Wi-Fi but uses its own (not the existing) wireless network. Examples are Z-Wave, ZigBee, and Thread.

Both IR and RF are the most common transmission methods. It is important to research prior to recommending an accessory or device that uses IR whether or not the device has the necessary codes built-in that will allow it to transmit the necessary actions to the target. If not, the device needs to be capable of "learning" the codes. This can be complicated and referencing the instruction manual or calling the manufacturer are sometimes needed. Wi-Fi and wireless transmission methods are quickly rising in popularity. They work with a variety of equipment and provide great opportunities for improved independence and participation. However, be cautious of the quality of network when recommending equipment. Private Internet with no data cap is ideal, but not often the case (especially in rural areas). The speed of the Internet service makes a difference to products working efficiently and whether or not the service can sustain numerous products working simultaneously. Public Wi-Fi networks are not considered stable or secure, and devices on these networks may be kicked off often, requiring reconnection to work. In an area with data caps or public Internet access, clinicians should consider products that do not use wireless transmission methods (non-Smart devices).

Assessing for EADLs requires consideration of the person's environment as well. Responsible occupational therapists should observe the physical layout, family/caregiver support, and other assistive devices when evaluating for EADL access and consider safety when providing equipment recommendations.

Platforms for EADLs

Remember that a platform is an operating system. Examples of platforms commonly used for EADL devices include tablet operating systems such as iOS (Apple) and Android, and computer operating systems such as Windows (Microsoft) and Macintosh (Apple). Very simple EADL devices that control only one or two items, such as the Powerlink 4 (*AbleNet Inc.*) and LinkSwitch (*Adaptivation*), do not have platforms. They act as the interface between the wired device and the switch interface. Simple EADLs may use operating systems though, such as the Phillips Hue products and Belkin WeMo products. The Phillips Hue iOS or Android app, when installed on the appropriate model phone, can act as an interface between the human and the target.

EADL platforms are often commercial, but the EADL software and accompanying accessories may be produced commercially for the entire population or specifically for people with disabilities. If the product was produced commercially, pay attention to the brand names. For example, Samsung products tend to work best with Google platforms and may not be available or compatible with Apple accessories. For example, it is a long process for an Amazon Prime movie app to become available on Microsoft Xbox. Typically, people have brand preferences that don't significantly impact recommended equipment, but brand compatibility should be considered during the selection process.

Disability-specific products tend to be more stable because they are generally not as affected by updates. This allows the person to use the device consistently to control his or her environment (once it is set up and the person is trained), with less interruptions or changes from software updates. If interruptions do occur, the product manufacturers often understand the context of disability better than a commercial manufacturer and may provide better customer support. Disability-specific products often emphasize accessibility and accommodate a variety of access methods; and the display interfaces are often simpler or can be adjusted for the user. However, this flexibility and customizability comes at a price. The research and development that contributes to a disability-specific device is significant, and when combined with the potential smaller population, increases the price tag of the device and accessories. Technology compatible with disability-specific devices may also fall behind the commercial products because the manufacturers often respond to the commercial market. Therefore, if a person has a new smart television and the latest home theater system, there may be difficulty controlling it through a disability-specific EADL device. Researches, through instruction manuals and manufacturer support, are available resources to help guide product choice.

Customizing EADL Devices

People with disabilities often need devices customized to improve efficiency with accessing electronics. Learning IR codes, and the ability of the EADL device to put one or more IR codes together to form a **macro**, may be an important feature. Making macros can improve the efficiency of the person navigating to specific television channels, by enabling the device to emit IR codes for two- or three-digit channel numbers with one selection. The EADL device display is also important to consider. Icons supporting text and/or symbols may be important so that the device doesn't appear too young or too old for the user. Icon placement should be intuitive. For example, an icon for "TV Power" in the upper left-hand corner, and arrow buttons in a compass format, makes sense to many people. The most frequently used icons should be placed in an area that the person is able to access easily. If the person uses direct access with his or her right pointer finger, the icons may be best placed in the right lower quadrant. If he or she using switch scanning, perhaps the upper left quadrant, where the scanning box initiates the scan pattern. Intuitive icon placement results in greater efficiency and endurance with EADL device use.

Single-purpose EADLs

EADL devices that control one object, such as a bed, door, fan, lights, blinds, or remote door lock, are considered single-purpose EADLs. Many single-purpose EADLs control the power of the target. A simple test can be used to determine whether the target (e.g., plug-in fan or light, or even radio) can be used for power control. Plug the target into a powered electrical outlet and turn it on into the desired configuration (e.g., specific radio station). Keeping the target on, unplug the target, and then plug it back in. If the target, once plugged back in, returns automatically to the desired configuration, it will work with a simple EADL device. However, if it remains off (as some digital devices do), it will not.

Commercial products for EADLs are often wireless in nature and require a hardware component and software for control. For example, the Wemo Insight Smart Plug (*Belkin*) can be used to control a plug-in fan or desk lamp. The fan or desk lamp plugs into the Smart Plug, which plugs into the wall. The person must have a smartphone or tablet, download the WeMo app, and pair the Smart Plug, which enables control of the light or fan through the phone display. The phone could be controlled with a variety of access methods, making the phone the person's EADL device. However, as it is not a native Apple or Android app, the access method should be trialed directly with the app to make sure it will work. Other commercial products exist that may work with various access methods to provide occupational competence. For example, bed control may be accomplished through with a smart bed (see the Sleep Number products). Door management requires consideration of the door itself and the lock, both onsite and remote. Door openers are often disability specific (such as *Open Sesame*) and are managed through wired transmission (using a wall plate) or RF (using a door opener). However, the locking mechanism needs to unlock or lock for safety and security. A smart lock (such as the August Smart Lock Pro from *August Home Secure Access*) may be useful, which enables lock control through an app. Additionally, onsite or remote surveillance may be accomplished through the Ring or other similar commercially available products. Mixing and matching single-purpose products may be necessary for occupational performance.

Disability-specific options for single-purpose EADLs are often wired or RF, such as in the door management example in the previous paragraph. The Powerlink 4 (*AbleNet*) or LinkSwitch (*Adaptivation*) are two examples of devices that work with wired targets, such as plug-in lamps and appliances, to offer momentary, timed, or latched control, through switch access (see Fig. 26-10). Momentary and timed switch activations only require one-switch activation for an action to occur, but vary in the length of time that they activate the target. A **momentary switch activation** activates the target for the length of time that the witch is pressed and

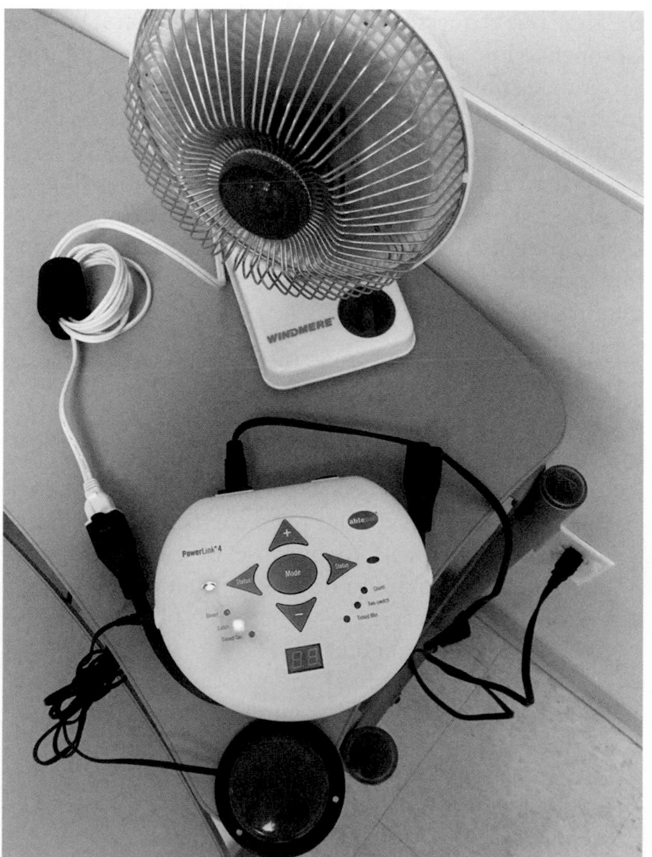

Figure 26-10. Powerlink 4 and Jelly Bean switch (AbleNet Inc.) setup with commercial fan.

is most common in a 1:1 format. A **timed switch activation** will maintain the connection for a specified (often adjustable) amount of time, then turn off automatically. The **latched switch activation** requires two-switch presses, one to start the target activation and another to stop the action.

This section provided examples of only a few single-purpose EADLs. This area changes quickly with advancing technology, so specific examples provided are few. When matching people with single-purpose EADLs, research is required. See the content in Considerations with Recommending Equipment for more information on choosing quality products.

Multi-purpose EADLs

Multi-purpose EADL devices enable access to more than one target and often communicate in more than one transmission method. Commercial products that work as multi-purpose EADLs are often home automation in nature. For example, SmartHome accessories can manage plug-in appliances such as lights and fans, thermostat, and peripherals such as home theater systems and surveillance, all of which can be managed by their software or an app, after initial setup. Addition of other technology, such as the Amazon Echo Dot, enables voice control of these products. Similarly, the Wemo (*Belkin*) products and *August Smart Lock Pro* can be managed through the HomeKit (Apple) app. In this situation, the HomeKit app on an iOS device serves as the person's EADL. Commercial EADLs are created with the goal of home automation for the user, so compatibility with access methods must be verified.

Disability-specific multi-purpose EADLs range from moderately complex to significantly complex. Midlevel disability-specific devices have fewer customizable features (they may not support changes to the display, such as names or placement of the icons), control less products, but still enable access through multiple features and are less costly ($299 through around $5,000) than significantly complex disability-specific EADLs. Examples of moderately complex EADLs include the EyeR (*TobiiDynavox*), Relax, Primo!, and HouseMate for iOS (each from *AbleNet*), and PocketMate (Saje Technology). All of the devices come on their own proprietary platform, except the EyeR (Fig. 26-11) and HouseMate. The EyeR comes with software and hardware (USB IR emitter) that turn a tablet or computer into an IR EADL, and the HouseMate turns an iOS device into an IR remote control.

Significantly complex disability-specific EADLs may be stand-alone or built into an Augmentative Communication device. EADLs may cost from $7,000 through $15,000, depending on the device and access method used (eye gaze augmentative communication systems are expensive). These powerful stand-alone EADLs are often built on a computer platform. For example, the REACH (available through *AbleNet, Break* Boundaries) as well as the autonoME (*Accessibility Services, Inc.*) utilize Windows tablets. Various accessories can be purchased to enable independence with environmental control, including light switches (that work using an X-10 transmission method), door openers, and blinds. These accessories should be customized to meet the person's goals. Complex disability-specific EADL device displays should be configured for each individual person.

Augmentative Communication devices may have built-in EADL capabilities as well. Devices including the I-12+ and I-15+ (*TobiiDynavox*) (see Fig. 26-11), Accent devices (*Prentke Romich*), and Eyegaze Edge (*LC Technologies, Inc.*) have EADL features built-in to the software program, but may require accessories or upgrades to utilize the IR capabilities.

Each complex EADL should be configured for the person in two main ways. First, the aesthetics of icon and page, including the symbols and text on each icon and background of the software set, can be changed to reflect the person's wants and needs. For example, if the person has figure ground issues, a plain background can be set, using contrasting colors to the icons. If the person often watches NBC, an icon can be added or changed to state "NBC" and even a picture of the NBC symbol. Intentional software configuration is important. For example, creating or programming at least two TV pages is helpful. The first for TV controls (such as power, guide, menu, info, arrow, and ok/select buttons), and the second with icons programmed with macros that give the person quick access to often watched TV channels. Thinking further, it is often helpful to have volume up/down and/or mute on both pages, giving quick access to the volume in case someone comes into the room to talk to the person, or the phone rings. These purposeful design principles lead to the second modification that each icon must be programmed with meaningful actions. Each icon holds a set of hidden actions. These actions may be navigation actions, such as "go back to previous page" or "go back to home page" or may be IR commands such as "Power on" or "Volume up." Programing the numbers into the IR database in the device allows for multiple numbers to be programmed on one icon, to be sent out as a macro. These IR commands may be built-in the device or trained if the device accepts IR learning (which most significantly complex EADL devices will). Considering how the person controls the environment, his or her familiarity with technology, and routines when watching movies and shows should guide the way that the device is set up.

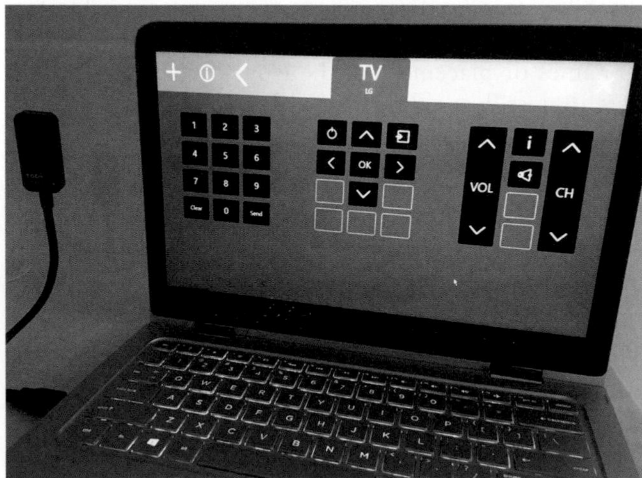

Figure 26-11. EyeR (TobiiDynavox) USB dongle with infrared emitter pair with the Virtual Remote computer software to create a computer-based electronic aids to daily living (EADL).

Funding for EADL

Health care insurance is not usually an option for AT devices that are not considered a medical necessity. In some situations, EADL may be funded by a health care insurance if the system is built into the AAC system at the time it is requested. In certain circumstances, Worker Compensation insurance, Vocational Rehabilitation programs, the Veterans Administration, or no-fault insurance may be able to fund some AT devices if the equipment is specifically needed for employment.

When an occupational therapist is requesting an employer, family, organization, or foundation to consider funding AT, some or all of the following information may be helpful (depending on to whom you are making the request):

- *Client information:* Name, birthdate, physician name, date of evaluation, and diagnosis
- *Purpose of evaluation:* Client's goals
- *Background information:* Including prior medical history, therapy experience, experience with AT, description of the person's routines and environments, current technology pertinent to purpose of evaluation (e.g., computer, electronics in home environment)
- *Performance analysis:* The person's physical, cognitive, and perceptual abilities
- *AT trials:* Description of the person's various equipment trials (most funding sources require a minimum of three)
- *Recommendations:* Numerical list of specific recommended equipment, including a short statement describing the purpose of the equipment.

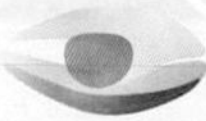

CASE STUDY

Patient Information

James is a 57-year-old, right-handed male. He presents with a diagnosis of brainstem stroke, locked-in syndrome, with an onset 8 weeks ago. Prior medical history included hypertension; prior surgical history included G-tube placement and tracheostomy. Prior to the stroke, James worked as an architect and owned his own company. He was very active and enjoyed playing golf and cards with his friends.

Directly after the cerebrovascular accident (CVA), James was admitted to intensive care unit (ICU). After medical stabilization, James was transferred to inpatient rehabilitation and then was discharged to home 5 weeks later. Inpatient rehabilitation focused on training of his wife and daughter for care and attempting to facilitate volitional movement.

During the evaluation, James demonstrated the ability to answer yes/no questions with eye blink. Owing to significant physical and psychosocial limitations that were expected to persist over time, AT, specifically a communication device, was trialed with both eye gaze and switch scanning access methods. James demonstrated switch scanning with row-column intact with Micro Light switch with left thumb when his hand was in a fisted position, ulnar side lying on the bed; but he required moderate assistance to maintain thumb position against gravity. James trialed eye gaze for increased independence and efficiency with communication; however, the inpatient therapist documented inaccurate selections 8/10 trials and difficulty calibrating the James' eyes to the eye gaze unit. At discharge, James' only active movement was right thumb adduction in a gravity eliminated plane. He went home with a loaner Micro Light switch and beeper device, a switch-enabled device that sounded upon activation.

Assessment Process and Results

James was transferred home where he lived with his wife and grown daughter who are his primary caregivers. Home health occupational therapy assessment included an occupational profile, which focused on James' interests, recovery, adaptive equipment, and profile of existing technology within the home. Precautions included allergy to penicillin and to monitor pulse oxygen (maintain above 92%).

Upon arrival, James is in a front room of the home, laying in a hospital bed with the head of bed raised at about 30°. The occupational therapist notes a tilt-in-space manual wheelchair in the hallway. There is a bathroom off to the left of the room, and an LG television setup across from James. There is a Comcast cable box below the television. James' daughter verifies that they have Comcast cable and wireless Internet throughout the home. James mainly watches cable television shows and does not record shows on the DVR. Currently, James and his daughter and wife are communicating using the Micro Light switch and the beeper device, but they report that they are having trouble setting the switch up for independent use; they often resort to yes/no questions using one blink for "no" and two for "yes." However, James' cannot reach his wife and daughter with urgent needs if they leave the room, and this makes them uneasy. James' wife and daughter are great advocates for him to engage in any activities, and they note that he enjoys watching sports, especially golf and poker on television.

The performance analysis assessed cognition and physical motor skills. James was able to answer yes/no questions accurately about demographic and historical information. He followed commands for the visual motor screen, where the occupational therapist noted his left eye tracking slower than his right eye in the horizontal plane. Active range of motion of bilateral upper extremities demonstrated right thumb adduction 0° to 20° with forearm pronated and resting on the bed; no other active movement was noted other than eye blinks. Passive range of motion of bilateral upper extremities was intact in all joints and planes, and sensation was intact for light touch except on his left upper extremity below elbow in the ulnar nerve innervation. James was dependent for transfers using a Hoyer lift and dependent for all basic activities of daily living. James' receives all nutrition through G-tube. James actively engaged visually with the therapist for 15 minutes of the session before falling asleep. The family verified that this was typical for James' activity tolerance at this time.

Occupational Therapy Problem List

- James is unable to spontaneously call caregivers for help because of an inability to speak.
- James is unable to participate with basic ADLs because of dependent functional mobility and lack of active upper extremity control.
- James is unable to control the television and cable by standard remote control because of only active movement in right thumb 0° to 20°.
- James attends to task for 15 minutes prior to sleeping because of difficulty regulating level of arousal.

Occupational Therapy Goal List

- James will activate Micro Light switch modified independence × 5 to call caregiver in other room in one treatment session in 2 weeks.
- James will create and speak one five-word phrase modified independence with a maximum of one inaccurate activation per word on speech-generating device utilizing appropriate access method in 5 minutes in 4 weeks.
- James will control television, demonstrating power on, review the guide, and change the channel × 2 modified independence in 4 weeks.
- James will attend to therapy task for 30 minutes without falling asleep in 4 weeks.

Intervention

James was treated in occupational therapy 1 to 2 times a week. James was seen first with the occupational therapist to explore

(continued)

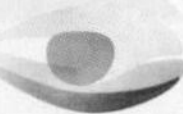

CASE STUDY *(continued)*

access methods. The occupational therapist found that resting James' hand on a towel in a fisted position, palm down, allowed James to abduct and adduct his thumb independently in a gravity eliminated position. James was then able to activate the Micro Light independently, when placing the Micro Light switch in between his pointer finger and thumb. Once James demonstrated competence with this task in the session, his family was trained in the setup and use of the switch outside occupational therapy for caregiver call. They reported that this setup worked well and provided them with a level of peace, knowing that James could activate the switch to beep if he needed them.

Once James was proficient with the single switch, the occupational therapist and speech therapist met to trial speech-generating devices. The Tobii I12 (TobiiDynavox) and Eyegaze Edge (LC Technologies) were trialed with James. Eyegaze continued to be difficult to configure with James' incongruent eye movement, but James' was able to follow directions for switch scanning on the Tobii I12. First, the occupational therapist trialed the Scanning Wizard with James' to introduce him to row-column scanning and to identify optimal switch settings to initially program into the Tobii I12. Second, the occupational therapist duplicated the switch settings, lowering the time slightly to accommodate for James' learning the software, and trialed the Tobii I12 with single switch scanning, with the Micro Light placed at James' right thumb. James demonstrated typing three words at three to four letters each, with five inaccurate selections on his first trial. Over the next 2 weeks, James improved to typing 10-word novel phrases using word prediction and completion with one to two inaccurate selections overall in 3 to 4 minutes. The Tobii I12 was identified, in collaboration with James, his wife and daughter, and the speech therapist, to be the optimal device for his communication needs. The Daessy Rolling Mount was recommended as well, to enable secure and consistent positioning of the Tobii I12 when James was in bed or up in his wheelchair.

The television and cable IR commands were programmed into the EADL pages. Custom pages were made to improve access. First, the power, volume up and down, mute, guide, up, down, right, left, ok, and exit were programmed. Second, 10 of James' most frequently watched stations were programmed. James demonstrated accessing the commands appropriately to watch television with only two inaccurate selections upon initial trial, progressing to zero inaccurate selections.

Given James' proficiency with the Micro Light switch and James' daughter and wife's advocacy for his participation, the occupational therapist inquired about James' recommended wheelchair. A tilt-in-space wheelchair was in process for James'; however, if the family and James agreed, the occupational therapist felt that James might be able to operate a power wheelchair with single switch scanning. James and the family agreed to trial a power wheelchair.

Over time, James progressed significantly. James trialed power wheelchairs and was able to drive through single switch scanning. The wheelchair was recommended with single switch scanning, but also a joystick, to accommodate for progression. When received, James demonstrated an ability to drive the wheelchair using the joystick with a t-handle.

James' increased hand movement related to other functional tasks as well. James' returned to AT to trial computer access 1 year later. James' trialed wheelchair access using his joystick to control the mouse pointer, but preferred to use the computer from bed level. James trialed the laptop touchpad, touchscreen (as his right upper extremity gross and fine motor had improved) with right powered arm support, and a trackball mouse. When lying in bed, James' preferred method for navigation and selection was the trackball mouse using preprogrammed mouse and page up and down clicks with right his hand suspended over the mouse (his wrist propped on a towel).

Vendors of Assistive Technology

Vendor	Website
Accessibility Services, Inc.	https://asi-autonome.com/
Adaptivation	https://www.adaptivation.com/
Abilitations	https://store.schoolspecialty.com/OA_HTML/xxssi_ibeCategoryPage.jsp?docName=V700839&minisite=10206
AbleNet, Inc.	https://www.AbleNetinc.com/
Access Ingenuity	https://www.accessingenuity.com/
Adaptive Switch Laboratories, Inc.	http://www.asl-inc.com/
August Home Secure Access	https://august.com/products/august-smart-lock-wifi/
Belkin	www.belkin.com
BigKeys Company	http://www.bigkeys.com/
Compusult Solutions for Assistive Technology	http://www.compusult.net/assistive-technology-solutions
EnableMart	http://www.enablemart.com/
Ergoguys	http://www.ergoguys.com/quadjoy-mouse.html
Freedom Scientific	http://www.freedomscientific.com/
Grammarly	www.grammarly.com
Greystone Digital	http://www.bigkeys.com/
Infogrip	www.infogrip.com
Kensington Technology Group	http://www.kensington.com/
Koester Performance Research	http://www.kpronline.com/
Kurzweil Education	https://www.kurzweiledu.com/default.html
LC Technologies, Inc.	http://www.eyegaze.com/
Nuance Communications, Inc.	www.nuance.com/dragon.html
Open Sesame Door Systems Inc.	www.opensesamedoor.com
Quadstick	http://www.quadstick.com/
Patterson Medical	https://www.healthproductsforyou.com/m-patterson-medical.html

(continued)

Vendors of Assistive Technology (*continued*)

Vendor	Website
Prentke Romich	https://www.prentrom.com/
Saje Technology	http://www.saje-tech.com/
School Health	https://www.schoolhealth.com/special-education
TextHelp	https://www.texthelp.com/en-us/
TobiiDynavox	www.tobiidynavox.com/en-us/
Traxys	www.traxsys.com/AssistiveTechnology/Joysticks/RollerIIJoystick/tabid/1409/Default.aspx
ST4 Learning	https://www.quillsoft.ca
Words+	http://words-plus.com/

Best Evidence for Assistive Technology Used in Occupational Therapy

Intervention	Description	Participants	Dosage	Research Design and Evidence Level	Benefit	Statistical Significance and Effect Size
Systematic review and meta-analysis of randomized controlled trial (RCT) and quasi-randomized clinical trials of interactive gaming and/or interactive engagement with hardware or software[13]	Data pooled from 11 studies; 7 outcomes of interest	466 participants with diagnosis (dx) of multiple sclerosis (MS) (65.8% female)	Most 1:1 with physical therapy (PT); two studies were home-based; one telerehabiliation. Frequency: 1–5×/week. intensity: 20–60 minutes duration: 3–12 weeks; 10–48 sessions.	Systematic review and meta-analysis; Level I evidence; quality assessment with PEDro scale; Preferred Reporting Items for Systematic Reviews and Meta-Analyses (PRISMA) guidelines	VR training is at least as effective as convention training and more effective than no intervention for balance and gait for people with MS.	Postural control improvement when compared to no intervention: standardized mean difference (SMD) = −0.64; 95% confidence interval (CI) = −1.05 to 0.24; $p = 0.002$. No significant overall effect compared with conventional training: SMD = −0.04; 95% CI = −0.70, 0.62; $p = 0.90$.
Systematic review of RCT using VR for people with stroke dx[19]	All 54 trials/studies had intervention protocol and follow-up, focus on upper limbs and or lower limbs and/or balance.	1,811 participants; 14 trials body structure, 20 body functions, 17 activity, 8 participation; personal and one environmental factor	Upper extremity (UE) (arm, hand) ranged from 3 to 7 times/week for 4–6 weeks, mean dose of 17.6 hours. For self-care, an average intervention time of 13 hours. Household tasks ranged from 10 to 15 hours.	Systematic review of RCT with PRISMA; Level I evidence	Positive results were seen for VR for UE (arm, hand) with immersive, semi-immersive, and nonimmersive VR in people with subacute and chronic stroke. For self-care, 5 of the 12 trials found positive effects, whereas 7 found no difference between control and experimental groups.	Statistical results not reported in article.

(continued)

Best Evidence for Assistive Technology Used in Occupational Therapy *(continued)*

Intervention	Description	Participants	Dosage	Research Design and Evidence Level	Benefit	Statistical Significance and Effect Size
Meta-analysis of 33 RCT studies comparing VR rehabilitation for upper limb function poststroke with conventional therapy (CT)[12]	VR (user–computer interface) (real-time simulation with patient interaction) and CT addressing upper limb motor, cognitive or ADL; CT = PT or occupational therapy (OT)	971 total participants, 492 VR (mean [M] = 14.9, standard deviation [SD] = 10.9/study); 479 participants received CT; average age 60; time poststroke varied 1.9–427.8 weeks	Mean doses in minutes; intensity: overall: 685 daily: 42 minutes weekly: 153.9 frequency/week 3 sessions (range = 1–5). Median duration: 18 sessions (range 4–36 sessions)	Systematic review and meta-analysis using the PRISMA	Benefits of VR over CT for immediate- and longer-term gains in motor function and cognitive and motor activities poststroke	Average effect size for VR interventions small to medium, but significant benefit for VR compared to CT. Upper limb: small-to-medium overall effects were seen for body structures/function and activity outcomes, whereas participation outcomes were insignificant.
Comparison of purposeful movements in the UE between video games and traditional therapy for people with stroke[20]	Individuals with chronic stroke wore wrist accelerometers to measure purposeful and nonpurposeful repetitions of weaker and stronger UE while playing video games with a partner or in traditional therapy (perform movement and functional tasks).	RCT: 29 participants with chronic stroke, mean age 59 years, 1–7 years poststroke. 15 in traditional therapy TTG, 14 played video games in group VGG	1–2 sessions with OT; 30 minutes videotaped sessions	RCT Level II evidence	Video games elicit more UE purposeful repetitions and higher acceleration of movement than traditional therapy.	Compared number of purposeful movement and activity counts between two groups; VGG: 271 and 37,970; TTG: 48 and 14,872 $z = -3.0, p = 0.001$ and $z = -1.9, p = 0.05$ Video games elicit more UE purposeful repetitions and higher acceleration of movement than TTG in people with stroke.
Survey questionnaire on perception of Environmental Control Units (ECUs)[16]	Veterans Affairs (VA) hospital; surveys distributed to current patients or recently discharge patients	150 VA patients with spinal cord injury/disorder (SCI/D); 70 inpatients; 80 discharged patients completed questionnaires for perceptions of ECU	One-time questionnaire for either inpatients or recently discharged patients	Survey research; Level VII evidence	ECUs well accepted	Descriptive stats: inpatient/discharged watching TV/movies (81%), using a call button (i.e., for nurse 85%)

Explored subjective meaning of ECU for people with high cervical SCI[17]	In-depth interviews regarding meaning of using an ECU	Five participants with high cervical SCI, ranged in age from 22 to 55 years old; all at least 3 years following rehab discharge were provided ECU devices and training.	Participants provided with ECS starter pack. ECS was fitted, customized, and left for trial of unspecified period of time. 41–56-minute in-depth interviews at conclusion of trial	Qualitative: Interpretive Phenomenological Analysis (IPA) to explore personal meaning of ECU according recommended IPA guidelines. Level VI evidence	Using an ECU helps a person reclaim a little of what he or she can do and helps him or her to feel enabled—supports value of widespread access to ECU.	Yardley's guidelines for ensuring quality and rigor followed for sensitivity to context, commitment and rigor, transparency, coherence, and impact and importance.
Systematic review of AT access interfaces used for text entry rates (TER) for common interfaces[15]	39 studies met criteria—7 interfaces included and TER reported in either WPM or could be converted to WMP.	295 individuals with physical impairments (majority SCI quadriplegia or cerebral palsy) control sites for interface included: hands, head, mouthstick, chin, tongue, neck, and eye.	All studies meeting criteria collected TER via WPM for a user on a type of interface	Systematic review of descriptive studies Level V evidence	Average TER for different interfaces can be used as a comparison with individual TER to help with decision-making process for best interface for person.	Averages for TER for each type of interface were based on at least four studies and 30 subjects.
Exploration of rates, barriers, and facilitators of electronic assistive technology (EAT) users[21]	Semi-structured interviews and published measures of support need, EAT satisfaction, and psychosocial impact	22 identified EAT users with acquired brain injury (ABI); 72.7% male, mean age 43.7. All were living in shared supported homes in Australia.	EAT users identified and recruited. Research data included semi-structured interviews, Care and Needs Scale (CANS), Psychosocial Impact of Assistive Devices Scale (PIADS), and Quebec User Evaluation of Satisfaction with Assistive Technology (QUEST).	Mixed-method design Level VI evidence	EAT can positively influence everyday function and participation for people with ABI if given a skilled prescription and ongoing support for use.	Descriptive stats used for QUEST and PIADS. Qualitative analysis for barriers to effective use of EAT

References

1. American Occupational Therapy Association. Assistive technology and occupational performance. *Am J Occup Ther.* 2016;70:7012410030p1–7012410030p9. doi:10.5014/ajot.2016.706S02.
2. Cook AM, Polgar JM. *Assistive Technologies: Principles and Practice.* 4th ed. St. Louis, MO: CV Mosby Co; 2015.
3. Baum CM, Christiansen CH. Person-environment-occupation-performance: an occupation-based framework for practice. In: Christiansen CH, Baum CM, Bass-Haugen J, eds. *Occupational Therapy: Performance, Participation, and Well-being.* 3rd ed. Thorofare, NJ: SLACK Incorporated; 2005.
4. World Health Organization. International classification of functioning, disability and health (ICF). 2001. http://www.who.int/classifications/icf/en/
5. Cook AM, Hussy SM. *Assistive Technologies Principles and Practice.* 2nd ed. St. Louis, MO: Mosby; 2002.
6. Anson D. Assistive technology. In: Pendleton HM, Schultz-Krohn W, eds. *Pedretti's Occupational Therapy: Practice Skills for Physical Dysfunction.* 7th ed. St. Louis, MO: Elsevier; 2012:427–449.
7. Scherer MJ. The matching person and technology model. In: Scherer MJ, eds. *Connecting to Learn: Educational and Assistive Technology for People with Disabilities.* Washington, DC: American Psychological Association; 2004:183–201.
8. American Occupational Therapy Association. Occupational therapy practice framework: domain and process [3rd ed.]. *AJOT.* 2017;68:S1–S48. doi:10.5014/ajot.2014.68.
9. RESNA. Professional specialty groups. https://www.resna.org/professional-development/volunteer-and-leadership-opportunities/special-interest-groups/professional. Accessed July 3, 2018.
10. Csikszentmihaly M. *Finding Flow: The Psychology of Engagement with Everyday Life.* New York, NY: Basic Books; 1997.
11. Rakoski DR, Ferguson RC. The virtual context of occupation: integrating everyday technology into everyday practice. *OT Practice.* 2013;18:CE.1–CE.8.
12. Aminov A, Rogers JM, Middleton S, Caeyenberghs K, Wilson PH. What do randomized controlled trials say about virtual rehabilitation in stroke? A systematic review and meta-analysis of upper-limb and cognitive outcomes. *J Neuroeng Rehabil.* 2018;15(29). doi:10.1186/s12984-018-0370-2.
13. Casuso-Holgado MJ, Martin-Valero R, Carazo AF, Medrano-Sánchez EM, Cortés-Vega MD, Montero-Bancalero FJ. Effectiveness of virtual reality training for balance and gait rehabilitation in people with multiple sclerosis: a systematic review and meta-analysis. *Clin Rehabil.* 2018;1-15. doi:10.1177/0269215518768084.
14. Proffitt R, Foreman M. Low-cost virtual reality and game-based technologies in rehabilitation. *Technol Spec Inter Sect Quart.* 2014;24(3):1–3.
15. Koester HH, Arathnat S. Text entry rate of access interfaces used by people with physical disabilities: a systematic review. *Assist Technol.* 2018;30:151–163. doi:10.1080/10400435.2017.1291544.
16. Etingen B, Martinez RN, Vallette MA, et al. Patient perceptions of environmental control units: experiences of Veterans with spinal cord injuries and disorders receiving inpatient VA healthcare. *Disabil Rehabil Assist Technol.* 2018;13:325–332. doi:10.1080/17483107.2017.1312574.
17. Verdonk M, Nolan M, Chard G. Taking back a little of what you have lost: the meaning of using an Environmental Control System (ECS) for people with high cervical spinal cord injury. *Disabil Rehabil Assist Technol.* 2018;13:785–790. doi:10.1080/17483107.2017.1378392.
18. Little R. Electronic aids for daily living. *Phys Med Rehabil Clin N Am.* 2010;21:33–42. doi:10.1016/j.pmr.2009.07.008.
19. dos Santos Palma GC, Freitas TB, Vonuzzi GMG, et al. Effects of virtual reality for stroke individuals based on the International Classification of Functioning and Health: a systemic review. *Top Stroke Rehabil.* 2017;24(4):269-278. doi:10.1080/10749357.2016.1250373.
20. Rand D, Givon N, Weingarden H, Nota A, Zeileg G. Eliciting upper extremity purposeful movements with traditional therapy for stroke rehabilitation. *Neurorehabil Neural Repair.* 2014;28(8):733-739. doi:10.1177/1545968314521008.
21. Jamwal R, Callaway L, Ackerl J, Farnworth L, Winkler D. Electronic assistive technology used by people with acquired brain injury in shared supported accommodation: implications for occupational therapy. *Br J Occup.* 2017;80(2):89–98. doi:10.1177/0308022616678634.

Chapter 27

Restoring Activities of Daily Living

Rochelle J. Mendonca, Susan Santalucia, Taliah Cook, and Colleen Maher

LEARNING OBJECTIVES

This chapter will allow the reader to:

1. Describe the components of activities of daily living (ADLs) and their relationship to the Occupational Therapy Practice Framework (OTFP-3).
2. Describe the procedures for client-centered ADL evaluations including occupational profiles and assessments to document client priorities and functional independence.
3. Describe how functional physical, visual-perceptual, and cognitive limitations can impact ADL performance.
4. Modify task performance techniques for clients with functional limitations to support ADL engagement.
5. Describe principles of altering the task environment to enable maximal participation in ADLs.
6. Evaluate the need for and recommend adaptive equipment to enable safe and independent ADL performance for clients with functional limitations.
7. Train clients with functional limitations in modified task performance techniques and adaptive equipment use to progress toward occupation-based goals and functional independence.

CHAPTER OUTLINE

TERMINOLOGY

Activities of daily living (ADLs): activities oriented toward taking care of one's body and include bathing and showering, toileting and toilet hygiene, dressing, swallowing and eating, functional mobility, personal device care, personal hygiene and grooming, and sexual activity. They are also referred to as personal activities of daily living (PADLs) or basic activities of daily living (BADLs).[1]

Adaptive equipment: devices, tools, or products that are used to assist individuals with disabilities to engage in occupations within their natural contexts and environments; also referred to as assistive technology, assistive devices, or adaptive devices.

Client-centered approach: an approach to service delivery that includes respect for and collaboration with clients (individuals, groups, agencies, governments, or corporations). Therapists involve clients in decision-making, advocate for and with clients to meet needs, and recognize clients' experience and knowledge.[2]

Durable medical equipment (DME): supplies that provide therapeutic benefit to clients experiencing difficulty or functional deficits resulting from medical conditions or illnesses. DME must be prescribed by physicians or health care providers authorized by state law. DME must be reusable and primarily used in the home.

Occupational profile: a component of the occupational therapy evaluation that provides information about clients' occupational histories and experiences, daily living patterns, interests, values, needs, reasons for seeking services, and concerns related to occupational performance and disruption.[1]

Occupations: activities that individuals, groups, or populations engage in that are meaningful and include activities of daily living, instrumental activities of daily living, rest and sleep, education, work, play, leisure, and social participation.[1]

Activities of Daily Living

Occupations are defined as activities that provide a sense of identity and meaning to individuals, groups, and populations.[1,3] The American Occupational Therapy Association's official practice document, the *Occupational Therapy Practice Framework*, Third Edition (OTPF-3), identifies eight areas of occupation, including **activities of daily living (ADLs)**, instrumental activities of daily living (IADLs), rest and sleep, education, work, play, leisure, and social participation.[1] Individuals who are satisfied with their life roles have the resources and capabilities needed to accomplish everyday tasks, whether they perform tasks themselves or seek assistance. Difficulties in occupational engagement lead to loss of functional independence and reduced quality of life.[4,5] Occupational therapists are skilled in evaluating, remediating, and restoring occupational performance limitations due to injury, disease, or disability.

ADLs are defined as activities needed to care for one's body[1]; they are also referred to as personal activities of daily living (PADLs) and basic activities of daily living (BADLs). ADLs include nine different categories: (1) bathing and showering, (2) toileting and toilet hygiene, (3) dressing, (4) swallowing and eating, (5) feeding, (6) functional mobility, (7) personal device care, (8) personal hygiene and grooming, and (9) sexual activity.[1] This chapter describes strategies and intervention techniques used by occupational therapists to restore ADL performance for individuals with impairments. Intervention strategies for eight ADLs are addressed: (1) bed mobility (part of functional mobility), (2) bathing and showering, (3) toileting and toilet hygiene, (4) personal hygiene and grooming, (5) dressing, (6) feeding, (7) personal device care, and (8) sexual activity.

Challenges or difficulties in ADL performance can occur secondary to disability, illness, or injury[1] and lead to activity limitations and participation restrictions.[6] This chapter addresses the above noted ADLs for clients with weakness, low endurance and fatigue, limited or restricted range of motion (ROM), incoordination and poor dexterity, decreased sensation, lost use of one upper extremity (UE) or one body side, lower extremity (LE) amputation, low or limited vision, bariatric considerations, and memory deficits.

Evaluation of Activities of Daily Living

The occupational therapy (OT) process begins with an evaluation that informs intervention and defines therapy outcomes. The goal of evaluation and intervention is to promote occupational function through remediation of client skills and adaptation of tasks and environments. Occupational therapists use a **client-centered approach** involving collaboration with clients and caregivers to prioritize therapy outcomes.[7]

Chart Review

Evaluation begins with a thorough chart review. It is important to determine the exact prescription for OT evaluation and intervention. The chart will inform therapists about any restrictions or contraindications including other comorbidities, current ambulation or weight-bearing status, and current equipment use. The chart will also provide preliminary information about clients' prior ADL status, home environment, and support system. Therapists should review notes from other professionals, including, but not limited to, physical therapists, speech therapists, social workers, dieticians, and nurses. Prior to beginning a detailed evaluation, it is often useful to complete a quick screening, including a brief interview and observation of some ADLs to determine whether further evaluation and intervention are warranted.

Occupational Profile

If, after screening, it is determined that an evaluation is needed, therapists complete **occupational profiles** to gain information about client factors, performance skills and patterns, contexts, and occupations.[1] Occupational profiles help therapists to understand client abilities, capacities, interests, values, roles, habits, routines, environments, and needs related to occupational engagement. It is important to ask the following questions:

- What is the client's current lifestyle?
- What was the client's ADL status prior to injury, disease, or illness?
- What are the client's current occupational challenges?
- What comprises the client's typical day-to-day routines?
- What occupations are meaningful to the client?
- In what environments does the client currently navigate to complete occupations?

Assessment of Activity of Daily Living Performance

A critical component of evaluation is ADL observation and analysis. Therapists can evaluate ADL performance by asking clients to provide a self-report of their performance or use performance-based ADL assessments. It is often important to assess client factors and skills such as ROM, strength, sensation, balance, and cognition prior to beginning ADL assessments. Ideally, ADL performance should be assessed in the environments in which they are typically done, or the environment should closely simulate clients' natural environments. ADL tasks to be assessed should range from simple to complex and should be based on the information obtained from the referral, chart review, and occupational profile. Therapists may use standardized ADL assessments such as the Functional Independence Measure (FIM); the Klein-Bell Activities of Daily Living Scale; the Katz Index of Independence in Activities of Daily Living; Performance Assessment of Self-Care Skills (PASS); Disabilities of the Arm, Shoulder, and Head (DASH) Assessment; and the Barthel ADL Index; or nonstandardized measures such as ADL checklists.[8–13] These standardized assessments can be used for re-evaluation to measure outcomes and to determine whether clients met their goals.

Levels of Independence

When evaluating ADL performance, occupational therapists use terminology to describe the level or amount of assistance required to perform ADLs. The following are general categories and definitions to categorize levels of independence.

- *Independent:* Clients can perform the activity independently; without modification of technique, assistive devices, or aids; and within a reasonable time frame.
- *Modified independence:* Clients either require an assistive device to complete the activity, the activity takes more than a reasonable time, or safety considerations exist.
- *Supervision (standby assistance):* Clients require a therapist to stand by for safety in case of balance loss. Therapists may provide verbal cues for safety.
- *Contact guard:* Therapists place one or two hands on the client's body to maintain balance, dynamic stability, or safety; however, they do not assist in task performance.
- *Minimal assistance:* Therapists provide 25% of assistance (physical or verbal), and clients are able to perform 75% or more of the activity.
- *Moderate assistance:* Therapists provide 50% of assistance (physical or verbal), and clients are able to perform 50% to 74% of the activity.
- *Maximal assistance:* Therapists provide 75% of assistance (physical or verbal), and clients are able to perform 25% to 49% of the activity.
- *Dependent:* Therapist provides more than 75% of assistance (physical or verbal), and clients are able to perform less than 25% of the activity.

When assessing ADLs using levels of independence, it is important to note whether clients require assistance from more than one person, and the amount of assistance provided by each person. Also note clients' ability to direct their care despite physical dependence. If clients are satisfied with their ability to direct their care, they may be considered independent.[1]

Other Factors to Consider in Activities of Daily Living Evaluations

It is important to consider the contextual and environmental factors that might impact client performance. Physical environmental factors such as clutter, barriers to access, rugs, steps, or stairways should be eliminated or adapted for safe ADL performance. Cultural and social factors also impact ADL performance and should be incorporated in evaluation and intervention when possible and desired by clients. Therapists should determine whether clients desire family and caregivers to be present and should comply with Health Insurance Portability and Accountability Act of 1996 (HIPAA) regulations.

Therapists working in acute or intensive care settings must consider the client's medical complexity. When evaluating and intervening with clients in these settings, therapists should understand and monitor lab values, vital signs, and code status repeatedly, as well as documented precautions for clients. Therapists should be familiar with equipment typically encountered in this setting, including electrocardiogram (EKG) monitors, ventilators, lines, catheters, tubes, dialysis equipment, pacemakers, mechanical circulatory devices, and respiratory care equipment. Isolation precautions, if applicable, should be reviewed and followed. This information is usually available in client charts and posted on hospital room doors.

Settings for Activities of Daily Living Evaluation and Intervention

ADLs are the focus of evaluation and intervention in most settings in which occupational therapists work including intensive care, acute care, acute rehabilitation, subacute rehabilitation, skilled nursing facilities, outpatient facilities, home care, and hand therapy. ADLs are typically assessed through observation of task performance in all of the abovementioned settings. In the practice area of hand therapy, ADLs may sometimes be assessed through self-report or interview.

Activities of Daily Living Intervention Techniques

Evaluation information—including interviews, occupational profiles, and assessment instruments—are integrated to develop intervention plans, goals, and outcomes. Long- and short-term goals should focus on remediating client skills, modifying performance techniques, altering the environment, or using **adaptive equipment**, to maximize independent ADL performance. Prior to beginning ADL intervention sessions, it is important to plan therapy sessions, set up the environment, and ensure that chosen activities provide the "just right challenge."[14] The complexity of ADL intervention should be increased gradually over time.

OT interventions can include preparatory methods and tasks such as physical agent modalities, ROM exercises, or strengthening approaches. Preparatory methods can be followed by purposeful activities, such as donning button-down shirts or cooking family meals.[1] Restoration and modification approaches are most often used in ADL interventions.[1] The restoration approach focuses on remediating client skills, which may have been lost due to injury or disease, to promote occupational resumption.[1] Sometimes, clients do not regain full capabilities and require modification to participate in ADLs. In these situations, the modification approach is used involving either (1) modification of the task performance technique (e.g., leaning against a sink when clients fatigue easily while brushing teeth) or (2) using adaptive equipment and altering the environment (e.g., using toothbrushes with built-up handles for clients with decreased grasp strength). Often, adaptation involves the use of **durable medical equipment (DME)**, which provides therapeutic benefits to clients with functional deficits resulting from medical conditions or illnesses. With the advent of 3-D printing, creating adaptations that enable ADLs has become easier. The following section addresses ADL modifications as they apply to the 10 conditions.

Weakness

Weakness in the limbs, trunk, or overall body can result in difficulty in dynamic and static balance, posture, transfers, functional mobility, reaching, and grasping. The techniques used and the amount of assistance provided to clients will differ based on upper and lower body weakness, trunk weakness, or overall body weakness. Some modifications and adaptive equipment used to enhance ADLs for clients with weakness are outlined in the subsequent sections.

Bed Mobility

Bed mobility is the ability to bridge in bed, roll from supine to side-lying, scoot up and down in bed, move from supine to sitting and sitting to supine, and sit at the edge of the bed. Teaching bed mobility skills to clients with weakness promotes ADL participation.

Modification of Technique

- *Bridging in bed:* For clients with weakness, bridging in bed can assist with strengthening the back, abdominals, quadriceps, and gluteal muscles. Bridging enables clients to move their hips to allow independence or assistance with ADLs in bed such as lower body dressing, toileting, and perineal hygiene (Video 27-1).

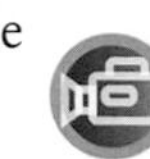

  - Clients should lay flat on their back, bend the knees, and bring the feet flat on the bed.
  - Lift the buttocks, upper legs, and lower back on the bed using the back and hip extensors. Move the hips toward the desired position.
  - Therapists can help stabilize the knees and feet if clients have difficulty holding the lower extremities (LEs) in position.
  - Clients can place their hands flat on the bed for stabilization if required.
- *Rolling in bed:* Rolling in bed is a critical component of bed mobility. It allows clients to change position by shifting weight in bed, assists with lower body dressing, and prepares the body to sit up in bed (Video 27-2).

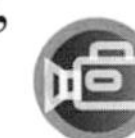

  - Clients should bend both knees by sliding their heels toward their buttocks.
  - Abduct one UE to 90° or less and horizontally adduct the other UE.
  - Lower the knees on the side of the abducted UE and turn the hips and shoulder to roll onto the side.
  - If clients have weakness on one side, have them reach across their body with their unaffected side to grip the bedrail or halo. Lower the knees on the affected side and turn the hips and shoulder to roll onto the affected side.
  - If clients have weakness secondary to spinal disease or injury, and have precautions to avoid twisting the spine, have them hold onto a bedrail and drop the knees while turning their shoulders and hips at the same time like a log (log rolling).
  - If clients require assistance to roll in bed, therapists can assist clients with shoulder protraction, grabbing the bedrail, flexing the knees, and guiding the roll.

- *Scooting in bed:* Scooting allows clients to be mobile in bed and build strength in the trunk and LE muscles (Videos 27-3 and 27-4).

  - To scoot to the head of the bed, clients should flex the hips and knees with feet flat on the bed. Bring the heels close to the buttocks. Shoulders should be slightly abducted and elbows should be flexed so that hands are flat on the bed next to the waist. Clients should raise their pelvis using bridging techniques and push on the LEs, while depressing and adducting their shoulders simultaneously to move up in bed.
  - To move down in bed, clients should flex their hips and knees with feet flat on the bed. Shoulders should be adducted, and elbows flexed with hands flat on the bed next to the buttocks. Clients should pull on their LEs to push their buttocks closer to their heels while simultaneously pushing up with the shoulders and abducting the shoulders to move down in bed.
  - For clients who need more assistance because of weakness, therapists can assist by stabilizing the knees and feet.
  - Alternatively, to scoot to the head of the bed, lower the head of the bed to make it flat, place a sheet under the client, and use a two-person assist to pull the sheet toward the head.

- *Side-lying to sitting at the edge of the bed:* Sitting at the edge of the bed allows clients to prepare to stand, transfer to a mobility device, and complete ADLs such as grooming, feeding, and hygiene in a seated position. To move from a side-lying position to sitting in bed, ask the client to:

  - Bring their legs over the side of the bed.
  - Use forearms and hands to push up to a sitting position with legs over the side of the bed.
  - To scoot to the edge of the bed, clients should place both hands flat on the bed and weight shift to one side of the body, while moving the opposite buttock forward. Then move the weight to the other side of the body, while moving the opposite buttock forward. Repeat until clients are comfortably seated at the edge of the bed.
  - If clients have weakness on one side of the body, they should roll onto the affected side, reach across the chest with the unaffected UE and use the unaffected hand to push up to a sitting position.
  - For clients who have whole-body weakness, or one-sided weakness but still require help to move to a seated position, therapists should bring the clients' legs to the edge of the bed and stabilize their knees between their legs. Then assist clients to an upright position by guiding the scapula and the hips.
  - For seated clients with one-sided, lower body, or whole-body weakness who require help to move the buttocks toward the bed edge, therapists can stabilize the clients' legs between their knees, and place both hands under the clients' buttocks or behind their knees to gradually move their body forward.

- *Sitting at the edge of the bed to supine:*

  - Clients should sit close to the head of the bed. They should scoot back further in the bed by placing both hands flat on the bed and weight shifting on one side while pulling their opposite pelvis backward until they are seated with their thighs fully supported in bed.
  - Lift LEs with knees slightly bent onto the bed, while simultaneously leaning down on one forearm or holding the handrail with the hand closest to the head of the bed.
  - Clients should then roll onto their back using their UEs and LEs to guide the roll.
  - For clients with one-sided weakness, therapists should place both hands under the clients' buttocks to scoot them back in the bed, while stabilizing their LEs between their knees. To move to side-lying, have clients lay down on their affected side in the bed by holding onto the handrail with the unaffected UE and placing the forearm of the affected UE on the bed for support. Hook their unaffected LE below the affected LE to simultaneously lift both legs onto the bed.
  - For clients with LE or whole-body weakness, therapists can place both hands under the clients' buttocks to move them back into the bed. When moving to a side-lying position, therapists can guide clients by placing one hand under the scapula of the side closer to the head of the bed to lower clients in bed; the other hand guides the LEs onto the bed.

Use of Adaptive Equipment or Altering the Task Environment

- Use bed rope ladders or overhead trapeze bars for clients with LE/trunk weakness.
- Electric or adjustable beds with powered head and knee controls assist with moving from supine to sitting and sitting to supine in bed.
- Bedrails or halos provide support for changing bed position (Fig. 27-1A to D).
- Leg lifters assist with lifting clients' legs into or out of bed, one leg at a time (Fig. 27-2).
- Transfer sheets or draw sheets help with rolling and moving to the edge of the bed; two people should always assist with transfers for safety.
- Hoyer lifts move clients out of bed into seated positions. Two people should always assist with Hoyer lift transfers to ensure safety.

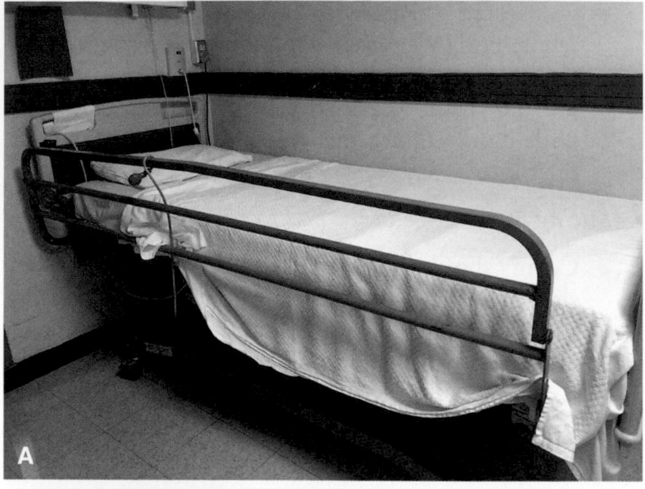
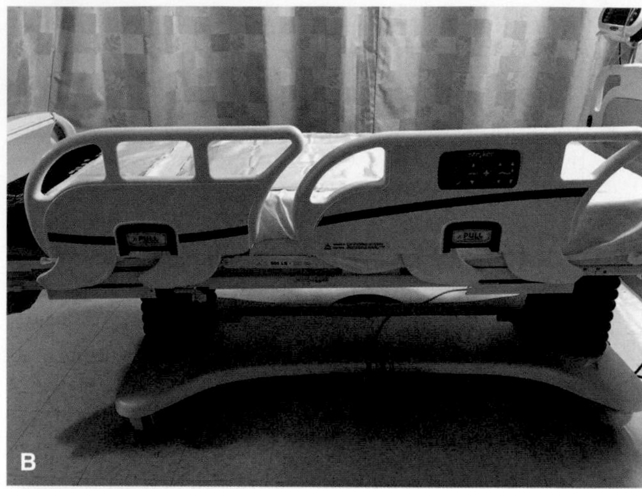
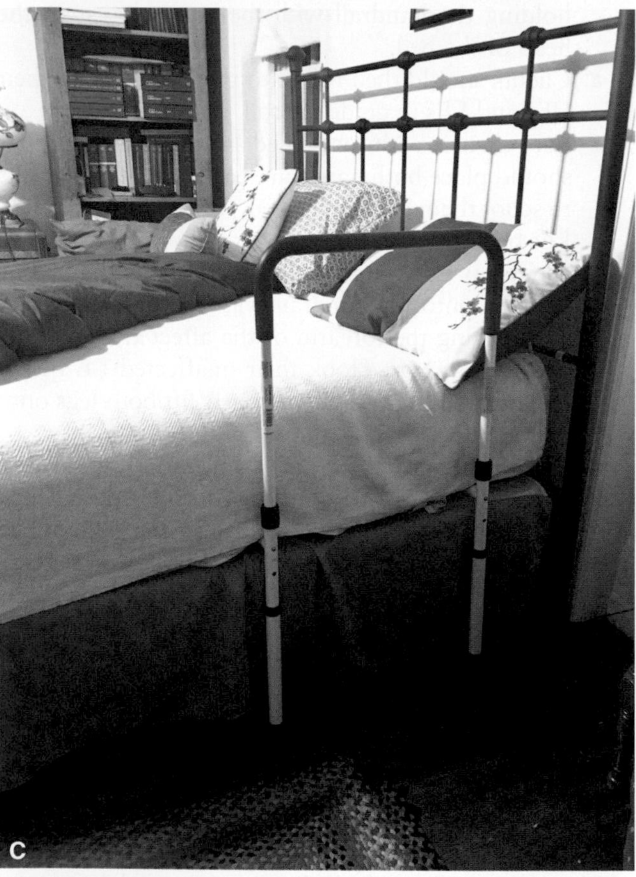
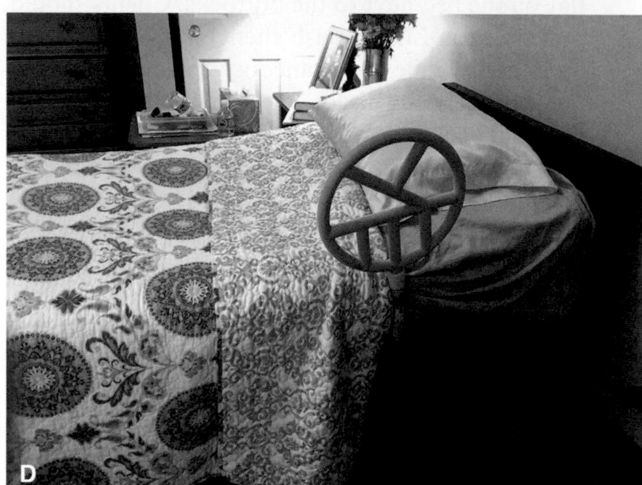

Figure 27-1. Bedrails or halos provide support for changing bed position. **A.** Single full-length hospital bedrail. **B.** Two part full-length hospital bedrail. **C.** Portable hand bedrail. **D.** Halo.

Bathing and Showering

Clients with weakness may have difficulty transferring into the bathtub or shower, standing or sitting in the shower, and grasping and holding onto items such as soap.

Modification of Technique

- Start with sponge bathing in bed (clients may need to begin with the upper body and progress to the whole body as tolerated). Clients should roll on their side to wash their back or allow caregivers to assist. Progress to bedside sponge bathing, then bathing at the bathroom sink, followed by a walk-in shower with a shower chair, and finally showering in a tub with a bath bench.
- Crossing one leg over the other while seated to wash alternate lower limbs is easier than bending down to wash limbs.
- If clients have a back brace, ensure that there is a second set that can be worn in the shower.

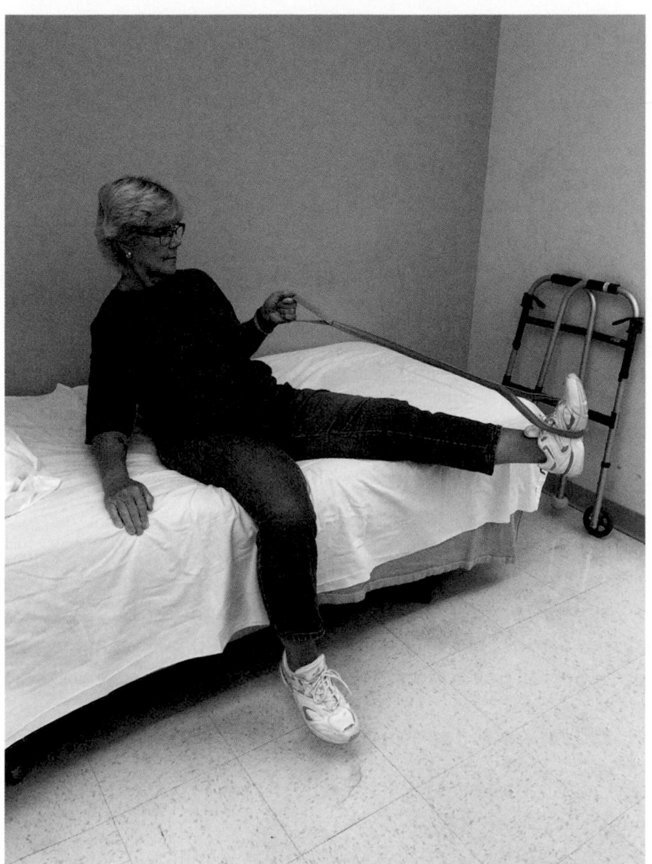

Figure 27-2. Leg lifters assist with lifting clients' legs into or out of bed.

Use of Adaptive Equipment or Altering the Task Environment

- Use 3-in-1 commodes that can be used as a shower chair, shower chair only (Fig. 27-3A and B), transfer tub bench with or without arm rests depending on trunk control and if arms are needed for transfers (Fig. 27-4), wheeled shower chair for clients who have difficulty ambulating to the shower (Fig. 27-5) or bath lifts.
- Walk-in bathtubs eliminate the need to transfer over the bathtub.
- Grab bars or portable safety rails assist with standing showers or transfers (Fig. 27-6).
- Nonslip mats provide stability in the shower.
- Soap on a rope or wash mitts with soap inserted in pocket reduce the need for grip strength.
- Use pump or automatic soap dispensers for clients who are unable to lift and squeeze.
- Long-handled sponges, brushes, and toe brushes allow clients to reach all body parts with minimal effort (Fig. 27-7).
- Use long, large, or lever shower handles for easier grip or touchless faucet adapters.
- Handheld adjustable shower hose or shower slide bars reduce the amount of movement needed in the shower.
- Use shower wraps to dry body for clients who have difficulty manipulating and using towels.

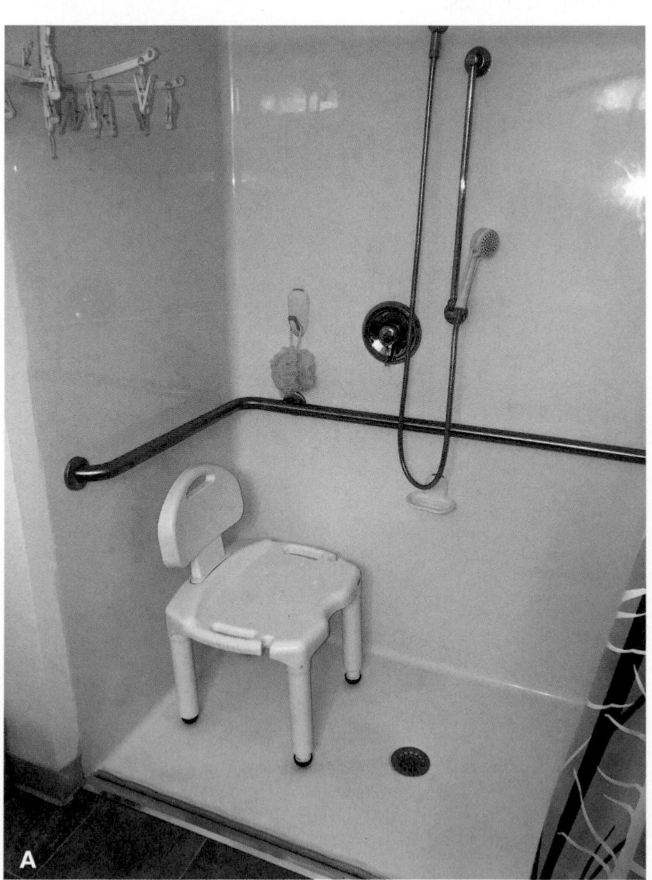

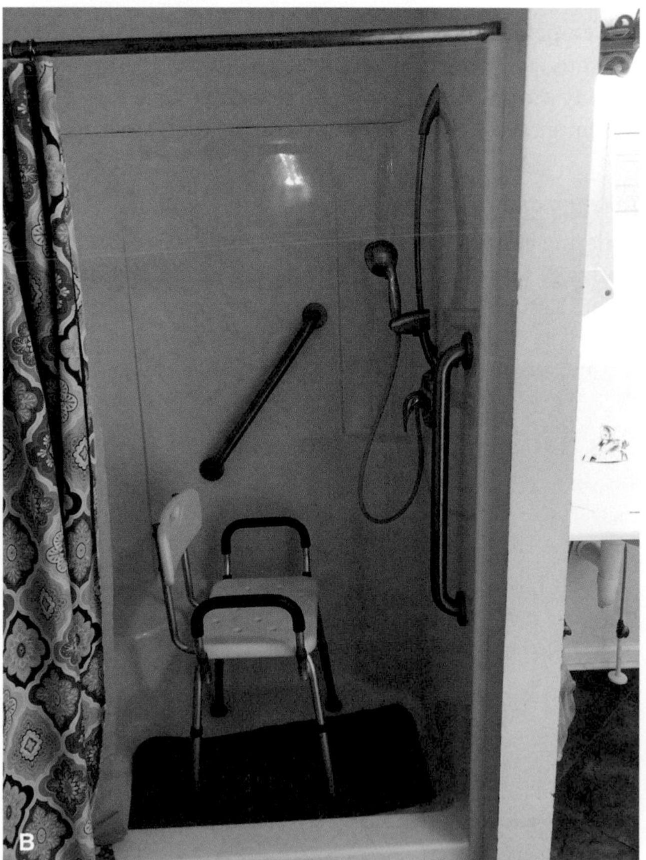

Figure 27-3. A. Shower chair. **B.** Shower chair with arm rests.

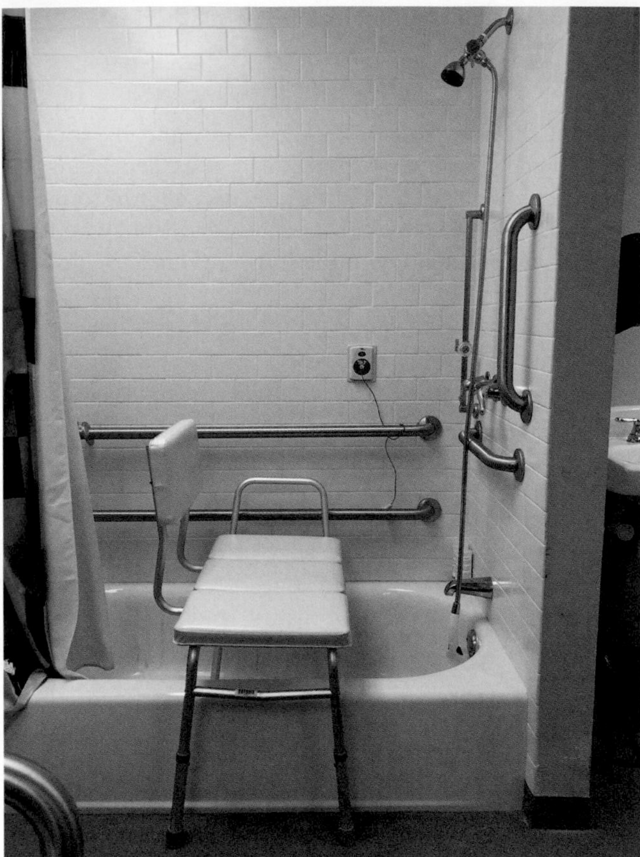

Figure 27-4. Transfer tub bench.

- Temperature-control shower valves eliminate sudden water temperatures changes. Avoid hot water as this may cause a temporary increase in weakness. Water temperature can also be lowered at the water heater.

Toileting and Toilet Hygiene

Toileting requires a person to be able to don and doff clothing, sit on and rise from the toilet, reach and grasp toilet tissue, and clean perianal areas. Clients with weakness may have difficulty grasping and holding onto clothes and cleaning supplies, as well as transferring onto and off of toilets.

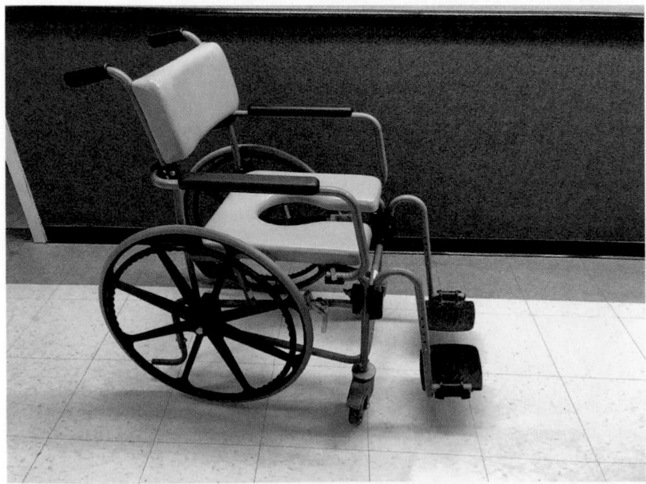

Figure 27-5. Wheeled shower chair.

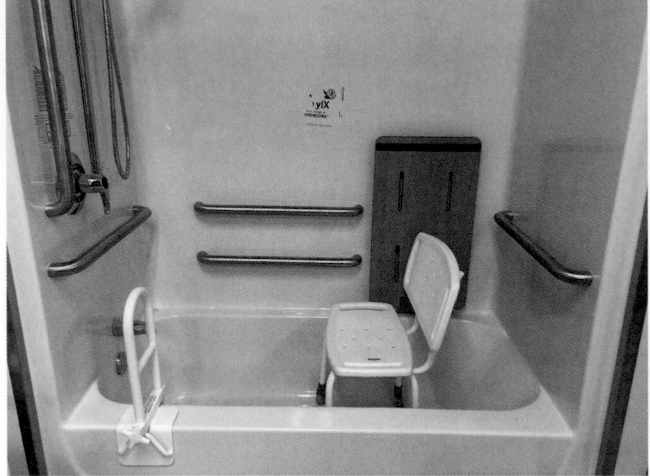

Figure 27-6. Grab bars.

Modification of Technique

- Establish routines or use alarms for regular bowel and bladder voiding.
- Use bed pans or adult diapers for clients who have difficulty getting to the toilet in time or completing toileting activities.

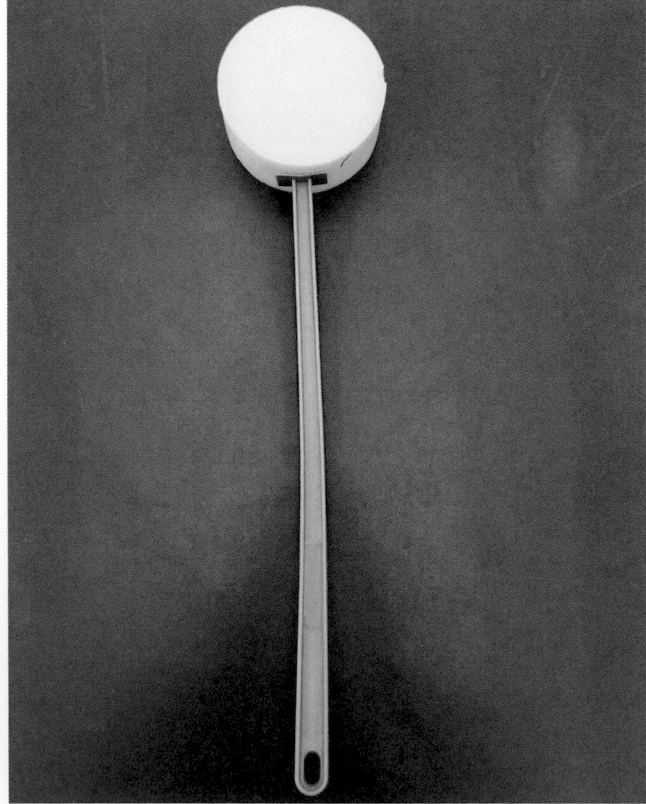

Figure 27-7. Long-handled sponges.

- Clients who have weakness due to spinal cord injury may have loss of bowel and bladder control. Specific bowel and bladder management techniques are described in Chapter 39.

Use of Adaptive Equipment or Altering the Task Environment

- Use raised toilet seats (Fig. 27-8) and grab bars or arm rests for easier transfer on and off toilets.
- Use 3-in-1 bedside commodes with pails to avoid the need to ambulate to the bathroom (Fig. 27-9).
- Use toilet seat lifts to mechanically move clients from sitting on a toilet seat to standing or moving to a mobility device.
- Use floor-to-ceiling grab bars to increase safety while transferring.
- Use drop-arm commodes for clients who need to reach behind for toilet hygiene.
- Bidet-toilet combos or bidet-toilet seats eliminate the need for toilet paper.
- Comfort-wipe extended-handle toilet paper holder or tongs reduce the amount of effort required to reach perianal areas for toilet hygiene.

Personal Hygiene and Grooming

Clients with weakness, especially of the UE, will have difficulty grasping and holding onto grooming supplies, such as combs, brushes, makeup, and shampoo.

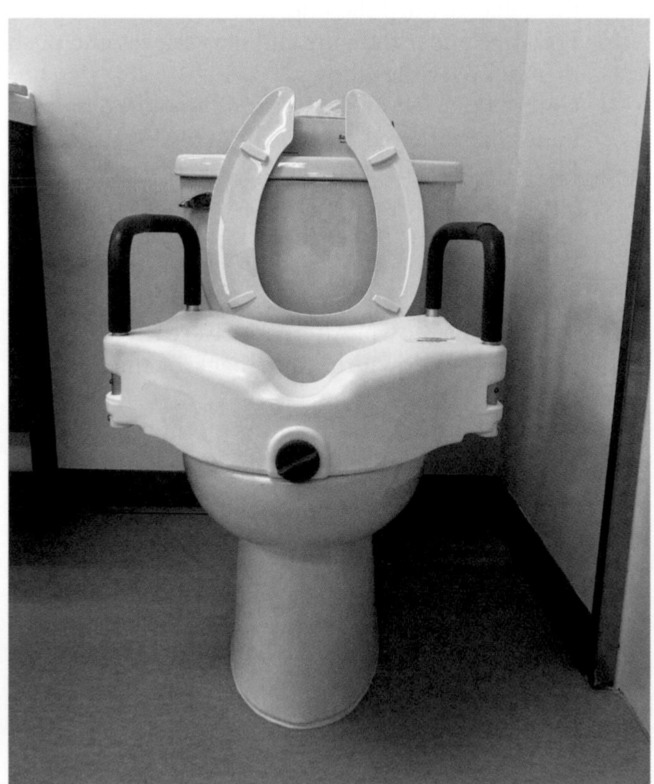

Figure 27-8. Raised toilet seat.

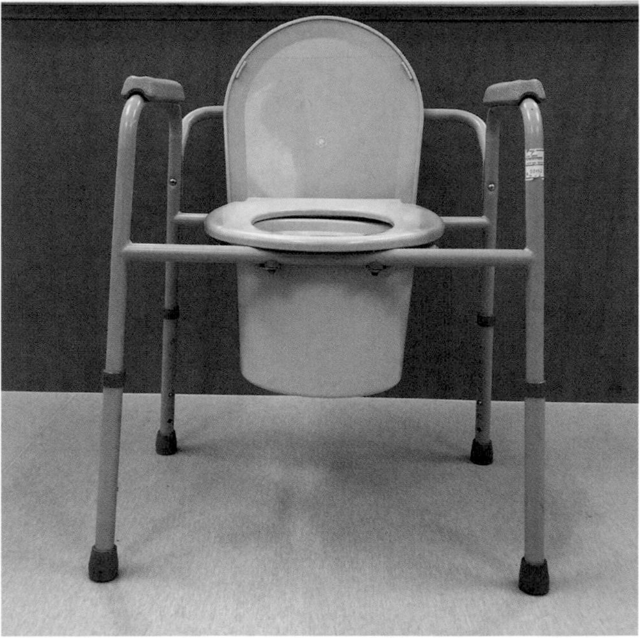

Figure 27-9. 3-in-1 commode with pail.

Modification of Technique

- Sit at the sink or vanity with arms supported on the surface.
- Organize and place required supplies in close proximity to avoid excessive reaching.

Use of Adaptive Equipment or Altering the Task Environment

- Use built-up handles on toothbrushes for individuals with reduced grasp (Fig. 27-10).
- Electric toothbrushes reduce the effort required to brush teeth.
- Toothpaste dispensers require less strength to dispense toothpaste on a toothbrush.
- Use waterpiks or dental floss holders for easier teeth flossing.
- Suctioned denture brushes and cleaners (in which dentures soak overnight) allow one-handed cleaning.
- Use pump or automatic dispensers for shampoos and lotions.
- Use dry shampoo and conditioners.
- Use flip-top bottles for easier opening and closing.
- Use built-up handles on combs and brushes (Fig. 27-10).
- Use wall-mounted hair dryers to dry hair.
- Use built-up tubing on manual or electric razors.
- Use hair removal cream to eliminate the need for razors.
- Use jar openers for twist-off caps on lotions or makeup supplies.
- Use universal cuffs to hold combs, brushes, toothbrushes, razors, and lipstick.

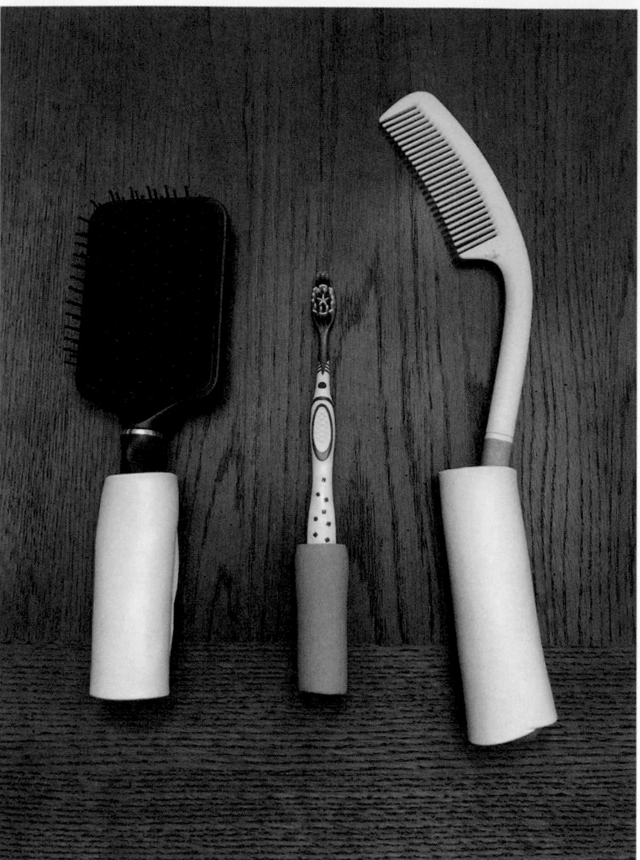

Figure 27-10. Built-up handles on toothbrushes and hair brushes.

- Applying friction material to tool surfaces can reduce the need for grasp strength.
- For deodorants, replace fingertip dispensers with long trigger nozzles to allow clients to spray themselves using all fingers, palm, or fist. Modified nozzles can be used for hair care products as well.
- For nail care, mount the nail clipper and/or nail file to a friction resistant or emery board to allow one-handed use (Fig. 27-11). Nails can be clipped using the palm or fist of the opposite hand. Clients can also use one-handed nail clippers, long-handled and pistol-grip LE toenail clippers, and suction nail brushes.

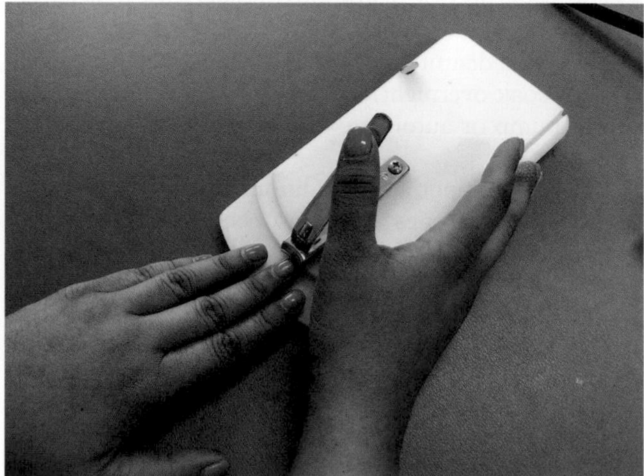

Figure 27-11. Mounted nail clipper.

Dressing

Clients with weakness or paralysis may have difficulty obtaining clothing, moving extremities into clothing, and manipulating buttons or zippers because of decreased grip and pinch, and decreased sitting balance.

Modification of Technique

The following modification techniques were developed for clients with spinal cord injury, but can be adapted for people with weakness secondary to other diagnoses.[15–18]

- Organize closets so that commonly used clothes are placed within easy reach.
- Lower closet pole height to allow easier clothing access.
- Remove closet doors if opening and closing requires too much effort.
- Easy-glide dresser drawers that only require a light push to slide open require less UE strength.

Upper Body Dressing—Shirts and Blouses

- *Donning shirts and blouses: Technique 1*

1. The client should be seated either in a bed or wheelchair (Video 27-5).
2. Position the shirt with the label facing down and the collar toward the knees.
3. Put arms under the shirt and into sleeves and push them up over the elbows.
4. Gather the back of the shirt and hook the thumbs under the gathered back using wrist extension.
5. Place the shirt over the head.
6. Shrug to get the shirt across the shoulder and hook the wrists into each sleeve to straighten them across the UEs.
7. Lean forward and reach back with one hand to pull the shirt down. Alternatively, reach across the body to pull down the shirt back of the opposite side.
8. Line the shirt fronts up and begin buttoning from the bottom up. A buttonhook or Velcro fasteners can be used.

- *Donning shirts and blouses: Technique 2*

1. The client should be seated either in a bed or wheelchair (Video 27-6).
2. Position the shirt with the label facing up and the collar toward the abdomen.
3. Put the arms into the sleeves, and push them up over the elbows.
4. Place the hands under the back of the shirt, tuck the chin, and flip shirt over the top of the head.

5. Once the shirt is flipped, straighten the arms and allow the shirt to fall around body.
6. Align the shirt fronts and begin buttoning from the bottom up. A buttonhook or Velcro fasteners can be used.

- *Doffing shirts and blouses*

1. Push one side and then the other side of the shirt off the shoulders by bending the elbows and using the fingers, fist, or chin to push the sleeve-off shoulder (Video 27-7).
2. Alternately, elevate and depress (shrug) the shoulders to allow gravity to assist in lowering the shirt down the arms.
3. Hook one thumb into the opposite sleeve to pull the shirt over the elbow and remove the arm from the shirt. Then, similarly remove other shirt arm.

- *Donning and doffing pullover shirts*

1. An overhead shirt is put on in the same manner as Technique 1.
2. To doff the pullover shirt, hook one thumb in the back of the neckline, gather the shirt back and pull it over the head. The sleeves are then pulled off each arm. Note: This is an alternate method for a button-down shirt (after shirt is unbuttoned).

Lower Body Dressing—Slacks and Pants

- *Donning slacks and pants: Technique 1*

1. Client sits in bed with legs extended and the head of the hospital bed elevated, if available (Video 27-8).
2. Position pants with the front up and pant legs over the bottom of the bed.
3. Lift one leg by hooking the opposite wrist or forearm under the knee and put the foot into the pant leg. Hook the thumb of the other hand into a belt loop or pocket to hold the pant leg open. This cross-body position of donning pants provides stability for those with poor balance. Return the knee to extension.
4. Insert the other foot in a similar manner.
5. Use the hands or palms to pat and slide the pants up over the calves, and get the cuffs over the feet.
6. Hook the wrists under the waistband or in the pockets to pull pants up over the knees.
7. Continue to pull on the waistband while moving to a supine position to pull the pants up to the thighs. Hooking the wrist or thumb in the crotch also helps to pull the pants up.
8. If UE strength is good, return to a sitting position and weight shift while leaning on one hand or elbow to pull the pant leg up the opposite buttock. Repeat the process for the other side.
9. If clients are unable to weight shift in a seated position, have them move from a supine to a side-lying position. Hook the thumb of the top arm in the back belt loop and pull the pants over the buttocks. Then roll onto the other side and repeat the process.
10. In a supine position, fasten the pants using a zipper pull loop, Velcro tab, or buttonhook.

- *Donning slacks and pants: Technique 2*

1. This method is useful for clients who have limited forward reach (Video 27-9).

2. Position the pants parallel to the client's legs.
3. Lift one leg by hooking the opposite wrist or forearm under the knee or calf and cross over the other leg.
4. Slide the pant leg all the way over the foot and up to the knee.
5. Uncross the leg and similarly slide the other leg in the pant leg.
6. To pull pants up and over buttocks, use steps 5 to 10 from Technique 1.

- *Doffing pants and slacks*

1. Pants are removed by reversing the steps of either technique described earlier and pushing the pants off.

- *Donning and doffing bras:* Either front or back closure bras can be used. The hook and eye fasteners can be replaced with Velcro for easier fastening.

1. If using a back closure bra, position the bra with the cups in the back and hook the fasteners in the front at waist level. Use the fingers, palm, or wrist to rotate the bra so the hooks move to the back and the cups to the front. Place both arms through the shoulder straps. Hook the opposite thumb under a strap and pull it over the shoulder. Repeat for the other shoulder.
2. For front-opening bras, position the bra with the cups in front and hook the bra. Place both arms through the shoulder straps. Hook the opposite thumb under a strap and pull it over the shoulder. Repeat for the other shoulder.
3. To doff the bra, reverse the steps for donning.

- *Donning and doffing socks*

1. To don socks, clients can be seated in a bed or wheelchair. Cross one leg over the other. Grasp the sock to put it over the foot and use patting movements with the palm to pull it on.
2. If clients cannot cross their legs, the foot can be placed on a stool or chair.
3. To doff socks, clients can be seated in a wheelchair or bed with legs crossed.

4. Hook the thumb over the sock edge and move the sock off the foot. Clients can also be seated with legs extended in bed and hips flexed to hook thumb over the sock edge and remove socks.

- *Donning and doffing shoes*

1. To don shoes, have the client seated with one leg crossed over the other. Balance the shoe sole in the palm and pull the shoe onto the foot. Use the palm to pull the shoe over the heel. Alternatively, place the foot on the floor or the foot pedal of the wheelchair, and push the foot down in the shoe by pushing on the knee.
2. A dressing stick can be used to get the shoe over the toes, and a long-handled shoehorn can be used to get the heel into the shoe (Fig. 27-12).
3. To doff shoes, clients can be seated with the legs crossed. Push on the heel of the shoe with the palm, and let the shoe fall off or use palm to push the shoe off the foot. A shoehorn can be used to push on the heel of the shoe and remove it from the foot.
4. Wearing slip-on shoes that are half to one size larger are easier to don and doff.

Additional Considerations for Dressing

- Knit shirts and looser shirts are easier to get on. Avoid shirts with tight necks.
- Pull-on pants are easier to put on. For women, skirts are easier to put on than pants.
- Step-in bras or sports bras are easier to don and doff.

Use of Adaptive Equipment or Altering the Task Environment

- Long-handled dressing sticks with an S-hook on one end can be used to pull pants on or tug clothing into place (Fig. 27-13).
- Use bras with Velcro front clasps or step-in bras.
- Use loops of fabric attached to the zipper pull of pants, shirts, or jackets to pull the zipper up or down with one finger.
- Use buttonhooks (with built-up handles or placed in universal cuffs) to manipulate buttons (Fig. 27-14).
- Replace buttons with Velcro to avoid the need to button.
- Use elastic instead of buttons for shirt cuffs.
- Use reachers to pick up clothing or shoes, or to retrieve clothing from closets.
- Use long-handled shoehorns to reach feet while seated.

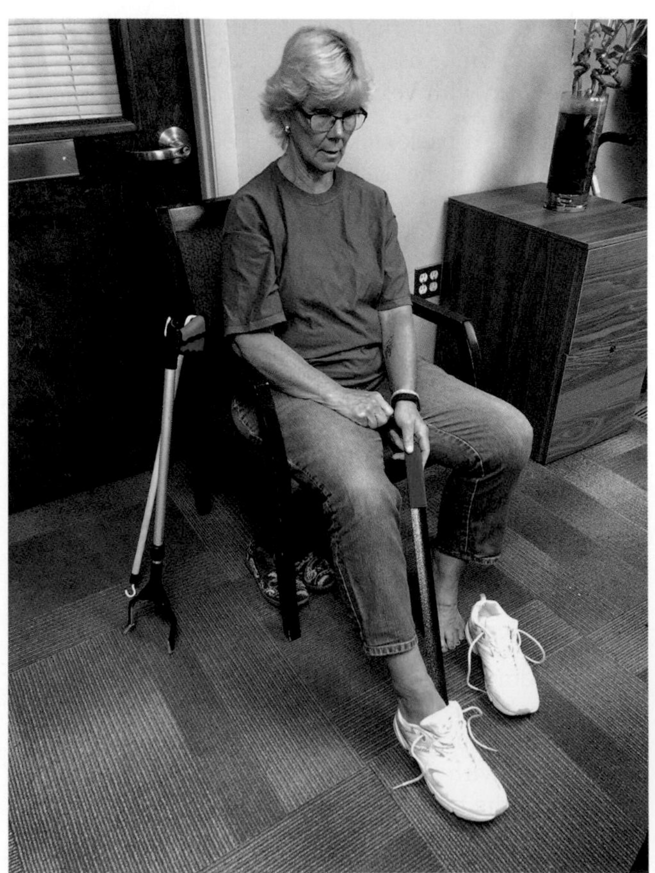

Figure 27-12. Long-handled shoehorn.

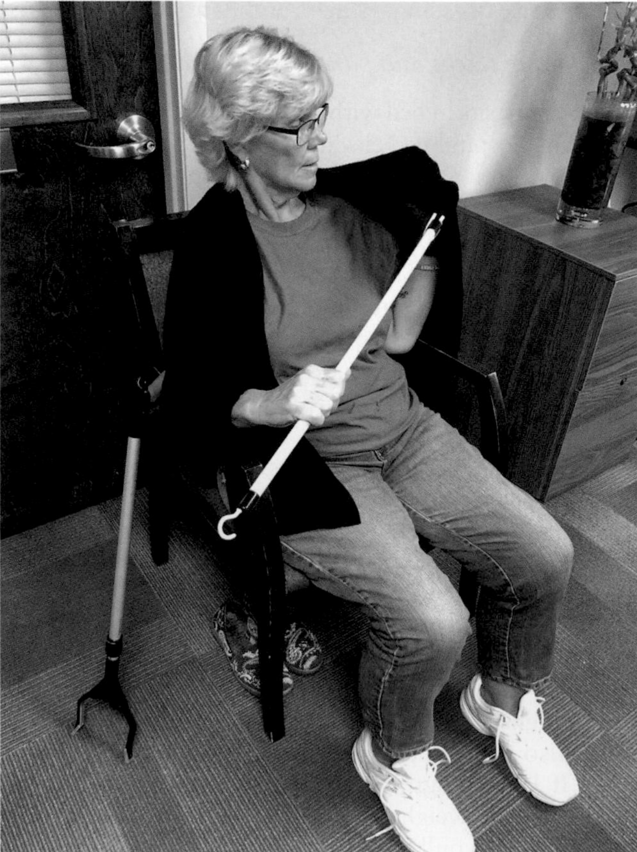

Figure 27-13. Dressing stick.

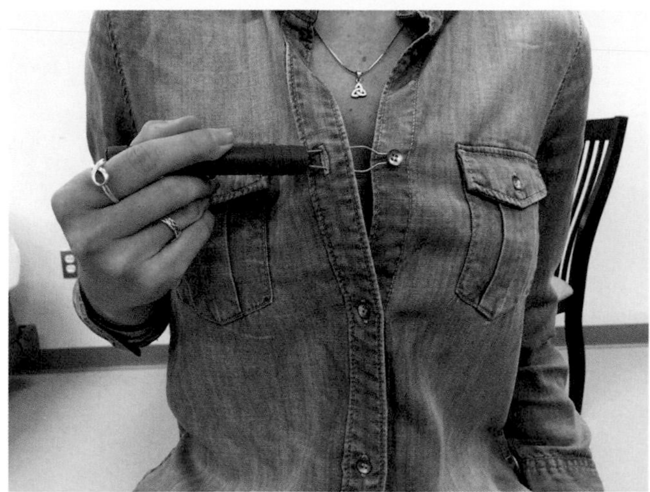

Figure 27-14. Button hook.

- Use shoes with Velcro or shoelaces with lace locks that do not require tying.
- Use sock or stocking aids to reach feet and pull socks up (Fig. 27-15).
- Use fabric loops around sock cuffs to pull socks up by hooking fingers in the loop.

Feeding

Feeding concerns for clients with weakness are caused by difficulty grasping utensils, cutting food, and bringing food from plate to the mouth.

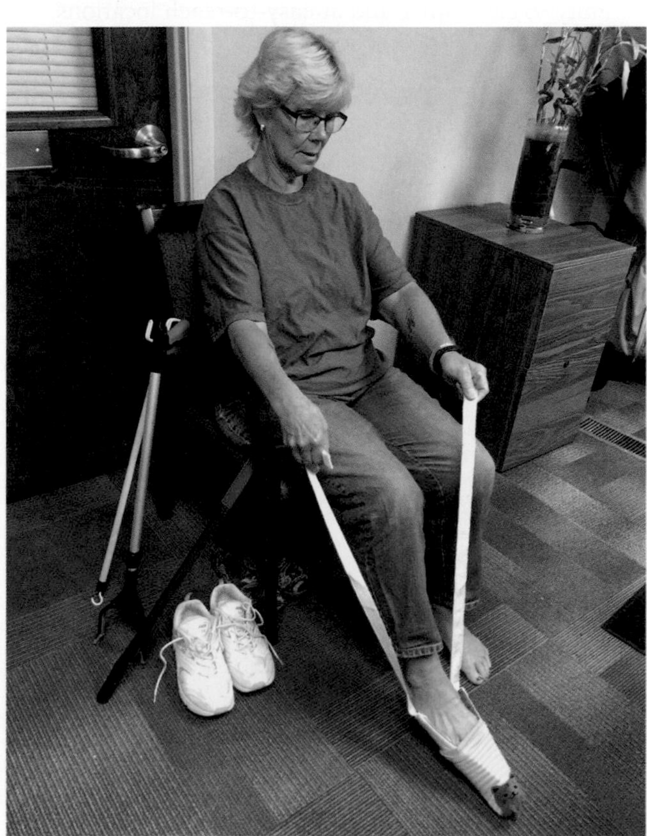

Figure 27-15. Sock or stocking aid.

Modification of Technique

- Position the client close to the table and use the table surface to support the arms while eating.
- Use precut meats and vegetables for eating or have caregivers cut food.

Use of Adaptive Equipment or Altering the Task Environment

- Use lightweight utensils such as heavy-duty plastic eating utensils.
- Built-up utensils allow clients with limited grasp to hold onto utensils (Fig. 27-16).
- Sporks, which combine spoons and forks, eliminate the need to change utensils while eating.
- Swivel utensils reduce the amount of rotation required to bring food from plate to mouth.
- Rocker knives with or without T-handles allow clients with UE weakness to cut their food with a rocking motion (Fig. 27-17A and B).
- Glasses or cups with lids prevent spillage.
- Large-handled or two-handled cups reduce the need for a strong grasp.
- Drink-mounting devices for beds or wheelchairs allow clients to drink without holding onto cups.
- Long or flexible straws reduce the need to lift and tilt cups.

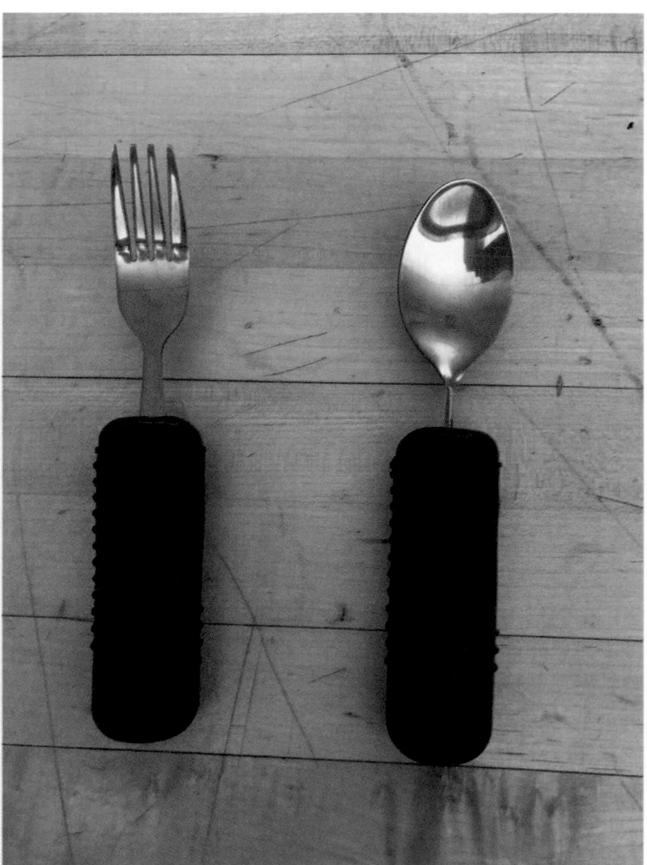

Figure 27-16. Built-up eating utensils.

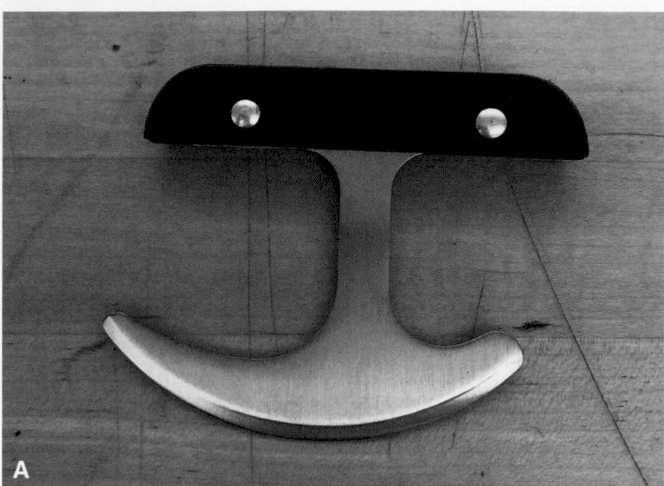

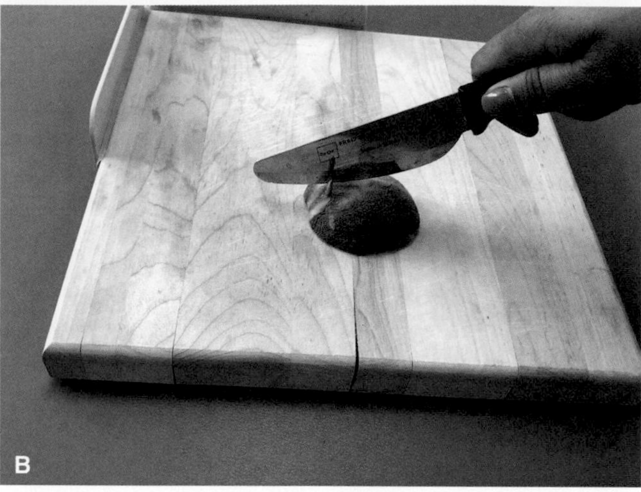

Figure 27-17. Rocker knife. **A.** With T-handle. **B.** Without T-handle.

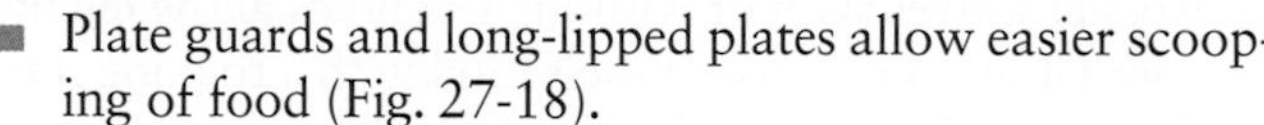

- Plate guards and long-lipped plates allow easier scooping of food (Fig. 27-18).
- Universal cuffs with eating utensils reduce the need to grasp (Fig. 27-19).
- Mobile arm supports promote client horizontal and vertical arm movements to reach plates and mouth. These can be mounted to sinks, wheelchairs, or tables and are portable.
- Food can be stored in containers with easy-to-open lids for one-handed use.

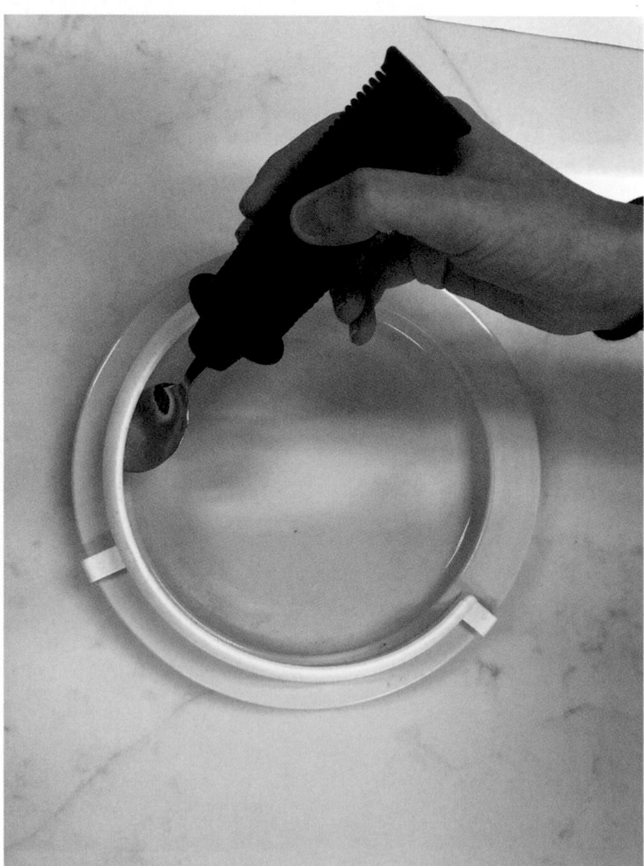

Figure 27-18. Plate guards and long-lipped plates.

Personal Device Care

Managing and using personal devices such as contact lenses, glucose monitors, and orthotics may arise because of difficulty grasping, pinching, and positioning devices.

Modification of Technique

- Clients should sit at a table with arms supported while using, cleaning, and maintaining personal devices.
- Place commonly used personal devices in close proximity to each other and at easy-to-reach locations.

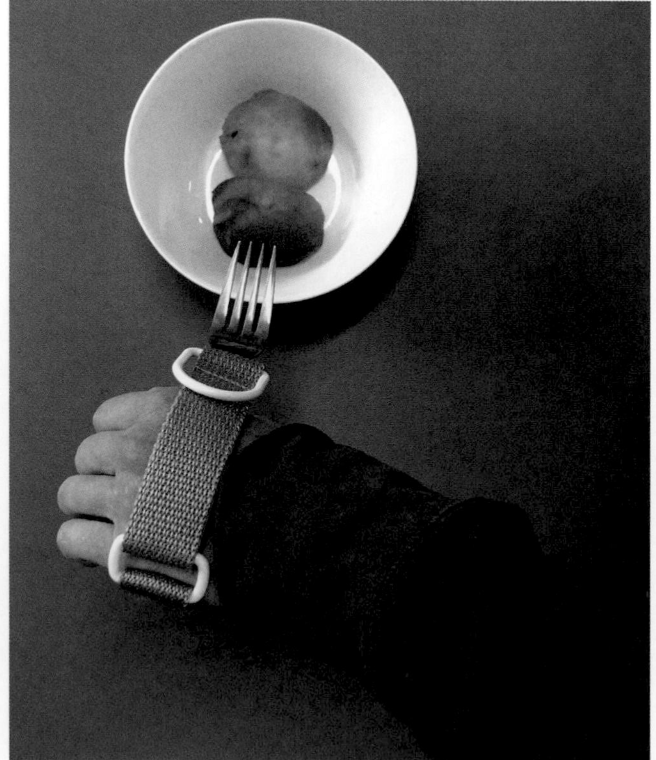

Figure 27-19. Universal cuffs with eating utensils.

- LE orthotics should be donned and doffed similarly to donning and doffing socks as described in dressing.
- Use gravity to assist with using and maintaining personal devices.

Use of Adaptive Equipment or Altering the Task Environment

- Optiwand soft contact lens insertion and removal tools hold lenses until placed on the cornea for clients who have limited grasp and pinch. Handles can be built up for weak grasp.
- Large flip-top contact lens cases can be opened and closed with fist movements.
- Use larger eye drop bottles for easier grasp. Or use an autosqueeze eye drop bottle dispenser with a larger grasp area that makes bottle squeezing easier by providing extra leverage.
- The Opticare Arthro eye dropper has extended handles and is easy to squeeze for clients with arm and hand ROM limitations.[19]
- Automatic glucose and blood pressure monitors have fewer buttons to use (e.g., automatic on/off and no coding) and have multiple strips filled in the drum to eliminate strip reinsertion with each use.
- Larger hearing aids are easier to grasp and insert into the ear.

Sexual Activity

Sexual activity is often an area of concern for individuals with disabilities. Depending on the extent of their weakness, clients may need help identifying positions that best support engagement in sexual expression. In addition to identifying different positions, it is important to discuss the scope of intimacy (including increasing opportunities to touch, hug, and kiss), to shift the focus from function to pleasure, and to consider the impact of impairment on body image and fears about resuming sex. Several publications describe sexual expression and activity for individuals with weakness.[20,21]

Modification of Technique

- For clients with weakness of the LEs, trunk, and/or UEs, it is often easier to engage in intercourse while in a wheelchair or while seated and supported by a backrest with the partner positioned on top of them.
- For clients with paralysis, it is better to be positioned below the partner in a missionary position, with a rolled towel or small pillow to support the lumbar spine.
- When clients have hemiparesis, positioning both partners in a side-lying position with the client lying on the affected side allows free movement of the unaffected side.
- Alternatively, clients with hemiparesis can position themselves in a missionary position with their partner on top and supporting some of their weight on the surface on which they are lying.
- Rear entry positions may be used with both partners kneeling and both sets of forearms on the bed or supporting surface; this reduces both partners' energy expenditure.
- For clients with spinal cord injury, it is necessary to complete preparatory activities prior to engaging in sexual activity, such as emptying the bladder and managing catheters.

Use of Adaptive Equipment or Altering the Task Environment

- Use pillows and wedges to assist with positioning during sexual activity.
- Use bedrails or overhead trapezes to reposition self in bed.

Low Endurance and Fatigue

Endurance is the ability to sustain physical activity over time. General endurance is a reflection of cardiopulmonary function and overall fitness. Fatigue is not simply low endurance, but a subjective experience of feeling tired or exhausted.[22] Fatigue is multidimensional and includes cognitive, behavioral, and emotional components,[23] as well as physical factors. A person with low endurance and fatigue may experience difficulty initiating or completing ADLs. Therapists should understand the importance of assessing and monitoring endurance and fatigue during ADL performance such as heart rate (HR)/vitals, metabolic equivalent for task (MET) levels, number or repetitions over a period of time, and scales of perceived exertion. A compendium of physical activities based on MET levels is available in Chapter 40; however, this should always be used in combination with monitoring vital signs.[24] Therapists should also be aware of precautions and contraindications when performing ADLs for persons with low endurance and fatigue such as holding one's breath during ADLs; isometric contractions for clients with active cardiac histories; significant changes in blood pressure, O_2 rate, and HR (>20 beats over resting HR); shortness of breath (dyspnea); and angina. When determining ADL interventions for clients with low endurance and fatigue, therapists should carefully consider the client, the activity, and the environment in which the ADL will be performed.[25] Modification techniques and use of adaptive equipment to enhance ADLs for clients with low endurance and fatigue should include energy conservation techniques, as outlined in the subsequent sections.

Bed Mobility

Modification of Technique

- Preplan: Prepare the surface to which the patient will transfer and/or the ambulatory device needed.
- Perform bed mobility tasks in steps and take breaks.

- Supine to sit: Log roll independently or, depending on low endurance level, use assistance of one or two persons (see Weakness).
- Bed mobility techniques for weakness apply to clients with low endurance and fatigue.

Use of Adaptive Equipment or Altering the Task Environment

- Adjustable beds assist in bringing patients upright or lowering to supine.
- Use portable bedrails at home.
- Use Hoyer lifts.

Bathing and Showering

Modification of Technique

- Pace activities and incorporate rest breaks.
- If sponge bathing bedside, set all items on tray table or nearby within easy reach.
- It is preferable to take showers instead of baths. Baths require too much energy to get in and out of the tub basin.
- When showering, preplan: Prepare all items needed for showering (place soap, shampoo, clothing, and towels within reach).
- Delegate aspects of the task to be completed by caregivers.
- Use lukewarm water because hot water may increase fatigue level.
- Cross legs to bathe feet while seated on a tub bench (it takes less energy) or use long-handled equipment.

Use of Adaptive Equipment or Altering the Task Environment

- Use tub benches for clients who do not have the endurance to step in and out of the tub.
- Use shower chairs for clients who have the endurance to step in and out of the tub, but who fatigue easily.
- Use long-handled equipment (long-handled bath and toe sponges).
- Use shower hoses or adjustable mounted shower hoses.
- Use shower caddies with all needed items within reach.
- Use soap on a rope placed nearby and bath mitts with soap inserted in pockets to eliminate having to hold soap and washcloths.
- Use walk-in showers or tubs.

Toileting and Toilet Hygiene

Modification of Technique

- Don't strain during a bowel movement.
- Set a routine for bowel management.

Use of Adaptive Equipment or Altering the Task Environment

- Use raised toilet seats.
- Use stools (squatty potty) that raise the feet in a squatting position to promote effortless bowel movements.
- Use toilet-bidet combos for toilet hygiene.

Personal Hygiene and Grooming

Modification of Technique

- Sit to perform grooming activities, including brushing teeth, shaving, hair care, and makeup.
- Rest upper arms/elbows on vanity/counter.
- Preplan needed items and position them in easy reach.
- Take rest breaks.

Use of Adaptive Equipment or Altering the Task Environment

- Use electric razors.
- Use electric toothbrushes.
- Use standing or wall-mounted hair dryers.

Dressing

Modification of Technique

- Pace dressing activities, and other ADLs completed before and after dressing, so that clients do not perform multiple ADLs in a row without breaks.
- Incorporate rest breaks.
- Sit to perform dressing.
- Preplan and gather needed items: Organize clothes within easy reach in dressers and closets.
- Crossing the legs to don socks and shoes requires less energy than bending down.
- Wear light, loose clothing (microfiber stretches).
- Dressing techniques for weakness apply to clients with low endurance and fatigue.

Use of Adaptive Equipment or Altering the Task Environment

- Use dressing sticks, reachers, and sock aids.
- Use slip-on shoes or shoes with elastic laces or Velcro.
- Use Velcro closure and zipper pulls.

Feeding

Modification of Technique

- Delegate caregivers to precut food and place meals on table.
- Take rest breaks between courses.
- Consider multiple small meals throughout the day.
- Rest upper arms/elbows on table when feeding.
- Keep all condiments within reach: Consider a Lazy Susan.

Use of Adaptive Equipment or Altering the Task Environment

- Use long-handled and lightweight utensils.
- Mobile arm supports and deltoid aids assist with bringing the hand to the mouth.
- Consider feeding robots (iEat) or electric feeding devices (Mealtime Partner).[26]
- Use chairs that support the trunk and neck.
- Mount cups with straws to wheelchairs.

Personal Device Care

Modification of Technique

- Rest upper arms on vanity table for support.

Use of Adaptive Equipment or Altering the Task Environment

- See section on Weakness and Limited or Restricted Range of Motion.

Sexual Activity

The American Heart Association provides information on cardiovascular changes that occur during sexual intercourse, guidelines for resuming sex after myocardial infarction or heart surgery, other facts that influence sexual interest and capacity, and actions to take if symptoms arise during sex.[27] Sexual activity should be preplanned to provide rest time before and after. Sexual intercourse for the client with low endurance and fatigue is less stressful when positioned on the bottom and laying supine. Positions that require the least movement should be chosen. Sexual activities should be planned for day and week times when energy levels are highest. For additional information, see section on Sexual Activity in Weakness.

Limited or Restricted Range of Motion

Limited or restricted ROM of the limbs, trunk, or overall body could result in difficulty reaching body parts to perform self-care, reaching for objects at different heights, transferring or sitting on surfaces with different heights, functional mobility, and grasping items to complete ADLs. Occupational therapists should understand the functional ranges needed to perform common ADLs.[28,29] When determining ADL interventions for persons with limited or restricted ROM, therapists should carefully consider the client, the degree of ROM limitation/restriction, the activity, and the environment in which the ADL is performed.[25] Modification techniques to enhance ADLs for clients with limited or restricted movement are outlined in the subsequent sections.

Bed Mobility

Modification of Technique

- Use log rolling for clients with restrictions on spine ROM.
- When clients have hip ROM restrictions such as total hip arthroplasty (THA) and hip fracture:
  - To exit bed: Transfer from stronger side (client should learn to transfer from both sides), prop upper body on forearms, and slowly move LEs to bed edge (avoid hip adduction), followed by the trunk (avoiding hip flexion > 90°) (Video 27-10).

  - To enter bed: Using rolling walker, back up to the middle or upper one-third of bed, reach back for bed with both hands, and slowly lower buttocks to the bed while extending the affected LE (do not flex hips >90°). Slide back to the middle of the bed and slowly bring legs onto the bed (keeping them abducted) while turning to face the bed end. Scoot buttocks toward the head of bed so that legs are supported comfortably on the bed. Lower upper body onto forearms and then lay down flat onto bed (Video 27-11).

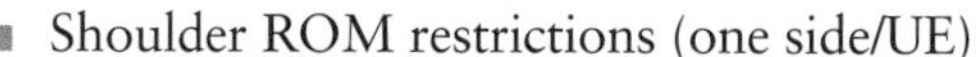

- Shoulder ROM restrictions (one side/UE):
  - To exit bed: Roll toward stronger side and then move legs so that they hang over the bed edge and, at the same time, use the stronger arm to prop trunk upright at the bed edge.
  - To enter bed: Sit on bed edge (middle to upper one-third of bed) with stronger side toward head of bed. Move to a side-lying position by lowering the upper body onto the forearm of the unaffected UE while at the same time bringing legs onto bed. Slowly move from side-lying to supine. Make certain there is a pillow for the affected extremity to roll onto.
- Shoulder ROM restrictions (both sides/bilateral upper extremities [BUEs]) such as radial artery (RA) and status-post (s/p) coronary artery bypass grafting (CABG).
  - To exit bed: Log roll to side (for sternal precautions, hug a pillow), then move legs so that they hang over the bed edge. At the same time, move the trunk up to the bed edge. Do not pull on bedrail or push off bed.
  - To enter bed: Sit on bed edge (middle to upper one-third of bed). Move to a side-lying position by lowering the upper body to the bed (for sternal precautions, hug a pillow), while at the same time bring legs onto bed. Slowly move from side-lying to supine.

Use of Adaptive Equipment or Altering the Task Environment

- Use leg lifters for clients with limited active or passive LE ROM.
- Electric or adjustable beds can assist with sitting up in bed and sit-to-supine movements.
- Home care therapists can place risers or blocks beneath the bed legs to raise bed height.
- Ladder ropes can assist moving from supine to sitting (requires good UE strength).
- Clients can sleep in adjustable recliner chairs.

Bathing and Showering

Modification of Technique

- Clients can sponge bathe bedside using adjustable tray tables with items at waist level.
- Showering is preferred over tub baths for ROM restrictions of the spine.

- With restricted shoulder ROM of one extremity, a grab bar for the unaffected extremity or a tub bench should be used for safety. When showering, place the affected shoulder in a passive pendulum position to wash the axilla with the unaffected extremity.
- With restricted ROM in both UEs, a tub bench should be used for safety.

Use of Adaptive Equipment or Altering the Task Environment

- Use soap on a rope or bath mitts for limited finger ROM.
- Use adjustable bath benches for clients with LE ROM limitations or restrictions.
- Use adjustable handheld shower hoses.
- Use lever faucet handles.
- Towel racks should be placed so that reaching remains below shoulder level.
- Faucet controls should be at waist level for clients with ROM restrictions of the spine and/or shoulder.
- Use long-handled sponges to bathe feet for clients with hip limitations or restrictions.
- Use long-handled toe brushes to wash toes.
- Use built-up handles on bathing devices for limited finger ROM.
- Bath caddies and shower racks decrease the need to reach.
- Use shower wraps to dry body after bathing.

Toileting and Toilet Hygiene

Use of Adaptive Equipment or Altering the Task Environment

- Use automatic toilet paper dispensers within easy reach.
- Use comfort-wipe extended-handle toilet paper holders or wiping tongs.
- Raise toilet height or use raised toilet seats for limited or restricted hip ROM.
- Use bidet-toilet combos or bidet-toilet seats for clients with limited UE ROM.
- Place toilet paper holders in easy reach or use long-handled toilet paper holders.
- Toilet seat incline lifts assist with sit-to-stand transfers.
- Sanitary napkins with adhesive strips are easier to use than tampons.

Personal Hygiene and Grooming

Modification of Technique

- Limited shoulder ROM: While seated, support proximal UEs on tabletop/vanity (add book/block to increase elevation) and perform grooming/makeup.
- Restricted shoulder ROM: Use a one-handed technique or perform with upper arm adducted to side and use only the distal extremity (elbow and hand).

Use of Adaptive Equipment or Altering the Task Environment

- Use hair dryer stands.
- Use hair removal creams in place of shaving.
- Using the palm, use pump bottles for shampoo, lotions, and makeup.
- Use long- and curved-handled tools for shaving, hair brushing and combing, and applying lotion.
- For limited finger ROM, use built-up handles for toothbrushes, combs, and brushes. For makeup, select large diameter makeup brushes, lip glosses, and eye pencils. Small-diameter makeup items can be built up with duct tape or pencil grips that can be easily cleaned.[30]
- Use aerosol bottles for deodorants, hair sprays, powders, and perfumes.
- For limited reach, use long-handled clippers for toenails and one-handed mounted clippers for finger nails.
- Use water flossers and electric toothbrushes.

Dressing

Modification of Technique

- Organize closets so that items are within reach (may require lowering closet pole and adding shelves at waist level). Use reachers to gather clothing. Consider open concept by removing closet doors for easy access. Easy-glide dresser drawers that only require a light push to slide open help to address limited finger and UE ROM. Organize dressers so that commonly worn clothing is placed in drawers at waist level or within easy reach.
- LE ROM limitations:
  - Donning: While seated, use a reacher to grasp the waist of pants or skirt and lower toward the floor to dress the affected LE first, then the unaffected leg. Raise garment above the knees toward the hips. Stand (with ambulatory device) and pull garment above hips. Sit to button or zip garment.
  - Doffing: Unzip or unbutton while seated or standing. While standing, push pants below hips toward knees. Sit and use dressing stick to push the affected leg out of pants, followed by the unaffected leg.
  - Socks: Don with sock aid, doff with dressing stick.
  - Shoes: Use long-handled shoehorns, elastic laces, and slip-on shoes. For posterolateral approaches to total hip arthroplasty (THA), position shoehorn on the medial aspect of the foot, which reduces the chance that clients will move the foot into internal rotation while donning shoes. For anterolateral approaches to THA, position shoehorn on the lateral aspect of the foot to reduce the possibility that clients will move the foot into external rotation while donning shoes.
- UE ROM restrictions on one side (status post rotator cuff repair, shoulder fracture):
- Button-down shirt: For one-handed technique, see section on Loss of Use of One UE or One Side of Body.

Also clients can don by placing the affected extremity in a semi-passive pendulum position and bringing the sleeve up the arm to the shoulder. Walk the collar around the neck and place the unaffected arm through the sleeve. To button, start at the bottom button to align the button holes. If clients have limited finger ROM, consider a buttonhook.

- ROM limitations of both UEs: Button-down shirts are easier to don and doff (consider a shirt one size larger or made of stretchable microfiber materials). Use a dressing stick or reacher to bring garment around back. Gradually turn bras around so the cups are in front and slip the hands through the straps.
- Use front-opening bras, step-in bras, or sports bras. Replace hook and eye fasteners with Velcro. For UE ROM limitations, hook a back-opening bra in the front at the waist.

Use of Adaptive Equipment or Altering the Task Environment

- Use long-handled equipment (reachers, dressing sticks, sock aids, and long-handled shoehorns) for LE ROM limitations.
- Use elastic laces or slip-on shoes for restricted or limited ROM and clients who can't bend to touch feet.
- Use front-hook bras or step-in bras for limited shoulder internal rotation.
- Use buttonhooks or Velcro closures for limited finger ROM.
- Use loops on pants waist to pull up pants.

Feeding

Modification of Technique

- Eat with one hand if ROM limitation is specific to one side.

Use of Adaptive Equipment or Altering the Task Environment

- Use built-up utensils for clients with limited finger ROM.[31]
- Use long-handled or curved-handled utensils for clients with limited reach.
- Use rocker knives for clients to cut food with one hand.
- Use universal cuffs for clients with moderate-to-severe grasping limitations.
- Use cups with cut-outs for the nose for clients with limited cervical ROM.
- Use cups with long straws for clients with limited elbow flexion.
- Use T-handle cups for clients with limited finger ROM.
- Use long plastic straws for clients with neck, elbow, and shoulder limitations.
- Use adjustable height tray tables.
- Use electric feeding devices.

Personal Device Care

Modification of Technique

- Clients should sit at a sink or vanity with all required items placed within easy reach.
- For clients with limited shoulder ROM, eye drops can be administered lying supine, keeping the affected extremity near side and using elbow flexion while holding bottle horizontally to administer drops.[19]

Use of Adaptive Equipment or Altering the Task Environment

- Deep-well, easy flip-top and easy-grip, large ridge contact cases help clients with limited finger ROM.
- Rechargeable In-The-Ear hearing aids are larger and easier to insert for clients with limited finger ROM. Remotes with push-button volume controls are better than dial controls.
- The Opticare Arthro eye dropper has extended handles and is easy to squeeze for clients with arm and hand ROM limitations.[19]

Sexual Activity

Modification of Technique

- There are many ways to be intimate with a partner if a client experiences ROM limitations or restrictions, such as kissing, hugging, caressing, and sexual device use. Prior to sexual activity, a warm shower and pain medication can be effective for clients with ROM and pain issues such as arthritis.[32] Surgeons must approve the following for clients postsurgery:
  - Face-to-face missionary positions are safe for clients with ROM restrictions from hip and knee replacements. The client with the hip or knee replacement should position a pillow between the knees and lie beneath the partner. The partner on top should limit the amount of weight on the operated hip or knee and facilitate most of the movement.
  - Side-lying positions (client in front and partner entering from behind) can be used for clients with hip ROM limitations. Face-to-face side-lying can also be used with the partner facilitating most of the movement when clients have back problems.
  - Positions described in weakness can apply to clients with ROM restrictions; however, clients must adhere to precautions.

Use of Adaptive Equipment or Altering the Task Environment

- Use abduction pillows.
- Use electric blankets for clients with painful stiff joints.

Incoordination and Poor Dexterity

Incoordination is the loss of precise smooth movements and can result from central nervous system disorders. Incoordination may present as ataxia, dysmetria, dyssynergia, dysdiadochokinesis, tremors, and involuntary movements.[33] Incoordination leads to poor dexterity, which is loss of fine and nimble manipulation, and motor coordination skills.[34,35] Clients who have incoordination disorders or poor dexterity have difficulty stabilizing body parts and safely coordinating movements and objects to complete ADLs. Stabilizing the body as much as possible by sitting during ADL activities, bearing weight on the UEs, holding the UEs close to the body, or using splints to stabilize selected joints can improve clients' extremity control.[36]

Bed Mobility

Modification of Technique

- Clients can delegate assistance for bed mobility, especially for safety.

Use of Adaptive Equipment or Altering the Task Environment

- Use bedrails or halos for safety.
- Use Hoyer lifts.
- Adjustable beds can elevate clients to a seated or supine position. Adjustable turning beds can be used if incoordination interferes with turning/rolling in bed.
- Bed hand blocks are helpful when beds are too soft for clients to push off from.

Bathing and Showering

Modification of Technique

Note: Safety precautions must be closely adhered to.

- Clients should shower in a seated position for safety.

Use of Adaptive Equipment or Altering the Task Environment

- Use grab bars for safety.
- Use adjustable mounted shower hoses.
- Use tub benches or shower chairs (both with arms for safety).
- Use bath mitts with soap in a pocket or soap on a rope to prevent soap slippage.
- Use suctioned shower caddies with pump soap or suctioned bottles.
- Use temperature-control shower valves to control water temperature.
- Use nonskid mats in and outside the shower/tub.
- Preset water temperature.

Toileting and Toilet Hygiene

Modification of Technique

Note: Safety precautions must be closely adhered to.

- Weighted wrist cuffs may assist with stabilizing the UEs during toileting.

Use of Adaptive Equipment or Altering the Task Environment

- Use toilet seats with arms for safety.
- Bidet-toilet combos or bidet-toilet seats reduce difficulty with wiping.
- Use comfort-wipe extended-handle toilet paper holders or wiping tongs.
- Use toilet seat incline lifts to assist with sit-to-stand transfers.
- Sanitary napkins with adhesive strips are easier to use than tampons.

Personal Hygiene and Grooming

Modification of Technique

- Weighted cuffs on wrists may help with accuracy of grooming activities (Fig. 27-20).
- Clients can delegate assistance with makeup application (eyeliner, mascara).
- Tattooed eyeliner and eyebrows eliminate coordination demands.
- Clients should rest elbows on vanities for proximal stability or hold upper arms close to chest when performing grooming activities.
- Standing in a corner enables clients with incoordination to stabilize their trunk and head on the wall of the clients' side, and their forearms on the wall in front for activities involving the face (e.g., brushing teeth, shaving, applying makeup).[36]
- Using a strap attached to grooming tools that are stabilized around the wrist prevents them from falling.

Use of Adaptive Equipment or Altering the Task Environment

- Electric razors are safer to use and provide more stability.
- Electric toothbrushes are heavier and can be held steady during head movement.
- Use standing hair dryers.
- Large-handled makeup brushes, hair brushes, and toothbrushes facilitate grasp.
- Large lipstick tubes are easier to use than small ones with stabilization of the arms.

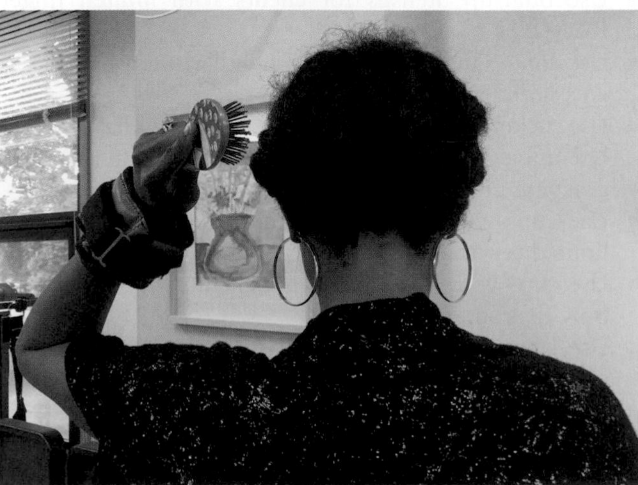

Figure 27-20. Weighted wrist cuffs for grooming activities.

- Stick deodorants are preferable to spray deodorants to avoid accidently spraying the eyes.
- Cutting nails can be unsafe for clients with incoordination. Instead, file nails using an emery board mounted to a flat surface and move nails over the emery board.

Dressing

Modification of Technique

- Button-down shirts are easier to don and doff (consider shirts one size larger or shirts with stretchable microfiber material).
- Velcro closures, zipper pulls, and large buttons are easier to open and close than snaps and hooks.
- Elastic waist pants are easier to don and doff.
- Wrinkle-resistant and stain-shedding materials enable clients to appear well groomed throughout the day.
- Sports bras, step-in bras, and elastic straps on bras make donning and doffing bras easier.

Use of Adaptive Equipment or Altering the Task Environment

- Buttonhooks with enlarged or weighted handles can be used instead of fingers for buttoning.
- Zipper pulls allow ease of pulling zippers up and down.
- Slip-on shoes, shoes with elastic laces, and shoehorns assist with easier shoe donning and doffing, especially for clients with LE ataxia.
- Use sock aids to don and doff socks.

Feeding

Modification of Technique

- Clients should rest elbows on tables for proximal stability.
- Use precut food or have caregivers cut food.
- Use weighted wrist cuffs and/or weighted utensils to improve food-to-mouth time and minimize tremors.[37,38] Recent studies show that weighted utensils and cuffs may not be as effective in decreasing tremors as previously thought[39,40]; however, they are still common practice for clients with tremors.
- Avoid sharp utensils for safety.
- Consider food types being eaten—for example, liquids easily spill and ravioli easily slide off forks.
- Provide hand-over-hand assistance as needed.

Use of Adaptive Equipment or Altering the Task Environment

- Dycem or nonskid surfaces stabilize plates and cups (Fig. 27-21).
- Plate guards and scoop dishes prevent food from falling off plates.
- Use large-handled eating utensils to facilitate grasp, weighted or swivel utensils for stability, and plastic-coated utensils to protect clients' teeth.
- Use universal cuffs for severe incoordination.
- Use cups and water bottles with lids, sipping spouts, or straws to prevent spills.

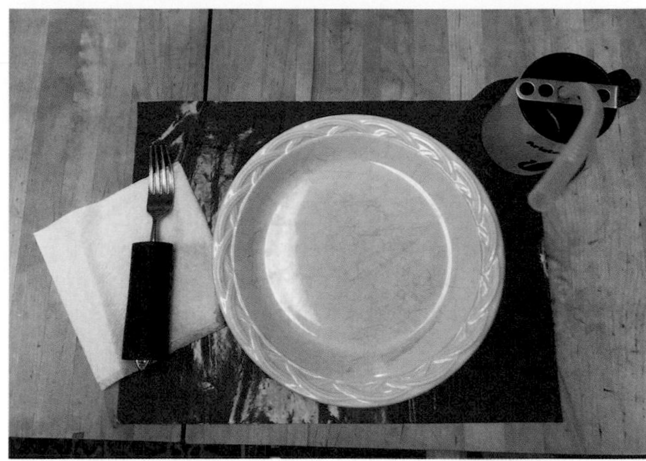

Figure 27-21. Dycem or nonskid surfaces stabilize plates and cups.

- Adaptive utensils accommodate tremors and prevent spillage.
- Cups with long straws that are mounted to wheelchairs and beds prevent spillage and reduce the need to grasp (Fig. 27-22).

Personal Device Care

Modification of Technique

- When applying or removing contacts and hearing aids, stabilize the UEs. Approach eyes from the sides so that the hand can rest on the cheek when applying contacts.
- Wrists weights may minimize tremors.

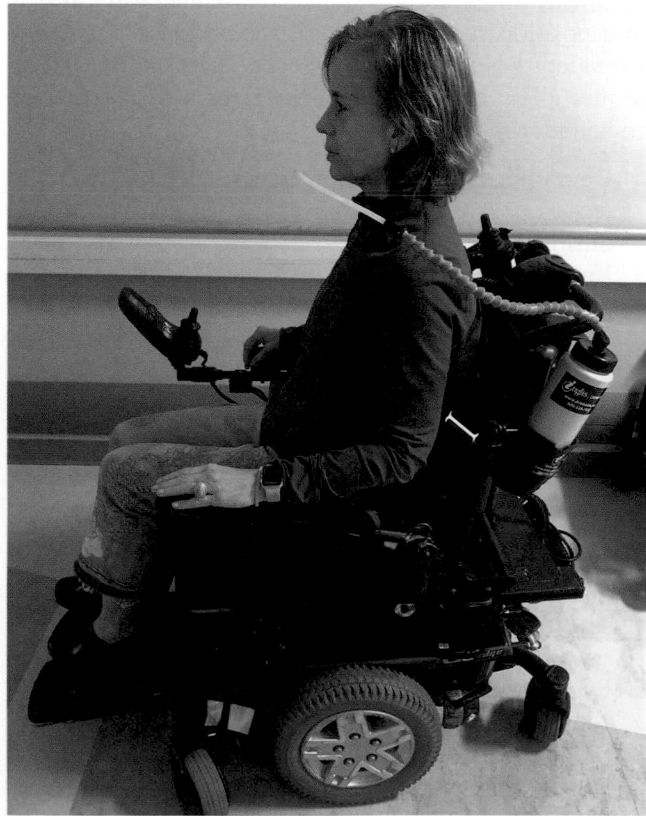

Figure 27-22. Cups with long straws that are mounted to wheelchairs prevent spills and reduce grasp needs.

Use of Adaptive Equipment or Altering the Task Environment

- Use eye drop guides.
- Use eyeglasses on a chain to prevent dropping.

Sexual Activity

Muscle tremors and incoordination can interfere with clients' ability to engage in sexual activity. Physical pain that might accompany uncoordinated and involuntary movements can make sexual activity painful or uncomfortable. The following modifications allow clients with incoordination and poor dexterity to engage in sex:

- Wrist and ankle weights reduce tremor intensity.
- Both partners can stand against a wall or high table. Clients rest the forearms against the table or wall to stabilize the UEs and use their body weight while standing to stabilize the LEs.
- Both partners can kneel with arms resting on a low stool, sofa, or bed, which stabilizes the UEs. Body weight while kneeling stabilizes the LEs.
- Clients can use pillows for comfort and support.

Decreased Sensation

Absent or impaired sensation affect ADL and IADL performance because of the lack of sensory information provided to the motor system. Modification of technique and adaptive equipment to prevent injury is particularly important when interacting with hot or sharp items. Clients with impaired or absent pain, temperature, touch, and position sense should use compensatory strategies for safety when performing ADLs. The following techniques allow clients with impaired or absent sensation to be independent in ADLs:

- Develop habits of attending to the affected part to protect against burns, cuts, pressure sores, and bruising during ADLs.
- Visually inspect the skin for injury and redness regularly during ADLs. Long-handled mirrors can be used to view areas outside the visual field.
- Protect impaired body parts from sharp items or cold/heat. Avoid placing insensate hands in locations outside the visual field.
- Use vision to compensate for decreased sensation and limb position awareness/mobility when using the hands for ADLs.
- Feeding: For loss of sensation in the hands, use built-up handles for feeding to distribute pressure over a greater surface area. Be cautious when holding hot foods right out of the oven or microwave.
- Reduce the amount of force used to grip objects to prevent breaking them and injuring the hand.
- Bathing: Always start and end with cold water when running a bath. Install an anti-scald valve or temperature-control shower valve in the shower to control water temperature and volume. Adjust the water heater thermostat to below 120°F (49°C).[41] Use body parts with intact sensation or bath thermometers to test water temperature.
- Dressing: Select clothes that are snug enough to prevent bunching, but loose enough to avoid binding or excessive pressure. Inspect clothes visually or with an area of intact sensation to avoid wrinkles. Dress warmly in cold weather to prevent frostbite. Fine manipulation needed for fasteners may be affected by decreased hand sensation. Clients can learn to compensate visually or may benefit from larger fasteners or adaptive devices described for people with impaired coordination, such as buttonhooks or Velcro closures.
- Grooming: Use electric razors for safe shaving. Avoid using electric hair curlers, irons, and straighteners.

Loss of Use of One Upper Extremity or One Side of Body

Individuals who have lost use of one UE or one body side (hemiplegia) are taught one-handed techniques to facilitate ADL independence. Clients with cognitive–perceptual disorders, however, may have difficulty learning and retaining information. Many clients who sustained stroke may also have apraxia, a motor perception disorder that affects motor planning and the ability to learn new or perform previously learned motor skills.[42] Clients who do not have cognitive–perceptual disorders will find it easier to complete one-handed ADLs.

Bed Mobility

For clients with lost use of one UE or one body side, it is essential to teach bed mobility techniques that are safe and that protect the affected shoulder. It is possible for such clients to roll in bed, move from a supine to seated position, and move back to supine independently with some modifications in technique. If required, adaptive equipment can be used to increase safety and provide support.

Modification of Technique

See section on Weakness.

Use of Adaptive Equipment or Altering the Task Environment

- Bedrails or halos provide support to allow clients to change positions in bed.
- Electric or adjustable beds with powered head and knee controls assist with sitting in bed.
- Leg lifters assist with lifting the affected LE.

Bathing and Showering

Individuals with lost use of one UE or one body side may have difficulty obtaining and opening supplies for bathing, washing all body parts, and maintaining stability and balance while bathing.

Modification of Technique

- Progress from sponge bathing in bed with assistance from family or caregiver, to sponge bathing at the sink, and then bathing in a walk-in or tub shower.
- It is always recommended to shower instead of bathe because getting up and down from the tub floor is difficult.
- Sitting on a tub bench or shower chair provides more stability than standing in the shower.
- Ensure that all supplies are gathered and placed within easy reach before showering.
- Avoid hot water when bathing because it can temporarily increase weakness, if present.

Use of Adaptive Equipment or Altering the Task Environment

- 3-in-1 commodes allow clients to transfer in and out of the tub without the need to stand. They also allow clients to reach all body parts and bathe in a seated position.
- Grab bars provide support by allowing clients to change positions safely.
- Adjustable handheld shower hoses allow clients to bathe in a seated position and reach all body parts.
- Nonslip mats reduce falls.
- Long-handled sponges, brushes, and toe cleaners allow clients to bathe difficult-to-reach areas.

Toileting and Toilet Hygiene

Donning and doffing clothing to complete toileting activities, sitting on the toilet and maintaining balance, and completing toilet hygiene activities may be difficult for clients who have lost use of one UE or one body side.

Modification of Technique

- Use toilet paper dispensers that are located on the unaffected side.
- Use the unaffected hand to obtain the desired amount of toilet paper.
- Use the unaffected UE to complete toilet hygiene activities.
- Adult diapers or bed pans may also be used to prevent toileting accidents.

Use of Adaptive Equipment or Altering the Task Environment

- One-handed toilet paper dispensers allow clients to retrieve toilet paper with one hand.
- Raised toilet seats allow clients to get on and off the toilet safely.
- 3-in-1 or bedside commodes with or without drop arms allow clients quicker and easier toilet access.
- Grab bars provide stability for clients to change position.
- Comfort-wipe extended-toilet paper holders or tongs allow for perianal hygiene.
- Bidet-toilet combos eliminate the need for toilet paper.

Personal Hygiene and Grooming

Individuals who have lost use of one UE or one side of the body will have difficulty manipulating bottles, grasping, and holding onto grooming supplies.

Modification of Technique

- Clients should complete grooming activities in a seated position.
- Apply toothpaste to brush while it rests on the sink.
- Put toothpaste in the mouth instead of on the toothbrush.
- Arrange needed items within easy reach.
- Stabilize containers with the ulnar digits. Use the radial digits of the same hand to unscrew containers.

Use of Adaptive Equipment or Altering the Task Environment

- Electric razors are easier to use with one hand compared to manual razors.
- Shampoo pumps and automatic dispensers allow clients to wash hair without having to open containers.
- Flip-top bottles for shampoo, lotions, creams, and toothpaste are easier to use with one hand compared to screw-top containers.
- Lightweight and wall-mounted hair dryers allow the unaffected extremity to brush or comb hair while hair is being dried.
- Long-handled combs or brushes can reach all parts of the head.
- Curling brushes allow clients to dry, curl, and brush hair with one device instead of multiple devices.
- Use suction nail brushes or one-handed nail clippers attached to the sink or counter; use long-handled and pistol-grip LE toenail clippers.
- Use suction emery boards to file nails.
- Use dental floss holders or water flossers.
- Use one-handed pump toothpaste dispensers.
- Use electric toothbrushes.
- Use suctioned denture brushes and cleaners (soaking dentures overnight).
- Spray-on instead of roll-on deodorants require less effort and do not require applicators to contact the body.

Dressing

For clients who have lost use of one UE or one body side, dressing activities can be done while seated or standing. If clients present with muscle weakness and decreased balance, safety awareness, or endurance, dressing should be completed while seated. Clients can be seated in standard chairs with arm rests or in wheelchairs with their feet on the floor. Clothes should be placed within the client's reach. Clients with lost use of one UE or body side require compensatory techniques and adaptive equipment to dress themselves independently.[43–45] Clients should always don clothing on the affected extremity first and remove clothing from the unaffected extremity last.

Modification of Technique

Following are modification techniques for upper body dressing and lower body dressing.

Upper Body Dressing

- *Donning and doffing shirts and blouses: Technique 1 (Over-the-Shoulder Method)*

1. Place the shirt on the lap, label facing up, collar toward the abdomen, with the sleeve of the affected arm hanging between the knees (Video 27-12).
2. Use the unaffected hand to put the affected hand into the sleeve and lean forward to let gravity extend the elbow. Using the unaffected hand, slide the sleeve onto the affected arm while holding onto the shirt.
3. Grasp the collar at the point closest to the unaffected side.
4. Hold tightly to the collar, lean slightly forward, and bring the collar and shirt around the affected side and behind the neck to the unaffected side.
5. Put the unaffected hand into the other armhole and raise the arm out and up to push through the sleeve.
6. To straighten the shirt, lean forward slightly, and use the unaffected arm to work the shirt down over the shoulders. Reach back and pull the tail down; straighten the sleeve under the affected axilla with the unaffected UE.
7. To button the shirt or blouse, align the shirt fronts and match each button with the correct buttonhole. Use one-handed buttoning or a buttonhook, beginning from the bottom up.
8. To doff, unbutton the shirt and use the unaffected hand to throw the shirt off the unaffected shoulder. Work the shirt sleeve off the unaffected arm, pressing the shirt cuff against the leg to pull the arm out. Lean forward slightly and use the unaffected hand to pull the shirt across the back and off the affected arm (Video 27-13).

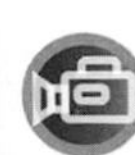

- *Donning and doffing shirts and blouses: Technique 2 (overhead method):* This method is less confusing for patients with selected perceptual impairments or limited unaffected UE reach.

1. Place the shirt on the lap, label facing up, and collar next to the abdomen; drape the shirttail over the knees.
2. Pick up the affected hand and put it into the sleeve.
3. Pull the sleeve up over the elbow to avoid the hand falling out when continuing to don the shirt.
4. Put the unaffected hand into the armhole. Raise the arm and push it through the sleeve as far as possible.
5. Gather the back of the shirt from tail to collar.
6. Hold the gathered shirt up, lean forward, tuck chin, and put the shirt over the head.
7. To straighten the shirt, lean forward and work the shirt down over the shoulders. Often, shirts get caught on the affected shoulder and must be pushed back over the shoulder.
8. Reach back and pull the shirt down.
9. To button the shirt or blouse, align the shirt fronts and match each button with the current buttonhole. Start buttoning one handed or with a buttonhook from the bottom up.
10. To doff, unbutton the shirt, lean forward, and use the unaffected hand to gather the shirt up over the back of the neck. Tuck chin, pull shirt over the head, then take the shirt off the unaffected arm first.

- *Donning and doffing pullover garments*

1. Place the pullover garment on the lap, bottom toward chest, and label facing down.
2. Using the unaffected hand, roll up the bottom edge of the shirt back, all the way up to the sleeve on the affected side.
3. Spread the armhole opening as large as possible. Using the unaffected hand, place the affected arm into the armhole and pull the sleeve up onto the arm past the elbow. Alternatively, the sleeve may be positioned between the legs as described in Technique 1 for shirts and blouses.
4. Insert the unaffected arm into the other sleeve.
5. Gather the shirt back from the bottom edge to the neck, lean forward, tuck the chin, and pass the shirt over the head.
6. Adjust the shirt on the unaffected side up and onto the shoulder, and remove twists.
7. To doff a pullover garment, start at the top back, gather the shirt up, lean forward, tuck chin, and pull the shirt forward over the head. Remove the unaffected arm and then the affected arm.

- *Donning and doffing bras*

1. For back closure bras, position the bra with the cups in the back and pull the straps in front. The bra on the affected side can be held in position by tucking it between the trunk and the affected arm. Hook the fasteners in the front at waist level. Use the unaffected side to rotate the bra so the hook moves to the back and the cups in front. Place the strap over the affected shoulder with the unaffected side. Hook the unaffected thumb under the strap on the unaffected side and pull it over the shoulder.

2. For front-opening bras, position the bra with the cups in the front. The bra on the affected side can be held in position by tucking it between the trunk and the affected arm. Hook the fasteners in the front at waist level. Place the strap over the affected shoulder with the unaffected side. Hook the unaffected thumb under the strap on the unaffected side and pull it over the shoulder.
3. Step-in bras and sports bras can be easier to use and should be donned and doffed using Technique 2, overhead method described for shirts and blouses.
4. A heavier woman may need an adapted front-closing bra if she cannot approximate the two edges of the bra to fasten it. The bra is adapted with a D-ring on the side of the bra opening on the affected side and a pile Velcro strap on the opposite side. After the bra is around the waist, the strap is threaded through the D-ring and pulled to bring the two bra ends together. Hook Velcro must be stitched onto the bra so the strap can be fastened.

Lower Body Dressing

The following techniques described for donning and doffing pants that can be used for underwear.

- *Donning and doffing pants in a seated position*

1. The client should be seated on a firm surface with feet on the floor and unaffected limb beyond the midline of the body for balance.
2. Grasp the ankle or calf of the affected leg with the unaffected UE and cross the affected leg over the unaffected leg. Alternatively, cup under the affected knee with clasped hands to lift and cross the leg.
3. Pull the pant over the affected leg up to but not above the knee.
4. Uncross the legs.
5. Put the unaffected leg into the other pant leg.
6. Remain sitting. Pull the pants up above the knees as far as possible.
7. To prevent the pants from dropping when standing, put the affected hand into the pant pocket or the thumb into a belt loop. Alternatively, use a pant clip to attach the pants to the shirt so they do not slide down. Pants with elastic waistbands are also less likely to slide when standing up.
8. Stand up. Pull the pants over the hips; button and zip pants while standing. If clients need support while standing, have them lean against a wall or table. Alternatively, clients with poor balance may remain seated and pull the pants up over the hips by shifting from side to side; they should button and zip pants while seated.
9. To doff pants, unfasten the pants while sitting. Stand and let the pants drop past the knees or push the pants down if wearing elastic waist garments. Sit and remove pants from the unaffected leg. Cross the affected leg over the unaffected leg. Remove the pants from the affected leg. Uncross the legs.
10. For clients with poor balance, pants should be doffed in a seated position. Unfasten the pants. Work the pants down on the hips as far as possible by shifting weight from side to side in the chair. Use the unaffected arm to work the pants down past the hip. Remove the pants from the unaffected leg. Cross the affected leg over the unaffected leg. Remove the pants from the affected leg and uncross the legs.

- *Donning and doffing pants in bed*: See section on Weakness.
- *Donning and doffing socks or stockings*

1. The affected leg is crossed over the unaffected leg using the technique described for donning pants in a seated position.
2. The sock is opened by inserting the thumb and index finger of the unaffected hand into the top of the sock and spreading the fingers.
3. Put the sock on the foot by slipping the toes into the opening made under the spread hand. The sock is then pulled over the heel and over the whole leg. Wrinkles are smoothened.
4. Repeat the process for the unaffected leg.
5. To doff socks, the legs are positioned in the same position required for donning, and the socks are pushed off the foot using the unaffected hand.
6. Sock aids are not useful for people who have lost use of one UE because it is difficult to get the sock onto the aid with only one UE.

- *Donning and doffing shoes*

1. Loafers are put on the affected foot with shoes on the floor. Lift the affected leg by clasping the unaffected hand under the knee. Then place the foot into the shoe. Shoehorns are used to ease the foot into shoes.
2. For tie shoes, cross the affected leg over the unaffected leg. Put the shoe on by grasping the shoe heel with the unaffected hand and work it back and forth over the heel until it goes on completely. Adapted shoe closures such as elastic laces or Velcro ties can be used. Alternatively, one-handed shoe-tying techniques can be used, but require good cognitive, perceptual, and motor planning skills.
3. To doff shoes, either cross the affected leg over the unaffected leg and pull the shoe up with the unaffected hand, or place the unaffected foot behind the shoe heel on the affected side and push the affected leg forward while pushing on the shoe heel to pull it off.

- *Donning and doffing ankle-foot orthoses*
  1. Place the ankle-foot orthosis in the shoe.
  2. The shoe laces or ties should be loose enough to allow maximum room for inserting the foot into the orthosis and shoe.
  3. Use the techniques described for donning shoes to get the foot into the orthosis and shoe.
  4. Apply pressure on the knee with the foot flat on the floor to insert the heel into the shoe.
  5. The orthosis acts as a shoehorn as the foot slides into the shoe.
  6. To doff orthosis, use the techniques described for removing shoes, while pushing down on the orthosis with the unaffected hand to assist with getting the shoes and orthosis off.

Use of Adaptive Equipment or Altering the Task Environment

- Long-handled dressing sticks assist clients in donning and doffing LE clothing.
- Use bras with Velcro front clasps.
- Use buttonhooks to manipulate buttons with one hand or Velcro strips in place of buttons.
- Clip-on neck ties or pretied conventional ties are easier to use than tying a tie.
- Use shoes with elastic laces or Velcro strap shoes.
- Use long-handled shoehorns to reach shoes while seated.
- Use reachers to retrieve clothing from closets.
- Use stocking aids to reach feet and pull up socks.
- Use fabric loops around sock cuffs to pull up socks by hooking fingers in the loop.

Feeding

The following modification techniques were developed for clients with spinal cord injury. Clients with lost use of one UE or one body side may experience difficulty with tasks such as simultaneously holding a fork and cutting foods with a knife.

Modification of Technique

- Place the affected UE on the table and use the table surface to support the arm while eating.
- Use precut meats and vegetables or have caregivers cut them.

Use of Adaptive Equipment or Altering the Task Environment

- Use of a spork, which combines a spoon and fork, reduces the need to change utensils while eating.
- Rocker knives with or without T-handles allow clients with UE weakness to cut food with one hand using a rocking motion (reduces strength requirements).
- Plate guards and long-lipped plates allow easier scooping of food.
- Dycem or nonskid mats prevent plate movement while eating.
- Food can be stored in containers with easy-open lids for one-handed use.

Personal Device Care

The following modification techniques were developed for clients with spinal cord injury. Clients who have lost use of one UE or one body side may have difficulty using and managing personal devices with one hand.

Modification of Technique

- Sit at a table with the affected arm supported while using, cleaning, and maintaining personal devices.
- Place needed personal devices in close proximity to each other and in easy-to-reach locations.

Use of Adaptive Equipment or Altering the Task Environment

- Large flip-top contact lens cases can be opened and closed with one hand.
- Autosqueeze eye drop bottle dispensers can be operated with one hand.
- Automatic glucose and blood pressure monitors can be used with one hand, have fewer buttons to use (e.g., automatic on/off and no coding), and have multiple strips filled in the drum that eliminate strip reinsertion at each use.

Sexual Activity

The following modification techniques were developed for clients with spinal cord injury. Several resources discuss sexuality after stroke.[21,45,46] It is important to consider clients' sexuality and body image, fears about resuming sex, bowel and bladder control, birth control, pregnancy, decreased endurance, erectile dysfunction, alternative positions, and sexual activity other than intercourse. For a description of compensatory strategies and adaptive devices for clients having sustained a stroke, see the section on Sexual Activity under Weakness.

Lower Extremity Amputation

The following modification techniques were developed for clients with spinal cord injury. LE amputation is the removal of all or part of the LE on one or both sides.[47] Clients with LE amputations can benefit from many of the adaptations described for people with limited mobility caused by weakness or limited ROM; however, lower body dressing is unique owing to prosthetic device use. Prior to dressing, clients should change the shoe and/or sock on their prosthesis to match the day's clothing.

- Clients with transtibial (below knee) amputations with pants wide enough to pull up to the knee should dress while seated using the following steps:
  1. Place the pants over the unaffected and amputated leg, pulling pants as far up as possible.
  2. Clients who are stable standing on one leg can stand to pull pants up over the hips and fasten them. They can then sit down to don the residual limb stocking and prosthesis, exposing the area by sliding the pant leg up over the knee.

3. Clients who are not stable standing on one leg should remain seated and don the prosthesis before standing to pull up their pants. This allows stability of both LEs when standing to pull up pants over the hips.

- Clients with transfemoral (above knee) or transtibial amputations who wish to wear fitted pants that cannot slide over the knees should use the following steps to dress:

1. Slide the end of the pant leg for the amputated limb over the top of the prosthesis so that the prosthesis is dressed first. The shoe and limited ankle mobility will prevent the pants from sliding over the prosthetic foot.
2. Don the stocking and prosthesis.
3. Place the unaffected leg into the pants, stand to pull pants over the hips, and fasten.

Low or Limited Vision

The following modification techniques were developed for clients with spinal cord injury. Low vision is defined as visual acuity of 20/70 or worse in the better eye that is not correctable through surgery, pharmaceuticals, glasses, or contact lenses.[48] It can be caused by eye diseases, inherited conditions of the eye, aging conditions of the eye, and trauma. Eye diseases that cause low vision include, but are not limited to, age-related macular degeneration (ARMD), glaucoma, diabetic retinopathy, and retinitis pigmentosa.[49] Depending on the disease or causative factor, vision loss may include blurred vision, lost sight in certain visual fields, blind spots called scotomas, tunnel vision, low-contrast sensitivity, or lack of glare modulation.[49] Low vision can impact people of all ages but is primarily associated with older adults, although it is not a normal part of aging.[50] Low vision places people at risk for falls and other injuries and decreases ADL performance. Impaired psychosocial adaptation, social isolation, and depression frequently occur in older adults with low vision.[51] Many compensatory strategies and techniques can be taught, including the use of residual vision, modifying the environment, and using adaptive equipment to support safe ADL performance.

Meyers[52] outlined four intervention steps for clients with low vision to assist clinical decision-making. Therapists should move through steps 1 to 4 for each intervention task.

1. Maximize visual functioning. Refer the client to the eye doctor to obtain best-corrected vision. Therapists should work with clients to identify and use remaining best vision to compensate for areas of lost vision.
2. Modify the task or environment to enhance visual performance. Use bigger items and magnification devices, increase contrast, simplify or increase visual cues, sit closer, increase or change lighting, decrease glare, and decrease clutter.
3. Modify tasks or environments to reduce or eliminate visual performance. Use tactile cueing or touch, use smell to identify items, use auditory output devices, store items in the same location and order to enhance memory, and substitute different tools or items that do not require vision to accomplish the task.
4. Eliminate tasks or ask caregivers to complete tasks.

The following modification techniques were developed for clients with spinal cord injury. For clients with substantial vision loss, consider referring individuals to low vision optometrists, certified low vision specialists, rehabilitation teachers, orientation and mobility specialists, or specialized low vision occupational therapists for expert guidance in obtaining the appropriate magnification devices and technology.

General recommendations to support clients with low vision include:

- Increase lighting: Use higher watt bulbs and additional room lighting. Use floor or table lamps with hoods (over lights) and adjustable necks to increase illumination directly onto ADL task areas and away from the eyes to avoid glare.
- Reduce glare: Use blinds, curtains, or tinted windows to control outside glare, cover shiny surfaces, and avoid too much lighting (which can create glare).
- Maximize contrast: Increase contrast on objects and surroundings compared to backgrounds (as shown in table arrangement in Fig. 27-21).
- Organize and label items: Reduce clutter in drawers, shelves, and closets. Organize items by maintaining commonly used items together. Label items with markers on high-contrast backgrounds.
- Use tactile cues (e.g., Velcro, buttons, raised marker pens) to identify and differentiate objects, or indicate orientation.
- Use auditory cues on devices such as blood pressure cuffs, glucometers, and alarms.
- Use sense of smell to identify products.
- Remove hazards such as clutter in walkways. Organize furniture consistently to support safe movement.

Bathing and Showering

The following modification techniques were developed for clients with spinal cord injury. Clients with low vision may have difficulty locating and identifying similarly sized bottles and supplies and being safe in the bathroom. The following techniques enable clients with low vision to be safe and functional while bathing and showering.

- Use high contrast in the bathroom between tubs, floors, showers, and bathing equipment to enhance safety.
- Maintain bathing supplies in the same area and order.

- Use visual cues, such as different colored bottles and caps/lids, or adhere different colored tapes to bottles and supplies.
- Use visual or tactile cues to identify hot/cold water faucets or to identify direction in a unilevered faucet.
- Use color-contrasted soap.
- Feel for water level when filling the tub, use talking bath thermometers, lower hot water temperature to below 120°F (49°C), or use temperature-control shower valves.

Toileting and Toilet Hygiene

The following modification techniques were developed for clients with spinal cord injury. Clients with low vision may have difficulty locating the toilet, transferring safely onto the seat, locating grab bars for sit-to-stand support, and locating toilet paper. Modifications to the toilet include the following:

- Select toilet seats or toilets that contrast with the floor color.
- Place contrasting colored tape or nonskid mats on the floor around the toilet base.
- Maintain toilet paper in the same, easy-to-reach, clutter-free area against a contrasting colored surface.
- Use bidet-toilets or toilet seat-bidet combos to ensure thorough cleaning.

Personal Hygiene and Grooming

The following modification techniques were developed for clients with spinal cord injury. Grooming often includes the use of small tools and the application of materials to small areas, which can be difficult for clients with low vision. Techniques that enable clients with low vision to complete grooming activities independently include the following:

- Use magnifiers, lighted magnifiers, or magnified mirror stands to identify small objects or see the face.
- Use labeled tray dividers to hold items like cosmetics and hygiene supplies.
- Organize supplies in the same order using a technique that is intuitive to the client.
- Group commonly used items together. For example, put hair dryers, curling irons, brushes, and other related supplies in a one-handled basket that fits beneath the sink.
- For safety, use electric razors, electric nose and ear hair trimmers, and hair removal creams.
- Use smell to identify supplies.
- Place toothpaste on a finger and then on the toothbrush. Or, squeeze toothpaste into mouth or a cup, and dip toothbrush in.
- Use fingers to apply cosmetics to face area.
- Use the fingers of one hand as a guide when shaving sideburns or applying eyebrow pencil.
- Use emery boards to file nails.
- Avoid aerosol sprays; clients with low vision cannot see the extent of spray.

Dressing

- Increase closet lighting.
- Label drawers with large print or tactile cues.
- Use large colored ribbons tied to closet poles to divide garments into sections for the identification of color, type, and specific outfits.
- Maintain adaptive dressing devices in the same place.
- Maintain shoes in their original boxes, label boxes in large print or tactile cues for identification, and store in a systematic way. When storing shoes, tie them together in pairs, or slip one inside the other.
- Pin dirty socks together so that socks stay matched when laundered.
- Place small safety pins or other tactile cues inside clothing so that it is worn in the correct orientation.
- Place tactile labels (e.g., Hi-Marks pen dots, iron-on tape) inside clothes to identify colors and match clothing.
- Talking "color identifiers" or phone apps are available in several models from low vision dealers. When pointed at objects, they verbally identify colors.
- An inexpensive voice labeling system called "Pen Friend" allows easy recording onto self-adhesive labels.
- Ask caregivers to place accessories in bags and hang them with appropriate outfits.
- Ask caregivers to hang matching outfits together.

Feeding

The following modification techniques were developed for clients with spinal cord injury. Clients with low vision may have difficulty setting up, arranging, and identifying the location of cups, plates, and utensils. Understanding the location of food on plates, cutting food, and spearing food with a fork may be challenging. Feeding adaptations for clients with low vision include the following:

- Use dishes, cups, and napkins that contrast with the table or table linens.
- Pour liquids into contrasting colored cups (e.g., coffee in a white mug). When pouring liquids, the correct amount can be determined by inserting a clean finger over the cup rim to feel when the liquid is near the top. Liquid-level indicators placed on cup rims provide auditory signals when cups are nearly full.
- Caregivers can use the clock method to describe food location on plates (e.g., meat at 6:00, vegetables at 3:00). Different food items (e.g., meats, vegetables) can be served in consistent locations on plates.
- To locate utensils, plates, and glasses, use a place mat and set items in a grid form. Ensure high contrast between placemat and items.
- To cut food, find food edges with a fork. Move the fork a bite-sized amount into the meat, and then cut the food, keeping the knife in contact with the fork.
- Place main dishes, side dishes, seasonings, and condiments in a semicircle or straight line just outside

the client's place setting area. Place items in the same order at each meal. Shake seasonings into the palm; then apply to food in pinches. Pour ketchup, mustard, sauces, and liquid seasonings in small side bowls or on the side of plates for dipping or spooning as needed.

- Use tactile cues to identify similarly shaped or colored containers, like salt and pepper shakers.
- Use dinner plates with raised lips to avoid spills while eating.
- When reaching for table items, curl fingers and move them slowly along the table until they reach items.

Personal Device Care

- Use tactile cues, visual cues, and olfaction to identify personal care products and cleaners.
- Substitute medical devices with audio output devices such as glucometers and blood pressure cuffs.
- Use handheld or tabletop magnification aids with or without lights.

Bariatric Considerations

The following modification techniques were developed for clients with spinal cord injury. The World Health Organization defines overweight and obesity as abnormal or excessive fat accumulation that may impair health.[53] Body mass index (BMI), calculated as body weight in kilograms divided by height in meters squared (kg/m^2), is commonly used to identify overweight and obesity in adults.[53] In adults, BMIs between 18.5 and 25 are desirable. BMIs between 25 and 30 are classified as overweight, 30+ are obese, and 40+ are morbidly obese. Bariatrics is a health care field that relates to or specializes in the investigation, prevention, and treatment of obesity.[54,55]

Obesity can aggravate osteoarthritis, damage joint structures, destroy cartilage, and cause spinal and peripheral nerve compression—which can lead to difficulty moving and reaching, decreased activity tolerance and mobility, and difficulty accessing the environment. Excessively large individuals with a medical condition may have more occupational performance deficits than are typically seen because of preexisting limitations in strength relative to body mass, limited reach, and decreased endurance.

It is important to complete a thorough functional assessment to identify all occupational performance challenges and to determine the most appropriate adaptive equipment.[56] Most standard DME is manufactured to serve individuals weighing approximately 250 to 300 lb. Individuals weighing more must have specialized equipment ordered. Bariatric equipment is made extra wide and with materials to provide stable support for obese and morbidly obese individuals. It is important to identify body type and fat distribution to determine the proper equipment that fits the client and environment. Some modifications that can assist in functional activities in bariatric care are outlined in the subsequent sections.

Bed Mobility

- Use handrails, halos, or overhead trapeze bars for repositioning and moving from supine to sitting in bed.
- Electronic bariatric beds are designed to allow for capacities of up to 1,000 lb. They can also be electronically adjusted to assist bed mobility and positioning.
- Overhead lifts and Hoyer lifts used with slings can mechanically assist with turning and repositioning.

Bathing and Showering

- If clients have difficulty standing, bathe while seated on bariatric shower commode chairs, tub seats, tub transfer benches, or shower chairs with or without backs. If back support is required, choose seats with an open area in the lower back to accommodate posterior body mass when seated.
- Use long-handled sponges to wash LEs, back, and buttocks.
- Use long-handled sponges in different sizes to wash between skin folds and difficult-to-reach areas.
- Heavy-duty grab bars can be installed to provide assistance for sit-to-stand transfers to wash and rinse the body.
- Use of adjustable handheld shower hoses allows clients to bathe safely without the need to stand to access areas between skin folds and difficult-to-reach body parts.
- Clients should rinse well and end with cool water to lower skin temperature.
- Use clean towels to dry off. Extra care is needed on areas where skin contacts skin. Use fans or hair dryers (set on cool) to dry skin.
- If clients cannot get into the tub or shower, sponge bathe with assistance at the sink, while seated in a wheelchair or bed. Caregivers can assist to reach and lift skin folds and to access difficult-to-reach places.

Toileting and Toilet Hygiene

- Use reachers and dressing sticks to pull up garments after toileting.
- Use comfort-wipe extended-handle toilet paper holders or toilet tongs to hold/release tissue and extend reach for hygienic cleaning.
- Toilet seat-bidets or toilet-bidet combos eliminate the need for wiping.
- Use raised toilet seats that can accommodate weight.
- Use heavy-duty bariatric commodes that stand alone or over the toilet as a safety frame. Extra wide seats can be ordered. Drop-arm commodes allow transfers when clients cannot stand.

Personal Hygiene and Grooming

- Use spray products such as dry shampoo, hair spray, and deodorant to compensate for decreased reach.
- Wall-mounted hair dryers allow hair to be dried without holding and raising the hair dryer.
- Use long-handled mirrors for skin inspection (Fig. 27-23).
- Use long-handled brushes and combs.
- Portable and inflatable wash basins allow hair to be washed in bed by caregivers.

Dressing

The following modification techniques were developed for clients with spinal cord injury. Clients with obesity have many body areas with skin folds where skin consistently contacts skin. Air cannot circulate in these areas, and moisture builds, creating irritation and an environment for bacteria and yeast growth.

- Clients should wear natural fibers (such as cotton or rayon) that breathe and pull moisture away from the body, allowing it to evaporate.
- Washable liners should be placed under bras and abdominal liners between skin folds to absorb perspiration and prevent skin irritation.
- For the upper body, wear pullover or front-opening clothing that is stretchable and nonconstrictive. Dressing sticks can be used to assist upper body dressing.
- Wear pants with elastic waists to eliminate the need to reach for zippers and buttons. Use dressing sticks or reachers to don and doff lower body clothing.
- Wear nonbinding extra-width socks. Cotton and polypropylene are best for absorbing perspiration.
- To don socks, use a deluxe sock aid that is flexible, soft, and made larger.

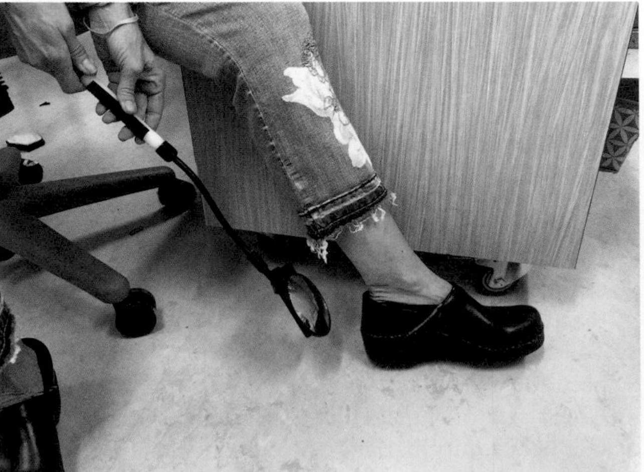

Figure 27-23. Long-handled mirrors for skin inspection.

- Slip-on shoes, elastic laces, and Velcro strap shoes can compensate for difficulty reaching the feet. Long-handled shoehorns assist with donning shoes.
- Reachers can be used to retrieve items from the floor and surrounding areas.

Sexual Activity

The following modification techniques were developed for clients with spinal cord injury. Studies of sexual function in obese patients in clinical settings show a relationship between obesity and lower levels of sexual functioning, especially erectile dysfunction.[57] Positioning can be challenging with larger body sizes and cause increased joint pain. Experiment with positions that alleviate each partner's joint stress. Use large firm pillows for support and positioning. For sexual intercourse, suggested positions include spooning, rear entry, and modified missionary positions with pillows supporting the hips and back.

Memory Deficits

The following modification techniques were developed for clients with spinal cord injury. Cognition involves the ability to perceive, understand, and make use of information.[58] An important component of cognition is memory, which includes storing and retrieving information for use. Memory deficits can have significant impact on clients' ability to remember ADL steps and sequences. Strategies that can assist clients with memory deficits in independent ADL performance include:

- Use of graded cueing strategies beginning with verbal, then visual, and finally tactile cues.
- Simplifying activities by breaking them into small steps.
- Reducing the amount of physical, visual, and auditory clutter in the environment.
- Developing lists of needed ADL and the order in which they should to be completed.
- Posting large, visual, step-by-step instructions in the areas where ADLs are performed (such as toileting instructions in front of the commode).
- Using alarms to remind clients when ADLs need to be completed (such as toileting routines, and eating and medication schedules).
- Journaling to remember tasks that need to be or have been completed.
- Using labels on containers, bottles, and cupboards as organizational reminders.
- Lists, alarms, journals, and reminders can be configured on smartphones and tablets because of programming ease and information portability.
- Intelligent assistive technologies help clients with memory deficits in ADL performance, such as the Archipel (assists with cooking) and COACH (assists with hand washing).[59–61]

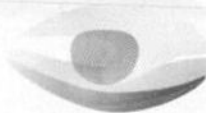

CASE STUDY

Patient Information

Lena is an 82-year-old Asian female who lives with her husband in a one-floor, elevator apartment in Chinatown. She has two grown children who live over 4 hours away by car. Every morning, Lena participates in a Tai Chi class in her apartment building. On her way to class, she lost her balance while descending a curb and fell onto the asphalt. She was helped to stand by several people but was unable to bear weight on her right leg. Lena was taken to the hospital where an x-ray revealed a nondisplaced fracture of the right femoral head. Her medical management at the acute care hospital included surgical open reduction, internal fixation (ORIF) of the right hip (hip pinning). The next morning and throughout the day after surgery, Lena's nurses reported that she was very lethargic and had reduced motor activity, confusion, and incoherent speech. She was diagnosed with postoperative hypoactive delirium. At post-op day 3, Lena was still lethargic and had difficulty with short-term memory, but was less confused and spoke coherently. When asked, Lena could not recall her hip precautions. She was discharged to a skilled nursing facility the next day.

Reason for Occupational Therapy Referral

Lena was referred for subacute rehabilitation services that included OT to increase ADL independence. She was weight bearing as tolerated (WBAT) and was required to follow hip precautions. Her cognitive status was of concern as it impacted her safety and judgment during ADLs. Prior to falling, Lena was independent in ADLs. She cooked both lunch and dinner daily for herself and husband. Lena was very active in her community and participated in the occupations of gardening, Tai Chi, and Chinese sword dancing without assistance. Her medical history included osteoporosis and depression.

Assessment Process and Results

The subacute OT evaluation began with an occupational profile interview. Lena revealed that she lives with her husband in a step-free, elevator apartment. She was able to identify her meaningful occupations and could describe a typical day in her life. Lena told the therapist that she does not use any equipment and has one bathroom with a tub/shower without grab bars, and a small kitchen. She was oriented to her name, but not to date. Lena knew that she was in a hospital but did not know the hospital name. She could not recall any of her hip precautions.

Assessment showed Lena's UE ROM and muscle strength to be within functional limits (WFL). Sensation of BUEs was intact. Pain was a 7/10 for the right hip. Moderate assistance (FIM 3) was needed to move from supine to sitting at bedside. A bed-to-chair transfer using a rolling walker required maximum assistance (FIM 2). Upper body dressing required minimal assistance (FIM 4). Lower body dressing using long-handled devices required maximum assistance (FIM 2). Upper body bathing (at sink) required modified independence. Lower body bathing (at sink) using long-handled devices required maximum assistance (FIM 2). Lena required verbal cues to maintain hip precautions during the evaluation.

Occupational Therapy Problem List

- Decreased independence in BADLs and IADLs
- Decreased performance in transfers
- Decreased memory (leading to safety concerns during ADLs/IADLs)
- Pain in right hip

Occupational Therapy Goal List (By Discharge in 2 Weeks)

- Modified independence with lower body dressing using long-handled devices
- Modified independence with lower body bathing using long-handled devices and tub bench
- Decreased pain in hip to 3/10 during ADLs
- Independence in bed mobility
- Modified independence in all transfers using a rolling walker/cane
- Communicate and demonstrate an understanding of hip precautions during all ADLs
- Modified independence in small meal preparation

Intervention

The first day of treatment began in Lena's room with bed mobility (supine to sit) while adhering to hip precautions. Lena appeared more upbeat and reported her pain at a 3/10, which she attributed to a good night sleep and taking pain medication 30 minutes before therapy. The therapist reviewed hip precautions with Lena and described supine-to-sit movements before beginning. Lena was then instructed to roll onto her left side, push up with her arms, and bring her legs off the bed to a sitting position. She required minimal assistance to move the right leg off the bed.

The therapist adjusted the bed height to assist with transfers from sit to stand to rolling walker. Once seated on the bed edge, Lena was instructed to push off with both hands, making certain not to flex her hip above 90° by straightening the right affected leg out in front when standing. Once standing, she grasped the walker and took small steps toward a chair. Lena required standby assistance and two verbal cues for correct hand placement as she reached for the walker before standing. She walked 10 feet to the chair with close supervision. Lena was instructed to feel the chair on the back of her legs before sitting. When lowering herself to the chair, the therapist instructed her to reach back for the chair arm with one hand and hold onto the walker with the other hand. When lowering herself to the chair, she was instructed to slide the involved leg out in front. Lena was able to follow these steps with one verbal cue to remind her to reach back with one hand.

(continued)

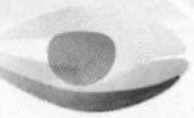

CASE STUDY *(continued)*

The treatment session concluded with Lena practicing lower body dressing from the chair. When asked, Lena was able to recall two-thirds hip precautions. Lena required minimal assistance to don her socks using a sock aid. To don her elastic pants, Lena was instructed to use a reacher to grasp and lower her pants waist toward the floor to dress the affected LE first, followed by the unaffected leg. Then, using the reacher, she raised her pants above her knees toward her hips. Lena then stood with her walker and pulled her pants above her hips. Lena required minimal assistance to stand to pull up her pants, and verbal cues to use the reacher and maintain hip precautions. She was able to don her slip-on shoes with a long-handled shoehorn.

In subsequent sessions, the therapist worked with Lena to further improve her ADL status to modified independence while adhering to hip precautions. Lena became more oriented and interactive in therapy sessions. The therapist also worked with Lena on Tai Chi from a seated position and asked Lena to teach her several movements. This helped prevent deconditioning of Lena's UEs and began reengagement in one of her identified meaningful occupations. Lena was very excited to show the therapist Tai Chi movements and decided to perform Tai Chi in a chair every morning after breakfast. Because Lena cooks at home, Lena and the therapist practiced using her walker to retrieve kitchen items from the refrigerator, cabinets, and oven. At the end of her stay, Lena prepared a small side dish for a traditional Chinese meal while using her rolling walker with a tray to transport cooking items. By discharge, Lena demonstrated safety during all ADLs, and her mild cognitive confusion and decreased memory resolved. Discharge plans included recommendations for home care OT to address safety during ADLs in the home, and ordering of a tub bench and raised toilet seat.

Evidence Table of Studies for ADL Interventions

Intervention	Description	Participants	Dosage	Research Design and Evidence Level	Benefit	Statistical Significance and Effect Size
Use of everyday life occupations and a client-centered approach in stroke rehabilitation[62]	Varied OT interventions that used a client-centered approach or occupation. Interventions included therapeutic occupations or adaptive or compensatory occupations for stroke rehabilitation.	Twenty-five studies with a total of 2,792 patients, relatives, and staff; 75 OTs or staff members; and 9 systematic reviews/ meta-analyses	Use of client-centered approaches and everyday occupations varied across included studies.	Systematic review Level I	Using a client-centered approach and/or every day occupations in OT intervention resulted in improved outcomes in ADLs and participation.	No statistical analysis
Comparison of two groups of adults with stroke. Control group received a predischarge home visit only and intervention group received additional training in bathing assistive devices (ADs)[63]	Both groups received prescription and training for bathing ADs in the hospital. Control group received a predischarge home visit, but no treatment postdischarge. Intervention group received additional home-based training in AD use by occupational therapists upon discharge including AD use in home and safety.	Fifty-three older adults with stroke randomly assigned to intervention ($n = 30$) and control ($n = 23$) groups	At least two, but not more than three follow-up home services, were provided to intervention group. Control group received one predischarge home visit, but no intervention at home.	Randomized controlled trial Level I	Home visits and training in bathing ADs improved independence level, AD use, and satisfaction with AD use for older adults with stroke.	FIM pretest–posttest total mean difference (MD) and motor MD were higher in intervention than control group ($p < 0.001$). At 3 months, FIM motor scores were higher in intervention than control group ($p = 0.051$). QUEST mean score was higher in intervention (4.63) than control group (3.72).
Efficacy of OT interventions in clients with dementia to recover or strengthen residual functional capacities[64]	Both groups received OT ADL interventions to recover or improve function including washing, personal hygiene, dressing, sanitary services, and eating.	Thirty-five clients with dementia and moderate-to-severe cognitive impairment (14 = vascular dementia, 20 = Alzheimer dementia)	ADL interventions for 40 days including washing, personal hygiene, dressing, sanitary services, and eating	Two group pretest–posttest design Level II	OT ADL interventions improved functional performance in ADLs for individuals with dementia.	Clients in both groups showed statistically significant improvements in washing, sanitary services use, and dressing ($p < 0.00$) measured on the RBEB. No significant differences between groups. Improvements seen in personal hygiene and nutritional functions, but not statistically significant.

References

1. American Occupational Therapy Association. Occupational therapy practice framework: domain & process 3rd edition. *Am J Occup Ther*. 2014;68(suppl 1):S1–S48. doi:10.5014/ajot.2014.682006.
2. Canadian Association of Occupational Therapists. *Enabling Occupations: An Occupational Therapy Perspective*. 2nd ed. Ottawa, ON: CAOT Publication ACE; 2002. https://www.caot.ca/client/product2/68/itemFromIndex.html.
3. World Federation of Occupational Therapists. Position statement: activities of daily living. ///C:/Users/sg2422/Downloads/Activities-of-Daily-Living.pdf. Published 2012. Accessed July 6, 2018.
4. Lyu W, Wolinsky F. The onset of ADL difficulties and changes in health-related quality of life. *Health Qual Life Outcomes*. 2017;15(1):217. http://search.proquest.com/docview/1972096864/.
5. Williams JS, Egede LE. The association between multimorbidity and quality of life, health status and functional disability. *Am J Med Sci*. 2016;352(1):45–52. doi:10.1016/j.amjms.2016.03.004.
6. World Health Organization. Towards a common language for functioning, disability and health: ICF. http://www.who.int/classifications/icf/training/icfbeginnersguide.pdf. Published 2002. Accessed May 25, 2018.
7. Boyt Schell B, Gillen G, Scaffa M. Glossary. In: Boyt Schell B, Gillen G, Scaffa M, eds. *Willard and Spackman's Occupational Therapy*. 12th ed. Philadelphia, PA: Lippincott Williams & Wilkins; 2014:1229–1243. https://shop.lww.com/Willard-and-Spackman-s-Occupational-Therapy/p/9781451110807.
8. Ottenbacher KJ, Hsu Y, Granger CV, Fiedler RC. The reliability of the functional independence measure: a quantitative review. *Arch Phys Med Rehabil*. 1996;77(12):1226–1232. doi:10.1016/S0003-9993(96)90184-7.
9. Klein RM, Bell B. Self-care skills: behavioral measurement with Klein-Bell ADL scale. *Arch Phys Med Rehabil*. 1982;63(7):335–338.
10. Katz S, Downs TD, Cash HR, Grotz RC. Progress in development of the index of ADL. *Gerontologist*. 1970;10(1):20. doi:10.1093/geront/10.1_part_1.20.
11. Chisholm D, Toto P, Raina K, Holm M, Rogers J. Evaluating capacity to live independently and safely in the community: performance assessment of self-care skills. *Br J Occup Ther*. 2014;77(2):59–63. doi:10.4276/030802214X13916969447038.
12. Hudak PL, Amadio PC, Bombardier C. Development of an upper extremity outcome measure: the DASH (disabilities of the arm, shoulder and hand) corrected. The Upper Extremity Collaborative Group (UECG). *Am J Ind Med*. 1996;29(6):602.
13. Collin C, Wade DT, Davies S, Horne V. The Barthel ADL index: a reliability study. *Int Disabil Stud*. 1988;10(2):61–63. doi:10.3109/09638288809164103.
14. Yerxa EJ. An introduction to occupational science: a foundation for occupational therapy in the 21st century. *Occup Ther Health Care*. 1990;6(4):1–17. doi:10.1080/J003v06n04_04.
15. Runge M. Self-dressing techniques for clients with spinal cord injury. *Am J Occup Ther*. 1967;21:367.
16. International Spinal Cord Society. E-Learn SCI's videos. http://www.elearnsci.org/. Published 2012. Accessed May 29, 2018.
17. Thomas Jefferson University Hospital and Magee Rehabilitation. Activities of daily living-spinal cord injury manual. In: *Spinal Cord Injury Manual* (English). Manual 10. 2009. https://jdc.jefferson.edu/spinalcordmanual_eng/10/.
18. Hall CA. *Occupational Therapy Toolkit: Treatment Guides and Handouts for Physical Disabilities and Geriatrics*. 6th ed. Scotts Valley, CA: CreateSpace Independent Publishing Platform; 2013. http://www.ottoolkit.com/.
19. International Glaucoma Association. Opticare Arthro 5 (Light Blue). https://www.glaucoma-association.com/shop/patient-support-compliance-aids/opticare-arthro-5-ref-103.html.
20. Consortium for Spinal Cord Medicine. Sexuality and reproductive health in adults with spinal cord injury: a clinical practice guideline for health-care professionals. *J Spinal Cord Med*. 2010;33(3):281–336. doi:10.1080/10790268.2010.11689709.
21. Kaufman M, Silverbery C, Odette F. *The Ultimate Guide to Sex and Disability: For All of Us Who Live with Disabilities, Chronic Pain & Illness*. San Francisco, CA: Cleis Press; 2007.
22. Stout K, Finlayson M. Fatigue management in chronic illness. *OT Pract*. 2011;16:16–19.
23. Matuska K, Mathiowetz V, Finlayson M. Use and perceived effectiveness of energy conservation strategies for managing multiple sclerosis fatigue (Report). *Am J Occup Ther*. 2007;61(1):62. doi:10.5014/ajot.61.1.62.
24. Ainsworth BE, Haskell WL, Herrmann SD, et al. 2011 Compendium of physical activities: a second update of codes and MET values. *Med Sci Sport Exerc*. 2011;43(8):1575–1581. doi:10.1249/MSS.0b013e31821ece12.
25. Rogers JC, Holm MB, Perkins L. Trajectory of assistive device usage and user and non-user characteristics: long-handled bath sponge. *Arthritis Rheum*. 2002;47(6):645–650. doi:10.1002/art.10788.
26. Assistive Innovations. Feeding supports. https://assistive-innovations.com/news/217-the-improved-ieat-feeding-robot. Published 2016. Accessed June 5, 2018.
27. American Heart Association. Sex and heart disease. https://www.heart.org/en/health-topics/consumer-healthcare/what-is-cardiovascular-disease/sex-and-heart-disease. Published 2012. Accessed May 29, 2018.
28. Magermans DJ, Chadwick EKJ, Veeger HEJ, van Der Helm FCT. Requirements for upper extremity motions during activities of daily living. *Clin Biomech*. 2005;20(6):591–599. doi:10.1016/j.clinbiomech.2005.02.006.
29. Gates D, Walters L, Cowley J, Wilken J, Resnik L. Range of motion requirements for upper-limb activities of daily living. *Am J Occup Ther*. 2016;70(1):1–50. doi:10.5014/ajot.2016.015487.
30. Wheeler RB. 8 smart makeup tricks for women with arthritis. https://www.everydayhealth.com/news/makeup-tricks-women-with-arthritis/. Published 2015. Accessed June 18, 2018.
31. McDonald SS, Levine D, Richards J, Aguilar L. Effectiveness of adaptive silverware on range of motion of the hand. *PeerJ*. 2016;4(2):e1667. doi:10.7717/peerj.1667.
32. American College of Rheumatology. Sex and arthritis. https://www.rheumatology.org/I-Am-A/Patient-Caregiver/

Diseases-Conditions/Living-Well-with-Rheumatic-Disease/Sex-Arthritis. Published 2017. Accessed June 8, 2018.

33. Ropper AH, Samuels MA, Klein JP. Ataxia and disorders of cerebellar function. In: Ropper AH, Samuels MA, Klein JP, eds. *Adams and Victor's Principles of Neurology*. 10th ed. New York, NY: The McGraw-Hill Companies; 2014. accessmedicine.mhmedical.com/content.aspx?aid=57610681.
34. Chan T. An investigation of finger and manual dexterity. *Percept Mot Skills*. 2000;90(2):537–542. doi:10.2466/pms.2000.90.2.537.
35. Ittyerah M. Hand. In: Dautenhahn K, Cangelosi A, eds. *Hand Preference and Hand Ability: Evidence from Studies in Haptic Cognition*. Amsterdam, The Netherlands: John Benjamins Publishing Company; 2013:35–66. https://ebookcentral.proquest.com/lib/templeuniv-ebooks/reader.action?docID=1375110&query=#.
36. Gillen G. Improving activities of daily living performance in an adult with ataxia. *Am J Occup Ther*. 2000;54(1):89. doi:10.5014/ajot.54.1.89.
37. Mcgruder J, Cors D, Tiernan AM, Tomlin G. Weighted wrist cuffs for tremor reduction during eating in adults with static brain lesions. *Am J Occup Ther*. 2003;57(5):507. doi:10.5014/ajot.57.5.507.
38. National Multiple Sclerosis Society. Tremor: the basic facts—Multiple sclerosis. https://www.nationalmssociety.org/NationalMSSociety/media/MSNationalFiles/Brochures/Brochure-Tremor-The-Basic-Facts.pdf. Published 2016. Accessed June 18, 2018.
39. Ma H-I, Hwang W-J, Tsai P-L, Hsu Y-W. The effect of eating utensil weight on functional arm movement in people with Parkinson's disease: a controlled clinical trial. *Clin Rehabil*. 2009;23(12):1086–1092. doi:10.1177/0269215509342334.
40. Li K-Y, Hsiao Y-P, Chen R-S, Wu C-Y. Effects of wrist weights on kinematic and myographic movement characteristics during a reaching task in individuals with Parkinson disease. *Arch Phys Med Rehabil*. 2018;99(7):1303–1310. doi:10.1016/j.apmr.2017.11.009.
41. Shields WC, Mcdonald EC, Frattaroli SC, Perry EC, Zhu JC, Gielen AC. Still too hot: examination of water temperature and water heater characteristics 24 years after manufacturers adopt voluntary temperature setting. *J Burn Care Res*. 2013;34(2):281–287. doi:10.1097/BCR.0b013e31827e645f.
42. Koski L, Iacoboni M, Mazziotta J. Deconstructing apraxia: understanding disorders of intentional movement after stroke. *Curr Opin Neurol*. 2002;15(1):71–77. doi:10.1097/00019052-200202000-00011.
43. Ryan PA, Sullivan JW, Gillen G. Activities of daily living adaptations: managing the environment with one-handed techniques. In: Gillen G, ed. *Stroke Rehabilitation: A Function-Based Approach*. 4th ed. St. Louis, MO: Elsevier Inc.; 2016:136–154. https://www.elsevier.com/books/stroke-rehabilitation/9780323172813.
44. Brett G. Dressing techniques for the severely involved hemiplegic patient. *Am J Occup Ther*. 1960;14:262–264.
45. American Heart Association. Sex after stroke: our guide to intimacy after stroke. https://www.rheumatology.org/I-Am-A/Patient-Caregiver/Diseases-Conditions/Living-Well-with-Rheumatic-Disease/Sex-Arthritis.
46. Farman J, Friedman JD. Sexual function and intimacy. In: Gillen G, ed. *Stroke Rehabilitation: A Function-Based Approach*. 4th ed. St. Louis, MO: Elsevier Inc.; 2016:280–295. https://www.elsevier.com/books/stroke-rehabilitation/gillen/978-0-323-17281-3.
47. Arya S, Escobar GA. Principles of lower extremity amputation: etiology, goals, limb length decisions, and impact on prosthetic management. In: Davis A, Kelly B, Spires MC, eds. *Prosthetic Restoration and Rehabilitation of the Upper and Lower Extremity*. New York, NY: Demos Medical Publishing; 2013. http://web.a.ebscohost.com.libproxy.temple.edu/ehost/detail/detail?vid=0&sid=d89f4078-c512-4474-9ee3-2d6feda29f-c9%40sessionmgr4009&bdata=JnNpdGU9ZWhvc3Qt-bGl2ZSZzY29wZT1zaXRl.
48. Scheiman M. Epidemiology, history, and clinical model for low vision rehabilitation. In: Scheiman M, Scheiman M, Whittaker S, eds. *Low Vision Rehabilitation : A Practical Guide for Occupational Therapists*. Thorofare, NJ: SLACK Inc.; 2007:3–22. https://www.healio.com/books/health-professions/occupational-therapy/%7B92ba610a-82d6-49d2-b583-dccd09195ee4%7D/low-vision-rehabilitation-a-practical-guide-for-occupational-therapists-second-edition.
49. Scheiman M. Eye diseases associated with low vision. In: Scheiman M, Scheiman M, Whittaker S, eds. *Low Vision Rehabilitation: A Practical Guide for Occupational Therapists*. Thorofare, NJ: SLACK Inc.; 2007:55–74. https://www.healio.com/books/health-professions/occupational-therapy/%7B92ba610a-82d6-49d2-b583-dccd09195ee4%7D/low-vision-rehabilitation-a-practical-guide-for-occupational-therapists-second-edition.
50. Schulz R, Wahl H-W, Matthews JT, De Vito Dabbs A, Beach SR, Czaja SJ. Advancing the aging and technology agenda in gerontology. *Gerontologist*. 2015;55(5):724–734.
51. Burmedi D, Becker S, Heyl V, Wahl H-W, Himmelsbach I. Emotional and social consequences of age-related low vision. *Vis Impair Res*. 2002;4(1):47–71. doi:10.1076/vimr.4.1.47.15634.
52. Meyers J. Addressing low vision in the older adult: a model for clinical decision making. *Gerontol Spec Interes Sect Q*. 2004;27(2):1–4.
53. World Health Organization. Obesity and overweight. http://www.who.int/news-room/fact-sheets/detail/obesity-and-overweight. Published 2018. Accessed June 5, 2018.
54. Forhan M, Bhambhani Y, Dyer D, Ramos-Salas X, Ferguson-Pell M, Sharma A. Rehabilitation in bariatrics: opportunities for practice and research. *Disabil Rehabil*. 2010;32(11):952–959. doi:10.3109/09638280903483885.
55. Reingold F, Jordan K. Obesity and occupational therapy. *Am J Occup Ther*. 2013;67(6):S39–S46. doi:10.5014/ajot.2013.67S39.
56. Foti D, Littrell E. Bariatric care: practical problem solving and interventions. *Phys Disabil Spec Interes Sect Q*. 2004;27(4):1–4. https://higherlogicdownload.s3-external-1.amazonaws.com/AOTA/PDSISDEC04.pdf?AWSAccessKeyId=AKIAVRDO7IERBJP4KSQZ&Expires=1567958021&Signature=r2hCkBKJ6LbwLIKmE41uzCn9hQc%3D..

57. Kolotkin RL, Zunker C, Østbye T. Sexual functioning and obesity: a review. *Obesity*. 2012;20(12):2325–2333. doi:10.1038/oby.2012.104.
58. Brown C. Cognitive skills. In: Brown C, Stoffel V, eds. *Occupational Therapy in Mental Health a Vision for Participation*. Philadelphia, PA: F.A. Davis Co.; 2011:241–261. https://www.fadavis.com/product/occupational-therapy-mental-health-vision-participation-brown-stoffel.
59. Boger J, Mihailidis A. The future of intelligent assistive technologies for cognition: devices under development to support independent living and aging-with-choice. *NeuroRehabilitation*. 2011;28(3):271–280. doi:10.3233/NRE-2011-0655.
60. Bauchet J, Giroux S, Pigot H, Lussier-Desrochers D, Lachapelle Y. Pervasive assistance in smart homes for people with intellectual disabilities: a case study on meal preparation. *IJARM*. 2008;9:42–54.
61. Hoey J, Poupart P, Von Bertoldi A, Craig T, Boutilier C, Mihailidis A. Automated handwashing assistance for persons with dementia using video and a partially observable Markov decision process. *Comput Vis Image Underst*. 2010;114(5):503–519. doi:10.1016/j.cviu.2009.06.008.
62. Kristensen HK, Persson D, Nygren C, Boll M, Matzen P. Evaluation of evidence within occupational therapy in stroke rehabilitation. *Scand J Occup Ther*. 2011;18(1):11–25. doi:10.3109/11038120903563785.
63. Liu C-J, Brost MA, Horton VE, Kenyon SB, Mears KE. Occupational therapy interventions to improve performance of daily activities at home for older adults living with low vision: a systematic review. *Am J Occup Ther*. 2013;67(3):279–287. doi:10.5014/ajot.2013.005512.
64. Baldelli MV, Boiardi R, Ferrari P, Bianchi S, Bianchi MH. Dementia and occupational therapy. *Arch Gerontol Geriatr*. 2007;44(suppl 1):45. https://www-sciencedirect-com.libproxy.temple.edu/science/article/pii/S0167494307000076.

Chapter 28

Restoring Family, Parenting, and Social Roles

Sharon A. Gutman and Marianne H. Mortera

LEARNING OBJECTIVES

This chapter will allow the reader to:

1. Understand how disability impacts family, parenting, and social roles.
2. Understand how occupational therapists use remediation, adaptation, and compensation in client role restoration and assumption.
3. Understand how occupational therapists help clients restore or newly assume parenting roles after disability onset.
4. Identify adaptive strategies and equipment that support parenting roles.
5. Understand how occupational therapists help clients restore or newly assume caregiving of pets and animals assistants after disability onset.
6. Identify adaptive strategies and equipment that support animal caregiving roles.
7. Understand how occupational therapists help clients restore or newly assume dating and courtship roles after disability onset.
8. Identify adaptive strategies that support dating and courtship roles.

CHAPTER OUTLINE

TERMINOLOGY

Adaptation: an intervention method in which an activity or environment is modified to promote client performance of desired activities and roles.

Compensation: an intervention method in which strategies and devices are used to substitute for impaired client skills that have minimal or no recovery potential after disability.

Family roles: positions in a family unit that support the maintenance of individual member and family functions, including feeding, bathing, clothing, housing, health care provision, companionship, nurturing, and financial assistance.

Remediation: an intervention method in which impaired client skills that have recovery potential are addressed through therapeutic activities designed to restore lost or diminished function after disability.

Role conflict: discordance in role performance resulting from (1) the opposing demands of several different roles held by one individual, or (2) contrasting role performance expectations perceived by the individual, significant others, and larger community.

Role disruption: a temporary or permanent interruption in the ability to carry out and perform the functions associated with a specific family and/or social role as a result of disability, illness, injury, and aging.

Role distress: the occurrence of anxiety and stress resulting from an inability to carry out the perceived essential functions associated with specific desired family or social roles as a result of skill deficits; lack of needed knowledge; or disability, illness, and aging.

Social roles: positions within a social system that are characterized by a set of behaviors intended to fulfill role expectations defined by the individual, significant others, and larger community and that support community participation.

Role Disruption after Physical Disability

Illness, disease, and injury commonly result in disabilities that disrupt a client's participation in desired family and **social roles**. For example, sustaining traumatic brain injury (TBI) that causes mild-to-severe cognitive, visual perceptual, emotional regulatory, and physical impairments can significantly impede a client's ability to carry out the activities associated with spousal roles, parenting, and elder caregiving, including[1]:

- Overseeing bathing, feeding, and clothing of children
- Managing a family home or an elderly parent's residence
- Participating in joint decision-making regarding family concerns
- Earning an income that supports the family's material needs
- Managing a family's financial decisions and assets
- Overseeing health care and medical decisions of an elderly parent
- Maintaining intimate and healthy interpersonal relationships with all family members
- Providing caregiving, nurturance, and companionship

Depending on the severity, **role disruption** resulting from disability can have devastating effects on the ability to maintain the roles that clients constructed prior to disability. Consequently, it is estimated that 50% to 75% of individuals sustaining severe and permanent disability—such as TBI, spinal cord injury (SCI), and cerebrovascular accident—commonly experience family and social role disruption, including divorce, loss of primary parenting responsibilities, and lost connection with predisability friends and social support systems.[2–4]

Our primary roles as occupational therapists are to help clients restore desired roles that have been lost as a result of disability and assume new roles desired postdisability. Evaluation should begin with an assessment of the role changes that clients have experienced or are likely to experience when discharged from the hospital. Once role changes postdisability are understood, an assessment of the client's ability to engage in the specific activities supporting each desired role should be made. A client's activity participation will depend on (a) the requirements of the activity (i.e., activity demands), (b) client skills (i.e., cognitive, sensory–motor, musculoskeletal, visual perceptual, and psychosocial skills), and (c) environmental supports and barriers that impede or facilitate activity participation.

Restoring former roles and assisting in the assumption of new roles postdisability requires:

1. **Remediation** of skill deficits having the potential for improved function (e.g., increasing muscular strength, joint range of motion, cognitive executive functions, visual scanning)
2. Adapting an activity or modifying the environment to enhance client performance (e.g., using built-up handles on eating utensils to increase grasp, and installing grab bars and toilet rails to increase safe bathing)
3. Using compensatory strategies and devices to substitute for impaired client functions that have minimal to no potential for recovery (e.g., using electronic reminder systems and voice activated computer features).

Family Roles

A family system is defined as a small group of individuals who are connected to each other by birth, legal union, and/or self-proclaimed feelings of loyalty and reciprocal affection.[5,6] Although family systems have traditionally been defined in Western society as small units comprised of people related by birth and legal designations (e.g., parents, children, siblings, grandparents, aunts and uncles, extended relatives), such formal relationships have loosened in recent decades, allowing for the broader inclusion of unmarried partners having children, people of the same sex who have either legally married or are in committed partnerships, blended families comprised of parents and children from separate birth families in which the spouses have divorced and remarried, and individuals who are considered as family members because of reciprocal closeness and affection but who are neither related by birth or legal designations. In recent decades, family pets have been elevated to a unique status equivalent, in many instances, to human members. Family members enter through birth, adoption, marriage, or other legal union (e.g., domestic partnership); maintain their membership over time; and leave by death, divorce, mutual consent, and sometimes abandonment. Regardless of the family type noted earlier, most families deal with the similar issues of caregiving and providing nurturance, managing a communal home, earning money sufficient to provide for the family's material needs, child rearing, elder caregiving, sustaining healthy interpersonal relationships, and supporting each members' participation in the larger community.[7]

The most common **family roles** disrupted by adult disability include spousal roles, parenting, and elder caregiving.[8–11] Restoring the activities associated with spousal and elder caregiving roles—providing emotional support and nurturance, self-care and medical assistance, home management and meal preparation, and working to financially support family material needs—is addressed in Chapters 27 and 29. This chapter addresses restoration of parenting roles and caring for pets and animal assistants who are considered to be family members.

Restoring or Newly Assuming Parenting Roles

Approximately 6 to 9 million adults with moderate-to-severe disability (e.g., TBI, SCI, progressive neurological disorders such as multiple sclerosis) have young children under the age of 10 and must seek help for or modify activities needed for parenting.[12] Parenting activities that are commonly impacted by disability include bathing, feeding, and dressing infants and children; engaging in play and recreational activities; and providing affection and healthy limit setting.[13–16] When clients need to resume or newly assume parenting roles with disability, therapists must first collect information regarding (1) the infant or child's age and any special needs, (2) the type and amount of support available for childcare assistance (e.g., financial resources for equipment and hired caregivers, and the existence of family members who can participate in infant and child care), and (3) the presence of environmental barriers (e.g., inability to access a standard floor tub in which to bathe children).

Therapists should then determine the specific parenting activities for which the client desires resumption or new assumption and implement an activity analysis to understand each task's unique requirements (see Chapter 3). Clients should be observed while attempting to perform each activity in order to evaluate whether they possess sufficient abilities with regard to cognitive, sensory–motor, musculoskeletal, visual perceptual, and psychosocial skills.

Performance should be observed in natural contexts whenever possible and in simulated environments when not possible. Intervention should address (1) remediation of skill deficits having the potential for recovery, (2) **adaptation** or modification of the activity or environment to facilitate performance, and (3) **compensation** using alternative strategies and devices when recovery of skill deficits is not possible.

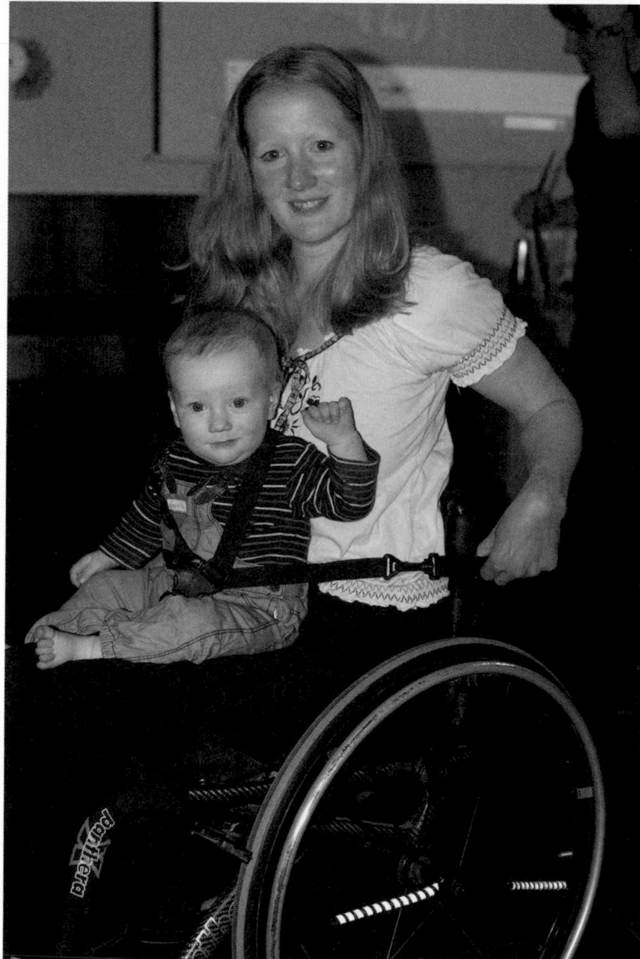

Figure 28-1. Mother using a safety harness to transport her infant. (Printed with permission from Dorothee Riedel, Spinalisttips, http://www.spinalistips.se)

Transitional Activities: Holding, Carrying, and Transferring

The transitional activities of holding, carrying, and physically transferring infants and toddlers are components embedded within all other caregiving activities (e.g., bathing, feeding, dressing) and must be addressed to support parenting roles. There are a number of adaptive devices designed to aid in the assistance of transitional activities for parents with physical disabilities.

Safety Straps, Harnesses, and Front Packs

Safety straps, harnesses, and front packs allow infants and toddlers to be safely secured to a parent's lap or trunk for transport (see Fig. 28-1). These devices enable a parent's arms and hands to be freed for other activities or to be freed from use when hand function is impaired. When fine motor ability is limited, safety straps, harnesses, and front packs must either be secured by another individual or adapted to match the parent's hand function. These devices allow parents in wheelchairs to transport infants and toddlers with ease and safety.

Fabric Carriers

Fabric carriers are similar to small cradles in which the infant is positioned (see Fig. 28-2). A secure strap is placed over the shoulders to hold the carrier in place as it is positioned on the parent's lap. Fabric carriers allow hands-free transport of infants, particularly for parents using wheelchairs. Such devices, however, may be contraindicated for parents with poor trunk control or chronic back pain because infant weight is supported in part by the shoulder strap positioned around the parent's upper back and shoulders.

Adjustable Wheeled Infant Carriers

Adjustable wheeled infant carriers are similar to small cradles on wheels and can be raised or lowered in height to accommodate parent needs (see Fig. 28-3). The infant is strapped securely in the cradle area and can be transported easily by parents in wheelchairs who possess sufficient upper extremity (UE) strength and mobility. This device is particularly beneficial for parents with limited hand function, UE and trunk weakness, lower extremity

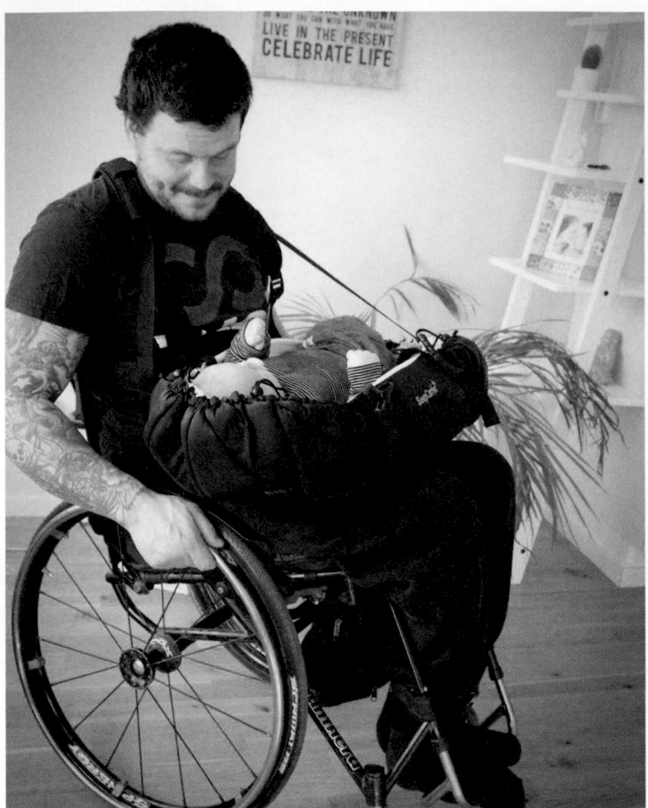

Figure 28-2. Father transporting an infant in a carrier on lap. (Printed with permission from Dorothee Riedel, Spinalisttips, http://www.spinalistips.se)

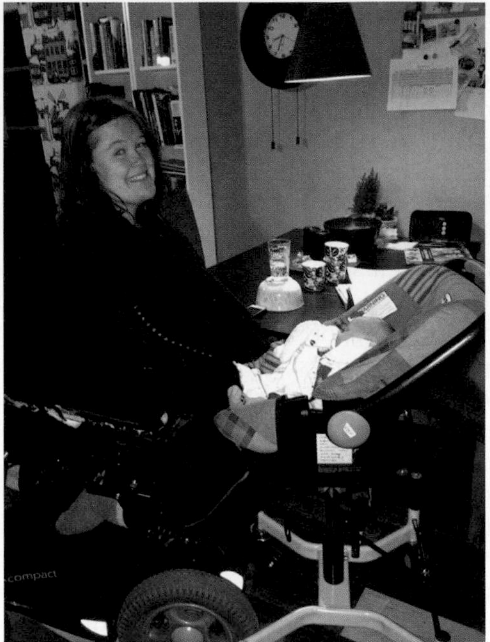

Figure 28-3. Adjustable-height wheeled infant carrier. (Printed with permission from Dorothee Riedel, Spinalisttips, http://www.spinalistips.se)

(LE) paralysis, and who fatigue easily with activity (e.g., multiple sclerosis).

Wrist Supports

Parents with limited arm and hand movement secondary to weakness and pain (e.g., rheumatoid arthritis) may benefit from the use of wrist supports to reduce joint stress when lifting and carrying their infants and toddlers. Wrist supports should be customized for parents with regard to their specific hand impairments and activity needs.

All of the abovementioned equipment and adaptive devices can be trialed using weighted dolls in order to provide practice opportunities that enhance client performance, safety, and confidence. Additionally, therapists should provide client education regarding safe body mechanics and proper positioning when lifting, holding, and carrying infants and toddlers. Remediation approaches may address activities designed to increase UE strength, trunk control, and dynamic sitting or standing balance when the potential for improvement exists. For example, to enhance functional endurance and activity tolerance, clients could practice lifting and transporting weighted dolls in varying adaptive infant carriers for progressively longer periods. To enhance functional UE strength, clients could practice reaching for infant supplies spread across a table area using proper body mechanics while seated in a wheelchair or standing. To increase task demands, clients could be fitted with weighted wrist cuffs, or retrievable items could be selected to provide a progression of weights and sizes.

Bathing

Parents using wheelchairs, those who cannot stand for long periods of time secondary to LE weakness and balance deficits, and parents with insufficient trunk control to reach toward the floor will have difficulty bathing infants and toddlers in portable baby bathtubs placed within standard floor tubs or on kitchen/bathroom counters. In these cases, bathing infants and toddlers can be achieved by positioning a portable baby bathtub on a secure table (28"-34" [~71-86 cm] high in accordance with the American with Disabilities Act [ADA] standards), allowing wheelchair access near a sink. If the baby bathtub does not possess rubber grips, a nonskid mat can be positioned beneath the tub to safely secure it to the table surface. The tub can be filled and drained using a portable hose connected to the sink faucet and drained into the sink basin; parents, however, must either possess sufficient hand function to attach the hose or depend on another individual for set up. For parents with UE sensory loss, baby bath temperature readers can be used to reduce possible scalding and ensure safety. C-shaped plastic handles can be attached to infant care products (e.g., shampoo and soap bottles) to enhance grasp when parents possess limited hand mobility; shampoo and liquid soap can also be transferred to pump-style dispensers to reduce the need for functional grasp. Similarly, wash towels can either be sewn into the shape of a mitt or purchased in this form for parents with limited hand function and coordination.

Remediative strategies would include, when possible, activities designed to increase UE strength, trunk control, dynamic sitting balance, functional endurance, and activity tolerance. For example, clients in wheelchairs could practice reaching for, lifting, and transferring a weighted doll into and out of a portable baby bathtub. Clients could also practice retrieving and transporting infant bath supplies having a progression of weights and sizes, and positioned from the client at varying distances. Activity participation time could also be progressively extended as skill proficiency increases.

Diapering and Dressing

Most commercially available changing tables do not provide sufficient wheelchair access and are commonly too high for parents using wheelchairs. Several companies have designed adjustable-height changing tables that allow wheelchair access, are built with side frames to prevent infant falls, and have wheels for easy transport of infants when needed (see Fig. 28-4). Sturdy tables that allow wheelchair accessibility can be adapted to serve as changing tables by securing a standard changing table mattress atop the surface using a nonskid mat to prevent slippage. For safety, Velcro straps can be attached to the mattress to secure the infant in place and prevent possible falls.

Infant and toddler clothing can be purchased or adapted with Velcro fasteners to reduce the need for fine motor coordination. Velcro-closure cloth or disposable diapers can be used and further adapted with loop closures that may be more easily manipulated by parents with fine motor limitations. Clothing such as pullover tops, elastic waistbands, and slip-on shoes (instead of buttons, zippers, and snaps) reduce the need for fine motor abilities. Clothing can be additionally modified by widening neck, waist, arm, and leg openings that can be tightened with adjustable Velcro straps.

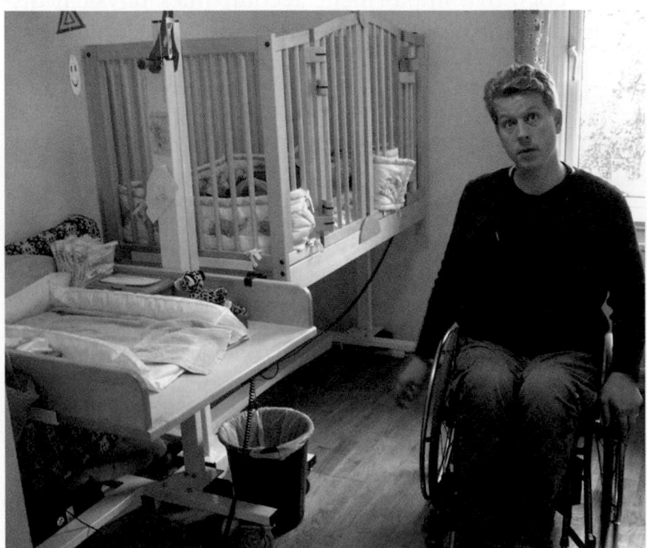

Figure 28-4. Adjustable-height changing table. (Printed with permission from Dorothee Riedel, Spinalisttips, http://www.spinalistips.se)

As noted earlier, when recovery potential is possible, remediative strategies would include activities designed to increase UE strength, fine and gross motor control, dynamic sitting balance, functional endurance, and activity tolerance. Compensatory strategies could involve work simplification and energy conservation techniques in which all items needed for an activity would be gathered and placed in one accessible location. Clothing can be stored in closets with lowered or drop-down clothing racks to increase accessibility for those using wheelchairs, or in drawers with pull-strap handles for parents with limited hand function. Therapists should also help patients redesign activities to increase efficiency and reduce step number.

Feeding

Mothers with physical disabilities who breastfeed their infants can use commercially available nursing pillows designed to position the infant at the breast to support latching. Nursing pillows sit on top of the mother's lap and wrap around her waist, providing a stable and comfortable surface for the infant; some pillows can be positioned directly in a wheelchair if needed. The infant's weight is supported by the pillow, reducing the amount of UE strength needed to hold the infant in the arms. Nursing pillows can be adapted with Velcro straps with loop closures to more securely stabilize the infant and prevent possible falls. These types of pillows are particularly beneficial for mothers with UE weakness, poor trunk control, and diminished fine motor control.

Parents with the above-noted physical impairments who bottle feed infants can use adjustable infant carriers that can be raised to accommodate the parent's seated position and can tilt to elevate the infant's head during feeding (see Fig. 28-3). C-shaped handles can be attached to bottles to reduce the need for fine motor control. For parents with UE sensory loss, baby bottle temperature readers can be used to ensure safety. Older infants and toddlers can be spoon fed using universal cuffs with inserted spoons; spoons should be rubber coated or made of flexible plastic to protect the toddler's gums and teeth if accidentally contacted during feeding. Baby food jars can be opened with a number of adaptive devices requiring minimal hand function, including nonskid rubber jar openers, and electronic automatic push-button jar openers that latch to and open jar lids. Adjustable-height high chairs with swing-away trays can be purchased for parents using wheelchairs and those with reduced UE strength and grasp who have difficulty lifting toddlers into standard high chairs.

As noted earlier, when recovery potential is possible, remediative strategies would include activities designed to increase UE strength, fine and gross motor control,

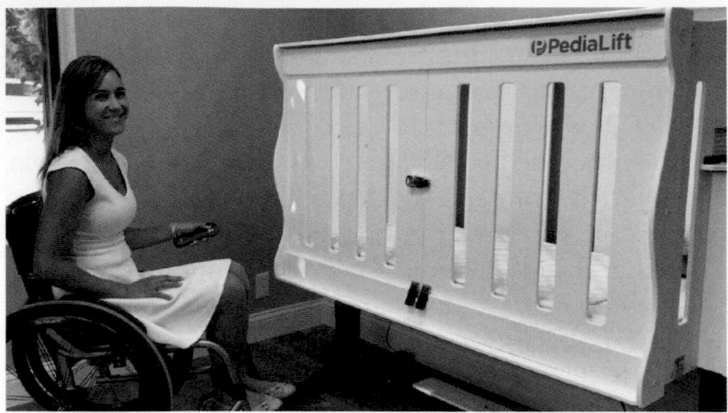

Figure 28-5. Mother raising an adjustable-height crib. (Printed with permission from PediaLift, https://www.pedialift.com)

dynamic sitting balance, functional endurance, and activity tolerance. Compensatory strategies could involve work simplification and energy conservation techniques in which all items needed for an activity would be gathered in one accessible location, and activities redesigned to reduce step number to a minimum.

Crib Use

Most standard cribs are inaccessible to parents using wheelchairs who can neither stand to reach over crib rails or negotiate wheelchairs sufficiently close to cribs for safe infant and toddler transfers. Traditional drop-down crib rails further prevent wheelchair accessibility. Several adaptive cribs are commercially available for parents using wheelchairs and offer an array of features designed to provide accessibility and safe infant handling. Many adaptive cribs have electronically adjustable heights that can accommodate the specific height requirements of parents using wheelchairs (see Figs. 28-4 and 28-5). This type of obstruction-free undercarriage crib design allows wheelchair users to position their chairs close to the crib while maintaining stable trunk control against the wheelchair backrest. In this position, parents are not forced to lean forward and risk balance loss, and the UEs are freed for safe infant and toddler handling. Common adaptive crib rail designs include double-door rails that swing (see Fig. 28-6) or horizontally slide open (see Fig. 28-7). Both style rails allow parents to easily and safely access and transfer their infants. If funding for adaptive cribs is not available, standard cribs can be adapted using leg extenders or wood blocks to raise crib height to allow wheelchair accessibility beneath the crib carriage. Raising the crib height would require the additional security measures of stabilizing the crib legs and anchoring the crib to the wall. Standard crib rails can be adapted by converting traditional drop-down rails to double-door swing or slider rails.

Playing with Toddlers and Small Children

Parents using wheelchairs and those unable to bend or reach to the floor may experience difficulty physically playing with toddlers. If funding is available, electronically adjustable-height playpens can be purchased that allow wheelchair access beneath the playpen carriage. Many adaptive playpens are designed with double swing-open or sliding doors that allow parents using wheelchairs to reach into the playpen while maintaining trunk control against the wheelchair backrest. Adaptive playpens allow infants and small toddlers sufficient space in which to practice gross motor skills, while offering accessibility for parents using wheelchairs or who cannot bend to the floor. Parents with older toddlers may find that children's tables, approximately 18 inches (46 cm) high, are at a height sufficient for interactive play. Some parents with adequate trunk and UE strength may be able to transfer from wheelchairs to lower height sofas or chairs to further enhance play accessibility.

Parenting with Cognitive Impairment

When cognitive impairment accompanies physical disability, parents will need support to understand and

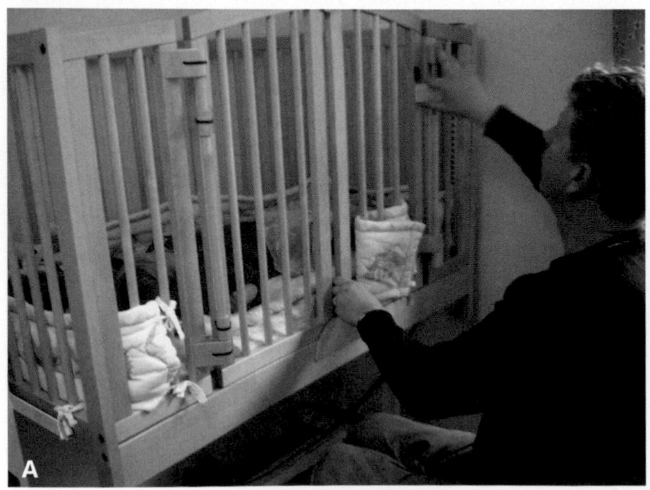

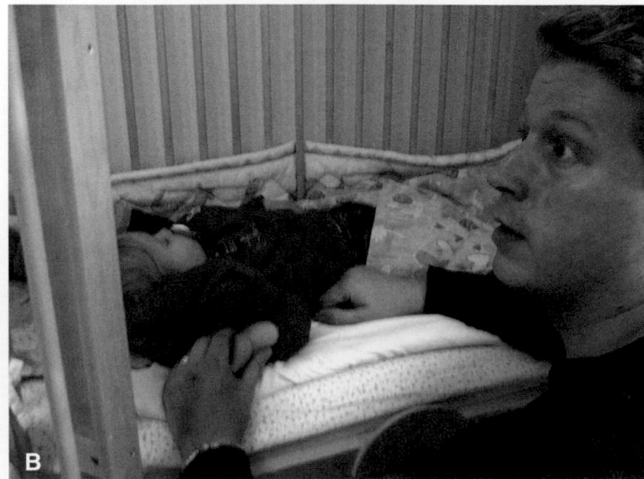

Figure 28-6 A, B. Father opening swing-away crib rails. (Printed with permission from Dorothee Riedel, Spinalisttips, http://www.spinalistips.se)

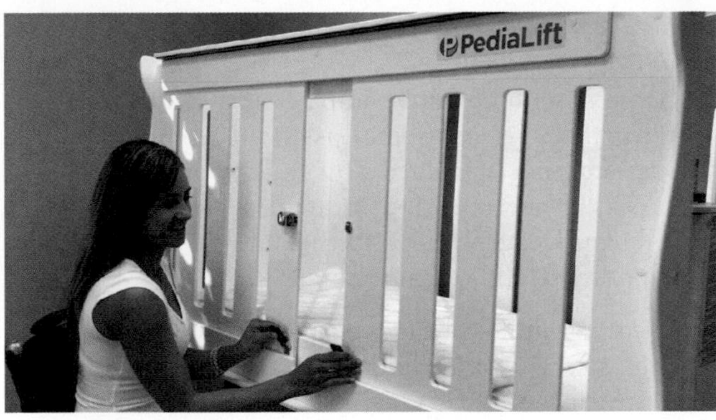

Figure 28-7. Mother opening horizontally sliding crib rails. (Printed with permission from PediaLift, https://www.pedialift.com)

organize the steps of many needed activities. Beneficial compensatory strategies include:

- Posting the steps for all activities in written and/or pictorial form in the location in which they will be performed
- Creating and teaching the parent to use checklists for all essential activities and providing opportunities for practice and return demonstration
- Teaching the parent to use preprogrammed smartphone and tablet cuing systems to facilitate activity performance
- Labeling drawers, cabinets, and closets (in written and/or pictorial form) to enhance organization and memory of supplies stored within
- Gathering and locating the supplies for each activity in easily accessible organizational systems (e.g., self-care dispensers, plastic storage shelves and trays) maintained in the area in which the activity will be performed
- Teaching a family member or caregiver in the above compensatory strategies to monitor their use and correct errors.

Restoring or Newly Assuming Caregiving Roles of Pets and Animal Assistants

As noted previously, pets have become elevated to the status of human family members in recent decades, largely because of the emotion, affection, and companionship that they readily offer to owners when positively treated.[17,18] The perception of pets as family members may be more pronounced for individuals who, as a result of traumatic disability, may have experienced loss of significant others including spouses, friends, and access to a larger support community.[19] Pets may provide the first experience of acceptance after disability and may counter feelings of stigmatization encountered in the larger human community.[20] Pets also commonly provide a bridge across which recently disabled individuals may begin to connect and interact with others.[19,20] Clients who obtain animal assistants to help with the performance of daily activities after disability commonly develop intimate and intense bonds with their animals based on emotional and physical dependence.[21] In the previous instances, pets and animal assistants likely assume primary emotional and survival roles in client lives, and their ongoing care must be addressed by occupational therapists. The following section provides an overview of the ways in which therapists can adapt animal care routines—particularly of dogs and cats—for clients with physical and/or cognitive disabilities.

Feeding

Pet owners using wheelchairs should store food supplies at an accessible height, preferably in a low cabinet or on a counter that accommodates a wheelchair. Large food bags should be avoided as clients using wheelchairs and having UE weakness and/or chronic back pain will be unable to lift or reach down into them to access food. For pet owners with limited hand function, food bags can be opened with an adaptive scissors. Bagged food should be transferred to and stored within small, lightweight containers with easy-open plastic lids (such as lids with pull straps and C-shaped handles). Dry food can then be retrieved from containers using a universal cuff with an attached scooper. Canned food can be opened with easy-touch electric can openers requiring minimal hand control to place the device atop the can. A single light touch then latches the device to the can top and opens it without further hand use. Owners can then scoop moist food using a universal cuff with an attached spoon. For large dogs, food should be placed on a standard raised dog tray that is easily accessible for clients using wheelchairs. For smaller dogs and cats, food can be placed on a raised platform with a stool positioned for the animal's easy access.

Toileting

There are a number of commercially available pooper-scoopers that require minimal hand mobility (but do require UE gross motor function) and retrieve dog waste either electronically or through spring action. Such devices are typically inexpensive, lightweight, eliminate the need for bagging waste, and can be secured to a wheelchair with Velcro if needed. Similarly, electronic cat litter box cleaning systems that automatically clean and store waste for up to several weeks (at which time waste removal requires proficient UE mobility) are available. When electronic cat litter boxes are not an option, traditional litter boxes can be located on raised platforms for pet owners using wheelchairs. Those with limited hand function can use a universal cuff with an attached cat litter scooper to remove waste.

Walking and Playing

Most dogs need to be walked a minimum of 30 minutes, twice per day. Pet owners using wheelchairs can secure the lead to the metal frame to free the hands for wheelchair propulsion. In this case, the dog must be trained to

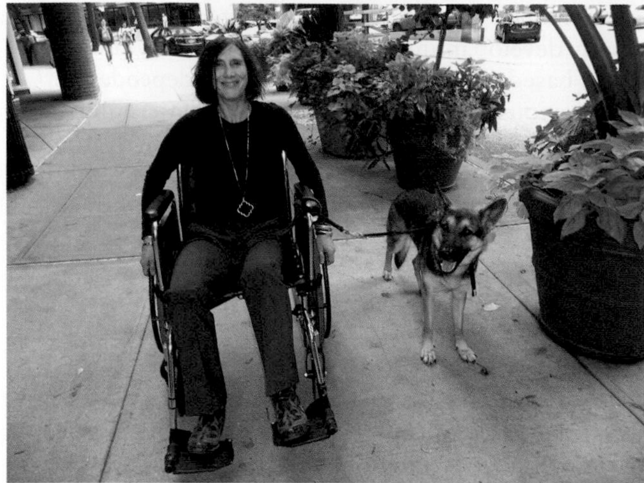

Figure 28-8. Pet owner in wheelchair walking her dog.

walk at the owner's wheelchair side to avoid tangling the leash in the wheels or inappropriately pulling the chair (see Fig. 28-8). For pet owners with limited fine motor ability, slip-dog leashes can be used that easily slide over the animal's head and tighten to fit around the neck. Dog toys, such as balls and tugs, can be adapted with Velcro C-shaped loops and straps for pet owners with limited hand function. Interactive cat toys can be adapted in similar ways by attaching toy handles to universal cuffs, allowing owners to swing stringed, catnip-stuffed mice or birds. Laser pointers can also be secured to universal cuffs, allowing owners to engage their cats in play and exercise with limited fine motor requirements.

Bathing and Grooming

Although cats are self-grooming (and can maintain trimmed nails with regular scratching post use), dogs require regular bathing, fur trimming, and nail clipping—the frequency of which depends on breed. Professional grooming can be obtained inexpensively and can maintain the animal's health with no physical requirements of the owner. This is particularly true of mobile groomers who provide services in the animal's home. Pet owners who wish to bathe their dogs, but who cannot bend to the floor, can use a basin on a raised platform. The basin can be filled and drained with a hose attached to an indoor sink or outdoor faucet. Dog shampoo bottles can be adapted with C-shaped handles, or liquid shampoo can be transferred to pump-style containers to allow use with limited hand function. Washcloths can be purchased or sewn into the shape of a mitt to reduce hand mobility requirements. For owners with UE sensory loss, bath temperature readers can be used to reduce possible scalding and ensure safety. Dog brushes can be inserted into universal cuffs for owners with limited fine motor ability. Owners with UE weakness but good fine motor skills can use electronic nail clippers and fur shears to accomplish these specific grooming activities.

Providing Animal Care When Pet Owners Have Cognitive Impairment

Pet owners with cognitive impairment can still provide care for their pet or animal assistant using compensatory strategies established and taught by occupational therapists. The following strategies can help owners with cognitive deficits to participate in pet care with minimal setup and ongoing supervision:

- The steps for all pet care activities noted previously can be posted in written and/or pictorial form in the area in which the activity will be performed. Steps should be written as simply as possible and include photos or illustrations where possible.
- A checklist for all daily pet care activities should be created and maintained in one location in which the owner commonly accesses. The therapist should teach the owner checklist use, and opportunities for practice with return demonstration should be provided.
- Drawers, cabinets, and closets in which pet supplies are stored should be labeled (in written and/or pictorial form) to enhance organization and ease of item retrieval.
- Electronic cuing systems on smartphones and tablets can be programmed to remind the owner to carry out daily pet care activities such as walking and feeding.
- Automated food dispensers can be programmed to reduce the need for the owner to remember this essential task; however, the owner must be cued or depend on a family member to fill the dispenser when needed.
- An electronic smartphone calendar can be programmed to alert the owner to schedule regular veterinary and grooming appointments.
- A family member or caregiver should be educated to oversee all of the above to ensure optimal animal care.

Social Roles

Social roles are positions within a social system that are characterized by a set of behaviors intended to meet role expectations that support community participation.[6,22] Role expectations are shaped by both individuals holding specific roles and the larger community in which expected roles are carried out. Common social roles in Western society include family roles as noted earlier, and worker, student, friend, neighbor, coach or facilitator, group participant (e.g., sports team and religious participant), volunteer, consumer or patron, and patient or client roles. The duration of one's social roles varies as a factor of personal need, desire, and interest; family and larger societal demands; and the availability of resources and support needed to maintain specific roles.[6,22] The behaviors associated with a specific role can also change over time as people age, children mature into adulthood, partners separate or pass away, and societal norms change.[23]

It is common for individuals to hold multiple roles and to experience **role conflict** resulting from the opposing demands of several different roles. Role conflict may also occur when individuals' expectations of role behaviors differ from those held by significant others and the larger community.[24,25] **Role distress** occurs when individuals desire to assume and carryout the specific behaviors characteristic of a role, but are unable to as a result of skill deficits, lack of needed knowledge, or disability and illness.[26] Most social roles are equated with a particular status and value by the larger society, and individuals who lose a desired role can often experience depression and decreased self-esteem.[27] For example, when individuals experience divorce as a result of disability and lose their roles as spouse and primary parent, depression and lost life meaning may ensue.[28]

One social role that is commonly impacted by disability, particularly for young adults, is that of dating and courtship roles. As noted previously, severe disability—such as TBI and SCI—is commonly accompanied by divorce, loss of predisability dating partners, and lost connection to a larger social group of friends. Many individuals with severe disabilities report that loneliness and lost emotional connection are among their most devastating postdisability experiences.[29] Clients with severe disabilities who have lost spouses, dating partners, and connection to their social groups commonly desire to resume and sometimes newly assume dating roles. This section addresses the unique ways in which occupational therapists can help clients to enter or restore desired dating and courtship roles, particularly in outpatient and community care settings, after the impact of disability on such roles has become clearer. The restoration of other social roles, such as worker, student, community member, and leisure participant, is explored in Chapter 29.

Restoring Dating and Courtship Roles

When occupational therapists find, through the construction of an occupational profile, that clients have lost spousal and dating roles as a result of disability, and wish to regain such roles, therapists should engage in the evaluation of activity demands and client skills that are needed to support role resumption. Therapists may also find with young adults, whose disabilities occurred in adolescence, that desired skills for dating roles were never acquired and that dating experiences have been limited or nonexistent. In such cases, therapists may need to newly teach and practice underlying skills with clients. Underlying skills primarily address (a) knowledge of where and how to meet potential partners; (b) how to interact through online communication, and in-person verbal and nonverbal skills; and (c) how to navigate dating events given physical and/or cognitive disability.

Meeting Potential Partners

Clients whose disabilities have resulted in diminished self-esteem, particularly when loss of spouse or predisability dating partners has occurred, may feel apprehensive when attempting to meet potential partners. Through discussion, therapists should attempt to understand how clients feel about dating after disability onset, and meeting and describing their disability to potential dating partners. Depending on disability severity and comfort level, some clients may desire to date others with similar disabilities. A number of online dating sites and meet-up groups are available that provide opportunities for people with disabilities to meet similar others. When clients wish to use these types of meeting venues, therapists should help clients identify specific websites and local meet-up events. Other clients may feel comfortable meeting and dating both people with and without disabilities, and therapists must determine client preferences.

Most opportunities to meet potential partners for both people with and without disabilities occur through online dating sites and chat rooms, and in-person local meet-up groups. To access online sites, clients with UE and/or visual perceptual impairment will need assistance to configure adaptive keyboards, screens, smartphones, tablets, and/or computer systems (such adaptive equipment is discussed in Chapter 29). Clients with cognitive impairment will likely require assistance to identify and bookmark online dating sites, create membership accounts, construct dating profiles, upload one or more photographs, and evaluate and select other members with whom to communicate. Such clients will also likely benefit from the posting of written steps to remember how to access the site, view member profiles, and message members. It will also likely be important to assess clients' judgment, insight, awareness, and inhibition with regard to Internet safety. Clients with cognitive impairment may require assistance to understand the need to identify signs of and protect against possible abuse and predation. Basic protective information regarding privacy—such as refraining from providing residential, work, and email addresses, and newly meeting dates in public places—should be conveyed. Opportunities through which to practice the identification of possible signs of predation should be provided in simulated role-play between the therapist and client.

Communication Skills: Online and In-person

Online communication requires knowledge of specific etiquette that may or may not be understood by clients, particularly those with cognitive impairment. Therapists should provide client education about the following etiquette skills and allow opportunities for practice in simulated role-play together:

- Initial messages should be brief, neutral, and invite response.
- A period of 24 hours in which to receive a response should be allowed; clients with impulsivity and lack of inhibition should be coached to wait for response without sending further messages.
- Clients should be provided with opportunities to practice messaging appropriately neutral questions about another's interests and dating objectives that broach conversation and maintain it in a reciprocal way. Clients with diminished insight and impulsivity control should be helped to understand and avoid personally invasive or intrusive questions (e.g., about religion, politics, salary, sexually related topics). Clients should also practice constructing messages that avoid disclosing too much and oversharing.
- Rejection is difficult for everyone, particularly for people who have lost confidence as a result of disability. Clients with emotional dysregulation and diminished impulse control will need to practice skills to appropriately deal with rejection and to identify and avoid unsuitable behaviors such as perseverative messaging and verbal attacks.
- Clients will also need to identify inappropriate communications from others and understand the procedures for blocking, unmatching, and reporting improper communication to site managers. Such skills should be practiced in simulations with the therapist.

Clients who attend in-person meet-up events or who decide to meet online dates may need to learn and/or practice the skills required to initiate social contact, sustain reciprocal turn-taking conversations, and interpret verbal and nonverbal cues. Nonverbal skills accompany verbal skills in conversation and are used to convey messages through eye contact, personal space, and body language and orientation. Clients will need to practice skills such as maintaining eye contact and others' personal space during interaction, orienting one's body to face others during conversation, and refraining from touching others. Such nonverbal skills may be difficult for clients with diminished inhibition, and opportunities to practice these behaviors within role-play with the therapist will likely be warranted.

Verbal interpersonal skills include knowledge of socially accepted forms of greetings when meeting potential dates, being able to introduce oneself, and engaging in socially appropriate conversation beyond formal introduction. Clients with diminished impulse control may have difficulty engaging in reciprocal, turn-taking conversation and may instead monopolize interactions; have difficulty refraining from verbalizing inappropriate content; and may perseveratively maintain a conversation without allowing it to end. These skills should be practiced in role-play between the therapist and client until performance reaches a socially acceptable level. Such clients will also need to practice verbal skills for expressing interest in future social contact, as well as skills to appropriately deal with rejection if a person of interest declines the client's social invitation.

Intervention should provide opportunities for clients and therapists to role-play the abovementioned skills in one-to-one interactions in simulated scenarios that closely mirror the natural contexts in which clients will use the identified skills. Opportunities to practice desired behaviors in increasingly more natural, unstructured environments should also be provided when possible. Feedback should be offered by therapists to enhance client performance to socially acceptable and personally desired levels.

Navigating Dating Events with a Disability

Clients who reach a stage in which in-person dating events occur must consider and prepare for environmental and emotional variables that can impact dating events. For example, although clients attending initial dates should obtain their own transportation to and from the event for safety, later stage dating may involve situations in which both partners travel together. In such situations, individuals using wheelchairs must ensure that transportation modes are able to safely accommodate one or more wheelchairs. Similarly, although public places (such as restaurants, movie theaters, and dance clubs) are required to be compliant with the ADA, clients should contact business owners to ensure that doorway entrances, restrooms, aisle spaces, ramps, and tables are wheelchair accessible. For example, although a restaurant owner may perceive the environment to be ADA compliant, there may be a disproportionate number of booths to tables (tables are easier than booths for people using wheelchairs), aisle space between tables may be inadequate for wheelchair use, tables may be too small to accommodate two wheelchair users, and ramps to enter the restaurant may be inaccessible if they do not meet ADA specifications or are located on unlevel surfaces. It would be equally important for individuals with low vision or visual perceptual impairment to ensure that the environment was adequately lit, that floor transitions were level and adequately lighted, and that any printed text (e.g., menus, playbills, bills, receipts) could be read with adaptive aids. Therapists should help clients to understand the environmental factors that could impact dating events and the steps needed to research a specific location's safety and accessibility.

It may be important, as well, to provide opportunities in which clients can practice discussing their disability to gain comfort in preparation for real-life conversations with dating partners. As relationships grow more intimate, questions about sexuality, reproductive abilities, and procreative desires as they are impacted by disability will emerge, and clients will benefit from opportunities to practice these discussions in role-play with therapists in simulated scenarios. As a relationship advances to a level of sexual intimacy, clients may need assistance to understand physical positions and adaptive aids that can allow sexual activity despite factors such as UE and LE weakness or paralysis, fatigue and lack of endurance, joint mobility restrictions, sensory loss, and incoordination and poor dexterity. Interventions for such impairments can be found in Chapters 27 and 39.

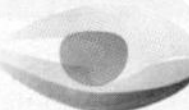

CASE STUDY

Patient Information

Ellie is a 28-year-old white female who sustained a T3 SCI 12 years ago in a diving accident and is presently 6 months pregnant. After Ellie and her wife, Maddie, decided to conceive a child through artificial insemination, Ellie agreed to carry and give birth to the baby, who through ultrasound was determined to be a girl. Maddie, a 26-year-old Asian American female, also sustained an SCI at T5 7 years ago. Ellie reported that she understands her increased risk of pressure ulcers, urinary tract infection, and the formation of LE blood clots and has taken appropriate precautions to maintain her health and that of the pregnancy. The pregnancy has thus far been typical, and Ellie is expected to give birth in 3 months. Both women have been focused on Ellie's and the baby's health and have not had time to consider needed adaptive equipment and supplies. Ellie's obstetrician has referred Ellie for an occupational therapy consultation to help determine needed adaptive equipment and to teach both parents about adaptive infant care strategies.

Assessment Process and Results

Because both Ellie's and Maddie's SCIs are in the high thoracic regions, they each possess innervation of the UE muscles (with full fine motor abilities) and long muscles of the back, allowing for moderate trunk control. Ellie reports that her trunk control has decreased in the past 3 months of her pregnancy. Both women possess UE range of motion and strength within normal limits. Muscle innervation below the mid trunk has been lost, resulting in LE paralysis, and both women use wheelchairs for mobility and are independent in self-care, grooming, meal preparation, and home management with adaptive equipment and environmental modifications. The couple lives in a two-bedroom, elevator apartment building with a standard tub/shower and bathroom space sufficient for wheelchair transfers. No modifications have been made to the kitchen to enhance meal preparation from a wheelchair position, although tilted mirrors have been positioned above the stove to better view foods atop the stove burners. The kitchen sink does not accommodate a wheelchair user to position directly beneath the counter. A standard infant crib, changing table, high chair, baby bathtub, and playpen have been donated by Ellie's mother; however, these items are not accessible for parents using wheelchairs. Both women work, have health insurance, and have been provided 6 months of parental leave once the baby is born. Ellie has been provided an additional 1 month in her last trimester. Both sets of grandparents live nearby and are eager to provide assistance in their grandchild's care.

Occupational Therapy Problem List

Both parents will have difficulty using the standard infant equipment that has been donated.

- Neither mother can access the baby bathtub if placed in the tub or on the kitchen counter.
- The standard crib has a drop-down rail and does not permit a wheelchair to be positioned beneath the crib basin. Neither mother is able to stand and reach over the crib rails.
- The changing table sits atop a set of drawers and is inaccessible from a wheelchair, which cannot be positioned directly beneath the changing area.
- The high chair will be too high for Ellie and Maddie to lift the baby into once she is older.
- Neither mother will be able to transfer her infant into or retrieve the baby from the playpen while seated in a wheelchair.

Occupational Therapy Goal List

- Explore funding options to purchase needed adaptive infant equipment.
- Explore resources needed to adapt standard infant equipment to enhance accessibility for both mothers.
- Provide instruction in and practice opportunities to use adapted equipment for bathing, feeding, diapering and dressing, and crib and playpen use.

Intervention

Both sets of in-laws combined their financial resources and purchased an adjustable-height crib with horizontally sliding rails so that Ellie and Maddie could position their wheelchairs directly beneath the crib carriage, slide the rails open, and access their infant safely without the risk of balance loss or infant falls. Ellie's father, who possesses carpentry skills, built a changing table that is wheelchair accessible and has side frames to prevent infant falls. The changing table mattress was secured to the surface with a nonskid mat to prevent slippage. An adjustable Velcro strap, to secure the infant in place while changing, was attached to the mattress as an additional safety feature. Ellie and Maddie purchased an adjustable-height high chair with a swing-away tray for easy infant lifting into the seat area. Both women were fitted with infant harnesses and carriers to enhance easy and safe infant transport using a wheelchair. Ellie, who will be breastfeeding her infant daughter until she returns to work, was instructed in the use of a nursing pillow and purchased one that fits within the width of her wheelchair. The therapist also helped the mothers set up the portable baby bathtub on their kitchen table (which is wheelchair accessible) near the sink. A detachable hose was secured

(continued)

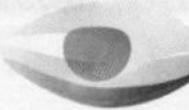

CASE STUDY *(continued)*

to the sink faucet to both fill the baby bathtub and empty the bath water into the sink drain once used. Ellie's father also built a raised platform on which to stabilize the playpen so that both mothers could obtain access from their chairs. The therapist adapted the playpen netting on one side so that it opens and closes with a zippered fastener. These adaptations allow both mothers to retrieve and place their infant in the playpen without risking balance loss or infant falls. Ellie, Maddie, and the therapist practiced the use of all adaptive equipment with a weighted doll until both mothers demonstrated safe use, comfort, and mastery.

At a 3-month follow-up visit after their infant daughter, Kenzie, was born, both mothers reported that they were able to care for their baby independently with the above-noted adaptations and were eager to begin community exploration with Kenzie in tow.

Evidence Table of Studies Assessing Role Restoration for Adults with Disabilities

Intervention	Intervention Description	Participants	Dosage	Research Design and Evidence Level	Benefit	Statistical Significance and Effect Size
Examination of the perceived benefits of occupational therapy services designed to help mothers with arthritis[16]	Mothers received ongoing occupational therapy services in the United Kingdom to address parenting with arthritis, including adaptive equipment and compensatory strategies.	Four mothers with diagnoses of severe arthritis; all having children under the age of 11 years; age range 26–28 years. Two occupational therapists	One-hour occupational therapy sessions in mothers' homes, followed by 1-hour interview with mothers, and separate 1-hour interviews with therapists	Qualitative case series using observation of occupational therapy sessions, interviews with mothers and therapists, and analysis of clinical documentation	The following interventions were perceived by mothers to be the most beneficial in promoting parenting roles: lightweight infant carriers and slings, supportive infant feeding cushions, preparing and storing milk for 24-hour periods, adjustable-height changing tables, wrist splints, energy conservation techniques, work simplification, and pain management.	No statistical analysis
Examination of the adaptive methods used by mothers with physical disabilities[14]	Nine of 22 mothers received occupational therapy services to assist with adaptive strategies for parenting roles.	Twenty-two mothers with physical disabilities with children under the age of 10 years. Mean age = 34.8, standard deviation (SD) = 5.3	Not provided	Qualitative semi-structured, open-ended interviews were carried out with 22 mothers with physical disabilities. Each mother participated in a 2-hour one-time phone interview.	The following adaptations were reported as most beneficial (whether derived from occupational therapy services or independently): infant carriers, and modifying standard cribs and changing tables for wheelchair accessibility. Participants who received occupational therapy services reported that services were most beneficial in helping resolve issues with infant feeding, bathing, and carrying.	No statistical analysis
Occupational therapy intervention designed to help adult men with TBI to regain lost preinjury roles, including dating and courtship roles[26]	Three tiered intervention in which Tier 1 addressed identifying desired roles after injury, Tier 2 addressed regaining participation in activities supporting role resumption, and Tier 3 addressed attaining desired rites of passages such as living independently and engaging in a committed relationship.	Four men with TBI ranging in age from 27 to 48 (mean = 37), residing in a community-assisted living facility	Intervention was carried out in 3 weekly individual sessions, 1–2 hours in length, over 4 months.	Case series with qualitative analysis through focused interviews and participant observation	All four participants reported greater participation in and satisfaction with desired roles postinjury, including dating and courtship roles. Desired rites of passages—such as participation in a committed relationship—were not attained, but still desired after intervention end.	No statistical analysis

References

1. Juengst SB, Adams LM, Bogner JA, et al. Trajectories of life satisfaction after traumatic brain injury: influence of life roles, age, cognitive disability, and depressive symptoms. *Rehabil Psychol.* 2015;60(4):353–364. doi:10.1037/rep0000056.
2. Ma VY, Chan L, Carruthers KJ. Incidence, prevalence, costs, and impact on disability of common conditions requiring rehabilitation in the United States: stroke, spinal cord injury, traumatic brain injury, multiple sclerosis, osteoarthritis, rheumatoid arthritis, limb loss, and back pain. *Arch Phys Med Rehabil.* 2014;95(5):986–995. doi:10.1016/j.apmr.2013.10.032.
3. O'donnell ML, Creamer M, Elliott P, Atkin C, Kossmann T. Determinants of quality of life and role-related disability after injury: impact of acute psychological responses. *J Trauma.* 2005;59(6):1328–1335. doi:10.1097/01.ta.0000197621.94561.4e.
4. Olsen R, Wates M. *Disabled Parents: Examining Research Assumptions.* Dartington: Research in Practice; 2003.
5. Walsh F. Family resilience: a framework for clinical practice. *Fam. Process.* 2003;42(1):1–18. doi:10.1111/j.1545-5300.2003.00001.x.
6. Mosey AC. *Psychosocial Components of Occupational Therapy.* New York: Raven; 1986.
7. Furstenberg FF. On a new schedule: transitions to adulthood and family change. *Future Child.* 2010;20(1):67–87. https://repository.upenn.edu/cgi/viewcontent.cgi?article=1009&context=sociology_papers.
8. Kitzmüller G, Häggström T, Asplund K. Living an unfamiliar body: the significance of the long-term influence of bodily changes on the perception of self after stroke. *Med Health Care Philos.* 2013;16(1):19–29. doi:10.1007/s11019-012-9403-y.
9. Kitzmüller G, Asplund K, Häggström T. The long-term experience of family life after stroke. *J Neurosci Nurs.* 2012;44(1):E1–E3. doi:10.1097/JNN.0b013e31823ae4a1.
10. Johnson CL, Resch JA, Elliott TR, et al. Family satisfaction predicts life satisfaction trajectories over the first 5 years after traumatic brain injury. *Rehabil Psychol.* 2010;55(2):180–187. doi:10.1037/a0019480.
11. Post MW, Van Leeuwen CM. Psychosocial issues in spinal cord injury: a review. *Spinal Cord.* 2012;50(5):382–389. https://www.nature.com/articles/sc2011182
12. Through the Looking Glass. How many parents with disabilities are there in the US? https://www.lookingglass.org/national-services/research-a-development/126-current-demographics-of-parents-with-disabilities-in-the-us. Published 2012. Updated 2018. Accessed August 1, 2018.
13. Pakenham KI, Samios C. Couples coping with multiple sclerosis: a dyadic perspective on the roles of mindfulness and acceptance. *J Behav Med.* 2013;36(4):389–400. doi:10.1007/s10865-012-9434-0.
14. Wint AJ, Smith DL, Iezzoni LI. Mothers with physical disability: child care adaptations at home. *Am J Occup Ther.* 2016;70:7006220060. doi:10.5014/ajot.2016.021477.
15. Farber RS. Mothers with disabilities: in their own voice. *Am J Occup Ther.* 2000;54(3):260–268. doi:10.5014/ajot.54.3.260.
16. Grant M. Mothers with arthritis, child care and occupational therapy: insight through case studies. *Br J Occup Ther.* 2001;64(7):322–329. doi:10.1177/030802260106400702.
17. Walsh F. Human-Animal bonds II: the role of pets in family systems and family therapy. *Fam. Process.* 2009;48(4):481–499. doi:10.1111/j.1545-5300.2009.01297.x.
18. Friedmann E, Son H. The human–companion animal bond: how humans benefit. *Vet Clin N Am Small Anim Pract.* 2009;39(2):293–326. doi:10.1016/j.cvsm.2008.10.015.
19. Oliver K. Service dogs: between animal studies and disability studies. *PhiloSOPHIA.* 2016;6(2):241–258. doi:10.1353/phi.2016.0021.
20. Walther S, Yamamoto M, Thigpen AP, Garcia A, Willits NH, Hart LA. Assistance dogs: historic patterns and roles of dogs placed by aDi or igDF accredited facilities and by non-accredited us facilities. *Front Vet Sci.* 2017;4:1. doi:10.3389/fvets.2017.00001.
21. Irvin S. The healing role of assistance dogs: what these partnerships tell us about the human–animal bond. *Anim Front.* 2014;4(3):66–71. doi:10.2527/af.2014-0024.
22. Hogg MA, Reid SA. Social identity, self-categorization, and the communication of group norms. *Commun Theory.* 2006;16(1):7–30. doi:10.1111/j.1468-2885.2006.00003.x.
23. Turner RH. Role change. *Annu Rev Sociol.* 1990;16(1):87–110. doi:10.1146/annurev.so.16.080190.000511.
24. Evandrou M, Glaser K. Family, work and quality of life: changing economic and social roles through the lifecourse. *Ageing Soc.* 2004;24(5):771–791. doi:10.1017/S0144686X04002545.
25. Carlson DS, Kacmar KM, Williams LJ. Construction and initial validation of a multidimensional measure of work–family conflict. *J Vocat Behav.* 2000;56(2):249–276. doi:10.1006/jvbe.1999.1713.
26. Gutman SA. Brain injury and gender role strain: rebuilding adult lifestyles after injury [Special issue]. *Occup Ther Mental Health.* 2000;15(3/4). doi:10.1300/J004v15n03_03.
27. Gutman SA. The transition through adult rites of passage after traumatic brain injury: preliminary assessment of an occupational therapy intervention. *Occup Ther Int.* 1999;6(2):143–158. doi:10.1002/oti.94.
28. Gutman SA. The alleviation of gender role strain in adult men with traumatic brain injury: an evaluation of a set of guidelines for occupational therapy. *Am J Occup Ther.* 1999;53:101–110. doi:10.5014/ajot.53.1.101.
29. Obst P, Stafurik J. Online we are all able bodied: online psychological sense of community and social support found through membership of disability-specific websites promotes well-being for people living with a physical disability. *J Commun Appl Soc Psychol.* 2010;20(6):525–531. doi:10.1002/casp.1067.

Chapter 29

Restoring Home, Work, and Recreation Roles

Mary W. Hildebrand

LEARNING OBJECTIVES

This chapter will allow the reader to:

1. Understand essential home, work, and recreation roles.
2. Identify assessments for home, work, and recreation.
3. Identify barriers and challenges for clients to engage in home, work, and recreational activities.
4. Apply remediation, compensation, and adaptation principles to occupations in the home, workplace, and recreational setting.
5. Apply work simplification and energy conservation principles to occupations in the home, workplace, and recreational setting.
6. Identify adapted methods and equipment that enable persons to regain competence in occupations in the home, workplace, and recreational setting.
7. Define functional capacity evaluations (FCE) and describe an FCE format.
8. Describe resources for job descriptions and job adaptations.
9. Describe components of and differences between work readiness, work hardening, and work conditioning programs.

CHAPTER OUTLINE

TERMINOLOGY

Energy conservation: an essential intervention for clients with low endurance or fatigue that is comprised of simple principles that clients may adopt to save energy to perform occupations that are most important to them.

Functional capacity evaluation: standardized batteries of work-related tests that consider the person's body functions and structures, environmental factors, personal factors, and health status used to make recommendations for participation in work.

Home management: activities that involve obtaining and maintaining personal and household possessions and environment (e.g., home, yard, garden, appliances, vehicles), including maintaining and repairing personal possessions (e.g., clothing, household items) and knowing how to seek help or whom to contact.

Job analysis: part of a functional work assessment that includes a systematic evaluation of the physical, cognitive, social, and psychological requirements of a job.

Leisure: free time or "non-obligatory activity that is intrinsically motivated and engaged in during discretionary time—that is, time not committed to obligatory occupations such as work, self-care, or sleep."[1]

Recreation: activities that people do to relax, have fun, or that provide amusement or enjoyment.

Work conditioning: work treatment program focused on basic physical conditioning such as restoration of flexibility, strength, coordination, and endurance; typically conducted after completion of acute care and before work hardening.

Work hardening: multidisciplinary structured, graded return-to-work treatment program that progressively introduces greater rehabilitation requirements to achieve full capability of the worker to meet job demands; includes psychosocial, communication, physical, and vocational needs and incorporates work simulation as treatment modalities.

Work readiness: work programs to help individuals identify work goals, interests, and skills.

Work simplification: strategies to reduce the amount of energy expended in occupations by clients with low endurance or fatigue; similar to energy conservation.

Introduction

Adults experience higher quality of life and life satisfaction when they participate in self-reported meaningful activities, including **home management**, active community participation, paid employment or volunteerism, and recreational activities. Adults with disabilities or chronic conditions, however, often withdraw from engaging in productive, leisure, and social activities as a result of physical, emotional, and psychological impairments associated with disability or environmental barriers.

Researchers have examined the effect of disability severity and participation in productive activities (e.g., work, volunteer, home management) and recreation (e.g., sports) on self-reported well-being of adults with disabilities. They found that performing productive and recreational activities is integral to maintaining well-being and postulated that these activities offer adults with disabilities the opportunity to fulfill essential productive and social roles.[2]

Participation in home management, recreation, and community activities contributes to personal identity, well-being, and quality of life and is a vital source for social interaction. People with disabilities, however, are less likely to participate in such activities and, thus, are more socially isolated. Community participation has been found particularly beneficial to people with disabilities and older adults by increasing their sense of empowerment and their number of social interactions. When people with disabilities or older adults participate in civic or religious organizations, not only do they benefit, but their communities do as well.[3] Volunteer contributions from older adults, for example, help to maintain a functioning society.[4]

Similar to home management and community participation, work is the occupation from which people receive meaning and spend most of their time. Work is a source of personal identity, income, and social interaction and offers psychological well-being. Conversely, the relationship between work and health can be negative. When a disability disrupts participation in productive activities, the emotional and financial costs are significant to persons unable to work, their families, employers, and society. The majority of people who experience work disability want to return to work.[5]

Recreation is often seen as the adult version of play. Like play, **recreation** or **leisure** has positive effects on physical and emotional health by improving physical fitness, creating opportunities for social interaction, coping with stress, improving cognitive skills, and increasing quality of life. A disabling event, such as a brain injury, typically leads to decreased participation in former leisure activities, particularly those with greater physical or cognitive demands.[6] Given the benefits of participation in recreation, it is important that occupational therapists address recreation with clients with disabilities and chronic conditions.

Therapists provide interventions to clients that target remediation of client factors, and performance skills and patterns that limit participation in desired occupations. Therapists also recommend compensatory strategies and adaptations to occupations or the environment to support occupational performance. This chapter provides an overview of common assessments and interventions to improve client involvement in the roles of home manager, worker, and recreational participant—which overlap with and support larger community member roles.

Occupational Performance Assessments for Home Management, Work, and Recreation Roles

The first step in the occupational therapy process is performance of a top-down assessment to identify the occupations that the client, a person after a disabling event or with a chronic condition, wishes to perform.

Top-down assessment in these categories begins with participation measures that assess a client's desire to perform home management, work, and recreational activities. Examples of these assessments include the Activity Card Sort (ACS),[7] the Canadian Occupational Performance Measure (COPM),[8] and the Occupational Performance History Interview-II (OPHI-II).[9] The ACS, an interview-based assessment, consists of full-color photographs of adults performing 20 instrumental, 35 low-demand leisure, 17 high-demand leisure, and 17 social activities. It is used to compare an adult's premorbid participation in activities with their current participation level and is useful for goal setting, intervention planning, and monitoring changes in participation.[7] The COPM is a semi-structured interview that asks clients to identify and prioritize occupations with which they are experiencing difficulty in the categories of self-care, leisure, and productivity. Clients are asked to choose their top five priorities and to rate their performance of and satisfaction with the five activities. The COPM is an outcome measure, is useful for goal setting and intervention planning, and may be administered in all types of rehabilitation settings and with clients with a wide variety of conditions.[8] The OPHI-II is also interview based. It has a rating scale of occupational function and elicits the client's life history narrative. The OPHI-II provides information with which to develop client occupational profiles, identify their strengths and weaknesses, and create an intervention plan[9] (see Assessment table at the end of this chapter).

The ACS, COPM, and OPHI-II provide therapists with an opportunity to build rapport and gain a deeper understanding of the client and, thus, guide treatment planning. These measures motivate clients to participate in occupational therapy because client priorities are heard and addressed in treatment. The assessments provide evidence of the benefits of therapy by assessing outcomes. In addition, they guide the therapist's next steps in further assessment of occupational performance.

Selecting the Intervention Approach: Remediation, Compensation, or Adaptation

Intervention to improve performance or increase participation in home management, work, and recreation roles includes remediation and compensation or adaptation. Remediation techniques, such as improving range of motion (ROM), strength, endurance, motor control, or cognition, change the client in order to develop or restore a skill. When using remedial techniques with appropriate clients, it is important for clients to understand that practicing occupations will aid in remediation and improve performance. For example, when strength is impaired, the preparatory method of exercise should be followed by real-life activities impacted by client weakness (e.g., laundry, cooking) to improve client strength needed to perform those occupations. Compensation or adaptation involves finding ways to change the context, environment, tools, or occupation to allow clients to participate in desired occupations with greater independence. It does not focus solely on changing client factors.

Compensation or Adaptation

Basic principles of compensation or adaptation depend on the client's functional limitations and can be applied in home management, work, or recreational occupations.

- *Limited ROM:* Increase the client's reach with extended handles or reorganize workspace to place frequently used items within reach.
- *Weakness and low endurance:* Use lightweight and/or power equipment and allow gravity to assist. Use work simplification and energy conservation techniques.
- *Chronic pain:* Use proper body mechanics, work simplification, and energy conservation techniques.
- *Unilateral loss of motor control and limb function:* Use affected limb to stabilize objects when possible. Use one-handed adaptive techniques or equipment for bilateral activities.
- *Incoordination:* Stabilize at proximal joints to reduce the degrees of freedom of movement necessary for control. Use weighted objects to minimize distal incoordination.
- *Visual impairments:* Use senses of smell, touch, and hearing to substitute for vision. With low vision impairments, improve lighting, reduce glare, or increase contrast.
- *Cognitive limitations:* Employ visual and auditory aids to enhance memory and organization. Work in familiar environments and reduce distractions.

Work Simplification and Energy Conservation

Therapists teach the principles of **work simplification** and **energy conservation** when home management, work, and recreational occupations are too demanding for those with physical impairments. Basic principles of work simplification and energy conservation include:

- *Limit the amount of work:* Ask others to perform heavier tasks when possible. When financially feasible, use prepared items or power tools to decrease time and energy expenditure.
- *Plan ahead:* Schedule and evenly distribute energy-demanding tasks throughout the week.
- *Prioritize:* Schedule important activities and tasks first to complete them before fatiguing.
- *Organize:* De-clutter and reorganize work areas; store frequently used items within reach.
- *Sit to work:* Avoid standing when an activity or task can be performed while sitting.

- *Use efficient methods:* Identify and gather items needed before beginning a task. Instead of carrying items, use a utility cart to move them or slide them along a work surface.
- *Use correct equipment and techniques:* Use good body mechanics in all tasks, assistive equipment to decrease bending and reaching, and power equipment or tools to reduce work.
- *Balance physical tasks with rest breaks:* Perform physically demanding tasks early in the day and take frequent rest breaks (5–10 minutes) throughout the day.

Therapists also teach clients ergonomic guidelines for home management, work, and recreational activities. Ergonomics help to reduce muscle fatigue and injury risk and are important work simplification and energy conservation interventions. Chapter 21 provides a detailed discussion of ergonomic assessment and intervention for workplace settings.

Restoring Home Management Roles

Restoring competence in home management roles following a disabling event can enhance self-efficacy and esteem. This section reviews assessment of and interventions to restore instrumental activities of daily living (IADLs) that involve home management roles for people with disabilities and temporary or chronic health conditions. These occupations include meal preparation and cleanup, shopping, and home and financial management. They are categorized as IADLs because they support daily life within the home but may be more complex than activities of daily living (ADLs) or self-care. Although home management can be addressed at any time in the rehabilitation process, it is typically addressed after clients approach or achieve ADL independence.

Performance-Based Measures of Home Management Occupational Roles

After identifying the client's priorities in home management occupations, the next step should be evaluation of the client's performance of those occupations. In practice, this often occurs through informal observation to determine where client performance fails.

A standardized, quantitative measure of the client's progress in goals—including home management occupations and the efficacy of the therapist's interventions—is Goal Attainment Scaling (GAS).[10] GAS has been used in rehabilitation settings to construct personalized client goals and measure client outcomes. Examples of successful implementation of GAS have been reported in home health with patients with complex needs,[11,12] an intensive aphasia program,[13] and in outpatient rehabilitation clinics with clients with traumatic brain injury (TBI).[14] Using GAS, the therapist creates a five-point graded series or scale for each client goal composed of treatment outcomes from least favorable to most favorable. Box 29-1 shows an example of GAS with a meal preparation goal.

Other standardized evaluations assess home management occupations (see Assessment table). The Performance Assessment of Self-Care Skills (PASS), version 3.1 is an observational, performance-based assessment of mobility, self-care, and IADL tasks. Home management occupations include housework, home maintenance, and cooking safety.[15]

Box 29-1

Goal Attainment Scaling (GAS): Home Management Example

Goal: Client will prepare a simple meal with supervision using adaptive equipment, such as a one-handed jar opener, a rocker knife, and Dycem, and minimal verbal cueing to use energy conservation techniques in two sessions.

Predicted Attainment	Score	Goals
Most favorable outcome likely	+2	Client prepares a simple meal with adaptive equipment without assistance and independently uses energy conservation techniques.
Greater than expected outcome	+1	Client prepares a simple meal with adaptive equipment without assistance and one verbal cue to use energy conservation techniques.
Expected outcome	0	Client prepares a simple meal with adaptive equipment with supervision and two verbal cues to use energy conservation techniques.
Less than expected outcome	−1	Client is provided instruction on use of adaptive equipment for making a simple meal and on energy conservation techniques.
Least favorable outcome	−2	Client is unable to prepare a simple meal with adaptive equipment and requires maximum physical assistance and three or more verbal cues to use energy conservation techniques.

The Assessment of Motor and Process Skills (AMPS) is an observational assessment in which clients choose three to five activities that they wish to perform from a list of 85 ADLs and IADLs. Therapists rate client performance of the chosen activities on 16 motor and 20 process skills.[16]

The Executive Function Performance Test (EFPT) assesses functional cognition in four IADL tasks: simple cooking, telephone use, taking medication, and paying bills.[17] The EFPT determines which executive functions are impaired and the type and amount of assistance clients require to complete tasks.

The final step in assessment of occupational performance in home management roles involves selected analysis of clients' performance skills (e.g., motor or process skills), performance patterns (e.g., habits, routines), context or environment (e.g., cultural, natural, built), and client factors (e.g., body functions or structures, activity demands).[18] These assessments are discussed in depth in other chapters of this textbook.

Intervention to Restore Home Management Occupational Roles

Included in IADLs and discussed here are meal preparation and cleanup, and home and financial management. Remediation to restore or prevent limitations in these occupations for clients with an impairment includes home exercise programs and exercise classes to improve balance, strength, ROM, and activity tolerance or endurance. Therapists may also recommend home programs and group activities to remediate cognitive skills that have been affected by disabling events such as brain injury.

Following the basic principles of compensation and adaptation techniques, therapists provide education in adaptive techniques, training in adaptive equipment use, and recommendations and training in home modifications. Therapists will also analyze occupations and provide education in work simplification and energy conservation techniques.

Meal Preparation and Cleanup

Meal preparation and cleanup is defined as "Planning, preparing, and serving well-balanced, nutritious meals and cleaning up food and utensils after meals."[18] Efficient kitchen work areas and storage, adaptive techniques, and assistive devices will enhance client safety and participation in meal preparation and cleanup.

Kitchen Work Areas and Storage

Cost-effective home modifications include placing frequently used kitchenware and cookware within easy reach: from the floor, between 15 and 48 inches (38–122 cm) for wheelchair users and between 30 and 60 inches (76–152 cm) for those who are ambulatory. Reducing clutter and clearing pathways may decrease client accident risk and conserve energy. High-end home modifications to enhance meal preparation might include installing wheelchair accessible counters (28–34 inches [71–86.36 cm] from the floor and with a depth clearance of 24 inches [61 cm] underneath for wheelchair leg rests[19]), pullout shelves or turntables in cabinets, and appliances with accessible controls.

Gathering and Transporting Items

To transport multiple or larger items, a wheeled utility cart is useful in the kitchen (Fig. 29-1). For wheelchair users, lap trays and cup holders can attach to armrests. Optional walker accessories include attachable trays, baskets, and walker bags for transporting small items (Fig. 29-2). Long-handled reachers may be useful for retrieving lightweight, unbreakable items from high or low cabinets (Fig. 29-3). Attaching a reusable grocery bag or basket to a walker may help with transporting small, lightweight items and is inexpensive.

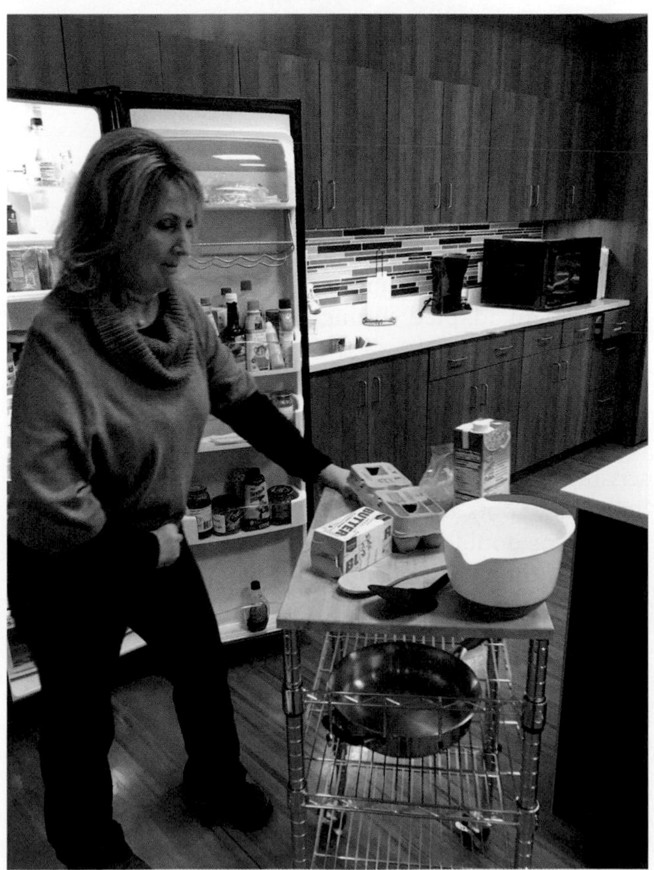

Figure 29-1. To transport multiple or larger items, a wheeled utility cart is useful in the kitchen.

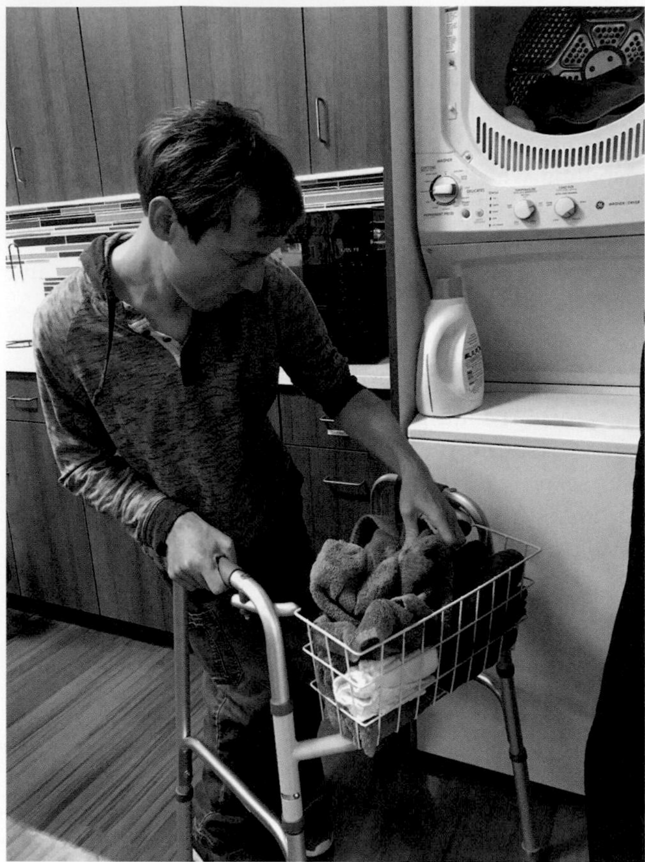

Figure 29-2. Optional walker accessories include attachable trays, baskets, and walker bags for transporting small items.

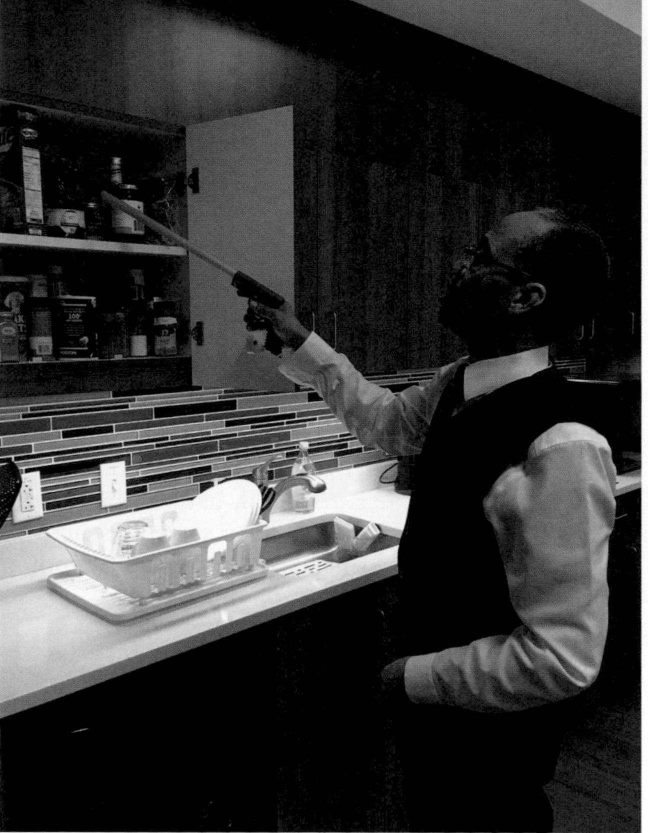

Figure 29-3. Long-handled reachers may be useful for retrieving lightweight, unbreakable items from high or low cabinets.

Food Preparation and Cooking

There are many assistive devices on the market that can make food preparation easier. For one-handed performance after a stroke, upper extremity injury, or an amputation, an adapted cutting board with spikes is useful for holding vegetables or fruit to cut (Fig. 29-4).

For clients with weak, or otherwise impaired grip, there are kitchen utensils that have ergonomic handles, freestanding and mounted jar openers, adapted kitchen scissors for opening packaging or cutting foods, and lightweight pots and pans with easy-to-grip heat-resistant handles or double-handled pots. Attaching a rope, cord, or zip-tie loop to appliance door handles is an inexpensive way to allow clients to pull the door open with a weak grip. Loops can be added to other kitchenware to aid in retrieval from shelves or cabinets (Fig. 29-5).

To reduce the amount of work and save time in meal preparation, there are a variety of small electric appliances from which to choose such as can openers, blenders, food processors, and knives. For wheelchair users, a typical range (i.e., stovetop and oven) should have accessible front-operated controls and a wall-mounted mirror angled to see food cooking on the stovetop. If it is not economically feasible to replace the range, small electrical appliances may substitute if placed safely on a stable wheelchair accessible surface (i.e., electric griddles, skillets, toaster ovens, or microwaves).

Cleanup and Dishwashing

Energy conservation techniques for cleanup include lining baking pans with foil to reduce washing, serving food directly from cooking pots, organizing tasks to flow in a single direction, sitting on a stool to wash dishes, using electric dishwashers, and air-drying dishes.

If washing dishes at wheelchair level, place a wooden rack on the sink bottom to reduce its depth, making it easier to reach dishes, and remove cabinet doors under the sink to provide knee and footrest space. A swing-away, lever-handled faucet is easier to control with limited hand function; installing it on the sink's side rather than the back is easier to reach. Clients with limited grasp can also use terry cloth mitts to wash dishes. For one-handed dishwashing, there are bottle brushes and scrub brushes for cleaning glasses, bottles, and utensils that can be suctioned to the sink's side.

Grocery Shopping

Planning ahead is the key to successful grocery shopping and energy conservation. Organizing the shopping list by grocery store layout will minimize the time and effort

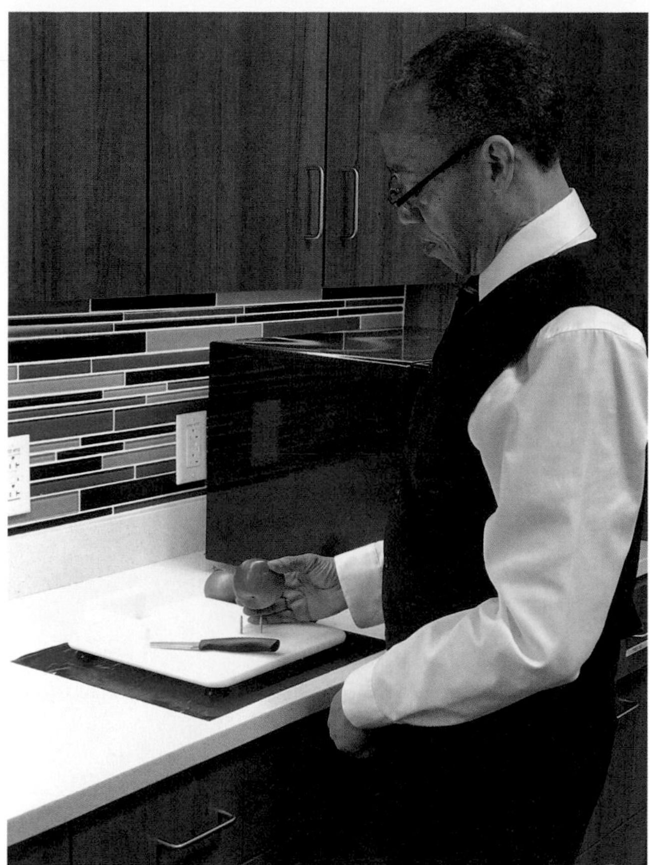

Figure 29-4. For one-handed performance after a stroke, upper extremity injury, or an amputation, an adapted cutting board with spikes is useful for holding vegetables or fruit to cut.

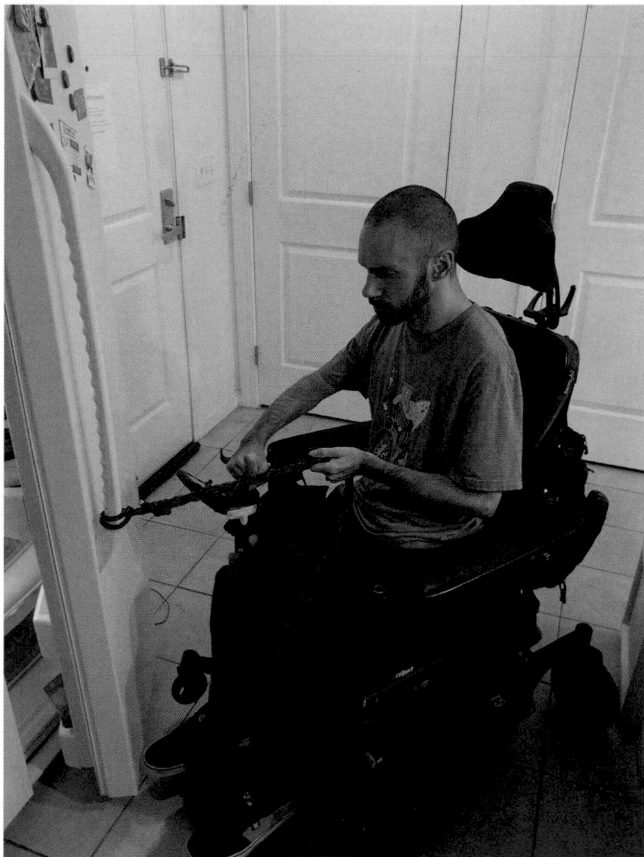

Figure 29-5. Attaching a rope, cord, or zip-tie loop to appliance door handles is an inexpensive way to allow clients to pull the door open with a weak grip. Loops can be added to other kitchenware to aid in retrieval from shelves or cabinets.

needed to search for groceries. Many printable grocery shopping lists are available online and have space for weekly menus and food items by category. Shopping lists can be printed or laminated and items to be bought the next week checked off. The client can then photograph the shopping list with a smart phone. There are also smart phone applications (apps) on which the client can add and organize items by category. While shopping, the apps check off items when acquired. When shopping in-person, it is best to shop during off-peak hours when there are fewer customers, aisles are not crowded, and store employees are available to help as needed.

A shopping cart may be used by clients who are ambulatory. Adapted shopping carts for wheelchair users and motorized scooters for clients with poor endurance and mobility are also available at most large grocery stores (Fig. 29-6).

Many stores offer online shopping with either home delivery or store pickup. Home delivery, though expensive, is convenient for clients who lack access to transportation or are physically unable to go to the store. When clients can drive or have someone who can drive them to the store, curbside pickup service is convenient and costs less than home delivery. There are also newer options for home food delivery such as food plan services that create menus and deliver ingredients and instructions for each recipe.

Home Management

Home management is defined as "Obtaining and maintaining personal and household possessions and environment (e.g., home, yard, garden, appliances, vehicles), including maintaining and repairing personal possessions (e.g., clothing, household items) and knowing how to seek help or whom to contact."[18]

Laundry and Clothing Care

Sorting soiled laundry is a step that can be eliminated by placing it in separate hampers or bags when undressing. Use of in-home appliances, self-service laundries, or laundry services is dependent on client living situation and financial resources. In-home washers and dryers may be front-loading and top-loading. Top-loading appliances require less bending, whereas front-loading appliances are better for persons who perform laundry while seated. A knob turner may make it easier to turn

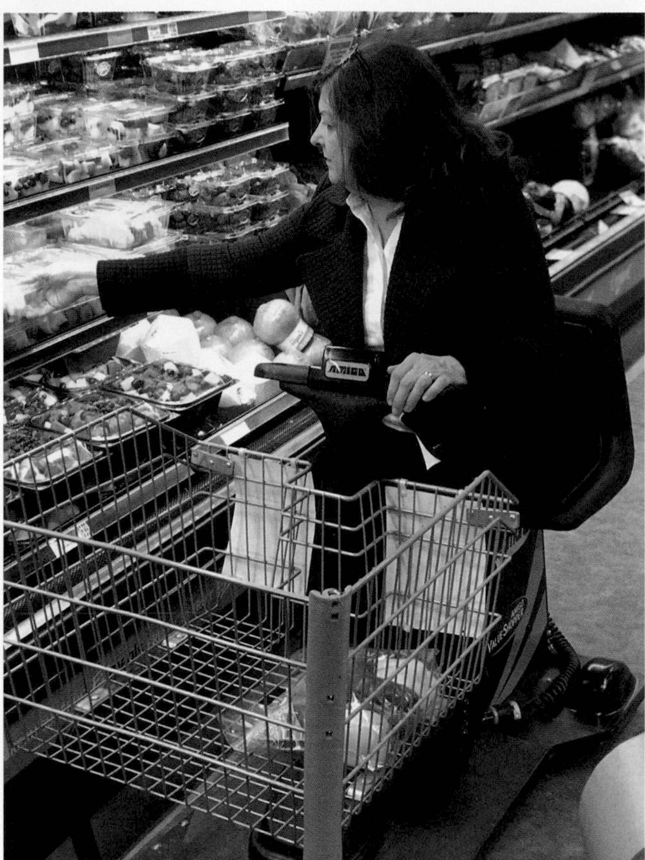

Figure 29-6. Adapted shopping carts for wheelchair users and motorized scooters for clients with poor endurance and mobility are also available at most large grocery stores.

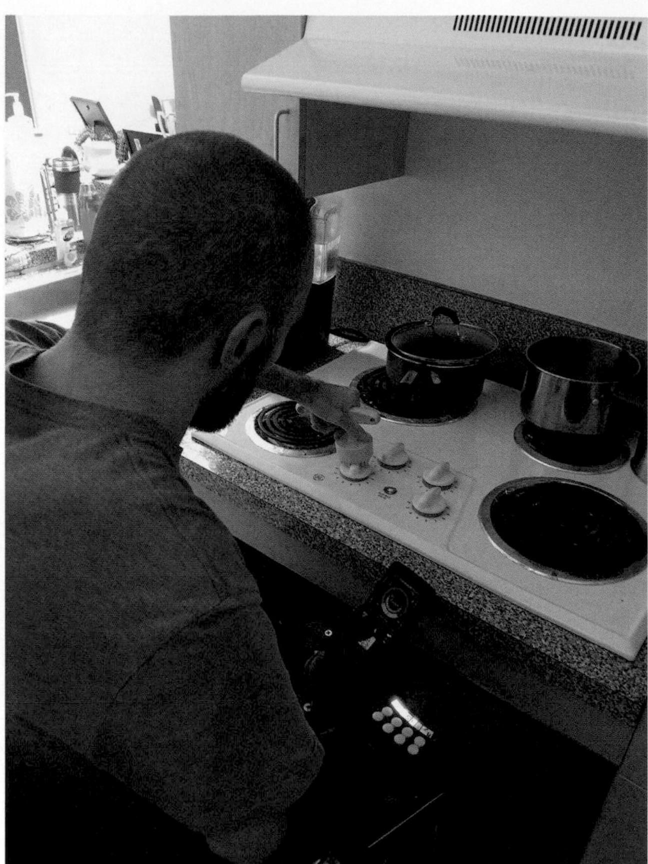

Figure 29-7. A knob turner may make it easier to turn appliance knobs for clients with weak grip.

appliance knobs for clients with weak grip (Fig. 29-7). If taking clothing to a self-service or commercial laundry, a rolling basket to transport laundry and premeasured detergent save energy. Clothes can be folded while sitting or standing at a table, and sheets can be reused immediately to bypass folding. If clothing is not permanent press and ironing is required, it should be performed with a lightweight iron and board that can be adjusted for sitting or standing. A tabletop ironing board may also be an option.

Indoor Household Maintenance

Many tasks are involved in maintaining a home. Bedmaking can be simplified by straightening sheets and blankets before getting out of bed or by adjusting one side of the bed before moving to the other side. Loose fitted sheets and lightweight blankets or comforters may be easier to manage for persons with poor strength or endurance. Dusting can be adapted using long-handled, lightweight dusters. For persons with poor grip, a mitt can be used as a dusting cloth. When clients have poor hand strength, they can purchase adapted spray handles for household cleaning products. Floor care is a heavy cleaning task, but there are available products that make it easier, such as lightweight vacuums, long-handled brush and dustpans, self-wringing mops, and mops that spray cleaning fluid. Bathroom care is also a heavy household cleaning task. Spray-on products for the bathtub and sink, and drop-in toilet cleaning tablets reduce heavy scrubbing demands. To safely clean bathtubs, clients can use long-handled brushes and scrubbing sponges. Sliding glass doors may get in the way of bathtub cleaning. Replacing them with shower curtains provides better tub access for both bathing and cleaning.

Outdoor Household Maintenance

Lawn care and gardening are important occupations for many clients. Self-propelled or riding lawn mowers and lightweight or battery-powered lawn tools, such as weed trimmers and edgers, may aid those with poor endurance or strength. Ergonomic shovels and gardening tools, long-handled gardening tools, and gardening stools can also be purchased. Tools can be transported around the garden in apron pockets or a child's wagon. Raised beds for flowers and vegetables can increase a person's access to gardening from a wheelchair. Container gardening is also an option for those with limited mobility.

For all home management occupations, therapists should always address work simplification, energy conservation, proper body mechanics, and safety.

Financial Management

Financial management is defined as "Using fiscal resources, including alternate methods of financial transaction, and planning and using finances with long-term and short-term goals."[18] Being unable to manage their own finances places people with disabilities at risk for being exploited. Basic financial management typically includes money handling and banking tasks. Traditional ways to pay bills consisted of handwriting checks, keeping track of bank account balances by recording credits and debits in check registers, and mailing checks. Adaptive aids are available to help clients with conditions such as low vision, poor fine motor skills, and cognitive impairment—for example, pocket check writing guides, writing aids to hold pens for poor grip, low vision check registers, preprinted envelopes, and signature ink stamps.

Online and mobile banking are gaining popularity and have the potential to provide greater access to financial management for people with disabilities.[20] Financial institutions' websites should follow the Web Content Accessibility Guidelines (WCAG) and be compatible with input devices and screen readers.[20] Mobile phone banking has unique features that persons with disabilities may find useful. For example, assessable banking apps are available that take and upload photos of checks for remote check deposits. Persons with hearing impairment can utilize text messaging or video conferencing with sign language interpreters for communicating with bank employees. Online and mobile banking technologies continue to advance quickly, and therapists must maintain knowledge of such devices.

Home Management with Cognitive Impairment

When cognitive impairment accompanies physical disability, clients will need support to understand and organize the steps of many of the abovementioned activities. Beneficial compensatory strategies include:

- Posting the steps for all activities in written and/or pictorial form in the location in which they will be performed.
- Creating and teaching clients to use checklists for all essential activities and providing opportunities for practice and return demonstration.
- Teaching clients to use preprogrammed smartphone and tablet cuing systems to facilitate activity performance.
- Labeling drawers, cabinets, and closets (in written and/or pictorial form) to enhance organization and memory of supplies stored within.
- Gathering and locating the supplies for each activity in easily accessible organizational systems (e.g., self-care dispensers, plastic storage shelves and trays) maintained in the area in which the activity will be performed.
- Teaching a family member or caregiver in the abovementioned compensatory strategies to monitor their use and correct errors.

Efficacy of Interventions for Home Management

There is little evidence of the efficacy of interventions to improve home management roles specifically as broader assessments of IADL are typically used as outcomes measures in research. A systematic review of occupational therapy interventions to improve IADL performance in community-dwelling older adults found that four types of interventions were effective.[21] Home management was not the sole focus of this review but was included, and some of the same interventions discussed earlier were implemented. Strong evidence was found for IADL improvement after cognitive interventions with a focus on functional task exercises. There was moderate evidence indicating that self-management interventions or Stanford University's Chronic Disease Self-Management Program led by an occupational therapist improved activity participation, quality of life, and self-efficacy for older adults with multimorbidities. Strong evidence was found for interventions to prevent deterioration in IADL performance, including education regarding depression, problem-solving, health promotion behaviors, and energy conservation. Other interventions that prevented IADL deterioration were exercise, home modifications, follow-up visits when transitioning from hospital to home, and a Tai Chi program. Home-based rehabilitation had strong evidence that indicated improvement in IADL performance. These studies included both occupational and physical therapy in client-centered home rehabilitation programs, addressing daily activity participation, task modification, assistive devices, falls prevention, chronic disease self-management, and mobility (see Evidence table at the end of this chapter).

A common occupational therapy intervention for improving participation in home management roles is energy conservation. Sometimes called fatigue management, much research, particularly with people with multiple sclerosis, has been conducted on Managing Fatigue using energy conservation interventions. The presumption is that managing one's fatigue will improve participation in meaningful occupations. The Managing Fatigue program was developed for people with chronic conditions and has been successful in multiple research studies when presented in group and teleconference formats. In a one-to-one, 6-week long format with adults with chronic conditions, the Managing Fatigue course resulted in statistically significant decreases in fatigue and increases in self-efficacy and quality of life.[22] Participants reported that they implemented energy conservation strategies in their everyday activities.

Home modifications are another commonly used intervention to improve participation in home management roles. A systematic review found strong evidence to support that home modifications improved function of frail older adults, adults aging with a disability, adults after hip repair, those with low vision, and those with schizophrenia. Moderate evidence was found for using home modifications to support caregivers of people with dementia. Studies of fall risk reduction also found strong evidence supporting home modifications by occupational therapists[23] (see Evidence table).

Restoring Work Roles

Background

The components of work include employment interests and pursuits, employment seeking and acquisition, job performance, retirement preparation and adjustment, and volunteer exploration and participation.[18] Work meets multiple needs. In addition to being an economic necessity to finance essentials, such as food and shelter, and nonessentials such as leisure activities, work may also bestow identity, provide meaning or a sense of purpose, give structure to the day, provide social opportunities, and confer status within one's community.[5] These benefits of work may not be realized for persons whose health impairments prevent or interrupt their work.

In 2017, unemployment for adults with disabilities between the ages of 16 and 64 years was over twice as high as for adults without disabilities (10% and 4.2%, respectively).[24] Occupational therapists must be aware that racial disparities in work participation exist for persons with disabilities. Blacks with disability have a higher unemployment rate (13.8%) than Hispanics (10.2%), whites (8.5%), and Asians (6.6%).[24] The unemployment rate is defined as the percentage of persons in the workforce who had no employment at the time they were interviewed, were available to work, and were actively seeking employment. The unemployment figure, however, may understate the problem because 80% of persons with disabilities are not in the workforce compared to 30% without disabilities. A more revealing statistic is that only 29.3% of adults with disabilities in the prime working age range, 16 to 64, were employed compared to 73.5% for those without disabilities.[24]

Adults aged 65+ may also want to remain in the workforce for financial reasons, to be active, for personal fulfillment, or health care access. However, only 7.3% of adults aged 65+ with disabilities are working compared to 23.4% of adults older than 65 years without disabilities.[24] Volunteering has many benefits for people with disabilities and their communities and may lead to employment, but volunteering is also less common in people with disabilities.[3]

Many people with disabilities want to work. A scoping review found that work remains meaningful and important to the lives of those with disabilities. For people with cancer, HIV/AIDS, brain injury, musculoskeletal disorders, and spinal cord injury, work provided many benefits: a sense of identity, activity and social engagement, structure in their day, decreased boredom, financial independence, fulfillment, and self-worth.[5]

In spite of their desire to work, people with disabilities find many barriers to joining or returning to the workforce. Pain, fatigue, headaches, weakness, medication side effects, bodily changes, cognitive difficulties, illness susceptibility, and numerous medical appointments act as barriers to work participation and result from health conditions or medical treatment.[5] There are also environmental barriers such as lack of accommodations, inaccessible workplace, loss of social security benefits and income support, mismatches in physical or cognitive job demands, poor relationships with supervisors or coworkers, and stigmatization.[5]

A challenge for occupational therapists in the assessment process is to discover the meaning and importance of work to clients both before and after illness or injury. Focusing intervention on the meaning of their work can be a strong motivator for clients.[5] Further, therapists must also identify the complex barriers to work that clients face and provide interventions and recommendations to help them overcome those barriers.

Performance-Based Measures of Worker Roles

Once the client's priorities for work are identified with an assessment such as the ACS, COPM, or OPHI-II, performance-based measures should be administered. The assessments discussed here focus on those that target adults with disabilities or injuries who may or may not return to their former vocation.

Functional Work Assessments

Functional work assessments typically have two steps: (1) a job analysis and (2) a client evaluation.

Job Analysis

A **job analysis** is a systematic evaluation of the physical, cognitive, social, and psychological requirements of a job. It is an important first step in becoming familiar with a job's demands and should be performed early in the work rehabilitation process so that the occupational therapist is aware of the skills required in order to tailor therapy appropriately.[25] A job analysis requires going to the job site; observing workers performing tasks; interviewing workers and supervisors; and writing detailed descriptions of tools, equipment, services or materials produced, and environmental characteristics of the worksite. A helpful source of information about occupations is the US Department of Labor/Employment and Training Administration's Occupational Information Network (O*NET).[26] O*NET replaced the Dictionary of Occupational Titles (DOT) and is a publicly available, free database that has descriptions of approximately 1,000 occupations. For each occupation in O*NET, there is a report that includes details about technology skills, knowledge, abilities, activities and tasks, context, education, tools, styles, and values that are needed to perform the occupation. It lists core and supplemental tasks for each occupation with core tasks defined as those that are critical and supplemental tasks as less important to the occupation. O*NET may also be utilized for career exploration, determining career interests, writing job descriptions, or identifying skills for advancement.[26]

Uses of job analysis data or O*NET information may include:

- Involve the employer in the work rehabilitation process.
- Develop or select a functional capacity evaluation (FCE).
- Develop preplacement, post-job offer screenings that enable companies to place new hires in positions that minimize potential future injuries.
- Tailor goals and intervention to job demands.
- Match the injured workers' capabilities to job task requirements.
- Place previously injured workers on light duty or return to work.
- Identify risk factors associated with work-related musculoskeletal disorders.
- Identify essential functions.
- Write job descriptions using Americans with Disabilities Act (ADA) of 1990 terminology.
- Describe and advertise jobs.

Functional Capacity Evaluations

A **functional capacity evaluation (FCE)** is a performance-based measure of a person's ability to participate in work. It compares a person's health status, body functions, and body structures with the demands of a job.[27] An FCE may also be known as a functional capacity assessment (FCA), a physical capacity assessment (PCA), a physical capacity evaluation (PCE), a work capacity assessment (WCA), or a work capacity evaluation (WCE). FCEs can be used in industrial settings for preemployment and postoffer screenings, in clinical settings for developing goal and treatment plans, and for determining workers' ability to return to their job duties.

An FCE consists of two parts: (1) a general evaluation of the physical and cognitive abilities of the client and (2) a job-specific evaluation. This is analogous to assessment in traditional occupational therapy settings in which the client's physical and cognitive abilities and occupational performance are assessed, and from which goals and interventions are developed. FCEs include a review of a client's medical record, a work and educational history interview, a basic musculoskeletal evaluation, performance evaluations, and a comparison of the results with the client's job requirements.

The general evaluation of a client's physical abilities consists of measures of flexibility, strength, balance, coordination, cardiovascular condition, and body mechanics. It may include assessment of the person's ability to sit, stand, walk, squat, kneel, carry, bend, climb, reach, stoop, and perform fine motor or repetitive motions. The evaluator should document weight lifting/pushing/pulling limits, activity tolerance, environmental restrictions, side effects of medications, and note any report of pain or observations of pain behaviors. The general evaluation of cognitive abilities may include observations about following instructions, safety, memory, communication skills, or decision-making. Psychosocial behavioral assessments are not consistently included in FCEs, but occupational therapists should administer brief depression and anxiety screenings. These mood disorders commonly coexist with and may exacerbate physical and cognitive problems.

The second part of the FCE is analysis of the client's ability to perform job-specific tasks. Therapists begin by identifying the most difficult and important task components of the job. For example, if a carpenter is required to lift 10-lb tools and a 50-lb toolbox, the more difficult and important task component to be assessed will be lifting a 50-lb toolbox. Work simulations are also performed. They are more complex and have greater face validity than assessing a person's ability to perform a task component because they combine multiple constructs such as strength, balance, and fine motor skills. Using the carpenter as an example, a work simulation may involve standing on a stepladder (balance) while using a 4-lb cordless power drill overhead for 15 minutes (strength and activity tolerance) and then changing the drill bit (grip strength and fine motor coordination).

The results of an FCE can be used to match a client's residual capacities with the demands of a specific job, as evidence to determine disability status, and as a baseline for new employees. However, choosing the appropriate FCE can be difficult. There are many FCEs available; they differ in the physical, cognitive, and psychosocial factors assessed and in the training required to administer and interpret them.

FCEs are primarily conducted in artificial environments with engineered physical work tasks. The Assessment of Work Performance (AWP) was developed by occupational therapists and may be used in real-life work situations or in artificial environments with clients who have different kinds of work-related problems and diagnoses.[28] It does not target specific work tasks but assesses work skills in three domains: motor, process, and communication and interaction skills. Each of the 14 AWP test items is rated by the observer on a four-point Likert scale, ranging from incompetent to competent performance (see Assessment table).

Intervention

AOTA lists the goals of work rehabilitation as maximizing work function, facilitating safe and timely return to work through remediation, and assisting workers to retain or resume their worker role and prevent future impairments following injury or illness.[29] There are different types of work rehabilitation programs: work readiness, work conditioning, and work hardening. These interventions principally employ techniques to establish or remediate the client's ability to work by changing client variables (e.g., strength, activity tolerance).

Work Remediation

Work Readiness

Work readiness programs allow clients to explore other options if they cannot return to a previous occupation. These programs help individuals to identify work goals, interests, and skills. Clients may be referred to their state Department of Rehabilitation for job training and placement after participating in a work readiness program.

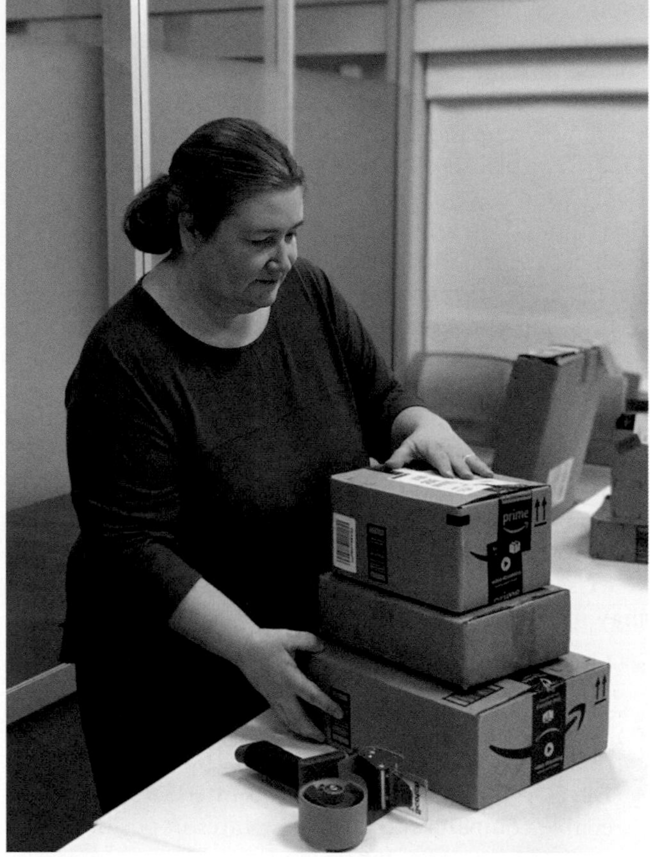

Figure 29-8. Work conditioning may include warm-up exercises, conditioning exercises based on job requirements, and job-related tasks that replicate essential task components.

Work Conditioning

Work conditioning generally follows acute care and precedes work hardening. It focuses on remediation of physical or cognitive deficits to improve work function. It may include warm-up exercises, conditioning exercises based on job requirements, and job-related tasks that replicate essential task components (Fig. 29-8). A program may begin with hour-long sessions and progress to 8 hours per day as the client's condition improves.

Work Hardening

Work hardening is a multidisciplinary structured treatment designed to maximize a client's ability to return to work. The psychosocial, communication, cognitive, and physical components of a job are addressed. Work hardening aims to replicate a specific job or classification of jobs, and differs from work conditioning in that it uses graded real or simulated work activities. The work hardening environment should replicate the workplace as closely as possible in aspects such as space, equipment, interactions with others, hours, breaks, and performance standards. Other disciplines that may be included in work hardening programs are physical therapy, vocational rehabilitation, psychology, social work, social services, drug and alcohol counseling, nutrition, and education.

Work Adaptation or Compensation

The ADA prohibits discrimination on the basis of disability and requires an employer to provide reasonable accommodations to a qualified person with a disability who is an employee or an applicant for employment.[30] However, to reiterate, barriers to employment remain with only 29.3% of adults with disabilities in the prime working age group, 16 to 64, employed compared to 73.5% for those without disabilities.[24] Identifying and recommending reasonable accommodations is a common compensation or adaptation intervention by occupational therapists who specialize in work-oriented therapy or return to work. Identifying reasonable accommodations requires collaboration between the client, employer, and occupational therapist. The best resource for identifying appropriate accommodations for a worker with a disability is the Job Accommodation Network (JAN) funded by the US Department of Labor, Office of Disability Employment Policy.[31] JAN provides menus of accommodations in four categories: disability (e.g., stroke), limitation (e.g., pain), work-related function (e.g., manipulate items), and topic (e.g., accessibility).

Some adaptations for the current computer-based work environment are explained in the subsequent sections.

Voice Recognition Software

Voice recognition software (VRS) identifies words and phrases in spoken language and converts them to a readable format. When using a keyboard is physically difficult, an individual can use VRS to take notes, send emails, or perform other computer-related work tasks. VRS has been used for individuals with motor impairment conditions, such as cerebral palsy, Parkinson disease, TBI, and motor neuron diseases.[32]

Screen Reader Software

Screen reader software (SRS) programs read text that is displayed on computer, tablet, or smartphone screens with a speech synthesizer, sound icons, or a Braille display. SRS programs can be beneficial for clients with vision impairments who have difficulty reading a computer screen, thus enabling access to digital information and computer-related work tasks. An SRS program can also benefit clients with a learning disability or a cognitive impairment that slows their reading speed, including persons with TBI and stroke.

Browsers That Provide User-Friendly and Customizable Web Interface

Computers have settings that allow users to adjust the screen lighting, contrast, mouse size and speed, and other accessibility features to enhance computer and Internet use. There are also web browsers that further provide user-friendly and customizable web interface, such as Web Trek and MozBraille. Web Trek is a web browser designed for individuals with intellectual impairment. To reduce the complexity of the web browser and eliminate barriers for individuals with cognitive impairments, Web Trek has a built-in SRS, enlarged images, and minimizes clutter on the page.[33] MozBraille is designed specifically for individuals with visual impairments and is customizable. Users can transform Mozilla or Firefox with an SRS, large character view, or a Braille terminal to access the Internet.[34]

Color-Coded Keyboards

A color-coded computer keyboard or keyboard cover is designed to provide a high-visibility keyboard option by designating specific colors on certain keys (e.g., red vowels, yellow shift key). Persons with vision impairments may find this helpful in locating important keys or in finger placement on the keyboard. Color-coded keyboards may also help persons with cognitive impairments to more easily learn how to use a keyboard.

Efficacy of Interventions for Restoring Work Roles

Blas et al. performed a scoping review of occupational therapy interventions that targeted work-related outcomes.[35] They found 46 articles with 163 different occupational therapy interventions. The interventions included altering the work activities, the environment, and body functions and structures. The most frequently used interventions included acquisition of new skills; using health services, products, and technology; handling psychosocial demands; and work preparation. The most often targeted work-related outcomes they identified were remunerative employment, sensation and pain perception, ability to handle psychosocial demands, emotional function, economic self-sufficiency, and muscular and cardiovascular endurance.

Four systematic reviews examined remediation interventions for work-related injuries, including low back[36]; conditions of the forearm, wrist, and hand[37]; elbow injuries[38]; and shoulder injuries.[39] However, only one reported results of return-to-work interventions.[36] Snodgrass performed a systematic review of interventions for work-related lower back injuries and found that therapeutic exercises, client education in body mechanics, work reconditioning and graduated return to work, ergonomic modifications, cognitive behavioral strategies such as progressive relaxation, and physical agent modalities were supported in the literature.[36]

A systematic review for effective return-to-work interventions after acquired brain injury (ABI) found strong evidence that adaptation of working tasks, hours, and the environment; vocational counseling; person-centered goals; supported employment; and access to support and education increased the likelihood of return to work.[40]

Restoring Recreation Roles

Background

Balancing work with recreation is essential for mental and physical health and promotes a less stressful and more satisfying life. In the literature, the terms recreation and leisure are often used interchangeably. However, leisure is more properly defined as free time or time that is not spent in obligatory occupations, whereas recreation indicates an activity that is performed for pleasure or amusement. Law and colleagues[41] used the term leisure rather than recreation and described three categories of leisure activities: quiet leisure or activities such as reading or sewing, active leisure or activities that require physical exertion such as wheelchair rugby, and socialization or activities that involve interaction with other people such as going out to a restaurant.

Adults with physical disabilities tend to engage in quiet leisure and to reduce their participation in physically demanding recreational activities. After a disabling event such as stroke, research has shown that there is a significant decrease in participation in high-demand leisure activity.[42] Participating in physically demanding recreational activities is important to physical and mental health and wellness for people with disabilities. Occupational therapists can encourage clients by providing physically demanding activities and experiences, recommending adaptive techniques or adaptive equipment, and providing resources for existing activity programs in their community. One such resource is recreational programming offered by therapeutic recreation specialists. Similar to occupational therapy's beginnings after World War I, therapeutic recreation is a field that has gained prominence since World War II when they used recreational activities for treatment of war veterans with disabilities. Therapeutic recreation specialists have played a major role in developing leisure programs in medical settings, such as rehabilitation hospitals. The distinguishing difference between the two professions is that therapeutic recreation specialists always use recreational activity as their primary form of treatment.

Assessment of Recreation Roles

To identify appropriate leisure interests and activities for the client, there are many leisure exploration assessments that occupational therapists may administer. As noted previously, one of the COPM categories asks clients about their leisure interests and the ACS explores pre- and postdisability participation in high- and low-demand leisure and social activities. There are interest checklists available from both the occupational therapy and therapeutic recreation professions. Beard and Ragheb have developed a series of leisure questionnaires that may be used by therapeutic recreation specialists or occupational therapists. The Leisure Interest Measure can determine the level of interest in types of leisure activities and can be used to monitor change.[43] The Leisure Satisfaction Measure assesses whether clients perceive their leisure activities as meeting their needs or benefiting them[44] (see Assessment table). Based on the results of the assessments discussed, occupational therapists can help clients resume premorbid recreational interests or explore new options.

Intervention for Quiet and Active Leisure or Recreational Pursuits

Quiet Leisure

Basic principles of compensation or adaptation also apply to enabling participation in recreation activities. The quiet leisure activities of needlecrafts, reading, table games, playing cards, drawing or painting, puzzles, or writing may be performed with limited ROM by organizing and placing items within reach and building up tool handles in the case of poor grip or pinch. Persons with weakness, low endurance, or incoordination may use proximal stabilization (i.e., sitting with feet on the floor, trunk supported, and elbows or forearms supported on a table to limit the degrees of freedom of movement) as an adaptive technique for performing quiet leisure activities involving fine motor skills. With unilateral loss of motor control and limb function, objects should be stabilized with the weaker side or adaptive equipment used to hold the craft or card. An embroidery hoop holder and/or a playing card holder are examples. For visual impairments, there are many tools on the market for increased lighting and magnification of needlecrafts and handcrafts. There are enlarged print cards and games and items with Braille symbols. With chronic pain, clients should be instructed in proper body mechanics, work simplification, and energy conservation techniques. Visual aids or simplified instructions may facilitate participation in crafts or games for those with cognitive impairment.

Active Leisure

Compensatory techniques and adaptation of the environment, tools, or activity may also be necessary to facilitate participation in active leisure for clients with disabilities. For example, many high-demand sports activities have their counterpart for wheelchair users. Wheelchair users with specialized wheelchairs or equipment may participate in racing, rugby, basketball, tennis, soccer, snow skiing, water skiing, mountain biking, sailing, kayaking, canoeing, golf, and swimming, to name some of the most popular sports (Fig. 29-9). Chair yoga and Tai Chi have gained popularity for people with many types of disabilities who may be unable to assume certain poses. Specialized wheelchairs for rough terrain allow users to go hiking and access the beach. There are often precautions for clients with certain conditions that must be observed when participating in active leisure. For example, a client with rheumatoid arthritis may be prohibited from strenuous physical activity during an acute phase or may need to practice joint protection strategies when performing a sport. Condition-specific precautions are discussed in later chapters.

Resources for Recreational Activities

There are many resources for participation in active leisure and recreational pursuits. The National Center on Health, Physical Activity and Disability (NCHPAD) is a health promotion resource to help people with disabilities and chronic health conditions achieve health benefits from participation in physical and social activities.[45] The NCHPAD website has links to programs, organizations, equipment, parks, and personal trainers for

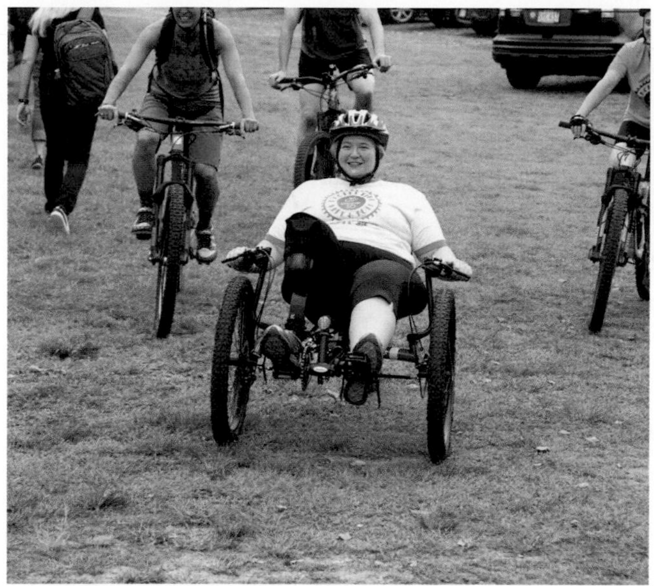

Figure 29-9. Wheelchair users with specialized wheelchairs or equipment may participate in a variety of leisure sports.

people with disabilities and health conditions by state, city, or zip code.

The National Sports Center for Disabled,[46] Disabled Sports USA,[47] and Adaptive Sports USA[48] are organizations that provide leadership, opportunities, and expertise in adaptive sports. They offer a wide variety of active sports and recreational activities year-round for people of all ability levels. Sports camps, clinics, and events have also been developed to introduce active leisure to people with disabilities. These may specialize in specific sports, or they may be aimed at people with certain diagnoses. Occupational therapists are often involved in directing, working for, or volunteering for sports camps or clinics. Volunteering for them is an excellent service learning opportunity for occupational therapy students.

Efficacy of Interventions for Restoring Recreation Roles

Smallfield and Molitor performed a systematic review of the evidence for the effectiveness of occupational therapy interventions to address leisure participation in older, community-dwelling adults.[49] They found strong evidence in support of leisure education programs by occupational therapists targeting increased leisure activity participation by this population. Moderate evidence supported a self-management of chronic disease program that was led by occupational therapists in promoting an increase in leisure performance and satisfaction. A study of assistive device use to facilitate leisure participation found that assistive devices increased the likelihood of older adults attempting leisure activities; however, further research on this intervention is required.

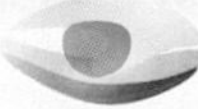

CASE STUDY

Patient Information

Tom is a 68-year-old white male who is a farmer with 200-acres of soybeans. He returned home 1 month ago from a 2-day acute care hospitalization for a left total knee arthroplasty (TKA) as a result of knee osteoarthritis (OA). Tom also has OA in the lower lumbar spine and right thumb. Prior to the TKA, Tom complained of back pain when driving his tractors and soybean combine, pain in his right thumb when gripping tools, and pain in both knees when ambulating and working in his equipment workshop. Tom received 3 weeks of home health care physical therapy to increase his left knee ROM and ability to ambulate safely for longer distances on uneven terrain.

Reason for Occupational Therapy Referral

The physical therapist has referred Tom to the local AgrAbility program, a state affiliate of the National AgrAbility Project.[50] The state program contracts with an occupational therapist to perform worksite farm visits to evaluate farmers with disabilities, assess their work tasks and farm and home environments, and make recommendations for worksite and homesite modifications.

Assessment Process and Results

The occupational therapist prepared for Tom's initial evaluation by reviewing the treatment notes provided by the physical therapist and the O*NET core tasks for the occupation of farmer. O*NET listed several core tasks including operating irrigation equipment and tractors and tractor-drawn machinery to plow/plant/harvest crops and repairing and maintaining farm vehicles and equipment. The occupational therapist first administered the COPM and found that Tom's top five priorities were as follows:

Occupation	Importance	Performance	Satisfaction
1. Operate tractor and soybean combine to harvest crops (Work)	10	2	1
2. Maintain farm vehicles and equipment (Work)	10	3	1

(*continued*)

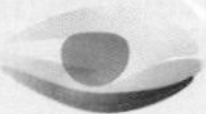

CASE STUDY (continued)

Occupation	Importance	Performance	Satisfaction
3. Resume leading his 4-H group of teens who raise lambs (Community participation)	9	2	1
4. Drive into town and grocery shop with his wife (Home management)	7	2	2
5. Go bass fishing (Recreation)	7	3	1

Because the visit was to Tom's home and farm, the occupational therapist scored the AWP while observing Tom perform two work tasks: (1) climb onto his tractor and drive it in a field and (2) change the oil in the tractor in his workshop. In motor skills, Tom scored 2 of 4 (limited performance) in mobility, strength, and physical energy. In process skills, he scored 3 of 4 (questionable performance) in organization of space and objects and adaptation. In communication and interaction skills, he scored 4 of 4 (competent performance) in all areas. On the AWP, the therapist analyzed Tom's limitations and concluded that he had limited knee ROM, decreased lower extremity strength, and poor physical energy that impaired his ability to climb the four vertical ladder rungs into the tractor. He also reported bilateral knee pain (5 on a 10-point pain scale) when climbing the four rungs. When driving the tractor, Tom complained of knee pain when using foot pedals, thumb pain (3 on a 10-point pain scale) while gripping the steering wheel, and back pain (4 on a 10-point pain scale) after 30 minutes of driving on rough terrain. When changing the oil in the tractor, he complained of back pain while standing on the concrete floor and bending over to pickup tools (5 on a 10-point pain scale) and hand pain when using a socket wrench (3 on a 10-point pain scale).

The therapist assessed the worksite, vehicles, and equipment while Tom was performing the work tasks. She noted that Tom did not utilize adaptive techniques or equipment for access and seating in farm vehicles, tool adaptations, or pain and fatigue management techniques.

The occupational therapist also questioned Tom about his work, volunteer, and leisure schedules. As with most farmers, she found that during planting and harvest seasons, Tom reported working very long hours on heavy equipment with few rest breaks. He also reported that pain was exacerbating his fatigue and that he had no energy for those things he enjoyed such as working with teenagers in 4-H and going bass fishing. His wife was present for the interview and stated that she missed having him along for trips into town for grocery shopping and visiting their grandchildren. He agreed with her, but he stated that his priority was work and that he was too tired to go.

Occupational Therapy Problem List

- Significant difficulty climbing tractor rungs and into soybean combine due to pain, decreased knee ROM, and decreased lower extremity strength as a result of left TKA and right knee OA.
- Pain from carpometacarpal OA in right thumb reduces Tom's ability to perform tasks that require a tight grasp such as hand tool use to repair farm equipment.
- Lower back pain from OA of the lumbar spine limits his ability to operate heavy farm vehicles, stand on concrete workshop floor, and bend and lift when repairing farm equipment.
- Tom is unable to resume his 4-H volunteer position or go trout fishing due to fatigue.
- Tom is unable to accompany his wife to shop and visit family due to fatigue.

Occupational Therapy Goal List

- Tom will climb onto his tractor and soybean combine with Modified Independence using adaptive equipment in 4 weeks.
- Tom will operate his tractor, soybean combine, and truck while reporting decreased back pain, from a self-rating of 5 to 2 on a 10-point pain scale, while using adaptive equipment and pain management strategies in 2 weeks.
- Tom will repair and drive farm vehicles and equipment with Modified Independence while utilizing adaptive equipment for reducing OA pain in 2 weeks.
- Tom will participate in volunteer and leisure activities for 2 hours per week while using energy conservation strategies by 4 weeks.
- Tom will grocery shop with his wife one time per week while using energy conservation strategies in 2 weeks.
- Tom will be able to perform work, volunteer, and leisure activities with report of decreased pain and fatigue by following a home exercise program three times per week to increase strength and activity tolerance in 1 month.

Intervention

The occupational therapist began the intervention process by researching adaptive equipment options for arthritis and pain in the Job Accommodations Network. She also searched the National AgrAbility Project Toolbox[51] for adaptive equipment specific to farm tasks and equipment.

To aid in climbing onto tractors and the soybean combine, the therapist recommended two possible modifications, add-on tractor steps for the bottom of each vehicle's

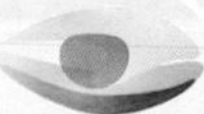

CASE STUDY *(continued)*

ladders to shorten the distance and reduce the strength needed for climbing onto the first rung[52] or installing a power standing platform lift for each vehicle.[53] To reduce back and hand pain when driving the farm vehicles, the therapist provided resources for antivibration seat cushions, lumbar support cushions, and padding and antivibration steering wheel covers. Vibration dampening gloves can also reduce pain and protect joints when driving heavy equipment or using power tools.

The occupational therapist recommended antifatigue standing mats for the workshop concrete floor to reduce back and lower extremity pain and fatigue while working. She recommended pain and fatigue management strategies such as reorganizing the workshop to reduce bending and reaching by placing tools at waist level on a rolling cart, using a power socket wrench and other power tools rather than manual tools, and padding handles of other tools to reduce contact with hard surfaces that cause pain in his hand.

The therapist provided education in energy conservation and pain management techniques to reduce his pain and fatigue. These included taking brief rest and stretch breaks throughout his workday. Planning ahead is often difficult for farmers because of unpredictable conditions, but the therapist worked with Tom to make a weekly schedule with lighter work tasks on 1 day per week so that he had energy to go shopping with his wife and on 2 days per month to go fishing. She discussed saving energy when shopping such as planning the grocery list by the layout of the store. The therapist explored ways that Tom could share responsibility for his 4-H club, and he was able to identify another community member he could mentor and with whom he could alternate club activities. The therapist emphasized the importance of exercise as an energy conservation technique and of continuing to follow a home exercise program to improve his strength and ROM. Finally, the therapist provided information for grants and loans to pay for equipment through the US Department of Agriculture and other farm and rural support organizations.

Assessment Table of Instruments for Home Management, Work, and Recreation Roles

Instrument and Reference	Intended Purpose	Administration Time	Validity	Reliability	Sensitivity	Strengths and Weaknesses
Occupational Performance Assessments for ADLs						
Activity Card Sort (ACS)[7]	Interview-based, card sorting task for older adults in four categories: instrumental, low-demand leisure, high-demand leisure, and social activities	20–60 minutes	Concurrent validity was established by comparing versions with other assessments. Content validity was based on consultation with community living older adults.	Test–retest reliability = 0.74 Internal consistency with Cronbach α from 0.71 to 0.93	Not established	Strengths: May be used in many types of settings to determine retention of premorbid activities and for planning of occupation-based intervention Weaknesses: Does not provide information regarding the length of time spent engaged in activities, frequency of activity participation, social interactions during activities, nor difficulty experienced performing an activity.
Canadian Occupational Performance Measure (COPM)[8]	Semi-structured, interview-based rating scale to identify and prioritize self-care, leisure, and productivity occupations	30–40 minutes	COPM scores were responsive to self-perceived changes in performance. Other instruments used COPM as a valid measure of occupational performance.	Test–retest reliability ranged from 0.63 to 0.89 for performance and 0.76 to 0.88 for satisfaction.	A two-point change in score is considered clinically significant.	Strengths: Problem list serves as guide for client-centered intervention. Can be used in many settings with variety of conditions. Weaknesses: Dependent on interview style of administrator. Only used in limited clinical fields and disciplines. Not suitable depending on the practice setting or if clients lack insight.
Occupational Performance History Interview-II (OPHI-II), Version 2.1[9]	Semi-structured interview, rating scale, and life history narrative to elicit a detailed history of a client's work, play, and self-care and the impact of impairment	60 minutes	Validated using Rasch analysis	Test–retest reliability not available	Not established	Strengths: Used to develop an occupational profile to guide intervention. Can be used with adult clients who are able to perform an in-depth interview. Weaknesses: Dependent on client's willingness to share information; clients could feel vulnerable if no rapport is built. Often cannot be administered in single session.

Home Management Assessments						
Assessment of Motor and Process Skills (AMPS)[16]	Observation-based rating, designed to measure quality of performance in basic ADLs and IADLs	30–40 minutes	Established validity across age, culture, ethnic, and diagnostic groups and genders through various studies. Also used widely to examine ADL differences between different diagnostic groups.	Test–retest reliability for motor scale ranged from 0.88 to 0.91 and the process scale ranged from 0.86 to 0.90	Not established	Strengths: Assist in intervention planning and used to compare reevaluation results to assess intervention success. Weaknesses: Measures reflecting normal variation overlap for many age groups. Items needed are dependent on task patient wishes to perform. Time commitment and cost for administrator training
Performance Assessment of Self-Care Skills (PASS) version 3.1[15]	Observation based to determine performance for daily living skills in the clinic or home	1.5–3 hours	Content validity was established by an investigation of ADL/IADL categories and tasks in relationship to ADL and functional assessment tools in rehab. Construct validity was based on a comparison of scores with controls and persons with dementia.	Inter-observer reliability scores ranged from 0.80 to 0.99. Test–retest reliability ranged from 0.82 to 0.97.	Not established	Strengths: Establishes baseline functional status; can assist in treatment planning. Aids in discharge planning by identifying type and amount of support required. Weaknesses: Time required to complete assessment is lengthy.
Work Assessments						
DSI Work Solutions Functional Capacity Assessment (DSI FCA)[55]	Designed as an objective measure of an individual's ability to perform various work-related tasks	Three-hour administration for one-part FCA, 5-hour administration for two-part; FCA over the course of 2 days	Validity was demonstrated by comparing performances health clients and clients with chronic nonspecific back pain.	Intraclass correlation coefficient was ≥ 0.75. Test–retest reliability is considered acceptable based on analysis of ceiling and criterion tests.	Not established	Strengths: Supported by extensive research on kinesiophysical approach; report focuses on evaluee's abilities; report is brief. Weaknesses: Extensive time to complete

(*continued*)

Assessment Table of Instruments for Home Management, Work, and Recreation Roles (*continued*)

Instrument and Reference	Intended Purpose	Administration Time	Validity	Reliability	Sensitivity	Strengths and Weaknesses
Work Assessments						
Assessment of Work Performance (AWP)[28]	Based on the model of human occupation; assesses a patient's observable work performance skills	Not predetermined; can vary from a few hours to weeks	Adequate face validity and acceptable content validity have been established based on principal component analysis.	High-item separation reliability (0.99) indicates good internal consistency.	Statistically sensitive and discriminated between clients	Strengths: Observation based; theory based; comprehensive assessing motor, process, and communication/interaction skills; instructions were clear. Weaknesses: Further assessments are necessary to determine client's abilities; use of ordinal scoring psychometrically questionable; administrators stated they had to spend time to become comfortable administering.
Recreation Assessments						
Leisure Satisfaction Measure[44]	Questionnaire-based rating scale; measuring the amount to which a person feels that his or her general needs are being met through leisure activities	5–25 minutes	Validity was established based on a factor analysis to which conventional item and test analysis techniques fell within an acceptable range.	Reliability coefficient (α) = 0.96	Not established	Strengths: Can be used to explore new areas of leisure to increase satisfaction; includes current or existing leisure programs. Weaknesses: Requires quiet room to administer; patient must be Level 7 or above on Rancho Los Amigos Scale.
Leisure Interest Measure[43]	Questionnaire based, designed to determine the level of interest in leisure activities and what activities they are interest in	5–25 minutes	Measures both intensity of breadth of leisure interest; Pearson correlation coefficients evaluated whether domains were interrelated—physical and outdoor domains did not show any statistically significant interrelationships.	Internal consistency (α) = 0.87	Not established	Strengths: Assesses various domains of leisure; can be used to ensure individual has activities available that are interesting to him or her; used to point out areas where therapist can provide education to create new leisure activities. Weaknesses: Domains are not all interrelated; does not assess current leisure participation satisfaction.

Evidence Table of Intervention Studies for Restoring Home Management, Work, and Recreation Occupational Roles

Intervention	Description	Participants	Dosage	Research Design and Evidence Level	Benefit	Statistical Significance and Effect Size
Home Management Roles						
Interventions within the scope of occupational therapy practice aimed at IADL performance[21]	Interventions since 2012 were investigated for efficacy in improving or slowing the decline in IADL performance of older adults with disabilities: cognitive, self-management, prevention, and home-based multidisciplinary rehabilitation, client centered.	Fourteen peer-reviewed, scientific articles (13 Level I and 1 Level III) examining community-dwelling individuals aged 65 years and older		Systematic review Level I	Four areas of intervention were found to improve or slow the decline in IADL performance: cognitive, self-management, prevention, and home-based multidisciplinary rehabilitation, client centered. Chronic Disease Self-Management Program improved participation and perceived performance.	No statistical analysis
One-to-one fatigue management course delivered by occupational therapy practitioners or students[22]	Five modules were as follows: basics of fatigue, communication and fatigue, body mechanics and environment, analyzing and modifying environment, and living a balanced lifestyle.	Forty-nine adults with chronic disease and moderate or severe fatigue as dictated by an average score of 4/7 or higher on the Fatigue Severity Scale	1–2-hour sessions for 4–6 weeks until all modules were completed.	One-group, pretest–posttest, follow-up design	Participants experienced significant decreases in fatigue and significant increases in self-efficacy and most components of quality of life from pretest to posttest.	Large effect size was mentioned.
Work Roles						
Interventions within the scope of occupational therapy aimed at increasing work participation[54]	Evidence-based interventions within occupational therapy's scope of practice that have been studied because the enactment of the ADA were investigated for efficacy in increasing participation in work for individuals with disabilities.	Forty-six peer-reviewed, scientific articles (27 Level I, 6 Level II, 12 Level III, and 1 Level IV) studying work-related interventions for individuals with a variety of disabilities including mental, physical, cognitive, and hearing		Systematic review Level I	Most effective interventions for physical disability were peer mentorship and multidisciplinary health care for work-related satisfaction and self-efficacy; for neurological disability were one-on-one intervention in supported competitive employment and assistive technology; and for intellectual disability, using apps and telehealth services. Overall, technology, coaching, peer mentorship, and work accommodations were most effective.	No statistical analysis

(*continued*)

Evidence Table of Intervention Studies for Restoring Home Management, Work, and Recreation Occupational Roles (*continued*)

Intervention	Description	Participants	Dosage	Research Design and Evidence Level	Benefit	Statistical Significance and Effect Size
Return-to-work interventions[40]	Return-to-work interventions delivered in four continents were analyzed to find those most effective for individuals with acquired brain injuries of both a traumatic and nontraumatic nature. Combinations of the following were studied: work-directed intervention, education and coaching, skills training, cognitive rehabilitation, and supported employment.	Twelve studies (5 Level I and 7 Level IV) with return to work as a primary or secondary outcome for employed adults with nonprogressive acquired brain injuries		Systematic review Level I	Strong evidence supports the efficacy of combining work-directed intervention, such as task adaptation, with education or coaching. Complementing those interventions with skills training involving the employee and the employer was also indicated. Overall, the best return-to-work outcomes involved workplace support and employer collaboration.	No statistical analysis
Recreational Roles						
Interventions within the scope of occupational therapy practice aimed at social participation and leisure engagement[49]	Interventions within the scope of occupational therapy practice were investigated for efficacy in improving social participation and leisure engagement for community-dwelling older adults.	Fourteen articles (11 Level I, 1 Level II, 1 Level III, and 1 Level IV) studying interventions within the scope of occupational therapy practice aimed at social participation and leisure engagement for individuals with an average age of 65 years or older living in the community, a retirement home, an assisted living facility, or a medical setting being discharged home. Individuals with chronic conditions were included in the studies.		Systematic review Level I	Effective and recommended interventions to promote social participant and leisure engagement for older adults are as follows: leisure education programs and chronic disease self-management programs aimed at leisure participation. Based on individual client factors, community-based group interventions and electronic games aimed at social participation are also supported.	No statistical analysis

References

1. Parham LD, Fazio LS, eds. *Play in Occupational Therapy for Children*. St. Louis, MO: Mosby; 1997.
2. Freedman VA, Carr D, Comman JC, Lucas R. Impairment severity and evaluative and experienced well-being among older adults: assessing the role of daily activities. *Innov Aging*. 2017;1:igx010. doi:10.1093/geroni/igx010.
3. Rak EC, Spencer L. Community participation of persons with disabilities: volunteering, donations and involvement in groups and organisations. *Disabil Rehabil*. 2016;38(17):1705–1715.
4. Wolverson C. Volunteering. In: Hunt LA, Wolverson CE, eds. *Work and the Older Person: Increasing Longevity and Well-Being*. Thorofare, NJ: Slack Inc; 2015:101–111.
5. Saunders SL, Nedelec B. What work means to people with work disability: a scoping review. *J Occup Rehabil*. 2014;24:100–110. doi:10.1007/s10926-013-9436-y.
6. Wise EK, Mathews-Dalton C, Dikmen S, et al. Impact of traumatic brain injury on participation in leisure activities. *Arch Phys Med Rehabil*. 2010;91(9):1357–1362.
7. Baum CM, Edwards D. *ACS: Activity Card Sort*. Bethesda, MD: AOTA Press; 2008.
8. Law MC, Baptiste S, Carswell A, McColl MA, Polatajko H, Pollock N. *Canadian Occupational Performance Measure: COPM*. Ottawa, Ontario, Canada: CAOT Publications ACE; 1998.
9. Kielhofner G, Mallinson T, Crawford C, et al. *Occupational Performance History Interview-II (OPHI-II), Version 2.1*. Chicago, IL: Model of Human Occupation Clearinghouse; 2004.
10. Kiresuk TJ, Sherman RE. Goal attainment scaling: a general method for evaluating comprehensive community mental health programs. *Community Ment Health J*. 1968;4(6):443–453.
11. Grant M, Ponsford J. Goal attainment scaling in brain injury rehabilitation: strengths, limitations and recommendations for future applications. *Neuropsychol Rehabil*. 2014;24(5):661 677.
12. Dickson KL, Toto PE. Feasibility of integrating occupational therapy into a care coordination program for aging in place. *Am J Occup Ther*. 2018; 72(4):7204195020p1–7204195020p7.
13. Escher AA, Amlani AM, Viani AM, Berger S. Occupational therapy in an intensive comprehensive aphasia program: performance and satisfaction outcomes. *Am J Occup Ther*. 2018;72(3):7203205110p1–7203205110p7.
14. Radomski MV, Giles G, Finkelstein M, Owens J, Showers M, Zola J. Implementation intentions for self-selected occupational therapy goals: two case reports. *Am J Occup Ther*. 2018;72(3):7203345030p1–7203345030p6.
15. Holm MB, Rogers JC, Hemphill-Pearson B. The performance assessment of self-care skills (PASS). *Assess Occup Ther Ment Health*. 2008;2:101–110.
16. Fisher A. *The Assessment of Motor and Process Skills (AMPS)*. Vols 1 & 2. 7th rev ed. Fort Collins, CO: Three Star Press; 2012.
17. Baum CM, Connor LT, Morrison T, Hahn M, Dromerick AW, Edwards DF. Reliability, validity, and clinical utility of the executive function performance test: a measure of executive function in a sample of people with a stroke. *Am J Occup Ther*. 2008;62:446–455. doi:10.5014/ajot.62.4.446.
18. Amini DA, Kannenberg K, Bodison S, et al. Occupational therapy practice framework: domain & process 3rd edition. *Am J Occup Ther*. 2014;68:S1–S48.
19. ADA Accessibility Guidelines. 2010 ADA standards for titles II and III facilities: 2004 ADAAG. https://www.ada.gov/regs2010/2010ADAStandards/2010ADAstandards.htm#c1. Accessed September 10, 2018.
20. Global Initiative for Inclusive Information and Communication Technologies (G3ict). Inclusive financial services for seniors and persons with disabilities: global trends in accessibility requirements. https://g3ict.org/publication/inclusive-financial-services-for-seniors-and-persons-with-disabilities-global-trends-in-accessibility-requirements. Published February. 2015. Accessed September 25, 2018.
21. Hunter EG, Kearney PJ. Occupational therapy interventions to improve performance of instrumental activities of daily living for community-dwelling older adults: a systematic review. *Am J Occup Ther*. 2018;72(4):7204190050p1–7204190050p9.doi:10.5014/ajot.2018.031062.
22. Van Heest KNL, Mogush AR, Mathiowetz VG. Centennial topics—effects of a one-to-one fatigue management course for people with chronic conditions and fatigue. *Am J Occup Ther*. 2017;71(4):7104100020p1–7104100020p9 doi:10.5014/ajot.2017.023440.
23. Stark S, Keglovits M, Arbesman M, Lieberman D. Effect of home modification interventions on the participation of community-dwelling adults with health conditions: a systematic review. *Am J Occup Ther*. 2017;71(2):7102290010p1–7102290010p11. doi:10.5014/ajot.2017.018887.
24. Bureau of Labor Statistics. News Release—persons with a disability: labor force characteristics-2017 (USDL 18-1028, p. 1–11). U.S. Department of Labor. https://www.bls.gov/news.release/disabl.nr0.htm. Published June 21, 2018. Accessed September 28, 2018.
25. Joss M. The importance of job analysis in occupational therapy. *Br J Occup Ther*. 2007;70(7):301–303.
26. U.S. Department of Labor. O*NET OnLine. https://www.onetonline.org. Updated August 7, 2018. Accessed September 1, 2018.
27. Kuijer PP, Gouttebarge V, Brouwer S, Reneman MF, Frings-Dresen MH. Are performance-based measures predictive of work participation in patients with musculoskeletal disorders? A systematic review. *Int Arch Occup Environ Health*. 2012;85(2):109–123.
28. Sandqvist J, Tornquist KB, Henriksson CM. Assessment of work performance (AWP): development of an instrument. *Work*. 2006;26(4):379–387.
29. American Occupational Therapy Association. Occupational therapy services in facilitating work participation and performance. *Am J Occup Ther*. 2017;71(suppl 2): 7112410040. doi:10.5014/ajot.716S05.
30. U.S. Equal Employment Opportunity Commission. Enforcement guidance: reasonable accommodation and undue hardship under the Americans with Disabilities Act. https://www.eeoc.gov/policy/docs/accommodation.html. Updated October 22, 2002. Accessed September 5, 2018.

31. U.S. Department of Labor, Office of Disability Employment Policy. Job accommodation network. https://askjan.org. Accessed September 15, 2018.
32. Hird K, Hennessey NW. Facilitating use of speech recognition software for people with disabilities: a comparison of three treatments. *Clin Linguist Phon.* 2007;21(3):211–226.
33. AbleLink Smart Living Technologies. Solutions: Web trek. https://www.ablelinktech.com/index.php?id=222. Accessed November 27, 2018.
34. GPII Unified Listing. MozBraille. https://ul.gpii.net/content/mozbraille. Accessed November 27, 2018.
35. Blas AJT, Beltran KMB, Martinez PGV, Yao DPG. Enabling work: occupational therapy interventions for persons with occupational injuries and diseases: a scoping review. *J Occup Rehab.* 2018;28:201–214.
36. Snodgrass J. Effective occupational therapy interventions in the rehabilitation of individuals with work-related low-back injuries and illness: a systematic review. *Am J Occup Ther.* 2011;65(1):37–43.
37. Amini D. Occupational therapy interventions for work-related injuries and conditions of the forearm, wrist, and hand: a systematic review. *Am J Occup Ther.* 2011;65(1):29–36.
38. Bohr PC. Systematic review and analysis of work-related injuries to and conditions of the elbow. *Am J Occup Ther.* 2011;65(1):24–48.
39. von der Heyde RL. Occupational therapy interventions for shoulder conditions: a systematic review. *Am J Occup Ther.* 2011;65(1):16–23.
40. Donker-Cools BHPM, Daams JG, Wind H, Frings-Dresen MHW. Effective return-to-work interventions after acquired brain injury: a systematic review. *Brain Inj.* 2016;30(2):113–131. doi:10.3109/02699052.2015.1090014.
41. Law M, Polatajko H, Pollock MA, Carswell A, Baptiste S. Pilot testing of the Canadian occupational performance measure: clinical and measurement issues. *Can J Occup Ther.* 1994;61:191–197.
42. Hildebrand M, Brewer M, Wolf T. The impact of mild stroke on participation in physical fitness activities. *Stroke Res Treat.* 2012;2012:6. doi:10.1155/2012/548682.
43. Ragheb MG, Beard JG. *Leisure Interest Measure.* Enumclaw, WA: Idyll Arbor; 1991.
44. Ragheb MG, Beard JG. *Leisure Satisfaction Measure.* Enumclaw, WA: Idyll Arbor; 2002.
45. National Center on Health, Physical Activity and Disability. https://www.nchpad.org. Accessed September 29, 2018.
46. National Sports Center for Disabled. https://nscd.org. Accessed September 29, 2018.
47. Disabled Sports USA. https://www.disabledsportsusa.org. Accessed September 29, 2018.
48. Adaptive Sports USA. https://adaptivesportsusa.org. Accessed September 29, 2018.
49. Smallfield S, Molitor WL. Occupational therapy interventions supporting social participation and leisure engagement for community-dwelling older adults: a systematic review. *Am J Occup Ther.* 2018;72(4):190020p1–190020p8.
50. National AgrAbility Project. AgrAbility: cultivating accessible agriculture. http://www.agrability.org/. Accessed October 10, 2018.
51. National AgrAbility Project. The toolbox assistive technology database. http://www.agrability.org/toolbox/. Accessed October 10, 2018.
52. National AgrAbility Project. The toolbox assistive technology database: add-on tractor steps. http://www.agrability.org/toolbox/?solution=495. Accessed October 10, 2018.
53. National AgrAbility Project. The toolbox assistive technology database: coachlift person lift. http://www.agrability.org/toolbox/?solution=1211. Accessed October 10, 2018.
54. Smith D, Atmatzidis K, Capogreco M, Lloyd-Randolfi D, Seman V. Evidence-based intervention for increasing work participation for persons with various disabilities: a systematic review. *OTJR (Thorofare N J).* 2017;37(2S):3S–13S.
55. Isernhagen SJ. *DSI Work Solutions Functional Capacity Assessment.* Duluth, MN: DSI Work Solutions; 2004.

Chapter 30

Restoring Transfers and Functional Mobility

Anita Perr

LEARNING OBJECTIVES

This chapter will allow the reader to:

1. Select and describe the most appropriate transfers as a result of an assessment and in collaboration with the client depending on the abilities, preferences, environmental conditions, and support available.
2. Describe treatment approaches, potential risks, and documentation of transfers.
3. Describe the occupational therapy assessment for manual and power wheelchair mobility.
4. Describe intervention approaches for manual and power wheelchair mobility.

CHAPTER OUTLINE

TERMINOLOGY

Lateral transfer (popover transfer): moving from one surface to another in a mostly seated position, and using the arms to lift from the surface on which they sit to the landing surface; such transfers may be performed in one movement where the person moves from the original surface to the landing surface in one movement or they may be performed in increments where the person moves in multiple, short movements, repositioning his or her body, hands, and arms or to rest.

Manual wheelchair: a wheeled mobility device that is propelled by physical exertion by the user and/or an assistant.

Modified stand pivot transfer: similar to a stand pivot transfer, but the person does not stand fully, instead remaining in a crouched position.

Power wheelchair: a wheeled mobility device that has a motor and battery and is controlled electronically via a joystick or other control.

Sliding board transfer: a seated transfer performed with a transfer aid, such as a sliding board or Beasy Board placed under the person providing a surface upon which he or she may slide.

Stand pivot transfer: the person moving from one surface to another stands fully, or nearly fully, upright, then pivots his or her feet to back up to the landing surface, and then sits on that surface.

Transfer: the process of moving from one surface to another without standing and/or walking and usually refers to movement performed by people with disabilities who are unable to easily stand or move from one surface to another.

Wheelchair: a wheeled mobility device comprised of a sitting surface atop wheels.

Wheelie: a position assumed by manual wheelchair users, whereby the casters (front wheels) are lifted off the ground and maintained by the wheelchair user by holding his or her center of gravity over the rear wheels axle position; partial wheelie is lifting the casters of a manual wheelchair off of the ground momentarily to navigate over small obstacles.

Introduction

People move routinely throughout the day. These movements are critical aspects of functional mobility and allow people to get from point A to point B in order to participate in preferred activities. This chapter focuses primarily on two areas of functional mobility: **transfers** and **wheelchair** use. In each of these two areas, you will learn about the reasons for deficits in these areas and the principles of assessment and interventions to improve function through remediation and adaptation.

Transfers

Deficits in the ability to move from one surface to another occur for various reasons including impairments in body functions such as mental, sensory, cardiovascular, respiratory, neuromuscular, and movement-related functions or impairments in body structures such as the nervous system, cardiovascular and respiratory systems, and structures related to movement. The skin and related structures are also addressed during transfers as pressure, abrasion, and shearing encountered during the transfer can lead to damage to skin and the structures below the skin, resulting in pressure injuries.[1] The level of importance is raised in people at risk for pressure injury development.

Assessment for Transfers

The assessment for transfers comprises many other assessments that are often completed in the course of the occupational therapy (OT) evaluation. Such assessments included those for cognitive function, visual acuity and perception, motor function, and sensory function. Identifying these underlying deficits helps to guide goal writing and treatment planning. For instance, deficits in memory or problem-solving may portend unsafe movements during transfers, such as attempting to move prior to engaging wheelchair wheel locks or placing the feet on the floor rather than wheelchair footrests.

In addition to identifying these underlying impairments, the assessment also includes performance of the transfers themselves. By having the person perform the transfer, the occupational therapist determines how the interactions of the underlying impairments impact the movement in each transfer environment. The therapist can then determine the level of function: whether a seated or standing transfer is most appropriate; the amount and location of hands-on assistance; and the type, frequency, and style of verbal and nonverbal cues or instructions. As with all decisions, this is determined with input from the person transferring. Depending on the person's abilities, he or she may have more or less input.

Environmental attributes also influence the person's abilities during the transfer and should be assessed in each new transfer environment. The most common are transfers to and from the bed, toilet and bathing equipment, a car seat, or other transportation system. When assessing the environment, it is important to note whether there is space for the wheelchair or other equipment to be placed in optimal locations and whether obstacles or barriers can be removed or eased.

After completing the assessment and the activity analysis of the transfer, goals are written in collaboration with the person transferring and others involved in his or her care. Transfer goals should include the type of transfer to be completed, the location where the transfer will take place, the amount and type of assistance needed, any alternative techniques or equipment to be used, and the timeline for attaining the goal. Sample goals include the following:

- The client will perform stand pivot transfers to and from the wheelchair and bed, including wheelchair setup, with distant supervision and occasional verbal cues for safety and technique within 2 weeks.
- The client will demonstrate good safety techniques during a controlled fall from the wheelchair and when regaining a seated position in the wheelchair within 1 week.
- The client will perform a popover transfer to and from surfaces that are up to 3 inches (7.62 cm) difference in height within two sessions.
- The client will perform wheelchair safety skills and transfer setup with three to four verbal reminders for memory loss and problem-solving difficulties by 1 week.
- The client will direct assistance in **sliding board transfers** including wheelchair setup, sliding board placement and removal, and the actual transfer by 1 week (see Fig. 30-1).

Other qualifiers of performance that can be used to document progress are the amount of time required for the transfer, the number of cues required for setup and transfer, and the amount of assistance provided. Documentation regarding the transfer assessment is usually very brief and may be part of the activities of daily living (ADLs) or functional mobility status.

The assessment documentation includes your findings in the areas that are crucial for any given person, including visual acuity and perception, cognition, and motor function. The documentation should clearly identify how difficulties in these areas lead to difficulty in transfers. Documentation should include the following points:

- Type of transfer
- Locations: Starting surface and ending surface
- Amount and type of assistance required
- Amount and type of cuing/direction required
- Ambulation and/or wheeled mobility devices used

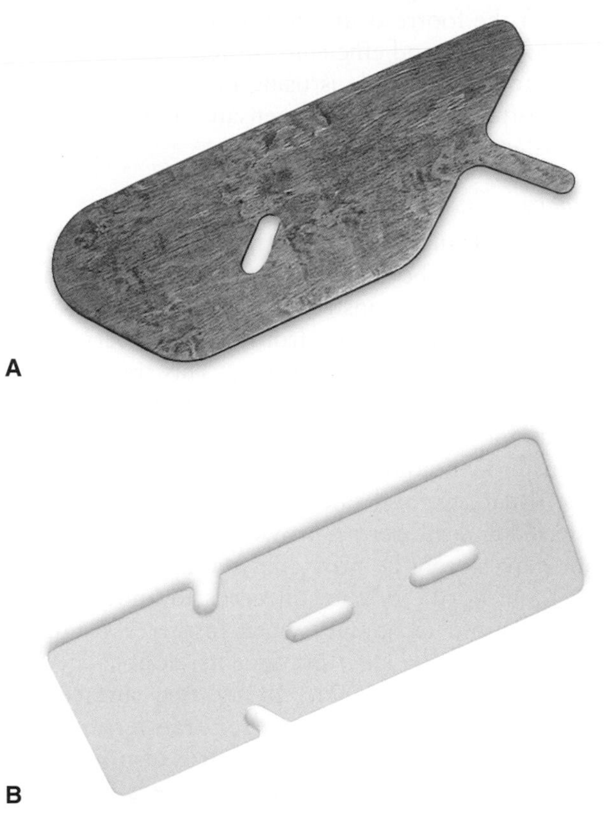

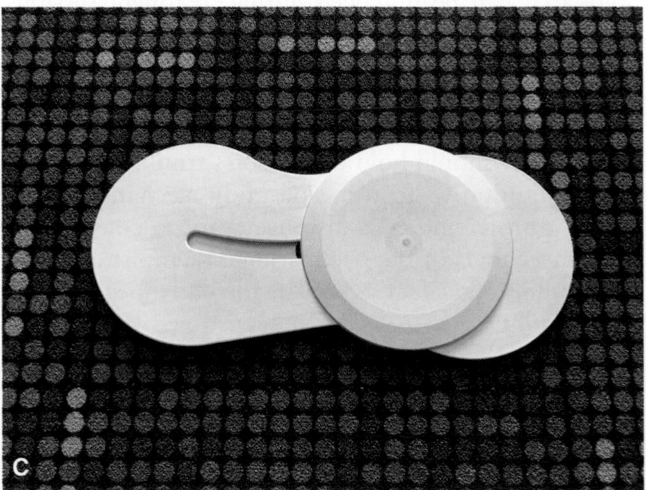

Figure 30-1. Examples of different sliding boards. **A.** Offset transfer board fits around the wheel of the wheelchair when the armrest is removed. (Courtesy of North Coast Medical, Morgan Hill, CA.) **B.** Transfer board with hand holes and notches allows transfers from either side. **C.** Beasy Board has a disc that the person sits on. The disc rides in a groove, making it easier for some people to move from one surface to the other.

Intervention for Transfers

The intervention for improving transfers comprises two approaches: remediation and adaptation. For example, if the person demonstrates impaired attention, the occupational therapist should focus part of the therapy sessions on activities to improve attention, a remedial approach. Transfer training should take place initially in a quiet environment, free of distractions; an adaptive strategy whereby changing the context in which treatment takes place allows the person to focus intently on the task. If the assessment reveals difficulty following verbal directions and impaired safety judgment, then the intervention focuses on improving these skills. The intervention can include practicing during transfers, but any other activities addressing these cognitive skills are also useful. For instance, an occupational therapist might develop a multiple step scavenger hunt that even includes identification of unsafe situations in pictures, such as a transfer setup with too much distance between the two surfaces, the wheelchair positioned at a poor angle, and the wheel lock disengaged.

If the assessment reveals impaired standing balance, strength, and coordination, activities that target these skills can be developed for the intervention. The same goes for any other difficulties identified. Of course, creativity in intervention planning will help keep the person interested and may allow him or her further improvement without realizing it. It is important to explain how the chosen activities relate to the person's priorities and relate directly to achievement of goals. Interventions themselves should be upgraded or downgraded based on the person's performance. As with other interventions, finding the balance between challenge and success is part of the key to making progress.

Interventions for improving transfers may include addressing the underlying impairments as well as direct transfer training. Each underlying impairment can be addressed alone or in combination. They should be addressed in a variety of activities in addition to practicing the actual transfers. Environmental attributes can also be varied during transfer training such as varying the heights of the transfer surfaces.

Transfer Principles

There are a few basic principles underlying most transfers. For ease of explanation, the following information refers to transfers between a wheelchair and another seating surface. Beyond the principles discussed in this chapter, there are typical transfer methods, but these are often adapted depending on the person's abilities and the environmental constraints.

The first principle is making sure the equipment is set up appropriately. The optimal setup puts the feet in a position where they can just pivot without having to take any steps. In order for the feet to be in this position, the wheelchair should be set up at about a 45° angle from the other transfer surface (Fig. 30-2). People who have more advanced skills may not need to focus as highly on setup. They are more able to compensate for

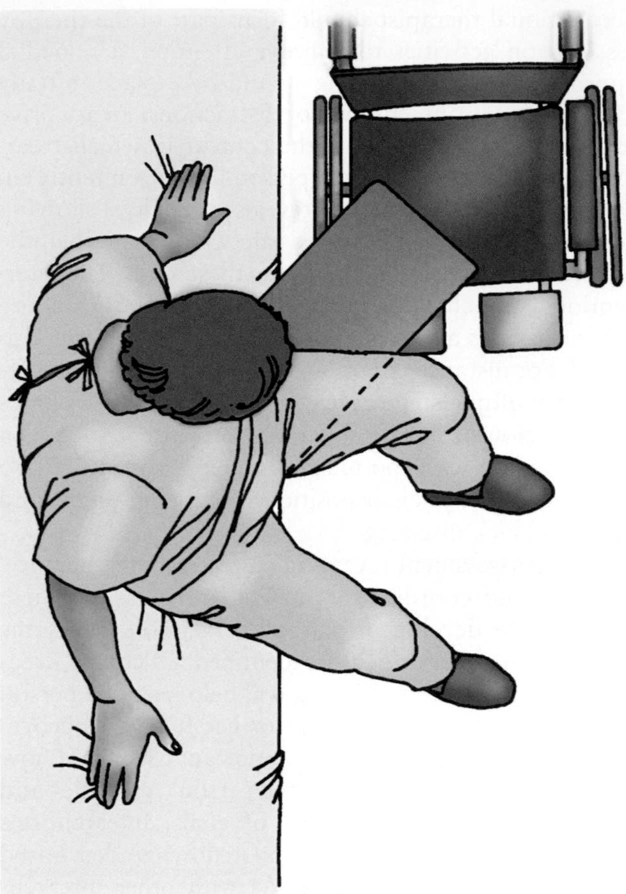

Figure 30-2. Setup for transfer. Wheelchair is positioned at approximately 45° to transfer surface. Wheel locks are engaged. Foot rests are out of the way.

less than optimal setups. For instance, people who are adept at and experienced with transfers may not lock their wheel locks or take their feet off the wheelchair footrests prior to transferring.

Clients with more safety concerns, less experience, or less ability should attend to setup more critically. Such concerns are especially relevant for people who are attached to medical lines. This might be a person in a hospital intensive care unit or a hospital room that is hooked up to a ventilator or oxygen, urinary catheters with collection devices on the person or on a transfer surface, and/or intravenous (IV) lines. Assistance should be provided to insure that all of the lines are in a position where the will not impede the transfer.

The second principle has to do with weight shifts and body mechanics. Transfer movements are eased when the person shifts his or her weight forward bringing his or her center of gravity over his or her feet. Depending of the person's abilities and conditions, he or she should maintain the best positions attainable. Insuring that low back muscles are not overstretched and that the tenodesis hand grip is preserved are the types of body mechanics principles to which the person should adhere.

The third principle is preparing for the transfer. Double-checking the setup, ensuring that the wheelchair's wheel locks are engaged, and positioning oneself (such as feet off the footrests and in position) all prepare the person for a safe and efficient transfer.

The fourth principle is using momentum. Momentum can often be used to compensate for weakness during transfers.

Assistance

If the person transferring needs help, it is important for the assistant(s) to be trained and for the person transferring to know how to instruct others in assistance. The amount of assistance varies from distant supervision to maximal (or dependent) assistance. This training often includes wheelchair parts management and mobility as well, but for transfers, the areas of concentration are the transfer techniques themselves, problem-solving for unique situations, and safety of both the person being transferred and the person providing assistance. The assistant may merely be providing standby assistance or supervision, but he or she still needs to know the best hand holds and techniques when further assistance is needed. Reinforcing slow movements, double-checking the setup, including stability of the two surfaces and training the assistant and the person transferring in coordinated movements, is beneficial. It is also important for the assistant to know the specific needs of the person. Some people need specialized instructions and hand holds that can be practiced during treatment sessions, and it is important to teach client-specific safety concerns, such as protecting the upper limbs on the affected side of a stroke survivor to prevent overstretching or even subluxation. Instead of holding the person's arms, the assistant should hold the person's trunk.

In addition to focusing on body mechanics of the person transferring, it is also necessary to consider the body mechanics of the occupational therapist assessing and training the client as well as the body mechanics of the assistant.

During these training sessions, the person transferring should also be trained in instructing others in how to assist them. This is useful for regular assistance, but is also very helpful when someone not associated with the person must assist. This can take practice because many people do not like to ask for help and many are reticent to correct helpers or give very specific instructions. The specificity is quite helpful, however, because most people are unaware of how to offer assistance.

Variations by Age and Ability/Disability

It is important to consider each person's abilities and conditions during transfers and training. Conditions such as orthostatic hypotension may influence the person's ability to change positions as he or she moves from supine to sitting at the edge of bed to moving from sit to stand. He or she might need rest breaks to acclimate to the changes in position. People with arthritis may need to take extra care to position their bodies and limbs safely and in a position that does not cause joint irritation or pain.

Addressing cognition is also imperative for safety. Assistants, as well as the person transferring, may need to slow down and use simple instructions in order to transfer. Quiet environments are suggested for training sessions so that the person does not get distracted.

Some people have difficulty shifting their weight forward to make the transfer to standing easier. If the difficulty is caused by fear of falling forward, care should be taken to work on that forward movement until the person feels more comfortable. This can be addressed during a variety of intervention activities.

If the person is unable to shift his or her weight forward because of hip flexion range of motion limitations or owing to the presence of heterotopic ossification, the technique may need to be altered. For instance, because the weight shift predisposes the person to be able to unweight his or her buttocks, he or she may need to use a sliding board or use more assistance that might otherwise be needed.

Optimal Techniques

During **stand pivot transfers**, the person pushes up from the seating surface to rise to standing and regains his or her balance. The person then pivots his or her feet such that he or she is standing with his or her back to the surface to which he or she is transferring. At that point, the person reaches back and slowly sits. In a **modified stand pivot transfer**, the person stays in a somewhat crouched position. He or she may reach for or hold on to the surface to which he or she is transferring.

People who transfer while remaining in a seated position often both push from the transfer surface and pull to the destination surface while leaning forward to shift their weight over their feet. Seated transfers may be performed in a single step or in multiple smaller steps. When a sliding board is used, the person shifts his or her weight to the side opposite the destination surface in order to unweight his or her buttocks to place the board under his or her buttocks and thigh. The board should be placed far enough forward under the thigh so that he or she does not slide forward off of the board during the transfer. After transferring to the destination surface, the person should shift his or her weight away from the original surface in order to unweight his buttocks and remove the sliding board. The sliding board should then be stowed in the location where it will be accessible the next time it is needed.

Seated transfers can lead to pressure ulcer development if the person is unable to unweight is buttocks sufficiently. During the seated transfer, the skin may be abraded as it scrapes along the transfer surfaces. Even more damage can occur if the person drags his or her buttocks over the top of the wheelchair wheel during the transfer. Shearing can also occur between the tissue under the skin of the buttocks and the body prominences if the person drags himself or herself across the sliding board or other surfaces. The greater the friction between the buttocks and the transfer surface, the more likely it is for these kinds of injuries to occur. In order to lessen the likelihood of this occurrence, intervention should include activities to strengthen the upper body and improve balance so that the person is able to lift himself or herself farther off the seating surfaces, unweighting the buttocks and making the transfer easier.

The abrasion and shearing that occurs during these sliding transfers can be even worse if the person's skin is unclothed and wet, such as during transfers to the toilet, commode, tub bench, or bath seat. Some people place a towel on the sliding board to ease the slide. Others place powder or cornstarch on the surface to make it slipperier. Using sliding boards on these slick surfaces of toileting and bathing equipment is also a bit more dangerous because the sliding board may shift during the transfer. Care must be taken to insure proper placement and to insure that the sliding board does not shift during use.

A dependent person may use a mechanical lift that offers dependent assistance, such as a mobile lift or ceiling-mounted lift. These are usually comprised of a single sling or a sling system that is placed under the person being lifted, often while he or she is supine in bed. The slings are then attached to the hoist that is controlled electronically, hydraulically, or mechanically. These lifting aids are also used within facilities and at home to help the assistant avoid musculoskeletal injuries[2] (see Fig. 30-3).

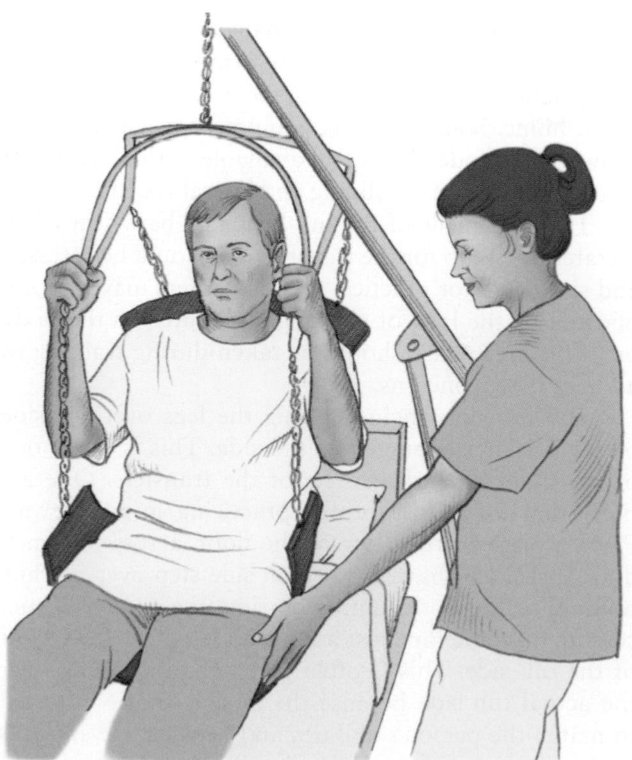

Figure 30-3. Client using mobile lift with assistance.

Special Considerations by Transfer Location

People transfer to and from a variety of surfaces and in a variety of locations. There are certain considerations that can ease the difficulty of these transfers.

Bed

Transfers from the bed to the wheelchair are often the first to be addressed by occupational therapists working on inpatient hospital units. Considerations for the bed include:

- Making sure the wheel locks are secured so the bed does not shift during the movement
- Raising or lowering the bed height to the same height of the wheelchair's seating surface. This height should allow the person to place his or her feet on the floor for stability. If standing transfers are being performed, it is important that person be able to reach the floor when seated at the edge of the bed. If the bed cannot lower far enough to be even with the wheelchair, the transfer to the lower surface may be easier and the transfer to the higher surface more difficult. In any case, practice is important, and activities that simulation these changes in level are suggested during treatment sessions.

Bathroom

Transfers to and from a toilet or commode may require the person to stand from and sit to a rather low surface. The person's ability to do this should be considered when making suggestions for environmental adaptations. The bathroom is often the smallest space in the person's home, so practicing maneuvering the wheelchair into position, moving the armrests or footrests, and placing any transfer equipment can ease the transition home. Some toileting equipment, such as rolling shower commode chairs, are available with a drop-arm feature that can make sliding and **lateral transfers** easier.

The placement of the tub bench or bath seat often dictates the setup for the transfer and should be assessed and simulated for practice. These transfers may be complicated by the lack of clothing and water on the body or in the area. Care should be taken during training to address these concerns.

Tub transfers include lifting the legs over the side of the tub or stepping over the side. This is often one of the more difficult aspects of the transfers. One activity that may be helpful is practicing in a doorway. Place a piece of tape low to the floor, across the open door space, and have the person side step over it while holding to the door jam. Each time the person is successful, raise the tape just a bit until it is near the height of the tub side. This is often easier than stepping over the actual tub side because the height can be adjusted to match the person's abilities and because the surfaces on both sides of the tape are level and the same height where many tub surfaces are higher inside the tub than outside. This activity is very easy to grade depending on the person's abilities. It can be set up to simulate transfers in the same direction and those that the person will do at home. Practicing in an actual tub and as part of the bathing process should occur concurrently. It is not uncommon that the person needs additional instruction and assistance for wet transfers. By working simultaneously in the actual tub setting and in the simulated setting of the doorway, the person is able to practice the different steps in the transfer process.

Car

Car transfers can be difficult because the space between the wheelchair and the car is often larger than that encountered during a typical transfer. The two seating surfaces are rarely level, and many car seats have a bucketed shape. If the person has a choice in the car's upholstery, leather or leatherette is easier to slide on than fabric seats. In addition, the car door itself limits the space for maneuvering. Some car doors open wider than others, and some wheelchair users select their cars based, in part, on the space available when the door is open. The wheelchair should be positioned adjacent to the seat where the person will ride. It may be necessary to move or remove the footrests prior to pulling the wheelchair into the small space. Finding secure hand holds to use during the transfer, both on the original surface and the destination surface, helps make this transfer easier. The person should use nonmoving surfaces such as the car seat or dashboard to hold to rather than moving car parts, like the door. The door may swing, causing the person to lose his or her hold or balance, and the fingers may be pinched if the hands slip or the door mistakenly closes.

Many wheelchair users drive. People who are able transfer to the driver's seat and lift their equipment into the car either onto the passenger seat or the back seat. Riding in the vehicle's own seat is safer than being transported or driving from the wheelchair. This option is not always the best, especially if the repeated transfers throughout the day limit the person's energy for other activities. Most **power wheelchairs**, including scooters, are too heavy for this maneuver.

If the person can walk short distances, he or she can place the wheelchair in the trunk or back seat of the car and walk the short distance to the driver's seat. If the person travels with a companion or assistant, he or she can transfer to the driver's or passenger's seat and have the assistant stow the equipment.

There are electronic, hydraulic, and mechanical devices to assist with placement of wheelchair and other mobility aids on the car. These include lifts that place the wheelchair inside the automobile's trunk, on a rack outside the back of the car, or on a stowage device on the roof of the car.

Buses, Trains, and Subways

Transfers to and from seats in public transportation should be assessed, and intervention should be provided as needed. Being transported in the vehicle's own seat is safer than riding in the wheelchair, whenever possible. Transferring to or from a bus or train seat is complicated because tight spaces limit the person's ability to set up his or her wheelchair in its optimal position. Some bus and train seat armrests move out of the way for lateral transfers. For transfers to bus or train seats, the person may need closer supervision or more assistance than is usually required. Bus drivers and train conductors are often able to assist with securing the wheelchair, but not with the transfer itself. These transfers will also be complicated if they are performed while the transportation device is moving.

Whether the wheelchair user rides on the transport system in his or her wheelchair or in the vehicle's seat, it is important that securement be available for both the rider and the device. Tie-down and lock-down systems are used to secure wheelchairs to the vehicle's floor. This securement is necessary so the wheelchair does not become a projectile in the event of an accident.

Airplanes

When accessing an airplane, some **manual wheelchair** users are able to use their own wheelchairs as some have wheels at the end of the antitip bars and when the large wheels of the wheelchair are removed, the mobility device can be rolled on the casters and small antitipper wheels. Manual wheelchair users who are independent in propulsion often need help with navigation when relying on the small wheels only. On entering the plane and rolling in the aisle, the person's wheelchair should be placed in the optimal position for transfers. This is often parallel to the seat and facing forward because of the limited space on board the plan. Many manual wheelchair users can perform this transfer, but some may need help because of the limited space for optimal wheelchair placement.

Other manual wheelchair users and powered wheelchair users must transfer to a transport chair (or aisle chair) supplied by the airline. If the person is using a transport chair, the transfer from the wheelchair will take place in the gate area. The person may need assistance because the transport chair is very small and unstable. The transport chair and the user are then wheeled onto the plan. The transport chair is then placed parallel to the passenger's airplane seat, facing in the same direction as the seat. A stand pivot, lateral, or dependent transfer can then be performed to the airplane seat. Aisle seats on airplanes have locked armrests, but these can often be released by airline personnel, freeing up space for the transfer. Care must be taken that the person is positioned well in the seat, that his or her clothing is smoothed so as not to cause pressure under the buttocks and thighs. Reclining the seat and using positioning aids may also be necessary.

Floor

Not everyone needs or wants to learn to transfer to or from the floor, but it should be discussed with most people, especially those at risk for falling. These transfers are especially useful for people who wish to spend time on the floor, such as for exercise routines or leisure, and for children who play on floor surfaces. It is also helpful for the most active wheelchair users because the environments they frequent and their own wheelchair skills may put them at risk for falling.

For power wheelchair users who want or need access the floor, the transfer is quite similar. Once the person is on the floor, it will be nearly impossible to move the wheelchair so he or she will need to be able to crawl or scoot to the wheelchair for the return transfer. An assistant may be needed to help with the setup and to help with the transfer. There are pediatric power wheelchairs that have a seat-lowering function to bring children to the floor level for playing, exploration, and participation in school activities.

Ambulation Aids

Ambulation aids, such as canes, crutches, and walkers, are used to help people move from one place to another. They may assist with ambulation or compensate for the inability to stand and walk to meet the needs of a given person and are often useful during transfers. A straight cane offers the least stability of the ambulation aids. During a standing transfer, the person may hold one hand on his or her cane while pushing up from the sitting surface with the other. The same strategy may be used with a four-prong or quad cane.

A standard walker with four legs gives the user bilateral support for balance and stability while walking. When used during standing transfers, the person may hold one handle of the walker while pushing up from the seating surface with the other arm (Fig. 30-4). Once he or she is able, that arm is moved to the walker. Once the person is standing and steady, he or she pivots while moving the walker in an arc, step-by-step, until he or she can back up against the second surface. He or she then reaches back for the destination surface and sits. A similar strategy is used with a rolling walker, except that walker may pivot more smoothly. When an ambulation aid is used, it must be included in the associated documentation.

Functional Mobility

If the person is unable to walk, with or without an ambulation aid, or is unable to walk to meet all of his or her needs, a wheelchair should be considered. If the person can walk short distances or for short periods of

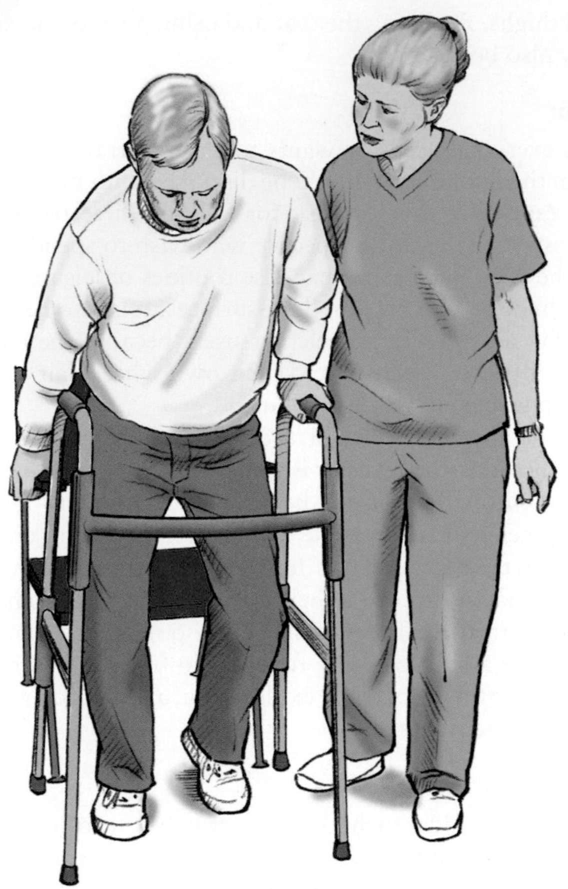

Figure 30-4. Teaching safe use of a walker: Sitting down: First, tell the patient to stand with the back of his stronger leg against the front of the chair, his weaker leg slightly off the floor, and the walker directly in front. Tell him to grasp the armrests on the chair one arm at a time while supporting most of his weight on the stronger leg. (In the illustrations, the patient has left leg weakness.) Tell the patient to lower himself into the chair and slide backward. After he's seated, he should place the walker beside the chair.

time or on certain days, depending on how he or she is feeling, a wheelchair should be provided for longer excursions or for whenever it is needed. One important point of the mobility aid is to enable the person to have sufficient energy to participate in desired activities. If the transit from one location to the other uses the person's energy, he or she will be unable to participate as fully as desired. This can be a difficult conversation to have because some people are concerned that moving from walking with an ambulation aid to using a wheelchair is a sign of deterioration or failure. By focusing the conversation on the activities in which the person wishes to participate, he or she may be more willing to consider using a wheeled mobility device.

The primary purpose of a wheelchair is to facilitate movement within and between environments and to allow exploration of those environments. Some wheelchair users independently navigate their wheelchairs through environments, whereas others need assistance for some or all of their maneuvers. Efficiency, body mechanics, planning and judgment, and safety are a few of the principles that underlie effective navigation. These are all intertwined. For instance, efficiency is using the most efficient route of travel over the surfaces that are navigable to reserve energy for participation in the desired activities at the destination. Efficiency also refers to the person's technique for manual propulsion so that he or she uses the most efficient body movements to reserve energy and prevent overuse or injury. For power wheelchair users, efficiency is related to the battery life of their wheelchair. Depending on the usage, a power wheelchair user may select short routes and turn off his or her wheelchair when stopped in order to conserve battery power.

Assessment for Functional Mobility

As with transfers, the assessment for wheelchair navigation comprised of many other assessments that are often completed in the course of the OT evaluation. Such areas include assessment of the nervous system, vision and hearing, and structures related to movement. Besides assessing the structures, the assessment should include actual wheelchair propulsion. Environmental conditions should also be assessed. This includes environments where training will take place, such as a patient's hospital room and therapy area. It should also include environments where the person is expected to participate in his or her chosen activities.

Body mechanics and posture need to be considered during navigation. Of primary importance is maintaining optimal posture for function. If the wheelchair user loses his or her position during navigation, his or her function will likely be limited, and the seating and positioning aids may need to be adjusted to provide sufficient support. Besides maintaining posture for function, it is also important for manual wheelchair users to feel comfortable with moving his or her own body position in relation to their wheelchair, or knowing their center of gravity. This is important for skills such as popping a **wheelie** and rolling up and down ramps. The assessment also determines the method the wheelchair user will use to propel his or her wheelchair. If upper extremity strength, endurance, and coordination are sufficient, the person may be able to use a manual wheelchair to meet his or her needs. If he or she is able to use one hand and one foot, such as following a stroke, this will indicate wheelchair propulsion using those extremities. If the person is unable to propel a manual wheelchair sufficiently, a power wheelchair should be considered. In addition to physical abilities, cognitive function, the person's social support, and the environments the person uses should also be assessed.

Planning and judgment are two cognitive skills that influence a wheelchair users ability to get to and from his or her desired locations. This might include getting from home to work taking public transportation, or it might include navigating around an obstacle, such as in sidewalk construction. In order to demonstrate good judgment, people need to have insight into their abilities and strengths in order to compensate for difficulties. For instance, a person with good insight will likely be better able to know how close he or she can roll to a curbside without tipping into the street. The assessment reveals this information. There are additional considerations for power wheelchair users, such as the ability to perform regular maintenance including charging the battery as needed. Manual and power wheelchair use is complicated, and the assessment for the use of these wheeled mobility devices often takes multiple sessions. At the completion of the assessment, the occupational therapist should be able to determine the best strategies for navigation and a plan to improve performance via goals. The goals are developed in collaboration with the wheelchair user and others in the social support system. Goals might address endurance for propulsion, speed, accuracy, obstacle climbing abilities, and so on. Goals also must include consideration of safety, planning, and judgment.

Intervention for Functional Mobility

Safety, of course, is the priority. In many wheelchair mobility training programs, the first skill that is taught is falling safely. People with paraplegia, for instance, can hold one arm across their thighs and the bend their heads forward and protect their head with their other arm so that (1) their legs do not bend and their knees hit their face and (2) they do not hit the back of their heads if the wheelchair tips backward, as may happen when popping a wheelie.

The initial stages of mobility training take place inside the rehabilitation facility where the person learns how to maneuver on a smooth surface in an open space. Training continues focusing on more difficult skills and depending on the person's intended use. This might include negotiating surfaces such as sand or gravel and navigating over or around obstacles like curbs, steps, and railroad tracks. Training also includes navigation through tight spaces, such as a busy restaurant or office. The occupational therapist can incorporate wheelchair mobility goals within other ADL intervention. For example, if a power wheelchair user is taken to the grocery store to shop for food in preparation for cooking a meal, there is the opportunity to explore wheelchair mobility in a public environment while also carrying items or pushing a shopping cart.

As the person thinks about and attempts community-level mobility, it is also helpful to provide resources regarding accessibility guidelines. In the United States, changes in access to public places often result from advocacy and self-advocacy. Asking for help and providing information about access are skills that most wheelchair users need at one time or another, and some wheelchair users may embrace more fully. The Americans with Disability Act Accessibility guidelines address indoor and outdoor access for people with varying needs, including those who use wheelchairs or ambulation aids, those with hearing or vision impairments and those with cognitive limitations.[3]

It is important to address the psychosocial impact of using a wheelchair or other mobility device. Focusing on success and practicing skills in community spaces gives the wheelchair user the opportunity to build his or her esteem and is an important component of participation in community-based activities.

Part of the training in the use of a mobility device like a wheelchair is its care and maintenance. Such operations as cleaning the wheelchair, adjusting the wheel locks, adjusting air in tires, charging batteries, or even replacing spokes in the wheels can be performed by the user or assistant. During intervention, occupational therapists should make sure that the wheelchair user and/or assistant can perform wheelchair parts management and everyday care and maintenance. They should also be instructed about whom to contact for repairs and replacement.

There are some terrific resources for clinicians and for wheelchair users. Clinicians can learn the skills they will be teaching at training courses and using manuals and related materials. Materials from the Wheelchair Skills Program can be downloaded at https://wheelchairskillsprogram.ca/en/. Associated with this training program is a skills test that can be used to identify each user's skill level.[4] The skills listed in this test can also be used to determine interventions for individual clients. There are also very useful manuals for wheelchair users and clinicians that describe independent as well as assisted power and manual wheelchair mobility skills.[5,6]

Manual Wheelchair Navigation

Propulsion

Manual wheelchair propulsion usually occurs by pushing on the push rims that are attached to the outer surface of the rear wheels. According to Boninger et al.,[7] there are four common propulsion patterns. The least efficient is in an arc moving back and forth from about 12:00 to 2:00. This pattern is often seen when the wheelchair seating surface is too high in relation to the push rims and/or when the rider has limited sitting balance in his or her wheelchair. The pattern that is most efficient and most likely to prevent repetitive stress is semicircular, "with the hand traveling below the pushrim in recovery" (Fig. 30-5). Using this strategy may improve wheelchair propulsion and decrease the tendency for pain and repetitive stress that is shown to occur in the shoulders of people with paraplegic spinal injuries.[8]

Using both hands/arms is not the only method of propulsion. Manual wheelchairs can also be propelled using both feet; using one arm/hand and one

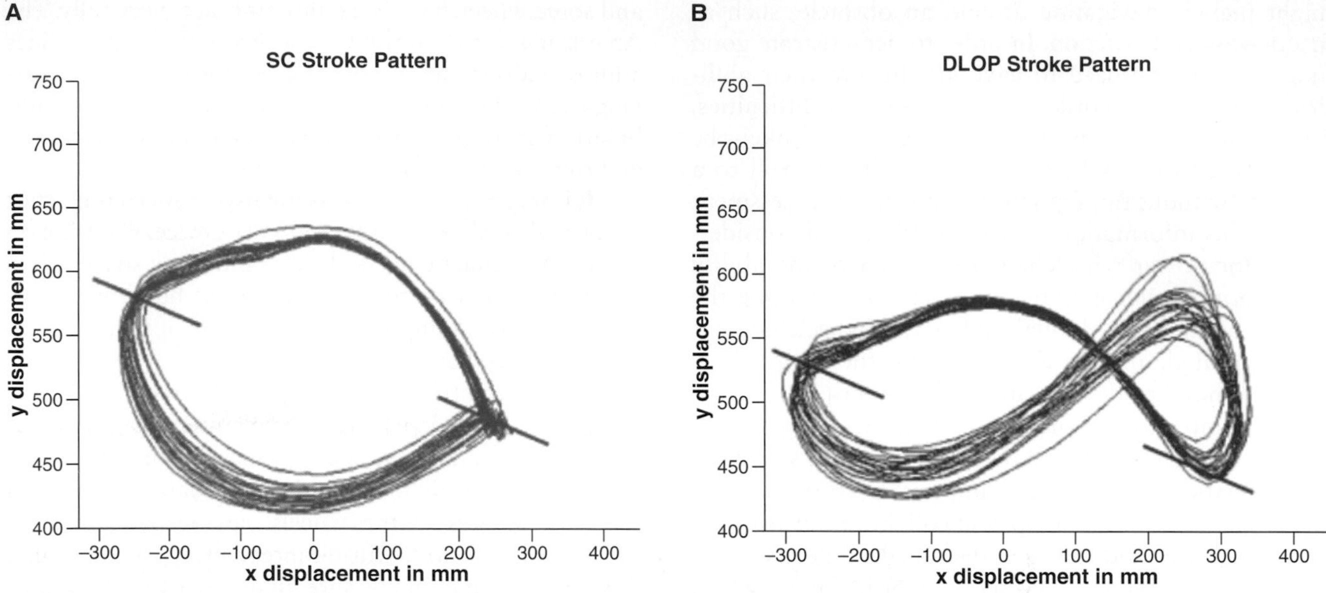

Figure 30-5. Manual wheelchair propulsion patterns. **A.** Results from the optimal propulsion pattern. **B.** Results from the least efficient propulsion pattern. DLOP, double-looping; SC, semicircular.

foot, as is common for people who are hemiplegic such as following a stroke; or with one arm/hand. And of course, manual wheelchairs can also be propelled by an assistant, although some of the most highly adjustable wheelchairs may not have push handles as they often impede self-propulsion. If the person is propelling the wheelchair with one or both feet, it is important to insure that the seat height is low enough so the person can reach the floor while maintaining an optimal seated posture. This may require selecting a specially designed low wheelchair or adapting the seat surface so that it is low.

Propulsion on smooth, level surfaces is accomplished by pushing on both push rims evenly. Wide turns can be made by "dragging the hand" on the push rim on the side to which the person wants to turn. For example, if the person wants to turn right to continue down a hallway, he or she could merely hold his or her hand against the right push rim. That slows the roll of that wheel while the left wheel continues at its speed, causing the wheelchair to veer or turn to the right. If a sharp right turn is needed, the person can continue pushing forward on the left push rim and slowing the roll of the right wheel. A very tight turn is accomplished by pushing forward on one wheel and rearward (pulling back) on the other, allowing the person to turn his or her wheelchair on its own axis (Fig. 30-6).

Ramps and Slopes

The Americans with Disabilities Accessibility (ADA) guidelines state that any change in level over ½ inch (1.27 cm) should be ramped and that ramps should be 5° or less.[9] For every 1 inch (2.54 cm) of rise (height), the ramp must have 12 inches (30.48) of length (1:12 slope). For example, a 4-inch (10.16 cm) step will require the ramp length to be 48 inches (121.92) in order for a most people to navigate it using a wheelchair. A ramp in a public place must have a surface with a detectable texture for persons with visual impairments. It must have railings and a curb to keep wheelchair wheels from rolling over the edge. There must be 4 feet (1.22 m) of level landing at the top of the ramp.[3] Leaning in the uphill direction, whether ascending or descending the ramp, helps to keep the wheelchair from tipping (Fig. 30-7).

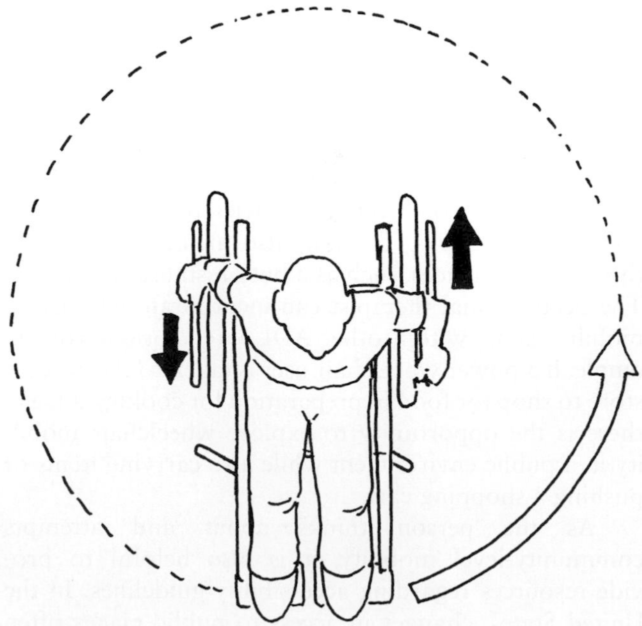

Figure 30-6. View from above: By pulling back on one wheel while pushing forward on the other, the wheelchair and user can make their tightest turn. (Courtesy of Beneficial Designs.)

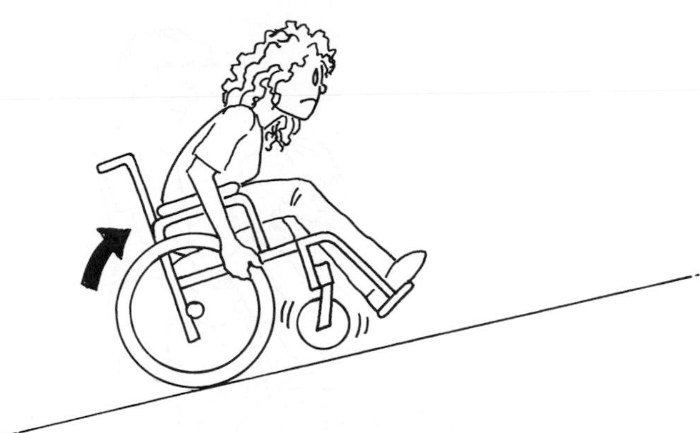

Figure 30-7. Leaning forward when ascending a ramp helps to prevent the wheelchair and user from tipping backward. (Courtesy of Beneficial Designs.)

Skilled manual wheelchair users may descend ramps in a wheelie to prevent falling forward (Fig. 30-8).

Unlike ramps that people negotiate in the forward or backward direction, side slopes impact forward propulsion as the wheelchair continuously veers in the downhill direction. Thus, the downhill arm works much harder to keep the wheelchair moving straight. In the United States, sidewalks are built with a side slope toward the street so that rain drains to the gutter rather than into businesses and homes. Manual wheelchair users traveling long distances on sidewalks and people with low endurance may need to switch sides of the street so they can rest the downhill arm.

Wheelies

Wheelies are an important skill for manual wheelchair users to master, allowing them to propel more easily over uneven surfaces, and providing a seating system where position changes are possible. Even if the wheelchair user cannot complete a full wheelie, leaning back in the wheelchair lightens the load over the front casters, allowing more maneuverability. A pop-up or partial wheelie is very useful for navigating low obstacles like door sills and uneven sidewalks.

To pop a partial wheelie, the user rolls the wheelchair backward a short distance and then grabs the back of the push rims and pushes forward, while weight shifting rearward[5] (Fig. 30-9). Once the pop-up is achieved, further training and practice can lead to finding the balance point and sustaining a wheelie.

Changes in Level

Since the passage of the ADA Standards in 1990, curbs on sidewalks at street intersections are becoming less of a problem as curb ramps proliferate; however, at times, the wheelchair user may encounter a curb. In order to ascend a curb, it is easier if the manual wheelchair user can perform a wheelie while moving forward. If that is not possible, the person approaches the curb or step, facing it, pops up to place the casters on the curb, leans forward to redistribute the weight, and propels the large rear wheels up the curb or step with a hearty push. A person must have good balance, upper extremity strength, and hand function to perform this maneuver. To go down a curb or a step, the person approaches it backward, leans forward in the chair, and slowly rolls the rear wheels over the step or curb. An assistant can help by slowing the movement (Fig. 30-10A). Once the rear wheels are lowered, he or she can spin to the left or right, maintaining his or her casters up and turns then bringing the casters to lower surface. An alternative method for going down a curb is to approach the curb facing it, move into the wheelie position, and roll slowly down the curb using the back wheels. The person must have an excellent sense of the balance point of the wheelchair to perform this technique safely. As with all other actions, if a wheelchair user cannot move up or down a curb or step or roll through grass or over uneven surfaces, another person can provide assistance (Fig. 30-10B).

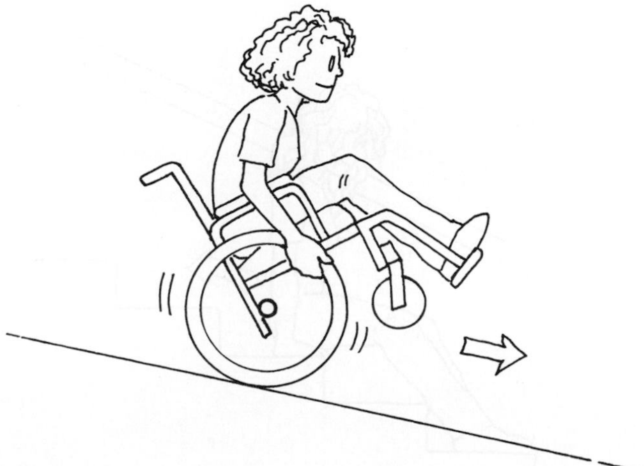

Figure 30-8. Descending a ramp in a wheelie position. (Courtesy of Beneficial Designs.)

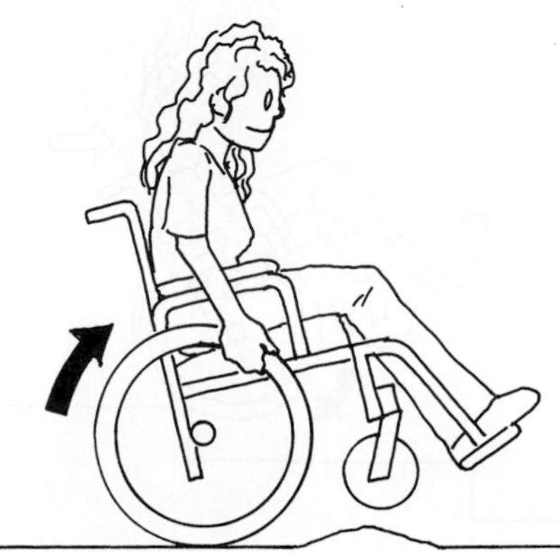

Figure 30-9. Popping a partial wheelie makes rolling over small bumps easier. (Courtesy of Beneficial Designs.)

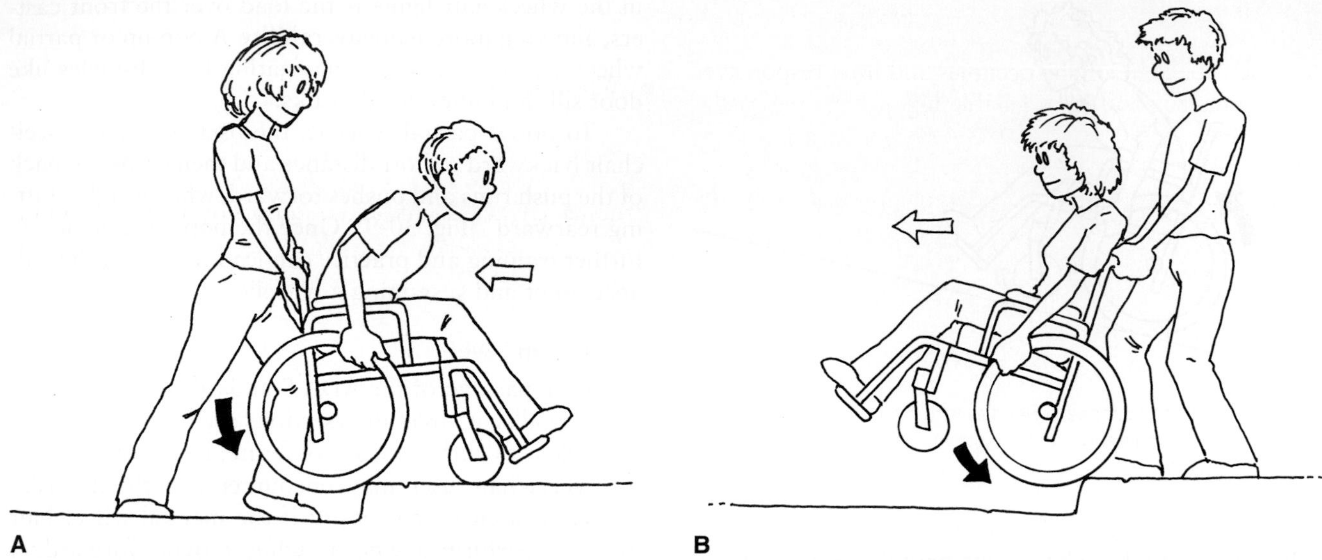

Figure 30-10. A. Descending a curb in the rearward direction with an assistant. **B.** Descending a curb in the forward direction with an assistant. (Courtesy of Beneficial Designs.)

Stairs

A skilled manual wheelchair user may be able to descend a couple of steps, especially if they have deep platforms, safely by performing a wheelie bouncing down the steps (Fig. 30-11). Some people perform a wheelchair-to-floor transfer and "bump" up or down the steps while pulling the chair along. Skin protection during this task must be understood and practiced (Fig. 30-12).

Power Wheelchair Navigation

Power wheelchair navigation has many of the same considerations as manual wheelchair mobility. Power wheelchair training should begin in an open, barrier-free environment so that the user can make mistakes without hitting obstacles. As with other OT interventions, arranging the environment and the equipment so the person can be successful is important. This may mean setting the speed of the power wheelchair at a slow setting or giving single-step directions rather than complex directions. Grading the task/activity can then help build the user's skills and confidence in his or her skills and may lead to success in more complex navigation.

Training often begins with orientation to the mobility device and the controller. The wheelchair user may practice moving the joystick or other controller without moving the wheelchair. It may even be possible to use similar joysticks or switches to activate other devices such as computer games to learn how the controller works. The wheelchair user should also learn how to turn the power wheelchair on and off and to switch between their own various settings. Moving the wheelchair should ideally begin on smooth surfaces with wide open spaces and then move to more constricted environments so the user can master steering and speed. Moving to environments with distractions or small obstacles might be the next step. Giving the wheelchair user the opportunity to

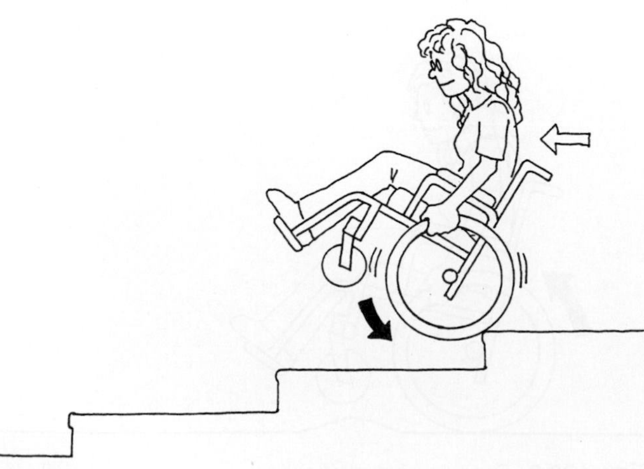

Figure 30-11. People with exceptional skills can "bump" down a few steps. Deep steps make this maneuver easier. (Courtesy of Beneficial Designs.)

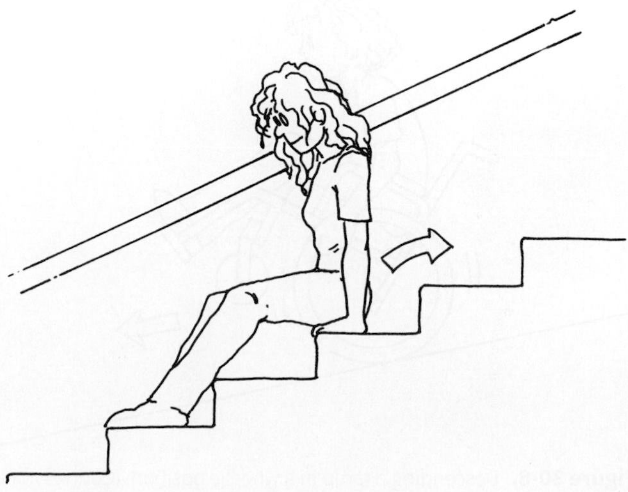

Figure 30-12. Bumping up steps one at a time. (Courtesy of Beneficial Designs.)

explore the dimensions of his or her own wheelchair and how it moves in the environment allows the user to know how much space he or she occupies and how responsive the equipment is and how reliable his or her own skills are. This will help with navigation around/over/behind obstacles. All of these skills can be performed with the occupational therapist providing support, or spotting, in case the wheelchair user needs assistance.

As the person's abilities improve, he or she can attempt more difficult navigation. Practicing these skills with a spotter or assistant is a good idea. More challenging navigation includes riding over soft surfaces, crossing gaps like on a train or subway platform, and riding over larger obstacles like small curbs. Whenever possible, obstacles like gaps and small curbs should be approached head-on, with the wheelchair perpendicular to the gap or curbs. This helps to prevent a caster or drive wheel from sliding into the space or tipping on a curb.

It is also important for the wheelchair user to be able to instruct others in the procedures for wheelchair skills, especially those that are more challenging. This is especially necessary when the wheelchair breaks down in some way. Most power wheelchairs stop working at some point or another, such as when the battery drains. Power wheelchairs can be moved from their "power mode" to a "manual mode" so the wheelchairs can be pushed manually. This involves disengaging the motors. Each power wheelchair works differently, so it is important to refer to the owner's manual for instruction on engaging and disengaging motors of specific makes and models of power wheelchair.

As of yet, drivers' tests are not required for power mobility use as they are elsewhere in the world. Some therapists working in rehabilitation or specializing in wheelchair use have developed their own checklists for power wheelchair use that act as a driver's test.

Documentation for wheelchair use should include the following information:

- Wheelchair used.
- Method of propulsion.
- Speed and accuracy of navigation in each environment, such as indoors over smooth surfaces, indoors in congested environments, and outdoors over rough terrain.
- Training of assistants should also be documented as should the wheelchair rider's ability to direct his or her care during navigation.
- Safety in performance of each skill. Safety, or safe navigation, is the most important aspect to document.

Emergency Evacuation

Areas of refuge (or rescue) should be located on every floor of every building (other than street level).[10] Local emergency responders are provided with these locations by the building's owner/manager so that the first responders can rescue anyone who is unable to leave the building. Emergency responders should know to check these areas to help people who are unable to evacuate on their own.

Manual and power wheelchair users, as well as people who use ambulation aids or have difficulty negotiating stairs and long distances, should be trained in safe evacuation locations and techniques so that they may instruct assistants when needed. If there are only a few steps and if there are strong and able helpers, the wheelchair user can be bumped down the steps. This can be very tiring and requires two people to lower the wheelchair. If the assistants are unable to manage those techniques, the wheelchair user can be carried out. Emergency evacuation chairs or mats can be used, so the wheelchair user does not have to be carried bodily (Fig. 30-13A and B).

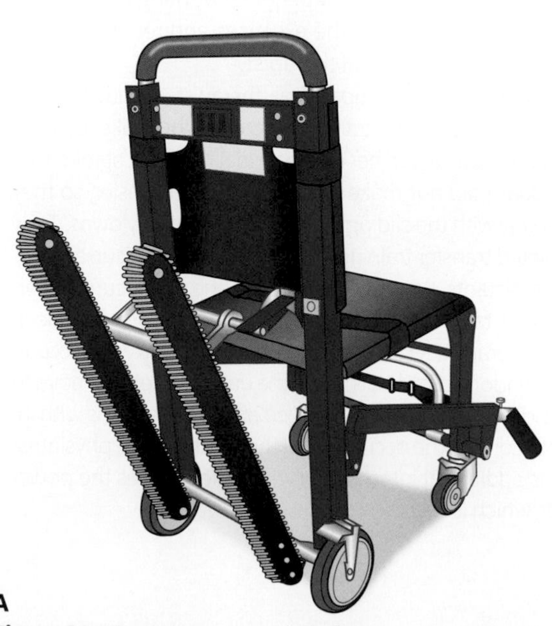

A

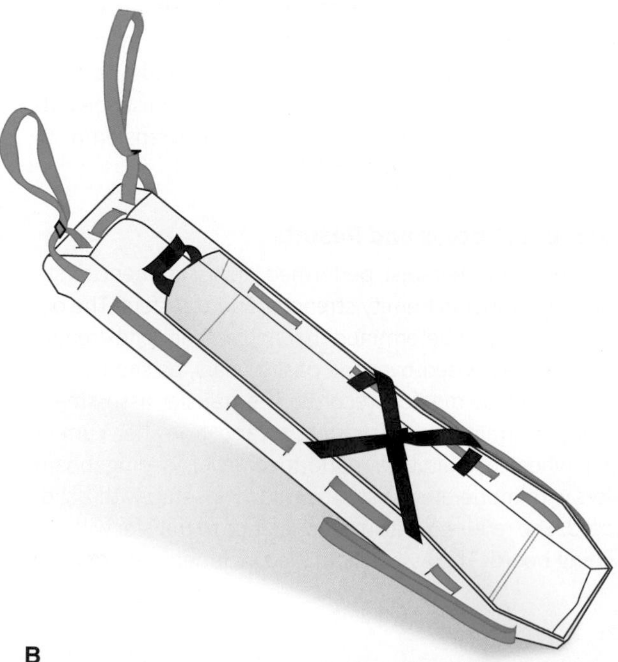

B

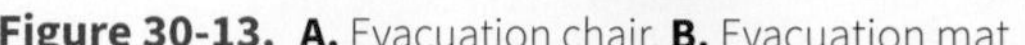

Figure 30-13. **A.** Evacuation chair. **B.** Evacuation mat.

Documentation of Wheelchair Mobility Skills

As with other OT documentation, the goals include the method of performance, the amount of assistance or other qualifiers such as the amount of time needed for a task or the environment where the task performance occurs, and the timeline. Many mobility skills are incorporated into other goals such as for ADLs, instrumental ADLs, work, and leisure. Kirby's wheelchair training program and test can also provide a framework for documentation.[4]

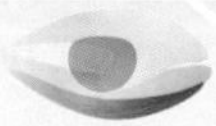

CASE STUDY

Patient Information

Louisa is a 32-year-old woman, s/p C5-6 spinal cord injury (SCI) × 8 years. She owns and lives in a three-story home. The first floor is accessible via a ramp to her back deck and has been adapted with a bedroom equipped with a hospital bed and environmental control unit. The bathroom has been renovated for wheelchair maneuverability and with a roll-in shower. Louisa works full time. She drives an accessible van adapted with hand controls and low-effort acceleration and braking. She has an assist dog that performs difficult tasks for her, such as retrieving objects from the floor, opening and closing doors, and acting as a buffer with other people, thereby increasing Louisa's socialization. She is seen by her physiatrist on an annual basis and during, her last visit, complained about shoulder pain and fatigue, especially when propelling her manual wheelchair and at the end of her workday. Louisa reported that when she was at her best, she needed occasional minimal assistance for level, sliding board transfers. She reports being concerned about transfers with the powered wheelchair because the seat height is about 3 inch (7.62 cm) higher than her current, manual wheelchair. She is also concerned that her personal care assistants need to be retrained in transfer assistance using the powered wheelchair.

Reason for Occupational Therapy Referral

Louisa was seen in the outpatient seating clinic for evaluation for powered mobility. The assistive technology professional in the seating clinic arranged for the physiatrist to prescribe outpatient OT for transfer training in preparation for transferring to and from her new, powered wheelchair.

Assessment Process and Results

The occupational therapist performed an assessment of sitting balance, upper extremity strength, and transfers. The occupational therapist determined that Louisa's upper extremity strength has decreased over the past 2 years, as she has full access to previous medical records. The transfer assessment includes performing level transfers to and from her current manual wheelchair. Louisa performed level, sliding board transfers with moderate assistance following setup with a sliding board. She required maximal assistance to transfer without the sliding board. The assessment also included performance of transfers to and from higher and lower surfaces, using an adjustable height mat table. Louisa required verbal directions and maximal assistance to perform these transfers. A brief, nonstandardized cognitive assessment revealed Louisa to have high function in both specific cognitive skills and executive functioning.

Occupational Therapy Problem List

- Decreased upper extremity strength and endurance
- Decreased independence wheelchair transfers

Occupational Therapy Goal List

- Increase strength and endurance for moderate assistance for sliding board transfers to and from higher and lower surfaces sufficiently by 2 weeks.
- Able to instruct care takers in safe techniques during transfers from wheelchair to higher and lower surfaces, including her bed and shower commode chair by 2 weeks.

Intervention

Louisa received outpatient OT twice weekly for 2 weeks. Louisa's assets included being highly motivated and having intact cognition with good problem-solving and judgment. The occupational therapist provided Louisa with recommendations for a strengthening program that Louisa plans to continue to use. During her time in OT, she contacted a personal trainer with whom she works and who has experience working with people with SCI. The trainer will use the exercises and techniques established by the occupational therapist.

During therapy, the occupational therapist introduced the Beasy Board because this transfer board might make Louisa's transfers easier. Louisa and her occupational therapist agreed that the Beasy Board did not make any of the transfers easier, so they decided to stay with the sliding board that she already owns. They also completed transfer training and practice with the current personal care assistants. Louisa realized that none of her current personal care assistants were with her early-on and none had been trained by a therapist. All of the therapy interventions were acceptable to and endorsed by Louisa with the exception of the move to the Beasy Board. Louisa was discharged after four sessions with instructions to contact the occupational therapist and the physiatrist if she needs additional intervention when she receives the power wheelchair, which is expected in 4 to 6 weeks.

Evidence Table of Intervention Studies for Manual Wheelchair Propulsion

Intervention	Description	Participants	Dosage	Research Design and Evidence Level	Benefit	Statistical Significance and Effect Size
Wheelchair skills training program[11]	Training in indoor and outdoor skills	Thirty-five wheelchair users (15 = treatment group; 20 = control group)	Six sessions, 30 minutes each	Two group controlled study; Level II	Wheelchair skills training program is effective.	Control group scores on wheelchair skills test improved by 8% ($p = 0.01$). Treatment group scores on wheelchair skills test improved by 25% ($p = 0.000$).
Wheelchair skills training[12]	Individualized wheelchair skills training	Hundred and six community-dwelling, manual wheelchair users, Veterans (53 = treatment group; 53 educational control group) began. Eighty-two completed (40 = treatment group; 42 = control group)	Five 1:1 training sessions over 5-week time period	Two group controlled study; Level II	Wheelchair skills improved in testing group. Retention of skills was evident for up to 3 months.	Significant improvement noted in advanced skills for treatment group ($p < 0.0001$) and for the overall wheelchair skills test ($p < 0.0001$).
Wheelchair skills training to impact wheelchair use self-efficacy, skills capacity and performance, and life space mobility[13]	Peer-led training using WheelSee to pairs of manual wheelchair users	Twenty-eight community-based manual wheelchair users (16 = treatment group; 12 = control group)		Pilot, two group controlled study; Level II	Wheelchair use self-efficacy and wheelchair skill capacity/performance improved in treatment group more than in control group.	Improvement in wheelchair use self-efficacy significant higher in treatment group over control group (Cohen $d = 1.4$). Wheelchair skills capacity and performance were significantly higher in treatment group over control group (Cohen $d = 1.3$, $d = 1.0$, respectively).

References

1. Hanson D, Langemo DK, Anderson J, Thompson P, Hunter S. Friction and shear considerations in pressure ulcer development. *Adv Wound Care.* 2010;23(1):21–24.
2. VISN 8 Patient Safety Center. Safe patient handling and movement instructions: assessment/algorithm document. *Medline.* https://www.medline.com/media/mkt/clinical-solutions/safe-patient-handling-program/tools/tools-pdf/OTH_Safe-Patient-Handling-Movement-Instructions.pdf
3. Department of Justice. *2010 ADA standards for accessible design.* 2010. https://www.ada.gov/2010ADAstandards_index.htm
4. Kirby RL, Dupuis DJ, MacPhee AH, et al. The wheelchair skills test (version 2.4): measurement properties11No commercial party having a direct financial interest in the results of the research supporting this article has or will confer a benefit on the author(s) or on any organization with which the author(s) is/are associated. *Arch Phys Med Rehabil.* 2004;85(5):794–804.
5. Axelson P, Chesney DY, Minkel J, Perr A. *Manual Wheelchair Training Guide.* Santa Cruz, CA: PAX Press; 1998.
6. Axelson P, Chesney DY, Minkel J, Perr A. *Powered Wheelchair Training Guide.* Minden, NV: Pax Press; 2013.
7. Boninger ML, Souza AL, Cooper RA, Fitzgerald SG, Koontz AM, Fay BT. Propulsion patterns and pushrim biomechanics in manual wheelchair propulsion. *Arch Phys Med Rehabil.* 2002;83(5):718–723.
8. Samuelsson KA, Tropp H, Gerdle B. Shoulder pain and its consequences in paraplegic spinal cord-injured, wheelchair users. *Spinal Cord.* 2004;42(1):41–46.
9. United States Access board. Chapter 4: Ramps and curb ramps. *Guide to the ADA Standards.* https://www.access-board.gov/guidelines-and-standards/buildings-and-sites/about-the-ada-standards/guide-to-the-ada-standards/chapter-4-ramps-and-curb-ramps
10. United Spinal Association. Fire safety for wheelchair users at work and at home. 2011. https://www.unitedspinal.org/pdf/WheelchairFireSafety.pdf
11. MacPhee AH, Kirby RL, Coolen AL, Smith C, MacLeod DA, Dupuis DJ. Wheelchair skills training program: a randomized clinical trial of wheelchair users undergoing initial rehabilitation. *Arch Phys Med Rehabil.* 2004;85(1):41–50.
12. Kirby RL, Mitchell D, Sabharwal S, McCranie M, Nelson AL. Manual wheelchair skills training for community-dwelling veterans with spinal cord injury: a randomized controlled trial. *PLoS One.* 2016;11(12):1–20.
13. Best KL, Miller WC, Huston G, Routhier F, Eng JJ. Pilot study of a peer-led wheelchair training program to improve self-efficacy using a manual wheelchair: a randomized controlled trial. *Arch Phys Med Rehabil.* 2016;97(1):37–44.

Chapter 31

Restoring Driving and Community Mobility

Sherrilene Classen and Beth Pfeiffer

LEARNING OBJECTIVES

This chapter will allow the reader to:

1. Conceptualize a definition of driving as an instrumental activity of daily living.
2. Understand the implications of motor vehicle crash statistics and trends over a decade in the United States.
3. Articulate the roles of the occupational therapist generalist and specialist in driver rehabilitation, specifically related to screening, assessment, and intervention.
4. Integrate and synthesize the knowledge on assessment and intervention via a case study example.
5. Understand the impact of community mobility on participation in essential and meaningful activities.
6. Identify the role of occupational therapist in addressing community mobility issues.
7. Understand assessment and intervention processes to improve the person–environment fit for community mobility.

CHAPTER OUTLINE

TERMINOLOGY

Community mobility: moving around in the community and using public or private transportation, such as driving, walking, bicycling, or accessing and riding in buses, taxi cabs, or other transportation systems.[1]

Community participation: active involvement in activities that are intrinsically social and either occur outside the home or are part of a nondomestic role.[2]

Comprehensive driving evaluation: a complete evaluation of an individual's driving knowledge, skills, and abilities by a health care professional that includes (1) medical and driving history; (2) clinical assessment of sensory/perceptual, cognitive, or psychomotor functional abilities; (3) on-road assessment, as appropriate; (4) an outcome summary; and (5) recommendations for an inclusive mobility plan including transportation options.[3]

Driver rehabilitation specialist (DRS): professional who provides clinical driving and driving mobility equipment evaluations and intervention to develop or restore driving skills and abilities[1]; may or may not have a health professional background; with a health professional background, a DRS can provide the comprehensive driving evaluation.

Driver rehabilitation specialist, certified: a DRS certified by the Association for Driver Rehabilitation Specialists (ADED) to hold a specialty certification in driver rehabilitation.

Fitness to drive: a characteristic of a driver, defined by the absence of any functional (sensory/perceptual, cognitive, or psychomotor) deficit or medical condition that significantly impairs an individual's ability to fully control the vehicle while conforming to the rules of the road and obeying traffic laws and/or that significantly increases crash risk.[4]

Occupational therapist generalists: professional who provides clinical driving evaluations or applies specific assessment tools in order to assess fitness to drive as an instrumental activity of daily living and intervention to develop or restore driving abilities.[5]

Paratransit: a supplemental form of transportation required by the American with Disability Act (ADA) provided by public transit agencies for individuals with disabilities who cannot use fixed-route transit services because of a disability.[6]

Personal mobility devices: devices used for community mobility when a person cannot walk or has limited walking ability such as a manual or electric wheelchair.

Driving as an Instrumental Activity of Daily Living

Driving is an instrumental activity of daily living (IADL) that requires intact visual, visual attention, visual perceptual, cognitive, executive, other sensory, and motor functions; all executed in a coordinated manner within a complex, dynamic, and unpredictable environment, while achieving control over the vehicle to steer it cautiously and safely in the flow of traffic and while observing the rules of the road and traffic regulations. This task, therefore, represents an integration of the person, the vehicle, and the environment domains and, as such, is embedded in the scope of occupational therapy practice. Driving is considered a privilege, not a right, and is one of the few IADLs that can lead to death or serious injury. But the benefits of being able to drive are multiple. Mainly, driving is an occupation enabler and a mediator of autonomy, freedom, and independence. For older drivers, studies associate mobility afforded by driving with increased life satisfaction, quality of life (QoL), autonomy, and well-being.[7–9] In contrast, driving cessation is associated with poor health trajectories, including increased rates of depression, limited life-space mobility, early nursing home admissions, and premature death.[10–14]

Our society is standing on the brink of a transportation revolution with the advent of the autonomous vehicles into our society. Although the highly autonomous vehicles may not be available for societal use for another decade or more,[15] we can anticipate that the task of driving, as well as the role of the driver, will change accordingly. Specifically, in the future, the task of driving will be executed by the autonomous vehicle, and the driver will, therefore, have to surrender personal control, show confidence in technology, and trust in the autonomous system. The role of the driver may change from a driver in a standard vehicle, to an operator in a semi-autonomous vehicle, or a passenger in a highly autonomous vehicle. Moreover, drivers and occupational therapists who may assess such drivers will have to be savvy and understand the lingo related to the evolving vehicle technology. Until such time, however, occupational therapists need to understand that driving has inherent risks and that they can make a difference in detecting at-risk drivers. To contextualize the scope of such risk, we will provide an overview of the crash statistics in the United States.

Overview of Crashes in the United States

According to the National Highway Traffic Safety Association (NHTSA), 35,092 road fatalities occurred in the United States in 2015, which is a 7.2% increase over 2014.[16] This is the largest percentage increase recorded in nearly 50 years with a fatality rate of 10.9 per 100,000 inhabitants. Provisional data from the first 9 months of 2016 indicate an additional 8% increase in traffic fatalities over the same period in 2015. Notwithstanding the loss of life, the number of injury crashes, and those who were seriously injured, also increased substantially. The NHTSA estimated that the cost associated with these road fatalities and injuries accounted for 242 billion dollars in 2010. When societal harm is factored in, then the cost increases to 836 billion dollars, which is about 6% of the gross domestic product in the United States.[16] The most vulnerable road users are the teens and the older drivers, as can be seen from Figure 31-1. Since 2010, teens (18–20 years of age) had the highest fatality rates per 100,000 population, followed by older persons (65 years and older).

Occupational therapists are positioned to help turn these statistics around though early detection and intervention. Specifically, human error accounts for 94%

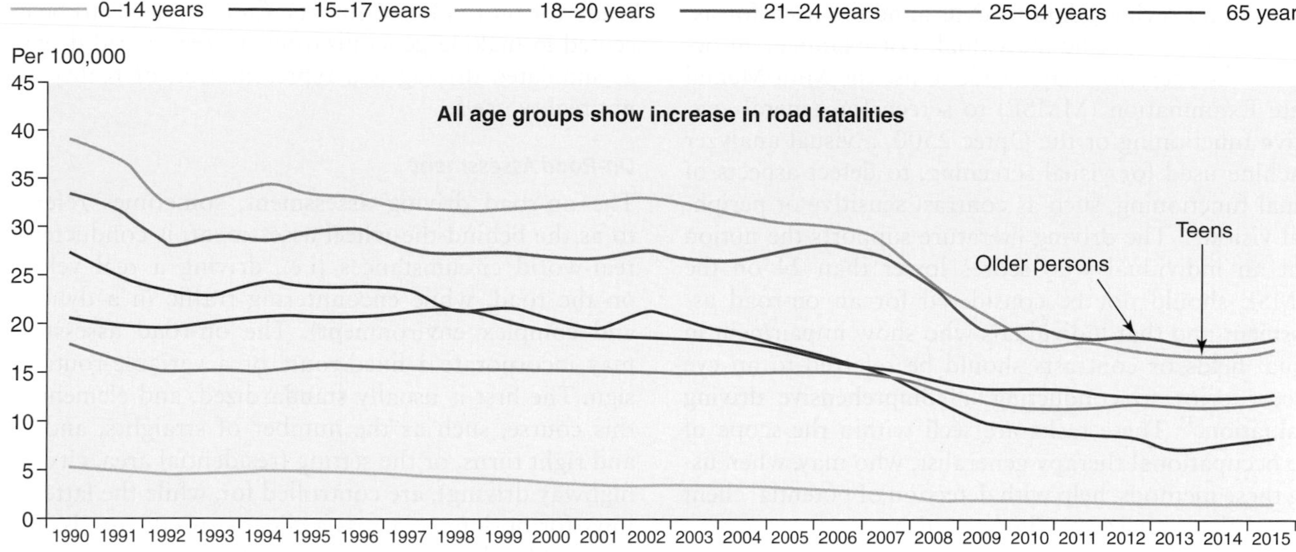

Figure 31-1. Road fatality rates by age group. Deaths per 100,000 inhabitants in a given age group, 1990 to 2015.[74]

of crash-related fatalities or injuries.[16] Human errors, which may include speeding, yielding, gap acceptance, lane maintenance, visual scanning, signaling, and adjustment to stimuli errors, occur, for example, in drowsy drivers, drunk drivers, older driver, and distracted drivers. Because occupational therapists work with people representative of these groups, practice opportunities exist for general client education, and/or screening, assessment, and intervention.

Driver Rehabilitation

Driver rehabilitation entails a process of intervention intended to ameliorate impairments or deficits related to the driving task or alternative methods of mobility.[4] The outcome of driver rehabilitation is successful implementation of an intervention or course of action that facilitates safe mobility and transportation. Driver rehabilitation usually starts with screening, assessment, intervention, and discharge.

Screening

Screening is the process preceding an assessment and entails obtaining and reviewing data, personal, social, and medical history, to determine the need for assessment and can be done by the person themselves, a proxy rater, or an evaluator.[4]

Self-Screening

For self-screening, an individual obtains and reviews his or her own data to determine the need for further assessment.[17–19] A limited number of valid and reliable screening tools for identifying at-risk older drivers exists.[20] For example, Roadwise Review, a self-screening, lacks predictive validity to detect at-risk drivers.[21] The DriveSafe and DriveAware self-screening accurately predicts the on-road performance of older drivers,[22] but as standardized in a country where driving occurs on the left side of the road. A drawback of self-screening tools is an overestimation of the client's driving abilities.[23]

Proxy Screening

For proxy screening, an individual may obtain and review data to determine the need for assessment of another person.[19,24] The Fitness-to-Drive Screening Measure (FTDS),[24–30] a free, web-based screening tool with established reliability and concurrent criterion validity, identifies at-risk older drivers using a proxy rater that includes family members, close friends, or caregivers who have been passengers in the past 3 months and who are able to rate the driver's skills. The FTDS measure takes approximately 20 minutes to complete and generates one of three driver-risk classifications, indicating that *critical safety concerns* exist that must be addressed immediately; or *some safety concerns* exist with early signs of needing intervention; or *no safety concerns* are present and the driver can continue driving. Based on the specific driver-risk classification, the FTDS provides risk mitigation resources, including a listing of all **driver rehabilitation specialist (DRS)**, as well as recommendations indicating the next logical step to pursue. For more information on the FTDS, see http://fitnesstodrive.phhp.ufl.edu/us/.

Evaluator Screening

Evaluator screening is the process through which a professional, skilled in using a specific screening tool, obtains and reviews data to determine the need for assessment for a specific individual. For example, an occupational therapist may decide to use the Mini-Mental State Examination (MMSE) to screen for general cognitive functioning or the Optec 2500, a visual analyzer machine used for visual screening, to detect aspects of visual functioning, such as contrast sensitive or peripheral vision.[31] The driving literature supports the notion that an individual who scores lower than 24 on the MMSE should not be considered for an on-road assessment and that individuals who show impairment in visual fields or contrasts should be referred to an eye doctor prior to conducting a **comprehensive driving evaluation.**[31] These tasks are well within the scope of the occupational therapy generalist, who may, when using these methods, help with detection of potential client factors that may impair **fitness to drive.**

Driving Assessment

Assessments may include clinical assessments, simulated driving assessments, or on-road assessments.

Clinical Assessment

Occupational therapist generalists or (certified) DRSs use clinical assessments to quantify and better understand client factors pertaining to visual (e.g., visual acuity or contrast sensitivity), cognitive (e.g., executive functions or working memory), motor (e.g., range of motion or upper extremity coordination), and other sensory (e.g., proprioception or stereognosis) functions. All of these functions, to a greater or lesser extent, are important for the task of driving. Although it is beyond the scope of this chapter to provide a comprehensive discussion on evidence-based clinical assessments that may be correlated to, or predictive of, driving performance in medically at-risk populations through the life span, the reader is referred to the text on Driving and Community Mobility that contains an excellent chapter on this topic.[31]

Driving Simulator Assessment

The driving simulator, a clinical tool, with excellent face, content and construct validity, as well as reliability for real-world driving performance, is increasingly used in occupational therapy practices.[32] This technology uses a computer-controlled environment that presents selected aspects of the driving experience considered representational of real-world driving.[4] Clients may "drive" a scenario in which their accelerator, brake, and/or steering responses are being assessed. Usually, the data obtained from the assessment allow for objective measurements of the users' responses to designated driving tasks.[33] This method is particularly appropriate for clients who want to return to driving, but who may still pose considerable risk on the road, and who are, therefore, not ready for on-road assessments. Caution needs to be executed in making generalizations to real-world driving, as simulated driving is a representation of reality and not reality itself.

On-Road Assessment

The on-road driving assessment, sometimes referred to as the behind-the-wheel assessment, is conducted in real-world circumstances (i.e., driving a real vehicle, on the road, while encountering traffic in a dynamic and complex environment). The on-road assessment may incorporate a fixed-route or a variable-route design. The first is usually standardized, and elements of this course, such as the number of straights, and left and right turns, or the setting (residential area, city and highway driving), are controlled for, while the latter allows for options to assess a client's specific needs, such as an older driver who only wants to drive in daylight and in the absence of peak traffic hours to a selected setting in the community. This assessment, conducted by a **certified DRS**, is the criterion standard for evaluating a driver's fitness-to-drive abilities.[34–36] The assessment can be performed in closed road or open on-road conditions. The first may entail no-traffic such as a closed road circuit, or limited traffic such as experienced in a deserted parking lot. These venues allow the driver to become comfortable with the assessment vehicle and the vehicles controls and to perform basic maneuvers in preparation for on-road driving. Each condition has its own innate characteristics pertaining to setting, traffic density, maneuvers (e.g., left turn, stop, yield, straight driving), or other road users that provide challenges for achieving a reliable and valid approach to determine a client's fitness to drive. Inability to control for these and other environmental conditions (i.e., time of the day, weather, roadway conditions, or other drivers' behaviors) may increase error during the evaluation.[37] As such, the final outcome of the on-road assessment (e.g., a pass/fail determination) may be prone to subjectivity. Table 31-1 illustrates selected on-road assessments and the percentage agreement between the driving maneuvers/behaviors and the driving environment. In a study by Odenheimer et al.,[35] the percentage representation of each on-road assessment against the components (driving maneuvers/behaviors and the driving environment) varies from 58% with minor representation of the environment to a 100% representation of the driving environment.[36]

Naturalistic Driving Assessment

To overcome the deficits associated with the on-road assessment, naturalistic driving studies have emerged.[40–42] These studies are using a methodology to monitor or evaluate driving behavior via instruments or sensors installed in a driver's own vehicle. Such instruments provide an objective driver identification (ID), as well as

Table 31-1. Selected Fixed Based Road Courses Matching Driving Maneuvers and Behaviors with Environmental Components[36]

		ENVIRONMENT COMPONENTS												
	DEMOGRAPHICS	PARKING LOT	RESIDENTIAL AREA	SUB-URBAN AREA		CITY		HIGHWAY						PERCENTAGE OF COMPONENT (BASED ON DRIVING MANEUVER/BEHAVIOR AND ENVIRONMENT) REPRESENTED IN EACH OF THE SOURCES
Driving maneuvers/behaviors	Course length and/or distance in time	Familiarize with test vehicle; basic maneuvers; angle/perpendicular parking; backing up	Low traffic/speed <35 km/hr (22 mph); R/L turn; adjust to stimuli; straight drive; school zones	Med. traffic with speed <70 km/hr (44 mph); changes, straight drive, traffic signals, pedestrian traffic	Four-lane road with med.-high traffic and speed >70 km/hr (44 mph)	Specific inter. include: yield, right of way, stop sign, four-way stop, two-way stop, traffic light protected/ unprotected; traffic circle	Busy shopping center, pedestrians, grocery carts, other obstacles	Vehicle maneuvers such as parking, adjusting speed, backing up, stopping	Follow structured/unstructured directions for way finding	Negotiating construction	Entering/exiting a ramp	Staying in the flow of traffic	Changing lanes	
Source														
Michon[38]	NA	x	x	x	x	x	X	x	x	x	x	x	x	100%, no environment
Odenheimer et al.[35]	16 km (10 miles) 45 minutes	X	X	–	–	x	X	x	–	–	x	x	–	58%, minor environment
Justiss et al.[34]	24 km (15 miles) 52 minutes	X	X	X	X	X	–	x	–	–	X	X	X	75%, major environment
Korner-Bitensky et al.[39]	– km 45–60 minutes	X	x	x	–	x	x	x	x	–	x	x	x	83%, no environment
UWO On-Road assessment[36]	36 km (23 miles) 60 minutes	X	X	X	X	X	X	X	X	X	X	X	X	100%, with environment

R, right; L, left; Med., medium; inter., intersection; – km, no documented kilometers; X, driving maneuvers/behaviors and environment; x, driving maneuvers/behaviors no mention of environment; "with/major/minor/no environment" denotes the source mentioned all/major/minor/no environmental descriptions; % of components (driving maneuver, behavior, or environment) represented in each source; NA, not applicable; "–", information is not available; UWO, University of Western Ontario.

driving data for each trip, and operate in a passive manner, requiring no interaction from the driver. Of course, collaboration with skilled team members is necessary to instrument the vehicle, activate the sensors, extract the data, and interpret the data. The main benefit of this method pertains to the objectivity inherent to the assessment process.

Comprehensive Driving Evaluation

This method entails a thorough assessment of an individual's personal, medical and driving history, driving knowledge, driving skills, and driving abilities by a DRS who may or may not be certified. The comprehensive driving evaluation generally includes clinical assessments of sensory/perceptual, cognitive, or psychomotor functional abilities; an on-road assessment; an outcome summary; and recommendations for an inclusive **community mobility** plan.[3,31] The outcome of the comprehensive driving evaluation results in a determination of whether the person is fit to continue to drive, requires rehabilitation prior to continued driving, or needs to consider driving cessation and alternative sources of community mobility. This information is usually related to the driver, who is accompanied by a caregiver, within the context of the multidisciplinary team. Clinicians need to be familiar with their state policies, as some states (e.g., California or Oregon) require mandatory reporting to the Department of Motor Vehicles, whereas others (e.g., Florida or Michigan) require voluntary reporting.

Interventions to Support Driving

Although evidence exists to support visual, cognitive, motor, and other sensory assessments in driver rehabilitation,[31] less is known about the efficacy and effectiveness of driving interventions across medically at-risk populations.[43,44] As such, occupational therapists are encouraged to design interventions based on best practices and sound clinical reasoning.[3] As is the case for other rehabilitation interventions, occupational therapists who are interested in driver rehabilitation make use of interventions pertaining to remediation, compensation, and adaptation.

- *Remediation of driving skills:* Drivers who show a lack of the necessary driving skills or a deterioration of driving skills may be referred to a DRS for behind-the-wheel training. In this case, the DRS may want to work on tactical skills (i.e., those maneuvers necessary for stopping, going, turning, yielding, overtaking, backing up, parking, or other general vehicle control maneuvers).
- *Compensation:* Imagine an older driver with depth perception challenges who stops too close to the lead vehicle at a traffic light. In this case, the occupational therapist may suggest improving the stopping maneuver, via teaching the client a compensatory method of "tire stopping." This means that the client needs to stop at a distance from the lead vehicle so that he or she can see the back tires of that vehicle. Such a compensatory method ensures safe vehicle positioning, while also overcoming the depth perception challenge.
- *Adaptation:* Much has been written on vehicle adaptations, and the reader is referred to the text on Driving and Community Mobility for an expansive overview of adaptive equipment used in the vehicle.[45] Such adaptations enable drivers to continue to manipulate the primary (i.e., steering, accelerator, and brake) and secondary (e.g., wind shield wipers, emergency brake, headlights) controls. Such adaptations are particularly helpful for clients with medical conditions impairing their function necessary to operate the vehicle and its controls. For example, orthopedic conditions, such as upper limb deficiencies and amputations; neurological conditions, such as hemiparesis, hemiplegia, or Parkinson disease; or spinal cord injuries, such as paraplegia, pose severe functional limitations on the client's abilities to safely operate a motor vehicle. Table 31-2 illustrates examples of diagnostic groups, the potential limitations in function, and the adaptive equipment necessary to overcome the functional deficit. Note that most all vehicle adaptations need to be implemented with great caution, requiring the clinical reasoning skills of a DRS and the technical installation skills of a vehicle modifier who meets the industry safety standards. Because this area of practice requires specialty knowledge, we are only introducing the occupational therapist to the concepts of vehicle adaptation and encourage referral of the client to a DRS for all vehicle modifications.

Community Mobility

Community mobility is defined as "moving around in the community and using public or private transportation, such as driving, walking, bicycling, or accessing and riding in buses, taxi cabs, or other transportation systems."[1] Access and availability of transportation is a critical facilitator for **community participation** and inclusion.[54–56] The National Council on Disabilities reported in 2015 that the lack of "accessible transportation represents one of the chief barriers to participating in economic and community life."[57] Research examining community participation defines this construct as "active involvement in activities that are intrinsically social and either occur outside of the home or are part of a nondomestic role."[2] Community participation can include integrated employment, health services, social events, education, and religious activities.[58] Recent research identified that perceived transportation and community mobility were predictors of participation restrictions in individuals with physical disabilities.[56] Older adults associated a sense of freedom and independence to participate in essential and desired activities with driving and

Table 31-2. Examples of Adaptive Equipment for the Vehicle Based on the Client's Diagnosis, Limitation in Function, and Function of the Adaptive Equipment to Overcome the Limitation

DIAGNOSIS	LIMITATION IN FUNCTION	ADAPTIVE EQUIPMENT	FUNCTION OF THE ADAPTIVE EQUIPMENT
Left upper limb deficiencies	Inability to use bilateral hands for turning maneuver	Spinner knob	Enables adequate steering wheel maneuvering with right hand
Right lower extremity amputation	Inability to manipulate gas and brake with the right lower extremity	Left foot accelerator and brake pedal	Enables client to manipulate accelerator and brake with the left lower extremity
Hemiparesis or paraplegia	Inability to use right lower extremity for accelerator and gas control	Push left-angled hand control or a push-rock hand control	Accelerator is controlled by pulling backward and brake is controlled by pushing forward on the hand control.
Parkinson	Rigidity in the neck and trunk with difficulty in turning to perform a backing up maneuver	Wide angled mirrors or back-up camera to	Provides a rear view scene without the need to turn the trunk
Quadriplegia	Inability to be securely positioned due to limited trunk control	Torso strap for injuries at or above T-12	Torso strap secures the position of the client during driving and especially during turning maneuvers.

community mobility.[59] As community participation is related to overall QoL,[60,61] self-determination,[60,61] and independence,[62] it is essential to identify needed supports and minimize barriers such as transportation to community participation. Transportation is integral to getting to many activities that are considered essential in the everyday lives of people, such as work, school, errands, medical appointments, and socialization with friends and family.

Types of transportation options for community mobility include personal, public, commercial, and supplemental transportation. Personal transportation involves moving around in the community using one's body and vehicle.[63] This includes traveling in a private automobile (i.e., being driven or driving), using other motorized or nonmotorized mobility devices (e.g., wheelchairs, scooters, biking), and walking. Driving oneself is often a preferred mode of transportation for many, although it may not be a viable option, because of newly acquired or progressing physical and/or sensory disabilities. Whereas driving is considered a privilege, community mobility using other forms of transportation is often considered a right. **Personal mobility devices** are used for community mobility when a person cannot walk or has limited walking ability. Public transportation options are available to everyone and involve moving more than one person at a time.[63] This includes both fixed-route transportation such as buses, trains, subways, and ferries, and **paratransit** services for individuals who have impairments that limit access to the fixed-route services. Supplemental transportation is an option for certain individuals, although availability can vary based on type of disability, age, and location. This type of transportation is often offered through volunteers from nonprofit or community-based services for individuals who are unable to use existing transportation services or need flexible travel options.[64] Finally, commercial transportation services are provided as for-profit entities most often paid by the individual. These can include taxis, transportation network companies (e.g., Uber/Lyft), shuttle/van services, and commercial carriers of airlines and trains. For shorter distances, commercial transportation options are now more affordable with the inception of transportation network companies and can provide greater flexibility than public transportation options. Although, for some of these options, there are accessibility issues for certain consumers when the transportation companies do not meet American with Disability Act (ADA) standards.

The physical environment often serves as a facilitator or barrier for community mobility.[56,65] The ADA, established in 1990, included guidelines for public and private transportation for individuals with disabilities.[6] According to the ADA, public transportation systems are required to provide information on services in accessible formats for individuals with disabilities, as well as needed equipment and facilities (i.e., lifts, ramps, securement devices, signage, communication devices) that are in good operating condition.[57,66] Additionally, public transportation systems must (1) provide adequate time to board and exit a vehicle, (2) allow service animals, (3) provide designated seating and signs on fixed-route

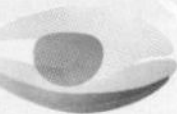

CASE STUDY: JULIO

To best illustrate the interplay of deficits in client factors, the assessment process, as well as the interventions necessary to address driving or community mobility, we introduce the reader to Julio via the following case study.[46,47]

Patient Information

Julio is a 15-year-old male, in the ninth grade, and living in the community with his parents and four siblings. He has never had a learner's permit or a driver's license. His parents are curious to know if he is ready to start driving. Currently, he is walking to school with his siblings, and although independent in way finding, he needs safety cues for scanning traffic before crossing the streets. Julio has a diagnosis of autism spectrum disorder (ASD) and shows characteristics consistent with attention-deficit hyperactivity disorder (ADHD). He has received occupational and speech therapies for the past 6 years and is taking medications to manage the symptoms of his medical conditions. His parents reported no medication side or adverse effects.

Clinical Assessments

Julio completed clinical assessments, summarized in Table 31-3, to assess his visual, cognitive, and motor functions. The results indicated that he had intact visual acuity, peripheral vision, depth perception, color discrimination, and phorias. He had intact central vision processing speed, divided visual attention, and selective visual attention skills. His overall ability to integrate visual information with a specific motor response was mildly impaired. Julio had poor skills for simple sequencing, was mildly impaired with complex sequencing and had limitations in attention shifting and planning, and showed difficulty with gross motor coordination and strength.

Driving Simulator

Julio became confident and comfortable with the driving simulator via return demonstration of understanding and using the vehicle controls. Then, he drove a basic scenario with minimal traffic in an interactive driving simulator with a 180° field of view that afforded an immersive experience, as displayed in Figure 31-2. The DRS sat in the passenger seat and recorded his driving errors throughout the drive. Julio drifted beyond the limits of his lane multiple times on straight roads and showed mild impairments with motor coordination when turning the steering wheel. Although ***lane maintenance*** errors are common among novice drivers, the frequency of Julio's errors and lack of his awareness to correct for such errors suggested significant impairments related to visual motor integration and attention shift, which are critical abilities for the task of driving. Julio did not perform ***visual scanning*** for traffic at cross streets or during lane changes. He approached all intersections with excessive ***speed,*** causing him to make wide turns to the right and encroaching into oncoming traffic on the left. He was unable to learn from his errors. Julio drove through two red lights and reported that he did not think it was necessary to stop, reflecting his poor understanding of traffic flow as a cause for collisions, and showing ***adjustment to stimuli errors***. He made two ***gap acceptance errors*** related to being overcautious, potentially owing to being a novice driver. Although he had severe difficulty with recognizing the ***divided attention*** symbols, his speed of response on the one divided attention task was good.

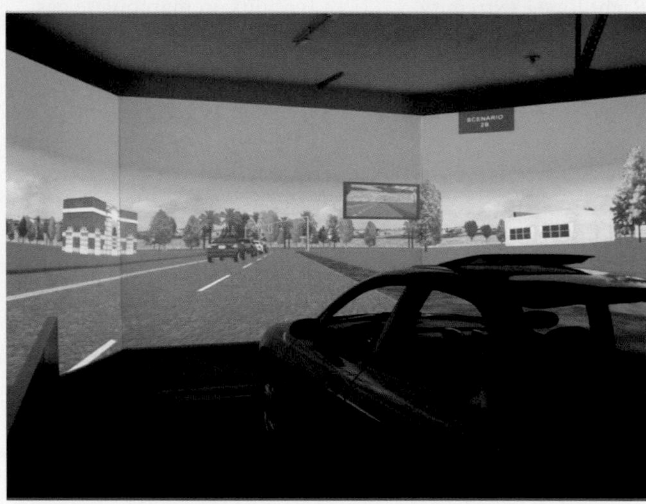

Figure 31-2. The University of Florida's STISIM M 500W interactive driving simulator with life-size images projected on the screen and simulator controls integrated with a 1997 Dodge Neon.

Occupational Therapy Recommendations

Based on the results of the clinical assessments and Julio's simulated driving performance, the Certified Driver Rehabilitation Specialist (CDRS) had to make a decision regarding Julio's readiness to drive. Relevant questions that the CDRS asked to decide if Julio was a candidate for driver training are:

- Was it appropriate to begin driver training?
- If driver training was appropriate, were there skill deficits that require occupational therapy intervention for remediation of underlying skills prior to driver's education?
- If no occupational therapy was required, would traditional driver's education be recommended?
- If driver training (with or without occupational therapy) was not recommended, is driving a possibility in the future?
- If driving was an appropriate future goal, what predriving skills needed to be further developed before learning how to drive?
- If driving was not a likely goal, what community mobility goals should be recommended?

Summary of the Short-Term Goals and Intervention

Based on Julio's personal and medical history, as well as the findings of the clinical assessments and simulated driving performance, the CDRS recommended that Julio was not ready to start driving. The short-term goal is to refer Julio to an occupational therapist to address a community mobility plan and the use of alternative transportation options.

In the next section, the reader will learn more about community mobility as a facilitator for participation.

Table 31-3. Julio's Clinical Tests, Description, and Scoring

CLINICAL ASSESSMENTS	DESCRIPTION AND SCORING	JULIO'S RESULTS
***/**Vision: Optec 2500 Visual analyzer (Stereo Optical, Inc.)[48]**		
Six tests on vision	Acuity, peripheral vision, phorias, depth perception, and color discrimination	Intact for all tests
***/**Visual Attention and Processing Speed[49]**		
UFOV risk index	Categories 1–5; 5 = very high risk for motor vehicle crashes	Intact: very low risk: category 1
Visual Motor Integration[50]		
Beery visual motor integration test[50]	30 possible points (30 = adequate age-based visual motor functioning)	Impaired at the 32nd percentile: 26/30 correct
Cognitive Assessments		
**Comprehensive trail making test[51]	Five trails tests measuring simple to complex sequencing	Overall impaired at the second percentile level
Symbol digit modalities test[52]	Measures motor, visual, speech, and executive functions and attention skills with the highest possible score of 110	Impaired: completed 39/110 symbols; 37/39 symbols were recorded with correct numbers
Motor Assessments		
Bruininks-Oseretsky test of motor proficiency (BOT-2): brief form[53]	Eight subtests of fine motor precision, motor integration, manual dexterity, bilateral coordination, balance, running speed and agility, upper limb coordination, and strength, with a total possible score of 88 points	Intact: percentile rank 38th Average score: 76 points
***Driving Simulator Assessment**		
****Simulator Operational Skills[a]**	Measured return demonstration of understanding and using vehicle controls on a VAS (0–10, where 10 = perfect demonstration)	Impaired: mild coordination deficits total VAS = 7.35/10
Driving Errors[34]		**Number of Driving Errors**
Lane maintenance errors: including wide turns or encroachments	The lateral lane position of the vehicle	30
Visual scanning errors	Visual scanning monitored at intersections and during lane changes	6
Lane position errors	The anterior and posterior position of the vehicle in relationship to the stop line	0
Speed error: over or under	Intact speed measured within 5 mph of the posted speed limit, or appropriate speed regulation required by maneuver (e.g., turn)	11 over speeding 0 under speeding
Signaling	Correct use of turn signal: timing, direction of signal, and appropriate use for the maneuver	0
Attention to stimuli	Correct response to changes in traffic light, posted signs, and traffic	2
Gap acceptance: overcautious or unsafe	Appropriate gap acceptance during the five unprotected left turns	2 over cautious 0 narrow
Divided attention (DA) responses	Five tasks of DA measured by the client honking when a diamond on the simulated scenario changed to a triangle	1
Speed of response to DA	Speed (norm < 11 seconds) at which the subject honks after the stimuli is presented	1.60 seconds
Number of collisions	Collisions involve either driving off road or hitting a vehicle or a pedestrian.	0
Number of errors at intersections	All errors across the 11 intersections	Impaired at the 50th percentile. Errors: 52

*No adolescent norms available; **percentile data based on the total driving errors of 18 neurotypical peers in the parent driving study.[46]
[a]The questionnaire measuring operational skills can be obtained from the primary author of this study.
UFOV, useful field of view; VAS, visual analog scale; WFLs, within functional limits.

systems, and (4) ensure training for operators to provide safe operation of vehicles and equipment, as well as assistance for individuals with disabilities. Specific architectural requirements exist (e.g., lifts and ramps; stop announcements; illumination of stepwells and doorways; slip-resistant surfaces for door and steps) for fixed-route transportation systems to improve accessibility.[66] Architectural requirements are also required for transit facilities (e.g., accessible paths of travel, boarding ramps, bus shelters). Transit agencies must provide paratransit services, an origin to destination service, where fixed-route services exist for individuals with disabilities who qualify. Private transportation entities (e.g., airport/hotel shuttles, private buses, taxis) that provide services to the public are required by the ADA to meet accessibility requirements. If the vehicles are not accessible to an individual with a disability, the transportation entity must have an equivalent service that provides an accessible vehicle to travel to the same place at the same time and at the same cost. Taxis are not required to purchase accessible automobiles, although they cannot discriminate against individuals with disabilities by refusing service, use of assistant animals, stowing of mobility devices, or charging higher fares.

The ADA provides specific guidelines to promote environmental access to transportation. Environmental factors are some of the most significant barriers to community mobility for individuals with a variety of physical disabilities.[56,65] A fit between the unique characteristics of the person and the environment is essential for successful community mobility. Although there are many environmental barriers to community mobility that must be considered during the occupational therapy assessment and intervention process, in 2010, the Beverly Foundation identified five A's that were common barriers for the aging population and those with disabilities.[67] These included availability, accessibility, affordability, acceptability, and adaptability (see Table 31-4). All of these are important considerations when evaluating the fit between the environment and the person.

Assessment of Community Mobility

Although assessment and intervention to promote community mobility is not a new area of practice for occupational therapists working with individuals with physical disabilities, it continues to be an emerging area where roles and needs have expanded significantly in recent years. This is likely due to the increased awareness of transportation as a primary barrier to community participation and engagement.[54,56] Occupational therapy assessments and interventions for community mobility are diverse and varied based on the types of transportation, service delivery model, and the unique needs of the individual with physical disabilities, although all have common elements (Fig. 31-3).

As in any occupational therapy evaluation, it is essential to obtain an occupational profile of the client to determine community mobility needs specific to the individual.[68] A person-centered approach in which the client is maximally engaged in the assessment and goal development process is essential. This includes identifying the person's important and meaningful activities and providing detailed information about their typical routines in order to understand the necessary mobility requirements and intervention for participation. Typical modes of transporting oneself or being transported by another person may change after an acquired physical disability or a change in a health-related condition making it necessary to reassess the way in which one travels in the community. This could include a change in the type of transportation mode (e.g., using paratransit instead of the taking the bus to get to a medical appointment) or the way in which the person travels in a previously used transportation mode (e.g., using hand devices to operate a car after sustaining an injury resulting in paraplegia).

Once community mobility needs are identified in the occupational profile, it is important to analyze the client and activity demands of the preferred or chosen types of travel modes. This will help determine individualize interventions based on the demands of the type(s) of travel and common environmental factors associated with specific types of travel. An example is an individual using a manual wheelchair due to a recent acquired physical injury who wants to use public transportation to visit his or her family or go shopping for essential items. After leaving home, he or she will need to be able to mobilize the wheelchair safely through the neighborhood to the bus stop and get on and off the bus. Environmental factors are an essential consideration when assessing the activity demands and can serve as either a facilitator or

Table 31-4. Environmental Factors Impacting Transportation Usability[67]

ENVIRONMENTAL FACTOR	DESCRIPTION
Availability	Existence of transportation when needed
Accessibility	Transportation is reached and used in light of riders' abilities/disabilities.
Affordability	The costs are within the users means or reimbursable.
Acceptability	Meets standards of cleanliness, safety, courteous/helpful operators
Adaptability	Modification can be made for disabilities and special needs.

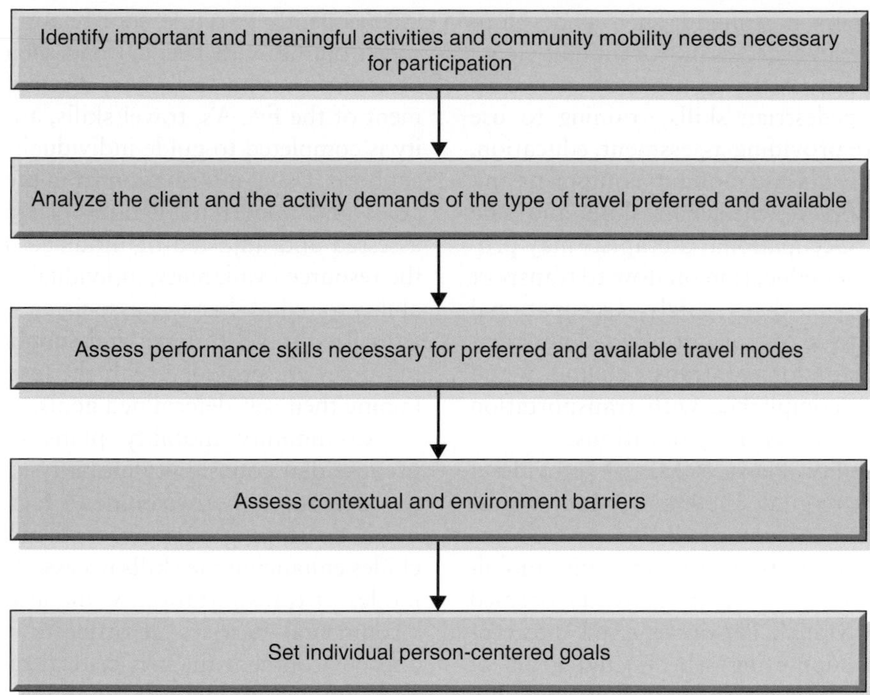

Figure 31-3. Assessing community mobility.

a barrier. For example, the presence of curb cuts on the pavements and a life with a wheelchair securement system on the bus could determine whether the use of a bus from the home is a safe and feasible option.

The evaluation process needs to consider both person factors (i.e., sensory issues, decreased balance, and motor deficits) and environmental barriers and facilitators to community mobility.[69,70] This allows the therapist and person to develop community mobility goals that match the strengths and needs of the person to environments that promote successful community mobility. The type of transportation often determines the necessary skills needed by the person. Although this can vary significantly, person factors[68] such as cognitive (i.e., attention, perception, memory, executive functions), sensory (i.e., vision, hearing, balance), and motor functions (i.e., endurance, control of voluntary movement, gait patterns) are often necessary skills for successful community mobility outcomes. Tools available that assess specific aspects of community mobility includes the Functioning Everyday with a Wheelchair (FEW),[71] a criterion-referenced tool that assesses how wheelchair features help the client complete ADLs in situations such as outdoor mobility and use of personal/public transportation. The Life-Space Assessment documents where and how often clients travel and any assistance needed.[72] The Community Mobility Assessment evaluates physical and cognitive abilities of individuals with traumatic brain injuries to determined safe community mobility.[73] Finally, the Assessment of Readiness for Mobility Transition[74] provides a method to assess the emotional and attitudinal perceptions of aging adults who acquire a health condition that requires a transition from driving to other methods of transportation for community mobility. Many of these tools assess both person and environmental factors.

Environmental factors consist of both physical and social aspects of the environment that impact on community mobility.[58] The five A's (i.e., availability, acceptability, accessibility, adaptability, and affordability, see Table 31-4) identify a set of environmental factors that impact transportation usability in the senior and general disability population. This may provide helpful guidelines to assess common environmental factors that can serve as barriers or facilitators to transportation for individuals with disabilities. Observations of the person in the community environments and using preferred transportation is an important component of the assessment and intervention process. For occupational therapy provided in inpatient settings, including community mobility screenings in the assessment process can help prepare a person for discharge and transition back into the home and community environments. Additionally, occupational therapists can complete evaluations for public and private community-based organizations to identify barriers to safe and accessible transportation in these environments.

Interventions to Support Community Mobility

Occupational therapist's role in community mobility interventions varies, based on the unique needs of his or her clients and the service delivery model.[75–77]

Interventions can be person-centered, such as developing specific foundation skills necessary for mobility (e.g., balance, motor planning, sensory awareness); providing travel training (e.g., pedestrian skills, training to use public transportation); providing assessment, education, and training to acquire and use mobility equipment and devices; and instruction in wheelchair skills and safe wheelchair transport. Occupational therapists may provide parent and caregiver education on how to transport family members and guardians safely. Occupational therapists can also provide organization-based interventions such as assessments for paratransit eligibility and consultation for ADA compliance with transportation providers and community-based organizations.

Community Mobility Plans (CMPs)[78] provide a conceptual framework to guide the intervention process (Fig. 31-4). The intended outcome of CMPs is to facilitate more independent transportation for community mobility necessary for participation in life activities deemed important by the individual. Person-centered interventions are integral to supporting self-directed goals of the individual that result in better community mobility and outcomes.[79,80] Community mobility plans outline a person-centered intervention in which the individual first identifies their community mobility goal(s) (e.g., traveling independently to work, coordinating transportation to a social outing with friends) and their preferred methods of transportation (e.g., bus, driving). A targeted assessment of the five A's, travel skills, and resource availability is completed to guide individualized intervention and supports. Using information from the assessment process, goals and preferred methods of transportation are reassessed and adjusted or modified as needed, based on the resource availability, individual's travel skills, and the ability to reduce barriers associated with the five A's. Individualized travel training and supports to obtain needed resources are provided with the targeted outcome of attaining their self-determined goals.

Community mobility plans are founded on the premise that community mobility is attained when both the person and environment factors are considered when developing supports and interventions. This includes enhancing the skills necessary to use the preferred modes of transportation, while also addressing the environmental barriers in order to improve the person and environment fit. It is critical to support the ability and skill development of the individual to use available transportation options, but other environmental barriers must also be addressed as part of the assessment and intervention process.

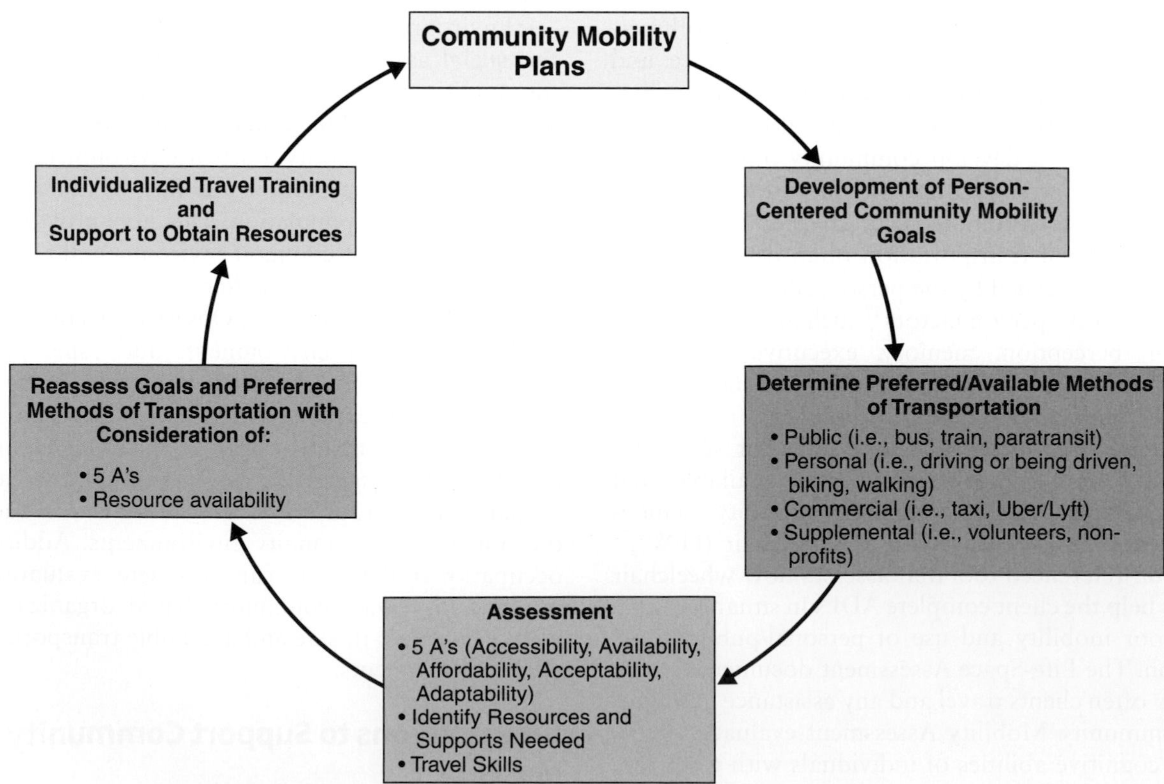

Figure 31-4. Community mobility plans.

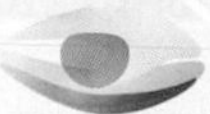

CASE STUDY: TRISTEN

Patient Information

Tristen is a 19-year-old female who is graduating from high school. She was diagnosed with cerebral palsy at birth and uses an electric wheelchair for functional mobility. She is able to independently mobilize in her house and around the neighborhood using the wheelchair. She has functional use of both his hands for all activities of daily living and most fine motor tasks. Tristen excels academically in school and enjoys reading and watching movies. She has strong verbal communication skills. Tristen is planning on starting courses at the local community college and will be continuing her part-time job at a bookstore located in a nearby mall upon graduation. She identified transportation as a main concern upon her graduation in her most recent Individual Education Planning meeting. She currently uses the school bus to get to classes each morning and is dependent on her parents to drive her to work on the weekend. Her work hours will expand after graduation and include weekdays. Tristen wants to be able to travel independently to work and school when needed, as both of her parents work during the day. She identified that she would like to learn to use the bus because there is a bus stop near her house that drops her off at the mall and a few blocks from the community college. She has taken a public transportation bus with a family member in the past, but has never done this on her own.

Occupational Therapy Recommendations

The school occupational therapist who provides transitional services completed an evaluation to assess Tristen's community mobility. She was able to navigate safely to cross streets and maneuver on pavements that had curb cuts. She was not familiar with how to purchase bus passes and plan a trip using the bus (i.e., find schedules, locate routes specific to her travel destinations). Her local transit system has accessible buses that include a lift and securement system for wheelchairs. The bus operators assist patrons in wheelchairs to use a lift to get on and off the bus and ensure proper securement. There were some streets that did not have proper curb cuts, resulting in a need for Tristen to mobilize further to another street to get to her destination. During bad weather days (e.g., rain or snow), Tristen was not able to maneuver her wheel chair safely to get to bus stops.

Summary of Short-Term Goals, Intervention, and Progress

Based on the evaluation of Tristen's community mobility and her self-identified priorities, additional occupation therapy services were added to her IEP to address the following community mobility goals: (1) Tristen will be able to plan and implement a fixed-route trip to the mall using a public transit bus when provided with supervision and environmental adaptations successfully in four out of five trips. (2) Tristen will obtain conditional paratransit eligibility and schedule trips when needed to get to work or school with minimal assistance 90% of the time.

After exploring available transportation options and resources, Tristen and the occupational therapist identified bus transportation as the preferred method of travel to get to work and school. She also wanted to obtain conditional paratransit eligibility for days when she was not able to use the bus because of environmental barriers related to the weather (e.g., inability to mobilize in wheelchair safety when the pavement was wet or had snow on it). Additionally, she needed paratransit services to travel to other destinations that were not easily accessible with public transportation (e.g., medical appointments). Tristen worked with the occupational therapist and transition team at the school to identify the necessary resources and contacts to obtain eligibility for paratransit. This involved completing intake paperwork, obtaining medical documentation, and participating in an in-person assessment with staff at the transit agency. She participated in travel training with the occupational therapist once a week. The occupational therapist used an established travel training curriculum[81] that focused on use of public transportation and worked on foundational skills necessary to travel in the community (e.g., safe wheelchair navigation/securement, safety awareness). This involved direct instruction in the following six core areas, along with individual travel training: (1) Interacting with Individuals in the Community; (2) Signs and Traffic Symbols; (3) Pedestrian Safety and Awareness of Surroundings; (4) Preparing for Your Trip; (5) Travel Practice; and (6) Expect the Unexpected: Dealing with the "What Ifs."

Tristen made significant progress toward her goal after consistent intervention over a 2- to 3-month period of time. She was able to plan trips (e.g., identify the appropriate buses and the schedules; plan out enough time to get to the bus stop) to both the local community college and her part-time job at the mall using public transportation. She worked with the occupational therapist to identify routes to the bus stops that had curb cuts for accessibility purposes. Tristen was able to physically get on and off the bus but continued to work on recognizing when her stop was nearing so she could pull the cord that indicated when she needed to get off. She was demonstrating awareness of safety 90% of the time but continued to need supervision when there were unexpected changes (e.g., construction on a typical pedestrian route, unfamiliar types of interactions with people in the community). Tristen obtained eligibility for paratransit services. She worked with the therapist on how to schedule trips on paratransit and was able to implement a trip without supervision. By the end of the school year, Tristen was using fixed-route bus transportation to get to work at the mall and was able to independently get to the local community college. She started to explore other routes on the bus and other modes of transportation (e.g., Uber and Lyft) to get to the houses of family members and friends.

References

1. Stav WB, McGuire MJ. Introduction to community mobility and driving. In: McGuire MJ, Schold-Davis E, eds. *Driving and Community Mobility: Occupational Therapy Strategies Across the Lifespan*. Bethesda, MD: AOTA Press; 2012:1–18.
2. Chang FH, Coster WJ, Helfrich CA. Community participation measures for people with disabilities: a systematic review of content from an international classification of functioning, disability and health perspective. *Arch Phys Med Rehabil*. 2013;94(4):771–781. doi:10.1016/j.apmr.2012.10.031.
3. Classen S, Lanford DN. Clinical reasoning process in the comprehensive driving evaluation. In: McGuire MJ, Schold-Davis E, eds. *Driving and Community Mobility: Occupational Therapy Strategies Across the Lifespan*. Bethesda, MD: AOTA Press; 2012:321–344.
4. Transportation Research Board. A taxonomy and terms for stakeholders in senior mobility. *Transp Res Circ*. 2016;E-C211:1–32.
5. Schold-Davis E, Dickerson A. The gaps and pathway project: meeting the driving and community mobility needs of OT clients. *OT Practice*. 2012;17(21):9–13, 19.
6. Americans With Disabilities Act of 1990. In Pub. L. No. 101-336. Vol. 104 Stat. 3281990. http://library.clerk.house.gov/reference-files/PPL_101_336_AmericansWithDisabilities.pdf. Accessed July 19, 2018.
7. Dickerson AE, Meuel DB, Ridenour CD, Cooper K. Assessment tools predicting fitness to drive in older adults: a systematic review. *Am J Occup Ther*. 2014;68(6):670–680. doi:10.5014/ajot.2014.011833.
8. Musselwhite C. The importance of driving for older people and how the pain of driving cessation can be reduced. *J Dementia Ment Health*. 2011;15(3):22–26. http://eprints.uwe.ac.uk/14060. Accessed July 19, 2018.
9. Dickerson AE, Molnar L, Bedard M, Eby DW, Classen S, Polgar J. Transportation and aging: an updated research agenda for advancing safe mobility. *J Appl Gerontol*. 2017:1–19. doi:10.1177/0733464817739154.
10. Chihuri S, Mielenz TJ, DiMaggio CJ, et al. Driving cessation and health outcomes in older adults. *J Am Geriatr Soc*. 2016;64(2):332–341. doi:10.1111/jgs.13931.
11. Edwards JD, Lunsman M, Perkins M, Rebok GW, Roth DL. Driving cessation and health trajectories in older adults. *J Gerontol A Biol Sci Med Sci*. 2009;64A(12):1290–1295. doi:10.1093/gerona/glp114.
12. Marottoli RA, Mendes de Leon CF, Glass TA, et al. Driving cessation and increased depressive symptoms: prospective evidence from the New Haven EPESE. Established Populations for Epidemiologic Studies of the Elderly. *J Am Geriatr Soc*. 1997;45(2):202–206. doi:10.1111/j.1532-5415.1997.tb04508.x.
13. Marottoli RA, de Leon CFM, Glass TA, Williams CS, Cooney LM Jr, Berkman LF. Consequences of driving cessation: decreased out-of-home activity levels. *J Gerontol B Psychol Sci Soc Sci*. 2000;55(6):S334–S340. doi:10.1093/geronb/55.6.S334.
14. Freeman EE, Gange SJ, Munoz B, West SK. Driving status and risk of entry into long-term care in older adults. *Am J Public Health*. 2006;96(7):1254–1259. doi:10.2105/AJPH.2005.069146.
15. Bhuiyan J. The complete timeline to self-driving cars: self-driving cars are coming. The question is when and how. 2016. https://www.recode.net/2016/5/16/11635628/self-driving-autonomous-cars-timeline. Accessed October 15, 2017.
16. National Highway Traffic Safety Administration. Traffic safety facts: data 2015. 2015. https://crashstats.nhtsa.dot.gov/Api/Public/ViewPublication/812372. Accessed October 15, 2017.
17. Decina LE, Staplin L, Lococo K. *Literature Review: Self Evaluation Guides/Materials for Older Drivers*. Kulpsville, PA: The Scientex Corporation; October 10, 1997. Penn DOT Project 96-13.
18. Eby DW, Molnar LJ, Kartje PS. SAFER driving: self-screening based on health concerns. *The Gerontologist, Special Issue*. 2008;47:86.
19. Wild K, Cotrell V. Identifying driving impairment in Alzheimer disease: a comparison of self and observer reports versus driving evaluation. *Alzheimer Dis Assoc Disord*. 2003;17(1):27–34. doi:10.1097/00002093-200301000-00004.
20. Classen S, Medhizadah S, Alvarez L. The fitness-to-drive screening measure©: patterns and trends for Canadian users. *Open J Occup Ther*. 2016;4(4):1–17. doi:10.15453/2168-6408.1227.
21. Bédard M, Riendeau J, Weaver B, Clarkson A. Roadwise review has limited congruence with actual driving performance of aging drivers. *Accid Anal Prev*. 2011;43(6):2209–2214. doi:10.1016/j.aap.2011.05.025.
22. Kay L, Bundy A, Clemson L. Validity, reliability and predictive accuracy of the Driving Awareness Questionnaire. *Disabil Rehabil*. 2009;31(13):1074–1082. doi:10.1080/09638280802509553.
23. Blanchard RA, Myers AM, Porter MM. Correspondence between self-reported and objective measures of driving exposure and patterns in older drivers. *Accid Anal Prev*. 2010;42:523–529. doi:10.1016/j.aap.2009.09.018.
24. Classen S, Velozo CA, Winter SM, Bédard M, Wang Y. Psychometrics of the fitness-to-drive screening measure. *OTJR (Thorofare NJ)*. 2015;35(1):42–52. doi:10.1177/1539449214561761.
25. Classen S, Wang Y, Winter SM, Velozo CA, Lanford DN, Bedard M. Concurrent criterion validity of the safe driving behavior measure: a predictor of on-road driving outcomes. *Am J Occup Ther*. 2013;67(1):108–116. doi:10.5014/ajot.2013.005116.
26. Classen S, Wen PS, Velozo C, et al. Psychometrics of the self-report safe driving behavior measure for older adults. *Am J Occup Ther*. 2012;66(2):233–241. doi: 10.5014/ajot.2012.001834.
27. Classen S, Winter SM, Velozo CA, et al. Item development and validity testing for a safe driving behavior measure. *Am J Occup Ther*. 2010;64(2):296–305. doi:10.5014/ajot.64.2.296.
28. Classen S, Winter SM, Velozo CA, Hannold EM. Stakeholder recommendations to refine the fitness-to-drive screening measure. *Open J Occup Ther*. 2013;1(4):1–14. doi:10.15453/2168-6408.1054.

29. Classen S, Yarney A, Monahan M, Platek K, Lutz A. Rater reliability to assess driving errors in a driving simulator. *Adv Transport Stud.* 2015;Section B(36):99–108. doi:10.4399/97888548856608.
30. Winter SM, Classen S, Bédard M, et al. Focus group findings for the self-report safe driving behavior measure. *Can J Occup Ther.* 2011;78(2):72–79. doi:10.2182/cjot.2011.78.2.2.
31. Classen S, Dickerson AE, Justiss MD. Occupational therapy driving evaluation: using evidence-based screening and assessment tools. In: McGuire MJ, Schold-Davis E, eds. *Driving and Community Mobility: Occupational Therapy Across the Lifespan.* Bethesda, MD: AOTA Press; 2012:221–277.
32. Classen S, Akinwuntan AE. Validity and reliability issues in driving simulation In: Classen S, ed. *Driving Simulation for Assessment, Intervention, and Training: A Guide for Occupational Therapy and Healthcare Professionals.* Bethesda, MD: AOTA Press; 2017:95–103.
33. Evans D, Akinwuntan A. Driving simulation as a clinical intervention tool. In: Classen S, ed. *Driving Simulation for Assessment, Intervention, and Training: A Guide for Occupational Therapy and Healthcare Professionals.* Bethesda, MD: AOTA Press; 2017:133–142.
34. Justiss MD, Mann WC, Stav WB, Velozo CA. Development of a behind-the-wheel driving performance assessment for older adults. The older driver, part 2. *Top Geriatr Rehabil.* 2006;22(2):121–128. doi:10.1097/00013614-200604000-00004.
35. Odenheimer GL, Beaudet M, Jette AM, Albert MS, Grande L, Minaker KL. Performance-based driving evaluation of the elderly driver: safety, reliability, and validity. *J Gerontol.* 1994;49(4):M153–M159. doi:10.1093/geronj/49.4.M153.
36. Classen S, Krasniuk S, Alvarez L, Monahan M, Morrow S, Danter T. Development and validity of Western University's on-road assessment. *OTJR (Thorofare NJ).* 2017;37(1):14–29. doi:10.1177/1539449216672859.
37. Hunt LA, Murphy CF, Carr DB, Duchek JM, Buckles V, Morris JC. Environmental cueing may effect performance on a road test for drivers with dementia of the Alzheimer type. *Alzheimer Dis Assoc Disord.* 1997;11(suppl 1):13–16.
38. Michon JA. A critical view of driver behavior models: what do we know, what should we do? In Evans EL, Schwing R, eds. *Human Behavior and Traffic Safety.* New York, NY: Plenum; 1985:485–520.
39. Korner-Bitensky N, Gélinas I, Man-Son-Hing M, Marshall S. Recommendations of the Canadian Consensus Conference on driving evaluation in older drivers. In Mann W, ed. *Community Mobility: Driving and Transportation Alternatives for Older Persons.* Binghamton, NY: Haworth Press; 2005:123–144.
40. Myers AM, Trang A, Crizzle AM. Naturalistic study of winter driving practices by older men and women: examination of weather, road conditions, trip purposes and comfort. *Can J Aging.* 2011;30(4):1–16. doi:10.1017/S0714980811000481.
41. Ott BR, Papandonatos GD, Davis JD, Barco PP. Naturalistic validation of an on-road driving test of older drivers. *Hum Factors.* 2012;54(4):663–674. doi:10.1177/0018720811435235.
42. Neale VL, Klauer SG, Knipling RR, Dingus TA, Hollbrook GT, Peterson A. *The 100 Car Naturalistic Driving Study: Phase I—Experimental Design.* Washington, DC: National Highway Traffic Safety Administration; December 2002. DOT HS 808 536. https://www.nhtsa.gov/sites/nhtsa.dot.gov/files/100carphase1report.pdf. Accessed July 19, 2018.
43. Classen S, Monahan M, Auten B, Yarney AK. Evidence-based review of rehabilitation interventions for medically at-risk older drivers. *Am J Occup Ther.* 2014;68(4):107–114. doi:10.5014/ajot.2014.010975.
44. Alvarez L, Classen S, Medhizadah S, Knott M, He W. Pilot efficacy of a DriveFocus™ intervention on the driving performance of young drivers. *Front Public Health.* 2018;6(125):1–9. doi:10.3389/fpubh.2018.00125.
45. Hegberg A. Use of adaptive equipment to compensate for impairments in motor performance skills and client factors. In: McGuire MJ, Schold-Davis E, eds. *Driving and Community Mobility: Occupational Therapy Strategies Across the Lifespan.* Bethesda, MD: AOTA Press; 2012:279–319.
46. Classen S, Monahan M, Brown KE, Hernandez S. Driving indicators in teens with attention deficit hyperactivity and/or autism spectrum disorder. *Can J Occup Ther.* 2013;80(5):274–283. doi:10.1177/0008417413501072.
47. Monahan M, Classen S, Helsel P. Case report: pre-driving skills of a teen with attention deficit hyperactivity and autism spectrum disorder. *AOTA Special Interest Section.* 2012;34(3):1–4.
48. Stereo Optical Company Inc. Reference and instruction manual: OPTEC® vision tester; unknown date. http://www.stereooptical.com. Accessed July 19, 2018.
49. Ball K, Owsley C, Sloane ME, Roenker DL, Bruni JR. Visual attention problems as a predictor of vehicle crashes in older drivers. *Invest Ophthalmol Vis Sci.* 1993;34(11):3110–3123.
50. Beery KE, Beery NA. *The Beery-Buktenica Developmental Test of Visual-Motor Integration: Administration, Scoring, and Teaching Manual.* 6th ed. Minneapolis, MN: Pearson; 2010.
51. Reynolds CR. *Comprehensive Trail Making Test.* Austin, TX: Pro-Ed; 2002. doi:10.1177/0734282905282415.
52. Smith A. *Symbol Digits Modalities Test: Manual.* Los Angeles, CA: Western Psychological Services; 1982.
53. Bruininks R, Bruininks B. *Bruininks-Oseretsky Test of Motor Proficiency.* 2nd ed. Minneapolis, MN: NCS Pearson; 2005.
54. Chang FH, Liu CH, Hung HP. An in-depth understanding of the impact of the environment on participation among people with spinal cord injury. *Disabil Rehabil.* 2017:2192–2199. doi:10.1080/09638288.2017.1327991.
55. Jonasdottir SK, Polgar JM. Services, systems, and policies affecting mobility device users' community mobility: a scoping review: services, systemes et politiques influencant la mobilite dans la communaute des utilisateurs d'aides a la mobilite: examen de la portee. *Can J Occup Ther.* 2018;85(2):106–116. doi:10.1177/0008417417733273.
56. Vaughan MW, Felson DT, LaValley MP, et al. Perceived community environmental factors and risk of five-year

participation restriction among older adults with or at risk of knee osteoarthritis. *Arthritis Care Res (Hoboken)*. 2017;69(7):952–958. doi:10.1002/acr.23085.

57. National Council on Disability. Transportation update: where we've gone and what we've learned. 2015. https://ncd.gov/rawmedia_repository/862358ac_bfec_4afc_8cac_9a02122e231d.pdf. Accessed May 5, 2018.
58. World Health Organization. *International Classification of Functioning, Disability, and Health*. Geneva, Switzerland: World Health Organization; 2001.
59. Gardezi F, Wilson K, Man-Son-Hing M, et al. Qualitative research on older drivers. *Clin Gerontol*. 2006;30:5–22. doi: 10.1300/J018v30n01_02.
60. Bramston P, Bruggerman K, Pretty G. Community perspectives and subjective quality of life. *Int J Disab Develop Educ*. 2002;49(4):385–397. doi:10.1080/1034912022000028358.
61. Lachapelle Y, Wehmeyer ML, Haelewyck MC, et al. The relationship between quality of life and self-determination: an international study. *J Intellect Disabil Res*. 2005;49(Pt 10):740–744. doi:10.1111/j.1365-2788.2005.00743.x.
62. Carmien S, Dawe M, Fischer G, Gorman A, Kintsch A, Sullivan JJ. Socio-technical environments supporting people with cognitive disabilities using public transportation. *ACM Trans Comput Hum Interact*. 2005;12(2):233–262. doi:10.1145/1067860.1067865.
63. Womack J, Silverstein N. The big picture: comprehensive community mobility options. In: McGuire M, Davis ES, eds. *Driving and Community Mobility: Occupational Therapy Strategies Across the Lifespan*. Bethesda, MD: AOTA Press; 2012:19–47.
64. American Occupational Therapy Association. Driving and community mobility. *Am J Occup Ther*. 2010;64(suppl):S112–S124. doi:10.5014/ajot.2010.64S112.
65. Chudyk AM, McKay HA, Winters M, Sims-Gould J, Ashe MC. Neighborhood walkability, physical activity, and walking for transportation: a cross-sectional study of older adults living on low income. *BMC Geriatr*. 2017;17(1):82. doi:10.1186/s12877-017-0469-5.
66. The American with Disabilities Act Network. The ADA and accessible ground transportation; 2017. http://adainfo.us/ADAtransportation. Accessed May 3, 2018.
67. The Beverly Foundation. The 5 A's of senior friendly transportation. *Fact Sheet Series*. 2007;70(5). https://www.fhwa.dot.gov/publications/publicroads/07mar/03.cfm. Accessed September 18, 2019.
68. American Occupational Therapy Association. Occupational therapy practice framework: domain and process (3rd ed.). *Am J Occup Ther*. 2014;68(suppl 1):S1–S48. doi:10.5014/ajot.2014.682006.
69. Law M, Cooper B, Strong S, Stewart D, Rigby P, Letts L. The person environment occupation model: a transactive approach to occupational performance. *Can J Occup Ther*. 1996;63:9–23. doi:10.1177/000841749606300103.
70. Crist P, Royeen C, Schkade J. *Infusing Occupation into Practice*. 2nd ed. Bethesda, MD: American Occupational Therapy Association; 2000.
71. Mills T, Holm MB, Trefler E, Schmeler M, Fitzgerald S, Boninger M. Development and consumer validation of the Functional Evaluation in a Wheelchair (FEW) instrument. *Disabil Rehabil*. 2002;24(1–3):38–46. doi:10.1080/09638280110066334.
72. Peel C, Sawyer Baker P, Roth DL, Brown CJ, Brodner EV, Allman RM. Assessing mobility in older adults: the UAB Study of Aging Life-Space Assessment. *Phys Ther*. 2005;85(10):1008–1119. doi:10.1093/ptj/85.10.1008.
73. Brewer K, Geisler T, Moody K, Wright T. A community mobility assessment for adolescents with an acquired brain injury. *Physiother Can*. 1998;50:118–122.
74. Meuser TM, Berg-Weger M, Chibnall JT, Harmon AC, Stowe JD. Assessment of Readiness for Mobility Transition (ARMT): a tool for mobility transition counseling with older adults. *J Appl Gerontol*. 2013;32(4):484–507. doi:10.1177/0733464811425914.
75. Carlstedt E, Iwarsson S, Stahl A, Pessah-Rasmussen H, Mansson Lexell E. BUS TRIPS: a self-management program for people with cognitive impairments after stroke. *Int J Environ Res Public Health*. 2017;14(11). doi:10.3390/ijerph14111353.
76. Lindsay S, Lamptey DL. Pedestrian navigation and public transit training interventions for youth with disabilities: a systematic review. *Disabil Rehabil*. 2018:1–15. doi:10.1080/09638288.2018.1471165.
77. Price R, Marsh A, Fisher M. Teaching young adults with intellectual and developmental disabilities community-based navigation skills to take public transportation. *Behav Anal Pract*. 2018;11:46–50. doi:10.1007/s40617-017-0202-z.
78. Pfeiffer B. Transportation and community participation for individuals with developmental disabilities. Paper presented at: American Occupational Therapy Annual Conference; 2018.
79. Ryan RM, Deci EL. Self-determination theory and the facilitation of intrinsic motivation, social development, and well-being. *Am Psychol*. 2000;55(1):68–78. doi:10.1037/0003-066X.55.1.68.
80. Vallerand RJ, Salvy SJ, Mageau GA, et al. On the role of passion in performance. *J Pers*. 2007;75(3):505–533. doi:10.1111/j.1467-6494.2007.00447.x.
81. Kennedy Center I. *Travel Training Guide*. Trumbull, CT: Kennedy Center, Inc; 2012.

Chapter 32

The Biomechanical Frame of Reference

Kimatha Oxford Grice

LEARNING OBJECTIVES

This chapter will allow the reader to:

1. Describe the theoretical bases of the Biomechanical Frame of Reference.
2. Apply the Biomechanical Frame of Reference for the evaluation of persons who have limitations in occupational performance because of physical impairments.
3. Apply the principles of the Biomechanical Frame of Reference for planning and implementing treatment for persons with physical impairments.
4. Explain the relationship of the Biomechanical Frame of Reference to the occupational therapy practice framework and occupation-based intervention.
5. Describe occupational therapy methods and modalities that are employed in treating persons from a Biomechanical Frame of Reference.

CHAPTER OUTLINE

TERMINOLOGY

Edema: the swelling of soft tissues as a result of excess fluid accumulation.

Endurance: the ability of muscles to exert their effort or force for extended periods of time.

Functional range of motion: the amount of range of motion that is required, at joints of the arm for instance, to enable an individual to perform requisite functional tasks.

Impairment: a state of reduced quality or function in a physical characteristic of the body, such as strength, motion, and endurance; can be partial or complete.

Kinematics: the science of describing the positions and motions of the body in space.

Kinetics: the study of forces that affect motion and the results they have on a body.

Physical agent modalities (PAMs): procedures and interventions that are applied to modify specific client factors that may be limiting occupational performance; using various forms of energy to modulate pain, modify tissue healing, increase tissue extensibility, modify skin and scar tissue, decrease edema and inflammation, or decreased function secondary to musculoskeletal conditions; are used as adjunctive or preparatory methods to engagement in occupation.

Range of motion (ROM): the pathway of movement possible at a joint; typically measured in degrees of motion.

Strength: the ability of a muscle or group of muscles to create a contractile force against a resistance in a single contraction or effort.

Therapeutic activities: tasks, including arts, crafts, sports, self-care, home management, and work related, that are used or adapted to meet a functional objective.

Therapeutic exercise: body movement or muscle contraction used to prevent or correct a physical impairment or improve musculoskeletal function; typically repetitive in nature.

Introduction

As a profession, occupational therapy was established and built on theories that support occupation as both a means and an end to enable humans to lead meaningful and productive lives.[1] These theories have helped define what occupational therapists do, how they do it, and why they do it. A theory is a system of ideas intended to explain something and puts forth a set of principles on which the practice of that activity is based; it justifies a course of action.[2] Frames of Reference (FORs) are based on theoretical principles that guide the evaluation and treatment of deficits. An FOR is a set of criteria or stated values in relation to which measurements or judgments can be made[2]; it helps determine how something will be approached, perceived, or understood.[3] In occupational therapy, FORs help therapists translate theory into intervention methods and approaches through applying clinical reasoning. A FOR is more specific in scope than a model and guides the clinician in the selection of appropriate ways to address the needs and goals of the client.

In the management of physical dysfunction, the more commonly used FORs include the Biomechanical, Sensorimotor, and Rehabilitation.[4] The Biomechanical FOR is used with musculoskeletal problems and orthopedic conditions; the Sensorimotor FOR is used for individuals with neurological conditions and involvement of the central nervous system; the Rehabilitation FOR can be used with anyone and is focused on returning individuals to their highest level of independence and function, in spite of any residual **impairments**. It is important to note that a therapist may employ more than one FOR with any one individual. For instance, for someone who has experienced a stroke, the therapist most likely would employ a Sensorimotor FOR, and also the Rehabilitation FOR, in choosing appropriate interventions. This chapter will address the Biomechanical FOR.

The Biomechanical Frame of Reference Theoretical Base

Biomechanics is the study of mechanical laws relating to the movement or structures of living bodies[2]; it is a discipline that uses principles of physics to study how forces interact within a living body.[5] More specifically, in the human body, principles of **kinetics** and **kinematics** are applied to understand normal movement. Movement is necessary for occupational performance and engagement in most occupations. Loss of motion can limit participation in occupation and, therefore, occupational performance. It is through knowledge and understanding of biomechanics, as well as the anatomy and physiology of the human body and the cardiopulmonary system, that a clinician can assess limitations in movement and occupational performance and prescribe interventions that will alleviate or compensate for this loss.

This FOR is applied to individuals who demonstrate limitations in moving freely, with adequate strength, or in motion sustained over time.[6] These limitations may be as a result of problems with the musculoskeletal system, the peripheral nervous system, the cardiopulmonary system, or as a result of injury or surgical procedures that require periods of immobilization for tissue healing.

Function/Dysfunction Continua

All occupational performance requires stability and mobility of the human body in varying amounts. Whether turning over in bed, standing at the sink to brush one's teeth, dressing, eating, or writing, some muscles are providing stabilization and others are allowing movement for performance of that activity. The capacity for motion involves three components: the potential for motion at a joint (joint range of motion [ROM]), muscle strength, and endurance. Limitations in any of these, or a combination, result in biomechanical impairments that can affect performance of one's occupations.[6] In addition, a clinician must look at the force, leverage, and torque required by the body to perform a task or an activity. Assessment of all of these components will help determine where the limitation lies, as well as what intervention is needed to overcome it.

Range of Motion

All joints in the human body have a normal **range of motion** (ROM) that is possible. This is determined by the structure of specific joints and the elasticity of the connective tissues, muscles, tendons, skin, and other soft tissues that surround that joint. A clinician must know what is "normal" or expected, to be able to recognize deficits, or what is not normal. Limitations in the available ROM at a joint may be caused by damage from injury or disease, **edema** in the surrounding tissues, pain, tightness or shortening of the muscles, tendons, skin, or surrounding tissues, muscle spasticity, or contracture of connective tissues such as the ligaments and joint capsule as a result of immobilization. Common conditions that can affect joint mobility include arthritis, fractures that create swelling and immobilization to allow for healing, and shortening of soft tissues such as the skin after a burn or laceration. ROM is usually measured in degrees of movement.

Strength

Muscles provide the forces necessary for maintaining a posture or position and moving the body in space, both of which are required for participation in occupations. Muscles create movement and stability through the force they exert on the bones of the body. A force can be a push or a pull that can produce, arrest, or modify movement.[5] The amount of force can vary depending on the size of the muscle, the number of muscle fibers recruited, and the capacity of that muscle. Muscles work simultaneously to provide stability or control at the same time others are causing motion. A deficit in strength, or weakness, has many causes. Primary weakness is a direct result of a condition or disease such as amyotrophic lateral sclerosis or muscular dystrophy or because of disruption of innervation secondary to injury to a peripheral nerve. It can be a secondary symptom as a result of disuse or immobilization such as after a fracture, or from restrictions of soft tissues such as contracture of the skin after a burn injury. **Strength** is usually measured in pounds of force exerted, or by the amount of force a muscle can withstand.

Endurance

The ability of muscles to sustain their effort over time is **endurance**.[4] Occupational therapists are concerned with endurance for occupational performance to determine whether a person will be able to carry out a certain activity. In addition to the normal capacity of the muscle and its condition, there are other factors that affect endurance. These include the cardiovascular and pulmonary systems of that individual. Limitations or deficits in endurance can be a result of diseases that directly affect the muscles, the cardiovascular or respiratory systems, or loss of normal conditioning from disuse or extended lack of activity.[6] Endurance is typically measured in time or duration, by repetitions, or by completion of an activity.

A decrease or deficit in any of the abovementioned components: ROM, strength, or endurance, can interfere with occupational performance and normal functioning. An individual may demonstrate a deficit in only one component, or in a combination, that will create dysfunction for him or her. A person with arthritis in the shoulder joint may not be able to wash or groom his or her hair because of the inability to move the shoulder to a position that would allow this activity. This is a result of decreased ROM. An individual who had a heart attack and was confined to bed for some days may not be able to get out of bed without assistance as a result of a decrease in strength and endurance. Someone who was casted following a fracture of the distal radius would have decreased movement at the wrist as well as weakness in the wrist musculature from being immobilized.

Evaluation: Indicators of Function and Dysfunction

In order to determine the extent of a limitation and its effect on function, these components of movement must be evaluated. In addition, through the evaluation process, the therapist will be able to determine the cause of the limitation and subsequently what intervention is needed to alleviate the problem. For example, if a client presents with decreased ROM at a joint and it is determined that there is edema present, the therapist may conclude that the edema is creating the limitation in joint movement and that intervention to lessen the edema will lead to an increase in the ROM. These measurements, taken in evaluation of the different components, will be used by the therapist to develop goals that will then be used to measure progress.

Range of Motion

ROM is usually measured with a goniometer in degrees of movement. There are accepted "norms" that allow the clinician to determine the extent of a deficit when compared to this norm. For instance, the norm for shoulder flexion is 0° to 180°.[7] If a client presents with 0° to 90° of shoulder flexion, this is only about half of the normal range. As mentioned previously, there are many factors that can cause a limitation in movement at a joint, such as edema or pain. If the therapist determines one of these causes is present, then evaluation of that particular cause would be done as well. Edema can be measured using a volumeter and water displacement or circumferentially with a measuring tape. Pain can be assessed using verbal and visual analog scales as well as questionnaires.

Strength

Strength is evaluated primarily with manual muscle testing in which a muscle or group of muscles is assigned a muscle grade based on the amount of resistance provided by the clinician. Grip strength is tested using a dynamometer that measures the amount of force, in pounds, that one can exert grip force on the instrument. Pinch strength is measured using a pinch gauge, which also measures the amount of force exerted in pounds. Strength can also be measured on equipment such as the BTE work simulator. This is useful for evaluating a client's capacity for certain tasks such as turning a screwdriver or lifting.

Endurance

Endurance can be evaluated in several ways. One way is by the number of repetitions that a person can perform an exercise or activity before fatiguing, such as counting the number of cones a patient can move from the table to the cabinet before tiring. It can also be measured by the length of time that a task can be carried out before tiring, such as cooking a meal. It can be measured in distance; for instance, how far an individual can propel his wheelchair before fatiguing.

Intervention: Postulates Regarding Change

The ultimate outcome for occupational therapy intervention is to enable an individual to be as independent as possible in the performance of his or her desired occupational roles and occupations. In the treatment of physical dysfunction, intervention may address performance skills as outlined in the Occupational Therapy Practice Framework,[8] including motor skills, process skills, and social interaction skills. The Biomechanical FOR focuses most on motor skills and the client factors of body functions and body structures. Within body functions, sensory function, pain, functions of joints and bones, and movement are specifically addressed.

In addition, occupational therapy intervention for physical dysfunction takes place along a "treatment continuum."[9] This continuum represents the progression of occupational performance and intervention from dependence to independence. There are four stages in the continuum that help define the types of intervention needed at that level of performance. The stages are adjunctive methods, enabling activities, purposeful activities, and performance of occupational roles[10] (Fig. 32-1).

Adjunctive methods prepare the client for occupational performance but are preliminary and preparatory to purposeful activity. They may include **physical agent modalities (PAMs)**, exercises, positioning, sensory stimulation, and use of devices such as braces and splints/orthoses.

Enabling activities simulate purposeful activities and may involve the use of devices and equipment that facilitate the specific performance skills necessary to carry out an occupation. Examples might include driving simulators, work simulators, tabletop activities, and exercise equipment.

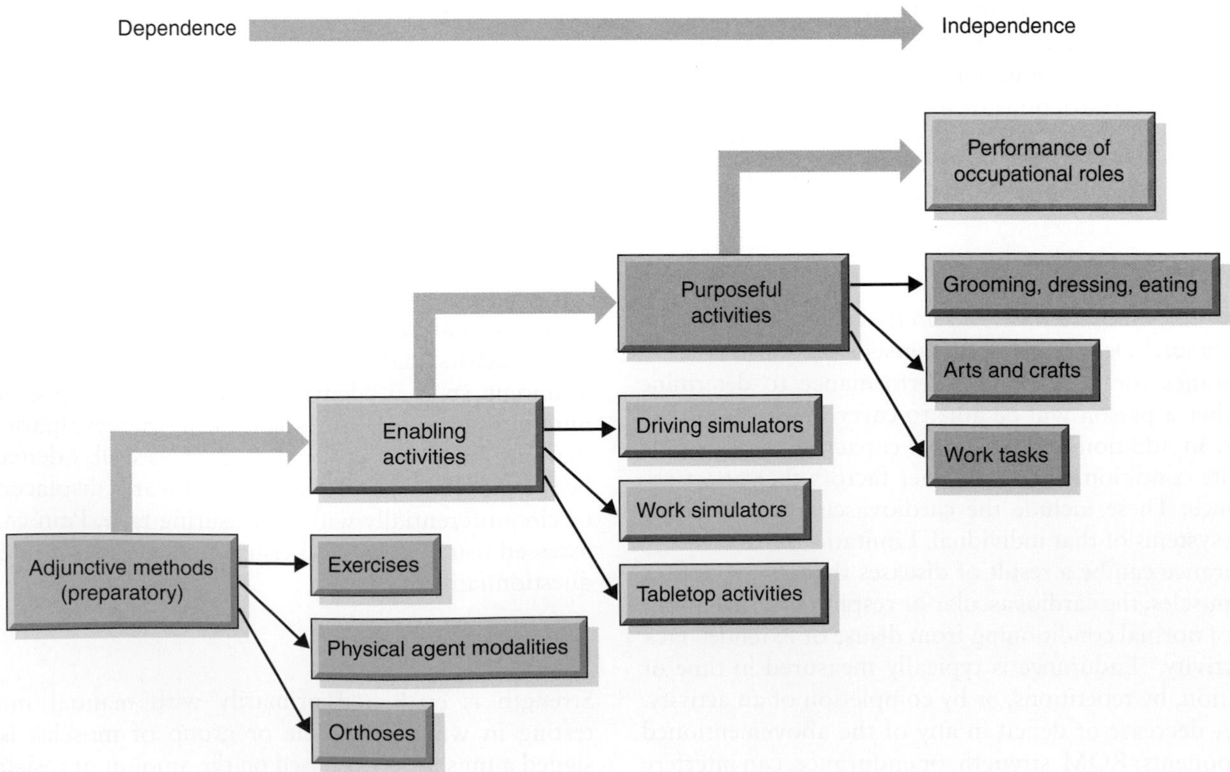

Figure 32-1. Treatment continuum in physical dysfunction.

Purposeful activities are part of daily-life routines and are relevant and meaningful to the client. They may include dressing, eating, mobility, arts and crafts, communication, and work. Purposeful activities are used to enhance performance in the occupations of activities of daily living (ADLs), education, rest and sleep, work, play, and social participation, as defined in the Occupational Therapy Practice Framework.

The last stage on the treatment continuum is performance of occupational roles. At this point, the client resumes or assumes his or her occupational roles at home and in the community.

When providing treatment from a Biomechanical FOR, many interventions will fall within the adjunctive and enabling methods and many purposeful activities apply biomechanical principles.[3] The final goal is for the client to regain the ability to engage in occupation, and this should be kept in mind when choosing interventions along the continuum.

Another aspect of treatment to consider is that the focus of intervention occurs along a continuum as well.[11] At one end of the continuum of focus is remediation and at the other end is occupational performance. When the focus is remediation of impairments, the goal is to restore the previously mentioned client factors of body functions and structures and motor skills. When enhanced occupational performance is the focus, then adaptive or compensatory occupation may be used to enable the client to engage in an occupation in spite of impairments that might be present. For example, a person who has limited shoulder motion might not be able to reach his or her back to bathe it. Remediation of the impairment might include exercises to increase the degrees of motion possible (Biomechanical FOR), whereas an adaptive or compensatory method would be to provide the client with a long-handled bath sponge so he or she can bathe his or her back, regardless of whether or not shoulder movement improves (Rehabilitation FOR).

Many times, the focus of intervention may be prevention—attempting to prevent a problem that would require remediation or compensation. For example, many postoperative protocols allow early motion and activity versus prolonged immobilization, in an attempt to alleviate stiffness and weakness from immobility.

Range of Motion

Occupational therapists want to ensure that an individual achieves the maximum amount of movement of his or her joints. Sometimes, normal movement may be possible, and other times, **functional ROM** may be the goal. They are also concerned with preventing loss of movement. Three concerns for preserving and changing the capacity for functional motion are prevention of deformity, restoration or improvement in the capacity for motion, and compensation for limited motion (which is usually permanent).[6]

Prevention

Ideally, normal active movement at a joint will keep it mobile and prevent stiffness. If active movement is not possible, then assisting the joint in movement or providing passive movement will keep the structures mobile and gliding and prevent loss of motion. Therefore, active, active assistive, and passive ROM exercises can be employed to prevent loss of joint motion.

Deformities can change the normal kinematics of a joint and, therefore, limit or change normal movement. Preventing these changes will ensure maintenance of normal movement. One way to accomplish this is through applying joint protection principles, especially in cases where joint and soft-tissue structures may be damaged by normal forces exerted in everyday activities, as a result of a disease process such as rheumatoid arthritis.

Orthotics can be used to prevent deformities and contractures at joints such as an anticlaw splint for someone who has loss of ulnar nerve function. The splint will prevent a claw deformity and subsequent loss of motion at the finger joints, as well as improve functional use of the hand by keeping it positioned appropriately. Early motion protocols following many surgical procedures use orthoses that will allow controlled movement to prevent scar formation and tissue shortening that would lead to stiffness and contractures from immobilization during healing.

In some instances, modification to the environment can prevent injury to tissues that can lead to pain and other movement limiting issues. Employing ergonomic principles, which in simplest terms means making the environment fit the person, can be used by clinicians to prevent and correct problems with engagement in occupations.

Edema and pain can limit movement, so preventing their occurrence or reducing them if they are present will help prevent loss of ROM.

Remediation/Correction

When loss of motion is present at evaluation, the clinician will need to determine what has contributed to the limitation in order to employ the appropriate intervention to improve the available ROM. For instance, edema may be present after an injury or surgical procedure. Methods that include elevation, massage, compression, and the use of PAMs such as heat, cold, and electrical stimulation can reduce the edema, therefore allowing greater mobility of the joints. ROM exercises, as possible, will help reduce the edema and maintain joint mobility. In addition, active and passive stretching exercises can be used, when not contraindicated, to elongate tissues in preparation for ROM and functional use. All of these fall under the stage of adjunctive or preparatory methods on the treatment continuum. Encouraging functional use of the hand or extremity with

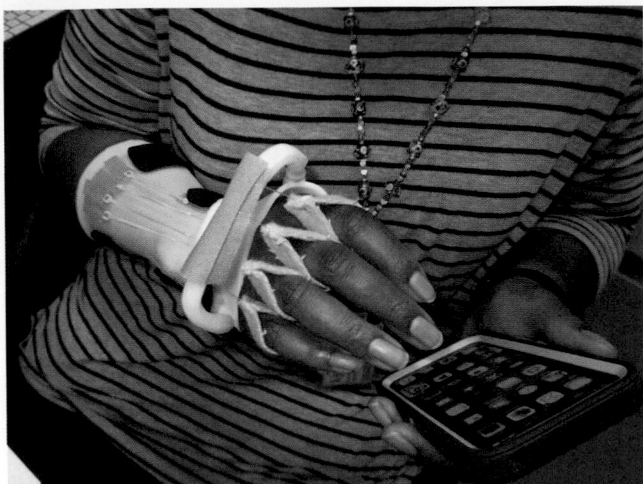

Figure 32-2. Use of a dynamic extension outrigger to compensate for loss of finger extension caused by radial nerve palsy following an injury to the radial nerve.

simulated and purposeful tasks will help reduce edema and increase ROM as well.

Orthotics, particularly dynamic orthoses, can provide forces that will create lengthening in the muscles, tendons, and other soft tissues that are shortened and limiting normal gliding and movement.

Compensatory/Adaptive

When limitations exist in movement that cannot be remediated, or existing motion is functional, then the clinician's focus with the patient may be on compensatory methods and independence in occupations in spite of decreased ROM. Many times, this will include the use of adaptive devices and equipment or orthoses (Fig. 32-2). Sometimes, it may require a modification to the environment.

Strength

Strengthening is defined as any intervention that involves an attempt at repetitive, effortful, muscle contraction for the purpose of increasing the capacity of work that the muscle can perform.[12] Activities and occupations require certain amounts of strength in order to perform them. Many times, a minimal amount will be needed for an individual to perform an activity or task independently. Occupational therapists may need to employ interventions for strengthening to enable their clients to have that ability.

Prevention

Participation in daily activities and occupations can serve to maintain existing levels of strength and prevent weakening of muscles. Many individuals choose to also engage in exercise as an occupation, such as jogging, walking, or working out at a gym. Therapists can prescribe a **therapeutic exercise** program that can achieve the same for individuals who have conditions that can lead to loss of strength and, therefore, function. Examples include those with chronic conditions such as arthritis and cardiopulmonary conditions.

Remediation/Correction

Once an individual has lost strength, due to illness, injury, or immobilization, intervention will be used in an attempt to restore and increase strength. In addition to actual participation in occupations, a therapist might use graded **therapeutic activities** and therapeutic exercises to achieve this goal. In using therapeutic exercises, the amount of force, number of repetitions, speed of the exercise, or length of time it is done can be varied to start with a level the client can perform and progress to a more challenging level as tolerated. Examples include the use of resistive bands, graded putty, free weights, and weighted pulleys. In using therapeutic activities, purposeful tasks can be used in targeted ways to increase strength. An example might be to engage the client in a tabletop activity with weights on his arms to increase resistance to the movement while performing the activity. Another example would be to use electrical stimulation to reinforce a movement while performing a particular task, such as weak wrist and finger extensors for opening and releasing objects.

Other options that are more purposeful and functional than therapeutic exercise include the use of equipment like the BTE work simulator which allows simulation of tool use, tasks such as jar opening, driving, and turning door knobs, with grading of the resistance and amount of time the activity is done (Fig. 32-3).

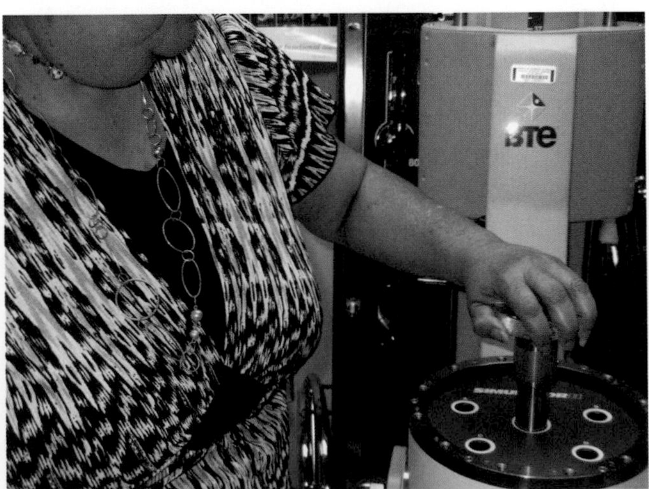

Figure 32-3. Use of the BTE work simulator to increase functional use and strength of the left hand following a distal radius fracture. This client complained of not being able to open jars, so the large jar lid tool is being used.

For an injured worker, work hardening can provide a program in which the worker carries out his or her specific job tasks in a work environment, gradually reaching his maximum potential, in preparation for safely returning to his or her job.

Compensatory/Adaptive

Like with ROM, many conditions may result in a permanent loss of strength. In these instances, activities and occupations will need to be adapted to enable the individual to continue to perform them as independently as possible. For instance, someone with a neuromuscular disease resulting in generalized weakness may not have enough strength in his or her trunk musculature to assume a sitting position from lying in bed. The use of a bed with a feature that brings the head of the bed upright would enable him or her to come to sit without assistance. An individual with chronic weakness in his or her hands due to rheumatoid arthritis and cannot open jars or cans, could use an adaptive jar opener and electric can opener to achieve these tasks independently.

Endurance

Sustaining the strength of a muscle over time is endurance. Varying lengths of time are required for different tasks and occupations. A person may be able to carry out a light task such as folding clothes for a longer period of time than he or she is able to for a more demanding task such as raking leaves. Interventions to improve endurance must grade the resistance and the time. The use of lighter resistance over increasing time has been advocated for endurance training.[13]

Prevention

As previously stated, engagement in normal occupations can help prevent loss of strength. It would follow that this can also prevent decreases in endurance as well.

Remediation/Correction

An individual who fatigues before being able to complete a particular task or occupation demonstrates a deficit in endurance. The therapist can grade therapeutic exercises and activities in such a way as to gradually increase the amount of time involved in the task. With therapeutic exercise, the number of repetitions can be increased incrementally. In an activity such as knitting, the individual can increase endurance by knitting for a few minutes longer each day. For example, a runner may build up his endurance by running a little farther each week.

Compensatory/Adaptive

The same conditions that may permanently limit strength may also limit endurance. In these cases, the therapist can use the Rehabilitation FOR to teach compensatory techniques for completing desired activities, such as energy conservation and the use of adaptive devices, that will allow completion of the activities. An individual with chronic obstructive pulmonary disease (COPD) may be limited in the distance he or she can walk before becoming fatigued. The use of a wheelchair may allow him or her to cover more distance with less energy expenditure. If this person is able to walk from his or her car to the door of the store, but not farther, the use of a motorized cart or a wheelchair may allow completion of shopping without any other assistance.

Evidence Regarding the Biomechanical Frame of Reference

Evidence-based practice (EBP) is the conscientious use of current best evidence in making decisions about patient care.[14] The goal of EBP is to eliminate unsound or risky practices in favor of those that have better outcomes. This has become more imperative for occupational therapists in recent years. Owing to higher caseloads and limited therapy visits, therapists have less time with each client; in addition, third-party payers have become less inclusive of the treatment for which they will reimburse. Increasingly, their emphasis is on improved functional outcomes. Therefore, clinicians have to choose wisely the interventions they will use in order to optimize the outcomes for their clients. The profession has to look at the evidence for the models, FORs, and treatment methods and modalities that have always been embraced and decide objectively whether they are effective or not.

Historically, the Biomechanical FOR has been shown to be effective in the prevention and remediation of physical impairments, such as ROM, strength, and endurance. However, improvements in these impairments do not necessarily equate to improved occupational performance or function. Third-party payers are no longer likely to reimburse treatment purely for biomechanical gains. Therefore, research is needed that can demonstrate the correlation between biomechanical interventions and improved functional outcomes.

Occupational therapists who work in orthopedic and hand therapy settings have been identified as having a tendency to follow a reductionist biomechanical approach in their practice, potentially losing the occupational focus in their interventions with these populations.[15] Reasons given for less occupation-based intervention are many and include time limitation, space limitation, and lack of resources.[16] Owing to these observations, there has been an increase in the use of functional outcomes, reporting that many achieved by self-report of the patient. In addition, there has been an increase in the research and studies being done to demonstrate the effectiveness of biomechanical interventions for improving function and increased occupational performance. Examples of these types of studies can be found in the Evidence table at the end of this chapter.

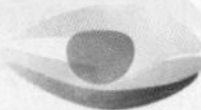

CASE STUDY

Patient Information

Selena is a 20-year-old right hand dominant college student who was living with her mother during summer break and working as a bar tender at a local restaurant/bar. She enjoys working out at the gym, walking her dog, and spending time with friends. While at work, she tripped over a box behind the bar while holding a glass goblet in her left hand. When she fell to the floor, the glass shattered, lacerating her left wrist/forearm on the volar surface. She was taken to the emergency room (ER) where the laceration was dressed, and she was told to seek the attention of a surgeon. All flexor tendons and the ulnar nerve were cut, and the median nerve was "nicked." Two weeks after the accident, a local general surgeon (no hand surgeons practiced in this area) repaired the tendons and placed her in a cast for 4 weeks. After cast removal, she was returning to college and was encouraged to get therapy in that city.

Her first treatment session was approximately 9 weeks after her injury and 7 weeks after surgery. Selena presented with flexion contractures of all fingers, thenar and hypothenar atrophy, and lack of sensation in the ring and small fingers. She had received no therapy or intervention once the cast had been removed. Based on initial evaluation findings, the occupational therapist/certified hand therapist questioned whether the ulnar nerve was intact. In communication with the surgeon, it was discovered that the ulnar nerve had not been found or repaired.

Assessment Process and Results

Selena had no pain at rest, but had discomfort with any passive ROM of the fingers and wrist. She had no measureable active ROM of the fingers and thumb, and her fingers were in fixed flexion contractures (Fig. 32-4). Sensation testing with the Semmes Weinstein was 2.83 for thumb and index finger, 3.61 for middle finger, and 6.65 for ring and small fingers. She reported being unable to use her left hand for ADLs or other activities because of the inability to grasp or "feel." She was unable to work out at the gym, except for one-handed exercises. She expressed extreme worry about her hand and the fact that she could not use it. She also expressed embarrassment and reported that she kept it covered or hidden when out in public since the cast was removed.

Occupational Therapy Problem List

- Decreased active and passive movement in left fingers, thumb, and wrist
- Contractures/shortening of soft tissues of left fingers and wrist
- Decreased sensation in the left hand; lack of protective sensation in ring and small fingers
- Hard, rigid scar tissue at injury and surgery sites
- Lack of functional use of left hand to perform ADLs or leisure activities

Occupational Therapy Goal List

Selena will:

- Demonstrate passive ROM within normal limits and active ROM within functional limits to facilitate functional use of the left hand.
- Demonstrate knowledge of safety techniques for prevention of tissue injury because of loss of ulnar nerve function in left hand.
- Achieve softening and increased extensibility of the scar tissue to promote gliding of flexor tendons and wrist mobility.
- Demonstrate a gross functional grasp with left hand for assisting with ADLs and leisure tasks.
- Independently perform home program of scar management, ROM.
- Exercises, use of orthoses, and safety measures for lack of sensation.
- Gain confidence in the use of her left hand and acceptance of its appearance to.
- Facilitate a decrease in emotional stress.

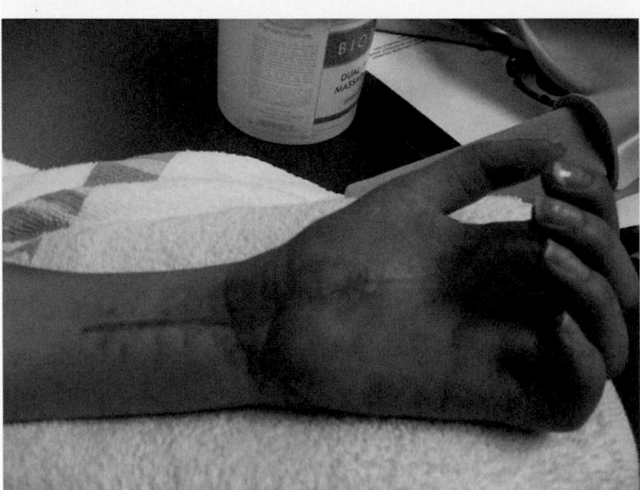

Figure 32-4. Case example at initial evaluation.

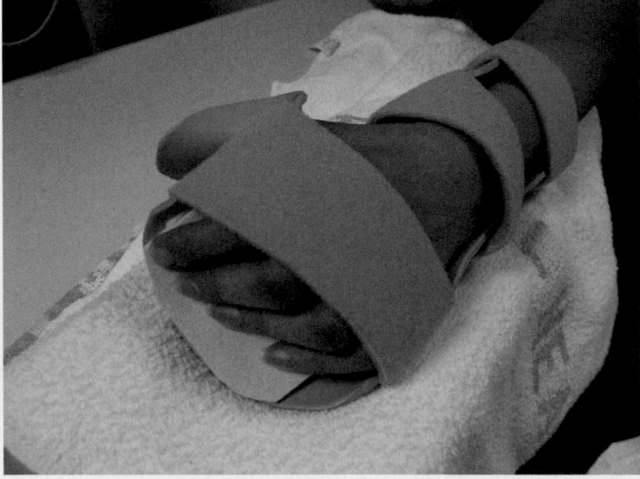

Figure 32-5. Functional position orthosis for night and rest periods.

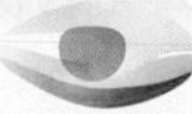

CASE STUDY (continued)

Intervention

At the first visit, in addition to an initial evaluation, Selena was educated about her injury, especially loss of ulnar nerve function and protective sensation, the surgery, and what to expect from therapy sessions. She was instructed in a home exercise program of active and passive ROM for her hand and wrist, gentle stretching techniques, and scar massage to soften and desensitize her scars. A functional position orthosis was fabricated for wear at night and during the day when she was not using her hand, to attempt to begin tissue lengthening of the extrinsic finger flexors and reduce the flexion contractures that had developed (Fig. 32-5). Encouragement was provided to help reduce her anxiety about ever being able to use her hand again.

Over the next 4 weeks, Selena was treated by the occupational therapist two times per week. Once increased extension of the proximal interphalangeal (PIP) joints was achieved, a dynamic extension splint was fabricated for day use to further increase digital extension. She continued to wear her resting splint at night, with the pan serially extended as appropriate. Therapy sessions included manual therapy techniques to increase elasticity of the scar tissue and other soft tissues to allow greater passive and active ROM; therapeutic activities to facilitate functional use of her left hand, including different simulated tasks on the BTE work simulator such as gripping, pinching, and jar opening; strengthening exercises for grip and pinch; and wrist and forearm movements.

Selena was diligent in her home program and progressed well. Her flexion contractures improved to the point that she had functional opening and closing of her fingers (Fig. 32-6). A resting splint (with a ball pan for finger abduction) was fabricated to continue to stretch the extrinsic finger flexors and provide abduction of

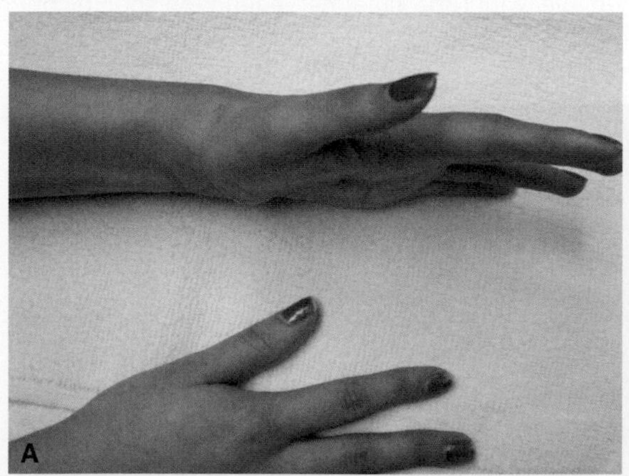

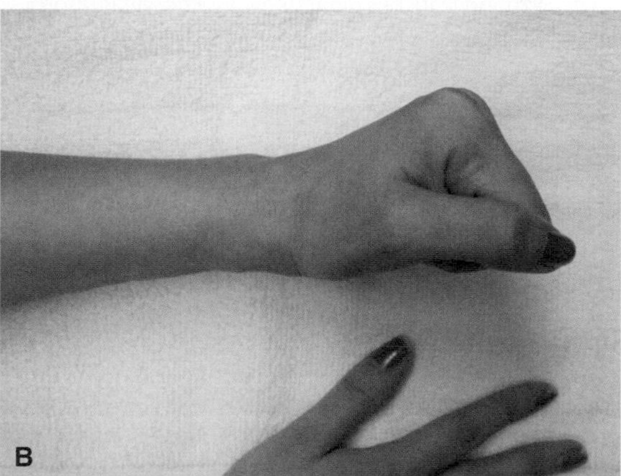

Figure 32-6. Active extension (**A**) and flexion (**B**) of injured hand after several months of therapy (about 3 months postinjury).

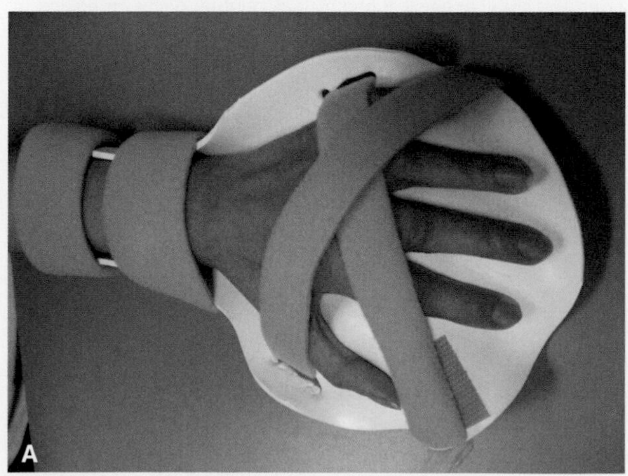

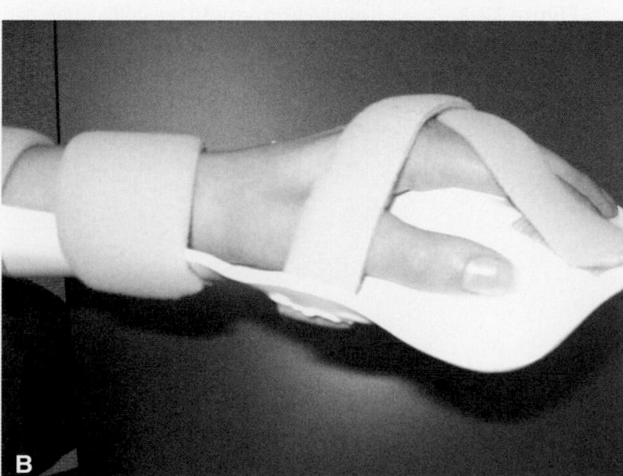

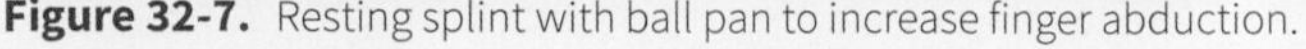

Figure 32-7. Resting splint with ball pan to increase finger abduction. (**A**) Dorsal View and (**B**) Radial View.

(continued)

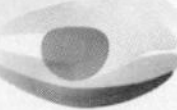

CASE STUDY *(continued)*

the fingers, which was limited because of the lack of ulnar nerve innervation to the finger intrinsics (Fig. 32-7). Selena gained confidence in the ability to use her left hand and returned to her work outs at the gym, using her left hand as much as possible. Her emotional health improved, and she no longer hid her hand, but jokingly called it her "claw," demonstrating that she had progressed through the grief process to acceptance. She was referred to a local hand surgeon for assessment of further surgery that might be appropriate. It was determined that she would undergo a sural nerve graft for the ulnar nerve so therapy sessions were continued one time per week for the next 6 weeks to prepare for that procedure.

Six months after her original injury, Selena underwent the nerve graft for the ulnar nerve of her left hand. Therapy sessions resumed for two times per week for the next several months to address wound and scar management and continue exercises and activities to increase strength and functional use of her left hand. An anticlaw deformity splint was fabricated to allow greater functional use of her hand until her ulnar nerve function was improved (Fig. 32-8). At discharge, Selena had met all of her goals and had reintegrated the use of her left hand into her daily tasks and life. As she stated, "I don't have to think about my hand anymore—I just use it normally like I did before." She was pleased with the appearance and the ability to use her hand.

Discharge assessment results demonstrated increased ROM, increased grip strength, and the return of sensation after the nerve graft. Results of the Semmes Weinstein revealed 4.56 for the ring and small fingers. It was hoped that eventually, she would have at least protective sensation in the ulnar nerve distribution of her left hand.

Next Steps

One year following nerve graft, Selena demonstrated protective sensation in the ulnar nerve distribution of the left hand; could extend the ring and small fingers without clawing and had quit using her anticlaw splint; atrophy of the thenar and hypothenar musculature was only apparent to the expert eye. With time, ulnar nerve function should continue to improve.

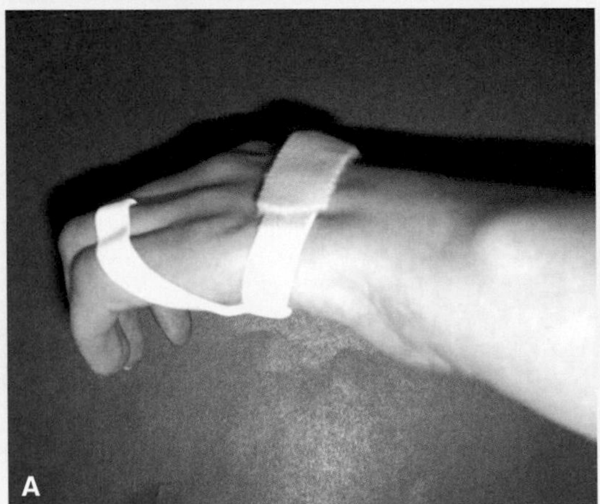

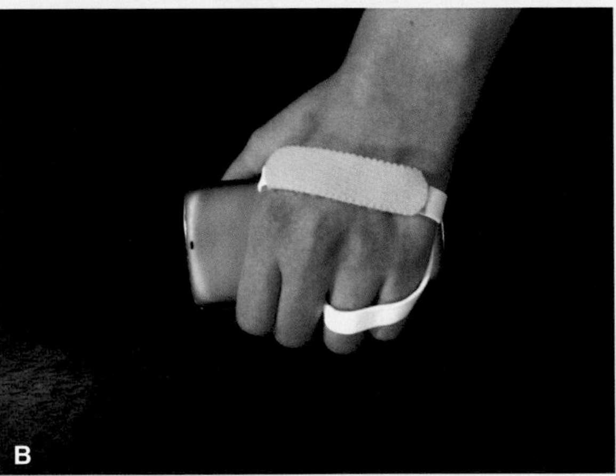

Figure 32-8. Use of anticlaw orthosis to prevent hyperextension of ring and small fingers caused by lack of ulnar nerve innervation and to allow greater functional use of hand. (**A**) Ulnar View and (**B**) Dorsal View.

Best Evidence for the Biomechanical Frame of Reference Regarding Occupational Therapy Process and Functional Outcomes

Intervention	Description	Participants	Dosage	Research Design and Evidence Level	Benefit	Statistical Significance
Use of superficial and deep heat for decreasing pain, increasing ROM and ADL performance in frozen shoulder (adhesive capsulitis)[17]	Three groups received intervention three times per week for 4 weeks: 1—stretching alone 2—superficial heat plus stretching (HP) 3—deep heat plus stretching (SWD).	Thirty subjects, 10 in each group, randomly assigned.	Both HP and SWD groups received treatment three times per week for 4 weeks (12 visits); all groups received standard set of shoulder stretching exercises.	Single-blinded randomized controlled study Level 1B	All groups made improvement in pain, ROM, and function, but deep heat more than the other two groups.	Between-groups shoulder score index was significant ($p = 0.046$); deep heat shoulder score was improved more than stretching alone ($p = 0.036$), and no significant difference between superficial heat and stretching alone.
Multimodal intervention (exercises, splinting, joint protection, use of assistive devices) for thumb carpometacarpal (CMC) osteoarthritis (OA) to reduce pain and increase activity participation[18]	Subjects received three visits—initial, 3-week follow-up, and 6-week follow-up; intervention included prescribed home exercise program (HEP), thumb spica orthosis, education in joint protection and use of adaptive devices.	Seventy-two adults with diagnosis of CMC OA who were not receiving other therapy, had no history of surgery or other inflammatory diseases	Initial visit to establish baseline, instruct in exercises, joint protection, and fabricate orthosis; second visit to review excess and reassess orthosis; third visit to reevaluate	Pre–post design Level 2B	Significant improvement in all outcome measures: pain, ROM, Canadian occupational performance measure (COPM) scores, disabilities of the arm, shoulder, and hand (DASH) scores	Statistically significant ($p = <0.0001$) positive association between pain scores with changes in activity and participation (DASH score); also strength measures statistically significant ($p = 0.05$) association with changes in activity and participation (DASH score)
Use of functional electrical stimulation (FES) to induce beneficial changes in proprioception, functional recovery of the paretic upper limb, and the patient's quality of life[19]	Daily 1-hour sessions over 10 consecutive workdays; FES to the wrist extensor muscles of affected limb while she performed functional movements of grasp, grip, pinch, and gross movement at a workstation; also, during prescribed ROM exercises, FES was applied alternately to the flexor and extensor muscles by the therapist.	Individual case study of a woman who was 11 months following cerebrovascular accident (CVA)	Patient was assessed before and after 10 consecutive therapy sessions.	Individual case control study Level 3B	Favorable change in magnitude of end-position errors in affected wrist, as well as scores for each task (grasp, grip, pinch, and gross); improved quality of life as demonstrated by changes in the SF—36, v. 2.0 scores.	Proprioception: linear regression analysis revealed a significant decrease in time taken to position the segments assessed ($p = <0.05$); upper limb function: all scores improved, but no statistical significance reported; quality of life: patient reported perceived improvement in bathing, dressing, and lifting or carrying bags.

References

1. Royeen CB. Occupation reconsidered. *Occup Ther Int.* 2002;9(2):111–120. doi:10.1002/oti.159.
2. Oxford University Press. English Oxford living dictionaries. https://en.oxforddictionaries.com/definition. Accessed February, 2018.
3. Merriam-Webster Dictionary. https://merriam-webster.com/dictionary. Accessed February, 2018.
4. Schultz-Krohn W, Pendleton HM. Application of the occupational therapy practice framework to physical dysfunction. In: Schultz-Krohn W, Pendleton HM, eds. *Occupational Therapy—Practice Skills for Physical Dysfunction.* 7th ed. St. Louis, MO: Elsevier; 2013:28–54.
5. Neumann D. *Kinesiology of the Musculoskeletal System.* 2nd ed. St. Louis, MO: Mosby; 2010.
6. Kielhofner G. *Conceptual Foundations of Occupational Therapy.* 3rd ed. Philadelphia, PA: F. A. Davis Company; 2004.
7. Greene WB, Heckman JD. *The Clinical Measurement of Joint Motion.* Rosement, IL: American Academy of Orthopedic Surgeons; 1994.
8. American Occupational Therapy Association. Occupational therapy practice framework: domain and process, 3rd edition. *Am J Occup Ther.* 2017;68:S1–S48. doi:10.5014/ajot.2014.682006.
9. Pedretti LW. Occupational performance: a model for practice in physical dysfunction. In: Pedretti LW, ed. *Occupational Therapy—Practice Skills for Physical Dysfunction.* 4th ed. St. Louis, MO: Mosby; 1996:3–12.
10. American Occupational Therapy Association. Occupational therapy practice framework: domain and process, 2nd edition. *Am J Occup Ther.* 2008;62(6):625–688. doi:10.5014/ajot.62.6.625.
11. Fisher AG. Uniting practice and theory in an occupational framework. *Am J Occup Ther.* 1998;52(7):509–521. doi:10.5014/ajot.52.7.509.
12. Fabrizio A, Rafols J. Optimizing abilities and capacities: range of motion, strength, and endurance. In: Radomski MV, Latham CA, eds. *Occupational Therapy for Physical Dysfunction.* 7th ed. Baltimore, MD: Lippincott Williams & Wilkins; 2014:589–613.
13. Ratamess NA, Alvar BA, Evetoch TK, et al. Progression models in resistance training for healthy adults. *Med Sci Sports Exerc.* 2009;41:687–708. doi:10.1097/00005768-200202000-00027.
14. Sackett DL, Strauss SE, Richardson WS, Rosenberg W, Haynes RB. *Evidence-Based Medicine: How to Practice and Teach EBM.* London, England: BMJ Publishing Group; 2000.
15. Fitzpatrick N, Presnell S. Can occupational therapists be hand therapists? *Br J Occup Ther.* 2004;67:508–510. doi:10.1177/030802260406701107.
16. Colaianni D. Standardized values for occupation-based hand therapy. *Adv Occup Ther Pract.* 2011;27(26):8.
17. Leung SF, Cheing G. Effects of deep and superficial heating in the management of frozen shoulder. *J Rehabil Med.* 2008;40:145–150. doi:10.2340/16501977-0146.
18. Shankland B, Beaton D, Ahmed S, Nedelec B. Effects of client-centered multimodal treatment on impairment, function, and satisfaction of people with thumb carpometacarpal osteoarthritis. *J Hand Ther.* 2017;30:307–313. doi:10.1016/j.jht.2017.03.004.
19. Bustamante C, Brevis F, Canales S, Millon S, Pascual R. Effect of functional electrical stimulation on the proprioception, motor function of the paretic limb, and patient quality of life: a case report. *J Hand Ther.* 2016;29: 507–514. doi:10.1016/j.jht.2016.06.012.

Chapter 33

The Rehabilitation Frame of Reference

Sunny R. Winstead

LEARNING OBJECTIVES

This chapter will allow the reader to:

1. Describe the key features of the Rehabilitation Frame of Reference, including the client situations and settings in which this approach is most commonly used.
2. Differentiate among remedial, compensatory, and adaptive approaches to occupational therapy services.
3. Understand key theoretical components of the Rehabilitation Frame of Reference, and how this approach aligns with other frames of reference.
4. Identify characteristics of function and dysfunction consistent with the Rehabilitation Frame of Reference, and understand how these continua influence the evaluation process.
5. Identify proposed mechanisms of change consistent with the Rehabilitation Frame of Reference, and be able to articulate common intervention strategies consistent with these postulates.
6. Summarize the key evidence that supports and challenges the use of the Rehabilitation Frame of Reference in occupational therapy practice.

CHAPTER OUTLINE

TERMINOLOGY

Adaptation: the process of modifying items, activities, and environments to promote function.

Assistive technology: items, equipment, and systems designed to promote function; may be commercially available, modified, or customized.

Compensation: the use of techniques that allow an individual to complete a desired activity in a modified way.

Compensatory techniques: intentional ways of performing an activity differently; also called *compensatory strategies*.

Continuum of care: a comprehensive range of health-related services provided over time and across levels of intensity.

Environmental modification: a change to the physical or human environment designed to promote function.

Orthotic: a device designed to stabilize a body part, prevent deformity, protect against injury, or assist with function.

Prosthetic: a device designed to replace the function of a missing body part.

Remediation: the process of improving or correcting a deficit.

Overview of the Rehabilitation Frame of Reference

One clinical question faced by therapists in physical disability practice is whether to focus on **remediation, compensation, adaptation**, or a combination of these approaches. Remedial approaches, such as the biomechanical frame of reference (see Chapter 32) or the motor learning frame of reference (see Chapter 34), focus on restoring or improving a client's functional abilities by directly addressing impairments in body functions. Remedial approaches are appropriate when it is feasible and desirable to restore abilities such as strength, range or motion, or coordination. In contrast, compensatory and adaptive approaches such as the Rehabilitation Frame of Reference are appropriate when remediating impairments is not possible or is not the immediate goal. The Rehabilitation Frame of Reference promotes the use of **assistive technology**, compensatory strategies, and environmental modifications to maximize clients' abilities to engage in meaningful occupations and to achieve the fullest quality of life. This approach emphasizes clients' strengths rather than their limitations[1] and helps clients make the most of those strengths. The Rehabilitation Frame of Reference aligns with the "modify" approach to intervention outlined in the third edition of the Occupational Therapy Practice Framework (OTPF-3), which also emphasizes compensation and adaptation.[2]

Although this chapter focuses on the use of the Rehabilitation Frame of Reference for individuals with physical dysfunction, it should be noted that this approach also has wider application. First, it can also be used for clients with cognitive and psychosocial deficits. People with conditions such as dementia, severe and persistent mental illness, and intellectual disabilities have the potential to achieve greater occupational engagement and quality of life through compensatory and adaptive approaches. Second, this frame of reference can be used in the provision of services to groups and populations. Examples could include providing adaptive equipment at an emergency shelter to meet the needs of homeless individuals with disabilities, or adapting the environment of a senior living facility to promote the safety of residents with low vision.[3]

Background

The Rehabilitation Frame of Reference can guide occupational therapy (OT) services for individuals across the life span and in a range of situations and settings. It can be used alone or in combination with other frames of reference. The following sections identify characteristics of clients, settings, and situations in which this approach is appropriate.

Characteristics of Clients

Individuals with Conditions That Are Considered Chronic, Permanent, or Progressive

Chronic conditions such as arthritis, diabetes, congestive heart failure (CHF), and chronic obstructive pulmonary disorder (COPD) persist or recur over time and can dramatically impact occupational participation. Conditions associated with long-term or permanent physical impairments include amputation, severe acquired brain injuries, spinal cord injuries, and more. Progressive conditions such as Parkinson disease, multiple sclerosis, and dementia also result in impairments that are not likely to improve and will in fact usually get worse over time. These chronic, permanent, and progressive conditions may not be "fixable," but individuals with these conditions can experience significant improvements in occupational participation through the use of assistive technology, compensatory strategies, and modifications to the environment. Following the 2013 *Jimmo vs. Sebelius* court decision (No. 11-cv-17 [D.VT]), the Centers for Medicaid and Medicare (CMS) clarified that an expectation of improvement is not required for payment of skilled therapy: "…the Medicare program covers skilled nursing care and skilled therapy services under Medicare's skilled nursing facility, home health, and outpatient therapy benefits when a beneficiary needs skilled care in order to maintain function or to prevent or slow decline or deterioration (provided all other coverage criteria are met)."[4] This means that individuals who need skilled therapy to maximize occupational engagement and quality of life can receive these services even when improvement is not the expected outcome. With its focus on compensating for impairments rather than trying to correct them, the Rehabilitation Frame of Reference can guide services for these individuals.

This client category also includes individuals who have limited (or no) ability to actively engage in therapy services, such as people with advanced medical conditions like late-stage dementia, advanced amyotrophic lateral sclerosis (ALS), or late-stage cancer. When working with these individuals, therapists often use the Rehabilitation Frame of Reference in combination with client-centered, psychosocial, and cognitive frames of reference consistent with quality of life and end-of-life concerns. Interventions could include training caregivers in the use of adaptive equipment and adaptive techniques for activities of daily living (ADLs), recommending assistive mobility devices such as power wheelchairs and vehicle lifts, and modifying the environment to promote safety and social/occupational engagement.

Individuals Who Have Undergone Remediation-Focused Treatment but Still Have Residual Impairments

According to Trombly, "the rehabilitative approach aims to make people as independent as possible in spite of any residual impairment."[5(p13)] For example, an individual who has had a severe stroke may receive OT in an acute rehabilitation setting for a number of weeks, with an emphasis on restoring upper extremity (UE) motor coordination, strength, and endurance. After several months, however, this individual may still not have regained full UE function, and the treatment emphasis (e.g., in a community-based setting, such as home health or an outpatient clinic) may, therefore, shift to include adaptive equipment and compensatory strategies to maximize ADL and instrumental activities of daily living (IADLs) performance.

It is important to note that remediation and compensation/adaptation are not mutually exclusive. They can be used sequentially, but often these approaches are used concurrently, with the emphasis shifting from remediation to compensation and adaptation as time passes and residual impairments become apparent. Compensation is sometimes used as an interim approach to maximize function, improve motivation, and limit frustration while a client engages in remediation-focused services. It also introduces strategies that may be needed in the long run if impairments do not resolve or do not resolve fully. For example, following a traumatic brain injury (TBI), a young man may temporarily switch to Velcro sneakers because he values dressing independently. If his strength, balance, and coordination are restored, he may no longer need this compensatory technique and will return to his preferred footwear. However, if residual deficits remain after intervention, the young man may continue to use this useful modification.

Individuals (or Families and Caregivers) Who Prefer a Compensatory or Adaptive Approach

Occupational therapists work collaboratively with clients to understand their experiences and desired goals, and the client's identified roles and priorities become the focus of OT intervention.[6] The Rehabilitation Frame of Reference can guide services in those cases where the client, family, or other support persons choose to work specifically on re-establishing function as quickly and efficiently as possible. Participating in a remediation-focused intervention program can be difficult, frustrating, and time-consuming. It, therefore, requires a significant level of motivation on the part of the client, and client motivation can directly impact therapy outcomes. Clients' motivation and readiness to learn can be negatively impacted by low self-efficacy, depression, cognitive impairment, communication barriers, values, and goals.[7] If the client prefers a quicker, more functionally oriented approach, or if she or he lacks the motivation for remediation-based intervention, then a compensatory and/or adaptive approach may be appropriate. For example, a client seen in the home health setting following a heart attack may simply prefer to reorganize his kitchen rather than work on strengthening his upper body and regaining endurance to reach the high cupboards. The therapist must always balance clinical judgment, an understanding of relevant evidence, knowledge of client and conditions factors, and the client's choice when making decisions about the best treatment approach.

Individuals Who Lack Access to Remediation-Focused Treatment

In some cases, a remedial approach may not be practical because of financial constraints or lack of access to therapy.[8,9] For example, an individual may have inadequate (or no) health insurance to cover the cost of rehabilitation services, or may live in an area where access to comprehensive services is limited. In these cases, the therapist and the individual may collaboratively decide to focus intervention on a compensatory and/or adaptive approach that will allow the individual to achieve maximum function with as little time and cost as possible.

Settings and Situations

Individuals with physical impairments can receive services across a variety of settings, each geared to specific needs and referred to collectively as a **continuum of care**. Depending on the client's needs, OT services may be provided in inpatient acute care, inpatient rehabilitation, subacute rehabilitation, skilled nursing facilities, intermediate care facilities, assisted living units, outpatient clinics, home health care, day treatment, or work site programs.[10] The Rehabilitation Frame of Reference can guide therapy in any of these settings, but it is often most useful later in the continuum of care. The early stages of rehabilitation (acute care and inpatient rehabilitation settings) tend to focus on restoring as many performance skills as possible. The Rehabilitation Frame of Reference may be an adjunctive approach during this stage, but if the client has the potential for improvement, the therapy focus is typically on remediation.

As clients move to later levels of care, it is common for services to shift toward maximizing function and quality of life using compensatory and/or adaptive approaches. In describing the community stage of recovery after TBI, Wheeler stated "clients increasingly use compensatory strategies as they increasingly recognize their long-term residual impairments."[11(p269)] One compensatory strategy described in the TBI literature is the use of electronic portable assistive devices (EPADs) such as smartphones, personal digital assistants (PDAs), and paging systems to compensate for impaired memory. Baldwin and Powell[12] reported on an experimental case study in which a man received an EPAD (Google Calendar with text alerts) to compensate for severe memory loss following a TBI. The client was seen in an outpatient setting 6 months after his initial injury, and he recognized that residual memory deficits were negatively impacting his life.[12] The client achieved improved functional outcomes after 12 weeks, even though his underlying deficits remained unchanged.[12] This case highlights the potential for functional improvement in the community phase of rehabilitation, using assistive technology that fits a client's personal context. Figure 33-1 shows athletes using specialized wheelchairs in competition, another example of assistive technology being used to compensate for residual impairments.

It should be noted that most clients do not move through all settings within the continuum of care. Clients may enter the continuum at any point. Ideally, referral decisions at each stage should be based on careful weighing of the options and a determination of which setting best aligns with the client's most valued goals.[13] Some clients with physical impairments may skip acute and inpatient rehabilitation altogether and receive therapy in an outpatient or home setting. For example, a college athlete recovering from arthroscopic surgery to repair a rotator cuff tear will likely receive physical therapy and OT in an outpatient setting. A compensatory approach could be used to promote function while the shoulder is immobilized, but the overall goal of rehabilitation would be to fully restore shoulder function using a biomechanical approach.

Some individuals with very serious conditions and limited ability to engage in direct therapy may return to a long-term care setting and receive services to maintain their current status and prevent complications. Although compensatory training for the client may not be appropriate, the Rehabilitation Frame of Reference can guide adaptive intervention focused on staff and family education and environmental modifications for safety and dignity. Figure 33-2 shows the use of a mechanical lift to safely transfer a nursing home resident who is dependent in mobility. The ability to move safely in and out of bed using adaptive equipment will improve this resident's quality of life, even if he does not have the potential to acquire independent transfer skills.

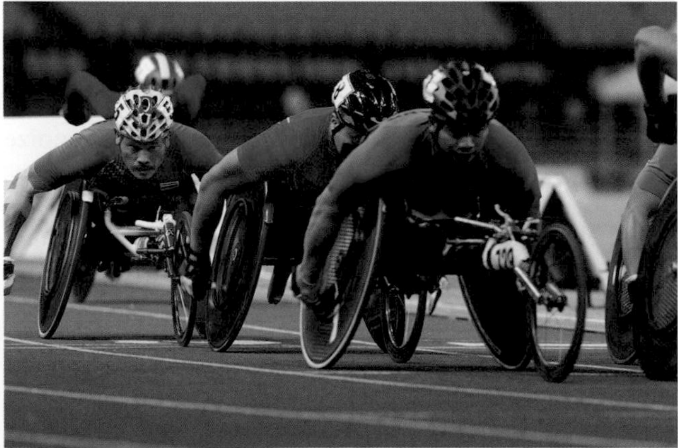

Figure 33-1. Use of assistive technology to promote occupational engagement.

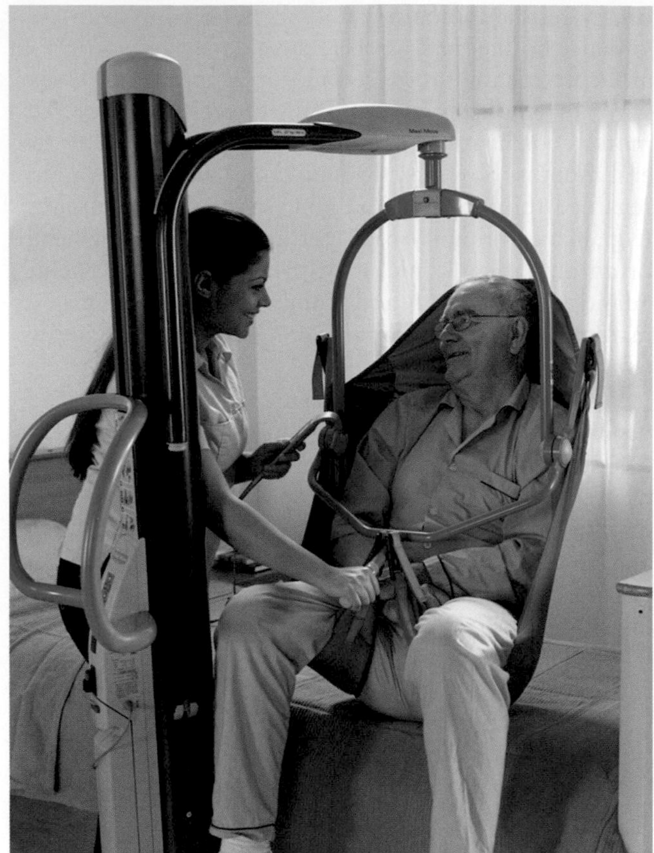

Figure 33-2. Use of a mechanical lift to promote safety.

Theoretical Base and Related Models

A frame of reference is a system of theoretical concepts that guides evaluation and intervention within OT domains,[6] or in Mosey's words, "A frame of reference is a link between theory and practice."[14(p5)] According to Seidel, the Rehabilitation Frame of Reference draws on the knowledge bases of the medical, physical, and social sciences and embraces the philosophy of rehabilitation.[15(p238)] Trombly stated that the theoretical basis for this approach includes both systems theory and learning theory.[16]

The Rehabilitation Frame of Reference has ties to a number of models, including the medical model; the rehabilitation model; the International Classification of Functioning, Disability, and Health (ICF) model; and the client-centered model. It also incorporates principles consistent with the OTPF-3 and other models that emphasize occupation-based practice, client-centered practice, and the importance of environmental and contextual factors.

The Medical Model and the Rehabilitation Model

The term *medical model* refers broadly to a practice approach that focuses on the management of trauma and disease and in which the clinician is viewed as the authority.[17] This model proposes that disability is the direct result of disease and, therefore, requires treatment by medical professionals.[18] While the medical model is most directly related to a remediation-focused approach to therapy, it is also foundational to the rehabilitation model. The rehabilitation model arose primarily after World War II, when there was an enormous need for physical and vocational rehabilitation services for returning service members.[19] Early rehabilitation programs focused on task analysis, compensatory strategies, and adaptive equipment to support function in daily activities.[6] Using compensatory strategies to help clients regain function, "occupational therapists took over where medicine left off."[6(p24)] Interestingly, despite the long history of the rehabilitation model, Dutton noted that rehabilitation was not identified as a specific frame of reference in an entry-level OT textbook until 1986.[20]

The International Classification of Functioning, Disability, and Health Model

In developing the ICF model, the World Health Organization contended that neither the medical model nor the social model could adequately describe disability and its impact on participation and health.[18] Medical diagnosis alone was seen as insufficient to predict service needs or functional outcomes, and the ICF was proposed to provide a new way of framing disability.[18] Intervention under the ICF model can be either remediation based or adaptation based. The ICF also includes language emphasizing the importance of environmental context, stating that functional outcomes are the result of interactions between health conditions, environmental factors, and personal factors.[18] The Rehabilitation Frame of Reference and the ICF share a number of similarities, most notably (1) the idea that intervention goes beyond remediation to include strategies to promote function even if impairments remain unchanged, and (2) the emphasis on context, which underlies environmental modification principles used in the Rehabilitation Frame of Reference.

The Client-Centered Model

Occupational therapists view the client as actively engaged and motivated to achieve personally meaningful goals.[21] The client is typically an individual, but may also be a group or organization.[2] In contrast to the medical model, in which the patient is often regarded as a passive recipient of services, the client-centered model promotes an active collaboration between client and professional in which the professional strives to understand the client holistically within her or his context.[6,21] The Rehabilitation Frame of Reference is inherently client centered because it teaches clients to compensate for temporary or permanent impairments by modifying valued activities and occupations.

Theoretical Assumptions

Dutton identified the following five assumptions underlying the Rehabilitation Frame of Reference[20(pp166,167)]:

1. Individuals can regain independence using compensation when underlying deficits cannot be remediated.
2. Regaining independence is closely tied to the individual's motivation, which is influenced by values, roles, preferences, and sense of purpose.
3. Motivation for independence cannot be separated from the environmental context, which includes characteristics of the setting, the individual's previous life, family and social support and resources, and cultural background.
4. Certain psychosocial and cognitive skills are needed for the individual to achieve independence because implementing adaptive techniques requires motivation and understanding.
5. The therapist's clinical reasoning should follow a top-down approach.

Evaluation (Function/Dysfunction Continua and Indicators)

OT evaluation includes the development of an occupational profile and an analysis of occupational performance that may include records review, interview with the client or caregiver, observation of the client during activities, observation of the environment, and the use of standardized and/or nonstandardized assessments.[2] Any of these evaluation techniques can be used with the Rehabilitation Frame of Reference. In some cases, the setting or the client's prognosis may dictate a compensatory or adaptive perspective from the start, but it is also common for the initial evaluation to be performed without a specific expectation of a frame of reference. As noted previously, frame of reference selection can evolve as a client progresses through the continuum of care, and multiple frames of reference can be used simultaneously.

Dutton identified the following components of a top-down approach to evaluation using the Rehabilitation Frame of Reference: (1) identify environmental demands and resources; (2) evaluate motivation, habits, and roles; (3) determine functional abilities; and (4) identify impairments affecting function.[20(pp167,168)] By integrating these components, an occupational therapist gains an understanding of what is important to the client, what the client can and cannot do, and how the client's context supports or limits function.

This understanding allows the occupational therapist to identify compensatory and/or adaptive approaches to address the functional areas of greatest concern to the client and/or caregiver.

Function and Dysfunction Continua

According to Mosey, a *function–dysfunction continuum* is "a delineation of the component parts of the specified area addressed in the frame of reference."[14(p13)] Although there is no set number of continua required, Mosey noted that continua should be mutually exclusive and should cover all the elements of function to which the frame of reference applies.[14] Individuals with physical impairments may experience dysfunction in any of the occupations identified in the OTPF-3. Therefore, function–dysfunction continua in the Rehabilitation Frame of Reference include:

1. ADLs
2. IADLs
3. Work and education
4. Play and leisure
5. Social participation
6. Rest and sleep

Each of these occupations is discussed in detail in other chapters, along with specific assessment tools and techniques that can be used in the evaluation of each occupation.

Indicators of Function and Dysfunction

During the evaluation process, the occupational therapist can use interview, observation, and assessment to determine a client's location on the continuum between function and dysfunction for each area of occupation. It is important to note that "function" is not the same for every client. Function is relative to the client's age, medical condition, health status, cultural and contextual background, environment, and personal values and priorities. That said, the following are general indicators of function in occupations, consistent with the Rehabilitation Frame of Reference. These indicators of function apply to each of the six continua identified earlier.

1. The client is able to engage in activities of choice in a way that she or he finds satisfying and meaningful.
2. The client is able to complete activities with an acceptable level of independence.
3. The client is able to complete activities with an acceptable level of safety.
4. The client is able to complete activities with an acceptable level of timeliness or efficiency.
5. The client is able to complete activities with an acceptable level of performance or accuracy.

Table 33-1. Examples of Dysfunction and Function within Each of Six Continua

CONTINUUM	DYSFUNCTION	FUNCTION
ADLs	William has Parkinson disease and is no longer able to safely shower as a result of impaired dynamic balance. He requires his spouse's assistance, which he finds unacceptable.	William showers safely and independently with the use of a transfer shower bench, grab bars, handheld shower, and long-handled sponge.
IADLs	Sam has relapsing-remitting multiple sclerosis (MS). She lives alone, except for her miniature poodle Suzy. Some days, Sam is so fatigued that she is not able to walk Suzy. Sam feels guilty and depressed when she cannot fully care for her pet.	Sam hires a contractor to fence her backyard. This allows Sam to let Suzy outside for safe exercise on days when she feels too tired to take Suzy for a walk.
Work and education	Jing has returned to work as a paralegal following a spinal cord injury, but it takes significant time for her to propel back and forth to the copy room. Jing worries that she is no longer as efficient as she used to be.	Jing receives a reasonable accommodation to have her work area relocated so that she is closer to the copy room and can perform her job more efficiently.
Play and leisure	Owing to age-related loss of visual acuity, Evelyn is no longer able to complete the intricate needlework projects she loves.	Using a lighted stand magnifier, Evelyn returns to this valued leisure activity and creates needlework projects with a level of detail that she finds satisfying.
Social participation	As his COPD has worsened, Draven has become reluctant to leave his home because of increased difficulty breathing. He misses the weekly card games with friends at his church.	Draven uses a portable oxygen concentrator that allows him to leave the house and enjoy social activities with friends.
Rest and sleep	Mateo has late-stage Alzheimer disease and is experiencing increased restlessness at night and difficulty sleeping.	Mateo's caregivers modify his bedroom to make it more conducive to sleep. By addressing temperature, lighting, and noise in the environment, the caregivers are able to help Mateo sleep more soundly.

ADLs, activities of daily living; COPD, chronic obstructive pulmonary disorder; IADLs, instrumental activities of daily living.

Dysfunction is considered to be present when these indicators are absent or limited. Table 33-1 provides examples of dysfunction and function for each of the six continua. Each example of function incorporates an intervention consistent with the Rehabilitation Frame of Reference.

Intervention (Postulates Regarding Change)

OT intervention is informed by the results of initial and ongoing evaluation, the client's goals, the chosen frame of reference, and the clinician's synthesis of the available evidence. OT intervention focuses on the interaction of the client, the environment, and the client's occupations or activities.[2] While remediation-based frames of reference focus on decreasing deficits in body function, the Rehabilitation Frame of Reference focuses primarily on modifying activities and the environment to allow clients to make the best use of their strengths.

According to Mosey, *postulates regarding change* are statements, consistent with a theoretical base, that explain how change is expected to occur.[14] In other words, how and why does a client move from dysfunction to function? The first postulate regarding change in the Rehabilitation Frame of Reference is that the use of compensatory and adaptive approaches can improve the client's ability to participate in desired occupations with greater independence, safety, efficiency, accuracy, and satisfaction. Occupational therapists using this approach assume that a client's deficits cannot be remediated (at least at the present time) by therapeutic interventions. This does not mean, however, that the client's functional status cannot be improved. Compensatory techniques such as one-handed dressing or energy conservation strategies can and do improve function, even when the underlying deficits are not likely to change. Adaptive approaches such as assistive technology or environmental modifications can substitute for lost abilities, thereby moving the client toward greater function in a given continuum. For example, in the continuum of ADLs, a teenage boy with hemiplegia following TBI may experience dissatisfaction and embarrassment when his mother helps with his toilet hygiene. A bidet toilet seat can increase his functional independence and satisfaction with this task, even though the underlying deficit (loss of motor function) remains unchanged.

The second postulate is that a compensatory or adaptive approach is client centered. Therapists using the Rehabilitation Frame of Reference teach clients to recognize and maximize their own strengths as a way to compensate for impairments that cannot be changed. According to Kramer and Hinojosa,[22] the process of *occupational synthesis* is critical to OT practice. These authors define occupational synthesis as the process through which the client internalizes activity modifications that have been implemented in OT.[22] Once clients are able to do this, they can expand on principles learned in therapy and apply compensatory and adaptive strategies to new problems that arise over time; clients become their own problem solvers. This process is inherently client centered because it requires both the client and therapist to collaboratively develop strategies that reflect the client's values, goals, and context. Kramer and Hinojosa noted that in some cases, the client is not able to articulate goals and choices, and in these instances, the therapist must seek other sources of information in order to maintain a client-centered approach.[22]

The third postulate is that compensatory and adaptive approaches require collaboration that recognizes client context and motivation. This final principle builds on the concept of client-centeredness. In order for the occupational therapist to understand which occupations are most important to the client or caregiver, she or he must have the ability to create a meaningful occupational profile and to augment that profile over time. A comprehensive occupational profile not only identifies client needs and priorities and guides intervention decisions; it also forges a relationship between the client and the therapist that is critical to the success of a compensatory and/or adaptive approach. If the client and occupational therapist cannot communicate honestly and effectively, it will be difficult for the therapist to design interventions that address the activities that the client really cares about in a way that recognizes the client's unique context. For example, the nicest shower bench will fail to promote independence if it does not fit in the client's bathroom. And a perfectly designed orthosis will fail to improve performance at work if the client is embarrassed to wear it. Clients and therapists must communicate effectively to avoid recommendations that do not align with the client's values and context.

Intervention Techniques

Common intervention techniques consistent with the Rehabilitation Frame of Reference include (1) assistive technology, (2) compensatory techniques, (3) environmental modifications, and (4) orthotics and prosthetics. Each intervention technique has the potential to address the characteristics of dysfunction identified earlier. Please see the relevant chapters in this textbook for more information about the application of each technique to specific conditions.

Assistive Technology

Although different definitions exist, *assistive technology* has been formally defined in the Assistive Technology Act of 1998, as amended in 2004 as "any item, piece of equipment, or product system, whether acquired commercially, modified, or customized, that is used to increase, maintain, or improve functional capabilities of individuals with disabilities."[23(sect 3,line 4)] This is a broad definition, inclusive of both specific rehabilitation technology and mainstream technology. This term encompasses *adaptive equipment* as well as *assistive devices*, and *adaptive technology*. In practice, therapists may use these terms in slightly different ways, but for the purposes of this chapter, the broad term assistive technology is used.

Assistive technology includes everything from low-tech, low-cost items such as reachers and sock aids, to high-tech, high-cost items such as wheelchairs, communication systems, and electronic aids for daily living (EADLs). What these items all have in common is that they help individuals be more independent using a device to compensate for an underlying impairment that is limiting function. The use of assistive technology as a therapeutic intervention requires significant training and education to make sure the client understands how and why to use the device. Figure 33-3 shows several pieces of adaptive equipment designed to increase independence with self-care in a home or institutional environment.

Compensatory Techniques

Compensatory techniques, or *compensatory strategies*, are intentional ways of performing an activity differently. Common ways in which activities or occupations can be modified include (1) position of the activity, (2) position or location of the person, (3) materials and tools used to complete the activity, (4) sequence of steps, (5) time requirements, and (6) performance requirements. For example, an occupational therapist working with an older adult with CHF in a home environment might educate the client about compensatory techniques to reduce fatigue during self-care. The therapist might suggest that the client gather all her clothes in one place rather than walk back and forth, that she sit rather than stand while dressing, or that she reduce the number of steps in her grooming routine. Each of these is a compensatory technique that modifies the client's self-care tasks so they require less energy and can, therefore, be completed with greater independence and efficiency.

Environmental Modifications

Environmental modifications are changes to a client's environment, most commonly the physical environment, but sometimes the social (human or nonhuman) environment as well. See Table 33-2 for examples of each. These interventions can include changes designed to address any of the indicators of dysfunction discussed previously: problems with participation, independence, safety, efficiency, performance, or satisfaction. For example, an occupational therapist might recommend that the bed of a nursing home resident with dementia be repositioned so that the resident can more easily see visitors who enter her room. This modification to the environment has both physical and social components, and it helps to address the dysfunction in participation that may result if the resident is unable to visually engage with visitors, or if she becomes agitated when people approach her bed unexpectedly. It should be noted that environmental modifications are an example of an adaptive intervention that can be implemented even if the client is not able to actively engage in therapy.

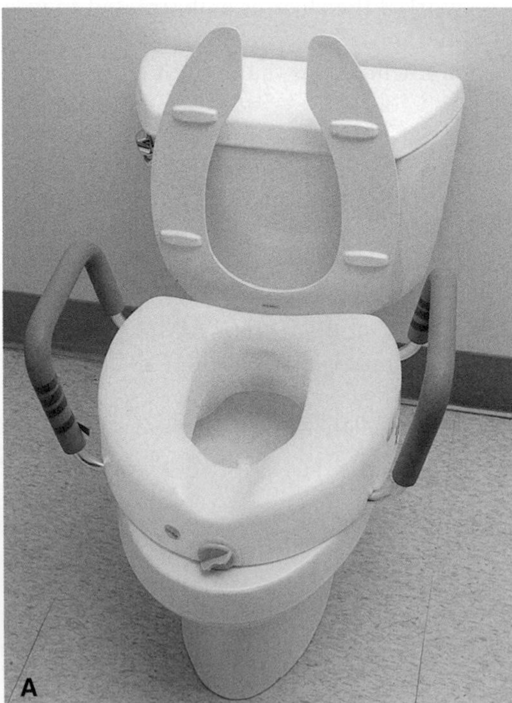

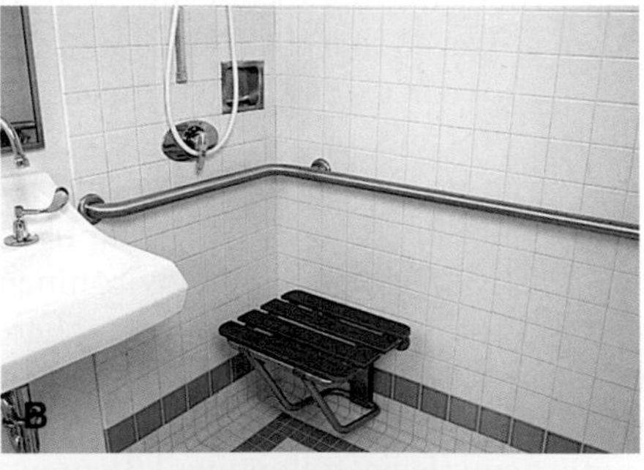

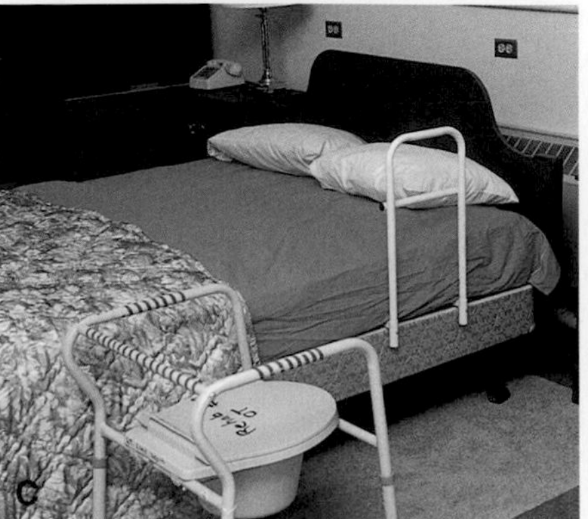

Figure 33-3. Adaptive equipment to increase self-care independence. (**A**) Raised toilet seat; (**B**) Shower bench and (**C**) Commode and bed rail.

Table 33-2. Examples of Modifications to the Physical and Social Environments to Improve Function

PHYSICAL ENVIRONMENT	SOCIAL ENVIRONMENT
Increasing lighting levels to compensate for decreased visual acuity	Limiting visitors for an agitated individual following traumatic brain injury
Reorganizing spaces for greater efficiency and safety	Providing a referral for respite services to decrease strain on a caregiver
Limiting clutter to compensate for decreased attention to task	Providing pet therapy services to decrease depression in a long-term care setting
Installing a wheelchair ramp to allow independent access to the home	Participation in group services or activities to promote social engagement and motivation

Orthotics and Prosthetics

An orthosis is "any of a class of external orthopedic appliances, braces, or splints applied to the body to stabilize, control, limit, or immobilize a body part, prevent deformity, protect against injury, or assist with function."[24] Orthoses can have both remedial and compensatory purposes. For example, a dynamic hand splint could be used to restore range of motion following tendon surgery; this would be a remedial use of an **orthotic.** A wrist cock-up could be used to substitute for function in an individual with a cervical level spinal cord injury; this would be a compensatory use of an orthotic. Figure 33-4 shows a customized orthosis with a universal cuff used to promote independence in eating.

A prosthesis is a "replacement of a missing part by an artificial substitute, such as an artificial extremity."[25] Prostheses are one component of the intervention approach for many individuals with amputations. Independence with ADL is a common goal after amputation, and occupational therapists can recommend adaptive equipment, compensatory techniques (such as switching hand dominance or using one-handed techniques), environmental modifications, and **prosthetics** to help clients achieve this goal.[26]

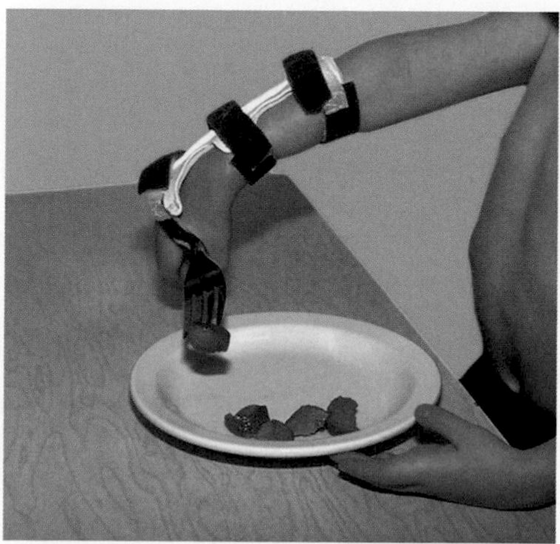

Figure 33-4. Use of an orthosis to promote independence with eating.

Evidence

Current research supports the use of compensatory and adaptive approaches for a variety of conditions. There is evidence that assistive technology, compensatory strategies, and environmental modifications can have beneficial impacts on function, although some of the studies conducted have had relatively small samples or less rigorous designs. See the Evidence table at the end of this chapter for an overview of the best evidence. Compensatory and adaptive interventions are also consistent with the current literature that validates the importance of using real activities to engage people more effectively and to promote carryover of skills and techniques taught during therapy. The Rehabilitation Frame of Reference guides therapists toward the use of "occupation as ends," because the focus is on changing task demands or aspects of the environment, rather than on changing the person.[27]

Although most of the interventions consistent with the Rehabilitation Frame of Reference are evidence based, the use of orthoses such as splints and slings either to improve function or to remediate deficits such as pain, spasticity, and limited range of motion is more controversial. This is especially true in the treatment of stroke. In AOTA's Occupational Therapy Practice Guidelines for Adults with Stroke, the authors wrote, "In conclusion, the evidence to support the use of positioning devices, orthoses (splints), and stretching seems to be limited. All of the included studies report nonsignificant findings for improving UE function and activity participation."[28(p50)] This conclusion is consistent with several systematic reviews that have analyzed the effectiveness of UE splints and slings and found little or no evidence that these devices improved function for people with strokes.[29–31]

Clinically, there are several important cautions to keep in mind when using the Rehabilitation Frame of Reference. First, although compensatory and adaptive approaches can improve function, they should be used with consideration of the client's condition and prognosis. In neurological rehabilitation, focusing on compensation when there is still the potential for remediation can suppress full recovery and contribution to the development of learned non-use.[32] In these cases, it may be best for therapists to use the Rehabilitation Frame of Reference in combinations with remediation-based interventions. It is also important for therapists to be aware of the potential psychosocial impacts of a compensatory or adaptive approach. Some clients may perceive assistive technology as a sign of disability and may fear stigma associated with completing daily occupations in a modified way.[33] Other clients may view the use of assistive technology and compensatory techniques as an admission that little or no further recovery is possible.[33] Occupational therapists should use the principles of collaboration and client-centered practice to address these issues.

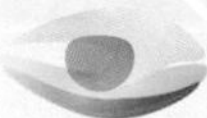

CASE STUDY

Client Information

Ray is a 78-year-old man with COPD, diabetes, and a recent history of depression. His wife of many years died 4 years ago, and Ray now lives with his two small dogs in a ranch-style house in a rural area. His oldest daughter lives nearby and comes several times a week to help Ray with housework and errands. Although Ray has a car and a license, he rarely drives. He spends most of his time sitting indoors and watching TV, but he does prepare simple meals, care for his dogs, manage his self-care, and occasionally work on Sudoku puzzles. Ray was hospitalized a week ago for exacerbation of his COPD symptoms. He has now returned home and is receiving home health OT, physical therapy, and nursing services. He uses supplemental oxygen at home.

Assessment Process and Results

Process

On her first visit, the occupational therapist completed Ray's occupational profile through interview and talked with him about his priorities and goals. Ray said his top priority was to stay in his own home and take care of himself and his dogs. He said he liked to get outside and "putter" in his shop, but had not been able to do this lately because of fatigue and difficulty managing his oxygen. Next, the occupational therapist completed a quick screening of UE function (range of motion, strength, and sensation), followed by an assessment of ADLs. This assessment was modified to some extent because of Ray's fatigue. Ray was observed during a transfer from bed to chair, simple grooming at the sink, and partial dressing (donning a jacket and attempting to don socks and shoes). Ray stated he had not been able to get into the bathtub to take a shower since returning home. The therapist was able to complete an observational assessment of functional mobility as Ray moved around the bedroom and bathroom using a rolling walker. She also completed an informal assessment of the home environment, including a survey of adaptive equipment and safety elements. Further conversation helped her gather information about how much assistance Ray was currently requiring with IADL tasks such as shopping, cooking, pet care, and getting to appointments. Owing to Ray's low activity tolerance, the occupational therapist decided to complete screenings of cognition and depression at a later visit.

Results

Ray ambulated with a rolling walker and was able to complete functional transfers. Shortness of breath and evident fatigue were observed during functional mobility, and the client required supplemental oxygen. UE range of motion was within functional limits and strength was generally 3+ to 4. Ray was independent with simple grooming (at sink) and dressing (seated), but was not able to don socks and shoes due to dyspnea when bending down. He was not able to shower and had no shower equipment. He reported that he was able to prepare simple meals with difficulty, take care of his dogs with difficulty, and do a very small amount of housework, but that he relied on his daughter for shopping, errands, appointments, housework, and socialization.

Occupational Therapy Problem List

- Fatigue and shortness of breath, made worse by activity
- Low endurance and limited activity tolerance
- Decreased UE strength
- Limited functional mobility due to fatigue, weakness, and limited endurance. Using a rolling walker at the time of evaluation
- Independent in most basic self-care, but with extra time and difficulty
- Unable to take shower due to fatigue, shortness of breath, and inability to transfer into the tub
- Requires support with IADLs (laundry, shopping, community mobility)
- Difficulty with IADLs he or she does complete, including meal preparation and pet care
- Difficulty bending down, such as to reach dogs and put on socks and shoes
- Difficulty completing skin inspection and diabetic foot care
- Loss of previously valued occupations
- Limited social interactions

Occupational Therapy Goal List

- Client will complete daily grooming and dressing with modified independence using energy conservation techniques, a reacher, and a sock-aid.
- Client will safely complete bathing with modified independence using energy conservation techniques, a transfer tub bench, grab bars, and a long-handled sponge.

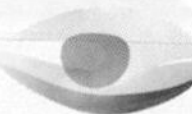

CASE STUDY (continued)

- Client will safely complete toileting with modified independence using energy conservation techniques and a bedside commode over the toilet.
- Client will complete tub and toilet transfers with modified independence using adaptive equipment and techniques.
- Client will complete skin inspection and diabetic foot care with modified independence using a long-handled inspection mirror, reacher, and long-handled sponge.
- Client will complete simple meal preparation and cleanup using an assistive mobility device (rollator walker), energy conservation techniques, and environmental modifications to improve safety and efficiency.
- Client will complete daily pet care with modified independence using energy conservation techniques and environmental modifications to improve safety and efficiency.

Intervention

Because of the chronic nature of Ray's primary conditions, the Rehabilitation Frame of Reference is an appropriate guide for OT intervention. Ray's goals focus on those tasks that he considers most important for his independence and safety at home. Intervention would begin with basic ADL tasks, incorporating adaptive equipment and education on energy conservation and task simplification. As Ray begins to master these compensatory techniques, OT intervention can progress to addressing more complex occupations, such as showering, toileting, cooking, and caring for his pet. The longer term goal would be to help Ray maximize his participation in valued occupations and to improve his quality of life.

1. ***Adaptive equipment:*** Reacher, sock-aid, long-handled sponge, long-handled inspection mirror, handheld shower, tub bench, three-in-one bedside commode, and rollator walker
2. ***Compensatory strategies:*** Energy conservation techniques including pacing, taking breaks, sitting, and breaking tasks down; and task simplification techniques to make valued occupations as easy as possible (e.g., modifications to his pet-care routine could include automatic feeder, a riser for food and water bowls, or the use of a pet-walking service)
3. ***Environmental modifications:*** Reorganize furniture and/or personal items for improved mobility, safety, and efficiency; place chairs strategically for breaks; reduce clutter and trip hazards (especially important with use of home oxygen); improve lighting in bathroom and hallway; install bathroom grab bars; consider emergency response options

Best Evidence for Rehabilitation Interventions in Occupational Therapy

Intervention and Reference	Intervention Description	Participants	Dosage	Research Design and Evidence Level	Benefit	Statistical Significance and Effect Size
Activity modification for dementia[34]	Activity modification categories included (1) matching client skills and interests, (2) cuing, and (3) compensatory and environmental strategies.	Ten studies addressing self-care and leisure occupations for older adults with Alzheimer disease (7 Level I and 3 Level III)	Varied by study	Systematic review Level I	Yes. Strong evidence that compensatory strategies including environmental modifications and simple adaptive equipment were effective for outcomes, including independence, quality of life, affect, and caregiver burden.	Not reported
Home modification for community-dwelling adults[35]	A variety of home modification interventions within the OT scope of practice were provided to community-dwelling adults with health conditions. Outcomes included functional performance, caregiving, and falls.	Thirty-six studies (25 Level I, 3 Level II, and 8 Level III)	Varied by study	Systematic review Level I	Yes. Strong evidence that home modification improved function and reduced fall rate and risk for adults with various health conditions. Moderate evidence that home modifications reduced caregiver burden.	Not reported
EPADs for acquired brain injury (ABI)[36]	Intervention studies evaluating the effectiveness of various EPADs for adults with ABI. EPADs included mobile phones, smartphones, PDAs, voice memos, pagers, and laptops. Multiple outcomes.	Twenty-three studies (1 Level I study, 18 Levels II/III, and 4 Level IV); total $N = 357$ (77% male)	Varied by study	Systematic review Level II because of lower levels of evidence of the included studies	Yes. Moderate evidence to support the use of EPADs as a compensatory device to support function for people with ABI. More high-quality studies are needed.	Eight studies reported or allowed calculation of effect size (six "large" and two "medium").
Home modification for fall prevention[37]	Various interventions within the OT scope of practice to reduce falls for community-dwelling adults. Interventions were classified as (1) multifactorial, (2) physical activity, and (3) home assessment and modification.	Thirty-three studies (31 Level I and 2 Level II)	Varied by study	Systematic review Level I	Yes. Strong evidence that a multifactorial approach reduced number of falls, reduced fear of falling, and helped preserve independence. Moderate evidence that physical activity or home assessment/modification used alone had these benefits.	Not reported
Adaptive devices after total hip replacement (THR)[38]	Patients in the experimental group received additional OT training and monitoring of adaptive equipment use (in person and by phone) over the 6 weeks following THR. Outcomes included pain, muscle strength, independence in ADL.	$N = 40$; diagnosis of osteoarthritis and THR, aged > 60	Three home visits and 18 phone calls to monitor adaptive equipment use over the 6-week postoperative period	Randomized controlled trial Level I	Yes. Both intervention and control groups achieved statistically significant improvements in pain, muscle strength, and ADL independence between pretest and posttest. However, the improvements made by the experimental group were significantly greater than those of the control group.	Within-group and between-group differences were statistically significant for all outcomes ($p < 0.001$).

References

1. Gillen G. Motor function and occupational performance. In: Boyt Schell BA, Gillen G, eds. *Willard and Spackman's Occupational Therapy*. 13th ed. Baltimore, MD: Wolters Kluwer, 2019:870–900.
2. American Occupational Therapy Association. Occupational therapy practice framework: domain and process, 3rd ed. *Am J Occup Ther*. 2014;68(suppl 1):S1–S48. doi:10.5014/ajot.2014.682006.
3. Scaffa ME. Occupational therapy interventions for organizations, communities, and populations. In: Boyt Schell BA, Gillen G, eds. *Willard and Spackman's Occupational Therapy*. 13th ed. Baltimore, MD: Wolters Kluwer, 2019:436–447.
4. Centers for Medicare and Medicaid. (n.d.). Jimmo settlement. https://www.cms.gov/Center/Special-Topic/Jimmo-Center.html. Accessed June 25, 2018.
5. Trombly CA. Conceptual foundations for practice. In: Trombly CA, Vining Radomski M, eds. *Occupational Therapy for Physical Dysfunction*. 5th ed. Baltimore, MD: Lippincott Williams & Wilkins; 2002:1–15.
6. Cole MB, Tufano R. *Applied Theories in Occupational Therapy: A Practical Approach*. Thorofare, NJ: SLACK, 2008.
7. James AB, Pitonyak JS. Activities of daily living and instrumental activities of daily living. In: Boyt Schell BA, Gillen G, eds. *Willard and Spackman's Occupational Therapy*. 13th ed. Baltimore, MD: Wolters Kluwer; 2019:714–752.
8. Gillen G. Occupational therapy interventions for individuals. In: Boyt Schell BA, Gillen G, eds. *Willard and Spackman's Occupational Therapy*. 13th ed. Baltimore, MD: Wolters Kluwer; 2019:413–435.
9. Trombly Latham CA. Conceptual foundations for practice. In: Vining Radomski M, Trombly Latham CA, eds. *Occupational Therapy for Physical Dysfunction*. 7th ed. Baltimore, MD: Lippincott Williams & Wilkins; 2014:338–359.
10. Schultz-Krohn W, McHugh Pendelton H. Application of the occupational therapy frame of reference to practice. In: McHugh Pendleton H, Schultz-Krohn W, eds. *Pedretti's Occupational Therapy Practice Skills for Physical Dysfunction*. 8th ed. St. Louis, MO: Elsevier; 2018:24–26.
11. Wheeler S. Community recovery and participation. In: Golisz KM, Vining Radomski M, eds. *Traumatic Brain Injury (TBI): Interventions to Support Occupational Performance*. Bethesda, MD: American Occupational Therapy Association Inc; 2015:231–299.
12. Baldwin VN, Powell T. Google Calendar: a single case experimental design study of a man with severe memory problems. *Neuropsychol Rehabil*. 2015;25(4):617–636.
13. Kane RL. Finding the right level of post-hospital care: "We didn't realize there was any other option for him." *JAMA*. 2011;305(3):284–293. doi:10.1001/jama.2010.2015.
14. Mosey AC. *Psychosocial Components of Occupational Therapy*. New York, NY: Raven Press; 1986.
15. Seidel AC. Rehabilitative frame of reference. In: Crepeau EB, Cohn E, Boyt Schell BA, eds. *Willard and Spackman's Occupational Therapy*. 10th ed. Philadelphia, PA: Lippincott Williams & Wilkins; 2003:238–240.
16. Trombly CA. Conceptual foundations for practice. In: Trombly CA, ed. *Occupational Therapy for Physical Dysfunction*. 4th ed. Baltimore, MD: Lippincott Williams & Wilkins; 1995:15–27.
17. Kielhofner G. *Conceptual Foundations of Occupational Therapy Practice*. 4th ed. Philadelphia, PA: F. A. Davis Company; 2009.
18. World Health Organization. Toward a common language for functioning, disability, and health: The International Classification of Functioning, Disability, and Health. WHO. http://www.who.int/classifications/icf/en/. Updated March 2, 2018. Accessed June 7, 2018.
19. Barker Schwartz K. History and practice trends in physical dysfunction intervention. In: McHugh Pendleton H, Schultz-Krohn W, eds. *Pedretti's Occupational Therapy Practice Skills for Physical Dysfunction*. 8th ed. St. Louis, MO: Elsevier; 2018:16–23.
20. Dutton R. *Clinical Reasoning in Physical Disabilities*. Baltimore, MD: Williams & Wilkins; 1995.
21. Boyt Schell BA, Scaffa ME, Gillen G, Cohn ES. Contemporary occupational therapy practice. In: Boyt Schell BA, Gillen G, Scaffa ME, eds. *Willard and Spackman's Occupational Therapy*. 13th ed. Baltimore, MD: Wolters Kluwer; 2019:56–70.
22. Kramer P, Hinojosa J. Activity synthesis as a means to structure occupation. In: Hinojosa J, Blount M, eds. *The Texture of Life: Occupations and Related Activities*. 4th ed. Bethesda, MD: AOTA Press; 2014.
23. Assistive Technology Act of 1998, as amended, PL 108-346, §3, 118 stat 1707, 2004.
24. Tabers Medical Dictionary Online. Orthosis. https://www.tabers.com/tabersonline/view/Tabers-Dictionary/769094/all/orthosis?q=orthosis. Accessed June 25, 2018.
25. Tabers Medical Dictionary Online. Prosthesis. https://www.tabers.com/tabersonline/view/Tabers-Dictionary/742272/all/prosthesis?q=prosthesis. Accessed June 25, 2018.
26. Orr AE, Glover JS, Cook CL. Amputations and prosthetics. In: McHugh Pendleton H, Schultz-Krohn W, eds. *Pedretti's Occupational Therapy Practice Skills for Physical Dysfunction*. 8th ed. St. Louis, MO: Elsevier; 2018:1083–1116.
27. Trombly Latham CA. Occupation: philosophy and concepts. In: Vining Radomski M, Trombly Latham CA, eds. *Occupational Therapy for Physical Dysfunction*. 7th ed. Baltimore, MD: Lippincott Williams & Wilkins; 2014:1–23.
28. Wolf TJ, Nilsen DM. *Occupational Therapy Practice Guidelines for Adults with Stroke*. Bethesda, MD: American Occupational Therapy Association; 2015.
29. Ada L, Foongchomcheay A, Canning CG. Supportive devices for preventing and treating subluxation of the shoulder after stroke. *Cochrane Database Syst Rev*. 2005;(1):CD003863. doi:10.1002/14651858.CD003863.pub2.
30. Harvey LA, Katalinic OM, Herbert RD, Moseley AM, Lannin NA, Schurr K. Stretch for the treatment and prevention of contractures. *Cochrane Database Syst Rev*. 2017;1:CD007455. doi:10.1002/14651858.CD007455.pub3.
31. Tyson SF, Kent RM. The effect of upper limb orthotics after stroke: a systematic review. *NeuroRehabilitation*. 2011;28:29–36. doi:10.3233/NRE-2011-0629.
32. O'Sullivan SB. Interventions to improve motor control and motor learning. In: O'Sullivan SB, Schmitz TJ, eds.

Improving Functional Outcomes in Physical Rehabilitation. Philadelphia, PA: F. A. Davis Company; 2010:12–41.

33. Gutman SA, Mortera M. Interventions to improve upper extremity skills. In: O'Sullivan SB, Schmitz TJ, eds. *Improving Functional Outcomes in Physical Rehabilitation*. Philadelphia, PA: F. A. Davis Company, 2010:216–231.
34. Padilla R. Effectiveness of interventions designed to modify the activity demands of the occupations of self-care and leisure for people with Alzheimer's disease and related dementias. *Am J Occup Ther*. 2011;65(5):523–531. doi:10.5014/ajot.2011.002618.
35. Stark S, Keglovits M, Arbesman M, Lieberman D. Effect of home modification interventions on the participation of community-dwelling adults with health conditions: a systematic review. *Am J Occup Ther*. 2017;71(2):7102290010p1–7102290010p11. doi:10.5014/ajot.2017.018887.
36. Charters E, Gillett L, Simpson GK. Efficacy of electronic portable assistive devices for people with acquired brain injury: a systematic review. *Neuropsychol Rehabil*. 2014;25(1):82–121. doi:10.1080/09602011.2014.942672.
37. Chase CA, Mann, K, Wasek S, Arbesman M. Systematic review of the effect of home modification and fall prevention programs on falls and the performance of community-dwelling older adults. *Am J Occup Ther*. 2012;66(3):284–291. doi:10.5014/ajot.2012.005017.
38. Asghar Jame Bozorgi A, Ghamkhar L, Hossein Kahlaee A, Sabouri H. The effectiveness of occupational therapy supervised usage of adaptive devices on functional outcomes and independence after total hip replacement in Iranian elderly: a randomized controlled trial. *Occup Ther Int*. 2016;23:143–153. doi:10.1002/oti.1419.

Chapter 34

Motor Learning and Task-Oriented Approaches

Dawn M. Nilsen and Glen Gillen

LEARNING OBJECTIVES

This chapter will allow the reader to:

1. Define motor learning and understand the differences between changes in performance, learning, and generalization of learning.
2. Describe the similarities and differences between various motor learning theories.
3. Define the various types of feedback and practice conditions, and compare and contrast their impact on retraining/training of motor skills.
4. Describe the theoretical underpinnings and assumptions of the occupational therapy task-oriented approach (OT-TOA).
5. Describe and apply evaluation and intervention strategies that are consistent with the OT-TOA.

CHAPTER OUTLINE

TERMINOLOGY

Augmented feedback: information about task performance that is fed back to the patient by artificial means; sometimes called extrinsic feedback.

Blocked practice: a practice schedule in which many trials on a single task are practiced consecutively and uninterrupted by practice of other tasks.

Continuous task: a task in which the action is performed without a recognizable beginning or end.

Discrete task: a task that has a recognizable beginning and end.

Distributed practice: a practice schedule in which the duration of rest between practice trials is equal to or greater than the time spent in practice.

External focus of attention: attention directed outside the body to an object or environmental goal.

Inherent feedback: information that is normally received during performance of a task; sometimes called intrinsic feedback.

Internal focus of attention: attention directed to locations inside the body (e.g., motor or sensory information).

Knowledge of performance (KP): augmented feedback about the nature of performance (movement patterns).

Knowledge of results (KR): augmented feedback about the outcome of the performance with respect to the task goal.

Massed practice: a practice schedule in which the amount of rest between practice trials is relatively short, often less than the length of the practice trial.

Serial task: a task consisting of several discrete tasks strung together to make a whole; order of the actions is usually critical for successful performance.

Introduction

As indicated in Chapter 16, task-oriented approaches (i.e., task-specific training, repetitive task practice, functional task practice) are considered the most current approaches used to address occupational performance deficits related to impaired motor function and motor control for those living with neurological impairments as a consequence of brain damage.[1] These approaches are guided by current understandings of motor control, motor development, recovery of function, and contemporary motor learning principles. In these approaches, it is assumed that movement emerges from a dynamic interaction between multiple systems in the brain, is organized around a specific goal, and is constrained by the environment.[2]

Task-oriented approaches assume that people learn or relearn motor skills by actively attempting to solve motor problems during the performance of functional tasks. Thus, effective movement strategies and patterns emerge from the interaction of persons with the environment as they attempt to achieve a specific task goal.[1,2] The occupational therapy task-oriented approach (OT-TOA), originally developed by Mathiowetz and Bass-Haugen in 1994, is an example of one such approach.[3] This chapter provides an overview of motor learning theories and key motor learning principles, as they are generally regarded as a common component of task-oriented approaches. Afterwards, the theoretical base, and evaluation and intervention principles associated with the OT-TOA are highlighted to provide specific examples of task-oriented approaches.

Motor Learning

Practitioners are faced with the challenge of assisting patients to learn or relearn motor skills that facilitate engagement in occupation. Motor learning is defined as "a set of processes associated with practice or experience leading to relatively permanent changes in the capability for skilled movement."[4] The notion of a relatively permanent change in skilled movement distinguishes learning from changes in motor performance, which are temporary changes in motor behavior seen during practice.[4] It is the retention of motor skills and the transfer of these skills to novel situations, known as generalization, that indicates learning.[2,4] The field of motor learning has provided valuable insights about how skilled actions are acquired, modified, retained, and transferred as the result of practice. These insights can guide practitioners as they assist patients to both reacquire motor skills that were lost due to disease or injury and acquire new motor skills in order to compensate for lost function.

Motor Learning Theories

Overtime, various motor learning theories have been proposed. These theories were informed by current theories of motor control and were developed based on the current knowledge of the structure and function of the nervous system.[2,4] Table 34-1 provides a brief overview of common motor control and motor learning theories. It should be pointed out that no one motor control or motor learning theory accounts for all

Table 34-1. Summary of Motor Control and Motor Learning Theories

THEORY	KEY COMPONENTS OF THEORY
Motor Control Theories[2,4]	
Reflex theory	• Stimulus–response view of motor control • Complex patterns of movement are the result of combining individual reflexes.
Hierarchical theory	• Top–down organizational control of movement with higher levels always exerting full control over lower levels
Motor programming theory	• *Central motor program* contains the "rules" for generating an action. • Program can be activated by sensory input or by central processes.
System theory	• Describes the body as a *mechanical system* that is subject to both external (e.g., gravity) and internal forces (e.g., inertial forces) • *Self-organization*: movement emerges from an interaction of multiple systems—no need for "higher centers" or "central motor program" • *Nonlinearity:* motor output is not proportional to input—variability expected and needed in the system • *Control parameters:* a variable that regulates a change in behavior (e.g., velocity may be considered the control parameter that shifts the action of walking to running) • *Attractor states:* preferred patterns of movements that are highly stable • *Attractor wells:* the degree of flexibility to change an attractor state: *shallow well*—unstable pattern that is easy to change; *deep well*—stable pattern that is difficult to change
Ecological theory	• Motor control evolved so that animals can cope with their environment: *perception–action coupling*. • Gibson's theory of affordances—perception of environmental factors that are critical to the task

Table 34-1. Summary of Motor Control and Motor Learning Theories (*continued*)

THEORY	KEY COMPONENTS OF THEORY
Motor Learning Theories[2,4]	
Schmidt's schema theory	• Draws heavily on *motor programming theory* of motor control • Emphasize on open-loop control processes and the development of the *generalized motor program* (GMP), which contains the *rules* for creating the pattern of muscle activity needed to perform the movement • After a movement is made, there are four elements available for short-term memory storage: (1) initial movement conditions, (2) parameters used in the GMP, (3) outcome of the movement (knowledge of results), and (4) sensory consequences of the movement (knowledge of performance). This information is stored as two schemas: *recall schema* (motor) and *recognition schema* (sensory). • *Recall schema* is used to select a specific set of responses and the *response schema* is used to evaluate the responses. • *Learning* occurs as a result of the updating of the two schemas each time a movement is attempted, and it is augmented by the amount of practice and variability of practice.
Ecological theory	• Draws heavily on *systems* and *ecological theories* of motor control • During practice, there is a search for *optimal strategy* to solve the task problem—search for most salient perceptual cues and optimal motor response. • *Learning* occurs as a performer searches for the optimal solution; this process strengthens perception–action coupling, and is augmented by helping the learner understand the nature of the perceptual/motor workspace, identifying the natural search strategies employed by the learner, and using augmented feedback to aid the search for the optimal solution.
Fitts and Posner three-stage model	• *Cognitive stage:* learner is figuring out what is to be done; determining appropriate strategies to complete the task. Effective strategies are maintained and ineffective ones are discarded. Performance is variable, but improvements are large. High cognitive demands are placed on the learner. The therapist uses instructions, models, feedback, etc., to assist in learning the task at hand. • *Associative stage:* learner determines the best strategy for the task and is now refining it. Performance is less variable and improvements are slower. Cognitive demands decrease. • *Autonomous stage:* skill is performed automatically requiring little attention.
Bernstein's three-stage model	• Draws heavily on the *systems theory* of motor control and solving the *degrees of freedom* problem • *Stage 1:* reduction in the number of degrees of freedom that must be controlled—learner will constrain the degrees of freedom and develop an *effective strategy* for task performance, but the *strategy is not energy-efficient or flexible.* • *Stage 2:* release of additional degrees of freedom and muscle synergies are used across multiple joints resulting in *well-coordinated movement* that is more efficient and flexible. • *Stage 3:* release of all the degrees of freedom needed for task performance; performer has *learned to exploit external and internal forces* acting on the system to produce the most coordinated and efficient movement pattern.
Gentile's two-stage model	• *Initial stage:* learner develops an understanding of the task and generates a movement pattern that enables some degree of success; key element of this stage is learning to discriminate between *regulatory features* (characteristic of environment that determine movement requirements) and *nonregulatory features* in the environment; high cognitive load. • *Later stage:* (aka: *fixation/diversification*) learner is refining the movement so that it can be performed to meet the demands of any situation, and so that it is performed consistently and efficiently. • *Closed tasks:* environmental conditions are stable and little variability is needed—*fixation.* • *Open tasks:* environmental conditions are changing requiring multiple movement patterns—*diversification.*
OPTIMAL (optimizing performance through intrinsic motivation and attention for learning) theory	• Goal-action coupling: learning is associated with structural brain changes and task-specific neural connections across brain regions (functional connectivity). • Evidence demonstrates strong motivational and attentional focus influences motor performance and learning—enhances goal-action coupling. • Key motivational variables include enhanced expectancies for future performance (need high expectancies of success) and learner autonomy (choices and a sense of control). • External focus of attention (concentration on task goal) is critical during practice.

Note: No single theory accounts for all of the experimental evidence to date.

Adapted from Table 57-7 in: Gillen G, Nilsen DM. Motor function and occupational performance. In: Schell B, Gillen G, eds. *Willard and Spackman's Occupational Therapy, Centennial Edition.* 13th ed. Philadelphia, PA: Wolters Kluwer; 2018.

experimental evidence compiled to date. Nonetheless, key principles related to the promotion of skill acquisition and generalization of learning have emerged from these theories and motor learning research. The following sections highlight key motor learning principles and provide examples of the practical application of these principles.

Key Principles

Generally speaking, key motor learning principles include taking into account the type of task to be learned (task specificity), the stage of the learner, the type of feedback provided during the learning process, and how best to structure practice conditions to optimize learning. Each of these are considered in turn and summarized in Table 34-2.

Task Specificity

Discrete, Continuous, and Serial Tasks

Different types of tasks pose different constraints with respect to the information that must be processed, as well as the movement strategies or patterns that must be organized for the patient to be successful.[4,5] There are multiple ways in which tasks can be categorized. When considering how tasks are organized, tasks can be categorized as discrete, continuous, or serial in nature (Fig. 34-1).[4,5] Tasks that have a recognizable beginning and end (e.g., kicking a ball or writing one's name) are considered **discrete tasks.** Discrete tasks are often very brief in duration.[4,5] Tasks that do not have a recognizable beginning and end are considered **continuous tasks.** Tasks that are rhythmical or repetitive in nature, such as walking and driving, are examples of continuous

Table 34-2. Key Motor Learning Principles

PRINCIPLES/CONSIDERATION[2,4]	EXAMPLE
Stage of the Learner: How Practice is Structure Is Dependent of the Stage of the Learner	
• Early stages of learning: focus is on understanding the action goal in a functionally relevant context, identifying key regulatory features in the environment, and attempting to generate a movement strategy that leads to goal attainment.	• During retraining of drinking from a cup, the therapist uses a cup filled with a desired beverage and makes sure the patient is aware of the task goal (i.e., drinking a cup of coffee using his or her right hand); prior to initiating an attempt to drink from the cup, the therapist asks the patient to describe the size, shape, and weight of the cup, as well as its location on the table surface. The therapist then models the performance of the activity for the patient and asks the patient to perform the task. Feedback is provided (see below) and task attempts are repeated.
• Later stages of learning: focus is on developing skill; cognitive demands are lower; the general movement strategy is refined through practice so that there is consistency in goal attainment and efficiency in the movement.	• During retraining of drinking from a cup, the therapist now uses multiple types of cups that are placed in various locations on the table surface and the patient is encouraged to practice drinking from the various cups. Feedback is provided as needed (see below).
Task Specificity: Learning is Contingent on the Type of Task Being Learned	
• Discrete tasks: tasks with a recognizable beginning and end.	• Kicking a ball, pushing a button, standing up from a chair, writing your name
• Continuous tasks: tasks without a recognizable beginning or end; the task is performed until arbitrarily stopped.	• Walking, swimming, driving
• Serial tasks: tasks that contain a series of movements linked together to make a "whole".	• Playing an instrument, dressing, making a sandwich, lighting a fire
• Closed tasks: performed in predictable and stable environments; movements can be planned in advance.	• Oral care, signing a check, bowling
• Open tasks: performed in constantly changing environments that may be unpredictable.	• Driving in traffic, walking down a busy street, playing a game of soccer
• Variable motionless tasks: involve interacting with a stable and predictable environment, but specific features of the environment are likely to vary between performance trials.	• Performing ADLs outside of the home environment
• Consistent motion tasks: involve interacting with environmental features that are in motion, but the motion is consistent and predictable between trials.	• Stepping onto an escalator, assembly line work, retrieving luggage from an airport carousel

Table 34-2. Key Motor Learning Principles (*continued*)

PRINCIPLES/CONSIDERATION[2,4]	EXAMPLE
Feedback: Information Learners Receive about Their Attempts to Learn a Skill can Enhance Learning	
• Inherent (intrinsic) feedback: information that is normally received during performance of a task.	• Seeing and feeling water spill from a cup as you are attempting to drink
• Augmented (extrinsic) feedback: information about task or motor performance that is fed back to the patient by artificial means; supplements intrinsic feedback (can be verbal or nonverbal).	• Therapist provides verbal information to a patient "you need to lock your wheelchair breaks before standing up" or nonverbal information (e.g., using a mirror to show the patient their sitting posture).
• Concurrent feedback: information that is provided during task performance.	• While the patient is reaching for the toothpaste, the therapist says, "Don't hike your shoulder."
• Terminal feedback: information that is provided after task performance.	• After the patient reaches for the cup the therapist says, "You didn't open your hand wide enough."
• Immediate feedback: information that is provided immediately after performance.	• Right after the patient attempts a tub transfer, the therapist says, "That was perfect."
• Delayed feedback: information that is delayed by some amount of time.	• At the end of the day the therapist says to the patient, "Your transfers were better today, keep checking your wheelchair brakes."
• Accumulated feedback: information that represents an accumulation of past performance.	• The therapist says, "Your feet were placed perfectly during 3 out of 5 of your transfers today."
• Distinct feedback: information that represents each performance separately.	• The therapist says, "Your feet were placed perfectly during that transfer."
• Knowledge of results: information about the outcome of the task performance.	• The therapist says, "Your shirt is on backwards." or "You dropped the cup."
• Knowledge of performance: information about the nature of the task performance.	• The therapist says, "Next time dress your right arm first." or "Your elbow was bent."
Practice Variables: Learning is Contingent on the Amount and Type of Practice Provided	
• External focus of attention: learner's attention is directed outside the body to an object or environmental goal.	• Therapist instructs the patient to focus on keeping his or her cup straight prior to practicing the task of drinking.
• Internal focus of attention: learner's attention is direct inward toward body movements.	• Therapist instructs the patient focus on his or her wrist position prior to practicing the task of drinking.
• Massed practice: practice time is greater than rest time.	• Patient practices the task of typing on a computer for 15 minutes, takes a brief rest for 2 minutes, and then practices typing again for 15 minutes.
• Distributed practice: practice time is equal to or less than rest time.	• Patient practices transferring to and from a commode for 10 minutes, takes a rest for 10 minutes, and then practices transferring again for 10 minutes.
• Blocked practice: repetitive practice of the same task, uninterrupted by practice of other tasks.	• Patient practices moving from sit to stand multiple times in a row. Practice sequence of tasks "A," "B," and "C": AAAAABBBBBBBCCCCC.
• Random practice: tasks being practiced are ordered randomly; attempt multiple tasks or variations of a task before mastering any one of the tasks.	• Patient practices transferring to multiple surfaces (couch, toilet, bench, chair, stool, car) in one occupational therapy session. Practice sequence of tasks "A," "B," and "C": ACBACABCCBACABCACABBACCACB.
• Whole practice: task is practiced in its entirety and not broken into parts.	• Patient practices dressing.
• Part practice: task is broken down into its parts for separate practice.	• Patient practices donning/doffing shirt.
• Motivational influences: o Enhancing learner's expectancy of success; practice conditions that enhance self-efficacy or confidence enhance learning. o Autonomy: giving the learner control over certain aspects of practice conditions enhances learning.	• Therapist sets up a just-right-challenge task, highlights the learnability of the task and provides information that helps reduce the perceived difficulty of the task. • Therapist provides the patient with choices over tasks to be practiced, when feedback is provided, or choices over irrelevant aspects of the task (e.g., color of a cup).

ADL, activity of daily living.

Adapted from Table 57-8 in: Gillen G, Nilsen DM. Motor function and occupational performance. In: Schell B, Gillen G, eds. *Willard and Spackman's Occupational Therapy, Centennial Edition*. 13th ed. Philadelphia, PA: Wolters Kluwer; 2018.

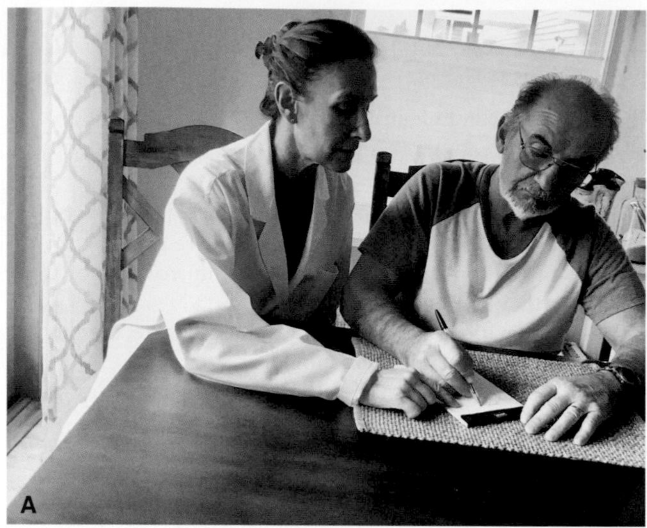

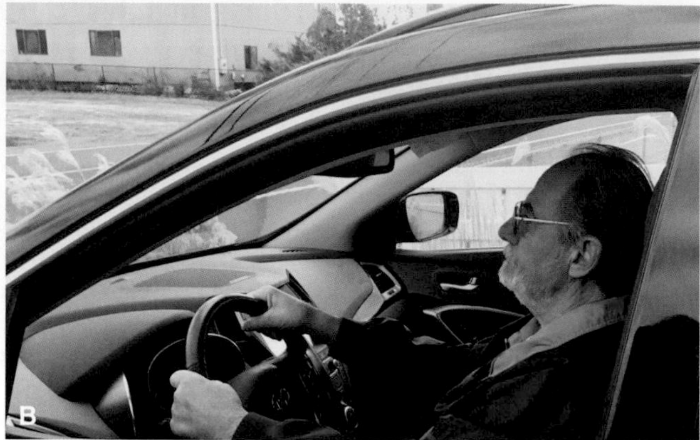

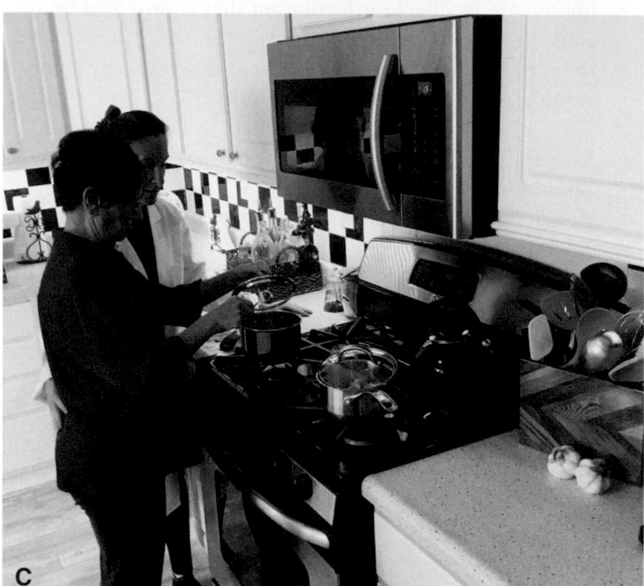

Figure 34-1. Examples of tasks categorized based on their organization. **A.** Discrete task: writing one's name. **B.** Continuous task: driving. **C.** Serial task: cooking a meal.

tasks.[4,5] **Serial tasks** consist of a series of discrete tasks that are linked together to make a "whole." Serial tasks are longer in duration and more complex, and the precise ordering of the discrete tasks is an important element of successful task performance.[4,5] Getting dressed in the morning or cooking a family meal are examples of serial tasks.

Closed versus Open Tasks

When considering the level of predictability in the environment during task performance, tasks can be categorized along a continuum with the end points being designated as closed or open (Fig. 34-2).[4,5] Closed tasks are performed in environments that are stable (lacking motion) and predictable (little variability between trials). When performing closed tasks, patients do not have to cope with moment-to-moment variability in the environment. Under these conditions, environmental demands can be evaluated in advance and movements are self-paced.[4,5] Brushing one's teeth or signing a check are examples of closed tasks. Conversely, open tasks are performed in environments that are variable and unpredictable. When performing open tasks, patients often need to adjust their movement to changing environmental demands.[4,5] Walking down a busy street or playing a game of soccer are examples of open tasks.

Variable versus Consistent Motion Tasks

When the task involves interacting in a relatively stable and predictable environment, but specific features of the environment are likely to vary between performance trials, the task is classified as a variable motionless task.[5] Performing activities of daily living (ADL) outside the normal home environment are an example of variable motionless tasks. When a task involves motion in the environment, but this motion is consistent and predictable between one trial and the next, the task is classified as a consistent motion task.[5] Stepping onto an escalator or assembly line work are examples of consistent motion tasks.

Practitioners should be cognizant of the type of task they are attempting to retrain (e.g., open or closed), as research suggests that motor abilities and functional connectivity within the brain are specific to particular tasks.[2,4] Therefore, training should be task-specific. For example,

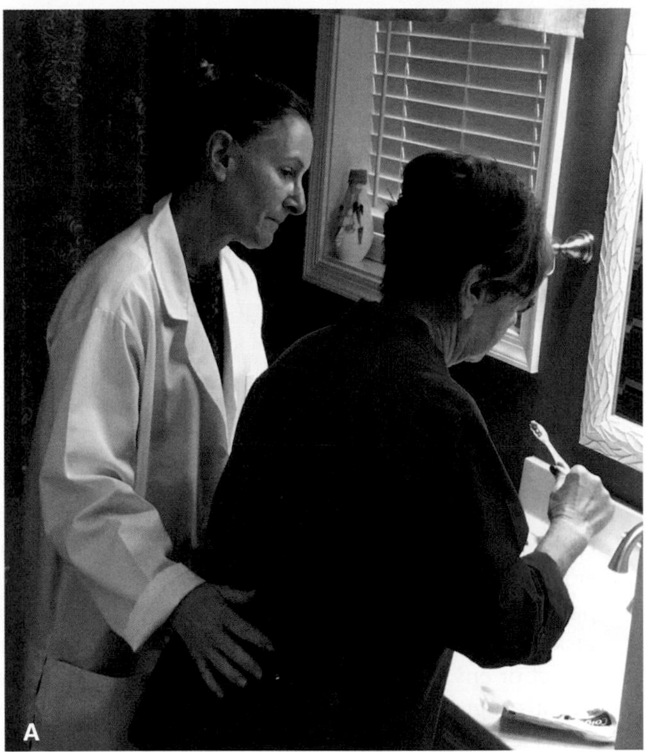

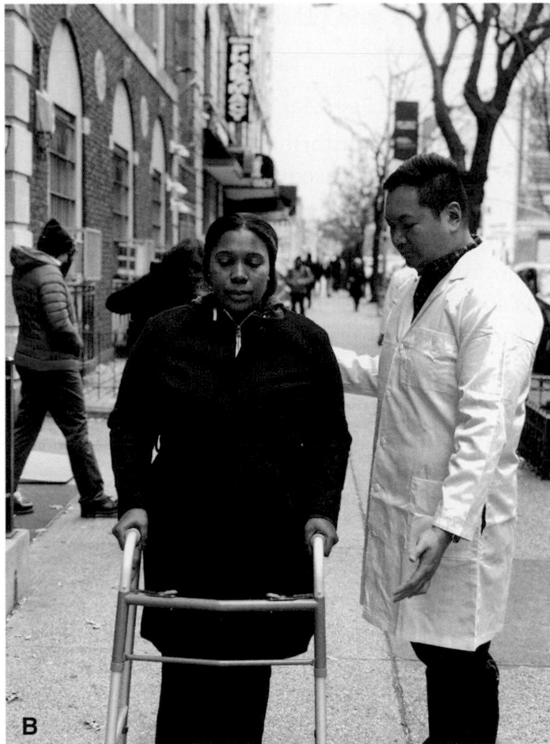

Figure 34-2. Examples of tasks categorized based on predictability in the environment. **A.** Closed task: brushing one's teeth. **B.** Open task: walking down a busy street.

if a patient's goal is to be able to feed himself, and upper limb function is a barrier to task engagement, the practitioner should focus on retraining upper limb movements within the context of a feeding task (e.g., reaching; grasping; transporting/manipulating utensils, cups, napkins, and food items while seated at a table), rather than stacking cones while seated at the edge of a therapy mat.

Stage of the Learner

Motor learning theorists propose that learners move through distinct stages when practicing a skill (see Table 34-1).[2,4] When structuring task practice, it is important to consider the stage of the learner.

During the early stages of learning when patients are new to a task or attempting to relearn a task under new constraints, they need to identify an effective strategy to accomplish the task goal. Cognitive demands are considered to be high during this stage of learning as patients are engaged in problem-solving to determine the best approach. As patients work to identify critical regulatory features in the environment and explore various movement strategies/patterns to attain the task goal, effective strategies are retained and ineffective ones are discarded. Through a "trial and error" process, the person identifies a movement strategy that accomplishes the goal. Gains in performance are typically rapid and large during this phase; however, performance is inconsistent and the movement pattern is not refined in terms of efficiency.[4,5]

During the later stages of learning, the focus is on adjusting how the skill is performed. The general movement strategy is refined through practice so that there is consistency in goal attainment and efficiency in movement. Cognitive demands are considerably lower during the later phases of learning and performance improvements are more gradual. Overtime, performance becomes more automatic and attention can be directed to other activities (e.g., listening to music or talking on the phone while preparing lunch).[4,5]

Practitioners should take into account the stage of learning when deciding how to structure practice. For example, during the early stages of learning, patients may benefit from clear instructions to identify the goal of an action, cueing to identify important regulatory features in the environment, and practice conditions that allow patients to explore task-specific movement strategies.[2,4] During the later stages of learning, the focus may be on setting up practice conditions that allow the patient to repeat the task performance under varying conditions, so that task performance becomes more consistent and the movement becomes more efficient.[2,4]

Feedback

Feedback includes all of the information that is available to patients while they are attempting to learn a skill, and it is instrumental to the learning process.[4] Feedback is generally divided into two broad types: (1) inherent or intrinsic feedback and (2) augmented or extrinsic feedback (see Table 34-2).[4]

Inherent (Intrinsic Feedback)

Inherent feedback is information that is available to patients as a natural consequence of task performance.[4] For example, when patients attempt to feed themselves breakfast, they receive visual information about whether they successfully scooped their eggs onto the fork, as well as somatosensory information about their arm and hand movements. Injury or disease processes that impact the ability to receive or process sensory information can impose limitations on the type and amount of intrinsic feedback that is available to patients.

Augmented (Extrinsic Feedback)

Augmented feedback is information about some aspect of task performance that is fed back to the patient by artificial means.[4] It is considered to be supplemental to intrinsic feedback. This type of feedback is provided by sources that are external to the person.[4] For example, when a therapist tells a patient that she needs to hold the fork tightly when attempting to scoop up eggs, extrinsic feedback is provided. This type of feedback may benefit learning by providing[4]: (1) information about what was wrong with the previous performance and (2) suggestions about how to change performance to achieve the goal. Augmented feedback can either be verbal (form that is either spoken or capable of being spoken) or nonverbal (form not capable of being spoken).[4]

Additional dimensions of augmented feedback include the following[4]:

- Whether the feedback is delivered during the movement (concurrent feedback) or after the movement has been completed (terminal feedback)
- The timing of delivery (immediate or delayed)
- Whether the feedback describes the average performance over a period of time (accumulated) or represents each performance separately (distinct)

Practitioners should consider each of these dimensions independently.[4] For example, after completion of a commode transfer the therapist immediately says, "You had your feet in the perfect position," or "That was a perfect transfer." Both of these are examples of verbal, terminal feedback that was provided immediately. However, notice that the first statement provides information about the nature of the performance, whereas the second statement provides information about the outcome of the performance. Augmented feedback that targets the outcome of the movement or goal achievement (e.g., "you spilled your juice") is termed **knowledge of results (KR)**, whereas feedback about the nature of performance (e.g., "you didn't grip the cup firmly enough") is termed **knowledge of performance (KP)**.[4] Research suggests that augmented feedback benefits motor learning in patient populations[4,6–9]; however, the optimal type and delivery schedule remains unclear (see the Evidence table at the end of the chapter).[8]

Practice Conditions

One of the most important things practitioners do when assisting patients to learn or relearn motor skills is structuring practice sessions to optimize learning.[2] To do this successfully, it is important to understand the practice variables that influence performance and learning. The subsequent paragraphs and Table 34-2 highlight key practice variables.

Attentional Focus

Whether patients' attention should be directed toward the intended movement effects (external focus) or whether their attention should be directed inwardly toward their body movements (internal focus) is an important consideration when structuring practice.[4] When instructing a patient to maintain an **external focus of attention** during task practice, attention is focused outside the body on an object or environmental goal.[4] Research on healthy individuals suggests that an external focus of attention optimizes learning, leading to greater automaticity and better performance outcomes as compared to an **internal focus of attention**[4]; however, results with patient populations are less conclusive. While several studies have provided evidence supporting the premise that an external focus is optimal,[10–13] others have failed to find superiority of an external focus over an internal focus of attention.[14,15]

Distribution of Practice: Mass versus Distributed Practice

Another important consideration is how practice should be distributed with regard to the amount of time spent practicing a task versus rest periods. Researchers investigating the effects of practice-distribution describe two main types of practice: massed and distributed practice.[4] **Massed practice** is a practice schedule in which the amount of rest between practice trials is relatively short, often less than the length of the practice trial. **Distributed practice** is a practice schedule in which the duration of rest between practice trials is equal to or greater than the time spent in practice.[4] Generally speaking, research suggests that lots of practice is needed to learn or relearn a skill, and that a distributed schedule may be optimal for learning.[4,16,17]

Practice Variability: Blocked versus Random Practice

When structuring practice, therapists also need to take into account how much variability should be introduced during task practice. There are two main types of practice described in the literature, blocked and random practice (Fig. 34-3).[4] **Blocked practice** is when the same task is practiced repeatedly and uninterrupted by practice of other tasks (e.g., practicing drinking from a single type of cup repeatedly). Random practice is when the tasks being practiced are randomly ordered so that multiple

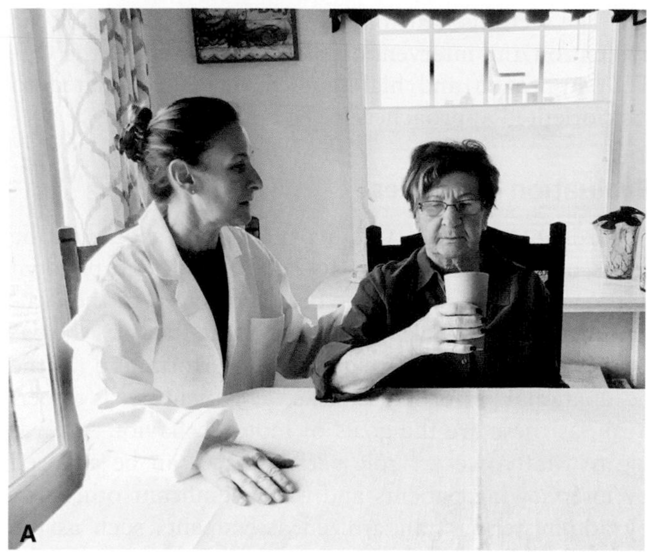

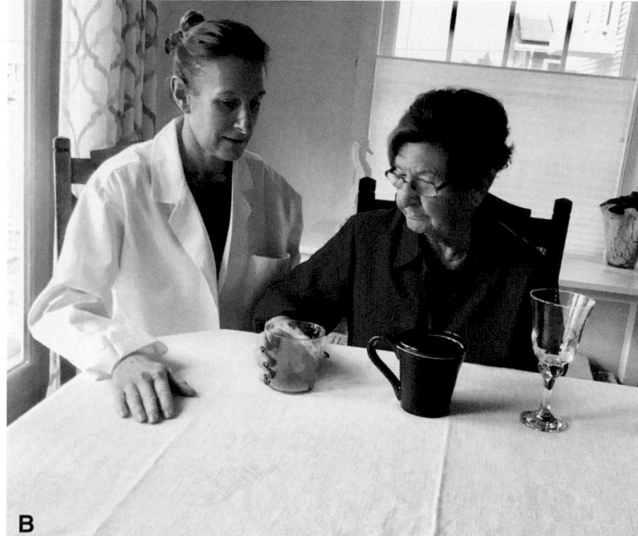

Figure 34-3. Practice variability. **A.** Blocked practice: practicing drinking from a single type of cup repeatedly. **B.** Random practice: practicing drinking from multiple types of cups placed at different locations on the table.

tasks or variations of the task (e.g., practicing drinking using multiple types of cups) are attempted before any one task or variation is mastered.[4] A large body of research suggests that blocked practice improves performance during skill acquisition, while random practice is optimal for learning (retention and generalization).[4,17,18]

Whole versus Part Practice

Decisions also need to be made with respect to whether a patient should practice a task in its entirety (whole practice) or whether the task should be broken down into smaller parts (part practice).[4] Generally speaking, if a task cannot be divided into component parts (e.g., discrete tasks like standing up from a chair) and the patient has the requisite motor capacity, the task should be practiced in its entirety. However, if a task can naturally be divided (e.g., serial tasks like making a family meal) into component parts, then part practice is reasonable to consider.[2,4,5]

Motivation

Finally, motivational influences on learning should be considered. In the past, motivation was thought to have an indirect effect on motor learning. It was thought that motivating practice conditions encouraged a person to practice more and that a greater amount of practice enhanced learning.[4] However, recent research suggests that motivation may directly influence the learning process as conditions that enhance a learner's performance expectancies or support the need for autonomy have been shown to enhance motor learning. The following have been shown to enhance learning[4]:

- Provision of positive feedback
- Providing information that reduces the perceived difficulty of the task
- Providing information that reduces the learner's concerns about their abilities
- Providing the learner with choices over certain aspects of practice conditions (self-controlled practice)

Occupational Therapy Task-Oriented Approach

In the early 1990s, Mathiowetz and Bass-Haugen argued for a shift away from the traditional neurophysiologic approaches that were commonly used in occupational therapy.[3] They proposed the OT-TOA that continues to develop.[3,19–21] The approach is based on current understandings of motor control, recovery, and development as well as contemporary motor learning principles (see Tables 34-1 and 34-2).[21]

Theoretical Foundation

The theoretical basis of the OT-TOA is the systems model of motor behavior, which according to the authors was heavily influenced by the systems model of motor control and development and contemporary motor learning principles.[21] The model emphasizes the dynamic interaction between the person (client factors, performance skills, and performance patterns), environment (context and activity demands), the occupational performance task (e.g., basic ADL, instrumental ADL, work), and role performance (social participation), and it suggests that behavior emerges from this dynamic interaction. Changes in any one subsystem can influence changes in any of the other subsystems.[21] Box 34-1 highlights the major assumptions of the OT-TOA based on a systems model of motor behavior.[1]

Box 34-1

Assumptions of the Occupational Therapy Task-Oriented Approach Based on a Systems Model of Motor Behavior

- Functional tasks help organize behavior.
- Personal and environmental systems, including the central nervous system, are heterarchically organized.
- Occupational performance emerges from the interaction of persons and their environment.
- Experimentation with various strategies leads to optimal solutions to motor problems.
- Recovery is variable because patient factors and environmental contexts are unique.
- Behavioral changes reflect attempts to compensate and to achieve task performance.

Adapted from Box 57-2 in: Gillen G, Nilsen DM. Motor function and occupational performance. In: Schell B, Gillen G, eds. *Willard and Spackman's Occupational Therapy, Centennial Edition*. 13th ed. Philadelphia, PA: Wolters Kluwer; 2018.

The sections that follow and Box 34-2 describe the evaluation and intervention principles based on the OT-TOA approach and highlight the evidence related to task-oriented approaches.[1]

Evaluation Principles

According to the OT-TOA, five main areas should be the focus of assessment (Box 34-2).[1,21] Using a top–down approach to assessment, the beginning steps of the evaluation process involve[21]: (1) determining the roles the patient wants, needs, or is expected to perform and (2) the occupational performance tasks the patient needs to perform, as these are the goals of motor behavior. According to Mathiowetz,[21] role performance can be assessed by interviewing patients and their significant others, or by administering standardized assessments such as the Role Checklist[22] or the Occupational Performance History Interview-II.[23] Likewise, identification of important

Box 34-2

Evaluation Procedures and Interventions Based on the Occupational Therapy Task-Oriented Approach

Occupational Therapy Task-Oriented Approach Evaluation Framework

Five Main Areas to Assess

1. Role performance (social participation)
   Roles: Worker, student, volunteer, home maintainer, hobbyist/amateur, participant in organizations, friend, family member, caregiver, religious participant, and other
   - Identify past roles and whether they can be maintained or need to be changed.
   - Determine how future roles will be balanced.
2. Occupational performance tasks (areas of occupation)
   - Activities of daily living: bathing, feeding, bowel and bladder management, dressing, functional mobility, and personal hygiene and grooming
   - Instrumental activities of daily living: home management, meal preparation and cleanup, care of others and pets, community mobility, shopping, financial management, and safety procedures
   - Work and/or education: employment seeking, job performance, volunteer exploration and participation, retirement activities, and formal and informal educational participation
   - Play/leisure: exploration and participation
   - Rest and sleep: preparation and participation
3. Task selection and analysis
   - What client factors, performance skills and patterns, and/or contexts and activity demands limit or enhance occupational performance?
4. Person (client factors; performance skills and patterns)
   - Cognitive: orientation, attention span, memory, problem-solving, sequencing, calculations, learning, and generalization
   - Psychosocial: interests, coping skills, self-concept, interpersonal skills, self-expression, time management, and emotional regulation and self-control
   - Sensorimotor: strength, endurance, range of motion, sensory functions and pain, perceptual function, and postural control
5. Environment (context and activity demands)
   - Physical: objects, tools, devices, furniture, plants, animals, and built and natural environment
   - Socioeconomic: social supports: family, friends, caregivers, social groups, and community and financial resources
   - Cultural: customs, beliefs, activity patterns, behavior standards, and societal expectations

Intervention Principles

- Interventions are occupation based and client focused.
- Keep clients active during treatment.
- Use natural objects and environments.
- Help patients adjust to role and task performance limitations.
- Create an environment that uses the common challenges of everyday life.
- Practice functional tasks or close simulations to find effective and efficient strategies for performance.
- Provide opportunities for practice outside of therapy time.
- Structure practice of the task to promote motor learning.
- Minimize ineffective and inefficient movement patterns.
- Remediate a client factor (impairment) if it is the critical control parameter.
- Adapt the environment, modify the task, use assistive technology, and/or reduce the effects of gravity.
- For persons with poor control of movement, constrain the degrees of freedom.
- For persons who do not use returned function in their involved extremities, use constraint-induced movement therapy (CI therapy).

Adapted from Box 57-3 in: Gillen G, Nilsen DM. Motor function and occupational performance. In: Schell B, Gillen G, eds. *Willard and Spackman's Occupational Therapy, Centennial Edition*. 13th ed. Philadelphia, PA: Wolters Kluwer; 2018.

occupational performance tasks (e.g., ADL, IADL, work education) can be determined by interviewing patients or by administering standardized assessments such as the Canadian Occupational Performance Measure (COPM).[24]

Once relevant tasks have been identified by the patient, actual task performance should be assessed.[21] For example, if a patient identifies the desire or need to return to the role of "home maintainer" and he indicates that the tasks of meal preparation and cleanup are instrumental to fulfilling this role, then the tasks of meal preparation and cleanup should be assessed. According to the OT-TOA, when evaluating task performance, the therapist must attend to both the outcome as well as the process to determine which person or environmental subsystems interfere with task performance, as these are considered the critical control parameters that have the potential to shift behavior.[21] Use of standardized assessments such as the Assessment of Motor and Process Skills[25] may assist with this process.[21]

Once critical control parameters have been identified, the therapist may need to perform specific assessments of client factors, performance skills, performance patterns, and the environment as appropriate.[21] Armed with the results of a comprehensive evaluation, the therapist can target intervention to address these critical control parameters.

Intervention Principles

Mathiowetz (2016) outlined the main intervention principles for the OT-TOA, which are summarized in Box 34-2.[21]

Help Patients Adjust to Role and Task Performance Limitations

It is common for individuals with acquired brain injuries such as stroke to be unable to return to their previous roles or perform meaningful tasks in the same way before injury or event. It is important to discuss this with patients and collaborate to develop strategies to adjust to these limitations. The inability to return to previous roles may be a factor in the development of depression (see Chapter 52).

An individual who previously embraced her role as homemaker may not be able to complete the task of shopping for the family secondary to an acquired inability to drive. The therapist may work with that individual to teach strategies to participate in shopping. This may include teaching online shopping skills, investigating grocery store delivery options, and using prepared food delivery services. A young parent with hemiplegia will likely experience difficulty maintaining a parenting role. The therapist must thoroughly investigate potential assistive devices and durable medical equipment that can allow the parent to independently perform parenting tasks, albeit using new methods and procedures.

Create an Environment that Uses the Common Challenges of Everyday Life

Unless occupational therapists are working in home care or performing onsite work evaluations, they will be working in contrived settings such as hospitals, outpatient clinics, and skilled nursing facilities. Contrived environments are not conducive to occupation-based (task-oriented) interventions. In fact, they most likely lead to the use of contrived activities as main intervention approaches.

Environments where occupational therapy takes place must be creatively configured to support the use of the OT-TOA. Suggestions include[21]:

- Replace contrived activities and objects with naturalistic objects that are found in a patient's home, place of business, or recreational environment.
- Create functional areas within the clinic. These may include an office, mini-apartment, meal preparation area, and leisure station (Fig. 34-4).

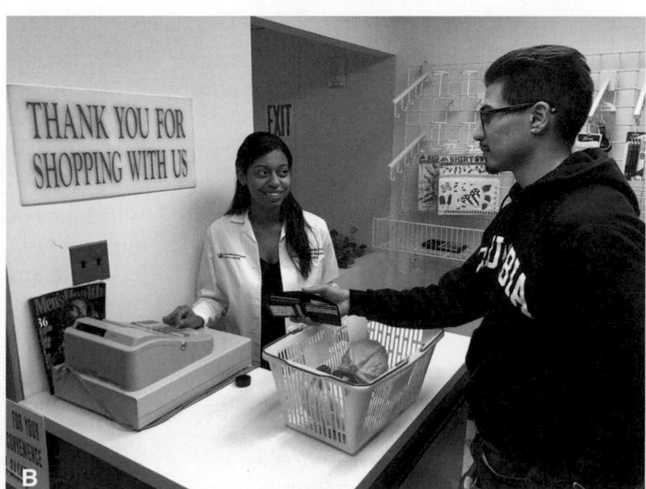

Figure 34-4. Creating functional settings in the clinic: simulated grocery store. **A.** Simulated grocery aisles with appropriate food items. **B.** Simulated grocery checkout area.

- In instances where this may be difficult in certain facilities, use other functional environments within the facility. This may include the cafeteria, gift store, office space, and chapel.
- Encourage family members to bring in the client's own clothing, grooming equipment, leisure items, and any other commonly used items such as iPads, diaries, and photo albums.

Practice Functional Tasks or Close Simulations to Find Effective and Efficient Strategies for Performance

The OT-TOA is completely consistent with traditional OT principles. The OT-TOA clearly states that the basis of intervention must be the practice of client-chosen tasks, components of those tasks, or close simulations of those tasks. The research is clear that this approach is effective[26,27] (see the Evidence table at the end of the chapter). On the other hand, little to no evidence exits demonstrating that rote exercise translates into meaningful changes in task performance and the resumption of life roles.

Provide Opportunities for Practice Outside of Therapy Time

As described above, practice is a potent variable in the development of motor skills and skill acquisition. Unfortunately, it has become clear that the amount of time allotted for therapy by insurance may not be sufficient to make these meaningful changes. Therapists must place as much emphasis on structuring client's time use outside of therapy as they do on developing in-clinic intervention plans. Suggestions include[21]:

- Encouraging homework. This may include practicing specific tasks or parts of specific tasks. Identifying tasks that remain challenging. Continuing to participate in tasks that have been mastered.
- For hospital-based therapists, encourage bedside practice of tasks that are safe in between therapy sessions. Tasks can be brought in by family members or low-cost tasks are provided by the therapist. Tasks may include playing cards, practicing manipulating cutlery, practice of rolling and bridging, and bedside ADLs.

Use Contemporary Motor Learning Principles in Training or Retraining Skills

As described above in this chapter and summarized in Table 34-2, integrating motor learning principles into intervention plans based on the OT-TOA is critical to train or retrain skills after an acquired brain injury. Research also supports the use of these principles[4,7,17] (see the Evidence table at the end of the chapter).

Minimize Ineffective and Inefficient Movement Patterns

After acquired brain injury, it is common for clients to use ineffective and inefficient movement patterns in the limbs and trunk. Mathiowetz identified several strategies that therapists can use to reduce ineffective and inefficient movement (Table 34-3 and Fig. 34-5).

Table 34-3. Strategies to Reduce Ineffective and Inefficient Movement Patterns Based on the Occupational Therapy Task-Oriented Approach

GENERAL STRATEGY	SPECIFIC EXAMPLES
Remediate a client factor (impairment) if it is the critical control parameter.	Multiple client factors can limit the learning or relearning of tasks. Examples include decreased balance, pain, depression, apraxia, visual impairment, weakness, decreased attention, etc. If the therapist determines that a specific client factor is a critical control parameter, remediation may be in order. See Chapters 8, 9, 11, 12, 14, and 17 for more details.
Adapt the environment, modify the task, use assistive technology, and/or reduce the effects of gravity.	Many examples fall under this strategy: prescription of power wheeled mobility, adapting bathrooms and outfitting them with durable medical equipment, using reminder functions on smart phones, educating in the use of adaptive dressing or feeding devices, using mobile arm supports for upper limb retraining, etc.
For persons with poor control of movement, constrain the degrees of freedom.	When movement is complex and requires the control of multiple joints simultaneously, movements tend to become more difficult, less efficient, and less fluid. Strategies to simplify movement and decrease the number of joints moving simultaneously (decreasing the degrees of freedom) may include using orthotics to stabilize or immobilize joints, providing external postural support, retraining movement patterns such as sliding the hand across a surface as opposed to reaching in space, increasing the diameter on the handles of daily living equipment, etc. See Chapters 21, 22, 25, 26, and 27 for more details.
For persons who do not use returned function in their involved extremities, use constraint-induced movement therapy (CIMT).	CIMT is an evidence based upper limb training approach that includes restraint of the unimpaired upper limb, repetitive massed task practice and shaping of the involved limb, and a transfer package to assure carryover of training in real world situations. See Chapters 16 and 36 for more details.

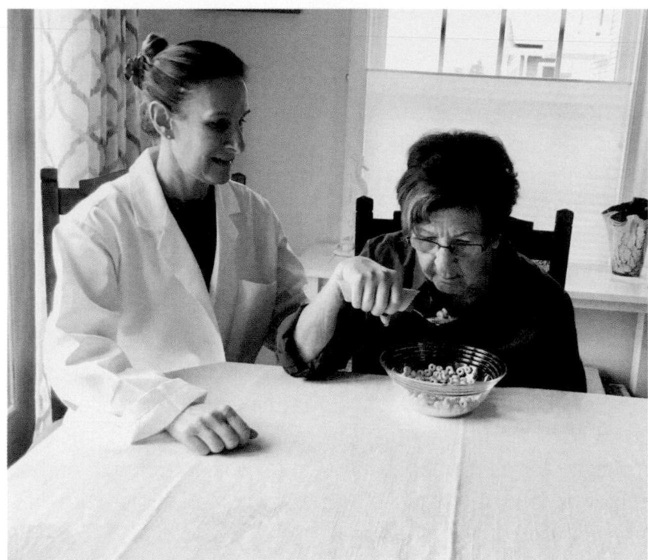

Figure 34-5. Minimizing ineffective and inefficient movement patterns during feeding: task is modified by using a built-up handled utensil and degrees of freedom are reduced by maintaining the elbow in contact with the table surface.

Evidence

When the principles of the OT-TOA approach were first developed and disseminated, several case studies were published demonstrating the early success of this approach and the practical clinical application. Flinn successfully demonstrated the use of the approach to improve occupational performance for an adult living with hemiplegia.[28] Gillen published two separate case studies demonstrating how the approach could be utilized to improve ADL[29] and functional mobility[30] for individuals with ataxia. More recently, Preissner[31] published a case study demonstrating the use of the OT-TOA for a person with significant cognitive limitations after stroke in which the client successfully met her personal goals.

Almhdawi et al.[20,32] present the strongest evidence to date regarding the OT-TOA. Their study evaluated functional and impairment efficacies of the OT-TOA on the more-affected upper extremity (UE) of persons post-stroke. The authors used a randomized single-blinded cross-over trial and recruited 20 participants post-stroke (mean chronicity = 62 months) who demonstrated at least 10° active more-affected shoulder flexion and abduction and elbow flexion-extension. Participants were randomized into immediate ($n = 10$) and delayed intervention ($n = 10$) groups. Immediate group had 6 weeks of 3 hours per week TOA intervention followed by 6 weeks of no-intervention control. The delayed intervention group underwent the reverse order. The authors utilized functional measures (Canadian Occupational Performance Measure [COPM], Motor Activity Log [MAL], and Wolf Motor Function Test [WMFT]) as well as impairment measures (UE active range of motion and handheld dynamometry strength). Measurements were obtained at baseline, cross over, and study end. The OT-TOA intervention showed statistically higher functional change scores. COPM performance and satisfaction scores were 2.83 and 3.46 units greater, respectively ($p < 0.001$), MAL amount of use and quality of use scores were 1.1 and 0.87 units greater, respectively ($p < 0.001$), WMFT time was 8.35 seconds faster ($p = 0.009$). The OT-TOA impairment outcomes were not significantly larger than control ones. The authors concluded that the OT-TOA appears to be an effective UE post-stroke rehabilitation approach inducing clinically meaningful functional improvements.

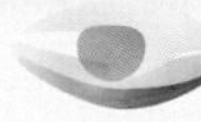

CASE STUDY

Patient Information

Angelina is a 70-year-old Italian-American female who is a retired seamstress. She lives with her husband, Giovani, in a three-bedroom, single-level home in a suburban area. They have two adult children and four grandchildren. Angelina and Giovani babysit for their eldest daughter's children, ages 5 and 7, after school 3 days per week. Angelina also performs the majority of the daily household duties, such as cooking, cleaning, and doing laundry.

Angelina was discharged home after receiving intensive inpatient rehabilitation for residual deficits associated with a left-middle cerebral artery stroke. Home occupational therapy services were recommended to assure that Angelina was safe and that she was beginning to generalize strategies she had learned in inpatient rehabilitation to the home environment. Eventually, Angelina would transition to outpatient services.

Assessment Process and Results

Following the evaluation framework of the OT-TOA, the occupational therapist used the Role Checklist to determine what roles Angelina performed prior to the stroke, what roles she feels she is currently capable of performing, and what roles she would like to perform in the future. Angelina identified the roles of "home maintainer" and "caregiver" as being the most important to her and her family. The therapist also administered the Canadian Occupational Performance Measure (COPM) to identify the important occupations that Angelina associated with those roles. She identified the following five occupations as being most important: (1) preparing meals, (2) doing laundry, (3) grocery shopping, (4) getting her grandchildren a snack after school, and (5) playing catch with her 7-year-old grandson. Out of a possible score of 10 (higher scores indicate better

(continued)

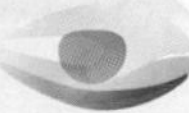

CASE STUDY *(continued)*

performance and greater satisfaction), she scored her present performance in and satisfaction with these five occupations as follows:

- Preparing meals: performance = 3, satisfaction = 2
- Doing laundry: performance = 3, satisfaction = 1
- Grocery shopping: performance = 2, satisfaction = 1
- Getting her grandchildren a snack: performance = 3, satisfaction = 2
- Playing catch: performance = 2, satisfaction = 1

Guided by the COPM results, the therapist evaluated Angelina's ability to engage in the identified tasks using direct observation of task performance focusing on both the performance outcome and the process in order to identify motor behaviors used to accomplish the task goal and to identify environmental supports and barriers to task performance.

The following client factors were identified as significant limiting factors during task performance:

- Sensorimotor: weakness and impaired joint coordination impacting the right dominant upper extremity resulting in reduced upper limb motor skills and impaired dynamic standing balance
- Cognitive: mild word finding deficits impacting verbal communication
- Psychosocial: easily frustrated by limitations

The following environmental factors were identified as barriers to task performance:

- Location of items in the kitchen and in the laundry room—outside of Angelina's current motor capabilities (e.g., reaching and balance abilities)
- Uneven terrain in the backyard where Angelina typically plays catch with her grandson—creates further demands on postural control
- Family's limited understanding of Angelina's challenges
- Angelina's belief that she should be able to do everything just as she has always done in the past without assistance from anyone.

Occupational Therapy Problem List

- Weakness and difficulty combining joint motions of the right UE resulting in inefficient forward, side, and overhead reaching and a reduced ability to transport and manipulate objects with the right hand
- Decreased dynamic standing balance resulting in the upper limbs being yoked to the postural system during upright activities
- Decreased verbal communication impacting her ability to communicate with family members
- Decreased coping skills

Occupational Therapy Goal List

- Angelina will be able to prepare a simple family meal with minimal family support by 6 weeks.
- Angelina will be able to assist her husband with unpacking the groceries by 6 weeks.
- Angelina will be able to fold the laundry while seated at the kitchen table by 6 weeks.
- Angelina will be able to play a modified game of catch with her grandson by 6 weeks.

Intervention

As Angelina was receiving occupational therapy services in her home, two guiding principles of the OT-TOA were embedded into the intervention plan: (1) create an environment that uses the common challenges of everyday life and (2) practice functional tasks or close simulations to find effective and efficient strategies for performance. What follows is an example of the implementation of the OT-TOA intervention principles with reference to one of Angelina's goals.

Angelina was initially treated in her kitchen to work on her meal preparation goal and to attempt to remediate her decreased standing balance and dominant upper limb weakness that the therapist identified as critical control parameters.

In her first session, the therapist allowed Angelina to select, out of a choice of three, which simple meal preparation task she would like to perform. Angelina selected making a pitcher of iced tea from powder and a bowl of ramen noodles. The therapist had Angelina standing at her kitchen counter with a chair behind her to begin the simple meal preparation activity. While standing, Angelina was taught to use her impaired upper limb as a stabilizer to compensate for her poor balance. Angelina was provided with an adapted one-handed scissors with suction cups, an adapted cutting board, and a rocker knife. She was taught to open the ice tea powder and ramen package with the adapted scissors and to cut lemons with the adapted cutting board and rocker knife. The therapist instructed Angelina to focus her attention on the closure of the scissors when cutting open the packages, and the position and direction of the movement of the rocker knife when cutting the lemons. The therapist instructed Angelina to cut one of the lemons in half for squeezing and the other lemon into slices and wedges that would be used for garnishing. This allowed Angelina the opportunity to practice using the rocker knife in several different ways. After this simple meal preparation task, the therapist encouraged Angelina to use her impaired arm to wipe down the counter. The therapist provided verbal feedback regarding Angelina's task performance after the session. As Angelina progressed, she was able to stabilize the lemon with her impaired limb without the cutting board and was able to bilaterally squeeze the juice out of the lemon using a standard juicer. The first meal that Angelina prepared for her family was a garden salad and traditional pizza from premade dough. Angelina was able to make both the salad and the pizza while in the standing position. She utilized her impaired limb to stabilize the vegetables while slicing and dicing them in preparation of making the salad, and she rolled out the premade pizza dough with both arms using a rolling pin with one built-up handle. For safety, Giovanni transferred the pizza to the oven and eventually to the table. Angelina was able to walk to the table to serve the salad with a rolling kitchen cart.

Evidence Table of Interventions Studies

Intervention	Description	Participants	Dosage	Research Design	Benefit	Statistical Significance
Contextual interference can facilitate motor learning in older adults and in individuals with Parkinson disease (PD).[18]	Study evaluated the effects of blocked practice (BP) versus random practice (RP) conditions on the learning of a peg sequencing task using a Nine-Hole Pegboard. Three patterns were practiced under BP conditions and three patterns under RP conditions. Time to complete the patterns (MT) and the number of errors were recorded. After completing the acquisition phases, participants completed a free and cued recall test as well as a transfer test 24 hours and 1 week later.	Fourteen people with PD (M age = 62.1 years, SD = 7.7 years) and 14 healthy age-matched control participants (M age = 63.2 years, SD = 6.6 years). Participants with PD had a Hoehn and Yahr stage of I–III, and a unified Parkinson Disease Rating Scale average motor score of 19.14. Participants were excluded if they had any neurological disease other than PD, a musculoskeletal problem of their dominant arm, color blindness, a Mini-Mental State Examination score of <24 of 30.	Both for BP and RP acquisition phases, participants completed 18 trials in each of three movement patterns for a total of 54 trials in each practice schedule. BP: the same movement pattern was practiced for 18 trials in a block for each of the three patterns. RP: in each block of 18 trials, 6 trials of each of the patterns were presented in a random order.	Nonrandomized controlled trial with follow-up. Level 2	For both groups, performance during skill acquisition was superior during BP rather than RP; however, RP was superior to BP for delayed recall and transfer of training to a novel task. Thus, both patients with PD and elderly healthy controls may benefit from RP conditions.	Acquisition phase: mean MT during BP was significantly shorter than that observed during RP ($p = 0.006$). Delayed recall: main effect of schedule: MT was significantly shorter following acquisition that consisted of RP as opposed to BP ($p < 0.001$) MT during the cued recall test was essentially unchanged from the 24-hour to 1-week delay, whereas mean MT for free recall decreased from 24 hours. Fewer errors were committed following RP than following BP ($p < 0.001$). Delayed transfer tests: MT was significantly less following RP as opposed to after BP ($p = 0.001$). In all conditions, MT was significantly slower for the group with PD as compared to controls.
Does provision of extrinsic feedback result in improved motor learning in the upper limb (UL) post-stroke? A systematic review of the evidence[8]	Review evaluated the effects of extrinsic feedback as opposed to no feedback on UL motor learning in adults post-stroke.	Included nine studies: six randomized controlled trials (RCTs), two pre–post designs, and one cohort study.	Varied in each study	Systematic review of published RCTs and pre–post designs. Studies were evaluated for methodological quality and the overall strength of the evidence was graded. Level 1	Stroke survivors are able to use explicit feedback to improve motor performance of both the more-affected and less-affected UL; KP may produce greater long-term benefits. However, further research is required to determine optimal type, delivery medium, and schedule of feedback.	Strong (Level 1) evidence for the effectiveness of feedback for motor learning using more-affected limb and Level 2b evidence using the less-affected limb.

(*continued*)

Evidence Table of Interventions Studies (*continued*)

Intervention	Description	Participants	Dosage	Research Design	Benefit	Statistical Significance
Influence of task-oriented training (TOT) content on skilled arm–hand performance in stroke: a systematic review[7]	Review evaluated the underlying training components currently used in TOT and assessed the effects of these components on skilled arm–hand performance in patients after a stroke.	Included 16 RCTs; total of 528 patients, all adults post-stroke.	Interventions ranged from 20 to 120 minutes per day; frequencies of sessions per week ranged from 3 to 7; intervention lengths ranged from 3 to 20 weeks.	Systematic review of RCT published through 3/2009. Studies were evaluated for methodological quality. Level 1	The total number of components used in an intervention was not associated with the posttreatment ES. "Distributed practice" and "feedback" were associated with the largest postintervention ES. "Random practice" and "use of clear functional goals" were associated with the largest follow-up ES.	Fifteen TOT components thought to contribute to motor learning were identified. All but three components were associated with large postintervention and follow-up MESs ($d > 0.533$). Components that were associated with the largest postintervention ES are "distributed practice" (MES = 2.39), "feedback" (MES = 1.95), "within task exercise variability" (MES = 1.72), "random practice" (MES = 1.72).
Efficacy of OT-task-oriented approach in UE post-stroke rehabilitation[32]	Individualized, client-centered approach applying motor learning and motor control principles; Canadian Occupational Performance Measure (COPM) results guided task selection for practice. Tasks were intensively practiced for 70% of therapy time. Remaining 30% of time was spent on supplemental exercises. Log book was used to monitor compliance.	$N = 20$, adults, $M = 62.1 \pm 46.11$ months post-stroke with some movement in affected UL	Task-oriented intervention was provided in two 1.5-hour sessions/week for 6 weeks. Plus, homework functional and impairment exercises (1–1.5 hours day on average)	Randomized cross-over trial. Level 1	Clinically, significant improvements in UE function noted postintervention and significant improvements noted in perceived performance and satisfaction with performance of client-chosen tasks	Mean change scores (SD) favored the treatment group for five out of six functional measures as follows: COPM: performance = 2.83 (1.70), $p < 0.001$; $d = 1.66$. COPM: satisfaction = 3.46 (2.17), $p < 0.001$; $d = 1.59$. Motor activity log: AOU = 1.11 (0.79), $p < 0.001$; $d = 1.41$; HW = 0.87 (0.65), $p < 0.001$; $d = 1.34$. Wolf motor function test: time = −8.35 (12.46) $p < 0.009$; $d = -0.67$. Function: 0.20 (0.52), $p < 0.126$; $d = -0.39$. No significant differences noted on impairment outcome measures.

Repetitive task training (RTT) to improve functional ability after stroke[27]	Review evaluated the effects of RTT on the primary outcomes of upper limb (UL) function and lower limb (LL) function/balance, and secondary outcomes of activities of daily living (ADL), global motor function and quality of life of adults post-stroke.	Included 33 studies (32 RCTs) with 1,853 participants. All adults post-stroke. Studies included a wide range of tasks to practice, including lifting a ball, walking, standing up from sitting, and circuit training with a different tasks at each station.	The number of hours of task practice varied from $<$10 hours of training to $>$40 hours of training and intervention lengths ranged from 2 to 20 weeks.	Systematic review of RCTs or quasi-RCTs published through June 2016. Studies were evaluated for methodological quality and the overall strength of the evidence was graded. Level I	In comparison to usual care, people who practiced functional tasks showed small improvements in UL function and walking. Improvements in UL and LL function were maintained up to 6 months. Further research is needed to determine the best type of task practice, and whether more sustained practice could show better results.	Low-quality evidence that RTT improves arm function (standardized mean difference (SMD) 0.25, 95% confidence interval (CI) 0.01–0.49); hand function (SMD 0.25, 95% CI 0.00–0.51), and lower limb functional measures (SMD 0.29, 95% CI 0.10–0.48). Moderate-quality evidence that RTT improves walking distance (mean difference (MD) 34.80, 95% CI 18.19–51.41) and functional ambulation (SMD 0.35, 95% CI 0.04–0.66). Small effect size that was statistically significant (SMD 0.28, 95% CI 0.10–0.45) suggesting RTT improves ADL.

References

1. Gillen G, Nilsen DM. Motor function and occupational performance. In: Schnell BG, ed. *Willard and Spackman's Occupational Therapy, Centennial Edition.* 13th ed. Philadelphia, PA: Wolters Kluwer; 2019.
2. Schumway-Cook A, Woollacott M. *Motor Control: Translating Research into Clinical Practice.* Baltimore, MD: Lippincott Williams & Wilkins; 2017.
3. Mathiowetz V, Bass-Haugen J. Motor behavior research: implications for therapeutic approaches to CNS dysfunction. *Am J Occup Ther.* 1994;48:733–745.
4. Schmidt R, Lee TD, Winstein C, Wulf G, Zelaznik. *Motor Control and Learning a Behavioral Emphasis.* 6th ed. Champaign, IL: Human Kinetics; 2019.
5. Schmidt R, Wrisberg, CA. *Motor Learning and Performance.* 3rd ed. Champlain, IL: Human Kinetics; 2014.
6. Chen JL, Fujii S, Schlaug G. The use of augmented auditory feedback to improve arm reaching in stroke: a case series. *Disabil Rehabil.* 2016;38(11):1115–1124.
7. Timmermans AA, Spooren AI, Kingma H, Seelen HA. Influence of task-oriented training content on skilled arm-hand performance in stroke: a systematic review. *Neurorehabil Neural Repair.* 2010;24(9):858–870.
8. Subramanian SK, Massie CL, Malcolm MP, Levin MF. Does provision of extrinsic feedback result in improved motor learning in the upper limb poststroke? A systematic review of the evidence. *Neurorehabil Neural Repair.* 2010;24(2):113–124.
9. Ghai S, Ghai I, Schmitz G, Effenberg AO. Effect of rhythmic auditory cueing on Parkinsonian gait: a systematic review and meta-analysis. *Sci Rep.* 2018;8(1):506.
10. Landers M, Wulf G, Wallmann H, Guadagnoli M. An external focus of attention attenuates balance impairment in patients with Parkinson's disease who have a fall history. *Physiotherapy.* 2005;91(3):152–158.
11. Wulf G, Landers M, Lewthwaite R, Tollner T. External focus instructions reduce postural instability in individuals with Parkinson disease. *Phys Ther.* 2009;89(2):162–168.
12. Fasoli S, Trombly CA, Tickle-Degnen L, Verfaellie MH. Effect of instructions on functional reach in persons with and without cerebrovascular accident. *Am J Occup Ther.* 2002;56:380–390.
13. Beck EN, Intzandt BN, Almeida QJ. Can dual task walking improve in Parkinson's disease after external focus of attention exercise? A single blind randomized controlled trial. *Neurorehabil Neural Repair.* 2018;32(1):18–33.
14. Kim GJ, Hinojosa J, Rao AK, Batavia M, O'Dell MW. Randomized trial on the effects of attentional focus on motor training of the upper extremity using robotics with individuals after chronic stroke. *Arch Phys Med Rehabil.* 2017;98(10):1924–1931.
15. Kal EC, van der Kamp J, Houdijk H, Groet E, van Bennekom CA, Scherder EJ. Stay focused! The effects of internal and external focus of attention on movement automaticity in patients with stroke. *PLoS One.* 2015;10(8):e0136917.
16. Page SJ, Hade EM, Pang J. Retention of the spacing effect with mental practice in hemiparetic stroke. *Exp Brain Res.* 2016;234(10):2841–2847.
17. Krakauer J. Motor learning: its relevance to stroke recovery and neurorehabilitation. *Curr Opin Neurol.* 2006;19:84–90.
18. Sidaway B, Ala B, Baughman K, et al. Contextual interference can facilitate motor learning in older adults and in individuals with Parkinson's disease. *J Mot Behav.* 2016;48(6):509–518.
19. Mathiowetz V, Bass-Haugen J. Assessing abilities and capacities: motor behavior. In: Radomski MV, Trombly Latham CA, eds. *Occupational Therapy for Physical Dysfunction.* 6th ed. Philadelphia, PA: Lippincott Williams & Wilkins; 2008:187–211.
20. Almhdawi K, Mathiowetz V, Bass JD. Assessing abilities and capacities: motor planning and performance. In: Radomski MV, Trombly Latham, CA, eds. *Occupational Therapy for Physical Dysfunction.* 7th ed. Philadelphia, PA: Wolters Kluwer; 2013:242–275.
21. Mathiowetz V. Task-oriented approach to stroke rehabilitation. In: Gillen G, ed. *Stroke Rehabilitation: A Function-Based Approach.* 4th ed. St. Louis, MO: Elsevier; 2016:59–78.
22. Barris R, Oakley F, Kielhofner G. The role checklist. In: Hemphill B, ed. *Mental Health Assessment in Occupational Therapy.* Thorofare, NJ: Slack; 1988.
23. Kielhofner G. *User's manual for the OPHI-II.* Chicago, IL: Model of Human Occupation Clearing House; 1988.
24. Law M. *The Canadian Occupational Performance Measure.* 4th ed. Ottawa, Canada: CAOT Publications ACE; 2005.
25. Fisher A. *Assessment of Motor and Process Skills.* 4th ed. Fort Collins, CO: Three Star Press; 2001.
26. Nilsen D, Gillen G, Geller D, Hreha K, Osei E, Saleem GT. Effectiveness of interventions to improve occupational performance for adults with stroke. *Am J Occup Ther.* 2015;69(1):6901180030p1–6901180030p9.
27. French B, Thomas LH, Coupe J, et al. Repetitive task training for improving functional ability after stroke. *Cochrane Database Syst Rev.* 2016;11:CD006073.
28. Flinn N. A task-oriented approach to the treatment of a client with hemiplegia. *Am J Occup Ther.* 1995;49(6):560–569.
29. Gillen G. Improving activities of daily living performance in an adult with ataxia. *Am J Occup Ther.* 2000;54(1):89–96.
30. Gillen G. Case Report—Improving mobility and community access in an adult with ataxia. *Am J Occup Ther.* 2002;56:462–466.
31. Preissner K. Case Report—Use of the occupational therapy task-oriented approach to optimize the motor performance of a client with cognitive limitations. *Am J Occup Ther.* 2010;64:727–734.
32. Almhdawi KA, Mathiowetz VG, White M, delMas RC. Efficacy of occupational therapy task-oriented approach in upper extremity post-stroke rehabilitation. *Occup Ther Int.* 2016;23(4):444–456.

Chapter 35

Functional Uses of Neurological Approaches: Rood, Brunnstrom, Proprioceptive Neuromuscular Facilitation, and Neuro-Developmental Treatment

Kris M. Gellert and Karen Halliday Pulaski

LEARNING OBJECTIVES

This chapter will allow the reader to:

1. Describe the following sensorimotor frames of reference that shape evaluation and treatment for clients with neurological insults: Rood, Brunnstrom, Proprioceptive Neuromuscular Facilitation (PNF), and Neuro-Developmental Treatment (NDT).
2. Demonstrate an appreciation for the historical impact and the evolution of these four major frames of reference.
3. Compare and contrast the frames of reference and how they guide occupational therapy practice.
4. Apply the principles of Brunnstrom, PNF, and NDT to the evaluation process.
5. Formulate a basic treatment plan based on PNF and NDT.

CHAPTER OUTLINE

TERMINOLOGY

Associated reactions: movements on one side of the body that are facilitated by providing resistance on the other side of the body; for example, resistance to the arm in flexion on the intact side will facilitate flexion in the arm on affected side; Brunnstrom used this as treatment technique.

Facilitatory: treatment that increases increase muscle tone/activation.

Inhibitory: treatment that reduces tone/decrease muscle activation.

Limb synergies: patterns of movement acting as a "bound" unit in a primitive, reflexive manner in both the upper extremity (UE) and the lower extremity (LE); in this chapter, we focus on the UE (e.g., UE extension limb synergy and UE flexor limb synergy).

Proprioception: the ability to sense the position and location and orientation and movement of the body and its parts.

Introduction

Occupational therapy (OT) is in part defined, supported, and explained by the various frames of reference in which the profession is grounded. This chapter provides a review of four major sensorimotor frames of reference that have shaped and continue to shape the practice implemented currently with clients with neurological impairments. OT has its own unique way of translating, understanding, and using these frames of reference to guide assessment and treatment. For OT, the overall goal is always to assist our clients to engage in meaningful activities tied to the roles that define who the client is and what the client values. Because of this, for OT, these frames of reference are far more encompassing than the goal of restoring more normal movement. The occupational therapist should always be asking "why" the patient needs to move better—in order to do what? In other words, the goal isn't for more normal movement in and of itself; the goal is to move more normally in order to allow the client to do something meaningful. It is the meaningful activities that are the structure of the client's life roles. These roles take place within a psychosocial and temporal context. These approaches for OT should always be embedded in this concept.

The individuals who developed these frames of reference were able to begin to define and give structure to a new model of assessment and/or intervention for helping clients with stroke or brain injury. They were pioneers in their respective fields, and many of the concepts that they initiated in the 1940s and 1950s are still used today. Many of the earlier frames of reference were based on hierarchical and reflexive theories of motor control. As the body of scientific research has grown for motor control, motor learning, and motor development, the profession has moved to using dynamic systems theory (DST) to understand in part the complexity of motor mastery. The reflex hierarchy refers to the belief that normal motor development was attributed to the refinement of cortical networking in the central nervous system (CNS). This hierarchical system results in the emergence of higher levels of control over lower level reflexes. The belief at the time was that when CNS damage occurred, an individual would revert to reflexive over cortical processing. Today, in rehabilitation, many of the techniques are supported by DST, which recognizes a constant interplay and interaction among many systems in the body (e.g., sensory, motor, cognitive, pulmonary, perceptual) and with the external world (e.g., gravity, inertia, fear, excitement).[1,2] When there is interference in one system, other systems have some ability to adapt or compensate for that change.

In practice, occupational therapists use many frames of reference for assessment and/or treatment and do not limit themselves to any one frame of reference.[3] Some of these frames of reference are used far less frequently today. As our understanding of neuroplasticity and recovery from a neurological insult grows, rehabilitation efforts have shifted toward inclusion of remediation of the impairments to restore as much functional ability as possible rather than just focusing on compensation. Although these frames of reference are applicable to children, adolescents, and adults, the scope of this chapter focuses primarily on the rehabilitation of the adult client. This chapter provides an overview of the following frames of reference: Rood, Brunnstrom, Proprioceptive Neuromuscular Facilitation (PNF), and Neuro-Developmental Treatment (NDT). A more in-depth review is provided for PNF and NDT because these frames of reference are more widely used today.

Rood Frame of Reference

Background and Historical Significance

Margaret Rood (1909–1984) was a pioneer in providing one of the earliest attempts at developing a formal, systematic way to understand and organize rehabilitation efforts and interventions with children and adults with neurological impairment.[4] She was trained initially as an occupational therapist and then earned her degree in physical therapy as well. She was considered a master clinician and educator and has been formally recognized by both the physical and OT professions.

Much of Rood's approach, developed in the 1950s, is not currently practiced in clinics today as the growing body of motor learning research does not necessarily support many of her early assumptions; however, it is important to understand the impact that Rood has had on the development of the rehabilitation profession as well as to recognize that other major frames of reference evolved out of her initial efforts.

Evaluation and Intervention Principles

Key Concepts

1. Normalized muscle tone (which is influenced by sensory input) is required in order to develop motor control and mastery of a desired movement. Rood's original approach emphasized the importance of normalizing muscle tone first before there could be an ability to elicit a specific motor response.
2. Flexion and extension patterns of movement are evident in our daily occupations. Rood emphasized the importance of using a specific developmental sequence of movement in order to achieve these patterns of movement.
3. Repetition of muscular responses is crucial to learning movement patterns.
4. The ability for clients to engage in occupations or meaningful functional activity is required for development of normal movement. In other words, clients need to learn motor patterns within the context of functional activity, not just in isolation of a learned movement pattern.

Rood's approach was employed predominantly as a preparatory approach used before the client engaged in purposeful activities. She used a variety of sensorimotor techniques that she believed influenced tone and, therefore, the development of normal movement. She identified two types of sensorimotor techniques—**facilitatory** (those that would increase muscle tone/activation) and **inhibitory** (those that would reduce tone/decrease muscle activation).

Facilitatory Techniques

1. Heavy joint compression
2. Manual resistance to a body part
3. Quick stretch
4. Tapping
5. Vibration
6. Fast brushing
7. Vestibular stimulation (fast movement)

Inhibitory Techniques

1. Neutral warmth
2. Slow stroking
3. Light joint compression
4. Vestibular stimulation (slow movement)
5. Tendon pressure
6. Prolonged stretch

Four Components of Motor Control

Rood described four main components of motor control that she considered essential for movement during purposeful, directed activity:

1. ***Reciprocal innervation:*** Simply put, this implies that whereas the agonist muscle is contracting, the antagonist muscle is relaxing (e.g., to bend your elbow to wash your face, the biceps would contract, whereas the triceps would relax).
2. ***Co-contraction:*** The agonist and antagonist muscles co-contract at the same time to provide stability (e.g., the biceps and triceps co-contract to allow you to lean on your arm while putting on your mascara at a mirror with your other hand). This provides a basis for postural control.
3. ***Heavy work:*** This allows for mobility to be superimposed on stability.[5] Proximal muscles co-contract, whereas distal segments (i.e., arm, legs, hands, and feet) are fixed. Examples Rood provided were lifting, moving, pulling, and pushing.
4. ***Skill:*** Rood considered this the most advanced level of controlled movement. This requires that mobility and stability be combined. Proximal muscles (i.e., trunk) act as stabilizers, whereas distal segments are allowed to move freely (i.e., arms, legs, hands, and feet). Examples Rood provided were painting on an upright canvas, writing on a blackboard, and dancing.

Developmental Sequence

Finally, Rood believed that the way to master these four components of movement was through the progression of a developmental sequence. She based this assumption on her observations of how an infant develops and masters movement and theorized that clients with neurological impairment could also master movement in the same way. She used the previously identified facilitatory and inhibitory techniques to assist a client in progressing through this sequence. She theorized that each developmental sequence allowed the client to master various specific movement patterns and thus becomes a building block for the next posture. Because she viewed this as sequential, she believed each step must be mastered to allow the achievement of the next level of control. This sequence consisted of:

1. Supine withdrawal/flexion (total flexion in supine)
2. Rollover
3. Prone extension (prone with upper trunk/head extension)
4. Neck co-contraction (prone with isolated head extension)
5. Prone on elbows
6. All fours (quadruped)
7. Static standing
8. Walking

Use of the Rood Frame of Reference Today

Several assumptions and assertions in Rood's frame of reference are no longer empirically supported. Current motor theory suggests:

1. Neuromuscular function is complex and constantly changing, not linear. It is no longer viewed as simply a system where sensorimotor input leads to motor output.[6–8]
2. Tone is only one variable that impacts movement, and tone is constantly changing due to various factors such as demand of the task, temperature, and a client's emotional response.
3. In general, many of the facilitatory and inhibitory techniques are viewed as unpredictable. Therapists still use some of the techniques, and the reader will note this in other frames of reference. However, many of the initial techniques Rood discussed are no longer embraced in today's clinics. While Rood and others established guidelines for the use of many of these techniques, the sensorimotor input described is generally considered relatively passive in nature, short lasting, and unpredictable.[8] With today's current health care climate and its emphasis on short lengths of stays, efficiency, and efficacy, many of these techniques are no longer used in clinics.
4. Motor development for an adult following a neurological insult does not require a sequential developmental progression for mastery of a motor skill.[9] Many of these postures are still used today to develop specific motor control. For example, a therapist may choose to use prone on elbows to encourage development of neck extension, head control, and upper thoracic extension required for postural control in sitting and standing, as well as proximal shoulder stability. The position of kneeling may be used to facilitate trunk control, address postural control, and develop balance reactions. It is, however, no longer used in today's clinic with adult rehabilitation as a sequential progression. Adults have a mature system that has already "learned" these skills; and as such, an adult system differs from that of an infant.

There are several important assertions developed by Rood that do still impact the delivery of rehabilitation services today. It is important to keep in mind that Rood developed this frame of reference without the benefit of current research:

1. Rood was one of the first therapists to see the importance of having a theoretical-based approach for evaluation and treatment.
2. Rood identified the importance of engaging in purposeful, meaningful activity to promote motor learning. This is a cornerstone belief in the profession of OT for many reasons, not just motor learning.
3. Rood recognized the importance of repetition as being critical to motor learning. Repetition of a motor response for learning is empirically supported,[10,11] and this concept is widely used in physical rehabilitation today. Research helps to guide therapists on the types of repetition (such as blocked or random), as well as the need for variation within that repetition, frequency and intensity of repetition/practice, and how to cue and guide clients.[8,12–18]
4. Rood also recognized a deep connection between the sensory system and skilled movement.
5. Rood discussed the importance of the "art" of OT, which we now refer to as the therapeutic use of self.
6. Rood articulated the premise that therapists have the ability to influence the variables that impact movement, which is a one of the basic building blocks for neuromuscular education.
7. Rood developed a systematic way to begin to categorize movement that influences the language still used today (i.e., stability, mobility, postural control, and skill).

Brunnstrom Frame of Reference

Background and Historical Significance

The Brunnstrom approach was initially developed by Signe Brunnstrom (1898–1988), a physical therapist, in the 1950s. She was also one of the first therapists and researchers involved in developing a comprehensive approach to understanding stroke recovery and rehabilitation of the stroke survivor. Her approach encompassed both evaluation and treatment interventions and was based on her numerous years of providing care to survivors of stroke as well as the early work of Twitchell[19] who first described patterns of recovery following stroke. She designed a framework that describes what she viewed as a common progression or stages of motor recovery poststroke as well as a systematic approach to assessment and treatment based on her understanding of stroke recovery patterns. Brunnstrom theorized that effective and meaningful evaluation and treatment is based on understanding what she viewed as a "normal" motor response to a cerebral vascular event. This is often also called movement theory.[20]

Evaluation and Intervention Principles

Brunnstrom theorized that normal development of motor control in infants is first dominated by primitive reflexive movement patterns (e.g., tonic neck reflex, righting reflex, stepping reflex). These are involuntary mass patterns of movement that are in response to a specific stimulus. Gradually, as the brain and CNS develop, these reflexive movement patterns are modified by higher control centers of the brain and result in the development of isolated, voluntary control of motor movement (e.g., as a baby develops, she can flex her right arm when her head is turned to the right, thus overriding the tonic neck reflex). Brunnstrom theorized that when a client suffers a stroke, it results in damage to the CNS and thus disrupts the higher centers of CNS control. This disruption then causes the client to undergo what she termed revolution in reverse. In other words, without higher level central control to modify the primitive reflexes, the client reverts back to movement dominated by primitive reflexive movement patterns. The clients lose the ability for isolated, voluntary, controlled movement. While others viewed the loss of volitional control as abnormal, Brunnstrom viewed this reversal to primitive reflexive movement as a "normal response" relative to the damage caused to the CNS by the cerebral vascular event. Based on this belief, she theorized that movement dominated by reflexive, synergistic movement patterns and other supposed "abnormal" motor responses were actually a part of the normal process or progression that a client must go through to regain normal movement. She believed that the overall goal of rehabilitation, and therefore the role of the therapist, was to enhance the progression through very specific, predictable stages of recovery to achieve the ability for more normal and complex movement patterns. She developed a scale of stages of recovery for the upper extremity (UE) and the lower extremity (LE) based on the presence of **limb synergies** as well as the amount of isolated controlled movement at any given time in stroke recovery. She also developed very specific treatment goals and interventions based on each stage to facilitate the client's progression from one stage to the next.

Additional Assumptions of Brunnstrom Theory

1. Motor return is always proximal to distal.
2. Progress can be slow or rapid through stages, and progress can cease at any stage.
3. Clients gain flexion of primitive movement patterns first, then extension.
4. Clients first recover reflexive movement and then progress to isolated movement.
5. Clients achieve gross motor movement and then progress to isolated, selective movement.
6. Use of cutaneous (skin) and proprioceptive stimulus as well as reflexes will help facilitate a client as he or she progresses through the stages of recovery.
7. Stages of recovery are not necessarily discrete—a client may show movement patterns of two different stages at once.
8. Practice of movement patterns within the context of daily activities promotes motor recovery.

Assessment Based on Brunnstrom

Assessment should include, but is not necessarily limited to:

- *Sensory testing:* Specifically, **proprioception** and light touch as Brunnstrom advocated the use of these stimuli in particular to influence motor recovery. A therapist would need to understand the client's ability to use these inputs during treatment.
- *Associated reactions and reflexes* (tonic reflexes in particular): Brunnstrom also used these as a way to promote progression through the stages of recovery (e.g., she may use a tonic neck reflex stimulus or **associated reaction** to facilitate flexion in the affected UE).
- *Presence of limb synergies:* Brunnstrom assessed this both to determine stage of recovery and to assess if they could be used in treatment (both to facilitate progression to the next stage and during functional activity by the client).
- *Amount of voluntary movement a client can generate:* This would provide information to allow the therapist to identify the stage of recovery as well as for use in treatment for functional use.
- *Tests of motor speed* (i.e., bring hand to chin, then down to opposite knee rapidly)
- *Prehension ability in the hand* (e.g., wrist stabilization, mass grasp, prehension, fine motor)

Table 35-1 outlines a general description of the stages of recovery for both the UE and LE.

Table 35-1. Brunnstrom: Stages of Recovery for the Upper/Lower Extremity

STAGE	GENERAL DESCRIPTION
I	Tone is flaccid, no voluntary movement, muscle or reflexive responses.
II	Synergies can begin to be elicited reflexively, spasticity is developing.
III	Begin voluntary movement but only in synergy, spasticity may be significant.
IV	Spasticity begins to decrease; movement starting to deviate from synergy patterns.
V	Further decreased tone, increased ability to perform more complex movement patterns independent of synergy patterns
VI	Tone nearly normal with ability to do complex combinations of isolated movement
VII	Normal speed and coordination of motor function

Intervention Based on Brunnstrom

Clinicians today employ a limited use of Brunnstrom's approach because rehabilitation professionals try to prevent the development of abnormal and synergistic movements; reflexive movement is no longer considered a precursor to isolated, volitional movements.[21] Therefore, only a brief review of treatment approaches based on the stages of recovery are included in the scope of this chapter. The intention of the review is to briefly familiarize the therapist with the historical significance and impact of this frame of reference from a treatment intervention standpoint. Treatment goals and techniques are outlined in Table 35-2.

Early Stage of Recovery (Stages I–III)

The goal of therapy is to aid the client in developing and gaining full control over limb synergies; clients are encouraged to use this limb synergies within the context of functional activity. For example, a client may use a UE flexion pattern to carry a bag, attempt to brush his or her hair or drink from a cup.

Middle to Late Stages of Recovery (Stages IV–VI)

Once the client reaches the ability to fully perform and use limb synergies in functional ways (stage III), the goal of therapy is to aid the client in learning to modify these synergies and to work toward the development and use of simple and complex movement that deviates from synergistic movements. For example, the focus for a client moving from a stage III (control of full flexion synergy) to a stage IV (beginning to break away from synergistic movements) may include encouraging extension patterns in the UE via functional activity (such as wiping a table) through the use of facilitatory techniques. Assuming the client progresses through each stage, this would result in the client being able to perform isolated, voluntary movement of the UE and LE.

The following are some of the treatment interventions Brunnstrom used:

1. Tonic reflexes (e.g., having a client turn his head toward or away from his affected arm will facilitate different movement patterns)
2. Associated reactions
3. Cutaneous and stretch (proprioceptive) stimuli such as skin stimulation and weight bearing of the extremity
4. Positioning (e.g., side-lying on the affected side to discourage excessive tone in the extremities)
5. Facilitation of balance reactions and use of trunk rotation to either encourage or discourage limb synergies.

Table 35-2. Brunnstrom: Treatment Goals by Stage

STAGES	TREATMENT GOALS
Stages I–II	Goal: To try to facilitate increased muscle tone as well as promote the beginning development of limb synergies. Tone should be increasing during these stages.
Stages II–III	Goal: To assist the client in achieving full voluntary control of limb synergies and to learn to use these in functional activities. Tone will be at its peak at the end of stage III. For example, to use a flexion synergy pattern to bring a washcloth to the face.
Stages IV–V	Goal: To assist the client in beginning to break away from limb synergies and to begin to move to more isolated and complex patterns of movement. Tone should be decreasing. For example the ability to extend the elbow when doing shoulder flexion to reach into a cabinet.
Stages V–VI	Goal: Continue to assist the client in developing more complex isolated movements as well as increase the speed of movement. For example, to be able to use normal isolated movement to bring a washcloth to the face.
Stage VII	Client demonstrates normal isolated complex movement.

Use of Brunnstrom Frame of Reference Today

Much of Brunnstrom's assumptions are no longer believed to be absolutes for every client as clients recover from cerebral vascular events in a multitude of ways:

1. Motor recovery is not always proximal to distal.[22] For example, clients can demonstrate movement in their hand while having little to no movement proximally. Clients often present with mixed patterns of return in the affected UE.
2. Depending on the location and size of the stroke, clients may not exhibit any reflexive movement at all.
3. Current research would not support facilitation of progressing a patient through the stages of recovery.[9] Clients may use compensatory limb synergies to complete tasks if they do not have isolated control (e.g., UE flexion synergy to hold an object). However, this is no longer the "goal" of neuromuscular re-education.
4. As stated before, cutaneous and proprioceptive inputs can be unpredictable, passive in nature, and short lived. There are no real guidelines empirically developed for the use of many of Brunnstrom's interventions. This does not mean that therapists never use them but rather that there may be a need for further research to guide best practice.

Perhaps, the most widespread influence of Brunnstrom's work is the recognition that survivors of stroke have a unique recovery course; this course is individualized and varies from client to client. There are general patterns of movement, however, that clients with stroke may exhibit. These stages of recovery have allowed for the development of standardized assessment tools that are widely used today. Although current treatment approaches no longer embrace the concept of encouraging the development of reflexive, synergistic movement patterns, research is focusing on the assessment tools relative to consistent categorization, prognosis, and prediction for functional outcomes for motor recovery and independence with functional activities. One of the most commonly used tools today is the Fugl-Meyer assessment,[22] which is based on Twitchell's original work regarding motor return following hemiplegia[19] as well as Brunnstrom's stages of recovery.[20] This assessment tool is widely supported by research in terms of inter-rater reliability and validity.[23–28] This tool also allows therapists to "speak" a common language when discussing clients and their recovery from stroke. This assessment tool thus influences the treatment approach and goals that therapists may choose when developing a plan of care.

Proprioceptive Neuromuscular Facilitation Frame of Reference

The term Proprioceptive Neuromuscular Facilitation (PNF), in its literal sense, means techniques that use an awareness of body position and movement, through specific commands and cues directed at muscles and nerves, to help a client achieve new movement patterns. PNF is a useful tool to assist with both the assessment and intervention for clients with orthopedic or neurological diagnoses, which lead to movement problems.[29]

Background and Historical Significance

Developed initially by neurophysiologist and physician, Dr. Herman Kabat, the underlying philosophy of PNF is that all human beings, including those with disabilities, have untapped existing potential.[30] Kabat's goal was to develop a hands-on treatment approach that enabled therapists to analyze and assess a client's movement while at the same time facilitating more efficient strategies of functional movement, thus untapping the existing potential.

Dr. Kabat's early work was influenced by the work of Sister Kenny, a nurse who worked with clients with polio, and who used unique stretching and strengthening techniques. Kabat was also familiar with the work of Dr. Charles Sherrington relating to the functioning of the neuromuscular system; concepts of the reflex hierarchy, facilitation, and inhibition and the phenomenon of irradiation, which will be defined later in this chapter. Dr. Kabat, influenced by these abovementioned practitioners, also believed intervention directed at encouraging combinations of movements would be more effective than the traditional interventions of moving one joint at a time. When a person performs daily living skills, he or she moves with many combinations of movements, through many planes of movement, using rotational and diagonal movement components. Therefore, Kabat's frame of reference is based on functional human anatomy, as well as neurophysiology. Dr. Kabat combined the manual techniques used by Sister Kenny and the scientific concepts of Dr. Sherrington and began his Proprioceptive Facilitation. It was in the mid- to late 1940s that Dr. Kabat began his search for physical therapists, thus Margaret Knott, and later Dorothy Voss, became the first physical therapists to work closely with him. Voss later completed the current moniker by adding Neuromuscular to the title to highlight the emphasis on sensory input and motor output. Kabat, Knott, and Voss combined their analysis of functional movement with theories from motor development, motor control, motor learning, and neurophysiology in the development of the PNF approach.

Initially, the techniques were used to treat those with poliomyelitis and multiple sclerosis, but it soon became clear that these techniques could be applied to a much broader group. Today, the PNF frame of reference is widely used throughout the world,[31] and it has shown to be effective for clients with orthopedic, traumatic, and neurological insults or injuries.[29] Intensive postgraduate training courses are available in many countries today.

Evaluation and Intervention Principles of PNF

Dr. Kabat believed that all human beings, including those with disabilities, have untapped existing potential,[29] and as such, a therapist using the PNF approach would structure his or her therapy interventions in a manner to maximize that potential as related to human occupation. We know today that as human beings, we use movement as way to interact with our surroundings, and movement is critical to our ability to engage in daily occupations. The PNF approach encourages the treatment of the entire human being, not just the problem areas. This approach is always positive with an emphasis on what the client is able to do and building from that point. The goals of PNF treatments are developed to help a client perform at his or her highest functional level.

PNF assessment and treatment strategies are based on specific diagonal and rotational patterns of movement throughout the entire body, including the head/the neck (as vision is always combined with diagonal patterns), the trunk, and the limbs. Those using the PNF frame of reference understand that the trunk is the foundation for limb movement and function. The patterns of movement encouraged with the PNF frame of reference incorporate all three planes of movement (sagittal, frontal, and horizontal) simultaneously.

The clinician using PNF employs a multisensory approach:

- *Visual:* Vision assists in initiation and coordination of patterns of movement.
- *Auditory:* Tone of voice and specific verbal commands. A calm, quiet voice may soothe; whereas a loud, direct tone may excite.
- *Tactile:* Manual contacts and client's own touch provide tactile stimulation for movement. The facilitation of specific movement patterns provides consistent proprioceptive input to improve functional movement patterns for each client.

Critical PNF Concepts

- *Resistance:* Resistance is used to improve muscle contraction. Older terminology was "maximal" resistance, but this created confusion. Current literature suggests using the right amount of resistance for the desired muscle contraction. This will vary for each client, and even within one body may vary among different muscle groups. Resistance may be used to guide or strengthen movement patterns and can help to reinforce the specifics of each pattern, so eventually the client can replicate movements without (or with less) facilitation.
- *Stretch:* In PNF, the use of quick stretch is applied to all three elements of the movement pattern with emphasis on the rotational components. This may be applied in the client's available range of motion, even in the absence of full range of motion. Using the PNF quick stretch technique, the application of quick stretch is done using therapist's entire body, not just the arms and hands. This delivers a safer experience for the client.
- *Irradiation:* Also referred to as overflow or the spread of a response to stimulation—can be excitatory or inhibitory.
- *Traction or approximation:* The elongation or compression of the limbs and trunk to facilitate motion or stability.[29]
- *Body position/mechanics:* The therapist using PNF considers a starting position that will initially offer the most stability to the client, advancing to more challenging positions as skills are mastered. Therapists must also consider their own body positions relative to the movement sequence being facilitated.

Examples of PNF Techniques for Strengthening

- *Rhythmic initiation:* Cue "relax and let me move you" passive range of motion (PROM) repeat movement active assisted range of motion (AAROM) several times, then cue "Now you do it." Active range of motion (AROM)[32]
- Repeated contraction
- *Slow reversal:* The reverse of the diagonal movement. If D1 flexion is desired movement, reversal is D1 extension.
- Slow reversal hold
- *Rhythmic stabilization:* mid-range isometric contraction of the agonist followed by an isometric antagonist (co-contraction). No movement occurs. Effective for static strengthening and for clients with pain[32]

Examples of PNF Techniques for Stretching

- Contract relax
- Hold relax

PNF Movement Patterns

In all PNF patterns, movement occurs in a straight line with diagonal direction and rotational component. Each pattern is comprised of three movement components: flexion/extension, abduction/adduction, and rotation, as shown in Figures 35-1 through 35-5.[32]

- *Chopping:* Bilateral asymmetrical D1 extension. One arm performs the chop, and the other hand is placed on the lateral extensor surface of the distal forearm. The reversal of this pattern is the reverse of the chop.[32]
- *Lifting:* Bilateral asymmetrical D2 flexion. One arm performs the lift, whereas the other arm maintains contact on the lateral flexor side of the forearm. The opposite of this pattern is called the reverse of lift.[32]
- *Controlled mobility:* The ability to perform fluid reversing motions necessary to perform skilled activity.[32]
- *Reciprocal inhibition:* The mechanism whereby contracture of an agonist muscle produces inhibition of its antagonist.[32]

PNF Positions

When using PNF, careful consideration is given to the choices for starting and subsequent positions for

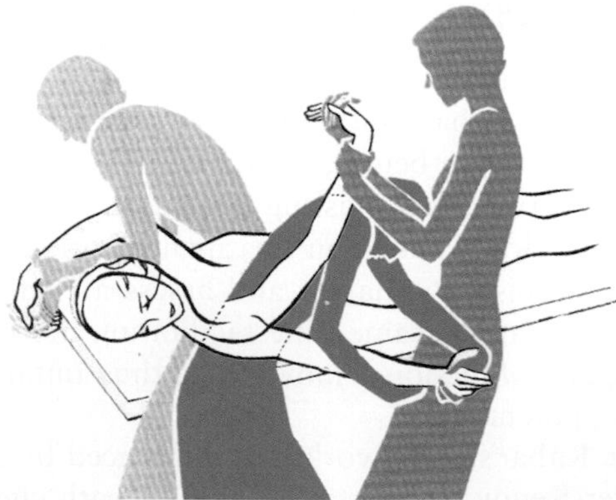

Figure 35-1. D1 Flexion: The final position of D1 flexion is shoulder flexion, adduction, and external rotation; elbow flexion; and supination so that the hand passes close to the ear on the opposite side of the head. Wrist, fingers, and thumb flex; and fingers and thumb adduct. (Used with permission of Voss DE, Iota MK, Myers BJ. *Proprioceptive Neuromuscular Facilitation: Patterns & Techniques*. 3rd ed. New York, NY: Harper & Row; 1985 and Rust K. Managing deficits of first level motor control capacities using Rood and proprioceptive neuromuscular facilitation techniques. In: *Occupational Therapy for Physical Dysfunction*. 7th ed. Philadelphia, PA: Lippincott Williams and Wilkins; 2014.)

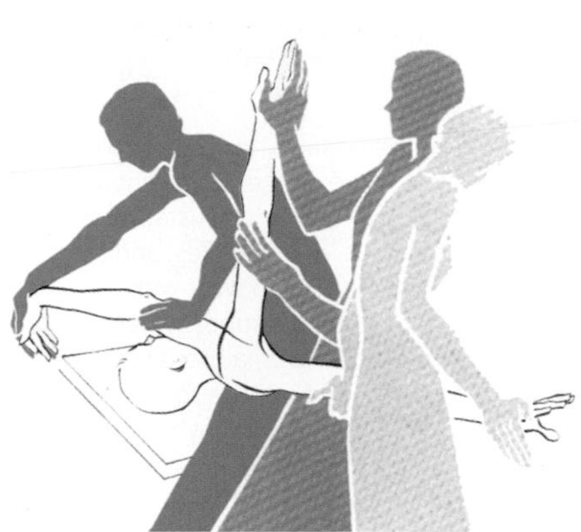

Figure 35-2. D1 Extension: The final position of D1 extension is shoulder extension, abduction, and internal rotation; elbow extension; and pronation so that the hand passes the hip on the same side of the body. The wrist, fingers, and thumb extend; and fingers and thumb abduct. During range of motion exercises, D1 extension is combined with its reciprocal D1 flexion. (Used with permission of Voss DE, Iota MK, Myers BJ. *Proprioceptive Neuromuscular Facilitation: Patterns & Techniques.* 3rd ed. New York, NY: Harper & Row; 1985 and Rust K. Managing deficits of first level motor control capacities using Rood and proprioceptive neuromuscular facilitation techniques. In: *Occupational Therapy for Physical Dysfunction*. 7th ed. Philadelphia, PA: Lippincott Williams and Wilkins; 2014.)

intervention (e.g., side-lying, prone on elbows, long sitting, tailor sitting, hands and knees, kneeling, half kneeling, short sitting, plantigrade). Positions are chosen when starting a treatment session to determine where the client will be supported, but also challenged to complete a task. Movement in and out of these positions may also be stressed within a treatment session because clients need to be able to adjust and change positions within a functional activity. For example, when getting

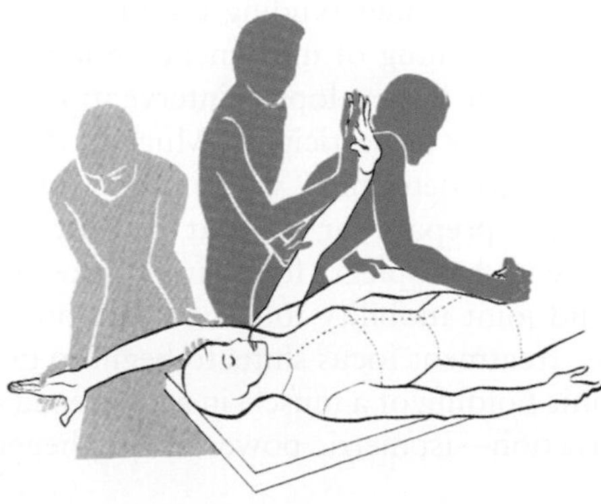

Figure 35-3. D2 Flexion: The final position of D2 flexion is shoulder flexion, abduction, and external rotation; elbow flexion; and supination so that the hand comes close to the ear on the same side of the head. Wrist extends, and fingers and thumb extend and abduct. (Used with permission of Voss DE, Iota MK, Myers BJ. *Proprioceptive Neuromuscular Facilitation: Patterns & Techniques.* 3rd ed. New York, NY: Harper & Row; 1985 and Rust K. Managing deficits of first level motor control capacities using Rood and proprioceptive neuromuscular facilitation techniques. In: *Occupational Therapy for Physical Dysfunction*. 7th ed. Philadelphia, PA: Lippincott Williams and Wilkins; 2014.)

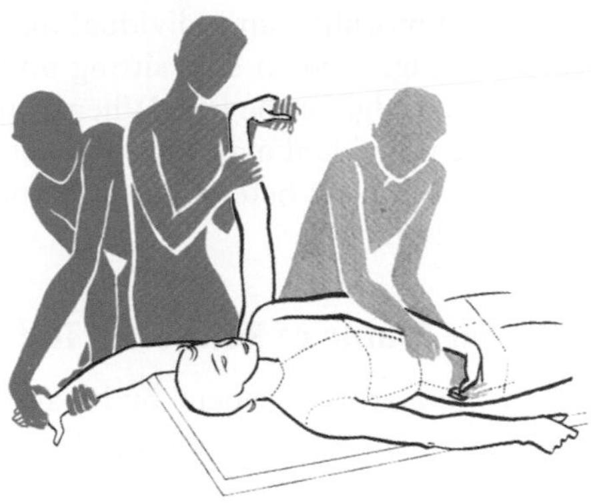

Figure 35-4. D2 Extension: The final position of D2 extension is shoulder extension, adduction, and internal rotation; elbow extension; and pronation so that the hand moves past the opposite hip. Wrist flexes; fingers flex and adduct; and thumb opposes. During range of motion exercises, D2 extension is combined with its reciprocal, D2 flexion. (Used with permission of Voss DE, Iota MK, Myers BJ. *Proprioceptive Neuromuscular Facilitation: Patterns & Techniques*. 3rd ed. New York, NY: Harper & Row; 1985 and Rust K. Managing deficits of first level motor control capacities using Rood and proprioceptive neuromuscular facilitation techniques. In: *Occupational Therapy for Physical Dysfunction*. 7th ed. Philadelphia, PA: Lippincott Williams and Wilkins; 2014.)

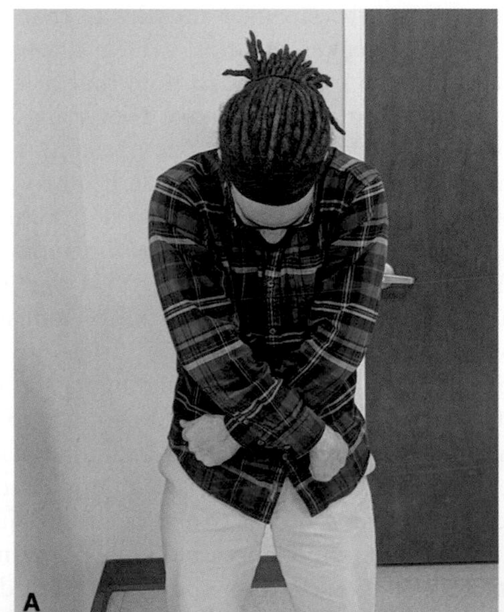

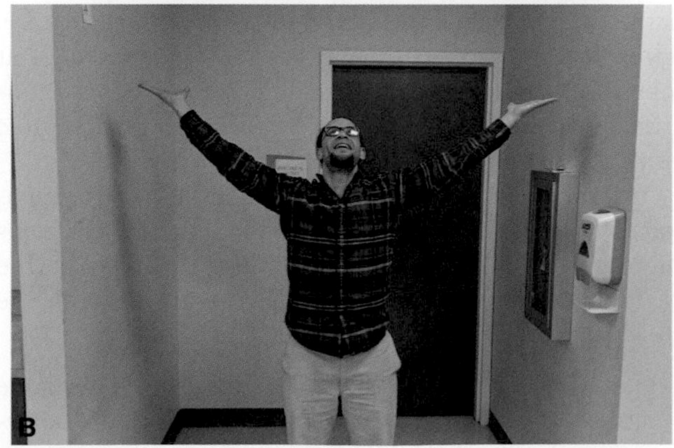

Figure 35-5. (**A**) Bilateral symmetrical D2 with shoulder extension, adduction, and internal rotation. (**B**) Bilateral symmetrical D2 with shoulder flexion, abduction, and external rotation.

out of bed in the morning, an individual may roll from supine to side-lying, then to side sitting and finally to short sitting at the edge of the bed. When putting on his or her pants, the individual may sit to don clothing over feet and pull up to thighs before transitioning to standing to pull up over hips.

Use of the PNF Frame of Reference Today

It is necessary to learn movement by breaking it down into its simplest parts. A novice therapist initially learns which movements and which directions for movement are available at each joint. However, in function, an individual moves at multiple joints, in multiple planes of motion simultaneously, and often at great speed. Functional movement is typically a combination of movements versus movement in one plane at a time. Consider being seated and reaching down with both hands to place a sock on the left foot. This functional activity uses a D1 flexion and extension pattern of the UE, with significant flexion at the hips and rotation in the trunk.

The therapist using PNF considers that patterned movement allows the stronger muscles in that pattern to influence the weaker muscles, a term known as irradiation. It is also important to note that in the PNF frame of reference, all patterns have a reversing pattern. Therefore, in a functional context, one may consider that when lifting an arm to reach overhead to pull the chain of a ceiling fan, it is also necessary to return that arm back to its starting position. This functional reversal requires a balance between the agonist and antagonist muscles for smooth, controlled movement in both directions.

The PNF frame of reference highlights the importance of the role of the trunk as a basis for limb movement and function. In the case of an individual with hemiplegia following a stroke, this is an important concept because recovery after a stroke or brain injury often includes muscle imbalances between prime movers (agonists and antagonists) that should be relaxed when the agonist is active. This muscle imbalance leads to an inefficient, ineffective, and limited movement repertoire. Shinde et al. outlined how PNF treatment directed at improving trunk control for clients with stroke demonstrated favorable results in both static and dynamic trunk skills needed for functional activity.[33]

In training for improved motor control, the occupational therapist using PNF needs to prioritize the goals for intervention. Consideration must be given to the stages of recovery. Consider a continuum of available ROM, stability, and controlled mobility.

- First, it is necessary to determine the client's available motion as well as the movements required for the desired task (PROM/AROM).
- The next step is to determine the client's stability needs: Does client need more stability or mobility to be able to engage in the activity? To determine this, the therapist must understand the stability requirements for this task.
- Finally, the therapist must identify if the client demonstrates sufficient controlled mobility to meet the demands to engage in this activity.

Box 35-1

PNF Treatment

Susan is 40-year-old homemaker who is eager to return to cleaning her kitchen after meal time. Since her recent stroke, Susan has left-sided hemiparesis, poor ability to sustain activity in her left shoulder, reported "heaviness" in her left leg, and profound sensory loss in her left hand. Susan is able to walk with a walker, although she relies heavily on her arms for support when walking; she has full PROM and AROM in her left arm, although she rarely uses this arm functionally, reporting "she forgets about it." Her occupational therapist starts with a standing activity where Susan is emptying the dishwasher. The therapist positions Susan at the counter to the left of the dishwasher to allow her to rotate and reach with her left hand, forward and downward to the right in front of her body to obtain dishes, and then place them up and to the left side of her head to place them in the over counter cabinets. (She is encouraging and facilitating a D2 flexion/and reversing D2 extension pattern.) She encourages Susan to turn her head and locate the dishes visually, then reach downward to grasp lightweight saucers, then move items upward prior to releasing them onto the shelf. The therapist guides Susan by standing behind and placing hands on Susan's pelvis on either side to help her shift weight from left to right foot and then back as activity requires. She allows Susan to keep her right hand on the countertop throughout this movement sequence to help provide balance stability.

Box 35-1 is an example of using PNF in a patient with a stroke.

Occupational therapists have specialized training in task analysis. Understanding the movement requirements and the timing of movements in a given activity is a critical skill in developing interventions to address the client's ability to participate. Much of the therapist's challenge is to determine where intervention is warranted and to prepare for the next stage of recovery. Individuals with hemiplegia following stroke need muscle length and joint mobility to ensure motion is possible. Then, the treatment focus shifts to begin to develop stability, tonic holding of a muscle in a shortened range and co-contraction—isometric power in lengthened range.

Neuro-Developmental Frame of Reference

Background and Historical Significance

Neuro-Developmental Treatment (NDT) originated in the 1940s by husband and wife team, Dr. Karel and Berta Bobath, for treatment of individuals with neurological disorders of posture and movement, such as stroke, brain injury, or cerebral palsy. Berta Bobath was a remedial gymnast who studied dance and movement, later became a physiotherapist, and worked with clients with CNS damage that leads to posture and movement problems.

Berta rejected the widespread belief that people with upper motor neuron lesions could not regain function. She would assess a client's asymmetrical postures and place him or her into a more neutral alignment. By putting her hands on the client at key points, and by moving him or her in a way that could encourage (facilitate) or discourage (inhibit) aspects of the movement, she helped to create more natural movement patterns. These early concepts still exist today. Specific key points of control encourage the therapist to contact the client's body purposefully and specifically to produce changes in alignment before a movement sequence, or to control the speed direction or effort the client uses during movement.[34]

Berta observed that by positioning and using various handling techniques, she could alter muscle tone. A client who demonstrated a significant amount of spasticity may experience a reduction of the hypertonicity in his or her limbs, more so than the current passive stretching techniques used at the time. Berta took her results from the clinic and shared them with her husband, Karel, who was a physician, to learn why she was able to influence movement in this way. Karel provided the scientific rationale to support her clinical experiences. Thus, the clinical practice of NDT preceded the scientific support for its intervention.

The Bobaths were frequently quoted for the idea that this theory was a "living concept." They recognized that in the mid-1900s, medical science was evolving, and health care was changing. They had expectations that their theory, initially called the Bobath approach, would also evolve as more scientific evidence became available.[35] The current model of NDT is supported by advances in the areas of neuroscience and motor learning, as well as DST. It requires an in-depth knowledge of the way movement is controlled and executed, the way in which feedback is used,[36] and the way our body systems interact with each other internally and with the outside world.

Definition of Neuro-Developmental Treatment

"NDT is a holistic and interdisciplinary clinical practice model informed by current and evolving research that emphasizes individualized therapeutic handling based on movement analysis for habilitation and rehabilitation of individuals with neurological pathophysiology. The therapist uses the International Classification of Functioning, Disability, and Health (ICF) model in a problem-solving approach to assess activity and participation, thereby to identify and prioritize relevant integrities and impairments as a basis for establishing achievable outcomes with clients and caregivers. An in-depth knowledge of the human movement system, including the understanding of typical and atypical development, and expertise in analyzing postural control, movement, activity, and participation throughout the lifespan, form the basis for examination, evaluation, and intervention. Therapeutic handling, used during evaluation and intervention, consists of a dynamic, reciprocal interaction between the client and therapist for activating optimal sensorimotor processing, task performance, and skill acquisition to enable participation in meaningful activities."[37]

There are not prescribed movement patterns with NDT. NDT is a problem-solving approach, with an emphasis on helping clients improve motor control to restore movement and participation in meaningful activities. Therefore, interventions are developed based on the very specific and unique needs of the client. Every client has his or her own personality, motivations, fears, goals, body type, prior level of activity, and supportive resources, and each has had a unique neurological event (no stroke or brain injury is alike—each has its own compilation of sequelae). The NDT frame of reference guides the clinician to identify, prioritize, and specifically address the underlying impairments that affect the client's ability to move and engage in meaningful life skills.

Key concepts of the NDT frame of reference that have stood the test of time include:

- Treating the individual as a whole: Since its inception, the NDT approach has stressed the importance of treating the whole person and the whole body.
- Individualized intervention
- Human movement is organized around functional activity.
- Hands-on intervention process to enhance functional outcomes
- Interdisciplinary approach
- Active participation: Passive motion, although helpful as a preparatory step, will not suffice for NDT intervention. Active participation by the client is necessary to improve motor performance and participation in life skills.

Evaluation and Intervention Principles for NDT

Assessment: Skilled Observation as well as Handling

The *International Classification of Functioning, Disability, and Health* (*ICF*) is a framework that organizes and categorizes biological and social aspects of health and disability.[38] The NDT model for assessment is based on the *ICF* with an added domain to guide the clinician to carefully analyze posture and movement as it directly relates to the client's level of participation, functional abilities, and body system strengths or impairments.

In the *ICF* framework, the clinician asks the following questions to determine an individual client's disability and health:

- ***Who*** the client is. What is his or her level of *participation* in life roles?
- ***What*** is the client able to do or not do? *Functional abilities/limitations*
- ***Why*** does he perform these tasks, or struggle to perform these tasks following a stroke or brain injury? Body *system integrities and impairments*

For the NDT model, the clinician also considers one additional question to determine the posture and movement abilities and limitations of the client:

- **How** does the client perform the functional task? The clinician uses an in-depth knowledge of the *human movement system* and understands movement problems that may develop following a stroke or brain injury.

This question of HOW precedes the question of WHY which identifies particular body systems that are intact or have been disrupted.

When assessing a client who has had a stroke or brain injury using the NDT frame of reference, the occupational therapist will use both skills of observation as well as handling to gather needed information regarding the manner in which he or she completes functional activities.

During assessment, through the use of skilled clinical observation, the occupational therapist can note:

- Alignment of whole body, or body part—symmetrical/asymmetrical
- Position of body parts relative to each other
- Coordination or fluidity of movement
- Direction of movement relative to the task
- Facial expressions (attention, fear, effort, frustration, etc.)

From these observations, the occupational therapist begins to appreciate the client's posture and movement abilities, and challenges.

One of the hallmarks of the NDT frame of reference is the use of individualized therapeutic handling for assessment of both client's typical and atypical movement patterns, and also for intervention to facilitate change in these patterns of movement.

The occupational therapist can further enhance the assessment using handling to gather information such as:

- *Amount of muscle recruitment:* Too active, not active enough for task
- *Quality of muscle contraction:* Flickering or sustained contraction
- *Timing of movement:* What moves first and what follows?
- *Client's reaction to being moved:* Passive, resistive
- *Breathing:* Breath holding, coordinating breathing with movement

Combining observation skills and handling skills, and comparing how client moves in contrast to the understanding of normal movement, helps the therapist identify specific strengths and impairments that lead to a direct plan for treatment.

Intervention: Hands-on and Problem-Solving Approach

Assessment and intervention are closely interwoven in every interaction when using the NDT frame of reference. When an NDT trained occupational therapist observes and feels how a client is controlling posture and movement to complete a particular functional task, he or she begins to determine whether the client's movement patterns differ from normal movement. From this, the therapist begins to prioritize the treatment interventions. When providing treatment interventions, it is essential to assess the effectiveness of each aspect of intervention and make further modifications. In this way, assessment and intervention have constant interplay within a session.

Using the NDT frame of reference, the occupational therapist's goal for intervention is to improve the client's postural control and movement to allow more efficient and effective patterns during activities of daily living (ADLs). The therapist will use a hands-on approach using either proximal or distal key points of control to facilitate new motor patterns at times within a functional activity, and at times separate from the activity itself. Putting hands on the client allows the therapist to realign the base of support, and the segments of the body to prepare for the task. The clients poorly aligned position places some muscles in an ineffective shortened or over-lengthened position. Realigning the base of support and body parts specific to the task allows optimal joint position and muscle length for best motor recruitment. It helps prepare the joints and muscles of the body to work at their greatest biomechanical advantage. Keeping hands on the client allows a dynamic interplay between gathering immediate feedback about the movement (assessment) and guiding and facilitating new patterns of movement (intervention).

Weight bearing is an important consideration for treating the individual with CNS dysfunction. An intervention applying weight bearing into a body part is directed at regaining muscle length, normalizing muscle tone whether it is too high (hypertonic) or too low (hypotonic), and/or creating a demand in the muscles to work.[39] Weight bearing to neutralize muscle tone happens naturally through the LEs when a client is assisted to stand on his or her legs. In the UE, this becomes more challenging, and the occupational therapist needs to explore options to safely allow the client to accept weight on the arms. This may begin by having client accept weight on forearm, while seated at table, or as a greater challenge, to facilitate the client to accept weight through an extended arm. In the NDT frame of reference, weight bearing is a dynamic, not passive, process with the goal of increasing muscle activity in the trunk as well as in the UE.

Individualized handling is a key concept used to change the way each client manages his or her body, but the ultimate goal is to teach the individual to move more naturally with less input from the therapist. The therapist is frequently considering changing the amount of support and the level of cueing to give the client the experience of moving more of himself or herself. With all of the emphasis on improving alignment and motor control, the occupational therapist must keep in mind that the overall goal for the client is to improve his or her functional abilities and help to restore participation in life roles.

Occupational therapists using the NDT approach need to have an appreciation and an excellent understanding of typical posture and movement. People who have not had a neurological insult develop thousands of movement patterns that are common. For example, when moving from a seated position to a standing position, there is a need to have weight shift forward at the hip joint to move the base of support from the backs of the thighs, to the feet on the floor. Once the body weight is shifted forward, there is an element of bilateral knee and hip extension to rise up from the sitting surface. The body stays fairly symmetrical throughout this motion. Most people would perform this movement using these common components of movement (see Fig. 35-6).

The occupational therapist also needs to understand how movement patterns are altered after a neurological event, such as a stroke or brain injury. When a neurological insult impedes a client's ability to maintain a posture or to move as he or she did prior to the event, the body adapts with its best attempt to solve the motor problem. In Figure 35-6, the individual first shifted weight forward onto the feet and then extended knees and hips nearly simultaneously to transition to stand. An individual who has had a stroke, which has affected his or her ability to move and control the entire left side of the body, left hemiplegia, and diminished somatosensory awareness on the left side, may use an atypical pattern of movement to rise from a seated position. This individual may first attempt to shift his or her trunk backward and not forward and then may shift the majority of his or her weight to the right leg, which he or she can feel and can control, as seen in Figure 35-7.

The occupational therapist needs to be able to recognize that this is an ineffective and potentially unsafe movement pattern and create interventions to directly influence the specific components of the asymmetry, and the weight shift forward to help the individual achieve a more natural transition to standing. The therapist would facilitate a more normal pattern using his or her hands to realign the body parts and by matching his or her own body's transition from sitting to standing with that of the client (see Fig. 35-8).

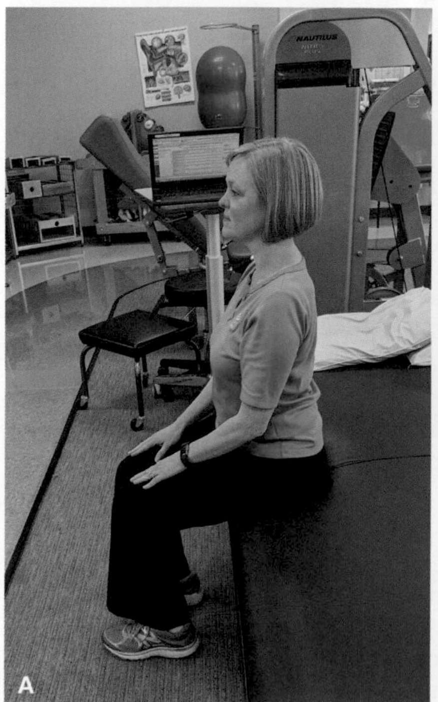

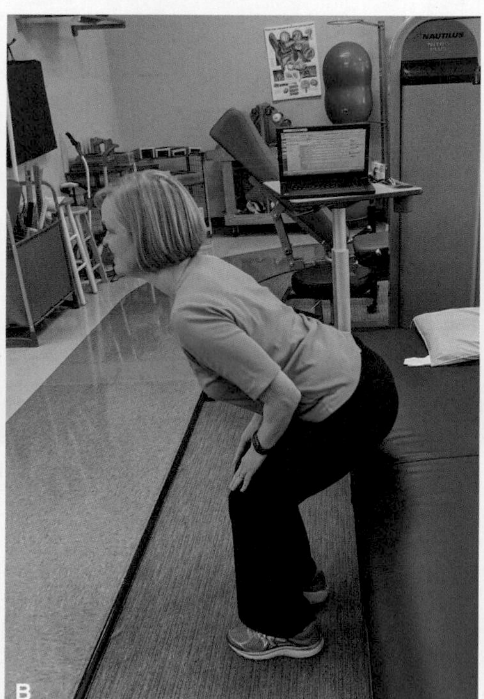

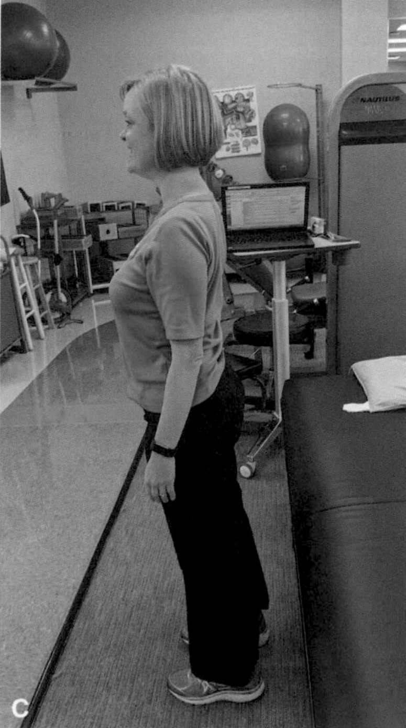

Figure 35-6. Sitting posture and sit to stand with normal subject. (**A**) Sitting; (**B**) Sit to stand and (**C**) Standing.

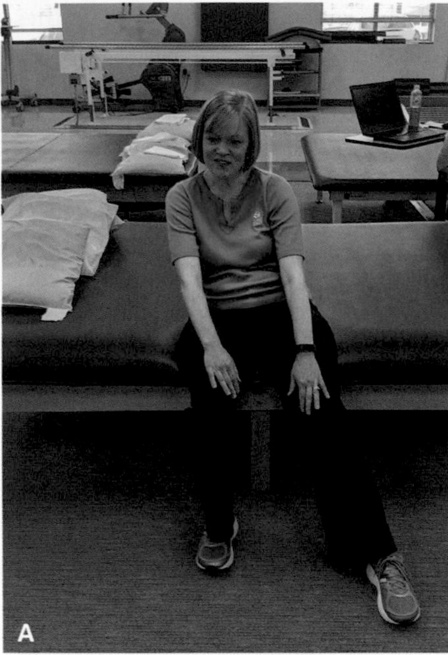
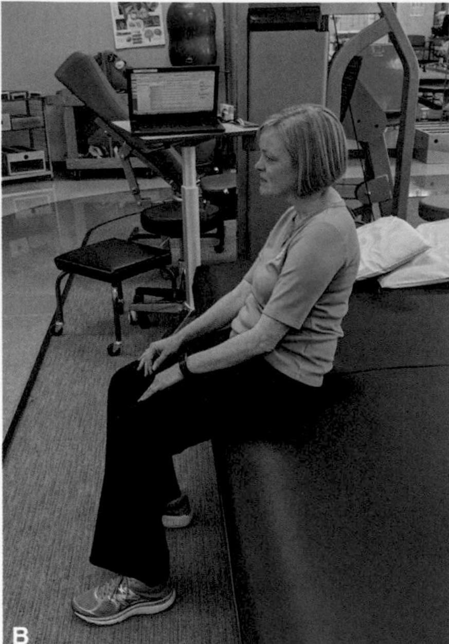
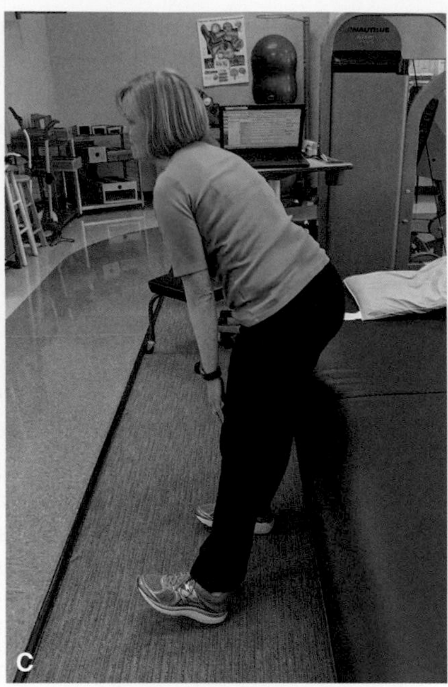

Figure 35-7. Ineffective sitting posture and sit to stand pattern as may be seen in client with stroke. (**A**) Asymmetrical sitting; (**B**) Dorsal leaning; and (C) Asymmetrical sit to stand.

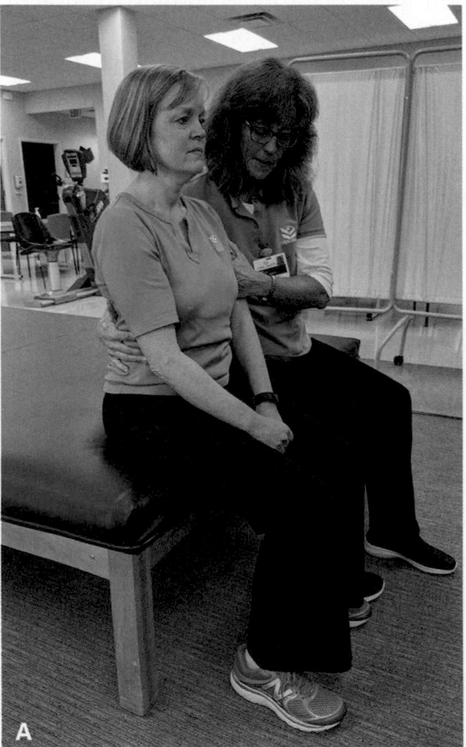
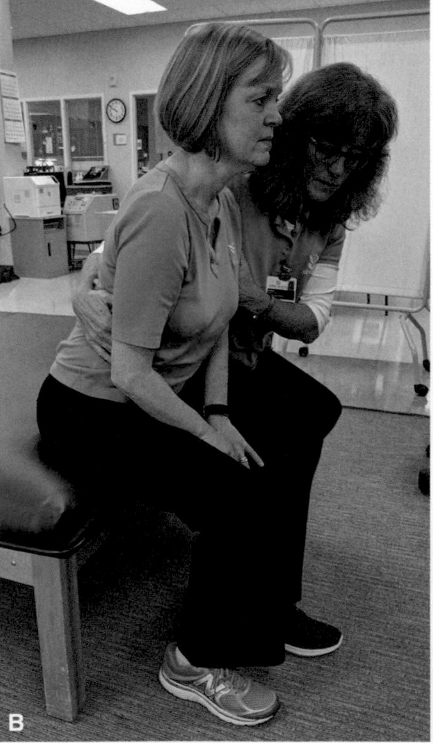
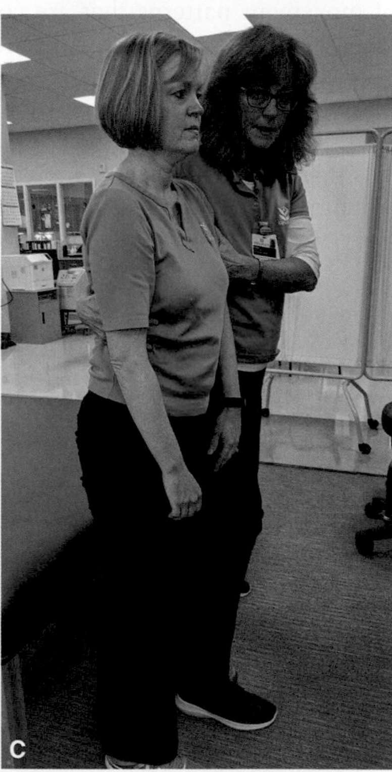

Figure 35-8. Facilitation of more effective transition from sit to stand. (**A**) Facilitation of sitting; (**B**) Facilitation of sit to stand and (**C**) Facilitation of standing.

Use of the NDT Frame of Reference Today

Today, the NDT approach is one of the most commonly used interventions for individuals with cerebral palsy, stroke, or brain injury and is used internationally. Although this frame of reference was initially developed in the 1940s, the theory has evolved over the years as has science relating to motor development, motor control, motor learning, and neuroplasticity.

Occupational therapists using the current NDT frame of reference add a strong understanding of movement patterns both typical and atypical—after a neurological event, to their expert analysis of task performance to help clients learn to move and perform daily-life functions in a more effective way.

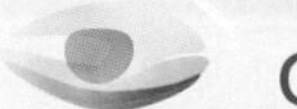

CASE STUDY

Patient Information

Lisa is a 38-year-old married mother of two who was working part time as a radiology technician. Her children are 7 years and 5 months of age. Lisa suffered a significant stroke 3 days after giving birth to her son. She had significant medical complications, including having two major seizures, resulting in a prolonged hospital stay that included inpatient rehabilitation. Lisa has returned home where she is living with her husband and her children. Her mother has also moved in to assist Lisa, provide care for her children, and manage her home. Lisa has a history of anxiety that she has actively managed with counseling and medication. She has no other significant medical history. Prior to her stroke, Lisa enjoyed running, spending time with her family, boating and water activities, and volunteering at her children's school.

Assessment Process and Results

Use of patient interview, skilled observation of movement during functional activities related to life roles, Fugl-Meyer assessment, and other formal and informal OT assessments including ROM, sensation, trunk control, balance, cognition, perception, and visual assessments.

Impairments in Client Factors/Performance Skills

1. Spastic dominant right hemiplegia
2. Brunnstrom stage IV for right upper extremity (RUE) and stage IV/V for right lower extremity LE (RLE)
3. Absent sensation on right side to midline
4. Impaired perception of body in space
5. Impaired postural alignment, trunk control, and postural control in sitting and standing
6. Impaired attention and memory
7. Decrease PROM/AROM and pain of the RUE
8. Mild expressive/receptive aphasia
9. Anxiety

Occupational Therapy Problem List

Lisa and the occupational therapist choose to focus primarily on these areas:

- Decreased ability to perform ADL, such as bathing, toilet hygiene, and donning her bra.
- Decreased independence in functional mobility such as shower transfers, functional ambulation, and transitioning from sit to stand without losing her balance. Lisa is currently using a wide based quad cane and is falling frequently in her home.
- Decreased ability to care for her 5-month-old son; in particular unable to pick him up from a crib, walk and carry him, and assist him in and out of the bathtub.

Lisa verbalizes that while she appreciates her mother's help, it is "time for my mom to move out."

Occupational Goal List

- Patient will be independent with shower transfers.
- Patient will be independent with toilet hygiene.
- Patient will demonstrate the ability to lift her son in and out of the bathtub from a kneeling position.

Intervention

1. Postural alignment/control in sitting and standing to improve balance, reduce spasticity in the RUE and RLE, reduce pain in the RUE, and facilitate voluntary combinations of functional patterns of movement in the trunk and extremities.

Techniques: Stability (maintain and recover a posture)—slow rhythmic weight shifts initially in sitting progressing to standing. Head and trunk with emphasis on rotational and diagonal movement patterns. Focus on alignment over the base of support (sitting and standing) with emphasis on progressing small controlled weight shifts in all directions. Practice unloading the dishwasher.

2. PROM/AROM and pain in the RUE in preparation for low to mid-reach during functional activities, such as holding a grab bar while entering shower, reaching for toilet paper, reaching behind body, and bilateral low reach to pick up items.

Techniques: PNF D1 flexion/extension, D2 flexion/extension, asymmetrical progressing toward bilateral symmetrical pattern to facilitate low reach. As client progresses, incorporate diagonals into functional tasks as listed in goals.

3. Ability to weight shift in standing initially to midline and then right to left with ease and without fear to improve balance, trunk control, alignment, and use of the extremities for activities such as stepping over the tub edge or leaning over to pick something up.

Techniques: Handling with an emphasis on assisting the client in active, aligned weight shifting on to her hemiplegic leg in preparation for single leg stance for shower transfers. Emphasis on larger controlled weight shifts in standing. Start with slow speed given client's fear of shifting on to hemiplegic side because of absent sensation. Therapist positions himself or herself to move with the patient for smoother, more controlled normal movement. Practice stepping over ledge of shower and picking up laundry off the floor.

4. Build strength in core and extremities to allow for increased demand with functional mobility, lifting, and caregiving.

Techniques: Quadruped: Tonic holding transitioning to side sitting (static to dynamic) to allow RUE to initially stay in weight-bearing progressing toward more controlled mobility that allows client to use RUE out of weight bearing against gravity in smooth controlled manner. Practice getting on and off the floor to play with the baby. Starting in supine and moving toward sitting and then standing, resistance through the UE into the trunk with dynamic weight shifting. Practice picking up the baby.

Summary of Results

At discharge from OT services, Lisa had met all three goals. Her mother has moved out and only helps with driving, grocery shopping, and more difficult home management tasks. Lisa is able to fully care for her children and is no longer experiencing falls. She has decided not to return to work but is volunteering at school in a limited manner. She and her family recently enjoyed a vacation at a lake where Lisa participated in boating and lake activities.

Best Evidence for Occupational Therapy Practice Regarding PNF and NDT

Intervention	Description	Participants	Dosage	Research Design and Evidence Level	Benefit	Statistical Significance and Effect Size
The Effects of trunk stability exercise using PNF on the functional reach test and muscle activities of stroke patients[40]	This study was performed to investigate the effects of trunk stability exercise using PNF for stroke patients' muscle activation and their results in the functional reach test (FRT).	Adult hemiplegia patients ($n = 40$) were randomly allocated to two groups: an experimental group and a control group.	The experimental group performed a trunk stability exercise using PNF, while the control group performed only a general exercise program for 6 weeks (5 times a week). Pre- and postexperiment measurements were made of the FRT. For measuring muscle activation, the quadriceps, hamstring, tibialis anterior, and soleus muscles were recorded by electromyography (EMG) in the FRT.	Level I evidence Randomized controlled trial	The results of this study show that after performing the therapeutic exercise program, the experimental group showed significant improvements in FRT, activities of quadriceps, hamstring, and soleus muscles on the affected side, and activities of the quadriceps, and soleus muscles on the nonaffected side. The control group showed significant improvements only in activities of the quadriceps, and soleus muscles on the nonaffected side. These results indicate that trunk stabilizing exercises using PNF performed by stroke patients were effective at improving FRT and the muscle activities of the soleus and quadriceps.	Paired t-tests $p < 0.05$ for FRT and soleus and quadriceps
Does physiotherapy based on the Bobath concept, in conjunction with a task practice, achieve greater improvement in walking ability in people with stroke compared to physiotherapy focused on structured task practice alone[41]	To compare the short-term effects of two physiotherapy approaches for improving ability to walk in different environments following stroke: (i) interventions based on the Bobath concept, in conjunction with task practice, compared to (ii) structured task practice alone.	Twenty-six participants between 4 and 20 weeks poststroke able to walk with supervision indoors.	Both groups received six 1-hour physiotherapy sessions over a 2-week period. One group received physiotherapy based on the Bobath concept, including 1 hour of structured task practice. The other group received 6 hours of structured task practice.	Level 1 evidence Randomized controlled trial	This pilot study indicates short-term benefit for using interventions based on the Bobath concept for improving walking velocity in people with stroke.	Walking velocity showed significantly greater increases in the Bobath group (26.2 [SD 17.2] m/minute vs. 9.9 [SD = 12.9] m/minute, $p = 0.01$) A sample size of 32 participants per group is required for a definitive effect size.
Concept vs. constraint-induced movement therapy to improve arm functional recovery in stroke patients[42]	To compare the effects of a Bobath intervention and constraint-induced movement therapy on arm functional recovery among stroke patients with a high level of function on the affected side.	A total of 24 patients were randomized to constraint-induced movement therapy or Bobath intervention group.	The Bobath intervention group was treated for 1 hour, whereas the constraint-induced movement therapy group received training for 3 hours/day during 10 consecutive weekdays.	Level 1 evidence Single-blinded randomized controlled trial.	Constraint-induced movement therapy and the Bobath intervention have similar efficiencies in improving functional ability, speed, and quality of movement in the paretic arm among stroke patients with a high level of function. Constraint-induced movement therapy seems to be slightly more efficient than the Bobath intervention in improving the amount and quality of affected arm use.	There were no significant differences in Wolf Motor Function Test "functional ability" ($p = 0.137$) and "performance time" ($p = 0.922$), Motor Evaluation Scale for Arm in Stroke Patients ($p = 0.947$) and Functional Independence Measure scores ($p = 0.259$) between the two intervention groups. Significant improvements were seen after treatment in the "amount of use" and "quality of movement" subscales of the Motor Activity Log-28 in the constraint-induced movement therapy group over the Bobath group ($p = 0.003$; $p = 0.01$, respectively).

References

1. Howle J. Motor control. In: Bierman JC, Franjoine MR, Hazzard CM, Howle JM, Stamer M, eds. *Neuro-Developmental Treatment: A Guide to Clinical Practice.* Stuttgart, Germany: Thieme; 2016:248–262.
2. Howle J. *Neuro-Developmental Treatment Approach: Theoretical Foundations and Principles of Clinical Practice.* Laguna Beach, CA: NDTA; 2002.
3. Schriner M, Thome J, Carrier M. Rehabilitation in the upper extremity after stroke: current practice as a guide for curriculum. *Open J Occup Ther.* 2014;2(1):1–14. doi:10.15453/2168-6408.1056.
4. Rood MS. Neurophysiological mechanisms utilized in the treatment of neuromuscular dysfunction. *Am J Occup Ther.* 1956;10:220–225.
5. Stockmeyer S. An interpretation of the approach of Rood to the treatment of neuromuscular dysfunction, NUSTEP proceedings. *Am J Phys Med.* 1967;46(1):900–961.
6. Cano-de-la Cuerda R, Molero-Sanchez A, Carratala-Tejada M, et al. Theories and control models and motor learning: clinical applications in neuro-rehabilitation. *Neurologia.* 2015;30(1):32–41.
7. Schaal S, Mohajerian P, Ijspeert A. Dynamic systems vs. optimal control—a unifying approach. *Prog Brain Res.* 2007;165:425–455. doi:10.1016/S00123(06)65027-9.
8. Schmidt CA. *Motor Learning and Performance: A Problem Based Learning Approach.* Champaign, IL: Human Kinetics; 2000.
9. Sabari JS, Capasso N, Feld-Glazner R. Optimizing motor planning and performance in clients with neurological disorders. In: Radomski MV, Trombly Latham CA, eds. *Occupational Therapy for Physical Dysfunction.* 7th ed. Philadelphia, PA: Lippincott Williams & Wilkins; 2014:614–674.
10. Kleim JA, Jones TA. Principles of experience-dependent neural plasticity: implications for rehabilitation after brain damage. *J Speech Lang Hear Res.* 2008;51(1):S225–S239. doi:1092-4388/0815101-S225.
11. Kawahira K, Shimodozono M, Ogata A, Tanaka A. Addition of intensive repetition of facilitation exercise to multidisciplinary rehabilitation promotes motor functional recovery of the hemiplegic lower limb. *J Rehabil Med.* 2004;36:159–164. doi:10.1080/16501970410029753.
12. Lohse KR, Lang CE, Boyd LA. Is more better? Using metadata to explore dose-response relationships in stroke rehabilitation. *Stroke.* 2014;45(7):2053–2058. doi:10.1161/STROKEAHA.114.004695.
13. Combs SA, Kelly SP, Barton R, Ivaska M, Nowak K. Effects of an intensive, task specific rehabilitation program for individuals with chronic stroke: a case series. *Disabil Rehabil.* 2010;32(8):669–678. doi:10.3109/09638280903242716.
14. Wulf G, Shea C, Lewthwaite R. Motor skill learning and performance: a review of influential factors. *Med Educ.* 2010;44(1):75–84. doi:10.1111/j.1365-2923.2009.03421.x.
15. Conti GE, Schepens SL. Changes in hemiplegic grasp following distributed repetitive intervention: a case series. *Occup Ther Int.* 2009;16(3–4):204–217. doi:10.1002/oti.276.
16. Hubbard IJ, Parsons MW, Neilson C, Carey LM. Task-specific training: evidence for and translation to clinical practice. *Occup Ther Int.* 2009;16(3–4):175–189. doi:10.1002/oti.275.
17. Cauraugh JH, Kim SB, Summers JJ. Chronic stroke longitudinal motor improvements: cumulative learning evidence found in the upper extremity. *Cerebrovasc Dis.* 2008;25(1–2):115–121. doi:10.1159/000112321.
18. Richards L, Senesac C, McGuirk T, et al. Response to intensive upper extremity therapy by individuals with ataxia from stroke. *Top Stroke Rehabil.* 2008;15(3):262–271. doi:101310/tsr1503-262.
19. Twitchell TE. The restoration of motor function following hemiplegia in man. *Brain.* 1951;74(4):443–480.
20. Brunnstrom S. *Movement Therapy in Hemiplegia.* New York, NY: Harper and Row; 1970.
21. Schultz-Krohn SA, Ope-Davis JM, Jourdan JM. Traditional sensorimotor approaches to intervention. In: Pendleton HM, Schultz-Krohn, SA, eds. *Pedretti's Occupational Therapy Practice Skills for Physical Dysfunction.* 7th ed. St. Louis, MO: Mosby; 2013:796–830.
22. Beebe JA, Lang CE. Absence of a proximal to distal gradient of motor deficits in the upper extremity early after stroke. *Clin Neurophysiol.* 2008;119:2074–2085. doi:10.1016/j.clinph.2008.04.293.
23. Fugl-Meyer AR, Jaasko L, Leyman I, Olsson S, Steglind S. The post-stroke hemiplegic patient. A method for evaluation of physical performance. *Scand J Rehabil Med.* 1975;7:13–31.
24. Page S, Fulk G, Boyne P. Clinically important differences for the upper extremity Fugl-Meyer scale in people with minimal to moderate impairment due to chronic stroke. *Phys Ther.* 2012;92(6):791–798. doi:10.2522/ptj.20110009.
25. Sullivan K, Tilson J, Cen S, et al. Fugl-Meyer Assessment of sensorimotor function after stroke: standardized training procedure for clinical practice and clinical trials. *Stroke.* 2011;42:427–432. https://www.ahajournals.org/doi/full/10.1161/STROKEAHA.110.592766
26. Woodbury ML, Veloza CA, Richards LG, Duncan PW, Studenski S, Lai SM. Dimensionality and construct validity of the Fugl-Meyer Assessment of the upper extremity. *Arch Phys Med Rehabil.* 2007;88(6):715–723. doi:10.1016/j.apmr.2007.02.036
27. Gladstone DL, Danells CJ, Black SE. The Fugl-Meyer assessment of motor recovery after stroke: a critical review of its measurement properties. *Neurorehabil Neural Repair.* 2002;16(3):232–240.
28. Duncan PW, Propst M, Nelson SG. Reliability of the Fugl-Meyer assessment of sensorimotor recovery following cerebral vascular accident. *Phys Ther.* 1983;63:1606–1610.
29. International PNF Association website. Historical perspective of PNF. http://www.ipnfa.org. Updated August 26, 2014. Accessed August 20, 2018.
30. Adler S, Beckers D, Buck M. *PNF in Practice: An Illustrated Guide.* 3rd ed. Heidelberg, Germany: Springer Medizin Verlag; 2008.
31. Smedes F, Heidmann M, Schäfer C, Fischer B, Stępień A. The proprioceptive neuromuscular facilitation concept; the state of the evidence, a narrative review. *Phys Ther Rev.* 2016;21(1):17–31. doi:10.1080/10833196.2016.1216764.

32. Rust K. Managing deficits of first level motor control capacities using rood and proprioceptive neuromuscular facilitation techniques. In: *Occupational Therapy for Physical Dysfunction*. 7th ed. Philadelphia, PA: Lippincott Williams and Wilkins; 2014.
33. Shinde K, Ganvir S. Effectiveness of proprioceptive neuromuscular facilitation techniques after stroke: a meta-analysis. *Natl J Med Allied Sci*. 2014;3(2):29–34. www.njmsonline.org
34. Bierman J, Franjoine M, Hazzard C, Howle J, Stamer M. *Neuro-Developmental Treatment: A Guide to Clinical Practice*. Stuttgart, Germany: Thieme; 2016:538.
35. Bierman J, Franjoine M, Hazzard C, Howle J, Stamer M. *Neuro-Developmental Treatment: A Guide to Clinical Practice*. Stuttgart, Germany: Thieme; 2016:4.
36. McLaughlin-Gray J. Traditional sensorimotor approaches to intervention. In: Pendleton HM, Schultz-Krohn W, eds. *Pedretti's Occupational Therapy Practice Skills for Physical Dysfunction*. 7th ed. St Louis, MO: Mosby; 2014:822–827.
37. Cayo C, Diamond M, Bovre T, et al. The NDT/Bobath (Neuro-Developmental Treatment/Bobath) approach. *NDTA Netw*. 2015;22(2):1.
38. World Health Organization. International classification of functioning, disability and health (ICF). Geneva, Switzerland: WHO; 2001. http://www.who.int/classifications/icf/en. Updated January 10, 2014. Accessed August 20, 2018.
39. Levit K. Optimizing motor behavior using the NDT approach. In: *Occupational Therapy for Physical Dysfunction*. 7th ed. Philadelphia, PA: Lippincott Williams and Wilkins; 2014.
40. Kim Y, Kim E, Gong W. The effects of trunk stability exercise using PNF on the functional reach test and muscle activities of stroke patients. *J Phys Ther Sci*. 2011;23(5):699–702. doi:10.1589/jpts.23.699.
41. Brock K, Haase G, Rothacher G, et al. Does physiotherapy based on the Bobath concept, in conjunction with a task practice, achieve greater improvement in walking ability in people with stroke compared to physiotherapy focused on structured task practice alone. *Clin Rehab*. 2011;25(10):903–912. doi:10.1177/0269215511406557.
42. Huseyinsinoglu B, Ozdincler A, Krespi Y. Bobath Concept versus constraint-induced movement therapy to improve arm functional recovery in stroke patients. *Clin Rehabil*. 2012;26(8):705–715. doi:10.1177/0269215511431903.

Chapter 36

Cerebrovascular Accident

Dawn M. Nilsen and Glen Gillen

LEARNING OBJECTIVES

This chapter will allow the reader to:

1. Describe the etiology and risk factors associated with cerebrovascular accidents (CVA, stroke).
2. Describe the classic signs and symptoms associated with stroke.
3. Identify common impairments in client factors and performance skills that impact engagement in occupation after stroke.
4. Describe how impairments in body function (e.g., motor impairments) impact daily functioning.
5. Apply a client-centered approach to evaluation and treatment.
6. Describe evaluation procedures to assess limitations after stroke.
7. List and describe standardized assessments that are commonly used to assess impairments in body functions and performance skills after stroke.
8. Describe evidence-based treatment approaches commonly applied during stroke rehabilitation.
9. Develop targeted occupation-based treatment plans designed to remediate or compensate for underlying impairments.
10. Describe health promoting behavioral changes designed to prevent secondary strokes.

CHAPTER OUTLINE

TERMINOLOGY

Acalculia/Dyscalculia: the inability or impaired ability to perform simple mathematical calculations previously mastered.

Agnosia: the inability to recognize objects, persons, smells, or sounds despite having normal sensory functions (e.g., vision or hearing).

Agraphia/Dysgraphia: the inability or impaired ability to produce written language.

Alexia/Dyslexia: the inability or impaired ability to read written language despite preservation of other aspects of language.

Aneurysm: a weakening of an artery wall, resulting in a bulge or distension of the artery.

Anomia: the inability to name objects or persons.

Anosognosia: an unawareness or denial of a neurological deficit that is clinically evident.

Aphasia: an acquired multimodality language disorder that results from damage to the language centers of the brain.

Apraxia: the inability to perform purposeful actions despite having normal muscle function.

Arteriovenous malformation: a tangle of abnormal blood vessels connecting arteries and veins without an intervening capillary bed.

Contracture: an abnormal shortening of muscle tissue, rendering the muscle highly resistant to passive stretching; typically results in permanent restrictions in joint motion.

Contralateral homonymous hemianopia: an ocular condition in which vision has been lost in the same field halves of both eyes.

Dysarthria: a speech disorder resulting from paralysis, weakness, or incoordination of the muscles involved in speech production.

Dysphagia: an eating disorder involving difficulty manipulating and transporting solids/liquids from the oral cavity to the pharynx.

Hemianesthesia: a loss of sensation in either half of the body.

Spasticity: a velocity-dependent increase in tonic stretch reflexes; also denotes a form of muscular hypertonicity with exaggeration of tendon reflexes.

Subluxation: an incomplete or partial dislocation of a joint.

Introduction

A cerebrovascular accident (CVA) or stroke is an acute neurological event of vascular origin that impacts brain functioning. According to the World Health Organization (WHO), a stroke is an "acute focal neurological dysfunction lasting more than 24 hours (or leading to death in <24 hours)."[1] A stroke in one hemisphere of the brain often results in upper motor neuron dysfunction, leading to contralateral weakness (hemiparesis) or paralysis (hemiplegia) of the body, and possibly the face and oral motor structures. For example, a left hemisphere lesion (left CVA) may result in right hemiplegia, whereas a right hemisphere lesion (right CVA) would result in left hemiplegia. In addition to motor deficits, a variety of other impairments may result from stroke. These include the following:

- Sensory impairment
- Cognitive and perceptual impairment
- Visual disturbances
- Behavioral changes
- Difficulty swallowing
- Speech and language function impairment

These client factor deficits can significantly impact an individual's ability to engage in chosen occupations, limiting participation and quality of life.

This chapter provides an overview of (1) stroke epidemiology, (2) common stroke syndromes, (3) medical management of stroke, (4) the impact of stroke on occupational engagement, and (5) evidence-based assessment and intervention for individuals sustaining stroke. Although the focus of this chapter is on patients with stroke, it should be noted that other types of brain injuries and disease processes, such as head injuries, neoplasms, and infectious diseases, can produce similar impairment patterns. Thus, some treatment approaches presented in this chapter may apply to other diagnoses.

Stroke Epidemiology

According to the American Heart Association/American Stroke Association (AHA/ASA),[2] stroke continues to be the number one cause of long-term disability in the United States. AHA/ASA stroke statistics indicate that 795,000 individuals sustain a new or recurrent stroke each year. An estimated 7.2 million Americans over the age of 20 self-report having had a stroke. Projections show that an additional 3.4 million Americans aged greater than or equal to 18 years will sustain a stroke by 2030, representing a 20.5% increase in prevalence from 2012.[2]

The incidence of stroke is 1.25 times higher in men than in women, although women have a higher lifetime risk of stroke. More than half of all patients hospitalized for acute neurological disease have sustained a stroke, and the impact of stroke on function is compelling. Among long-term patients who sustained a stroke, 50% have hemiparesis, 30% are unable to walk without assistance, 26% are dependent in activities of daily living (ADLs), 19% are aphasic, 35% are clinically depressed, and 26% require home nursing care.[2]

In addition, evidence suggests that long-term health-related quality of life is decreased in patients having sustained stroke.[3,4] Given the scope and long-term nature of the problems resulting from stroke, it is clear why stroke rehabilitation is an important practice area within occupational therapy.

Stroke Etiology

The vascular syndromes that cause stroke can be divided into two broad categories: ischemic and hemorrhagic. Ischemic strokes account for approximately 87% of all strokes.[2] Age, gender, race, ethnicity, and genetic factors are considered nonmodifiable risk factors for stroke[2]; however, there are several modifiable risk factors that are often targeted in stroke prevention and education programs. Important modifiable risk factors include[2]:

- Hypertension
- Diabetes mellitus
- Disorders of heart rhythm such as atrial fibrillation
- High blood cholesterol and other lipids
- Cigarette smoking

- Obesity
- Lifestyle factors such as physical inactivity, and poor diet and nutrition

Ischemia

Ischemia results when there is insufficient blood flow to meet metabolic demands. The most common cause of an ischemic stroke is an obstruction of the blood vessels supplying the brain.[2,5] Obstruction may result from a thrombus (blood clot) or an embolism.[5] A cerebral thrombosis is a blood clot that forms within a cerebral vessel. An embolism is a blood clot that originates in the heart (cardiac source) or arterial sources outside the brain.[5] These clots become dislodged from their origin sites and subsequently block vessels supplying the brain. While vessel obstruction is the most common stroke cause, ischemia can also result from systemic blood flow reduction (such as occurs during cardiac arrest).[2,5]

Hemorrhage

Hemorrhagic strokes are caused by rupture of a weakened blood vessel and include intracerebral (within the brain) and subarachnoid (within the subarachnoid space) hemorrhages.[5] The most common causes of weakened vessels are **aneurysms** and **arteriovenous malformations.**[5] Intracerebral hemorrhages account for approximately 10% of all strokes, whereas subarachnoid hemorrhages occur less frequently.[2]

Transient Ischemic Attack

A transient ischemic attack (TIA) is an event that results in neurological symptoms resembling a stroke.[2] Although these symptoms develop suddenly and may last up to 24 hours, they resolve completely, leaving no discernable symptoms or deficits.[2] TIAs are considered a "warning sign" of an impending stroke and precede approximately 12% of all strokes.[2]

Common Stroke Syndromes

Based on location, strokes are broadly categorized as either cortical or subcortical[5] and involve either the anterior (internal carotid artery and its branches) or posterior (branches of the vertebrobasilar system) circulations of the brain[6] (see Fig. 36-1). As the name suggests, cortical strokes impact areas of the cerebral cortex, such as the frontal, parietal, temporal, or occipital lobes. Subcortical strokes impact structures below the cortex, such as the internal capsule, basal ganglia, thalamus, brainstem, and cerebellum.[5,6] Strokes may also occur at the junction between two main arteries. These types of strokes are known as border zone or watershed infarcts.[6] Stroke outcomes largely depend on lesion size and location.[5]

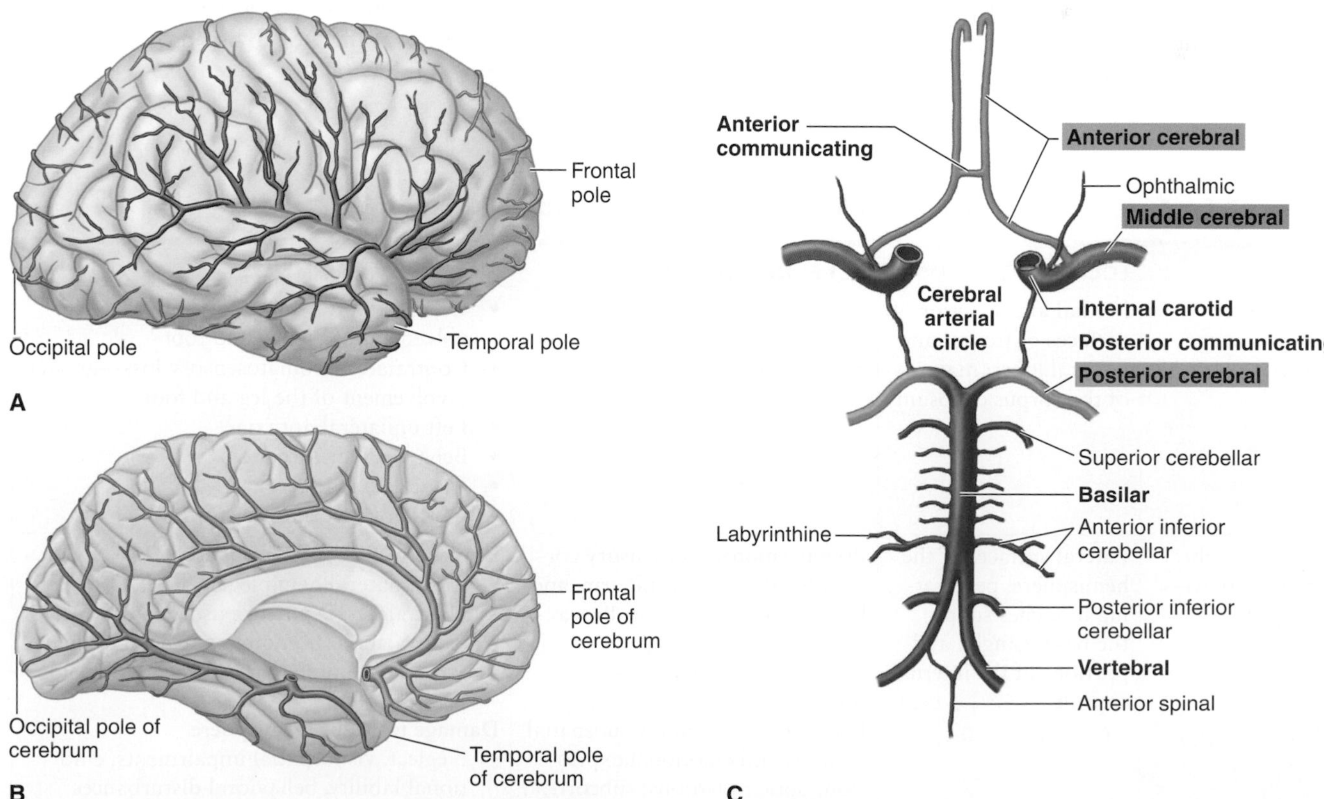

Figure 36-1. The anterior and posterior circulations of the brain. Note the internal carotid artery, the vertebral arteries, basilar artery, and the distribution patterns of the anterior (*green*), middle (*purple*), and posterior cerebral (*orange*) arteries. **A.** Right lateral view of right cerebral hemisphere. **B.** Medial view of left cerebral hemisphere. **C.** Inferior view.

Diagnostic imagining assists in determining stroke cause and location. Techniques such as computed tomography, magnetic resonance imagining, positron emission tomography, and single-photon emission computed tomography can provide information (e.g., lesion size and location) that may be used to assist with assessment and intervention planning.[5] Diagnostic testing results are usually accessible in the medical record and can be obtained during the information-gathering stage prior to patient evaluation.[5] A brief overview of common stroke syndromes is presented in the following section, and a summary of common impairments resulting from anterior and posterior circulation strokes is presented in Tables 36-1 and 36-2.

Anterior Circulation Strokes

The internal carotid arteries and their two main branches, the anterior cerebral arteries and middle cerebral arteries, supply approximately two-thirds of the brain, constituting the brain's anterior circulation.[6] Stroke in the territory of the middle cerebral artery is the most common type of anterior circulation infarct, accounting for approximately 70% of all first strokes.[7] The clinical presentation of anterior circulation strokes will vary depending on the branches involved and the extent of the occlusion.

Occlusion of the internal carotid artery commonly results in contralateral hemiplegia, **hemianesthesia**, homonymous hemianopia, changes in mental functions, and behavioral disturbances.[5] If the stroke occurs in the dominant hemisphere (i.e., hemisphere containing the representation of speech and controlling the extremities used to perform skilled movements such as writing and kicking a ball; the left hemisphere in the majority of individuals), the patient may also present with **aphasia**, **agraphia** or **dysgraphia**, **acalculia** or **dyscalculia**, and **apraxia**.[5] If the nondominant hemisphere is involved, the patient may present with visual perceptual impairments, unilateral body or spatial neglect, **anosognosia**, and dressing apraxia.[5]

An occlusion of the anterior cerebral artery typically produces contralateral hemiparesis and somatosensory loss, impacting the leg to a greater degree than the arm.[5] Behavioral disturbances, apraxia, and mental changes—such as confusion, disorientation, decreased initiation, and impairments in attention and short-term memory—are often present.[5]

An occlusion of the middle cerebral artery typically produces contralateral hemiplegia, impacting the upper extremity (UE), trunk, face, and tongue; contralateral somatosensory loss; and **contralateral homonymous hemianopia** with a strong gaze preference toward the lesion side observed acutely.[5] If the stroke involves the dominant hemisphere, aphasia is common. If the stroke involves the nondominant hemisphere, perceptual disturbance—such as unilateral neglect, anosognosia, and visual-spatial deficits—are common.[5] In addition, different patterns of deficits will be seen with a stroke involving the superior or inferior divisions of the middle cerebral artery (see Table 36-1).

Table 36-1. Anterior Circulation Strokes: Areas Supplied and Common Impairments

ARTERY	LOCATION	KEY FUNCTIONAL AREAS[6]	POSSIBLE IMPAIRMENTS[5]
Anterior cerebral artery (ACA)	Medial and superior surfaces of frontal and parietal lobes; majority of the corpus callosum	Primary motor and sensory cortices for the leg and foot; motor planning areas; prefrontal cortex	• Contralateral hemiparesis—greater involvement of the leg and foot • Contralateral somatosensory loss—greater involvement of the leg and foot • Left unilateral apraxia • Behavioral disturbances • Mental changes • Inertia of speech or mutism
Middle cerebral artery (MCA)—complete	Lateral surfaces of the hemisphere; penetrating branches supply the basal ganglia and portions of the internal capsule	Primary motor and sensory cortices for the face, trunk arm, and hand; frontal eye fields; Broca and Wernicke areas; parts of the frontal and parietal lobes important for motor planning, lateralized attention, visuospatial analysis and emotional expression; optic radiations; subcortical white matter (corticobulbar and corticospinal tracts); basal ganglia	**Damage to Either Hemisphere** • Contralateral hemiplegia • Contralateral somatosensory loss • Contralateral homonymous hemianopia • Strong gaze preference toward lesion side (acutely) **Damage to Right Hemisphere** • Neglect, visuospatial impairments, emotional lability, behavioral disturbances **Damage to Left Hemisphere** • Apraxia • Global aphasia

Table 36-1. Anterior Circulation Strokes: Areas Supplied and Common Impairments (*continued*)

ARTERY	LOCATION	KEY FUNCTIONAL AREAS[6]	POSSIBLE IMPAIRMENTS[5]
MCA—superior division	Lateral surfaces of frontal and parietal lobes	Primary motor and sensory cortices for the face, trunk, and UE; Broca area; frontal eye fields; parts of the frontal and parietal lobes important for motor planning, lateralized attention, visuospatial analysis, and emotional expression	**Damage to Either Hemisphere** • Contralateral hemiparesis: greater involvement of the face, arm, and hand • Contralateral somatosensory loss: greater involvement of the face, arm, and hand • Visual field impairment • Poor contralateral conjugate gaze • Ideational apraxia • Lack of judgment • Perseveration • Impaired organization of behavior • Depression • Lability • Apathy **Damage to Right Hemisphere** • Left unilateral body neglect • Left unilateral visual neglect • Anosognosia • Visuospatial impairment • Left unilateral motor apraxia **Damage to Left Hemisphere** • Bilateral motor apraxia • Broca aphasia • Frustration
MCA—inferior division	Lateral surfaces of temporal lobe, and portions of parietal and occipital lobes	Wernicke area; parts of temporal and parietal lobes important for visuospatial analysis and emotional expression; optic radiations	**Damage to Either Hemisphere** • Contralateral visual field deficit • Behavioral abnormalities **Damage to Right Hemisphere** • Visuospatial dysfunction **Damage to Left Hemisphere** • Wernicke aphasia
Internal carotid artery—source of the ACA and MCA	Combination of the anterior and middle cerebral artery distributions	Combination of the key functional areas supplied by the ACA and MCA	Impairments as indicated above for both ACA and MCA

UE, upper extremity.

Table 36-2. Posterior Circulation Strokes: Areas Supplied and Common Impairments

ARTERY	LOCATION	KEY FUNCTIONAL AREAS[6]	POSSIBLE IMPAIRMENTS[5,8–10]
Posterior cerebral artery (PCA)	Medial and inferior surfaces of temporal and occipital lobes; posterior corpus callosum; penetrating branches to midbrain and thalamus	Primary visual areas; optic radiations; parts of the temporal lobe important for memory formation; multimodal association areas important for visuospatial analysis, writing, reading, and so on	**Damage to Either Hemisphere** • Contralateral hemiparesis • Sensory loss • Homonymous hemianopia or quadrantanopia • Visual agnosia • Memory impairments **Damage to Right Hemisphere** • Cortical blindness • Visuospatial impairment • Impaired left-right discrimination **Damage to Left Hemisphere** • Finger agnosia • **Anomia** • Agraphia • Acalculia • Alexia/Dyslexia

(*continued*)

Table 36-2. Posterior Circulation Strokes: Areas Supplied and Common Impairments (*continued*)

ARTERY	LOCATION	KEY FUNCTIONAL AREAS[6]	POSSIBLE IMPAIRMENTS[5,8–10]
Vertebral-Basilar Artery System *Branches of the vertebral arteries:* • Anterior and posterior spinal arteries • Posterior inferior cerebellar artery (PICA) *Branches of the basilar artery:* • Anterior inferior cerebellar artery (AICA) • Pontine arteries • Superior cerebellar artery • PCA (terminal branch)—see above	Majority of the thalamus; hypothalamus; brainstem (BS) structures; cerebellum	Cranial nerve (CN) nuclei and CN roots (refer to Chapter 20); ascending and descending tracts as they travel through BS; areas important for balance, coordination, and motor learning; areas important for the regulation of vital functions (e.g., wakefulness, cardiorespiratory activities, swallowing)	Damage involving this system can produce specific BS syndromes that often produce crossed motor and sensory deficits and a complex set of signs and symptoms secondary to the involvement of multiple areas of the brain. See above for PCA strokes. The following select BS syndromes are presented as examples: **Wallenberg Syndrome** (aka lateral medullary syndrome) vascular territory of the PICA: • Contralateral loss of pain and temperature sensation—body • Ipsilateral loss of pain and temperature sensation—face • Dysphonia, dysphagia, and deviation of the uvula to the opposite side of the lesion on phonation • Vertigo, nystagmus, nausea, vomiting • Ataxia **Dejerine Syndrome** (aka medial medullary syndrome) vascular territory of the vertebral artery/anterior spinal artery: • Contralateral hemiplegia • Contralateral loss of touch, vibration, and proprioception—body • Ipsilateral deviation of the tongue on protrusion **Millard–Gubler Syndrome** (aka ventral pontine syndrome) vascular territory of the basilar artery • Contralateral hemiplegia • Contralateral impairments in pain and temperature sensation—body • Ipsilateral impairments in pain and temperature sensation—face **"Locked-in" Syndrome:** vascular territory of the basilar artery impacting the pons • Quadriplegia • Paralysis of all muscles innervated by CNs, except for the muscles of the eye. • Anarthria with preservation of consciousness • Dysphagia • May require assistance with ventilation **Weber Syndrome:** vascular territory of the penetrating branches of the PCA impacting the midbrain • Contralateral hemiplegia • Contralateral Parkinson tremor, akinesia • Contralateral weakness of the lower muscles of facial expression, deviation of the tongue to the contralateral side on protrusion, and ipsilateral weakness of the trapezius and sternocleidomastoid muscles • Ipsilateral oculomotor palsy (down and out position of the eye), dilated pupil, and diplopia

Posterior Circulation Strokes

The vertebrobasilar artery system (i.e., vertebral and basilar arteries and their many branches) constitutes the posterior circulation of the brain, which supplies the brainstem, diencephalon, cerebellum, parts of the temporal lobe, and the majority of the occipital lobe.[6] Strokes involving the posterior circulation are less common, accounting for approximately 20% of all ischemic strokes.[8] The clinical presentations of these strokes vary considerably, and specific subcortical stroke syndromes, such as Weber, Dejerine, and Wallenberg syndromes, are well described in the literature[8,9] (see Table 36-2). Common presenting signs and symptoms of posterior circulation strokes include vertigo, impaired balance, slurred speech, double vision, headache, nausea, vomiting, unilateral limb weakness and numbness, gait and limb ataxia, **dysarthria**, **dysphagia**, and nystagmus.[5,8,9]

Occlusion of the posterior cerebral artery may result in a variety of deficits depending on the extent of occlusion and the involved arterial branches. Possible deficits include sensory and motor impairments, visual field deficits (contralateral hemianopia or quadrantanopia), cortical blindness, **agnosia**, memory impairments, and **alexia/dyslexia**.[5,8,10]

Boarder Zone (Watershed) Infarcts

Border zone infarcts are thought to be the result of hemodynamic failure produced by repeated episodes of hypotension in the presence of severe arterial stenosis or occlusion, microemboli originating from the heart or atherosclerotic plaques in major arteries, or a combination of hypoperfusion and embolization.[11] They account for approximately 10% of all strokes and are classified as cortical (external) or subcortical (internal).[11] Common locations of cortical watershed infarcts are along the borders of the anterior and middle cerebral arteries, and the middle and posterior cerebral arteries.[6,11]

The clinical presentation of border zone infarcts will vary according to the involved vessels and areas of compromised cerebral tissue. Typically, damage to the anterior and middle cerebral artery border zone will result in LE contralateral hemiparesis, expressive language impairments, and behavioral disturbances. Damage to the middle and posterior cerebral artery border zone will typically result in partial visual loss and a variety of language impairments.[6]

Medical Management

The medical management of stroke will depend on multiple factors, including, but not limited to, lesion type, location, and extent; neurological deficits and associated medical problems; availability of technology; access to trained medical personnel; and ability and willingness of patients and their supportive network to cooperate with treatment recommendations.

According to the *AHA/ASA 2018 Guidelines for the Early Medical Management of Patients with Acute Ischemic Stroke*,[12] acute medical management should encompass prehospital care, urgent and emergency evaluation, treatment with intravenous (IV) and intra-arterial therapies as appropriate to restore blood flow, and in-hospital management focused on prevention measures instituted within the first 2 weeks after stroke onset.

The guidelines indicate the need to enhance public awareness of stroke warning signs and access medical care in a timely manner. It is recommended that first aid providers use a stroke assessment system and that emergency medical personnel begin initial stoke management in the field, including use of valid and standardized stroke screenings such as the FAST (Face, Arm, Speech Test) scale. Patients with a positive stroke screen and/or a strong suspicion of stroke should be transported to the nearest Certified Stroke Center, or health care facility capable of administering IV alteplase (aka IV tPA: tissue plasminogen activator), a medication that dissolves blood clots.[12]

Emergency evaluation and treatment should focus on determining the type and location of stroke and preventing mortality and/or progression of the brain lesion. The guidelines recommend the following[12]:

- Use of a stroke severity rating scale, preferably the National Institutes of Health Stroke Scale (NIHSS), to quantify the degree of neurological deficit
- Brain imaging evaluations to determine the type and location of stroke
- Additional diagnostic tests, as needed, to determine the cause of stroke
- Establishment of an open airway, maintenance of breathing, and appropriate oxygenation
- Maintenance of appropriate blood pressure, body temperature, and blood glucose levels
- Administration of IV alteplase or mechanical thrombectomy (i.e., removal of blood clots) as appropriate

After emergency management and treatment, in-hospital management should include the following[12]:

- Dysphagia screening before the patient begins eating, drinking, or taking oral medications
- Establishment of appropriate nutrition, which may necessitate the placement of a nasogastric tube (feeding tube that is placed through the nose and into the stomach)
- Continued maintenance of appropriate blood pressure, body temperature, and blood glucose levels
- Cardiac evaluation and monitoring as needed
- Treatment of any acute complications that may arise (e.g., edema, pneumonia)

Treatment of bowel and bladder incontinence; assessment, prevention, and treatment of hemiplegic shoulder pain; fall prevention; skin integrity maintenance; and prevention of deep vein thrombosis (DVT) (clots that form in the deep veins, frequently in the LEs) are also important during the acute phase.[12,13] Prolonged bed rest and immobilization place patients at risk for the development of decubitus ulcers (skin breakdown) and DVTs. Proper positioning and early mobilization may prevent the development of these secondary complications. In immobilized patients without contraindications, intermittent pneumatic compression in addition to routine care is recommended to reduce DVT risk.[12]

Finally, the guidelines recommend routine screening for poststroke depression, that patients diagnosed with depression be treated with antidepressants in the absence of contraindications, and that early rehabilitation for hospitalized patients be provided by trained personnel at an intensity appropriate to anticipated benefit and tolerance.[12] High-dose very early mobilization (within 24 hours of stroke onset) should be avoided because it can reduce the odds of favorable long-term outcomes.[12]

The course and prognosis for each patient will vary based on residual deficits, but the majority will require postacute care. In fact, more than two-thirds will receive rehabilitation services after initial hospitalization.[13] Rehabilitation services are typically delivered by a multidisciplinary team consisting of physicians, nurses, occupational therapists, physical therapists, and speech language therapists. Social workers, psychologists, psychiatrists, and counselors may also play a role in the rehabilitative process. Rehabilitative treatment intensity will vary depending on the setting. The most intensive treatment is provided in inpatient rehabilitation facilities (occupational, physical, and speech language therapy administered at a minimum of 3 hours per day, 5 days per week), followed by skilled nursing facilities delivering subacute care.[13,14]

For patients with continued needs who are discharged directly home after hospitalization, therapy is often provided in the community by home health agencies or outpatient clinics.[13,14] Although formal rehabilitation commonly ends 3 to 4 months after stroke, unmet needs persist in areas such as social reintegration, health-related quality of life, maintenance of activity, and self-efficacy.[13] Therefore, patients may require continued monitoring for needed therapy services for years after stroke onset.

The Impact of Stroke on Daily Occupation

Each patient having sustained stroke will have a unique set of impairments as a result of lesion location and extent (see Tables 36-1 and 36-2). These impairments can impede the patient's ability to engage in chosen activities. Hemiparesis is the most common consequence of stroke,[15] resulting in decreased ability to effectively move one side of the body. These motor impairments can pose significant barriers to occupational engagement. For example, impairment in trunk and postural control may limit the patient's ability to perform functional activities in sitting or standing, whereas UE weakness may limit use of the arm and hand in daily activities. Likewise, concomitant somatosensory impairment, cognitive and perceptual deficits, language production and comprehension impairment, visual impairment, and psychosocial limitations can negatively impact occupational engagement. The following sections and Table 36-3 highlight the most common problems experienced after stroke.

Trunk and Postural Control Impairments

Appropriate trunk and postural control (the ability to maintain equilibrium in a gravitational field by maintaining or returning body mass center over its base of support[16]) are needed for engagement in a broad range of activities, such as walking and wheelchair propulsion, morning self-care routines, work-related tasks while seated at a desk, and meal preparation. It is common for patients having sustained stroke to exhibit impairments in trunk and postural control.

Specific deficits related to stroke include:

- Multidirectional trunk weakness[17]
- Reduced and delayed activation of trunk muscles on the paretic side in anticipation of limb movements[18,19]
- Reduced and delayed activation of postural control muscles on the paretic side in response to postural perturbations[20,21]
- Loss of automatic postural reactions such as ankle, hip, and stepping strategies during standing[22]
- Asymmetrical trunk movements during walking[23]
- Asymmetrical weight bearing in sitting[24] and standing (favoring the nonparetic LE)[25]
- Soft-tissue **contractures** that limit spine mobility[26]
- Inability to perceive midline as a result of spatial relationship dysfunction[26]

These impairments may manifest as an inability to sit or stand in proper alignment, an inability to engage the upper limbs in functional tasks, an inability to reach beyond arm's length while sitting or standing, gait impairments, an inability to transfer or climb stairs, and balance loss and fall risk during functional activities. In fact, studies have found trunk and postural control to be strongly associated with poststroke UE function,[27] gait, and balance[28]; and trunk control to be a predictor

Table 36-3. Impact of Stroke on Occupational Engagement

COMMON LIMITATIONS	EXAMPLES OF IMPACT OF LIMITATIONS ON FUNCTION
Trunk and Postural Control	
• Multidirectional trunk weakness • Impairments in appropriate activation of trunk and postural control muscles • Assumption of abnormal static sitting postures (i.e., posterior pelvic tilt, kyphosis, lateral flexion) • Asymmetrical weight bearing in sitting and standing • Decreased ability to shift weight through the pelvis and legs • Inability to perceive the midline as a result of spatial relationship dysfunction	• Increased risk of falls • Decreased independence in ADL and IADL • Inability to use the more functional arm during chosen activities secondary to the arm being used for postural support • Visual dysfunction secondary to malalignment of the head and neck in sitting and standing • Swallowing difficulties secondary to poor proximal alignment
Upper Extremity	
• Weakness • Loss of selective motor control • Changes in muscle tone • Contractures • Joint subluxation • Pain • Somatosensory loss	• Decreased ability to reach, grasp, transport, and manipulate objects during ADLs • Decreased independence in ADL and IADL • Development of pain syndromes that can impact sleep patterns and decrease motivation to engage in activity
Cognition and Perception	
• Apraxia • Unilateral neglect • Memory loss • Attention deficits • Executive dysfunction • Spatial dysfunction	• Inability to use or manipulate utensils correctly • Difficulty locating a clock on the left side of the room • Forgetting a shopping list • Not able to sustain the task of reading a recipe • Difficulty multitasking • Difficulty aligning/orienting clothing to the body
Vision	
• Diplopia • Decreased acuity • Visual field cut • Strabismus	• Double vision impairs reading, mobility, and so on • Difficulty with medication management • Will require mobility options other than driving • Poor depth perception results in spilling milk when pouring into cup
Psychosocial	
• Depression • Anxiety • Lability	• Decreased engagement in leisure activities • Fearful to leave the home • Not able to maintain social relationships

ADL, activity of daily living; IADL, instrumental activity of daily living.

of comprehensive ADL function (as measured by the Barthel Index and Frenchay Activities Index)[29] and gait recovery.[30]

Upper Extremity Impairments

The majority of the daily activities in which we engage require interaction with objects in the environment. Thus, the ability to use the arm and hand to reach, grasp, transport, manipulate, and release objects is critical for daily functioning. A majority of patients experience UE dysfunction poststroke, with the most common impairment being paresis.[13] In addition to weakness, loss of selective motor control, changes in muscle tone, and somatosensory loss can impact the patient's ability to engage the UE during functional activities.[31,32]

Also problematic are secondary complications that may develop as a consequence of abnormal muscle activity. For example, profound muscle weakness and loss of muscle tone (flaccidity) during poststroke early phases, coupled with the dependent nature of the arm and hand, may cause the following[33]:

- Edema (predominantly in the hand)
- Overstretching of the glenohumeral joint capsule
- Establishment of muscle imbalances caused by shortening of some muscle groups and overlengthening of others (e.g., shortening of shoulder internal rotator and overlengthening of external rotators)

- Shoulder joint subluxation
- Risk of joint and soft-tissue injuries during the performance of daily tasks

After the initial period of profound weakness, hypertonia (increased muscle tone), stereotypical limb posturing, hyperactive stretch reflexes, and **spasticity** may develop. If spasticity is not appropriately managed, complications such as joint deformities and contractures, skin breakdown on the palmar hand surface, and the development of pain syndromes may arise.[32,33]

In fact, according to the *AHA/ASA Guidelines for Adult Stroke Rehabilitation and Recovery*,[13] shoulder pain is common after stroke, with a reported incidence of up to 22% within the first year after the onset. The development of pain is commonly associated with shoulder **subluxation** and motor weakness; however, spasticity is also thought to contribute to shoulder pain in some patients. Other predictors of shoulder pain include[13]:

- Older age
- Left hemiplegia
- Presence of tactile extinction (i.e., impaired ability to sense sensory stimuli applied to the affected limb when stimuli are simultaneously applied to the unaffected limb) and reduced proprioception
- Reduced passive abduction and external rotation at the shoulder joint
- Shoulder pain with passive shoulder abduction with the arm internally rotated
- Tenderness to palpation over the biceps and supraspinatus tendons

Few patients make a full recovery, and the vast majority must contend with UE limitations. It is estimated that approximately 65% of patients cannot incorporate their affected hand into daily activities at 6 months poststroke onset.[34] This decreased ability to use the arm and hand during ADLs results in activity limitations and participation restrictions that impact quality of life.[13,35]

Cognitive and Perceptual Impairments

Most patients having sustained stroke present with some deficits related to cognitive and perceptual processing.[36] Deficits can range from mild to severe and substantially impact activity and role performance. It is generally agreed that patients with cognitive and perceptual deficits have suboptimal outcomes compared to those without such deficits.[36] It is common for deficits to appear in clusters based on the stroke lesion site. For example, those with left hemispheric strokes may present with ideational apraxia, motor apraxia, poor organization, decreased ability to sequence, and impaired judgment. Those with right hemispheric strokes may present with unilateral spatial neglect, unilateral body neglect, decreased attention, and spatial dysfunction.

Depending on the type and severity of cognitive and perceptual deficits, multiple aspects of daily life can be impacted including:

- Decreased independence in basic ADLs and functional mobility[37]
- Decreased independence and efficiency performing instrumental activities of daily living (IADLs)[38]
- Inability to return to work[39]
- Inability to drive[40]

Language Impairments

Deficits in speech and language functions are common problems, particularly in strokes involving the left hemisphere. Disorders of aphasia, dysarthria, and speech apraxia can impair an individual's ability to communicate impacting engagement in daily occupations and overall quality of life.[41] The speech language therapist is the member of the rehabilitation team who evaluates and treats speech and language disorders. These therapists provide valuable information to the treatment team and members of the patient's social network regarding the best methods for communicating with the patient. Practitioners should incorporate these recommendations when working with their patients. Common disorders of speech and language functions are described in the subsequent sections. It is important to note that these disorders may range in severity and may occur in isolation or in combination with each other.

Aphasia is an acquired multimodality language disorder that results from damage to the brain's language centers.[41] As such, it can impair the understanding and expression of both oral and written language modalities. Aphasias are frequently classified according to verbal fluency, auditory comprehension, and repetition ability. According to Cherney and Small,[41] "non-fluent aphasia is characterized by output that is slow, labored, and effortful." Phrase length (i.e., number of words produced continuously without a pause) is short, and normal grammar is lacking. Conversely, fluent aphasia is characterized by speech that is easily produced and prosody (i.e., patterns of stress and language intonation) that is normal. Phrase length is adequate, and sentences are grammatically correct. The most common types of nonfluent and fluent aphasias are described as follows.[41]

Broca Aphasia

Nonfluent aphasia is characterized by speech that is slow and effortful, with disrupted prosody. Phrase length is short (<4 words), and sentences are simplified. Apraxia of speech may also be present. Comprehension is relatively intact, and repetition ability is poor.[41]

Wernicke Aphasia

Fluent aphasia is characterized by speech that is well articulated, but often produced at an increased rate. Phrase length is greater than four words. Oral expression contains paraphrasing (i.e., sound substitutions), neologisms (i.e., newly coined word), or often lacks content words. Comprehension and repetition ability are poor.[41]

Anomic Aphasia

Fluent aphasia is characterized by word-finding pauses that may interrupt speech flow. Phrase length is within normal ranges and sentences are grammatically correct. Circumlocution or use of nonspecific words to cope with word-finding difficulties is noted. Comprehension and repetition ability are good.[41]

Global Aphasia

Nonfluent and severely impaired aphasia are characterized by stereotypical utterances that may be present. Comprehension and repetition ability are severely impaired.[41]

Dysarthria is a term used to describe speech disorders that result from paralysis, weakness, or incoordination of the muscles involved in speech production.[41] These deficits impact various dimensions of speech, including articulation, pitch, loudness, vocal quality (e.g., harsh, hoarse, breathy, strained/strangled, hyponasality or hypernasality), ventilation, and prosody. Overall, speech intelligibility is affected to varying degrees from mildly impaired to unintelligible.[41]

Speech apraxia is a disorder of motor programming or planning impacting speech articulation and prosody.[41] Common symptoms of speech apraxia include difficulty producing correct sounds, inconsistent or variable errors in sound production with more consonant than vowel errors, difficulty producing consonants that are adjacent to each other (e.g., str, bl), incorrectly using sounds or words that approximate the target sound or word, and disruptions in prosody. Clients with speech apraxia are aware of their errors and may be frustrated by them.[41]

Visual Impairments

Approximately 25% of patients present with visual impairment poststroke.[42] Visual impairment after stroke is associated with older age, higher NIHSS scores on admission, higher modified Rankin Scale scores, and lower Barthel Index scores at day 7.[42] As compared to patients without visual impairment, those with such impairment present with lower quality of life, higher levels of depression and anxiety, higher fatigue severity, and lower levels of ADL and mobility function.[42]

Specific examples of occupations impacted by visual impairment include:

- Inability to drive secondary to visual field cut or impaired depth perception
- Impaired functional mobility and potential fall risk
- Inability to read or balance a checkbook
- Inability to access electronic communication methods
- Difficulty locating objects in the environment required to perform basic ADL and/or IADL

Psychosocial Impairments

Psychosocial impairments are common after stroke. Depression and anxiety are frequently observed and are associated with increased mortality and suboptimal functional outcomes.[13] It is important for occupational therapists to monitor and screen for signs and symptoms of psychosocial disorders. The impact of these disorders can be substantial and may include:

- Decreased or inability to participate in the rehabilitation process
- Suboptimal functional recovery
- Decreased overall social participation
- Interference with social relationships
- Altered sex drive
- Altered appetite

Evaluation and Intervention of Functional Skill Deficits Secondary to Stroke

Evaluation and intervention procedures will vary depending on the impairment pattern resulting from stroke, the recovery stage (i.e., acute, subacute, or chronic), and the treatment setting (e.g., hospital, inpatient rehabilitation facility, home environment). During the acute recovery stage, the patient is considered medically stable, the lesion is nonprogressing, and residual impairments are typically most severe. For example, a patient with a left hemisphere lesion may exhibit little or no movement of the right body side because of profound weakness, little or no response to sensory information from the right body side, and severe language impairment.

Over time, it is anticipated that the patient will improve both neurologically and functionally; however, the extent and course of improvement are difficult to predict. Some patients make only slight improvements slowly over time, whereas others regain almost full function. It is generally accepted that the majority of improvement occurs within the first 3 to 6 months[13,15] poststroke onset (acute to subacute stages of recovery). As indicated earlier, stroke should be considered a chronic condition because >30% of patients continue to report participation restrictions 4 years poststroke onset and evidence suggests that patients can make functional improvements several years after onset (chronic stage).[13]

When determining which specific evaluations and interventions to use, and how best to implement them to address a given patient's needs, therapists should use evidence-based practice principles. To determine the best evidence available from systematic research, practitioners must remain up to date with occupational therapy and related professional literature. Systematic reviews and meta-analyses provide a synthesis of evidence related to a specific topic. Evidence-based libraries and search engines, such as the Cochrane Library, are excellent resources for locating these types of reviews.

In addition, published practice guidelines and comprehensive evidence-based reviews are available to aid therapists in the selection of appropriate evaluations and interventions when working with patients having sustained stroke. The *American Occupational Therapy Association's Occupational Therapy Practice Guidelines for Adults with Stroke*[14] (AOTAPG), *AHA/ASA Guidelines for Adult Stroke Rehabilitation and Recovery*[13] (*AHA/ASA Guidelines*), and *Evidence-Based Review of Stroke Rehabilitation*[43] are highly recommended resources. These resources provide an overview of the care continuum and provide comprehensive recommendations regarding evidence-based evaluations and interventions that address patient needs. The following sections provide an overview of evidence-based evaluations and interventions that are commonly used with patients having sustained stroke.

Evaluation Approaches

The concepts of client-centered assessment and care have been discussed in occupational therapy for over 30 years[44] and are considered best practice. Client-centered approaches are particularly useful owing to patient variability in the presentation of poststroke function. The completion of an occupational profile, collaborative goal setting, and establishing a therapeutic partnership are important client-centered care components.

When evaluating a patient having sustained stroke, therapists may use a top-down, bottom-up, or combination approach.[45] A top-down approach begins with inquiry into role performance after stroke, followed by an evaluation of the activities required for desired roles, and finally determination of which client factors support or limit occupational performance. In contrast, a bottom-up approach begins with an evaluation of patient skill impairment, followed by an evaluation of daily activities, and finally inquiry into role performance limitations resulting from stroke.[46] Although both approaches are potentially useful, the authors recommend beginning with a top-down approach followed by bottom-up evaluations as needed. Beginning with a top-down approach ensures client-centeredness, individualized goals and is consistent with performance-based assessment.

Evaluation of Areas of Occupation

Stroke may impact a patient's ability to engage in a variety of desired occupations. Guided by a top-down approach, occupations that have been identified by the patient as desired and important should be the target of evaluation. Areas of occupation evaluated may include ADLs (e.g., grooming, bathing, toileting, dressing, feeding, functional mobility), IADLs (e.g., care of others, home management, meal preparation), rest and sleep activities, educational and work activities, leisure activities, and social participation.

Direct observation of task performance and use of activity analysis allow the therapist to determine those activities for which the patient is having difficulty and to identify the factors interfering with occupational performance. Both standardized and nonstandardized methods of evaluating areas of occupation may be useful depending on the context. Standardized assessments provide reliable and valid data that can be used to guide treatment planning and evaluate changes in performance over time. Examples of standardized assessments that can be used to evaluate areas of occupation include the Activity Card Sort,[47] the Canadian Occupational Performance Measure,[48] the Barthel Index,[49] and the Functional Independence Measure.[50]

Evaluation of Performance Skills and Client Factors

Residual deficits in performance skills and client factors that limit occupational performance are common after stroke. For example, impairments in arm and hand function, balance and mobility, processing skills, communication, and emotional expression are common performance skill deficits observed after stroke. These deficits typically occur secondary to underlying client factor impairments. As indicated earlier, neuromusculoskeletal impairments, sensory impairments, and changes in mental functions are common stroke consequences. Key skills and factors to be evaluated, and common instruments used to evaluate these areas, are presented in the sections that follow. In the case of strokes impacting the brainstem, cranial nerve assessment may be needed (see Chapter 20).

Balance and Mobility

Impairment in trunk and postural control limits a client's ability to assume and maintain balance in sitting and standing positions, and reduce overall functional mobility (e.g., bed mobility, transfers, walking). Trunk and postural control can be assessed during observation of task performance in sitting (see Fig. 36-2) and standing positions. This allows the therapist to determine the patient's isometric, concentric, and eccentric trunk muscle control; symmetry of weight bearing through the pelvis and LEs; limits of stability; and the use of postural strategies (ankle, hip, and stepping strategies) to maintain balance.[22,26] There are several standardized assessments available that can be used by occupational therapists to evaluate trunk control, balance, and functional mobility after stroke. Examples include the Postural Assessment Scale for Stroke Patients (PASS),[51] Timed Get Up and Go,[52] Berg Balance Scale,[53] Functional Reach Test (see Chapter 15),[54] Trunk Control Test,[55] and Tinetti Test.[56]

Upper Extremity Function

As indicated earlier, the ability to integrate the UE in ADLs is a significant problem after stroke. A comprehensive

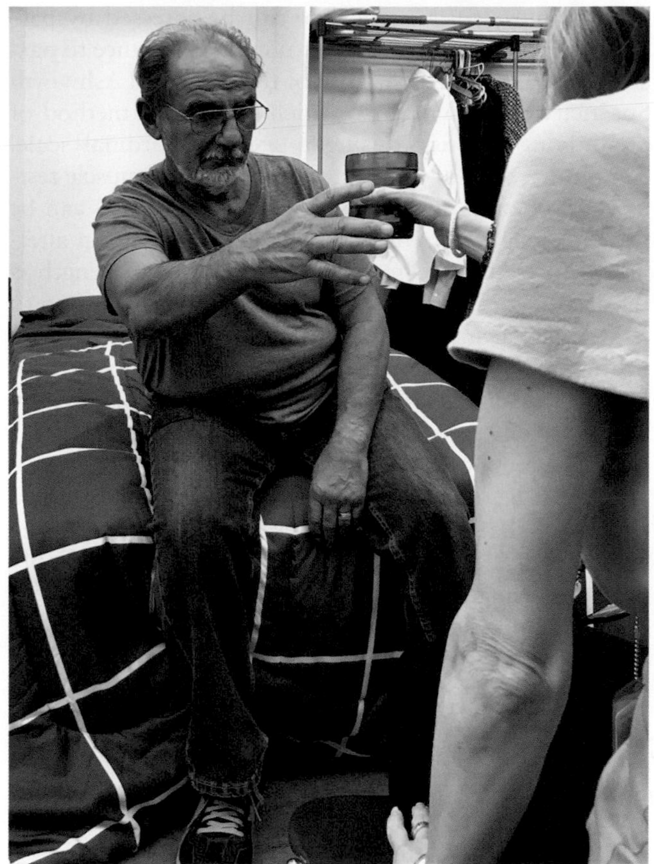

Figure 36-2. Observation of the patient reaching for a cup with the noninvolved upper extremity, while seated at the edge of the bed. Note the asymmetrical weight bearing through the pelvis favoring the intact (***right***) side.

evaluation of motor skills and client factors that may limit UE engagement during function should be undertaken. The main focus of this evaluation should be to determine the capacity to use the arm and hand in daily activity performance.

There are a variety of valid and reliable performance-based and self-report measures to evaluate the capacity of the arm and hand after stroke. Performance-based measures involve the therapist rating and/or timing UE movements during the performance of simple tasks (e.g., pouring water, transporting items from one location to another, flipping cards) or more complex activities (e.g., sentence copying, shoe tying, sandwich making, or laundry folding).[32] Standardized performance-based measures such as the Action Research Arm Test (see Fig. 36-3),[57] Jebsen-Taylor Test of Hand Function,[58] Wolf Motor Function Test,[59] Functional Test for the Hemiparetic UE,[60] and the Assessment of Motor and Process Skills[61] can provide objective measures of arm and hand function after stroke (see Chapter 15).

Conversely, self-report measures are typically semi-structured, Likert-scale questionnaires through which the therapist queries the patient or caregiver about the client's UE use during common daily activities.[32] Such self-report questionnaires provide important subjective information that can be used to compliment the objective findings of performance-based measures. Examples of self-report measures that can be used to evaluate UE function poststroke include the 30-, 28-, and 14-item Motor Activity Log (see Chapter 15)[62–64]; the hand and ADL subsections of the Stroke Impact Scale (SIS)[65]; the 36-item Manual Ability Measure[66]; and the 23-item ABILIHAND.[67]

Once UE capacity for engagement in daily activities has been determined, it may be necessary to evaluate specific client factors to gain a clearer understanding of the underlying factors limiting functional arm and hand use. For example, the inability to effectively reach, grasp, and transport objects from one location to another may be due to several factors, including, but not limited to, decreased hand sensation, restricted joint mobility, insufficient grip strength, or an inability to

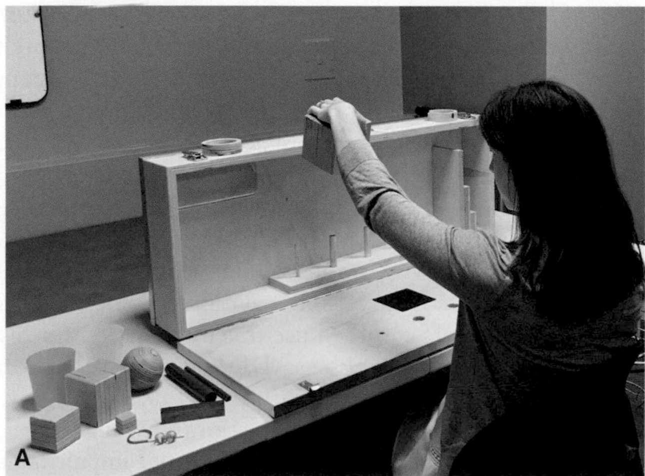

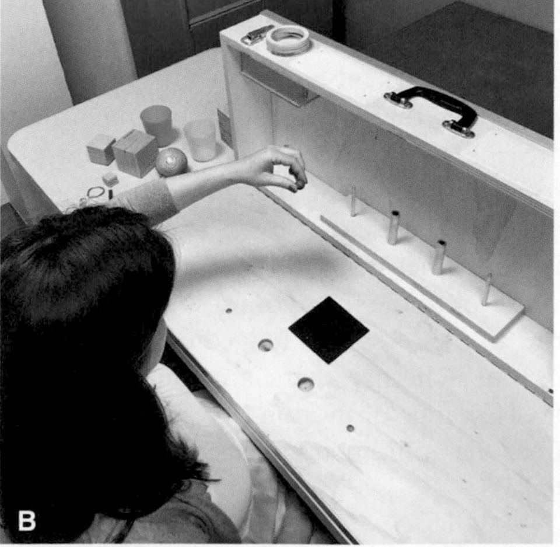

Figure 36-3. A and B. Action Reach Arm Test. This test consists of 19 items grouped into four subscales: grasp, grip, pinch, and gross movement. **A.** Patient performing hardest item of grasp subsection—moving a 10-cm block from the brown square to the top of the board. **B.** Patient performing easiest item of the pinch subscale—moving a marble (using the thumb and index finger) from the brown square to the top of the board.

selectively control and coordinate distal and proximal limb segment movement. Evaluations of sensation, joint alignment and mobility, muscle tone and strength, and the ability to isolate and coordinate various joint movements should be selectively performed if the therapist suspects that deficits in these areas may underlie difficulty using the arm and hand during functional activities. Each of these is discussed as follows.

Somatosensory Function

Standard procedures for assessing somatosensory functions (e.g., ability to sense touch, vibration, temperature, pain, and proprioception) are outlined in Chapter 12. The majority of these procedures can be used to assess UE sensation in patients having sustained stroke. It is important, however, to note that most of these tests require attention and the ability to follow directions, which may be impaired after stroke. It is, therefore, important to determine the patient's ability to follow assessment procedures prior to testing. Patients with language impairments impacting expressive abilities (e.g., Broca aphasia) may require modification of testing procedures (e.g., head nod or an agreed-upon gesture to indicate yes/no responses). In patients with severe language or cognitive impairments, standard testing is not possible. In these cases, gross information may be obtained via observation of limb movements (i.e., withdrawing of a limb) or facial grimacing in response to pinprick. Conversely, in patients with very mild impairments, more comprehensive sensory testing may be required to determine subtle deficits, such as impairment of two-point discrimination or the ability to distinguish light touch on the finger tips (see Chapter 12).

Joint Alignment and Mobility

It is important to assess the integrity of the shoulder joint because it is estimated that 50% of patients have inferior subluxation of the glenohumeral joint poststroke.[68] Alignment can be assessed by palpating the subacromial space while the patient is in a seated position with the arm hanging freely at the side. In this position, the therapist determines the location of the humeral head with respect to the glenoid fossa. Subluxations are typically classified according to the position of the humeral head with respect to the glenoid fossa as (a) inferior: humeral head is below the glenoid fossa; (b) anterior: humeral head is anterior to the fossa; or (c) superior: humeral head is superior to the fossa and lodged under the acromion.[33] To determine whether there are joint mobility restrictions, passive range of motion (ROM) measurements can be obtained via goniometric measurements as needed (see Chapter 13).

Muscle Tone, Strength, and Selective Motor Control

Changes in muscle tone should be assessed to determine the presence of hypotonicity or hypertonicity/spasticity (see Chapter 15). Muscle tone can be assessed by passively moving the limb to determine its resistance to passive stretch, coupled with use of the Modified Ashworth Spasticity Scale (MASS),[69] which provides a method of quantifying spasticity using a six-point ordinal scale. Traditional tests of strength such as manual muscle testing (MMT) and dynamometry (see Chapter 13) can be used to quantify strength deficits after stroke. An alternative to traditional methods of measuring strength is the use of the Motricity Index,[55,70] which is similar to MMT in that it involves grading strength on the basis of the patient's ability to activate muscles, move a limb segment against gravity, and tolerate resistance given by an examiner.[70]

The ability to isolate and coordinate UE joint movements can be objectively measured using the UE motor section of the Fugl-Meyer Assessment[71] (FMA-UE, see Chapter 15). The FMA-UE has been used to reliably measure change in UE motor impairment in a variety of stroke intervention trials[72] and has clinical utility.[73] It was developed from Brunnstrom stages of motor recovery and consists of 33 items that progress from reflexive muscle activity to the ability to selectively combine and fractionate movements. Evidence suggests that scores on the FMA-UE are valid and reliable indicators of motor impairment severity across poststroke stages of recovery. Scores on the FMA-UE have been correlated with spontaneous use of the UE in a variety of common daily activities.[74] In addition, a key form recovery map was developed for use with the FMA-UE.[73] Use of the form allows therapists to quickly identify those movements for which the patient is having difficulty. This information can then be used to tailor UE training to target missing motor components in the context of patient selected activities.[73]

Cognition and Perception

Because of the variability in cognitive and perceptual deficit presentation, occupational therapists must be familiar with a variety of instruments that measure the impact of these deficits on daily living skills. This approach differs from interprofessional colleagues who tend to assess cognitive skills outside the context in which they are typically performed.

The Kettle Test[75] is an example of a performance-based assessment that uses an IADL task (making two hot beverages with varying ingredients using an electric kettle) to assess cognitive skills within a functional context. Practitioners can then use this information for discharge planning. Similarly, the ADL-focused Occupation-based Neurobehavioral Evaluation (A-ONE; formerly, Árnadóttir OT-ADL Neurobehavioral Evaluation)[76] identifies specific cognitive and perceptual impairments (e.g., apraxia, unilateral neglect, spatial dysfunction, memory loss, poor organization and sequencing, decreased insight) during basic ADL and functional mobility.

There are also domain-specific performance-based assessments. Executive dysfunction is common after stroke and requires specific attention during the evaluation process. The Executive Function Performance Test[77] examines components of executive functioning such as initiation, organization, judgment, and safety while observing a patient performing IADL tasks such as cooking, money management, and bill paying. The Multiple Errands Test[78] examines the impact of executive dysfunction during a multitasking situation. The task can be performed in the community or in a public area such as a hospital lobby. Finally, the Weekly Calendar Planning Activity[79] examines executive functions performed as clients insert multiple appointments onto a weekly paper calendar using specific rules (e.g., "Do not schedule appointments on Wednesday").

The Catherine Bergego Scale[80] (CBS) is a standardized behavioral assessment of unilateral neglect. It is based on direct observation of the patient's behavior in 10 everyday situations such as grooming, dressing, eating, and wheelchair mobility. More recently, the Kessler Foundation Neglect Assessment Process (KF-NAP)[81] was developed based on the CBS. Because the authors found that additional instructions were needed for reliable CBS administration, they developed the KF-NAP, which provides detailed administration instructions and a scoring chart for the original 10 CBS behavioral categories (for further information regarding cognitive and perceptual evaluation, see Chapters 9 and 10).

Vision

Examples of visual screening components include near and far acuity, visual field testing, ocular ROM or control, ocular alignment, and contrast sensitivity. These skills are often considered the foundation skills for visual processing. Specific visuomotor abilities that should be assessed include fixation, pursuits, saccades, accommodation, and convergence (see Chapter 7). The Brain Injury Visual Assessment Battery for Adults (biVABA)[82] is an example of a standardized assessment of vision and perceptual processing, including visual acuity (distant and reading), contrast sensitivity, visual field function, oculomotor function, and visual attention and scanning.

Psychosocial

As mentioned earlier, a variety of psychosocial disorders can occur after stroke and negatively impact occupational performance. Similar to other domains, therapists should be familiar with a variety of psychosocial instruments based on individual patient needs. The Beck Depression Inventory[83] is one of the most widely used screening instruments to measure depression severity in both adults and adolescents over the age of 13. Items relating to depressive symptoms include hopelessness, irritability, cogitations such as guilt or feelings of being punished, as well as physical symptoms such as fatigue, weight loss, and lack of sexual interest. The Patient Health Questionnaire (PHQ)-2 and PHQ-9[84] are also commonly used instruments for those with psychosocial impairment. The 9-item PHQ is based on the *Diagnostic and Statistical Manual of Mental Disorders* criteria for major depression. Sample items include little interest or pleasure in doing things; feeling down, depressed, and hopeless; and poor appetite or overeating.[85] The Hospital Anxiety and Depression Scale[86] (HADS) is a self-administered measure used to screen for the presence of depression and anxiety. The HADS includes 14 total items that ask patients to reflect on their mood in the past week. Seven items assess depression, and two concern appearance and feelings of slowing down. Seven items assess anxiety, of which two assess autonomic anxiety (panic and butterflies in the stomach), and the remaining five assess tension and restlessness.

Intervention Approaches

As indicated earlier, intervention procedures used with patients having sustained stroke will vary depending on impairment pattern, recovery stage, and treatment setting. The general focus of occupational therapy intervention during the three primary recovery phases (acute, rehabilitation, and subacute-chronic) is outlined as follows.

Acute Stage

In the acute stage (hospital setting), therapists should address:

- Appropriate positioning to prevent secondary complications such as subluxation, muscle imbalances, joint contractures, skin breakdown, and the development of pain syndromes (see subsequent section on motor impairments)
- Dysphagia management (see Chapter 19)
- Fall prevention (see Chapter 30)
- Early mobilization and the beginning of self-care activity retraining (see Chapter 27)
- Initial remediation of client factor impairments that interfere with activity engagement (see subsequent sections on intervention and Chapters 8, 9, 11, 12, 14, 16, 17, and 20)

Rehabilitation Stage

In the rehabilitation stage (inpatient rehabilitation setting):

- The focus of treatment shifts to restoration of or compensation for performance skill deficits that continue to interfere with daily occupations (e.g., limitations in UE function, balance and mobility, and mental functions) (see subsequent section on intervention).
- Maximizing independence in ADLs and IADLs for discharge to the community is a key focus of treatment

during this recovery stage (see subsequent section on intervention and Section 4, Restoration of Independent and Community Living Roles).

Subacute-Chronic Stage (Home and Community Environments)

In this recovery phase, therapists should focus on:

- Maximizing independence in IADLs (see Chapter 28)
- Addressing skills needed for return to work (see Chapter 29)
- Resumption of driving (see Chapter 31)
- Promoting engagement in leisure activities and socialization (see Chapters 28 and 29).

When selecting appropriate interventions, therapists should be guided by evidence-based practice principles. Intervention approaches that use task-specific training or functional task practice to promote change in patients having sustained stroke are supported by both research and clinical perspectives.[87] For example, both the *AOTAPG*[14] and the *ASA/AHS Guidelines*[13] recommend practicing functional tasks to improve balance and mobility, UE function, and ADLs/IADLs.

Motor learning and intervention principles espoused in the Occupational Therapy Task-Oriented Approach[88] (OT-TOA) can serve as useful guidelines for developing appropriate treatment interventions for patients poststroke. These principles are discussed in detail in Chapter 34 and are briefly presented as follows:

- Assist patients to adjust to role and task performance limitations by exploring alternative ways to perform tasks associated with desired roles.
- Create a treatment environment that mirrors the common challenges that patients experience in daily life.
- Practice functional tasks (identified by the patient) or close simulations to identify effective and efficient strategies for task performance.
- Provide opportunities for practice outside therapy sessions.
- Use contemporary motor learning principles in training or retraining skills, including minimizing ineffective and inefficient movement patterns, the use of random and variable practice conditions, providing decreasing amounts of physical guidance and verbal feedback, and developing task analysis and problem-solving skills in patients so they can find their own solutions to occupational performance problems.

In addition to the OT-TOA, components of other approaches may help guide treatment of patients having sustained stroke. For example, application of a biomechanical approach may be useful for addressing impairments such as decreased strength, muscle imbalances, decreased joint mobility, edema, and pain (see Chapter 32). In contrast, the rehabilitative approach can guide the use of adaptation, compensation, and environmental modifications to maximize independence in daily activities when residual impairments continue to interfere with performance (see Chapter 33). The remainder of this section highlights evidence-based interventions that can be used with patients to address ADL and IADL impairments; motor impairments; cognitive, visual, and perceptual impairments; and psychosocial impairments poststroke.

Interventions that Address ADL and IADL Impairments

Evidence suggests that activity- and occupation-based interventions improve ADL and IADL performance after stroke.[14] According to the *ASA/AHA Guidelines*,[13] all patients with stroke should receive ADL and IADL training tailored to individual needs and the eventual discharge setting. This functional training should be task specific, repetitive, graded to challenge the patient's individual capabilities, and progressed as appropriate.[13,14]

For example, in the acute recovery phase, a patient may indicate a desire to self-feed without assistance from significant others or staff. In this case, the patient should be engaged in self-feeding activities to allow for learning and practice of such tasks (e.g., drinking from a cup, using a spoon, or cutting food). Grading of this task-specific training may begin with the relatively simple task of sandwich eating or drinking from a cup, progress to the appropriate use of utensils with a variety of food types (cereal, vegetables, meats), and finally advance to eating a variety of full meals unaided. In later recovery phases, this same patient may wish to prepare his or her own meals when discharged home. In this case, the patient should be engaged in meal preparation activities that are graded in complexity.

Depending on the degree of impairment, recovery stage, patient preferences, and the anticipated discharge environment, it may be appropriate to teach compensatory strategies (e.g., one-handed techniques performed with the intact UE, energy conservation, work simplification techniques) or introduce adaptive equipment during ADL/IADL training. According to the *ASA/AHA Guidelines*, adaptive and assistive devices should be used for safety and function when other methods of activity performance are unavailable or cannot be learned, or when patient safety is a concern.[13] For example, in patients with severe sensory and motor impairment impacting the arm and hand, remediation of UE function to allow independent daily activity performance may not be possible. In this case, instruction in one-handed techniques and/or the use of adaptive equipment for engagement in daily activities would be needed. See Figure 36-4 for an example of one-handed dressing techniques and Table 36-4 for adaptive equipment commonly used with patients poststroke.

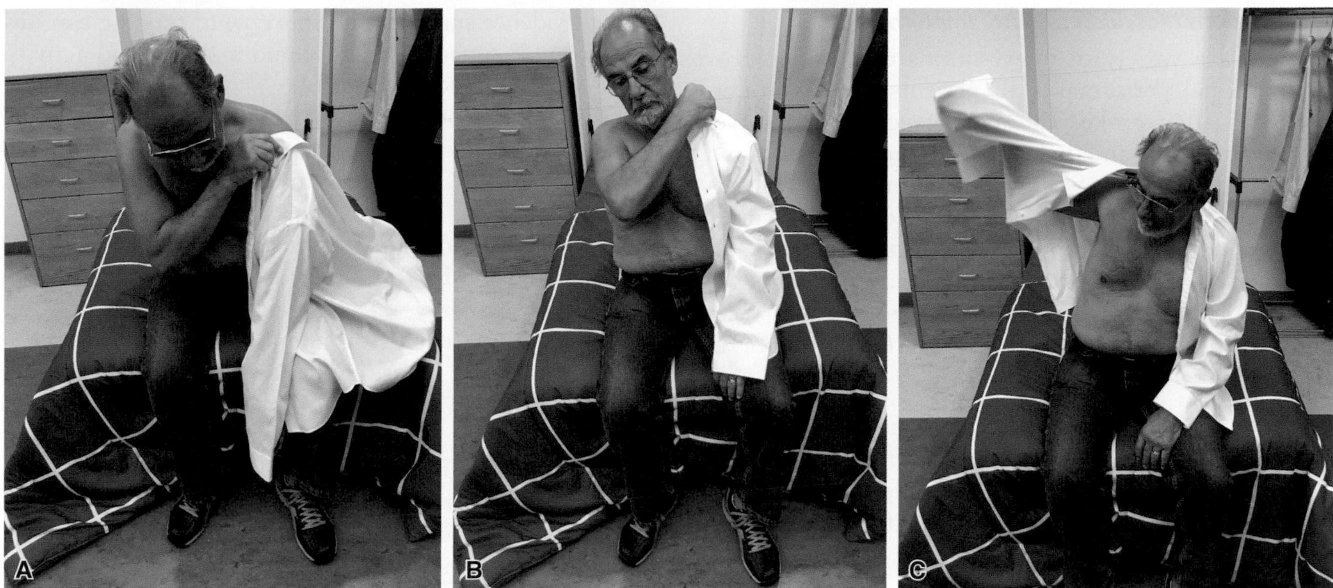

Figure 36-4. A to C. Sequence for one-handed dressing technique. **A.** Pulling shirt sleeve over affected arm. **B.** Pulling the shirt sleeve over the affected shoulder and swinging the shirt over back until the other sleeve hangs down over the back. **C.** Reaching to the back with unaffected arm and placing unaffected arm into the opening of the sleeve and pushing unaffected arm through sleeve.

Table 36-4. Examples of Commonly Used Adaptive Equipment

ADL/IADL	ADAPTIVE EQUIPMENT/DURABLE MEDICAL EQUIPMENT
Feeding	• Nonskid mats to hold plates/bowls steady on the table surface • Plate guards and scoop dishes to eliminate food spillage off plate when using utensils • Rocker knife to aid with cutting foods • Built-up handled utensils to aid weak grasp
Grooming	• Toothpaste dispenser • Electric toothbrush • Suction denture brush for one-handed cleaning of dentures • One-handed finger nail clipper • Long-handled brushes or combs to extend reach
Bathing	• Nonskid mats for inside and outside tub/shower for safety • Handheld shower head with control of water flow • Tub or shower seat to allow bathing in the seated position • Grab bars • Long-handled sponge to extend reach • Bath mitt with soap pocket to aid weak grasp
Dressing	• Reacher for clothing retrieval or to aid LB dressing • Dressing stick to aid LE and UE dressing • Long-handled shoe horn • Elastic shoe laces • Button hook
Toileting	• Commode • Raised toilet seat • Toilet safety frame • Toilet tissue aids to extend reach for wiping
Kitchen activities	• Jar opener to aid weak grasp • Box toppers to allow for opening of boxes one-handed • Pan/pot holders to stabilize pots on the stove top • Adapted cutting boards to allow for one-handed cutting, peeling, chopping, and spreading • Suction bottle brushes that allow for one-handed cleaning of glasses

ADL, activity of daily living; IADL, instrumental activity of daily living; LB, lower body; LE, lower extremity; UE, upper extremity.

Interventions that Address Motor Impairments

There are a variety of interventions that can improve occupational performance of patients with motor impairment after stroke. The majority of these interventions target UE and balance and mobility retraining within the context of activity performance.[87] The following is a brief description of various interventions found to effectively improve UE function, balance and mobility, and activity and participation in patients with motor impairment after stroke as reported in a recent evidence-based review,[87] the *AOTASPG*,[14] and/or the *AHA/ASA Guidelines*.[13]

- ***Task-oriented training:*** Are interventions that involve practicing functional tasks that are graded to challenge the patient's current motor capabilities. Tasks are practiced repeatedly and progressed in difficulty so that the patient is continuously challenged as gains are made.[14] Researchers and clinicians use a variety of names to describe this type of training:
  - Repetitive Task Practice
  - Repetitive Task Training
  - Task-specific Training
  - Meaningful Task-specific Training
  - Task-related Training

  Evidence suggests that this type of training can improve UE function, balance and mobility, and activity and participation after stroke[14,87] (see Evidence table). Training can be tailored to various impairment levels and administered in a variety of practice settings (see Fig. 36-5 and Chapters 16 and 34).

- ***Constraint-induced movement therapy (CIMT) or modified CIMT (mCIMT):*** Is a form of task training that involves (1) restraint of the unimpaired limb, forcing use of the impaired limb during daily activities; (2) repetitive task practice with the affected limb in the form of whole task practice and "shaping" for approximately 6 hours a day for 2 weeks[89] (see Fig. 36-6). mCIMT is a modification of the original protocol in which the restraint time of the unimpaired limb, and/or the amount of time for intensive training of the impaired limb, is reduced and/or distributed over a longer period of time.[90] Evidence suggests that both forms of training improve UE function in patients that have some residual wrist and hand function.[14,87] mCIMT appears to have similar efficacy (see Evidence table), and given the reduced practice schedule, greater clinical utility as compared to CIMT.[90]

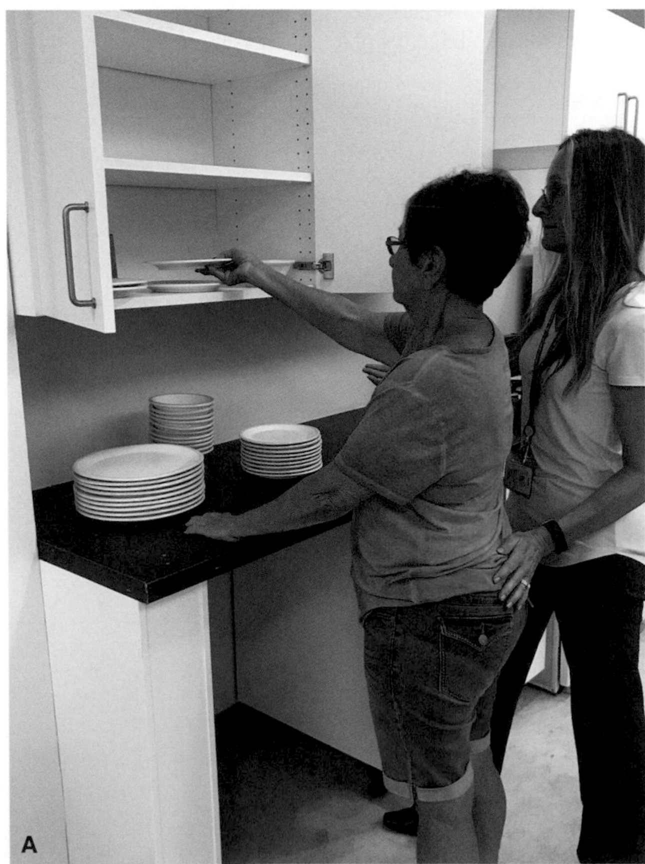

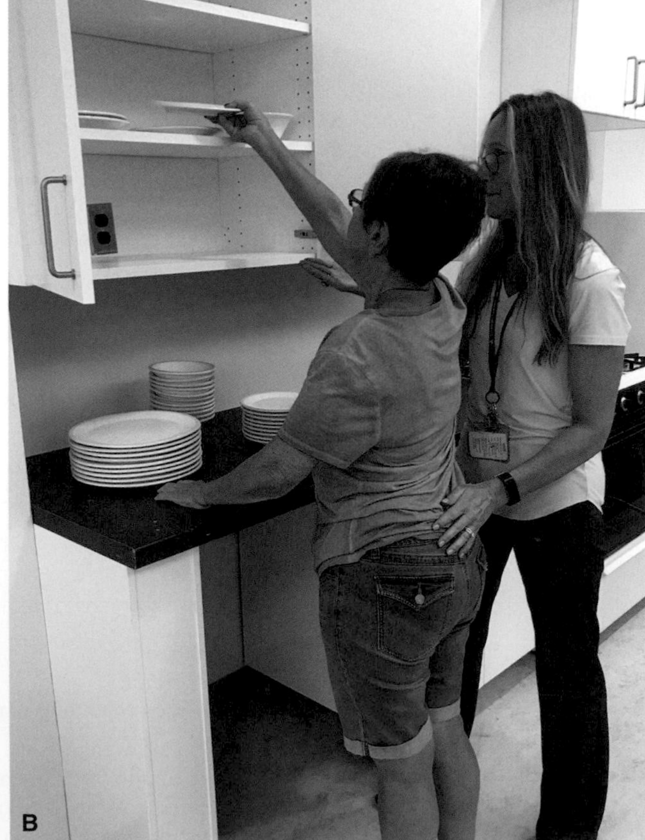

Figure 36-5. A and B. Example of task-oriented training targeting upper extremity (UE) function and standing balance. **A.** Using involved UE to place dishes in the cabinet, while noninvolved UE helps support balance. Note that dishes differing in size, shape, and weight are placed in various locations on the countertop to encourage variability in movement patterns. **B.** Graded up version of the activity.

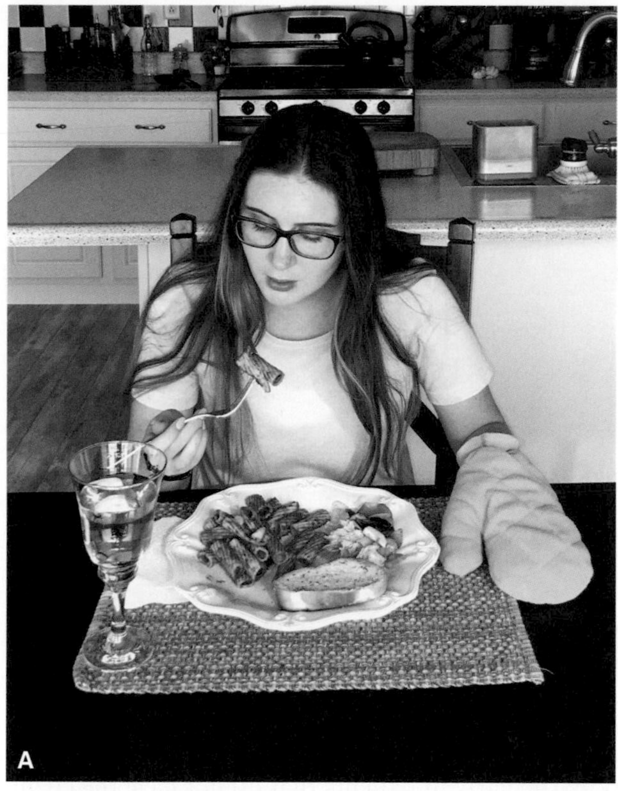
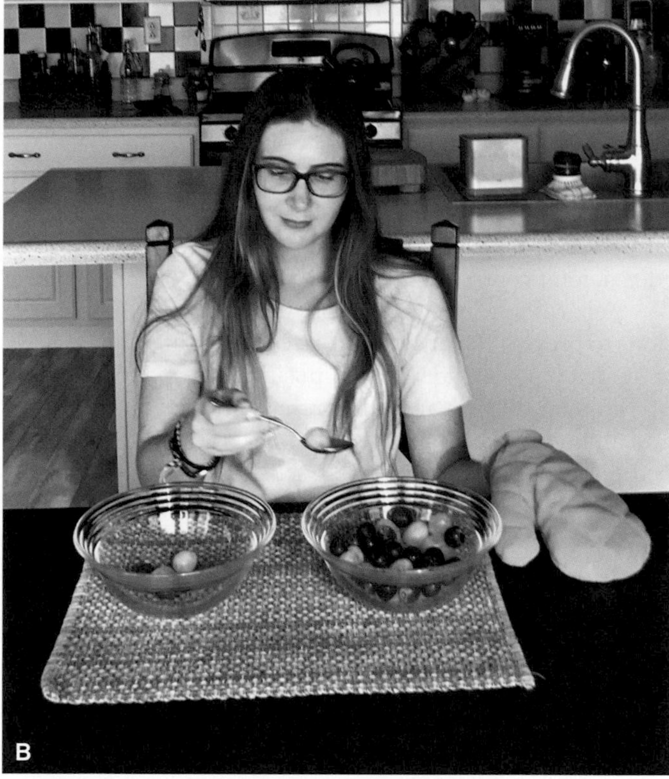

Figure 36-6. A and B. Constraint-induced movement therapy. **A.** Eating a meal. **B.** Shaping activity: using a spoon to transfer grapes between bowls with the impaired upper extremity, while the unimpaired hand is restrained in a mitt.

- *Bilateral upper limb training:* Involves the patient engaging both limbs in the simultaneous execution of identical activities. Evidence suggests that this type of training can improve UE function.[14]

Interventions that Combine Task Practice with Cognitive Strategies

Interventions that combine task practice with cognitive strategies, or use alternative methods of delivering task practice, are appropriate for use as adjuncts to task-oriented training.[14,87] These interventions can be tailored to various impairment levels (which may be especially useful for low functioning patients), and the majority of them can be administered in a variety of practice settings. Examples are:

- *Mental practice (MP):* In which the patient cognitively rehearses an activity (e.g., drinking from a cup, folding laundry, standing up from a chair) in the absence of actual movements. MP can be performed prior to a treatment session as preparation for the physical performance of an activity, or embedded within repetitive task practice sessions. Evidence suggests that MP improves UE function,[14,87] balance and mobility, and activity and participation after stroke.[14]
- *Mirror therapy (MT):* In which the patient performs movements and simple activities with the unimpaired limb while watching its mirror reflection superimposed over the (unseen) impaired limb. Evidence suggests that MT can improve UE function, and activity and participation after stroke.[14]
- *Virtual reality (VR):* In which the patient participates in goal-directed activities in a computer-based, interactive, simulated environment designed to replicate the real-world environment. These environments can be immersive or nonimmersive. Evidence suggests that VR training can improve UE function[14] and can be used as a method for delivering UE movement practice.[13] Evidence also suggests that VR training may improve gait,[13] and activity and participation after stroke.[14]
- *Action observation (AO):* In which the patient first watches another person perform an activity (most often on a prerecorded video) and then performs the activity himself or herself. Evidence suggests that AO may improve UE function.[14]
- *Robotic therapy*: There is evidence that robotic training can provide some benefit for UE motor abilities and activity participation and can be used to deliver intensive UE practice for patients with moderate-to-severe UE paresis.[13]
- *Strengthening and exercise:* Evidence suggests that strengthening exercises can be considered as an adjunct to functional task practice for improving UE function, balance and mobility, and activity and participation after stroke.[14,87]

- *Neuromuscular electrical stimulation (NMES):* Evidence suggests that NMES may improve UE function and can be considered for patients with minimal voluntary movement after stroke or for individuals with shoulder subluxation.[13]

In addition to the abovementioned interventions, it may be necessary to incorporate adjunctive treatments that prevent the development of secondary complications, such as edema, joint contractures, shoulder subluxation, and pain.

According to the *AHA/ASA Guidelines*,[13] interventions to prevent the onset of and treatment for hemiplegic shoulder pain include proper positioning, maintenance of shoulder ROM, and motor retraining. The patient and all involved caregivers should be educated in proper bed positioning (see Box 36-1), self-ROM exercises (see Fig. 36-7), and proper handling of the hemiparetic UE (see Box 36-2) during ADLs. Positioning devices such as wheelchair lap trays and arm troughs may help UE positioning during wheelchair mobility.[13,33] The use of a sling can be considered to support the UE both when the patient is upright and during transfers[13,33]; evidence for preventing or reducing long-term shoulder subluxation, however, is unclear.[33]

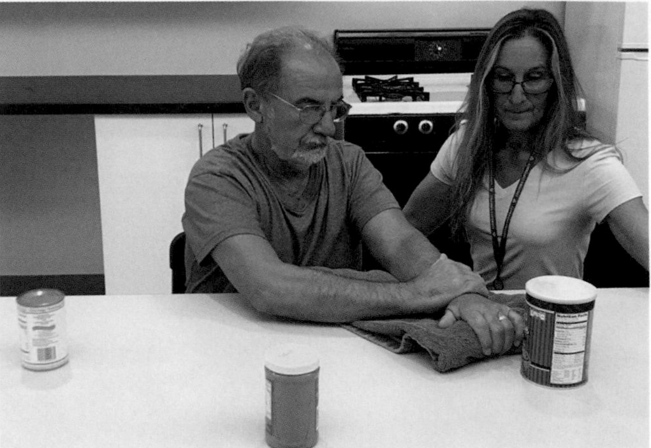

Figure 36-7. Example of self-range of motion exercises for the hemiplegic upper extremity. Patient places the affected arm on a towel and pushes the affected arm toward specific target locations (items located on the table) to encourage shoulder range of motion.

Finally, it may be necessary to use orthotic devices to properly position the hemiparetic hand to maintain appropriate biomechanical alignment and to prevent injury, particularly in patients that do not have the cognitive and perceptual abilities required to maintain ROM or properly manage their hemiparetic UE.[91] A variety of orthotic devices can be considered (see Chapters 22 and 23) for use with patients having sustained stroke. The type of device chosen and the device wearing schedule will vary according to the patients' individual needs. Regardless of the type of orthotic device used, wearing tolerance should be assessed and the need for continued use of the device periodically reevaluated.[91] In addition, the patient and caregiver should be educated regarding the goals of the device (e.g., maintain proper joint alignment, prevent hand injury, maintain palmar skin integrity), how to properly don and doff the device, how to care for the device, and the wearing schedule.[91]

Box 36-1

Procedures for Proper Bed Positioning of Patients with Hemiplegia

Supine Positioning

- Head and neck slightly flexed
- Trunk straight and aligned
- Involved upper extremity supported behind scapula and humerus with a small pillow or towel, shoulder protracted and slightly flexed and abducted with external rotation, elbow extended or slightly flexed, forearm neutral or supinated, and wrist neutral with hand open
- Involved lower limb with hip forward on pillow, nothing against soles of feet

Lying on the Unaffected Side

- Head and neck neutral and symmetrical
- Trunk aligned
- Involved upper extremity protracted with arm forward on pillows, elbow extended or slightly flexed, forearm and wrist neutral, and hand open
- Involved lower extremity with hip and knee forward, flexed, and supported on pillows

Lying on the Affected Side

- Head and neck neutral and symmetrical
- Trunk aligned
- Involved upper extremity protracted forward and externally rotated with elbow extended or slightly flexed, forearm supinated, wrist neutral, and hand open
- Involved lower extremity with knee flexed
- Uninvolved lower extremity with knee flexed and supported on pillows

Based on information from Carr EK, Kenney FD. Positioning of the stroke patient: a review of the literature. *Int J Nurs Stud*. 1992;29:355–369.

Box 36-2

Procedures for Proper Handling of the Hemiparetic Upper Extremity

- Teach the patient as early as possible to be responsible for the positioning of the arm during transfers, bed mobility, and other activities involving change of position.
- Use gait belts or draw sheets, rather than the affected arm, to assist the patient in moving his or her body.
- Avoid shoulder range of motion beyond 90° of flexion and abduction unless there is upward rotation of the scapula and external rotation of the humerus.
- Avoid overhead pulley exercises, because they appear to increase the frequency of pain in the shoulder because neither scapular nor humeral rotation occurs, and the force may be excessive.

Interventions that Address Cognitive, Visual, and Perceptual Impairments

Recent reviews[36] and practice guidelines[13,14] have examined the existing research literature to determine which interventions effectively improve function in patients with cognitive, visual, and perceptual impairments. Suggestions from these evidence-based reviews follow.

Apraxia

The Cognitive Strategy Training intervention is a compensatory method that teaches patients with apraxia internal and external strategies to overcome daily challenges. Internal strategies may consist of verbalizing the activity steps and internal rehearsal. External strategies include viewing pictures illustrating task performance and using listed instructions.[14,36]

Gesture Training has also been recommended for this population and consists of three categories: (1) transitive gesture training using common objects such as a spoon or comb, (2) intransitive symbolic gesture training such as the gesture of eating, and (3) intransitive nonsymbolic gesture training including imitating meaningless gestures.[14,36]

Executive Dysfunction

Time Pressure Management interventions have been used for those with mental slowness. This intervention provides patients with strategies to overcome daily challenges experienced secondary to external time pressure. The intervention consists of three stages: (1) identifying the problem, (2) teaching the strategy (analyzing the task for time pressure, making an emergency plan), and (3) generalization to other situations.[14,36]

There is limited but emerging evidence for interventions such as exercise and recreation programs, and training patients within VR environments to improve executive functioning and daily activity participation.[14,36]

Memory Loss

Interventions are limited for those with memory loss after stroke. While computer-based training has been evaluated with some success, this intervention should be monitored to determine whether memory gains actually generalize to everyday activities. Based on available evidence, remediation of memory has not been successful with the exception of very mild memory loss cases. Compensatory strategies such as memory books, diaries, checklists, and alarm systems may result in better outcomes.[92]

Unilateral Neglect

Several interventions have been identified to decrease the negative impact of unilateral neglect on daily life. These include[14,36]:

- *Visual scanning training:* Which involves teaching systematic and organized visual scanning patterns (see Fig. 36-8 and Evidence table)

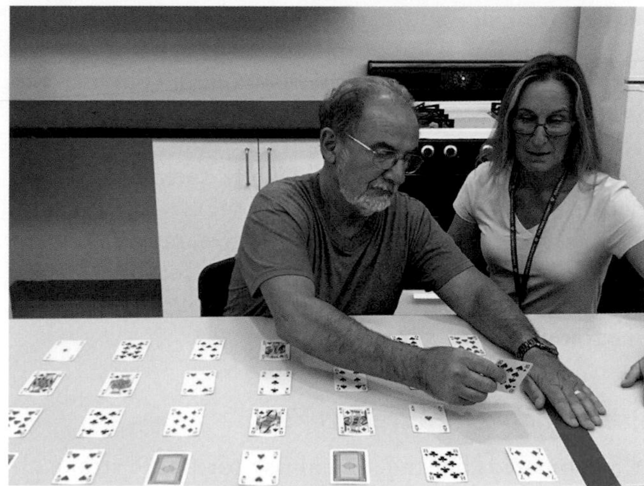

Figure 36-8. Example of visual scanning training. Red tape is used as a marker to aid the patient in locating the left side of space, and the patient is instructed in the use of an organized and systematic scanning strategy to locate and turn over cards of a specific suit.

- *Limb activation:* Involving active or passive limb movements contralesional to the brain lesion
- *Prisms/prism adaptation:* Involving the use of prismatic lenses to induce an optical shift (see Evidence table)
- *Vibration:* In which vibratory stimulation is provided to the neck muscles

Visual Field Deficits

There is general consensus that visual field deficits are not amenable to remediation. Therefore, compensatory approaches such as head/trunk turning and using wider saccades are encouraged in conjunction with environmental adaptations.

The reader should note that many of the identified evidence-based interventions for patients with cognitive and perceptual deficits after stroke fall under the category of strategy training. In order to successfully use strategy training approaches, the patient must have insight into his or her deficits, as well as the functional implications of these deficits. Therefore, awareness training should start early and be used consistently. If a patient does not respond to awareness training, the intervention approach must shift to environmental modification. Environmental modifications are usually taught to caregivers to apply in home and community settings (for more details on cognitive interventions, see Chapter 11).

Interventions that Address Psychosocial Impairments

A body of research has demonstrated the effectiveness of psychosocial intervention after stroke.[13,93] Several studies have examined the effect of exercise training on psychosocial impairments such as anxiety and depression. These programs may be single or multiple component and include interventions such as resistance training, tai chi, walking, and early mobilization in acute care. Behavioral therapy programs and stroke education programs have been used in isolation and in combination. Specific interventions in these categories include problem-solving therapy, motivational interviewing, and cognitive–behavioral therapy. Finally, there is emerging evidence that community-based programs led by occupational therapists may have a positive impact on mental health after stroke. These programs focus on leisure and recreation, community mobility, and/or community integration.

Prevention of Future Strokes

It is estimated that the annual risk for future stroke after an initial ischemic stroke or TIA is between 3% to 4%.[94] Given the morbidity associated with recurrent brain ischemia, preventing a future stroke is important for all patients having experienced a TIA. Education targeting modifiable risk factors should be considered as an important component of a patient's overall treatment program (refer to the section on Stroke Etiology of this chapter).

According to Schmid and colleagues,[95] prevention of a second stroke requires identification and control of modifiable risk factors—the majority of which are best managed through a combination of medication management and changing unhealthy lifestyle choices. Although all members of the health care team can play a role in the prevention of secondary strokes, occupational therapists can make a unique contribution by helping patients to understand and identify the facilitators and barriers to health promotion behaviors.[95] The *AHA/ASA Guidelines for the Prevention of Stroke in Patients with Stroke and Transient Ischemic Attack*[94] is an excellent resource that contains evidence-based recommendations that practitioners can use to develop preventive education programs.

Generally speaking, education programs should include identification of modifiable risk factors; teaching patients appropriate medication management; discussing the importance of a healthy diet, regular exercise, and the need for sufficient sleep; the need to eliminate or reduce unhealthy lifestyle choices such as smoking and the use of drugs and alcohol; and identifying perceived supports, facilitators, and barriers as they relate to engagement in healthy promotion behaviors.[94] In addition, preventive education should include increasing awareness of the signs and symptoms of stroke (i.e., FAST: **F**ace asymmetry, **A**rm weakness, **S**peech impairments, **T**ime to get to the hospital) and be designed to reach racially, ethnically, and age-, and sex-diverse populations.[12]

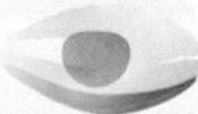

CASE STUDY

Patient Information

Jorge is a 45-year-old Hispanic man who owns a dog-walking business with two employees. He lives with his male partner, Luis, in a two-bedroom elevator-apartment in an urban area. Although Jorge and Luis have no children, they have a large social network. Jorge was transferred from the acute care floor to the inpatient rehabilitation unit with a diagnosis of right middle cerebral artery stroke. His past medical history is significant for hypertension. Jorge and Luis indicated that discharge to the current home environment is desired and that their extended support network can provide assistance as needed.

Assessment Process and Results

The occupational therapist used the Canadian Occupational Performance Measure (COPM) to identify occupations that were meaningful and important to Jorge. He identified the following five occupations as being most important: (1) bathing and dressing, (2) taking care of bathroom needs, (3) preparing simple meals, (4) returning to work, and (5) socializing with friends during their regular monthly poker game. Out of a possible score of 10 (higher scores indicate better performance and greater satisfaction), he scored his present performance in and satisfaction with these five occupations as follows:

- Bathing: performance = 5, satisfaction = 2
- Taking care of bathroom needs: performance = 3, satisfaction = 1
- Preparing simple meals: performance = 3, satisfaction = 1
- Returning to work: performance = 1, satisfaction = 1
- Socializing with friends: performance = 2, satisfaction = 2

Guided by the COPM results, the occupational therapist evaluated Jorge's ability to engage in the identified activities using the Functional Independence Measure (FIM) and observation of a simple meal preparation activity. Out of a possible score of 7 (higher scores indicate greater independence), the therapist scored Jorge as follows on the FIM:

- Feeding: 4
- Grooming: 4
- Bathing: 3
- UE Dressing: 4
- LB Dressing: 3
- Toileting: 3
- Bladder/bowel function: 7
- Transfers: 4
- Locomotion: 3

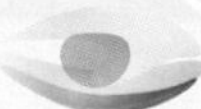

CASE STUDY *(continued)*

Decreased use of the left dominant UE, impaired standing balance during reaching, and left unilateral spatial neglect were significant limiting factors during task performance. Performance skills and client factors were evaluated using the following assessments:

- FMA-UE motor and sensory sections to assess motor and sensory impairments
- Action Research Arm Test (ARAT) to assess UE capacity
- CBS to assess the impact of unilateral spatial neglect on daily functioning
- PASS to assess balance
- Beck Depression Inventory-II (BDI-II) to assess psychosocial status

Scores on the abovementioned assessments were as follows:

- FMA-UE motor: 39/66 indicating moderate motor impairments of the left UE
- FMA-UE sensory: 8/12 indicating mild sensory impairments of the left UE
- ARAT: 37/57 indicating limited capacity of the left UE
- PASS: 29/36 with limitations noted in standing balance
- CBS: 15/30; self-awareness score: 2/30 indicating moderate left unilateral neglect with poor self-awareness of neglect
- BDI-II: 2/63 indicating minimal evidence of emerging depression

Occupational Therapy Problem List

- Difficulty combining joint motions of the left UE, resulting in inefficient forward, side, and overhead reaching
- Decreased ability to reach, grasp, transport, and manipulate objects with the left UE
- Diminished tactile sensation of the left arm and hand
- Decreased standing balance
- Moderate left unilateral spatial neglect with poor self-awareness of neglect
- Minimal evidence of emerging depression

Occupational Therapy Goal List

- Jorge will be able to bathe, dress, and toilet himself with supervision by 2 weeks.
- Jorge will be able to prepare a simple meal with supervision by 2 weeks.
- Jorge will be able to play a poker game with Luis and friends by 2 weeks.
- Increase left UE capacity to notable (score of ≥43 on ARAT) to allow for use of the left UE as a functional assist during self-care, meal preparation, and computer tasks by 2 weeks.
- Increase standing balance as evidenced by a 3-point increase on the PASS to allow for greater independence during self-care, meal preparation, and computer tasks by 2 weeks.
- Decrease left unilateral neglect and increase awareness of neglect as evidenced by a 5-point score change on the CBS to allow for increased independence during self-care, meal preparation, and computer activities by 2 weeks.

Intervention

Applying the principles of evidence-based practice, the following treatment interventions were chosen to address Jorge's needs:

- Occupation-Based Interventions to improve ADL/IADL
- Task-Oriented Training (TOT) to enhance arm and hand function, and improve standing balance to support engagement in chosen activities
- Visual Scanning Training (VST) to improve performance and compensation for unilateral neglect
- MP combined with task practice to promote self-directed independent practice outside regular therapy sessions

Three occupational therapy sessions are presented in the following to illustrate how the abovementioned interventions were implemented.

- Session 1 targeted specific practice of two of Jorge's chosen occupations (bathing and dressing) in his hospital room. The therapist began the session by describing the two activities that would be practiced. After describing the activities, Jorge was asked to predict (awareness training) how long each would take and how much assistance he would need. He predicted that each task would take approximately 8 minutes and that he would need someone close by, but no "real help." The therapist proceeded to engage Jorge in task practice, providing verbal and physical prompting as needed. Prompts were needed to encourage left limb use, locate items on the left side of the environment, and complete tasks. Occasional physical support was required to prevent loss of balance while standing. After task completion, the therapist helped Jorge to reflect on his performance and compare his actual and predicted performance by highlighting discrepancies between the two. It became clear that Jorge needed improved awareness to use strategies such as VST. Therefore, awareness training became an integral part of the overall intervention plan.
- Session 2 took place in the occupational therapy clinic and focused on improving arm and hand function, and VST for engagement in chosen activities. Jorge's interests drove the selection of tasks used for TOT. The goal was to maximize repetitions of reaching, grasping, transporting or manipulating, and releasing various meaningful task objects as follows:
- Manipulation of a computer mouse while seated at a table: Organizing icons on the screen of Jorge's work laptop, entering data onto a spreadsheet, and accessing email and social media.
- Manipulation of bathing items and kitchen utensils: Organizing (1) bathing items in a basin while seated at a table and (2) kitchen utensils in a drawer while standing at the countertop.

(continued)

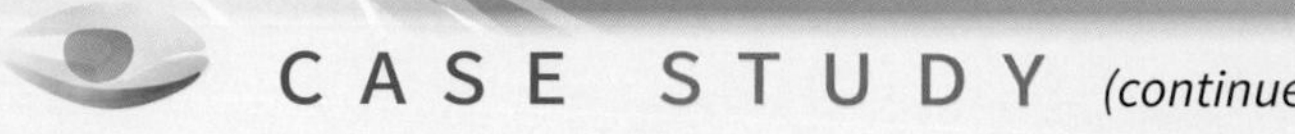

CASE STUDY (continued)

- Playing cards: Dealing cards, flipping cards, stacking cards, and manipulating poker chips.

Performance of a high number of repetitions of each task was encouraged, and tasks were graded to challenge Jorge's current motor skills. Examples of gradation included increasing the number of items manipulated; changing the location of items in the environment to encourage reaching over greater distances and in different planes of motion; changing the size, shape, and weight of objects; and varying speed requirements. VST was introduced, and Jorge was taught a structured scanning strategy to use while engaged in each of the abovementioned activities.

- Session 3 took place in the ADL kitchen and focused on preparing a simple meal while standing. Jorge identified a favorite afternoon meal, and the occupation-based intervention of making a chopped salad was chosen. Awareness building continued to be addressed using task prediction methods and review of discrepancies between predicted performance and actual performance. The task was set up to encourage the use of VST—for example, necessary items were placed on both sides of the table, and Jorge was verbally cued to engage in an organized visual search of the table for specific items. He was also encouraged to use his left arm and hand to assist throughout the session. A vegetable peeler and knife with built-up handles were provided, along with a cutting board with suction cups. Jorge was encouraged to use his left hand to peel vegetables; perform multiple repetitions required for chopping vegetables; place food items into a large bowl; and assist with washing, drying, and putting away meal preparation items.

In addition to individual sessions described earlier, the therapist provided Jorge with specific opportunities for self-directed independent practice. An individualized structured program was designed that Jorge carried out with the help of Luis outside of individual therapy session.

- Mentally practicing (1) manipulation of the computer mouse; (2) manipulation of bathing and grooming items; and (3) kitchen utensil use, followed by actual practice of these activities.
- Provision of an occupation box with items related to Jorge's identified goals, such as a deck of cards, dog brush, can opener, pen and paper, poker chips, and kitchen utensils that Jorge used to engage in TOT.
- Use of organized visual scanning strategies to locate specific items in a pet catalog, entries on an excel spreadsheet, and cards of specific suits spread out over a table.
- Provision of a practice log to record daily practice sessions that would be regularly reviewed to determine the need to modify the self-directed practice program.

By discharge, Jorge met the majority of his goals as evidenced by improved COPM performance and satisfaction scores, and improved performance scores on the noted selected objective measures. Prior to discharge, the therapist educated Jorge about his increased risk for a second stroke. They discussed common stroke signs and symptoms, the importance of monitoring his high blood pressure, medication management, the need to monitor his diet, and how to engage in regular exercise. In addition, Jorge and Luis were educated about the signs and symptoms of depression and were provided with community resources if depression emerged.

Jorge's additional occupational performance goals were addressed by outpatient occupational therapy, including community mobility and return to work.[96]

Evidence Table of Intervention Studies for Stroke

Intervention	Intervention Description	Participants	Dosage	Research Design and Evidence Level	Benefit	Statistical Significance and Effect Size
Meaningful Task-specific Training[97]	UE task-specific training program involving repetitive practice of meaningful unilateral and bilateral tasks	103 inpatients with hemiparesis after stroke; mean age, 50.93 ± 7.78 years; mean TPS, 12.15 ± 6.54 weeks	Dose-matched training for 1 hour/day, 4–5 day/week for 4 weeks	Assessor-blinded randomized controlled trial (RCT); Level I	Reduction in UE motor impairment as measured by the FMA Improvement in UE capacity as measured by the ARAT and WMFT Improvements in self-perceived UE function as measured by the MAL	FMA: $p < 0.001$ WMFT (time): $p < 0.001$ WMFT (quality): $p < 0.001$ ARAT: $p < 0.001$ MAL-AOU: $p < 0.001$ MAL-QOU: $p < 0.001$
mCIMT[90]	UE intensive task training with the impaired limb and restraint of the non-impaired limb	278 patients; age range: 31–83; TPS range: 2 days to 60 who met specific criteria for mCIMT (some residual wrist and hand function)	Intensive training of the paretic UE: 30 minutes to 3 hours a day, and restraint of the nonparetic UE was <6 hours a day in the mCIMT	Systematic review and meta-analysis of 13 RCT; Level I	Reduction in UE motor impairments as measured by the FMA Improvements in UE capacity as measured by the ARAT Improvements in self-perceived UE function as measured by the MAL Improvement in ADL as measured by the FIM	FMA: Mean difference (MD) = 7.8; 95% confidence interval (CI), 4.21–11.38 MAL-AOU: MD = 0.78; CI, 0.37–1.19 ARAT: MD = 14.15; 95% CI, 10.71–17.59 MAL-QOU: MD = 0.84; 95% CI, 0.42–1.25 FIM: MD = 7.0; CI, 0.75-13.26

(*continued*)

Evidence Table of Intervention Studies for Stroke (*continued*)

Intervention	Intervention Description	Participants	Dosage	Research Design and Evidence Level	Benefit	Statistical Significance and Effect Size
Cognitive Orientation to daily Occupational Performance (CO–OP)[98]	A cognitive-oriented intervention that uses client-driven cognitive strategies The Goal–Plan–Do–Check problem-solving strategy is the main global cognitive strategy.	20 stroke survivors with a mean age of 60.4, mean NIHSS of 7. 57.9% were women. The 12 subjects who withdrew had significantly lower scores on a variety of neuropsychological tests.	10 one-hour individualized interventions sessions in which the participant received training in two types of strategies: Goal–Plan–Do–Check and domain-specific strategies	Pilot RCT with a blind assessor; Level I	Improved Performance Quality Rating Scale Improved performance on the COPM	$U = 0.0$ $p = 0.02$ $U = 0.0$ $p = 0.02$
Visual Scanning Training (VST) and Prism Adaptation (PA)[99]	VST includes four structured tasks: visual-spatial scanning, reading and copying training, copying of line drawings, and description of scenes. PA consists of the repetition of exercises in which the patient points to targets placed in front of them, while wearing prismatic lenses.	20 subjects with right CVA and documented neglect based on objective testing Exclusion criteria were as follows: previous brain injury, previous substance abuse or dependence, a history of psychiatric disturbances, the presence of cognitive impairment and dementia, left brain lesion, severe hemianopia, and visual impairment.	20 sessions, 1/day, 5 days a week for 4 weeks	Pre–post design with alternating assignment; Level III	Reduced personal/body neglect (Fluff Test) Reduced peri-personal/near space neglect (Behavioral Inattention Test: Conventional scale)	$p < 0.05$ $p < 0.05$ Note: Both groups presented with significant changes with no difference between the groups, indicating both interventions are effective.

References

1. World Health Organization. *International Classification of Diseases (ICD-10)*. Geneva, Switzerland: WHO; 2007.
2. Benjamin EJ, Virani SS, Callaway CW, et al. Heart disease and stroke statistics—2018 update: a report from the American Heart Association. *Circulation*. 2018;137(12):e67–e492. doi:10.1161/CIR.0000000000000558.
3. Leach MJ, Gall SL, Dewey HM, Macdonell RA, Thrift AG. Factors associated with quality of life in 7-year survivors of stroke. *J Neurol Neurosurg Psychiatry*. 2011;82(12):1365–1371. doi:10.1136/jnnp.2010.234765.
4. Suenkeler IH, Nowak M, Misselwitz B, et al. Timecourse of health-related quality of life as determined 3, 6 and 12 months after stroke. Relationship to neurological deficit, disability and depression. *J Neurol*. 2002;249(9):1160–1167. doi:10.1007/s00415-002-0792-3.
5. Bartels M, Duffy CA, Beland HE. Pathophysiology, medical management, and acute rehabilitation of stroke survivors. In: Gillen G, ed. *Stroke Rehabilitation: A Function Based Approach*. 4th ed. St. Louis, MO: Elsevier; 2016:1–45.
6. Haines DE, Lancon JA. A survey of the cerebrovascular system. In: Hanies DE, ed. *Fundamental Neuroscience for Basic and Clinical Applications*. Philadelphia, PA: Elsevier; 2013:109–123.
7. Aminmansour B, Rezvany M, Sharifi D, Shemshaki H. Effect of decompressive hemicraniectomy on mortality of malignant middle cerebral artery infarction. *J Res Med Sci*. 2010;15(6):344.
8. Nouh A, Remke J, Ruland S. Ischemic posterior circulation stroke: a review of anatomy, clinical presentations, diagnosis, and current management. *Front Neurol*. 2014;5:30. doi:10.3389/fneur.2014.00030.
9. Balami JS, Chen RL, Buchan AM. Stroke syndromes and clinical management. *QJM*. 2013;106(7):607–615. doi:10.1093/qjmed/hct057.
10. Ng YS, Stein J, Salles SS, Black-Schaffer RM. Clinical characteristics and rehabilitation outcomes of patients with posterior cerebral artery stroke. *Arch Phys Med Rehabil*. 2005;86(11):2138–2143. doi:10.1016/j.apmr.2005.07.289.
11. Mangla R, Kolar B, Almast J, Ekholm SE. Border zone infarcts: pathophysiologic and imaging characteristics. *Radiographics*. 2011;31(5):1201–1214. doi:10.1148/rg.315105014.
12. Powers WJ, Rabinstein AA, Ackerson T, et al. 2018 Guidelines for the early management of patients with acute ischemic stroke: a guideline for healthcare professionals from the American Heart Association/American Stroke Association. *Stroke*. 2018;49(3):e46–e110. doi:10.1161/STR.0000000000000158.
13. Winstein CJ, Stein J, Arena R, et al. Guidelines for adult stroke rehabilitation and recovery: a guideline for healthcare professionals from the American Heart Association/American Stroke Association. *Stroke*. 2016;47(6):e98–e169. doi:10.1161/STR.0000000000000098.
14. Wolf TJ, Nilsen DM. *Occupational Practice Guidelines for Adults with Stroke*. Bethesda, MD: AOTA Press; 2015.
15. Krakauer JW. Arm function after stroke: from physiology to recovery. Paper presented at: Seminars in Neurology; 2005.
16. Horak FB. Clinical measurement of postural control in adults. *Phys Ther*. 1987;67(12):1881–1885.
17. Bohannon RW, Cassidy D, Walsh S. Trunk muscle strength is impaired multidirectionally after stroke. *Clin Rehabil*. 1995;9(1):47–51. doi:10.1177/026921559500900107.
18. Dickstein R, Shefi S, Marcovitz E, Villa Y. Anticipatory postural adjustment in selected trunk muscles in post-stroke hemiparetic patients. *Arch Phys Med Rehabil*. 2004;85(2):261–267. doi:10.1016/j.apmr.2003.05.011.
19. Dickstein R, Shefi S, Marcovitz E, Villa Y. Electromyographic activity of voluntarily activated trunk flexor and extensor muscles in post-stroke hemiparetic subjects. *Clin Neurophysiol*. 2004;115(4):790–796. doi:10.1016/j.clinph.2003.11.018.
20. Ikai T, Kamikubo T, Takehara I, Nishi M, Miyano S. Dynamic postural control in patients with hemiparesis. *Am J Phys Med Rehabil*. 2003;82(6):463–469. doi:10.1097/01.PHM.0000069192.32183.A7.
21. de Kam D, Kamphuis JF, Weerdesteyn V, Geurts AC. The effect of weight-bearing asymmetry on dynamic postural stability in people with chronic stroke. *Gait Posture*. 2017;53:5–10. doi:10.1016/j.gaitpost.2016.12.019.
22. Dontao S, Halliday Pulaski K, Gillen G. Overview of balance impairments: functional limitations. In: Gillen G, ed. *Stroke Rehabilitation: A Function Based Approach*. 4th ed. St. Louis, MO: Elsevier; 2016:394–415.
23. Tyson SF. Trunk kinematics in hemiplegic gait and the effect of walking aids. *Clin Rehabil*. 1999;13(4):295–300. doi:10.1191/026921599666307333.
24. Karthikbabu S, Chakrapani M, Ganesan S, Ellajosyla R. Pelvic alignment in standing, and its relationship with trunk control and motor recovery of lower limb after stroke. *Neurol Clin Neurosci*. 2017;5(1):22–28. doi:10.1111/ncn3.12092.
25. Eng JJ, Chu KS. Reliability and comparison of weight-bearing ability during standing tasks for individuals with chronic stroke. *Arch Phys Med Rehabil*. 2002;83(8):1138–1144. doi:10.1053/apmr.2002.33644.
26. Gillen G. Trunk control: supporting functional independence. In: Gillen G, ed. *Stroke Rehabilitation: A Function-Based Approach*. 4th ed. St. Louis, MO: Elsevier; 2016:360–393.
27. Wee SK, Hughes AM, Warner MB, et al. Impact of trunk control on upper extremity function in subacute and chronic stroke patients and healthy controls. *Physiotherapy*. 2015;101. doi:10.1016/j.physio.2015.03.1635.
28. Verheyden G, Vereeck L, Truijen S, et al. Trunk performance after stroke and the relationship with balance, gait and functional ability. *Clin Rehabil*. 2006;20(5):451–458. doi:10.1191/0269215505cr955oa.
29. Hsieh CL, Sheu CF, Hsueh IP, Wang CH. Trunk control as an early predictor of comprehensive activities of daily living function in stroke patients. *Stroke*. 2002;33(11):2626–2630. doi:10.1161/01.STR.0000033930.05931.93.
30. Veerbeek J, Van Wegen E, Harmeling-Van der Wel B, Kwakkel G; EPOS Investigators. Is accurate prediction of gait in nonambulatory stroke patients possible within 72 hours poststroke? The EPOS study. *Neurorehabil Neural Repair*. 2011;25(3):268–274. doi:10.1177/1545968310384271.
31. Hatem SM, Saussez G, della Faille M, et al. Rehabilitation of motor function after stroke: a multiple systematic

review focused on techniques to stimulate upper extremity recovery. *Front Hum Neurosci*. 2016;10:442. doi:10.3389/fnhum.2016.00442.

32. Lang CE, Bland MD, Bailey RR, Schaefer SY, Birkenmeier RL. Assessment of upper extremity impairment, function, and activity after stroke: foundations for clinical decision making. *J Hand Ther*. 2013;26(2):104–114. doi:10.1016/j.jht.2012.06.005.
33. Gillen G, Nilsen DM. Upper extremity function and management. In: Gillen G, ed. *Stroke Rehabilitation: A Function-Based Approach*. 4th ed. St. Louis, MO: Elsevier; 2016:424–485.
34. Dobkin BH. Rehabilitation after stroke. *N Engl J Med*. 2005;352(16):1677–1684. doi:10.1056/NEJMcp043511.
35. Morris JH, van Wijck F, Joice S, Donaghy M. Predicting health related quality of life 6 months after stroke: the role of anxiety and upper limb dysfunction. *Disabil Rehabil*. 2013;35(4):291–299. doi:10.3109/09638288.2012.691942.
36. Gillen G, Nilsen DM, Attridge J, et al. Effectiveness of interventions to improve occupational performance of people with cognitive impairments after stroke: an evidence-based review. *Am J Occup Ther*. 2015;69(1):6901180040p1-6901180040p9. doi:10.5014/ajot.2015.012138.
37. Árnadóttir G, Löfgren B, Fisher AG. Difference in impact of neurobehavioural dysfunction on activities of daily living performance between right and left hemispheric stroke. *J Rehabil Med*. 2010;42(10):903–907. doi:10.2340/16501977-0621.
38. Marom B, Jarus T, Josman N. The relationship between the Assessment of Motor and Process Skills (AMPS) and the Large Allen Cognitive Level (LACL) test in clients with stroke. *Phys Occup Ther Geriatr*. 2006;24(4):33–50. doi:10.1080/J148v24n04_03.
39. Van Patten R, Merz ZC, Mulhauser K, Fucetola R. Multivariable prediction of return to work at 6-month follow-up in patients with mild to moderate acute stroke. *Arch Phys Med Rehabil*. 2016;97(12):2061.e1–2067.e1. doi:10.1016/j.apmr.2016.06.006.
40. Akinwuntan AE, Feys H, De Weerdt W, Baten G, Arno P, Kiekens C. Prediction of driving after stroke: a prospective study. *Neurorehabil Neural Repair*. 2006;20(3):417–423. doi:10.1177/1545968306287157.
41. Cherney LR, Small SL. Aphasia, apraxia of speech, and dysarthria. In: Stein J, Harvey RL, Winstein CJ, Zorowitz RD, Wittenberg GF, eds. *Stroke Recovery and Rehabilitation*. 2nd ed. New York, NY: Demos-Medical; 2015:181–206.
42. Sand K, Wilhelmsen G, Naess H, Midelfart A, Thomassen L, Hoff J. Vision problems in ischaemic stroke patients: effects on life quality and disability. *Eur J Neurol*. 2016;23:1–7. doi:10.1111/ene.12848.
43. Canadian Partnership for Stroke Recovery. Evidence-based review of stroke rehabilitation. http://www.ebrsr.com/evidence-review. Accessed June 28, 2018.
44. Pollock N. Client-centered assessment. *Am J Occup Ther*. 1993;47(4):298–301.
45. Weinstock-Zlotnick G, Hinojosa J. Bottom-up or top-down evaluation: is one better than the other? *Am J Occup Ther*. 2004;58(5):594–599.
46. Trombly C. Anticipating the future: assessment of occupational function. *Am J Occup Ther*. 1993;47(3):253–257.
47. Baum C. *Activity Card Sort*. 2nd ed. Bethesda, MD: AOTA Press; 2008.
48. Law M. *The Canadian Occupational Performance Measure*. 4th ed. Ottawa, Canada: CAOT Publications ACE; 2005.
49. Barthel D. Functional evaluation: the Barthel Index, Maryland State. *Med J*. 1965;14:16–65.
50. Keith RA. The functional independence measure: a new tool for rehabilitation. In: Eisenberg M, Grzesiak RC, eds. *Advances in Clinical Rehabilitation*. Vol 1. New York, NY: Springer-Verlag; 1987.
51. Benaim C, Pérennou DA, Villy J, Rousseaux M, Pelissier JY. Validation of a standardized assessment of postural control in stroke patients: the Postural Assessment Scale for Stroke Patients (PASS). *Stroke*. 1999;30(9):1862–1868. doi:10.1161/01.STR.30.9.1862.
52. Mathias S, Nayak U, Isaacs B. Balance in elderly patients: the "get-up and go" test. *Arch Phys Med Rehabil*. 1986;67(6):387–389.
53. Berg K, Wood-Dauphinee S, Williams J. The Balance Scale: reliability assessment with elderly residents and patients with an acute stroke. *Scand J Rehabil Med*. 1995;27(1):27–36.
54. Duncan PW, Weiner DK, Chandler J, Studenski S. Functional reach: a new clinical measure of balance. *J Gerontol*. 1990;45(6):M192–M197. doi:10.1093/geronj/45.6.M192.
55. Collin C, Wade D. Assessing motor impairment after stroke: a pilot reliability study. *J Neurol Neurosurg Psychiatry*. 1990;53(7):576–579. doi:10.1136/jnnp.53.7.576.
56. Köpke S, Meyer G. The Tinetti test. *Zeitschr Gerontol Geriatr*. 2006;39(4):288–291. doi:10.1007/s00391-006-0398-y.
57. Lyle RC. A performance test for assessment of upper limb function in physical rehabilitation treatment and research. *Int J Rehabil Res*. 1981;4(4):483–492.
58. Jebsen RH, Taylor N, Trieschmann R, Trotter MJ, Howard LA. An objective and standardized test of hand function. *Arch Phys Med Rehabil*. 1969;50(6):311–319.
59. Wolf SL, Catlin PA, Ellis M, Archer AL, Morgan B, Piacentino A. Assessing Wolf motor function test as outcome measure for research in patients after stroke. *Stroke*. 2001;32(7):1635–1639. doi:10.1161/01.STR.32.7.1635.
60. Wilson DJ, Baker LL, Craddock JA. Functional test for the hemiparetic upper extremity. *Am J Occup Ther*. 1984;38(3):159–164.
61. Fisher A. *Assessment of Motor and Process Skills*. 4th ed. Fort Collins, CO: Three Star Press; 2001.
62. Hammer AM, Lindmark B. Responsiveness and validity of the Motor Activity Log in patients during the subacute phase after stroke. *Disabil Rehabil*. 2010;32(14):1184–1193. doi:10.3109/09638280903437253.
63. Uswatte G, Taub E, Morris D, Light K, Thompson P. The Motor Activity Log-28 assessing daily use of the hemiparetic arm after stroke. *Neurology*. 2006;67(7):1189–1194. doi:10.1212/01.wnl.0000238164.90657.c2.
64. Uswatte G, Taub E, Morris D, Vignolo M, McCulloch K. Reliability and validity of the upper-extremity Motor Activity Log-14 for measuring real-world arm use. *Stroke*. 2005;36(11):2493–2496. doi:10.1161/01.STR.0000185928.90848.2e.

65. Lai S-M, Studenski S, Duncan PW, Perera S. Persisting consequences of stroke measured by the Stroke Impact Scale. *Stroke.* 2002;33(7):1840–1844. doi:10.1161/01.STR.0000019289.15440.F2.
66. Chen CC, Bode RK. Psychometric validation of the Manual Ability Measure-36 (MAM-36) in patients with neurologic and musculoskeletal disorders. *Arch Phys Med Rehabil.* 2010;91(3):414–420. doi:10.1016/j.apmr.2009.11.012.
67. Penta M, Tesio L, Arnould C, Zancan A, Thonnard J-L. The ABILHAND questionnaire as a measure of manual ability in chronic stroke patients: Rasch-based validation and relationship to upper limb impairment. *Stroke.* 2001;32(7):1627–1634. doi:10.1161/01.STR.32.7.1627.
68. Yu DT. Shoulder pain and others musculoskeletal complications. In: *Stroke Recovery and Rehabilitation.* New York, NY: Demos-Medical; 2008:437–451.
69. Bohannon RW, Smith MB. Interrater reliability of a modified Ashworth scale of muscle spasticity. *Phys Ther.* 1987;67(2):206–207. doi:10.1093/ptj/67.2.206.
70. Bohannon RW. Motricity index scores are valid indicators of paretic upper extremity strength following stroke. *J Phys Ther Sci.* 2001;11(2):59–61. doi:10.1589/jpts.11.59.
71. Fugl-Meyer A, Jaasko L, Leyman I, et al. The Post Stroke hemiplegic patient: a method for evaluation of physical performance. *Scand J Rehabil Med.* 1975;7(1):13–31.
72. Bushnell C, Bettger JP, Cockroft KM, et al. Chronic stroke outcome measures for motor function intervention trials: expert panel recommendations. *Circ Cardiovasc Qual Outcomes.* 2015;8(6 suppl 3):S163–S169. doi:10.1161/CIRCOUTCOMES.115.002098.
73. Velozo CA, Woodbury ML. Translating measurement findings into rehabilitation practice: an example using Fugl-Meyer Assessment-Upper Extremity with patients following stroke. *J Rehabil Res Dev.* 2011;48(10). doi:10.1682/JRRD.2010.10.0203.
74. Sullivan KJ, Tilson JK, Cen SY, et al. Fugl-Meyer assessment of sensorimotor function after stroke: standardized training procedure for clinical practice and clinical trials. *Stroke.* 2011;42(2):427–432. doi:10.1161/STROKEAHA.110.592766.
75. Hartman-Maeir A, Harel H, Katz N. Kettle Test—a brief measure of cognitive functional performance: reliability and validity in stroke rehabilitation. *Am J Occup Ther.* 2009;63(5):592–599.
76. Arnadoittir G. *The Brain and Behavior: Assessing Cortical Dysfunction Through Activities of Daily Living.* St. Louis, MO: Mosby; 1990.
77. Baum CM, Connor LT, Morrison T, Hahn M, Dromerick AW, Edwards DF. Reliability, validity, and clinical utility of the Executive Function Performance Test: a measure of executive function in a sample of people with stroke. *Am J Occup Ther.* 2008;62(4):446–455.
78. Morrison MT, Giles GM, Ryan JD, et al. Multiple Errands Test–Revised (MET–R): a performance-based measure of executive function in people with mild cerebrovascular accident. *Am J Occup Ther.* 2013;67(4):460–468. doi:10.5014/ajot.2013.007880.
79. Toglia J. *Weekly Calendar Planning Activity.* Bethesda, MD: AOTA; 2015.
80. Azouvi P, Olivier S, De Montety G, Samuel C, Louis-Dreyfus A, Tesio L. Behavioral assessment of unilateral neglect: study of the psychometric properties of the Catherine Bergego Scale. *Arch Phys Med Rehabil.* 2003;84(1):5157. doi:10.1053/apmr.2003.50062.
81. Chen P, Hreha K, Kong Y, Barrett A. Impact of spatial neglect on stroke rehabilitation: evidence from the setting of an inpatient rehabilitation facility. *Arch Phys Med Rehabil.* 2015;96(8):1458–1466. doi:10.1016/j.apmr.2015.03.019.
82. Warren M. *Brain Injury Visual Assessment Battery for Adults.* Birmingham, England: VisABILITIES Rehab Services; 1999.
83. Beck A, Steer RA, Brown GK. *Beck Depression Inventory: Second Edition Manual.* San Antonio, TX: The Psychological Corporation; 1996.
84. Turner A, Hambridge J, White J, et al. Depression screening in stroke: a comparison of alternative measures with the structured diagnostic interview for the diagnostic and statistical manual of mental disorders, fourth edition (major depressive episode) as criterion standard. *Stroke.* 2012;43(4):1000–1005. doi:10.1161/STROKEAHA.111.643296.
85. Spitzer RL, Kroenke K, Williams JB, Patient Health Questionnaire Primary Care Study Group. Validation and utility of a self-report version of PRIME-MD: the PHQ primary care study. *JAMA.* 1999;282(18):1737–1744. doi:10.1001/jama.282.18.1737.
86. Snaith RP. The hospital anxiety and depression scale. *Health Qual Life Outcomes.* 2003;1(1):29.
87. Nilsen DM, Gillen G, Geller D, Hreha K, Osei E, Saleem GT. Effectiveness of interventions to improve occupational performance of people with motor impairments after stroke: an evidence-based review. *Am J Occup Ther.* 2015;69(1):6901180030p1-6901180030p9. doi:10.5014/ajot.2015.011965.
88. Mathiowetz V. Task-oriented approach to stroke rehabilitation. In: Gillen G, ed. *Stroke Rehabilitation: A Function-Based Approach.* 4th ed. St. Louis, MO: Elsevier; 2016:59–78.
89. Wolf SL, Winstein CJ, Miller JP, et al. Retention of upper limb function in stroke survivors who have received constraint-induced movement therapy: the EXCITE randomised trial. *Lancet Neurol.* 2008;7(1):33–40. doi:10.1016/S1474-4422(07)70294-6.
90. Shi YX, Tian JH, Yang KH, Zhao Y. Modified constraint-induced movement therapy versus traditional rehabilitation in patients with upper-extremity dysfunction after stroke: a systematic review and meta-analysis. *Arch Phys Med Rehabil.* 2011;92(6):972–982. doi:10.1016/j.apmr.2010.12.036.
91. Gillen G. Orthotic devices after stroke. In: Gillem G, ed. *Stroke Rehabilitation: A Function-Based Approach.* 4th ed. St. Louis, MO: Elsevier; 2016:529–552.
92. Gillen G, Brockmann-Rubio K. Treatment of cognitive-perceptual impairments: a function-based approach. In: Gillen G, ed. *Stroke Rehabilitation: A Function-Based Approach.* 4th ed. St. Louis, MO: Elsevier; 2016:612–646.
93. Hildebrand MW. Effectiveness of interventions for adults with psychological or emotional impairment after stroke: an evidence-based review. *Am J Occup Ther.* 2015;69(1):6901180050p1-6901180050p9. doi:10.5014/ajot.2015.012054.

94. Kernan WN, Ovbiagele B, Black HR, et al. Guidelines for the prevention of stroke in patients with stroke and transient ischemic attack: a guideline for healthcare professionals from the American Heart Association/American Stroke Association. *Stroke.* 2014;45(7):2160–2236. doi:10.1161/STR.0000000000000024.
95. Schmid AA, Butterbaugh L, Egolf C, Richards V, Williams LS. Prevention of secondary stroke in VA: role of occupational therapists and physical therapists. 2008. http://hdl.handle.net/1805/5122
96. Nilsen D, Gillen G, Arbesman M, Lieberman D. Occupational therapy interventions for adults with stroke. *Am J Occup Ther.* 2015;69(5):6905395010p1-6905395010p3.
97. Narayan Arya K, Verma R, Garg R, Sharma V, Agarwal M, Aggarwal G. Meaningful task-specific training (MTST) for stroke rehabilitation: a randomized controlled trial. *Top Stroke Rehabil.* 2012;19(3):193–211. doi:10.1310/tsr1903-193.
98. Polatajko HJ, McEwen SE, Ryan JD, Baum CM. Pilot randomized controlled trial investigating cognitive strategy use to improve goal performance after stroke. *Am J Occup Ther.* 2012;66(1):104–109. doi:10.5014/ajot.2012.001784.
99. Spaccavento S, Cellamare F, Cafforio E, Loverre A, Craca A. Efficacy of visual-scanning training and prism adaptation for neglect rehabilitation. *Appl Neuropsychol Adult.* 2016;23(5):313–321. doi:10.1080/23279095.2015.1038386.

Acknowledgment

The case study was reprinted with permission from the American Occupational Therapy Association.

Chapter 37

Acquired Brain Injury

Alicia Flores Lohmann and Asha K. Vas

LEARNING OBJECTIVES

This chapter will allow the reader to:

1. Describe the similarities and differences in the typical course of recovery for persons with mild, moderate, and severe traumatic brain injury.
2. Select appropriate assessment tools and strategies for persons with acquired brain injury during acute medical management, inpatient, and postacute rehabilitation.
3. Apply information from related chapters of this text to the treatment of motor, cognitive, behavioral, and emotional aspects of acquired brain injury.
4. Analyze the needs of family members during recovery and occupational therapy's role in the adaptation of life after brain injury.
5. Address occupational therapy's role in the long-term needs of survivors of acquired brain injury.

CHAPTER OUTLINE

TERMINOLOGY

Acquired brain injury (ABI): head injury that can include traumatic and nontraumatic injuries caused by cardiovascular defects, tumors, substance abuse, environmental exposure, anoxia, bacteria, viruses, nutritional deficiencies, genetic, congenital, and degenerative diseases.[1]

Agitation: excessive behavior including varied degrees of aggression, disinhibition, restlessness, and confusion. Person may present in an altered state of consciousness.

Concussion: a type of traumatic brain injury (TBI) usually caused by a blow to the head, usually reported in sports activities including direct blow, bump, or jolt to the head; effects are usually temporary but can include headaches and problems associated with concentration, memory, balance, and coordination.[2]

Diffuse axonal injury (DAI): extensive lesions in white matter tracts over a widespread area following traumatic acceleration/deceleration or rotational injuries; DAI often results in loss of consciousness and could result in persistent vegetative state after severe head trauma.[3]

Disorder of consciousness (DOC): a state of reduced wakefulness and awareness due to brain damage.[4]

Mild brain injury: a traumatically induced physiological disruption of brain function, as manifested by at least one of the following: (i) any period of loss of consciousness; (ii) any loss of memory for events immediately before or after the accident; (iii) any alteration in mental state at the time of the accident (e.g., feeling dazed, disoriented, or confused); or (iv) focal neurological deficit(s) that may or may not be transient; but where the severity of the injury does not exceed the following: loss of consciousness of approximately 30 minutes or less; after 30 minutes an initial Glasgow Coma Scale (GCS) of 13 to 15; and post-traumatic amnesia (PTA) not greater than 24 hours.[5]

Moderate brain injury: a brain injury resulting in a loss of consciousness from 20 minutes to 6 hours and a GCS of 9 to 12; moderate TBI is characterized by loss of consciousness for 1 to 24 hours, PTA for 1 to 24 hours of the TBI, and abnormal brain imaging results.[6]

Severe brain injury: a brain injury that results in loss of consciousness or coma for more than 24 hours, PTA for more than 24 hours of TBI, and abnormal brain imaging results.[6]

Spasticity: a continuous state of muscular contraction that if left untreated can limit muscle and joint motion.[7]

Traumatic brain injury (TBI): a form of ABI following an external trauma to the head; a TBI occurs when the head suddenly and violently hits an object, or when an object pierces the skull and enters brain tissue.[2]

Introduction

Acquired brain injury (ABI) can be due to internal or external causes. ABI is a public health problem. It is defined as "Damage to the brain, which occurs after birth and is not related to a congenital or a degenerative disease. These impairments may be temporary or permanent and cause partial or functional disability or psychosocial maladjustment."[8] ABIs are caused by one or more of the following: traumatic forces (e.g., traumatic brain injury [TBI], falls, assaults, gunshot wounds), stroke (e.g., hemorrhage, embolus), brain bleeds (e.g., hemorrhage, hematomas), lack of oxygen (e.g., anoxia, cardiac arrest), brain infections (e.g., meningitis), brain tumors, or environmental causes (e.g., toxic exposure).

This chapter focuses on the various levels of ABI that occur as a result of external or internal damages to the brain. Consequently, varying degrees of impairments occur in cognitive, behavioral, emotional, and/or physical functioning. These alterations in functioning result in changes in valued roles, tasks, and activities, which affect virtually every area of life for the survivor and his or her family.[9] For the many individuals, especially younger adults at the time of injury, changes in physical, cognitive, and psychosocial abilities may affect their occupational functioning for months, years, or decades. The complex interaction of factors associated with impairment, context, and environment requires an interprofessional approach to assessment and treatment. Therefore, occupational therapists who work with patients with ABI must appreciate the contributions and expertise of other team members in the best interest of the patient.

Incidence, Prevalence, and Causation

Each year, **traumatic brain injuries (TBIs)** contribute to a substantial number of deaths (30%) and cases of permanent disability in the United States.[10] In 2013, approximately 2.5 million people sustained a TBI.[2] Individuals with more severe injuries are more likely to require hospitalization. The estimated economic cost of TBI in 2010, including both direct and indirect medical costs, is estimated to be approximately $76.5 billion in the United States. Additionally, the cost of fatal TBIs and TBIs requiring hospitalization, many of which are severe, accounts for approximately 90% of the total TBI medical costs.[11,12] Each year, approximately 1.7 million civilians in the United States sustain a TBI.[13] Of these, 3% (52,000) die, 16% (275,000) are hospitalized, and 80% (1.4 million) are treated in an emergency room (ER) and released. The Centers for Disease Control and Prevention (CDC) measures incidence by combined emergency visits, hospitalizations, and deaths. The incidence has steadily risen from 2001 to 2010, from 521 to 616 per 100,000 population (between 2001 and 2005) to 824 per 100,000 population.[14] This steady increase is secondary to TBI-related ER visits that increased by 70% from 2001 to 2010, while hospitalization rates increased by only 11%. In addition, deaths related to TBI decreased by 7% over the same 10-year span.[14]

Factors such as automobile safety, seat belt use, helmet use, and better overall treatment for severe TBI in prehospital and hospital settings, although unable to prevent TBIs entirely, have mitigated their severity and thus mortality. In addition, there are an unknown number of individuals with TBI who are not included in these estimates because they are seen in an ER but discharged without a diagnosis of TBI.[15] Between 3.2 and 5.3 million persons (1.1%–1.7% of the US population) live with long-term disabilities that result from TBI.[16,17]

Estimated average annual numbers of TBI-related ER visits, hospitalizations, and deaths, by external cause, the United States, 2002 to 2010, are outlined in Table 37-1.[18]

Mechanisms of Injury and Clinical Implications

External mechanical forces that cause TBI include blow to head (e.g., fall onto pavement, head impacting windshield in a car accident, assault, baseball striking head), acceleration–deceleration forces, wherein no direct impact is required (e.g., a restrained passenger coming to

Table 37-1 Mechanisms of Average Annual Traumatic Brain Injuries

MECHANISM OF INJURY	EMERGENCY DEPARTMENT VISITS	HOSPITALIZATIONS	DEATHS
Falls	658,668	66,291	10,944
Struck by or against an object	304,797	6,808	372
Motor vehicle/traffic	232,240	53,391	14,795
Assault/homicide	179,408	15,032	5,665
Self-inflicted/suicide	*	*	14,713
Other	122,667	25,478	4,990
Unknown	97,018	113,172	0

*Estimate not reported because of small numbers.

a sudden stop when a car strikes a tree or telephone pole), projectile missile (e.g., bullet), and concussive forces (e.g., blast waves from an explosion). Neurological events that occur as a result of trauma to the head include bruising (contusion) to surface brain tissue or trauma to the blood vessels of the brain causing bleeding (hematoma). A hematoma can damage the brain tissue it contacts and can increase pressure in the brain. As a consequence of contusions and bleeding, intracranial pressure (ICP) may rise, which can shift and put pressure on brain tissue owing to the confined space of the skull. Adding to the building pressure is the possibility of edema or swelling of brain tissue due to trauma (see Fig. 37-1).

Typically associated with acceleration–deceleration injuries, there may be shearing or twisting of axonal fibers (white matter tracts) in the brain. This occurs most often in the frontal and temporal lobes. Midline structures (e.g., corpus callosum, anterior commissure) may also be affected, which can disrupt communication between left and right cerebral hemispheres. Extensive shearing can cause **diffuse axonal injury** (DAI), a serious condition that may be associated with coma and poor outcome. Changes in neurotransmitter (i.e., chemical

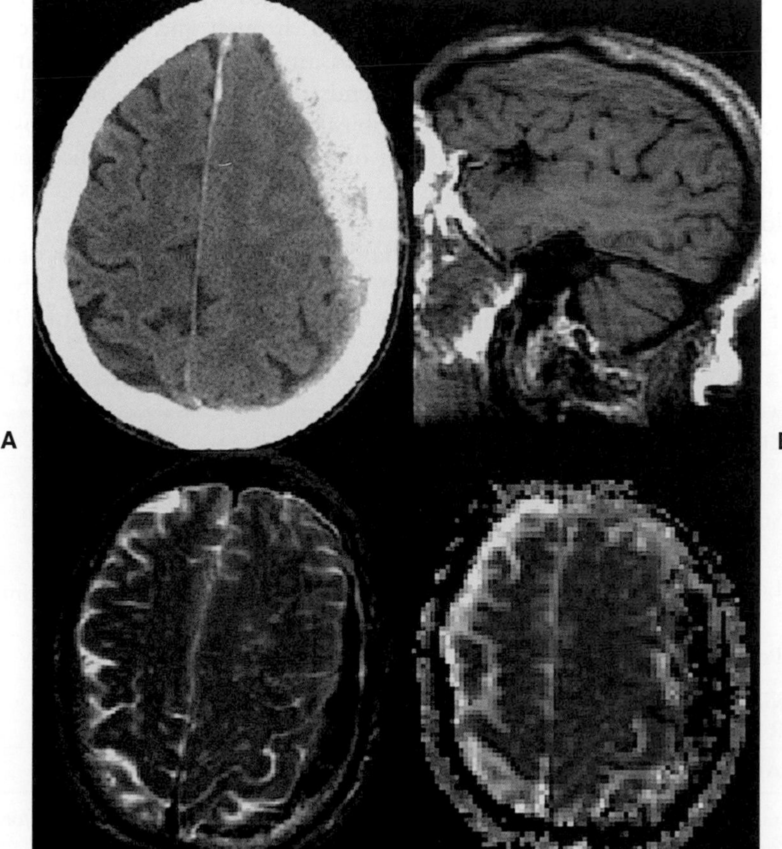

Figure 37-1. Subdural hematoma computed tomography (CT) images. Acute subdural hematoma, CT versus magnetic resonance (MR). **A.** Acute subdural hematoma in the left frontal region. **B, C.** Respective sagittal T1-weighted and axial T2-weighted MR images show an extra-axial clot consistent with intracellular deoxyhemoglobin (i.e., acute subdural hematoma). **D.** The calculated apparent diffusion coefficient map demonstrates marked hypointensity, indicating restricted diffusion within acute hematoma.

communicative agents in the brain) also occur as a result of an ABI. Increase in glucose metabolism in the context of decreased cerebral blood flow leads to an energy deficit in the brain. Hypoxia (i.e., decreased oxygen to the brain) as a result of drug overdose or toxic exposure leads to impaired blood supply to the brain that could lead to brain tissue damage or death. Coup/contracoup is a common mechanism to explain a TBI. Coup refers to damage occurring at the point of head trauma impact (e.g., where the head hit the ground in a fall) as the brain slides forward within the skull and impacts the inside of the skull. This can occur even if there is no direct external impact to the head (e.g., sudden deceleration in a motor vehicle accident). Countercoup injury refers to damage occurring when the head/brain rebounds from the initial force and either impacts an object (e.g., headrest in a motor vehicle accident) or simply rapidly moves in the opposite direction and hits the inside of the skull. The frontal lobes rest on bony prominences of the skull just above the eyes. When the brain moves within the skull, these prominences can cause a grating action against the brain tissue, leading to injury (Fig. 37-2).

A TBI can be classified as either open or closed based on the biomechanics of the injury.[19] In an open brain injury, an object, such as a bullet, enters the cranial cavity. Some classification systems categorize all open injuries as penetrating injuries.[6] Other systems differentiate between penetrating and perforating injuries depending on whether the object remains lodged within the cranial cavity (penetrating) or passes through and exits the cranial cavity (perforating). In an open brain injury, the extent of the damage depends on the shape, mass, direction, and velocity of the object.[19]

A TBI that results from a direct or indirect impact, without penetration of the brain tissue, is classified as a closed brain injury. Closed head injuries can result from dynamic or static loading.[19] A dynamic loading injury occurs when there is rapid acceleration and deceleration of the brain. A static loading injury, also termed crush injury,[6] occurs when a slow mechanical force is applied to the brain, for example, if the head were trapped for an extended time under heavy debris after an earthquake. This type of injury is uncommon. The damage from a closed brain injury is directly related to the type (e.g., shear, tensile) and amount of forces generated during the traumatic event. In the case of crush injuries, there tends to be more damage to the skull than to the brain.[6]

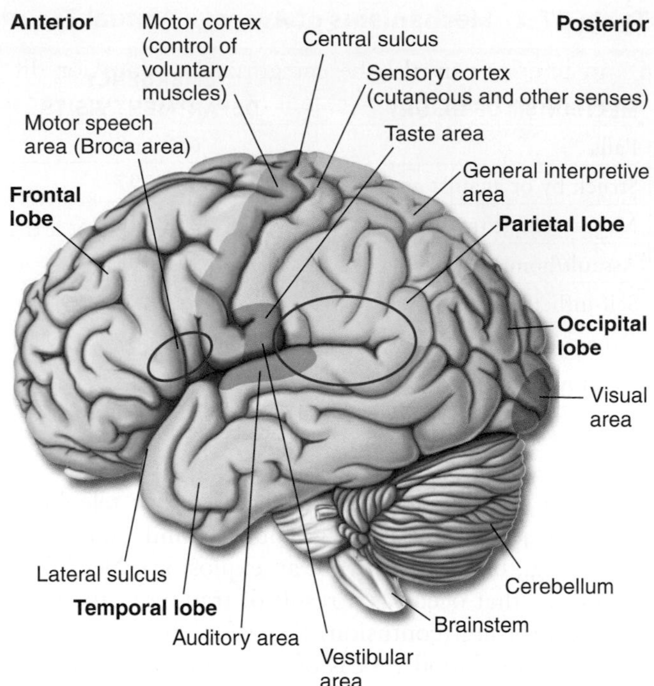

Figure 37-2. Anatomy of the cerebral cortex with areas of potential damage indicated.

Blast injuries have recently been recognized as a specific type of TBI.[6] A blast injury results from any type of blast explosion, including improvised explosive devices (IEDs). A blast injury can occur in conjunction with an open or a closed brain injury.

Table 37-2 shows criteria used to classify the severity of TBI.[20]

Table 37-2 Traumatic Brain Injury Severity Classification Criteria

CRITERIA USED TO CLASSIFY TBI SEVERITY	TBI SEVERITY		
	Mild	Moderate	Severe
Structural imaging	Normal	Normal or abnormal	Normal or abnormal
Loss of consciousness	<30 minutes	30 minutes to 24 hours	>24 hours
Post-traumatic amnesia	0–1 day	>1 and <7 days	>7 days
Glasgow Coma Scale (GCS) score (best available score in 24 hours)	13–15	9–12	3–8
Abbreviated Injury Scale score: head	1–2	3	4–6

Brasure M, Lamberty GJ, Sayer NA, et al. *Multidisciplinary Postacute Rehabilitation for Moderate to Severe Traumatic Brain Injury in Adults.* Rockville, MD: Agency for Healthcare Research and Quality (US); 2012.

Focal Versus Diffuse Injuries

Brain injuries can also be categorized as focal or diffuse injuries based on the extent of the pathology. Focal injuries result from brain contusions, lacerations, and masses of blood called hematomas.[21] Focal lesions are usually seen at the anterior poles and inferior surfaces of the frontal and temporal lobes. They occur when the brain hits the skull and scrapes over the irregular bony structures at these locations.[22] The occipital and parietal lobes, which have smooth surfaces, are less likely to incur damage. Focal lesions to the prefrontal and anterior temporal areas interrupt connections to subcortical limbic structures and affect modulation of memory, emotion, and drive.[23] Damage to the orbitofrontal areas generally results in impulsivity that is greater than with diffuse damage, whereas damage to the frontolateral cortex results in hemiparesis, impulsivity, and attentional impairments as well as decreased mental flexibility.[24]

Diffuse injuries typically occur in motor vehicle crashes where there is rapid movement of the head.[25] Traumatic axonal injury (TAI), previously termed diffuse axonal injury (DAI), is a type of diffuse injury that results when the brain accelerates, decelerates, and rotates inside the skull. The brainstem is more stable than the cerebrum, which rotates around the brainstem during impact. The rotation places a stretch or shear force on the long axons that transmit information throughout the brain and brainstem.[26] Although the mechanisms for TAI are not completely understood, contributing factors include altered permeability of the axonal cell membrane, which impedes axonal transport. This results in focal swelling of the axon and, ultimately, detachment of the axon at the point of the swelling.[27] These injuries are likely to result in coma.[17]

Coma due to axonal injuries may quickly reverse if the axonal damage was mild or may continue as a vegetative state if axons were ruptured. Recovery from coma progresses to a period of confusion with impaired attention and post-traumatic amnesia (PTA). When confusion clears, any cognitive impairments become more evident. Impairments may include diminished mental processing speed and efficiency and difficulty with divided-attention tasks, which require the patient to respond simultaneously to two sources of information. Memory, not only post-traumatic memory, but short- and long-term memory, may be reduced. There may also be a reduced capacity for higher level cognitive functions, including abstract reasoning, planning, problem-solving, organization, and self-awareness. Typical behavioral outcomes range from impulsivity, irritability, and exaggerated premorbid traits to apathy and poor initiative. Diffuse injuries often include damage to the brainstem and cerebellar pathways, resulting in ataxia, diplopia, and dysarthria.[24] It is common to find both focal and diffuse damages with a TBI, especially in more severe cases. In both types of injuries, secondary pathogenic events at the cellular, biochemical, and molecular levels contribute to widespread damage beyond the effect of the primary insult.[19]

Cranial Nerve Damage Associated with Brain Injury

Cranial nerves can be torn, stretched, or contused. The olfactory nerve (I) is often abraded or torn when the frontal lobes scrape across the orbital surface of the skull.[28] The optic nerve (II) may be damaged directly, or vision can be compromised by injury to the eye, the optic tracts, or the visual cortex. Cranial nerves III, IV, and VI, which control eye movements, are all vulnerable to injury. The oculomotor nerve (III) can be stretched when edema or bleeding expands the contents of the skull, causing the uncus of the temporal lobe to herniate into the foramen magnum and compress the brainstem. The abducens nerve (VI) is very long and consequently vulnerable to injury. The facial and vestibulocochlear nerves (VII and VIII, respectively) may be damaged if the temporal bone is fractured at the base of the skull. Cranial nerves V and IX to XII are rarely damaged.[29]

Brain Tumors

In the words of Victoria Lynn Johnson, "A diagnosis of brain tumor confirms at some point you WILL need assistance. Asking for assistance has always been difficult; however I soon realized two things: I needed to get over my own interpretation of independence so that I could ask for assistance and that if I expected anyone to assist me I must be an active participant in my own well-being."[30]

A tumor is a mass of abnormal cell growth. More than 200,000 people in the United States are diagnosed with a brain tumor each year.[31] According to the Central Brain Tumor Registry of the United States, nearly 80,000 new brain and central nervous system tumors are expected to be diagnosed in 2018. Over 90% of primary brain tumors are diagnosed in people over 20 years old; people over 85 have the highest incidence. The average age at diagnosis is 57. Family history of brain tumors is not very common. Only a very small number of families have several members with brain tumors.

There are over 100 different types of brain tumors. The World Health Organization (WHO) classifies brain tumors by cell origin and the rate of growth of cells.[32] Brain tumors are classified in multiple ways, including benign versus malignant, primary versus secondary, and different stages (0–IV) and grades (I–III).[33] The stage of a cancer describes the size of a tumor and the degree of progression from its original site. The grade describes the appearance of the cancerous cells. Stage 0 indicates that the cancer is at its site of origin (in situ) and hasn't spread. In stage I, the cancer is small and hasn't spread either. In stage II, the cancer has grown, but hasn't spread. However in stage III, the cancer is larger and may have spread to the surrounding tissues and/or the lymph nodes. Spread of cancer to another body organ represents stage IV. This stage of cancer is also known as secondary or metastatic cancer. With regard to cancer grades, a lower grade indicates a slower-growing cancer and a higher grade indicates a faster-growing one. In grade I cancer, cells resemble normal cells and aren't growing rapidly. In grade II, cells don't look like normal cells and are growing faster than normal cells. In grade III, cancer cells look abnormal and may grow or spread more aggressively.

Benign brain tumors are noncancerous in nature and usually grow slowly. These tumors do not spread to other organs or surrounding tissues. Most benign brain tumors seldom recur after surgical removal. Benign brain tumors can have an impact on function (or can be life-threatening), especially if the tumor is compressing on vital structures inside the skull. An example of a benign brain tumor is meningioma (tumor arising from the meninges). Meningiomas account for 20% to 30% of brain tumors. The risk of developing a meningioma increases with age, and they occur about twice as often in women.[34,35] Another example of a benign tumor is schwannoma (tumor of the nerve sheath that grows slowly and pushes nerve fibers aside). Schwannomas can arise from any peripheral nerve containing Schwann cells, including cranial nerves. The cranial nerve VIII is the most susceptible to schwannomas, referred to as acoustic neuroma.[36] Schwannoma accounts for about 9% of all brain tumors. Malignant primary brain tumors are cancers that originate in the brain, typically grow faster than benign tumors, and aggressively invade surrounding tissue including other parts of the brain or the spinal cord. Malignant tumors are also sometimes called brain cancer.

Brain tumors are also classified as primary and secondary tumors. Primary brain tumors originate in the brain. In the United States, primary brain tumors are among the top 10 causes of cancer-related death. Some of the more common types of primary brain tumors include:

- *Astrocytomas:* The most common type of cancer brain tumor that affects the astrocytes (star-shaped brain cells)
- *Oligodendrogliomas:* Is a slow-growing transformation of oligodendrocytes, cells that wrap around axons. Oligodendrogliomas account for 3% of primary brain tumors. They usually occur in young adults and range from grade II to grade III. Because oligodendrogliomas are less likely than other gliomas to spread into normal brain tissue, surgery alone is frequently very beneficial, especially for grade II tumors.
- *Medulloblastoma:* A malignant tumor that forms in the cerebellum. It can spread to the spinal cord and cause spinal fluid to back up into the brain (hydrocephalus).
- *Ependymomas:* Tumors formed in the lining around the cerebral ventricles. These tumors account for nearly 6% of intracranial gliomas and about 60% of all newly diagnosed spinal cord tumors.
- *Gliomas:* Brain tumors arising from glial cells. Mixed gliomas have cells and characteristics of more than one type of glioma, usually astrocytomas and oligodendrogliomas.

Secondary (metastatic) tumors start as a cancer in another part of the body, such as the lungs or breast. The cancer then spreads to the brain, where it forms a new tumor. Metastatic brain tumors occur in 20% to 40% of people with cancer. Breast, lung, colon, kidney, and melanoma cancers are the most common cancers to metastasize to the brain. Metastatic brain tumors are more common than primary brain tumors in adults. Numerical grading of brain tumors is based on the growth of the tumors.

- *Grade I:* These tumors are considered benign in nature and are often slow growing. Surgical removal of these tumors is common. Prognosis, with regard to longevity and quality of life (QoL), is favorable.
- *Grade II:* These tumors also grow slowly and are less likely to spread. However, relapse and reoccurrence can happened with grade II tumors even following treatment.
- *Grade III:* These tumors are cancerous and tend to spread to other parts of the brain. Relapse of tumors can happen, as grade IV tumors.
- *Grade IV:* These are the most malignant tumors. They grow and spread most rapidly. Response to treatment is minimal, so prognosis is negative.

Classifications of Brain Injury

Regardless of the cause, the primary goal after a diagnosis of ABI centers on surviving, achieving medical stability, and preventing or minimizing the impact of secondary insults and effects on the injured central nervous system.[37] Upon arrival to a medical facility, the patient who has been assessed a score on the Glasgow Coma Scale (GCS) will receive complete examinations including computed tomography (CT) scanning, neurosurgical assessment, ICP monitoring, and procedures to limit thromboembolic complications (Table 37-3).[44] Assessment of the spinal cord is necessary because spinal cord injury is associated with 4% to 8% of TBIs.[38] Airway protection is of utmost importance; therefore, many times, a tracheostomy is performed to secure the airway. The interprofessional team will observe and monitor vital signs and assess neurological function. The primary goals at this stage are to avoid further

Table 37-3 Glasgow Coma Scale

Eye opening (E)	Spontaneous To speech To pain Nil	4 3 2 1
Best motor response (M)	Obeys Localizes Withdraws Abnormal flexion Extensor response Nil	6 5 4 3 2 1
Verbal response (V)	Oriented Confused conversation Inappropriate words Incomprehensible sounds Nil	5 4 3 2 1
Coma score = $E + M + V$		

Jennett B, Teasdale G. *Management of Head Injuries*. Philadelphia, PA: F.A. Davis; 1981. doi:10.1093/bja/54.3.371-a.

neurological damage and to stabilize critical extracranial injuries.[38] The role of the physician is to prevent secondary medical complications such as sepsis, stress ulcers, and symptoms of "storming," a result of sympathetic hyperactivity.[39]

After appropriate evaluation and treatment for life-threatening injuries, the patient with a severe TBI is taken to the intensive care unit (ICU). Medical treatment in the ICU aims to optimize cerebral perfusion and brain tissue oxygenation, minimize brain swelling, and maintain all other physiological variables requiring advanced cerebral monitoring, including seizure prophylaxis.[40]

A physiatrist is typically consulted within the first few days of admission to the ICU to make decisions for appropriate rehabilitative care. Along with occupational therapists, interprofessional members of the rehabilitation team often see the patient for rehabilitative consult and contribute the results of their assessments. The physiatrist orders rehabilitation services, including occupational therapy (OT), for the patient who is in a coma and that treatment may begin in the ICU. Generally, patients with more severe injuries move from the ICU to acute inpatient rehabilitation facilities.[41]

Severe Disorders of Consciousness

A person with severe brain injury may exhibit any of a number of altered states of consciousness, depending on the severity of the injury. Various terms are used to describe the continuum from complete consciousness to complete absence of consciousness. These patients begin in coma as a result of loss of consciousness, which is characterized by the inability to open their eyes in response to any stimuli and absence of the sleep–wake cycle based on electroencephalogram (EEG) readings. Vegetative state is a result of cerebral hemisphere dysfunction and presents with complex reflexive movements such as eye movements, yawning, and withdrawal to noxious stimuli. These patients, however, still do not demonstrate ability to interact with their environment. A minimally responsive state presents with the person emerging from coma. These patients are severely disabled, yet demonstrate inconsistent abilities to purposely interact with their environment depending on the stimuli presented. These interactions are recorded through observation and further testing.[42] The ability to open eyes and sustain visual pursuit eye movement, along with evidence of a sleep–wake cycle, appears to be the first signs of the transition out of coma according to Coma Recovery Scale–Revised (CRS-R). Medical management goals include improving physical stability of the individual for future participation in daily routines and therapeutic activities.[43] Rehabilitation may also occur in acute medical or subacute units, such as long-term acute care or skilled nursing facilities. The decisions for ongoing care are made based on the degree and rate of recovery, as well as logistical factors such as insurance coverage and social factors important to the patient and their support system. During the rehabilitative process, occupational therapists, along with other team professionals, use a number of objective assessments to monitor changes in function as a response to physical, cognitive, pharmacological, environmental, and behavioral interventions.

Moderate Brain Injury

As stated in Table 37-2, a person has sustained a moderate brain injury if loss of consciousness has occurred between 30 minutes and 24 hours, imaging shows either normal or abnormal structures, PTA is greater than 1 day but less than 7 days. The patient has a GCS of 9 to 12 and an Abbreviated Injury Scale score of 3. Symptoms may consist of headache, nausea, and vomiting, along with increased confusion, restlessness, **agitation**, or increased sleepiness. A patient with moderate brain injury may present with functional impairments in the areas of motor, sensory, and/or cognition.[44] Interprofessional assessment of cognition and function is important and may include the Rancho Los Amigos Scale of Cognitive Functioning Scale (Table 37-4), Functional Independent Measure (FIM), Berg Balance, and the CRS-R. Outcomes vary depending on the cerebral structures that are injured, and each patient is treated based on his or her individual presentation of symptoms. The rehabilitation treatment provided is similar to that for those with severe injuries; however, prognosis is considered to be better because of original scores at time of injury.

Rancho levels I to VIII are widely used in brain injury rehabilitation. The addition of levels IX and X in 1998 describes higher level cognitive, behavioral, and emotional barriers to optimal functioning.[45,46]

Table 37-4 Rancho Los Amigos Levels of Cognitive Functioning Scale

LEVEL	DESCRIPTION
I	No response: unresponsive to stimuli
II	Generalized response: nonspecific, inconsistent, and nonpurposeful reaction to stimuli
III	Localized response: response directly related to type of stimulus but still inconsistent or delayed
IV	Confused—agitated: response heightened, severely confused, may be aggressive
V	Confused—inappropriate: some response to simple commands, but confusion with more complex commands; high level of distractibility
VI	Confused—appropriate: response more goal directed but cues necessary
VII	Automatic—appropriate: response robot-like, judgment and problem-solving lacking
VIII	Purposeful—appropriate (with standby assistance): response adequate to familiar tasks, subtle impairments require standby assistance with acknowledging other people's needs and perspectives, modifying plans
IX	Purposeful—appropriate (with standby assistance on request): responds effectively to familiar situations but generally needs cues to anticipate problems and adjust performance; low frustration tolerance possible
X	Purposeful and appropriate (modified independent): responds adequately to multiple tasks but may need more time or periodic breaks; independently employs cognitive compensatory strategies and adjusts tasks as needed

Mild Brain Injury

Mild brain injuries can occur without hospitalization and are often referred to as **concussions**. According to Levin and Diaz-Arrastia,[47] the terms concussion and mild TBI are considered interchangeable. Impact on the cranium from any type of mechanical force can result in mild TBI.[13] Mild TBI is estimated to account for the majority of all TBI cases in civilian and military populations.[47] The American Congress of Rehabilitation Medicine (ACRM) defines mild TBI to include at least one of the following: any loss of consciousness up to 30 minutes, PTA lasting no more than 24 hours, any period of confusion or disorientation; transient neurological abnormalities such as focal signs, seizures, and intracranial lesions; or GCS score of 13 to 15. Post-concussion symptoms may be physical, cognitive, or behavioral/emotional in nature. Physical symptoms occurring in mild TBI may include nausea, dizziness, headache, blurred vision, fatigue, and difficulty sleeping. Cognitive deficits may present with decreased memory and executive functioning, whereas behavioral or emotional symptoms may present in the form of anxiety, depression, or agitation. The prognosis of mild TBI is relatively good as patients seem to obtain complete recovery, in approximately 12 weeks after time of injury.

Phases of Recovery

Although management of ABI is typically an interprofessional enterprise, the following description of each level is based on a typical recovery with emphasis on OT evaluation and treatment. Note how the role of OT changes with each level of severity, increasingly focusing on occupational functioning the further the patient progresses in recovery.[41] Recovery after ABI is lifelong. Depending on the severity, the patient may require several hospitalizations and treatment in a variety of settings throughout this lifelong journey. Care after ABI requires interprofessional collaboration and constant communication in the best interest of the patient.

Table 37-5 explains the possible phases of hospitalization and the recovery process throughout the continuum of care. Movement throughout the system is based on the patient's medical changes, funding, physician, rehabilitation team recommendation, as well as patient and family advocacy.

Occupational Therapy Assessments

The level of severity is determined by the physician and medical team. As occupational therapists, the clinician needs to consider the overarching condition of the patient, estimated prognosis, length of stay, funding, and the lives of both the patient and families in efforts to service the needs of this population after brain injury.[48] Table 37-6 identifies the areas of concentration during assessment and intervention as a quick guide for occupational therapists. Table 37-7 lists the assessments used by occupational therapists to meet the needs of patients in specific areas of practice. Descriptions of each of the tests follow.

Physical Assessments

Range of Motion

Range of motion (ROM) is a musculoskeletal assessment that addresses the flexibility or range that a joint is capable of moving. The assessment is typically conducted with a goniometer measuring tool. Common joints that are assessed include the shoulders, elbows, neck, wrists, and fingers. ROM assessments can be used

Table 37-5 Phases of Hospitalization, Recovery, and Continuum of Care

CARE SETTING	CARE TEAM
Intensive care unit	Follow-up with Primary Care Physician (PCP), Neurologist, Physiatrist, all specialists, Nursing
Acute medical hospitalization	Follow-up with PCP, Physiatrist, Neurologist, all specialists, Nursing, Neuropsychology, Occupational Therapy (OT) and Physical Therapy (PT), Chaplin, Social Worker
Acute rehabilitation	Follow-up with PCP, Physiatrist, Neurologist, Medical Specialists, Nursing, OT, PT, Speech and Language Pathology, Social Worker, Neuropsychologist, Chaplin (Rehab Team)
Acute specialty inpatient rehabilitation	Follow-up with PCP, Physiatrist, Neurologist, Rehab Team
Skilled nursing facility (SNF)/long-term care facility (LTAC)	Follow-up with PCP, Physiatrist, Neurologist, Rehab Team
Outpatient rehabilitation	Follow-up with PCP, Physiatrist, Neurologist, Rehab Team
Residential specific for brain injury	Full team on location with follow-up of PCP, Physiatrist, Neurologist, Rehab Team
Home health	Follow-up with PCP, Physiatrist, Neurologist, Rehab Team
Community resources/support groups/advocacy	Respite care, PCP, Neurologist

Table 37-6 Occupational Therapy Assessments and Interventions

LEVEL OF INJURY	ASSESSMENTS	INTERVENTIONS
Severe	Coma Recovery Scale–Revised (Interprofessional) Modified Ashworth Scale Assessment of static head control Pain Skin integrity Seating and positioning Assistive technology needs Possible home assessment	Promote sensory stimulation, pain and or motor responses, positioning, muscle re-education, family/caregiver training, home modifications, and equipment trials
Moderate	Motor observations Range of motion Rancho Los Amigos of cognition Modified Ashworth Scale Pain Skin integrity ADLs FIM scoring Custom seating and positioning assessment Assistive technology needs Behavioral agitation scale Depression Equipment needs Home assessment	Target basic ADLs, cognition, physical, psychosocial and behavioral goals; equipment trials, family/caregiver training, home modifications
Mild	Motor Cognitive assessments aimed at memory IADLs FIM scoring Executive functioning Self-awareness Pain Depression Behavior Preinjury behavior Home assessment Equipment needs	Target areas with IADLs, higher cognitive skills, family, caregiver training, return to work, driving, sports

ADLs, activities of daily living; FIM, Functional Independence Measure; IADLs, instrumental activities of daily living.

Table 37-7 Assessments at Different Levels Used by Occupational Therapists

ASSESSMENT	MILD IMPAIRMENT	MODERATE IMPAIRMENT	SEVERE IMPAIRMENT
Physical Assessments			
Range of motion (ROM)	✓	✓	✓
Modified Ashworth Scale (MAS)	✓	✓	✓
9 Hole Peg Test	✓	✓	✓
QuickDASH	✓	✓	
Box and Blocks Test	✓	✓	✓
Berg Balance Scale	41–56	21–40	0–20
6-Minute Walk Test	✓	✓	
Activities of Daily Living (ADLs)			
A-One	✓	✓	
Activity Card Sort	✓	✓	
Assessment of Motor and Process Skills (AMPS-9)	✓	✓	
Barthel Index			✓
Functional Independence Measure (FIM)	✓	✓	✓
Performance Assessment of Self-care Skills (PASS)	✓	✓	✓
Cognitive Assessments			
The Kettle Test	✓	✓	
Montreal Cognitive Assessment (MoCA)	✓	✓	
Neurobehavioral Cognitive Status Examination	24–30	18–23	0–17
St. Louis Mental Status Examination (SLUMS)	26–30		
Lowenstein Occupational Therapy Cognitive Assessment (LOTCA)	✓	✓	✓
Rancho Levels of Cognitive Functioning Scale–Revised (RLCFS)	✓	✓	✓
Emotional Assessments			
Canadian Occupational Performance Measure (COPM)	✓	✓	
Sickness Impact Profile	✓		
Beck Depression Inventory	✓	✓	
Behavioral Assessments			
Agitated Behavioral Scale	✓	✓	✓
Motivations for TBI Rehabilitation Questionnaire	✓		
Quality of Life After Brain Injury (QoLIBRI)	✓		

TBI, traumatic brain injury.

to track ranges in joint mobility over time and determine whether an individual's ROM is within the expected range.[49]

Modified Ashworth Scale

The Modified Ashworth Scale (MAS) is used to measure the degree of **spasticity** in individuals with central nervous system lesions. Examples of populations include brain injury, cerebral palsy, stroke, and multiple sclerosis. The MAS is scored on a 6-point scale, ranging from 0 to 4. A score of 0 indicates no increase in muscle tone. A score of 1 indicates a slight increase in muscle tone, manifested by a catch and release or minimal resistance at the end of the ROM when the affected part(s) is moved in flexion or extension. A score of 1+ indicates a slight increase in muscle tone, manifested by a catch, followed by minimal resistance throughout the remainder (less than half) of the ROM. A score of 2 indicates more marked increase in muscle tone through most of the ROM, but affected part(s) easily moved. A score of

3 indicates considerable increase in muscle tone, passive movement difficult. Lastly, a score of 4 indicates the affected part(s) rigid in flexion or extension.[50]

Nine-Hole Peg Test

The purpose of the Nine-Hole Peg Test is to measure finger dexterity. The test is administered by asking the client to take pegs out of a container and place them one by one into holes on the board, as quickly as possible. The client must then remove the pegs after all holes are filled. Clients are scored based on their total time to place pegs in and take pegs out of the board.[51]

QuickDASH

Also known as the Quick Disabilities of the Arm, Shoulder, and Hand. This test uses 11 items to measure physical function and symptoms in people with any or multiple musculoskeletal disorder in the upper limb(s). The QuickDASH is a self-report disability measure that asks clients to answer questions on a scale of 1 to 5, with 5 indicating great difficulty. The higher the total score, the more disabled a person reports to be.[52]

Box and Blocks Test

The Box and Blocks Test measures unilateral gross manual dexterity. The patient is seated at a table facing a box that contains 150 blocks. The goal of the test is to move as many blocks as possible, one at a time, into an empty adjacent compartment in 1 minute. Higher scores indicate better gross manual dexterity.[53]

Berg Balance Scale

Fourteen-item objective measure used to assess static balance and fall risk in adults. The tester observes the client perform 14 tasks that assess both static and dynamic balance. Items are score on a 0 to 4 scale, with 56 being the maximum score.[54]

6-Minute Walk Test

The 6-Minute Walk Test (6MWT) assesses distance walked over 6 minutes as a submaximal test of aerobic capacity and endurance. Prior to beginning the test, the client should begin in a seated position. The client is allowed to take as many rest breaks as required, but the time should not stop during the breaks. It is ideal to have the test performed in a hallway or open area at least 12 m long with a smooth, consistent surface, and clear pathways at either end.[55]

Activities of Daily Living Assessments

A-ONE

The A-ONE evaluates the impact of neurobehavioral impairment on functional performance of activities of daily living (ADLs). The measure allows observation of ADLs and evaluation of the level of assistance required for ADLs performance. The A-ONE provides the therapist with an ecologically relevant assessment of the consequences of neurobehavioral impairments through clinical observation of ADLs tasks using a "top-down" (occupation-based) approach.[56]

Activity Card Sort

Used by occupational therapists to help clients describe their social, instrumental, and leisure activities. The Activity Card Sort (ACS) can be used to identify lost activities, set goals, and monitor rehabilitation. The test uses 89 photographs of various activities that the client sorts into different categories based on engagement and interest in occupations.[57]

Assessment of Motor and Process Skills

The Assessment of Motor and Process Skills (AMPS-9) is an observational assessment that allows for the simultaneous evaluation of motor and process skills and their effect on the ability of an individual to perform complex or instrumental and personal ADLs. The AMPS is comprised of 16 motor and 20 process skill items.[58]

Barthel Index

The Barthel Index (BI) measures the extent to which somebody can function independently and has mobility in their ADLs (i.e., feeding, bathing, grooming, dressing, bowel control, bladder control, toileting, chair transfer, ambulation, and stair climbing). The index also indicates the need for assistance in care. The BI is a widely used measure of functional disability.[59]

Functional Independence Measure

The Functional Independence Measure (FIM) was developed to offer a uniform system of measurement for disability based on the *International Classification of Impairment, Disabilities and Handicaps* for use in the medical system in the United States. The level of a patient's disability indicates the amount of support needed to care for him or her and items are scored on the basis of how much assistance is required for the individual to carry out ADLs. The FIM consists of 18 items assessing 6 areas of function. The items fall into two domains: motor (13 items) and cognitive (5 items).[60]

Performance Assessment of Self-Care Skills

The Performance Assessment of Self-care Skills (PASS) is designed to measure occupational performance of daily-life tasks. The PASS is a client-centered, performance-based, criterion-reference, observational tool that objectively documents occupational performance and helps plan occupation-based interventions for adolescent, adult, and older adult populations in a variety of settings. The PASS consists of 26 core tasks, categorized in 4 domains. The PASS includes 5 functional mobility (FM) tasks, 3 basic activities of daily living (BADLs) tasks, 4 instrumental activities of daily living (IADLs) tasks with a physical emphasis, and 14 IADLs tasks with a cognitive emphasis.[61]

Cognitive Assessments

The Kettle Test

The Kettle Test is used to assess functional cognitive performance. The client is asked to complete a variety of daily tasks, which the clinician observes and assesses. The task assesses 13 areas of performance, whereas the client prepares a drink for the clinician and themselves. Total possible score of 52, with higher scores indicating greater performance deficits.[62]

Montreal Cognitive Assessment

Screen of cognitive abilities used to detect mild cognitive dysfunction. Sixteen-item measure that screens visuospatial abilities, executive function, naming, memory, language, attention, orientation, and abstraction. Total possible score of 30, with a score of 26 or higher considered normal function.[63]

Neurobehavioral Cognitive Status Examination

Assessment of neurocognitive functioning in three general domains: (1) consciousness, (2) orientation, (3) simple attention; and five major domains: (1) language, (2) constructional ability, (3) memory, (4) calculation skills, and (5) executive skills.[64]

SELF-AWARENESS Assessment

Interprofessional assessment used to assess a person's degree of self-awareness using guidelines for building a collaborative relationship, and applying intervention, which aims at restoring self-awareness in a confidence and skill-building manner.[65]

St. Louis Mental Status Examination

Administered by the clinician to identify persons who have dementia or mild cognitive impairment. St. Louis Mental Status Examination (SLUMS) is a quick screening that can be completed in approximately 7 minutes.[66]

Lowenstein Occupational Therapy Cognitive Assessment

Used to measure basic cognitive skills needed to perform ADLs/IADLs, including orientation, visual perceptual/psychomotor abilities, problem-solving skills, and thinking operations. Scores on a 1 to 4 scale, with higher scores indicating less impairment.[67]

Rancho Levels of Cognitive Functioning Scale–Revised

This evaluation tool identifies patterns of recovery for people with brain injury. The scale describes behavioral characteristics and cognitive deficits associated with brain injury to help the team understand and focus on the person's abilities in designing an appropriate treatment program. Scores range from level I to level VIII, with higher levels indicating higher levels of cognitive functioning.[68]

Emotional Assessments

Canadian Occupational Performance Measure

Assesses an individual's perceived occupational performance in the areas of self-care, productivity, and leisure. The assessment takes place in a semi-structured interview setting. The information obtained can be used to create goals for therapeutic interventions.[69]

Sickness Impact Profile

Assessment of QoL and level of dysfunction that results from disability or illness. Provides a valid and sensitive assessment of outcomes that result from health care–related services. Assesses four areas: (1) behavior, (2) life participation, (3) mental health, and (4) social relationships.[70]

Beck Depression Inventory

The most widely used instrument for detecting depression, takes just 5 minutes to complete, and is clinically sensitive.[71]

Behavioral Assessments

Agitated Behavior Scale

The Agitated Behavior Scale (ABS) measures behavioral aspects of agitation during the acute phase of recovery from ABI, including aspects of aggression, disinhibition, and lability. The ABS measures 14 statements on a scale of 1 to 4. The maximum score is 56, and the minimum score is 14. Higher scores indicate greater levels of agitation.[72]

Motivations for Traumatic Brain Injury Rehabilitation Questionnaire

Designed to assess motivation to participate in postacute rehabilitation, including factors of denial, anger, apathy, compliance, medical information seeking, and excessive enthusiasm. Thirty-one items that are scored by Likert-style scoring, ranging from −2 to 2. Maximum possible score of 62.[73]

Quality of Life After Brain Injury

Health-related QoL instrument for survivors of TBI that includes the person's subjective perspective. The scores range from 0 to 100. 0 means worst possible QoL, and 100 means the best possible QoL.[74]

Assessments Used by the Interprofessional Team

Assessments used by interprofessional teams are outlined in Table 37-8.[75]

Table 37-8 Assessments Used by the Interprofessional Team

ASSESSMENT	DESCRIPTION
Abbreviated Injury Scale (AIS)	One-time tool used to measure the severity of brain injury. The AIS differs from other measures in that it represents the threat a brain injury presents to an individual's life rather than assessing the severity of the injury.
Glasgow Coma Scale	Measures severity of brain injury by objectively measuring conscious state, initially at time of injury and periodically afterward.
Glasgow Outcome Scale–Extended (GOS-E)	Extension of the GOS designed to address the original scale's insensitivity to changes or progress over time. The GOS-E extends the original five categories in the GOS to eight: ranging from Dead to Good Recovery.
JFK Coma Recovery Scale–Revised (JFK CRS-R)	Used to assess individuals who are emerging from a minimally conscious or vegetative state. The CRS-R addresses 23 items, including auditory, visual, motor, communication, arousal functions, and automatic body functions. It also measures communication and arousal functions.
Galveston Orientation and Amnesia Test (GOAT)	Measures post-traumatic amnesia. The test features 10 questions that assess the patient's temporal and spatial orientation (*Where Am I?*), biographical recall (*Who Am I?*), and memory (*What Happened?*).
Orientation Log (O-LOG)	Measures post-traumatic amnesia. The O-LOG measures the individual's orientation to time, place, and circumstance over a period of time.
Westmead Post-Traumatic Amnesia Scale (WPTAS)	Administered at bedside by a member of his or her treatment team. The WPTAS measures the length of post-traumatic amnesia.
Rancho Los Amigos Levels of Cognitive Functioning Scale	Ten levels of cognitive function based on behavioral observations and responses to environmental stimulation.

Data from Academy of Certified Brain Injury Association Web site. https://www.biausa.org/. Accessed November 2018; Radomski MV and Trombly Latham C, Lippincott Williams & Wilkins, Baltimore, MD;2014:1042–1075.

Functional Impairment in Daily Occupations

"Every day I wake up is a good day. Even the bad days are now good" (Alice Torres, 2018).[76] ABI is disruptive to a person's normal routine and interrupts many, if not all, areas of daily life in the context of physical, emotional, cognitive, psychosocial, behavioral, intimacy, and sexuality. The degree of severity and the areas of the brain affected impact overall independence in occupations such as ADLs, work, and social participation; client factors such as vision and cognition; and performance skills in motor control, physical agility, stamina, and mobility.[42,77] The person with a brain injury must learn a new way and modify his or her approach to living the remainder of life using new strategies to accomplish routine tasks. Some adjustments are temporary, whereas others are permanent and lifelong. Occupational therapists are the professional experts in developing rapport through therapeutic use of self. Through this relationship, occupational therapists gather information using the occupational profile, perform activity analysis, assess and predict the positive functional potential of the patient, and access patient personal motivation to assist in modification of the environment, and/or tasks as needed to enhance daily occupations.

Occupational Therapy Interventions

Many researchers have attempted to assess the predictive power of age; clinical observations such as the GCS, duration of unconsciousness, and length of PTA; and neuroimaging evidence of structural damage in efforts to predict recovery outcomes.[78,79] Despite all the medical and technological advances, the ability to predict outcomes on an individual basis remains complex. In the writing of new guidelines by the ACRM for managing vegetative and minimally conscious states, Joseph T. Giacino, PhD writes "People are sometimes misdiagnosed due to underlying impairments that can mask awareness. An inaccurate diagnosis can lead to inappropriate care decisions and poor health outcomes."[80] Although the occupational therapist does not diagnose or predict outcomes, he or she is a valuable team member in considering predictive factors that contribute to the overall recovery process of the patient. These predictive factors are used to determine goals, length of stay, course of interventions, equipment needs, and ability to move directionally within the continuum of care. It is imperative that occupational therapists use their keen observation skills to report changes and their therapeutic skills to empower changes regarding patient performance. Interventions chosen by the clinician are generally driven by areas of training, evidence-based practice, and the desire to apply new knowledge. As always, interventions chosen are patient centered and occupationally based.

Physical Interventions

Positioning

As an occupational therapist, it is important to work collaboratively with all professions regarding patient positioning. The patient's position must be reevaluated frequently with close monitoring of his or her reactions, including facial expression, changes in muscle tone, and vocalizations. Minor adjustments can make a difference between comfort and discomfort. Assistive positioning supports are to be removed as the patient's neuromuscular status improves.[41] When considering bed positioning, communication between the nursing staff, physical therapy (PT), and the patient's family must be good to make an informed decision regarding desired bed positioning, its purpose, and the schedule. Daily skin assessment is critical to protect from the development of skin breakdown or pressure wounds. Development of pressure wounds will require the occupational therapist to make necessary adjustments in collaboration with the medical team. Patient positioning is dependent on the medical condition of the patient and any precautions that may be on board. Refer to the patient chart, the physician, and the nursing team to guide you during your review for bed positioning. The standard practice in bed positioning is 2 hours on back and then alternate to each side. If the patient has a severe brain injury, swallowing precautions may need to be considered regarding bed of head angle and degree of elevation.

Supine

Lying supine may trigger an extensor response if not properly supported at lower extremities (LEs) with slight hip and knee flexion, feet supported with heels off the bed and in neutral dorsiflexion.[40] Collaboration with PT regarding LE positioning is in the best interest of the patient. Head is positioned in neutral with only one pillow for support. Depending on the degree of head control, more support may be needed with conscious effort to protect the ears from constant pressure. The trunk is in alignment with shoulders. Upper extremities (UEs) are positioned in partial abduction away from the body, with elbows extended, forearms elevated on pillows or wedges to decrease any edema, wrists are in extension, and hands are open in abduction. Hand splints may be in place to promote functional hand positioning, and the type of splinting used will be determined on whether the tone in the UEs is flaccid or increased. If increased abnormal flexor tone is present in the hand, custom splinting is the best option. Do not use soft towels in the hands because soft materials will elicit abnormal flexion reflexes.

Side-Lying

In side-lying, the head, resting on a small pillow, should be in neutral alignment with the trunk; the bottom UE should be in moderate scapular protraction and humeral external rotation; the top UE should be in scapular protraction, slight shoulder flexion, and resting on a pillow to avoid horizontal adduction; the bottom elbow should be flexed; the top elbow should be extended; wrists should be in extension; and hand splint should be placed to decrease spasticity and maintain thumb web spaces and finger abduction. A pillow between the knees decreases hip internal rotation and adduction. The lower leg also may need pillow support to align it with the thigh. If necessary, place a firm pillow or foam wedge in the space between the thigh and the calf to prevent excessive knee flexion. The foot should not be placed higher than the knee and hip because this can result in torque on the knee and cause the hip to go into internal rotation. Elongation of the lower side of the trunk between the shoulder and the pelvis is desirable. A pillow or foam wedge behind the back and shoulder will assist in maintaining trunk position in side-lying and may also need to be tucked in front of the trunk in maintaining the alignment.[40] If a long body pillow is used, it can often be positioned to maintain some abduction in the LEs and support the calf and foot of the upper leg. Avoid positioning the feet near the footboards because this may elicit extensor thrust. There are many options for foot orthotic devices used to avoid pressure to the heel of the foot, while maintaining ankle dorsiflexion to 90°, in efforts to prevent foot drop. The orthotic devices may also be used to avoid stimulating an extensor thrust from the foot. If the pelvis is retracted on one side, a small folded towel is placed behind it, and that leg is positioned in neutral. Some knee flexion should be encouraged with care to avoid prolonged knee flexion to prevent development of a contracture. A semi-recumbent bed position with head-of-bed angle maintained at 45° is recommended for patients on mechanical ventilators, tracheostomies, or swallowing issues, to minimize risk of aspiration and pneumonia.[81]

Wheelchair Positioning

Early and correct upright wheelchair positioning helps to facilitate arousal by stimulating the visual and vestibular systems, inhibiting abnormal tone, providing normal proprioceptive input, and reducing the likelihood and/or extent of contractures and complications from prolonged bed rest. The pelvis must be positioned correctly before other areas can be addressed. The pelvis should be in a neutral position or have a slight anterior tilt if needed to decrease extensor thrust. The pelvis should be symmetrical, without one side retracted or elevated.[40] Custom seating and positioning becomes valuable as equipment trials begin using solid seat inserts, solid backs, and cushions to gain optimal alignment. Because the spine and rib cage are the essential connecting parts between the shoulders and the pelvis, it is important to obtain alignment in these structures to facilitate shoulder and trunk stability. Positioning the trunk with thoracic extension and neutral scapulae is critical for improved function. The trunk should be symmetrical and in midline with shoulders over the pelvis in sagittal, frontal, and horizontal planes. Lateral trunk supports can be used in the wheelchair to better position the trunk in an upright manner and to decrease lateral trunk flexion. Experimentation with the positioning is essential because trunk control varies among patients and is the key to achieving reach. The therapist must not overcompensate with too much trunk support, but rather facilitate and challenge the patient's normal movement and control. With a solid seat, supportive cushion, and solid-custom wheelchair back, the patient may not require additional trunk support. Dependent trunk control may require a chest harness, shoulder straps, or a chest strap to enhance functional potential by keeping the patient from falling forward or limiting forward trunk flexion. Positioning of the extremities is also crucial. Hips, knees, and ankles are flexed to 90°. Heels are slightly behind the knees in sitting, with feet in neutral pronation-supination and inversion-eversion. The footplate should be large enough to support the whole foot. If abnormal tone presents in the ankles, wheelchair accessories such as foot wedges, heel loops, shoe holders, or custom bracing may be required to properly reach 90° of ankle flexion. The ideal UE position for wheelchair propulsion begins with scapulae in slight protraction, and slight shoulder abduction. Elbows are in comfortable flexion, and the forearm is in partial pronation. The wrists are in extension with neutral ulnar–radial deviation, the fingers are relaxed, and the thumb is radially abducted with the mobility coming from the first carpometacarpal (CMC). The height and angle of the solid back for trunk support impacts the shoulder position and must be considered for efficient wheelchair propulsion. In addition, a lap tray may be used to allow for UE weight bearing and serves as a support for an extremity with limited mobility. Head position also needs to be considered. Ideally, the head should be in midline with cervical elongation posteriorly and the chin tucked in slightly. It is important that positioning eliminates chin jutting and neck hyperextension. The position of the patient's pelvis, trunk, and shoulders all influence head position. When prescribing a wheelchair, keep in mind that the wheelchair is an extension of the person. "People are not confined by their wheelchairs. They are in fact liberated by their wheels."[82]

Passive Range of Motion

Passive range of motion (PROM) programs are used in conjunction with positioning to minimize the development of contractures from abnormal tone and static postures. PROM can be difficult when muscle tone is increased. Inhibitory movements opposite the abnormal tone are performed slowly, holding the stretch until muscles relax. Flexor muscle groups tend to present with higher risk of developing contractures than the extensor group muscles. Sudden quick stretch or noxious stimulation and handling should be avoided. Scapular mobility should be addressed before UE PROM to free the scapula and facilitate normal scapular and humeral movement during the rest of PROM.[83] Awareness of joint limitations along with increased pain and increased spasticity may be a sign of heterotopic ossification. Occupational therapists use PROM and positioning to minimize the development of contractures.[43]

Splinting and Casting

The goals of splinting and casting are to decrease abnormal tone and increase the patient's functional movement. Custom splinting focuses on inhibiting flexion or extensor patterns as a result of abnormal tone. Splinting can be used as a means to promote or inhibit motion. Plaster or fiberglass serial casting may be indicated when there is severe spasticity in the elbow and/or wrist.[84] Serial casting along with the use of neurolytic procedures such as BOTOX injections and intrathecal baclofen (ITB) pumps can be very effective in treating ROM limitations or motor issues as a result of spasticity, in the UE.[82,85] Dropout casts, which leave a portion of the limb exposed; bivalve casts, which are split in two, can be removed during therapy and nursing procedures; and weight-bearing inhibitory casts, which are fabricated to approximate the ideal weight-bearing posture of the foot or hand, can also be used.[41] Casting is contraindicated with uncontrolled hypertension, major open wounds, unhealed fracture, impaired circulation, acute inflammation, a recent episode of autonomic dysreflexia, or if professionals need access to the extremity for lines or monitoring of vital signs.[86] "When spasticity interferes with comfort, function, ADLs, mobility, positioning, or caregiver assistance, patients should be considered for ITB therapy."[85]

Occupational therapists work collaboratively with other professionals in this decision-making process. The treatment of spasticity is complex and challenging. It requires an investigative and continuous reassessment approach, while tapping into different therapeutic interventions. An interprofessional approach is critical as both occupational and physical therapists join with nurses and physicians in addressing secondary complications, during attempts to prevent risk of contracture and skin breakdown.[43] Because OT uses a client-centered approach, remember that the patient and/or supportive persons should be empowered to assist in all decisions in the best interest of the patient.

Sensory Stimulation

Although studies do not present reliable evidence of support regarding sensory stimulation for persons with **disorders of consciousness (DOCs)**, structured use of these techniques is generally accepted as a practice model. The goals of a sensory stimulation programs are to promote arousal from coma while stimulating the reticular activating system, prevent sensory deprivation by facilitating appropriate patterns of movement from prolonged immobility, and interaction with the environment, while facilitating ability to increase responses to stimuli and also encouraging the ability to follow commands.[43] Therapists use consistent protocols to standardize the administration of stimuli and data sheets to record observations regarding rate of response and changes in respiration, pulse, blood pressure, head movements, eye opening, eye movements, eye fixations, mimic responses, aimed and non-aimed motor reactions, and articulations in response to tactile, vestibular, olfactory, kinesthetic, proprioceptive, auditory, and visual stimuli. Therapists hope to see an increase in consistent responses, which is an indication of improvement.

Vision and Visual Perception

Vision and visual-perception issues present in most cases of ABI. Vision is another area that is dependent on communication between team members. Occupational therapists should include vision as part of their assessment protocols in identifying visual impairments that can impact function such as ADLs, IADLS, daily life, and QoL.[87,88] Assessments and interventions should include the areas of visual acuity, oculomotor, visual fields, binocular vision, vergence, and vestibular interactions. Patients with visual deficits will have damage to the areas of occipital and/or parietal lobes. Visual perceptual deficits may occur as a result of sensory interference and the inability to accurately respond to sensory information. Visual perceptual deficits include form discrimination, depth perception, figure–ground perception, topographical orientation, and spatial relations. Due to the fact that visual-perception difficulties interact with cognition, it is often important to rule out cognitive impairments.[43] As an occupational therapist addressing visual deficits, collaboration with other team members such as ophthalmologist, neuro-ophthalmologist, and neurologist is important when distinguishing between a visual function issue and/or a visual perceptual issue.[89] Mary Warren's Hierarchy Model of Visual Perception states that the foundation of visual function is based on oculomotor control, visual fields, and visual acuity. The highest order of the visual perceptual process is visual cognition. According to Warren, the role of OT in determining appropriate interventions is to identify the functional impairment and to link the presence of the functional impairment to the presence of the visual impairment.[89,90] Many clinicians today choose to use a combination of remedial, compensatory, and adaptive approaches when treating patients who have visual deficits from ABI. Generalization of cognitive and perceptual rehabilitation techniques has a higher ability to be transferred into function if training is done in a variety of settings.[91]

Management of Agitation

Post-traumatic agitation is reported to occur in the acute setting in 33% to 70% of patients with ABI and may last for up to 10 days or less. Agitation is a subtype of delirium in the coma-emerging patient that is associated with frontotemporal injury, disorientation, comorbid medical complications, and/or use of anticonvulsant medication.[92] Management of agitation is an interprofessional team process. The aggressive behavior may present in bizarre, unpredictable, and impulsive manners.[43] The main purpose of the team during this phase is to provide the patient with a safe environment. The role of clinicians is to determine which factors are contributing to the problem, considering client factors, social context, and the physical environment.[41] Interventions such as decreasing stimulation, implementing consistent behavior techniques, psychotropic medications, and one-on-one coaching with continuous supervision, including telemonitoring, may be warranted.[93]

Cognition

There are currently several million Americans living with long-term disabilities due to ABI.[2] In today's health care model, patients with ABI typically move quickly within the continuum of care. There has been much discussion in recent years about the role of OT in the assessment and treatment of cognition. Much of the confusion is surrounded by reimbursement issues and billing codes. The profession of OT has been involved in treating cognitive issues since the inception of the profession. Salvador Bondoc informs occupational therapists to justify the use of cognitive rehabilitation by applying clinical reasoning and describing how cognitive deficits influence occupational performance.[94] Occupational therapists use remedial, compensatory, and adaptive approaches to improve cognition. Activities and exercises combined with functional, client-centered purposeful challenges stimulate primary cognitive domains (attention, memory, and executive function). While past cognitive training methods have consisted of card or board games, puzzles, paper-and-pencil drills, and computer programs, increasing clinician involvement in occupation-based treatments with transfer ability to a variety of contexts is recommended.[95] During the 2018 AOTA Slagle Lecture, Gordon Giles speaks of evidence-based practice where occupational therapists have a unique role in skill development for patients with ABI. Although many professionals have the capacity to address cognition, the profession of OT has a unique position in assessing functional cognition. Functional cognition is the ability to use and integrate thinking and performance skills to accomplish ADLs and IADLs in both the dynamic clinical environment and the community to which patients will return. Giles discusses the neurofunctional approach to achieving functional cognition. The neurofunctional approach concentrates on incorporating principles of skill learning and promotes the development of routines and competencies in the practical activities required for daily living. Giles goes on to state that occupational therapists must increase confidence in their ability to clearly articulate the profession's unique approach to assessment during collaboration with the interprofessional team. Furthermore, he states, "Our unique vision is needed to improve client care and outcomes. If we fail to meet this need, another discipline will do so."[96]

Self-Awareness

The rehabilitation process is a journey for all those involved. The key to a full recovery includes intact self-awareness. The presentation of impaired self-awareness creates a significant barrier to successful rehabilitation.[65] The profession of OT emphasizes the importance of consideration between empathy, personal beliefs, dignity, and the interrelationships between the person, the occupations, and the environment.[97] As occupational therapists, the ability to integrate art and science while fostering self-awareness in an empathetic and dignified manner can be accomplished using the Self-Awareness Enhancement through Learning and Function (SELF) practice guide. This practice guideline is an interprofessional collaborative example merging the latest theoretical perspectives from disciplines such as neuroscience, psychology, computer science, and OT. Use of the SELF for assessment and treatment encompasses clear direction, while demonstrating therapeutic alliance, occupation, belief perspectives, neurological education, and compensatory strategies for the purpose of enhancing self-awareness. The SELF differs from traditional methods of cognitive retraining by providing "occupational therapists with guidelines for building a collaborative relationship with the client, using an intervention that restores self-awareness in a manner that builds confidence and skills," rather than focusing on poor performance-based feedback.[65]

Functional Training

The ability to develop rapport with a patient is imperative for safety and progression in treatment. Depending on the severity of the injury and the area in the continuum of care, the focus of therapy in the area of daily living begins with reestablishing routine self-care tasks. If the patient has a severe impairment, training is initiated with family or support system. All self-care is simplified until skills are successfully mastered. Activities are client centered, and distractions are minimized. Using the neurofunctional cognitive approach, training is performed by implementing the following steps: (1) task analysis, (2) whole task method, (3) cue experimentation, (4) consistent time delay cuing, (5) self-generation, (6) reinforcement, (7) errorless learning, and (8) overlearning. Practice is essential.[96] Occupational therapists may need to assist with establishing consistent and automatic self-care routines at home by documenting the sequence of steps for which the patient is successful. Clinicians must consider the patient's previous knowledge or familiarity with the task prior to attempting to reestablish habits and routines.[41] When choosing interventions, occupational therapists should be leaders in using authentic occupations by engaging patients in purposeful activities. Purposeful activities are meaningful tasks that are part of daily routines, such as personal care, home management, school, and work. Research has shown that using purposeful, occupation-based interventions is an intrinsic motivator for patients.[98]

Psychosocial

The consequences and effects associated with brain injury can be lifelong. ABI sequelae include impairments in the areas of cognition, emotions, behavior, and sensorimotor function. Many individuals experience increased life complexity after ABI. There are many factors such as prior premorbid personality, personal relationships, marital discord, work-related issues, and financial instability that contribute to further development of neuropsychiatric symptoms.[99] Patients recovering from mild brain injuries tend to experience more symptoms such as headaches, pain, cognitive, emotional, or even personality changes. Additional life stressors may contribute to anxiety or even depression. It is important that after discharge from inpatient rehabilitation services that the patient continue to be followed by neurology and even neuropsychology.[43] Ylvisaker et al.[100] recommend focusing on antecedents associated with positive behavior and less on consequences related to problems. The following are examples of strategies that contribute to the patient's ability to learn effective behaviors during inpatient rehabilitation and beyond:

- Redesign the environment.[100] For example, if noise and distractions seem to contribute to a patient's irritability and aggressiveness, provide treatment and care in areas that are calm and quiet.
- Capitalize on the superiority of procedural over declarative memory after brain injury by helping patients learn context-sensitive routines rather than broader transfer-dependent strategies.[100]
- Use of neurofunctional approach by incorporating task analysis with functional activity participation using cues, repetition, and errorless training to encourage success.[91]
- Provide successful experiences to reduce frustration-induced maladaptive behavior.

The discharge from inpatient status can often be anxiety producing for both the patient and the individual's support system. Patients will continue to focus on improvement in all areas of cognition, visual and visual-perception, and self-maintenance roles such as ADLs, IADLs, leisure and social participation, work, and behavioral and emotional adaptation. As patients and families attempt to resume and reintegrate into their prior lives, the ability to escape the awareness that change has occurred in some manner is difficult.[41]

Support Systems

With changes in health care, more families are assuming a participatory role in caring for individuals affected by brain injury. Patients' families continue to require information and support to understand the recovery and rehabilitation process. This information is to assist in making informed decisions and actively participating in discharge planning. Much has been stated about team and interprofessional collaboration. The support system is part of this collaborative team. Owing to shorter length of stays, family involvement should begin immediately, as allowed, to begin the training process. Families must be provided with information regarding the continuum of care system, home programs, equipment, and community resources to prepare for discharge options as soon as possible. Training should occur over the duration of hospitalization or length of stay in whatever setting the patient is being treated. Many times, occupational therapists are working closely with social work and case managers to provide a smooth transition for the patient and family to the next destination in the recovery process. Family members must consider developing support outside the immediate family unit because caregiver burden is estimated to occur in nearly 90% of caregivers of individuals with ABI.[101]

The survivorship phase of life for persons with ABI presents opportunities for clinicians to employ all that is truly unique to OT, synthesizing the totality of our education, philosophy, and values to enhance occupational functioning in society. Readers are challenged to consider the following ways to poise themselves for action:

- Recommend that a life care plan be prepared for survivors of moderate-to-severe ABI. A life care plan delineates the services and items required for the current and long-term care of the survivor as well as the costs of these services. A life care plan can be used clinically to plan appropriate long-term care, including intermittent follow-up, and for forensic purposes, such as determination of an appropriate settlement that will provide for the lifetime needs of the injured person.
- Promote to possible referral sources to enhance community integration and QoL for persons with ABI. Join the local brain injury association, connect with the state's vocational rehabilitation division, and become familiar with key personnel supporting disabled students at local colleges and universities.
- Establish the kind of therapeutic relationship with patients and family members that will make them want to return for help. Respecting the patient's readiness for treatment means sometimes not intervening, but making sure that he or she knows that the door is open in the future.

Make sure that the discharge from outpatient OT incorporates plans for follow-up and clear information regarding possible circumstances in the future when further OT services may be helpful. Provide information to the patient and his or her family regarding mechanisms to reinstate services. Remember that the nature of ABI interferes with patients' ability to advocate for themselves (e.g., lack of initiation, impaired memory), and so the therapist must build in opportunities to discern and respond to their needs.[41]

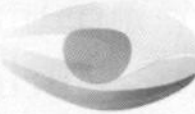

CASE STUDY

Patient Information

Nathan is a 16-year-old high school student who sustained a TBI from falling out of the back of a pickup truck after a high school football game. Nathan was previously an extrovert who loved music, worked at a local grocery store on weekends, and was excited about starting high school. Nathan is part of a blended family whose parents are very involved with their children, and who also work full time. Upon arrival to the trauma center, Nathan was still unresponsive. The assessment in the ER revealed the following:

- Initial GCS of 3
- Open wound to the back of the head with large hematoma
- Increased ICP
- Intubation requiring tracheostomy necessary to sustain breathing
- C4–C5 spinal processes hairline fracture
- Right posterior humeral fracture
- Left femur fracture
- Bleeding into all ventricles

Nathan was treated in the ICU for 21 days where he underwent surgery for fractures with internal pinning for right UE (RUE) and left LE (LLE) and was on non–weight-bearing status for both. Surgical placement of gastrostomy tube (G-tube) was also performed for feeding purposes prior to transfer to the acute floor. Nathan remained on the acute unit for 7 days while undergoing medical treatment for pain, continued monitoring of ICP, feeding,

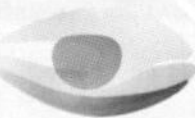

CASE STUDY (continued)

and further stabilization procedures. He was to wear a Miami J Collar at all times to protect his cervical spine. OT orders were initiated, along with PT and speech-language pathologist (SLP). OT received orders as part of the interprofessional team to assess and provide ROM, positioning, sensory stimulation, and caregiver education. At the time the patient was transferred to the acute care unit, he presented with abnormal flexor posturing in bilateral UEs (BUEs) and extensor posturing in bilateral LEs. RUE humeral and LLE femur were casted, PROM was still within normal limits at this time. Nathan also presented with spasticity in UEs scoring 0 to 2 throughout BUEs on the MAS. Nathan was still unresponsive to any stimuli, nonverbal, and not moving neither on command or involuntarily. While still on the acute care unit, the patient contracted methicillin-resistant *Staphylococcus aureus* (MRSA) in his urine and was placed on contact-isolation. Once stabilized, although he remained unconscious, he was transferred to acute inpatient rehabilitation for further DOC management. At 5 weeks after onset, Nathan was now receiving rehabilitation on the inpatient brain injury unit. He was referred to an interprofessional team consisting of OT, PT, SLP, neuropsychology, dietary, social work, and pharmacology. He is being followed by a medical team inclusive of physiatrist, orthopedic surgery, neurosurgery, gastroenterology, and infectious disease. OT received orders to assess and treat for responsiveness to stimuli, cognition, bed positioning, seating and positioning, ADLs, spasticity management, neuromuscular re-education, and caregiver training.

Assessment Process and Results

The CRS-R2 was administered jointly by OT and neuropsychology. Nathan's scores demonstrated emergence of coma in the following areas: eye movement but no eye opening, response to auditory stimuli, and response to pain.

PROM is still within normal limits; however, right elbow was not assessed due to cast from distal humeral fracture. Manual muscle test (MMT) is zero not only because of patient unable to follow commands but also because of spasticity. MAS reported increased tone of RUE shoulder internal rotators, adductors, and wrist and finger flexors bilaterally. He is dependent in all ADLs and mobility. Skin is intact; however, stage I redness is occurring on sacrum. Nathan's parents hope to take him home depending on status at discharge.

Occupational Therapy Problem List

- Decreased arousal and attention
- Inability to visually track
- Decreased ability to follow basic commands
- Poor head control
- Decreased ability to sit unsupported
- Dependent in ADLs
- Increased risk for skin breakdown
- Non–weight-bearing RUE and LLE

Occupational Therapy Goal List

OT goals are set for 4 weeks for long term (LTG) and 2 week for short term (STG). Length of stay varies depending on progress of Nathan and funding source. Discharge options are dependent on status at time of discharge as to whether it will be home or community based. Insurance requires updates every 2 weeks.

- ***LTG:*** Nathan will improve in level of arousal from severe to moderate level of consciousness.
- ***STG:*** Nathan will open eyes on command to stimuli 3/5 attempts. Nathan will tolerate sitting upright, with support, for 60 minutes daily.

Interventions

Nathan received inpatient OT for a total of 90 minutes, a day with one session being 60 minutes and another 30 minutes session. Focus of therapy was to increase sensory stimulation and deep pressure through the hips, pelvis, and left UE (LUE) joints while in upright posture to increase level of arousal and physical demands against gravity. Sessions start in supine to perform stretching, abnormal tone inhibitory techniques, and PROM to all UE joints with the exception of right elbow. Patient is placed in a tilt-in-space manual wheelchair that provides good head and trunk support. Patient is then transferred and placed in sitting with total support for trunk and head control. OT co-treats with music therapy to attempt to increase arousal and his ability to follow commands during weight-bearing activities. As Nathan's level of arousal improved to being alert throughout the day, OT continued to focus on head and trunk control, along with consistency in following verbal commands and increased ability to regain the use of UEs for the purpose of BADLs.

Upon discharge from inpatient rehabilitation, Nathan remained alert and could follow basic commands with eye blinks for "yes and no." Head control was fair, and he could sit upright in his manual wheelchair for 2-hour intervals three times a day with appropriate wheelchair accessories for head and trunk control. The OT was responsible for ordering necessary equipment, training parents on BADLs, PROM and stretching program, tone inhibition techniques, bed and wheelchair positioning splint wear and care, and follow-up care.

Best Evidence for Interventions Used for Acquired Brain Injury in Occupational Therapy

Intervention	Description	Participants	Dosage	Research Design and Evidence Level	Benefit	Statistical Significance and Effect Size
Neurofunctional approach[102]	Comparison of randomized controlled trial between cognitive and functional approaches over 10 years	Participants with moderate-to-severe TBI ($N = 360$)		Systematic Level I	Neurofunctional approach as compared to traditional rehabilitation can improve cognitive performance.	$p = 0.01$
Efficacy of activities of daily living[103]	ADL retraining was manualized, followed errorless and procedural learning principles with individualized goals.	Participants with severe TBI ($N = 104$)	Participants received individual ADL skills retraining for nine modules, using a structured format by occupational therapists.	Systematic review Level I	Individuals in PTA can benefit from skill retraining.	$p = 0.001$
Cognitive ehabilitation[95]	Various cognitive rehabilitation approaches	Participants (number not specified) with TBI or stroke from 112 studies	Varied by study	Systematic review Level I	Recommendations for practice standard for attention remediation in postacute rehab, metacognition strategy training; practice guidelines for use of memory compensations in severe TBI	Not calculated

References

1. Ontario Brain Injury Association Web site. http://obia.ca/?option=com_content&view=category&layout=blog&id=31&Itemid=41.
2. Centers for Disease Control and Prevention. Traumatic brain injury & concussion. Basic information about traumatic brain injury. https://www.cdc.gov/traumaticbraininjury/basics.html. Updated 2016. Accessed October 5, 2018.
3. Vieira RC, Paiva WS, de Oliveira DV, Teixeira MJ, de Andrade AF, de Sousa RM. Diffuse axonal injury: epidemiology, outcome and associated risk factors. *Front Neurol.* 2016;7:178.
4. Bruno M, Laureys S, Demertzi A. Chapter 17—Coma and disorders of consciousness. *Handbook of Clinical Neurology.* Vol. 118. Amsterdam, The Netherlands: Elsevier; 2013:205–213. doi:10.1016/B978-0-444-53501-6.00017-2.
5. American Congress of Rehabilitation Medicine. Brain injury interdisciplinary special interest group, mild traumatic brain injury task force definition of mild traumatic brain injury. *J Head Trauma Rehabil.* 1993;8:86–87.
6. Maas AIR, Stocchetti N, Bullock R. Moderate and severe traumatic brain injury in adults. *Lancet Neurol.* 2008;7(8):728–741. doi:10.1016/S1474-4422(08)70164-9.
7. National Institute of Neurological Disorders and Stroke. Spasticity information page. National Institute of Neurological Disorders and Stroke Web site. https://www.ninds.nih.gov/Disorders/All-Disorders/Spasticity-Information-Page. Updated 2018. Accessed October 5, 2018.
8. World Health Organization. *The World Health Report 1996—Fighting Disease, Fostering Development.* Geneva: World Health Organization; 1996.
9. Pagulayan K, Temkin N, Machamer J, Dikmen S. A longitudinal study of health-related quality of life after traumatic brain injury. *Arch Phys Med Rehabil.* 2006;87(5):611–618. doi:10.1016/j.apmr.2006.01.018.
10. Centers for Disease Control and Prevention. Traumatic brain injury & concussion. Severe TBI. Centers for Disease Control and Prevention Web site. https://www.cdc.gov/traumaticbraininjury/severe.html. Updated 2017. Accessed October 5, 2018.
11. Corso P, Finkelstein E, Miller T, Fiebelkorn I, Zaloshnja E. Incidence and lifetime costs of injuries in the United States. *Inj Prev.* 2006;12(4):212–218. doi:10.1136/ip.2005.010983.
12. Coronado VG, McGuire LC, Sarmiento K, et al. Trends in traumatic brain injury in the U.S. and the public health response: 1995–2009. *J Safety Res.* 2012;43:229–307.
13. Faul M, Xu L, Wald MM, Coronado VG. Traumatic Brain Injury in the United States: Emergency Department Visits, Hospitalizations and Deaths 2002–2006. Atlanta, GA: Centers for Disease Control and Prevention, National Center for Injury Prevention and Control. 2010.
14. Centers for Disease Control and Prevention. TBI: get the facts. Centers for Disease Control and Prevention Web site. www.cdc.gov/traumaticbraininjury/get_the_facts.html. Updated 2014. Accessed October 5, 2018.
15. Powell JM, Ferraro JV, Dikmen SS, Temkin NR, Bell KR. Accuracy of mild traumatic brain injury diagnosis. *Arch Phys Med Rehabil.* 2008;89(8):1550–1555. doi:10.1016/j.apmr.2007.12.035.
16. Selassie A, Zaloshnja E, Langlois J, Miller T, Jones P, Steiner C. Incidence of long-term disability following traumatic brain injury hospitalization, United States, 2003. *J Head Trauma Rehabil.* 2008;23(2):123–131.
17. Zaloshnja E, Miller T, Langlois J, Selassie A. Prevalence of long-term disability from traumatic brain injury in the civilian population of the united states, 2005. *J Head Trauma Rehabil.* 2008;23(6):394–400.
18. Centers for Disease Control and Prevention. *Report to Congress on Traumatic Brain Injury in the United States: Epidemiology and Rehabilitation.* Atlanta, GA: National Center for Injury Prevention and Control; Division of Unintentional Injury Prevention. 2015.
19. IOM (Institute of Medicine). *Gulf War and Health, Volume 7: Long-Term Consequences of Traumatic Brain Injury.* Vol. 7. Washington, D.C.: The National Academies Press; 2009.
20. Brasure M, Lamberty GJ, Sayer NA, et al. *Multidisciplinary Postacute Rehabilitation for Moderate to Severe Traumatic Brain Injury in Adults.* Rockville, MD: Agency for Healthcare Research and Quality (US); 2012.
21. Duff D. Review article: Altered states of consciousness, theories of recovery, and assessment following a severe traumatic brain injury. *Axone.* 2001;23(1):18–23.
22. Andriessen T, Jacobs B, Vos P. Clinical characteristics and pathophysiological mechanisms of focal and diffuse traumatic brain injury. *J Cell Mol Med.* 2010;14(10):2381–2392.
23. Katz DI. Neuropathology and neurobehavioral recovery from closed head injury. *J Head Trauma Rehabil.* 1992;7(2):1–15. doi:10.1097/00001199-199206000-00004.
24. Zappalà G, Thiebaut de Schotten M, Eslinger PJ. Traumatic brain injury and the frontal lobes: what can we gain with diffusion tensor imaging? *Cortex.* 2012;48:156–165.
25. Smith DH, Meaney DF, Shull WH. Diffuse axonal injury in head trauma. *J Head Trauma Rehabil.* 2003;18(4):307–316. doi:10.1097/00001199-200307000-00003.
26. Leech RW, Shuman RM. *Neuropathology: A Summary for Students.* Philadelphia, PA: Harper & Row; 1982.
27. Povlishock JT, Katz DI. Update of neuropathology and neurological recovery after traumatic brain injury. *J Head Trauma Rehabil.* 2005;20(1):76–94. doi:10.1097/00001199-200501000-00008.
28. Eaten B, Shaw T, Gallant J, Jaramillo C. Cranial nerve, visual and hearing dysfunction in disorders of the CNS. PM&R Knowledge NOW Web site. https://now.aapmr.org/cranial-nerve-visual-and-hearing-dysfunction-in-disorders-of-the-cns/. Updated September 20, 2014. Accessed October 5, 2018.
29. Coello A, Canals A, Gonzalez J, Martín J. Cranial nerve injury after minor head trauma. *J Neurosurg.* 2010;113(2):547–555.
30. In a conversation with V. L. Johnson. Surviving brain tumors (November 2019).
31. Metastatic brain tumors. American Association of Neurological Surgeons Web site. https://www.aans.org/Patients/Neurosurgical-Conditions-and-Treatments/Metastatic-Brain-Tumors. Updated 2018. Accessed Novemeber 18, 2018.
32. Louis D, Perry A, Reifenberges G, et al. The 2016 World Health Organization classification of tumors of the

central nervous system: a summary. *Acta Neuropathol.* 2016;131(6):803–820.

33. National Health Service. What do cancer stages and grades mean? National Health Service Web site. https://www.nhs.uk/common-health-questions/operations-tests-and-procedures/what-do-cancer-stages-and-grades-mean/. Updated 2018. Accessed November 18, 2018.
34. Perry A, Stafford S, Scheithauer B, Suman V, Lohse C. Meningioma grading: an analysis of histologic parameters. *Am J Surg Pathol.* 1997;21(12):1455–1465.
35. Harter P, Braun Y, Plate K. Classification of meningiomas – advances and controversies. *Chin Clin Oncol.* 2017;6(suppl 1):S2.
36. Louis D, Ohgaki H, Wrestler O, Cavemen W. *WHO Classification of Tumors of the Central Nervous System.* Lyon, France: IARC; 2007.
37. Hartl R, Ghajar J. Does following the recommendations in the guidelines for the management of severe traumatic brain injury make a difference in patient outcome? *Neurotrauma: Evidence-Based Answers to Common Questions*; 2005:120.
38. Baron E, Jallo J. Acute care management. *Brain Injury Medicine: Principles and Practice.* New York, NY: Demos; 2007.
39. Vincent J, Berré J. Primer on medical management of severe brain injury. *Crit Care Med.* 2005;33(6):2157.
40. Carney N, Totten AM, O'Reilly C, et al. Guidelines for the management of severe traumatic brain injury, fourth edition. *Neurosurgery.* 2017;80(1):6–15. doi:10.1227/NEU.0000000000001432.
41. Powell J. Traumatic brain injury. *Occupational Therapy for Physical Dysfunction.* 7th ed. Baltimore, MD: Wolters Kluwer; 2014:1042–1075.
42. Reed K. Nervous system disorders. *Quick Reference to Occupational Therapy.* 3rd ed. Austin, TX: Pro-Ed; 2014:306–311.
43. Kolakowsky-Hayner SA, Reyst H, Abashian MC, eds. *The Essential Brain Injury Guide.* 5th ed. Vienna, VA: Brain Injury Association; 2016.
44. Jennett B, Teasdale G. *Management of Head Injuries.* Philadelphia, PA: F.A. Davis; 1981. doi:10.1093/bja/54.3.371-a.
45. Hagen C. *The Rancho Los Amigos Scale of Cognitive Functioning.* Downey, CA: Rancho Los Amigos Medical Center. 1998;3.
46. Hagen C, Malkmus D, Durham P. Levels of cognitive functioning. In: *Rehabilitation of the Head Injured Adult; Comprehensive Physical Management.* Downey, CA: Professional Staff Association of Rancho Los Amigos National Rehabilitation Center; 1979.
47. Levin HS, Diaz-Arrastia RR. Diagnosis, prognosis, and clinical management of mild traumatic brain injury. *Lancet Neurol.* 2015;14:506–517. doi:10.1016/S1474-4422(15)00002-2.
48. Copley J, Kuipers K. *Extremity Across the Lifespan Neurorehabilitation of the Upper Managing Hypertonicity for Optimal Function.* Oxford: Wiley Blackwell; 2014.
49. Cerebral Palsy Alliance. Range of motion (ROM) assessment. Cerebral Palsy Alliance Research Foundation Web site. https://research.cerebralpalsy.org.au/about-cerebral-palsy/assessments-and-outcome-measures/range-of-motion-rom-assessment/#1487190336625-60de19c1-f020. Updated 2016. Accessed October 10, 2018.
50. Shirley Ryan AbilityLab. Rehabilitation measures database. Ashworth scale/modified Ashworth scale. https://www.sralab.org/rehabilitation-measures/ashworth-scale-modified-ashworth-scale. Updated 2016. Accessed October 10, 2018.
51. Shirley Ryan AbilityLab. Rehabilitation measures database. Nine-hole peg test. https://www.sralab.org/rehabilitation-measures/nine-hole-peg-test. Updated 2014. Accessed October 10, 2018.
52. Shirley Ryan AbilityLab. Rehabilitation measures database. Quick disabilities of arm, shoulder, and hand. https://www.sralab.org/rehabilitation-measures/quick-disabilities-arm-shoulder-hand. Updated 2015. Accessed October 10, 2018.
53. Shirley Ryan AbilityLab. Rehabilitation measures database. Box and block test. https://www.sralab.org/rehabilitation-measures/box-and-block-test. Updated 2012. Accessed October 10, 2018.
54. Shirley Ryan AbilityLab. Rehabilitation measures database. Berg balance scale. https://www.sralab.org/rehabilitation-measures/berg-balance-scale. Updated 2013. Accessed October 10, 2018.
55. Shirley Ryan AbilityLab. Rehabilitation measures database. 6-minute walk test. https://www.sralab.org/rehabilitation-measures/6-minute-walk-test. Updated 2013. Accessed October 10, 2018.
56. Canadian Partnership for Stroke Recovery. Arnadottir OT-ADL neurobehavioural evaluation (A-ONE). Stroke Engine Web site. https://www.strokengine.ca/en/indepth/a_2d_one_indepth/. Updated 2018. Accessed October 10, 2018.
57. Shirley Ryan AbilityLab. Rehabilitation measures database. Activity card sort. https://www.sralab.org/rehabilitation-measures/activity-card-sort. Accessed October 18, 2018.
58. Zeltzer L. Assessment of motor and process skills (AMPS). Stroke Engine Web site. https://www.strokengine.ca/en/assess/amps/. Updated 2018. Accessed October 10, 2018.
59. Marvin K, Zeltzer L. Barthel index (BI). Stroke Engine Web site. https://www.strokengine.ca/en/assess/bi/. Updated 2015. Accessed October, 10, 2018.
60. Zeltzer L. Functional independence measure (FIM). Stroke Engine Web site. https://www.strokengine.ca/en/assess/bi/. Updated 2011. Accessed October 10, 2018.
61. Rogers JC, Holm MB, Chisholm D. Performance assessment of self-care skills (PASS). University of Pittsburgh School of Health and Rehabilitation Sciences Web site. https://www.shrs.pitt.edu/ot/about/performance-assessment-self-care-skills-pass. Updated 2018. Accessed October 10, 2018.
62. Shirley Ryan AbilityLab. Rehabilitation measures database. Kettle test. https://www.sralab.org/rehabilitation-measures/kettle-test. Accessed October 18, 2018.
63. Shirley Ryan AbilityLab. Rehabilitation measures database. Montreal cognitive assessment (MoCA). https://www.sralab.org/rehabilitation-measures/montreal-cognitive-assessment. Updated 2012. Accessed October 18, 2018.

64. Shirley Ryan AbilityLab. Rehabilitation measures database. Cognistat cognitive assessment/neurobehavioral cognitive status examination. https://www.sralab.org/rehabilitation-measures/cognistat-cognitive-assessment-neurobehavioral-cognitive-status-examination. Updated 2017. Accessed October 18, 2018.
65. Dirette D. Self-awareness enhancement through learning and function (SELF): a theoretically based guideline for practice. *Br J Occup Ther*. 2010;73(7):309–318.
66. Shirley Ryan AbilityLab. Rehabilitation measures database. Saint Louis University mental status exam. https://www.sralab.org/rehabilitation-measures/saint-louis-university-mental-status-exam. Updated 2013. Accessed October 18, 2018.
67. Shirley Ryan AbilityLab. Rehabilitation measures database. Loewenstein occupational therapy cognitive assessment. https://www.sralab.org/rehabilitation-measures/loewenstein-occupational-therapy-cognitive-assessment. Updated 2016. Accessed October 18, 2018.
68. Shirley Ryan AbilityLab. Rehabilitation measures database. Rancho levels of cognitive functioning. https://www.sralab.org/rehabilitation-measures/rancho-levels-cognitive-functioning-3rd-edition-1998. Accessed October 18, 2018.
69. Shirley Ryan AbilityLab. Rehabilitation measures database. Canadian occupational performance measure. https://www.sralab.org/rehabilitation-measures/canadian-occupational-performance-measure. Updated 2013. Accessed October 18, 2018.
70. Shirley Ryan AbilityLab. Rehabilitation measures database. Sickness impact profile. https://www.sralab.org/rehabilitation-measures/sickness-impact-profile. Updated 2016. Accessed October 18, 2018.
71. Shirley Ryan AbilityLab. Rehabilitation measures database. Beck depression inventory. https://www.sralab.org/rehabilitation-measures/beck-depression-inventory. Updated 2012. Accessed October 18, 2018.
72. Shirley Ryan AbilityLab. Rehabilitation measures database. Agitated behavior scale. https://www.sralab.org/rehabilitation-measures/agitated-behavior-scale. Updated 2012. Accessed October 10, 2018.
73. Chervinsky, A. B., Ommaya, A. K., deJonge, M., Spector, J., Schwab, K., & Salazar, A. M. (1998). Motivation for traumatic brain injury rehabilitation questionnaire (MOT-Q): Reliability, factor analysis, and relationship to MMPI-2 variables. *Archives of Clinical Neuropsychology*, 13(5), 433–446. doi: 10.1016/S0887-6177(97)00016-4.
74. Shirley Ryan AbilityLab. Rehabilitation measures database. Quality of life after brain injury. https://www.sralab.org/rehabilitation-measures/quality-life-after-brain-injury. Updated 2012. Accessed October 10, 2018.
75. Academy of Certified Brain Injury Association Web site. https://www.biausa.org/. Accessed November, 2018.
76. In a conversion with A. Torres (June 2018).
77. American Occupational Therapy Association. Occupational therapy practice framework: domain and process. *Am J Occup Ther*. 2014;68(suppl 1):S19–S26.
78. Healey C, Osler TM, Rogers FR, et al. Improving the Glasgow Coma Scale score: motor score alone is a better predictor. *J Trauma*. 2003;54:671–680.
79. Nakase-Richardson R, Sherer T, Seel RT, et al. Utility of post-traumatic amnesia in predicting 1-year productivity following traumatic brain injury: comparison of the Russell and Mississippi PTA classification intervals. *J Neurol Neurosurg Psychiatry*. 2011;82:494–499.
80. Giacino JT, Trott CT. Rehabilitative management of patients with disorders of consciousness. *J Head Trauma Rehabil*. 2004;19(3):254–265.
81. Helman DL, Sherner JH, Fitzpatrick TM, Callender ME, Shorr AF. Effect of standardized orders and provider education on head-of-bed positioning in mechanically ventilated patients. *Crit Care Med*. 2003;31:2285–2290.
82. Christopher & Dana Reeve Foundation. https://www.christopherreeve.org/living-with-paralysis/wheelchairs/how-to-pick-the-right-wheelchair-for-you. Accessed September 19, 2019.
83. Roehrig SM. Use of neurodevelopmental treatment techniques in a client with kyphosis: a case report. *Physiother Theory Pract*. 2006;22;22(6):337–343. doi:10.1800959398060102371.
84. Mortenson PA, Eng JJ. The use of casts in the management of joint mobility and hypertonia following brain injury in adults: a systematic review. *Phys Ther*. 2003;83(7):648.
85. Saulino M, Ivanhoe CB, McGuire JR, Ridley B, Shilt JS, Boster AL. Best practices for intrathecal baclofen therapy: patient selection. *Neuromodulation*. 2016;19(6):607–615.
86. Stoeckmann T. Casting for the person with spasticity. *Top Stroke Rehabil*. 2001;8:27–35.
87. Suter PS. Rehabilitation and management of visual dysfunction following traumatic brain injury. In: Ashley M, ed. *Traumatic Brain Injury, Rehabilitative Treatment and Case Management*. 2nd ed. Boca Raton, FL: CRC Press;2004:209–249.
88. Smith T. LVIM 2014 [supplemental material]. In: Whittaker SG, Scheiman M, Sokol-McKay DA, eds. *Low Vision Rehabilitation: A Practical Guide for Occupational Therapists*. 2nd ed. Thorofare, NJ: Slack; 2016. http://www.healio.com/books/form-sites/lowvisionrehab2e/forms. Accessed October 27, 2018.
89. Warren M. Evaluation and treatment of visual deficits following brain injury. In: Pendleton HM, Schultz-Krohn W, eds. *Pedretti's Occupational Therapy: Practice Skills for Physical Dysfunction*. 7th ed. St. Louis, MO: Elsevier Mosby; 2013: 590–626.
90. Zoltan B. *Vision, Perception, and Cognition: A Manual for the Evaluation and Treatment of the Adult with Acquired Brain Injury*. 4th ed. Thorofare, NJ: Slack; 2007: 47–108.
91. Gillen G. *Cognitive and Perceptual Rehabilitation Optimizing Function*. St. Louis, MO: Mosby; 2009.
92. Edward K. Agitation, aggression, and disinhibition syndromes after traumatic brain injury. *NeuroRehabilitation*. 2002;17(4):297–310.
93. Tipton-Burton M, McLaughlin R, Englander J. Traumatic brain injury. In: Pendleton HM, Schultz-Krohn W, eds. *Pedretti's Occupational Therapy Practice Skills for Physical Dysfunction*. 7th ed. St. Louis, MO: Mosby Elsevier; 2013:590–915.
94. Brown, EJ. OT's role in cognitive rehabilitation. *Advance*. 2013;29(7):10.

95. Cicerone KD, Langenbahn DM, Braden C, et. al. Evidence based cognitive rehabilitation: updated review of the literature from 2003 through 2008. *Arch Phys Med Rehabil.* 2011;92:519–530.
96. Giles G. 2018 Eleanor Clarke Slagle lecture—neurocognitive rehabilitation: skills or strategies? *Am J Occup Ther.* 2018 Nov/Dec;72(6):7206150010p1-7206150010p16. doi: 10.5014/ajot.2018.726001.
97. Peloquin SM. The issue is: a reconsideration of occupational therapy's core values. *Am J Occup Ther.* 2007;61(4): 474–482.
98. Richardson H. Glen Gillen on non-purposeful intervention activities. *OT Pract.* 2018;23(16):16.
99. Rao V, Lyketsos C. Neuropsychiatric sequelae of traumatic brain injury. *Psychosomatics.* 2000;41(2):95–103.
100. Ylvisaker M, Jacobs HE, Feeney, T. Positive supports for people who experience behavioral and cognitive disability after brain injury. *Journal of Head Trauma.* 2003;18:7-32.
101. Hanks RA, Rapport LJ, Vangel S. Caregiving appraisal after traumatic brain injury: the effects of functional status, coping style, social support, and family functioning. *NeuroRehabilitation.* 2007;22:43–52.
102. Vanderploeg R, Schwab K, Walker W, et al. Rehabilitation of traumatic brain injury in active duty military personnel and veterans: defense and veterans brain injury center randomized controlled trial of two rehabilitation approaches. *Arch Phys Med Rehabil.* 2008;89(12): 2227–2238. doi:10.1016/j.apmr.2008.06.015.
103. Trevena-Peters J, Mckay A, Spitz G, Suda R, Renison B, Ponsford J. Efficacy of activities of daily living retraining during posttraumatic amnesia: a randomized controlled trial. *Arch Phys Med Rehabil.* 2018;99(2):329.e2–337.e2. doi:10.1016/j.apmr.2017.08.486.

Acknowledgments

With great love and gratitude, I thank my parents Joe and Frances Flores for their belief in the power of education; Candy, whose love and support allows me to accomplish anything life slings at me; Erica, Thomas, Maddi, and Zach, your constant support and tolerance of mountains of paper is remarkable. Thank you for allowing your mother to "just be." To Dr. Lee Mountain, what an inspiration you always are. Dawn Phillips and Rachel Sieber, your professionalism and collaboration have been invaluable. To the TIRR/Memorial Hermann Brain Injury Team OTs of 2018, thank you for allowing me pick your brain. To Bridget Furlong for your many hours of input. To all the OT students of Texas Woman's University, thank you for your support and inspiration.

Chapter 38

Neurodegenerative Diseases

Susan J. Forwell, Lucinda L. Hugos, and Setareh Ghahari

LEARNING OBJECTIVES

This chapter will allow the reader to:

1. Appreciate the complex considerations when approaching and working with a client with neurodegenerative disease.
2. Describe the epidemiology, etiology, course and prognosis, and medical management of multiple sclerosis (MS), Parkinson disease (PD), amyotrophic lateral sclerosis (ALS), and Guillain-Barré syndrome (GBS).
3. Describe the signs and symptoms of MS, PD, ALS, and GBS and the role of occupational therapy in their management.
4. Synthesize the functional impairment in daily occupation experienced by persons with MS, PD, ALS, and GBS.
5. Select standardized occupational therapy assessment and evaluation tools for clients with neurodegenerative diseases based on individual clients' characteristics and requirements.
6. To achieve client-centered goals, determine interventions for clients with MS, PD, ALS, and GBS based on their individual characteristics, the social context and physical environment, the occupational therapy evaluation, and current research evidence.

CHAPTER OUTLINE

TERMINOLOGY

Akinesia: initiation impairment of voluntary and spontaneous motor responses that interrupts performance to engage in voluntary activity.

Bradykinesia: slowness or poverty of movement such as lack of facial expression or "mask face" and reduced eye blink, arm swing during walking, and decreased postural stability.

Cogwheel rigidity: series of catches through passive range of motion much like a second-hand jerks on a clock face.

Demyelination: a process by which myelin, the covering on nerves that enables conduction speed, is lost or damaged and results in an absence or impairment of impulse conduction typically manifesting in functional limitations.

Festinating gait: small rapid steps when the posture of the head and trunk involuntarily lean forward ahead of the feet. One's center of gravity (COG) shifts forward and is compensated by small shuffling steps and increased gait resulting in "chase" the COG.

Intention tremor: an oscillating tremor that occurs during visually guided, goal-directed movements. Amplitude increases as the target is approached and when increased precision is demanded.

Lower motor neurons (LMN): neurons located in the brainstem and cranial nerves that allow voluntary muscle movement and link to upper motor neurons (UMN) and muscles; damage to LMN can lead to flaccidity, muscle atrophy, loss of swallowing, and vocalization ability.

Rigidity: hypertonicity of agonist and antagonist muscles that offers a consistent, uniform resistance to passive movement.

Upper motor neurons (UMN): neurons located in the brain that function to transmit motor signals to the spinal cord activating LMN to activate muscles; damage to UMN can result in weakness and paralysis, decreased motor control, and spasticity.

Introduction

Neurodegenerative diseases are chronic, potentially progressive, and frequently require coping with disability and the threat of functional loss. The underlying pathologies of neurodegenerative diseases are shown to have mechanisms that attack the peripheral and central nervous system, resulting in impairments and limitations that affect all aspects of life. Although, not curable, research, including rehabilitation interventions, has led to treatments that allow people to live longer, productive lives.

Occupational Therapy for Neurodegenerative Diseases

The unique contribution of occupational therapy (OT) for persons with neurodegenerative diseases is the consistent focus on participation in occupations that are valued in their lives. There is no script, because the nature, type, intensity, and context of these occupations are as individual as each person with the neurodegenerative disease. By listening to each individual coupled with professional expertise in occupation, occupational therapists support individuals and families by providing a repertoire of systematic processes and sensitive diverse solutions.

OT frequently begins at diagnosis and continues throughout the continuum of comprehensive care, taking place in inpatient acute care, inpatient rehabilitation, and in outpatient, in-home, or long-term care settings. Inpatient acute treatment usually follows a major relapse or deterioration in the disease, is short, and is limited to safety considerations and stabilizing symptoms with medical interventions. Inpatient rehabilitation may last one to several weeks, with daily therapy sessions to deal with changing symptoms. Outpatient therapy is usually weekly or biweekly, with 45- to 60-minute individual sessions to maximize independence in the home, minimize the effects of symptoms on chosen occupations, and identify and obtain needed equipment. OT in long-term care facilities may be related to adjusting to changing or deteriorating symptoms to ensure maintenance of function and control over their environment, or developing palliative care plans. Occupational therapists attend to their own coping and maintain objectivity, especially when treating individuals whose disease course portends increasing disability or death.

Occupational Therapy Evaluation

The OT evaluation with persons with neurodegenerative disease begins with an interview to gather information about the client's roles and occupations, relevant history of the neurodegenerative disease, previous and current strategies used to manage daily life, and the nature of present concerns or problems. This interview must be sensitive to the individual's changing function and fear of the unknown and should illuminate areas that clients may not naturally mention such as fatigue, depression, sexual function, and cognitive concerns that impact occupations and social network. With this information, the therapist selects assessments and measurement tools that will provide in-depth information on occupational areas of concern. For persons with neurodegenerative disease, the content of these measures may be limited to a few or cover a broad spectrum of occupational performance areas.

Occupational Therapy Intervention Process

The unplanned and profound impact of neurodegenerative disease frequently makes realistic goal setting and intervention complex and requires thoughtfulness, flexibility, and astute negotiation skills on the part of the occupational therapist. The therapist frequently helps the client modify behaviors and assumptions of a lifetime while assisting the person and significant others to move toward realistic goals. Given the progressive nature of many neurodegenerative diseases, regular reassessment and reordering of priorities may be necessary as intervention proceeds.

Because of the complexity of disability present with neurodegenerative disease, intervening in one area may affect several other symptoms or problems. Fatigue, for instance, may be related to pain, depression, and weakness. Interventions must be individually appropriate and may involve significant others, especially as the disease progresses. Depending on the setting, occupational therapists are involved with facilitating the maintenance of self-care (activities of daily living [ADLs] and instrumental activities of daily living [IADLs]), as well as employment, social and leisure occupations through the use of adaptations, appropriate planning, and credible websites and recommending new and emerging mainstream technology. For persons with neurodegenerative diseases, many of these advances have erased differences in participation, minimized the need for altered approaches, specialized adaptive equipment and environmental modifications, and have facilitated access to previously unavailable opportunities and personal connections.

Multiple Sclerosis

Epidemiology

Multiple sclerosis (MS) is the most commonly diagnosed neurological disease that can cause disability in young adults. An estimated 900,000 people in the United States have MS,[1] and worldwide that number is 2.3 million.[2] Onset of MS is typically between 15 and 50 years, although children are increasingly being diagnosed. Women are two to three times as likely to have MS. Caucasians of northern European descent have the highest risk of developing MS, whereas groups like the Norwegian Lapps, Inuit, and New Zealand Maoris who live in similar latitudes have no incidence of MS.[3]

Etiology

The precise cause of MS remains unknown. Research suggests that an environmental trigger, genetics, and infectious agents are among the factors that initiate the autoimmune response.[4] The *multiple* in multiple sclerosis refers to dissemination across both time and location of MS lesions and relapses. The *sclerosis* refers to the plaques on the axons and myelin covering that form scar tissue and interfere with nerve conduction.

Demyelinated axons may remyelinate and provide conduction of nerve impulses, though transected axons are permanently destroyed and lose potential for conduction. There is evidence that disease activity continues even during periods that are clinically quiet or when no change in symptoms is apparent.[5] Inflammation occurs with **demyelination** and axonal damage, which may explain the rapid improvement with corticosteroid anti-inflammatory agents used during relapses. Recent work has demonstrated that functional reserve influences the course (or phenotype) and prognosis of MS, suggesting that functional reserve may be important for future research.[5]

Course and Prognosis

Understanding of the initial neurological event and MS phenotypes has advanced over the past 30 years with imaging, biomarkers, and clinical observations. Currently, these are described as clinically isolated syndrome (CIS) and the phenotypes of relapsing-remitting, secondary progressive, and primary progressive MS.[6] CIS, or the first neurological episode that may go onto an MS diagnosis, is important to identify and follow so that early treatment can minimize disease progression prior to a confirmed MS diagnosis. The relapsing-remitting course, most common at diagnosis, produces clearly defined relapses of acute worsening followed by partial or complete improvement and then stable periods of remission between attacks. Secondary progressive MS starts with a relapsing-remitting course of up to 10 to 15 years and is typically diagnosed when there is continued deterioration and disability. People with primary progressive MS have continuously declining neurological function from onset without clear relapses.

Signs and Symptoms

OT intervention may reduce the impact of MS symptoms and ability to maintain desired occupations. Common signs and symptoms include fatigue, weakness, cognitive changes, pain, spasticity, tremor, dysphagia, sensory changes, balance disturbance, visual changes, bowel and bladder problems, vertigo, ataxic gait, sexual dysfunction, and depression.[4] A few of these are described here to exemplify therapy services.

Fatigue

Fatigue is the most common and pervasive MS symptom and a primary reason for referral to OT. It affects 60% to 80% of people with MS and is a significant contributor to unemployment and overall disability.[7] Fatigue augments other MS symptoms, varies from mild to severe with worsening typically in the afternoon, and may be related to increased ambient and core body temperature.[8]

Therapists must be aware of both the types and factors contributing to fatigue in MS[9] and know that multicomponent education programs and single component energy conservation programs have the strongest evidence of benefit for fatigue management.[10]

Types of fatigue in MS include the following:

- *Primary MS fatigue:* Fatigue caused by MS disease process, the cause of which is poorly understood.
- *Secondary MS fatigue:* Fatigue resulting from untreated MS problem(s) such as walking difficulties.
- *Physical fatigue:* Fatigue experienced in the limbs, torso, head, and neck such that the body is tired.
- *Cognitive fatigue:* Fatigue that affects one's thinking, planning, memory, word-finding, and decision-making processes such that the brain feels exhausted.
- *Local or focal fatigue:* Motor fatigue caused by inefficient nerve conduction to a selected area of the body, such as progressive foot-drop with extended walking.
- *Generalized fatigue:* An entire body experience; a complete exhaustion that is physical and cognitive.
- *Normal fatigue:* Fatigue experienced by humans after excessive energy output or several hours of being awake (a normal day) that benefits from rest or sleep.

Factors shown to contribute to fatigue in MS include the following:

- Other medical issues such as anemia, arthritis, cardiac problems, respiratory inefficiency, infection, and thyroid problems
- Sleep problems, often related to muscle spasms, depression, or urinary problems
- Depression
- Stress
- Anxiety
- Pain
- Deconditioning
- Side effects to medications
- Nutrition or caloric intake
- Ambulation difficulties

Weakness

Weakness may occur in all parts of the body, resulting in referral to OT. Weakness that increases after repeated muscle contractions is known as nerve fiber fatigue. The cause is unknown but likely related to the conduction impairment of demyelinated nerves. An example is dorsiflexion weakness, resulting in foot-drop that increases stumbling, particularly on uneven surfaces. Coupled with decreased balanced and gait impairment, the risk of falls is increased by 58%.[11] In some situations, with rest, conduction and muscle contraction can improved.

Cognition

Up to 60% of people with MS have cognitive problems that vary in severity and appear related to loss of brain volume, particularly gray matter.[12] It is estimated that 5% to 10% of those with MS have cognitive problems that interfere with participation in everyday occupations and employment in MS.[3]

Common cognitive problems include memory (acquiring and retaining new information); word-finding; attention, concentration, and executive function; and slowed information-processing speed.[3] Visual-spatial impairments may also occur. Cognitive issues do not correlate with physical disability in MS but are influenced by depression, stress, anxiety, and fatigue.[12] Individuals and their families may be unaware that cognitive problems such as reduced self-awareness and inflexible thinking are related to the disease and should not be mistaken for personality or psychological changes. By identifying cognitive impairments, compensation strategies can be recommended to benefit everyday function.

Pain

Pain is estimated to occur in 40% to 60% of people with MS, with 48% reporting chronic pain.[3] Pain negatively impacts quality of life (QoL) and independence[13] and is not related to age, length of time with MS, or degree of disability, although twice as many women report having pain than men. Pain in MS can be localized as in trigeminal neuralgia, Lhermitte sign (a stabbing, electric shock along the spine when neck forward flexes), or pain as a result of spasticity.[13] Pain directly caused by the neurological lesions is considered primary to MS and is treated with medications. Pain secondary to MS is often due to posture, gait, and positioning problems and can be relieved by therapy and proper mobility equipment.

Spasticity

Spasticity in MS is usually greater in the lower extremities and may be source of pain, interrupted sleep, and activity limitations. Up to 84% of people with MS deal with daily spasticity and 30% eliminate or modify activities because of spasticity.[14] Factors that may precipitate or augment spasticity include infections, distended bladder, and stress and disease progression. The assessment, MS Spasticity Scale with eight subscales, is a client-based measure that accounts for the physical, psychological, and functional experience of spasticity in MS.[15] Therapists should be familiar with standard medical management, particularly medications, such as baclofen and tizanidine, and their side effect of drowsiness. Botox (onabotulinumtoxin), a neurotoxin, results in relaxation of the targeted muscle and can last up to 3 months.[16] The intrathecal baclofen pump has been shown to reduce pain and improve function and QoL for people with MS with moderate-to-severe spasticity.[17] Should a baclofen pump be indicated, the therapist may be involved in assessment prior to and reevaluation following pump implantation. A recent systematic review has suggested that cannabis may reduce spasticity.[18]

Tremor and Ataxia

Intention tremor is the most common tremor seen in MS and is one of the most difficult problems to manage.[3] As an activity progresses and the extremity approaches the target (where greatest precision is required), the tremor is at its worse. Intention tremor occurs in the upper extremities, lower extremities, torso, and neck.

Ataxia presents in the trunk and lower extremities where postural responses tend to occur before upper extremity movements. The functional challenges of ataxia are further magnified because multiple joints are involved in ataxic movement.

Dysphagia

Research on swallowing problems in MS that did not use videofluoroscopy (VF) suggested that 34% to 43% of the individuals studied experienced dysphagia, although only half of these individuals reported swallowing difficulties.[19] When VF was used, however, swallowing abnormalities were identified that were not detected on non-VF swallow assessment. These studies suggest that the severity of disease and cerebellar or brainstem involvement are risk factors for dysphagia. Occupational therapists should routinely screen for choking, aspiration, and swallowing difficulties.

Medical Management

Diagnosing Multiple Sclerosis

The diagnosis of MS has evolved with the updated McDonald criteria based on the medical history, neurological examination, magnetic resonance imaging (MRI) results, and analysis of cerebrospinal fluid.[20] Additional tests including visual evoked potential and blood tests may be used to corroborate the MS diagnosis or exclude other diseases. Signs of MS include weakness, hyperreflexia, positive Babinski sign, dysmetria, nystagmus, and impaired vibratory or position sensation. The most common rating instruments for both clinical and research uses are the Expanded Disability Status Scale and the MS Functional Composite.

Medical Developments Changing Health Care for Multiple Sclerosis

The most significant medical advances consuming enormous research efforts and impacting clinical practice are the advent of disease-modifying therapies (DMTs).[21] There are five self-injectable immune-modulating medications approved in the United States[21]: interferon beta-1a (Avonex), interferon beta-1b (Betaseron), interferon beta-1b (Extavia), glatiramer acetate (Copaxone with generic version known as Glatopa), and interferon beta-1a (Rebif). These drugs have been shown to reduce the number of lesions evidenced on MRI and frequency and severity of relapses, although some studies suggest beta interferons do not impact long-term disability.[22] A newer interferon beta-1a known as peginterferon beta-1a (Plegridy). Natalizumab (Tysabri), a monthly injectable, is administered by qualified practitioners and is approved for relapsing-remitting MS. Mitoxantrone (Novantrone), an immunosuppressant rather than an immunomodulator, is rarely used because of significant side effects. Fingolimod (Gilenya) was the first oral medication and is generally used when the response to injectable DMTs has diminished. Another oral medication, dimethyl fumarate (Tecfidera), may have allergic and abdominal reactions as well as side effects associated with other immunosuppressant medications. Other immunosuppressant DMTs are teriflunomide (Aubagio) and alemtuzumab (Lemtrada). The first medication approved for progressive MS is ocrelizumab (Ocrevus). Another class of medications, neurofunctional modifiers, targets underlying pathophysiology and MS symptoms.[23] Of these drugs, dalfampridine has been shown to improve walking in any type of MS.[24]

Clients may want to discuss their medications with therapists, particularly DMTs, because they are designed to slow disease progression, not reverse disability. The therapist's responsibility is to understand and explain the importance of taking medications because the benefits may contribute to controlling the disease, thereby allowing continued employment and participation in priority occupations.

As MS is not curable, unproven remedies emerge periodically. The difference today is the presence of the Internet that enables diverse ideas to capture widespread attention. Occupational therapists must keep abreast of emerging remedies and relevant research. While communicating the evidence in a balanced way, sensitivity to clients' concerns and providing honest, compassionate, accurate responses without diminishing hope is essential.

Functional Impairment in Daily Occupation

A disease that strikes young adults has substantial economic, social, and emotional costs that influence all aspects of life. Between the ages of 20 and 40 years, when MS is typically diagnosed, people are entering the labor market, establishing careers, meeting life partners, and forming families. MS, with its common symptoms of fatigue, weakness, difficulties with prolonged walking, cognitive problems, and depression, can impede productivity at work and home and social engagement.

A body of research is developing that may influence family planning. The relapse rate in MS declines during pregnancy, increases in the first 3 months following childbirth, and thereafter returns to prepregnancy levels.[25] Therapists must be aware of this research to assist clients seeking information and refer as appropriate.

The uncertainty of the MS disease progression may explain an estimated lifetime prevalence of 50% for depression and 35% for anxiety.[26] It has been shown that persons with MS who leave employment have greater likelihood for social isolation, psychological distress, and great burden of disease, as well as lower incomes.[27]

Occupational Therapy Evaluation

OT evaluation begins with an interview about the person's goals for therapy, a brief history of symptoms and treatment since diagnosis, and life experience. This gives the therapist an understanding of the disease course and the person's coping style. Throughout the interview, the therapist listens for hints of cognitive difficulties, being mindful that there may be further hidden impairments. Brief questions regarding dizziness, thinking problems, motivation to engage in occupation, numbness and tingling, dexterity, walking and standing, employment, home physical and social environment, leisure interests, bladder problems, ADL, IADL, energy, sleeping pattern, cramping, pain, fine-motor activities, falls and balance problems, and vision can provide clues to the specific assessments needed.

Analysis of Occupational Performance: Tools and Methods

The initial interview gives the therapist an indication of the type of evaluation tools and methods to use.

There are a plethora of assessments that are used and developed for people with MS that are symptom-focused or function-focused or both. Examples include:

- Canadian Occupational Performance Measure
- Modified Fatigue Impact Scale or Fatigue Severity Scale to assess fatigue
- 6-Minute Walk Test to assess endurance
- Activities-specific Balance Confidence Scale
- Multiple Sclerosis Walking Scale or mobility section of the Functional Independence Measure to assess mobility concerns
- Pittsburgh Sleep Quality Index
- Home assessment
- Beck Depression Inventory-Fast Screen to assess depression
- Symbol Digit Modalities Test (SDMT) predictors MS cognitive impairment
- ADL, IADL, and dysphagia assessments
- Nine-Hole Peg Test to assess dexterity
- Semmes-Weinstein Monofilaments to test sensation
- Manual muscle test (MMT), range of motion (ROM) evaluation, and grip strength (dynamometry)

There are also composite assessment batteries that provide detailed or diverse estimation of an individual's ability. Examples include:

- The Brief International Cognitive Assessment for MS (BICAMS). The SDMT (above), one of its measures, is quick to administer and predicts unemployment.
- Comprehensive Fatigue Assessment Battery for MS (CFAB-MS) identifies factors contributing to MS fatigue, the functional implications, and is a guide for clinical decisions.
- Multidimensional Assessment of Tremor measures the severity and functional impact of intention tremor.
- MS Functional Composite measure provides a estimation of walking, hand function, and cognitive ability.

Administering such measures requires the therapist to accurately interpret findings in the context of the client's situation and the interrelationship between functional challenges and symptoms. For example, therapists must differentiate various types of fatigue by considering the results of several assessments. A high score on a depression index may indicate that depression is contributing to fatigue, whereas slow times on the 6-Minute Walk Test may suggest a nerve fiber or motor fatigue. Information from a sleep questionnaire may indicate that disturbed sleep caused by urinary frequency is a factor in daytime fatigue. Given this complexity, assessment selection must be sufficient to provide a nuanced understanding of the scope of concerns to make prudent clinical decisions.

Occupational Therapy Intervention Process

Client priorities are the cornerstone of goal setting and treatment planning, necessitating a collaborative process to achieve realistic and satisfying outcomes. Frequently, the person with MS and the referring provider mistakenly believe they must live with problems that, in fact, are treatable through therapy. For example, Finlayson[28] suggests that, for older adults with MS, the therapist must ensure they feel a sense of control over their future, work with families affected by the MS, and advocate for enhanced community support options. In addition, treatment focusing on isolated symptoms is unlikely to be effective, and thus working with and coordinating intervention of the health care team is often indicated. The first evidence table at the end of this chapter presents a sample of best evidence for OT intervention for MS. Considerations for activity strategies, equipment and environmental modifications, exercise programs, symptom management, and employment issues are discussed later in this chapter.

Self-Maintenance Roles

The occupational therapist assists the client to maintain independence in ADL and IADL priority activities, using specialized equipment, and participating in self-management strategies such as:

- Assisting in setting priorities
- Education about the disease process and effect on motor or cognitive changes
- Environmental modifications at home to promote safety
- Stretching and strength exercises to facilitate occupations like bathing
- Behavior modification strategies such as time management techniques
- Technology to assist many aspects of life, including environmental control, reminder systems, communications, and emergency alerts
- Balancing independence with assistance from others

Self-Advancement Roles

The onset of neurodegenerative diseases may affect employment in or outside the home. Many can and should continue to work rather than pursue disability benefits by seeking advice from an occupational therapist. Continued employment is beneficial for financial independence, access to health care, maintaining social network, and supporting a productive identity and healthy self-esteem. Therapists critically review job expectations; suggest modifications to the environment, behavior and routines, equipment, and resources; and make recommendations to the individual or employer.

Self-Enhancement Roles

Maintaining leisure pursuits as well as involvement in community, neighborhood, and family activities may be a priority but are often the first roles or occupations to be abandoned. Modifying activities, creative transportation solutions, and use of web-based interfaces enable continued involvement in meaningful occupations.

The tasks associated with self-maintenance, self-advancement, and self-enhancement roles are supported by technology, including smartphones, electronic tablets, and environmental controls. With technology, however, there are a number of challenges particularly related to the vast amount of information and misinformation.

Activity Strategies and Energy Conservation

Based on the comprehensive assessment, the fatigue intervention begins with the occupational therapist providing explanations about the underlying types of fatigue and contributing factor impacting the individual. The client then completes a detailed activity diary that can be done on paper or well-selected apps and identified goals and priorities. The therapist and client use the diary to analyze daily work, home, and leisure activities. Identifying activity and environmental modifications, equipment, and technology to address fatigue issues then follows. Energy conservation strategies and exercise routines will also be incorporated to help the individual perform valued occupations.

Research has demonstrated the effectiveness of a face-to-face OT-led group intervention in energy conservation strategies for MS.[10] The *Managing Fatigue* program[29] has shown positive results to improve energy that has both teleconference[30] and an online versions.[31] Further, there is a 6-week group video program called *Fatigue: Take Control* that has been tested with positive outcomes.[32] In addition to these programs, occupational therapists should collaborate with physical therapists who treat fatigue through obtaining gait equipment, recommending appropriate aerobic exercise routines, and educating on the difference between energy expenditure during functional activities and exercise to increase endurance. With any of these interventions, written recommendations and summaries should be provided. Clients then return to OT for a 2 to 3 month follow-up or sooner if changes in symptoms present or there are difficulties implementing strategies.

Equipment, Behavioral, and Environmental Modifications

Equipment, environmental, and behavioral modifications help persons with MS compensate for weakness, spasticity, tremor, fatigue, ataxia, and cognitive problems. Many pieces of adaptive equipment are helpful (e.g., scooters, electric wheelchairs, bath benches, shower chairs, bed poles) in limiting fatigue and mitigating functional limitations related to weakness and spasticity. Due to fatigue, self-propelling manual wheelchairs are usually not indicated. Carrying out physical tasks or doing activity that limits energy in the heat of the day may require a cool environment such as pool to do exercise or cooling garment to reduce one's body temperature (Fig. 38.1). Mainstream technology such as computers, motion sensors, and smart devices that have audio options reduce the impact of many MS limiting symptoms. When appropriate, the therapist identifies equipment and facilitates trials of consumer technology and adaptive equipment.

Behavioral changes, such as moving exercise from lunch to afterwork and incorporating a lunchtime nap, frequently improve productivity. Another example is using the elevator at work (rather than climbing stairs for exercise) to maximize energy for employment and engaging in exercise at another time. Environmental modifications may help in areas as diverse as maintaining independence in ADL to ensuring continued employment and involvement in the community. Home and/or work visits may be necessary to identify modifications. The combination of the right equipment, behavior changes, and environmental modifications depends on the individual's needs, resources, and personal preferences. Follow-ups are recommended to determine the need for new or further modifications as changes occur.

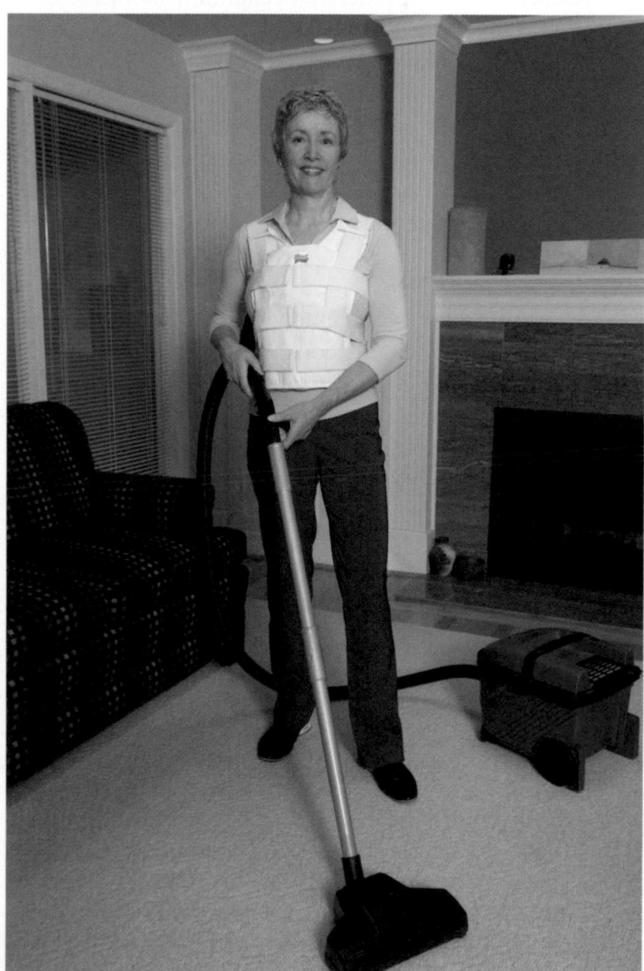

Figure 38-1. Woman in cooling vest vacuuming. Sensitivity to heat when participating in chosen occupation(s) can be mitigated by wearing cooling garments, such as cooling vests (as above) or cooling wraps comfortably worn on the neck or around the wrists.

Exercise Programs

Occupational therapists teach clients to monitor the effects of any MS exercise program on both fatigue and their ability to perform priority activities. Two MS symptoms, fatigue and spasticity, often decrease with regular exercise. A structured aerobic program has been shown to reduce fatigue and increase endurance,[33] and spasticity may be managed with rhythmic exercises such as walking or cycling and a stretching program.[34] Therapists can be instrumental in assisting the client to integrate exercise into weekly routines so that exercise does not reduce the ability to perform other activities. A realistic exercise program performed regularly is better than an ideal program that is never followed.

Spasticity Interventions

The appropriate intervention for spasticity depends on the severity and the extent to which it interferes with function and QoL. A recent study showed that education and daily stretching had a positive impact on self-reported spasticity, fatigue, depression, and physical health.[34]

Modifying the approach to occupation should be considered, such as using adapted dressing techniques (using a stool to maintain hip flexion to decrease extensor spasm). Another option may be using dressing sticks to compensate for inability to reach one's feet. A home standing program using a standing frame for 30 to 60 minutes per day may be beneficial. These are examples of modifying options, though the principle applies across occupations.

Cognitive Compensation

OT intervention for MS clients with cognitive problems focuses on education and compensation for deficits to manage everyday life. Education of clients and families is beneficial and brings awareness that these problems are due to MS and not personality, easing stress, and optimizing receptivity to modifications. Treating factors that reduce cognitive ability, such as fatigue, often improves cognitive performance. Caution should be exercised in disclosing cognitive issues to employers, with careful consideration given to each circumstance.

Interventions that include group therapy, stress management, personal digital assistants, electronic memory aids, and cognitive–behavioral therapy have been shown to have positive effects on cognitive function in MS.[35,36] Examples of cognitive techniques and strategies include:

- Scheduling work responsibilities and cognitively demanding tasks in the morning or after breaks to reduce the influence of the cognitive problems
- Maintaining a paper, smartphone, or electronic diary as a memory aid and to help identify the timing of cognitive and fatigue problems and the environment in which these occur
- Changing the environment to reduce distractions and interruptions and promote organization
- Using problem-solving strategies for decision-making rather than emotion-focused strategies
- Supporting involvement of social network to assist with problem-solving
- Using written step-by-step instructions for home and work routine tasks
- Doing one activity at a time, avoiding multitasking
- Incorporating assistive technology to improve high-order IADL, such as money management, family schedules, and transportation planning
- Increasing time for an activity and reducing the number of activities
- Delegating difficult tasks to others
- Using repetition in the learning process
- Assessing driving safety and recommending appropriate testing and interventions

Pain Intervention

For pain related to weakness or spasticity, interventions such as posture training, ergonomic seating, stretching, supportive splinting, and focal heat modalities on muscle trigger points may be effective. An ergonomic workstation (such as ergonomic chair with armrests, supportive back rest, headsets, and keyboard trays) tailored to the individual can be beneficial. Exercise and mobility equipment to correct gait problems may also minimize pain.

Tremor and Ataxia Intervention

The hallmarks of OT intervention for tremor and ataxia are proximal stabilization or support, modified approach to occupations, and adapted equipment and orthoses. Proximal stabilization includes supporting the trunk and larger joints of the upper and lower extremities. For example, at mealtime, position the client's torso against the table with arms resting on the table.[37] Because the position is sitting, the lower extremities are supported, the trunk is stabilized by leaning against the table, and the shoulders and elbows are supported. A modified approach may be the use of hand-over-hand guidance for writing or dialing a cell phone. If one hand is unaffected by tremor, consider retraining the unaffected hand as tolerated. Orthoses might include a cervical collar to reduce the travel of the head and neck or wrist splints to minimize travel and number of joints in motion. Weights on the wrist, for example, may also serve to dampen tremor[3] but may contribute to fatigue. Peripheral cooling of the forearm has been shown to reduce tremor amplitude and frequency and increase function for up to 30 minutes.[38] An OT intervention program, the Step-wise Approach to the Treatment of Intention Tremor,[37] developed specifically for MS was pilot tested and has shown some promising results.

Employment Modifications

The problems described in the preceding sections may affect the job performance of persons with MS. Additional modifications to maintain employment and satisfaction may include:

- Changing the time at which tasks are performed
- Limiting prolonged walking, standing, and travel using conference calls, Internet, and apps
- Using appropriate gait equipment and powered mobility devices
- Changing to an workspace that is convenient to frequent activities
- Modifying work hours
- Working completely or partly at home
- Arranging a space to rest periodically

Perspective on Intervention

Although referral to OT services can occur across the MS continuum, it is often those with relatively severe disability that are referred. Unfortunately, a tremendous window of opportunity has passed for interventions such as improving ambulation skills (and thereby reducing or delaying the need for wheeled mobility aids), attending to fatigue, and on-the-job modifications to support continued employment. It is essential that therapists educate referring practitioners about the need and benefit for early OT intervention for persons with MS.

It must also be recognized that people with MS, as well as those with other chronic conditions, play an integral role in the self-management of their conditions. Individuals with MS understand their unique circumstances and can provide information that is complementary to the health professionals' knowledge. There is evidence that people with MS with poorly developed self-management skills feel less control and, more uncertainty, have feelings of depression and hopelessness, and experience poor adjustment.[39] Self-management decisions for persons with MS involves taking control through planned strategies and routines and balancing the health providers' expectations and advice against the practicality in their lives.[40] It is for this reason that self-management is an important and critical for those living with MS.

Adjusting to Multiple Sclerosis

Although only a small percentage of people with MS are severely disabled, the diagnosis can be devastating. The need to adjust to changing symptoms and impairments affects self-esteem, relationships, sexuality, physical activities, vocation, and recreation. From questions about pregnancy to cognitive changes influencing competence or safety, MS affects every role and relationship. The variability of the disease and the hidden nature of symptoms such as cognitive changes, pain, and fatigue make it difficult to explain to friends, coworkers, and family.

Each person's reaction to MS varies and has implications for adjustment. Research has shown that emotion-focused coping techniques were used more often by those experiencing an MS relapse, whereas problem-solving and using one's social network were strategies used when in remission.[41] There is MRI evidence that emotional involvement was a marginal indicator of new MS lesions and that fewer lesions were found in persons who participated in a stress management program.[42]

Initially, people may be preoccupied with their diagnosis because it represents a change that may challenge assumptions about the future. As time passes, particularly if individuals with MS return to full function, they frequently ignore the diagnosis and MS issues. As long as the inattention does not result in adverse decisions, this may be a healthy attitude. The therapist helps clients process the implications of changes and identifies modifications to minimize their effects. Information about new symptoms may be all a person needs to make a successful adjustment.

Parkinson Disease

Epidemiology

Parkinson disease (PD), a progressive, variable condition, is the most common movement disorder[43] and the second most prevalent neurodegenerative condition of aging after Alzheimer disease. The onset is typically between 65 and 70 years and is slightly more frequent in men.[43] The incidence of PD is 1,000 per 100,000 persons (or 1%) in people older than 60 years.[43]

Etiology

The cause of PD is thought to stem from both hereditary and environmental factors. The link between hereditary factors and the condition is particularly marked in individuals with younger onset. A study by Bellou et al.[44] indicated that environmental factors related to PD included biomarkers, diet, drugs, exposure to toxic environments, lifestyle, and medical history. The authors noted that constipation and physical activity are risk factors for PD[44] and that gastrointestinal problems that start years before diagnosis are correlated with a lifetime risk of PD.[45] The pathogenesis is related to the loss of dopaminergic neurons of the substantia nigra that provide input to the corpus striatum and, in part, modulate the thalamus and its connections to the motor cortex.[46]

Course and Prognosis

PD has been described as having either five stages[47] (Table 38-1) or three stages[48] (Table 38-2). These stages are broadly described by the presence of symptoms, functional implications, and response to medications. PD is gradual at onset, and symptoms may take years to develop.

Table 38-1 Stages of PD as Defined by Hoehn and Yahr

STAGES	FEATURE
Stage I	Unilateral symptoms, no or minimal functional implications, usually a resting tremor
Stage II	Midline or bilateral symptom involvement, no balance difficulty, mild problems with trunk mobility and postural reflexes
Stage III	Postural instability, mild-to-moderate functional disability
Stage IV	Postural instability increasing, though able to walk; functional disability increases, interfering with ADL; decreased manipulation and dexterity
Stage V	Confined to wheelchair or bed

ADL, activities of daily living; PD, Parkinson disease.
From Hoehn MM, Yahr MD. Parkinsonism: onset, progression and mortality. *Neurology*. 1967;17(5):427–442.

Signs and Symptoms

PD is defined by the three cardinal motor signs of *T*remor, *R*igidity, and *A*kinesia and *P*ostural instability,[49] marked by the acronym TRAP. Tremor, often the first complaint, is a resting tremor that increases with stress and may present as pill-rolling. **Rigidity** tends to occur at more advanced stages of PD.[49] **Bradykinesia,** a type of **akinesia,** causes a lack of facial expression, or "masked face," and slowed movement of the limbs and occupational engagement. Postural instability begins with reduced arm swing, head and trunk leaning forward, and shorter strides that progress to a shuffling gait. Lack of postural reflexes and **festinating gait** results in 37% increase in falls and akinesia or episodes of motoric "freezing" that impedes spontaneous initiation of walking, turning, and crossing thresholds.

Other symptoms of PD are common, including cognitive impairment, word-finding difficulty, depression, apathy, fatigue, sensory symptoms, pain and paresthesia, urinary and sexual dysfunction, weight loss, and sleep disorders.[49] Swallowing problems can occur at any point and are unrelated to disease severity. These include delayed swallow reflex and abnormal tongue control that result in residue of food remaining in the mouth. Nonmotor symptoms are "recognized as a major source of disability in PD and treatment focus has shifted to quality of life and maintaining it in advanced disease."[49]

Table 38-2 Stages of PD as Described by Bradley

STAGES	DESCRIPTION
Early	Not disabling; monosymptomatic; responds well to medication; may remain at this level for years
Nonfluctuating	Some disability; levodopa added to medication regimen; 80% of function is restored
Fluctuating	Function limited; side effects to levodopa; difficult-to-control symptoms, postural instability, and gait disturbance become debilitating

PD, Parkinson disease.
From Bradley WE. *Neurology in Clinical Practice*. 2nd ed. Boston, MA: Butterworth-Heinemann; 1996.

Dementia occurs in 15% to 20% of persons with PD and tends to be among those who are older at diagnosis, a history of PD, and experience depression.[50] The cognitive functions most affected are attention, working and episodic memory, executive functions, word-finding, and visuospatial skills.[51] It has been shown that cognitive training using external cues, feedback, and repetition when learning new tasks has small-to-moderate effect on cognition for people with mild-to-moderate PD.[52]

Medical Management

Diagnosing Parkinson Disease

Diagnosis is based on clinical evidence using diagnostic criteria related to the cardinal signs of tremor, rigidity, bradykinesia, and postural stability and is complex in the early stages.[49] The clinical presentation can be very different from one person to another. The diagnosis must distinguish PD from other parkinsonian syndromes such as multiple system atrophy and corticobasal degeneration and from secondary causes resulting from drugs and neurotoxins. The presence of tremor predicts a more benign course, whereas older onset and initial symptoms of hypokinesia/rigidity are predictors of early cognitive impairments.[49]

Medical Interventions

Medical treatments can include medication and surgical procedures. Medications are used to compensate for dopamine loss throughout the course of PD and are effective for a limited period followed by "wearing off," particularly in later stages of PD, and may result in difficult "on/off" fluctuations and side effects. There are four types of medication for PD. L-Dopa, a first-line treatment, has not been shown to alter disease progression, though the standard formulation is efficacious as a monotherapy, whereas the catechol-O-methyltransferase (COMT) inhibitors as adjuncts to L-dopa appear to be clinical useful for treating motor symptoms. Monoamine oxidase B (MAO-B) inhibitors, particularly rasagiline, assist in reducing motor symptoms over 6 months in early PD. The numerous dopamine agonists, as an adjunct to L-dopa, are overall useful for controlling motor variability. It is recommended that the choice of medication be based on the person's lifestyle and choice.[49] It is essential that OT intervention accounts for fluctuations in medication effectiveness throughout the day to maximize therapeutic benefit. Surgical interventions are typically reserved for those with advanced disease with unilateral pallidotomy or deep brain stimulation deemed to be useful for improving motor challenges, particularly when the response to medications has diminished.[53]

Functional Impairment in Daily Occupation

In the initial stages of PD, the degree of physical disability is minimal. The emotional burden and social consequences, however, can be marked. Resting tremor, rarely resulting in motor disability, is a frequent source of distress, and reports suggest feeling embarrassed or self-conscious. In later stages, tremor and rigidity were highly correlated with distress and reduced QoL. Other predictors of poor QoL are depression, cognitive decline, social isolation, sleep disorders, mobility issues, fatigue, urinary incontinence, unpredictable on/off fluctuations, pain, and increasing dependence. Major depression was found in 58% of those with PD, whereas 84% demonstrated cognitive decline, suggesting that early identification and intervention are crucial.[54]

The social consequences of PD are striking. In early stages, handwriting may be shaky and micrographic, reducing legibility. In intermediate and later stages, the voice softens and becomes monotone, limited facial expression and hand gesturing contribute to reduced communication and negative messaging. The person with PD may have waning interest in social and previously enjoyed leisure activities challenging relationships and roles in families. Both the individual and family members, typically an elderly spouse or adult child, may have feelings of guilt, despair, and anger as caregiving increases.[55]

Economic implications of PD are frequently related to medications, wheeled mobility, accessibility modifications, self-care and safety equipment, and in-home support. If employed, increasing limitations may require employment modifications, early retirement, and application for disability benefits that accompany a loss of income.[56] People with PD stop working 5 to 6 years earlier than the normal population.[57] The caregiver may require assistance and respite, which has financial implications, and if required, long-term care placement is costly.

Occupational Therapy Evaluation

In the early stages of PD, OT is rarely indicated unless there are functional limitations or psychological issues. At this stage, it is recommended that interests and roles be maintained within and outside the home, including employment, social activities, and driving.[55] OT is most often required in the intermediate and later stages of the disease.[47] Evaluation should include a brief history and, in the intermediate stages, should identify occupational performance problems related to reduced mobility, safety, swallowing, incoordination, slowed movements, **cogwheel rigidity**, and depressed affect. A standardized QoL measure, the Parkinson Disease Questionnaire-39, may be a useful screening tool. Its 39 items are clustered into eight dimensions relevant to OT: mobility, ADL, emotional well-being, stigma, social support, cognition, communication, and bodily discomfort.[58] The therapist should also note occupations that have been eliminated. Examples of occupational limitations that may be included in evaluation are:

- Fine-motor activities at home and work (writing, eating, shaving, and fastening)
- Safe mobility, such as walking, stair climbing, driving, and moving from sit to stand
- Fatigue that affects most activities
- Work evaluation at early stages of PD to reduce the risk of unemployment or early retirement
- Bradykinesia, postural instability, and rigidity that limit participation in ADL and IADL
- Swallowing or other mealtime problems that prolong eating and reduce intake
- Cognitive problems that affect activities associated with usual roles
- Sexual activity limitations related to bradykinesia, fatigue, depression, and psychosocial issues
- Sleep disturbances

Occupational Therapy Intervention Process

When setting goals with the client with PD and significant others, the therapist must balance energy demands with motivation and frustration as well as caregiver time and abilities in the context of the dependence–interdependence–independence continuum. Participation of others in this process is crucial to the viability of interventions that vary, based on priorities and resources, stage of the disease, and occupational difficulties identified through the evaluation. Many of the interventions described in the subsequent section may be incorporated at home and in other relevant environments. Studies report an overall effectiveness of both OT and other rehabilitation interventions for PD.[59,60] A meta-analysis showed that 10 of the 15 studies reviewed demonstrated a positive effect for OT intervention, with 63% of persons with PD experiencing improvement as compared to 37% who did not receive therapy.[61] A randomized controlled trial showed the efficacy of a self-management rehabilitation program for persons with PD.[62] The second evidence table at the end of this chapter lists best evidence for OT interventions for patients with PD.

Interventions Related to Decreasing Isolation and Communication Problems

- Educate about timing activities to synchronize with optimal medication effectiveness.
- Modify leisure activities to encourage participation and decrease isolation.
- Provide information on support and advocacy groups.

- Educate caregivers about modifying communication and activities to support engagement.
- Recommend voice interventions such as the Lee Silverman Voice Treatment (LSVT) or RehabSelfCue-Speech programs to ensure continued social engagement.
- Use writing modifications such as an enlarged felt-tip pen and writing when rested.
- Use communication aids, including smart devices such as electronic tablets (mobile phone may be too small), large-key telephones, and electronic aids to daily living (EADL).
- Provide home exercise program to maintain facial movement and expression for socializing.

Interventions Related to Safety

- Instruct in sit-to-stand and bed mobility using the RehabSelfCue-Speech program.
- Manage motoric "freezing" while walking, including avoiding crowds, narrow spaces, and room corners; reducing distractions and not carrying items while walking; reducing clutter in path; focusing when changing directions; and using rhythmical beat or counting to maintain momentum.
- Recommend equipment to increase independence such as a raised toilet seat and grab bars.
- Prescribe walking aids (walker for festinating gait).
- Recommend, if required, a wheelchair having a proper seating system, cushion, and adjusted foot/leg rests and armrests that are appropriate for transporting within the community.
- Recommend good, uniform lighting, particularly in narrow spaces and at doorways.
- Provide home exercises to maintain mobility, coordination, posture, and tolerance.
- Perform home assessment and recommend modifications that might include alterations to the bathroom (e.g., nonskid surfaces, bath bench/chair) and flooring (e.g., eliminating throw rugs), horizontal strips on the floor where "freezing" episodes occur, and reducing furniture congestion.

Interventions to Maintain Independence and Participation

- Modify eating routine to include smaller portions, reduced distractions, schedule frequent meals that allow adequate time, and provide equipment such as nonslip surfaces for plates and built-up handles.
- Recommend use of adult absorbent underwear to reduce embarrassment should a bathroom be difficult to access.
- Recommend that sexual activity be engaged in following rest and urination and when medications are most effective.
- Encourage movement programs such as LSVTBIG that uses high-amplitude movements to assist in maintaining overall movement.[63]
- Instruct on energy effectiveness strategies in-home, leisure, and work activities.
- Reduce/eliminate the need for fine-motor control, such as minimal or no clothing fasteners.
- Reduce the impact of perceptual problems using visual cues and rhythmic music in a nondistracting environment; speak slowly using simple instruction.

Amyotrophic Lateral Sclerosis

Epidemiology

Amyotrophic lateral sclerosis (ALS) is most often a fatal motor neuron disease distinguished by changes to **upper motor neuron** (UMN) and **lower motor neuron** (LMN) functions as well as brainstem and multiple spinal cord regions. Amyotrophic is derived from Greek where *a* means no or without, *myo* refers to muscle, and *trophic* means to build or nourish—"No muscle building." "Lateral" locates the nerve cells signals and controls the muscles on the spinal cord. Sclerosis refers to the scarring that occurs as a result of degeneration.[64] The incidence of ALS is 2.7 per 100,000 people, with onset generally between the ages of 40 and 70 years and occurring more often in men.[65]

Etiology

The cause remains unknown, and it is widely believed that both genetics (several genes are identified) and environmental factors may play a role. It has been observed that oligodendrocyte degeneration, neuroinflammation, and mitochondrial impairment are implicated in the axonal retraction and cell denervation.[66] Other factors suggested to correlate with risk of ALS have not been established as causal.[65]

Course and Prognosis

ALS typically presents as either limb onset with a combination of UMN and LMN signs or bulbar onset with speech and swallowing difficulties,[67] the latter occurring in about 30% of cases. Despite the onset, muscle atrophy is initially focal and asymmetrical, then gradually widespread. It may begin in the hands, with wasting of the thenar and hypothenar eminences, as well as in the shoulders. Finger extension is usually affected earlier than grip strength because of dorsal and palmar interossei wasting. Falling and problems with walking and bed mobility are common because of leg weakness. Increasing difficulties with speech, swallowing, and breathing is common as the disease progresses. Six stages of ALS are recognized and described according to clinical features (Table 38-3). The median survival after diagnosis ranges from 20 to 48 months, although 10% to 20% survive more than 10 years.[64,68]

Table 38-3 Stages and Rehabilitation for Individuals with Activities of Daily Living

STAGE	CLINICAL FEATURES	ACTIVITIES TO MAINTAIN MOTOR FUNCTION	EQUIPMENT
I	Ambulatory, no problems with ADL, mild weakness	Normal activities, moderate exercise in unaffected muscles, active ROM, and strength exercise	None
II	Ambulatory, moderate weakness in certain muscles, increased fatigue	Modification in living; modest exercise; active, assisted ROM exercise	Assistive devices, use of hands-free devices, electronic tablet
III	Ambulatory, severe weakness in certain muscles, increased difficulty with ADL; marked fatigue	Adaptations to continue active life; active, assisted, passive ROM exercise; joint pain management	Smart technology, adaptive devices, home equipment and environmental controls
IV	Wheelchair confined, almost independent, severe weakness in legs	Passive ROM exercise, modest strength exercise in uninvolved muscles	Smart technology, adaptive devices, home equipment, environmental controls, wheelchair
V	Wheelchair confined, dependent, marked leg and arm weakness	Passive ROM exercise, pain management, decubitus ulcer prevention	Smart technology, adaptive devices, home equipment, environmental controls, wheelchair
VI	Bedridden, unable to perform ADL, maximal assistance required	Passive ROM exercise, pain management, prevention of decubitus ulcers and venous thrombosis	Smart technology, adaptive devices and home equipment to assist caregiver(s), environmental controls, wheelchair

ADL, activities of daily living; ALS, amyotrophic lateral sclerosis; ROM, range of motion.

From Mitsumoto H, Chad D, Pioro E. Amyotrophic lateral sclerosis. *Contemporary Neurology Series*. Philadelphia, PA: Davis; 1998; Sinaki M. Rehabilitation. In Mulder DW, ed. *The Diagnosis and Treatment of Amyotrophic Lateral Sclerosis*. Boston, MA: Houghton Mifflin; 1980:169–193.

The two primary forms of ALS are sporadic and familial. Sporadic occurs in 90% to 95% of those with ALS, whereas familial appears to have a genetic link occurring more than once in a family.[65] Age at onset and the pattern of symptom development are useful for determining an individual's prognosis, with a younger onset of UMN origin having a somewhat better prognosis.[69]

Signs and Symptoms

The primary symptoms of ALS are associated with motor dysfunction such as muscle weakness, spasticity, and dysphagia. Weakness occurs with a pronounced atrophy of muscle groups and leads to falling, dropping items, and difficulty performing self-care. Spasticity is associated to increased pain in ALS and interferes with daily activities. Dysphagia, a distinguishing symptom in ALS, is independent of disease course eventually occurring as a result of weakness and spasticity of the oral musculature with women experiencing greater difficulty.[69]

Although it has been thought that cognition is rarely affected in ALS, recent evidence suggests that up to 50% develop cognitive and/or behavioral difficulties, and 13% experience a frontotemporal dementia.[66] Of note, vision, bowel and bladder control, and sensation are commonly spared.

Medical Management

There is no single test or procedure to diagnosis ALS. Rather, several diagnostic tests are used in a careful, multistep system of exclusion of other diagnoses.[64] This may include combinations of a thorough neurological examination, use of electromyography and nerve conduction velocity tests, MRI, blood and urine analysis, spinal tap, and, possibly, muscle biopsy.

There are currently two ALS pharmacological treatments approved by the Food and Drug Administration (FDA). Riluzole (Rilutek), an antiglutamate agent taken in pill form, has been shown to slow the course of the disease though has side effects of dizziness, fatigue, and gastrointestinal and liver problems. In 2017, Edaravone (Radicava) was approved and shown to reduce the difficulty in daily activities associated with ALS and is taken by intravenous infusion. The side effects may include swelling, shortness of breath, walking difficulty, and hives as well as allergic reactions for those with sulfite sensitive.[70]

Medications for symptomatic management of difficulties with spasticity, anxiety, depression, insomnia, and excessive saliva are useful, but do not affect the progression of the disease. Assisted ventilation, tracheotomies, and gastrostomies ease problems with eating and breathing.[71]

Because of the disease progression, numerous symptoms, and potential interventions, a multidisciplinary team and clinics dedicate to the care of ALS have been shown to improve the QoL for those with ALS.[72]

Functional Impairment in Daily Occupation

As a result of the relatively fast progression, ALS is a devastating disease for individuals and their families. Because the disease quickly affects the ability to perform ADL, IADL, and employment, QoL is impacted, and significant depression results. One may feel an external locus of control and hopeless[73] and that this is not related to physical function or sociodemographic factors.[74]

People frequently withdraw from work soon after diagnosis and often confront economic instability and health insurance issues. Because those commonly affected are employed and actively involved in family and community activities, the abrupt change is devastating. Acceptance of the ALS diagnosis by family members may affect willingness to be involved in planning, incorporating necessary changes to maximize the independence, and making informed choices for intervention.[75]

Occupational Therapy Evaluation

OT is provided throughout the course of ALS and environments across the care continuum. Assessment is based on clearly defined levels of function and the individual's needs and priorities. It has been demonstrated that clients want to have control over health care services in order to enhance their feelings of control,[76] and thus, an interview to understand the ALS client and family's goals and changing needs is an essential mainstay throughout the care continuum. Early interventions should target the individual's symptoms as they affect their occupations. For example, facilitating continued employment can be a key contribution of OT to enable continuity with professional identity, meaningful occupation and financial benefits. As ALS progresses, interventions focus on individual function, as well as physical and social environment.

To assist with the evaluation process and to monitor ALS progression, the ALS Functional Rating Scale–Revised (ALSFS-R)[77] can be used. To determine functional ability, ADL and IADL assessments should be included in all evaluations. Functional limitations may be owing to reduced upper extremity ability; thus, the Purdue Pegboard, nine-hole peg test or other timed upper extremity function tests, and standard ROM and MMT are useful early in the disease to monitor disease progress. Fatigue affects physical activities and QoL and can be assessed with the Multidimensional Fatigue Inventory or other screening measures described earlier in this chapter. It is essential to evaluate mobility, seating, and positioning needs as ALS progresses in order to make appropriate occupational and equipment recommendations. As communication and swallowing decline,[78] ongoing assessment of social participation and nutritional needs should be maintained. Owing to disease progression, reevaluation at each visit is required.

Occupational Therapy Intervention Process

The progressive nature of ALS necessitates that rehabilitation be compensatory, focusing on adapting to disability and preventing secondary complications. Goals center on maintaining activity level and independence for as long as possible, resulting in interventions that focus on both individual function and physical and social environment. Examples of OT goals in the early stages include:

- Optimizing strength and ROM using home exercise programs[79]
- Maintaining function in ADL and IADL through use of assistive or adaptive devices
- Decreasing fatigue in the neck and extremities through use of splints and orthotics
- Managing pain and energy using joint protection and work simplification techniques

As function declines, mobility and self-care become increasingly difficult. Home evaluations and in-home therapy are important, and intervention focuses on enabling the caregiver to assist the client safely and effectively. The therapist helps the caregiver–client team to:

- Optimize safety and positioning, perform safe transfers, and maintain skin integrity
- Enable communication using augmentative communication equipment[75]
- Assess and manage dysphagia[78]
- Optimize social participation
- Identify and obtain equipment, such as a hospital bed to allow continued mobility and comfort
- Modify the environment to enhance participation, safety, and comfort
- Discuss differences with client and their caregivers about their view of emotional needs, caregiver burden, and QoL to make transparent any issues and allow for resolution of misunderstandings[80]

Throughout the stages of the disease, the occupational therapist must be sensitive to the client, family, and caregiver as physical demands, financial concerns, and transformation of the home into a hospital-like setting produce enormous stress and strain.[81] Despite this, it has been shown that the QoL of a person with ALS who has a supportive family and social network remains stable over time despite reduced health status.[82]

Open discussions and close collaboration with clients, caregivers, and the ALS team help to address the client and family's changing needs and goals in the face of this devastating illness.

Intervention Implementation

When treating clients with ALS, therapists must be aware of the client's level of gadget tolerance, financial resources, affective response, and social and cultural context. Evidence suggests that multidisciplinary intervention results in higher rates of receiving appropriate assistive devices and a 30% increase in survival as compared to general services. ALS clients also have better QoL and mental health when receiving care from multidisciplinary programs.[83]

The special considerations for persons with ALS to engage in meaningful occupation through movement programs, obtaining equipment and assistive technology, and with dysphasia management are reviewed in the subsequent sections.

Movement Programs

Moderate exercise of active and passive ROM, strengthening, endurance, stretching, and home breathing programs have been shown to maintain functional level and minimizing secondary complications when compared to a control group as measured by the ALSFS-R at various stages of the disease.[83] A client may initially be able to perform an independent home stretching program, but as the disease progresses and the program becomes too fatiguing or difficult, the caregiver may become involved.

Education and discussion about the importance of the client, family, and caregiver unit and perceived understanding about their experience will assist in improving overall QoL. This includes supporting client and caregiver spirituality, as appropriate, which has been shown to positively predict of QoL.[84]

Equipment and Assistive Technology

The therapist's role in providing information and assist with accessing assistive technology and adaptive equipment is essential and supports the client to achieve optimal level of independence at the various stages of ALS (see Table 38-3). Assistive devices such as a neck collar for improved positioning or universal cuff to enhance upper extremity function may be helpful. Mobility equipment, depending on the level of function, may include a foot-drop splint, cane, and/or walker. Because independent walking becomes difficult as ALS progresses, use of a wheelchair may need to be expedited. A study showed that 57% of those with moderate disability used a mobility device in addition to a wheelchair.[85] Among power wheelchairs users with ALS, there was a 77% satisfaction with comfort and 72% satisfaction with ease of use as well as an overall ability to participate in meaning occupation.[83] Other devices that were useful, depending on functional level, were raised toilet seat, shower seat, grab bars, transfer board, and communication boards.

Mainstream technology and environmental controls are extremely useful as the disease progresses. This technology, for example, includes lighting and call-alert systems, motion sensors, and remotes or keyless door (un)locking systems. Use of smart devices with voice activation (that can be adjusted if the voice is weak) to replace the need for touch typing is helpful to conserve energy and to maintain communication. Together, a home assessment and client–caregiver consultation inform selection of mobility and assistive devices for persons with ALS.

Dysphagia

Swallowing difficulties may be present at any stage of ALS, particularly when bulbar involvement is apparent. Depending on the dysphagia problem, interventions may include reducing distractions during mealtime (limit conversation and other activities), altering food consistency (i.e., thicken liquids), small bolus sizes,[86] teaching manual techniques to swallow, and ensuring adequate time for meals. Early introduction of an alternate route of nutrition may be indicated if nutrition and maintaining weight become issues. Occupational therapists should routinely screen for swallowing function in ALS.

Guillain-Barré Syndrome

Epidemiology

Guillain-Barré syndrome (GBS) or acute inflammatory demyelinating polyneuropathy results in axonal demyelination of peripheral nerves. Its distribution is worldwide, with a median incidence of 1.1 per 100,000[87] that increases with age such that those over 80 years have an incidence of 2.7 per 100,000. GBS is 1.5 times more common in men, and onset dominants in adults 20 to 24 years and 70 to 74 years.[88]

Etiology

The cause of GBS is unclear. No hereditary or environmental factors are known to increase susceptibility to GBS.[87] In the 2 to 4 weeks prior to GBS onset, however, most adults report a respiratory, gastrointestinal, or another infection.[89]

Course and Prognosis

GBS has three phases. In more than 95% of people with GBS, the onset, or acute inflammatory progressive phase, manifests as weakness in at least two limbs that progresses and reaches its maximum in 2 to 4 weeks accompanied by increasing symptoms.[88] Mechanical ventilation is required for 20% to 30% of individuals.[87] It is during this phase that GBS could be life-threatening; thus, appropriate treatment is essential. This is followed by the plateau phase of no significant change, which lasts for a few days or weeks, when the greatest disability is present. The third phase is progressive recovery, when remyelination and axonal regeneration occur and may last for up to 2 years, although the average length is 12 weeks.[88] Recovery generally starts at the head and neck and proceeds distally[90] with approximately 50% experiencing return of function, and another 35% experience some residual weakness that may not resolve. The remaining 15% experience more significant permanent disability,[91] of which fatigue is the most common problem. Subtle cognitive deficits in executive functions, short-term memory, and decision-making may also occur.[92]

Signs and Symptoms

Characteristics include a quickly progressing, symmetrical ascending paralysis starting with the feet; pain in the legs; the absence of deep tendon reflexes; mild sensory loss in glove-and-stocking distributions; cranial nerve dysfunction with possible facial palsy and swallowing problems; an autonomic nervous system response of postural hypertension and tachycardia; respiratory muscle paralysis; and pain, fatigue, and urinary dysfunction.[87,92] Cognition typically remains intact. Symptoms vary from being so mild that medical attention is unlikely to so severe that they may cause death in 1% to 10% of cases.[93]

Medical Management

Diagnosis of GBS entails a history of symptoms and a physical and neurological examination that includes nerve conduction tests and cerebral spinal fluid analysis to detect elevated fluid protein.[87] Features necessary for a GBS diagnosis include progressive weakness in legs and arms over 2 to 4 weeks and decreased tendon reflexes. The medical interventions for GBS attempt to lessen the severity but do not cure the disease, such that upon initial diagnosis, individuals may be admitted to hospital to monitor breathing and other functions until the GBS has stabilized.[87] Treatments in the acute phase include intravenous immunoglobulin, plasma exchange (or plasmapheresis), and steroids.[88] In the plateau phase, close monitoring is undertaken, and, like the recovery phase, symptomatic management along with OT and physical therapy are the treatment of choice.

Functional Impairment in Daily Occupation

Emotional and psychological reactions are in response to the rapid onset of symptoms and the mounting disability. As recovery progresses and improvement is slow, adjustment, impatience, and frustration may persist. At follow-up, GBS was reported to impact confidence and ability to live independently, with 18% having depression and 22% having anxiety.[91]

For young adults, the impact of GBS can have educational, employment, and economic implications. This age group is launching careers and may have only small savings. For those who develop GBS in later years, the economic effect may be less. For those returning to work after GBS, there may be a renewed value for work, a need to cope with losing and recovering a work identity, and dilemmas about work adaptations that require coping strategies. Lack of public awareness of GBS may be a barrier for returning to work.[94]

Occupational Therapy Evaluation

Referral to OT is common when the course of GBS is moderate to severe. Approximately 40% of all GBS clients require rehabilitation services.[95] The types of OT evaluation and intervention changes as improvement occurs through the three phases of GBS.

Assessment during the acute and plateau phases typically occurs in the intensive care unit, when the individual is undergoing extensive medical procedures and pain and abnormal sensations can be significant. Therapists should complete an interview to understand the client's feelings and fears[96] and evaluate communication, control of the environment, comfort, and level of anxiety and depression. A sensory assessment is essential because hypersensitivity is typical of acute GBS with the guiding principle to ask prior to touching the client.[96] Functional evaluation should be conducted based on the results of sensory tests, joint range, and muscle strength and may include communication, bed mobility, transfers and self-care during these early phases.

During the recovery phase, therapists evaluate self-care, communication, leisure, as well as mobility, sensation, strength, ROM and, as appropriate, reintegration into the workplace.

Occupational Therapy Intervention Process

Because the natural course of GBS is improvement, clients and caregivers tend to be optimistic about recovery. The long-term goal is full recovery, so that the individual performs at the same level as prior to the GBS onset with or without modification. Goals should focus on achieving optimal function at each level of recovery within tolerated pain levels.[96]

During the acute phase, the client may be actively involved in directing care rather than physically performing, providing the opportunity for educating the client and others about positioning and supports to maintain comfort in bed, protect against bed sores, and future therapy.[96]

In the recovery phase, goals are developed at the just-right challenge to increase involvement in occupation within safe parameters. Examples of goals include:

- Pacing occupations within energy and fatigue tolerance
- Grading therapy to be realistic and supporting continued progression
- Return to independence in self-care and communication with or without aids
- Maximizing mobility skills with or without aids
- Grading return to work with or without modifications
- Increasing re-engagement in leisure and recreational occupations

The therapist helps the caregiver–client team to closely collaborate to address concerns and encourage realistic expectations over the course of recovery.

Intervention Implementation

Modifications during the acute and plateau phases should be considered temporary and may include:

- Communication tools, such a picture board or voice-activated devices, if appropriate
- Access to the nurse call button, TV, and lights by remote control, as appropriate
- Use of hands-free telephone
- Modification of lying and sitting positions for optimal function, comfort, and reduced pain
- Positioning the trunk, head, and upper extremities for stability and comfort
- Introducing strategies to reduce anxiety for both the person with GBS and their families

Recovery-phase interventions are initially completed with few repetitions, punctuated with rest, and expanded gradually as persons with GBS should not be pushed to fatigue.[96] During this phase, OT services can be provided in an inpatient rehabilitation facility, through an outpatient program, and/or at home or work. It has been shown that with inpatient rehabilitation, individuals with GBS made meaningful improvements from admission to discharge in self-care, mobility, and cognition.[97]

The number and complexity of tasks should be increased gradually.[96] Examples of interventions include:

- Providing activities and dynamic splints to maintain ROM, particularly of the wrists, fingers, and ankle (hinged drop-foot orthosis)
- Slowly increase involvement in preferred occupations
- Instructing both caregiver and client on safe mobility and independent transfers
- Providing a sensory stimulation or desensitization program, as appropriate
- Training in modified self-care techniques and adapting other daily activities
- Using smart devices to facilitate communication and conserve energy
- Modifying and encouraging re-engagement in routine occupations, as appropriate
- Adapting equipment for home, leisure, and work occupations
- Instructing in energy conservation and fatigue management strategies
- Modifying employment roles, tasks, and environment, as indicated
- Recommending a fine-motor program to enhance strength, coordination, and sensation to engage in functional activities
- Undertaking a home assessment and modifications, as appropriate, to facilitate return to home

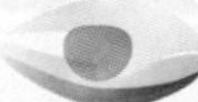

CASE STUDY

Client Information

Katie is a 34-year-old woman with relapsing-remitting MS. Two months prior to her first visit to OT, she resigned her position after 11 years as a human resources professional. Katie was distraught about leaving a job she enjoyed but believed she was no longer able to work due numerous problems, including (1) severe fatigue, resulting in her inability to do household tasks without becoming exhausted; (2) memory difficulties; (3) lower extremity weakness, resulting in falls and reduced ability to perform tasks requiring walking or standing; (4) stiffness in extremities, making tasks more difficult; (5) decreased manual dexterity; (6) daily headaches and dizziness; (7) bladder problems; and (8) disturbed sleep. Her adaptive strategies included use of a manual wheelchair and to stop driving. She was taking bladder medication and a DMT. Her husband was very supportive.

Assessment Process and Results

The OT evaluation revealed decreased strength and increased tone in Katie's lower extremities; decreased sensation, strength, and manual dexterity in the dominant upper extremity; severe dizziness with head movement; head, neck, and shoulder trigger points; and marked fatigue. She had no adaptations to reduce energy expenditure in daily activities.

(continued)

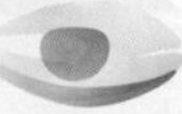

CASE STUDY *(continued)*

Katie was scheduled to have a neuropsychological evaluation to identify her current cognitive function and problems. Her self-selected adaptive strategies were inappropriate. She was not taking medications to manage spasticity or fatigue. Her seating at home and work was not supportive. Katie purposefully climbs the stairs in the morning and had a desk distant from the bathroom to get exercise, as she had no exercise program.

Occupational Therapy Problem List

The problems identified were:

- Minimal use of fatigue management strategies and use of inappropriate equipment
- Did not have cognitive compensation strategies
- Resigned from work without knowledge of options
- Had stopped driving without investigating options
- Is not involved in a home exercise program

Occupational Therapy Goal List

In collaboration with Katie, the goals established were to:

- Obtain appropriate power mobility equipment
- Incorporate energy-saving strategies in her day
- Withdraw resignation notice from employer
- Make changes to her work routines, that is, by taking the elevator
- Modify to work area by obtaining a headset, ergonomic chair, improved computer setup, and moved workstation closer to the bathroom
- Submit a request to her employer for automatic door on bathroom
- Apply to vocational rehabilitation and work with therapist and vendor to install hand controls for driving
- Educate Katie in head, neck, and shoulder exercises to relieve stiffness and reduce the impact of the headaches and dizziness

Occupational Therapy Intervention

The OT intervention included (1) instructing in the adoption of energy conservation techniques at home, work, and in the community[32]; (2) identifying and obtaining powered mobility equipment[28]; (3) identifying equipment to decrease energy expenditure and impact of cognitive issues at home and work; (4) decreasing headaches with head, neck, and shoulder stretching; (5) modifying workstation to decrease pain and energy consumption; (6) facilitating the use of hand controls to drive; (7) continuing full-time or part-time employment; and (8) educating on vestibular, stretching, and strengthening home exercise program to reduce dizziness, stiffness and weakness.[34]

Following the therapy, Katie withdrew her job resignation, returned initially part time, and made workstation modifications. She planned to resume driving with the appropriate hand control.

By 1 month, Katie had met her goals for energy conservation and felt more confident to manage her fatigue. However, she developed right foot-drop, which impacted her balance when fatigued. With prompting to use energy management strategies (use power chair for distances; managing schedule to reduce periods of extended walking), she was able to mitigate the impact of drop foot.

Best Evidence for Occupational Therapy Practice Intervention Related to Multiple Sclerosis

Intervention	Description	Participants	Dosage	Research Design and Level of Evidence	Benefit	Statistical Significance and Effect Size
An online fatigue self-management program for people with chronic neurological conditions[31]	Online fatigue program facilitated by occupational therapists. Included education, activities and discussions.	Ninety-five adults with MS, PD, and post-polio syndrome with access to the Internet 3×/week for at least 1 hour; minimum baseline score of 4 on Fatigue Severity Scale Excluded if scored >9 on the Memory Orientation Concentration Test.	One 2-hour asynchronized session/week for 7 weeks. Participants had access to the program anytime during the day.	Randomized controlled trial. Level I. Participants were in three groups: receiving the fatigue program, information only, and control (no intervention).	The online fatigue management group and the information-only group showed improvement in fatigue, whereas the control group did not improve.	Repeated-measures analysis of covariance (ANCOVA) ($p < 0.05$) with small effect size (ES)
Nintendo Wii Fit and its effect on physical activity behavior[100]	Exercise program (yoga, balance, strength, aerobic training) using Wii Fit. Participants were telephoned, monitored for adverse events and for duration and frequency of Wii Fit use.	Thirty participants with relapsing-remitting MS: 23 women, 7 men; 18–60 years; able to walk 25 feet with or without a cane. Excluded if doing 2.5+ hours of activity per week, had low vision, lower extremity amputation, severe fatigue or depression, cardiopulmonary disease, or were pregnant.	14-week Wii Fit exercise program for 3 days/week	One-group repeated-measures design with 5-week baseline period and 2-week Wii setup and training followed by 14-week intervention. Level IIIB3b	Balance and strength were significantly improved at week 7. By week 14, physical activity declined relative to week 7, and there was no difference compared with the baseline period.	Using multivariate analysis of variance showed physical activity improved at 7 weeks ($p = 0.001$; ES = 0.65) though declined at 14 weeks; self-efficacy improved to 14 weeks ($p = 0.025$); and no difference in QoL or the level of fatigue.
A self-management program that reduces spasticity in people with MS[34]	Spasticity self-management program: two groups sessions viewing and discussing stretching and education DVDs. Then stretches practiced with facilitator input. Participants recorded stretching and exercises for 4 weeks in diaries.	Forty participants with physician-confirmed MS, aged 18 years or older, who walked 25 feet independently with or without devices, lower extremity spasticity that interfered with daily activities, and agreed not to change medications during the study. Excluded if other conditions interfering with participation were present.	Two 2-hour facilitator-led group sessions 1 week apart	Randomized controlled, Level I, single-blinded, two-arm study of those who received the program and controls (usual care)	Mean total score and scores on two subscales of the MS Spasticity Scale-88 showed improvement for the program group compared to usual care ($p < 0.03$).	Signed test was used to evaluate the change following intervention within each group. The Wilcoxon rank-sum test was used to compare changes between groups.

Best Evidence for Occupational Therapy Practice Intervention Related to Parkinson Disease

Intervention	Description	Participants	Dosage	Research Design and Evidence Level	Benefit	Statistical Significance and Effect Size
Interdisciplinary self-management rehabilitation program for persons with PD[62]	Eighteen hours of group sessions included movement and speech exercises; ADL and gait training; discussions of cognitive strategies, stress management, and fall prevention.	One hundred and sixteen persons with PD: 30% were women; mean age of 66 years.	Six weeks of treatment. Participants divided into three groups: 1: 0 hours of rehab; 2: 27 hours having 18 in group and 9 social; 3: 27 hours having 18 in group and 9 in-home and community skill transfer training.	Randomized controlled trial Level: I	The two rehab groups improved in health-related QoL, with communication and mobility gains. There was no difference between intervention groups and no improvement for the untreated group.	Repeated-measures ANCOVA. Post-treatment effect at follow-up: $F = 3.98$, $p = 0.02$, and moderate ES ($\eta = 0.26$) A significant response ($p = 0.03$) was shown for the health-related quality of life (HRQOL) domains of communication (2-month follow-up) and mobility (6-month follow-up).
Exercise programs in PD—the Berlin LSVT-BIG study[63]	LSVTBIG uses intensive high-amplitude movements done 1 hour, 4× /week for 4 weeks with 15 reps/task.	Fifty-eight people with PD at Hoehn and Yahr stages I–III: 36 women, 22 men Mean weekly exercise time between baseline and final was 2.53 hours; in BIG, 2.10 (2.05) in WALK, and 2.6 (1.12) in HOME.	Participants were divided into three groups: BIG—training 1:1; WALK—Nordic group walking; HOME—non-supervised exercises.	Randomized controlled trial Level I	LSVTBIG group improved over other groups in motor performance, moving from sit to stand, and walking. No differences for QoL between groups.	ANCOVA for between-group comparison. BIG participants showed significant improvement on Unified Parkinson's Disease Rating Scale (UPDRS) ($F = 11.9$, $p = 0.001$) and timed up and go (TUG) ($F = 3.64$, $p = 0.033$), whereas 10-m walk approached significant benefit ($F = 2.97$, $p = 0.059$).

References

1. Wallin M, Culpepper W, Campbell J, et al. The prevalence of multiple sclerosis in the United States: a population-based healthcare database approach. *Mult Scler*. 2017.
2. Browne P, Chandraratna D, Angood C, Tremlett H, Baker C, Taylor BV, et al. Atlas of Multiple Sclerosis 2013: A growing global problem with widespread inequity. *Neurology*. 2014;83(11):1022–1024.
3. National Multiple Sclerosis Society. About MS. 2012. http://www.nationalmssociety.org. Accessed March 10, 2012.
4. Loma I, Heyman R. Multiple sclerosis: pathogenesis and treatment. *Curr Neuropharmacol*. 2011;9(3):409–416.
5. Krieger S, Sumowski J. New insights into multiple sclerosis clinical course from the topographical model and functional reserve. *Neurol Clin*. 2018;36(1):13.
6. Lublin FD, Reingold SC, Cohen JA, et al. Defining the clinical course of multiple sclerosis: the 2013 revisions. *Neurology*. 2014;83(3):278–286.
7. Julian LJ, Vella L, Vollmer T, Hadjimichael O, Mohr DC. Employment in multiple sclerosis: exiting and re-entering the work force. *J Neurol*. 2008;255(9):1354–1360.
8. Leavitt VM, Sumowski JF, Chiaravalloti N, Deluca J. Warmer outdoor temperature is associated with worse cognitive status in multiple sclerosis. *Neurology*. 2012;78(13):964–968.
9. Forwell SJ, Brunham S, Tremlett H, Morrison W, Oger J. Differentiating primary and non-primary fatigue in MS. *Int J MS Care*. 2008;10:14–20.
10. Asano M, Finlayson ML. Meta-analysis of three different types of fatigue management interventions for people with multiple sclerosis: exercise, education, and medication. *Mult Scler Int*. 2014;2014:798285.
11. Nilsagård Y, Gunn H, Freeman J, et al. Falls in people with MS—an individual data meta-analysis from studies from Australia, Sweden, United Kingdom and the United States. *Mult Scler*. 2015;21(1):92–100.
12. Rocca MA, Amato MP, De Stefano N, et al. Clinical and imaging assessment of cognitive dysfunction in multiple sclerosis. *Lancet Neurol*. 2015;14(3):302–317.
13. Ehde D, Osborne T, Hanley M, Jensen M, Kraft G. The scope and nature of pain in persons with multiple sclerosis. *Mult Scler*. 2006;12(5):629–638.
14. Rizzo M, Hadjimichael O, Preiningerova J, Vollmer T. Prevalence and treatment of spasticity reported by multiple sclerosis patients. *Mult Scler*. 2004;10(5):589–595.
15. Hobart J, Riazi A, Thompson A, et al. Getting the measure of spasticity in multiple sclerosis: the Multiple Sclerosis Spasticity Scale (MSSS-88). *Brain*. 2006;129(Pt 1):224.
16. Hyman N, Barnes M, Bhakta B, et al. Botulinum toxin (Dysport) treatment of hip adductor spasticity in multiple sclerosis: a prospective, randomised, double blind, placebo controlled, dose ranging study. *J Neurol Neurosurg Psychiatry*. 2000;68(6):707–712.
17. Erwin A, Gudesblatt M, Bethoux F, et al. Interthecal baclofen in multiple sclerosis: too little, too late? *Mult Scler*. 2011;17:705–713.
18. Koppel BS, Brust JC, Fife T, et al. Systematic review: efficacy and safety of medical marijuana in selected neurologic disorders: report of the Guideline Development Subcommittee of the American Academy of Neurology. *Neurology*. 2014;82(17):1556–1563.
19. Calcagno P, Ruoppolo G, Grasso MG, De Vincentiis M, Paolucci S. Dysphagia in multiple sclerosis prevalence and prognostic factors. *Acta Neurol Scand*. 2002;105(1):40–43.
20. Thompson AJ, Banwell BL, Barkhof F, et al. Diagnosis of multiple sclerosis: 2017 revisions of the McDonald criteria. *Lancet Neurol*. 2018;17(2):162–173.
21. National Multiple Sclerosis Society. Disease-modifying therapies for MS. 2018. http://www.nationalmssociety.org/NationalMSSociety/media/MSNationalFiles/Brochures/Brochure-The-MS-Disease-Modifying-Medications.pdf. Accessed June 1, 2018.
22. Shirani A, Zhao Y, Karim ME, et al. Association between use of interferon beta and progression of disability in patients with relapsing-remitting multiple sclerosis. *JAMA*. 2012;308(3):247–256.
23. Panitch H, Applebee A. Treatment of walking impairment in multiple sclerosis: an unmet need for a disease-specific disability. *Expert Opin Pharmacother*. 2011;12(10):1511–1521.
24. Goodman AD, Brown TR, Krupp LB, et al. Sustained-release oral fampridine in multiple sclerosis: a randomised, double-blind, controlled trial. *Lancet*. 2009;373(9665):732–738.
25. Vukusic S, Hutchinson M, Hours M, et al. Pregnancy and multiple sclerosis (the PRIMS study): clinical predictors of post-partum relapse. *Brain*. 2004;127(Pt 6):1353–1360.
26. Korostil M, Feinstein A. Anxiety disorders and their clinical correlates in multiple sclerosis patients. *Mult Scler*. 2007;13(1):67–72.
27. Coyne KS, Boscoe AN, Currie BM, Landrian AS, Wandstrat TL. Understanding drivers of employment changes in a multiple sclerosis population. *Int J MS Care*. 2015;17(5):245–252.
28. Finlayson M. Concerns about the future among older adults with multiple sclerosis. *Am J Occup Ther*. 2004;58(1):54–63.
29. Packer TL, Brink N, Sauriol A. *Managing Fatigue: A Six-Week Course for Energy Conservation*. Tucson, AZ: Therapy Skill Builders; 1995.
30. Finlayson M, Holberg C. Evaluation of a teleconference-delivered energy conservation education program for people with multiple sclerosis. *Can J Occup Ther*. 2007;74(4):337–347.
31. Ghahari S, Packer TL, Passmore AE. Effectiveness of an online fatigue self-management program for people with chronic neurological conditions: a randomized controlled trial. *J Clin Rehabil*. 2010;24(8):727–744.
32. Hugos CL, Copperman LF, Fuller BE, Yadav V, Lovera J, Bourdete DN. Clinical trial of a formal group fatigue program in multiple sclerosis. *Mult Scler*. 2010;16(6):724–732.
33. Kileff J, Ashburn A. A pilot study of the effect of aerobic exercise on people with moderate disability multiple sclerosis. *Clin Rehabil*. 2005;19(2):165–169.
34. Hugos CL, Bourdette D, Chen Y, Chen Z, Cameron M. A group-delivered self-management program reduces spasticity in people with multiple sclerosis: A randomized, controlled pilot trial. *Mult Scler J Exp Transl Clin*. 2017;3(1):2055217317699993.

35. Gentry T. PDAs as cognitive aids for people with multiple sclerosis. *Am J Occup Ther*. 2008;62(1):18–27.
36. Johnson KL, Bamer AM, Yorkston KM, Amtmann D. Use of cognitive aids and other assistive technology by individuals with multiple sclerosis. *Disabil Rehabil Assist Technol*. 2009;4(1):1–8.
37. Hawes F, Billups C, Forwell S. Interventions for upper-limb intention tremor in multiple sclerosis: a feasibility study. *Int J MS Care*. 2010;12(3):122–131.
38. Feys P, Helsen WF, Liu X, et al. Interaction between eye and hand movements in multiple sclerosis patients with intention tremor. *Mov Disord*. 2005;20(6):705–713.
39. Bishop M, Frain M, Tschopp M. Self-management, perceived control, and subjective quality of life in multiple sclerosis: an exploratory study. *Rehabil Couns Bull*. 2008;52(1):45–56.
40. Audulv Å, Ghahari S, Kephart G, Warner G, Packer TL. The Taxonomy of Everyday Self-management Strategies (TEDSS): a framework derived from the literature and refined using empirical data. *Patient Educ Couns*. 2018;102(2):367–375.
41. Briones-Buixassa L, Milà R, Mª Aragonès J, Bufill E, Olaya B, Arrufat FX. Stress and multiple sclerosis: a systematic review considering potential moderating and mediating factors and methods of assessing stress. *Health Psychol Open*. 2015;2(2):2055102915612271.
42. Mohr DC, Lovera J, Brown T, et al. A randomized trial of stress management for the prevention of new brain lesions in MS. *Neurology*. 2012;79(5):412–419.
43. Tysnes O-B, Storstein A. Epidemiology of Parkinson's disease. *J Neural Transm*. 2017;124(8):901–905.
44. Bellou V, Belbasis L, Tzoulaki I, Evangelou E, Ioannidis JPA. Environmental risk factors and Parkinson's disease: an umbrella review of meta-analyses. *Parkinsonism Relat Disord*. 2016;23:1–9.
45. Klingelhoefer L, Reichmann H. Parkinson's disease and gastrointestinal non motor symptoms: diagnostic and therapeutic options—a practise guide. *J Parkinson's Dis*. 2015;5(3):647–658.
46. Surmeier DJ. Determinants of dopaminergic neuron loss in Parkinson's disease. *FEBS J*. 2018;285(19):3657–3668.
47. Hoehn MM, Yahr MD. Parkinsonism: onset, progression and mortality. *Neurology*. 1967;17(5):427–442.
48. Bradley WE. *Neurology in Clinical Practice*. 2nd ed. Boston, MA: Butterworth-Heinemann; 1996.
49. Grimes D, Gordon J, Snelgrove B, et al. Canadian guidelines on Parkinson's disease. *Can J Neurol Sci*. 2012;39(4 suppl 4):S1–S30.
50. Savica R, Grossardt BR, Bower JH, et al. Survival and causes of death among people with clinically diagnosed synucleinopathies with parkinsonism: a population-based study. *JAMA Neurol*. 2017;74(7):839–846.
51. Papagno C, Trojano L. Cognitive and behavioral disorders in Parkinson's disease: an update. I: cognitive impairments. *Neurol Sci*. 2018;39(2):215–223.
52. Leung IH, Walton CC, Hallock H, Lewis SJ, Valenzuela M, Lampit A. Cognitive training in Parkinson disease: a systematic review and meta-analysis. *Neurology*. 2015;85(21):1843–1851. doi:10.1212/WNL.0000000000002145.
53. Goetz CG, Poewe W, Rascol O, Sampaio C. Evidence-based medical review update: pharmacological and surgical treatments of Parkinson's disease: 2001 to 2004. *Mov Disord*. 2005;20(5):523–539.
54. Jankovic J. Parkinson's disease: clinical features and diagnosis. *J Neurol Neurosurg Psychiatry*. 2008;79(4):368–376.
55. Baker MG, Graham L. The journey: Parkinson's disease. *BMJ*. 2004;329(7466):611–614.
56. Schrag A, Banks P. Time of loss of employment in Parkinson's disease. *Mov Disord*. 2006;21(11):1839–1843.
57. Dick S, Semple S, Dick F, Seaton A. Occupational titles as risk factors for Parkinson's disease. *Occup Med (Oxford, England)*. 2007;57(1):50–56.
58. Peto V, Jenkinson C, Fitzpatrick R, Greenhall R. The development and validation of a short measure of functioning and well being for individuals with Parkinson's disease. *Qual Life Res*. 1995;4(3):241–248.
59. Dixon L, Duncan DC, Johnson P, et al. Occupational therapy for patients with Parkinson's disease. *Cochrane Database Syst Rev*. 2007;(3):CD002813.
60. Rao AK. Enabling functional independence in Parkinson's disease: update on occupational therapy intervention. *Mov Disord*. 2010;25(suppl 1):S146–S151.
61. Murphy S, Tickle-Degnen L. The effectiveness of occupational therapy–related treatments for persons with Parkinson's disease: a meta-analytic review. *Am J Occup Ther*. 2001;55(4):385–392.
62. Tickle-Degnen L, Ellis T, Saint-Hilaire MH, Thomas CA, Wagenaar RC. Self-management rehabilitation and health-related quality of life in Parkinson's disease: a randomized controlled trial. *Mov Disord*. 2010;25(2):194–204.
63. Ebersbach G, Ebersbach A, Edler D, et al. Comparing exercise in Parkinson's disease—the Berlin BIG study. *Mov Disord*. 2010;25(12):1902–1908.
64. Amyotrophic Lateral Sclerosis Association. What is ALS? 2018. https://www.als.ca/about-als/what-is-als/. Accessed September 19, 2019.
65. Zarei S, Carr K, Reiley L, et al. A comprehensive review of amyotrophic lateral sclerosis. *Surg Neurol Int*. 2015;6:171.
66. Hardiman O, Al-Chalabi A, Chio A, et al. Amyotrophic lateral sclerosis. *Nat Rev Dis Primers*. 2017;3:17071.
67. Kiernan MC, Vucic S, Cheah BC, et al. Amyotrophic lateral sclerosis. *Lancet*. 2011;377(9769):942–955.
68. Chiò A, Logroscino G, Hardiman O, et al. Prognostic factors in ALS: a critical review. *Amyotroph Lateral Scler*. 2009;10(5–6):310–323.
69. Luchesi K, Kitamua S, Mourao L. Amyotrophic lateral sclerosis survival analysis: swallowing and non-oral feeding. *NeuroRehabilitation*. 2014;35(3):535–542.
70. Mayo Clinic. Patient Care & Health Information. Amyotrophic lateral sclerosis (ALS). 2018. https://www.mayoclinic.org/diseases-conditions/amyotrophic-lateral-sclerosis/symptoms-causes/syc-20354022. Accessed April 2, 2018.
71. Miller R. Practice parameter update: the care of the patient with amyotrophic lateral sclerosis: multidisciplinary care, symptom management, and cognitive/behavioral impairment (an evidence-based review). *Neurology*. 2009;73:1227–1233.
72. van den Berg JP, Kalmijn S, Lindeman E, et al. Multidisciplinary ALS care improves quality of life in patients with ALS. *Neurology*. 2005;65(8):1264–1267.

73. Foley G, Timonen V, Hardiman O. Exerting control and adapting to loss in amyotrophic lateral sclerosis. *Soc Sci Med.* 2014;101:113–119.
74. Plahuta JM, McCulloch BJ, Kasarskis EJ, Ross MA, Walter RA, McDonald ER. Amyotrophic lateral sclerosis and hopelessness: psychosocial factors. *Soc Sci Med.* 2002;55(12):2131–2140.
75. Ball LJ, Beukelman DR, Pattee GL. Acceptance of augmentative and alternative communication technology by persons with amyotrophic lateral sclerosis. *Augment Altern Commun.* 2004;20(2):113–122.
76. Soofi AY, Bello-Haas VD, Kho ME, Letts L. The impact of rehabilitative interventions on quality of life: a qualitative evidence synthesis of personal experiences of individuals with amyotrophic lateral sclerosis. *Qual Life Res.* 2018;27(4):845–856.
77. Miano B, Stoddard G, Davis S, Bromberg M. Inter-evaluator reliability of the ALS functional rating scale. *Amyotroph Lateral Scler Other Motor Neuron Disord.* 2004;5(4):235–239.
78. Higo R, Tayama N, Nito T. Longitudinal analysis of progression of dysphagia in amyotrophic lateral sclerosis. *Auris Nasus Larynx.* 2004;31(3):247–254.
79. Drory VE, Goltsman E, Goldman Reznik J, Mosek A, Korczyn AD. The value of muscle exercise in patients with amyotrophic lateral sclerosis. *J Neurol Sci.* 2001;191(1):133–137.
80. Johnson S, Alonso B, Faulkner K, et al. Quality of life perspectives of people with amyotrophic lateral sclerosis and their caregivers. *Am J Occup Ther.* 2017;71(3):7103190010p1–7103190010p7.
81. Mitsumoto H, Chad D, Pioro E. *Amyotrophic Lateral Sclerosis: Contemporary Neurology Series.* Philadelphia, PA: Davis; 1998.
82. Neudert C, Wasner M, Borasio GD. Individual quality of life is not correlated with health-related quality of life or physical function in patients with amyotrophic lateral sclerosis. *J Palliat Med.* 2004;7(4):551–557.
83. Arbesman M, Sheard K. Systematic review of the effectiveness of occupational therapy–related interventions for people with amyotrophic lateral sclerosis. *Am J Occup Ther.* 2014;68(1):20–26.
84. Calvo A, Moglia C, Ilardi A, et al. Religiousness is positively associated with quality of life of ALS caregivers. *Amyotroph Lateral Scler.* 2011;12(3):168–171.
85. Trail M, Nelson N, Van JN, Appel SH, Lai EC. Wheelchair use by patients with amyotrophic lateral sclerosis: a survey of user characteristics and selection preferences. *Arch Phys Med Rehabil.* 2001;82(1):98–102.
86. Leder SB, Novella S, Patwa H. Use of fiberoptic endoscopic evaluation of swallowing (FEES) in patients with amyotrophic lateral sclerosis. *Dysphagia.* 2004;19(3):177–181.
87. Willison HJ, Jacobs BC, Van Doorn PA. Guillain-Barré syndrome. *Lancet.* 2016;388(10045):717–727.
88. van Doorn PA, Ruts L, Jacobs BC. Clinical features, pathogenesis, and treatment of Guillain-Barré syndrome. *Lancet Neurol.* 2008;7(10):939–950.
89. Carroll Á, McDonnell G, Barnes M. A review of the management of Guillain-Barré syndrome in a regional neurological rehabilitation unit. *Int J Rehabil Res.* 2003;26(4):297–302.
90. Karavatas SG. The role of neurodevelopmental sequencing in the physical therapy management of a geriatric patient with Guillain-Barré syndrome. *Top Geriatr Rehabil.* 2005;21(2):133–135.
91. Khan F, Pallant JF, Ng L, Bhasker A. Factors associated with long-term functional outcomes and psychological sequelae in Guillain–Barré syndrome. *J Neurol.* 2010;257(12):2024–2031.
92. Gregory MA, Gregory RJ, Podd JV. Understanding Guillain-Barré syndrome and central nervous system involvement. *Rehabil Nurs.* 2005;30(5):207–212.
93. Khan F. Rehabilitation in Guillain-Barré syndrome. *Aust Fam Physician.* 2004;33:1013–1017.
94. Royal E, Reynolds FA, Houlden H. What are the experiences of adults returning to work following recovery from Guillain-Barré syndrome? An interpretative phenomenological analysis. *Disabil Rehabil.* 2009;31(22):1817–1827.
95. Meythaler JM, DeVivo MJ, Braswell WC. Rehabilitation outcomes of patients who have developed Guillain-Barré syndrome. *Am J Phys Med Rehabil.* 1997;76(5):411.
96. Hansen M, Garcia S. *Guidelines for Physical and Occupational Therapy.* Narberth, PA: GBS/CIDP Foundation International; 2012.
97. Andrews AW, Middleton A. Improvement during inpatient rehabilitation among older adults with Guillain-Barré syndrome, multiple sclerosis, Parkinson disease, and stroke. *Am J Phys Med Rehabil.* 2018;97(12):879–884.
98. Plow M, Finlayson M. Potential benefits of Nintendo Wii fit among people with multiple sclerosis: a longitudinal pilot study. *Int J MS Care.* 2011;13(1):21–30.

Chapter 39

Spinal Cord Injury

Deborah E. Budash

LEARNING OBJECTIVES

This chapter will allow the reader to:

1. Identify and understand the terminology and fundamental concepts related to spinal cord injury (SCI) and rehabilitation.
2. Appreciate the physical, psychosocial, and occupational challenges associated with SCI.
3. Recognize functional expectations of SCI at various neurological levels and the related factors that impact outcomes.
4. List the priorities and goals of the occupational therapist for each treatment phase and injury level.
5. Describe the tests and procedures appropriate for occupational therapy assessment.
6. Understand and adopt the perspective that focuses on the unique abilities of each patient and seeks individualized solutions to achieve goals.
7. Appreciate the long-term implications of SCI on the individual related to participation in valued roles and occupations.
8. Identify occupational therapy interventions for each treatment phase and injury level.
9. Understand how SCI care has evolved as a consequence of changing health care policies and the impact of these changes on the occupational therapy profession.
10. Perceive how the Occupational Therapy Practice Framework and the unique skills and knowledge of the therapist can support function and wellness of patients with SCI throughout the life span.

CHAPTER OUTLINE

TERMINOLOGY

Assessment: tool used to gather information during the evaluation process.

Catheterization: a bladder-emptying technique in which a flexible tube (catheter) is inserted into the urethra to drain urine.

Clonus: an alternating involuntary muscle contraction and relaxation in rapid succession, associated with changes in muscle tone as a consequence of neurological injury or disease.

Complete injury: a diagnostic label that represents an absence of sensory and motor function in the lowest sacral segments (S4–S5).

Crede method: a manual bladder-emptying technique that involves manual application of pressure superficial to the bladder.

Dermatome: the area of skin innervated by the sensory axons within each segmental nerve. A myotome is a group of muscles innervated by a single spinal nerve; myotomes are used in the diagnostic process of identifying the level of the spinal cord injury.

Ergometry: the study of physical work activity. In rehabilitation, ergometry often involves the use of a stationary bicycle or treadmill.

Functional electrical stimulation (FES): involves the application of electric current to paralyzed muscles in order to cause a muscle contraction.

Functional level: the lowest segment at which the strength of important muscles is graded 3+ or above out of 5 on a manual muscle test (MMT), and at which sensation is intact; the functional level has implications to functional rehabilitation outcomes.

Incomplete injury: a diagnostic label that represents the preservation of any sensory and/or motor function below the neurological level that includes the lowest sacral segments S4–S5.

Motor level: a diagnostic label that quantifies functional outcome expectations; the motor level is identified by the most caudal section of the spinal cord with normal motor function.

Paraplegia: the loss or impairment in motor and/or sensory function in the thoracic, lumbar, or sacral segments of the cord, resulting in impairment in the trunk, legs, and pelvic organs and sparing of the arms.

Sensory level: identified by the most caudal segment of the spinal cord possessing normal sensation to pin prick and light touch; it has implications for functional outcomes.

Tetraplegia: the loss or impairment in motor and/or sensory function in the cervical segments of the spinal cord, resulting in functional impairment in the arms, trunk, legs, and pelvic organs; previously known as *quadriplegia.*

Tracheostomy: a surgically created hole in the trachea through which the tracheostomy tube is inserted; the tracheostomy provides the connection to the ventilator for individuals who cannot breathe spontaneously.

Valsalva maneuver: method to facilitate a bowel movement; it involves holding one's breath while bearing down or pushing through the abdomen.

Zone of partial preservation: refers to the dermatomes and myotomes caudal to the neurological level that remain partially innervated; over time, strength and sensation improve, resulting in better functional outcomes.

Introduction

A spinal cord injury (SCI) is catastrophic and impacts every aspect of an individual's life.[1] Paralysis often results from SCI and is generally well understood, but there is also a corresponding loss of spontaneously occurring body functions that can seriously impact health in less-understood ways.[1,2] Contemporary medicine has facilitated the survival of SCIs, leaving those injured to cope with overwhelming loss.[3,4] Although the underlying objectives of SCI care have remained consistent over time—that is, to maximize the patient's abilities and minimize secondary complications—there is hope that future medical advances will achieve greater functional restoration for survivors of SCI and disease.[1,5,6]

Occupational therapists, with their unique skill set including knowledge of occupational performance, health and wellness, task analysis and adaptation, and psychosocial adjustment, play an important role in SCI rehabilitation.[7–9] This chapter provides a foundational understanding of SCI and the vital role that occupational therapists play in returning patients to meaningful occupations, despite the severity of their limitations. The chapter begins with the epidemiology and etiology of SCI. The medical management of SCI is reviewed with a focus on the sequelae that impact function—the primary focus for occupational therapists. An overview of the occupational therapy process with this unique group of patients follows, concluding with considerations for the profession's evolving role in SCI rehabilitation.

Description of Spinal Cord Injury

Epidemiology

Epidemiology provides information about SCI prevalence and incidence rate and offers insight into the typical characteristics of patients sustaining SCI. Such insights inform treatment, preventative initiatives, and proactive planning for the future of SCI care and rehabilitation.[3,10]

According to the National Spinal Cord Injury Statistical Center (NSCISC), about 17,500 people per year in the United States experience an SCI, or about 54 of every 1 million Americans.[11] The total number of people with SCI alive today in the United States is estimated to be in the range of 245,000 to 353,000. About 90% of SCIs are traumatic in nature, and the epidemiological data are present from the traumatic and nontraumatic perspectives, respectively.

Trends in SCI have evolved over time and generally align to demographic and societal trends.[10] As of 2017, the average age at injury is 42 years.[11] By contrast, the average age at SCI was 29 years in the 1970s. Considering SCI incidence from a life span perspective, the lowest incidence of SCI is seen in children at 3% to 5%,[5] is highest for the age range of late teens and early 20s, and generally declines as adults age.[5,10,12] Recent trends demonstrate an increasing incidence of SCI in elderly age groups.[5,10,13] This second peak in incidence is attributed to our aging population and is expected to continue.[10] The age groups most at risk for SCI are those 20 to 29 and 70+.[3,10]

Males account for about 81% of new SCIs.[11] However, SCI in children, the elderly, and of nontraumatic causes are more evenly distributed between genders.[5,10–12] The primary ethnicities of individuals incurring new SCIs includes non-Hispanic white (63%), non-Hispanic black (22%), and Hispanic (11%).[11] There are further trends to be considered within these data; for example, 22% of new SCIs occurring in non-Hispanic black populations is higher than the 12% representation of this group in the general population.

Most new SCIs are diagnosed as incomplete injuries, with 46% incomplete tetraplegia and 20% incomplete **paraplegia.**[11] Complete paraplegia is diagnosed in about 19% of SCIs, followed by 13% as complete **tetraplegia.** A recent increase in high cervical (C1–C4) and incomplete injuries has been observed.[10] Nontraumatic SCI (NTSCI) occurs more often in older patients and females and typically does not occur at the cervical level.[10,14]

The life expectancy of individuals with SCI is less than that of the general population.[3,10,11] This is particularly so within the first year following SCI. As explored later in this chapter, the nature of the SCI places individuals at risk for a number of life-threatening secondary conditions. As a result, about 33% of SCI patients will be rehospitalized within the first year of injury at least once.[11] If these conditions are not properly managed, they can escalate to become life-threatening. The most common cause of death for individuals with SCI is pneumonia followed by septicemia. These conditions have remained the primary causes of death for individuals with SCI for over 40 years. The mortality rates are higher for older patients with more severe SCIs.[10] One study found that increasing age, male gender, and lower functional independence scores at discharge were significantly related to decreased life expectancy.[15]

There are additional pertinent characteristics to consider related to patients with new SCI. Most individuals who experience a new SCI are single, but trends show that the number of individuals who marry over a lifetime increases, as does the divorce rate for those married at the time of injury.[3,11] Most individuals who incur an SCI (52%) possess a high school education.[11] About 11% of new patients with SCI are college or university-educated. The level of education slowly increases over time for those with SCI. Most individuals who experience an SCI are employed (60%) or are students (15%) at the time of injury. The rate of employment declines to 34% at 20 years postinjury.

On a global scale, similar trends are observed, but outcomes vary by country.[3] There is a higher incidence of SCI in the United States than throughout the rest of the world, but this may be due to the fact that, in underdeveloped countries, more of those injured do not survive.[3,10] The World Health Organization estimates that 40 to 80 SCI cases per million, or 250,000 to 500,000, occur annually throughout the world, and 90% are of a traumatic nature.[16] Many of the trends observed in SCI incidence in the United States are also noted throughout the world, with some regional variance. The incidence of SCI is higher for males than females, with a bimodal incidence by age groups, as noted previously.[3,17] Mortality is highest in the first year following injury and remains higher throughout the life span. Individuals with SCI possess a risk of premature death that is two to five times higher than the average population. As seen in the subsequent section, the causes of SCI are also similar globally.

Etiology

The overwhelming causes of SCIs, about 40%, are attributed to vehicular accidents.[18] Falls account for approximately 30% of incidence, followed by 14% due to violence, and 8% attributed to sports. SCI incurred by these causes are deemed traumatic and account for more than 90% of all SCIs. The remaining 8% are attributed to other causes and are considered nontraumatic. Nontraumatic causes include medical conditions related to the spinal cord, such as spinal stenosis, tumors, surgical complications, and other unclassified occurrences.[5,17,18] Falls are the leading cause of SCI in the elderly, with sports injuries and violence causing fewer SCIs in this group.[10] The most frequent causes of SCI in children include lapbelt injury, birth injury, and child abuse.[5,12] Violence is more often a cause of SCI in the African American population.[13]

Globally, the etiological trends are similar to those in the United States. Between the ages of birth and 5 years, the most common cause of SCI is vehicular crashes at a rate of 65%.[3,12] Violence is the cause of SCI in males more often in every age group.[3] Falls are the most common cause of SCI after the age of 60.

The most frequent causes of SCI are observed to be preventable, and successful public health campaigns have been developed to reduce the risk of injury.[3,10,16] Most remarkable in the United States are those related to sports activities, such as diving, football, and trampoline use.[10]

Course

To help guide and support their patients through the initial stage of injury, occupational therapists must be familiar with the usual course of events following SCI, the diagnostic process, and the factors relevant to prognosis.

SCI, depending on the level of spinal injury and accompanying injuries, can be a life-threatening situation, requiring intensive emergency and acute care.[13,19] Immediately following SCI, a period of spinal shock begins.[5,13] During this time, spinal reflexes and motor, sensory, and autonomic function cease below the lesion level.[13,20] The extremities below the lesion level become flaccid (or lose tone). Spinal shock is more extensive with lesions above T1, but even complete lower thoracic injuries are accompanied by some degree of spinal shock.[13] This is a temporary and variable phase that can last several days to weeks, during which the true extent of paralysis cannot be determined. Neurogenic shock (a life-threatening medical condition resulting from autonomic instability) can occur simultaneously with spinal shock because of a loss of sympathetically mediated peripheral vascular tone, causing hypotension and bradycardia. Increased bronchial secretions can also be experienced during this time as well as gastrointestinal motility issues, complicating the clinical scenario.[13] Resolution of spinal shock is characterized by the return of spinal reflexes and hyperreflexia (spasticity) as well as the return of voluntary motor function and sensation.[13,20]

A baseline neurological **assessment** is conducted during the provision of emergency care to establish the presence and nature of an SCI and thereafter periodically to quantify progress and healing.[13,19] The American Spinal Cord Injury Association (ASIA) assessment is the international standard for this assessment.[21] An SCI causes a disruption in the motor and sensory pathways at the lesion site.[13,21] Because the nerve roots are segmentally routed, a thorough evaluation of motor and sensory function can identify the lesion level, and this is the approach of the ASIA examination. The neurological level is diagnosed by the physician according to the findings.

The **motor level** is determined by testing 10 key muscles on each side of the body using manual muscle test (MMT), graded 0 (total paralysis) through 5 (normal).[21] The **sensory level** is determined by testing sensation of each of the 28 **dermatomes** at key sensory points on each side of the body (ASIA sensory examination). Sensation is assessed for pin prick and light touch and is graded on a scale of 0 (absent) to 2 (normal). The sensory examination includes the perianal area and external anal sphincter.[13,21]

Findings are classified in terms of bilateral sensory and motor levels, and neurological level.[13,21] The neurological level of injury (NLI) is the lowest segment of the spinal cord with preserved bilateral normal sensory and antigravity motor function. The level above must also have normal strength and sensation. The motor and sensory levels can differ; for example, sensory level may be higher than a motor level.[13] At the injury level, areflexia (loss of reflexes) may remain as the reflex arc is interrupted. The motor levels are identified by the injury location on the spinal cord, be it cervical (C1–C8), thoracic (T1–T12), lumbar (L1–L5), or sacral (S1–S5)[21] (Fig. 39-1).

Further classification of the injury can be made based on the results of the neurological examination.[21] Tetraplegia refers to a cervical injury causing sensory and/or motor loss in the arms, legs, pelvic organs, and trunk. Paraplegia refers to impairment or loss of motor and/or sensory function in the thoracic, lumbar, or sacral segments of the spinal cord. The upper extremities (UEs) are generally spared in paraplegia, and, depending on the lesion level, the trunk, legs, and pelvic organs are more or less affected[13] (see Fig. 39-1).

SCIs are further classified by whether they are complete or incomplete.[21] Complete injuries are those where there is no motor or sensory function preserved in S4–S5. Incomplete injures can be classified as motor or sensory incomplete, with sparing of sensory or motor function at S4–S5.[21] The ASIA Impairment Scale is used to clearly classify injuries by letter grade (Table 39-1).

During this assessment, the **zone of partial preservation** and the **functional levels** can be observed.[21] This information provides clues about functional outcomes and is of particular significance to the occupational therapist because the partially preserved neurological and sensory levels retain some innervation and imply possible strength and sensation improvements with time.[13,21]

Additional testing is included in the neurological examination, although it does not contribute to diagnosis but rather informs a comprehensive approach to care.[2] The autonomic assessment considers autonomic control of the heart, blood pressure, and the awareness and management of the bladder and bowel.[2] The monitoring of joint movement (proprioception, kinesthetic sense), deep pressure, and deep tendon reflexes are also assessed. The testing of deep tendon reflexes permits an appreciation of the evolution through spinal shock and has implications for bowel and bladder function.[13]

There are also a number of clinical syndromes that are not part of the International Standards examination

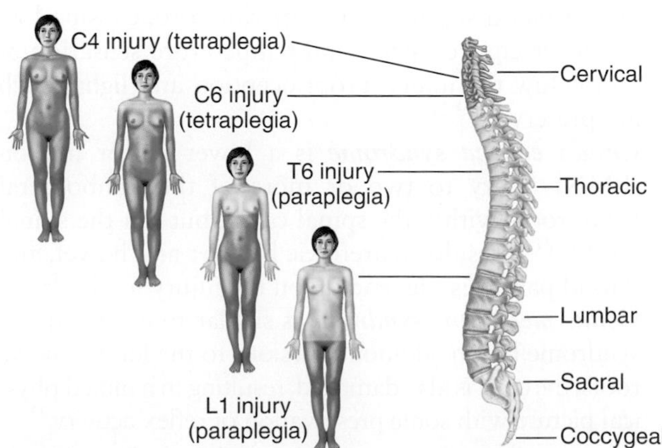

Figure 39-1. Spinal cord with segments: cervical, thoracic, lumbar, and sacral, with body areas affected by spinal cord injuries at C4, C6, T6, and L1 levels. (Reprinted with permission of Advancells.)

Table 39-1 ASIA Impairment Scale

STAGE	DESCRIPTION
A = Complete	No sensory or motor function is preserved in the sacral segments S4–S5.
B = Sensory incomplete	Sensory, but not motor, function is preserved below the neurological level and includes the sacral segments S4–S5 (LT or PP at S4–S5 or DAP), *and* no motor function is preserved more than three levels below the motor level on either side of the body.
C = Motor incomplete	Motor function is preserved at the most caudal sacral segments for voluntary anal contraction *or* the patient meets the criteria for sensory incomplete status (sensory function preserved at the most caudal sacral segments [S4–S5] by LT, PP, or DAP), and has some sparing of motor function more than three levels below the ipsilateral motor level on either side of the body. (This includes key or nonkey muscle functions to determine motor incomplete status.) For AIS C—less than half of key muscle functions below the single NLI have a muscle grade ≥3.
D = Motor incomplete	Motor incomplete status as defined above, with at least half (half or more) of key muscle functions below the single NLI having a muscle grade ≥3.
E = Normal	If sensation and motor function as tested with the ISNCSCI are graded as normal in all segments, and the patient had prior deficits, then the AIS grade is E. Someone without an initial SCI does not receive an AIS grade.

Using ND: To document the sensory, motor and NLI levels, the ASIA Impairment Scale grade, and/or the zone of partial preservation when they are unable to be determined based on the examination results.

AIS, ASIA Impairment Scale; DAP, deep anal pressure; LT, light touch; NLI, neurological level of injury; PP, pin prick; SCI, spinal cord injury.

or ASIA classification that should be recognized. All are incomplete injuries[21]:

- *Central cord syndrome* results from damage to the center of the spinal cord.[20] This is the most common syndrome resulting in more weakness in the UEs than the lower extremities (LEs). This injury is often caused by falls, occurs mostly to older people, and is often associated with cervical stenosis.[21]
- *Brown-Sequard syndrome* involves damage to one side of the cord, causing ipsilateral proprioceptive and vibratory sensory loss, loss of motor control at and below the lesion, and contralateral loss of pain and temperature sensation.[13,21] This syndrome is most often caused by a motor vehicle accident, gunshot, or stabbing wound.
- *Anterior cord syndrome* is rare and associated with absent blood supply to the anterior cord, causing loss of motor control, pain, and temperature sensation at and below the injury. Proprioception and light touch are preserved.[13,21]
- *Cauda equina syndrome* is a lower motor neuron (LMN) injury to two or more of the lumbosacral nerve roots within the spinal canal, but not the spinal cord.[13,21] It results in areflexic bladder and bowel, and flaccid paralysis (depending on the injury level).[13,20,21]
- *Conus medullaris syndrome* is similar to cauda equina syndrome but in addition to lesions to the lumbar nerve roots, the cord is also damaged, resulting in a mixed physical picture with some preservation of reflex activity.[21]

Once the patient's medical condition is stabilized, inpatient SCI rehabilitation is recommended to maximize function, strengthen preserved muscles, and teach the patient how to function given the effects of injury.[5,6,8,22] Active participation in interdisciplinary rehabilitation has been found to improve functional outcomes following SCI. At a minimum, the interdisciplinary team should include a physiatrist, rehabilitation nurse, physical therapist, occupational therapist, psychologist, and social worker/case manager.[23] The lengths of stay for both acute and subacute inpatient care have been greatly reduced.[11,24,25] Today, inpatient acute care lasts an average of 11 days (reduced from 24 days in the 1970s), and inpatient rehabilitation currently lasts an average of 35 days (reduced from 98 days in the 1970s). Outpatient services can continue from 3 to 12 months following the inpatient rehabilitation stay. This implies that patients may be weaker upon entering rehabilitation and that more of their rehabilitation is conducted in both outpatient and home/community settings than in the past.[24]

Prognosis

In the 1930s, an SCI was more likely to cause a terminal outcome in 80% of cases.[3] Today, an SCI causes great change to an individual's life, but is much less likely to mark the end of life, and many with SCI adapt and find new ways to lead meaningful lives.[3,26] This disparity in both function and mortality can be appreciated by comparing SCI outcomes in developed countries to underdeveloped countries, where outcomes are less positive.[3]

The prognosis of SCI can be inferred by the injury level.[5,13,21] Cervical injuries greatly impact more body functions and thus place individuals at higher risk for medical complications. Patients with lumbar or sacral injuries have better prognoses because they have less motor and sensory loss and lower risk of complications. The NLI is only one metric that impacts prognosis. The age at the time of injury, the extent of injury, the availability and timing of services, and the environment in which the patient lives all contribute to outcomes.[3] The patient's environment includes and is impacted by the physical, social, economic, and attitudinal surroundings. In addition, the patient's pre-injury level of health and functioning, past medical history and comorbidities, concurrent injuries, and physical build and gender all factor into ultimate outcomes.[25,27]

Neural recovery during rehabilitation is common and can result in significant improvement in function.[5] In patients with complete injuries, muscles in the zone of partial preservation strengthen, which may result in significant functional change. Most individuals with tetraplegia regain UE function within one to three motor segments below the initial injury.[5,6,28] This is true especially if a key muscle, such as extensor carpi radialis, strengthens enough to enable the person to extend the wrist and hold objects. Patients with **incomplete injury** have a better prognosis, but their recovery is less predictable than **complete injury.**[28] Most recovery occurs within 3 months of injury, but recovery can continue through 1 year or longer.[20,22,28] The longer that time passes without improvement generally lessens opportunities for improvement.[28] The prognosis for NTSCI is generally less favorable because patients tend to be older with comorbidities and possess less physical reserve.[10,14]

Functional outcomes resulting from SCI are critically important issues for patients and families. Table 39-2 provides an overview of functional outcomes

Table 39-2 Functional Outcomes by Neurological Level of Injury

WHAT ARE MY FUNCTIONAL GOALS?
There is a chart on the following pages that outlines common functional goals. These goals are daily activities that most people can manage with the control of muscle movement that they have with a complete injury. You may be able to do additional activities if you have an incomplete injury or if you regain control of more muscle movement. You will work with your rehab team to set your goals and find ways you can reach your goals. The following is a step-by-step guide to using the chart.

1. Find your level of injury in the Level of Injury column.
2. The Physical Abilities column shows what muscle movement is common for anyone with a complete injury at that level.
3. The Functional Goals column outlines how people might manage typical daily activities based at that level of injury.
4. The Equipment Used column suggests various equipment options that might be useful in accomplishing those functional goals.

LEVEL OF INJURY	PHYSICAL ABILITIES	FUNCTIONAL GOALS	EQUIPMENT USED
C1–C3	C3—Limited movement of head and neck	**Breathing:** Depends on ventilator for breathing	Suction equipment to clear secretions, two ventilators with back-up generator and battery
		Communication: Talking is sometimes difficult, very limited, or impossible. If the ability to talk is limited, communication can be accomplished independently, with adaptive equipment.	Mouth stick and assistive technology (e.g., computer, communication board) for speech or typing
		Daily tasks: Full assistance from caregiver for turning in bed, transfers, and all self-care (including bowel and bladder management). Assistive technology can allow for independence in tasks such as reading a book or newspaper, using a telephone, and operating lights and appliances.	Mouth stick, environmental control unit (ECU)
		Mobility: Can operate an electric wheelchair by using a head control, mouth stick, sip and puff, or chin control. Can also operate a power tilt wheelchair for independent pressure relief.	Power or manual lift, electric or semi-electric hospital bed, power wheelchair with pressure-relieving cushion

(continued)

Table 39-2 Functional Outcomes by Neurological Level of Injury (*continued*)

LEVEL OF INJURY	PHYSICAL ABILITIES	FUNCTIONAL GOALS	EQUIPMENT USED
C3–C4	Usually has head and neck control. At C4 level, may shrug shoulders.	**Breathing:** May initially require a ventilator for breathing; usually adjusts to breathing full time without ventilator assistance.	Cough-assist device
		Communication: Normal.	
		Daily tasks: Individual requires full assistance from a caregiver for turning in bed, transfers, and all self-care (including bowel and bladder management). Individual may be able to use adaptive equipment to eat independently. May also be able to operate an adjustable bed and perform other tasks, such as painting, writing, typing, and using a telephone with assistive technology.	**Eating:** Sandwich holder on a gooseneck, feeder, long straw for liquids **Other activities:** ECU for operating bed (e.g., head or voice activated, mouth stick controller), hands-free devices, mouth stick for typing, etc.
		Mobility: Can operate a power wheelchair using head control, a mouth stick, sip and puff, or chin control. Power tilt function on wheelchair allows for independence with pressure relief.	Power or manual lift, electric or semi-electric hospital bed, power wheelchair with pressure-relieving cushion
C5	Typically has head and neck control, can shrug shoulders, and has some shoulder control. Can bend elbows and turn palms face up.	**Daily tasks:** Individual can be independent with eating and grooming (e.g., face washing, oral care, shaving, makeup application) after setup from caregiver, with specialized equipment. Individuals will require total assistance from caregiver for bed mobility, transfers, and all other self-care. May be able to assist caregiver with upper body dressing and some bathing, with adaptive equipment.	**Eating:** Universal cuff for attachment of utensils, scoop plate, plate guard, long straw **Grooming:** Universal cuff for attachment of tooth brush, comb or brush, adapted or electric razor, makeup applicators; wash mitt for face **Bathing:** Roll-in padded shower and commode chair, or padded transfer tub bench; wash mitt; adapted loofah
		Health care: Individual will require assistance from caregiver for cough assist. Can perform pressure relief with power tilt in power wheelchair.	Cough-assist device
		Mobility: May have strength to push a manual wheelchair for short distances over level surfaces; however, a power wheelchair with hand controls will be required for daily activities. At this level, the individual may be able to drive with specialized hand controls in a modified van with a lift, but still may require attendant to assist with transportation.	**Wheelchair:** Power or manual lift, electric or semi-electric hospital bed, power wheelchair with pressure-relieving cushion **Bed:** Bed ladder, thigh straps, and bed rails used for bed mobility

Table 39-2 Functional Outcomes by Neurological Level of Injury (*continued*)

LEVEL OF INJURY	PHYSICAL ABILITIES	FUNCTIONAL GOALS	EQUIPMENT USED
		Bowel and bladder management: Individual requires total assistance from caregiver for bowel and bladder management. Individual may have indwelling catheter, or the caregiver may perform intermittent catheterization for bladder management. Bowel management can be performed with use of specialized equipment or medication.	**Bowel:** Roll-in padded shower and commode chair, or padded transfer tub bench **Bladder:** Leg-bag emptier
C6	Has movement in head, neck, shoulders, arms, and wrists. Can shrug shoulders, bend elbows, turn palms up and down, and extend wrists.	**Daily tasks:** With use of some specialized equipment and setup from a caregiver, an individual can be independent with most feeding, grooming, and upper body dressing. Will still require some assistance for lower body dressing and will be able to assist with upper body during bathing. Can perform sliding board transfers to padded shower commode chair and/or tub bench for toileting and bathing, with some to total assist from caregiver. Can perform some light meal preparation tasks. **Health care:** Can independently perform pressure relief with power tilt and may require some to no assist for forward or lateral lean pressure relief. **Mobility:** An individual may require some to no assist for turning in bed, with use of special equipment. May be able to perform sliding board transfers on level surfaces with some to no assistance from caregiver. Can use an ultra-lightweight manual wheelchair for mobility, but some may use a power wheelchair for greater ease over uneven terrain. Can be independent driving a vehicle from power or manual wheelchair with specialized equipment. **Bowel and bladder management:** Some to total assist with adaptive equipment for management of bowel and bladder.	**Feeding:** Universal cuff, built-up utensils, scoop plate, long straw, plate guard **Grooming:** Universal cuff, adapted electric razor, or toothbrush **Dressing:** Dressing stick, leg lifter, thigh straps, dressing hook splints; adapted or specialized clothing **Bathing:** Adapted loofah, long-handled sponge with universal cuff **Transfers:** Power or manual lift, sliding board, padded drop-arm bedside commode, padded tub bench with cutout, padded shower and commode chair **Bed:** Bed ladder, thigh straps, bed rails **Wheelchair:** Wheelchair pegs, specialized wheelchair gloves, and rubber tubing on wheels. Also, power-assist wheels can be used for independence with manual wheelchair propulsion. **Transportation:** Modified van with lift, specialized hand controls, tie-downs **Bowel:** Digital stimulation splint device, enema insertion device **Bladder:** Catheter inserter, penis positioner, thigh spreader with mirror

(*continued*)

Table 39-2 Functional Outcomes by Neurological Level of Injury (*continued*)

LEVEL OF INJURY	PHYSICAL ABILITIES	FUNCTIONAL GOALS	EQUIPMENT USED
C7–T1	Has movement similar to C6 level, with the added ability to straighten elbows. At the C8–T1 level, has added strength and precision of hands and fingers.	**Daily tasks:** Independent with all feeding, grooming, and upper body dressing, with equipment. Individuals may require some to no assistance with lower body dressing and bathing with equipment. Can perform sliding board transfers with some to no assistance to padded shower commode chair and/or tub bench for toileting and bathing.	**Feeding:** Universal cuff, built-up handles, curved utensils, long straw, plate guard, adapted techniques for grasp **Grooming:** Universal cuff, splint material to adapt devices **Dressing:** Leg lifter, dressing stick, zipper pull, hooks-on shoes **Bathing:** Adapted loofah, long-handled sponge with universal cuff **Transfers:** Sliding board, padded drop-arm bedside commode, padded tub bench with cutout, padded shower and commode chair
		Health care: Independent with wheelchair pushup or lateral lean for pressure relief.	
		Mobility: Independent with manual wheelchair propulsion and level surface sliding board transfers. Some assistance may be required from caregiver for uphill transfers. Can be independent with driving if able to load and unload wheelchair.	**Wheelchair:** Rigid or folding lightweight wheelchair, wheelchair pegs, wheelchair gloves **Transportation:** Hand controls, modified van if unable to perform transfer or load–unload chair
		Bowel and bladder management: Depending on hand function, some to total assist for bowel management, with use of adaptive equipment or medication. Can be independent or need some assist for bladder management with intermittent catheterization or condom catheter.	**Bowel:** Digital stimulation splint device, enema insertion device, toileting aid **Bladder:** Catheter inserter household (for men), thigh spreader with mirror (for women)
T2–T12	Has normal motor function in head, neck, shoulders, arms, hands, and fingers. Has increased use of rib and chest muscles, or trunk control. At the T10–T12 level, more improvements in trunk control because of increase in abdominal strength.	**Daily tasks:** Independent with all self-care, including bowel and bladder management, with adaptive equipment if necessary.	**Dressing:** Thigh straps, reacher, dressing stick, sock aid **Bathing:** Long-handled sponge **Transfers:** Sliding board, padded drop-arm bedside commode, padded tub bench with cutout, padded shower/commode chair **Bowel/bladder:** Mirror
		Health care: Independent with wheelchair pushup for pressure relief.	
		Mobility: Independent with all bed mobility and transfers, with or without use of equipment. Independent with wheelchair propulsion on uneven and even surfaces and up and down curbs. Able to load and unload wheelchair independently for driving with hand controls.	**Wheelchair:** Ultra-lightweight wheelchair **Transfers:** Sliding board, leg straps **Transportation:** Hand controls

Table 39-2 Functional Outcomes by Neurological Level of Injury (*continued*)

LEVEL OF INJURY	PHYSICAL ABILITIES	FUNCTIONAL GOALS	EQUIPMENT USED
L1–L5	Has additional return of motor movement in the hips and knees.	**Mobility:** Independent with all bed mobility and transfers with or without use of equipment. Independent with wheelchair propulsion on uneven and even surfaces and up and down curbs. Ambulation possible with use of specialized leg braces and walking devices. Functionality of ambulation depends on strength and movement in legs. Individuals' ability to ambulate depends primarily on their level household distances. Individuals may use a wheelchair for community mobility. Able to load and unload wheelchair independently for driving with hand controls.	**Wheelchair:** Ultra-lightweight wheelchair if necessary **Walking:** Leg braces that extend to the hip, the knee, or just the ankle/foot and varying assistive devices **Transportation:** Hand controls
S1–S5	Depending on the level of injury, various degrees of return of voluntary bladder, bowel, and sexual function	**Mobility:** Increased ability to walk with fewer to no bracing or assistive devices	**Walking:** Braces that support the ankle/foot

From *"Understanding Spinal Cord Injury: Part 2—Recovery and Rehabilitation"* was developed by Phil Klebine, M.A.; Olivia Smitherman, M.O.T.R./L.; and Laney Gernenz, P.T. in collaboration with the Model Systems Knowledge Translation Center.

Source: Portions of this document were adapted from materials developed by the UAB SCI Model System, Northwest Regional SCI System, Southeastern Regional Spinal Cord Injury Care System, Rocky Mountain Regional Spinal Injury System, and Paralyzed Veterans of America Consortium for Spinal Cord Medicine.

by neurological level. When clinicians are asked about patient outcomes, it is important to be factual but hopeful and make clear that many factors can impact ultimate outcomes.[5] The information widely disseminated about SCI outcomes are to be viewed as general guides only, not as final dictates. Best practice in this regard is to encourage open discussion of progress and possible outcomes as often as needed, acknowledge the fear and grief that the patient and families are experiencing, and provide for measured yet realistic hope for the future.[5]

Secondary Conditions

There are numerous secondary conditions associated with SCI.[5,13] The occupational therapist must understand the etiology and effect of these secondary conditions on function, as well as the unique contribution of occupational therapy services provided as part of a comprehensive interprofessional rehabilitation team.

Spinal Stabilization

Spinal surgery is indicated on an individual basis, depending on the level and severity of SCI, the mechanism of injury, and the extent of compression.[5] Closed reduction is a less invasive option to achieve spinal alignment, and realignment of the cervical spine is attempted using skeletal traction or via halo ring or cranial tongs.[13] Traction is typically begun with little weight and is gradually increased.[5]

If closed reduction is not an option, or when a progressive neurological deficit is present, spinal surgery is indicated.[13] Spinal surgery can involve reducing or realigning the spinal elements, decompressing compromised neural tissue, and/or stabilizing the spine.[5] Surgical goals include spinal stabilization, decreased pain, and a quicker return to activity.[1,5] Surgery can also serve to improve neurological recovery.

Following surgery, the use of a spinal orthosis may be ordered.[5] The spinal orthosis limits spinal motion; stabilizes, supports, and realigns the spine; and protects it after trauma and surgery. The duration of use may vary, but a spinal orthosis is generally worn for 10 to 12 weeks following spinal surgery. Spinal orthoses are named for body regions stabilized. Movement restrictions and discomfort are to be expected as braces and orthoses must be snug fitting. The spinal orthosis may make activities of daily living (ADLs) more cumbersome and should be monitored to ensure that it is not causing pressure areas on insensate skin.

Paralysis and Loss of Sensation

As noted earlier, much of SCI care is directed at the prevention of complications.[1] With the loss of active movement, there is risk of the development of joint stiffness and contractures.[5,9] Because loss of feeling is often associated with SCI, care must be taken to protect insensate areas at all times. It is possible to incur injury without awareness, which can aggravate other complications and cause needless progression of injury. Osteoporosis or bone loss is a complication of SCI caused, in part, by the lack of weight bearing.[5] As a result, fractures can occur unexpectedly with routine activities. Great care should be utilized at all times with regard to paralyzed extremities.

Respiration

Many patients with SCI have compromised breathing, but the extent to which breathing is impacted is directly related to the NLI.[5] Cervical injury, with regard to respiration, is the most involved. Patients with high cervical injuries will undergo **tracheostomy** early in the acute phase of care to provide for mechanical ventilation.[13] Patients with injures of C4 or lower may require tracheostomy depending on their age, comorbidities, or the extent of other injuries.

There are many muscles involved in breathing, and their innervations fall at different levels of the spinal column.[5] As a result, injuries above the level of T12 may involve some degree of respiratory compromise. The diaphragm is innervated at the level of C3–C5. The intercostals are innervated at the levels of T1–T11. The abdominal muscles are innervated at T6–T12, and various accessory muscles are innervated at the cervical or cranial nerve level. Ventilation is primarily as a result of the function of the diaphragm, the cervical accessory muscles, and the external intercostals. Cough is mainly a function of the abdominal muscles and the internal intercostals. When the chest does not expand during inspiration, vital capacity is lessened. With impaired sympathetic function, secretions are increased with accompanying bronchoconstriction. Vocal cord paralysis, tracheostomy, neck orthoses, and anterior surgical approaches can impair swallowing and cause aspiration, which can further impair breathing capacity.[5]

Autonomic Dysreflexia

Autonomic dysreflexia (AD), a sudden dangerous increase in blood pressure, is a possible life-threatening complication associated with lesions at the T6 level or above.[5,29] AD is brought on by an unopposed sympathetic response to noxious stimuli and does not occur until after spinal shock. Some of the more common causes of AD are distended bladder, urinary tract or other infection, bladder or kidney stones, fecal impaction, pressure ulcers, ingrown toenails, invasive procedures such as urinary catheterization or enema, and pain.[29] This condition qualifies as a medical emergency because of the dangerous elevation in blood pressure. AD may be asymptomatic, or it can be recognized by complaints of a pounding headache, profuse sweating and flushing of the skin above the lesion level, piloerection of the skin (goosebumps), blurred vision or spots in visual fields, nasal congestion, and/or feelings of anxiety or apprehension.[5,29]

Orthostatic Hypotension

Orthostatic hypotension (OH) is a sudden drop in blood pressure occurring when a person assumes an upright position.[5] It has been reported that as many as 74% of patients with acute SCIs experience OH, but the condition is less likely in injuries below T6 and incomplete injuries. The cause of OH is believed to be impaired autonomic regulation, specifically related to reflex vasoconstriction. The hypotension is caused by gravitational effects of venous pooling in the LEs and is aggravated by prolonged bed rest (cardiovascular deconditioning). The patient may complain of lightheadedness or dizziness and may faint when transitioning from reclined to upright. OH can be experienced when initially acclimating to a seated position, the tilt table, and/or to standing.[5]

Pressure Injuries

Individuals with SCI are at a high risk for developing pressure injuries.[5,30] Prolonged pressure, as a result of a lack of spontaneous movement and impaired sensation, compresses the skin and underlying muscles, occluding blood supply. Pressure injuries typically develop over bony prominences. The areas most vulnerable to pressure injuries include ischial tuberosities, sacrum, coccyx, greater trochanters, malleoli, knees, occiput, and calcaneous.[30] The causes of pressure injuries include decreased movement, loss or impaired sensation, and changes in the skin as a result of SCI. Prolonged pressure, friction, and shear are forces on the skin that can cause breakdown and ultimately ulceration. Moisture from incontinence and less-than-ideal nutritional status can also contribute to circumstances where pressure injuries can occur. Pressure injuries are a major cause of morbidity, hospitalization, and reduced engagement in activity for individuals with SCI.[5,30] As such, prevention is the best intervention because significant injuries can require surgical intervention and can be a source of serious infection.[5]

Neurogenic Bladder and Bowel

Bowel and bladder function is controlled in the S2–S5 spinal segments.[5] Therefore, all persons with complete lesions at and above the S2–S5 levels lose their ability to void and defecate voluntarily. As a consequence, there is a loss of overriding cortical control of these functions, and management of bowel and bladder function must be intentional.[5] Ultimately, a routine is established, individualized to the needs of each patient, which lessens the impact of these tasks on activities and improves patients' quality of life (QoL).[31,32] Management of the neurogenic bowel and bladder depends on the level and completeness of the injury.[5] For injuries above S2–S4, some level of reflex activity remains; this condition is deemed reflexic or upper motor neuron (UMN) bowel and bladder. If the injury is at or below S2–S4, the bowel and bladder are areflexic and referred to as an LMN bowel and bladder. Incontinence can occur in either instance but is lessened by implementation of a care routine (detailed in the section, Neurogenic Bowel and Bladder).[31,32] The care routine must be continually assessed to assure optimal efficacy for the patient so as to minimize impact on activities and QoL.

Sexual Function

The need for emotional and physical intimacy does not diminish after SCI, but the ways through which an individual with SCI can address these needs do.[5,33] SCI affects both sexual intercourse and reproduction, both of which are determined by the level of injury and its completeness. Most male patients with complete injuries are unable to have voluntary erections and ejaculations. They can, however, have reflex erections that may be facilitated by sensory stimulation. Patients with complete injuries at S2–S5 lose bowel, bladder, and genital reflexes and have a complete loss of erection. Male fertility is decreased after SCI; however, advances in technology provide ways for male patients to sustain an erection and improve the chances of fathering children.[33] Over 80% of men regain some erectile function within 2 years of their SCI.[5]

Sexual and reproductive functioning is less affected in women.[5] The menstrual cycle typically resumes between 6 and 12 months after SCI, and fertility is assumed to be unchanged. As pregnancy advances, a higher level of caregiving assistance may be needed. Premature delivery is relatively common, and because of sensory loss, the signs of impending labor should be regularly monitored after 28 weeks of gestation. Blood pressure must be monitored on an ongoing basis because the risk of AD is higher during this time.[5] Labor is affected depending on the level of injury, particularly with injuries above T10.[13] Most women with SCI have atypical labor symptoms and deliver by cesarean section with greater frequency.

Temperature Regulation

Related to disrupted autonomic function, particularly with injuries above T8, individuals with SCI have difficulty regulating their temperature, a condition referred to as poikilothermia.[12,34] As a consequence, their internal temperature acclimates to that of their surroundings, and care must be taken to avoid overheating, core cooling, and exposure to the elements.

Pain

Pain is a significant concern for patients with SCI[5] and can be related to acute injuries or can be chronic in nature (pain that has endured more than 6 months).[16] There are several causes for pain, and its presence greatly impacts QoL.[5] Musculoskeletal pain is described as dull and aching and is often caused by overuse in the UEs related to wheelchair propulsion. Visceral pain is described as cramping or tenderness and may be generalized. This type of pain is due to a visceral cause and can include fecal impactions, bowel obstruction, or gallstones. Neuropathic pain feels like burning, tingling, or shocking and can be related to damage to the spinal cord near the injury level. Pain is estimated to affect as high as 80% of patients with SCI.[5,34] Shoulder pain is estimated in 30% to 70% of individuals with SCI.[5] Studies vary greatly in estimating the prevalence of chronic pain, with the reported range of pain being 26% to 96%, regardless of SCI completeness and level.[35]

Fatigue and Sleep Disturbance

Many individuals with SCI experience difficulty with sleep and associated fatigue.[13,36] This phenomenon is not fully understood because there are many possible causes. Disordered sleep may be associated with the actual SCI and its consequences, or with the associated treatment, such as frequent repositioning for pressure relief, or bowel or bladder care. Additional causes could be infection, respiratory or cardiac failure, medication side effects, or depression.[5] Fatigue can impact the individual's ability to participate in his or her care and engage in activities. Individuals with SCI also have a higher incidence of sleep apnea.[5,36]

Changes in Muscle Tone

Spasticity is a motor disorder related to UMN syndrome.[5,12] It is characterized by a velocity-dependent resistance to passive range of motion (PROM) owing to exaggerated stretch reflexes.[12] Spasticity includes an increase in muscle tone, involuntary muscle spasms, and **clonus.**[5] The appearance of spasticity follows spinal shock days to weeks following injury, and 50% to 75% of individuals with SCI report spasticity.

Spasticity can be worsened by noxious stimuli, many of the same stimuli that can trigger AD.[5,37] Spasticity can be painful and limit mobility and ROM. As a result, spasticity can impair independence in ADLs and can make assisting patients difficult. Some spasticity can be functionally helpful, but effective management often proves challenging. Spasticity can lead to complications such as joint contractures, subluxations, and pressure ulcers.[5,37] By contrast, in LMN (areflexic) injuries, below the level of the spinal cord, the LEs remain flaccid.[21]

Thromboembolism

Thromboembolism (a blood vessel obstructed by a clot dislodged from another region), which includes deep vein thrombosis (DVT) and pulmonary embolus, is a common complication and accounts for significant morbidity and mortality in patients with SCI.[13] The signs and symptoms of DVT include swelling (typically in the LEs), warmth, and discoloration; patients may also be asymptomatic. DVT can be difficult to detect because chronic leg swelling is common following SCI because of the loss of mobility and venous status, and pain perception impairment due to the spinal injury.[38] As a result, the condition can be extensive before it is detected. A pulmonary embolus is a clot that has traveled to the lungs.[5,13] This condition presents with dyspnea, tachycardia, fever, or chest pain.[5] Owing to the gravity of this condition, thromboprophylaxis is initiated immediately in the care of SCI.[38] Thromboembolism occurs more frequently in paraplegia, older patients with SCI, complete SCI, and when there are concurrent fractures of the LEs and pelvis.

Psychosocial Adaptation

SCI, independent of its severity, is an emotionally traumatic event. In the days following injury and often during acute rehabilitation, paralysis, multiple medical problems, and the need to rely on others for basic functions can be overwhelming.[26] Patients and families may experience a myriad of feelings, such as confusion, anxiety, loss, hope, grief, depression, and helplessness.[19,26] Most people with SCI adapt well with time and reintegrate into their communities.[26] Many factors influence SCI psychological outcomes.[19,26] Premorbid lifestyle and interests, personality and coping styles, fewer medical complications, and the degree of social and economic support all contribute to outcomes. Weaknesses in any of these areas place individuals at risk for developing psychological syndromes, such as anxiety or depressive disorder, substance abuse, and a suicide rate five times higher than the general public.[26]

Medical Management

This section briefly describes the medical management of the secondary conditions noted in the previous section, with special emphasis on aspects that impact the services and contributions that occupational therapists make to patient care.

Paralysis and Impaired Sensation

Paralysis and a lack of sensation are the most common results of SCI. The therapist must be aware of the implications of these impairments to provide a safe therapeutic environment and educate patients about how to manage these concerns for optimal health maintenance.[7] Care in this regard involves proper positioning; early mobilization by active, active assisted, or passive means; and splints or orthotics to prevent contracture and loss of joint ROM.[5,9] Transitioning to an upright position as soon as medically tolerated conditions the cardiovascular system and permits the patient to engage in activities and socialization.[5] Daily visual inspection of the skin to identify reddened areas or bruising should be completed to compensate for the loss of sensation.[5,30] This task should become part of ADL routines, and the occupational therapist is a natural provider to reinforce this practice as a preventative and health maintenance activity.[7]

Respiration

Respiratory complications, specifically pneumonia, have been identified as the leading cause of death in the first year after SCI.[11] The occupational therapist typically does not provide care in this area but must be aware of possible difficulties and symptoms and should reinforce breathing interventions in daily routines.[20]

The goal of respiratory care is to maximize breathing, improve coughing ability, and minimize complications.[20] High tetraplegics require mechanical ventilation, and the occupational therapist must become familiar with these devices. Patients requiring long-term ventilator use will likely have a tracheostomy.[5,36] Suctioning may be required to clear secretions from the airway.[5] Nebulized medications (breathing treatments) may be used to improve breathing. The use of a rotating bed assists with postural drainage of fluids in the lungs. Respiratory and physical therapists may implement assisted coughs (like the Heimlich Maneuver, a forceful thrust to the abdomen while the patient attempts to cough); chest percussion, vibration, or cupping to break up secretions; or mechanical insufflation or exsufflation that provides for a machine-facilitated deep breath.[5,20] Physical therapists work with patients to strengthen the muscles associated with breathing and teach self-coughing. Patients may undergo the insertion of a phrenic nerve stimulator that provides an electrical stimulation to cause the diaphragm to contract to improve breathing.[20,36]

Occupational therapists can contribute to respiratory care by remaining vigilant related to positioning of the patient. The best seated position for breathing begins with an anterior pelvic tilt, an upright trunk, and a neutral head and neck.[20] Diaphragmatic breathing should be encouraged, and the patient's pattern of breathing should be noted including chest and diaphragm excursion, and the contraction of neck muscles so that variances can be identified.[20] In addition, adherence to proper infection control standards is important for respiratory care to minimize exposure to risks.

Autonomic Dysreflexia

The occupational therapist should be mindful of the symptoms of AD and, if the symptoms appear, respond immediately to this medical emergency.[5] If the eliciting cause of the AD can be identified, often of a urinary nature, it should be addressed. Medications can be administered to lower blood pressure.[13] Sitting the patient upright may lower blood pressure by venous pooling in the LEs. Any restrictive clothing should be loosened. Emergency attention should be sought if these interventions do not resolve the AD.

Orthostatic Hypotension

Medically, OH or postural hypotension can be managed by reviewing the medications utilized and their hypotensive effects.[5] Additional measures can be included in the daily routine to attempt to minimize OH. Simple routine-related interventions such as assuring adequate hydration and attending to the timing of meals related to activity can lessen the risk of OH (blood flow is diverted to the gut for digestion, making OH a higher risk after meals). Exercise later in the day may be tolerated better than early in the morning. Gradual elevation of the bed while sleeping may foster tolerance to the upright position, leading incrementally to longer periods of tilt table use, sitting upright in a reclining or tilt-in-space chair, using a standard wheelchair, and possible standing. Rapid position changes should be avoided as well as exercise in a hot environment. Abdominal binders and compression stockings are often used to increase venous pressure and decrease venous pooling in the LEs.[5,38]

Pressure Injuries

One of the main interventions in the prevention of pressure injuries is the implementation of routine positions changes.[5,30] This is begun in the emergency department with position changes every 2 hours as medical condition allows[19,30] and can involve pressure reduction mattresses. Efforts should be made to control skin exposure to moisture and heat, for example, changing clothing after incontinence. Shearing forces should be minimized during repositioning. Positioning with the use of pillows and other positioning aids to elevate (unweight) bony prominences should be part of routine care. Patients and their caregivers should be educated to visually inspect their insensate skin daily for areas of pressure.[5,30] Ideally, there will be no reddened areas enduring more than 15 minutes. If so, adjustment of the pressure redistribution regime may be indicated.

When the patient is strong enough, a weight-shifting schedule should be implemented and trained to be spontaneously completed.[30] It is recommended that every 30 minutes, at least 1 to 2 minutes is offloaded or unweighted. This can be done by weight-shifting forward or side to side, or by wheelchair push-ups. For patients who cannot weight shift manually, a tilt-in-space or reclining wheelchair may be indicated to provide pressure relief.

The prescription of a wheelchair seating system, customized to the needs of the individual, is recommended with the goals of redistributing pressure; minimizing shear; and providing comfort, stability, and mobility.[30] Specific body measurements are taken to facilitate proper prescription of the wheelchair seating system. Pressure mapping of the seated positions may be conducted to identify areas of high pressure and permit customization of the wheelchair seating system.[5] Wheelchair cushions are prescribed to assist with pressure distribution, and options include foam, gel, air, and alternating air. Regular assessment of the system's efficacy is important to insure ongoing efficacy of pressure relief.

Neurogenic Bowel and Bladder

Care of bowel and bladder function is generally a primary task of nursing, but the occupational therapist can be involved in training these new habits and adapting techniques to meet patient abilities.[31,32] Bowel and bladder regimens are individualized to each patient's unique needs and circumstances. The loss of cortical control, dyscoordination of sphincter function, and lack of sensation of the need to void, all imply the use of different techniques as part of the individualized routine. Factors impacting routines include the level and severity of injury, lifestyle, dexterity, caregiver willingness and ability, diet, and activity levels. Diligence to the established routine, and ongoing monitoring for effectiveness and side effects, should be considered as important as all other bowel and bladder care tasks.[31,32]

There are two bowel function scenarios that relate to the presence of bowel reflexes.[31] A reflexic bowel is the result of a cervical or thoracic SCI. Cortical control of the elimination process is lost due to the SCI, but the spinal reflexes continue to function. Reflex peristalsis provides for stool movement through the colon to the rectum, which can cause a reflex bowel movement. At other times, the anal sphincter is tight/spastic and requires digital or manual stimulation, or stimulant medications or enemas to relax and permit evacuation. For a UMN or reflexive bowel, a bowel training program includes defecation every 1 to 3 days at the same time each day.[5,31]

An areflexic or LMN bowel occurs with SCI to the lumbar or sacral sections, or to the nerve roots.[31] In this case, peristalsis is impaired, and there is no to little reflexive control over the anal sphincter. Here, the need to defecate is not appreciated and must be facilitated by mechanical stimulation and manual evacuation of the rectum. The areflexic bowel requires more facilitating of stool movement using the **Valsalva maneuver**, abdominal massage, seated push-ups, and leaning and forward-bending at the waist. Consistency in routine remains important, and bowel training is implemented daily to minimize incontinence.[5]

Both bowel care routines are ideally completed from a seated position over a commode.[31,32] Both require stimulation of the rectum to permit stool to pass. This can be done using one or two fingers if the patient has sufficient dexterity, or with a dil stick (a specialized device for this purpose). Mirrors and lighting may need to be arranged to facilitate task completion to compensate for sensory loss, and the occupational therapist can provide support in this area.

As with the bowel program, the goal of the bladder program is to achieve a simple and effective routine that minimizes the risk of complications, reduces incontinence, and permits engagement in valued activities.[5,32] Recurring urinary tract infection is a frequent complication and the most frequent cause of rehospitalization after SCI.[5] To avoid complications, patients must empty their bladder fully and routinely, and some of the options below provide for better emptying than other methods.

There are several options for managing the bladder, and the entry-level occupational therapist must have an understanding of each so as to support the patient's successful engagement in the task.[32] **Catheterization** can be done intermittently, usually at 4- to 6-hour intervals, or as needed.[32] Urine is drained through the catheter into the commode or a collection bag. This method is associated with fewer complications and is more convenient than indwelling catheterization where the catheter can remain in place for 2 to 4 weeks, but a collection device for the urine is needed (such as a leg bag). Indwelling catheters are associated with higher rates of infection. Reflex voiding (spontaneous voiding) is an option for males and utilizes a condom catheter that is connected to a leg or other type bag to collect urine. The **Crede method** and **Valsalva technique** can assist with bladder emptying, but are not effective at completely emptying the bladder. There are additional surgical and pharmacological interventions to assist with managing bladder function, but are beyond the scope of this chapter. The advanced options are generally utilized if traditional methods are chronically ineffective. With bowel and bladder training, the occupational therapist may assist in the management of clothing, practicing the bowel or bladder care routine in varied environments and circumstances, and modifying activities if the patient has additional needs caused by cognitive or perceptual deficits.[32]

Bladder care is classified in a similar manner, UMN (reflexive) and LMN (areflexive).[32] Intermittent catheterization is the preferred method of managing urinary function, but this implies that the patient has sufficient hand function to self-catheterize or has a caregiver willing to complete the task.

Diet and fluid intake and activity levels impact bowel and bladder care.[31,32] Complications related to bowel care include constipation, fecal impaction, diarrhea, rectal bleeding, and hemorrhoids.[5] For complicated and persistent bowel and bladder issues, medications, injections, and surgical options may be considered.[31,32] **Functional electrical stimulation (FES)** involves electrical stimulation of the nerve roots to cause contraction of muscles involved in bowel and bladder function and is also an option to improve routines.[20]

Sexual Function

The entry-level occupational therapist likely does not possess sufficient expertise to educate patients in the area of sexual function, but certainly can be alert to patients' readiness to learn more in this area.[5] Experienced occupational therapists may function as part of an interdisciplinary team specializing in sexual functioning and can facilitate candid discussion about the topic. If this expertise is not readily available, a referral for specialized providers may be appropriate. In this context, the role of the occupational therapist is to address varied individual needs such as grooming activities to improve appearance or to find equipment to either compensate for lack of hand function or to help with position to facilitate physical contact.[39] When addressing sexual function issues, the therapist must be particularly sensitive to the needs of the individual and discuss issues in a factual and nonjudgmental way.[5,33] In the ideal situation, counseling is offered to couples, the patient and the partner, to help both work through the complex issues related to intimacy.[33]

Temperature Regulation

The occupational therapist has a natural role in educating patients and caregivers to be aware of environmental conditions that can impact patients' impaired ability to regulate their internal temperature.[7] The occupational therapist provides education about the selection of clothing appropriate to environmental conditions, the importance of avoiding temperature extremes, and the protection of skin from environmental exposure (heat or cold).

Pain

Musculoskeletal pain is managed in a similar manner to individuals without SCI.[13] Joint protection, rest, flexibility, and strengthening exercises are prescribed for overuse injuries.[5,26] Splinting, home modifications, and alternate techniques may be introduced to facilitate healing.[5] Medications are utilized for neuropathic pain, but efficacy is inconsistent.[5,26] Visceral pain is also addressed by treating the underlying cause. Pain can impact function and the patient's ability or willingness to engage in rehabilitation.

Fatigue and Sleep Disturbance

Rest and sleep are identified as part of the occupational therapy scope of practice.[7] The occupational therapist can help to facilitate restorative rest and sleep by considering activity levels; modifying behaviors to facilitate restful sleep such as limiting screen time or liquid intake prior to bed time; and by evaluating the sleep environment for variables such as temperature, noise, and interruptions.

Changes in Muscle Tone

An injury to the spinal cord often results in an increase in transmission within the synaptic stretch reflex, causing spasticity.[5] Spasticity develops into clonic or tonic spasms triggered by sensory stimuli, such as sudden touch, infection, or other irritation. Management of spasticity is important in maximizing a patient's functional independence. Severe spasticity may hinder function.[37] For example, the hypertonicity of the hip and knee adductors can make donning pants difficult.

Medications are prescribed to manage spasticity and often include baclofen, dantrolene, and benzodiazepines, such as diazepam or clonazepam.[37] An intrathecal pump, a method of continual baclofen administration into the spinal canal, or motor point/nerve blocks (which provide temporary reduction in spasticity in specific muscles) may be used in severe cases.[12,37] Spasticity can lead to contractures necessitating attention to proper positioning in bed and in the wheelchair. Additional interventions can include ROM exercise, splinting, and weight-bearing activities.[5,13,37]

Thromboembolism

Thromboembolism is treated with blood thinning medications (heparin and warfarin).[5,38] Mobilization should occur as soon as is feasible after the SCI to lessen the risk of thromboembolism.[13] Compression stockings and pneumatic compression sleeves are used to improve venous return and limit venous pooling.[5,13,38] Combining the abovementioned methods has been found to be effective in the prevention of thromboembolism.[38] The use of vena cava filters is an option for patients with anticoagulation medication contraindication.[5,38]

The occupational therapist can contribute to the care of DVTs by observing for asymmetry in the LEs in color, size, and/or temperature. It is also noteworthy that an anticoagulant side effect is blood thinning, which can cause excessive bleeding in even minor injuries.[38]

Heterotopic Ossification

Heterotopic ossification (HO) is the pathological formation of bone in the soft tissues around the joints.[5] HO has been recorded in 25% to 30% of patients with SCI. HO typically appears 1 to 4 months after injury and presents as localized swelling and redness, fever, and/or loss of ROM. HO is most often seen in the hip (80%–90%), knee, elbow, and shoulder joints. Preventative interventions include nonsteroidal anti-inflammatory drugs (NSAIDs), attention to positioning in bed and in the wheelchair, and daily ROM.

Psychosocial Adaptation

The complexity and ramifications of SCI can leave the patient at risk for depression, post-traumatic stress disorder (PTSD), anxiety, substance abuse, and suicide.[26] Routine and ongoing screening is indicated and should include attention to biological, social, and psychological factors.[40] An antidote to these risks is active engagement in rehabilitation and social activities, as participation fosters mastery of new skills, growth, and self-efficacy, including better rehabilitation outcomes.[4,6,26]

Antidepressant medications may be used to manage psychological conditions when function is impaired.[40] The occupational therapist can share valuable observations about the efficacy of the prescribed pharmacological interventions and provide guidance and support to patients as their new reality is realized.[4,6] The occupational therapist may also reinforce cognitive–behavioral therapy strategies during patient interactions, help to educate families and caregivers, and work with patients in groups to foster socialization with peers.[5,26] When environmental or social concerns are identified in the patient with SCI, the occupational therapist may facilitate referrals for social work, rehabilitation counseling, or case management for additional support.

Polytrauma

Given the violent nature of traumatic SCI, it is common that the patient may have additional injuries that complicate outcomes.[5] The occupational therapist must pay particular attention to precautions and activity restrictions related to injuries. About 15% to 60% of patients with SCI have a concomitant traumatic brain injury (TBI). A TBI adds medical complexity and heightens issues with frustration, concentration, memory, and behaviors that can impair new learning.

Functional Impairment in Daily Occupations

SCI is incurable, and treatment is limited to minimizing secondary complications and maximizing remaining functional capabilities.[1] The SCI levels have been mapped to the functional expectations of injury at those levels. Although the mapping is generally accurate, functional outcomes ultimately depend on several variables including the completeness of the injury, the patient's age, preinjury function and health, past medical history and comorbidities, concurrent injuries, and psychosocial well-being.[25] For more detailed explanation of functional outcomes, refer to the section on Evaluation and Intervention of Functional Skill Deficits Secondary to Spinal Cord Injury and Table 39-2.

Evaluation and Intervention of Functional Skill Deficits Secondary to Spinal Cord Injury

The occupational therapy evaluation permits an understanding of the patient's baseline functional level, goals, and values.[41] The evaluation process also provides a method for measuring progress and gathering information to project outcomes.[41] Inherent to this process is the establishment and cultivation of the therapeutic relationship between the client and occupational therapist, where the occupational therapist leverages "therapeutic use of self" to facilitate the client's understanding of the implications of injury to his or her personal goals, valued activities, and roles.[7]

The Initial Occupational Therapy Evaluation

Completion of the comprehensive occupational therapy initial evaluation may require multiple interactions with the patient owing to the chaotic nature of transition in care.[7] If the client is not able to fully participate, valuable information may be gathered from caregivers or family members. In general, all evaluation follows a basic process, including a review of the medical record, meeting and interviewing the client to gather data about problems of concern, observation of functional activities with an evaluation of component skills, and analysis and summarization of the data.[42] Special attention must always be given to identify and adhere to prescribed activity or medical precautions, which are typically identified in the medical record.

Occupational therapy evaluations consider similar content areas, but the specific characteristics of focus vary by the needs of the client, the practice setting, and the therapist's practice model.[43] Areas of concern to the occupational therapist include ADLs, instrumental activities of daily living (IADLs), occupations (noted later), client factors, and body functions; client habits, roles, and routines; the impact of culture, spirituality, social support, and the environment on function; and specific performance skills.[43] The evaluation process may include the use of standardized and/or nonstandardized assessments.[7] Evaluation may proceed formally or informally. These considerations are encompassed in the two-part occupational therapy evaluation process that includes the occupational profile and the analysis of occupational performance.

Occupational Profile

The occupational profile section of the assessment provides information about the patient's occupational history, activity patterns, interests, values, and needs.[7] These data inform the client-centered perspective by acknowledging the client's priorities and providing a picture for the therapist of what the client's life was like prior to injury. With time, a deeper appreciation of the client's occupational profile is gained, prompting ongoing evaluation and refinement of goals throughout the occupational therapy process. There are many assessment instruments that can guide the gathering of this information, and use varies by facility and guiding philosophies.[43] Commonly noted assessments include the Canadian Occupational Performance Measure (COPM)[44] and the Occupational Performance History Interview Second Version (OPHI-II).[45]

Evaluation of Performance Skills

Occupational performance is the completion of occupations within the context of client factors, the occupational setting or environment, and the activity itself.[7] Client factors include the client's beliefs, values, and spirituality; and his or her body structures and functions. Body structures include vision and cardiovascular status (and the impact of these on the client's functional ability). Body functions include memory, ROM, and cognition. The client's contexts and environments are viewed from multiple perspectives, including the physical environment (architecture and accessibility), cultural influences (role in family structure), personal or demographic aspects (education level), temporal context (life span development issues), and virtual context (interactions that occur absent from physical contact). Activities or occupations within the scope of occupational therapy practice include ADLs, IADLs, rest and sleep, education, work, play, leisure, and social participation.[7]

The assessment of client factors includes UE ROM, strength, muscle tone, and sensation.[7] The therapist also observes the patient's endurance, transfer ability to and from varied heights and places, trunk balance, bed mobility, sensation, muscle tone, and pain. The MMT[46] is most widely used to measure strength. The Functional

Independence Measure (FIM)[47] is often used for grading the level of assistance required for ADLs. The Spinal Cord Independence Measure (SCIM) is a similar tool that provides sufficient sensitivity to demonstrate progress toward goals.[48]

The assessment of hand function is of special interest in tetraplegia levels C5–C8 because the ability to use the hands implies a higher level of independence.[22,27] A dynamometer and pinch meter may be used to measure strength, but some patients will need more sensitive tools to quantify strength and dexterity. Dexterity and grasp ability can be observed through manipulative tasks and the use of assessments such as the Sollerman Hand Function Test[49]; Graded Redefined Assessment of Strength, Sensibility, and Prehension (GRASSP)[50]; or the Jebsen Test of Hand Function.[51] Readers are encouraged to refer to assessment indices for a comprehensive index of assessments utilized in occupational therapy evaluation as utilization choices vary.[41]

The connection between evaluation and intervention is the identification of goals.[52] The hallmark of client-centered care is collaborative goal setting between the occupational therapist and client.[25,52] Goals guide the progression in therapy, foster positive coping skills and participation, and yield functional gains.[26,52]

Occupational Therapy Intervention

The manner in which occupational therapy intervention proceeds is client centered and designed to address the results obtained from the evaluation.[7,9] Intervention is influenced by the patient's level and severity of injury, support available, the phase of care (acute care, rehabilitation, outpatient/community), and the phase in the life span.[24,53] For example, a pediatric patient with SCI will need little rehabilitation time addressing home management tasks. Finally, each phase in the life span impacts the nature of SCI rehabilitation. SCI occurring during adolescence heightens the issues of personality development and puberty, and complicates transition to adulthood.[12,54] Patients incurring SCI in their 30s may have a high-priority goal of resuming their parenting role.[7] The greater frequency of SCI in the elderly presents concerns related to slower recovery and discharge planning.[10]

It is now estimated that more than half of SCI rehabilitation is conducted in the outpatient or community setting.[24,55] This shift of care setting implies that certain occupations may or may not be addressed in the early phases of rehabilitation. Medical stabilization, basic ADLs, and preventative measures are the main focus of acute care.[13] Often, occupational therapy in the acute care phase are of short duration and may serve to prepare the patient for the rehabilitation phase. Inpatient rehabilitation will likely explore more ADLs, IADLs, and discharge planning including a home evaluation.[39] Outpatient rehabilitation and beyond will address the occupations of education and work, leisure and play, and community reintegration and accessibility (in addition to those noted earlier). In areas where outpatient services are not available, ongoing rehabilitation services may be conducted through home care or in a transition placement (skilled nursing facility) prior to returning to the home environment. Social participation should be addressed throughout this continuum, but appropriate to the situation. For example, social engagement in the community may be appropriate postrehabilitation once the patient's status has stabilized and new functional routines have been established.

Another way to characterize occupational therapy intervention is by the underlying objective. Five strategies have been identified in all occupational therapy intervention: health promotion, remediation and restoration, maintenance, compensation and adaptation, and prevention. Each of these strategies means different things in each phase of the rehabilitation process. For example, promoting health and preventing isolation by fostering engagement with the environment and care providers in acute SCI rehabilitation is vitally important, and this intervention looks very different when addressing these same objectives in outpatient therapy sessions.

The following sections provide a brief overview of the occupational therapy intervention process addressing the functional capabilities of patients and the key tasks and interventions of therapy at these levels.

Patient with High Tetraplegia: C1–C4

Patients with SCI at C1–C3 have intact functionally relevant musculature of the sternocleidomastoid, cervical paraspinal, and neck accessory muscles.[13] As a consequence, active movement is limited to neck flexion, extension, and rotation. Patients with complete C1–C3 SCI require an external breathing device because their diaphragm is either paralyzed or only partially innervated (C3).[5,13] The most common device for assisted breathing is the ventilator, a pneumatic electric machine that forces room air into the lungs. This device is attached to the patient via tracheostomy.

Patients with SCI at the level of C4 possess function in the upper trapezius and diaphragm musculature, meaning that they can generally elevate the scapula and breathe in.[13] They require support with ventilation during acute care, but typically can be weaned eventually.

People with complete high tetraplegia are paralyzed from the neck down and require a high level of specialized care.[5,9,13] The occupational therapist who works with this population must be comfortable with nursing procedures and ventilators. The rehabilitation team must also be well coordinated, simultaneously caring for the patient and family while providing education in preparation for discharge.

The role of the occupational therapist is limited in the traditional sense because of the involved nature of this injury. Patients with these injuries are dependent in ADLs.[9,28] Occupational therapy may consist of teaching how to direct care, educating and engaging in decision making related to equipment, training in the use of a mouth stick, and exploring assistive technologies for environmental control[13] (Fig. 39-2). Tilt-in-space power wheelchairs are required at this level for mobility and pressure relief and are fitted with high back supports and a chest strap to provide positional security.[9]

Positioning and ROM are important interventions at this phase for the monitoring and prevention of secondary issues, particularly the maintenance of skin integrity and joint mobility.[5,22] To prevent ROM limitations, therapists use positioning techniques and ROM exercises. In bed, most persons with tetraplegia tend to lie with their arms adducted, internally rotated, and with elbows flexed and, over time, are at risk for contracture.[56] Positioning the UEs in either some abduction or external rotation, with elbow extension, within the patient's tolerance, provides passive stretch to the shoulder and UE joints (Fig. 39-3). Hands are fitted with resting hand splints.[9,13] There is also evidence in the literature of using FES with **ergometry** to maintain range, minimize muscle atrophy, and improve cardiovascular health.[22]

ROM to the hand of the patient with tetraplegia is performed in a special way to facilitate tenodesis grasp.[22] Specifically, this includes passive opening of the fingers when the wrist is flexed and closing of the fingers when the wrist is extended (Fig. 39-4A and B). The patient and all caregivers should be taught how to perform

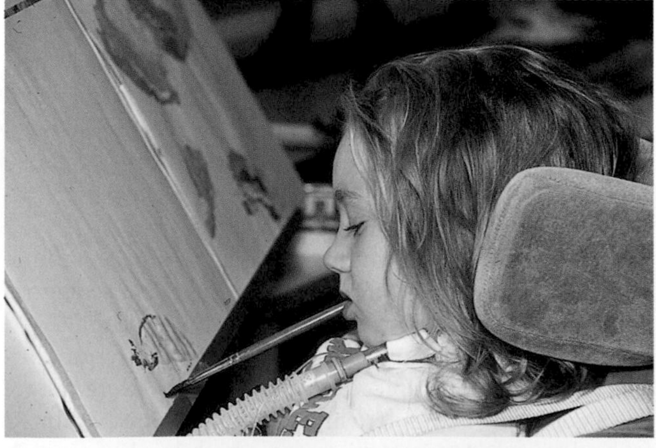

Figure 39-2. A 6-year-old girl with cervical spine injury using a mouth stick–paintbrush to engage in age-appropriate activities. Note the tracheostomy and attachment of portable ventilator and also the head rest on the electric wheelchair.

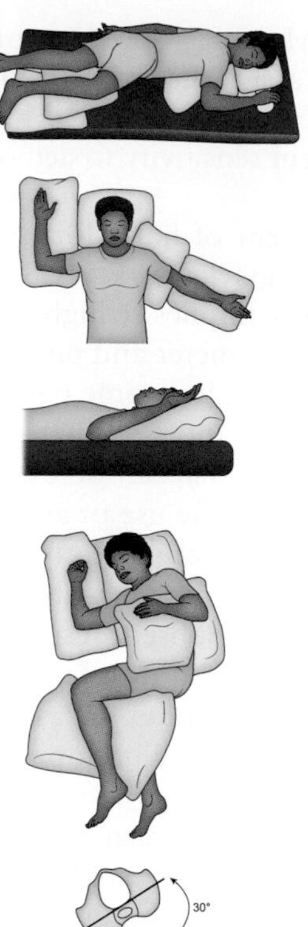

Figure 39-3. Positioning in bed (top image to bottom). Views of prone and supine lying with shoulder abduction and external rotation. Side-lying with alternate upper extremity in shoulder abduction and external rotation with pelvic rotation. (Adapted and reprinted with permission from Paralyzed Veterans of America, Washington, DC.)

ROM exercises to the UEs and hands, and positioning methods to hinder loss of joint mobility.

Patient with Lower Cervical Injuries: C5–C8

The lower the cervical injury, the more strength and function will be preserved in the UEs.[13] Patients with a complete C5 injury possess function in the deltoids, biceps, brachialis, brachioradialis, rhomboids, and part of the serratus anterior. This musculature permits active shoulder flexion, extension, and abduction; elbow flexion and supination; and scapular adduction and abduction. Patients with C5 tetraplegia lack elbow extension, pronation, wrist and hand movement, and trunk and LE movement. Patients with C6 tetraplegia possess scapular protraction, some horizontal adduction, forearm supination, and radial wrist extension. Wrist flexion and elbow extension are absent. At C7–C8, elbow extension, ulnar wrist extension, wrist flexion, finger and thumb flexion and extension, and thumb abduction are present. Dexterity and grasp release are limited, but greater function is possible by virtue of active hand and wrist motion.[13]

Occupational therapy intervention includes positioning, splinting, and exercise as noted earlier, with the addition of strengthening exercises as proximal strength is increased.[28] Strengthening can be performed by

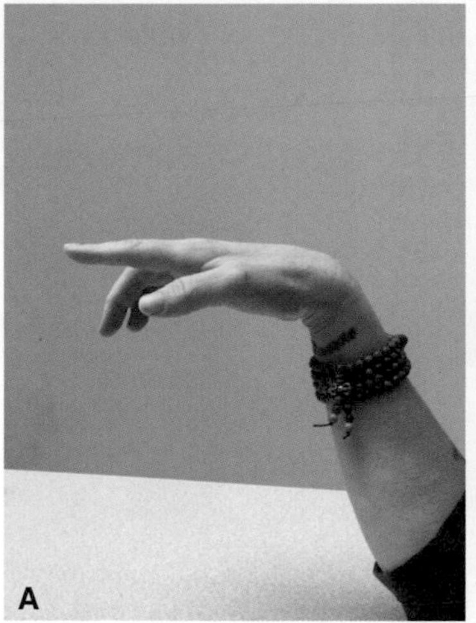

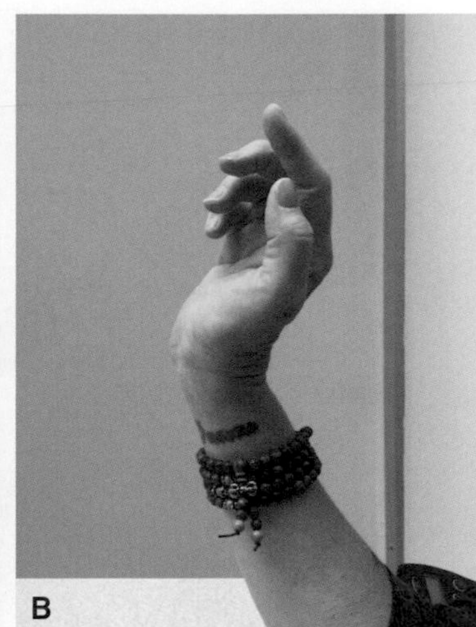

Figure 39-4. Tenodesis grasp. **A.** When the wrist is flexed, the fingers are extended. **B.** When the wrist is extended, the fingers are flexed. (Images courtesy DiSepio Institute, Saint Francis University.)

weights, pulley systems, tabletop skateboards, suspension slings, and mobile arm supports.[20,57] The mobile arm support, also called a ball-bearing feeder, is a mechanical device attached to the wheelchair that carries the weight of the arm and allows distal use of the UEs for task completion.[13,57]

Research has demonstrated that corticomotor reorganization or neuroplasticity can be fostered through mass practice task training, somatosensory stimulation (SS) (low-level continuous electrical stimulation), and FES.[22,58,59] Regimens of intense repetitive UE training using external FES devices or implants ("neuroprosthetic") can facilitate reach-and-grasp activities.[57–59]

Occupational therapists can effectively address patient functioning in the virtual realm and achieve functional goals through mass practice.[7] Video games can be used to provide repetitive motion with the aim of increasing function, particularly in the hands of patients with tetraplegia.[60] Another example is the implementation of compensatory interventions to permit use of a smartphone in patients with tetraplegia.[61] By modifying the environment (setup for phone use), adjusting phone settings, exploring wrist and hand compensatory techniques, using splints, and adapting styli, participation and socialization can be facilitated.[27,61]

Patients with C5 Tetraplegia

Initially, the deltoids and biceps—key muscles for this level of injury—are weak, so upper limbs require support to function.[13] The mobile arm support can assist the patient in driving the wheelchair, feeding, hygiene and grooming, and carrying out tabletop activities, such as writing.[57]

Patients with C5 complete tetraplegia need a way to grasp and hold objects because their wrists and hands are paralyzed.[28] A stable wrist is required for grasp, and this is achieved with a splint or orthosis.[13,20] A universal U- or C-shaped cuff can be secured to items (such as a phone or electric razor) to permit placement on the splinted hand for use[28,39] (Fig. 39-5). Experimentation with alternate grasp patterns should be conducted to permit gross utilization of the hands[27] (Fig. 39-6A to C). To maximize functional gain with any device, the patient must have adequate time and repeated training sessions to strengthen musculature and adopt new movement patterns. Most patients with C5 tetraplegia can master tabletop activities, basic grooming tasks, and can assist with upper body ADLs.[25,28]

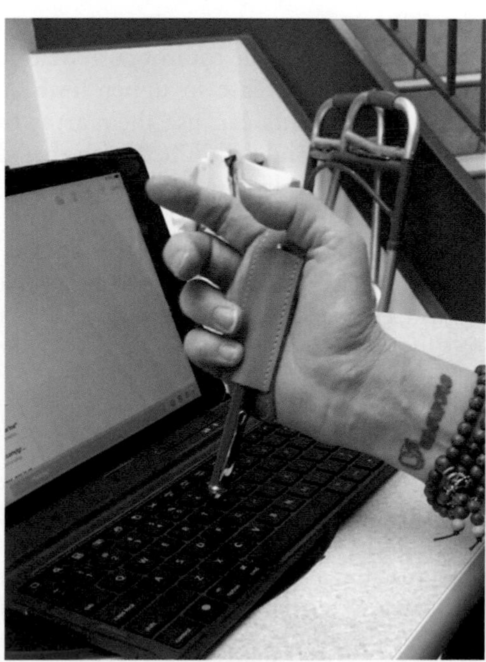

Figure 39-5. Universal cuff to type: using devices to compensate for lack of ability to point and isolate finger movements. (Image courtesy DiSepio Institute, Saint Francis University.)

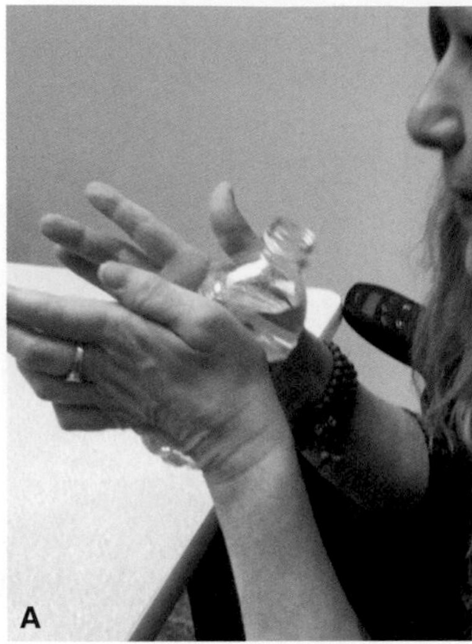

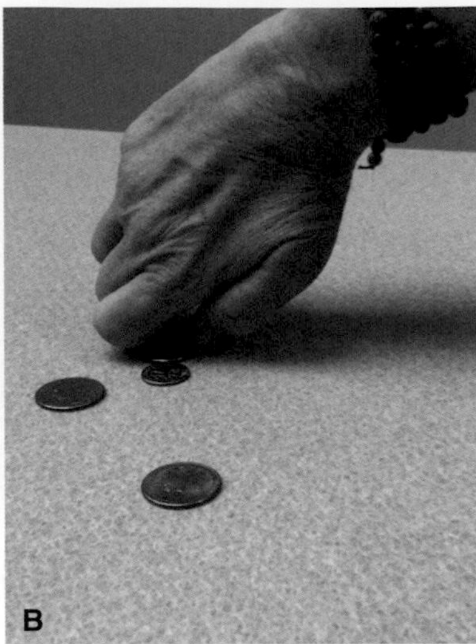

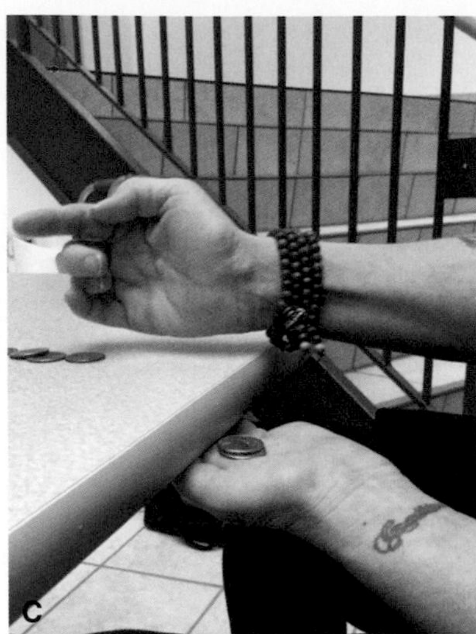

Figure 39-6. Hand compensatory techniques of an individual with incomplete C6 tetraplegia. **A.** Pressing one hand against the other to lift a bottle. **B.** Alternate grasp pattern to pick up coins. **C.** Dragging the coin to the edge of the table in order to pick it up. (Images courtesy DiSepio Institute, Saint Francis University.)

Patients with C6 and C7 Tetraplegia

Patients with C6 and C7 tetraplegia may attain significantly higher levels of independence than those with C5 injury.[5,13,28] The addition of radial wrist extensors allows patients to close their fingers with a tenodesis grasp. A tenodesis grasp allows patients to pick up and hold light objects—a critical functional movement. The wrist-driven wrist–hand orthosis (also called the flexor hinge splint or tenodesis splint) is a metal device that transfers power from the extended wrist to the radial fingers, allowing a stronger pinch.[13,25]

More fully innervated proximal scapular and shoulder muscles, such as the rotator cuff, deltoids, and biceps, allow for an increase in upper limb strength and endurance.[13] Patients can use their arms to cross the midline forcefully and roll in bed with the addition of the clavicular pectoralis muscle.[28] The ability to use the triceps, the key muscle for C7 tetraplegia, allows the patient to reach for objects above head level, transfer with greater ease, and push a manual wheelchair on level surfaces. Generally, upper body ADLs can be completed, but assistance is required for lower body ADLs.

Patients with C8 Tetraplegia

Hand function is significantly improved with the addition of extrinsic finger muscles and thumb flexors, but still lacks dexterity and strength because of the of absence of intrinsic finger and thumb muscles.[13] A patient with complete C8 tetraplegia grasps objects with the metacarpophalangeal joints in extension and the proximal interphalangeal and distal interphalangeal joints in flexion. This is called a claw hand or intrinsic minus hand.[13] Depending on the individual, lower body ADLs, transfers, and bowel and bladder care may require no assistance.[28] Wheelchair propulsion is functional on level surfaces.

Surgical Options for the Upper Extremities

The restoration of hand function is a top priority for all patients with tetraplegia.[22,58,59] Patients with C5, C6, C7, or C8 injuries may have surgical options to provide improved function in the hands.[22,62] Tendon transfer surgeries can be explored after all strength, and recovery has been realized following the SCI. These surgeries involve attaching a tendon from a functioning muscle to one that acts on the hand that is not functioning.[22,62] This is often accompanied by the stabilization of the interphalangeal joint of the thumb and can provide improved use of the hands. The procedure changes the anatomy and function of the hand and requires muscular retraining for grasp and release. The best outcomes are a result of multiple characteristics including target range of SCI level, patient and surgeon characteristics, an absence of spasticity, and investment in postsurgical rehabilitation. It is believed that surgical options are underutilized in SCI rehabilitation.[22,62]

Patient with Paraplegia

Typically, patients with paraplegia have fewer medical complications than those with tetraplegia.[13] The lower the injury level, the greater the trunk strength and ease in resuming ADLs. Discharge from inpatient rehabilitation comes quickly, and ongoing support is offered from and within the community (outpatient services).[24] These interventions often include reassessing routines such as ADLs/IADLs within the context of broader functional environments, facilitating return to school or work, and exploring leisure interests and mobility in the community[7] (Fig. 39-7).

Ambulation

Foremost in the minds of many with SCI is whether the ability to walk will be restored.[13,20] Viewing the SCI as a whole, the simple answer is that very few individuals with SCI will be able to walk again without restriction.[13] Walking potential is mainly determined by the level and completeness of the injury.[13,25] For example, at 1-year postinjury, no patients with ASIA level A (complete) tetraplegia and about 5% of patients with paraplegia can ambulate. The opposite extreme are patients with ASIA level D injuries, 95% of whom achieve community ambulation at discharge from rehabilitation services.[13] Additional factors that impact the ability to walk following SCI include body weight, age, prior ambulation status, UE involvement, and pain.[13]

Ambulation training with patients with complete SCI requires a great deal of effort, expense (orthoses), and energy on the part of patients, and many find the effort unreasonable for function.[20] Ambulation for those with incomplete SCI depends on the motor function below the lesion level; sensory sparing; strength and motor control in the UE, LE, and trunk; age; and the pattern of injury. Gait training may proceed in a more traditional manner utilizing FES, or utilizing robotics to support body weight while on a treadmill, and typically involves orthotics and assistive devices.[20]

The ability to ambulate has been classified in four ways, which is also pertinent to this discussion.[13] Community ambulators can ambulate 250 feet in a functional manner, with or without a device, and transfer from sit to stand independently. Household ambulators are able to ambulate within a safe structured home environment. Exercise ambulators walk short distances as a form of exercise and are not functional ambulators. Household, exercise, and nonambulators have progressively less ability to ambulate. The latter three categories require a wheelchair for mobility, in particular community mobility, and prescription of the right wheelchair is an important part of rehabilitation and discharge planning.

Ambulation carries unique challenges for the occupational therapist.[7] To properly inform treatment planning, the occupational therapist must clearly understand ambulation goals, and this requires collaboration with the physical therapist.[20] Clarity in terms of the type of ambulation expected, whether the UEs will be needed to use an ambulatory device, and whether LE braces will be utilized all have important implications on functional activities under the purview of occupational therapy (Fig. 39-8). Considerations related to falls and fall prevention should also be part of ambulation education and training.[13,20]

There are some additional tasks that are addressed at every level of occupational therapy in SCI rehabilitation, including patient and family education, wheelchair and equipment selection, and protecting the UEs.

Education and Personal Advocacy

Education is a vital part of SCI rehabilitation and should be prominent in every phase.[63] Education begins

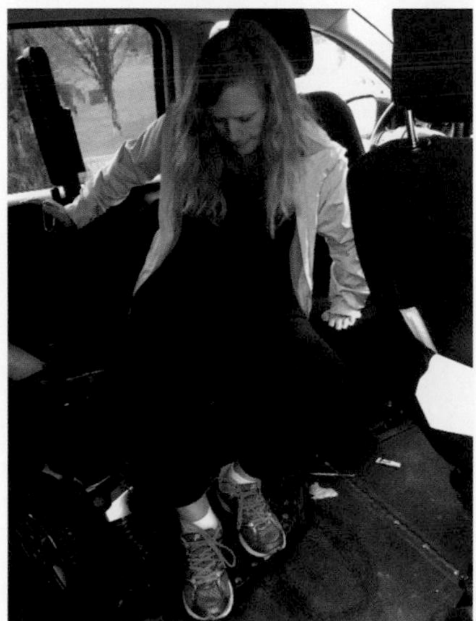

Figure 39-7. Vehicle transfer of an individual with incomplete C6 tetraplegia. (Image courtesy DiSepio Institute, Saint Francis University.)

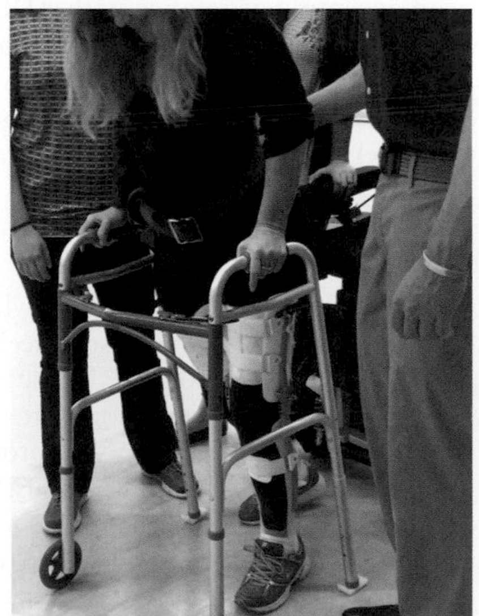

Figure 39-8. Ambulation with equipment and assistance for an individual with incomplete C6 tetraplegia. This individual is not a functional ambulator, but rather ambulates for exercise and other health benefits. (Image courtesy DiSepio Institute, Saint Francis University.)

with the injury and should involve the patient and significant others. The patient with SCI should be trained to give explicit instructions to caregivers because most caregivers do not possess requisite experience with SCI. But there are many factors that hinder learning. Shortened hospitalizations restrict the time available to learn a vast amount of information. The stress of the injury limits readiness to learn and with time, when readiness improves, patients have been discharged to community settings where access to SCI expertise is often lacking.[55,63]

It remains, however, that education is vital to maintaining health, improved QoL, and community integration.[63] Suggestions to facilitate learning in this fractured environment include the utilization of peer and group learning experiences, problem-based learning, using multiple teaching methods, and providing multiple opportunities to learn.[55,63,64]

Education is also key to personal development, empowerment, and self-advocacy for individuals with SCI.[64] The nature of SCI places patients and caregivers in a position in which they must depend on others and can foster feelings of helplessness.[4,64] Engagement has proven critical in successful outcomes for patients with SCI and must be part of the rehabilitation process.[26,64] Engagement can begin by offering simple choices, encouraging the expression of preferences, and involving patients in problem-solving. Rehabilitation should focus on the patient's individual strengths and empower patients to attend to what they can do and adapt to what they cannot. The patient will also need to weigh the value of activities and roles and identify those that provide the most personal gratification.[4] This can mean accepting assistance with ADL tasks in order to conserve energy for other more valued activities.[39] Working through this process, and with time, most patients grow to develop effective coping skills and achieve mastery navigating the lifelong care needs related to SCI.[4,26,55,64]

Wheelchair Use

Most patients with SCI require the use of wheelchairs for mobility.[13,20] Selection of the best wheelchair requires expertise and has important implications for mobility, accessibility, and participation. Often, a medical equipment vendor is involved in this process. The therapist, patient, and family/caregivers must consider many factors when weighing the advantages and disadvantages of specific chairs.[56] How and where the wheelchair will be used must be identified. The appearance of the wheelchair is a consideration as is its weight. The patient's endurance, posture, availability of assistance, and means of transportation are factors that must all be addressed in the selection of a manual or power wheelchair (Fig. 39-9).

Shoulder Overuse

Because patients with SCI rely on their UEs for mobility through manual wheelchair propulsion, preventative care of the shoulders and UEs has great implication for function, well-being, and independence.[22,56] Routine care, and patient and caregiver education, should address both frequent inspection of equipment to assure working order, and ergonomic review of transfers and the environment. Best practice dictates that risk of overuse be minimized by limiting the frequency of repetitive tasks and avoiding UE joint extreme position. Other recommendations include arranging for level transfers whenever possible—varying the technique so as to not stress one UE more than the other—and propelling the wheelchair using long, smooth strokes of the UE. For high-risk patients, consideration of a power wheelchair may be prudent.

Many trends are merging at this time in history related to the ability of the disabled to fully participate in society and live productive, meaningful lives. At the same time, shortened rehabilitation stays and access to and funding for care in the community remain real obstacles to optimal outcomes.[24,55,64] These factors, coupled with the philosophy of occupational therapy, provide exciting opportunities for our profession.[7] As experts in the science of occupation, therapists possess the knowledge and understanding that can inform public policy and lifelong wellness initiatives for our clients. With ongoing advances in SCI research and technology, new opportunities will continue to present themselves, facilitating both the growth and evolution of occupational therapy, and the empowerment and full participation of our clients in the world in which we live.[6,55]

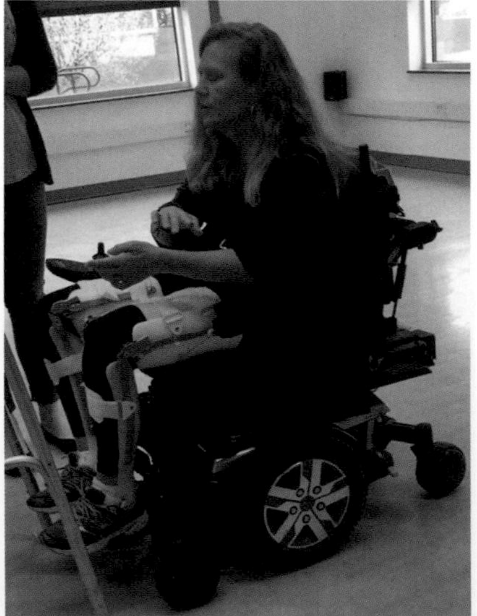

Figure 39-9. Individual with incomplete C6 tetraplegia in power wheelchair. The utilization of the power wheelchair saves wear and tear on shoulder joints. (Image courtesy DiSepio Institute, Saint Francis University.)

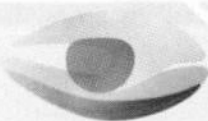

CASE STUDY

Patient Information

Sheniqua is a 21-year old, African American college student who was involved in a violent altercation resulting in a fall down a flight of stairs. She reportedly lost consciousness at the scene. When she awoke at the hospital, she could not feel or move her LEs, and she reported pain in her left wrist. Diagnostic testing showed a spinal fracture at T10 with an ASIA grade A SCI and a left Colles fracture. In addition, Sheniqua was diagnosed with a concussion. She underwent spinal stabilization surgery, and her left wrist was casted. She began occupational and physical therapy in the hospital, but did not initially tolerate either well. Sheniqua experienced headaches and had difficulty concentrating, presumably due to the concussion.

Reason for Occupational Therapy Referral

Sheniqua is right-hand dominant. Upper body ADLs were impeded by the fracture and cast; transfers were also difficult for this reason and the T10 SCI. She required maximal assistance for lower body ADLs, and bowel and bladder care. Attention to task was impaired, and Sheniqua was easily frustrated.

Assessment Process and Results

Two weeks following her injury, Sheniqua was transferred to a nearby inpatient rehabilitation hospital. Her occupational therapy assessment found Sheniqua to require full set up for grooming and UE ADLs. She required maximal assist with lower body dressing, bathing, and level transfers. Bowel and bladder care required maximal assistance due, in large part, to the casted wrist. Her headaches subsided, and her concentration, memory, and follow-through were within functional limits. She experienced fatigue with minimal activity and was fearful about her future. Sheniqua required education related to all aspects of the SCI. The discharge plan was to return home with her family with her mother serving as her primary caregiver, and a long-term plan of returning to campus to complete her final year of undergraduate studies.

Occupational Therapy Problem List

- Requires assistance for wheelchair propulsion indoors (throughout facility, during ADLs, etc.).
- Requires full setup with grooming and UE dressing tasks.
- Requires maximal assist with lower body dressing from a seated position.
- Requires maximal assist with managing LEs during transfers.
- Transfers require maximal assistance.
- Activity tolerance is fair.
- Easily frustrated with current limitations, particularly with the restricted use of her left hand.

Occupational Therapy Goal List

- Propel wheelchair indoors within facility with modified independence.
- Complete grooming and UE ADLs with modified independence.
- Complete level transfers with a transfer board and minimal assistance.
- Don and doff pants with minimal assistance.
- Complete shower ADL with equipment and minimal assistance.

Intervention

- Daily ADLs with emphasis on bed mobility, bed transfers, and LE dressing.
- Progress to shower ADL using durable medical equipment likely to be used in the home environment.
- Modify wheelchair push rims to permit easier propulsion.
- Practice wheelchair propulsion particularly negotiating indoor barriers (small spaces, door thresholds, etc.).
- Transport self within facility from room to therapy department and back, and throughout facility.
- Practice shower transfers using shower chair.
- Educate Sheniqua and mother about durable medical equipment needed for discharge to home, precautions and secondary conditions, and preventative measures.
- Prescription and ordering of wheelchair.
- Training in use and care of wheelchair.
- Schedule overnight stay in facility's training apartment for Sheniqua and her mother prior to discharge to identify any concerns and have time to problem solve.
- Schedule and complete home evaluation and make recommendations to improve accessibility.

Best Evidence for Intervention for Spinal Cord Injury Used in Occupational Therapy

Intervention	Description	Participants	Dosage	Research Design and Evidence Level	Benefit	Statistical Significance and Effect Size
Impact of clinical practice guideline for preservation of upper limb function on transfer skills of persons with acute spinal cord injury[65]	Participants were educated in transfer skills using structured protocol or provided standard care in these activities.	Volunteer sample of 70 full-time wheelchair users	Standard care or parallel training using structured protocol	Randomized controlled trial; Level I	Participants trained using the protocol performed higher quality transfers for stand pivot transfers and all dependent transfers.	At 1-year postdischarge, intervention group participants performed higher quality assisted sitting pivot transfers (mean ± standard error [SE]: 9.43 ± 0.55) compared with standard care group (mean ± SE: 7.81 ± 0.46) ($p = 0.026$).
Effectiveness of group wheelchair skills training for people with spinal cord injury: a randomized controlled trial[66]	Use of group training to train wheelchair mobility skills	114 manual wheelchair users with SCI	Six 90-minute group wheelchair skills sessions vs. two 1-hour active control group sessions	Randomized double-blind controlled trial; Level I	Group training can lead to improvement in wheelchair skills, particularly in those having attended more classes and possessing lower baseline skills.	Compared with control group, the wheelchair skills group improved in performance ($p = 0.02$).
A synthesis of best evidence for the restoration of upper extremity function in people with tetraplegia[22]	Electrical stimulation and surgical intervention to improve grasps function	43 studies	Dosage unspecified	Review; Level I	Both electrical stimulation (with assistive technologies) and surgical intervention enhance functional abilities for individuals with tetraplegia.	NA
Effects of practice combined with somatosensory or motor stimulation on hand function in persons with spinal cord injury[58]	FES, SS, and task training to improve hand function and cortical excitability	24 participants with chronic tetraplegia	Control group assignment or assignment utilizing FES or SS	Randomized controlled trial; Level I	Hand training associated with SS or FES was associated with improved hand use and cortical excitability.	Control group did not improve as demonstrated by an increase in time (mean [standard deviation or SD] change = 9.52 [45.55] seconds); the intervention group improved as demonstrated by a decrease in time (mean [SD] change = −71.63 [100.16] seconds); effect size = −81.14 seconds.

References

1. Ramer LM, Ramer MS, Bradbury EJ. Restoring function after spinal cord injury: towards clinical translation of experimental strategies. *Lancet Neurol.* 2014;13(12):1241–1256. doi:10.1016/S1474-4422(14)70144-9.
2. American Spinal Injury Association. *International Standards to Document Remaining Autonomic Function After Spinal Cord Injury.* Atlanta, GA: American Spinal Injury Association; 2015.
3. Bickenback J, ed. *International Perspectives on Spinal Cord Injury.* Geneva, Switzerland: World Health Organization; 2013.
4. Palmer S, Kriegsman KH, Palmer JB. *Spinal Cord Injury: A Guide for Living.* 2nd ed. Baltimore, MD: Johns Hopkins University Press; 2008.
5. Sabharwal S. *Essentials of Spinal Cord Medicine.* New York, NY: Demos Medical; 2014.
6. Steves JD, Fawcett JW, Tuszynski MH, et al. *Experimental Treatments for Spinal Cord Injury: What You Should Know (Version 2).* Richmond, VA: American Spinal Injury Association; 2012.
7. American Occupational Therapy Association. Occupational therapy practice framework: domain and process. 3rd ed. *Am J Occup Ther.* 2014;62:625–700.
8. Pallastrini P, Mugnai R, Bonfigliolo R, et al. Evaluation of an occupational therapy program for patients with spinal cord injury. *Spinal Cord.* 2008;46:78–81. doi:10.1038/sj.3102072.
9. Nas K, Yazmalar L, Sah V, Aydın A, Öneş K. Rehabilitation of spinal cord injuries. *World J Orthop.* 2015;6(1):8–16. doi:10.5312/wjo.v6.i1.8.
10. DeVivo MJ. Epidemiology of traumatic spinal cord injury: trends and future implications. *Spinal Cord.* 2012;50:365–372. doi:10.1038./sc.2011.178.
11. National Spinal Cord Injury Statistical Center. Spinal cord injury: facts and figures at a glance. National Spinal Cord Injury Statistical Center Web site. https://www.nscisc.uab.edu. Published 2017. Accessed December 30, 2017.
12. Powell A, Davidson L. Pediatric spinal cord injury: a review by organ system. *Phys Med Rehabil Clin N Am.* 2015;26:109–132. doi:10.1016/j.pmr.2014.09.002.
13. Lin VW, ed. *Spinal Cord Medicine: Principles and Practice.* 2nd ed. New York, NY: Demos Medical Publishing; 2003.
14. Ahn H, Bailey CS, Rivers CS, et al. Effect of older age on treatment decisions and outcomes among patients with traumatic spinal cord injury. *CMAJ.* 2015;187(12):873–879. doi:10.1503/cmaj.150085.
15. Hatch BB, Wood-Wentz CM, Therneau TM, Walker MG, Payne JM, Reeves RK. Factors predictive of survival and estimated years of life lost in the decade following nontraumatic and traumatic spinal cord injury. *Spinal Cord.* 2017;55:540–577. doi:10/1038/sc.2016.182.
16. World Health Organization. Spinal cord injury fact sheet. World Health Organization Web site. http://www.who.int/mediacentre/factsheets/fs384/en/. Published 2013. Accessed December 28, 2017.
17. van den Berg MEL, Castellote JM, Mahillo-Fernandez I, de Pedro-Cuesta J. Incidence of spinal cord injury worldwide: a systematic review. *Neuroepidemiology.* 2010;34:184–192. doi:10/1159/000279335.
18. National Spinal Cord Injury Statistical Center. Recent trends in causes of spinal cord injury. National Spinal Cord Injury Statistical Center Web site. https://www.nscisc.uab.edu/Public/Recent%20trends%20in%20causes%20of%20SCI.pdf. Published 2015. Accessed December 30, 2017.
19. Consortium for Spinal Cord Medicine. *Early Acute Management in Adults with Spinal Cord Injury: A Clinical Practice Guideline for Health-Care Professionals.* Washington, DC: Paralyzed Veterans of America; 2008.
20. Somers MF. *Spinal Cord Injury: Functional Rehabilitation.* 3rd ed. Upper Saddle River, NJ: Pearson Education; 2010.
21. American Spinal Injury Association. *International Standards for Neurological Classification of Spinal Cord Injury.* Atlanta, GA: American Spinal Injury Association; 2015.
22. Kalsi-Ryan S, Verrier MC. A synthesis of best evidence for the restoration of upper-extremity function in people with tetraplegia. *Physiother Can.* 2011;63(4):474–489. doi:10.3138/ptc.2009-46.
23. American Spinal Injury Association. Consumer guidelines for spinal cord injury rehabilitation. American Spinal Injury Association Web site. http://asia-spinalinjury.org/wp-content/uploads/2016/02/Consumer_Guidelines_SCI_Rehab.pdf. Accessed January 18, 2018.
24. Whiteneck GG, Gassaway J, Dijkers MP, et al. Inpatient and postdischarge rehabilitation services provided in the first year after spinal cord injury: findings from the SCIRehab Study. *Arch Phys Med Rehabil.* 2011;92:361–368. doi:10.1016/j.apmr.2010.07.241.
25. Consortium for Spinal Cord Medicine. *Outcomes Following Traumatic Spinal Cord Injury: A Clinical Practice Guideline for Health-Care Professionals.* Washington, DC: Paralyzed Veterans of America; 1999.
26. Craig A, Tran Y, eds. *Psychological Aspects Associated with Spinal Cord Injury Rehabilitation: New Directions and Best Evidence.* New York, NY: Nova Science Publishers; 2008.
27. Curtin, M. An analysis of tetraplegic hand grips. *Br J Occup Ther.* 1999; 62:444–450.
28. Klebine P, Smitherman O, Gemenz L. Understanding spinal cord injury: Part 2—The body before and after injury. http://www.msktc.org/sci/factsheets/Understanding_SCI_Part_2. Published 2015. Accessed December 30, 2017.
29. Consortium for Spinal Cord Medicine. *Acute Management of Autonomic Dysreflexia: Adults with Spinal Cord Injury Presenting to Health Care Facilities.* Washington, DC: Paralyzed Veterans of America; 2001.
30. Consortium for Spinal Cord Medicine. *Pressure Ulcer Prevention and Treatment Following Spinal Cord Injury: A Clinical Practice Guideline for Health-Care Professionals.* 2nd ed. Washington, DC: Paralyzed Veterans of America; 2014.
31. Consortium for Spinal Cord Medicine. *Neurogenic Bowel Management in Adults with Spinal Cord Injury: Clinical Practice Guidelines.* Washington, DC: Paralyzed Veterans of America; 1998.
32. Consortium for Spinal Cord Medicine. *Bladder Management for Adults with Spinal Cord Injury: A Clinical Practice Guideline for Health-Care Professionals.* Washington, DC: Paralyzed Veterans of America; 2006.
33. Consortium for Spinal Cord Medicine. *Sexuality and Reproductive Health in Adults with Spinal Cord Injury.* Washington, DC: Paralyzed Veterans of America; 2010.
34. Hagen EM. Acute complications of spinal cord injuries. *World J Orthop.* 2015;6(1):17–23. doi:10.5312/wjo.v6i1.17.
35. Dijkers M, Bryce T, Zanca J. Prevalence of chronic pain after spinal cord injury: a systematic review. *J Rehabil Res Dev.* 2009;46:13–30.

36. Consortium for Spinal Cord Medicine. *Respiratory Management Following Spinal Cord Injury: A Clinical Practice Guideline for Health-Care Professionals.* Washington, DC: Paralyzed Veterans of America; 2005.
37. Reyes MR, Chiodo A. Spasticity and spinal cord injury. Model Systems Knowledge Translation Center Web site. http://www.msktc.org/sci/factsheets/Spasticity. Published 2011. Accessed March 5, 2018.
38. Consortium for Spinal Cord Medicine. *Prevention of Venous Thromboembolism in Individuals with Spinal Cord Injury: A Clinical Practice Guideline for Health-Care Professionals.* 3rd ed. Washington, DC: Paralyzed Veterans of America; 2016.
39. Atkins MS, Bashar JC. Occupational therapy and the care of individuals with spinal cord injury. American Occupational Therapy Association Web site. https://www.aota.org/About-Occupational-Therapy/Professionals/RDP/spinal-cord-injury.aspx. Published 2015. Accessed January 8, 2018.
40. Consortium for Spinal Cord Medicine. *Depression following Spinal Cord Injury: A Clinical Practice Guideline for Health-Care Professionals.* Washington, DC: Paralyzed Veterans of America; 1998.
41. Asher IE, ed. *Asher's Occupational Therapy Assessment Tools: An Annotated Index.* Bethesda, MD: AOTA Press; 2014.
42. Neistadt ME. *Occupational Therapy Evaluation for Adults: A Pocket Guide.* Baltimore, MD: Lippincott Williams & Wilkins; 2000.
43. Hinojose J, Kramer P. *Evaluation in Occupational Therapy: Obtaining and Interpreting Data.* 4th ed. Bethesda, MD: AOTA Press; 2014.
44. Law M, Polatajko H, Pollock N, McCall MA, Carswell A, Baptiste S. Pilot testing of the Canadian Occupational Performance Measure: clinical and measurement issues. *Can J Occup Ther.* 1994;61(4):191–197.
45. Keilhofner G, Mallinson T, Forsyth K, Lai JS. Psychometric properties of the second version of the Occupational Performance History (OPHI-II). *Am J Occup Ther.* 2001;55:260–267. doi:10.5014/ajot.55.3.260.
46. Kendal FP, McCreary EK, Provance PG. *Muscles: Testing and Function.* Baltimore, MD: Lippincott Williams & Wilkins; 1993.
47. Deutsch A, Braun S, Granger C. The Functional Independence Measure (FIM instrument). *J Rehabil Outcome Meas.* 1997;1(2):67–71.
48. Catz A, Itzkovich M, Agranov E, Ring H, Tamir A. SCIM: spinal cord independence measure. A new disability scale for patients with spinal cord lesions. *Spinal Cord.* 1997;35:850–856. doi:10.1038/sj.sc.3100504.
49. Sollerman C, Ejeskar A. Sollerman hand function test: a standardized method and its use in tetraplegic patients. *Scand J Plast Reconstr Surg Hand Surg.* 1995;29:167–176. doi:10.3109/02844319509034334.
50. Kalsi-Ryan S, Curt A, Fehlings MG, Verrier M. Assessment of the hand in tetraplegia using the Graded Redefined Assessment of strength, sensibility and prehension (GRASSP): impairment versus function. *Top Spinal Cord Inj Rehabil.* 2009;12(4):34–36. doi:10.1310/sci1404.34.
51. Jebsen RH, Taylor N, Trieschmann RB, Trotter M, Howard L. An objective and standardized test of hand function. *Arch Phys Med Rehabil.* 1969;50:311–319.
52. Custer MG, Hueber RA, Freudenberger L, Nichols LR. Client-chosen goals in occupational therapy: strategy and instrument pilot. *Occup Ther Health Care.* 2013;27(1):58–70. doi:10.3109/07380577.2012.747120.
53. Foy T, Perritt G, Thimmaiah D, et al. Occupational therapy treatment time during inpatient spinal cord injury rehabilitation. *J Spinal Cord Inj Med.* 2011;34(2):162–175. doi:10.1179/107902611X12971826988093.
54. Grossenbacher NL. The trauma of spinal cord injury on the adolescent. *Occup Ther Health Care.* 2009;2(3):79–90. doi:10.1080/J003v02n3_09.
55. Goodridge D, Rogers M, Klassen L, et al. Access to health and support services: perspectives of people living with a long-term traumatic spinal cord injury in rural and urban areas. *Disabil Rehabil.* 2015;37(16):1401–1410. doi:10.3109/09638288.2014.972593.
56. Consortium for Spinal Cord Medicine. *Preservation of Upper Limb Function Following Spinal Cord Injury: A Clinical Practice Guideline for Health-Care Professionals.* Washington, DC: Paralyzed Veterans of America; 2005.
57. Herder JL, Vrijlandt N, Antonides T, Cloosterman M, Mastenbroek PL. Principle and design of mobile arm support for people with neuromuscular weakness. *J Rehabil Res Dev.* 2006;43(5):591–604. doi:10.1682/JRRD.2006.05.0044.
58. Hoffman L, Field-Fote E. Effects of practice combined with somatoesensory or motor stimulation on hand function in persons with spinal cord injury. *Top Spinal Cord Inj Rehabil.* 2013;19(4):288–299. doi:10.1310/sci1904-288.
59. Hoffman LR, Field-Fote EC. Upper extremity training for individuals with cervical spinal cord injury: functional recovery and neuroplasticity. In: Field-Fote EC, ed. *Spinal Cord Rehabilitation.* Philadelphia, PA: FA Davis; 2009:259–290.
60. Seco MP, Saldena BG, Sastre AR, García Carpintero MJ. Virtual reality in rehabilitation: WII™ as an occupational therapy tool in patients with spinal cord injuries. *J Access Design.* 2014;4(3):223–237. doi:10.17411/jacces.v4i3.54.
61. Verdonck M, Maye F. Enhancing occupational performance in the virtual context using smart technology. *Br J Occup Ther.* 2016;79(6):385–390. doi:10.1177/03082261559.1172.
62. Mohindra M, Sangwan SS, Kundu ZS, Gogna P, Tiwari A, Thora A. Surgical rehabilitation of a tetraplegic hand: comparison of various methods of reconstructing an absent pinch and hook. *Hand.* 2014;9:179–186. doi:10.1007/s11552-014-9615-0.
63. van Wyk K, Backwell A, Townson A. A narrative literature review to direct spinal cord injury patient education programming. *Top Spinal Cord Inj Rehabil.* 2015;21(1):49–60. doi:10.1310/sci2101-49.
64. Rohatinsky N, Goodridge D, Rogers MR, Nickel D, Linassi G. Shifting the balance: conceptualizing empowerment in individuals with spinal cord injury. *Health Soc Care Community.* 2017;25(2):769–779. doi:10.1111/hsc.12370.
65. Rice RA, Smith AR, Greenwald K, Hoelmer C, Boninger ML. Impact of clinical practice guideline for preservation of upper limb function on transfer skills of persons with acute spinal cord injury. *Arch Phys Med Rehabil.* 2013;94:1230–1246. doi:10.1016/j.apmr.2013.03.008.
66. Werebey LA, Kirby RL, Heinemann AW, et al. Effectiveness of Group Wheelchair Skills Training for people with spinal cord injury: a randomized controlled trial. *Arch Phys Med Rehabil.* 2016;97(10):1777–1784. doi:10.1016/j.apmr.2-16.04.006.

Chapter **40**

Cardiac and Pulmonary Diseases

Midge Hobbs

LEARNING OBJECTIVES

This chapter will allow the reader to:

1. Describe the most common cardiac and pulmonary diagnoses, including clinical presentation and symptoms.
2. Identify the role of occupational therapy in evaluating, planning, and treating individuals with cardiac and/or pulmonary disease.
3. Describe the common risk factors for cardiac and/or pulmonary disease and determine the most appropriate educational strategies to ameliorate their effect.
4. Define common terminology and procedures, including diagnostic tests, pertaining to cardiac and pulmonary rehabilitation.
5. Recognize the signs and symptoms of exercise/activity intolerance and its impact on occupational performance.
6. Determine the most appropriate interventions to maximize an individual's functional independence.

CHAPTER OUTLINE

TERMINOLOGY

Angiogram: diagnostic imaging technique used to evaluate arterial blockages and typically conducted under sedation; the most common interventions provided during an angiogram are stent placement and balloon angioplasty.[1]

Arterial blood gas (ABG): test to provide information about the acidity (pH) and the partial pressures of specific gases such as oxygen (PaO_2) and carbon dioxide ($PaCO_2$) in the blood.[2]

Atherosclerosis: slow progressive disease typified by arterial thickening and hardening commonly caused by hypertension, high cholesterol, tobacco use, diabetes, or obesity; atherosclerosis is a form of arteriosclerosis that specifically refers to increased lipids, cholesterol, or other substances that restrict arterial blood flow.[3]

Coronary artery bypass graft (CABG): cardiothoracic surgical procedure used to improve blood flow to the heart by diverting blood around narrowed or restricted arteries; a healthy artery or vein is harvested from the body and used as a graft to bypass blockages in the coronary arteries; surgery can be performed for multiple vessel disease.[4]

Dyspnea: shortness of breath or difficulty breathing that is commonly an indicator of airway, lung, or heart dysfunction.

Echocardiogram (echo): noninvasive test that uses sound waves to produce images of the heart and determine the cause of heart disease; often used to assess overall cardiac performance as well as more specific concerns such as unexplained chest pain, arrhythmias, or heart valve function.[5]

Ejection fraction (EF): measurement of the percentage of blood leaving the ventricles during each contraction, often used to diagnose and track heart failure; a normal EF reading is typically between 50% and 70%; an EF under 40% may be evidence of heart failure.[6]

Electrocardiography (ECG/EKG): painless diagnostic test used to measure the heart's electrical activity via electrodes attached to specified areas of the body; commonly performed to assess unexplained chest pain; to check the condition of the heart in the context of disease such as hypertension, high cholesterol, smoking, and diabetes; and to diagnose heart disease.[7]

Gas exchange: the primary role of respiration or gas exchange is to deliver oxygen from the lungs to the bloodstream; the process occurs via simple diffusion and takes place in the alveoli in the lungs and the surrounding capillaries; as oxygen moves from the alveoli to the blood, carbon dioxide is transferred from the blood in the capillaries to the alveoli and is breathed out via the lungs.[8]

Hypoxemia: abnormal low levels of oxygen (O_2) in the blood, typically below 90%, indicative of breathing or circulatory disorders; without sufficient O_2, the brain, liver, and other organs may be damaged.

Interstitium: lace-like network of supportive tissue that extends throughout both lungs; chronic inflammation of the interstitium changes the lung's ability to function well, impacting gas exchange.[9]

Noninvasive positive-pressure ventilation (NIPPV): a means of delivering ventilation without the need for invasive procedures like intubation or a tracheostomy; bilevel positive airway pressure (BiPAP) and continuous positive airway pressure (CPAP) are the most common options that deliver pressurized air via a tube to a nasal or facial mask worn over the nose and mouth.[10]

Oxygen saturation (O_2 sat): measurement of the amount of oxygen carried by the hemoglobin in the blood; a normal O_2 sat is greater than 95%.[11]

Percutaneous coronary intervention (PCI): nonsurgical reperfusion procedure, also known as coronary angioplasty, that uses a catheter to open an occluded vessel or place a stent in order to improve blood flow to the heart; most commonly used with an ST-segment elevation myocardial infarction (STEMI).[12]

Pneumothorax: accumulation of air, gas, or blood in the pleural space causing the lung to collapse or partially collapse causing chest pain and difficulty breathing.[14]

Pulmonary function test (PFT): an assessment of gas exchange, typically via a spirometer; lung volume measurements indicate lung elasticity and respiratory muscle strength; flow rates indicate the degree of airway narrowing or obstruction.[15]

Pursed-lip breathing: technique used to slow breathing rate by prolonging exhalation in order to manage shortness of breath; clients are encouraged to breathe in slowly and normally through the nose for a count of two before exhaling through pursed-lips while counting to four.[8]

Sternotomy: procedure used in open heart surgery; the sternum is split in two allowing the surgeon access to the chest cavity and is wired back together postsurgery.[16]

Introduction

Cardiovascular disease is an umbrella term that includes conditions affecting the blood vessels such as coronary artery disease (CAD), heart rhythm issues such as arrhythmias, and congenital defects. Although hospitalizations and deaths associated with heart disease have declined in the United States over the past decade—because of an increase in evidence-based practice and medications, as well as initiatives to promote heart-healthy lifestyles—it remains the number one cause of death for both men and women, killing more than 600,000 Americans annually and spanning most racial/ethnic groups.[17] Advancing age remains one of the most significant factors for increased risk of heart disease.[18] Although many occupational therapists may not work primarily in cardiopulmonary rehabilitation, many therapists working in physical medicine settings will encounter adults with limitations associated with cardiac or pulmonary disease; it is important to understand occupational therapy's (OT) role in these clinical areas and be prepared to provide appropriate services.[19]

Description of Cardiac Disease

Hypertension

Hypertension (HTN), or high blood pressure, is a common condition determined by a resting systolic blood pressure of 140 mm Hg or more, and/or a diastolic pressure of 90 mm Hg or more, on repeated examination. Without appropriate medical management, the persistent high force of blood pumping through the blood vessels places significant stress on the heart, increasing the risk of serious health problems such as CAD, myocardial infarction (MI), and stroke.[20] HTN is either the primary or contributing cause of almost 1,000 deaths each day in the United States[21] and is commonly called the silent killer because it is typically asymptomatic; a high blood pressure measurement is often the first indication of the condition. HTN is classified by its degree of severity, which guides treatment, but family history and additional risk factors, such as stress, sodium intake, obesity, excessive alcohol consumption, overuse of nonsteroidal anti-inflammatory drugs (NSAIDs), and corticosteroids must also be considered.[20] Treatment focuses on lowering blood pressure and includes a medication regimen and lifestyle changes.[22]

Coronary Artery Disease

CAD is one of the most common cardiac-related disorders. In the United States, approximately 370,000 deaths are attributed to the disease annually, with the majority of individuals affected over the age of 65.[23] CAD is an ischemic disease, commonly attributed to **atherosclerosis**, a buildup of fatty, fibrous plaque in the arteries that can progressively narrow vessels over time and occlude blood supply to the heart muscle, increasing the risk of significant health-related issues, including angina pectoris, MI, and heart failure. Restricted blood flow or blockage may also trigger a heart attack, and if blood supply is not restored promptly, cardiac tissue will begin to die, which may result in death. Genetic predisposition or a family history of heart disease may increase the likelihood of developing CAD, but additional risk factors include HTN, high cholesterol, diabetes mellitus, obesity, and smoking. Stress and the ability to manage stress may also contribute to the development of CAD—not only do these increase workload on the heart muscle, but they may also lead to unhealthy behaviors.[24]

CAD is commonly diagnosed through a detailed medical history, physical examination, and diagnostic tests that may include an **echocardiogram** (echo) to assess the heart's effectiveness, a stress test to determine the heart's response to increased activity demand, and/or cardiac catheterization or **angiogram** to determine potential blockages.[1,5] Individuals may be asymptomatic during the early stages of the disease, which is commonly treated by controlling risk factors.[25] Angina pectoris is a complication of CAD that may develop as arteries continue to narrow over time reducing blood supply. This causes the heart muscle to constrict with increased activity demand, such as exercise, eating, or stress, causing discomfort or pain in the chest or left shoulder, arms, neck, back, or jaw. Other symptoms include shortness of breath, nausea, a rapid or irregular heartbeat, diaphoresis, or a feeling similar to indigestion.[26] Typically, women's angina symptoms are less easily identified and may include significant fatigue, sleep disturbance, and anxiety.[27]

Angina is commonly classified as either stable or unstable. Stable angina occurs more predictably during periods of exertion or stress. Episodes last approximately 2 to 15 minutes and resolve with rest or medication. Unstable angina typically occurs when more than 70% of arteries are occluded, and symptoms can occur at rest without any notable cardiac demand. Treatment includes nitrates or beta-adrenergic blockers that dilate vessels. Symptoms of angina are similar to those of a heart attack, and immediate medical attention is imperative if symptoms persist longer than 15 minutes or there is no response to prescribed medication. With significantly narrowed or blocked vessels, a more invasive treatment may be indicated to alleviate angina and minimize the risk of MI. Treatment includes **coronary artery bypass graft (CABG)** surgery to circumvent blocked vessels. Alternately, **percutaneous coronary intervention (PCI)**, also known as coronary angioplasty, with or without stent placement may be indicated to open the artery.[16]

Acute Coronary Syndrome

Acute coronary syndrome (ACS) is an umbrella term that includes unstable angina and acute MI, which is the irreversible damage to heart muscle as a result of coronary artery obstruction or prolonged lack of oxygen to cardiac tissue (see Fig. 40-1).[28] If blood flow is not restored quickly, cardiac muscle begins to die and the infarction may be fatal.[29] In the United States, someone has a heart attack every 43 seconds. One in five infarctions is asymptomatic, and around 50% of individuals experiencing an MI die within an hour after onset before they reach the hospital. Men are more likely to experience an MI than premenopausal women, although the risk increases after menopause. About half of all Americans have at least one of the three risk factors that may contribute to heart disease and increase the possibility of an MI. These include HTN, high cholesterol, and smoking.[30]

Infarction is tissue death that occurs in response to one or more coronary occlusions. Infarction may occur as a result of an atherosclerotic rupture that leads to thrombus formation, which, in turn, plugs the artery and obstructs blood flow to the heart. In many cases, the vessels may already be narrower if there is underlying atherosclerosis. Classification of an acute MI is designed to assist rapid decision-making and is based on the presence of serum markers in the blood, symptoms of ischemia, and imaging results. The three classifications include unstable angina and two types of MI: non–ST-segment elevation MI (NSTEMI) and ST-segment

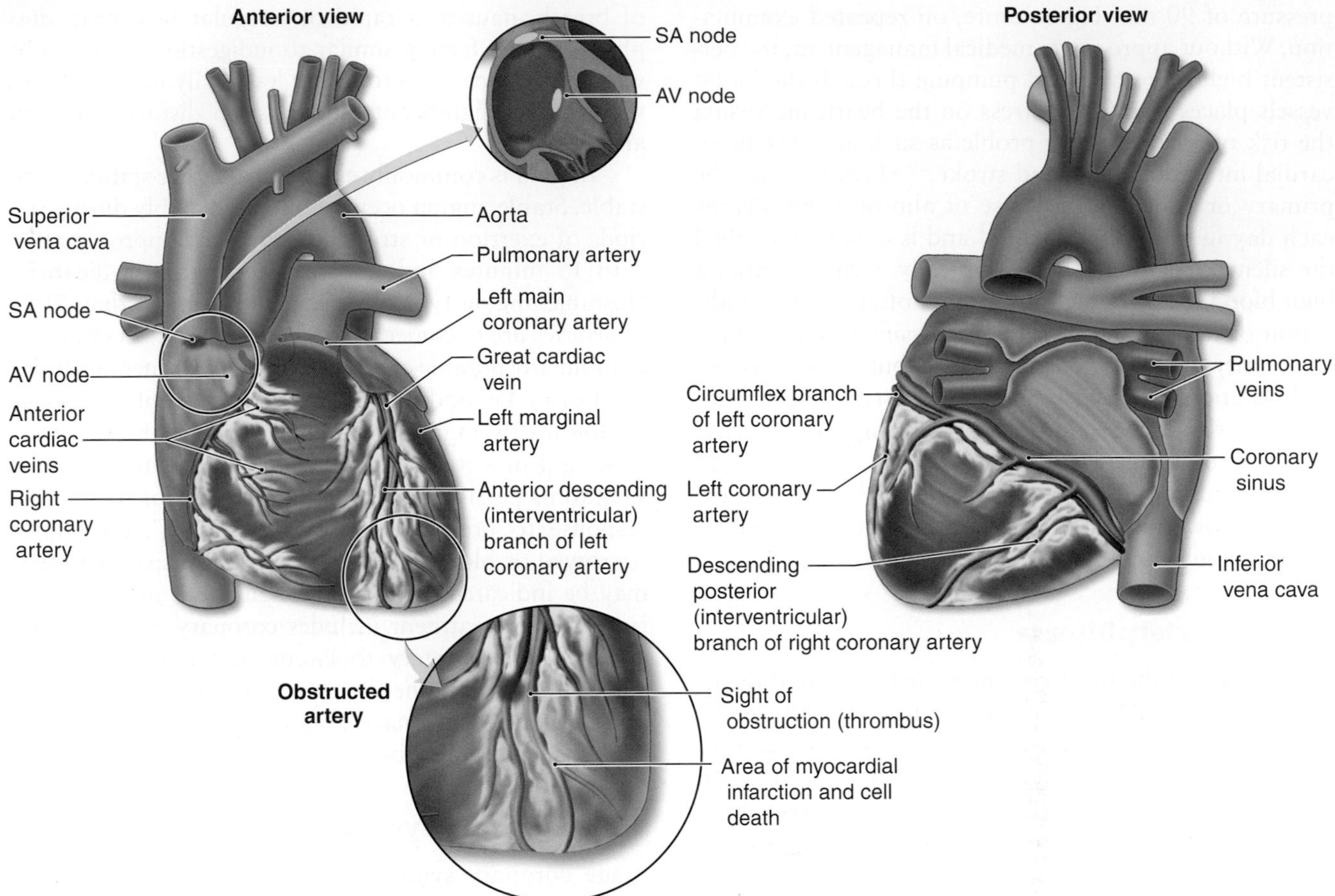

Figure 40-1. Coronary artery circulation. Lower inset shows a myocardial infarction resulting from coronary arterial blockage. AV, atrioventricular; SA, sinoatrial.

elevation MI (STEMI), which are determined by the presence or absence of ST-segment elevation or Q waves on an electrocardiogram (ECG/EKG) (see Fig. 40-2). In cases of NSTEMI, there may be ST-segment depression and/or T-wave inversion, and blood tests will show cardiac markers, troponin I or troponin T and creatine kinase-muscle/brain (CK-MB), to be elevated. In cases of STEMI, ECG changes will show ST-segment elevation

R wave
P wave
ST segment
T wave
Q wave I S wave

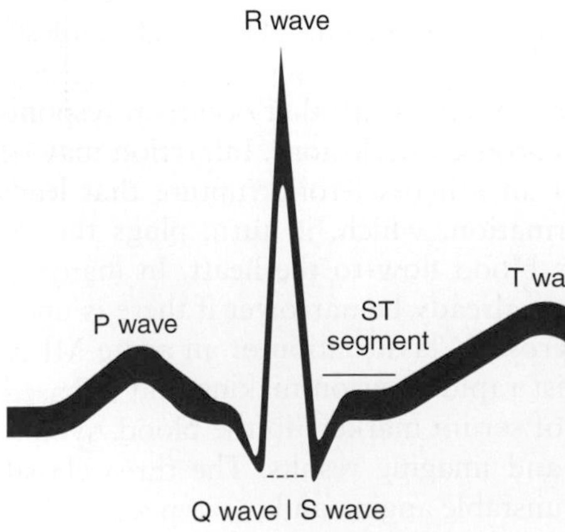

Figure 40-2. Electrocardiogram (EKG/ECG).

as well as elevated cardiac markers.[30] The severity of an infarction depends on several factors, such as the extent of the arterial occlusion, the duration of the blockage, and whether there is collateral circulation. Typically, the more proximal the blockage, the more likely there will be extensive myocardium tissue necrosis.[31] Although the immediate prognosis is better for individuals with an NSTEMI, they are often at higher risk for further cardiac events owing to the extent of the underlying heart disease.[31]

Some individuals are asymptomatic during a heart attack, but there are several characteristic warning signs associated with an infarction, although these often differ between men and women. Symptoms include significant chest pain often described as pressure, fullness, or a squeezing sensation that may radiate into the jaw, shoulders, left arm, and/or upper back. Additional symptoms may include **dyspnea**, diaphoresis, epigastric discomfort with nausea or vomiting, syncope, and impaired cognition. Evaluation begins with serial **electrocardiography (ECG/EKG)** that shows the electrical activity of the heart, identifies the location of damaged cardiac muscle, and helps to determine whether or not an individual is having a heart attack. An ECG will also help doctors differentiate between unstable angina, NSTEMI, or STEMI, in order to provide appropriate medical care.[30,31]

Treatment focuses primarily on restoring coronary blood flow and recovering functional myocardium. Once diagnosis is confirmed, intervention is determined by the clinical picture and prognosis. Medication is most often the mainstay of therapy. Typical drugs include thrombolytic agents to revascularize tissue, antiplatelet drugs to prevent new clots forming or existing clots from growing larger, and beta-blockers to relax cardiac muscle, decrease blood pressure and myocardial demand, and minimize heart muscle damage. Additional medications include angiotensin-converting enzyme (ACE) inhibitors to lower blood pressure and minimize the stress on the heart, antiarrhythmics to manage ventricular arrhythmias, and pain medication such as morphine to ease discomfort. Surgical interventions include PCI and stenting. PCI is the preferred reperfusion intervention for individuals with STEMI, provided it can be performed within 90 minutes of admission to the hospital. For others, CABG may be indicated when arterial disease is severe and an individual cannot undergo PCI.[12]

Even if blood flow is successfully restored, individuals who have experienced MI may remain in the hospital until medically stable. Additional treatment focuses on minimizing complications, restoring normal function, and exploration of lifestyle modifications to reduce risk factors. Once discharged, treatment may include cardioprotective medications, cardiac rehabilitation, and ongoing dietary/lifestyle education.[32] Several lifestyle modifications have been shown to strongly decrease risk for recurrent MI and minimize the progression of cardiac disease, including adoption of a low-fat and low-sodium diet, smoking cessation, and increased physical activity. However, prognosis varies according to age and clinical picture, including the presence or absence of risk factors. Many individuals continue to live full active lives with appropriate lifestyle changes and medical management.

Congestive Heart Failure

Congestive heart failure (CHF) is a complex diagnosis that results from impaired structure and/or function of the ventricles and affects the heart's ability to pump. The heart muscle becomes stretched beyond its ability to contract efficiently, resulting in the collection of fluid in the lungs or the extremities, hence the term congestive heart failure (CHF). The condition often affects both sides of the heart; however, one side may be more affected than the other. Although both left-sided and right-sided dysfunction share similar clinical traits, left ventricular dysfunction typically presents with increased fatigue, shortness of breath, and pulmonary edema; right-sided dysfunction is notable for peripheral and/or abdominal edema. Left-sided or right-sided heart failure may be the result of either systolic dysfunction, whereby the heart is unable to contract efficiently, or diastolic dysfunction when cardiac muscle is unable to relax.[33]

Seventy-five percent of individuals with CHF have a history of HTN that leads to diastolic dysfunction; as the heart pumps more forcibly at a higher pressure, the cardiac walls thicken, leading to ventricle hypertrophy, which makes oxygenating the heart muscle even more difficult and may lead to ischemic damage. Additionally, an acute ischemic event such as an MI may destroy tissue, contributing to cardiac inefficiency. The most common etiology for systolic dysfunction is CAD, typically caused by a combination of factors; as vessels narrow over time limiting the flow of oxygenated blood to the heart, cardiac muscle weakens impacting its ability to contract. Unhealthy lifestyle factors may also increase the risk for developing heart failure. Approximately 5.7 million American adults have a diagnosis of CHF, and each year, 1 million hospitalizations are attributed to the disease.[34]

Under stress, the body releases hormones designed to increase cardiac output. However, with sustained response to the stress of chronic conditions such as CAD or HTN, the heart ultimately becomes weaker with a notable impact on stroke volume and a further decrease in cardiac output. The body responds by triggering compensatory mechanisms that include structural changes to the heart muscle wall. As the heart works harder, its walls thicken and enlarge in order to contract more forcefully. Although this measure may increase stroke volume in the short term, the tissue ultimately stiffens with effort, thereby decreasing its effectiveness over time. Additionally, decreased renal perfusion causes a release of the renin–angiotensin–aldosterone–vasopressin system (antidiuretic hormone [ADH]), which promotes sodium and water retention, ultimately leading to volume overload. Initially, retaining salt and water instead of excreting it into urine helps to increase heart function and regulate blood pressure and organ perfusion, but chronic activation is detrimental to cardiac efficiency. Over time, the effort weakens cardiac muscle, worsening the heart failure.[34]

Heart failure may begin with an acute onset or progress slowly and become chronic, although many cases are initially asymptomatic. Heart failure symptoms are classified in stages from mild to severe. Even when both left and right sides of the heart are compromised, one side will likely dominate in terms of presentation. In the majority of cases, left-sided heart failure will lead to right-sided dysfunction. Although both right-sided and left-sided heart failure produce different symptoms, the most common symptoms associated with the disease are shortness of breath, fatigue, and muscle weakness. In severe cases, individuals may also experience a rapid or irregular heart rate, which should be considered a medical emergency requiring immediate help. Diagnosis is typically determined through a complete medical history with a thorough physical examination. Additional procedures are used to support the diagnosis, which typically includes an ECG to determine heart rhythm irregularities, ascertain whether there are structural changes in the ventricles, or assess valve function. An ECG may also help determine if heart failure is the result of systolic or diastolic dysfunction by assessing the thickness and stiffness of the heart wall and the **ejection fraction** (EF). A normal ventricle ejects approximately 60% of its blood. An EF below this percentage confirms systolic heart failure. A normal EF suggests diastolic dysfunction.[34]

Although CHF is considered a chronic condition that can be managed long term with appropriate medical care and lifestyle changes, much depends on the severity of the condition and which treatment options are applicable. Medications and lifestyle changes are often the cornerstone of treatment plans, while surgical interventions may also be indicated. In acute heart failure, such as the development of pulmonary edema, individuals commonly require supplemental oxygen alongside diuretics to decrease edema. Lifestyle changes can also help minimize symptoms and slow disease progression.[34]

Functional Impairment in Daily Occupation Resulting from Cardiac Disease

Whether cardiac disease presents as an acute health crisis or a chronic condition, symptoms can often limit function, leading to loss of independence and a decline in confidence.[35] Structural changes, or increased workload to the heart, are often characterized by the clinical symptoms of shortness of breath and fatigue, which may significantly impact an individual's ability to perform self-care activities, participate in instrumental activities of daily living (IADLs), including work and leisure activities, as well as fully engage in social relationships. In addition, edema, commonly associated with volume overload and CHF, may impact general mobility and sleep, particularly with increased fluid in the lungs. In the elderly, research indicates that heart failure also has an impact on memory and recall, attention, and the capacity for new learning. The effects on function may include an inability to manage the disease appropriately, or problem-solve daily routines and challenges. A decline in function may also lead to anxiety, decreased self-esteem, and depression.[9] In cases of open heart surgery or CABG where a **sternotomy** is performed, individuals may also be limited by precautions impacting function. These include weight-bearing restrictions, no excessive twisting or turning, and a lifting limit, all of which affect participation and ability to perform self-care tasks and IADLs, including driving.[36]

Evaluation and Intervention of Functional Skill Deficits Secondary to Cardiac Disease

Individuals with cardiac disease benefit from an interprofessional approach that may include physicians, nurses, occupational and physical therapists, dieticians, chaplains, psychologists, and social workers, depending on the availability. Collaborative practice is integral to providing safe, quality, accessible, and client-centered care and includes four competencies:

1. Understanding one's role and those of other professionals to assess and address the needs of clients and populations served
2. Maintaining a climate of mutual respect based on shared values and ethical principles
3. Providing responsible and timely communication with clients, caregivers, communities, and other health care providers
4. Applying relationship-building values to maintain healthy team roles in order to plan and deliver effective client-centered health care[10]

OT plays a distinct role in interprofessional practice to address cardiac disease across the continuum from acute care to inpatient rehab to home care.[37]

In order to understand an individual's performance strengths and limitations, an occupational therapist will use his or her clinical reasoning skills to perform an evaluation that may include a synthesis of formal standardized assessment tools, such as the Functional Independence Measure (FIM), to evaluate activities of daily living (ADLs) and medical data. Informal observation and interview of patients, along with information obtained through interprofessional communication, will also be used in evaluation. Many individuals who have experienced a life-threatening cardiac event or disease progression and undergone lifestyle changes also benefit from OT intervention to help with psychosocial adjustment to their new situation. Therefore, in addition to performance skills impacting motor, cognitive processing, and/or social interaction, it is also important to address client factors and performance patterns—such as values and beliefs, and roles and routines—as well as environmental and contextual factors to reflect OT's holistic approach to caring for the client with a history of cardiac disease.[38]

By synthesizing all pertinent data, the therapist is able to develop an occupational profile that will guide the plan of care. This includes collaborating with the client and/or caregiver to determine his or her priorities regarding outcomes in order to develop objective and measurable goals that are meaningful and client centered. Once goals have been established, interventions may be determined to execute the plan of care.[11] The occupational therapist's expertise in the rehabilitative process across the continuum, as well as knowledge of comorbid diseases, is extremely important when evaluating and adapting treatment for the individual needs of patients with cardiac disease.

The goals of inpatient cardiac rehabilitation are to prevent muscle loss from bed rest, monitor and assess the patient's ability to function, instruct the patient in appropriate home activities, educate the patient about individual risk factors, and teach methods to minimize risks.

Evidence indicates that limited mobility is a significant contributor to long-term health issues, including muscle weakness, delirium and cognitive impairments, and joint shortening. Research suggests that safe and appropriate early mobility can significantly improve functional outcomes.[39] Therapists treat each patient at least once a day as soon as the patient's medical status has stabilized, often within the first 24 to 48 hours after admission, and hospital stays for cardiac events have declined significantly in the past 10 years. The average hospital stay is 1 day for the uncomplicated NSTEMI, 2 to 3 days for STEMIs, and 3 to 7 days for open heart surgery. During any activity, physical measurements of heart rate, blood pressure, EKG response, and symptoms are noted. Many occupational therapists working in acute care or cardiac rehabilitation participate in training courses to read EKGs.[39]

Despite finding their ability to perform basic ADLs compromised by fatigue, dyspnea, and decreased activity tolerance, individuals with cardiac conditions are encouraged to participate in self-care re-training that will include energy conservation techniques and recommendations to modify tasks, such as adjusting body mechanics to minimize fatigue and work of breathing. Additionally, altering the environment to reduce extraneous effort and decrease activity demand, or using adaptive equipment to maximize functional independence, may be indicated. Dressing equipment may include items such as a long-handled shoe horn or sock aide, while a tub seat may be recommended to minimize time standing during a shower. In addition to encouraging participation in functional activities, an exercise routine may also be introduced. For example, individuals following bypass or with a diagnosis of CHF may begin with a program of mild calisthenics consisting of 2-minute bouts interspersed with 1-minute rest. As the patient progresses, the amount of exercise time typically increases to 8 to 10 minutes. For individuals who have had NSTEMIs, STEMIs, or PCI with stents, the therapist may incorporate hall walking or treadmill use in addition to ADLs. Regardless of the modality used, activity demand progression is based on the patient's tolerance and diagnosis with continued monitoring of vitals.

Upon discharge from the hospital or rehab facility, each patient is given a tailored home program based on diagnosis, individual needs, and circumstances. The general components of a home program are activity and exercise guidelines for all meaningful activities, including IADLs such as home management, shopping, meal preparation, leisure tasks, transportation, social activity, and sexual relations. Signs and symptoms of exercise intolerance and a discussion of disease risk factors are included in the educational process. Examples of recommendations include making larger meals to freeze, letting dishes air dry, grouping task items together to minimize unnecessary searches, sliding items on countertops rather than carrying them, shopping with someone who can carry bags, or using grocery home delivery services.

Individuals who have had open heart surgery, a diagnosis of CHF, or experienced an STEMI are often provided with more specific instructions. For example, individuals who have undergone a CABG often have pain and require analgesics, which may impact retention and application of new information. Postoperative patients will have specific precautions defined by the surgeon, which typically include avoiding lifting, pushing, or pulling greater than 10 lb for 6 to 12 weeks. Therapists should make recommendations for alternative ways of performing activities to avoid breaking sternal precautions, such as opening a heavy door or lifting objects such as a coffee pot with two extremities versus one (see Fig. 40-3). Patients who complain of feeling sternal shifting or clicking are told to avoid the activity that causes it and to stop any upper extremity (UE) exercises. In addition to the potential physical responses postsurgery, such as sternal discomfort and fatigue, individuals are also given information to highlight the possible emotional responses they may expect during the healing process, such as depression. Education may also address affection and intimacy. After open heart surgery, it is generally suggested that patients wait 6 to 8 weeks before resuming sexual intercourse and then begin with

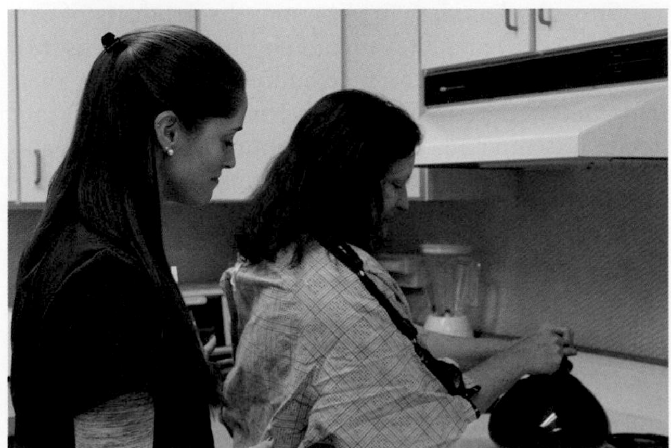

Figure 40-3. Sternal precautions: Lifting with two hands.

alternate positions to minimize strain on the sternum, such as side-lying or sitting in a chair facing each other.[40]

Patients with a diagnosis of CHF often experience significant endurance limitations. Consequently, home programs emphasize energy conservation strategies and work simplification in addition to light exercise programs. Education also includes daily monitoring signs and symptoms of worsening medical status, such as increased edema and shortness of breath.

A home program for a patient who has had an STEMI typically focuses on evaluating activity/exercise tolerance and determining the correct energy expenditure during recovery. Depending on the amount of damage sustained, heart muscle healing takes about 2 to 4 weeks, and patients are asked to restrict activities to the 2 to 4 MET range during this time. METs, or metabolic equivalents, are a unit of measure used to describe the amount of oxygen the body needs for a given activity. Values are approximate and do not include environmental factors or skill level. Generally, the more the body moves and has to work against resistance, the higher the MET (see Box 40-1).[41] Energy conservation and work simplification strategies are the cornerstone of cardiac education, which includes prioritizing tasks, reorganizing the environment to access necessary items with minimal exertion, and using adaptive equipment. Depression and sexuality are discussed because certain cardiac medications can significantly impact mood as well as sexual function and desire. The American Heart Association suggests that post-MI patients who can tolerate activities between 3 and 5 METs without symptoms are ready to resume sexual relationships.[40]

Many patients who have experienced a PCI, MI, CABG, or valve replacement/repair are often referred to outpatient cardiac rehabilitation to continue skilled monitoring of exercise, risk factor education, and modifications. Individuals may also benefit from home OT to support a safe transition as well as to ensure appropriate application of educational strategies for identified lifestyle changes. Goals vary according to individual needs and are often dependent on heart function, physical condition, and circumstances.

Stress and anxiety are common by-products of cardiac disorders and life-threatening events such as MI. Providing education to help individuals manage their symptoms in the context of daily routines is an important step in lessening anxiety and promoting participation in the treatment program, as well as improving outcomes.[42] Interventions include strategies to help clients prioritize activities and create a balanced lifestyle, increase awareness of body-and-mind interaction to manage stressors and perform daily activities with more confidence, and provide education on a variety of relaxation methods (e.g., guided imagery, progressive muscle relaxation, and diaphragmatic breathing). Many therapists use standardized questionnaires to determine depression or anxiety such as the Beck Depression Inventory or the Center for Epidemiological Studies Depression Scale.[43] Testing results will indicate whether a referral to a chaplain, social worker, or psychologist is needed based on patient circumstance or preference.

Cardiac rehabilitation education may also include medication management training, exploration of healthy leisure pursuits to promote lifestyle balance, and information regarding community resources. Emphasis should also be placed on managing controllable risk factors, such as smoking, hyperlipidemia, HTN, sedentary lifestyle, and obesity. Smoking is a major modifiable risk factor that contributes to heart disease in multiple ways. The incidence of heart disease is two to four times higher in people who smoke than in nonsmokers.[44] Smoking damages the endothelial lining of the coronary arteries, making them more susceptible to plaque formation. Nicotine causes arterial vasoconstriction and increases heart rate. Smoking makes the heart more susceptible to lethal ventricular arrhythmias and predisposes it to coronary artery spasm.[45] Carbon monoxide in cigarette smoke binds with hemoglobin faster than oxygen, resulting in decreased oxygen distribution to tissues. Nicotine alters the metabolism of fats, increasing the levels of atherogenic low-density lipoprotein (LDL) cholesterol and decreasing the levels of the heart-protective high-density lipoprotein (HDL) cholesterol. Smoking also causes the blood to coagulate more quickly and promotes thrombus formation.[45] Even those who are regularly exposed to secondhand smoke at work or home have a 25% increase in their risk of cardiovascular disease. However, the benefits of smoking cessation accrue quickly and the risk of heart disease may significantly decline over time.[45]

Hyperlipidemia or a high lipid level is also a major risk factor for cardiac disease. Cholesterol levels may be lowered through a low-fat diet, regular aerobic exercise, and weight loss. If these options are unsuccessful, the physician will place a patient on a lipid-lowering drug. A sedentary lifestyle is also a risk factor for heart disease and its impact is comparable with smoking, hypercholesterolemia, and high blood pressure.[45] Regular physical exercise assists with weight control, lowers blood pressure, and improves lipid profile and glucose tolerance.[46] In the United States, more than 37% of adults are considered overweight or obese.[46] Obesity is now the second leading preventable cause of death in the United States and negatively influences a number of risk factors for heart disease such as HTN, diabetes, hyperlipidemia, and physical activity. The distribution of body fat is important in disease promotion. For example, abdominal obesity is linked to increased risk of CAD. Even 5% to 10% weight loss, however, can have a positive influence on risk factors such as HTN, lipid levels, and sleep apnea.[47] Stress is also a significant risk factor for heart disease, but its effect is difficult to quantify. Several studies have shown that depression, limited social support, and

BOX 40-1

MET Values for Various Activities

Home	Leisure and Vocational	Exercise and Sports
1.0–2.5 METs		
Sweeping floors Dusting Straightening up Serving food Table setting Knitting and crocheting Putting away groceries Making bed Standing quietly in line Mowing lawn with a riding mower Sexual activity (general, moderate effort) Dressing and undressing Sleeping Watching TV Dish washing Bathing-sitting Changing light bulbs Hairstyling–Standing	Power boating Fishing from boat Pumping gas Typing, computer Sitting for light office work Card playing, sitting Board games Playing piano or organ Driving tractor Sewing with a machine Driving an auto or truck Sitting to study, read, or write Casino gambling–standing	Walking at slow pace Playing catch with a baseball or football Horseback riding, walking
2.6–4.0 METs		
Child care bathing and grooming Walk, run, and play with children (moderate) General house cleaning Walking downstairs Sweeping garage or sidewalk Raking lawn Walking and carrying load of 15 pounds	Pitching horseshoes Home auto repair Planting seedlings and shrubs Playing the drums Home wiring or plumbing Feeding small farm animals Standing doing light-to-moderate effort. Bartending–standing Walking and picking up yard Sailing Motorcycle riding	Very light stationary biking Weight lifting of light-to-moderate effort. Stretching, yoga Golf using a cart Snowmobiling Walking at moderate speed Water aerobics Walking pushing a wheelchair Bicycling (<10 mph) Activity videos moderate effort (i.e., Wii Fit™ aerobics and weight training) Curves™ exercise for women
>4.0–6.0 METs		
Major house cleaning, such as washing windows, vigorous effort Moving furniture Scrubbing floors on hands and knees Cleaning gutters Painting the outside of house Painting and wallpapering inside of house Weeding or cultivating Walking carrying a 15-pound load	Laying carpet or tile Slow wood chopping Farming, feeding cattle Carpentry on outside of house Carpentry, refinishing surfaces Hunting-general Road building, carrying heavy loads Roofing Golf, carrying clubs	General calisthenics, moderate effort Shooting hoops Softball, fast or slow pitch Low-impact or dance aerobics Dodgeball or hopscotch Bicycling (10-11.9 mph) Walk/jog (with jogging part less than 10 minutes) Elliptical, moderate effort.
6.0–10 METs		
Carrying groceries upstairs Moving household items in boxes Shoveling more than 16 pounds per minute (heavy) Walking or standing with objects weighing 50–74 pounds	Farming, bailing hay Concrete masonry Moving heavy objects such as furniture Firefighter carrying hoses	High-impact aerobics Running 10–12 minutes/mile Basketball game Jump roping Race walking Swimming laps at a moderate pace Bicycling at moderate pace (> 12 mph)

From Ainsworth, B. W., Haskell, W. L., Herrmann, S.D., Meches, N., Bassett, D. R., Jr., Tudor-Locke, C., Greer, J.L., Vezina, J., Whitt-Glover, M. C., & Leon, A. S. (2011). Compendium of physical activities: A second update of codes and met levels. Medicine & Science in Sports & Exercise, 43, 1575–1581; Ainsworth, B. W., Haskel, W. L., Leon, A., Jacobs, D., Jr., Montoye, H., Salis, J., & Paffenbarger, R. (1998). Compendium of physical activities: Classification of energy costs of human physical activities. In J. Roitman (Ed.), ACSM's resource manual for exercise testing and prescription (pp. 656–667). Baltimore, MD: Williams & Wilkins.

stress increase an individual's risk for developing CAD and other adverse life events.[48]

Description of Pulmonary Disease

According to the Centers for Disease Control and Prevention, 15% of adults in the United States live with chronic lung disease, such as asthma or chronic obstructive pulmonary disease (COPD). While approximately 10% of those adults report mild symptoms, more than one-third report persistent moderate-to-severe symptoms that greatly impact quality of life.[12] Each year, more than 614,000 inpatient admissions are attributed to chronic and unspecified bronchitis. Additionally, chronic lung disease greatly increases the risk of developing pneumonia, with critical episodes accounting for approximately 1.1 million inpatient admissions annually.[13] Critical illness or acute lung injury, such as acute respiratory distress syndrome (ARDS) commonly associated with sepsis, trauma, and severe pulmonary infections, account for approximately 15% to 18% of all ventilated patients in inpatient care.[14] Lung disease is now the third highest cause of mortality in the United States.[49]

Chronic Obstructive Pulmonary Disease

COPD is an umbrella term used to describe progressive lung diseases that include emphysema and chronic bronchitis. Although COPD is considered preventable, it is also a progressive, life-threatening disorder in which the lungs are irreparably damaged, making it difficult to breathe. Multiple factors may contribute to its onset and progression, including smoking, exposure to environmental pollutants, and a history of asthma. Prolonged exposure to toxic agents over time may result in increased mucous production (chronic bronchitis) and tissue breakdown (emphysema).[15] COPD is characterized by irreversible airflow obstruction impacting **gas exchange** and causing dyspnea, as well as limited reserve lung capacity with an increased risk of developing **hypoxemia**.[50]

Worldwide, 64 million people live with COPD with an estimated 3 million deaths attributed to the disease each year. According to the World Health Organization, 80% of deaths are a result of long-term smoking, which explains why COPD typically affects older adults who may have had a long-standing history of tobacco use. Additionally, more women than men are now being diagnosed with the disease as a result of increased tobacco use over the past 30 years. In 2010, the cost of hospital admissions attributed to COPD exacerbations was estimated at $32.1 billion dollars annually and was projected to reach $49 billion by 2020.[51]

Dyspnea with minor exertion is the most common symptom associated with COPD, along with a persistent cough, expiratory wheezing, and fatigue.[52] However, symptoms of COPD typically do not manifest until significant lung damage has already occurred. A diagnosis may be confirmed through a **pulmonary function test (PFT)**, chest x-ray, computed tomography (CT) scan, or **arterial blood gas (ABG)** analysis. Management of the disease focuses on lifestyle changes, including smoking cessation, and prescribed medication such as bronchodilators that relax the muscles around the airways and relieve coughing and dyspnea.[17] For more severe symptoms, inhaled corticosteroids may be prescribed to reduce airway inflammation and minimize the risk of worsening symptoms known as an exacerbation. In cases of moderate-to-severe COPD, doctors may also prescribe supplemental oxygen.[18] Immediate medical care is indicated for an acute exacerbation to minimize the risk of lung failure.[52]

Acute Respiratory Distress Syndrome

Acute respiratory distress syndrome (ARDS) is defined as an acute life-threatening inflammatory reaction to illness or trauma affecting approximately 200,000 people each year in the United States.[19] In many cases, ARDS is a complication of severe pneumonia, sepsis, or major trauma, with severity greatly influenced by age, comorbidities, and alcohol consumption. The inflammatory response causes injury to the lungs and fluid to build up in the alveoli, compromising gas exchange, making breathing difficult, and increasing the risk of respiratory failure.[20] Up to 40% of ARDS cases are fatal.[21] Lung injury associated with ARDS is characterized by tissue damage and narrowing of air space with fibrotic changes in the lungs, which is commonly a predictor of outcomes.[22,53]

Signs and symptoms vary in severity depending on the cause and presence of underlying heart or lung disease; however, the most common early symptoms include significant dyspnea, increased respiration rate, low blood pressure, extreme fatigue, and confusion.[23] Diagnosis is usually determined via a complete physical examination and diagnostic testing. These include an ABG test, a chest x-ray to assess fluid levels in the lungs, a chest CT scan to look for signs of pneumonia or tumors, a complete blood count (CBC), and a sputum culture to clarify the cause of the infection.[24,53]

Owing to its life-threatening nature, treatment is most commonly conducted in an intensive care unit (ICU) with the primary aim of improving oxygen levels and treating the underlying cause. Oxygen may be initially provided via nasal cannula or face mask, but if breathing is significantly difficult, **noninvasive positive-pressure ventilation (NIPPV)** may be trialed or mechanical ventilation may be required. Additional treatment focuses on fluid management and minimizing further complications such as **pneumothorax** and pneumonia. Medications may include vasodilators to improve gas exchange, as well as anti-inflammatories. Owing to the severity of ARDS, recovery from the condition may be protracted, and it is commonly associated with residual physical and cognitive challenges requiring additional pulmonary rehab or support for depression.[54]

Interstitial Lung Disease

Interstitial lung disease (ILD) is a group of disorders that share a similar clinical profile. The chief characteristic is scarring of the pulmonary **interstitium**, which includes the walls of the alveoli and the microscopic spaces around the blood vessels. Scarring causes progressive lung stiffness impacting the ability to breathe.[9] Disorders associated with ILD may be of known or unknown etiology.[25] It has not been possible to accurately estimate the prevalence of ILD given the diverse number of associated diseases and variation in etiology.[55]

ILD may be the result of exposure to toxic agents through occupation, such as asbestos and coal dust, or prolonged radiation as in cancer management. ILD may also develop as a complication of systemic disease, including rheumatoid arthritis, scleroderma, and systemic lupus erythematosus. Sarcoidosis, a multisystem inflammatory disease, is the most common ILD in the United States. In some cases, individuals with ILD belong in the idiopathic interstitial pneumonia (IIP) category. The most common IIP is idiopathic pulmonary fibrosis, a crippling disorder with minimal treatment options most commonly affecting individuals over the age of 60. Idiopathic pulmonary fibrosis has a poor prognosis because of rapid progressive scarring.[55]

Regardless of etiology and type, the clinical signs and symptoms of ILD are similar. These include dyspnea and a nonproductive cough. Additional symptoms, such as increased sputum production, hemoptysis associated with microscopic hemorrhages, and wheezing, as well as non–respiratory-related symptoms, such as myalgia and joint pain, may help to further classify the disease. A thorough physical examination is imperative to determine an accurate diagnosis.[26] Upon auscultation, many individuals with ILD will have bilateral respiratory crackles with inhalation indicating excess fluid in the lungs. Imaging, PFTs, and a lung tissue analysis are used to make a definitive diagnosis. Given that lung scarring is irreversible, treatment is typically associated with disease management—for example, minimizing exposure to known toxic agents, providing oxygen to assist breathing, and prescribing anti-inflammatory or immunosuppressing medications. In some cases, a lung transplant may be considered, although mortality risk is high.[56]

Functional Impairment in Daily Occupation Resulting from Pulmonary Disease

Common symptoms associated with lung disease include increased shortness of breath, deconditioning with general loss of muscle mass and strength impacting activity tolerance, chronic cough and increased sputum production, as well as anxiety and depression. Persistent shortness of breath and an inability to increase ventilation to meet physiological demand can greatly impact function, leading to a gradual loss of independence and a downward spiral in confidence based on the understanding that quality of life has been permanently compromised. Studies have indicated that individuals with a diagnosis of chronic disease, such as COPD, typically experience higher rates of depression than other comparable chronic conditions.[57] Eating is another necessary activity that individuals find challenging with compromised breathing due to lung disease. This may lead to inadequate nutrition and weight loss, which will, in turn, further impact endurance and function. In contrast, long-term use of steroids to manage inflammation associated with pulmonary disease may lead to weight gain requiring increased energy expenditure during functional tasks.

Evaluation and Intervention of Functional Skill Deficits Secondary to Pulmonary Disease

Interdisciplinary pulmonary rehabilitation is generally designed to alleviate and/or manage symptoms, increase strength and endurance to optimize function, and maximize quality of life.[27] Occupational therapists can be key members of the interprofessional team with our focus on providing client-centered care to maximize individual functional capacity through education and individual lifestyle recommendations, improve activity tolerance, and enhance psychosocial support.[57] Although many occupational therapists may not choose to specialize in pulmonary rehabilitation, therapists will encounter adults with limitations associated with lung disease in any setting, from acute rehabilitation to home care, and it is important to understand the occupational therapist's role and be prepared to provide appropriate services across the continuum.[28]

Individuals are typically admitted to acute care hospitals with significant or life-threatening health concerns requiring immediate medical diagnosis and/or intervention, as well as a 24-hour physician and nursing care. An ICU is indicated for those who require advanced medical support, which may include ARDS, respiratory arrest, threatened airway, and significantly low oxygen saturations, causing hypoxemia and risk of brain injury. Occupational therapists are increasingly assuming more active roles in acute care settings with an emphasis on early mobilization, monitoring of vitals with activity, client and caregiver education, restoring function, and performing evaluations to assist with the coordination of care and determine appropriate discharge recommendations. As successful critical care intervention increases and mortality rates decline, the number of individuals surviving, but experiencing long-lasting complications, is on the rise. In many instances, individuals who have experienced a prolonged and/or complex hospital course may remain significantly impaired requiring 24-hour care. In these cases, a long-term acute care facility may be indicated as a bridge between acute care and rehabilitation or home. Regardless of setting, the primary focus of OT is to (1) promote strength, endurance, and mobility within the context of ADL and IADL re-training and (2) provide client/caregiver education, including energy conservation strategies and stress management, to manage conditions at home and in the community.

Upon evaluation and throughout the intervention process, it is vital that oxygen levels are monitored via pulse oximetry, as well as an individual's respiratory pattern to determine work of breathing at rest and with increased activity demand. Often, individuals with chronic pulmonary disease will present with poor ventilation strategies such as shallow or fast breathing, as well as increased use of accessory muscles, which may further compound dyspnea and anxiety. Occupational therapists provide education that includes strategies to regulate breathing with activity, self-assess dyspnea with exertion, and independently apply appropriate techniques to minimize work of breathing as well as perform recovery breathing, if applicable. The most common technique employed to minimize shortness of breath in cases of COPD is **pursed-lip breathing**. Strategies are commonly embedded into ADL/IADL tasks and mobility.[29] Use of supplemental oxygen may also be necessary if **oxygen saturation (O_2 sat)** falls below 90% during activity. Clients should be provided with adequate education to manage O_2 equipment, including the O_2 cord, to increase functional independence, build confidence, and maximize safety.

Individuals experiencing respiratory disorders commonly find their ability to perform even basic tasks, such as bathing and dressing, compromised by dyspnea and decreased activity tolerance; energy conservation techniques are often incorporated into self-care re-training. Recommendations may include the modification of tasks, such as adjusting body mechanics to minimize the work of breathing, or altering the environment to reduce extraneous effort and decrease activity demand. Therapists will also educate clients in the use of adaptive equipment to maximize functional independence (e.g., long-handled sponge or dressing stick) or the use of durable medical equipment (e.g., tub seat for seated showers) (see Fig. 40-4). Similarly, recommendations are made to maximize participation and satisfaction in IADLs, such as home management, meal preparation, driving, leisure tasks, and social participation. Education emphasizes prioritizing, planning, and organizing tasks. This may include eliminating unnecessary steps, sitting versus standing if possible, setting up equipment in advance to minimize extraneous effort, and using lightweight tools or utensils. Additionally, clients are encouraged to self-assess dyspnea, pace themselves through activities, and take rest breaks before experiencing fatigue.

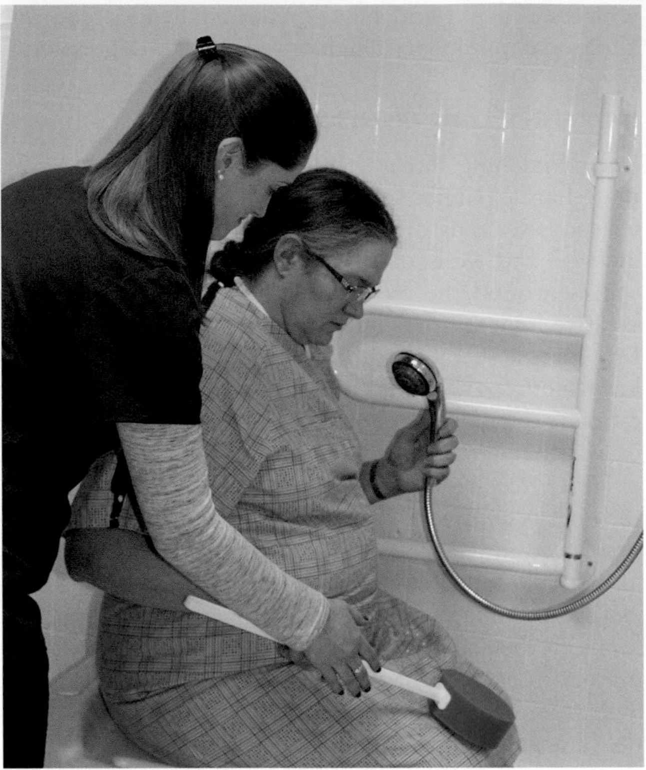

Figure 40-4. Tub seat for seated showers.

Stress and anxiety are common by-products of respiratory disorders. Educating individuals to manage dyspnea is integral to lessening anxiety and promoting participation in the treatment program. In addition to prioritizing activities, interventions include strategies to create a balanced lifestyle, increase awareness of body-and-mind interaction to manage breathing, identify stressors and perform daily activities with more confidence, and provide education on a variety of relaxation methods. These include guided imagery, progressive muscle relaxation, pursed-lip breathing technique, and diaphragmatic breathing.[30,31]

Prolonged hospitalization and chronic respiratory conditions frequently impact muscle strength and, in turn, may limit participation and/or performance in activities. Clients with a diagnosis of COPD, for example, often experience pain in the neck and shoulder region associated with overuse of accessory muscles, whereas individuals who have experienced critical illness may have significant muscle weakness. Providing education for body mechanics, stretching, and an appropriate exercise program can be invaluable to the process of improving aerobic capacity, reducing O_2 requirements, minimizing pain, and increasing performance in functional tasks. A tailored education plan may also include medication management training, exploration of healthy leisure pursuits to promote lifestyle balance, information regarding community resources (e.g., fitness groups, nutritional education), smoking cessation, and caregiver recommendations to support a safe transition.

CASE STUDY

Patient Information

Paul is a 58-year-old white male with a past medical history of HTN, CAD, hypercholesterolemia, obesity, and COPD with a history of tobacco use who developed chest pain due to angina while at work. He was treated on site with nitroglycerin and oxygen before being transported by emergency medical technicians (EMTs) to the emergency room. Upon admission, his blood pressure was 162/102 with a heart rate of 96 at rest, a respiration rate of 22, and an O_2 saturation of 90%. He underwent an EKG and cardiac catheterization to identify arterial blockages and subsequently underwent surgery for a CABG × 4. The left lower extremity great (long) saphenous vein (GSV) was harvested for grafting during the procedure. Paul initially tolerated the surgery well, but experienced lower extremity edema and pain that impacted his early mobilization and recovery. Once medically stable, Paul's interdisciplinary team determined that he would benefit from additional medical management and rehabilitation prior to discharge home.

Reason for Occupational Therapy Referral

In addition to decreased strength, endurance, and reduced functional mobility, Paul has ongoing discomfort at both sternal and graft sites, and he is functioning below his baseline for ADLs. He lives alone and must be independent with ADLs and many IADLs before returning home. His ultimate goal is to return to work.

Assessment Process and Results

The evaluation was conducted in Paul's room via informal interview, observation, and the FIM.[58] He reports fatigue and 4/10 pain at his graft site, but agrees to participate as tolerated. His sternum is covered with a protective dressing, whereas his lower extremity incision is open to the air with staples visible.

Paul states that he is in the process of a divorce, which has added to his recent stress. He works approximately 60 hours a week in the retail industry, which he reports is also highly stressful. He lives in a second floor single-level condo with one flight of stairs to enter and bilateral rails. His bathroom includes a tub/shower combo, but no equipment. Prior to surgery, he was independent with all mobility, ADLs, and IADLs. Paul admits to eating a large portion of fast food and leading a generally sedentary lifestyle, even though he knows he should be making healthier decisions because of his heart condition. He has not taken a vacation in 6 years and reports watching televised sports as his only leisure interest.

Throughout the assessment, Paul appeared fatigued with moderate increase in activity demand, although his vitals were stable and he only reported a mild increase in pain at his graft site with movement. He was able to perform mobility with a rolling walker (RW) and supervision, but benefited from verbal cues to refrain from pushing with his UEs to protect his sternum. He ambulated 15 feet to the bathroom and sponge-bathed sitting sink-side, but was able to stand for up to 1 minute at a time as needed. He required moderate assistance (Mod A) for both bathing and dressing tasks because of the sternal precautions impacting his ability to reach his lower extremities, and to bend and twist his torso. He reported significant fatigue with increased cardiopulmonary workload. A basic cognitive screen indicated that Paul was alert and oriented to person, place, and date; able to follow multistep directions; and demonstrated intact short- and long-term memory. At the end of the evaluation, Paul expressed his concerns regarding returning to work and how he would manage the lifestyle changes recommended by his cardiologist.

Occupational Therapy Problem List

- Limited activity tolerance impacting mobility and participation in ADLs/IADLs
- Limited knowledge of available adaptive equipment to assist with ADLs
- Limited knowledge of energy conservation education and effective pacing strategies
- Inconsistent application of sternal precautions with ADLs and mobility
- Limited knowledge of lifestyle modifications consistent with cardiologist's heart-healthy recommendations, including smoking cessation
- Increased signs of stress associated with life events and decline in function with limited knowledge of stress management strategies
- Limited knowledge of community-based resources

Occupational Therapy Goal List

Anticipated length of stay: 7 to 10 days

Duration and frequency of OT sessions: Approximately 45 to 60 minutes per day, 5 to 6x per week

- Complete ADL routine with modified independence (Mod I) sitting/standing as tolerated with appropriate use of adaptive equipment and application of energy conservation strategies and sternal precautions.
- Complete simple meal prep or laundry task with Mod I and appropriate energy conservation and work simplification strategies, and application of sternal precautions.
- Purchase adaptive equipment to maximize functional independence with ADLs upon discharge home.
- Explore stress management strategies, including healthy leisure pursuits, and plan to implement them in daily routine.
- Participate in disease management and lifestyle modification strategies.
- Explore community resources regarding smoking cessation.

Intervention

Paul's treatment plan consisted of increasing functional mobility and activity tolerance through ADLs and IADLs in order

(continued)

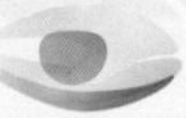

CASE STUDY *(continued)*

to maximize functional independence. It was of primary importance to include disease/stress management education, energy conservation skills, and adaptive equipment use via all tasks to better manage his condition and prepare for safe discharge. He was encouraged to pace himself throughout the day while gradually increasing tolerance for more demanding tasks in order to manage all necessary activities upon discharge. He was instructed in energy conservation strategies to perform tasks more efficiently and with less fatigue while continuing to build endurance. Discussion about the benefits of adaptive equipment was embedded into ADLs, and he was encouraged to trial recommendations during bathing and dressing tasks while maintaining sternal precautions. Once he had mastered his ADL routine, he more confidently participated in meaningful IADL. Energy conservation, work simplification strategies, and application of sternal precautions were included in kitchen activities, as well as light housekeeping, allowing Paul to perform tasks more efficiently and confidently.

Addressing disease management education to help implement lifestyle changes was an important step in empowering Paul to take responsibility for his health and minimize the risk of future cardiac events. Paul committed to smoking cessation and agreed to review the literature provided as well as follow up with community resources. He also agreed to explore stress management strategies and healthier leisure options. He completed both the Stress Management Questionnaire (SMQ)[59] and Interest Checklist[60] to understand his stressors and potential areas of interest. Paul identified the warning signs associated with burnout and anger, and was educated about the physical effects of high level and prolonged stress on his heart. He identified several healthier leisure tasks to explore and expressed an interest in relaxation strategies. He was introduced to progressive muscle relaxation strategies and guided imagery as an additional means of reducing stress.

Paul met all long-term goals by the anticipated date and was discharged home at an independent level for mobility, and at a Mod I level of function for ADLs and simple IADLs. He agreed to receive OT upon discharge to ensure a safe transition home, apply his new strategies in his own environment, and continue to build activity tolerance via higher level IADLs so that he could perform these meaningful tasks to a satisfactory level and ultimately return to work. As a short-term measure and although he was still unable to drive, he also agreed to a home delivery service for his groceries and a home health aide to assist with heavier household tasks.

Evidence Table of Intervention Studies for Cardiac and Pulmonary Disorders

Intervention	Description	Participants	Dosage	Research	Benefit	Statistical Significance
Early mobilization in mechanically ventilated patients vs. control group[39]	Sedated adults receiving mechanical ventilation in the ICU provided with mobilization to minimize long-term immobilization complications	One hundred and four participants randomly assigned to intervention or control group; 49 received mobilization during daily interruption of sedation; 55 received daily interruption of sedation only	Daily; duration of intervention varied	Randomized, double-blind, controlled trial Level II	Higher number of intervention group participants returned to independent level compared to control group.	Return to independence occurred in 59% of intervention group vs. 35% of control group ($p < 0.2$; odds ratio = 2.7 [95% confidence interval or CI 1.2–6.1]). Intervention group had shorter delirium duration (median 2 days, interquartile range [IQR] 0.0–6.0 vs. 4.0 days, 2.0–8.0; $p < 0.2$) and more ventilator-free days (23.5 days, 7.4–25.6 vs. 21.1 days, 0.0–23.8; $p < 0.05$).
Supervised or unsupervised structured exercise program vs. control group[28]	Inpatient, outpatient, or community-based setting exercise program	Six thousand one hundred and eleven participants	Varied from study to study. Minimum 2 weeks with minimum follow-up of 12 weeks	Systematic review and meta-analysis of 34 randomized controlled trials Level I	Participants in exercise-based cardiac rehab programs had a lower rate of re-infarction, cardiac, and all-cause mortality.	Reduction in all-cause mortality (odds ratio = 0.74; 95% CI 0.58–0.95). Reduction in cardiac mortality (odds ratio = 0.64); lower risk of re-infarction (odds ratio = 0.53); 95% CI 0.38–0.76.
Short-term pulmonary rehabilitation compared to brief advice[29]	Rehabilitation group included exercise and education. Brief advice group given instruction and advice on exercise with handout.	One hundred and three participants with severe COPD randomly assigned to pulmonary rehab or advice group. Fifty-four assigned to pulmonary group; 48 to the advice group.	Participants in rehabilitation group seen twice per week for 6 weeks. Advice participants received 1 hour individual advice and education.	Randomized controlled trial Level I Trial did not have blinded therapists or participants. Intervention time varied.	Rehabilitation group increased shuttle walking distance compared to advice group.	Statistically significant differences between group rehabilitation program and brief advice groups at 3 months in terms of shuttle walking distance (34.1 m; 3.0–65.3, $p < 0.05$)

References

1. Fuster V, Walsh RA, Harrington RA. Cardiac catheterization, cardiac angiography, and coronary blood flow and pressure measurements. In: *Hurst's the Heart*. 13th ed. New York, NY: The McGraw-Hill Companies; 2011.
2. Wood K. Measurement of gas exchange. Merck Manual Professional Version web site. https://www.merckmanuals.com/professional/pulmonary-disorders/tests-of-pulmonary-function-pft/measurement-of-gas-exchange. Updated October 2017. Accessed March 12, 2018.
3. World Health Organization. Cardiovascular diseases. World Health Organization web site. http://www.who.int/mediacentre/factsheets/fs317/en/. Updated May 2017. Accessed March 12, 2018.
4. Hawkes AL, Nowak M, Bidstrup B, Speare R. Outcomes of coronary artery bypass graft surgery. *Vasc Health Risk Manag*. 2006;2:477–484.
5. American Heart Association. Echocardiogram. American Heart Association web site. http://www.heart.org/HEARTORG/Conditions/HeartAttack/DiagnosingaHeartAttack/Echocardiogram---Echo_UCM_451485_Article.jsp#.WqrRayPMyCQ. Updated July 2015. Accessed March 8, 2018.
6. American Heart Association. Ejection fraction heart failure measurement. American Heart Association web site. http://www.heart.org/HEARTORG/Conditions/HeartFailure/DiagnosingHeartFailure/Ejection-Fraction-Heart-Failure-Measurement_UCM_306339_Article.jsp#.Wqvi-yPMxo4. Updated October 2017. Accessed March 7, 2018.
7. United States National Library of Medicine. Electrocardiogram. U.S. National Library of Medicine web site. https://medlineplus.gov/ency/article/003868.htm. Updated July 2015. Accessed March 12, 2018.
8. Tortora GJ, Derrickson BH. *Principles of Anatomy and Physiology*. Hoboken, NJ: John Wiley & Sons; 2008.
9. Chapman JT. Interstitial lung disease. Cleveland Clinic web site. http://www.clevelandclinicmeded.com/medicalpubs/diseasemanagement/pulmonary/interstitial-lung-disease/. Updated August 2010. Accessed March 14, 2018.
10. Alter A. Aboussouan LS, Mireles-Cabodevila E. Neuromuscular weakness in chronic obstructive pulmonary disease: chest wall, diaphragm, and peripheral muscle contributions. *Curr Opin Pulm Med*. 2017; 23(2):129–138. https://www.ncbi.nlm.nih.gov/pubmed/28079615.
11. Fahy B, Lareau S, Sockrider M. Pulse oximetry. *Am J Respir Crit Care Med*. 2011;184(1). Available from https://www.thoracic.org/patients/patient-resources/resources/pulse-oximetry.pdf. Online version updated December 2013. Accessed March 8, 2018.
12. National Heart, Lung, and Blood Institute. Percutaneous coronary intervention (PCI). National Heart, Lung, and Blood Institute web site. https://www.nhlbi.nih.gov/health/health-topics/topics/angioplasty. Published 2016. Accessed March 2, 2018.
13. Light RW. Pleural effusion. Merck Manual Professional Version web site. https://www.merckmanuals.com/professional/pulmonary-disorders/mediastinal-and-pleural-disorders/pleural-effusion. Updated October 2017. Accessed March 2, 2018.
14. Light RW. Pneumothorax. Merck Manual Professional Version web site. http://www.merckmanuals.com/professional/pulmonary-disorders/mediastinal-and-pleural-disorders/pneumothorax. Updated October 2017. Accessed March 2, 2018.
15. Scanlon PD. Respiratory function: mechanisms and testing. In: Goldman L, Schafer AI, eds. *Goldman's Cecil Medicine*. 25th ed. Philadelphia, PA: Elsevier Saunders; 2016:chap 85.
16. Shea MJ. Coronary artery bypass grafting (CABG). Merck Manual Professional Version web site. https://www.merckmanuals.com/professional/cardiovascular-disorders/cardiovascular-tests-and-procedures/coronary-artery-bypass-grafting-cabg. Updated September 2017. Accessed March 3, 2018.
17. American Heart Association. Hospitalizations, deaths from heart disease, stroke drop in last decade. American Heart Association web site. http://newsroom.heart.org/news/hospitalizations-for-heart-failure-on-the-decline-disparities-remain-for-blacks-and-men. Published June 2017. Accessed March 12, 2018.
18. American Heart Association. Statistical fact sheet 2013 update: Older Americans and cardiovascular disease. American Heart Association web site. https://www.heart.org/idc/groups/heart-public/@wcm/@sop/@smd/documents/downloadable/ucm_319574.pdf. Published 2013. Accessed March 2, 2018.
19. White CM, Buyting PL. Heart-happy occupations in a cardiac rehabilitation circuit. *OT Now*. 2011;13:11–13.
20. Bakris GL. Overview of hypertension. Merck Manual Professional Version web site. http://www.merckmanuals.com/professional/cardiovascular-disorders/hypertension/overview-of-hypertension. Updated February 2018. Accessed March 1, 2018.
21. Centers for Disease Control and Prevention. Blood pressure: make control your goal infographic. Centers for Disease Control and Prevention. https://www.cdc.gov/bloodpressure/infographic.htm. Updated September 2014. Accessed March 12, 2018.
22. Weber MA, Schiffrin EL, White WB, et al. Clinical practice guidelines for the management of hypertension in the community. *J Clin Hypertens*. 2014;16(1):14–26.
23. Centers for Disease Control and Prevention. Heart disease facts: heart disease in the United States. Centers for Disease Control and Prevention web site. https://www.cdc.gov/heartdisease/facts.htm. Updated November 2017. Accessed March 13, 2018.
24. Grech ED. Pathophysiology and investigation of coronary artery disease. *BMJ*. 2003;326:1027–1030.
25. Mayo Clinic. Coronary artery disease: diagnosis. Mayo Clinic web site. http://www.mayoclinic.org/diseases-conditions/coronary-artery-disease/diagnosis-treatment/diagnosis/dxc-20165331. Updated July 2017. Accessed March 12, 2018.
26. Cleveland Clinic. Coronary artery disease symptoms. Cleveland Clinic web site. http://my.clevelandclinic.org/health/articles/cad-symptoms. Published July 2017. Accessed March 12, 2018.
27. McSweeney JC, Cody M, O'Sullivan P, Elberson K, Moser DK, Garvin BJ. Women's early warning symptoms of acute myocardial infarction. *Circulation*. 2003;108(21):2619–2623.

28. Lawler PR, Filion KB, Eisenberg MJ. Efficacy of exercise-based cardiac rehabilitation post myocardial infarction: a systematic review and meta-analysis of randomized controlled trials. *Am Heart J*. 2011;162:571–584.
29. White RJ, Rudkin ST, Harrison ST, Day KL, Harve IM. Pulmonary rehabilitation compared with brief advice given for severe chronic obstructive pulmonary disease. *J Cardiopulm Rehabil*. 2002;22:338–344.
30. Heart disease facts. Centers for Disease Control and Prevention web site. https://www.cdc.gov/heartdisease/facts.htm. Updated November 2017. Accessed March 10, 2018.
31. Cannon C, Braunwald B. Unstable angina and non-ST-elevation myocardial infarction. In: Libby P, Bonow R, Mann D, Zipes D, Braunwald E, eds. *Braunwald's Heart Disease*. Philadelphia, PA: Sanders Elsevier; 2005:1183, 1319–1351.
32. Zafari AM, Abdou MH. Myocardial infarction treatment and management. Medscape web site. http://emedicine.medscape.com/article/155919-treatment#d5. Updated February 2018. Accessed March 2, 2018.
33. Shah SJ. Heart failure (congestive heart failure): Merck Manual Professional Version web site. http://www.merckmanuals.com/home/heart-and-blood-vessel-disorders/heart-failure/heart-failure. Updated March 2017. Accessed March 4, 2018.
34. Centers for Disease Control and Prevention. Heart failure fact sheet. Centers for Disease Control and Prevention web site. https://www.cdc.gov/dhdsp/data_statistics/fact_sheets/fs_heart_failure.htm. Updated June 2016. Accessed March 10, 2018.
35. Doherty RF. Cardiopulmonary dysfunction in adults. In: Crepeau EB, Cohn E, Schell BAB, eds. *Willard & Spackman's Occupational Therapy*. Philadelphia, PA: Lippincott Williams & Wilkins; 2003:807–819.
36. Cahalin LP, LaPier TK, Shaw DK. Sternal precautions: Is it time for change? Precautions versus restrictions—a review of literature and recommendations for revision. *Cardiopulm Phys Ther J*. 2011;22(1):5–15.
37. Interprofessional Education Collaborative Expert Panel. *Core Competencies for Interprofessional Collaborative Practice: Report of an Expert Panel*. Washington, DC: IPEC. https://nebula.wsimg.com/2f68a39520b03336b41038c370497473?AccessKeyId=DC06780E69ED19E2B3A5&disposition=0&alloworigin=1. Updated 2016. Accessed March 2, 2018.
38. American Occupational Therapy Association. *Occupational Therapy Practice Framework: Domain and Process*. 3rd ed. Bethesda, MD: AOTA Press/American Occupational Therapy Association; 2014.
39. Schweickert WD, Pohlman MC, Pohlman AS, et al. Early physical and occupational therapy in mechanically ventilated, critically ill patients: a randomised controlled trial. *Lancet*. 2009;373(9678):1874–1882.
40. Levine GN, Steinke EE, Backaeen FG, et al. Sexual activity and cardiovascular disease: a scientific statement from the American Heart Association. *Circulation*. 2012;125:1058–1072.
41. Ainsworth BW, Haskell WL, Hermann SD, et al. Compendium of physical activities: a second update of codes and met levels. *Med Sci Sports Exerc*. 2011;43:1575–1581.
42. Maden SK, Sivarajan Froelicher ES. Psychosocial risk factors: assessment and management interventions. In: Woods SL, Sivarajan Froelicher ES, Adams Motser S, Bridges EJ, eds. *Cardiac Nursing*. Philadelphia, PA: Lippincott Williams; 2010:769–782.
43. Ehrman JK, Dejong A, Sanderson B, Swain D, Swank A, Womak C, eds.; American College of Sports Medicine. *ACM's Resource Manual for Guidelines for Exercise Testing and Prescription*. Philadelphia, PA: Wolters Kluwer; 2010.
44. Sohn M, Hawk M, Martin K, Froelicher ESS. Smoking cessation and relapse prevention. In: Woods SL, Sivarajan Froelicher ES, Adams Motser S, Bridges EJ, eds. *Cardiac Nursing*. 6th ed. Philadelphia, PA: Lippincott Williams; 2010:783–798.
45. Ridker P, Libby P. Risk factors for atherothrombotic disease. In: Libby P, Bonow R, Mann D, Zipes D, Braunwald E, eds. *Braunwald's Heart Disease*. Philadelphia, PA: Saunders Elsevier; 2008:1419–1449.
46. Center for Disease Control and Prevention. Adult obesity facts. Center for Disease Control and Prevention web site. https://www.cdc.gov/obesity/data/adult.html. Updated March 2018. Accessed March 14, 2018.
47. Warzeski M, Choo J, Novak J, Burke LE. Obesity. In: Moser D, Reigel, B, eds. *Cardiac Nursing*. St. Louis, MO; 2008:446–462.
48. O'Connell-Edwards CF, York E, Blumenthal JA. Psychosocial risk factors and coronary disease. In: Durstine JL, Moore GE, LaMonte MJ, Franklin BA, eds. *Pollock's Textbook of Cardiovascular Disease and Rehabilitation*. Champagne, IL: Human Kinetics; 2008:235–245.
49. Center for Disease Control and Prevention. Chronic obstructive pulmonary disease (COPD) includes: chronic bronchitis and emphysema. Center for Disease Control and Prevention web site. http://www.cdc.gov/nchs/fastats/copd.htm. Updated May 2017. Accessed March 14, 2018.
50. MacNee, W. ABC of chronic obstructive pulmonary disease: pathology, pathogenesis, and pathophysiology. *BMJ*. 2006;332(7551):1202.
51. Ford ES, Murphy LB, Khavjou O, Giles WH, Holt JB, Croft JB. Total and state-specific medical and absenteeism costs of COPD among adults aged ≥ 18 years in the United States for 2010 and projections through 2020. *Chest*. 2015;147(1):31–45.
52. National Heart, Lung, and Blood Institute. What is COPD? National Heart, Lung, and Blood Institute web site. https://www.nhlbi.nih.gov/health-topics/copd. Accessed March 2018.
53. Pierrakos C, Karanikolas M, Scolletta S, Karamouzos V, Velissaris D. Acute respiratory distress syndrome: pathophysiology and therapeutic options. *J Clin Med Res*. 2012;4(1):7–16.
54. American Lung Association. Lung and health diseases: recovering from ARDS. American Lung Association web site. http://www.lung.org/lung-health-and-diseases/lung-disease-lookup/ards/recovering-from-ards.html. Accessed March 2018.
55. Lee J. Disease: diffuse parenchymal lung diseases. Merck Manual Professional Version web site. https://www.merckmanuals.com/professional/pulmonary-disorders/interstitial-lung-diseases/overview-of-interstitial-lung-disease. Reviewed April 2016. Accessed March 2, 2018.

56. Raghu G, Brown KK. Interstitial lung disease: clinical evaluation and keys to an accurate diagnosis. *Clin Chest Med*. 2004;25(3):409–419.
57. Schneider C, Jick S, Bothner U, Meier CR. COPD and the risk of depression. *Chest*. 2010;137:341–347.
58. Uniform Data System for Medical Rehabilitation. About the FIM system®. http://www.udsmr.org/WebModules/FIM/Fim_About.aspx. Accessed March 12, 2018.
59. Stein F, Bentley D, Natz M. Computerized assessment: the stress management questionnaire. In: Hemphill-Pearson B, ed. *Assessments in Occupational Therapy Mental Health: An Integrative Approach*. Thorofare, NJ: SLACK Incorporated; 1999:321–337.
60. Klyczek JP, Bauer-Yox N, Fiedler RC. The interest checklist: a factor analysis. *Am J Occup Ther*. 1997;51(10):815–823.

Chapter **41**

Orthopedic Conditions

Colleen Maher and Rochelle J. Mendonca

LEARNING OBJECTIVES

This chapter will allow the reader to:

1. Identify the role of the occupational therapist in assessing and planning treatment for persons with occupational dysfunction secondary to injuries, disease, or conditions affecting the musculoskeletal system.
2. Select appropriate assessments and plan treatment according to the stages of recovery following a musculoskeletal injury or conditions of the upper extremity.
3. Describe how to accomplish daily life tasks without causing adverse sequelae following fracture or surgery to the back, hip, and upper extremity.
4. Describe the phases of fracture management of the upper extremity and how to optimize occupational functioning at each stage.
5. State the principles of body mechanics and describe how to apply them to activities and tasks of daily life.

CHAPTER OUTLINE

TERMINOLOGY

Abduction pillow brace: a sling or brace that positions the shoulder in 30° to 45° of abduction to protect the repaired supraspinatus.

Codman's pendulum exercises: shoulder exercises in which the client stands or sits, bends over at the hips so that the trunk is parallel to the floor, and swings the arm passively or actively in various linear and circular motions.[1]

Controlled range of motion: active or passive movement within a predetermined safe arc.

Scapular plane: the midpoint between shoulder flexion and abduction. The majority of functional activities occur in this plane.

Shoulder immobilizer: adjustable elastic band that fits around the waist with two straps that position and secure the arm in a slightly abducted and internally rotated position.

Trendelenburg gait: ambulation pattern that results from a weakened gluteus medius muscle; the client lurches toward the injured side to place the center of gravity over the hip; it is characterized by dropping of the pelvis on the unaffected side at heel strike of the affected foot.

Volkmann's ischemia: increased compartment pressure in one anatomic area of the extremity as a result of a fracture or crush injury.

Introduction

Orthopedic conditions include injuries, diseases, and deformities of bones, joints, and their related soft tissue structures: muscles, tendons, ligaments, and nerves. In the United States, one out of two people aged 18 and older suffer from orthopedic conditions.[2] These conditions can be caused by traumatic events, such as motor vehicle, sports, recreational, or work-related accidents; by cumulative trauma; by obesity; or by congenital anomaly. This chapter provides an overview of the occupational therapy assessments and treatment interventions used with adult clients who have orthopedic conditions. Specifically, it reviews upper extremity and hip fractures and their sequelae, hip surgery for trauma and disease, and shoulder injuries and their effects on function.

Purpose and Role of Occupational Therapy in Orthopedics

The aim of occupational therapy in orthopedic rehabilitation is to help clients achieve maximal musculoskeletal functioning in order to perform their everyday activities. In the acute stage of recovery, the occupational therapist's role is to help relieve pain, decrease swelling and inflammation, assist in wound care, maintain joint or limb alignment, and restore function at the injury site. The therapist teaches the client to safely perform tasks and activities while protecting the injury site for healing. As healing progresses, the occupational therapist works with the client to restore activities of daily living (ADLs) and other occupational tasks.

For individuals who have a chronic joint disease, such as osteoarthritis, the occupational therapist's role depends on the stage of recovery and the directives of the treatment team. The occupational therapist may directly help relieve pain, realign structures, or reduce the stress on soft tissue, or work closely with the physical therapist to relate the functional program to the treatment offered in physical therapy. As the acute episode of pain decreases, the occupational therapist focuses on an individually tailored education program to help the client physically and psychologically make the required lifestyle changes to reach and sustain optimal occupational functioning.

Occupational Therapy Evaluation in Orthopedics

Evaluation is an ongoing process that is carefully coordinated with the stage of recovery. The occupational therapist selects assessments that will provide sufficient information to plan and to direct treatment but will not threaten the injured or inflamed structure during healing. The occupational therapist chooses assessments based on several factors that may include the postsurgical precautions provided by the surgeon, the level of bone healing, the chosen method of reduction and stabilization, and the plan for movement during soft tissue healing or the acute inflammatory episode. The therapist assesses participation in life roles, including areas of occupations, performance skills and performance patterns, as well as impairments of capacities and abilities.

Participation in Life Roles

Although resumption of life roles may not be possible at the start of the rehabilitation program, life roles regulate the choices made during treatment planning and serve as the end point for treatment planning. The therapist notes activities and tasks that can and cannot be accomplished.

Impairments of Abilities and Capacities

Physical impairments are directly measured by various assessment instruments. The surgeon's protocol may stipulate no movement or no force at or near the fracture or surgical site, or it may require **controlled range of motion** beginning immediately or within the first 2 to 6 weeks after stabilization. If the surgeon's protocol requires complete rest of the injured tendon, bone, or joint, range of motion (ROM) measurements are deferred until movement is permissible. If the client is on a specific program, such as controlled ROM, the therapist measures the joint, adhering to the precautionary boundaries, and does not allow the client to exceed the limits of the surgeon's prescription. The adjacent joints are measured, and a treatment program is designed for any adjacent joint that demonstrates less than normal function. Detailed strength testing with applied resistance is deferred until there is bony consolidation and tissue healing, or the acute inflammation has calmed. Because of the force required, grip and pinch testing are usually deferred for 2 to 4 weeks following cast removal in forearm fractures. The occupational therapist not only focuses on direct measurement of the injured and adjacent anatomical regions but also closely observes the client's total body response in terms of postural changes, pain responses, and psychological reactions. Assessing strength after a fracture or surgery should only be performed when ordered by the orthopedist.

Occupational Therapy Treatment in Orthopedics

The most important treatment goal is the restoration of occupational functioning. To achieve this, the client needs to be directed from the start of recovery to move and to use all joints that are not affected by the injury or the disease. For clients who have an upper limb fracture, rotator cuff repair, or a short-term inflammation, the therapist may recommend temporary use of the uninjured hand alone to perform some ADLs, assisted by adaptations such as pump bottles for toothpaste and shampoo, a button hook, or a rocker knife. Other ADLs may require the temporary assistance of another person so as not to disturb the healing region. When the client is medically ready, the occupational therapist, through careful activity analysis, ascertains how the client can safely resume tasks that correspond with the achieved recovery status to reintegrate the injured, postsurgical or inflamed limb into activity safely. Attention is directed toward redeveloping the function of the injured limb to resume its capacity in mobility, stability, weight bearing, and ultimately skilled activity. When a condition is chronic or has postsurgical precautions, such as a total hip replacement, the therapist recommends alternative methods, adaptive equipment, or environmental modification for safe task completion.

Upper Extremity Fractures

As long as orthopedic surgeons have been treating fractures, there has been a controversy between those who recommend movement and those who recommend rest. The surgeons prescribing rest as a fracture treatment keep their clients immobilized in traction, plaster, or fiberglass for long periods after stabilization. For many surgeons, however, the goal in fracture treatment is to mobilize the injured structures as quickly as is compatible with healing and return the client to work and leisure activities.[1]

The goal of fracture treatment is to achieve a precise and effective stabilization for optimal recovery and return to function. Closed fractures that are relatively undisplaced and stable may be managed by protection alone, without reduction or immobilization. Fractures that are undisplaced, but unstable, do not need reduction but do require positioning and immobilization by external fixation methods such as a sling, cast, or a fracture brace. Open reduction internal fixation (ORIF) surgically reduces open fractures, closed fractures that are unstable, and where the bone fragments cannot be approximated accurately by closed manual reduction alone. The bone fragments are brought into closer anatomical alignment during surgical reduction and are stabilized by insertion of an internal fixation device, such as a nail, pin, screw, rod, or compression plate or by an external fixator.[3] Surgical repair can also include prosthetic devices that are implanted to restore joint motion.

Fracture healing has a general timetable that is confirmed routinely by physical examination and x-rays to reveal the healing status before advancing the rehabilitation program. The estimated healing time for uncomplicated upper extremity fractures in adults is as follows: callus formation 2 to 3 weeks, union 4 to 6 weeks, and consolidation 6 to 8 weeks. For uncomplicated lower extremity fractures, the estimated healing time is as follows: callus formation 2 to 3 weeks, union 8 to 12 weeks, and consolidation 12 to 16 weeks.[4]

There are three phases of fracture healing: the inflammation phase, the reparative phase, and the remodeling phase.[5] The timing, amount, and kind of therapy depend on the location and kind of fracture, the method of fracture reduction selected by the orthopedic surgeon, and, in some instances, the age of the client. Early movement prevents the unwanted side effects of immobilization: stiff joints, disuse atrophy, and muscle weakness.

Shoulder Fractures

The shoulder complex comprises the glenohumeral joint, scapulothoracic joint, sternoclavicular joint, and acromioclavicular joint. The shoulder complex not only provides a wide range of movements for hand placement but also provides the important functions of stabilization for hand use, lifting, pushing, reaching, and weight bearing.[6] The shoulder is considered the most challenging portion of the body to rehabilitate. After a shoulder fracture, the therapy goals are delicately balanced to relieve pain, to restore movement and muscle strength, to allow for callus formation and the approximation of the bony fragments in the injured region, and to return to a maximal level of functioning. The progression of the exercise program and return to functional tasks is directed by the orthopedist based on radiographic imaging of the fracture site.

Immobilization of the shoulder results in stiffness and pain; therefore, nonoperative and postoperative therapy programs call for a specific regimen of passive range of motion (PROM), active-assisted range of motion (AAROM), or active range of motion (AROM) within a controlled, guarded range. The therapist must remember that PROM differs from passive stretching. PROM is movement of the limb by an external force to its available end range or prescribed end range. Passive stretching is movement of the limb by an external force to its available end range and then applying overpressure.

Passive stretching is contraindicated in the early stages of fracture healing. Emphasis is on the client resuming nonresistive functional activities and using the injured limb as soon as movement is allowed.

Conservative or Nonoperative Management

Because immobilization quickly results in stiffness, shoulder motion begins as soon as the acute pain diminishes in stable or minimally displaced shoulder fractures. Therapy begins with sling immobilization. Controlled exercise programs can begin as early as 1 to 2 weeks postinjury and include **Codman's pendulum exercises** and gentle PROM. PROM is performed in supine with shoulder forward flexion, abduction in the **scapular plane**, and internal rotation and external rotation (initially may be restricted). AROM of the uninvolved joints should begin at this time. ADLs are performed using one-handed techniques. Gentle submaximal isometrics may begin at 4 weeks for flexion, abduction, and internal rotation. At 6 weeks, the client can begin AROM.[7–9] AROM should begin in gravity-lessened positions and progress to against gravity, with the therapist making certain that there are no unwanted compensatory movements such as shoulder hiking. Light self-care activities can begin at this time. Self-care activities should be nonresistive and include only those in a gravity-lessened position (such as reaching for a salt shaker in the middle of a table while standing). The client can be weaned off the sling when AROM begins. At 8 to 12 weeks, the sling is usually discarded, and the client can begin isotonic strengthening. After 12 weeks, sports, leisure, and work activities are initiated.[7–9]

Postoperative Management

Unstable shoulder fractures usually require surgical intervention for fixation. The protocols are based on the classification of fracture, the type of surgical procedure, and the age and activity level of the client, and they often follow the guidelines as originally described by Neer.[10] Some postoperative protocols start with early mobilization programs, whereas others have a period of immobilization. A study found no difference in function between those who received early mobilization immediately versus those who started mobilization 3-weeks postsurgical fixation.[11] When approved by the surgeon, the sequence of exercise begins with Codman's pendulum exercises (see Fig. 41-1). Codman's pendulum exercises are performed with the client bending over so that the injured upper limb is perpendicular to the floor. In this gravity-assisted plane, the client does clockwise and counterclockwise circular movements and flexion, extension, abduction, and adduction. Codman's pendulum exercises may be contraindicated if the upper extremity is edematous.

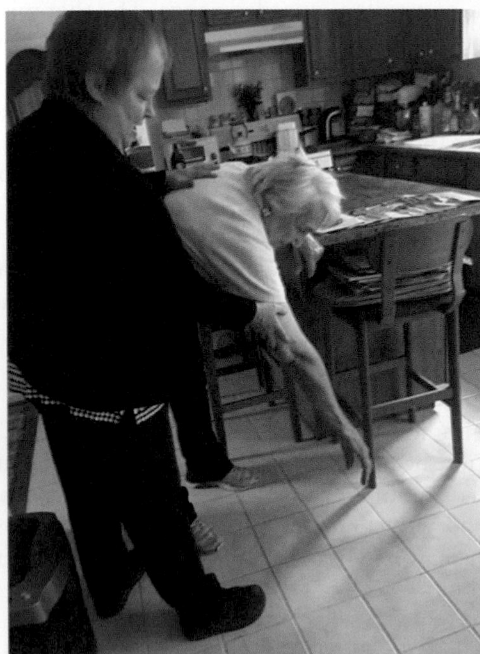

Figure 41-1. Codman's pendulum exercise.

Also, during the first 6 to 8 weeks, PROM of shoulder flexion and external rotation to 40° are started in supine, as are isometric exercises, a stimulant for fracture healing and callus formation. By 6 weeks, AROM, nonresistive therapeutic activities, and light ADLs begin. Strengthening starts at 12 weeks.[8,12]

Humeral head fractures that are unstable and significantly displaced are often surgically treated with humeral head replacement, known as hemiarthroplasty (see Fig. 41-2). A total shoulder arthroplasty is considered for clients with severe arthritis in combination with a proximal humerus fracture.[13] Another surgical approach is the reverse total shoulder replacement. This approach is used when there is significant damage to the rotator cuff or severe arthritis of the glenohumeral joint. The major limitation of this surgery is impaired shoulder rotation.[14,15]

Therapy for total shoulder arthroplasty varies with the design of the prosthesis and the surgical procedure. The rehabilitation program begins within the first 1 to 2 days after surgery. The exercises should not cause any pain. The key to a satisfactory functional result is early achievement of shoulder elevation and external rotation in the plane of the scapula. Passive shoulder elevation done lying supine with the opposite hand assisting the affected limb, and use of an exercise wand to perform passive external rotation, which may be restricted to 30°, are introduced during the first 3 to 5 days after surgery.[16,17] Codman's pendulum exercises are added at 1 week post-op.[8] The client is instructed to perform the exercises four to six times daily. Because the subscapularis tendon may be incised during surgery and the integrity of the rotator cuff may be disrupted, some surgeons introduce external rotation slowly in the first

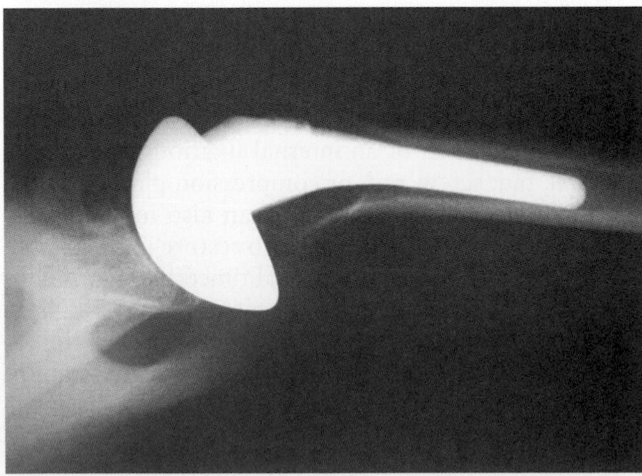

Figure 41-2. Hemiarthroplasty.

4 weeks; others incorporate passive external rotation on the second postoperative day. The preferred position for passive external rotation exercise is with the humerus in slight scaption. During this phase, the client is instructed to begin nonresistive everyday activities, such as brushing teeth and self-feeding, while keeping the shoulder adducted to the side. At 3 weeks, submaximal isometrics are added. AROM is added at 6 weeks. Progress AROM from supine to sitting, avoiding compensatory movements such as shoulder hiking.[16] At 8 to 12 weeks, Thera-band exercises, free weights, and purposeful activities that emphasize shoulder elevation and rotational movements are initiated. At 12 weeks, the client is instructed in sports and work activities. Weight bearing on the injured arm is not allowed for at least 6 months.[10,17] The goal is to achieve 135° of shoulder elevation (scaption), which is considered functional AROM, and 50° of internal and external rotation.

Following the initial treatment of closed reduction of fractures in the shaft of long bones, such as humeral shaft fractures, the surgeon may prescribe a functional fracture brace as popularized by Sarmiento,[18,19] as shown in Figure 41-3. The lightweight thermoplastic fracture brace allows for motion above and below the fracture site and minimizes the detrimental effects of prolonged immobilization. The client is closely monitored for biomechanical alignment and desired, controlled movement. The therapist adjusts the fracture brace to facilitate comfort, to respond to changes such as a reduction of limb volume, and to adjust the amount of movement the splint permits. Management of humeral shaft includes Codman's pendulum exercises and PROM exercises that are performed several times a day to prevent stiffness. The therapist must be careful to flare and roll the edges of the shell to prevent compromise to circulation and nerve impingement while allowing available movement.

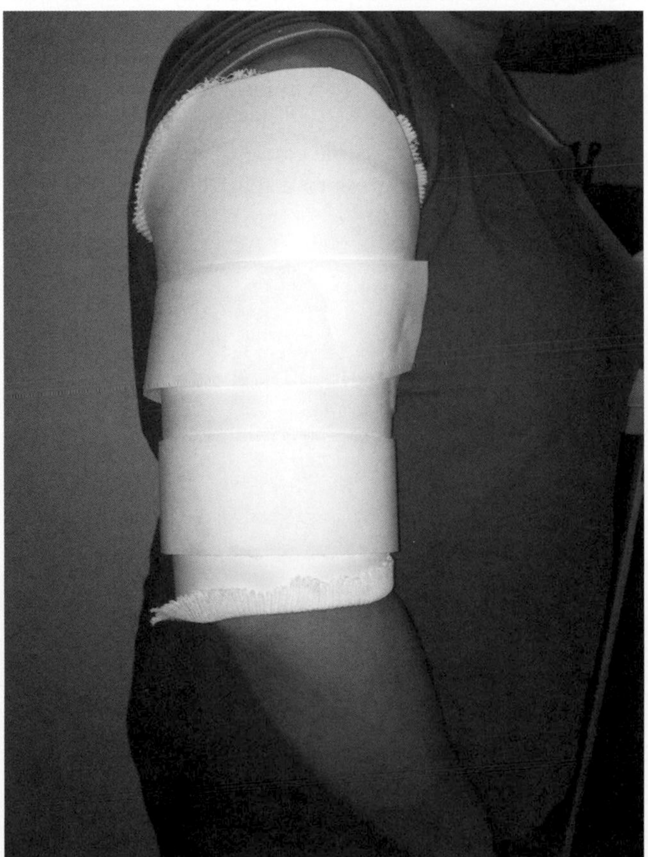

Figure 41-3. Thermoplastic humeral fracture brace to support the length of the humerus during healing.

In the case of humeral shaft fracture, there is a risk of radial nerve damage because of the location of the injury relative to the course of the radial nerve. Radial nerve injury is characterized by the inability to extend the elbow, wrist, and digits. Other complications that are common with humeral shaft fractures are delayed union and nonunion.

For phase II, the therapist encourages AAROM, progressing to AROM and lightly resistive exercises. The surgeon will guide the therapist on the timing to begin each of these exercises. These exercises often begin with the client supine and progress to seated, in which the weight of the extremity is first supported by the therapist. Phase III addresses both stretching and strengthening. As healing permits, the client can combine shoulder forward flexion with abduction with or without external rotation.[12]

Elbow Fractures

Elbow motion gives the individual the capacity to position the hand in space close to or far from the body for fine motor activities and to function as a stabilizer for strength activities.[20] These movements are accomplished by two degrees of freedom: flexion and extension at the ulnohumeral and radiohumeral joints, and pronation and supination at the proximal radioulnar joint. Intercondylar and supracondylar fractures (the extension type) are the most common of the distal humerus fractures that impact elbow function. These fractures are associated with complications that include malunion and peripheral nerve injury and have a risk of **Volkmann's ischemia**, a compartment syndrome of the forearm. Ischemia, considered an urgent medical matter, can be caused by an increase in pressure within a fascia-surrounded compartment. Signs of ischemia include severe pain with passive stretching; pale, bluish skin color; absence of forearm radial pulse; and decreased hand sensation and paralysis.[21] Report these signs immediately.

Immediate medical action is important if Volkmann's ischemia is suspected. The common surgical approach includes a decompressive fasciotomy. One unfortunate complication is Volkmann's ischemic contracture, which can be mild to severe and often requires additional surgeries. Under the close supervision of the surgeon, the occupational therapist will focus on restoring functional ROM, managing scar tissue, and regaining function.[21]

The nondisplaced or minimally displaced supracondylar fracture may be treated with closed reduction and immobilization in a removable cast or thermoplastic splint. After 1 to 2 weeks, the splint is removed daily for gentle AROM in a hinge splint.[22] The splint is discharged after 6 weeks and client is encouraged to use his or her extremity for light ADLs.

Complex elbow fractures, which include displaced supracondylar fractures and intercondylar fractures, are most often treated with open reduction and well-secured fixation.[23] Active motion begins 2 to 3 days after surgery. The elbow fracture is splinted in 90° of flexion rather than extension because flexion has greater functional importance. The splint is removed by the therapist to begin gentle AAROM. ROM of elbow flexion and extension is best performed in a supine or seated position with the distal humerus supported by a pillow or towel roll (see Fig. 41-4). Gravity will assist with flexion and extension. Adhere strictly to any ROM restrictions. If the client also injured the collateral ligaments, restrictions on forearm rotation during elbow flexion and extension may be prescribed by the orthopedic surgeon. Forearm ROM is performed in a seated position with the elbow flexed at 90°.[20] Gentle PROM and light isotonic exercises are usually initiated between 6 and 8 weeks. The client is encouraged to use his or her extremity for light self-care activities. At 8 weeks, there is an increased emphasis on restoring full ROM and increasing strength. In the elderly, elbow fractures are often treated with a sling alone, and active movement begins early to prevent stiffness and pain. A functional arc of motion for daily activities can be regained, but full ROM is not always achieved.

Radial head fractures can be treated with closed reduction or, depending on the severity, may require radial head excision. Radial head fractures seldom require more than a sling for immobilization. Active pronation and supination exercises are encouraged early. Emphasis should be placed on regaining active supination. Full supination is more difficult and painful than pronation.[20] Supination and pronation exercises should be performed seated or standing, with the shoulder adducted to the side and elbow flexed to 90° (see Fig. 41-5). Exercises should be performed several times daily, with a minimum of two sets of 10 repetitions. Exercises should be pain-free. Continuous passive motion (CPM), dynamic supination splint, and static progressive splinting can be used to further encourage forearm rotation.

Rotator Cuff Pathologies

The shoulder complex is the foundation of all upper extremity movements. The rotator cuff musculature plays an integral part in the function and control of the shoulder complex. The supraspinatus performs humeral elevation, the infraspinatus and teres minor perform external rotation, and the subscapularis performs internal rotation. Besides the actions they produce, the rotator cuff musculature functions as a force couple to control the head of the humerus on the glenoid fossa. Its anatomical location at the subacromial space, between the coracoacromial arch and the head of the humerus, makes the rotator cuff extremely vulnerable to compression (see Fig. 41-6). Charles Neer[10] described a hooked acromion (type 3) as a possible cause of impingement syndrome that could progress to a tear. The supraspinatus

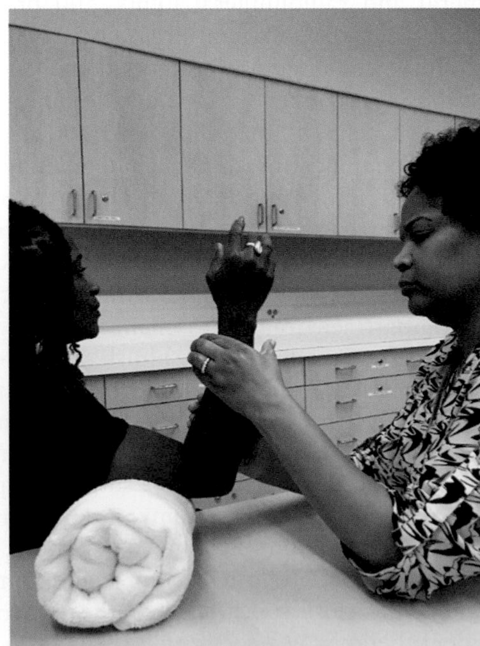

Figure 41-4. Range of motion of the elbow.

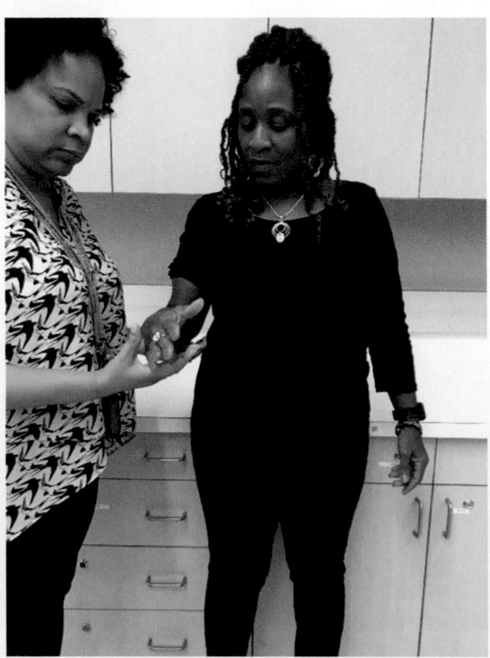

Figure 41-5. Forearm supination pronation.

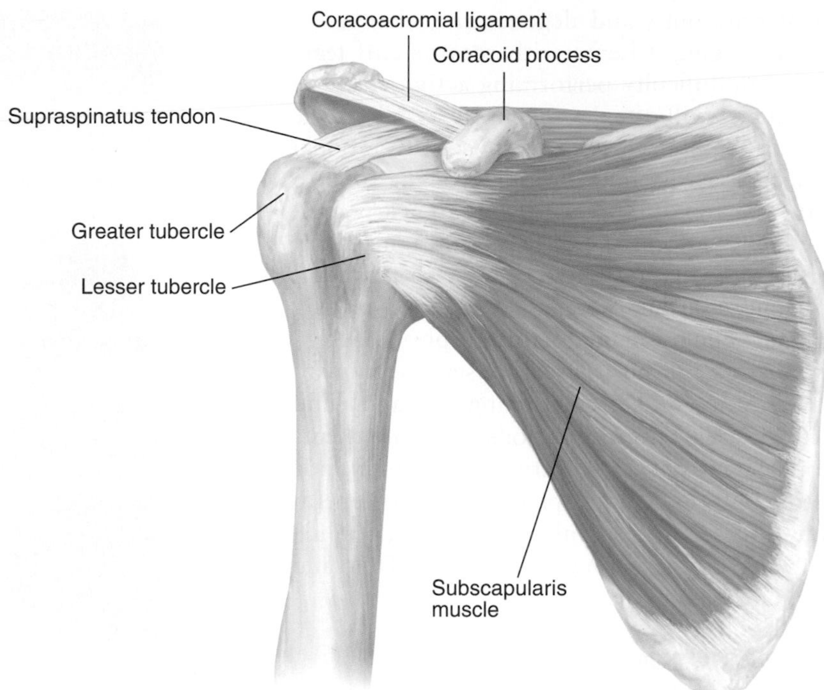

Figure 41-6. Subacromial space.

also has an area of hypovascularity known as the critical zone. This zone is where the supraspinatus tendon inserts on the greater tuberosity of the humerus. Because of its anatomical location and area of hypovascularity, the tendon of the supraspinatus is the most commonly impinged rotator cuff tendon. Clients with rotator cuff pathology are often faced with the inability to perform the most personal self-care tasks. Activities such as toileting, hair care, and hooking a bra are all dependent on a normally functioning rotator cuff.

Shoulder Impingement Syndrome

Shoulder impingement syndrome is a compression of the structures found in the subacromial space. Structures found in the subacromial space (superior to inferior) include the subacromial bursa, supraspinatus, joint capsule, and long head of the biceps. Shoulder impingement syndrome is most commonly caused by a hooked acromion and or repetitive or sustained elevation of the shoulder above 90°. If shoulder impingement syndrome goes untreated, it can result in a rotator cuff tear. Neer[10] developed a classification system to better understand the progression of shoulder impingement syndrome. Stage I is described as edema, inflammation, and hemorrhage. In this stage, the bursa and/or the tendons become irritated and inflamed. The symptoms can be reversed with occupational therapy intervention. The focus should be on activity modification. In stage II, the bursa and tendons become thick and fibrotic. At this stage, a person can be treated conservatively; however, recovery may take longer. In stage III, a person may present with bone spurs and partial- or full-thickness tears. A small tear is less than 1 cm, a medium tear is 1 to 3 cm, a large tear is 3 to 5 cm, and a massive tear is greater than 5 cm.[24]

Rotator Cuff Tendonitis and Bicipital Tendonitis

A person may have rotator cuff tendonitis and or bicipital tendonitis, but not shoulder impingement syndrome. The chief complaint of tendonitis is pain during humeral movement above 90°. In most cases, the client is independent with ADLs; however, the client will experience pain while performing these tasks. Common causes are repetitive overhead use, curved or hooked acromion, weakness of shoulder or scapula musculature, and capsular tightness. Tendonitis can be treated conservatively with pain modalities, activity modification, strengthening exercises, and occupation-based activities.

Bursitis

Shoulder bursitis is inflammation of the subacromial bursa. Subacromial bursitis can be differentiated from rotator cuff tendonitis if the client has pain during passive shoulder elevation and is pain-free during AROM and muscle testing of the rotator cuff. It is rarely a major source of pain and usually coexists with shoulder impingement syndrome.[25] See the section on shoulder impingement for causes.

Rotator Cuff Tear

Tears of the rotator cuff can be of partial or full thickness. Causes include trauma, progression of impingement syndrome, and degenerative changes of the tendon and aging. Clients with rotator cuff tears will present with difficulty performing activities above shoulder level and will often compensate by hiking the shoulder using the upper trapezius muscle. Rotational movements, such as reaching the small of the back to tuck a shirt in or remove a wallet from a back pocket, can also be limited. Rotator cuff tears can significantly limit a person's occupational functioning. Rotator cuff tears are diagnosed using magnetic resonance imaging (MRI) and magnetic resonance arthrography (MRA).[26] Some partial tears can be treated conservatively with activity modification and strengthening of scapula and rotator cuff muscles. Surgical options for those clients who do not benefit from conservative treatment include arthroscopic, mini-open, and open repairs. Postoperative therapy focuses on regaining full ROM, scapula and rotator cuff strengthening, practicing ADLs, and other meaningful tasks.

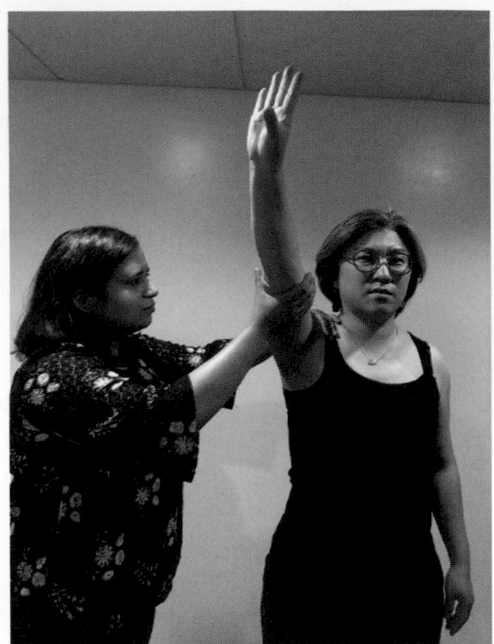

Figure 41-7. Neer impingement sign.

Evaluation of the Nonsurgical Client

The evaluation should begin with an occupational profile and a thorough history. Discuss the mechanism of injury. Was it a sudden onset or gradual onset? If it was a gradual onset, try to determine what activity or sustained posture led to the rotator cuff problem. Also discuss the client's level of pain (scale of 0–10). Is the pain localized or referred? What activities or occupations cause pain? Can the client sleep on the involved side? The therapist should also observe the client's posture and symmetry of the scapula at rest and during upward rotation. The physical assessments can then begin with asking the client to perform various functional movements such as reaching the small of the back, reaching the opposite axilla, and touching the top of the head. Active cervical ROM and sensory testing the C4 to T1 dermatomes should be performed to eliminate the possibility of cervical involvement. Palpation of the rotator cuff tendons will assess tenderness and swelling. Special tests should be administered to determine all the involved structures. Special tests for rotator cuff pathology include:

- *Neer impingement sign:* Forced forward flexion with the shoulder internally rotated. If the patient expresses pain, the sign is positive, indicating compression and/or inflammation of the supraspinatus and/or long head of the biceps (Fig. 41-7).
- *Hawkins test:* Shoulder and elbow are flexed to 90° followed by forced internal rotation. If the patient expresses pain (Fig. 41-8), the test is positive, indicating compression and/or inflammation of the supraspinatus and long head of the biceps.
- *Jobe's test (empty can test):* Shoulder elevation to 45° and internal rotation (thumb facing down). Therapist applies resistance to abduction (downward force) (Fig. 41-9). Positive sign is weakness or pain. This test indicates a tear of the supraspinatus tendon. Repeat the same test at 90°. If pain is only experienced at 90° position, suspect bursitis.
- *Drop arm test:* Patient's arm is positioned in 90° of abduction. The patient slowly lowers his or her arm to the side. The test is positive if the patient drops the arm to the side, indicating a supraspinatus tear (Fig. 41-10A and B).

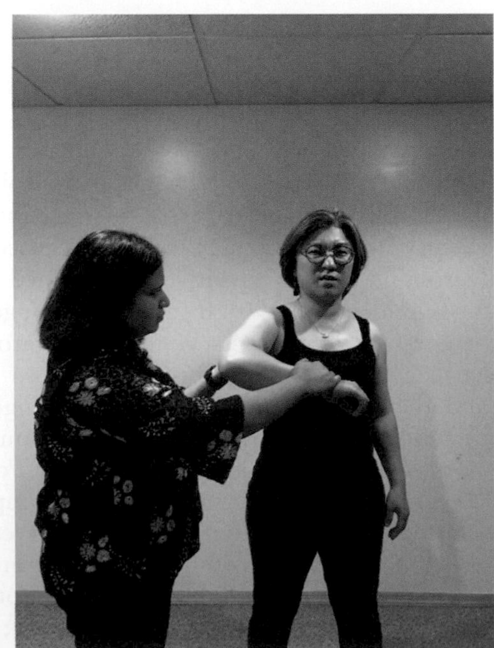

Figure 41-8. Hawkins test.

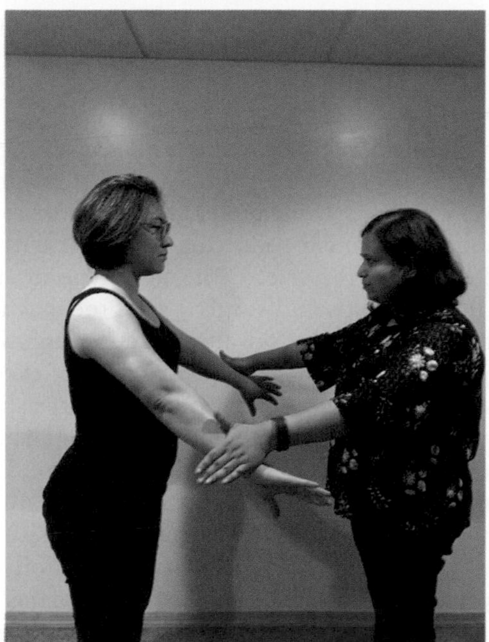

Figure 41-9. Jobe's/Empty can test.

- *Biceps Speed's test:* Shoulder flexed to 90°, forearm supinated, and elbow extended. Resistance is applied to flexion (downward force using a long lever arm). Positive sign is pain over bicipital groove (Fig. 41-11).[27–31]

ADLs should be assessed by observing the client using the involved extremity during activities that are within low range (waist level), mid-range (shoulder level), and high range (above shoulder level). The therapist should note any compensating or expressions of pain while performing the activities. There are also numerous standardized functional assessments specific to the shoulder, some of which should be included in the evaluation. Examples of standardized functional assessments that address World Health Organization International Classification of Functioning, Disability and Health (ICF) components: impairments, activity limitation, and participation restriction include the Disabilities of Arm, Shoulder and Hand (DASH), American Shoulder and Elbow Surgeons Self Report, Shoulder Disability Questionnaire, Shoulder Pain and Disability Index, and the Penn Shoulder Score.[32–36]

Treatment of the Nonsurgical Client

Conservative treatment should begin with educating the client on activity modification. The client should be instructed to avoid above shoulder level activities until pain subsides. Sleeping postures should also be addressed. The client should avoid sleeping with the arm above shoulder level or in an adducted and internally rotated position. Combined adduction and internal rotation for a long period of time can further compromise the blood supply of the supraspinatus tendon. Exercise should focus on pain-free ROM. Begin with PROM. As pain decreases, progress to AROM. Strengthening should include isometric and isotonic exercises for the rotator cuff and scapula musculature. Also improve ROM and strength through functional activities such as dressing (Fig. 41-12A to C). Investigate what occupations are most important to the client and have him or her bring in the necessary equipment

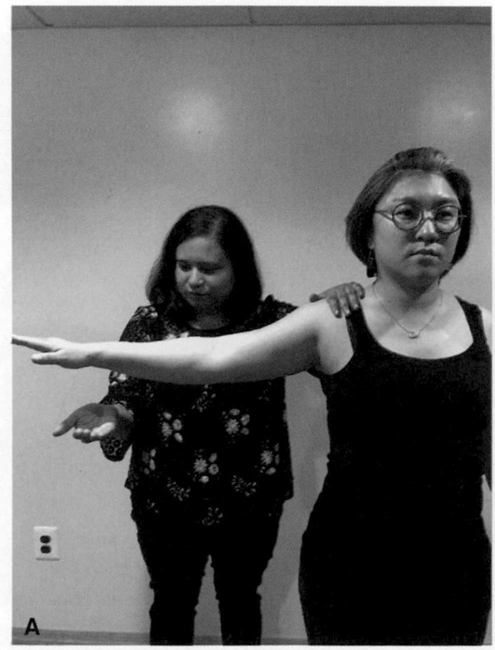

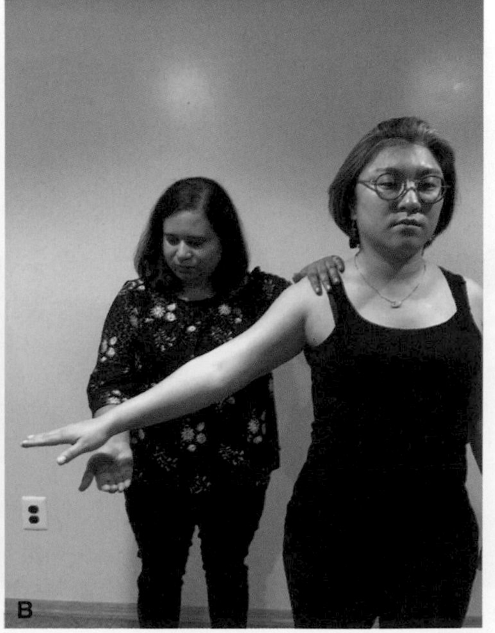

Figure 41-10. A, B. Drop arm test.

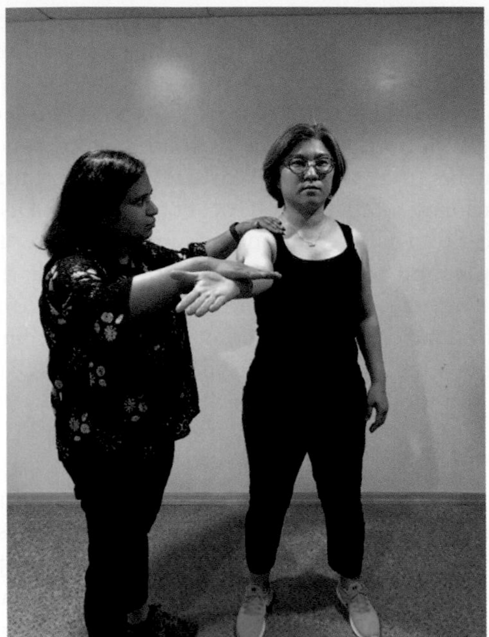

Figure 41-11. Biceps Speed's test.

such as a golf club or tennis racquet. The long-term goal is to return the client to unrestricted, pain-free occupational functioning.

Evaluation of the Postsurgical Client

The evaluation for the postsurgical client will be guided by the surgeon. Request for occupational therapy services can begin as early as 24 hours after surgery, but may be delayed up to 6 weeks after surgery. The decision to begin therapy and how to progress the client is based on many factors that include size and location of the tear, tissue quality, surgical approach, and the surgeon's protocol.[37]

Treatment of the Postsurgical Client

Early mobilization and delayed mobilization programs have been shown to have similar results in regard to improvement of tissue healing and functional return.[13] Initiation of treatment following a rotator cuff repair will be based on the size of the tear, type of surgical repair, tissue quality, and surgeon's protocol. After surgery, the client is placed in an **abduction pillow brace** or sling. The sling is to be worn at all times except for exercise. Clarify with the surgeon to see if the sling can be removed for bathing. Following repair of a small or medium tear, the client will begin with PROM/AAROM. The movements emphasized should include pain-free Codman's pendulum exercises, passive shoulder elevation, and internal/external rotation in the slightly abducted position in the scapular plane. An ice pack should be used before, during, and after exercise to decrease pain and swelling. The client should be instructed to perform these exercises at home using the uninvolved arm to supply the power. Internal and external rotation is performed with the client supine and the shoulder slightly abducted to 30° (in the scapular plane) and elbow flexed to 90°. A cane or stick is held in both hands, whereas the uninvolved arm supplies the power to move the involved extremity toward the stomach (internal rotation) and away from the stomach (external rotation) (see Fig. 41-13). Depending on the tension of the repair, the surgeon may set ROM limits. The client is also instructed to begin AROM of the elbow, forearm wrist, and hand. Overhead pulleys

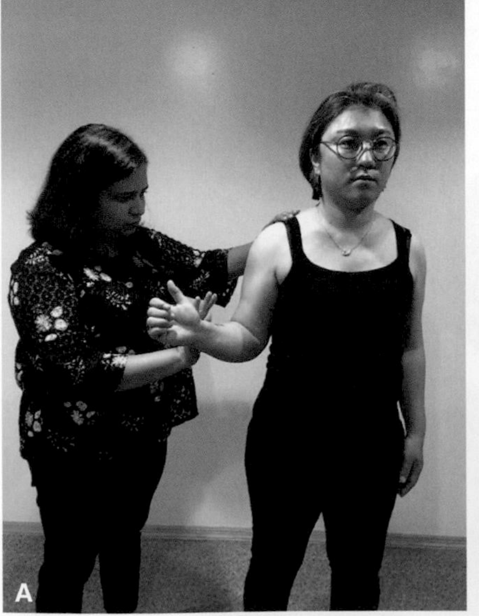

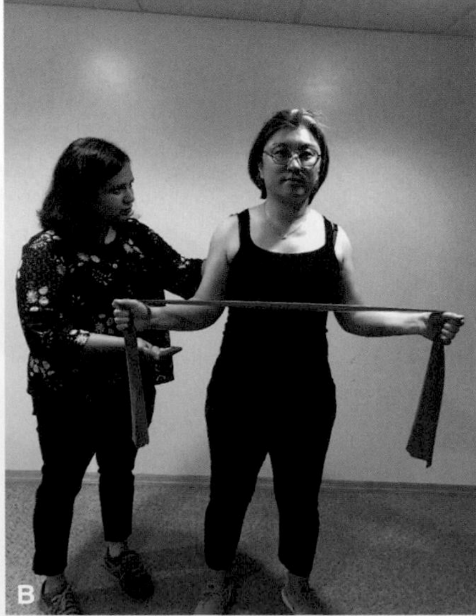

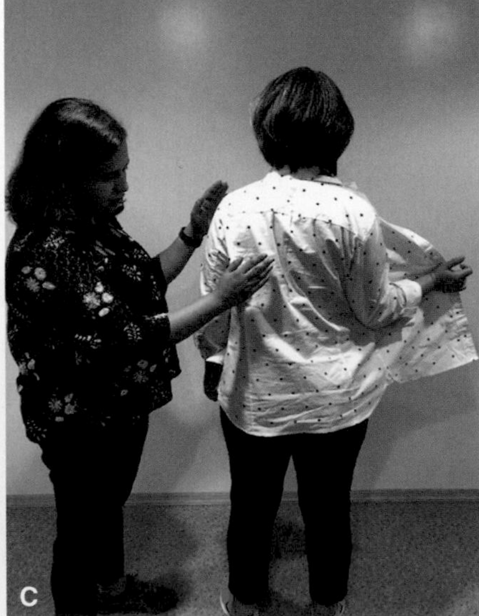

Figure 41-12. Progression of strengthening program. **A.** Isometric resistance to external rotation. **B.** Isotonic resistance to external rotation. **C.** Functional activity that incorporates external rotation.

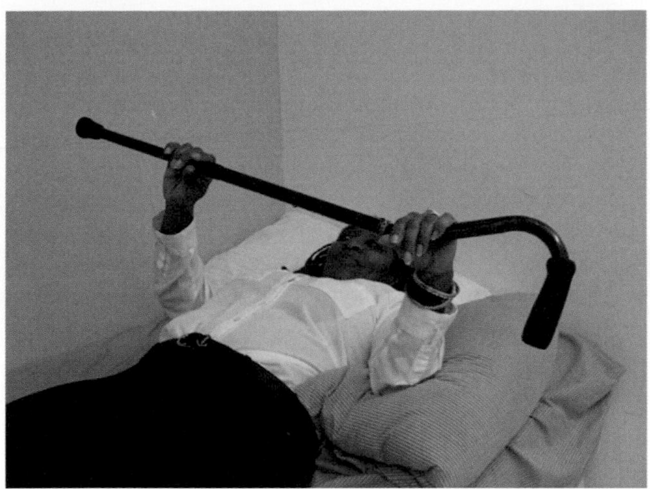

Figure 41-13. Cane exercise for internal and external rotation.

are only used if requested by the surgeon because repetitive shoulder elevation may irritate the repair.

During this time, the client should be instructed in one-handed techniques to perform ADLs. The involved shoulder should not be used for any activity at this time, unless indicated by the surgeon. At 6 weeks or later if following the delayed protocol, the client progresses to AROM. Begin in gravity-lessened positions and progress to against-gravity movements. Shoulder extension and internal rotation to the small of the back are added when approved by the surgeon. Encourage the client to achieve functional ROM. Engage the client in light nonresistive ADL. Avoid compensatory movements such as hiking the scapula or lateral bending of the trunk. Strengthening can be initiated 10 to 12 weeks postsurgery to prepare the client for functional activities. Initially, the strengthening program begins with isometric exercises for the rotator cuff and scapula stabilization exercises. The client then progresses to isotonic exercises using Thera-band and free weights.[16] All strengthening should be performed below 90° and be pain-free. Initially, exercises using free weights should begin supine to lessen gravity and prevent compensating. Then eventually increase to against-gravity strengthening remaining below 90°.[37–39] Later, light ADLs above shoulder level can be emphasized (if there is no hiking of the scapula), including cooking and folding laundry. At 12 weeks, the client can begin light-resistive occupation-based tasks. No lifting over 5 lb. Again, the long-term goal is to return the client to normal pain-free occupational functioning.

Following repairs of large and massive tears of the rotator cuff, the client is immobilized in an abduction brace.[40] ROM begins with pendulum exercises only. ROM restrictions vary depending on the surgeon's protocol. Some clients begin PROM within the first week, and others begin 6 weeks following surgery. AROM does not occur until 8 to 12 weeks post-op.[16] The preparatory interventions (exercise and ice) and purposeful activities are the same as for a small and medium tear, but the time frame of when they start are delayed. Time frames are determined by the surgeon. The treatment protocols given here are only guidelines; communication with the surgeon should be ongoing throughout the client's rehabilitation.

Hip Fractures

It is estimated that by the year 2030, there will be 289,000 individuals diagnosed with a hip fracture.[41] There are three types of hip fractures: femoral neck fracture, intertrochanteric fracture, and subtrochanteric fracture. Intertrochanteric hip fractures and femoral neck fractures are the most common fractures in adults older than 50 years of age.[42,43] Intertrochanteric fractures are more common in individuals with osteoporosis. Many of these clients have comorbidities that affect the duration and potential of the rehabilitation program.[44]

Hip fractures can be treated with closed reduction, which includes bed rest, traction, or early mobilization. The large majority of hip fractures are treated with open reduction internal fixation (ORIF) using pins, screws, plate, or rods[13,43] (see Fig. 41-14). Hemiarthroplasty is the treatment for some fractures of

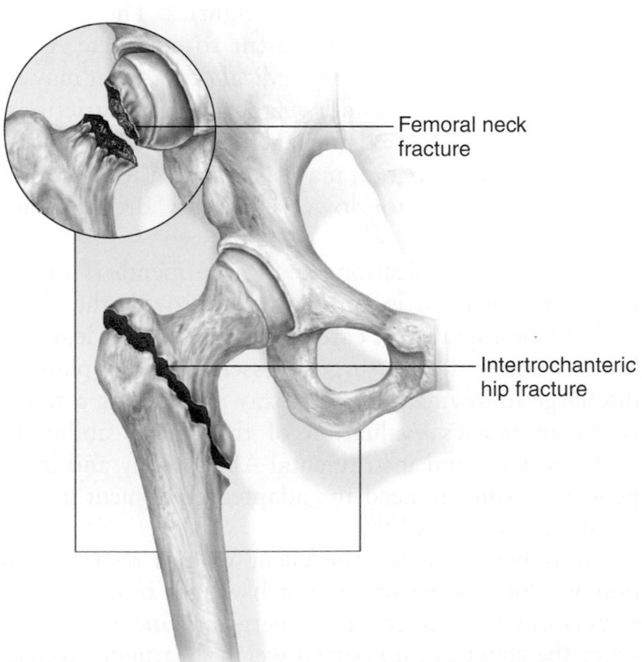

Figure 41-14. Intertrochanteric hip fractures and femoral neck fractures.

the neck and head of the femur. Hemiarthroplasty is a partial joint replacement in which the femoral head and neck are replaced by a prosthesis. After excision of the femoral head, the stem of the prosthesis is inserted distally into the medullary canal of the femur so that its head articulates with the normal acetabulum.[43] If destructive changes have taken place in both the femur and the acetabulum, a total hip arthroplasty (THA) is necessary.[13]

Occupational Therapy Following a Hip Fracture and Surgery

Occupational therapy should begin with an evaluation that includes an occupational profile to identify occupations that were meaningful to the client prior to the hip fracture. Incorporation of these meaningful activities in the acute care phase of the treatment is an important step in preparing the client for discharge.[45] The restrictions for weight bearing and hip movement on the operated leg are directly related to the severity and location of the fracture, the surgical approach, the ability of the fixation device or prosthesis to withstand stress, the integrity of the bone, the weight of the client, and the client's cognitive status.[46] The physical therapist teaches the client to use a walker or crutches, depending on percentage of body weight allowed on the operated limb, which ranges from non–weight bearing (0% weight), to touchdown weight bearing (10%–15% weight), to partial weight bearing (30% weight), to 50% weight bearing (50% weight), to full weight bearing (75%–100% weight).[46] The occupational therapist teaches the client to complete ADLs safely, corresponding to the medical orders that may or may not include ROM and weight bearing restrictions. For some clients, preexisting factors or the risk of dislodging the new hip joint may necessitate the assistance of another person for lower extremity dressing and for bathing.

Close communication among the members of the rehabilitation team is imperative to provide the client with the best quality of care and consistency in learning how to function after surgery. Essential to the planned discharge following a hospital stay of less than a week, is the therapist's evaluation of the client's ability to perform basic and instrumental ADLs safely and independently and the need for adapted equipment and/or assistance of others.[47,48]

It is best to teach the client who is restricted to non–weight bearing or toe-touch weight bearing to sit to perform ADLs to conserve energy and increase safety. Once the client can do partial weight bearing or weight bearing as tolerated (WBAT), he or she can safely stand while grooming. For at least 6 weeks, and for some clients longer, movement may be restricted. The therapist must be reminded to thoroughly review the chart for weight bearing status and possible ROM restrictions. Movement restrictions after hip surgery may include:

- No hip flexion beyond 90°, including movement of the trunk over the thighs
- No hip rotation (avoid internal rotation for posterolateral approach and external rotation for anterolateral approach)
- No crossing the operated leg over the unoperated leg
- No adduction of the operated leg

Because these restrictions preclude bending over or bringing the foot closer to the hands, adaptations are required to resolve performance challenges in bathing, dressing, functional mobility, and home management. Long-handled dressing and grooming devices are provided, and the therapist teaches the client to bathe and dress the operated side using these devices to avoid bending over (flexion) or crossing the operated leg (adduction). Some examples of adaptive devices include:

- Reacher or dressing stick to don and doff pants
- Sock aide to don and doff socks
- Extended-handled shoehorn (medial side for posterior surgical approach and lateral for the anterior approach) or elastic laces can be adaptations to don and doff shoes

For bathing, if permitted, some clients shower standing. Instructions for transferring in and out of the tub from a standing position include:

To Get Into the Bathtub

- Stand with feet parallel to the tub with the operated leg next to the bathtub.
- Shift body weight to unoperated leg.
- Hold onto a grab assist rail for support.
- Position the operated leg into hip extension and knee flexion; then abduct the hip to allow the leg to go over the edge of the bathtub.
- Extend the knee on the operated side once the leg is over the tub edge.
- Place the foot on the nonskid bath mat inside the tub.
- When balance is secure, transfer the body weight to the operated leg. Lift the unoperated leg over the edge of the tub and place the foot on the bath mat.

To Get Out of the Bathtub

- Position oneself so feet are parallel to the side of the tub and the operated leg leads (goes out of the tub first).
- Use the same procedure as for getting into the tub.

Others prefer to sit to conserve energy or feel secure, and they require a bath bench. The bath bench must be high enough so the hip does not flex more than 90°. To reduce hip flexion during sitting and rising, the client is instructed to use a raised toilet seat, bed, and chair. The client is encouraged to sit in a reclined position enhanced by a wedge cushion or a small rolled pillow or towel at the junction of the chair's seat and back, as originally described by McKee.[49]

The client who must sit in a regular-height chair is taught to stand up without overflexing the operated hip. In a chair with armrests, the client scoots to the front edge of the seat, keeping the operated hip extended, uses the armrests to push straight up without bending the trunk forward, and then stands upright holding onto a walker (Fig. 41-15A to C). In a chair without armrests, the client moves to the side of the chair so that the operated thigh is over the edge with the foot placed at the midline of the chair. This places the operated hip in extension, puts the foot close to the center of gravity, and enables the person to gain momentum to stand without excessive hip flexion. With this technique, the unoperated hip, knee, and ankle are in position for weight bearing. A cushion or folded blanket will increase the height of the chair.

By 6 weeks, almost all clients walk with a cane, and some walk unassisted; most can return to driving a car, swimming, and work.[46] Physical restrictions against bending to put on shoes or socks, sleeping on the operated side, and using a regular-height toilet seat are often lifted 8 to 12 weeks after surgery; however, the surgeon will determine this.

Degenerative Hip Disease

Some orthopedic conditions are chronic. One is progressive hip pain from degenerative disease. When that pain interferes with activities and tasks of daily life despite medication, rest, reduction in lower extremity loading by the use of a cane, walker, or crutches, and physical therapy, hip surgery is indicated.[1] After hip replacement surgery, therapists teach the clients to move the operated leg within the ordered weight bearing and movement restrictions.

Occupational Therapy after Elective Hip Surgery

A number of surgical procedures are used for the reduction of hip pain. They include osteotomy, arthrodesis or hip fusion, hip resurfacing, and partial or total hip arthroplasty. To select the procedure, the orthopedic surgeon considers not only the client's age and physical status but also his or her occupational requirements and lifestyle. The most common are partial or total hip arthroplasty (THA).

A THA surgically replaces the entire hip joint destroyed by disease or trauma. The main benefit of hip replacement is to resolve arthritic pain. Joint replacement surgery can also restore the length of the limb and its alignment, which has the potential to improve ROM and function.[50] This surgery replaces the arthritic acetabular cup with a titanium cup and polyethylene plastic liner. The femoral head is replaced with a femoral head implant made of ceramic and a titanium stem component (see Fig. 41-16).

The surgical approach to perform the THA varies among surgeons. The most common is the posterolateral approach.[51] With this approach, there is no disruption to the gluteus medius and minimus muscles, and therefore, hip abduction is not compromised. The risk

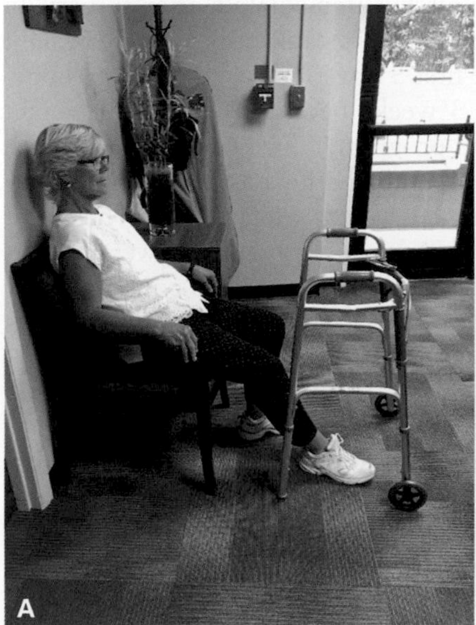

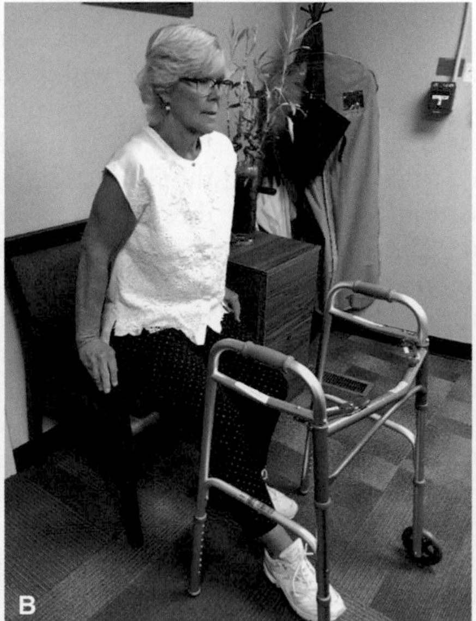

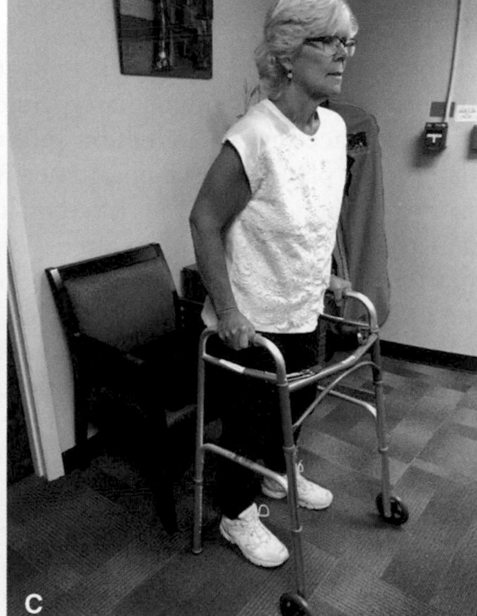

Figure 41-15. Sit-to-stand transfer for a client with partial weight bearing status after total hip arthroplasty. **A.** Extends knee and pushes off arms of chair. **B.** Avoids flexing hip past 90° while pushing off. **C.** Maintains partial weight bearing status when standing.

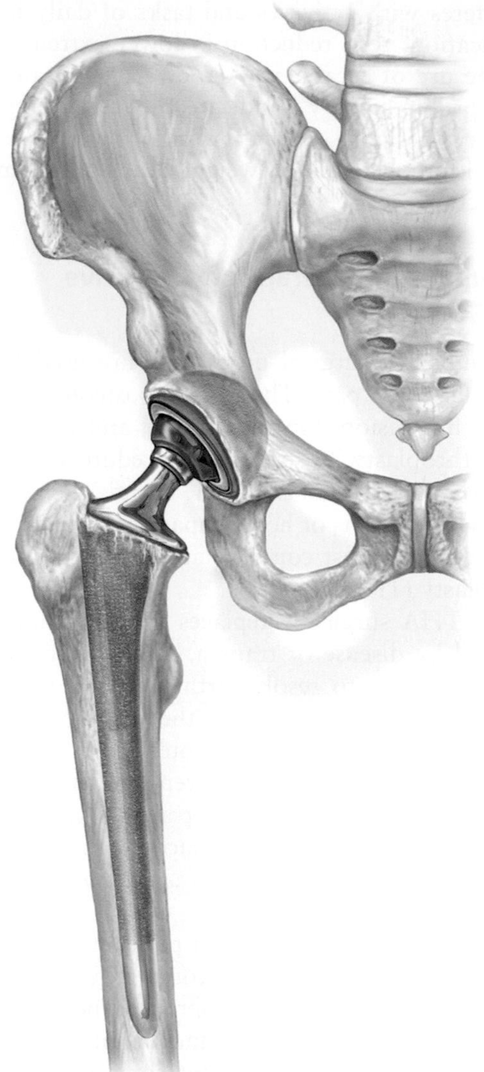

Figure 41-16. Total hip arthroplasty.

of the posterolateral approach is posterior dislocation. To avoid dislocation, immediately following surgery, the client is placed in an abduction pillow. Some surgeons also opt to place the ipsilateral knee in a knee immobilizer to further decrease the risk of dislocation. The client is instructed to avoid hip flexion beyond 90°, adduction, and internal rotation.[51,52] Another common approach is the anterolateral approach. With this approach there is a limited risk for dislocation. Some surgeons follow a no-restriction protocol,[53] whereas other surgeons have specific restrictions that may include avoiding flexion beyond 90°, avoid hip extension, adduction, and external rotation.[52,54]

Another decision the surgeon must make when performing a THA is what type of implant fixation he or she will use. The choices are cemented, cementless, or hybrid prostheses.[55] The cemented total replacement usually requires 4 to 6 weeks of WBAT using a standard or rolling walker, and then the client progresses to a straight cane. The cementless prosthesis, which depends on ingrowth of porous bone for stability, requires 6 to 12 weeks of partial weight bearing before a cane is used. Some surgeons may initially order non–weight bearing. In the case of the hybrid prosthesis, in which the femoral portion is cemented and the acetabulum is uncemented, 4 to 6 weeks of partial weight bearing precedes introduction of a cane.[51]

Early mobility and rapid recovery protocols start the client in therapy as early as postoperative days 0 to 1.[56] Preoperative education should be the first phase of occupational therapy for the client receiving a THA. Hip precautions, demonstration of long-handled equipment, and medically necessary durable medical equipment should be presented. Preoperative education has been linked to reducing anxiety.[57] The first 2 months after THA is critical for protection and function of the new hip joint. The postsurgical program is designed to allow for healing of the trochanter and soft tissues and for development of a capsule around the joint for future stability.

The client learns to transfer from supine to sitting to standing without flexing the operated hip beyond 90° by keeping the knees apart (hips abducted) and sliding out of a bed to take weight on the unoperated leg. Some clients use an overhead trapeze bar to assist this transfer. The client also needs to practice transferring from a variety of surfaces such as a high chair, tub bench, raised toilet seat, and a car seat using a walker. To protect the prosthesis, the occupational therapist instructs the client in adaptive procedures and in methods to modify the environment to allow for safe performance of ADLs and homemaking tasks.

The client with a cemented or hybrid total hip prosthesis usually begins partial weight bearing with a rolling walker or crutches immediately after surgery. In some instances, these clients can withstand full weight bearing within the first 3 days; however, many orthopedic surgeons wait 3 weeks before ordering full weight bearing.[46] The ADL program, which can be taught with the client standing, uses the bathing and lower extremity dressing techniques described for fractures. The client with a cementless THA is usually toe-touch weight bearing for the initial recovery phase and is conservatively progressed to partial weight bearing.[46] This necessitates learning ADLs from the seated position. Once 50% weight bearing is ordered, the ADL program is upgraded to allow for standing with a cane. The cane is used until the **Trendelenburg gait** disappears.

Usually, after a THA, clients do not receive outpatient therapy following inpatient rehabilitation, although many may receive home care occupational and physical therapy for safety assessment and/or treatment. Between the second and third month after surgery, clients usually resume all routine daily activities, with hip precautions still applicable.

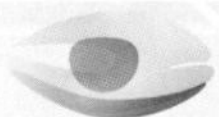

CASE STUDY

Client Information

Lucy is a 68-year-old female who has been discharged to home following a 2-week length of stay in an acute care rehabilitation hospital secondary to a car accident and resultant low back strain and right rotator cuff injury. Lucy's medical care included arthroscopic repair of the supraspinatus with a **shoulder immobilizer** and pain management for low back pain. The focus of her occupational therapy while in the rehabilitation hospital included ADL training, functional mobility, and pain management.

Reason for Occupational Therapy Referral

Lucy has been referred for outpatient occupational therapy services to increase independence in ADLs and instrumental activities of daily living (IADLs). Additional orders include remove shoulder immobilizer to begin gentle PROM to the right shoulder and AROM of the uninvolved joints. Prior to her accident she was independent (I) with all ADLs and IADLs.

Assessment Process and Results

The outpatient occupational therapy evaluation reveals that Lucy lives alone in a one-story condominium with two steps to enter. She has one bathroom that has a tub and shower unit with no grab bars. Lucy has a small kitchen and prior to her accident she cooked all her own meals. Lucy identified gardening and cooking as meaningful occupations.

Assessment of Lucy's range of motion revealed that she has full AROM of her left uninvolved upper extremity and of the uninvolved joints of the right upper extremity. PROM of the right shoulder included the following: shoulder elevation (scaption) 0° to 85°, internal rotation to stomach, and external rotation 0° to 10°. Right shoulder pain was rated as a 7/10 and is reported to be worse at night.

Lucy requires minimal assistance for upper body dressing. She is unable to place her right upper extremity through the sleeve of her shirt and instead wears loose T-shirt that she pulls overhead and over her arm while wearing her sling. She is unable to don her socks, however is modified independent for donning her pants. Lucy uses a tub bench that was given to her during her inpatient stay to transfer to-and-from the tub. She reports having difficulty washing her hair with one hand.

Lucy has identified cooking as an activity she is having difficulty with due to surgical precautions. She is unable to open containers, cut food, or lift pots and pans. She is presently unable to drive and is concerned about grocery shopping.

Occupational Therapy Problem List

- Decreased ROM secondary to right rotator cuff repair
- Decreased independence in basic ADLs
- Shoulder pain that interferes with sleep
- Decreased independence with IADLs

Occupational Therapy Goal List

- Increase PROM of right shoulder elevation (scaption) to 130° in preparation for participation in hair care in 2 weeks.
- Decrease pain to a 5/10 by proper positioning of the right UE in 1 week.
- Client will be modified (I) for cutting food using a rocker knife in 1 week.
- Client will be modified (I) for dressing upper body in 1 week.
- Client will be modified (I) for simple meal preparation using a one-handed technique in 1 week.

Intervention

Treatment began with a preparatory method using a hot pack × 15 minutes (skin checked and OK). This was followed by passive pendulum exercises and PROM (supine) for shoulder elevation (scapular plane), internal rotation, and external rotation. Lucy was instructed by the occupational therapist on how to correctly perform the pendulum exercises as a home program three times daily: 10 repetitions clockwise and 10 repetitions counter clockwise. The exercises were followed by proper positioning of Lucy's right upper extremity (supine) using a pillow in slight shoulder elevation and external rotation for comfort while sleeping. Lucy reported the change in position when sleeping has decreased her shoulder pain at night.

The therapist worked with Lucy on performing her ADLs using one-handed techniques. The therapist instructed Lucy to don a button down shirt by releasing her right arm from the sling and relaxing her arm in a pendulum position. Using her left uninvolved extremity, pull the sleeve gently onto the involved extremity and up to the shoulder, Lucy is then instructed to reach behind her neck with her left hand and grasp the collar to move the shirt around her back and place her uninvolved arm in the sleeve. To button her shirt one-handed, she is instructed to begin with the bottom button to help align the buttons and button holes correctly. Lucy is taught additional one-handed techniques to perform other ADLs such as one-handed cutting and opening containers needed for cooking. These one-handed techniques now enabled Lucy to only require modified independence to perform her ADLs.

At 6-weeks her PROM included shoulder elevation (scaption) 0° to 150°, internal rotation to stomach, and external rotation 0° to 50°. Right shoulder pain was rated as a 4/10. Lucy was able to perform all her ADLs with modified independence using one-handed techniques. The referring physician upgraded orders to begin AROM and progress to strengthening at 8 weeks. The occupational therapist started Lucy with AROM in supine to lessen gravity and prevent any substitutions. Other preparatory tasks included cane exercises and wall walking to prepare her to perform purposeful activities such as reaching into cabinets and the refrigerator for cooking items. At 8 weeks, the therapist instructed Lucy in isometrics and slowly progressed to isotonic exercises. Prior to discharge, the therapist progressed Lucy to perform an occupation-based activity of cooking a full meal, which she identified as meaningful. Lucy was able to perform the cooking activity independently using her involved extremity without any compensatory movements.

Best Evidence for Occupational Therapy Practice in Orthopedics

Intervention	Intervention Description	Participants	Dosage	Research Design and Evidence Level	Benefit	Statistical Significance and Effect Size
Comparison of a standard care group (SC) to a combined care group (CT) in patients hospitalized for hip fracture[58]	The SC group received standard medical, nursing and physical therapy treatment and the CT group received the standard care as well as individual occupational therapy.	Totally, 122 patients with hip fracture were allocated to two groups (CT = 61, SC = 61). After losses at follow-up, 116 were analyzed (CT = 57, SC = 59).	The SC group received physical therapy 5 days/week starting the day after surgery for 30 minutes daily. Patients in the CG group received the physical therapy treatment that the SC group received, in addition they received 20 minutes of occupational therapy 5 days/week starting the day after surgery.	Randomized controlled trial, level I	Integrating occupational therapy as a key component of hip fracture rehabilitation shows short- and long-term improvements in emotional distress, fatigue, and function.	CT group reported lower fatigue at 6 months ($p < 0.044$), whereas SC group had a greater increase in emotional distress at 1, 3, and 6 months ($p < 0.001$). At 6 months, the CT group showed better results in ADLs ($p < 0.048$). Both groups showed an increase in hip function throughout the intervention ($p < 0.001$).
Total shoulder arthroplasty (TSA) for degenerative osteoarthritis of the humeral head and glenoid[59]	TSA followed by a standardized postoperative rehabilitation protocol including range of motion exercises and gradual progression in active resistive movements.	Totally, 13 patients who received a TSA for degenerative osteoarthritis of the humeral head and glenoid and 10 matched controls (controls) with no shoulder problems.	TSA followed by a standard rehabilitation protocol with passive ROM, external rotation limited to 0° and abduction to 90° for 4 weeks. Progressive active resistive motion was allowed for 4–6 weeks and no limitations after 10–12 weeks.	Case-control study, level III	TSA with standard rehabilitation improves range of motion and performance in activities of daily living for individuals who have degenerative shoulder osteoarthritis.	No significant differences in ROMs between groups except in abduction/adduction while combing hair ($p = 0.001$) and reaching a high shelf ($p = 0.008$). Preoperatively to 6-months postoperatively, use of the arm in ADLs increased (31.5%–90.8%). Active flexion increased on average from 85O to 140.4O, and abduction from 67.5O to 122.7O.

Comparison of occupational therapy (OT) to home-based exercise program (EP) as a conservative treatment in patients with full-thickness isolated rotator cuff tears[60]	OT group received supervised exercises determined by the supervising therapist. EP group received an exercise booklet with detailed instructions and demonstrations for exercises to restore neuromuscular control at the shoulder as well as strength and ROM including type of exercises, repetitions, intensity, training, rest phases, and dairy for weekly planning.	Totally, 37 patients with unilateral, symptomatic, atraumatic rotator cuff tears (OT = 22, EP = 16)	The OT group received supervised exercises three times per week for 8 weeks. The EP group were required to participate in two training unites to be performed for 30 minutes, each once in the morning and once in the evening.	Randomized controlled trial, level I	Standardized home exercise programs have the same benefits as occupational therapy interventions in improving pain, strength, quality of life, and range of motion at the shoulder.	Both groups improved in pain, strength, impingement signs, and quality of life. EP group had higher subjective health status compared with OT group ($p < 0.049$). Shoulder ROM improved in both groups, with the highest gains in abduction. EP group showed more improvement in abduction peak torque compared with the OT group.
Early postoperative individualized occupational therapy[61]	Occupational therapy group (OTG): individual ADL and IADL training, including the use of technical aids plus one home visit Control group: conventional care	One hundred patients aged ≥65 years having undergone surgery for hip fracture. All lived independently, and none used walking or technical aids prior to hospitalization (randomized to group). Ninety completed the study (10% attrition).	After the third to fourth postoperative day, the OTG received 45–60 minutes of individualized training (including technical aids) each weekday morning for 3–33 days. The control group received conventional care from the nursing staff for 3–23 days. All patients received instruction in walking with mobility aids.	Randomized controlled trial, level IB1b	OT sped up the ability of patients to perform ADLs. At discharge, the OTG had significantly better ability to dress, complete personal hygiene, toilet, and bathe independently compared with the control group. No other factors explained the outcome. After 2 months, all patients had regained independence.	Klein–Bell ADL Scale subtests: Dressing: $F_{(2,91)} = 79.0$, $p = 0.0001$, $r = 0.79$.[a] Toileting: $F_{(2,90)} = 5.97$, $p = 0.02$, $r = 0.34$. Bathing/hygiene: $F_{(2,91)} = 17$, $p = 0.0001$, $r = 0.52$. Mobility: $F_{(2,91)} = 2.20$, $p = 0.1$, $r = 0.21$. 52% of the OTG needed technical aids and adaptation of their homes.

[a] r value was calculated from data reported, using a formula for F with $df_{numerator} > 1$. Effect size (r) is considered large if ≥0.50, medium if ≥0.30, and small if ≥0.10.

References

1. Salter RB. *Textbook of Disorders and Injuries of the Musculoskeletal System: An Introduction to Orthopaedics, Fractures, and Joint Injuries, Rheumatology, Metabolic Bone Disease, and Rehabilitation*. Philadelphia, PA: Lippincott Williams & Wilkins; 1999.
2. United States Bone and Joint Initiative. The Burden of Musculoskeletal Diseases in the United States. http://www.boneandjointburden.org. Published 2014. Accessed March 13, 2018.
3. von Keudell A, Collins M, Jupiter JB. Principles of fracture fixation: plates/screws and intramedullary nails. In: Frank RM, Forsythe B, Provencher MT, eds. *Case Competencies in Orthopaedic Surgery*. Philadelphia, PA: Elsevier; 2017:223–238.
4. Solomon L, Warwick DJ, Nayagam S. *Apley's Concise System of Orthopaedics and Fracture*. 3rd ed. Boca Raton, FL: Taylor and Francis Group, LLC; 2005.
5. Donovan S, Brechter J, Sueki D. Tissue injury and healing. In: Sueki D, Brechter J, eds. *Orthopedic Rehabilitation Clinical Advisor*. Maryland Heights, MO: Mosby Elsevier; 2010:3–16.
6. Greene D, Roberts S. *Kinesiology: Movement in the Context of Activity*. 3rd ed. St. Louis, MO: Elsevier Inc.; 2017.
7. Hodgson S. Proximal humerus fracture rehabilitation. *Clin Orthop Relat Res*. 2006;442:131–138. doi:10.1097/01.blo.0000194677.02506.45.
8. Lowry V, Bureau NJ, Desmeules F, Roy J-S, Rouleau DM. Acute proximal humeral fractures in adults. *J Hand Ther*. 2017;30(2):158–166. doi:10.1016/j.jht.2017.05.005.
9. Singleton E, Turner R, Gulotta L. Rehabilitation after proximal humeral fractures. *Tech Shoulder Elbow Surg*. 2014;15(1):46–50. doi:10.1097/BTE.0000000000000013.
10. Neer CS. *Shoulder Reconstruction*. Philadelphia, PA: Saunders; 1990.
11. Agorastides I, Sinopidis C, El Meligy M, Yin Q, Brownson P, Frostick SP. Early versus late mobilization after hemiarthroplasty for proximal humeral fractures. *J Shoulder Elbow Surg*. 2007;16(3 suppl):S33. doi:10.1016/j.jse.2006.07.004.
12. Basti JJ, Dionysian E, Sherman PW, Bigliani LU. Management of proximal humeral fractures. *J Hand Ther*. 1994;7(2):111–121. doi:10.1016/S0894-1130(12)80080-9.
13. Keenan ME, Mehta S, McMahon PJ. Rehabilitation. In: Skinner HB, McMahon PJ, eds. *Current Diagnosis & Treatment in Orthopedics*. 5th ed. New York, NY: McGraw-Hill; 2014.
14. Gallinet D, Clappaz P, Garbuio P, Tropet Y, Obert L. Three or four parts complex proximal humerus fractures: hemiarthroplasty versus reverse prosthesis: a comparative study of 40 cases. *Orthop Traumatol Surg Res*. 2009;95(1):48–55. doi:10.1016/j.otsr.2008.09.002.
15. Garrigues G, Johnston P, Pepe M, Tucker B, Ramsey M, Austin L. Hemiarthroplasty versus reverse total shoulder arthroplasty for acute proximal humerus fractures in elderly patients. *Orthopedics*. 2012;35:e703–e708. doi:10.3928/01477447-20120426-25.
16. de Herder E. *Evidence Based Hand and Upper Extremity Protocols*. In: Mattox S, Justice L, eds. Elizabeth de Herder; 2015.
17. Tan V, Leggin BG, Kelley MJ, Williams G. Surgical and postoperative management of the shoulder arthritis. In: Skirven TM, Osterman AL, Fedorczyk JM, Amadio PC, eds. *Rehabilitation of the Hand and Upper Extremity*. 6th ed. Philadelphia, PA: Elsevier/Mosby; 2012:351–360.
18. Colditz JC. Functional fracture bracing. In: Skirven TM, Osterman AL, Fedorczyk JM, Amadio PC, eds. *Rehabilitation of the Hand and Upper Extremity*. 6th ed. Philadelphia, PA: Elsevier/Mosby; 2011:1061–1074.
19. Mader K, Mader S, Berntsson P-O. The diaphysis: nonsurgical treatment. In: Castoldi F, Blonna D, Assom M, eds. *Simple and Complex Fractures of the Humerus*. Milan, Italy: Springer Milan; 2015:213–220.
20. Davila SA. Therapist's management of fractures and dislocations of the elbow. In: Skirven M, Osterman AL, Fedorczyk JM, Amadio PC, eds. *Rehabilitation of the Hand and Upper Extremity*. 6th ed. Philadelphia: Elsevier/Mosby; 2012:1061–1074.
21. Kistler JM, Ilyas AM, Thoder JJ. Forearm compartment syndrome: evaluation and management: evaluation and management. *Hand Clin*. 2018;34(1):53–60. doi:10.1016/j.hcl.2017.09.006.
22. Beredjiklian PK. Management of fractures and dislocations of the elbow. In: Skirven TM, Osterman AL, Fedorczyk JM, Amadio PC, eds. *Rehabilitation of the Hand and Upper Extremity*. 6th ed. Philadelphia, PA: Elsevier/Mosby; 2011:1049–1060.
23. Amir S, Jannis S, Daniel R. Distal humerus fractures: a review of current therapy concepts. *Curr Rev Musculoskelet Med*. 2016;9(2):199–206. doi:10.1007/s12178-016-9341-z.
24. Post M, Silver R, Singh M. Rotator cuff tear. Diagnosis and treatment. *Clin Orthop Relat Res*. 1983;(173):78.
25. McMahon PJ, Kaplan LD, Popkin CA. Sports medicine. In: Skinner HB, McMahon PJ, eds. *Current Diagnosis & Treatment in Orthopedics*. 5th ed. New York, NY: McGraw-Hill; 2014.
26. McGarvey C, Harb Z, Smith C, Houghton R, Corbett S, Ajuied A. Diagnosis of rotator cuff tears using 3-Tesla MRI versus 3-Tesla MRA: a systematic review and meta-analysis. *Skeletal Radiol*. 2016;45(2):251–261. doi:10.1007/s00256-015-2299-x.
27. Neer CS. Anterior acromioplasty for the chronic impingement syndrome in the shoulder: a preliminary report. *J Bone Joint Surg*. 1972;54(1):41–50. doi:10.2106/00004623-197254010-00003
28. Hawkins RJ, Kennedy JC. Impingement syndrome in athletes. *Am J Sports Med*. 1980;8(3):151–158. doi:10.1177/036354658000800302
29. Jobe FW, Moynes DR. Delineation of diagnostic criteria and a rehabilitation program for rotator cuff injuries. *Am J Sports Med*. 1982;10(6):336. doi:10.1177/036354658201000602
30. Codman EA. Rupture of the supraspinatus tendon. In: Codman EA, ed. *The Shoulder: Rupture of the Supraspinatus Tendon and Other Lesions in or about the Subacromial Bursa*. Boston, MA: Thomas Todd; 1934:123–177.

31. Crenshaw AH, Kilgore WE. Surgical treatment of bicipital tenosynovitis. *J Bone Joint Surg*. 1966;48(8):1496–1502. doi:10.2106/00004623-196648080-00003.
32. Mcqueen M, Johnston M, Dixon D, Court-Brown C. The Disabilities of the Arm, Shoulder and Hand Questionnaire (DASH) can measure the impairment, activity limitations and participation restriction constructs from the International Classification of Functioning, Disability and Health (ICF). *BMC Musculoskelet Disord*. 2008;9(1):114. doi:10.1186/1471-2474-9-114.
33. Silva DA, Ferreira SR, Cotta MM, Noce KR, Stamm TA. Linking the disabilities of arm, shoulder, and hand to the international classification of functioning, disability, and health. *J Hand Ther*. 2007;20(4):336. doi:10.1197/j.jht.2007.07.008.
34. Hudak PL, Amadio PC, Bombardier C. Development of an upper extremity outcome measure: the DASH (disabilities of the arm, shoulder and hand) corrected. The Upper Extremity Collaborative Group (UECG). *Am J Ind Med*. 1996;29(6):602. doi:10.1002/(SICI)1097-0274(199606)29:6<602::AID-AJIM4>3.0.CO;2-L.
35. Mcclure P, Michener L. Measures of adult shoulder function: The American Shoulder and Elbow Surgeons Standardized Shoulder Form Patient Self Report Section (ASES), Disabilities of the Arm, Shoulder, and Hand (DASH), Shoulder Disability Questionnaire, Shoulder Pain and Disability Index (SPADI), and simple shoulder test. *Arthritis Care Res (Hoboken)*. 2003;49(S5):S50–S58. doi:10.1002/art.11404.
36. Roy JB, Macdermid JC, Woodhouse LJ. Measuring shoulder function: a systematic review of four questionnaires. *Arthritis Care Res (Hoboken)*. 2009;61(5):623–632. doi:10.1002/art.24396.
37. Ghodadra NS, Provencher MT, Verma NN, Wilk KE, Romeo AA. Open, mini-open, and all-arthroscopic rotator cuff repair surgery: indications and implications for rehabilitation. *J Orthop Sports Phys Ther*. 2009;39(2):81. doi:10.2519/jospt.2009.2918.
38. Boissonnault WG, Badke MB, Wooden MJ, Ekedahl S, Fly K. Patient outcome following rehabilitation for rotator cuff repair surgery: the impact of selected medical comorbidities. *J Orthop Sports Phys Ther*. 2007;37(6):312. doi:10.2519/jospt.2007.2448.
39. Butler MW. Common shoulder diagnoses. In: Cooper C, ed. *Fundamentals of Hand Therapy: Clinical Reasoning and Treatment Guidelines for Common Diagnoses of the Upper Extremity*. 2nd ed. St. Louis, MO: 2014:219–255. doi:10.1016/B978-0-323-09104-6.00022-5.
40. O'Brien MY, Leggin BG, Williams GR. Rotator cuff tendinopathies and tears: surgery and therapy. In: Skirven T, Osterman AL, Fedorczyk J, Amadio PC, eds. *Rehabilitation of the Hand and Upper Extremity*. 6th ed. Philadelphia, PA: Elsevier/Mosby; 2011:1157–1173.
41. Centers for Disease Control and Prevention/National Center for Health Statistics. National Hospital Discharge Survey. https://www.cdc.gov/nchs/nhds/index.htm. Published 2015. Accessed July 8, 2018.
42. Altizer L. Hip fractures. *Orthop Nurs*. 2005;24(4):283–292. doi:10.1097/00006416-200507000-00010.
43. Lareau C, Sawyer G. Hip fracture surgical treatment and rehabilitation. *Med Health Rhode Island*. 2010;93(4):108–111. http://www.rimed.org/medhealthri/2010-04/2010-04-108.pdf. Accessed May 10, 2018.
44. Antanelov L, Dabai N. Hip fracture. *PM&R Knowledge Now*. 2017. https://now.aapmr.org/hip-fracture/. Accessed May 10, 2018.
45. Wong C, Fagan B, Leland NE. Occupational therapy practitioners' perspectives on occupation-based interventions for clients with hip fracture. *Am J Occup Ther*. 2018;72(4):7204205050p1. doi:10.5014/ajot.2018.026492.
46. Goldstein TS. *Geriatric Orthopaedics orthopaedics org/ers' perspectives on occupation*. Gaithersburg, MD: Aspen Publishers; 1999.
47. Sandell C-L. A multidisciplinary assessment and intervention for patients awaiting total hip replacement to improve their quality of life. *J Orthop Nurs*. 2008;12(1):26–34. doi:10.1016/j.joon.2007.11.002.
48. Dorsey J, Bradshaw M. Effectiveness of occupational therapy interventions for lower-extremity musculoskeletal disorders: a systematic review. *Am J Occup Ther*. 2016;71(1):7101180030p1–7101180030p11.doi:10.5014/ajot.2017.023028.
49. McKee JI. Foam wedges aid sitting posture of patients with total hip replacement. *Phys Ther*. 1975;55(7):767. doi:10.1093/ptj/55.7.767.
50. Drake C, Ace M, Maale GE. Revision total hip arthroplasty. *AORN J*. 2002;76(3):412–427. doi:10.1016/S0001-2092(06)61655-4.
51. Youm T, Maurer SG, Stuchin SA. Postoperative management after total hip and knee arthroplasty. *J Arthroplasty*. 2005;20(3):322–324. doi:10.1016/j.arth.2004.04.015.
52. Dutton M. *Dutton's Orthopaedic Examination Evaluation and Intervention*. 3rd ed. New York, NY: McGraw-Hill Education; 2012.
53. Restrepo C, Mortazavi S, Brothers J, Parvizi J, Rothman R. Hip dislocation: are hip precautions necessary in anterior approaches? *Clin Orthop Relat Res*. 2011;469(2):417–422. doi:10.1007/s11999-010-1668-y.
54. Peak EL, Parvizi J, Ciminiello M, et al. The role of patient restrictions in reducing the prevalence of early dislocation following total hip arthroplasty. A randomized, prospective study. *J Bone Joint Surg*. 2005;87(2):247. doi:10.2106/JBJS.C.01513.
55. Skinner HB, Sekiya JK, Jameel O, McMahon PJ. Adult reconstructive surgery. In: Skinner HB, McMahon PJ, eds. *Current Diagnosis & Treatment in Orthopedics*. 5th ed. New York, NY: McGraw-Hill Education; 2014.
56. Stambough JB, Nunley RM, Curry MC, Steger-May K, Clohisy JC. Rapid recovery protocols for primary total hip arthroplasty can safely reduce length of stay without increasing readmissions. *J Arthroplasty*. 2015;30(4):521–526. doi:10.1016/j.arth.2015.01.023.
57. Spalding NJ. Reducing anxiety by pre-operative education: make the future familiar. *Occup Ther Int*. 2003;10(4):278–293. doi:10.1002/oti.191.
58. Martin-Martin LM, Valenza-Demet G, Jimenez-Moleon JJ, Cabrera-Martos I, Revelles-Moyano FJ, Valenza MC. Effect of occupational therapy on functional and emotional outcomes after hip fracture treatment: a randomized controlled trial. *Clin Rehabil*. 2014;28(6):541–551. doi:10.1177/0269215513511472.

59. Kasten P, Maier M, Wendy P, et al. Can shoulder arthroplasty restore the range of motion in activities of daily living? A prospective 3D video motion analysis study. *J Shoulder Elbow Surg*. 2010;19(2):59–65. doi:10.1016/j.jse.2009.10.012.
60. Krischak G, Gebhard F, Reichel H, et al. A prospective randomized controlled trial comparing occupational therapy with home-based exercises in conservative treatment of rotator cuff tears. *J Shoulder Elbow Surg*. 2013;22(9):1173–1179. doi:10.1016/j.jse.2013.01.008.
61. Hagsten B, Svensson O, Gardulf A. Early individualized postoperative occupational therapy training in 100 patients improves ADL after hip fracture a randomized trial. *Acta Orthop Scand*. 2004;75(2):177–183. doi:10.1080/00016470412331294435.

Chapter 42

Rheumatoid Arthritis and Osteoarthritis

Anne Crites and Preethy S. Samuel

LEARNING OBJECTIVES

This chapter will allow the reader to:

1. Describe key features of rheumatoid arthritis and osteoarthritis.
2. Identify clinical sequelae that interfere with meeting occupational performance goals.
3. Select assessments to optimize occupational performance for clients with rheumatoid arthritis and osteoarthritis.
4. Describe interventions to enable clients with rheumatoid arthritis and osteoarthritis to continue, resume, and/or adopt new occupational performance goals.
5. Describe methods of helping clients with rheumatoid arthritis and osteoarthritis to understand and adopt self-management methods during occupational performance.

CHAPTER OUTLINE

TERMINOLOGY

Bouchard nodes: hard, bony outgrowths at the proximal interphalangeal (PIP) joints due to osteoarthritis (OA).

Boutonnière deformity: joint deformity characterized by flexion of the PIP joint and hyperextension at the distal interphalangeal (DIP) joint.

Cachexia: loss of muscle mass as the inflammatory processes affects muscles and the metabolism in rheumatoid arthritis (RA).

Chondropenia: loss of cartilage faster than the rate of repair in the osteoarthritic joint.

Crepitus: feeling or sound of crunching, creaking, or grating coming from the articular surface during range of motion.

Disease-modifying antirheumatic drugs (DMARDs): drugs that affect the immune response or suppress the disease process (e.g., methotrexate).

Fibrillation: the initial degenerative changes in OA, marked by softening of the articular cartilage and development of vertical clefts between groups of cartilage cells.

Heberden nodes: hard, bony outgrowths at the DIP joints caused by OA.

Joint protection techniques: the application of ergonomic principles in daily activities, work, and leisure to reduce internal and external stress on the joints and soft tissues.

Mallet finger deformity: deformity resulting from damage to the extensor tendon at the DIP joint.

Swan-neck deformity: hyperextension of the PIP joint and flexion at the DIP joint.

Synovitis: inflammation of the synovial membrane (which lines synovial joint capsules, the function of which is to produce synovial fluid, which lubricates joints).

Volumetry: a water displacement measure of hand volume, conducted by inserting the hand to a specified depth in a measuring cylinder containing a specified amount of water.

Z deformity of OA thumb: carpometacarpal (CMC) joint adduction, metacarpophalangeal (MCP) joint hyperextension, and interphalangeal (IP) joint flexion.

Z deformity of RA thumb: excessive hyperextension of the IP joint and flexion of the MCP joint of the thumb.

Rheumatoid Arthritis: Definition, Prevalence, and Background

Rheumatoid arthritis (RA) is an autoimmune, chronic, systemic inflammatory disease affecting the joints. It is the most commonly diagnosed type of inflammatory arthritis. In the United States, about 1.5 million adults are estimated to live with RA. Women are two to three times more likely than men to develop RA in their lifetime. The most common age of onset of RA is between 30 and 60 years, with younger age of onset for women.[1]

Rheumatoid Arthritis Etiology and Pathophysiology

The cause of RA is unknown. The disease process is initiated by an interaction between genetic, hormonal, environmental, and lifestyle factors. Joints can be damaged within months of symptom onset.[2] The pathological changes observed in the joints include the following:

- *Synovitis*: Thickening of the synovial membrane with increased synovial fluid causes edema around the joint. Edema-related pressure stretches nociceptors in surrounding tissues, causing pain.
- *Pannus*: Protein-degrading enzymes released from inflammatory cells lead to hypervascularization and thickening of synovial membrane to form pannus (inflammatory tissue) that invades the bone and cartilage at the joint margins, leading to chondral and subchondral erosions.
- *Cachexia*: Loss of muscle mass as the inflammatory processes affects muscles and metabolism.
- *Joint instability*: Prolonged joint swelling stretches and weakens joint ligaments and capsules, thereby disrupting the stability of the joint.
- *Joint deformity*: Abnormal movement in the joints with weak ligaments and disrupted structures leads to deformities.
- *Fatigue*: Inflammatory proteins (e.g., tumor necrosis factor alpha) that are released lead to marked fatigue.

Rheumatoid Arthritis Course and Prognosis

The progression of RA varies considerably among individuals. Except in rare cases of spontaneous remission within the first 6 months of symptoms, most people diagnosed with RA have periods of exacerbations and remissions. The three distinct disease courses of RA are as follows:

1. ***Monocyclic***: About 20% have one episode ending within 2 to 5 years of initial diagnosis without any recurrence. Early diagnosis and/or aggressive treatment with **disease-modifying antirheumatic drugs** (DMARDs) can arrest disease progression.
2. ***Polycyclic***: About 75% experience fluctuating disease activity over the course of the condition, which can last for many years.
3. ***Progressive***: About 5% RA continues to rapidly increase in severity and is unremitting.

Rheumatoid Arthritis Signs and Symptoms

Signs and symptoms of RA include symmetrical presentation of polyarticular pain, edema, early morning stiffness, malaise, and fatigue. The four stages of the inflammatory process in RA are *acute* characterized by red, hot swollen joints with pain, tenderness, and stiffness; *subacute* associated with morning stiffness but less pain and tenderness; *chronic active* and *chronic inactive* with reduced pain and increased tolerance but low endurance. RA can also affect the eyes, skin, lungs, heart, gastrointestinal system, kidneys, nervous system, and blood. RA typically has a gradual onset, with symptoms appearing first in the hands and feet. However, in about 20%, the onset is rapid, and clients wake one morning with multiple painful, stiff, and swollen joints, requiring emergency care. The upper limb joints that are usually affected are the wrists (85% of people with RA), metacarpophalangeal (MCP) joints (80%), elbows (70%), proximal interphalangeal (PIP) joints (65%), and shoulders (60%). In the lower limb, knees (80%), ankles (70%), metatarsophalangeal (MTP) joints (70%), and hips (30%) are affected. Additionally, the cervical spine (35%) and temporomandibular joint (25%) can also be affected.[3] Although there is no cure, early diagnosis and intervention can slow disease progression.

Rheumatoid Arthritis Hand

In women with early RA (<2 years), average losses are 20° of wrist extension, 30° wrist flexion, 15° MCP flexion, and 60% of normal power and pinch grip strength. A third develop hand deformities.[4] Early aggressive DMARD therapy, however, may be lowering such losses that have not been documented because of the absence of recent research on RA hand deformities. Deformities develop because of persistent synovitis, disrupted joint structures that alter joint mechanics, and both normal and abnormal forces over joints during daily use of hands.[5] For example, power grip to hold a hammer requires MCP ulnar deviation, especially in the fourth and fifth fingers, promoting ulnar deviation at weakened MCP joints. During lifting, external pressures in a volar or longitudinal direction increase strain on weakened wrist ligaments. Strong pinch grips increase intrinsic muscle pull, promoting imbalance at the IP joints (Fig. 42-1).

Rheumatoid Arthritis Wrist Joint Changes

The ulnar side of the wrist is an early site of inflammation. The triangular fibrocartilage is disrupted, allowing the proximal carpal row to rotate ulnarward. The distal row compensates by sliding radially, resulting in a gradually radially deviating wrist. Persistent synovitis promotes laxity of the wrist ligaments. Radioulnar ligament laxity allows rotation of the radius and ulna, with the ulnar styloid becoming more prominent. Extensor carpi ulnaris then displaces volarly, passing beneath the wrist joint axis, exerting a flexor pull. This, combined with wrist ligament laxity, and the natural volar incline of the distal radius, increases risk of wrist volar subluxation. Radial deviation at the wrist disrupts biomechanics of the extensor and flexor tendons, causing these to exert an ulnar pull at the MCP joints.

Rheumatoid Arthritis Metacarpophalangeal Joint Changes

Persistent synovitis weakens MCP collateral ligaments, volar plates, and dorsal hoods, leading to joint instability.

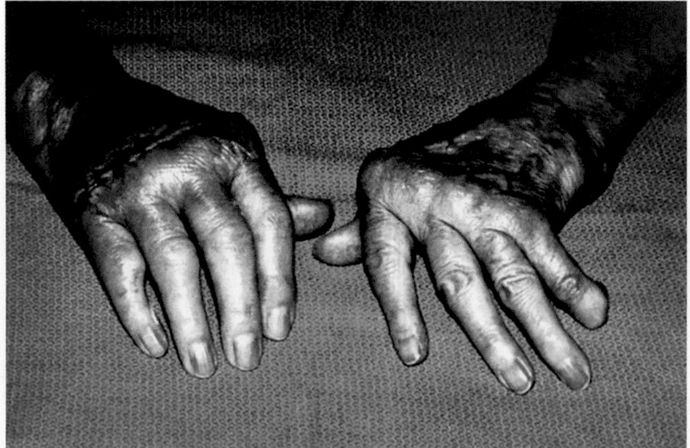

Figure 42-1. Rheumatoid arthritis: right-hand post-op metacarpophalangeal (MCP) arthroplasty, left-hand MCP subluxation and ulnar drifting.

The finger extensors can slip volarly and ulnarly, increasingly acting as weak flexors. Normal MCP joint features further contribute to ulnar deviation once joint structure is disrupted. These include (1) the flexor tendons normally approach the index and middle fingers from an ulnar direction exerting a significant ulnar torque, (2) the metacarpal head anatomically predisposes to tendons slipping ulnarward, and (3) the ulnar interossei exert a stronger pull than the radial ones. See Box 42-1 to observe this phenomenon in the middle finger.

Rheumatoid Arthritis Interphalangeal Joint Changes

Persistent synovitis can also disrupt positioning of the extensor tendon central slip and lateral bands at the PIP joints, allowing a **Boutonnière deformity** to develop. Similar changes can result in **Z deformity of the RA thumb.** MCP joint inflammation can also cause protective spasms in the interossei, causing MCP flexion during finger extension (the intrinsic plus position), which further contributes to Boutonnière and **swan-neck deformity** development. View the video listed in Box 42-1 representing the mechanics of a swan-neck deformity in active fisting. Appreciate the lateral bands as they have become overstretched and drop below the axis of the PIP joint and thus function to hyperextend the PIP in conjunction with the terminal tendon flexing the distal interphalangeal (DIP) joint.

View video of splinting for swan neck and appreciate the control of the hyperextension provided by the three-point pressure splint.

Rheumatoid Arthritis Medical Management

The goal of pharmacotherapy is to rapidly reduce inflammation to prevent or limit joint damage. The earlier the patient starts DMARDs such as methotrexate, the better the outcome. Combination of medicines (e.g., methotrexate,

Box 42-1

Links to Videos

Rheumatoid Arthritis Metacarpophalangeal Joint Changes
https://youtu.be/nS_tafjHxbg

Mechanics of Swan-Neck Deformity in Active Fisting; Splinting for Swan-Neck Deformity
https://youtu.be/fp3-OMOaZI8; https://youtu.be/nS_tafjHxbg

Gait Arms Legs Spine Examination
http://www.youtube.com/watch?v=9jTZ03CbZm0

Examination of Tender and Swollen Joints for Calculation of Disease Activity Score
http://www.youtube.com/watch?v=RnvsbD6NKoc

Occupational Therapist Making a Pattern and Fabricating a Custom Short Opponens Splint
https://youtu.be/0C51BRlnCfE

and/or leflunomide, sulfasalazine, or hydroxychloroquine) is recommended in moderate-to-severe disease and has better outcomes than monotherapy, with no difference in drug tolerability or toxicity.[6] Biologic drugs such as etanercept, infliximab, or adalimumab are used if DMARDs are ineffective, or if there are poor prognostic indicators.[7] Early aggressive use of combined DMARD therapy and biologics has improved outcomes of those newly diagnosed with RA. These medications decrease proliferation of synovial tissue, thereby reducing the incidence of severe wrist and hand deformities as seen in the past. Common surgical procedures of the wrist and hand joints include synovectomy, tenosynovectomy, tendon repair and transfers, joint arthroplasty, and arthrodesis.[8]

Rheumatoid Arthritis–Related Functional Impairments in Daily Occupation

The loss of productivity due to RA is substantial because many are diagnosed in their working years of adulthood. About 60% of those diagnosed with RA from the early stages have difficulty with hand function and challenges completing activities of daily living (ADL).[9] About 20% to 70% of working adults stop working within 7 to 10 years of initial diagnosis.[1] Once unemployed, they are unlikely to return to work. This suggests that two-thirds could benefit from occupational therapy (OT) for hand and ADL difficulties, and at least one-third could benefit from work rehabilitation. Although physical activity is known to decrease pain, improve physical function, and reduce 40% of health care costs, one in three adults with arthritis are inactive.[10]

Osteoarthritis: Definition, Prevalence, and Background

Osteoarthritis (OA) is a clinical syndrome of joint pain linked with degenerative joint changes. OA is the most common form of arthritis and the leading causes of pain and disability worldwide. OA affects 30.8 million adults in the United States.[1] OA is a metabolically active, dynamic process involving all joint tissues (cartilage, bone, synovium, capsule, ligaments, and muscle). It primarily affects the cartilage in the hands (thumb carpometacarpal [CMC], PIP, and DIP joints) and weight-bearing joints specifically, cervical and lumbar spine, hips and knees. The lifetime risk of developing symptomatic OA of the hip joint is 25%,[1] the knee joint 46%,[1] and the hand 40%.[11] OA is more prevalent among woman aged 50 years or older,[12] whereas among people aged 45 years or younger, OA is more prevalent among men.[1]

Osteoarthritis Etiology and Pathophysiology

OA is caused by the damage of joint cartilage attributed to multiple risk factors: genetic (heritability accounts for 40% to 60% of hand, knee, and hip OA), constitutional factors (more common in women, with age, and with higher body weight), and biomechanical factors (e.g., joint injury, greater occupational or leisure use of a joint, reduced muscle strength, joint laxity, or misalignment). Any synovial joint can develop OA, but structural changes do not always cause symptoms. Pathophysiological changes include **fibrillation**, loss of articular cartilage, and remodeling of adjacent bone with new bone formation (osteophytes). Focal synovial membrane inflammation can occur because of irritation from osteophytes and other joint changes. These changes suggest that OA is a repair process, which is initially effective, resulting in a structurally altered but symptom-free joint. However, continued damage or ineffective repair or **chondropenia** means symptomatic OA results.[13]

Osteoarthritis Course and Prognosis

OA may affect one joint or be multifocal. Onset is typically gradual, although the progression of OA can vary widely based on whether it was a result of an injury or insult to the joint such as a fracture or an insidious onset. Although OA is often viewed as a part of the aging process, types of OA have different prognoses. More than half of all individuals diagnosed with knee OA progress significantly to qualify for a knee replacement.[1] People with IP joint OA become asymptomatic after a few years, although structural joint changes such as nodes persist that can affect function. Thumb base OA frequently continues, causing pain and disability. Hip OA has the poorest outcome, with a significant number needing hip replacements after 1 to 5 years.[14]

Osteoarthritis Signs and Symptoms

Signs and symptoms of OA include joint pain, initially on activity that reduces with rest. Over time, pain is persistent and can disturb sleep. Pain is caused by the stretching of nociceptors in the joint capsule due to focal synovitis, increased vascular pressure in subchondral bone, and from spasm of muscles surrounding the involved joints. Joint stiffness occurs after sleep or prolonged inactivity known as the gel phenomenon, which typically lasts 5 to 30 minutes and reduces with movement. Postactivity flare-ups of edema and pain are common symptoms. Joint guarding and decreased willingness to move the painful joint contributes to muscle weakness and limitations in range of motion (ROM). **Crepitus** can occur in advanced cases during ROM with a feeling or sound of crunching, creaking, or grating coming from the articular surface. Hip OA often presents as groin pain.

In hand OA, the repair process can lead to osteophyte formation at joint margins and focal synovitis in affected joints. Hand OA most commonly affects the

DIP and CMC joints.[12] Bony enlargement and persistent synovitis can cause joint ligament laxity. Combined with forces exerted on the hands during daily use, deformities can result. At the PIP joints, bony enlargements are known as **Bouchard nodes**, and at the DIP joints, they are known as **Heberden nodes** (Fig. 42-2). **Mallet finger deformity** results at the DIP joint if the distal extensor digitorum communis tendon attachment is disrupted by bony enlargement. The classic thumb deformity in OA consists of squaring at the CMC joint, with **Z deformity of the OA thumb**, which results from CMC joint adduction, MCP joint hyperextension, and IP joint flexion. Muscle wasting is noticeable in the thenar eminence, and finger, thumb, and wrist movement reduces.

Osteoarthritis Medical Management

The goal of pharmacotherapy is to decrease pain and stiffness and to improve joint mobility and physical activity. Acetaminophen and topical nonsteroidal anti-inflammatory drugs (NSAIDs) (e.g., ibuprofen gel) are recommended for pain relief. If necessary, oral NSAIDs may be prescribed. Capsaicin cream or intra-articular steroid injections may be used if problems continue.[14] Early medications were found to have gastrointestinal complications. Newer medications target only the COX-2 enzymes while protecting the prostaglandins in the gastrointestinal tract. These COX-inhibiting nitric oxide donators (CINODs) have been demonstrated to control pain and reduce inflammation while maintaining gastrointestinal safety.[15] If conservative management fails to resolve pain and the degenerative nature of the disease causes further loss of mobility and function in ADLs, surgery may be recommended. Common surgical interventions include joint replacements, such as total hip arthroplasty (THA) and partial and total knee arthroplasty (TKA). The most common procedure of the CMC joint of the thumb is arthroplasty with ligament reconstruction with tendon interposition (LRTI). Arthrodesis, or joint fusion, is reserved for only the most painful joints that have not responded to all other interventions.[16]

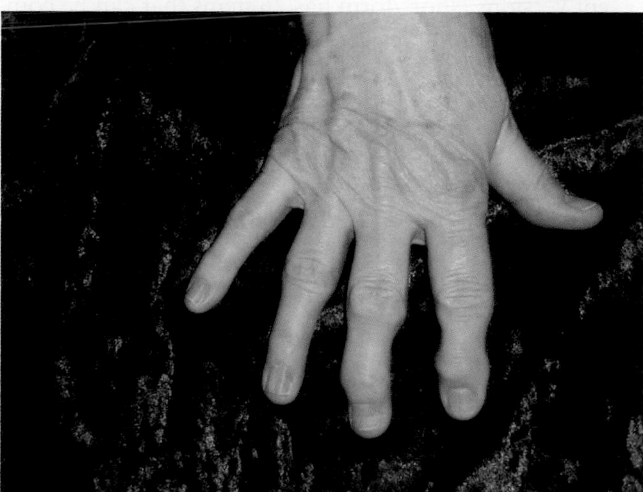

Figure 42-2. Osteoarthritis: the hand and osteoarthritis showing wrist, carpometacarpal, Bouchard nodes (proximal interphalangeal joint), and Heberden nodes (distal interphalangeal joint).

Osteoarthritis-Related Functional Impairments in Daily Occupation

People with combined finger and CMC OA have the poorest function. In women with hand OA, grip strength is only 57% of normal.[17] Estimates indicate that 80% of those with OA experience some degree of movement limitation and 25% cannot perform major ADLs.[18,19] One in five with OA have to give up work or retire early because of their condition, and four in five are in constant pain. About 5% of working-age adults with OA report arthritis-attributable work limitations with three lost workdays per year per person.[1]

Evaluation of Functional Skill Deficits Secondary to Rheumatoid Arthritis and Osteoarthritis

Assessment identifies client factors, performance skills, and impairments to participation in meaningful life activities. Treatment effectiveness can be evaluated if standardized, reliable, valid measures are used.

Initial Interview

A chart review of patients' medical history, comorbidities, and current medications will help with the history taking component of the interview. For RA, it is helpful to know how long the patient has been taking DMARD or biologic drugs because, if started recently, functional gains may be expected. The interview should also gather information about the social history, which should include whether patients live alone or with others; care of pets, children, and elderly parents; and type of home. It should include a summary of their prior level of function to the present episode of care. The initial interview should also focus on occupational performance: ADL (personal and instrumental); rest and sleep; work (paid or volunteer); education (formal or informal); and leisure, social, and community activities. For example, the Canadian Occupational Performance Measure (COPM) is a semi-structured interview requiring about 20 to 40 minutes to administer that focuses on activity limitations and participation.[20] COPM administration ends with identification of the five problems related to self-care, work, or leisure with ratings for each of them by importance, performance, and satisfaction with performance.

As problems are reported, it is essential to explore why they occur: Is it due to pain? Fatigue? Stiffness?

Physical limitations (e.g., in movement, strength, endurance)? Environmental factors (e.g., barriers, lack of equipment)? Psychological factors such as poor concentration, low mood, or lack of confidence or knowledge about their condition (self-efficacy)? Performing specific activities because of fears of pain and/or fatigue, or a lack of information about alternatives?

Ask how patients spend a typical weekday and weekend. How much time is spent in activity and in rest or leisure activities? Do patients take regular rest breaks or keep pushing themselves even though fatigued? How are they coping with competing demands of work and home life? How much do they understand about their condition, and what they could do themselves to make a difference? Objective and subjective assessments are selected according to client priorities.

Body Functions and Activity Limitations

ADL observation is more appropriate for those unable to self-report limitations because of comorbid cognitive problems and postsurgery, because changing circumstances can reduce self-awareness of limitations. Interview is more appropriate for those with low mood, which is prevalent among those living with RA and OA.[21] Using self-reported questionnaires saves time and indicates the need for comprehensive evaluations when required.

- *The Health Assessment Questionnaire (HAQ) and HAQ-DI (disability index)*[22] is a 20-item instrument that can be self-administered in approximately 5 minutes and is widely used in rheumatology clinics for quick screening of eight categories of functioning (dressing, rising, eating, walking, hygiene, reach, grip, and usual activities). Scores, however, worsen if assistive devices are used, and hence, the instrument is unsuitable as an OT outcome measure.
- *The Short-Form Valued Life Activities Scale (S-VLA)*[23] is a 14-item instrument that can be self-administered in 2 to 4 minutes and is reliable and valid for clients with RA. The S-VLA assesses a broad range of life activities (self-care, leisure, and social activities such as work, travel, caring, household tasks, and gardening) and use of behavioral accommodations to monitor disability.
- *Measure of Activity Performance of the Hand (MAP-Hand)*[24] is an 18-item instrument that can be self-administered in 3 minutes and has established reliability and validity for clients with RA. The MAP-Hand screens hand function deficits by evaluating performance in eight activities using a four-point rating scale. Total scores range from 0 to 54.
- *Patient Rated Wrist and Hand Evaluation (PRWE and PRWHE)*[25] is a 15-item instrument that can be self-administered in 5 to 10 minutes. The instrument was originally developed for distal radius fractures, but was later modified to include other hand conditions, and possesses validity and reliability data for clients with arthritis. The instrument evaluates pain and function to determine degree of disability; develop treatment goals; predict prognosis of injury from baseline scores; measure clinically important changes; and communicate limitations meaningfully to clients, other health care professionals, and insurance companies.
- *Michigan Hand Outcomes Questionnaire*[26] is a 37-item instrument that can be self-administered in 15 minutes and has established reliability and validity for clients with RA and OA. The instrument evaluates hand aesthetics, pain, ADL, work, function, and satisfaction with hand function. There is also a brief 12-item version[27] that is available and has validity for clients with OA and RA.
- *The Evaluation of Daily Activity Questionnaire (EDAQ)*[28] involves a comprehensive evaluation of common effects of arthritis on body functions (e.g., mood, pain, stiffness) using a 10-point rating scale and has the ability to perform 138 daily activities with and without ergonomic methods/assistive devices using a four-point rating scale. The EDAQ is available in multiple languages, can be self-administered in 30 to 60 minutes, and has established reliability and validity for clients with RA and OA.
- *The Arthritis Impact Measurement Scale-2 (AIMS2)*[29] is a 101-item instrument that can be self-administered in 20 to 30 minutes and assesses the negative impact of arthritis in the past 4 weeks with regard to arm function, mobility, physical activity (walking, bending, lifting), dexterity, household activity (managing money and medications, housekeeping), work, social activities, ADL, pain, depression, and anxiety. Total scores using the Guttman response scale range from 0 to 60, where lower scores represent better health status. The AIMS2 was psychometrically tested with clinical sensitivity to measure treatment effect in clients with RA and OA. AIMS2 is available in multiple languages and in different versions (short-form has 26 items that can be completed in 10 minutes; pediatric and geriatric versions).

Activity Diaries

A diary of how the client spends a typical weekday and weekend day, with each day divided into half-hour periods, helps identify occupational balance. Several designs exist. For example, the patient can write the main activity completed in each half hour, indicate level of pain and fatigue experienced using a 10-point rating scale, and note whether rest was taken.

Mobility and Upper Limb Function

Overall movement can be assessed, if necessary, using the Gait Arms Legs Spine (GALS), a reliable, valid musculoskeletal screening examination[30] that takes 5 to 10 minutes to administer. See Box 42-1 for the link to a video that shows the examination being conducted.

Hand and Upper Limb Assessment

In RA, a tender and swollen joint count can be conducted for hand splint assessment or to monitor progress over time. See Box 42-1 for a link to a video that shows this assessment performed as part of the Disease Activity Score-28.[31] **Volumetry** that measures hand girth can be used to measure hand edema. Although reliability of circumferential measurements has not been shown, they can be helpful for documenting the swelling of an isolated joint, especially when volumetry will not capture hand girth. Circumferential measurement of involved joints can be compared to the contralateral side, if uninvolved, or to adjacent joints in the case of the digits. In RA and OA, recording hand appearance (e.g., the presence of joint swelling, pain, and deformity) on a hand chart is particularly useful, as is digital photography. ROM should be measured using standard goniometric methods.

Grip strength can be assessed using the Jamar dynamometer, although this is less accurate for weak grip. Pinch strength can be measured with a B&L pinch gauge, which is also reliable. Normative data are published for grip and pinch measured using the Jamar and B&L gauges.[32] Other reliable and valid hand assessments include (1) the *Grip Ability Test*, which takes 5 minutes to administer and consists of pouring water from a jug, placing a paper clip on an envelope, and pulling Tubigrip over the hand and forearm[33]; (2) the *Sequential Occupational Dexterity Assessment* (SODA),[34] a more detailed assessment requiring about 15 to 20 minutes to measure bimanual dexterity activity in RA; and (3) the *Nine-Hole Peg Test* (NHPT), which measures unilateral fine manual dexterity, is compact, simple, and easy and takes 5 minutes to administer.[35]

Work Assessments

Evaluation of work is important in the rehabilitation of persons with arthritis. Interviews, screening tools, and self-assessments, such as the Work Environment Survey-Rheumatic Conditions,[36] Worker Role Interview,[37] and Manual Work Instability Scale,[38] are all effective tools for identifying employment-related problems and the client's perceptions of abilities, limitations, and expectations related to work.

- *Ergonomic Assessment Tool for Arthritis (EATA)*[39] documents task description, equipment used, typical activities at work during 1 day, work postures, work demands, and work station layout. The EATA helps guide observation and recording during a work site visit and job analysis, or can be conducted as an interview and/or client self-report.
- *Functional Capacity Evaluation (FCE)*[40] is an observational and functional assessment of work ability that describes a person's ability to perform work activities. FCE is an umbrella term that includes evaluation systems such as the WorkHab, WorkWell Systems, and Matheson systems.

Interventions for Functional Skill Deficits Secondary to Rheumatoid Arthritis and Osteoarthritis

The overarching goal of occupational interventions is to enable patients to improve their occupational performance and participation in daily-life roles and routines, despite the functional impairments due to arthritis. In the *acute stage* of inflammation, the focus of treatment should be on gentle passive and active ROM to the point of pain (without stretch). In the *subacute stage,* treatment can include both active and passive ROM, gentle passive stretch, and isotonic and graded isometric exercises with minimal stress to joints. In the *chronic active* and *inactive stages*, treatment focuses on stretch at end range, and resistive isotonic and isometric exercises that do not stress the joints. The key factors to consider when developing treatment plans are to respect pain, avoid fatigue, manage stress, prevent deformities when possible through avoidance of stress to inflamed tissues and joints or excessive activity/exercise during a flare-up or exacerbation, use thermal modalities with caution and limit the application of heat to 20 minutes, use resistive exercise with caution, and be aware of sensory impairments. Therapeutic programs should promote weight-bearing activities, and ROM as tolerated with affected joints and as much as possible with unaffected joints, and aerobic exercise. Interventions to reduce functional impairments associated with RA and OA in all stages can be broadly classified into five categories: client education, physical agent modalities, edema management, orthotic devices, and therapeutic activities and exercises. The focus of intervention varies by the stage of the inflammatory process. Interventions are summarized in Box 42-2.

Physical Agent Modalities

Nonpharmacological interventions that include physical agent modalities can be beneficial in reducing pain and stiffness, although extant research on their effectiveness is inconclusive.[12] Heat applications such as superficial hot-packs, infrared radiation, paraffin wax bath, fluidotherapy, and hydrotherapy have the potential to reduce pain, muscle spasms, and increase elasticity of periarticular structures.[12] Therefore, these applications are best used for 10 to 20 minutes before engaging in therapeutic exercises or activities.[15]

Cold applications such as ice-packs and cryotherapy are preferred over thermotherapy in active joints where intra-articular heat increase is contraindicated, such as during an exacerbation of RA symptoms. Care should be used in selection of heat and cold modalities with attention to the stage of the disease process and monitoring of vascular reactions, and skin and tissue responses. Heat is generally preferred for the effects on

Box 42-2

Comprehensive List of Occupational Therapy Interventions in Rheumatology

Activities of Daily Living (ADL) Rehabilitation

- Work rehabilitation: including on-site work assessments, ergonomics; work assistive devices; employer liaison; work environment adaptation; functional capacity evaluation; work hardening
- Avocational rehabilitation: voluntary work, adult education, and leisure opportunities; modifying leisure activities
- Stress and pain management
- Relaxation training
- Communication and assertiveness training

Counseling

- (may also include cognitive–behavioral therapy if the therapist has postgraduate training)
- Family/caregiver liaison and support
- Advice on social security benefits and community resources
- Exercise for health and well-being (e.g., Tai Chi, yoga, swimming, walking, low impact dance programs)
- Self-management education (individual and group work) using cognitive–behavioral approaches
- Activity/role planning, goal clarification, and setting
- Ergonomic education (joint protection), fatigue management

Assistive Technology and Adaptive Equipment

- Orthoses (e.g., resting and working hand splints, elbow and neck orthoses)
- Hand and upper extremity therapy and exercises (active range of motion [ROM], passive ROM, resistive and dexterity exercise)

Therapeutic Activities

- Home assessment, recommendations for environmental and housing adaptations
- Mobility aids prescription (including wheelchair/powered aids), driving/transport advice
- Total joint replacement postoperative management (ADL retraining, assistive technology)
- Foot care advice and simple orthoses (e.g., metatarsal pads, arch supports, insoles)

pain and periarticular structures. Warm water soaks and baths/showers can alleviate pain and stiffness for people with arthritis.

Ultrasound uses high-frequency sound waves to provide mechanical and thermal effects that can improve healing of soft tissue, decrease the inflammatory response, increase blood flow, increase metabolic activity, and decrease pain based on emerging evidence.[41,42] Electrostimulation such as transcutaneous electrical nerve stimulation (TENS) that involves noninvasive delivery of electrical signals via superficially placed skin electrodes can reduce pain for people with arthritis and improve hand grip strength.[12] Low-level laser therapy uses a single wavelength of light to produce not a thermal effect but photochemical reactions in the cells to promote soft-tissue healing, reduce inflammation, and reduce acute and chronic pain seen in OA and RA.[43]

Edema Management

Interventions to reduce edema focus on improving circulation to the affected limb. Increased use of the affected limb within pain limits must be strongly encouraged as well as elevation of the involved limb above the heart when at rest. Avoidance of the dependent position will reduce fluid retention within the extremity. Gentle hand pumping (fisting) combined with elevation should be encouraged to improve circulation. Contrast baths that involve immersing the swollen arm or leg alternatively in hot and cold water can also reduce edema.[44] Compression gloves can decrease edema, reduce nocturnal pain, and reduce pain and stiffness during daytime activities, because they are easily worn in activity, although the evidence is still inconclusive.[12] Kinesiotaping that involves the use of an elastic therapeutic tape can reduce edema and pain without restricting use of the affected limb in daily activities for those with RA[45] or OA.[46] Caution should be used with fragile skin.

Orthotics

Splints are used to reduce local inflammation, reduce soft-tissue and joint pain, correctly position joints, improve joint stability, and improve hand function. During the *acute stage* in the inflammatory process of RA, splints can be used to support the joints in their open-packed position, allowing the most space in the joint and reducing pain associated with swelling. Joint effusion can cause damage to the soft-tissue structures surrounding the joint. Therefore, joints should be placed as close to a functional position as possible. Splint wear regimen should include intermittent removal, gentle ROM, and use of the hand in daily activities.

Static Resting Splints

Resting splints can reduce localized pain and inflammation by providing support in an anatomically correct position at rest. They can be worn at night and/or during daytime rest periods. Although the research evidence can be mixed, there is clinical consensus on the value of using resting splints for those living with RA[5] and OA[15] (Fig. 42-3).

Wrist Orthoses

Wrist orthoses are widely used with many available designs. A close fit, not impeding MCP and thumb movement, is needed. They can be worn for nighttime pain relief if the person has wrist, but not MCP or IP pain. Their main aim is to reduce torque during heavy tasks involving the wrist and to stabilize the wrist in

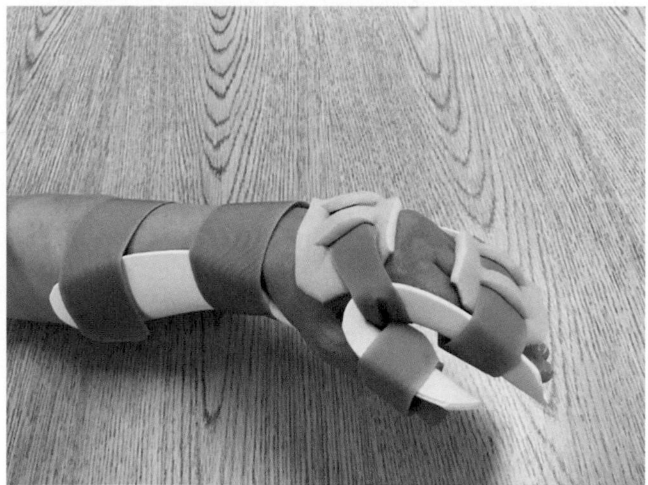

Figure 42-3. Resting pan splint.

a functionally effective position (i.e., 10°–15° of extension). Wrist orthoses are more effective in reducing hand pain than improving grip strength or hand function.[15] Supportive wrist splints can be beneficial when worn during heavy activities, such as ironing, gardening, housework, and at work.

Metacarpophalangeal Splints

Small palm-based splints can have a wrist and forearm component to reduce medial force on the MCPs and maintain fingers in correct alignment. These splints reduce ulnar deviation of the fingers and improve hand function in people with RA with established MCP deformities.[47]

Finger Splints

Swan-neck splints apply three-point pressure around the PIP joint to prevent PIP joint hyperextension and subsequent DIP flexion. They can be made or bought in thermoplastics or made in silver. Both types can improve dexterity and hand function, and many clients prefer prefabricated splints.[12] In the case of significant swelling at the PIP joint, custom thermoplastic three-point pressure splints can be fabricated. See Box 42-1 for a link to a video of three-point products' thermoplastic "ring" splint preventing swan-neck deformity in active fisting.

Thumb Splints

Short, hand-based splints are designed to immobilize the CMC joint only, the CMC and MP, or a longer hand/forearm splint if pain extends to the wrist. Evidence suggests that CMC joint splints can reduce pain, improve function, and avoid or delay surgery in OA.[48] Many prefer a short flexible splint to longer more rigid versions (Fig. 42-4). See Box 42-1 for a link to a video of an occupational therapist making a pattern and fabricating a custom short opponens splint.

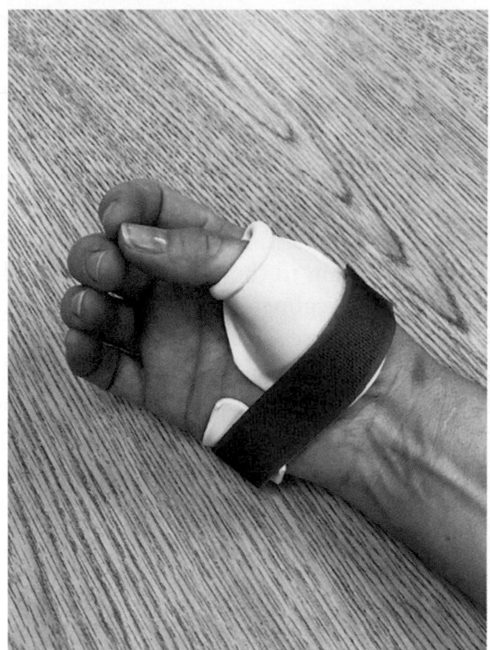

Figure 42-4. Short opponens splint.

Therapeutic Activities and Exercises

Physical activity for people with RA also has favorable effects on bone by slowing joint destruction and increasing bone mineral density as evidenced by radiographs.[49] Short-term aerobic exercise programs comprising activities such as cycling or running for 1 hour each day four to five times a week for about 5 days a week are effective in RA.[50] Resistance training not only increases muscle strength but reduces systemic inflammation. However, in the acute phase of inflammation or flare-up, resistive exercises are contraindicated. Aquatic aerobic programs are considered more effective for people with OA.[51] Engaging in physical activity for people with arthritis is associated with improved self-esteem, quality of sleep, reduction of pain, and depressive symptoms.[49] People with arthritis are often not physically active owing to low energy, fear of aggravating pain, and also because of low awareness of these benefits.

Occupational therapists should develop home programs that integrate physical activity into daily routines and teach home maintenance programs for ROM, strength, and aerobic exercises. People often need advice tailoring exercise and activity to suit their changing ability and to progress gradually, rather than overdoing it. Efficacy of home exercise programs is contingent on educating patients about the benefits of physical activity—how it reduces pain, improves fitness, and increases energy levels as muscle strength and aerobic capacity increase, and in RA and OA, how it helps protect joints as stronger muscles compensate for weakened ligaments. Working together with other specialists, such as physical therapists and recreational therapists, can maximize the outcomes of home programs.

Hand Exercises

Exercise is effective in improving hand strength (grip and pinch) and function and to reduce pain in RA[52] and OA.[15] The addition of an individually tailored resistive hand exercise program to the usual care of people with RA on a stable drug regimen led to improved hand function without any adverse effects.[52] In hand OA, exercises can improve grip by up to 25% and reduce pain.[53] However, exercise must be sustained, otherwise the benefits are lost. Exercise diaries and goal setting help people sustain exercising. Opportunities to remind people to restart, if they lapse, are essential. A simple home program is described in Box 42-3.

Ergonomics in Arthritis

The term *ergonomics* is most literally translated to mean "the laws of work." It is the science of addressing human performance in relation to occupational tasks and applying the most efficient use of equipment, tools, and the environment to promote health and safety. Related approaches are *joint protection*, *energy conservation*, and *body mechanics*. **Joint protection** aims to reduce loads on joints and reduce deforming forces, thus minimizing risks of injury. Patients with rheumatic conditions causing joint or soft-tissue pain and swelling, loss of motion, and deformities often have decreased energy and may require more energy for even basic activities. Energy conservation techniques function to conserve energy resources, so an individual can perform tasks at a higher level of function without expending more energy. Body mechanics focuses on minimizing strain on body structures by preserving a balance of musculature. The emphasis is on maintaining a neutral position through muscle co-contraction, thereby supporting the soft-tissue structures (joints, ligaments, muscles, and tendons) during daily activities. Ergonomic and joint protection principles are summarized in Box 42-4. For more information, consult the following resources: www.osha.gov/SLTC/ergonomics/ or http://ergo.human.cornell.edu/.

Goals of Ergonomics

The goals of the ergonomic approach in RA and OA are to:

1. ***Reduce pain*** during activity, and at rest, resulting from pressure on nociceptive endings in joint capsules, caused by inflammation and/or mechanical forces on joints
2. ***Reduce forces on joints***: Internal (i.e., from muscular compressive forces, e.g., during strong grip) or

Box 42-3

A Home Hand Exercise Program

Find a comfortable position: support the arm to avoid shoulder aching.

- Warm up by moving the joints a little first and/or soaking in warm water for a few minutes.
- Exercise 3 days the first week, increasing repetitions and number of days over 2 to 4 weeks, to 10 repetitions most daily.

Range of Motion

- Wrist extension/flexion
- Forearm pronation/supination
- Tendon gliding exercise
- Radial finger walk

Muscle Strength and Dexterity Exercise

Use a good handful of therapeutic putty. Five minutes initially, gradually increasing to 10 to 15 minutes. (Caution: Do not use during acute phase of inflammation or with unstable joints.)

- Gently knead and squeeze.
- Push fingers into dough and push out straight.
- Pinch off dough with each finger/thumb in turn.
- Roll into a sausage (two hands).
- Form a "ring doughnut" from the sausage. Put the fingers/thumbs in the hole; stretch out.

Grip a 0.5-L (16.9-fl oz) water bottle (with a "waist" filled with water or sand). Support the forearm.

- Lift bottle up and down slowly, first with palm facing down 10 times, and then with the palm facing up 10 times.
- Isometrically (statically) squeeze the bottle with a 10-second hold, repeat 5–10 times.

Box 42-4

Ergonomic (Joint Protection) Principles

- Respect pain.
- Distribute load over several joints.
- Reduce the force and effort required in activities.
- Use correct patterns of movement.
- Use good body positioning, posture, and moving and handling techniques.
- Use the strongest, largest joint available for the job.
- Avoid staying in one position for too long.
- Use ergonomic equipment, assistive devices, and labor-saving gadgets.
- Pace activities: balance rest and activity, alternate heavy and light tasks, and take microbreaks.
- Use work simplification: plan, prioritize, and problem solve.
- Modify the environment and equipment location to be ergonomically efficient.
- Maintain muscle strength and range of motion.
- Use adequate lighting.

external (i.e., forces applied to joints while carrying or pulling/pushing objects)

3. ***Reduce secondary inflammation*** and subsequent strain on soft tissues resulting from excess (i.e., beyond tolerability) force on already inflamed and/or disrupted joints
4. ***Reduce loading*** on articular cartilage and subchondral bone, thus preserving joint integrity and reducing risk of development and/or progression of deformities
5. ***Reduce pain resulting from overuse*** (i.e., beyond tolerability) of deconditioned muscles
6. ***Reduce fatigue,*** by reducing effort required for activity performance, thus improving function

Ergonomic Methods

Hand ergonomics in RA include changing movement patterns to limit strong grips, twisting movements, and sustained grips to reduce MCP forces; to limit lifting heavy objects and sustained wrist radial positioning to reduce wrist volar and radial forces; and to limit tight, prolonged key, tripod, and pinch grips to reduce volar and ulnar forces on the MCP, IP, and CMC joints. Approaches are similar in OA, although there is no need to emphasize reducing ulnar forces on the second through fifth MCPs, because these are not affected. The rapid decline of hand function often seen in early RA and hand OA suggests that effective ergonomic education should be provided early to improve and maintain function or prevent problems.

Ergonomics and Assistive Technology

According to the Assistive Technology Act of 1998 (amended in 2004), *assistive technology* is defined as "any item, piece of equipment or product system whether acquired commercially, modified, or customized that is used to increase, maintain or improve functional capabilities of individuals with disabilities." In RA and OA, the focus is to reduce the effort required using ergonomic equipment or products with *universal design*, that is, devices that are designed for an array of abilities and to be easy for all to use such as levered-handled faucets and doorknobs. Avoid lifting using wheels; put shopping in a folding hand cart, easily kept in the trunk of the car when not in use. Avoid bending and kneeling; sit on a garden kneeler/stool when weeding. Wear cushioned, shock-absorbing insoles in shoes to reduce pressure on foot and knee joints when walking and standing. At work, use voice-activated software to reduce keyboarding. Communicate using hands-free phones (headsets, speaker, or voice-to-text). There are many kitchen and household products available in stores and via the Internet, such as jar openers and electric can openers. Encourage people to consider features of good design when creating or selecting assistive technology and universal design products. Ergonomic products should be

- Lightweight, durable, compact
- Nonslip with larger handles
- Comfortable to hold and easy to maneuver
- Attractive and acceptable to the user
- Simple to operate, multipurpose (if appropriate)
- Reduce stress to all joints needed to operate the device
- Affordable

Altering Movement Patterns and Use of Proper Joint and Body Mechanics

In hand activities, two hands can be used, and the load can be spread over the palmar surface (Fig. 42-5). Movement patterns can be changed by, for example, turning a jar lid using the thumb, index, ring fingers, and thumb web space. The fingers are kept in correct anatomic alignment, and ulnar forces are avoided. Placing Dycem (nonslip matting) under items reduces effort to stabilize objects with the nondominant hand (Fig. 42-6). Using offset knife with built-up handle promotes a neutral wrist position with less effort for grip. Using an adapted cutting board with prongs to hold the food in place reduces effort to stabilize the food item (Fig. 42-7).

Objects should be kept closer to the body when lifting and carrying, and/or a stronger larger joint can be used. For example, avoid carrying a shopping bag using a hook grip in the hand (Fig. 42-8). Alternatively, use

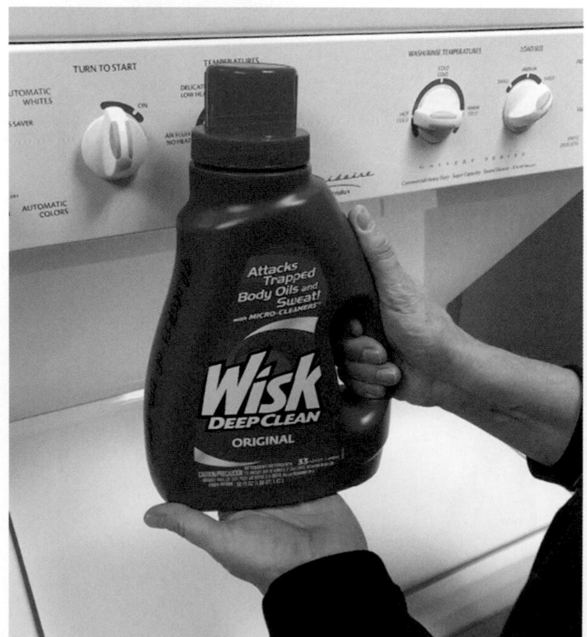

Figure 42-5. Distribute the load using two hands to carry laundry soap.

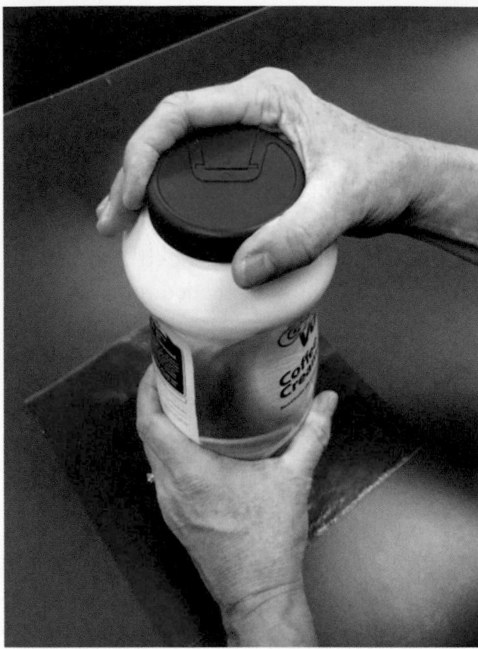

Figure 42-6. Altering movement patterns avoiding ulnar forces opening container, using Dycem to secure the object requiring decreased force to stabilize the object.

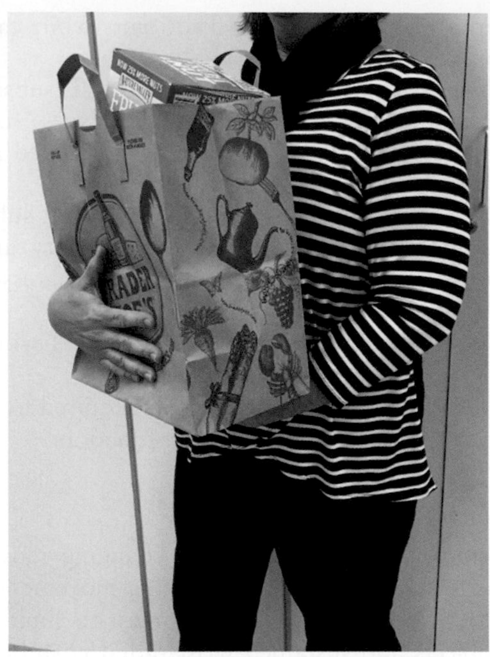

Figure 42-8. Using stronger, larger joints and holding closer to the body: carrying a grocery bag.

a bag with longer handles pulled over the shoulder or backpacks to distribute weight on both the shoulders. Avoid prolonged sitting and standing. Change position frequently. Smartphones and smartwatches have apps that offer intermittent reminders for such postural adjustments and movement breaks. For people with knee and foot pain, a counter-height chair or an adjustable perch stool reduces standing when preparing food or ironing. For postoperative hip and knee replacements or patients with limited ROM in hips, knees, or spine, assistive devices such as long-handled shoe horns and sock aids can assist with donning lower extremity clothing (Fig. 42-9). Work surfaces and items should be within the reach of the arms. Maintain efficient postures when working (e.g., avoid sitting with a forward head posture when working at a desk or reading). Book stands, writing slopes, and document holders help. Keep the back straight using supportive seating, such as ergonomic office chairs and higher back supportive sofas. Poor

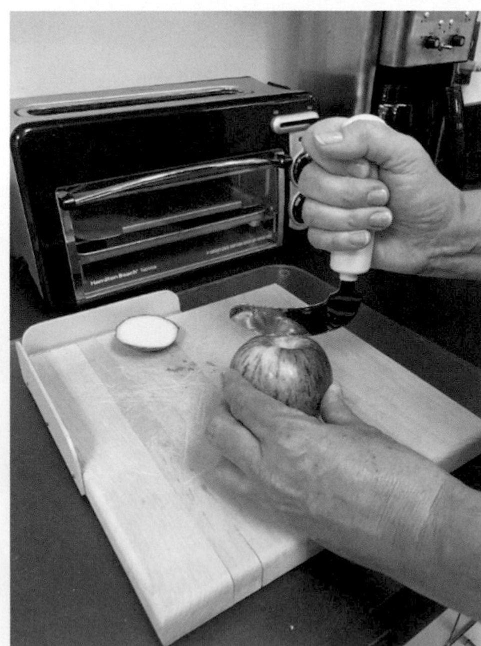

Figure 42-7. Assistive technology: offset knife w/ built-up handle, adapted cutting board stabilizes food.

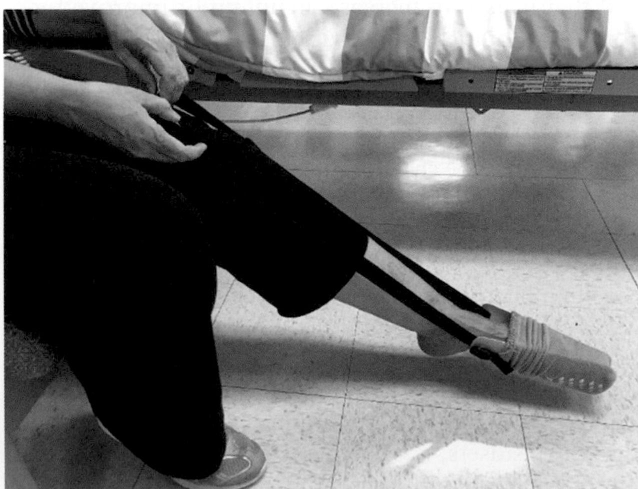

Figure 42-9. Sock aid to don socks caused by loss of motion in spine, hip, or knee, or post-op range of motion precautions.

posture and positioning increase muscle fatigue and pain because greater energy is used to maintain biomechanically inefficient postures.

Restructuring Activities, Work Simplification, and Altering the Environment

Can an activity be done differently? For example, rather than taking a sauce pan to the sink, holding it while it fills, and carrying it back across the kitchen, fill it with a lightweight measuring cup instead (Fig. 42-10). Use a pot/pan stabilizer to assist with the effort required to hold the pan in place. Could shopping be done via the Internet to save driving, walking, and carrying bags? Reorder the sequence of tasks within activities to increase efficiency. Eliminate unnecessary tasks: Do all items need to be ironed? Keep frequently used equipment easily accessible and within reach. Unclutter and reorganize work areas to streamline work processes. Locate equipment to promote correct joint positioning (e.g., keyboards). Raise or lower work surfaces to maintain good posture. Ensure storage is efficient (e.g., use stepped shelves in cupboards and sliding racks so that jars, cans, and boxes are easily reached).

Fatigue Management

Fatigue can be caused by physical and psychosocial factors. Physical factors include pain, increased physical demands because of altered joint biomechanics, deconditioning because of insufficient physical activity, and/or overdoing activities (the boom–bust cycle). In RA, the inflammatory process contributes to fatigue and also causes anemia and muscle cachexia. Psychosocial factors (e.g., depression, anxiety, helplessness, stress, poor self-efficacy), poor social support (e.g., lack of understanding from family and friends), and work pressures contribute to fatigue. A variety of strategies help reduce fatigue, including ergonomic approaches at home and work, activity pacing, increasing physical activity/exercise, and stress management. Encourage clients to manage stress using mindfulness therapy, relaxation, meditation, and cognitive–behavioral therapy.

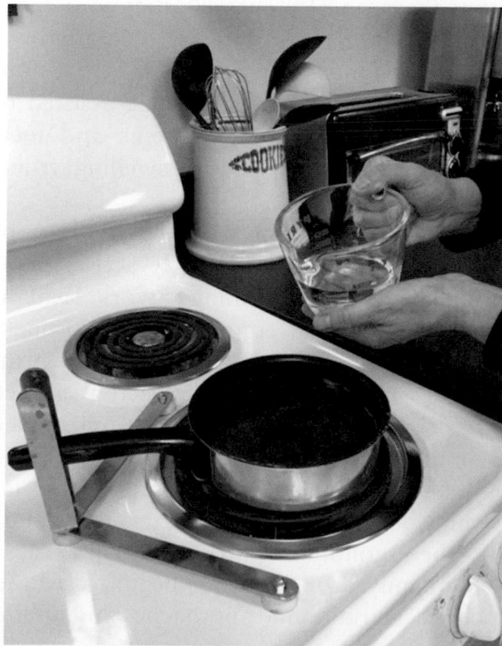

Figure 42-10. Restructuring activity: fill pan with measuring cup/use of pan holder to assist stabilizing pan.

Activity Pacing

Many find taking a rest break difficult because it can be seen as "giving in." Rest "recharges the batteries," allowing people to keep going for longer. Rest recommendations include taking microbreaks for 30 seconds every 5 to 10 minutes or so, stretching and relaxing joints and muscles being most used, or taking a rest break for up to 5 minutes every 30 to 60 minutes. Frequency depends on fatigue severity. Rest breaks allow muscle recovery time. Help develop habits by using computer screen prompts, a kitchen timer, or a mobile phone alarm (or set to vibrate) to remind the person to take the rest break.

Activity Planning

Balance activities to alternate between light, medium, and heavy tasks during the day and week. A "boom–bust" cycle is common, with people doing too much on good days and suffering the consequences for the next few. Breaking this habit requires attitudinal change. Many fear the consequences of failing to meet responsibilities. Activity diaries help people see boom–bust patterns. Use a diary with a line for each day of the week, each divided into 24 hours, showing 7 days on one page. The person completes this over a week, coloring the hours of high activity in red, medium in amber, and low in green, with rest colored blue. This graphical shows how clients are overdoing activity and why they are fatigued.

Sleep Hygiene

A sleep diary that could include apps on smartwatches or smartphones can help identify why sleep is problematic. Solutions can include change of mattress and pillow (e.g., memory foam); establishing a regular bedtime and relaxing evening routine (e.g., listening to a relaxation recording, warm bath, or hot milky drink); avoiding stimulants (coffee, tea, alcohol, nicotine, and caffeinated soft drinks) before bedtime; reducing stimuli in the bedroom (e.g., no TV or computer use) and black-out curtains; and muted colors. Improving sleep can help in fatigue management.

Vocational Rehabilitation

Vocational rehabilitation includes (1) job modifications or "accommodations" such as ergonomic changes (restructuring work tasks, assistive technology and adaptations, work station/place redesign, and splints); (2) psychosocial and informational strategies (increasing confidence to ask for job modifications, work rights, statutory [imposed by law] VR service availability, and coping strategies); and (3) liaising with employers (about job and hours flexibility and better understanding of the condition), occupational health, and statutory services. Evidence indicates that vocational rehabilitation when combined with comprehensive OT improved self-perceived ability to manage self-care, work and leisure, work instability, work satisfaction, and pain reduction.[54]

Postoperative Management

The postoperative management of surgical interventions of the wrist and hand due to RA and OA are most often managed by the occupational therapist who specializes in hand therapy. Treatment typically consists of custom thermoplastic splint fabrication to provide support to the surgical area protecting percutaneous pins and surgical scars in a position that is most conducive to recovery of motion without disruption of the procedure. There are specific postoperative protocols related to the various surgical procedures, which vary from surgeon to surgeon. Most often, the patient is initially immobilized followed by active and passive ROM to restore joint mobility and progressive strengthening, coordination retraining, and hand use to tolerance. Some procedures such as MCP joint arthroplasty with tendon repositioning include dynamic splinting to allow for controlled early mobilization of the joints and excursion of the tendons during the healing phase of recovery.

Postoperative management of hip and knee replacements include education of the various precautions for motion to prevent disruption of the joint prosthesis and training in lower body dressing and hygiene with adherence to motion restrictions. Assistive technology such as long-handled reachers, sponges, shoe horns, and sock aids are provided when necessary for independence in ADLs (see Fig. 42-9). Adaptations to typical movement patterns such as transferring in and out of bed, and up and down from the toilet or chairs are reviewed with the client and caregivers.

Theoretical Frameworks and Clinical Outcomes

All of the abovementioned interventions assist clients in adapting their lifestyle to improve self-management and occupational balance. However, changing habits and routines is not easy. On average, adherence rates are about 50% for many interventions. Theoretical frameworks such as the transtheoretical model, social cognitive theory, and cognitive–behavioral therapy can be invaluable in fostering long lasting change via the process of OT interventions.[55] According to the transtheoretical model, people cycle through five stages (precontemplation, contemplation, preparation, action, and maintenance) when modifying health behaviors with lapses possible at any of these stages. If the person is not yet ready to make changes, *motivational interviewing* can help to foster attitudinal changes. The following are examples of motivational interviewing questions that can be self-rated on a scale ranging from 0 to 10:

- How important is it for you to reduce these symptoms and continue these activities?
- How confident do you feel about making changes?
- How ready are you to make changes?

Let the client discuss his or her concerns, which are commonly about negative self-image, embarrassment, not wanting to use assistive devices, wanting to remain as he or she is, not wanting to take the time to change, or concerns that using ergonomics makes tasks slower and more difficult.

Enhance principles of social cognitive theory by encouraging clients to participate in self-help groups. Group interventions enable modeling, problem-solving, peer support, and idea exchange. Watching others like themselves successfully perform actions enhances their beliefs that they can also succeed, therefore encourage participating in support groups (virtual or in-person). Group members must be encouraged to reinterpret physiological signals; clients should be assisted to perceive differences in disease symptoms and increased symptoms (e.g., aches, fatigue, joint swelling) from overdoing activities.

Incorporate the cognitive–behavioral approach by helping clients set short (weekly action plan) and long-term goals such as remaining at work. Explain how assistive technology and ergonomics can propel them toward their goal. Encourage clients to apply principles of ergonomics in work and leisure activities. Between sessions, ask them to self-monitor: watch movements during common activities (e.g., making a meal, at work) as they normally do them. What forces occur? Is there aching, pain, or fatigue? Ask them to reflect and compare with the ergonomic approaches they are learning. Often, "the penny drops"; clients begin to see the connection between ergonomic approaches and a reduction in pain and fatigue.

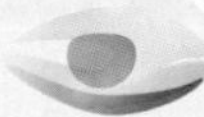

CASE STUDY

Patient Information

Aanya is 45-year-old Indian woman with a 3-year history of RA. She is stable on DMARDs. At her last 6 monthly rheumatology appointment, she complained of increasing pain in her right wrist, hand, shoulder, and feet. She is a full-time fourth-grade schoolteacher, the quality of her work is affected greatly because she is right handed, and she is unable to take time off work. She lives in a first floor, one-bedroom apartment.

Reason for Occupational Therapy Referral

Aanya was referred by her rheumatologist for assessment of hand function, help with work problems, and self-management education. She wants to keep working full time.

Assessment Process and Results

Because Aanya's priority is work, she was assessed using the Work Environment Survey-Rheumatic Conditions (WES-RC) and an activity diary. Every day, in the classroom, Aanya regularly uses an interactive whiteboard, desktop computer, tablet, and cell phone. She has to move round the classroom and bend frequently to help students with activities in small groups. She drives to work and has a full briefcase to carry to the car. She buys lunch at the school cafe. Work consumes all her time and energy, and she is unable to manage her housework. Aanya buys ready meals and seeks help from her friends and family. She spends weekends recovering, and the pain reduces, but she is often still tired. Her sleep is disturbed by hand pain at night. Her pain and fatigue decrease during school vacations. She enjoys her work very much despite the daily pain and fatigue, but has no energy left for leisure and community engagements.

Physical examination of Aanya's hands, wrist, shoulder and feet (using the Gait Arms Legs Spine [GALS]), and tender and swollen joint count showed a mild inflammatory process and no deformity. Bilateral grip strength was 30 lb (norm is about 60 lb). On a Visual Analog Scale (VAS) for pain and fatigue, Aanya scored 7 of 10 for both after workday. Self-administration of the EDAQ indicated that she had problems in cooking, meal preparation (such as opening jars, peeling vegetables, and lifting pots/pans), cleaning using the vacuum cleaner and mop, sewing, knitting, and social outings such as bowling.

Occupational Therapy Problem List

- Right wrist, MCP, shoulder, and foot pain worsen during the workday, especially when she is using the interactive whiteboard at work that requires prolonged standing.
- Difficulty with home maintenance
- Difficulty preparing meals
- Limited leisure activities
- Poor sleep because of nocturnal hand pain

Occupational Therapy Goal List

- Use ergonomic approaches to reduce wrist, MCP, shoulder, and foot pain during work, home, and meal preparation activities.
- Use fatigue management (activity pacing) to reduce fatigue.
- Wear right wrist orthosis to protect her hands during heavier activities and compression glove at night to reduce pain and morning stiffness.
- Perform hand exercises daily to improve grip strength and endurance.
- Identify leisure and community engagements that demand less energy consumption.

Intervention

- Identify activities that are most important to Aanya to accomplish each day at work, home, and in the community.
- Identify long-term goals and set priorities together; teach how to action plan short-term goals.
- Provide ergonomic education emphasizing self-analysis of activity, problem-solving, and practicing alternative methods to reduce joint stress. Practice each session.
- Explore alternative equipment to operate the interactive whiteboard to reduce shoulder movement (e.g., light pens); alternative mouse and keyboard designs; use voice-activated software to reduce keyboarding time.
- Explore adapted equipment for carrying heavy briefcase (e.g., wheeled briefcase, folding hand cart). Discuss use of online assessment with kids to reduce marking and getting books home.
- Explore using a stool with wheels around classroom to scoot between tables and reduce standing/bending.
- Discuss fatigue management, such as pacing activities and microbreaks. Discuss goals to practice and how to fit into routines.
- Review meal preparation activities, teach ergonomic methods, and review equipment available in shops to reduce wrist and MCP stress (e.g., easy jar, can openers, adapted cutlery with built-up handles such as Good Grip knives).
- Review driving such as padded steering wheel, and hand and arm positioning.
- Identify and fit appropriate right wrist splint, fit right compression glove. Explain wearing time of orthoses and purpose. Train in appropriate donning, doffing, and general care.
- Teach hand exercise program (ROM and strength): Practice and grade-up weekly.
- Review adaptive equipment/techniques to help with knitting and sewing.
- Recommend socialization by joining a book club (virtual or in-person).

Evidence Table of Intervention Studies for Arthritis

Intervention	Description	Participants	Dosage	Research Design and Evidence Level	Benefit	Statistical Significance and Effect Size
Ergonomics (i.e., joint protection [JP]) for adults with RA[56]	Standard arthritis education program versus a JP program using educational, behavioral, motor learning, and self-efficacy–enhancing strategies	$n = 65$ (JP); $n = 62$ (standard) programs; RA: Mean age: 50 years; 30 men, 97 women	Both study and control groups received 8 hours of intervention (4×2-hour weekly meetings). Study group received JP training in addition to the information that control group received on RA, exercise, pain, and foot care.	Randomized controlled trial (RCT) Level I	Four years post-treatment, JP group continued to have better ADL scores and JP adherence than control group.	Study group significantly improved in ADL ($p = 0.04$, effect size, $r = 0.15$), early morning stiffness ($p = 0.01$), and behavioral assessment ($p = 0.001$, $r = 0.27$) and fewer hand deformities: MCP ($p = 0.02$) and wrist joints ($p = 0.04$) in study group.
Wrist splints to support the wrist to permit functional use of the hand in adults with RA during daily activities[57]	Review of the effect of wrist splints on reducing pain, increase strength and dexterity, and in functional activities for adults with RA	Twenty-three studies from 1981 to 2009 were reviewed: with total sample 1,492 participants.	Wide variety of splints and variable disease duration lead to diverse splint wearing regimen. Use of splint was task specific, for example, greater use of splints in heavy tasks such as vacuuming.	Mixed-methods systematic review Level I	Working wrist splints reduced pain and improved grip in RA, but effect on function was unclear.	Strong quantitative evidence (including nine RCTs) supported by conclusions from two qualitative studies indicates that working wrist splints reduce pain ($d = 0.7$–0.8), moderately improve grip strength ($d = 0.3$–0.4), and decrease dexterity.
Assess the benefits and harms of exercise for people with hand OA to reduce pain, increase grip and pinch strength, increase dexterity, maintain joint stability and ROM[58]	Comparison of RCTs with and without exercise. Intervention content varied widely in content (i.e., type of exercises, adding lower and upper arm exercises), mode (i.e., group-based or home-based or both).	Pooled analyses of data from five trials ($n = 381$). Majority of participants are females: 66%–100% Mean age most frequently 60–65 years.	Dosage varied from three times daily to three times a week, and supervision ranged from full supervision of all sessions to all home based.	Meta-analysis Level I	Low-quality evidence that exercise improves hand pain, function, joint stiffness, and grip strength. Uncertain on changes in pinch strength, quality of life, adverse events between groups	Hand pain: Standardized mean difference (SMD): −0.27 (95% confidence interval [CI]: 0.47–0.07) Hand function: SMD: −0.28 (95% CI: 0.58–0.02) Stiffness: SMD: −0.36 (CI: −0.58 to −0.15) Grip strength: SMD: 0.34 (CI −0.01 to 0.69) Pinch strength: SMD: 0.20 (CI: −0.10 to 0.49)
Effect of assistive technology (AT) in people with hand OA[59]	Study group received informational materials and AT (splints and assistive devices). Control group received informational materials on hand OA, hand exercises, ergonomic suggestions.	Seventy participants: ($n = 35$) group, $n = 4$ (didn't complete all assessments). Mean age = −60.5 years 97% females	Total number of splints were 39 (8 right hand, 5 left hand, and 13 bilateral) and total devices of 347 (median = 11, range 1–17) were given.	Observer-blinded, RCT Level I	AT was well tolerated and used (92%) and significantly improved activity performance and satisfaction with performance.	*COPM Performance* Mean difference (MD) = 1.8 (95% CI: 1.1–2.6) *COPM satisfaction* MD = 1.7 (CI: 0.7–2.6), moderate-to-large treatment effect (effect size of 0.9)

References

1. Arthritis Foundation. *Arthritis by the Numbers*. https://www.arthritis.org/Documents/Sections/About-Arthritis/arthritis-facts-stats-figures.pdf. Accessed November 2, 2018.
2. Gibofsky A. Epidemiology, pathophysiology, and diagnosis of rheumatoid arthritis: a synopsis. *Am J Manag Care*. 2014;20(7 Suppl):S128–S135. http://www.ncbi.nlm.nih.gov/pubmed/25180621. Accessed November 8, 2018.
3. Hill J. *Rheumatology Nursing: A Creative Approach*. John Wiley & Sons; 2006. https://www.wiley.com/en-us/Rheumatology+Nursing%3A+A+Creative+Approach%2C+2nd+Edition-p-9780470019610. Accessed November 9, 2018.
4. Eberhardt KB, Rydgren LC, Pettersson H, Wollheim FA. Early rheumatoid arthritis—onset, course, and outcome over 2 years. *Rheumatol Int*. 1990;10(4):135–142. doi:10.1007/BF02274837.
5. Adams J, Burridge J, Mullee M, Hammond A, Cooper C. The clinical effectiveness of static resting splints in early rheumatoid arthritis: a randomized controlled trial. *Rheumatology*. 2008;47(10):1548–1553. doi:10.1093/rheumatology/ken292.
6. Singh JA, Saag KG, Bridges SL Jr, et al. 2015 American College of Rheumatology guideline for the treatment of rheumatoid arthritis. *Arthritis Care Res (Hoboken)*. 2016;68(1):1–25. doi:10.1002/acr.22783.
7. Combe B, Landewe R, Daien CI, et al. 2016 update of the EULAR recommendations for the management of early arthritis. *Ann Rheum Dis*. 2017;76(6):948–959. doi:10.1136/annrheumdis-2016-210602.
8. Riches PL, Elherik FK, Dolan S, Unglaub F, Breusch SJ. Patient rated outcomes study into the surgical interventions available for the rheumatoid hand and wrist. *Arch Orthop Trauma Surg*. 2016;136(4):563–570. doi:10.1007/s00402-016-2412-1.
9. Hammond A. What is the role of the occupational therapist? *Best Pract Res Clin Rheumatol*. 2004;18(4):491–505. doi:10.1016/J.BERH.2004.04.001.
10. Barbour KE, Helmick CG, Boring M, Brady TJ. Vital signs: prevalence of doctor-diagnosed arthritis and arthritis-attributable activity limitation—United States, 2013–2015. *MMWR Morb Mortal Wkly Rep*. 2017;66(9):246–253. doi:10.15585/mmwr.mm6609e1.
11. Qin J, Barbour KE, Murphy LB, et al. Lifetime risk of symptomatic hand osteoarthritis: the Johnston County osteoarthritis project. *Arthritis Rheumatol*. 2017;69(6):1204–1212. doi:10.1002/art.40097.
12. Beasley J. Osteoarthritis and rheumatoid arthritis: conservative therapeutic management. *J Hand Ther*. 2012;25(2):163–172. doi:10.1016/J.JHT.2011.11.001.
13. National Collaborating Centre for Chronic Conditions (UK). *Rheumatoid Arthritis: National Clinical Guideline for Management and Treatment in Adults*. London: Royal College of Physicians (UK); 2009. http://www.ncbi.nlm.nih.gov/pubmed/21413195. Accessed November 6, 2018.
14. National Clinical Guideline Centre (UK). *Osteoarthritis*. London: National Institute for Health and Care Excellence (UK); 2014. http://www.ncbi.nlm.nih.gov/pubmed/25340227. Accessed November 10, 2018.
15. Kloppenburg M. Hand osteoarthritis—nonpharmacological and pharmacological treatments. *Nat Rev Rheumatol*. 2014;10(4):242–251. doi:10.1038/nrrheum.2013.214.
16. Katz JN, Earp BE, Gomoll AH. Surgical management of osteoarthritis. *Arthritis Care Res (Hoboken)*. 2010;62(9):1220–1228. doi:10.1002/acr.20231.
17. Kjeken I, Dagfinrud H, Slatkowsky-Christensen B, et al. Activity limitations and participation restrictions in women with hand osteoarthritis: patients' descriptions and associations between dimensions of functioning. *Ann Rheum Dis*. 2005;64(11):1633–1638. doi:10.1136/ard.2004.034900.
18. Neogi T. The epidemiology and impact of pain in osteoarthritis. *Osteoarthr Cartil*. 2013;21(9):1145–1153. doi:10.1016/j.joca.2013.03.018.
19. CDC. Osteoarthritis (OA). https://www.cdc.gov/arthritis/basics/osteoarthritis.htm. Accessed November 10, 2018.
20. Carswell A, McColl MA, Baptiste S, Law M, Polatajko H, Pollock N. The Canadian Occupational Performance Measure: a research and clinical literature review. *Can J Occup Ther*. 2004;71(4):210–222. doi:10.1177/000841740407100406.
21. Matcham F, Gullick NJ, Hotopf M. The prevalence of depression and anxiety in a cross-section of rheumatological conditions. *Arthritis Rheumatol*. 2015. doi:10.1002/art.39448.
22. National Institute of Environmental Health Sciences. *The Health Assessment Questionnaire (HAQ) Disability Index (DI) of the Clinical Health Assessment Questionnaire (Version 96.4)*. https://www.niehs.nih.gov/research/resources/assets/docs/haq_instructions_508.pdf. Accessed November 21, 2018.
23. Katz PP, Radvanski DC, Allen D, et al. Development and validation of a short form of the valued life activities disability questionnaire for rheumatoid arthritis. *Arthritis Care Res (Hoboken)*. 2011;63(12):1664–1671. doi:10.1002/acr.20617.
24. Prior Y, Tennant A, Tyson S, Kjeken I, Hammond A. Measure of activity performance of the hand (MAP-Hand) questionnaire: linguistic validation, cultural adaptation and psychometric testing in people with rheumatoid arthritis in the UK. *BMC Musculoskelet Disord*. 2018;19(1):275. doi:10.1186/s12891-018-2177-5.
25. School of Rehabilitation Science at McMaster University. *The Patient-Rated Wrist Evaluation (PRWE) User Manual*. 2011. https://srs-mcmaster.ca/wp-content/uploads/2015/05/English-PRWE-User-Manual.pdf. Accessed November 21, 2018.
26. Shauver MJ, Chung KC. The Michigan hand outcomes questionnaire after 15 years of field trial. *Plast Reconstr Surg*. 2013;131(5):779e–787e. doi:10.1097/PRS.0b013e3182865d83.
27. Waljee JF, Kim HM, Burns PB, Chung KC. Development of a brief, 12-item version of the Michigan Hand Questionnaire. *Plast Reconstr Surg*. 2011;128(1):208–220. doi:10.1097/PRS.0b013e318218fc51
28. Hammond A, Tennant A, Tyson S, Nordenskiold U. *Evaluation of Daily Activity Questionnaire: User Manual v1 The Evaluation of Daily Activity Questionnaire (EDAQ) User Manual: Version 1*. 2014. https://core.ac.uk/download/pdf/19725860.pdf. Accessed November 21, 2018.

29. Meenan RF, Mason JH, Anderson JJ, Guccione AA, Kazis LE. Arthritis impact measurement scales—2. *Arthritis Rheum (Arthritis Care Res)*. 1992. doi:10.1037/t04214-000.
30. Plant MJ, Linton S, Dodd E, Jones PW, Dawes PT. The GALS locomotor screen and disability. *Ann Rheum Dis*. 1993;52(12):886–890. doi:10.1136/ard.52.12.886.
31. Prevoo MLL, Van'T Hof MA, Kuper HH, Van Leeuwen MA, Van De Putte LBA, Van Riel PLCM. Modified disease activity scores that include twenty-eight-joint counts development and validation in a prospective longitudinal study of patients with rheumatoid arthritis. *Arthritis Rheum*. 1995;38(1):44–48. doi:10.1002/art.1780380107.
32. Crosby CA, Wehbé MA. Hand strength: normative values. *J Hand Surg Am*. 1994;19(4):665–670. doi:10.1016/0363-5023(94)90280-1.
33. Dellhag B, Bjelle A. A Grip Ability Test for use in rheumatology practice. *J Rheumatol*. 1995;22(8):1559–1565.
34. van Lankveld W, van't Pad Bosch P, Bakker J, Terwindt S, Franssen M, van Riel P. Sequential occupational dexterity assessment (SODA): a new test to measure hand disability. *J Hand Ther*. 1996;9(1):27–32. doi:10.1016/S0894-1130(96)80008-1.
35. Feys P, Lamers I, Francis G, et al. The Nine-Hole Peg Test as a manual dexterity performance measure for multiple sclerosis. *Mult Scler*. 2017;23(5):711–720. doi:10.1177/1352458517690824.
36. Allaire S, Keysor JJ. Development of a structured interview tool to help patients identify and solve rheumatic condition-related work barriers. *Arthritis Rheum*. 2009;61(7):988–995. doi:10.1002/art.24610.
37. Lohss I, Forsyth K, Kottorp A. Psychometric properties of the worker role interview (Version 10.0) in mental health. *Br J Occup Ther*. 2012;75(4). doi:10.4276/03080 2212X13336366278095.
38. Gilworth G, Smyth MG, Smith J, Tennant A. The manual work instability scale: development and validation. *Occup Med*. 2016;66:300–304. doi:10.1093/occmed/kqv217.
39. Backman CL, Village J, Lacaille D. The ergonomic assessment tool for arthritis: development and pilot testing. *Arthritis Rheum*. 2008;59(10):1495–1503. doi:10.1002/art.24116.
40. Bieniek S, Bethge M. The reliability of workwell systems functional capacity evaluation: a systematic review. *BMC Musculoskelet Disord*. 2014;15:106. doi:10.1186/1471-2474-15-106.
41. Casimiro L, Brosseau L, Robinson V, et al. Therapeutic ultrasound for the treatment of rheumatoid arthritis. *Cochrane Database Syst Rev*. 2002;(3):CD003787. doi:10.1002/14651858.CD003787.
42. Loyola-Sánchez A, Richardson J, MacIntyre NJ. Efficacy of ultrasound therapy for the management of knee osteoarthritis: a systematic review with meta-analysis. *Osteoarthr Cartil*. 2010;18(9):1117–1126. doi:10.1016/J.JOCA.2010.06.010.
43. Brosseau L, Welch V, Wells G, et al. Low level laser therapy for osteoarthritis and rheumatoid arthritis: a metaanalysis. *J Rheumatol*. 2000;27(8):1961–1969. http://www.ncbi.nlm.nih.gov/pubmed/10955339. Accessed November 16, 2018.
44. Breger Stanton DE, Lazaro R, MacDermid JC. A systematic review of the effectiveness of contrast baths. *J Hand Ther*. 2009;22(1):57–70. doi:10.1016/j.jht.2008.08.001.
45. Szczegielniak J, Łuniewski J, Bogacz K, Sliwiński Z. The use of kinesiology taping method in patients with rheumatoid hand—pilot study. *Ortop Traumatol Rehabil*. 2012;14(1):23–30. http://www.ncbi.nlm.nih.gov/pubmed/22388357. Accessed November 16, 2018.
46. Kaya Mutlu E, Mustafaoglu R, Birinci T, Razak Ozdincler A. Does kinesio taping of the knee improve pain and functionality in patients with knee osteoarthritis? *Am J Phys Med Rehabil*. 2017;96(1):25–33. doi:10.1097/PHM.0000000000000520.
47. Goia DN, Fortulan CA, Purquerio BM, Elui VMC. A new concept of orthosis for correcting fingers ulnar deviation. *Res Biomed Eng*. 2017;33(1):50–57. doi:10.1590/2446-4740.02516.
48. Gomes CA, Jones A, Natour J. Assessment of the effectiveness of a functional splint for osteoarthritis of the trapeziometacarpal joint on the dominant hand: a randomized controlled study. *J Rehabil Med*. 2010;42(5):469–474. doi:10.2340/16501977-0542.
49. Verhoeven F, Tordi N, Prati C, Demougeot C, Mougin F, Wendling D. Physical activity in patients with rheumatoid arthritis. *Joint Bone Spine*. 2016;83(3):265–270. doi:10.1016/J.JBSPIN.2015.10.002.
50. Hurkmans E, van der Giesen FJ, Vliet Vlieland TP, Schoones J, Van den Ende EC. Dynamic exercise programs (aerobic capacity and/or muscle strength training) in patients with rheumatoid arthritis. *Cochrane Database Syst Rev*. 2009;(4):CD006853. doi:10.1002/14651858.CD006853.pub2.
51. Bartels EM, Lund H, Hagen KB, et al. Aquatic exercise for the treatment of knee and hip osteoarthritis. *Cochrane Database Syst Rev*. 2007;(4):CD005523.. doi:10.1002/14651858.CD005523.pub2
52. Lamb SE, Williamson EM, Heine PJ, et al. Exercises to improve function of the rheumatoid hand (SARAH): a randomised controlled trial. *Lancet*. 2015;385(9966):421–429. doi:10.1016/S0140-6736(14)60998-3.
53. Valdes K, Marik T. A systematic review of conservative interventions for osteoarthritis of the hand. *J Hand Ther*. 2010;23(4):334–351. doi:10.1016/J.JHT.2010.05.001.
54. Macedo AM, Oakley SP, Panayi GS, Kirkham BW. Functional and work outcomes improve in patients with rheumatoid arthritis who receive targeted, comprehensive occupational therapy. *Arthritis Rheum*. 2009;61(11):1522–1530. doi:10.1002/art.24563.
55. Niedermann K, Hammond A, Forster A, de Bie R. Perceived benefits and barriers to joint protection among people with rheumatoid arthritis and occupational therapists. A mixed methods study. *Musculoskeletal Care*. 2010;8(3):143–156. doi:10.1002/msc.177.
56. Hammond A, Freeman K. The long-term outcomes from a randomized controlled trial of an educational–behavioural joint protection programme for people with rheumatoid arthritis. *Clin Rehabil*. 2004;18(5):520–528. doi:10.1191/0269215504cr766oa.
57. Ramsey L, Winder R, McVeigh J. The effectiveness of working wrist splints in adults with rheumatoid arthritis: a mixed methods systematic review. *J Rehabil Med*. 2014;46(6):481–492. doi:10.2340/16501977-1804.
58. Østerås N, Kjeken I, Smedslund G, et al. Exercise for hand osteoarthritis: a Cochrane systematic review. *J Rheumatol*. 2017;44(12):1850–1858. doi:10.3899/jrheum.170424.
59. Kjeken I, Darre S, Smedslund G, Hagen KB, Nossum R. Effect of assistive technology in hand osteoarthritis: a randomised controlled trial. *Ann Rheum Dis*. 2011;70(8):1447–1452. doi:10.1136/ard.2010.148668.

Chapter 43

Hand Impairments

Debbie Amini

LEARNING OBJECTIVES

This chapter will allow the reader to:

1. Describe clinical features of common hand diagnoses.
2. Describe impact of hand impairments on occupational participation.
3. Identify elements of a client-centered and occupation-based evaluation of the hand.
4. Identify outcome measures used to identify goals of occupational therapy intervention.
5. Discuss assessment tools used to determine the status of client factors and performance skills impacting occupational performance.
6. Identify intervention approaches and techniques to enhance occupational participation of persons with hand impairment.
7. Recognize the impact of various interventions on client factors and performance skills affected by hand conditions.
8. Identify orthotics that can be applied to the wrist and digits to minimize, prevent, or correct hand deformity.
9. Explain the importance of occupation-centered intervention goals.
10. Discuss the evidence for occupational therapy interventions for hand impairments.

CHAPTER OUTLINE

TERMINOLOGY

Claw deformity: finger position of MP hyperextension and proximal interphalangeal (PIP) flexion associated with muscle imbalance in ulnar-innervated structures; also called *clawing.*

Contracture: lack of passive motion caused by tissue shortening.

Counterforce strap: support used over flexor or extensor muscle wads to support muscles and prevent maximum muscle contraction, decreasing load on the tendon; often used to reduce symptoms of lateral or medial epicondylitis.

End feel: quality of joint motion at end range when moved passively; can be hard, firm, or soft.

Extensor lag: inability to extend a joint actively when passive movement is available.

Froment sign: a symptom of ulnar nerve impairment in which a forceful lateral pinch elicits thumb IP flexion because of weakness of the adductor pollicis.

Intrinsic tightness: decreased IP flexion with MP extension as a result of imbalance in the extensor systems of the digits because of shortening of the lumbricals and interosseous muscles.

Joint traction: a treatment technique in which the ends of the bones that create the joint are gently pulled apart from each other to allow the bone ends within the joint to glide over each other.

Neuroma: disorganized mass of nerve fibers that can occur following nerve injury and may create significant nerve pain with associated hypersensitivity.

Wartenberg sign: a symptom of ulnar nerve impairment in which a client is unable to adduct the small finger with hand palm down on the table.

Description of Common Hand Diagnoses

Human hands function elegantly; they gesture and express, touch and care, and dress and feed. Conditions of the hand, which may be cosmetic or functional or both, can greatly affect the ability of clients to successfully participate in desired occupations. The purpose of this chapter is to introduce readers to the elements of hand rehabilitation, including knowledge of common diagnoses and basic techniques used in the clinical setting.

Tissue Healing

Scar tissue, a natural consequence of the tissue healing process, is a common focus of all hand rehabilitation intervention. Owing to the close proximity of the anatomical structures within the hand as well as their highly mobile nature, the impact of scar can be catastrophic when it creates blockages to movement in the form of adhesions, changes in density, alignment, and shape of surrounding soft tissue that change or block movement patterns and shift angles and lines of pull.

Tissue heals in the following phases: inflammation, fibroplasia, and maturation or remodeling. The inflammation phase lasts several days. It includes vasoconstriction followed by vasodilation, with white blood cell migration to promote phagocytic removal of foreign bodies and dead tissue. Depending on the diagnosis, rest is often recommended during the inflammation phase.

The fibroplasia phase starts at approximately day 4 and continues for 2 to 6 weeks. In this phase, fibroblasts synthesize scar tissue. The wound's tensile strength increases gradually with the increase in collagen fibers. At this time, active range of motion (AROM) and orthotics may be appropriate to protect healing tissues and promote balance in the hand.[1]

The maturation, or remodeling, phase may last for years, but tissue is usually more responsive early rather than late in this period. The remodeling phase reflects the changing architecture and improved organization of collagen fibers and the associated increased tensile strength. Although gentle resistive activity may be appropriate during maturation, its use should be monitored because it may also generate an inflammatory response leading to increased scar formation; gentle application of corrective dynamic or static orthoses may also be appropriate.[2]

Tolerance of tissues to controlled stress requires monitoring throughout all phases of intervention. As tissue continues to heal, the wound contracts, and the scar shrinks. Collagen continues to remodel because it is constantly doing in uninjured tissue.

Any upper extremity injury can result in the serious and sometimes irreversible problem of a function-limiting hand stiffness. Edema, the body's natural response to trauma, is the main culprit in the series of events, leading to a stiff hand. Crushing injuries that create diffuse edema and a significant inflammatory response are one example of a precipitating injury for a still hand. However, even an injury in the proximal upper extremity can cause serious stiffening of the digits when edema persists, scar is present, and the extremity is not mobile. The challenge for occupational therapy is to strike a balance between rest and movement. Too much rest may increase or maintain edema and allow for adhesion formation and the development of joint **contractures**. Too much movement may increase the inflammation and lead to more scar formation. The right amount of rest in an appropriate position reduces inflammation and promotes healing. Proximal motion plus well-tolerated functional use, particularly while elevated, help to reduce edema and restore motion. Various surgical interventions may be indicated to reduce stiffness of the hand and may include open or closed joint capsule or ligament release, scar removal, and tendon lengthening or release.[3]

Tendinopathy

Tendons are extensions of muscles made up of poorly vascularized connective tissues that primarily connect to bone to create changes in joint angle for function. Tendinopathy is a general term for conditions of tendons known as tendonitis or tendinosis. These conditions can occur anywhere along the length of the tendon and have varied pathophysiology ranging from overuse to inflammatory pathology due to systemic disorders such as rheumatoid arthritis (RA) or diabetes mellitus

(DM) among others, which result in tendon adhesions or thickening. Histological findings in the sheath associated with these underlying conditions include collagen breakdown, over vascularization, and fibrocartilage metaplasia, resulting from compression and shear during tendon gliding.[4]

Tendinosis refers to chronic degenerative changes in the tendon in which there is an absence of inflammatory cells. Prolonged repetitive stress of conditions such as stenosing tenosynovitis put mechanical strain on the tendon, causing micro ruptures. Because of a lack of a robust intrinsic blood supply and uneven strain, the healing and remodeling responses are altered.[4] Because the pathology is not primarily inflammatory, treatment approaches for this type of tendinopathy emphasize interventions that restore nourishment to collagen.[5]

The pain associated with tendinitis/tendinosis can be severe and can seriously impact performance in all areas of occupation. Biomechanical deficits include muscular weakness, inflexibility, and scar tissue; symptoms include pain with AROM, with resistance, and with passive stretch of the involved structures. Several specific tendon conditions are described in the subsequent sections.

Lateral Epicondylitis (Tennis Elbow)

Lateral epicondylitis involves the extrinsic extensors of the hand at their origin. The extensor carpi radialis brevis is most commonly involved. Pain is at the lateral epicondyle and extensor wad (the proximal portion of the extensor muscles) and can be at a level that significantly limits daily activity of the client (see Fig. 43-1). Pain is most pronounced with activities involving resisted wrist extension, but may be continuous and interfere with sleep. This diagnosis is differentiated clinically from radial tunnel syndrome, a painful nerve compression, in which tenderness occurs more distally over the radial tuberosity. Test for radial tunnel syndrome with the middle finger test (positive if there is pain secondary to resisting the middle finger proximal phalanx while the client maintains elbow extension, neutral wrist, and metacarpophalangeal [MP] extension) or by percussing distally to proximally over the superficial radial nerve. This percussion test is positive if it elicits paresthesia.[6]

Initial medical intervention may include a corticosteroid injection into the area surrounding the extensor muscle origins with surgical intervention reserved for unrelenting cases that have not responded to conservative approaches, including therapy, for 9 to 12 months.

Medial Epicondylitis (Golfer Elbow)

Medial epicondylitis involves the extrinsic flexors at their origin on the volar aspect of the medial elbow. The flexor carpi radialis (FCR) is most commonly involved. Pain is at the medial epicondyle and flexor wad (the proximal portion of the flexor muscles) and worsens with resisted flexion and pronation (see Fig. 43-2). Although not as common as lateral epicondylitis, medial epicondylitis can impede the ability of the client to engage in daily activities, particularly those involving resisted wrist flexion.

Medical intervention is same as for lateral epicondyle with corticosteroid injection and possible surgery for nonresponsive cases.

De Quervain Tenosynovitis

De Quervain tenosynovitis is tendinitis involving the abductor pollicis longus (APL) and extensor pollicis brevis (EPB) tendons at the first dorsal compartment of

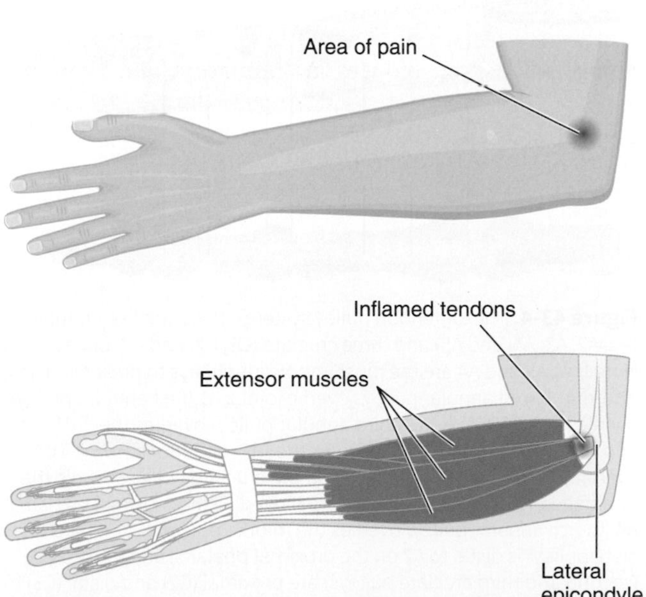

Figure 43-1. Lateral epicondylitis. (Shutterstock/Aksanaku.)

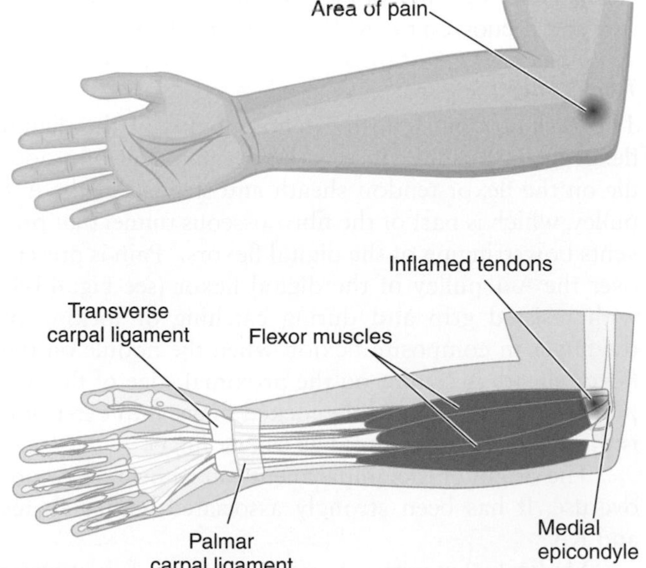

Figure 43-2. Medial epicondylitis. (Shutterstock/Aksanaku.)

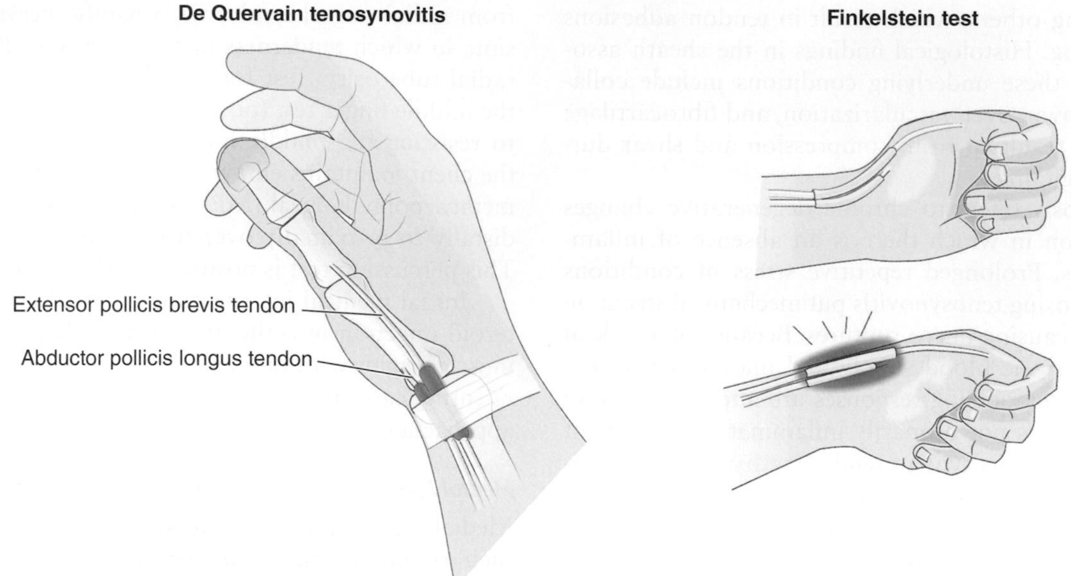

Figure 43-3. Finkelstein test for de Quervain disease. (Shutterstock/ellepigrafica.)

the wrist. It is the most common upper extremity tenosynovitis. Finkelstein test is positive if there is exquisite pain with passive wrist ulnar deviation while flexing the thumb (see Fig. 43-3). This diagnosis occurs frequently among golfers, knitters, new mothers, and racquet sports players. Thumb posture in sustained hyperabduction at the computer space bar or on a cellular phone may also cause or worsen de Quervain. Differential diagnosis is for carpometacarpal (CMC) arthritis, scaphoid fracture, intersection syndrome, and FCR tendinitis.[7]

Medical intervention typically involves the use of nonsteroidal anti-inflammatory drugs (NSAIDs) with possible corticosteroid injection into the first dorsal compartment. Cases that are nonresponsive to conservative methods, that also include immobilization and therapy, may require surgical release of the first dorsal compartment to relieve pressure and friction on the APL and EPB tendons.

Trigger Finger

Trigger finger or stenosing tenosynovitis of the digital flexor(s). The usual cause is the development of a nodule on the flexor tendon sheath and stenosis at the A-1 pulley, which is part of the fibro-osseous tunnel that prevents bowstringing of the digital flexors.[8] Pain is present over the A-1 pulley of the digital flexor (see Fig. 43-4) with resisted grip and during catching or locking of the finger in composite flexion when the nodule on the flexor sheath is caught on the proximal edge of the A-1 pully.[9] The snapping of the locked finger into extension is the "triggering," referred as trigger finger.

The origin of this impairment can be overuse or not overuse. It has been strongly associated with diabetes and RA.

Medical management often consists of a mixture of steroid and local anesthetic injected into the flexor sheath. If symptoms persist beyond conservative interventions, the surgeon may surgically release the A-1 pulley to stop the repeated inflammation caused by the triggering and reduce chance of recurrence. The nodule itself may or may not be removed and will eventually be reabsorbed once friction from the A-1 pulley is removed.

Nerve Injury

The terminal branches of the peripheral nervous system that innervate the upper extremity arise from the

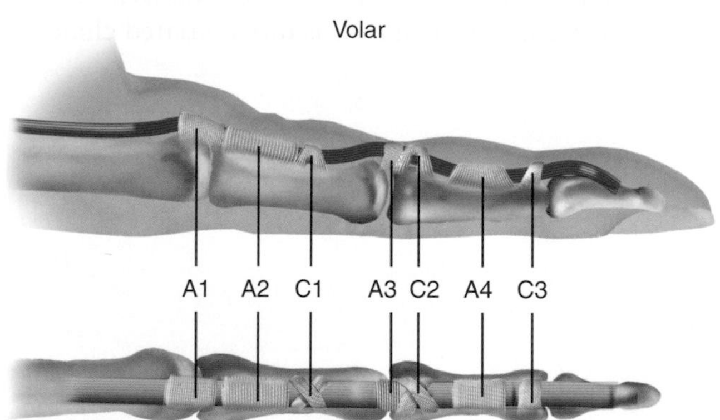

Figure 43-4. Flexor tendon pulley system—there are five annular (A1, A2, A3, A4, and A5) and three cruciate (C1, C2, and C3) pulleys. Note that A2 and A4 are the most important pulleys to preserve. The odd-numbered annular pulleys overlie joints: A1 (first annular pulley) overlies the MCP joint, A3 (third annular pulley) overlies the PIP joint, and A5 (fifth annular pulley) overlies the DIP joint (not shown). The even-numbered annular pulleys and the cruciate pulleys overlie the phalanges, A2 (second annular pulley) overlies the proximal phalanx, A4 (fourth annular pulley) overlies the middle phalanx, C1 (first cruciate pulley) is distal to A2 on the proximal phalanx, and C2 and C3 (second and third cruciate pulleys) are proximal (C2) and distal (C3) to the A4 pulley on the middle phalanx. DIP, distal interphalangeal; MP, metacarpophalangeal; PIP, proximal interphalangeal.

brachial plexus that originates from spinal segments C5 to T1. Several terminal nerves innervate the soft-tissue structures of the arm, but the major nerves responsible for movement and sensation of the forearm and hand are the median, ulnar, and radial nerves. The various mechanisms of nerve injury include acute or chronic compression, stretch ischemia, electrical shock, radiation, injection, and laceration.[10] When injury or disease occurs to a neural structure in the upper extremity, there is a high likelihood of the phenomenon known as double or multiple crush syndrome where damage to the physiology of one nerve impacts another.[11] All forms of nerve pathology can result in significant changes in sensory awareness, pain, and movement of the hand and arm, leading to significant impairments to functional performance.

Nerve Compression

Carpal Tunnel Syndrome

Carpal tunnel syndrome (CTS) is the most common upper extremity nerve entrapment. It results from compression of the median nerve within the carpal tunnel at the wrist. The carpal tunnel is formed by the carpal bones dorsally and the transverse carpal ligament (flexor retinaculum) volarly. The tunnel acts as a pulley for the nine long finger flexor tendons during gripping[12,13] (see Fig. 43-5). Because the space within the carpal tunnel is very small, swelling such as that seen in pregnancy or wrist fractures, or thickening of the tendons as seen in tendinopathy, can lead to circulation, compromising pressure on the nerve. The resulting ischemia results in sensory and, ultimately, motor dysfunction in the distribution of the median nerve.[14]

Typical complaints include hand numbness, particularly at night or when driving a car, along with pain and paresthesia in the distribution of the median nerve (thumb through radial ring finger pads), and clumsiness or weakness.[14] Medical intervention for CTS can include cortisone injection to reduce inflammation, provision of over-the-counter wrist orthosis, and surgery that includes cutting the transverse carpal ligament in two, thus reducing pressure on the nerve and tendons.[14]

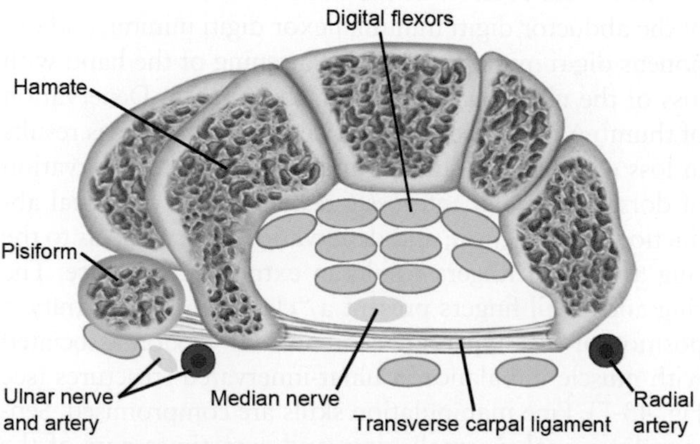

Figure 43-5. Carpal tunnel cross section.

Cubital Tunnel Syndrome

Cubital tunnel syndrome is the second most common upper extremity nerve entrapment and is the most commonly compressed site of the ulnar nerve, at its location between the medial epicondyle and the olecranon.[15] Typical complaints include proximal and medial forearm pain that is aching or sharp; decreased sensation of the dorsal and palmar surfaces of the small finger and the ulnar half of the ring finger; and weakness of interossei, adductor pollicis (AP), flexor carpi ulnaris (FCU), and flexor digitorum profundus (FDP) of the ring and small fingers. A **claw deformity** (*clawing*) may be more evident if the FDP is not involved because the long flexors are unopposed; **Wartenberg sign** and **Froment sign** may be seen. Grip and pinch strength are decreased, and clients complain of dropping things. Symptoms are worse when the elbow is flexed repeatedly or is held in flexion because this position dramatically reduces the volume of the cubital tunnel.[16] Understandably, symptoms may increase at night if the person sleeps with the elbow flexed.

Cubital tunnel syndrome may result from trauma, such as a blow to the elbow or fracture or dislocation of the supracondylar or medial epicondylar area, or it may be due to chronic mild pressure on the elbow. Associated diagnoses include osteoarthritis (OA), RA, diabetes, and Hansen disease. Medical intervention depends on the cause of the condition and typically involves cortisone injection to reduce swelling within the cubital tunnel or surrounding structures, surgical decompression of the cubital tunnel, and/or anterior relocation of the ulnar nerve superficially or under muscle tissue.[17]

Posterior Interosseous Nerve Syndrome

Posterior interosseous nerve syndrome (PINS) is purely motor. It presents two clinical pictures. In one, paralysis affects all muscles innervated by the posterior interosseous nerve, with inability to extend the MP joints of the thumb, index, long, ring, or small fingers. Wrist extension occurs only radially because of paralysis of extensor digitorum and extensor carpi ulnaris (ECU). In the other presentation of this syndrome, the person cannot extend the MP joint of one or more digits. Paralysis may spread to other digits if it is not treated on a timely basis.[18]

A common site of entrapment of the posterior interosseous nerve is at the supinator muscle, where it pierces the two heads of this muscle. Other causes include soft-tissue tumors, RA with synovial proliferation, and radial head fractures or dislocations. Therapy focuses on maintaining passive range of motion (PROM) and orthotic selection to prevent deformity and promote function. Medical intervention for PINS that is not managed with conservative techniques involves surgical decompression of the nerve.

Compression of the radial nerve more proximally can lead to "Saturday night palsy," which is an ischemic event caused with sustained reduction of the blood supply to the nerve at the level of the humerus and is seen when a person sleeps on his or her arm without movement or uses axillary crutches incorrectly.

Nerve Laceration

Peripheral nerves, unlike tendons, are vascular, have an internal metabolism, and must regenerate after significant injury or laceration. A tendon is more similar to a rope, in that if cut in two, it can be repaired and return to its primary function of moving joints within several weeks. However, when a nerve is cut, the portion distal to the laceration will die and eventually be reabsorbed by the body; the tunnel that houses it will atrophy and limit any potential for spontaneous reinnervation. To offer any potential for reinnervation, the distal portion of a severed nerve must be reattached to the proximal portion that contains the nucleus in as close to perfect alignment as possible. The desired outcome is for the axons to regrow into the existing nerve tunnels in hopes that they will reach the terminal end plates that are sensory or motor in nature.[19]

Nerve lacerations are categorized as complete or partial. Stretching and contusion injuries can occur along with the laceration. Nerve reconstruction is termed primary if within 48 hours, early secondary if within 6 weeks, and late secondary after 3 months. Nerve repairs have a better prognosis for recovery if they are repaired sooner and are located more distally. Axonal regeneration for a more proximal laceration places a great deal of stress on the nerve cell that may not be able to nourish full regrowth. After an initial period of proximal axonal degeneration from the trauma of the laceration, axons can regenerate at the rate of up to 3 mm per month.[19]

On occasion, a **neuroma** can develop along the nerve or at that anastomosis that causes significant pain when touched. Impaired functional use of the hand caused by the hypersensitivity of this nerve scar can be reduced with padding to protect the painful area or through surgical removal. Occupation dysfunction of varying degrees will occur as a result of nerve lacerations because of motor impairment and/or sensory impairment.

Median Nerve Lesions

Median nerve laceration at the wrist results in low median nerve palsy, with denervation of the opponens pollicis and abductor pollicis brevis of the thumb and of the lumbricals to the index and long fingers. Clawing of the index and long fingers does not usually occur because the interossei remain ulnarly innervated. Loss of sensation of the radial side of the hand is present. With the absence of thumb abduction and opposition, the thumb rests in adduction, where it may become contracted (see Fig. 43-6). Median nerve laceration creates serious functional loss of manipulation and sensibility of the thumb, index, and long fingers and leads to an "ape hand" deformity. Motor recovery usually occurs before sensory recovery.

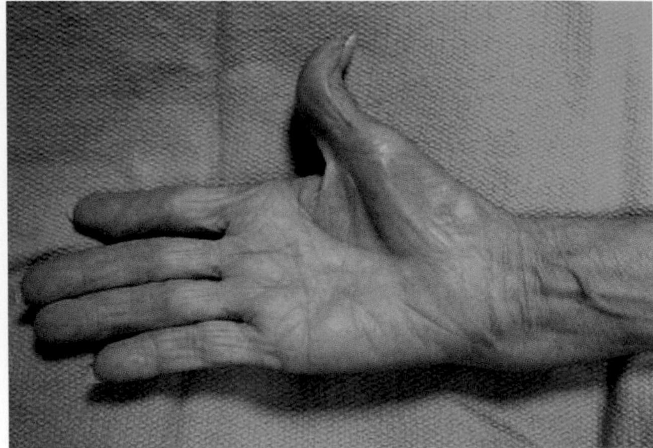

Figure 43-6. Thenar wasting (atrophy of thumb muscles) due to median nerve injury.

Injury near or at the elbow is called a high median nerve injury. Along with the motor loss identified earlier, there is denervation of FDP to the index and long fingers, flexor digitorum superficialis (FDS) to all digits, pronator teres, and pronator quadratus. The median nerve is considered the most important sensory nerve, and its loss severely compromises hand function. In therapy, prepare clients for probable tendon transfers by preventing deformity with orthotics and by maintaining PROM of pronation, digital MPs in flexion, digital IPs in extension, and thumb CMC abduction. Visual cues, adaptive devices, and modified handles may help compensate for the functional loss.

Ulnar Nerve Lesions

Laceration of the ulnar nerve at the wrist, a low ulnar lesion, results in loss of most of the hand intrinsics. Denervation of the abductor digiti minimi, flexor digiti minimi, and opponens digiti minimi results in flattening of the hand with loss of the ulnar transverse metacarpal arch. Denervation of thumb AP and deep head of flexor pollicis brevis results in loss of thumb adduction and MP support; denervation of dorsal and volar interossei results in loss of digital abduction or adduction; and denervation of lumbricals to the ring and small fingers results in extrinsic imbalance. The ring and small fingers present a "claw hand" deformity, a position of MP hyperextension and PIP flexion associated with muscle imbalance in ulnar-innervated structures (see Fig. 43-7). Fine manipulation skills are compromised. Sensory loss involves small, ring, and sometimes part of the long finger, known as the ulnar digits.

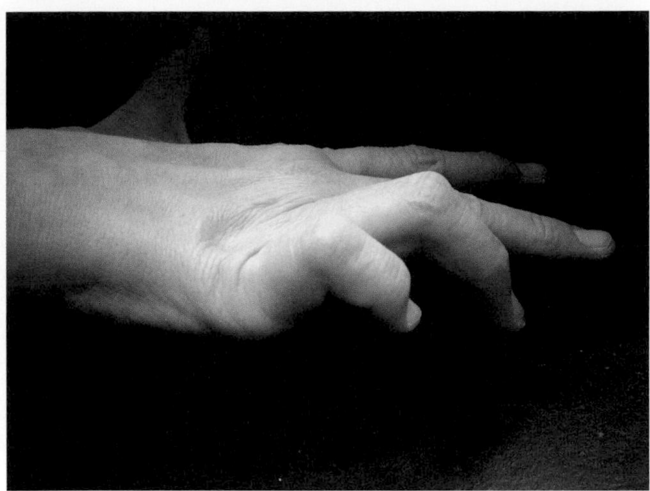

Figure 43-7. Clawing of digits due to ulnar nerve injury.

A high ulnar nerve lesion is often identified with trauma at or proximal to the elbow. There is involvement of the muscles listed earlier and denervation of FDP of the ring and small fingers and of FCU. Ring and small finger clawing is less apparent with the high lesion but becomes noticeable as the FDP are reinnervated and are unopposed by the still-absent intrinsics.

Radial Nerve Lesions

Low radial nerve injury of the deep motor branch is called posterior interosseous palsy. Presentations vary, but brachioradialis and extensor carpi radialis longus function are usually present. Efforts to actively extend the wrist yield strong radial deviation; MP extension is affected. Sensation on the dorsal radial hand is affected, although this may not significantly impact function as a result of the overlapping sensory input of the median nerve.

A high radial nerve injury commonly occurs with humeral fractures because this nerve spirals around the humerus. Damage to the radial nerve in this area leads to absent wrist and digital extensors and a "wrist drop" deformity (see Fig. 43-8). Sensory loss occurs on the dorsal–radial hand, which interferes less with function than does sensory loss on the palmar hand. Triceps function remains, but the supinator and all wrist and finger extensors lose function. Tenodesis, or the passive mechanical flexion of the MCPs and IP joints with active wrist extension, is lost as is the ability to stabilize the wrist in extension while using the digits for function.[19] **Intrinsic tightness** can occur, leading to difficulty with MP extension and IP flexion if length of interosseous and lumbrical muscles are not maintained during the period of lost extrinsic extension.

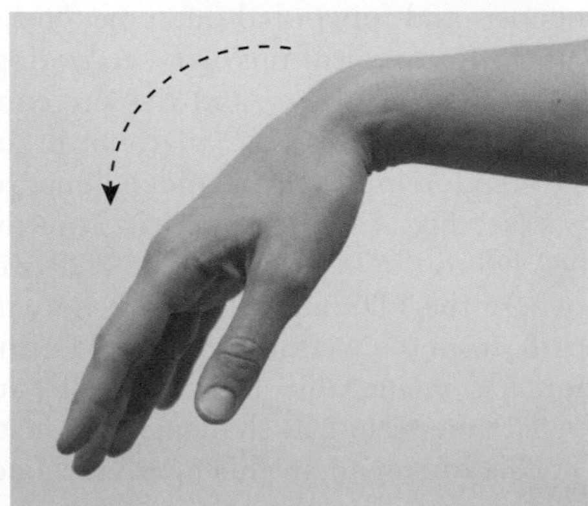

Figure 43-8. Wrist drop due to radial nerve injury.

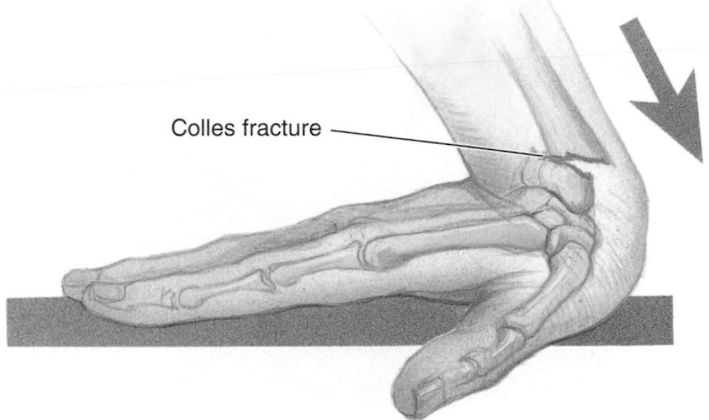

Figure 43-9. Colles fracture; dinner-fork deformity.

Fractures

Distal Radius Fracture

Distal radius fractures (distal radioulnar joint [DRUJ] fractures or wrist fractures) are among the most common upper extremity fractures.[20,21] DRUJ fractures are often caused by a fall on an outstretched or extended hand and are known as Colles fracture if the fracture has dorsal displacement leading to a dinner-fork deformity (see Figs. 43-9 and 43-10), or Smith fracture if the wrist was flexed at the time of injury and has a volar displacement leading to a garden-spade deformity (see Fig. 43-11). Medical management will depend on the severity and type of the fracture. Considerations include fragmentation, angulation, open fracture, concurrent ulnar fracture, and compression

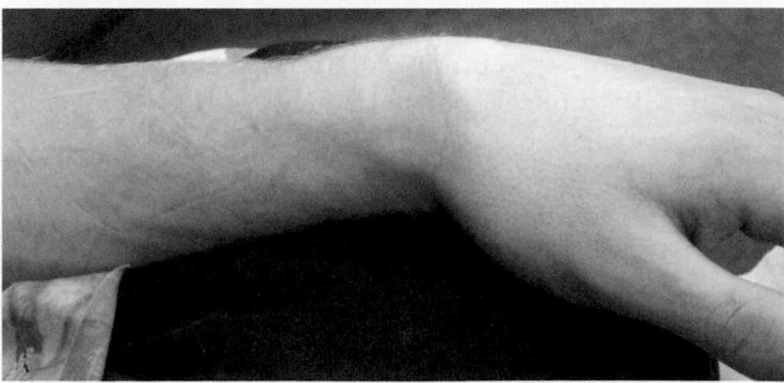

Figure 43-10. Dinner-fork deformity.

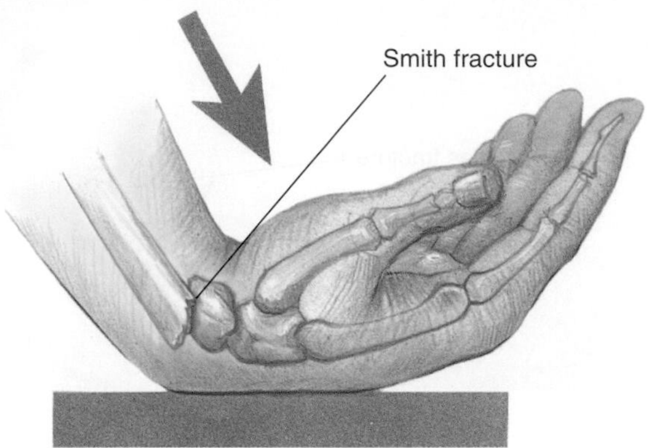

Figure 43-11. Smith fracture; garden-spade deformity.

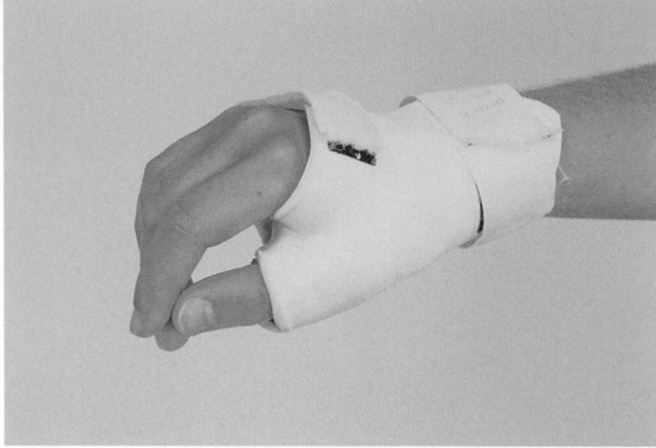

Figure 43-12. Hand-based thumb MP orthosis to immobilize grade I or II Skier thumb injury. MP, metacarpophalangeal.

of the distal fragment into the proximal bone. Plaster splints followed by circumferential casting with closed reduction (setting) of the bone, surgical open reduction, and internal fixation and closed reduction with percutaneous pinning are options for fixing and immobilizing DRUJ fractures. The main complication associated with distal radius fracture is traumatic arthritis caused by malunion or poor alignment of the distal portion of the bone when healing. Decreased wrist ROM, decreased grip strength, alteration of the carpal alignment, and instability may ensue. Other complications include extrinsic tightness, tendon rupture, compression of the median or ulnar nerve, and complex regional pain syndrome (CRPS).[22]

Ligament Injury

Ligament injuries are also known as strains and sprains. Their severity, which may be underappreciated, is described as grade I through grade III. In grade I, the ligament remains intact, but there is diffuse individual fiber disruption. In grade II, there is complete disruption of one of the joint capsule's major retaining ligaments. In grade III, there is complete disruption of one collateral ligament in addition to injury to dorsal and/or volar capsular structures. Pain, decreased ROM, and risk of flexion contracture are the most common problems associated with grades I and II injuries. Joint instability may occur with grade III injuries.[23]

Skier's Thumb

Disruption of the ulnar collateral ligament of the thumb MP joint occurs with acute radial deviation. This diagnosis, which may entail avulsion of bone fragment at the ligamentous insertion, is often seen among people who fall while skiing. Injury to the radial collateral ligament of the thumb MP occurs only one-tenth as often.[24] Grade III ulnar collateral ligament injuries require surgical repair with interosseous wire because an avulsed ligament will retract and not return to the original insertion on the bone, leaving joint instability (see Fig. 43-12).

Tendon Injury

The flexors and extensors of the fingers are relatively superficial and susceptible to lacerations, avulsions, and rupture. The finger tendons most at risk for damage are the extrinsic—so named because their muscle bellies are located outside the hand. The lack of large bulky muscle in the hand itself allows the fingers to complete precision movements and fine motor tasks. However, to accomplish fine movements so far from their origin, the tendons must glide over several joints through a tendon sheath and work in balance with each other and the small intrinsic muscle group within the hand. Injuries to the tendon are some of the most complex hand injuries resulting from their limited vascularity and the significant impact that scar tissue will have on their mobility.[25]

Flexor Tendon Injury

Surgical repair of flexor tendon injury is a complex undertaking performed by specialists in the field. Multiple structures are potentially involved including more than one tendon (FDP and FDS), the pulley system, digital arteries, and, possibly, digital nerves that can affect prognosis and functional outcome.[26] Many precautions and contraindications vary according to the details of the client's surgery and the surgeon's specifications and preferences. Five anatomical zones describe flexor tendon injury to the index, long, ring, and small digits (see Fig. 43-13). Zone I is from the insertion of the FDS to the insertion of the FDP. Zone II is the area where the FDS and FDP both lie within the flexor sheath, from the A-1 pulley to the FDS insertion. This region has memorably been dubbed "no man's land" to reflect the technical challenge and historically poor prognosis for repair in this area.[9,25] Zone III describes the area from the distal edge of the carpal tunnel to the A-1 pulley of the flexor sheath, including the lumbrical muscles. Zone IV is where the flexor tendons

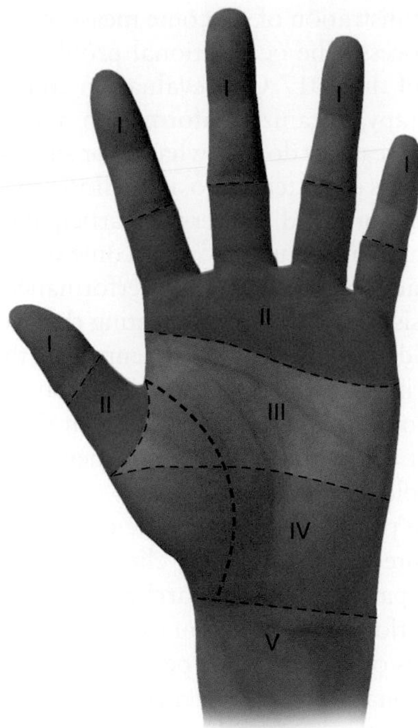

Figure 43-13. The five zones of the hand based on flexor tendon anatomy.

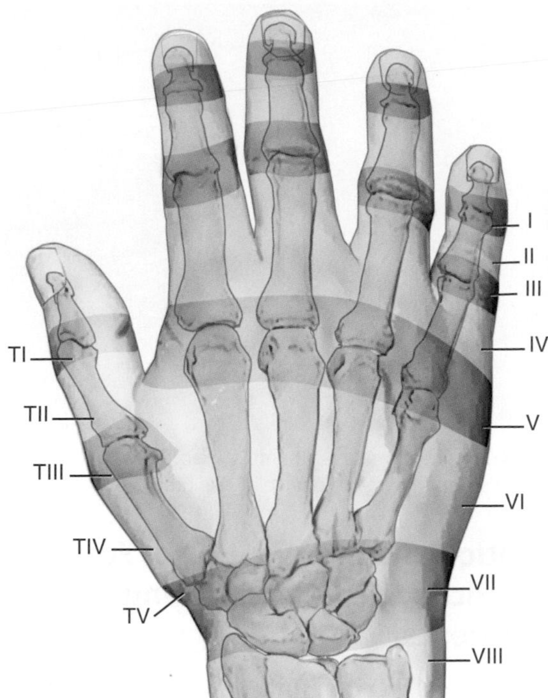

Figure 43-14. The seven zones of the hand based on extensor tendon anatomy.

lie under the transverse carpal ligament in the carpal tunnel. Injuries in this zone may include the median and ulnar nerves. Zone V is the area from the forearm flexor musculotendinous junction to the border of the transverse carpal ligament.[9,25]

Physicians usually indicate specific postoperative positioning guidelines to protect repaired structures following flexor tendon repair that serve to allow preservation of gliding but limit forces that can cause rupture of the repair.

Extensor Tendon Injury

Seven zones describe the digital extensors for the index, long, ring, and small fingers, and five zones describe the thumb extensors (see Fig. 43-14). Injury in zones I and II leads to a mallet deformity, which follows disruption of the terminal extensor tendon and manifests itself as distal interphalangeal (DIP) **extensor lag.** Depending on the nature of the problem, an injury to zone I or II may not require surgical intervention and will be referred to therapy or the surgeon will simply immobilize the DIP continuously in extension for 6 to 8 weeks.[26] Extensor injuries in zones III and IV lead to a boutonnière deformity and can be treated conservatively or through surgery depending on the extent of the tendon damage. Without intervention, the deformity becomes "fixed" or permanent because of volar displacement of the lateral bands secondary loss of the central slip and eventual volar plate contracture. Injury in zones V, VI, and VII will require surgical repair followed by either immobilization or controlled early motion protocols.

Functional Impairment in Daily Occupation Resulting from Hand Impairments

Regardless of the specific diagnosis, hand impairments have the potential to impact client factors in the areas of sensory functions and neuromusculoskeletal and movement-related functions that include tactile sensation, pain, joint mobility and stability and muscle strength, and endurance.[1] Impairments of these client factors will affect the ability of the hand and upper extremity to engage in activities involving motor skills and, ultimately, impact the ability of the client to engage in desired occupations the extent of which can be impacted by pain levels, the context and environment, and the adaptability of the client.[1]

For example, a flexor tendon laceration and repair of the dominant hand of an auto mechanic may impact his ability to complete work-related tasks for up to 12 weeks. Working on car engines requires force and precision and the environment where the work takes place does not allow for open wounds and may limit use of protective orthotics. This same individual may not have any difficulties with activities of daily living (ADLs) or instrumental activities of daily living (IADLs) because of some assistance received from his supportive spouse and ability to adapt to using his nondominant hand functionally. Conversely, a client with de Quervain stenosing tenosynovitis may find the condition so painful that she is unable to complete dressing activities that require small fastenings, cook dinners from scratch, or complete laundry tasks due to resisted grasping, but is able to work as an accountant-cum-computer data entry while using a customized orthotic device (see Fig. 43-15).

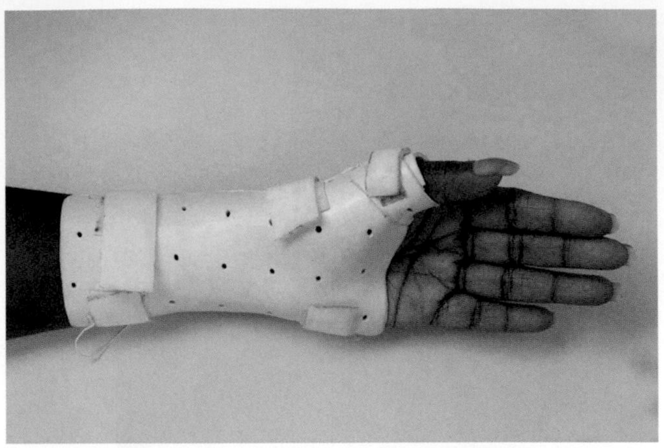

Figure 43-15. Forearm-based thumb spica orthosis for de Quervain tenosynovitis. Used to provide pain relief and promote functional pinch.

Evaluation and Intervention of Functional Skill Deficits Secondary to Hand Impairments

All occupational therapy evaluations must assess deficits in the various aspects of the domain, including occupations, through administration of outcome measures or use of an interview process. The occupational profile,[27] a required component of the 2017 CPT evaluation codes for occupational therapy, organizes information and documents what the client cannot do and what he or she wants to do, needs to do, or is expected to do, in addition to identifying additional supports and barriers to participation, such as the context and environment.[28] Outcome measures, such as the Canadian Occupational Performance Measure (COPM), assist the therapist in creating the occupational profile and identifying areas of occupation that will be targeted during the course of intervention.[29] Outcome measures also provide a way to document the amount of improvement and report that improvement to payers and other stakeholders such as physicians.

Once the profile is complete, the occupational therapist looks more specifically at the client factors, skills, and performance patterns that are barriers to the identified areas of occupation. This section of the evaluation is known as the analysis of occupational performance according to the Occupational Therapy Practice Framework (OTPF). Table 43-1 lists common assessment tools used in occupational therapy for the hand and their purpose.

Table 43-1. Common Assessment Tools for the Hand

ASSESSMENT TOOL	PURPOSE	TECHNIQUE	ASPECT OF THE DOMAIN
Visual Analog Scale (VAS)	Client report of pain level	Client chooses level on 1–10 scale.	Sensory function of pain
Observation of wound	To determine stage of healing and assess change	Determine size (length, width, depth), exudate color, odor, and tissue color (red, yellow, black) through observation and measurement	Skin integrity
Scar assessment	To determine the status and type of scar (hypertrophic, keloid) and possible impact on hand usage	Observe scar location, length, width, and height and suppleness. Determine whether banding is present, whether joint motion is limited, and hypersensitivity is present.	Skin integrity
Vascular assessment	Determine whether circulation is compromised	Cyanosis, erythema, pallor, gangrene, or grayish color indicates vascular compromise. To test digital capillary refill, apply pressure to the fingernail or distal pad of the involved digit. Color should return within 2 seconds of release of pressure. Compare the refill time to that of uninvolved digits.	Circulatory system
Circumferential measurements	Determine changes in size of the hand and fingers to note changes in edema	Wrap small tape measure around desired part of hand. Note placement and provide consistent force reading result. Document finding to the mm (e.g., 2.5 cm or 25 mm)	Circulatory system, skin integrity
Volumeter	Determine changes in hand volume to note changes in edema	Using a commercially available volumeter, immerse client hand as instructed and measure water displaced in milliliters	Circulatory system, skin integrity

Table 43-1. Common Assessment Tools for the Hand (*continued*)

ASSESSMENT TOOL	PURPOSE	TECHNIQUE	ASPECT OF THE DOMAIN
Goniometers (varying sizes and style)	Determine AROM and PROM of each joint to determine whether motion is compromised, indicating joint, tendon, muscle, or skin impairment. Comparison of active (muscle contacting active) vs. passive (outside force) motion are the same or different provide additional information on the status of tendon mobility and muscle strength	Use goniometer sized according to joint being measured. Use technique described in Chapter 13	Neuromusculoskeletal status
Grip and pinch strength	Determine grip and pinch strength to obtain baseline and determine level of strength compared to noninvolved hand. Norm tables can be used for general comparison, although functional strengths can vary client to client. There may be approximately 10%–15% difference in strength between dominant and nondominant hands, with dominant hands usually being stronger. It is routine to measure three pinch patterns: lateral, three-jaw chuck, and tip. As with grip, compare pinch scores with those of the contralateral extremity.	Jamar dynamometer and pinch meter or comparable reliable devices are used following recommended technique. When properly calibrated, the Jamar dynamometer is one of the best instruments to assess grip strength because of its reliability, face validity, and accuracy.	Muscle strength
Manual muscle testing	Manual muscle testing is particularly useful for monitoring progress following peripheral nerve lesions. Facilities usually have their preferred method of grading, which may be numerical or descriptive.	Follow standard testing methods described in the literature. Strength is graded on a scale of 1–5 (trace-poor-fair-good-normal) with specific criteria for determining each grade.	Muscle strength
Semmes monofilaments and observation	To determine tactile sensation of the hand to determine areas of degeneration or regeneration, determine specific nerve involvement, and ensure that client is aware of loss of protective sensation for safety with temperature and sharp objects	Inspect the client's hand for dryness, moistness, shiny skin, calluses, and possible reduced wrinkles and tissue bulk (see Chapter 12). The Semmes-Weinstein Monofilament Test assesses pressure threshold and provides a valid and reliable means of determining levels of protective sensation.	Tactile sensation
Moberg Pickup Test	Determine functional ability of hand with median nerve lesion	The Moberg Pickup Test is a structured assessment that measures the speed of picking up and placing small household items with vision and vision occluded. A difference in time and behavior of hand picking up items indicates possible median nerve sensory impairment.	Sensation
Box and Block Test	Measures gross manual dexterity	Client transfers 1-inch blocks from one side of box to the other. The score is the number of blocks transferred in 1 minute for each hand. Test–retest reliability and inter-rater reliability of the Box and Block Test is high, norms are available for persons aged 20–75 years and older.	Motor skills

(*continued*)

Table 43-1. Common Assessment Tools for the Hand (*continued*)

ASSESSMENT TOOL	PURPOSE	TECHNIQUE	ASPECT OF THE DOMAIN
The Purdue Pegboard Test of finger dexterity	Tests finger or fine motor dexterity	This standardized tool assesses picking up, manipulating, and placing little pegs into holes with speed and accuracy using a wooden board with two rows of tiny holes plus reservoirs for holding pins, collars, and washers. Four subtests are performed with the subject seated. The subtests for preferred, nonpreferred, and both hands require the client to place the pins in the holes as quickly as possible, with the score being the number of pins placed in 30 seconds. The subtest for assembly requires the client to insert a pin and then put a washer, collar, and another washer on the pin, with the score being the number of pieces assembled in 1 minute. The tool has normative data and is valid ad reliable.[30]	Motor and finger manipulation skills
Nine-Hole Peg Test	Measures finger dexterity among clients of all ages	Test administration is brief—only involving the time it takes to place nine pegs in holes in a 5-inch square board and then remove them. Found to have high test–retest reliability coefficients (0.95 for right hands and 0.92 for left hands). High inter-rater reliability has been reported.[47,48]	Motor skills
Upper Extremity Performance Test for the Elderly (TEMPA)	Assesses hand dexterity using nine tasks: (1) pick up and move a jar, (2) open a jar and take a spoonful of coffee, (3) pour water from a pitcher into a glass, (4) unlock a lock, (5) take the top off a pillbox, (6) write on an envelope and affix a postage stamp, (7) put a scarf around one's neck, (8) shuffle and deal cards, and (9) use coins, and pick up and move small objects.	Instructions are in the manual. The test takes about 15–20 minutes for an unimpaired elderly subject and about 30–40 minutes for an impaired elderly subject. Normative data for young adults have been determined TEMPA norms were established on adults aged 60 years or older (n = 360) by 10-year age groups and by gender. Inter-rater reliability of the TEMPA ranged from 0.96 to 1.00. Test–retest reliability was excellent.[49]	Motor skills
Manual Ability Measure (MAM-20)[50]	Offer clients the opportunity to discuss their injuries in the context of their daily lives lend insight into the needs that must be addressed	A 20-item self-report questionnaire. Tool consists of two parts: (1) a client demographic sheet and (2) a self-report task list consisting of items that the client rate on a 4-point scale based on his or her perceived ability to complete tasks. It also includes a VAS for pain and column for indicating if skill can be completed with the noninvolved hand.	Motor skills to complete functional activities
Canadian Occupational Performance Measure (COPM)	Client-centered approach to assessment of perceived functional abilities, interest, and satisfaction with occupations	Interview-based valid and reliable tool is scored and can be used to measure outcomes of treatment.	Participation in occupations
Disabilities of the Arm, Shoulder, and Hand (DASH) assessment	Assists with the development of the occupational profile through its valid and reliable measure of clients' functional abilities	Consists of 30 predetermined questions addressing function within performance areas. Clients are asked to rate their recent ability to complete skills on a scale of 1 (no difficulty) to 5 (unable).	Performance in predetermined activities Visit the DASH/ QuickDASH website at http://www.dash.iwh.on.ca

Psychosocial Factors Affecting Therapeutic Outcomes

Occupational therapists should be aware of the specific mental functions that underlie the ability of the client to cope and adapt to an injury or condition of the hand. If these client factors appear to contribute to occupational dysfunction, they must be assessed and addressed to ensure a positive treatment outcome that provides the client with the expected result. Adaptive responses to hand impairment are influenced by body image as well as individual functional needs and contextual elements. The personal or symbolic meaning of the hand, self-esteem, family and friend support systems, and coping strategies all influence outcome. Whenever possible, encourage clients to participate in their care and to return to their typical habits, roles, and routines as soon as possible. Empower clients by ensuring heath literacy, listen well, use nonmedical terminology and instructional diagrams, and encourage some amiable conversation as appropriate.[30]

Motivation is the most important variable favorably influencing recovery. Realistic expectations and appropriate communication that emphasizes participatory decision-making and education are also important. Psychological symptoms related to hand trauma resolve best when intervention occurs early.

Goal Setting

Identified occupational therapy outcomes and goals must reflect the desired occupational performance of the client. The number of degrees of motion achieved is less important than whether the client can open a door, get dressed, or return to work. To this end, all goals should have occupation as the focus. In hand rehabilitation, there is often a desire to follow a bottom-up approach to treatment—in other words, to measure factor and skill-level abilities and to write goals addressing these areas. One way to address these areas while keeping the documented goals as occupations is to create a list of behavioral objectives that represent the underlying factors needed to participate in the occupation addressed in long- and short-term goals. This third level of goal writing does not become part of the medical record, but can assist with clinical decision-making.[31] For example, for a long-term goal addressing self-care, with a short-term goals specifically addressing face washing, a behavioral objective may describe the expected outcome of forearm supination and hand strength.

Although some hand specialists do incorporate purposeful activity into intervention, more support is needed for an approach to hand therapy that leads with concepts of occupations as both the means and the ends of intervention.[32] One way to achieve this is to integrate client-directed goals and typical daily

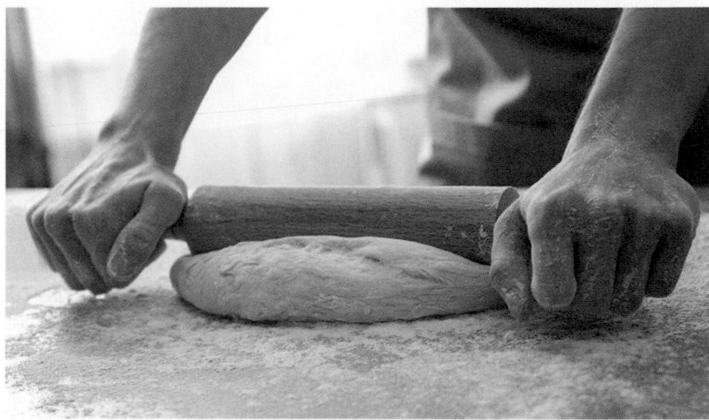

Figure 43-16. Using rolling pin as therapeutic activity to encourage flexion of digits. (Shutterstock/Africa Studio.)

activities and occupations into specialized hand therapy intervention planning and implementation. Occupation elicits adaptive responses that do not occur with exercise alone. Compared to isolated exercise, activities and occupations promote more coordination and better movement quality.[33] An example of isolated hand therapy exercise to increase grip strength is gross grasp with therapy putty or exercise grippers. An example of activity to increase strength would be putting away groceries, starting with light items, and progressing to heavier objects.

Occupation-as-means instills occupational therapy's heritage in what might otherwise be a less function-oriented context.[32] The examples cited earlier become therapeutic occupation with the use of activity that is meaningful to the particular person to accomplish the therapeutic goal. If the client enjoys baking, then rolling dough with a rolling pin would be a therapeutic occupation to promote grip function (see Fig. 43-16).

Basic Interventions

Edema Control

Elevation, active exercise and movement of the extremity, and compression have been the mainstays of edema control. Treatment of upper extremity edema has also historically included retrograde massage, string wrapping, compression garments, and modalities such as an intermittent pressure pump and therapeutic cold (see Fig. 43-17).

Prior to initiating an edema reduction plan, the therapist should determine the type of edema present in the limb. Peripheral edema of the hand can often be caused by the increase in blood supply with capillary leaking surrounding the inflammatory response of the healing mechanism. Lymphedema is a more chronic, pitting edema may be caused by impaired lymphatic function requiring a specialized approach to reduction include stimulating the lymphatic system to remove large plasma proteins.[34]

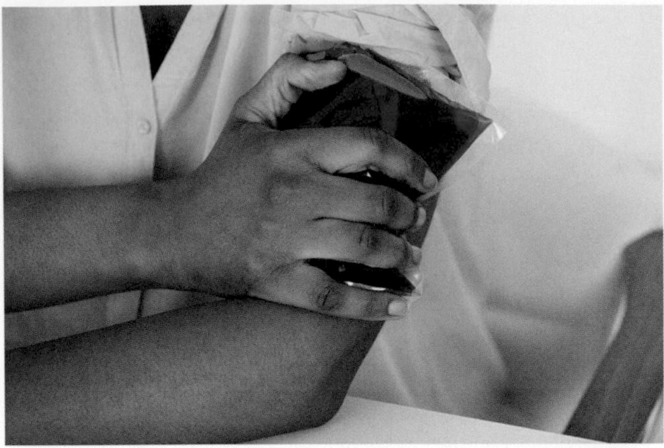

Figure 43-17. Ice pack for reduction of edema. (Shutterstock/Andrey_Popov.)

Scar Management

Compression (e.g., Isotoner gloves, Tubigrip, or Coban wrap) and mechanical forces of vibration are traditionally used to promote scar softening and maturation (see Fig. 43-18). Silicone gel applied over the scar and topical creams such as Mederma are effective in reducing the appearance of scar.[35,36] Other materials inserted in gloves and orthotic devices, such as padding, or elastomer can also be used to provide a more even custom distribution of compressive forces over the scar. Application of micropore tape over incision scars is gaining popularity. It has been shown to be very effective and is much more affordable than the other options.[34]

Differential Digital Tendon Gliding Exercises

Tendon gliding exercises maximize total gliding and differential gliding of digital flexor tendons at the wrist to reduce the risk of scar adhesions between the tendons and surrounding tissue that can occur following tendon injury and repair, crushing injury, and fractures, particularly of bones in the fingers (see Fig. 43-19). Because scar is one of the primary culprits leading to long-term hand dysfunction, tendon gliding exercises are a mainstay of most home exercise programs. Occupations that involve use of the hand in both hook and gross grasp positions can also encourage differential gliding of the tendons and lead to improved motion of digits through participation. Examples can include kneading bread dough, carrying grocery bags in the affected hand, and transferring clothing items from the washer to the dryer. It should be noted that activities requiring resistance must be avoided until the tensile strength of the repair allows (see Fig. 43-20).

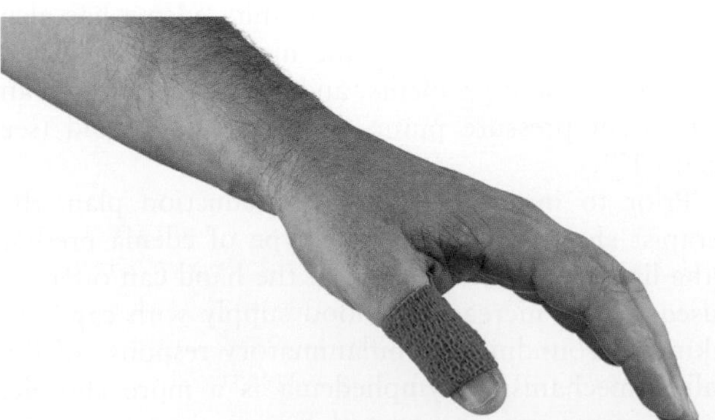

Figure 43-18. Elastic wrap providing compression to reduce scar on dorsal thumb IP. IP, interphalangeal. (Shutterstock/Melodia plus photos.)

Blocking Exercises

Blocking is a technique that also improved tendon gliding/excursion and that can assist with capsular stretch. The technique involves blocking finger joints from either flexing or extending in order to increase the tendon force at the impacted joint. The therapists' hand, the client's nonaffected hand, or a device such as a splint or scrap of splinting material or wood can block the desired joints. For example, when blocking to increase PIP extension, the MP joint is held in flexion while the client attempts to extend the PIP and DIP joints through activation of the extensor mechanism and intrinsic muscles responsible (see Fig. 43-21). Another example of blocking to increase DIP flexion would involve maintaining the MP and PIP joints in full extension with an external device or opposite hand while pulling the DIP into flexion (see Fig. 43-22).

Instruct clients who do blocking exercises to exercise comfortably into the end range to remodel the tissue. Teach him or her to do the exercises frequently and slowly, holding at the comfortable end range for 3 to 5 seconds. Occupations and activities that naturally block sets of joints and allow for force application to a specified tendon include holding onto a steering wheel of a car (block MCPs and flex IPs), playing guitar (affected hand changing chords), sweeping, or raking leaves (see Fig. 43-23).

Diagnosis-Specific Interventions

If not contraindicated by medical diagnosis, encourage the client to achieve gentle full arcs of available motion with functional use or exercise instead of performing quick or incomplete arcs of motion that are less effective. Use occupations or meaningful activities that target the structures requiring motion. If needed for preparation, preparatory tasks such as grasping and releasing various items can be used. If the client's hand is painful or more swollen after use or exercise,

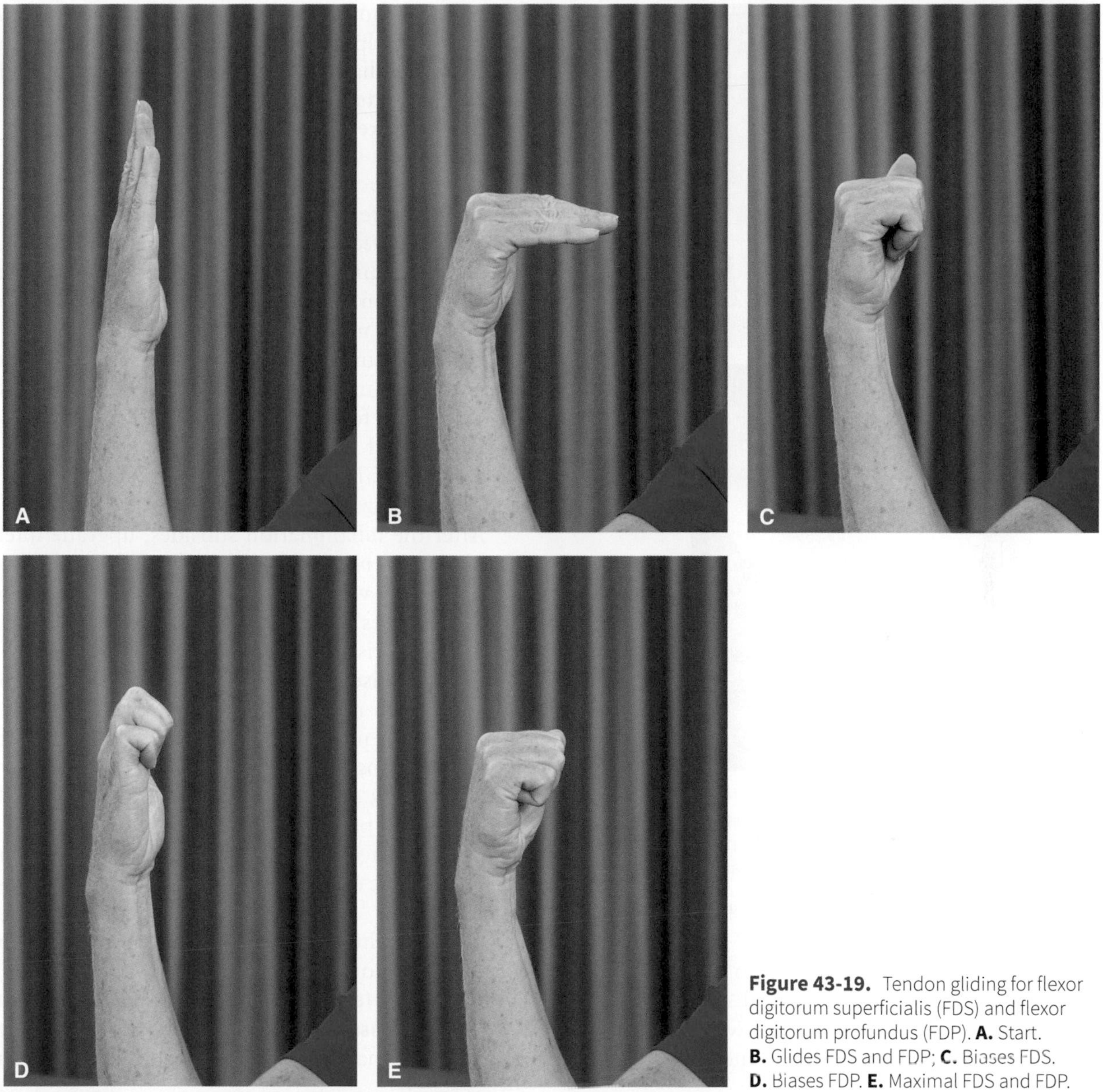

Figure 43-19. Tendon gliding for flexor digitorum superficialis (FDS) and flexor digitorum profundus (FDP). **A.** Start. **B.** Glides FDS and FDP; **C.** Biases FDS. **D.** Biases FDP. **E.** Maximal FDS and FDP.

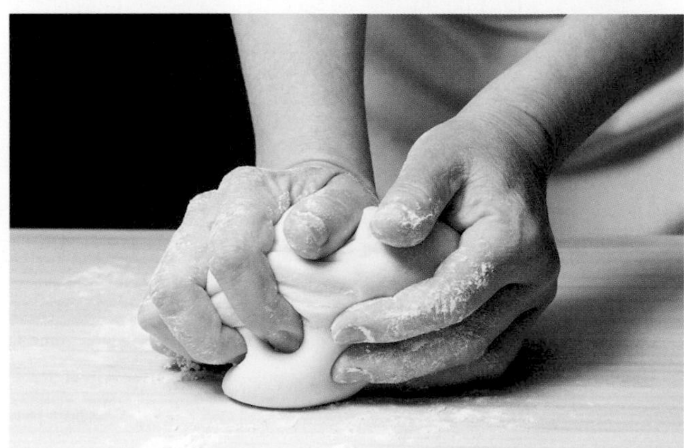

Figure 43-20. Using meaningful activity of kneading dough to improve hand strength and mobility. (Shutterstock/Vladimir Volodin.)

the amount of activity being performed should be decreased temporarily.[37]

Avoid aggressive PROM. It is okay to coax tissues to lengthen within their available comfortable range, but always respect the feeling of tissue resistance, and do not exceed it. Gentle passive motion, if indicated, should be accompanied by **joint traction** (a gentle pressure applied to pull the end of the bones apart) to promote gliding of the joint surfaces. Sustained holding of a position is much more effective than fast jerky stretches, which frequently add to the inflammation.

During the acute inflammatory stage, static splinting is usually most appropriate. After the inflammation has subsided and while the joint displays a soft **end**

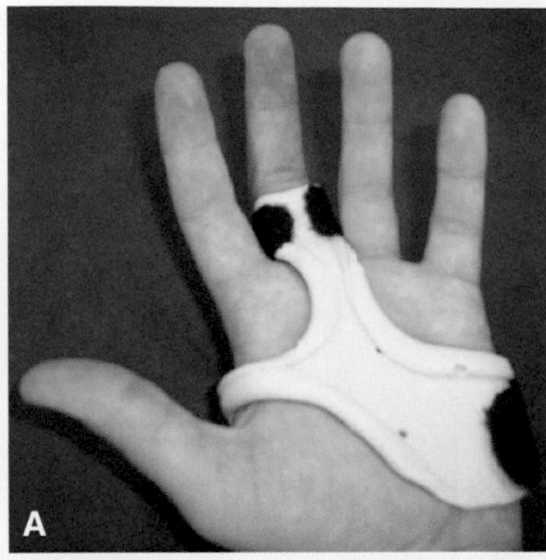

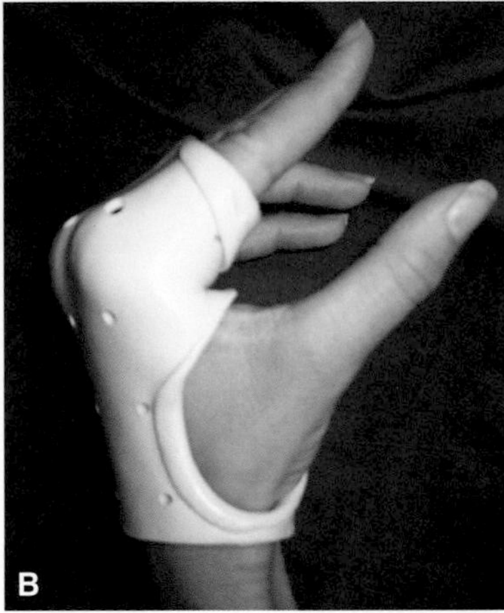

Figure 43-21. Blocking splints. MP splint blocks MP in flexion, promoting PIP and DIP extension. (**A**) Palmer view of a blocking splint, (**B**) Radial view of a blocking splint. DIP, distal interphalangeal; MP, metacarpophalangeal; PIP, proximal interphalangeal.

feel, dynamic splinting is productive. Inflamed tissue is not as flexible as uninflamed tissue.[37] Watch closely for signs of inflammation and return to static splinting as indicated. Later, if there is a hard **end feel**, serial static or static progressive splinting will most likely be needed.[37] Many clients with hand impairments complain of morning stiffness. Night splinting, which can be very helpful for this problem, also corrects tissue tightness that limits daytime use of the hand. Always ensure that no contraindications for dynamic splinting are present.

Tendinopathy

Treat the acute phase with ice, compression, elevation of the involved structures, and rest, if needed, to manage pain. Anti-inflammatory physical agent modalities, considered preparatory methods in the OTPF may be useful at this time, but remember that tendinitis/tendinosis may not be primarily inflammatory. Orthotic use is individualized to the client's and physician's preferences. Orthotic intervention may be most beneficial and least problematic at night. There are also clinical compromises associated with disuse from immobilization.

After the inflammation subsides, upgrade intervention to restore normal function through gradual use of hand balanced with rest; avoid pain. Instruct in tendon gliding exercises in a pain-free range and progress from isometric exercises with gentle contractions of involved structures to isotonic exercises. Gradually introduce low-load, high-repetition strengthening in short arcs of motion. Then increase the arc of motion and modify proximal positions to be more challenging if appropriate for work simulation. Instruct in gentle flexibility exercises in a pain-free range. It is often difficult for clients to learn to perform slow and pain-free passive stretch. Aerobic exercises and proximal conditioning are essential.

Prevent reinjury by teaching the client to avoid repetitive motions using muscles involved in the specific diagnosis (e.g., trigger finger caused by repetitive grasp and release). In addition, specific combination of motions that may not be highly repetitive but that put

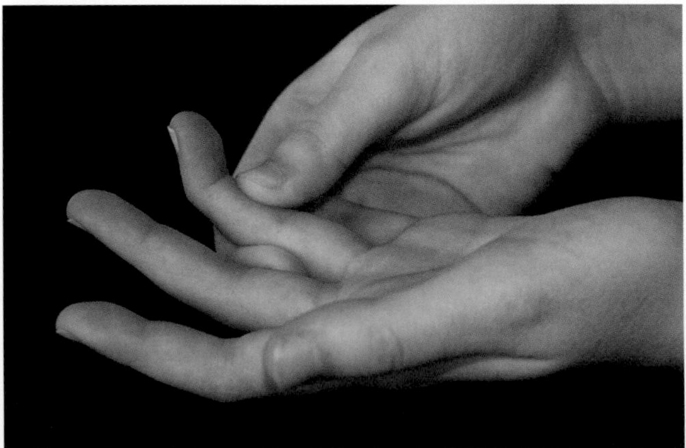

Figure 43-22. Actively flexing the DIP while blocking the PIP and MP joints. DIP, distal interphalangeal; MP, metacarpophalangeal; PIP, proximal interphalangeal.

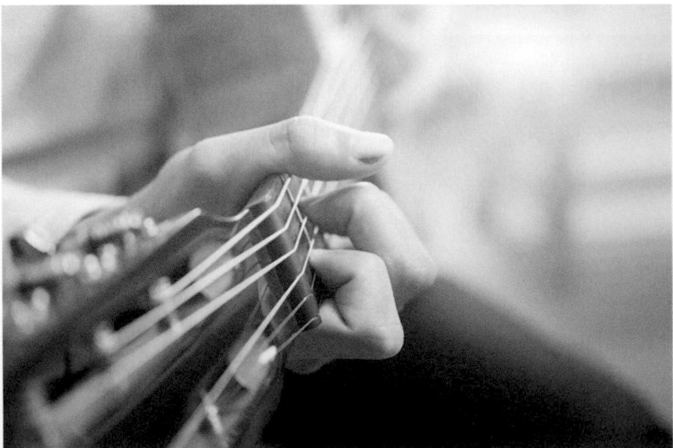

Figure 43-23. MP flexion blocked, while IPs flex to hold chords on guitar. MP, metacarpophalangeal; IP, interphalangeal. (Shutterstock/Have a nice day photo.)

significant stress on a tendon should be avoided (e.g., de Quervain tenosynovitis exacerbated by pinching while wrist is flexed and ulnarly deviated).

Easily recognizable issues, such as poor posture or trunk twisting with reaching and lifting, should be solved by working with the client to understand the goals of the activity and changes to position or technique that will allow the goal to be reached more efficiently. Instruct in pacing to avoid fatigue that leads to inflammation. Use of the upper extremities without support together or alone, in an asymmetrical manner, and lateral to trunk can be very taxing. People with distal symptoms recover well by focusing intervention on posture, conditioning, and proximal strengthening. Using handheld tools with ergonomic design can be helpful. Even a small ergonomic adjustment, such as learning to lift bilaterally with proper body mechanics or making use of a telephone headset instead of laterally flexing the neck and elevating the shoulder to hold the receiver, can often lead to dramatic improvement.

Lateral Epicondylitis (Tennis Elbow)

Exercises should include proximal conditioning and scapular stabilizing as well as eccentric loading of the wrist extensors to strengthen without exacerbating inflammation of the muscle origin. Eccentric loading consists of grasping a small dumbbell (1–2 lbs), supination of the forearm, dropping the wrist into extension with gravity assist, holding the wrist in extension, pronating the forearm, and slowly lowering the wrist into flexion—work up to 3 sets of 10 repetitions and repeat several times per day.[38] An orthosis to support the wrist in extension can be used at night and during arm-intensive activities during the day to rest the muscle origins at the lateral epicondyle; wrist position recommendations range from neutral to about 30°. A **counterforce strap**, which is a strap placed over the extensor wad to prevent full muscle contraction to reduce the load on the tendon during the day with activity, and KinesioTape (KT) can also be utilized as conservative approaches to reduce pain and inflammation[39] (see Fig. 43-24).

Medial Epicondylitis (Golfer Elbow)

Exercise should promote proximal conditioning. Avoid activity that requires force at end ranges. Provide built-up handles to reduce forces on flexor muscles. As with lateral epicondylitis, eccentric loading in reverse can assist in strengthening writs flexors without adding stress to the muscle origins. An orthosis maintaining the wrist in neutral or a counterforce strap over the flexor wad will assist in reducing forces on the muscle origin.

Modifications and alternatives to activities that are responsible for or exacerbate the diagnosis are made to reduce repetitive and/or forceful wrist flexion and grasping, especially when coupled with forearm pronation.

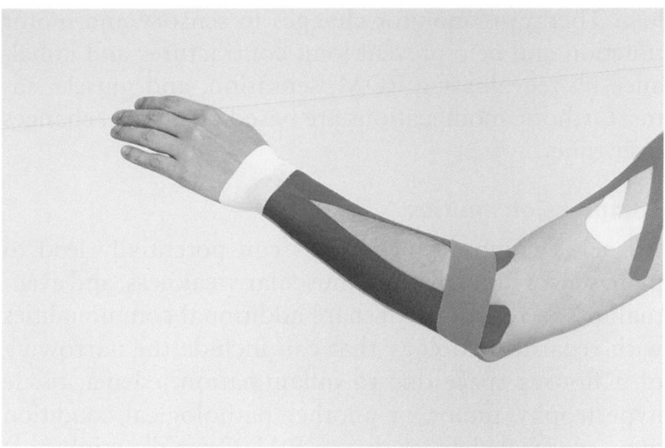

Figure 43-24. KinesioTape applied to the forearm to reduce symptoms of lateral epicondylitis and promote healing. (Shutterstock/staras.)

De Quervain Tenosynovitis

Teach clients to avoid wrist deviation, especially in conjunction with pinching. Provide built-up handles and a forearm-based thumb spica orthosis, leaving the IP free. Watch for irritation from the radial orthosis edge along the first dorsal compartment. Modify or suggest alternatives to activities that bring on or exacerbate condition. Physical agent modalities including ice and iontophoresis with dexamethasone can be applied to reduce inflammation.

Trigger Finger

Therapy for stenosing tenosynovitis consists of splinting the MP in neutral to prevent composite digital flexion (preventing triggering) while promoting tendon gliding and place-and-hold fisting to maintain motion and strength while preventing triggering. Built-up handles, padded gloves, and pacing strategies are helpful. The client must be instructed to avoid the triggering of the digit as much as possible, as abrupt tendon force re-inflames the tissue. Physical agent modalities such as ice to reduce inflammation and ultrasound to enhance circulation and reduce scar may be effective.

If surgery is required, postsurgical intervention will include early gently mobilization of digit with grading of activity to minimize inflammation and scar formation, tendon gliding, and activity modification if needed for discomfort and decreased finger flexion caused by tendon bowstringing.

Nerve Injury

Following nerve injury, therapy promotes functional performance in the areas of occupation with ADL training and adaptive equipment and assists in prevention of deformity with orthotics and appropriate PROM. Occupational therapy provides valuable education to clients about their diagnosis and general recovery sequence and teaches protective guidelines to compensate for sensory loss. Therapists monitor changes in sensory and motor function and help prevent joint contractures and imbalance by reevaluating ROM, sensation, and muscle status. Orthotic modifications are based on clinical changes over time.

Compression Injuries

All nerve compression injuries can potentially lead to pain, sensory impairment, muscular weakness, and eventual loss of function. All share additional commonalities with regard to etiology that can include the narrowing of a fibrous space due to inflammation, edema, tissue hypertrophy, tumor, or another pathological condition (e.g., synovial changes due to RA). Once the etiology is understood, both conservative and medical interventions can be determined. If conservative methods are an option, they may include immobilization with an orthotic to either provide positioning for optimal circulation to the nerve (e.g., CTS) or to rest the area surrounding the nerve to reduce inflammation (e.g., cubital tunnel syndrome). Myofascial-type massage to improve mobility of tissue within the fascial planes and nerve gliding exercises can also be trialed to improve circulation and free nerves from adhesions.

CARPAL TUNNEL SYNDROME. Conservative therapy for CTS includes night splinting with the wrist in neutral because this position minimizes pressure in the carpal tunnel, exercises for median nerve gliding at the wrist, differential flexor tendon gliding exercises, ergonomic modification, and postural training. Teach clients to avoid extremes of forearm rotation or of wrist motions and to avoid sustained pinch or forceful grip. For example, thick padded automobile steering wheel covers are helpful as are ergonomic computer keyboards that are split and angled to maintain forearms in slight supination. In the case of pregnancy-induced CTS, consider techniques to reduce edema, such as isotoner gloves, retrograde massage, and ice packs.

Postoperative therapy, when necessary, consists of edema control, scar management, desensitization as needed, nerve and tendon gliding exercises, and eventual strengthening. Many therapists postpone strengthening exercises until at least 6 weeks following carpal tunnel release to avoid inflammation. Pillar pain, or pain on the lateral aspects of the palm, may be present and can be minimized with deep pressure massage and padded gloves, if needed, during hand-intensive activities.

RADIAL TUNNEL SYNDROME. Conservative treatment of the radial nerve compression in the forearm includes wrist extension splinting to reduce pressure of extensor muscle mass and to limit contractions of the muscles that can cause exacerbation. Because radial nerve compression can be caused by resisted wrist extension with grasping, as is seen in forearm strengthening exercises, the client may be instructed to reduce the force or frequency of activities contributing to the condition. Radial nerve compression can also be caused by use of a tennis elbow strap that is applied incorrectly or used for extended periods of time. If the client is using a tennis elbow strap device, check to ensure that is not causing or contributing to the radial nerve compression. Radial nerve gliding and myofascial-type massage can also be trialed to reduce discomfort. A nonresponsive compression may require surgical decompression.

CUBITAL TUNNEL SYNDROME. Conservative therapy for cubital tunnel syndrome includes edema control, orthosis or padding the elbow, and positioning guidelines to avoid leaning on the elbow, elbow-flexed postures, and elbow-intensive activity. An elbow orthosis positioned at approximately 30° of flexion helps ensure circulation to the ulnar nerve while sleeping and, at other times, during the day. Types of orthotics include elbow pads or soft splints, pillows, and anterior or posterior thermoplastic orthoses. Additional therapy includes proximal conditioning, postural and ergonomic training, and ulnar nerve gliding exercises. Retrograde massage and gentle ice treatments can also be trialed to reduce any inflammation that may be contributing to the nerve compression.

Nerve Laceration

Repaired nerves require a period of protection to reduce stress on the delicate anastomosis that can be pulled apart or encounter traction forces that will create a gap, leading to a high likelihood of neuroma formation. Postoperative therapy for all hand nerve repairs includes fabrication of an orthosis that limits movement of the joint(s) crossed by the nerve in close proximity to the repair. For example, a digital nerve repaired at the level of the middle phalanx will require the MP and IP joints be secured in a flexed position. Although protected from extension forces, the client is instructed to remove straps from the orthotic to actively and passively flex the finger to maintain joint and tendon integrity. The dorsally based orthotic is not removed from the digit for added protection during the exercises. If the orthotic is removed for cleaning, the client is instructed not to straighten the finger. This same principle can be applied to other joints in the hand and arm depending on the nerve repair.

As the anastomosis heals, the angle of the orthosis will be increased to allow the nerve to gently lengthen. Once completely healed (approximately 6–8 weeks), the device will be discontinued and may be replaced by an antideformity orthosis, as described later in this section.

However, although the repair may have healed, the regrowth of the axons and reinnervation of motor and sensory end plates must still occur. The nerve will regrow at the rate of 1 inch per month; a radial nerve injury at the humeral level may take up to 18 months for regrowth.

The occupational therapist ensures that the client is aware of the location and degree of sensory loss and how to protect the area from temperature, pressure, and sharp objects. Clients are instructed not to use the unaffected hand to gauge the impact of even minimal temperature or pressure changes (e.g., an ill-fitting orthosis) on the insensate hand; because of damaged autonomic fibers, the insensate hand may not respond the same as a noninjured hand. The therapist should avoid the use of thermal modalities or forceful massage to the scar tissue. Silicone gel sheets provide scar reduction without mechanical pressure or friction to the skin.

As the nerve regrows, the therapist assists the client with grading of daily activities to ensure that strength is gradually increased, that function returns—with adaptations if needed—and that delicate healing tissues are not overstressed.

Injuries to the three major nerves of the hand may require long-term orthotic use to prevent permanent deformities. For the ulnar nerve, a dorsal hand–based device that maintains the MPs in flexion will direct the force of the intrinsic muscles to extend the IPs that are otherwise held in a clawed position from the loss of the balancing forces of the ulnar nerve innervated long finger flexors. In the case of a median nerve injury, an orthosis that secures the thumb in a position of abduction and opposition will maintain function of the hand and prevent an adduction contracture of the thumb. A radial nerve injury will benefit from a device that holds the wrist and MP joints in extension and includes the thumb. An orthosis that suspends the digits with soft-finger loops and dental floss and has a thermoplastic base that does not cross the wrist will utilize and preserve a tenodesis motion for grasp and release. A more simplistic and easy-to-manage prefabricated wrist extension splint can also work well to prevent the functional limitations of the drop-wrist deformity.

Distal Radius Fracture

Immobilization Phase

Appropriate early therapy intervention can make a huge difference in the client's overall functional recovery. If the digits are allowed to become swollen and stiff, the long-term functional results can be devastating. These fractures are common among older people with osteoporosis and balance problems. Temporary loss of independence following fracture can trigger an irreversible downward spiral in the client occupational functioning.

Typical medical management of Colles fracture is cast immobilization, usually above elbow with the elbow in 90° of flexion to prevent forearm rotation during the first 3 weeks. When the client is put in a short arm cast and the elbow is freed, begin elbow AROM for flexion and extension, but avoid resisted elbow motion so as not to stress the fracture healing. Do not perform elbow PROM without medical clearance, and be very gentle. Biceps tightness commonly follows elbow immobilization.

Certain fractures require some form of fixation. Some physicians delay the referral of clients to therapy, but postponing the initiation of therapy can result in significant problems with edema and decreased ROM. It is a good idea to communicate with referring physicians and encourage routine early therapy referral for this diagnosis.

While the client has percutaneous pins, provide pin site care as the physician prescribes using sterile technique and standard precautions. Teach the client digital ROM and tendon gliding exercises, and instruct in precautions related to cast wearing. It is critical to monitor for cast tightness because a tight cast can cause CRPS. Call the physician if the cast is too tight. Discourage the use of slings because they promote unnecessary proximal stiffness, guarded posture, and disuse.

The onset of shoulder restrictions, which can be attributed to additional trauma occurring at the time of the wrist fracture, is problematic and should be immediately ruled out or treated. Physicians most assuredly appreciate therapists' input regarding early signs of this problem. To prevent a frozen shoulder, proximal ROM is a high treatment priority. Instruct in shoulder flexion, abduction, internal rotation, and external rotation. Perform as thorough a physical assessment as tolerated and as cast constraints permit. This may have to be done in phases. Early identification of guarding, excessive pain, or autonomic signs can alert the team to the possibility of CRPS.

Following distal radius fracture, the recovery of function depends on restoration of motion and strength and on maximizing the length–tension relationship of the digital flexors and extensors.[34] Edema can contribute to decreased ROM at uncasted areas. Clients are often surprised that uninjured and uncasted areas can stiffen.

The goals of early therapy during immobilization are to normalize edema and achieve as nearly normal AROM of uncasted areas as possible. During this period, intrinsic tightness, extrinsic tightness, and digital joint tightness may occur. The chance of tendon adherence is increased following open reduction and its accompanying incisional scar. Various blocking splints may be used with functional activity and exercise to resolve joint or musculotendinous tightness. Differential tendon gliding exercises are extremely important. Frequent exercise throughout the day is better than a few long sessions. It is generally advised to perform exercises every hour or 2, perhaps 5 to 10 repetitions each, maintaining the end position comfortably for 3 to 5 seconds.

Incorporate exercises into occupations, including ADL, as much as possible.[37]

If extrinsic musculotendinous tightness persists, it may be appropriate to add night static progressive splinting or low-load, long-duration dynamic splinting in conjunction with exercise to normalize extrinsic length. Consult the physician before making this determination.

Mobilization Phase

When fracture immobilization is discontinued, physicians often recommend a custom-fabricated volar wrist orthosis. This is protective and can be corrective to help restore functional wrist motion (usually extension). This temporary support is particularly helpful if the client maintains habitual wrist flexion because this "doggy-paw" posture leads to development of the undesirable deformity position of MP extension, PIP flexion, and thumb adduction and extension discussed earlier. At this stage of therapy, there is usually measurable limitation in ROM, with clients reporting awkwardness and decreased function. Consult the physician for medical clearance and guidelines for forearm and wrist ROM. Teach the client to wean off the protective orthosis according to the physician's guidelines, which are individualized. Edema control continues to be the highest priority until it is resolved. AROM and ADL can help correct the edema. Guided motor imagery has also been shown to be effective with wrist fractures.[40]

At any time, but especially in this early stage, overzealous therapy is harmful. Clients and families who think they should be aggressive in their home programs need education and reinforcement to avoid overdoing it. Use written material and illustrations to teach them how to observe tissue responses and monitor inflammation. Temperature elevation or redness over the joints of digits may indicate that intervention is eliciting an inflammatory reaction and should be adjusted accordingly.[41]

It is extremely important to retrain the wrist extensors to function independently of the extensor digitorum. Have the client practice wrist extension with available composite digital flexion, being especially sure the MPs are flexed. Then have the client flex the wrist with the digits relaxed but extended to isolate the wrist flexors. It is also important to retrain the extensor digitorum to function independently of the intrinsics. Have the client extend the MPs with the IPs slightly flexed to isolate the extensor digitorum.

Gradually upgrade therapy with increasingly challenging motions, combined motions, and activities aiming to restore joint suppleness and musculotendinous lengths. Client selected dexterity activities, such as cat's cradle, and games, such as pick-up sticks, promote spontaneous functional movements. Sorting drawers and folding small items of clothing are good home activities (see Fig. 43-25). Initiate graded functional strengthening with medical clearance, usually after good motion has been achieved. Upgrade carefully, monitor client and tissue responses, and adjust the intervention accordingly.

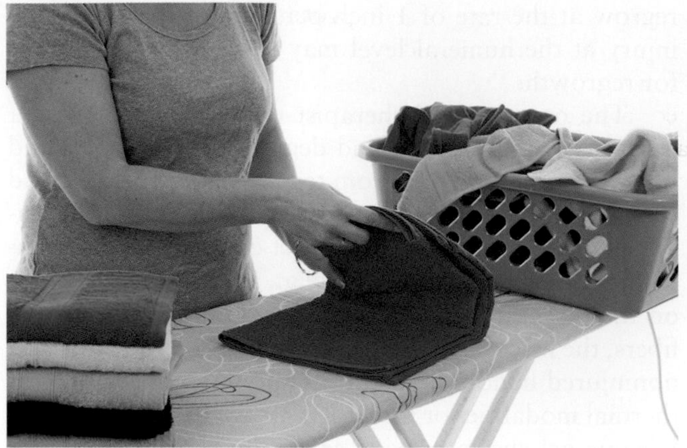

Figure 43-25. Sorting clothes as therapeutic activity to improve hand function. (Shutterstock/Sandra van der Steen.)

Ligament Injury

Grade I ligament injuries, also considered sprains, may produce enough discomfort during functional activities that they require rest, thermal modalities, and temporary modifications to work, ADL, and leisure activities. Rest may require the use of a customized orthotic device depending on the location of the injury and the painful dysfunction experienced. Therapeutic heat or cold can be recommended to the client depending on the acuity of the injury; cold will reduce pain and inflammation, and heat will reduce chronic pain and increase extensibility of a stiff joint. In addition to pain control and adaptations, grade II injuries will require longer immobilization until ligament fibers are healed enough to ensure stability of the joint. During immobilization, gentle protected active movement should be encouraged within anatomical lines of motion to maintain joint flexibility but prevent reinjury. As mobilization is discontinued, client should return to normal levels of activity within pain tolerance. Grade III injuries will require surgical intervention to reattach the ligament to bone with occupational therapy to improve functional use of hand following full healing.

Skier's Thumb

Skier's thumb (grade 3 ligament injury of the ulnar collateral ligament of the thumb MP) may require surgical intervention for ligament reattachment. During the post-op immobilization period, the occupational therapist can provide a protective hand- or forearm-based thumb spica orthosis and edema control techniques. ROM exercises for noninvolved joints and recommendations for use of the hand for light ADLs are initiated. After approximately 1 to 2 weeks, the client is instructed to complete gentle ROM exercises for the MP joint that will progress over time. Strength and motion of the IP joint are also addressed because full MP flexion may not be achieved, especially among older clients. Resistive exercise will be started at approximately 6 weeks; then lateral pinch and tip pinch (which may not be for 12 weeks owing to the strenuous nature of the tip pinch). The hand-based spica orthosis may be used beyond 12 weeks if needed for additional joint protection during strenuous activity. Scar hypersensitivity caused by the underlying radial sensory nerve is common.

Flexor Tendon Repair

Various protocols exist for controlled mobilization, using a dorsal orthosis with the wrist in 10° to 30° of flexion, MP joints in 40° to 60° of flexion, and IP joints ideally in full extension (unless there has also been a digital nerve repair). The involved IP joints may have to be in some flexion if a digital nerve has been repaired. The Duran protocol entails passive digital flexion and extension within the protective orthosis to achieve 3 to 5 mm of differential digital tendon excursion.[42,43] With this protocol, gentle active motion begins with medical clearance about 4 weeks after surgery.

Another popular protocol is known as the Kleinert protocol and involves passive flexion–active extension with rubber band attachments to the fingernails within the protective dorsal orthosis.[44] The client performs gentle active digital extension, and the rubber band provides passive digital flexion within the confines of the protective orthosis. Exercises are gradually increased to 10 repetitions comfortably every waking hour. At night, the digits may be strapped carefully and comfortably to the dorsal hood of the orthosis to counteract the tendency to develop PIP or DIP flexion contractures.

The Chow protocol uses a combination of the Duran and Kleinert techniques. With advances in suture techniques, flexor tendons protocols are incorporating early active motion in clients who are good candidates (see Fig. 43-26).[44]

With all three protocols, active flexion of the digits begins at approximately 4 to 6 weeks from initial repair and increases in frequency and intensity until the client can return to full function, usually 12 weeks or after repair. When the physician gives medical clearance to discontinue the dorsal protective orthosis, begin a graded program to promote functional movement. Edema control and scar management remain high clinical priorities. Assess closely and determine tissue-specific limitations that guide the therapy program. Tendon gliding exercises and place-and-hold exercises are typical early techniques. Corrective splinting is useful, along with ADL, graded activity, and upgraded exercise as appropriate.

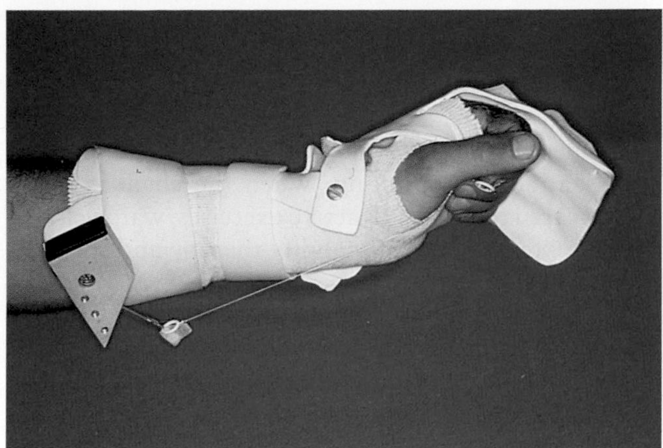

Figure 43-26. Early active motion protocol dorsal protective orthosis with elastic traction and hinged wrist.

Extensor Tendon Repair

Zone I or II extensor tendon injuries, also called mallet finger deformities, not requiring surgical intervention will be immobilized in slight hyperextension for a minimum of 8 weeks, leaving the PIP joint free. The occupational therapist may create a custom orthosis or fit a premade device. The physician may also provide this device. Once provided to the client, it is essential to instruct the client in use of the device, including cleaning of the digit and changing soiled tape or self-adhesive wrap applied to hold it in place. The therapist will also instruct the client in AROM and gentle PROM to noninvolved joints of the hand, especially the PIP joint of the digit.

Once the tendon has healed, the client will begin gentle active flexion activities to regain motion lost through immobilization. Flexion activities must be balanced with active extension to ensure that there is no recurrence of DIP extensor lag. Use of the extension orthosis should continue between exercise sessions and eventually reduced to times of sleep only. However, if a lag is noticed during the day or is getting more pronounced over time, the client should be instructed to resume splinting as needed to recover DIP extension.

Extensor injuries in zones III and IV lead to a boutonnière deformity, an imbalanced digital position of PIP flexion and DIP hyperextension. The deformity is caused by volar displacement of the lateral bands secondary to involvement of the central slip.

In nonoperative cases, splint the PIP in full extension for 6 weeks, and promote DIP active and passive flexion to prevent stiffness of the oblique retinacular ligament. In operative cases, follow the physician's guidelines, which may vary in timing and technique of mobilization and splinting. When the client is medically cleared to begin PIP active exercises, watch closely for PIP extensor lag, and modify therapy and splinting accordingly.

Injury in zones V and VI may be treated by immobilization or controlled early motion.[45] Specific positioning and motion guidelines vary from surgeon to surgeon and are modified according to each client's tissue responses. Multiple complex orthotics may be needed to achieve a program that balances rest and motion appropriately.

Injury in zone VII is likely to result in restrictions because of the development of adhesions. Communicate closely with the surgeon for specific positioning and motion guidelines.

Conclusion

Occupational therapists who work with individuals with hand injuries and conditions must have comprehensive knowledge of body functions and structures, including the musculoskeletal and nervous systems. In addition, they understand and appreciate the relationships of client factors to performance skills, performance patterns, occupations, and the context/environment of the client. Advanced levels of knowledge of diseases and conditions affecting the hand and upper extremity and their potential impact on occupational participation are also integral to this practice area. Therapists are also be well versed in a variety of assessment tools, outcome measures, and specialized treatment techniques that support occupational performance. The role of occupational therapy within hand rehabilitation as with all other specialized areas of practice is to ensure that the client can participate in the desired areas of occupation, regardless of the impact of conditions, disease, or the environment.

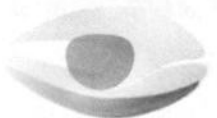

CASE STUDY

Sage: A Case Study of de Quervain Tenosynovitis

Patient Information

Sage is a 31-year-old who is married and recently adopted an infant. Sage began to experience pain in the radial side of the right dominant wrist that has caused significant difficulties with caring for the infant child. Activities such as diapering, connecting and disconnecting the car seat straps, opening and closing fastenings on all clothing, and preparing food are becoming impossible to complete because of significant pain and limited motion of the thumb into flexion and wrist into flexion and ulnar deviation. Sage was seen by a physician at the local hospital orthopedic clinic who diagnosed the condition as de Quervain tenosynovitis and provided a corticosteroid injection into the first dorsal compartment.

Reason for Occupational Therapy Referral

Owing to the difficulties in childcare and other basic ADLs, the physician ordered occupational therapy assessment and treatment following the injection. In addition, the therapy order included the provision of a thumb spica orthosis.

Assessment Process and Results

The occupational therapy evaluation took place the day of the doctor visit and began with the completion of the Occupational Profile.[27] The results of the profile indicated that Sage has significant concerns with the ability to care for the new baby and complete self and home care activities due to significant pain and stiffness. Although the cortisone injection made the wrist and thumb somewhat less painful immediately following, the doctor indicated that it may take several days for the de Quervain to be resolved. With regard to environmental supports, Sage indicated that her partner shares the childcare responsibilities, but that her partner works outside the home during the day and returns home later in the evenings. Sage does not have any knowledge of modifications to task completion and is not clear on the cause of the pain; no orthosis has been provided.

The analysis of occupational performance was conducted next and included assessments targeting active motion of the wrist and thumb and pain level. Results are as follows:

Assessment	Criteria	Results
Visual Analog Scale (VAS) for pain	At rest	4/10
	With activity	9/10
Goniometric assessment of AROM	Wrist flexion/extension (normal = 70°/75°)	10°/30°
	Radial deviation/ ulnar deviation (normal = 20/35)	15°/10°
	Thumb MP composite flexion with wrist neutral (opposite hand 55°)	12°
	Isolated thumb MP flexion with neutral wrist (opposite hand 56°)	20°

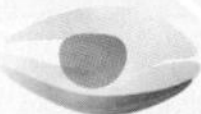

CASE STUDY (continued)

Visual inspection indicates swelling and fullness at the radial wrist in the area of the first dorsal compartment; bruising is apparent due to the injection several hours ago. Findings of the client factors of pain and motion limitations due to tenosynovitis of the first dorsal compartment are consistent with functional limitations being reported.

Occupational Therapy Problem List

- Difficulty caring for new infant
- Difficulty with clothing fasteners on self and infant
- Difficulty with cooking activities

Occupational Therapy Goal List

- Client will report pain-free abilities to bath, dress, and secure infant in car seat within 2 weeks.
- Client will report the ability to dress self fully including securing all fasteners within 2 weeks.
- Client will report the ability to prepare food for the family without pain within 2 weeks.

Intervention

Sage was provided with a prefabricated thumb spica orthosis for intermittent use during the immediate postinjection phase. Instructed to use splint whenever engaged in resistive child care and ADLs. Instructed to decrease orthosis usage as pain subsides and motion improves. Sage was also instructed in gentle AROM activities, including wrist flexion and extension, supination, pronation, and radial and ulnar deviation (with thumb flexion and without thumb flexion). Instruction in use of therapeutic ice to decrease pain as needed and gentle retrograde massage was also provided.

Sage was seen for a follow-up visit 2 weeks later, where ergonomics with regard to hand usage and childcare activities were reviewed. Sage was instructed to avoid resisted ulnar deviation and pinching with thumb whenever possible through attention to position of hand and wrist and to use built-up handles on cooking devices if needed. If pain appears to be returning, instruction to return to full-time splint usage and to use therapeutic cold to reduce inflammation was provided. At time of second visit, ROM had returned to normal, and pain was reduced to 2/10 with activity and 0 per the VAS at rest.

Evidence Table for Occupational Therapy Interventions for Hand Impairments

Intervention	Description	Participants	Dosage	Research Design and Level of Evidence	Benefit	Statistical Probability and Effect Size of Outcome
Effect of immobilization of metacarpophalangeal joint in thumb carpometacarpal osteoarthritis on pain and function[46]	Comparison of the effectiveness of two different static orthoses on pain and functional abilities on CMC OA.	Eighty-four patients, 91.7% females (mean standard deviation [SD] age, 60.1 ± 9.6 years), with thumb CMC OA were randomized into one of two groups. For group A, a Ballena orthotic was constructed, and for group B, a Colditz orthotic was constructed.	Both orthoses were worn for 3 months.	A quasi-experimental trial Level II	Both orthoses improved pain level and functional abilities (F[1.0] ¼ 413.327 and F[1.0] ¼ 211.742; both $p < 0.001$). There was no statistically significant difference between two groups regarding pain recovery and functional improvement (F[1.0] ¼ 0.075 and F[1.0] ¼ 7.248; both $P > 0.05$)	Sample size and power calculations indicated the number of participants needed in each group to be 40. Calculations were based on a difference on a 100-mm VAS, assuming an SD of 20 mm, a two-tailed test, an alpha level of 0.05, and a desired power of 80%. In all analyses, $p < 0.05$ were considered statistically significant.
The effects of Kinesio-Tape on the treatment of lateral epicondylitis[38]	Application of KT with and without tension on pain intensity, pain pressure threshold, grip strength, and disability in individuals with lateral epicondylitis (LE), and myofascial trigger points (MTPs) in forearm muscles.	Thirty women with LE and MTP in the forearm muscles were randomly assigned to KT with tension and placebo (KT without tension).	The treatment was provided three times in 1 week, and outcome measures were assess pre–post treatment.	Randomized clinical trial Level I	The application of KT produces a reduction in pain intensity and upper extremity disability in subjects with LE and MTP in the forearm muscles, and KT with tension was more effective than placebo group.	Study showed no significant difference between groups in variables either immediately or after 1 week. However, Disabilities of the Arm, Shoulder, and Hand (DASH) questionnaire and VAS during activity were statistically significant between the two groups.
Effectiveness of the graded motor imagery to improve hand function in patients with distal radius fracture: a randomized controlled trial[40]	To investigate the effectiveness of graded motor imagery (GMI) in hand function in patients with distal radius fracture	Thirty-six participants were randomly allocated to either GMI (n ¼ 17; 52.59 [9.8] years) or control (n ¼ 19; 47.16 [10.5] years) groups.	The GMI group received imagery treatment in addition to traditional rehabilitation, and the control group received traditional rehabilitation for 8 weeks.	Single–blinded, randomized controlled trial Level I	GMI appears to provide beneficial effects to control pain, improve grip strength, and increase upper extremity function in patients with DRFx.	Statistical power analyses were used to determine the optimum sample size using DASH score. The minimum necessary sample size was 15 subjects for each group, with a 20% absence rate. The alpha level used in determining the sample size was 0.05, and the ideal power was considered to be 80%.

Effectiveness of edema management techniques for subacute hand edema: a systematic review[34]	This systematic review examined the evidence of effectiveness of a range of hand edema treatments on hand volume.	Ten studies met the inclusion criteria. Study quality ranged from 23 to 41 of 48 points on the Structured Effectiveness Quality Evaluation Scale (SEQES). A total of 16 edema interventions were evaluated across the studies.	The following inclusion criteria were used for study selection: randomized controlled or controlled trials in adults who have subacute swelling after a recent upper limb musculoskeletal trauma or cerebral vascular attack or after surgery. Two independent assessors rated study quality and risk of bias using the 24-point MacDermid SEQES.	Systematic review Level IIb	Manual edema mobilization (MEM) techniques should be considered in conjunction with conventional therapies, in cases of excessive edema, or when the edema has not responded to conventional treatment. MEM is not advocated as a routine intervention.	Owing to heterogeneity of the patient characteristics, interventions, and outcomes assessed, it was not possible to pool the results from all studies. Therefore, a narrative best evidence synthesis was undertaken. There is low-to-moderate quality evidence with limited confidence in the effect estimate to support the use of MEM methods in conjunction with standard therapy to reduce problematic hand edema.
Comparison of effects of eccentric training, eccentric-concentric training, and eccentric-concentric training combined with isometric contraction in the treatment of lateral elbow tendinopathy[38]	The effectiveness of eccentric training, eccentric-concentric training, and eccentric-concentric training combined with isometric contraction in the treatment of lateral elbow tendinopathy.	A group of 34 patients with later elbow tendinopathy was randomly allocated to group A ($n = 11$) who underwent eccentric training, group B had eccentric-concentric, and group C who had eccentric-concentric and isometric training.	All patients received five treatments per week for 4 weeks.	A randomized clinical trial Level III	The eccentric-concentric training combined with isometric contractions was the most effective treatment.	The eccentric-concentric training combined with isometric contractions produced the largest effect in the reduction of pain and improvement of function at the end of the treatment ($p < 0.05$) and at any of the follow-up time points ($p < 0.05$).

References

1. Dreifke MB, Jayasuriya AA, Jayasuriya AC. Current wound healing procedures and potential care. *Mater Sci Eng.* 2015;1(48):651–662. doi:10.1016/j.msec.2014.12.068.
2. Fess EE, Gettle KS, Philips CA, Janson JR. *Hand and Upper Extremity Splinting: Principles and Methods.* 3rd ed. St. Louis, MO: Mosby; 2005.
3. Goodman AD, Got CJ, Weiss AP. Crush injuries of the hand. *J Hand Surg.* 2017;42(6):456–463. doi:10.1016/j.jhsa.2017.03.028.
4. Adams JE, Habbu R. Tendinopathies of the hand and wrist. *J Am Acad Orthop Surg.* 2015;23(12):741–750. doi:10.5435/JAAOS-D-14-00216.
5. Ashe MC, McCauley T, Khan KM. Tendinopathies in the upper extremity: a paradigm shift. *J Hand Ther.* 2004;17:329–334. doi:10.17/j.jht.2004.04.002.
6. Fedorczyk JM. Elbow tendinopathies: clinical presentation and therapist's management of tennis elbow. In: Skirven TP, Osterman AL, Fedorczyk JM, Amadio PC, eds. *Rehabilitation of the Hand and Upper Extremity.* 6th ed. Philadelphia, PA: Mosby; 2011:1098–1108.
7. Crop JA, Bunt CW. Doctor, my thumb hurts. *J Fam Pract.* 2011;60:329–332.
8. Taras JS, Martyak GG, Steelman PJ. Primary care of flexor tendon injuries. In: Skirven TP, Osterman AL, Fedorczyk JM, Amadio PC, eds. *Rehabilitation of the Hand and Upper Extremity.* 6th ed. Philadelphia, PA: Mosby; 2011:445–456.
9. Lee MP, Biafora SJ, Zelouf DS. Management of hand and wrist tendinopathies. In: Skirven TP, Osterman AL, Fedorczyk JM, Amadio PC, eds. *Rehabilitation of the Hand and Upper Extremity.* 6th ed. Philadelphia, PA: Mosby; 2011:569–588.
10. Smith KL. Nerve response to injury and repair. In: Skirven TP, Osterman AL, Fedorczyk JM, Amadio PC, eds. *Rehabilitation of the Hand and Upper Extremity.* 6th ed. Philadelphia, PA: Mosby; 2011:601–610.
11. Novak CB, Mackinnon SE. Evaluation of nerve injury and nerve compression in the upper quadrant. *J Hand Ther.* 2005;18:230–240. doi:10.1197/j.jht.2005.02.002.
12. Cooke ME, Duncan SF. History of carpal tunnel syndrome. In: *Carpal Tunnel Syndrome and Related Median Neuropathies.* Cham, Switzerland: Springer; 2017:7–11.
13. Tran TA, Szabo RM. Surgical release of the carpal tunnel. In: *Operative Dictations in Plastic and Reconstructive Surgery.* Cham, Switzerland: Springer; 2017:489–491.
14. Zhang W, Johnston JA, Ross MA, et al. Effects of carpal tunnel syndrome on adaptation of multi-digit forces to object weight for whole-hand manipulation. *PLoS One.* 2011;6(11):e27715. doi:10.1371/journal.pone.0027715.
15. Spies CK, Löw S, Langer MF, Hohendorff B, Müller LP, Unglaub F. Cubital tunnel syndrome: diagnostics and therapy. *Der Orthopade.* 2017;46(8):717–726. doi:10.1007/s00132-017-3453-z.
16. Staples JR, Calfee R. Cubital tunnel syndrome: current concepts. *J Am Acad Orthop Surg.* 2017;25(10):e215–e224. doi:10.5435/JAAOS-D-15-00261.
17. Strohl AB, Zelouf DS. Ulnar tunnel syndrome, radial tunnel syndrome, anterior interosseous nerve syndrome, and pronator syndrome. *J Am Acad Orthop Surg.* 2017;25(1):e1–e10. doi:10.5435/JAAOS-D-16-00010.
18. Antoniadis G. The peripheral nerve: neuroanatomical principles before and after injury. In: *Modern Concepts of Peripheral Nerve Repair.* Cham, Switzerland: Springer; 2017:1–10.
19. Patel S, Zhang D, Earp BE. Acute combined median and radial nerve palsies after distal humeral shaft fracture. *Arch Bone Joint Surg.* 2018;6(2):150–154. https://www.ncbi.nlm.nih.gov/pmc/articles/PMC5867360/
20. Medoff RJ. Distal radius fractures: classification and management. In: Skirven TP, Osterman AL, Fedorczyk JM, Amadio PC, eds. *Rehabilitation of the Hand and Upper Extremity.* 6th ed. Philadelphia, PA: Mosby; 2011:941–948.
21. George AV, Lawton JN. Management of complications of forearm fractures. *Hand Clin.* 2015;31(2):217–233. doi:10.1016/j.hcl.2015.01.010.
22. Garala K, Taub NA, Dias JJ. The epidemiology of fractures of the scaphoid: impact of age, gender, deprivation and seasonality. *Bone Joint J.* 2016;98(5):654–659. doi:10.1302/0301-620X.98B5.36938.
23. Ritting AW, Baldwin PC, Rodner CM. Ulnar collateral ligament injury of the thumb metacarpophalangeal joint. *Clin J Sport Med.* 2010;20:106–112. doi:10.1097/JSM.0b013e3181d23710.
24. Tang P. Collateral ligament injuries of the thumb metacarpophalangeal joint. *J Am Acad Orthop Surg.* 2011;19:287–296. doi:10.5435/00124635-201105000-00006.
25. Lutsky KF, Giang EL, Matzon JL. Flexor tendon injury, repair and rehabilitation. *Orthop Clin North Am.* 2015;46(1):67–76. doi:10.1016/j.ocl.2014.09.004.
26. Anderson D. Mallet finger. *Aust Fam Physician.* 2011;40:47–48.
27. American Occupational Therapy Association. Occupational therapy practice framework: domain & process. *Am J Occup Ther.* 2014;68:S1–S48. doi:10.5014/ajot.2014.682006.
28. Brennan C, McGuire MJ, Metzler C. New occupational therapy evaluation CPT® codes: coding overview and guidelines on code selection. *OT Pract.* 2016;21(22):CE1–CE8.
29. Law M, Baptiste S, Carswell A, McColl MA, Polatajko H, Pollock N. *Canadian Occupational Performance Measure.* 5th ed. Ottawa, ON: CAOT; 2014.
30. de la Llave-Rincon AI, Fernandez-de-las-Penas C, Perez-de-Heredia-Torres M, Martinez-Perez A, Valenza MC, Pareja JA. Bilateral deficits in fine motor control and pinch grip force are not associated with electrodiagnostic findings in women with carpal tunnel syndrome. *Am J Phys Med Rehabil.* 2011;90:443–451.
31. Amini D. *AOTA Documentation Series: Module 2: Occupation-Based Goal Writing for OT Practice.* AOTA Continuing Education; 2016.
32. Trombly CA. Occupation: purposefulness and meaningfulness as therapeutic mechanisms [Eleanor Clarke Slagle Lecture]. *Am J Occup Ther.* 1995;49(12):960–972. doi:10.5014/ajot.49.10.960.
33. Omar MT, Hegazy FA, Mokashi SP. Influences of purposeful activity versus rote exercise on improving pain and hand function in pediatric burn. *Burns.* 2012;38:261–268. doi:10.1016/j.burns.2011.08.004.
34. Miller LK, Jerosch-Herold C, Shepstone L. Effectiveness of edema management techniques for subacute hand edema:

a systematic review. *J Hand Ther.* 2017;30(4):432–446. doi:10.1016/j.jht.2017.05.011.
35. von der Heyde RL, Evans RB. Wound classification and management. In: Skirven TM, Osterman AL, Fedorczyk JM, Amadio PC, eds. *Rehabilitation of the Hand and Upper Extremity.* 6th ed. Philadelphia, PA: Mosby; 2011: 219–232.
36. Berman B, Nestor M. Observer-blinded, randomized study to determine the safety and efficacy of a silicone gel versus a gel containing onion extract for the appearance and symptoms of surgical scars. *J Cutan Med.* 2017;1(3.1):s123. doi:10.25251/skin.1.supp.122.
37. Moscony AMB, Shank TM. Wrist fractures. In: Cooper C, ed. *Fundamentals of Hand Therapy: Clinical Reasoning and Treatment Guidelines for Common Diagnoses of the Upper Extremity.* 2nd ed. St. Louis, MO: Mosby; 2014:312–335.
38. Stasinopoulos D, Stasinopoulos I. Comparison of effects of eccentric training, eccentric-concentric training, and eccentric-concentric training combined with isometric contraction in the treatment of lateral elbow tendinopathy. *J Hand Ther.* 2017;30(1):13–19. doi:10.1016/j.jht.2016.09.001.
39. Shakeri H, Soleimanifar M, Arab AM, Behbahani SH. The effects of KinesioTape on the treatment of lateral epicondylitis. *J Hand Ther.* 2018;31(1):35–41. doi:10.1016/j.jht.2017.01.001.
40. Dilek B, Ayhan C, Yagci G, Yakut Y. Effectiveness of the graded motor imagery to improve hand function in patients with distal radius fracture: a randomized controlled trial. *J Hand Ther.* 2018;31(1):2–9. doi:10.1016/j.jht.2017.09.004.
41. Michlovitz S, Festa L. Therapist's management of distal radius fractures. In: Skirven TM, Osterman AL, Fedorczyk JM, Amadio PC, eds. *Rehabilitation of the Hand and Upper Extremity.* 6th ed. Philadelphia, PA: Mosby; 2011:949–262.
42. Lalonde DH, Kozin S. Tendon disorders of the hand. *Plast Reconstr Surg.* 2011;128(1):1e–4e. doi:10.1097/PRS.0b013e3182174593.
43. Groth GN. Current practice patterns of flexor tendon rehabilitation. *J Hand Ther.* 2005;18:169–174. doi:10.1197/j.jht.2005.01.010.
44. Griffin M, Hindocha S, Jordan D, Saleh M, Khan W. An overview of the management of flexor tendon injuries. *Open Orthop J.* 2012;6:28–35. doi:10.2174/1874325001206010028.
45. Evans RB. Clinical management of extensor tendon injuries: the therapist's perspective. In: Skirven TM, Osterman AL, Fedorczyk JM, Amadio PC, eds. *Rehabilitation of the Hand and Upper Extremity.* 6th ed. Philadelphia, PA: Mosby; 2011:521–554.
46. Cantero-Téllez R, Villafañe JH, Valdes K, Berjano P. Effect of immobilization of metacarpophalangeal joint in thumb carpometacarpal osteoarthritis on pain and function. A quasi-experimental trial. *J Hand Ther.* 2018;31(1):68–73. doi:10.1016/j.jht.2016.11.005.
47. Higgins J, Salbach NM, Wood-Dauphinee S, Richards CL, Cote R, Mayo NE. The effect of a task-oriented intervention on arm function in people with stroke: a randomized controlled trial. *Clin Rehabil.* 2006;20:296–310.
48. Wang Y-C, Magasi SR, Bohannon RW, et al. Assessing dexterity function: a comparison of two alternatives for the NIH toolbox. *J Hand Ther.* 2011;24:313–321.
49. Rallon CR, Chen CC. Relationship between performance-based and self-reported assessment of hand function. *Am J Occup Ther.* 2008;62:574–579.
50. Chen CC, Bode RK. Psychometric validation of the Manual Ability Measure-36 (MAM-36) in clients with neurologic and musculoskeletal disorders. *Arch Phys Med Rehabil.* 2010;91(3):414–420. doi:10.1016/j.apmr.2009.11.012.

Chapter 44

Amputations and Prosthetics

Lisa Smurr Walters

LEARNING OBJECTIVES

This chapter will allow the reader to:

1. Design treatment programs for preprosthetic and prosthetic management of upper limb amputations.
2. Discuss upper limb amputation levels and respective prosthetic options.
3. Describe the psychological implications of amputation and the therapeutic management.
4. Discuss treatment program considerations for persons with lower limb amputations.
5. Discuss challenges of treating individuals with multiple limb loss.

CHAPTER OUTLINE

TERMINOLOGY

Body-powered (BP) prosthesis: an upper limb device that operates from an individual's proximal motions (typically the muscles of the shoulders, neck, and back).

Externally powered (EP) prosthesis: an upper limb device that operates through external power.

Functional envelope: the area of space in which the patient can effectively operate an upper extremity prosthesis.

Heterotrophic ossification: bone that abnormally grows in soft tissue where it should not exist and it commonly occurs after trauma to the musculoskeletal system, brain, or spinal cord.

Hybrid prosthesis: an upper limb device that combines two prosthetic options into one; the most common combination is with a transhumeral prosthesis with a BP elbow and EP terminal device.

Musculoskeletal pain: discomfort that occurs in other areas of the body, such as the back, neck, shoulder, or contralateral limb, as a result of overuse or poor body mechanics.

Myodesis: surgical technique that involves directly suturing muscle or tendon to amputated bone in order to provide optimal distal muscle stabilization.

Myoplasty: surgical technique that involves suturing muscle to muscle and then placing it over the end of the amputated bone before closing the wound; more commonly used in patients with poor vascular health.

Neuroma: an injured nerve in which severed nerve fibers form a disorganized mass of nerve cells (neuroma) that is painful with direct pressure.

Terminal device (TD): an upper limb prosthetic component that is inserted at the distal end of an upper limb prosthesis and is used to grasp and release objects; may be a hook or hand.

Amputation Epidemiology

There are nearly two million people living with upper or lower limb loss in the United States, and this is expected to increase to 3.6 million by 2050.[1] Annually, more than 185,000 persons in the United States have amputations.[2] Amputations are classified as major and minor amputations. Major limb amputation(s) are proximal to the wrist or ankle, whereas minor limb amputation(s) are distal to the wrist (hand and fingers) or ankle (foot and toes). The ratio of lower limb to upper limb amputation varies depending on the source cited. The estimated ratio of general lower limb amputations to upper limb amputation is 52:1.[1] Major lower to upper limb amputation ratio is estimated to be 40:1.[3] In all, 92% of all upper limb amputations occur below the wrist, whereas 65% of all lower limb amputations occur at or above the ankle.[1]

Levels of upper and lower extremity amputation are illustrated in Figures 44-1 and 44-2, respectively.

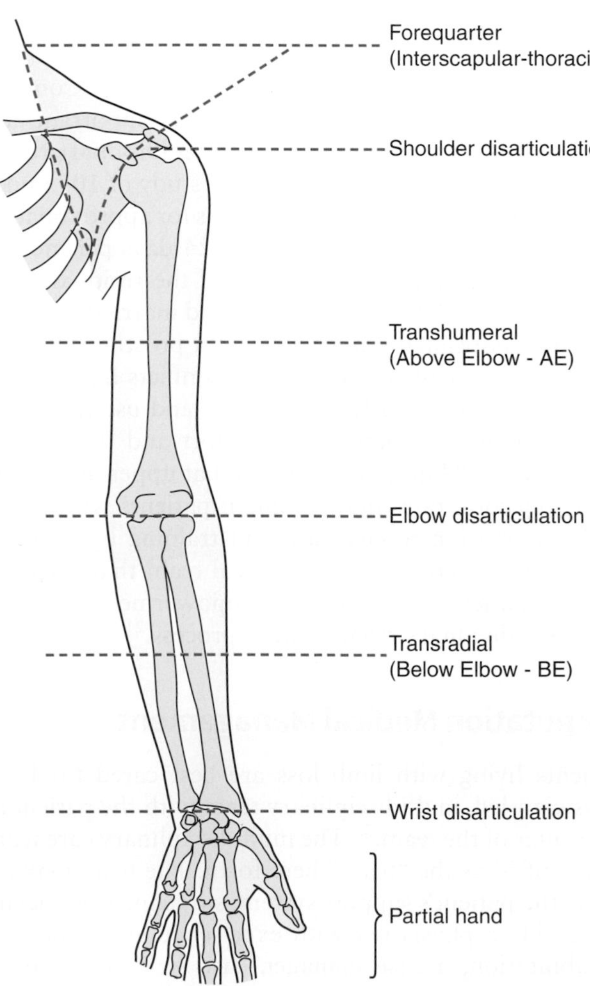

Figure 44-1. Levels of upper extremity amputations.

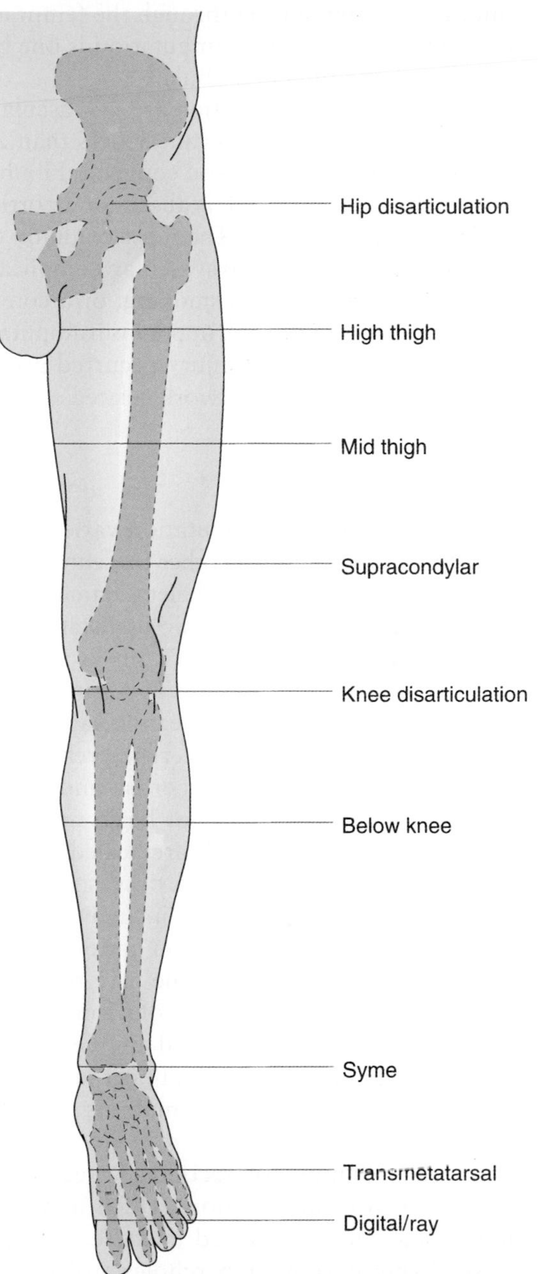

Figure 44-2. Levels of lower extremity amputations.

The term interscapulothoracic is an amputation of the arm, scapula, and clavicle, resulting in the loss of hand, arm, and scapular function. The term transhumeral is an amputation through the humerus, resulting in a loss of hand, wrist, forearm, and elbow function[4] and decrease in shoulder internal and external rotation. Transradial is an amputation through the radius and ulna, resulting in reduced forearm motion and loss of wrist and hand function.[4] Partial hand is an amputation through all or a portion of the metacarpals, and partial or complete amputations of the digits are referred to as digit or partial finger amputations. Partial hand and digit amputations result in complete loss or partial loss of grip function[4] and may impact dexterity and coordination. The term transfemoral is an amputation through the femur above the knee, whereas a transtibial amputation is one below the knee through the tibia and fibula.

The main causes of amputation are dysvascular disease (54%), trauma (45%), and cancer (less than 2%).[1] Other causes include infection and congenital limb deficiency in which a complete limb is absent or a portion of the limb is shortened at birth. The most common cause of lower limb amputation is dysvascular complications from diabetes, arteriosclerosis, smoking, or a combination of these.[5] Nearly 70% of all upper limb amputations are the result of trauma[6] and injury occurred primarily to males aged 15 to 45 years in work-related accidents.[7]

Sequelae

Course and prognosis after amputation varies based on the cause of limb loss as well as other present comorbidities (e.g., soft-tissue or musculoskeletal damage, neurovascular impairments, **heterotrophic ossification**). With acquired amputations, the surgeon's aim is to preserve as much limb length as possible. This aim, however, must be balanced against wound healing capability and residual limb coverage, patient preference, rehabilitation potential, and local prosthetic expertise and availability.[8] Fitting of a prosthesis does not begin until sutures are out and residual limb wounds are healed.

Signs and symptoms related to dysvascular disease that may lead to amputation may include nonexistent or failed medical or revascularization options of the extremity, significant loss of soft tissue as a result of the dysvascular condition, or complications from infections that can only be managed by surgical interventions.[9] Because trauma is the leading cause of upper limb amputations, there are often no signs or symptoms that lead up to the amputation.

There are a number of secondary health effects that may occur after amputation, which may include poor nutritional intake, reduced exercise, obesity, tobacco use, hypertension, hypercholesterolemia, skin issues, diabetes, and cardiac disease.[10] Patients who present with amputations related to dysvascular disease are at high risk for further complications about the residual limb and/or amputation of the contralateral limb because of the systemic nature of the disease process. They are also at higher risk for other health problems, such as cardiovascular disease, cerebrovascular accident, renal disease, and peripheral neuropathy.[5] Patient education should focus on the importance of engaging in a healthy lifestyle, including proper diet, regular exercise, avoidance of nicotine, and benefits of routine follow-up with medical providers for annual wellness examinations.

Individuals with major limb loss are at higher risk for the development of various medical and musculoskeletal complications.[11] Individuals with lower limb amputation are at higher risk for upper limb nerve entrapment.[12] According to research, individuals with unilateral upper limb amputation experience **musculoskeletal pain** in the neck, upper back, shoulders, and remaining limb,[13] but specific factors that lead to these conditions are not clear.[14] Preservation of the residual and contralateral limb, the individual's general health, and wellness are integral parts of ongoing care for these patients.[15]

Use of Prosthetic Devices

The level of amputation may affect the use of a prosthesis. The more proximal the amputation, the more difficult a prosthesis is to use. There are fewer joints and muscles available, so more complex suspension strategies are needed for control, device weight is greater, and more energy is required to use a device. The percentage increase in energy costs of prosthetic ambulation is 9% to 28% for unilateral transtibial, 40% to 60% for a unilateral transfemoral, 41% to 100% bilateral transtibial, and 280% for bilateral transfemoral amputations.[16]

Various reasons are cited in the literature why a patient decides to use or not use a prosthesis.[17] Comfort and function have long been accepted as important factors. Studies have attempted to reveal additional predictor variables of prosthetic use. In one study of 107 upper limb amputees, 56% wore a prosthesis for approximately 11 hours per day for an average of 24 days per month; this study identified longer length of the residual limb, the absence of phantom limb pain, and married status as variables associated with the use of a prosthesis.[18] Military service members from recent conflicts have higher than previously recorded acceptance and use rates that may be a result of improved comfort and function of prostheses.[19,20] Literature suggests that upper limb prosthetic rejection rates may decline if patients with upper limb amputation receive sufficient training by a highly specialized, interdisciplinary clinical team that provides focused patient education and empowerment throughout the individual's rehabilitation process.[21]

Amputation Medical Management

Patients living with limb loss are best cared for by a physician-led, multidisciplinary team with the patient at the center of the team.[5,6] The multidisciplinary care team is identified as the "team" here forth. The team may include the patient's support system; surgeon; a physician, preferably a physiatrist with experience in amputation rehabilitation; a case manager, case worker, or social worker; prosthetist; occupational therapist; physical therapist; behavioral health provider; trained peer support visitors or peer mentors;[5,6] and assistive technology specialist, if necessary.[22] Patients are active, equal members of the team and should be involved in a shared decision-making process in order to maximize their rehabilitation outcome with or without a prosthesis.[5,6,23] Ongoing, frequent, and routine open communication among the team members and the patient is imperative to ensure progress toward goals and for the patient to obtain higher levels of independence in both activities of daily living (ADLs) and instrumental activities of daily living (IADLs).[6]

Individuals with multiple limb loss present a unique set of challenges. Frequent team meetings regarding the initial focus of rehabilitation, achievable goals, and progression of prosthetic training for both upper and lower extremity amputations is highly recommended.[5,6] General considerations that will influence rehabilitation for this subset include (1) increased body temperature secondary to reduced body surface area; (2) increased risk of joint contractures, weight gain, deconditioning, and bone resorption as a result of immobility; (3) unique pain management needs, given architectural changes to the musculoskeletal system; (4) psychosocial issues, such as the importance of body image acceptance and return to work; and (5) likely ongoing medical risks, such as cardiovascular disease, metabolic dysfunction, musculoskeletal pain, and arthritis.[24–26]

Phases of Rehabilitation

In general, experts consider three phases of rehabilitation after amputation (see Table 44-1): perioperative, preprosthetic, and prosthetic training.[5,6] The beginning and end of each phase does not represent fixed points in time; they often overlap and, depending on the patient's recovery process, may be sequential. Additionally, throughout the patient's life as he or she learns to define a new normal, as well as receive different devices, he or she will move throughout these phases.[5,6] The focus of this chapter is primarily on management of individuals with upper limb amputation with general discussion on management of patients with lower limb loss. Therapists are encouraged to consult the appropriate Veteran's Administration/Department of Defense (VA/DoD) Clinical Practice Guidelines on upper[6] or lower extremity amputation[5] for more detailed information as well as other references when working with patients with multiple limb amputation.[27,52,58,63,66]

Patient Education

The team is charged with educating the patient and family throughout all phases of rehabilitation.[5,6] To facilitate informed decisions, clinicians should provide clear

Table 44-1. Phases of Rehabilitation

PHASE	BEGINNING EVENT MARKER	ENDING EVENT MARKER	INTERVENTION FOCUS
Perioperative[5,6] *(upper and lower limb amputations)*	Decision to amputate or after traumatic amputation	All wounds are healed, sutures are removed, the patient the patient has been medical cleared and has maximized independence in self-care ADL using adaptive strategies, assistive technology, or durable medical equipment.	• Wound care and healing • Edema control • Scar management • Pain control • Joint mobility and progressive physical conditioning • Psychological and emotional support • Connect with peer visitor or mentor.
Preprosthetic Training[6] *(upper limb amputations, only)*	Postsurgical period ends	Patient receives a preparatory (temporary) or definitive (permanent) prosthesis.	• Provide emotional support. • Stabilize limb volume, desensitize sensitive areas of residual limb, and optimize residual limb shape. • Progressive resistance exercises • Facilitate independence in ADL, change of dominance, and activities to strengthen motor patterns in preparation to operate the prescribed device. • Determine optimal type of prosthesis to meet patient's goals.
Prosthetic Training[6] *(upper limb amputations, only)*	Delivery of temporary or definitive prosthesis	Patient demonstrates a successful functional outcome with proper prosthetic use during desired functional activities.	• Control training • Repetitive drills • Functional training to learn to integrate the prosthesis as an assistive tool in daily activities that align with patient goals

ADL, activity of daily living.

and appropriate education that, at a minimum, includes surgical interventions when possible, amputation level, wound healing, residual limb management, pain management, rehabilitation programs and sequence of care, patient safety, potential psychological consequences and psychosocial adjustment issues, procedural and recovery issues, peer support groups, prosthetic types and options, and expected functional outcomes.[5,6] Patients with upper limb amputation should also be educated about overuse syndromes in the neck/upper back, the shoulders, and the remaining limb.[12,13]

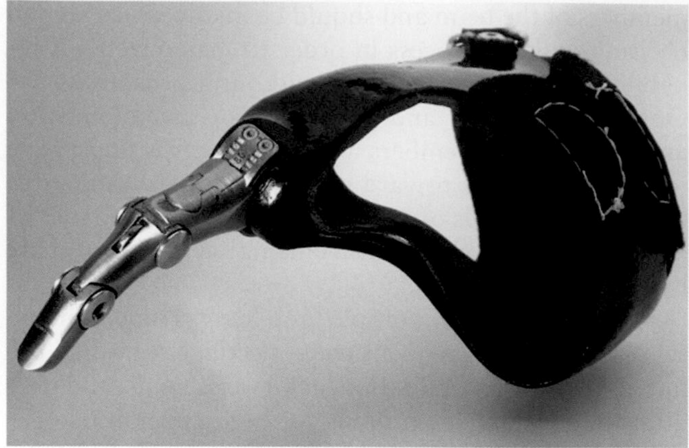

Figure 44-3. Heavy-duty positional locking index finger prosthesis by Point Designs, LLC (Louisville, CO) for a partial hand amputation.

Managing Expectations of an Upper Limb Prosthesis

The human hand executes numerous postures, prehension patterns, grip and pinch forces to engage in activity or with an object. Restoring functional capabilities of the hand through a prosthesis is an exceptional challenge because natural sensory feedback cannot be restored through any commercially available prosthesis. Many patients with upper limb loss have initial prosthetic expectations that are not realistic; no one device can restore human hand function, sensation, or appearance. Furthermore, a frequent goal of returning function and aesthetic appearance are often incompatible with each other in currently available prosthetic options.[23] It is critical that the team provide patient and family education to better manage device expectation.

An upper limb prosthesis is considered a tool to assist in the performance of a task or tasks and should not be considered a prime mover during any activity. Task performance can be achieved through activity modification, work simplification, compensatory strategies, commercially available adaptive aids, customized adaptive equipment design, and with the assistance of a prosthetic device. Success is unique to each individual patient,[28] and patients often benefit from the use of more than one type of prosthesis to regain independent function and restore quality of life.[6,23]

Upper Limb Prosthetic Options

The most common upper extremity prosthetic options currently available include passive, **body-powered (BP)**, **externally powered (EP)**, **hybrid**, and activity-specific prostheses. Passive prostheses do not have an active grasp but do provide functional benefits and can enhance individual recovery by restoring a sense of normalcy.[29] Depending on the level of amputation and prosthetic design, ratcheting passive joints may be used for heavy-duty activity (see Fig. 44-3) after a partial hand amputation. Passive prostheses are available to replace any part of a limb, from a single digit to a whole arm. A BP system operates through a cable and harness system that captures body motions proximal to the amputation to create tension through the cable and open or close the **terminal device (TD)**. There are BP options for major and minor amputations. With major amputations, BP TDs operate through one of two systems, voluntary-opening or voluntary-closing. In a voluntary-opening design, the TD remains in the closed position until force is exerted through the cable to open the TD. Terminal device often closes through force of rubber bands placed at the base of the TD. A voluntary-closing design remains open until force captured through the cable closes the TD; therefore, grip strength in this design is dependent on the strength of the prosthetic user. An EP system uses power external to the body for operation. A common type of EP prosthesis is known as myoelectric that requires electrical signals produced from muscle contractions to operate powered components. A hybrid system is a combination of two types of devices. Most commonly, this includes BP and electric components and is an option for patients with amputation at or above the elbow. An activity-specific prosthesis is designed for a specific function or activity, such as weight lifting or swimming.

A prosthesis is comprised of a socket, frame, and components. The socket encapsulates the residual limb and often has a very intimate fit to the skin. The frame encases the socket to provide stability and rigidity and serves to restore the length of the missing extremity. It may also house internal components, such as the wrist mechanism, batteries (if necessary), or electronics (if applicable). Components include prosthetic joints and TDs. Some prosthesis require harnessing to suspend the device from the residual limb. Some devices require use of socks or silicon sleeves that are placed over the residual limb before donning the device to enhance comfort or suspension. Some devices may include a cover such as a glove or sleeve that is external to the frame and some components. Often, these covers provide a more natural appearance of the missing limb.

Each prosthetic option has specific socket designs for various levels of amputation, as well as harnessing and suspension options, and available TDs. These topics are beyond the scope of this chapter; however when working with patients with upper limb amputation, the occupational therapist should meet with the fitting prosthetist to learn about device operation, appropriate device use, component information, and, if EP, control setup because all will impact prosthetic training.

Individuals with bilateral upper extremity amputations and amputation of three or more limbs present unique challenges when selecting the prosthetic systems. Early fitting with a temporary prosthesis on at least one upper limb is strongly recommended[30] to reduce dependency for self-care activities. One study identified that those with congenital amputation fit within 2 years of birth or those with acquired amputation fit within 6 months of amputation were 16 times more likely to continue prosthesis use.[17] Additional studies suggest that early fitting and prosthetic training may foster acceptance and use of the prosthesis.[21,31] If an early postoperative prosthesis is prescribed, daily communication between the patient, occupational therapist, and prosthetist is imperative to maintain proper fit and function.[6]

Functional Impairment in Daily Occupation after Amputation

Regardless of the level of limb loss or if the amputation is of the lower or upper extremity, every facet of an individual's life, as well as the family's, is impacted to some degree. Therefore, renegotiation is required. Consider how you would get up to go to the restroom at night if you did not have a leg. How would you dance at a wedding if you were missing an upper and lower limb, or cut food with a knife and fork if you were missing the radial portion of the hand?

Degree of impairment is influenced by the level of amputation, whether the patient has an upper or lower extremity amputation, the number of limbs amputated, and the presence of comorbidities. Additionally, level of functional impairment after an amputation or amputation(s), particularly of the upper extremity, is very individualized, because presentations uniquely vary. In general terms, those with more proximal amputations and multiple limb involvement tend to experience greater functional impairment in daily occupations than those who have unilateral distal amputations. Individuals with higher level of upper limb amputation (above the elbow) tend to experience greater challenges with accepting and using prostheses,[8] whereas those with partial hand amputation report greater perceived levels of disability than those with major upper limb amputation.[32] Patients with unilateral upper extremity limb loss experience difficulties with bimanual ADL and IADL. Limited evidence identifies that individuals with dominant hand injury have greater functional impairment,[33] and it has been the clinical experience of this author that individuals who sustain an amputation of the dominant hand demonstrate greater levels of impairment because the nondominant hand is forced to become the primary limb and executor of most activity.

Emotional Impact

Limb loss affects not only physical function but also the patient's competence and satisfaction in life roles: self-maintenance, family, and home; self-enhancement, such as engaging in leisure and community activities; and self-advancement as a worker or student.[34] Reactions to amputation are as complex as the unique nature of each human, and an individual's personality and belief system may influence how he or she responds to limb loss. Emotional reactions to the loss of a limb have been likened to grieving the loss of a loved one, and it impacts body integrity and sense of self.[22] Often, an initial response is shock and disbelief. Depression rates in those with lower limb amputations are higher than general population rates for up to two years after amputation.[35] Individual beliefs related to appearance and self-consciousness in public after lower limb amputation were associated with both distress and psychosocial adjustment difficulties.[35,36]

Patients with upper limb amputation are more likely than the general population to screen positive for depressive symptoms and post-traumatic stress disorder (PTSD).[37,38] Individuals with partial hand amputation are even more likely to screen positive for these psychological changes. Pain affects PTSD and depressive symptoms in this population because it impacts positive emotions and postinjury activity.[39] Furthermore, individuals who are less resilient tend to engage in avoidant coping behavior which is prospectively predictive of higher PTSD and depression.[40]

The patient may project negative feelings onto others so it's beneficial to encourage open discussion, develop a relationship based on trust and respect, and collaborate with the other team members to facilitate the patient's psychological adjustment and reintegration into previous roles. The therapist should communicate with and, when necessary, refer the patient to a behavioral health provider throughout the psychosocial adjustment periods of survival, recovery, and reintegration after limb loss.

The therapist should also provide the patient and caregiver(s) information about the therapy process and establish realistic goals and outcomes to help clarify expectations and reduce fear and anxiety, and reference materials on topics to include information on coping and adjusting to the amputation, information on prosthetic options, tips on how to manage ADLs independently, and a list of organizations as resources.

Actively listening to the patient and understanding life roles and future goals foster a sense of trust and control for the patient.

The therapist may introduce the patient to a peer visitor who has a similar amputation to facilitate discussion of stages of recovery, the rehabilitation process, and problem-solving strategies. Peer visits are most successful when the patient meets someone of the same sex, age, and with the same type of amputation.[6] Attendance to local or virtual amputation support groups may also be helpful for the patient to enhance his or her support structure.

Evaluation after Amputation

Evaluation of the patient with upper limb loss consists of a formal interview, physical evaluation, and observation of ADL and IADL performance, when possible. The evaluation is often ongoing and directed by the patient's recovery after amputation. The therapist notes the mechanism of injury and any comorbidities that occurred if the amputation is a result of trauma. If the surgical report is available, it is helpful to know if the residual limb muscles were surgically managed by **myodesis** or **myoplasty**.

The intent of the patient interview is to develop the patient's occupational profile to understand the personal, social, and cultural contexts and how he or she influences the individual response to injury. Key areas to discuss include vocational responsibilities, avocational interests, cultural factors, coping strategies, level of family or caregiver support, spiritual support, roles and responsibilities at home and in the community, accessibility to resources and services, as well as financial limitations or constraints. It is also helpful to learn if the patient has had previous exposure to individuals with amputation to assess his or her familiarity and to identify any language barriers, the patient's educational level, and the preferred learning style to effectively communicate and train the patient.[6]

Evaluation of Pain Associated with Amputation

The therapist should assess the presence, quality, intensity and duration of residual limb pain (RLP), associated musculoskeletal pain, phantom limb sensation (PLS), and phantom limb pain (PLP). The most often used pain assessment is the Visual Analog Scale (VAS) (0–100 mm), followed by the numeric rating scale (0–10) and verbal rating scale (0–3 = nil/mild/moderate/severe).[41] Both RLP and PLP occur more frequently and are more intense for those who have an upper limb amputation versus those with a lower limb amputation.[42] Postoperative RLP is expected and typically subsides as edema resolves and wound healing progresses. Recurrence or chronic RLP may be a result of several different causes and should be evaluated by the team to determine proper treatment.

Associated musculoskeletal pain occurs in other areas of the body, such as the back, neck, shoulder, or contralateral limb. This pain is often a result of compensatory motor patterns of the trunk and extremities from overuse and/or poor body mechanics because of fit and use of a prosthesis or no prosthesis use.[6] Other comorbidities may also be a source of this type of pain.

Nonpainful sensation experienced in the missing limb is PLS. PLS may be described as a sense of the phantom limb still being present, temperature changes, itching, pressure, and tingling. PLS is a universal phenomenon that is remarkably real to the patient and may last long term. The cause of PLS is still not clearly understood and is most common in adults with traumatic amputations, although it has been known to occur with congenital limb loss.[43]

PLP is any pain that is perceived in the amputated limb that is often described as an intense burning, stabbing, crushing, or shooting pain and is most common in traumatic amputations. PLP is exceptionally common after limb loss and is not clearly understood. Current theories suggest that the causes are related to central nervous system changes and peripheral nervous system damage.[44] Recent evidence specifically suggests that a substantial reorganization of the primary sensory and motor cortices occurs after hand amputation that is correlated with PLP.[45]

Evaluation of Neuromusculoskeletal and Sensory Impairments after Amputation

The therapist should measure residual limb length to the nearest bony landmark, measure edema through circumferential or figure-of-eight measurement, describe limb shape (i.e., cylindrical, conical, bulbous, or irregular), assess integrity of distal soft tissue, and assess any open or healing wounds (if present), as well as scar characteristics. Adherent scars can be problematic in the socket, resulting in a blister or skin breakdown.[46] The therapist should assess functional range of motion of the upper and lower extremities, proximal residual limb muscle strength, muscle strength in the contralateral limb, and observe unilateral and bilateral hand function. In the literature, the Modified Box and Blocks and the Jebsen-Taylor Test of Hand Function (JTHF) light- and heavy-can tests have been used to assess hand function with and without a prosthesis.[47–49] The therapist should assess proprioceptive, touch functions as well as residual limb sensitivity to pressure and temperature, as well as identify any areas of significant sensitivity about the residual limb that may be exceptionally tender to the touch, causing the patient to withdraw the limb. These may be signs of a **neuroma** or heterotrophic ossification, which may impact wear of prosthesis or use of the residual limb in ADLs. If the patient has lost a portion or all of the dominant hand and will be working on change of dominance training, assess dexterity of the nondominant hand.

Evaluation of ADL and IADL after Amputation

In an acute care setting, the Functional Independence Measure (FIM) may be used to determine ADL status after amputation. In outpatient settings, generic outcome measures are used, such as the Disabilities of the Arm Shoulder and Hand (DASH) or Canadian Occupational Performance Measure (COPM), although neither is validated with upper limb amputation. The QuickDASH was recently validated for use in this population,[50] and the Patient Specific Functional Scale (PSFS) has also been used,[47] but the measure is validated for individuals with upper limb musculoskeletal issues.[51] Regardless of setting, it's important to determine the individual's current level of functioning in bathing/showering, toileting and toilet hygiene, dressing, feeding, functional mobility, personal device care, personal hygiene and grooming, sexual activity, and rest and sleep.

The therapist should also assess the patient's abilities to navigate a healthy return to desired IADLs, areas of education, work, play, leisure, and social participation as the patient progresses through recovery. Return to IADL may be influenced by the patient learning his or her "new normal," so this may involve exploration of new occupations or return to prior occupations using different strategies or approaches. Returning to or integrating into new IADL is very individualized and may occur years after amputation, particularly if it is determined that the patient is not safe to return to his or her prior occupation and would benefit from vocational rehabilitation services.

Evaluation of the Prosthesis after Amputation

Initially, after device delivery, the occupational therapist evaluates the patient's ability to care and use prosthesis, specifically the ability to safely operate all components; ability to properly clean, maintain, wear, and use the device; and comfort and fit of the prosthesis. If the patient is fit with an EP prosthesis, the therapist must have a good understanding of the prosthetic control setup in order to assess and direct prosthetic controls training. Control setup refers to how the patient switches between components (i.e., elbow control, wrist control, and hand) as well as grip patterns, if available with the TD. The therapist should contact the prosthetist if there are any questions about the prosthesis setup.

Therapists may evaluate patient satisfaction with the prosthesis using standardized measurement tools as well as measuring performance while using a prosthesis; however, there is no gold standard for measurement. Adult patient satisfaction has been measured using the Trinity Amputation and Prosthetic Experience Scales (TAPES).[47] Unfortunately, there are few optimal functional clinical tests that assess upper limb prosthetic skill or performance in daily activity.[31] Generic time-based tests that reflect skill of device operation use[52] include the Southampton Hand Assessment Procedure (SHAP)[53] and the JTHF.[54] Others that demonstrate capacity of use[52] include the Assessment of Capacity for Myoelectric Control (ACMC)[55] and the Activities Measure for Upper Limb Amputees (AM-ULA).[56]

Intervention for Pain, Neuromusculoskeletal, and Sensory Impairment after Amputation

Occupational therapy treatment to address the abovementioned impairments will typically begin in the perioperative phase. Interventions involve residual limb management, range of motion and strengthening, and change of dominance training.

Residual Limb Management

Postoperatively, residual limb management includes wound healing, limb protection, edema control, residual limb shaping, pain management, and decreasing any areas of hypersensitivity.[6] In the upper limb, the residual limb is postoperatively wrapped in a figure-of-eight pattern with gauze and a compressive wrap. In the lower limb, postoperative dressings vary, depending on the level of amputation, surgical technique, healing requirements, patient compliance, and surgeon preference.[57] Dressings may include soft dressings similar to those used on the upper limb, nonremovable rigid dressings, immediate postoperative prostheses (IPOPs), removable rigid dressings, and prefabricated postoperative devices.[57] Soft dressings are typically used on patients with dysvascular disease.[57] Wound drains may be in place in either the upper or lower limb to help with edema.

Healing after an uncomplicated amputation follows a standard wound healing progression. If a skin or sheet graft is present, the therapist should follow wound care guidance provided by the surgeon or wound care team. Typically, sutures or staples are in place for 3 to 4 weeks, and the patient may be cleared to get the limb wet during this period. The limb may be cleaned with antibacterial soap and clean water and then gently dried. An appropriate dressing is applied, which may include use of a sterile nonadherent impregnated gauze, followed by gauze squares and gauze wrap applied in a figure-of-eight pattern. Once all sutures or staples are out, wounds are healed and maturing, the patient is instructed to wash the limb daily with water, mild soap, and dry thoroughly.

To facilitate wound healing, protect, shape, and reduce pain in the residual limb, the patient and caregiver

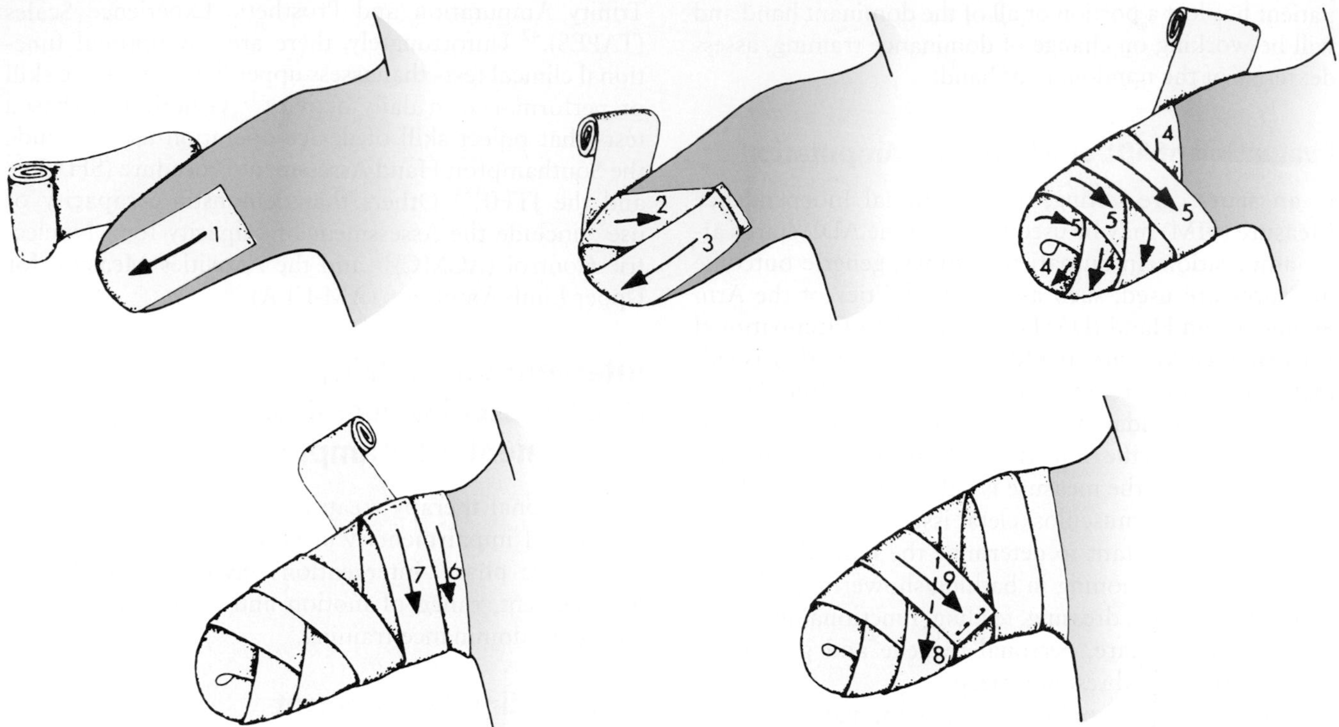

Figure 44-4. Wrapping technique for transhumeral amputation. Repeat diagonal turns as necessary to cover the limb with no constriction.

are instructed about the importance of figure-of-eight wrapping. The wrap must be applied in a figure-of-eight diagonal configuration, with the most pressure applied at the end of the limb to shape the residual limb into a conical shape if possible (Fig. 44-4). The bandage must conform firmly to the limb, be worn continuously, and reapplied immediately if it loosens. The patient or caregiver is advised to remove the wrap two to three times daily to examine the wound and assess skin for any redness or excessive pressure. The wrap is worn for 23 hours a day, and a clean bandage should be applied at least every 2 days.

Once wound drainage stops, use of an elastic compression shrinker or sock may be considered to replace the compression wrap if the residual limb skin can tolerate the shear forces from a shrinker application. Patients with diabetes often do not use a shrinker until 21 days postoperation.[57] The shrinker will be worn for the same duration as the compressive wrap and is worn after each prosthetic wear session and at night. It is recommended to continue to use the shrinker for up to 18 months until residual limb scars mature, shape, and size stabilize.[58]

Management of a patient's pain after amputation is complex and requires a team-based, patient-centric approach that blends pharmacological and nonpharmacological treatment strategies throughout all phases of rehabilitation. Nonpharmacological treatment strategies include transcutaneous electrical nerve stimulation (TENS), desensitization, graded motor imagery or mirror therapy[59] (Fig. 44-5), scar mobilization, relaxation, and biofeedback.[6] No single approach has proven to be clearly successful.[6]

Desensitization of the residual limb is necessary to prepare for fitting the socket or using the residual limbs in daily activities. Desensitization of the residual limb can be accomplished through percussion (tapping, rubbing, and vibration) with and without desensitization media and progressive loading against various surfaces. Loading begins with very resilient media, such as soft foam, to variously resistant and textured, such as layers of felt, a bucket of rice, and a mound of clay. Once

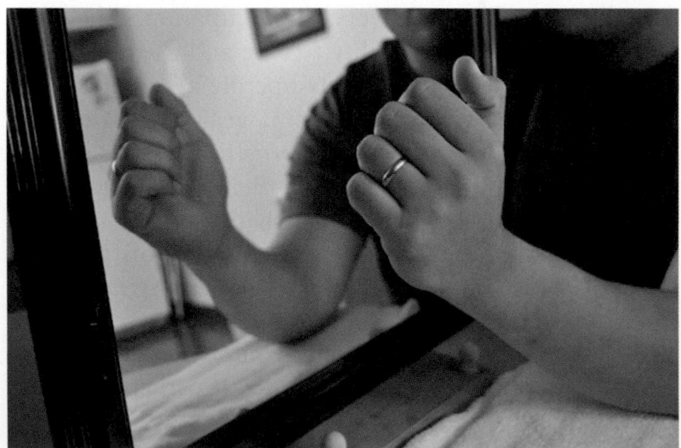

Figure 44-5. A patient with a transhumeral amputation performing mirror box therapy. Position the mirror at the patient's midline with the residual limb behind the mirror. Instruct him to continuously look at the reflection of the intact limb while performing mirror box therapy.

sutures are out, the patient and family receive instruction about scar massage to prevent or release adhesions and soften scar tissue, which can also help with pain.

Maintain or Increase Range of Motion and Strength

A physical conditioning program to increase or maintain the range of motion of all joints proximal to the amputation is initiated, which also increases circulation and reduces edema. Chronic limitation in shoulder external rotation on the side of limb deficiency is not uncommon,[60] so a structured shoulder stretching program in all planes of movement is initiated. The patient's anatomical sense of the phantom limb can be used to achieve motion in all planes. Bilateral horizontal adduction is beneficial for patients with bilateral limb loss to promote the use of the residual limbs at midline for self-care task performance.[58] In general, all patients with upper limb loss at any level are encouraged to incorporate the residual limb or digits into bilateral tasks during ADLs as much as possible.

A strengthening program focused on periscapular stabilization, rotator cuff strengthening, and strengthening of all major muscle groups proximal to the amputation is initiated bilaterally to increase endurance and prepare the limb for use or the weight of a prosthesis. Use of TheraBand CLX bands (Performance Health, Boiling Brook, IL) or lined weight-lifting cuffs such as Medicordz wrist cuffs (NZ Manufacturing, Tallmadge, OH) are recommended for residual limb resistance training. The contralateral side should be included if limitations are noted. A core strengthening program is initiated to promote postural control, balance, and endurance and to reduce asymmetry of the trunk and spine, which commonly occurs with upper limb loss.[60] Core stabilization during residual and upper limb strengthening promotes postural control in preparation for wearing and using a prosthesis, which may be perceived as heavy to the user.[58]

Change of Dominance

Change of dominance activities after dominant upper limb amputation must receive special attention.[61] The behavioral and neurological effects from long-term forced use of the nondominant hand are largely unknown.[62] *Handwriting for Heroes* (Loving Healing Press, Ann Arbor, MI; http://www.handwritingforheroes.com/) provides a structured 6-week program to change handwriting dominance. Education regarding one-handed techniques as well as recommend adaptive equipment[33] can greatly help the patient.

Intervention for Independence in ADLs after Amputation

A patient receiving a prosthesis must develop skills to be proficient with and without a prosthesis in his or her ADL because there will be times when the prosthesis will be in for repair. There are numerous adaptive strategies as well as adaptive equipment options available to assist patients with daily activities, such as:

- Nonslip grip materials
- Universal cuffs, Eazyhold universal cuff grip assist (EazyHold, Simi Valley, CA; www.eazyhold.com), or modified quadriplegic palmar clip with palmar pocket
- Built-up foam or Elastack (Sutton Scientifics, Inc., Star, NC) for handles or utensils
- Customized handles or tools with Allfit thermoplastic pellets (Orifit industries, Belgium)
- Modified long-handled sponges or wall-mounted back scrubbers
- Soap pockets or bath ropes
- Rocker knives (consider handle shape to maximize independence)
- Elastic shoelaces or Lock Laces (Positive Distribution, LLC, Durham, NC; www.locklaces.com)
- One-handed nail clippers and nail brushes
- Multipurpose bottle openers, electric can, and jar openers
- Pocket dresser (Performance Health Holdings, Inc., Warrenville, IL) or button hook
- Zipper pulls or key rings placed on zippers
- Pumps for bottles

Additionally, there are resources that discuss strategies to increase ADL independence after multiple limb loss, which are of great benefit to the occupational therapist.[6,63,66] Task analysis, creativity, and collaborative problem-solving between the occupational therapist and patient are paramount.

Intervention to Prepare for Prosthetic Fitting

Patients receiving a prosthesis will progress to the preprosthetic training phase while continuing necessary interventions initiated in the perioperative phase. Preprosthetic training focuses on acquiring necessary knowledge to operate the prescribed device and strengthening motor patterns so the patient is prepared to operate the prosthesis upon delivery. A collaborative relationship between the occupational therapist and prosthetist is critical during this and subsequent phases to properly prepare the patient for and train the patient on device use as well as problem solve prosthetic issue that may evolve during training.[63]

A patient fit with a BP device will use different body motions to operate the device depending on the level of amputation (see Table 44-2). Wrist-driven or hand-based prostheses use wrist flexion and extension or residual digit flexion and extension, respectively, to operate the prosthesis. Operation of transradial BP prosthesis is achieved through humeral flexion and scapular abduction. Function of a transhumeral BP prosthesis requires

Table 44-2. Motions to Operate Body-Powered Components Based on Level of Amputation

LEVEL	TERMINAL DEVICE OR DIGIT OPERATION	ELBOW COMPONENT OPERATION
Partial finger	PIP or MP flexion and extension	NA
Partial hand	Wrist flexion and extension	NA
Wrist disarticulation and transradial amputation	Humeral flexion and scapular protraction	NA
Elbow disarticulation and transhumeral	Humeral flexion and unilateral or biscapular protraction (see Fig. 44-6) Incorporating chest expansion may be used if necessary.	Combination of scapular depression, and humeral extension and abduction (see Fig. 44-7) to lock/unlock elbow

MP, metacarpophalangeal; NA, not applicable; PIP, proximal interphalangeal.

not only the same motion as a transradial prosthesis to operate the TD (Fig. 44-6) but also scapular depression and humeral extension and abduction to operate the elbow lock (Fig. 44-7). Strengthening of the serratus anterior, pectoralis major, and pectoralis minor on the side of the amputation is beneficial for a patient receiving a BP prosthesis.[58]

Muscle site testing and training is typically necessary for patients receiving an EP prosthesis. Testing is done by the prosthetist or therapist using a special myotester, such as Myolab II (Motion Control, Inc., Salt Lake City, UT) or Myoboy (Ottobock, Austin, TX), or a biofeedback computer program. With traditional direct control setup, prosthetic electrodes are applied to the residual limb typically over the agonist and antagonist muscles bellies. Figure 44-8 depicts a two-state direct control transradial system whereby two separate muscle groups are used to operate the TD. The intent is to choose muscle sites, or myosites, that are physiologically similar to the outcome motion and also produce strong electrical signals when contracted. Ideally, the two contractions can be isolated from one another. The preferred myosite is one in which the patient can maintain a steady contraction for at least 2 to 3 seconds and relax for the same amount of time. Wrist extensors and flexors are commonly chosen to achieve open and close of the TD or electric digits. For transhumeral amputations, the common choices are the biceps and triceps. For higher level amputations, as in shoulder disarticulation or interscapulothoracic amputations, the choices for control may be pectoralis or infraspinatus. To switch between prosthetic joint components, a co-contraction may be necessary or a strong versus light contraction may be used depending on the control set by the prosthetist. Once the optimal myosites are determined, the patient practices

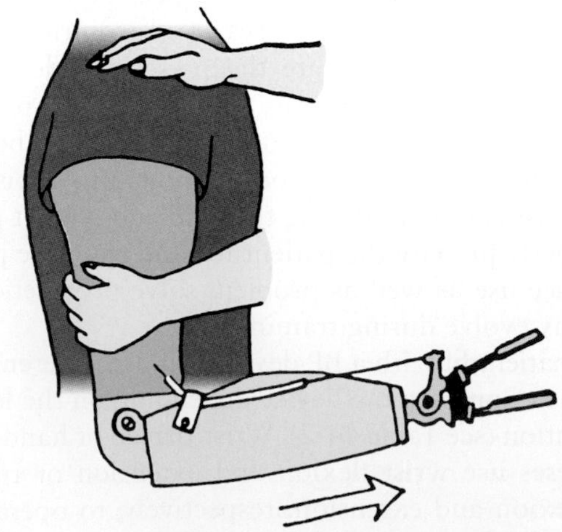

Figure 44-6. Teaching activation of voluntary-opening (*VO*) terminal device (*TD*). With elbow locked, the therapist guides the patient's upper arm forward to open *TD*. (Illustration by Gregory Celikyol.)

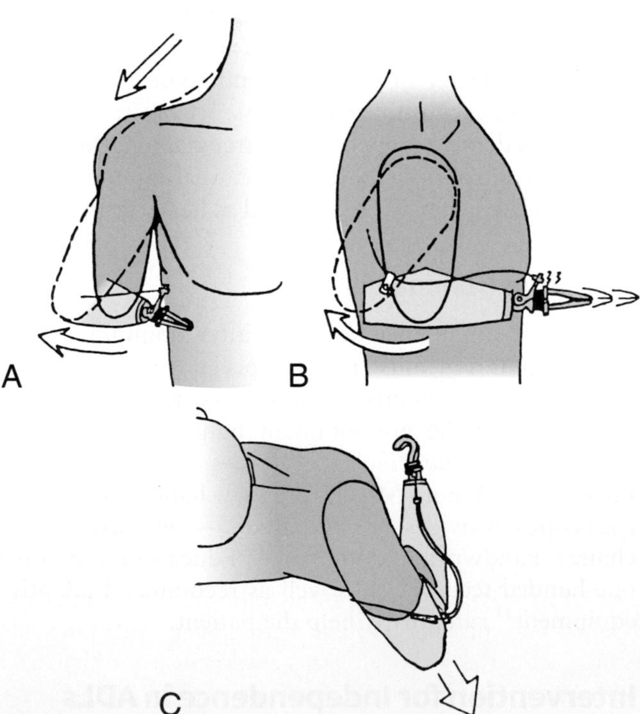

Figure 44-7. Motions (*arrows*) necessary to lock or unlock the elbow of a transhumeral prosthesis. **A.** Abduction with depression. **B.** Extension. **C.** Combined movement pattern of extension, depression, and abduction. (Illustration by Gregory Celikyol.)

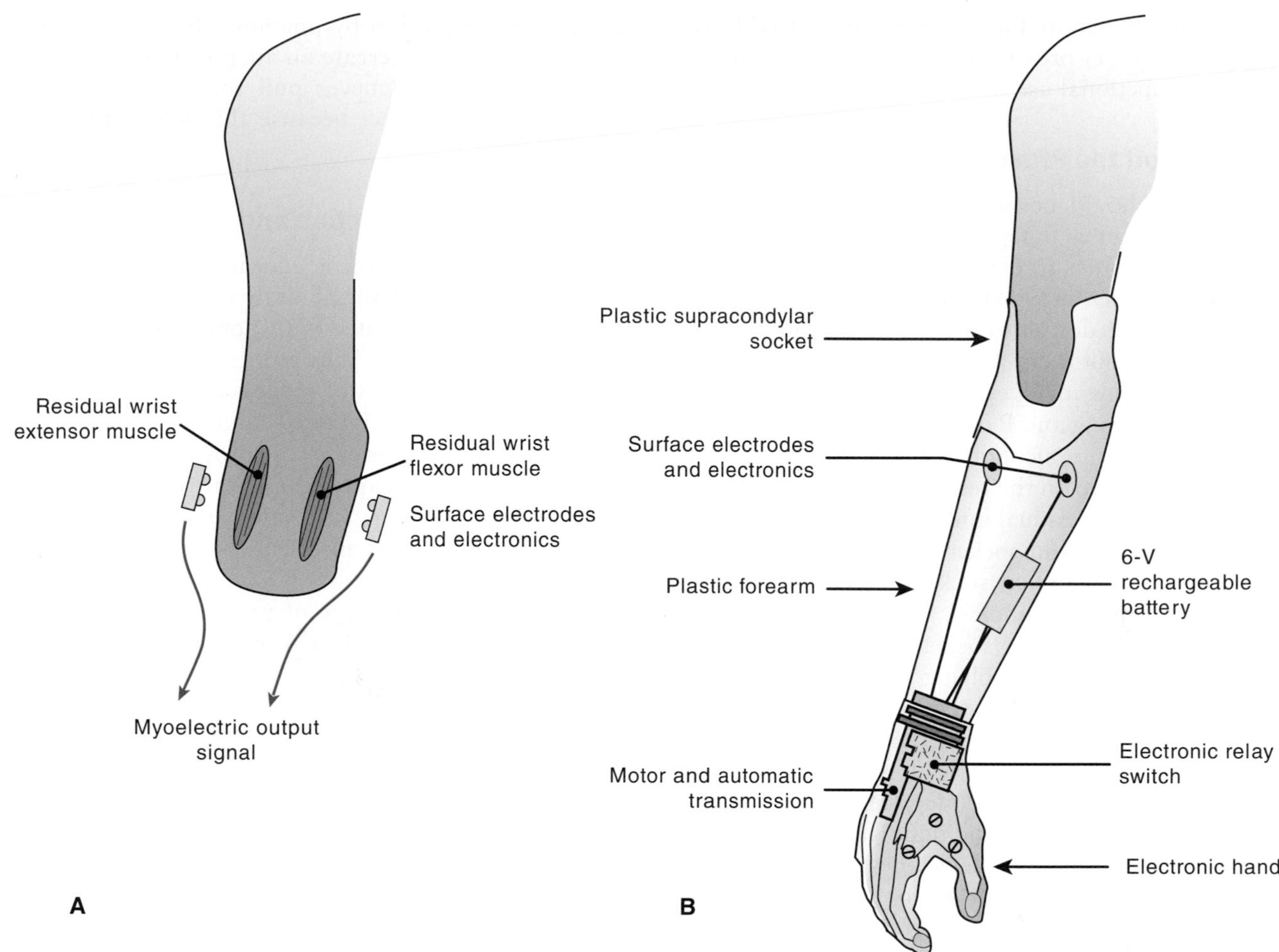

Figure 44-8. Myoelectric prosthesis, a direct control two-state system in which two separate muscle groups operate the terminal device. **A.** 1, The muscle contracts and creates an electrical signal that can be measured in microvolts (1 millionth of a volt). 2, The electromyography (EMG) signal is detected by the surface electrode. 3, The EMG signal is processed by the electronics and transmitted to the electronic relay in the hand. **B.** 1, When the electronic relay receives an EMG signal from the wrist flexors, the circuit is complete, and the electricity from the battery runs the motor to close the hand. 2, When the relay receives an EMG signal from the wrist extensors, the motor runs in the opposite direction to open the hand. (Illustration courtesy of Jack Hodgins, CPO, Kessler Institute for Rehabilitation, West Orange, NJ.)

with the feedback device to hone strength and isolate the skill of each myosite contraction. A single-case study is presented in the literature that describes utilization of a virtual reality environment to enhance motor learning for a patient training to use an advanced upper limb prosthesis in the preprosthetic phase of rehabilitation.[64]

Intervention with the Upper Limb Prosthesis

Use of a prosthesis is an important assistive tool, particularly because individuals with upper limb amputation tend to be younger, otherwise healthy individuals who have years of productivity remaining in life.[31] As previously discussed, some literature indicates a high abandonment rate in upper limb prosthetics. Proper training, however, may be helpful to improve compliance and use. Upper limb prosthetic training tends to be clinic dependent and is not grounded in evidence-based practice but rather expert opinion.[6] Recent literature has suggested the consideration of neurorehabilitation principles in the provision of prosthetic training because motor learning is a fundamental principle that must be considered when learning to integrate a prosthesis.[65]

Patients who are candidates for a prosthesis are fit with a device and then begin prosthetic training. The initial stage of treatment can generally be covered in one or two therapy sessions and should include the following:

- Evaluation to determine roles, tasks, and activity needs and preferences
- Evaluation of the prosthesis
- Explanation of the program goals to the patient
- Teaching the patient to don and doff the prosthesis
- Discussing the wearing schedule with the patient
- Teaching limb hygiene care
- Teaching care of the prosthesis

The therapy program for the prosthesis is addressed in two phases: (1) prosthetic controls training and (2) prosthetic functional use training.

Don and Doff the Prosthesis

The patient should be able to don and doff the full prosthetic system as independently as possible. The full prosthetic system may include a residual limb sock(s) or prosthetic liner, prosthetic socket, and harnessing as appropriate.[66] To don a prosthesis with a harness, the patient can either put it on like a coat or over the head like a pullover. Doffing involves reversal of the steps taken to don. When donning an EP or activity-specific prosthesis, the patient may use alcohol-based lubricant gels, powder, or a pull sleeve on the residual limb. The pull sleeve helps to guide the residual limb into the socket and provides the best skin and socket fit (Fig. 44-9, A–C). If a valve is used to maintain socket suspension, the valve is applied last when donning. Doffing requires release of the suction needed for socket suspension by removing the valve and either applying lubricant gel along the socket trim lines or working the residual limb soft tissue out of the socket. To promote the highest level of independence, the patient, therapist, and prosthetist may need to collaborate to determine the simplest or most ideal method for donning and doffing.

Donning of a passive device often involves use of an alcohol-based lubricant gel or use of special lotion. A thin layer of lubricant or lotion is applied to the inside of the device and to the residual limb. The patient pushes the limb into the socket and works all the air out to create a suction fit. Doffing also requires release of the suction by pinching the proximal edge of the prosthesis to create an air pocket in the socket. The patient should never pull the device off solely from the distal aspect because this may damage the prosthesis.

Residual Limb Inspection and Device Care

The patient or caregiver is educated about the importance of frequent residual limb inspection and signs and symptoms associated with poor residual limb tolerance, which include skin redness, irritation, or skin breakdown.[6] Any areas of redness on the residual limb that do not resolve within 20 minutes after device removal should be reported to the prosthetist, and the device should not be reapplied until after the patient has a prosthetic follow-up. Inspection of the residual limb after device removal is an essential part of the patient's daily routine.

Regardless of the type of prosthesis, the patient is expected to become proficient in basic prosthetic maintenance procedures for the device, as appropriate. These include (1) maintaining the socket daily (i.e., daily cleaning and socket inspection); (2) powering the device on and off and battery charging procedures, as applicable; (3) maintaining components (i.e., routine cleaning and lubrication); (4) adjusting the harness ; and (5) replacing the rubber band and changing the cable system for BP prosthesis.[66] The prosthetist is responsible for appropriate patient education and training of the abovementioned procedures, and the therapist ensures the patient can complete each task proficiently and with maximal independence within his or her everyday environment.

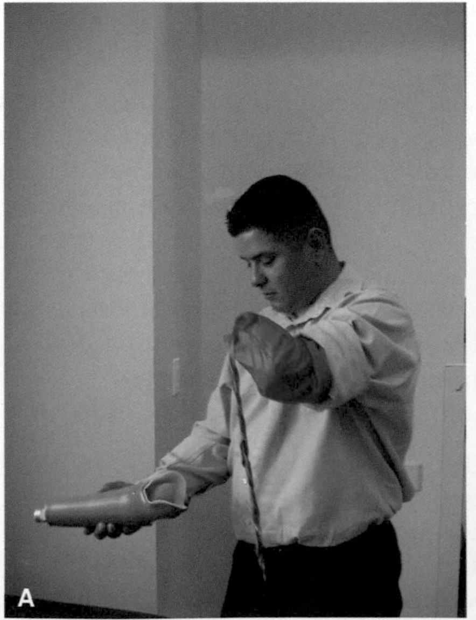

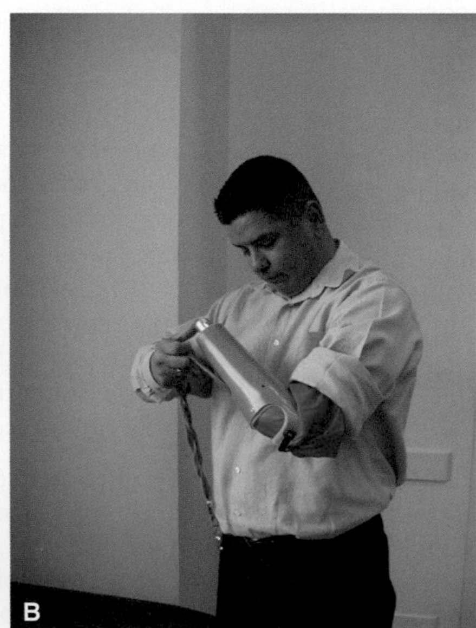

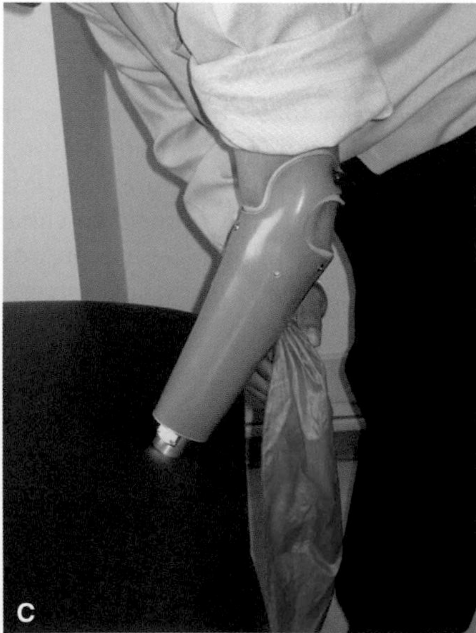

Figure 44-9. Transradial myoelectric prosthetic donning method with pull sock. This method can also be used to don transhumeral-level myoelectric prosthesis. **A.** Don the pull sock over the residual limb. **B.** Pull the lanyard of the pull sock through the socket opening. **C.** Pull the pull sock completely through to ensure good skin contact.

Prosthesis Wear Schedule

The patient and family are educated on the device wear schedule. Wear time is a gradual process to develop tolerance to the socket and device suspension. The importance of gradually increasing the wearing time cannot be overemphasized, particularly for patients with decreased sensation and scar tissue.[66] Initial wear time is for 30 minutes three times per day, followed by a residual limb skin inspection. If there are no signs of poor fit, wear time may be increased by 15 minutes each session and should be continued until the patient tolerates device wear all day or for the necessary amount of time to complete selected activities of the patient.

Prosthetic Controls Training

Controls training is necessary for patients fit with BP, EP, and passive positional devices. The prosthetist educates the patient how to control the device, and the therapist works with the patient to develop skill with control progressively grading the environment. Refer to Figures 44-10 and 44-11 for schematic overview of controls training for BP and EP prostheses by level of amputation, respectively. The intent of controls training is for the patient to correctly and consistently operate each device component(s), learn to preposition component(s) to reduce awkward body mechanics as appropriate during use, and hone skills in proportional control. Prepositioning refers to positioning components either passively (BP or passive) or actively (BP or EP) prior to task execution to reduce proximal compensatory movements during device operation. The therapist instructs the patient to determine the most natural and efficient device position before grasping an item. Proportional control involves the user learning to elicit ample force with the TD or prosthetic digits to grasp objects without dropping or

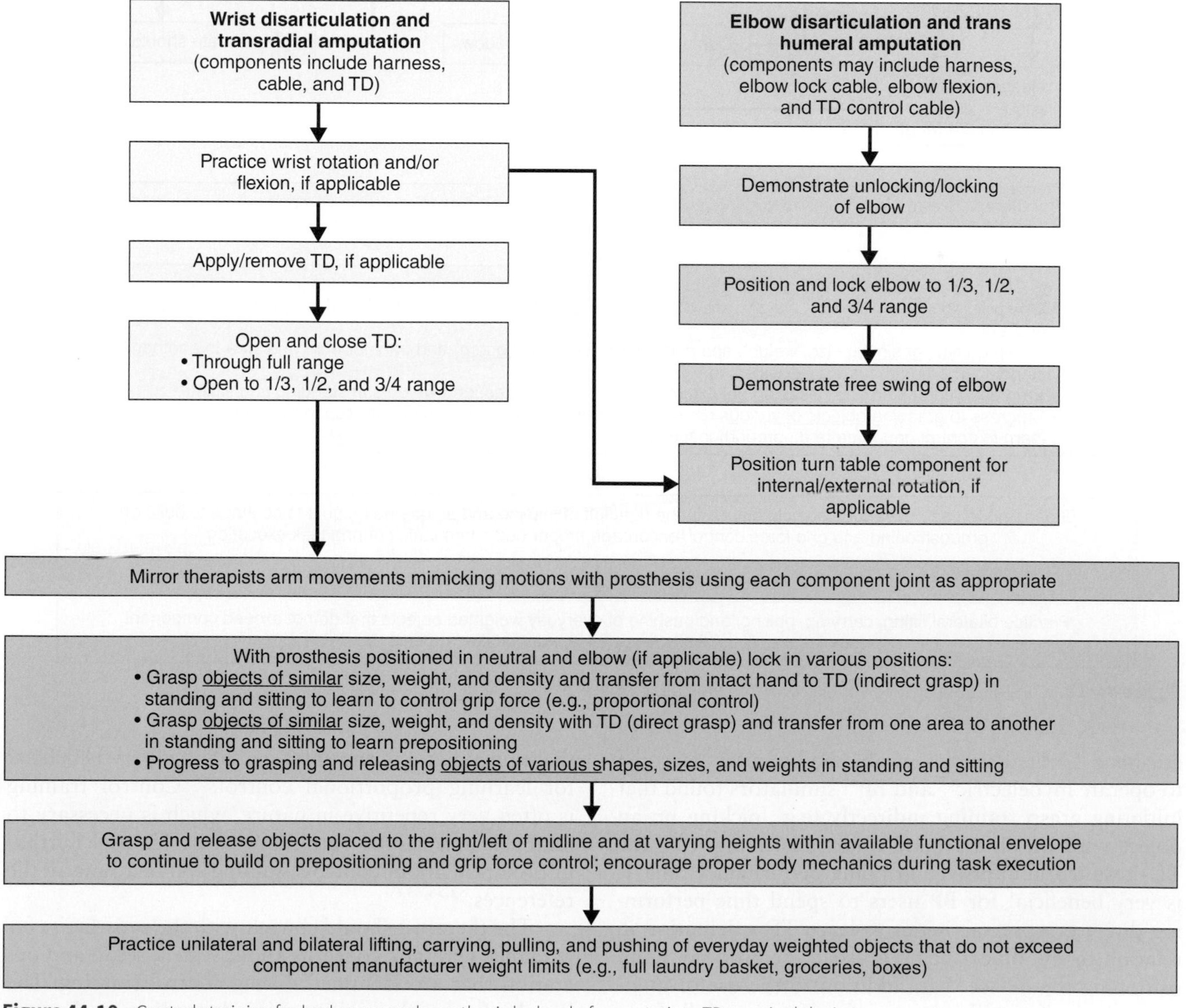

Figure 44-10. Controls training for body-powered prosthesis by level of amputation. *TD*, terminal device.

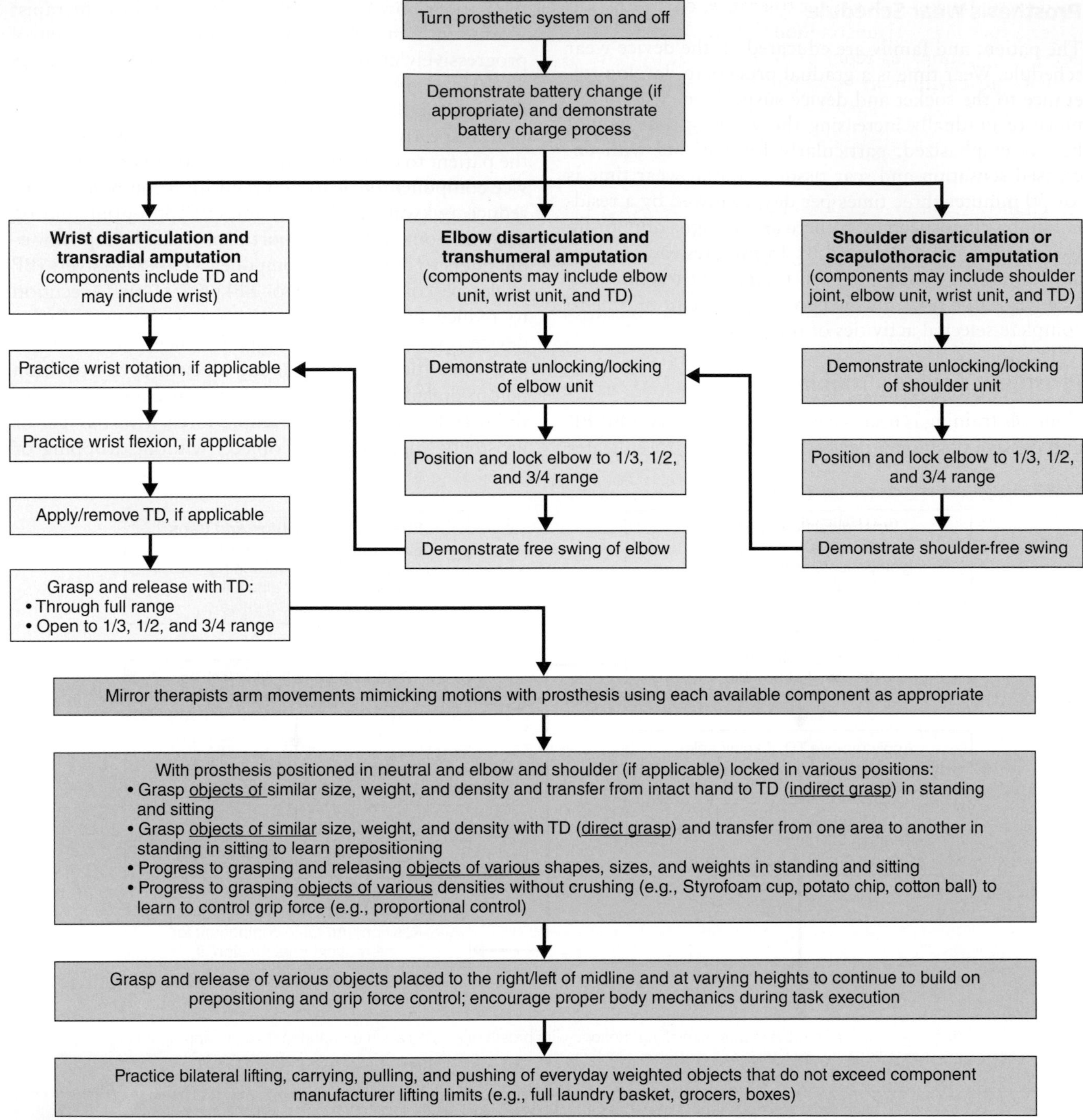

Figure 44-11. Controls training for externally powered prosthesis by level of amputation. *TD*, terminal device.

crushing. Limited studies of able-bodied users learning to operate myoelectric[67] and BP[68] simulators found that initiating grasp training indirectly (e.g., picking up an object with the intact hand and transferring it to the TD) resulted in improved gripping performance time. It is very beneficial for BP users to spend time performing direct grasping activities to learn TD orientation in relation to the object being grasped, or properly prepositioning the device.[68] In addition to the use of intermanual transfer skills, the transfer of motor skills from the trained hand to the untrained hand is very beneficial for learning proportional control.[69] Control training is often very repetitive in nature, which is necessary to establish new motor patterns with device use. Further information about controls training can be found in the references.[52,58,63,66]

The therapist should consult with the prosthetist for guidance with any concerns about system setup and operation that are identified during control training. The length of control training varies, depending on the type of device, the patient's gadget tolerance, cognition, and motivation. It is not uncommon for those with higher level amputations to require more control training as well as those with more advanced EP prosthesis.[21]

Functional Training with the Upper Limb Prosthesis

Spontaneous, automatic, skillful use of the prosthesis as an assistive tool during bimanual tasks is the hallmark sign of a skilled prosthetic user. The goal of functional training is to teach the patient how to use the device as a tool to maximize independence and reduce caregiver burden, safely integrate the device into daily bimanual activities appropriately, reduce learned compensatory motions from one-handed use during bimanual tasks, maintain proper body mechanics during device use, and instill patient confidence in the ability to operate and rely on the device for function.

A person with a unilateral amputation can be expected to use the prosthesis primarily for sustained holding or for stabilization. Table 44-3 suggests how some activities can be accomplished. A key component to successful training is deliberate practice using the prosthesis for realistic, functional tasks. Much of functional training involves repetition to help the patient develop new motor pathways in the brain to execute daily tasks with skill and efficiency using the prosthesis. A small case study used modified constraint-induced movement therapy as part of a 3-week home prosthetic training program and results showed a meaningful change based on objective performance measure scores whereas self-report outcome measures demonstrated mixed results.[70]

It is also important that the user complete activities within a reasonable length of time while using minimal extraneous movement and energy expenditure. The therapist encourages patients to analyze and see similarities among situations and reminds them of relevant principles. This prepares the patient to respond with a sense of control in unpredictable situations.

In the final stage, prosthetic functional use skills are further developed, and ADLs that are more demanding are

Table 44-3. Suggested Approaches for Functional Activities: Unilateral Upper Limb Amputation

TASK	PROSTHESIS	INTACT LIMB
Eating		
Cut food	Hold fork	Cut with knife
Butter bread	Stabilize bread	Spread toward body
Fill glass from faucet	Hold glass	Turn knob or lever
Carry tray	TD in midposition to hold	Hold in midposition
Peel fruit	Stabilize with TD	Peel
Dressing		
Don and doff shirt or blouse	Don: prosthesis in sleeve first; doff: remove intact arm first	Don: intact arm last; doff: remove prosthesis last
Put clothing on hanger	Hold hanger	Place clothing on hanger
Buckle belt	Stabilize belt	Push belt through buckle
Tie bow	Stabilize lace	Manipulate and make loops
Button cuff on intact side	Use buttonhook (or sew on button using elastic thread)	Hold cuff in place with fingertips while using buttonhook
Use zipper	Hold fabric with TD	Pull zipper
Desk skills		
Write	Stabilize paper	Write
Insert letter in envelope	Hold, stabilize envelope at end	Insert letter and seal
Use phone, dial, take notes	Hold receiver: TD or with chin and shoulder	Dial and write
Draw line with ruler; use paper clip	Stabilize ruler; hold paper	Draw line; apply clip
General skills		
Take bill from wallet	Hold wallet or stabilize on table	Manipulate wallet and remove bill
Wrap and unwrap package	Stabilize box and paper	Manipulate box, paper, tie
Thread needle	Hold needle	Thread needle

TD, terminal device.

introduced. Exploration of use of a prosthesis during IADL performance should also be considered and encouraged if use of a prosthesis is appropriate and not contraindicated for the type of device used. Advanced functional training centers on the patient's goals and is very individualized, so therapy should take place in the clinic as well as in relevant environments and contexts in which the patient engages in occupations. Visits to the community, home, school, and work are strongly advised. This brings the patient and therapist into the actual environment, away from simulated, static settings of a clinic. Figures 44-12 to 44-15 show sample functional ADL and IADL tasks.

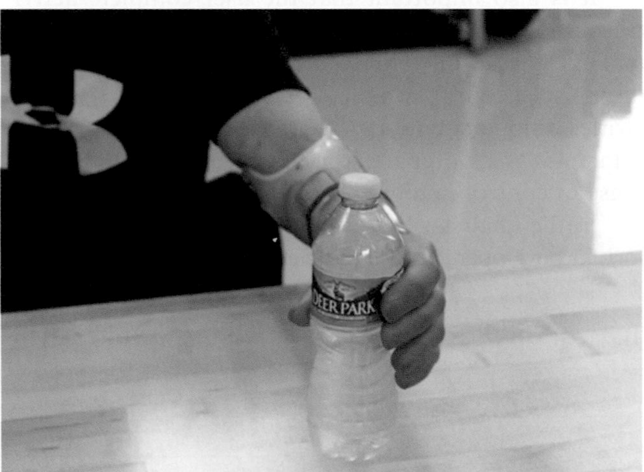

Figure 44-12. The practice of holding a bottle of water with a myoelectric prosthesis and electric hand is an excellent functional activity to learn proportional control and build individual confidence in the prosthesis.

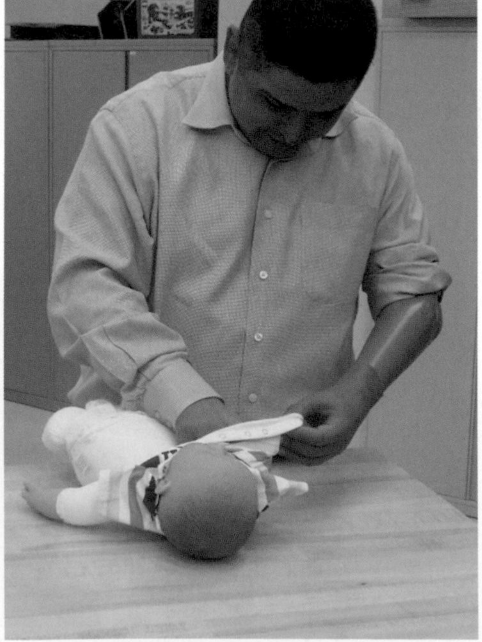

Figure 44-13. Practicing bimanual tasks with a myoelectric prosthesis and electric hand. This individual changing a diaper and dressing a doll using his prosthesis as an assist.

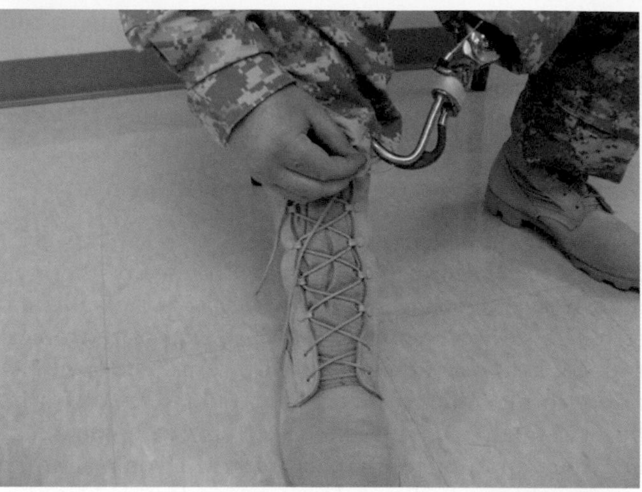

Figure 44-14. Tying military boots with a body-powered prosthesis. The individual is using the hook as an assist to hold the lacing during this task.

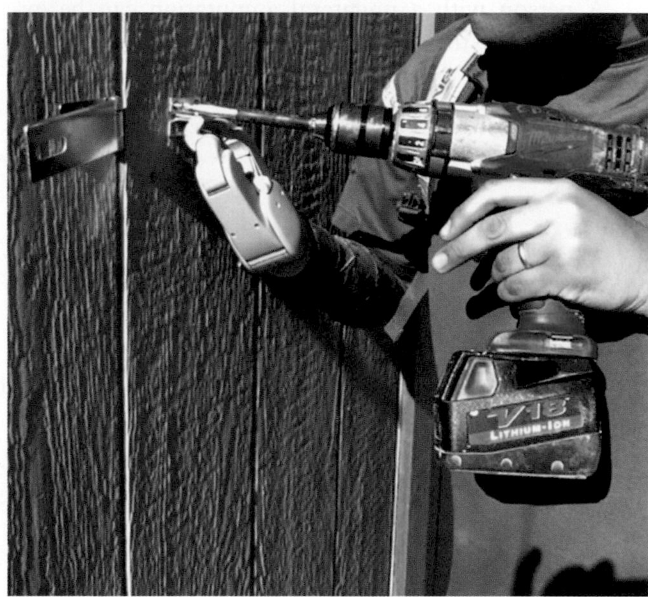

Figure 44-15. Using a hybrid prosthesis and electric hook for a bimanual home maintenance task. The individual has prepositioned the elbow and wrist to stabilize hardware with the electric hook and securing it with a drill using intact hand.

Driving and Community Mobility

Driving is usually of considerable importance. Many patients are eager to return to driving following either an upper and/or lower limb amputation. Safe and independent driving involves a complex interaction of multiple systems to include one's physical, visual, cognitive, and behavioral abilities. When appropriate, the patient should be referred for a comprehensive driving assessment. The driving rehabilitation specialist will complete an assessment and make recommendations for any needed adaptive equipment or vehicle modifications. For example, a spinner knob or driving ring may be recommended for patients with a unilateral upper extremity amputation. Installation of a left-foot accelerator bar and pedal may be necessary for a person with a right lower extremity amputation. Hand controls can be installed for patients with bilateral leg amputations. Patients are encouraged to contact their state licensing agency or department of motor vehicles to determine whether there are any limitations or driving restrictions for those individuals with amputations.

Rehabilitation after Lower Limb Amputation

The therapeutic program for patients with lower limb amputations requires collaboration between the physical therapist and the occupational therapist. This may occur in the acute care setting immediately following amputation, in an outpatient clinic, or in the patient's home. Both therapists will perform an evaluation of the patient. The physical therapist is typically responsible for limb wrapping, core and lower limb strengthening exercises, range of motion, preprosthetic, prosthetic, and gait training.

Initial patient treatment sessions by both professionals may focus on ADLs to include patient and family education on wound care, limb wrapping, bed mobility, transfers, and basic wheelchair propulsion and management skills. After lower limb amputation, the therapist must consider general health condition, strength, and endurance and how these influence patient safety when performing ADL or IADL. Safety is a major concern with lower limb amputations, particularly for patients with other comorbidities. Patient and family are educated on safety precautions with specific activities such as transfers. Treatment sessions may include safe transfers from the wheelchair to the bed, toilet, furniture, and car. Early patient education on desensitization of the residual limb is also addressed.

The occupational therapist may also include other self-maintenance skills, such as kitchen tasks, housecleaning, and bed-making during the treatment sessions. Home and community visits with the patient may be indicated. During standing activities and ambulation, special attention is paid to balance, posture, and equal weight bearing through both lower extremities. Visual or verbal cues should be used to correct these impairments, if necessary. The physical therapist or the occupational therapist will teach fall recovery to the patient and the family because safety after amputations is always important.

The occupational therapist may recommend home modifications and equipment. Equipment often includes a transfer tub bench or shower chair for use while showering and bathing and grab bars in the shower/tub and around the toilet. These rails provide a means of arm support that assists with lowering to the toilet and coming to the standing position safely.

The primary surgical or medical team will clear the patient to start wearing a shrinker on his or her lower residual limb prior to receiving the first prosthesis. The patient needs to be educated on the proper shrinker donning techniques and care of the shrinkers and liners. The shrinkers should have no wrinkles, and seams should not be over bony areas or the scar. The patient must inspect the skin on the residual limb daily to check for any changes in skin integrity before and after shrinker, liner, or prosthetic wear. If the patient has difficulty inspecting the residual limb, a long-handled mirror may be used to assist.

The physical therapist will assess and recommend the lower extremity prosthetic wearing schedule, the amount of assistance required, and assistive devices needed, as well as readiness for any standing or ambulation activities. A patient needs to be able to don and doff the lower extremity prosthesis independently. If unable, a family member needs to be educated and able to demonstrate the proper technique in donning and doffing the prosthesis. The occupational therapist continues to address ADLs with the patient both with and without the prosthesis. The occupational therapist works with the patient to identify how to incorporate the prosthesis into daily activities while assessing energy, effort, balance, transfer, and mobility skills. Energy conservation methods should be included in the program. Further information pertaining to rehabilitation strategies for individuals with lower limb amputations can be found in the reference.[46]

Conclusion

Rehabilitation of an individual with an amputation is best managed through a holistic, multidisciplinary approach with a team of clinicians highly specialized in amputation rehabilitation.[6] Rehabilitation after amputation is a process that takes time in order for the patient to accommodate the phases of adjustment, acceptance, healing, recovery, and ultimate mastery of skills needed to achieve higher levels of function and independence after such a life-changing event. The field of prosthetics is rapidly developing and necessitates expertise to remain abreast of new technologies; however, keystone principles of occupation-based, patient-centered rehabilitation remain the foundation for a successful rehabilitation experience.

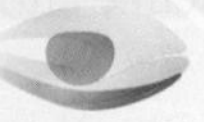

CASE STUDY

Patient Information

Alex is a 25-year-old, right-hand–dominant, married male injured in a work-related accident. He sustained a right partial hand amputation of digits 1 to 3 after a 1200-pound metal object crushed his hand. He works as a machinist, making heavy equipment engine parts. He has a GED and has worked for the company for 3 years. Attempts were made to salvage his fingers, and he was treated with multiple irrigation and debridement, but ultimately his fingers could not be saved. His right thumb, and index and middle fingers are amputated at the middle metacarpal level, and he had no impairments to the ring and small fingers.

Reason for Occupational Therapy Referral

Alex is referred to outpatient occupational therapy for evaluation and treatment of his right hand after amputation 4 weeks ago.

Assessment Process and Results

During his initial outpatient appointment, the goals and expectations of the patient and his family were determined. Alex's pain, neuromusculoskeletal, and sensory status, as well as his ability to participate in his roles and occupations were determined. The extent of education he and his family had received about rehabilitation after amputation and prosthetic options was identified. During the evaluation, he reported that he has burning electric-type pain in his phantom fingers that worsens at night. He has little tolerance for light touch or deep pressure to his residual hand. His incisions are well healed, and the sutures have been removed, but there is a layer of thick dead dermis over the incision. His motion in his remaining digits and proximal joints on the right arm and on the left are within functional limits. His strength in the right shoulder, elbow, and left arm are normal, but his right wrist and hand strength are limited by pain. He is not using his right hand in any activity. He gets help from his spouse to wash his back, left underarm, and dry off. He has difficulty applying deodorant to his left underarm, holding his razor and toothbrush with either hand, and managing buttons and zippers on clothing. He cannot floss his teeth, cut his nails, and needs his wife to cut his food because he cannot hold a knife and fork. He also has a difficult time stabilizing plates when he eats. He has difficulty holding his cell phone, texting or dialing phone numbers, and typing on his computer keyboard. He likes to work in his shop at home fixing up old cars, but he has not touched his shop since the accident. He and his wife enjoy going to dance halls on weekends, but he has not wanted to go out; he is afraid of what people will think of him, and he does not like to be asked about his hand. He is not sure that he can return to work and do his previous job. He is not sleeping well, identifying that his mind races about his future and the many unknowns. He has met with the local upper limb prosthetic specialist, looked at device options, and is going to get a passive positional finger prosthesis so that he can get back into his home shop.

Occupational Therapy Problem List

- Dependence in some ADL and IADL
- Residual limb sensitivity
- Phantom limb pain
- Decreased strength in right wrist and hand
- Loss of prehension of the dominant hand
- Disuse of right dominant hand in activity, resulting in performance of most tasks one handed
- Sleep problems
- Avoidant coping behaviors

Occupational Therapy Goal List

Long-term goal: Alex will be independent in ADL and actively participate in home management, meal preparation, and shopping in 3 months.

Initial short-term goals:

- Alex will be able to perform ADLs with modified independence using adaptive equipment and adaptive strategies with his left hand and residual right hand.
- Alex will demonstrate compliance with a prescribed home exercise program to manage his right residual hand sensitivity to optimize use and prepare for fitting of a prosthesis.
- Alex will increase his right wrist strength to 5/5 and increase his right-hand strength to 40% of the mean for his age to prepare his right hand for use in activity.
- Alex will demonstrate compliance with change of dominance training by completing the *Handwriting for Heroes* program within 6 weeks.
- Alex will self-select and use relaxation strategies to calm his mind in preparation for sleep five nights of the week.
- Alex will self-identify two positive coping strategies that he will use when participating in structured therapeutic community reintegration activities.

Intervention

Alex is seen two to three times per week for 4 weeks in the clinic. Treatment focuses on identifying adaptive equipment items that will help reduce pain and fatigue when using his right residual hand (e.g., built-up foam on handles) and increase his independence with ADL. A residual limb management program will be initiated to address hypersensitivity, adherent

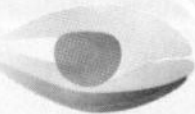

CASE STUDY *(continued)*

scar, and weakened musculature in the right wrist and hand. Strengthening exercises will involve isometric and kinetic exercise with use of a wrist cuff or TheraBand CLX (Performance Health Holdings, Inc., Warrenville, IL) resistance bands, despite not being able to comfortably hold weight in his right hand. Strengthening of the extrinsic and intrinsic muscles of the right hand will be addressed as well with resistive putty. Dexterity training of the left hand as well as change of dominance activities will be incorporated into treatment. Exploration of various relaxation strategies as well as active coping strategies will be explored with the patient. He will be expected to self-select one of each strategy during future treatment. He will also explore graded motor imagery to help self-manage his PLP. Once fit with his prosthesis, he will be trained on device care, wear, and safe use as an assistive tool in daily activities. Attention will be given to prepositioning the prosthesis to optimize secure grip of light objects and motor learning because his left hand will have to become the prime executor of tasks with the right hand providing support.

Next steps:

- Continue to assess and improve ADL and IADL status with and without prosthesis.
- Meet with a peer visitor who has a similar level amputation.
- Explore local support groups and support patient through psychological recovery process.
- Facilitate community reintegration.
- Educate patient and family in risks of developing overuse injuries, use of proper body mechanics during activity performance with and without the prosthesis, and training in work simplification and energy conservation strategies.
- Collaborate with multidisciplinary care team about vocational rehabilitation and support patient through exploration.
- Provide patient and family education about additional prosthetic options that may be useful tools in his future (e.g., passive silicone restoration or EP devices).
- Communicate results of discussion to multidisciplinary team and prosthetist.

Evidence Table of Intervention Studies for Amputation Rehabilitation

Intervention	Description	Participants	Dosage	Research Design and Evidence Level	Benefit	Statistical Significance and Effect Size
Mirror therapy to reduce PLP in unilateral males with upper limb amputations[59]	Experimental group ($n = 9$) completed mirror therapy. Control group ($n = 6$) completed covered mirror or mental visualization therapy.	Active duty service members, beneficiaries, or retirees between the age of 18 and 70 years with unilateral upper extremity amputation. Subjects were randomly assigned to either the mirror therapy group (MTG) ($n = 9$) or the control group (CG) ($n = 6$).	Both groups completed 15 minutes daily of structured movement of the intact and residual limbs using the assigned therapy (MTG vs. CG), 5 days/week for 4 weeks. Subjects in the CG were given option to switch to mirror therapy after 4 weeks (20 sessions).	Randomized controlled trial Level I	Eight (89%) subjects in MTG experienced a decrease in PLP and a decrease in the time spent experiencing PLP. Seven subjects in the MTG initially reported constant pain and five no longer reported this at the end of the intervention. Five in the CG who crossed over to the MTG all had a decrease in pain severity and time experiencing pain.	In the MTG, the group pain score decreased from a mean of 41.4 to 27.5 mm on a 100-mm VAS ($p = 0.001$), therapy had a large effect on pain reduction (Cohen's $d = 0.971$), and therapy had a large effect on time experiencing pain (Cohen's $d = 0.924$).
Comparison of (1) learning direct grasp tasks (DG); (2) learning indirect grasp (IG) tasks; (3) learning fixation (FIX) tasks (i.e., stabilize object with device and execute task with intact hand); (4) learning a combination (COM) of all three tasks; and (5) no practice to learn to grasp with myoelectric prosthetic simulator and an Ottobock VariPlus Speed hand[67]	The experimental group (EG) (1) practiced learning assigned tasks with a myoelectric simulator (2) to assess performance improvement, SHAP test administered at pretest, posttest, and two retention tests. The CG performed the SHAP two weeks apart with no training.	Able-bodied, right-handed participants with normal or corrected to normal vision, and no earlier experience with a prosthetic simulator were randomly assigned to the EG (DG, IG, FIX, COM) ($n = 31$). CG was 31 gender-matched participants.	EG learned each assigned task with simulator for five sessions over a 2-week period. The DG, IG, and FIX groups performed 15 trials with four objects in a random order. The COM group performed five trials per object per task (DG, IG, FIX), resulting in 20 trials per task.	Randomized controlled trial Level I	Training is necessary to improve skill in prosthetic use. Fine motor control of the myoelectric hand (e.g., adjusting opening and closing to different object characteristics) takes longer to learn than gross motor control (i.e., positioning the prosthesis in space). Begin myoelectric training with IG tasks in order to promote success with device use. Use a blocked, repeated order structure in training to improve overall function faster. Learning grip force takes a long time and requires special attention and use of deformable objects.	Significantly larger improvement on SHAP in EG as compared to CG ($F = 21.61, p = 0.00$). DG and COM regulated grip force better over sessions, whereas IG showed no improvement in object compression ($F = 3.22, p = 0.01$); however, IG had fastest performance. Shorter reach times were observed with hard resistance objects ($F = 11.66, p = 0.00$).

Comparison of (1) learning direct grasp tasks (DG), (2) learning indirect grasp (IG) tasks, (3) learning fixation (FIX) (i.e., passive object stabilization with the device and tasks), (4) learning a combination (COM) of all three tasks, and (5) no practice to learn to grasp with body-powered prosthetic simulator with TRS voluntary-closing Hook, Grip 3, and figure 9 harness[69]	The EG practiced learning the tasks they were assigned with a BP prosthetic simulator. The SHAP was administered at pretest, posttest, and two retention tests (2 weeks and 3 months) to assess performance improvement. The CG performed the SHAP with no training.	Training group of 30 right-handed able-bodied participants were randomly assigned to one of four training groups: DG $n = 7$, IG $n = 8$, FIX $n = 7$, and COM $n = 8$. CG of 17 right-handed able-bodied participants.	The EG learned each assigned task with simulator for five sessions over a 2-week period. The DG, IG, and FIX groups performed 15 trials with four objects in a random order. The COM group performed five trials per object per task (DG, IG, FIX), resulting in 20 trials per task.	Randomized controlled trial Level I	EG and CG improved on the SHAP at posttest and both retention tests. DG showed biggest improvement in functionality after training. IG used less force than the COM group while picking up objects, suggesting that IG benefits force control with BP device. DG training helps the user learn how to orientate the hook to the object to be grasped. Start BP training with IG tasks.	Shorter reach times in IG group ($p < 0.03$) Grip force control takes time to learn ($F = 4.21$; $p < 0.03$). Largest SHAP improvement in DG group (exact value not presented)

References

1. Ziegler-Graham K, MacKenzie EJ, Ephraim PL, Travison TG, Brookmeyer R. Estimating the prevalence of limb loss in the United States: 2005 to 2050. *Arch Phys Med Rehabil.* 2008;89:422–429. doi:10.1016/j.apmr.2007.11.005.
2. Owings MF, Kozak LJ. Ambulatory and inpatient procedures in the United States, 1996. *Vital Health Stat 13.* 1998;139:1–119.
3. Dillingham TR, Pezzin LE, MacKenzie EJ. Limb amputation and limb deficiency: epidemiology and recent trends in the United States. *South Med J.* 2002;95(8):875–883.
4. Amputation, Upper Extremity, in Adults: Occupational Therapy. Esbsco Web site. https://www.ebscohost.com/promoMaterials/September_2016_-_Amputation_Upper_Extremity.pdf. Published August 5, 2016. Accessed November 4, 2018.
5. US Department of Veterans Affairs and US Department of Defense. VA/DoD Clinical Practice Guideline for Rehabilitation of Individuals with Lower Limb Amputation. Version 2.0 2017. https://www.healthquality.va.gov/guidelines/Rehab/amp/VADoDLLACPG092817.pdf. Accessed May 21, 2018.
6. US Department of Veterans Affairs and US Department of Defense. VA/DoD Clinical Practice Guideline for the Management of Individuals with Upper Extremity Amputation Rehabilitation. Version 1.0 2014. https://www.healthquality.va.gov/guidelines/rehab/uear/index.asp. Accessed May 21, 2018.
7. Esquenazi A. Amputation rehabilitation and prosthetic restoration. From surgery to community reintegration. *Disabil Rehabil.* 2004;26(14-15):831–836. doi:10.1080/09638280410001708850.
8. Nanos GP. Wrist disarticulation and transradial amputation: surgical management. In: Krajbich JK, Pinzur MS, Potter BK, Stevens PM, eds. *Atlas of Amputations and Limb Deficiencies.* 4th ed. Rosemont, IL: American Academy of Orthopaedic Surgeons; 2016:221–231.
9. Swaminathan A, Vemulapalli S, Patel MR, Jones WS. Lower extremity amputation in peripheral artery disease: improving patient outcomes. *Vasc Health Risk Manag.* 2014;10:417–424. doi:10.2147/VHRM.S50588.
10. Pasquina PF, Hendershot BD, Isaacson BM. Secondary health effects of amputation In: Krajbich JK, Pinzur MS, Potter BK, Stevens PM, eds. *Atlas of Amputations and Limb Deficiencies.* 4th ed. Rosemont, IL: American Academy of Orthopaedic Surgeons; 2016:697–706.
11. Robbins CB, Vreeman DJ, Sothmann MS, Wilson SL, Oldridge NB. A review of the long-term health outcomes associated with war-related amputations. *Mil Med.* 2009;174(6):588–592. doi:10.7205/MILMED-D-00-0608.
12. Pyo J, Pasquina PF, Demarco M, et al. Upper limb nerve entrapment syndromes in veterans with lower limb amputations. *PMR.* 2010;2(1):14–22. doi:10.1016/j.pmrj.2009.10.002.
13. Ostlie K, Franklin RJ, Skjeldal OH, Skrondal A, Magnus P. Musculoskeletal pain and overuse syndrome in the adult acquired major upper-limb amputees. *Arch Phys Med Rehabil.* 2011;92(12):1967–1973. doi:10.1016/j.ampr.2011.06.026.
14. Burger H, Vidmar G. A survey of overuse problems in patients with acquired or congenital upper limb deficiency. *Prosthet Orthot Int.* 2016;40(4):497–502. doi:10.1177/0309364615584658.
15. Varma P, Stineman MG, Dillingham TR. Epidemiology of limb loss. *Phys Med Rehabil Clin N Am.* 2014;25(1):1–8. doi:10.1016/j.pmr.2013.09.001.
16. Shah SK. Cardiac rehabilitation. In: Frontera WR, Gans BM, Walsh NE, Robinson LR. eds. *DeLisa's Physical Medicine & Rehabilitation: Principles and Practice.* 5th ed. Philadelphia, PA: Lippincott Williams & Wilkins; 2010.
17. Biddiss EA, Chau TT. Upper limb prosthesis use and abandonment: a survey of the last 25 years. *Prosthet Orthot Int.* 2007;31(3):236–257. doi:10.1080/03093640600994581.
18. Raichle KA, Hanley MA, Molton I, et al. Prosthesis use in persons with lower- and upper-limb amputation. *J Rehabil R D.* 2009;45(7):961–973.
19. Gailey R, McFarland LV, Cooper RA, et al. Unilateral lower-limb loss: prosthetic device use and functional outcomes in service members from Vietnam war and OIF/OEF conflicts. *J Rehabil R D.* 2010;47(4):317–331. doi:10.1682/jrrd.2009.04.0039.
20. McFarland LV, Hubbard-Winkler SL, Heinemann AW, Jones M, Esquenazi A. Unilateral upper-limb loss: satisfaction and prosthetic-device use in veterans and service members from Vietnam and OIF/OEF conflicts. *J Rehabil R D.* 2010;47(4):299–316. doi:10.1682/jrrd.2009.03.0027.
21. Resnik L, Meucci MR, Lieberman-Klinger S, et al. Advanced upper limb prosthetic devices: implications for upper limb prosthetic rehabilitation. *Arch Phys Med Rehabil.* 2012;93(4):710–717. doi:10.1016/j.apmr.2011.11.010.
22. Pasquina PF, Miller M, Carvalho AJ, et al. Special considerations for multiple limb amputation. *Curr Phys Med Rehabil Rep.* 2014;2(4):273–289. doi:10.1007/s40141-014-0067-9.
23. Melton DH. Physiatrist perspective on upper-limb prosthetic options: using practice guidelines to promote patient education in the selection and the prescription process. *J Prosthet Orthot.* 2017;29(4S):40–44. doi:10.1097/JPO.0000000000000157.
24. Harvey ZT, Loomis GA, Mitsch S, et al. Advanced rehabilitation techniques for the multi-limb amputee. *J Surg Orthop Adv.* 2012;21(1):50–57.
25. Davidson JH, Jones LE, Cornet J, Cittarelli T. Management of the multiple limb amputee. *Disabil Rehabil.* 2002;24(13):688–699. doi:10.1080/09638280110115384.
26. Naschitz JE, Lenger R. Why traumatic leg amputees are at increased risk for cardiovascular disease. *Q J Med.* 2008;101(4):251–259. doi:10.1093/qjmed/hcm131.
27. Smurr Walters L, Yancosek KE, Acker D, Conyers D. Rehabilitation of the upper extremity amputation and prosthetic training. In: Skirven TM, Osterman AL, Fedorczyk J, eds. *Rehabilitation of the Hand and Upper Extremity.* 7th ed. Philadelphia, PA: Elsevier; in press.
28. NiMhurchadha S, Gallagher P, MacLachlan M, Wegener ST. Identifying successful outcomes and important factors to consider in upper limb amputation rehabilitation: an international web-based Delphi survey. *Disabil Rehabil.* 2013;35(20):1726–1733. doi:10.3109/09638288.2012.741138.

29. Maat B, Smit G, Plettenburg D, Breedveld P. Passive prosthetic hands and tools: a literature review. *Prosthet Orthot Int*. 2018;42(1):66–74. doi:10.1177/0309364617691622.
30. Uellendahl JE. Bilateral upper limb prostheses. In: Smith DG, Michael JW, Bowker JH, eds. *Atlas of Amputations and Limb Deficiencies: Surgical, Prosthetic and Rehabilitation Principles*. Rosemont, IL: American Academy of Orthopaedic Surgeons; 2004:311–325.
31. Østlie K, Lesjø IM, Franklin RJ, Garfelt B, Skjeldal OH, Magnus P. Prosthesis use in adult acquired major upper-limb amputees: patterns of wear, prosthetic skills and the actual use of prostheses in activities of daily life. *Disabil Rehabil Assist Technol*. 2012;7(6):479–493. doi:10.3109/17483107.2011.653296.
32. Davidson J. A comparison of upper limb amputees and patients with upper limb injuries using the Disability of the Arm, Shoulder and Hand (DASH). *Disabil Rehabil*. 2004;26(14-15):917–923. doi:10.1080/09638280410001708940.
33. Troianello T, Yancosek K, Rhee PC. Unilateral hand training on functional performance in patients with upper extremity trauma. *J Hand Ther*. 2017;32(1):25–34.e2. doi:10.1016/j.jht.2017.10.002.
34. Murray CD. The social meanings of prosthesis use. *J Health Psychol*. 2005;10(3):425–441. doi:10.1177/1359105305051431.
35. Horgan O, MacLachlan M. Psychosocial adjustment to lower-limb amputation: a review. *Disabil Rehabil*. 2004;26(14-15):837–850. doi:10.1080/09638280410001708869.
36. Atherton R, Robertson N. Psychological adjustment to lower limb amputation amongst prosthesis users. *Disabil Rehabil*. 2006;28(19):1201–1209. doi:10.1080/09638280600551674.
37. Desmond DM. Coping, affective distress, and psychosocial adjustment among people with traumatic upper limb amputations. *J Psychosom Res*. 2007;62(1):15–21. doi:10.1016/j.jpsychores.2006.07.027.
38. Reiber GE, McFarland LV, Hubbard S, et al. Servicemembers and veterans with major traumatic limb loss from Vietnam war and OIF/OEF conflicts: survey methods, participants, and summary findings. *J Rehabil R D*. 2010;47(4):275–298. doi:10.1682/jrrd.2010.01.0009.
39. Walsh MV, Armstrong TW, Poritz J, Elliott TR, Jackson WT, Ryan T. Resilience, pain interference, and upper limb loss: testing the mediating effects of positive emotion and activity restriction on distress. *Arch Phys Med Rehabil*. 2016;97(5):781–787. doi:10.1016/j.apmr.2016.01.016.
40. Elliott T, Hsiao Y, Kimbrel N, et al. Resilience, traumatic brain injury, depression, and posttraumatic stress among Iraq/Afghanistan war veterans. *Rehabil Psycho*. 2015;60(3):263–276. doi:10.1037/rep0000050.
41. Humble SR, Dalton AJ, Li L. A systematic review of therapeutic interventions to reduce acute and chronic postsurgical pain after amputation, thoracotomy or mastectomy. *Eur J Pain*. 2015;19(4):451–465. doi:10.1002/ejp.567.
42. Hanley MA, Ehde DM, Jensen M, Czerniecki J, Smith DG, Robinson LR. Chronic pain associated with upper-limb loss. *Am J Phys Med Rehabil*. 2009;88(9):742–751. doi:10.1097/PHM.0b013e3181b306ec.
43. Price EH. A critical review of congenital phantom limb cases and a developmental theory for the basis of body image. *Conscious Cogn*. 2006;15(2):310–322. doi:10.1016/j.concog.2005.07.003.
44. Flor H, Nikolajsen L, Staehelin Jensen TS. Phantom limb pain: a case of maladaptive CNS plasticity? *Nat Rev Neurosci*. 2006;7(11):873–881. doi:10.1038/nrn1991.
45. Raffin E, Richard N, Giraux P, Reilly KT. Primary motor cortex changes after amputation correlate with phantom limb pain and the ability to move the phantom limb. *Neuroimage*. 2016;130:134–144. doi:10.1016/j.neuroimage.2016.01.063.
46. Klarich J, Brueckner I. Amputee rehabilitation and preprosthetic care. *Phys Med Rehabil Clin N Am*. 2014;25(1):75–91. doi:10.1016/j.pmr.2013.09.005.
47. Resnik L, Borgia M. Reliability and validity of outcome measures for upper limb amputation. *J Prosthet Orthot*. 2012;24(4):192–201. doi:10.1097/JPO.0b013e31826ff91c.
48. Resnik L, Borgia M. Responsiveness of outcome measures for upper limb prosthetic rehabilitation. *Prosthet Orthot Int*. 2016;40(1):96–108. doi:10.1177/0309364614554032.
49. Resnik L, Borgia M, Silver B, Cancio J. Systematic review of measures of impairment and activity limitation for persons with upper limb trauma and amputation. *Arch Phys Med Rehabil*. 2017;98(9):1863–1892. doi:10.1016/j.apmr.2017.01.015.
50. Resnik L, Borgia M. Reliability, validity, and responsiveness of the QuickDASH in patients with upper limb amputation. *Arch Phys Med Rehabil*. 2015;96(9):1676–1683. doi:10.1016/j.apmr.2015.03.023.
51. Hefford C, Abbott JH, Arnold R, Baxter GD. The patients-specific functional scale: validity, reliability, and responsiveness in patients with upper extremity musculoskeletal problems. *J Orthop Sports Phys Ther*. 2012;42(2):56–65. doi:10.2519/jospt.2012.3953.
52. Hermansson LN, Turner K. Occupational therapy for prosthetic rehabilitation in adults with acquired upper-limb loss: body-powered and myoelectric control systems. *J Prosthet Orthot*. 2017;29(4S):45–50. doi:10.1097/JPO.0000000000000154.
53. Light CM, Chappell PH, Kyberd PJ. Establishing a standardized clinical assessment tool of pathologic and prosthetic hand function: normative data, reliability, and validity. *Arch Phys Med Rehabil*. 2002;83(6):776–783. doi:10.1053/apmr.2002.32737.
54. Jebsen RH, Taylor N, Trieschmann RB, Trotter MJ, Howard LA. An objective and standardized test of hand function. *Arch Phys Med Rehabil*. 1969;50(6):311–319.
55. Hermansson LM, Fisher AG, Bernspang B, Eliasson AC. Assessment of capacity for myoelectric control: a new Rasch-built measure of prosthetic hand control. *J Rehabil Med*. 2005;37(3):116–171. doi:10.1080/16501970410024280.
56. Resnik L, Adams L, Borgia M, et al. Development and evaluation of the activities measure for upper limb amputees. *Arch Phys Med Rehabil*. 2013;94(3):488–494.4e. doi:10.1016/j.apmr.2012.10.004.
57. Gailey RS, Gaunaurd IA, Laferrier J. Physical therapy management of adults with lower limb amputations. In: Krajbich JK, Pinzur MS, Potter BK, Stevens PM, eds. *Atlas of Amputations and Limb Deficiencies*. 4th ed. Rosemont, IL: American Academy of Orthopaedic Surgeons; 2016:597–620.
58. Fletchall S. Upper limb prosthetic training and occupational therapy. In: Krajbich JK, Pinzur MS, Potter BK, Stevens PM, eds. *Atlas of Amputations and Limb Deficiencies*. 4th ed. Rosemont, IL: American Academy of Orthopaedic Surgeons; 2016:351–362.

59. Finn SB, Perry BN, Clasing JE, et al. A randomized, controlled trial of mirror therapy for upper extremity phantom limb pain in male amputees. *Front Neurol.* 2017;8:267. doi:10.3389/fneur.2017.00267.
60. Postema SG, van der Sluis CK, Waldenlöv K, Norling Hermansson LM. Body structures and physical complaints in upper limb reduction deficiency: a 24-year follow-up study. *PLoS ONE.* 2012;7(11):e49727. doi:10.1371/journal.pone.0049727.
61. Yancosek KE, Howell D. Systematic review of interventions to improve or augment handwriting ability in adult clients. *OTJR (Thorofare NJ).* 2011;31:55–63. doi:10.3928/15394492-20100722-03.
62. Philip BA, Frey SH. Compensatory changes accompanying chronic forced use of the nondominant hand by unilateral amputees. *J Neurosci.* 2014;34(10):3622–3631. doi:10.1523/JNEUROSCI.3770-13.2014.
63. Swanson Johnson S, Mansfield E. Prosthetic training: upper limb. *Phys Med Rehabil Clin N Am.* 2014;25(1):133–151. doi:10.1016/j.pmr.2013.09.012.
64. Resnik L, Etter K, Klinger SL, Kambe C. Using virtual reality environment to facilitate training with advanced upper-limb prosthesis. *J Rehabil R D.* 2011;48(6):707–709.
65. Wheaton LA. Neurorehabilitation in upper limb amputation: understanding how neurophysiological changes can affect functional rehabilitation. *J Neuroeng Rehabil.* 2017;14(1):41–53. doi:10.1186/s12984-017-0256-8.
66. Smurr LM, Gulick K, Yancosek K, Ganz O. Managing the upper extremity amputee: a protocol for success. *J Hand Ther.* 2008;21(2):160–175. doi:10.1197/j.jht.2007.09.006.
67. Bouwsema H, van der Sluis CK, Bongers RM. Changes in performance over time while learning to use a myoelectric prosthesis. *J Neuroeng Rehabil.* 2014;11:16–31.
68. Huinink LH, Bouwsema H, Plettenburg DH, van der Sluis CK, Bongers RM. Learning to use a body-powered prosthesis: changes in functionality and kinematics. *J Neuroeng Rehabil.* 2016;13:90–102. doi:10.1186/s12984-016-0197-7.
69. Romkema S, Bongers RM, van der Sluis CK. Influence of the type of training task on intermanual transfer effects in upper-limb prosthesis training: a randomized pre-posttest study. *PLoS One.* 2017;12(11):e0188362. doi:10.1371/journal.pone.0188362.
70. Cancio J, Edmondson A, Yancosek KE. Modified constraint-induced movement therapy for persons with a unilateral upper extremity amputation. *J Hand Ther.* 2018;31(1):143–144. doi:10.1016/j.jht.2017.11.005.

Acknowledgments

The author wishes to acknowledge the work of the authors from previous editions of this chapter: Kathleen Yancosek and Sarah Mitsch (7th edition), and Kathy Stubblefield and Anne Armstrong (6th edition). The author also wishes to acknowledge Matthew Walters, DPT, for his review of this chapter. The author thanks Dr. Diane Dirette for her guidance and support for this chapter.

Chapter **45**

Diabetes

Brigette Vachon, Catherine Donnelly, and Setareh Ghahari

LEARNING OBJECTIVES

This chapter will allow the reader to:

1. Differentiate type 1 and type 2 diabetes and population-based risk factors.
2. Identify risk factors for diabetes and impact on population health.
3. Know the long-term medical complications of diabetes.
4. Understand how diabetes and other chronic conditions can influence occupational performance in youth and adults/elderly with type 1 and type 2 diabetes.
5. Understand diabetes self-management principles, behavioral change models, and evidence-based interventions.
6. Explain the importance of an interprofessional team care approach to support diabetes self-management.
7. Use occupational therapy interventions to help people with diabetes adapt to their chronic condition and adopt a healthy occupational lifestyle.

CHAPTER OUTLINE

TERMINOLOGY

Diabetes distress: emotional burdens and worries that are part of the person's experience when he or she needs to manage a severe and demanding chronic disease like diabetes.

Diabetes mellitus: a disease in which the body's ability to produce or respond to the hormone insulin is impaired, resulting in abnormal metabolism of carbohydrates and elevated levels of glucose in the blood and urine. There are two main types of diabetes: type 1 and type 2. People with type 1 diabetes don't produce insulin. People with type 2 diabetes don't respond to insulin as well as they should and later in the disease often don't make enough insulin.

Glycated hemoglobin (HbA1c): any derivative of hemoglobin in which a glucose molecule is attached to the hemoglobin molecule. The most abundant form of glycated hemoglobin is hemoglobin A1c (HbA1c), levels of which are significantly increased in diabetes.

Hyperglycemia: high level of blood glucose caused by the body's inability to properly use or make the hormone insulin that leads to symptoms such as increased urination, extreme thirst, and unexplained weight loss.

Insulin: a protein hormone, produced in the pancreas, that is crucial in regulating the amount of sugar (glucose) in the blood. Lack of this hormone results to diabetes mellitus.

Nephropathy: a kidney disease that affects the ability of the kidney to excrete any waste products and to regulate the water and acid–base balance of the body.

Neuropathy: a disease of the peripheral nerves, usually causing weakness and numbness. When blood glucose levels stay high for an extended period of time, it can damage the nerves, particularly the nerves in the lower limbs.[3]

Retinopathy: disease of the retina resulting in impairment or loss of vision. In the most serious cases, retinopathy can lead to blindness.

Self-management: a person's ability to manage the symptoms, treatment, physical and psychosocial consequences, and lifestyle changes inherent in living with a long-term disorder.

Diabetes Epidemiology

Diabetes: Prevalence and Importance of the Problem

The prevalence of diabetes has been steadily increasing in recent years, with up to a fourfold increase in the past 40 years.[1] The highest prevalence rates are found in the North American and Caribbean Regions, with an estimated 10.8% of the population. In low- and mid-income countries, there is a greater predominance of individuals with diabetes who are under 65 years old as compared to high-income countries where the greatest proportion of individuals with diabetes are over the age of 65 years.[1] It is anticipated that the prevalence of diabetes will continue to rise, most notably in those countries transitioning from low income to middle income.[1]

This growing epidemic of diabetes is related to multiple factors, including obesity, urbanization, aging populations, and sedentary lifestyles.[2] The impact of diabetes is tremendous. From an economic perspective, the global economic burden is 1.4 trillion dollars, and this number will rise substantially by 2030. Diabetes is estimated to result in 3.96 million deaths, accounting for 6.8% of the global mortality.[1]

Definition of Type 1 and Type 2 Diabetes

Diabetes is a chronic disease. It causes blood sugar levels to rise higher than normal because the body cannot produce **insulin** or cannot properly use the insulin it produces.[3,4] Insulin is a hormone produced by the pancreas that helps to regulate blood glucose levels and transport glucose from the bloodstream into the cells. In type 1 diabetes, the body does not produce insulin. Type 1 diabetes occurs most often in children, adolescents, or young adults and represents only 10% of people with diabetes.[3] The exact causes of type 1 diabetes are still unknown, but the body's immune system destroys the beta cells in the pancreas that produces insulin. Hypothesis is that it would be related to a genetic predisposition or certain environmental factors.[2,3] The risk of a child to develop type 1 diabetes is approximately of 5% if one parent is affected or 15% if they both have the disease. The risk is higher if the father is affected. There is also a small higher prevalence of type 1 diabetes in men, but reasons for the sex difference are still unknown.[2]

Type 2 diabetes is the most common form of diabetes, accounting for 90% of cases.[3] In type 2 diabetes, the body either does not produce enough insulin or does not use it properly, leading to a **hyperglycemia**. This phenomenon is called insulin resistance: the pancreas produces extra insulin to compensate, but over time is not able to produce sufficient insulin to keep blood glucose levels normal.[3] The body, then, cannot effectively use glucose as an energy source. The chronic hyperglycemia of diabetes is associated with relatively specific long-term microvascular complications affecting the eyes, kidneys, and nerves, as well as an increased risk for cardiovascular disease.[4]

Diabetes Diagnostic Criteria

The American Diabetes Association (ADA) recommends that individuals are diagnosed with diabetes when their fasting levels of glucose in the blood reaches 7.0 mmol/L or higher, and/or the level of **glycated hemoglobin** (HbA1c) in the blood is 6.5% or higher.[3] The term prediabetes is used for people whose HbA1c levels are between 6.0% and 6.4%.[3] These individuals are at high risk of developing diabetes and the diabetes-related complications. However, not all individuals with prediabetes will necessarily progress and develop diabetes. Prediabetes and type 2 diabetes are often manifestations of a broader underlying disorder called metabolic syndrome.[3,4] Metabolic syndrome is a highly prevalent, multifaceted condition characterized by a combination of medical conditions that increases the risk of heart disease. People with this syndrome present some or all of the following abnormalities: high blood glucose, abdominal obesity, hypertension, dyslipidemia, high triglycerides, and insulin resistance.[4]

Diabetes Risk Factors

There is a matrix of both genetic and lifestyle risk factors that interact within the broader physical and sociocultural environment.[2,5] Although there is noted to be a clear genetic predisposition to type 2 diabetes, there is also strong evidence to suggest that type 2 diabetes could be prevented and that lifestyle plays a substantial role. The single strongest risk factor for type 2 diabetes is a high body mass index (BMI), with up to 61% of cases attributed to BMI >25.[2] Physical activity level can also predict the development of type 2 diabetes. Activity and exercise can help prevent obesity and increase insulin sensitivity. Individuals who exercise most frequently were found to have 25% to 60% less risk of developing type 2 diabetes,[2] regardless of the presence of other risk factors. Diet and lifestyle factors play a significant role, and it has been clearly demonstrated that the incidence of **diabetes mellitus** can be reduced by up to 58% through lifestyle interventions.[2,6] Other known risk factors are dietary habits, high blood pressure, heredity, ethnicity (Aboriginals, Africans, Asians, Latin-Americans), and level of education.[2]

Complications

Individuals may experience several complications associated with both type I and type 2 diabetes that impact daily occupations (see Table 45-1). These complications can be categorized in two types: microvascular (small blood vessels) and macrovascular (large blood vessels).[7] Microvascular complications include **retinopathy** (eye damage), **nephropathy** (kidney damage), and **neuropathy** (nerve damage). Macrovascular complications include stroke, heart attack, and circulatory disease. Individuals with diabetes also have a high level of psychosocial stress with higher rates of anxiety and depression.

Impact of Diabetes on Daily Occupations across the Life Span

Because of the extent and nature of complications, people living with diabetes can experience a wide range of difficulties in their daily occupations, such as difficulty performing activities of daily living (ADLs), limited community mobility, decreased energy, social isolation, poor time usage, poor daily planning, lack of meaningful leisure activities, and diminished healthy habits.[8] The management of diabetes is complex and requires both medical monitoring and lifestyle management, including, but not limited to, monitoring blood glucose levels, injecting insulin, taking medications, healthy eating, and engaging in regular physical activity. **Self-management** of diabetes impacts occupations across the life span.[8,9]

Type 1 Diabetes

Type 1 diabetes is often diagnosed in childhood and can have a significant impact on daily routines and activities.[10] In young children, the impact is felt across the families as parents and caregivers support the medical management of diabetes. Childhood diabetes may be difficult to control, leading to multiple medical appointments and ultimately resulting in lost-school days and challenges participating in after-school activities. Research has found that children with diabetes have poorer school outcomes compared to those without diabetes.[11]

Table 45-1. Diabetes Complications, Prevention, and Treatment

COMPLICATION	SCREENING	PREVENTION	TREATMENT
Microvascular complications			
Retinopathy	Dilated fundus examination	Yearly eye screening examination Glycemic control Blood pressure control	Laser surgery Low-vision rehabilitation
Neuropathy	Clinical examination Monofilament test	Glycemic control Preventive foot care Appropriate footwear	Pain management Sensory rehabilitation Foot ulcer care
Nephropathy	Urine microalbumin test (proteins in urine)	Glycemic control Blood pressure control	Dialysis
Macrovascular complications			
Stroke Heart attack Circulatory disease	Risk factors screening	Diet and exercise Healthy daily routines and habits Smoking cessation	Medication to control blood pressure and lipids Stroke and/or cardiac rehabilitation Lifestyle redesign
Psychosocial complications			
Anxiety and depression	Symptoms screening	Social and health professional support Healthy daily routines and habits	Medication Psychotherapy Self-management support Physical activity

As children move to adolescents and take responsibility for their own management, there can be challenges with adherence to medical and lifestyle management.[10] Adolescents are faced with unique developmental challenges that can influence the ways in which they successfully manage the daily self-care activities of diabetes. Furthermore, hormonal changes during puberty may reduce adolescents' insulin and can require more attention and planning to maintain metabolic control.[12] This is a crucial time to develop self-management skills, particularly related to developing health habits and routines that will lay the foundation for management in adulthood.[13] Diabetes self-management activities can create feelings of being different from their peers and may lead to feelings of exclusion and isolation. Type 2 diabetes in children and youth is a more recent phenomenon, and there is a higher mean age at diagnosis and greater complications compared to children and youth with type 1 diabetes.[14] Less is written about this populations, but the impact on occupations will be similar.

Type 2 Diabetes

Type 2 diabetes is most often diagnosed in adulthood: a time that involves juggling multiple roles where finding the time for self-management and for implementing healthy eating and exercise can be a significant challenge. It is also a time within the life span where the worker role is dominant. Burda and colleagues[15] identified 10 broad areas of diabetes management behaviors to support people with diabetes applying for work and functioning in the workplace. These behaviors considered both the technical and medical management of diabetes at work, highlighting that some jobs will be more challenging to incorporate self-management activities than others, particularly those that have rigid schedules and long shifts. The authors also considered communication of health-related needs to coworkers, both related to incidents that may occur at work or potential health-related work absences.[15]

Other areas of occupation are also impacted. Marinho and colleagues[16] administered the Canadian Occupational Performance Measure (COPM)[17] to 475 individuals with type 2 diabetes. They found that the top three areas of difficulties related to mobility, self-care, and management of household activities. The authors also found that lack of physical activity, presence of diabetic neuropathy, depression, and pain were associated with these occupational performance challenges.[16]

In a survey conducted among 52 older adults with diabetes, work and leisure participation were identified as the top areas of occupation for which they experienced the most difficulties. Older adults with diabetes have a higher rate of functional decline, both related to the disease process itself and increasing diabetes complication with aging, as compared to those without diabetes.[18,19] Impaired cognitive and physical functions and low education level among the elderly can require more support to make lifestyle changes.[20] Also, as seen in the adult population, diabetes impacts mobility, and in older adults, this results in a higher risk of falls.[18]

There are a number of issues related to diabetes that impact occupation across the life span. Social stigma related to diabetes has been found to have social, occupational, and emotional consequences. For example, fear of social embarrassment, rejection, being treated differently, or damaging relationships with significant others are common concerns associated with injecting insulin.[21] In childhood and adolescents, there is stigma related to time away from school and school-related activities.[11] Adults with type 2 diabetes also report feeling embarrassed when they need to refuse unhealthy food options at social events.[22]

The use of technology in monitoring and managing diabetes integration of technology has evolved significantly, and the impact on the use and integration of technology across the life span needs to be considered.[23] In youth and children for whom technology is part of their everyday routines, technology is seen as something that can readily be incorporated into diabetes management.[24] In older adults, a recent qualitative study that examined the use of technology to provide real-time continuous glucose monitoring found that the technology provided a sense of safety and enabled them to engage in their daily routines with the knowledge that their sugars were under control.[25]

Fatigue was also found to be related to psychological factors, such as depression or emotional distress, and can be a barrier to self-management, such as engaging in healthy eating or participating in a regular exercise plan.[26,27]

Finally, it is critical to consider the sociocultural contexts because diabetes will have a unique impact on occupation depending on cultural beliefs, values, and practices.[28]

Psychosocial Adaptation

Because diabetes is a chronic condition, people with this disease will need to adapt to this new life situation. People with chronic diseases generally go through a transformation process that "seeks to make sense of their new self, their new illness, and their new life by participating in a process of interpretation and transformation of personal meaning perspectives."[29] Thus, people living with diabetes will need to gain new knowledge and skills and learn new ways of being to deconstruct their current ways and reconstruct new meaning perspective.[29] The Process of Transformation Model: Rehabilitation of Chronic Illness and Disability was developed by Dubouloz et al.[29] (see Fig. 45-1). It describes the various stages, steps, or phases that an

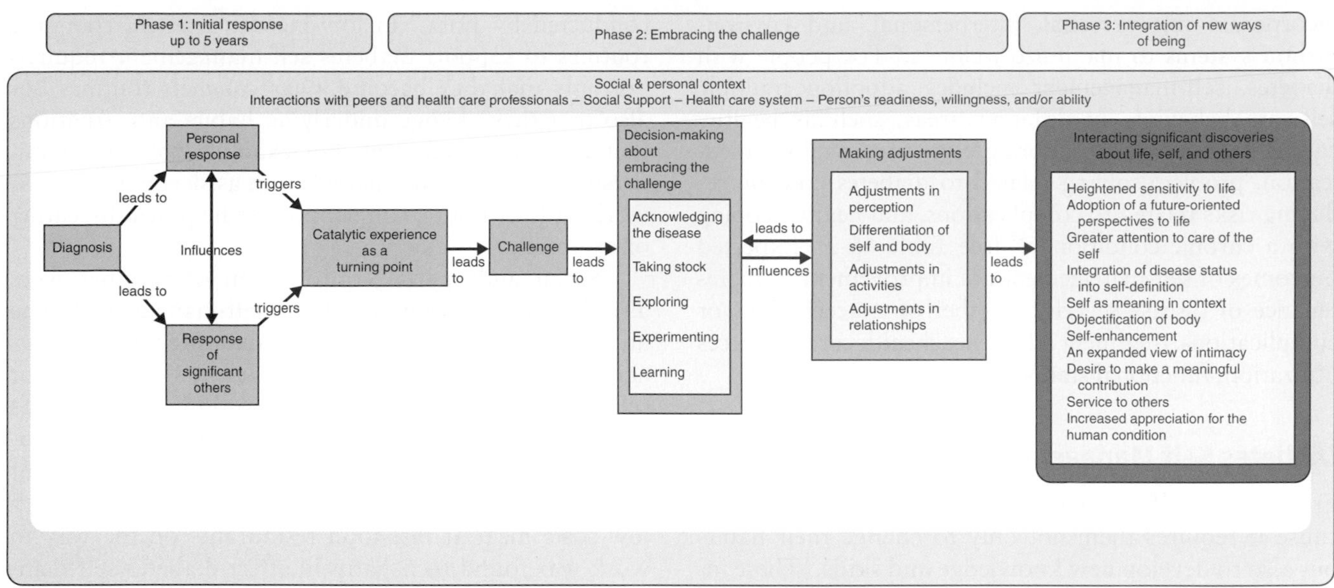

Figure 45-1. The Process of Transformation Model: Rehabilitation of Chronic Illness and Disability. (Reprinted with permission from Dubouloz CJ, King J, Paterson B, Ashe B, Chevrier J, Moldoveanu M. A model of the process of transformation in primary care for people living with chronic illnesses. *Chronic Illn.* 2010;6(4):282–293.)

individual can go through to adapt to a chronic condition. It is composed of three phases: the trigger phase, the process of changing phase, and the outcomes phase.

In the trigger phase, the person is suddenly faced with the limits and losses of disease. For diabetics, the symptoms are often described as silent in its early stages. Nevertheless, the onset of the diagnosis requires people to make important changes to their life habits to prevent important complications. The pressure felt to suddenly change these habits may cause some distress, resistance, or even denial of the disease.[30] This can last a few months to a few years before people describe being ready to engage in the change process. The trigger phase is a state of disorientation where clients try to make sense of what is happening to them. They rely on external sources of information, such as advices from professionals, to maintain hope for the future.

The process of changing phase comes with the development of readiness for change. People with chronic diseases usually find it difficult to explain why and how they became ready to change. Nevertheless, they report that it was prompted by the constant reminders and encouragements they received from health care professionals, family, and friends, but also by an inner reconciliation or confrontation with their reality.

Finally, in the outcomes phase, the individual has adopted new meaning perspectives, new feelings, new behaviors, or even a new identity. They learn to live with their conditions and are able to adopt a future-oriented perspective to life. People in this phase show behavioral and emotional stability. However, there is no final outcome, and people living with diabetes need to constantly develop and cope with change in their condition and, therefore, may require them to cycle through the model multiple times.

Self-Management of Diabetes

Self-management is a widely used term and is defined by the active participation and engagement of clients in the management of their health and treatment to live well with their long-term condition.[31,32] Thus, self-management is an active process and involves individuals taking necessary actions to meet their health, psychological, social, and emotional needs associated with living with one or more chronic disease.[31,32] Self-management places the responsibility with the individual, but requires managing his or her condition within his or her environment. In a concept analysis, Udlis[33] described that antecedents or prerequisite conditions for clients to engage in self-management are information regarding chronic disease, self-efficacy or the confidence in one's ability to engage in health behaviors, social, family and emotional support, intention, goal setting and planning, and partnering with health care professionals. She also described dimensions of self-management as the use of information and resources necessary to equip clients with the knowledge and tools to be successful in self-management behaviors; adherence to a plan of care, active participation, and responsibility for one's own care; and informed decision-making to provide clients the capacity to make individual best choices and used adapted self-management strategies on a day-to-day basis.

As defined by Miller et al.,[32] "chronic disease self-management is a fluid, iterative process during which clients incorporate multidimensional strategies that meet their self-identified needs to cope with chronic disease within the context of their daily living. Strategies are multidimensional because they require the individual to incorporate intrapersonal, interpersonal, and environmental systems to maximize wellness." For people with diabetes, self-management includes adopting multiple self-care behaviors in different areas, such as healthy eating, being active, monitoring blood sugar, taking medication, problem-solving related to diabetes control, reducing risks related to complications, and healthy coping with a chronic condition[34,35] (see Table 45-2). Expected outcomes of self-management are improvement or maintenance of disease severity, number of exacerbations or complications, treatment adherence, health care resources utilization, functional status, and quality of life.[35]

Diabetes Self-Management as an Occupation

Engaging in self-management is difficult for people because it requires them not only to change their habits but also to develop new knowledge and skills.[9] These individuals need to adopt a new routine that provides temporal organization and structure to daily life. In a study conducted by Fritz,[9] in low-income women, changing routines to support diabetes self-management required not only that they become aware of their routines but also that they change underlying habits and situations that shape these patterns. For example, this meant understanding how other habits, such as sleeping habits or working long hours, can support or help healthy eating or exercising.

Social and spatial coordination of routines were also found to be important for self-management time and resources.[9] For example, coordinating family or caregiver responsibilities was important to secure time for self-management tasks or getting support from friends and relatives for transportation. Geographical distribution of daily routines also impacted self-management habits. For example, a convenient and easy access to low-costs meal at fast-food restaurants on the way to work was found to negatively affect diabetes self-management. Furthermore, participants reported the importance of time to develop diabetes self-management.

Table 45-2. Diabetes Basic Self-Management Recommendations

RECOMMENDATION	GOAL	ACTIONS
Adopting healthy eating habits	Keep blood sugar level at target Reduce risk of diabetes complications	Eat three meals a day Count carbohydrates (approximately 45–60 g per meal) Limit sugar and sweets Limit high-fat food Drink water Limit alcohol consumption
Monitoring blood glucose level	Assess how lifestyle and medication affect blood glucose levels	Use a blood glucose meter to check blood sugar level at home as often as recommended by the health care team
Doing regular physical activity	Improve blood pressure control, level of energy, and body's sensitivity to insulin to help manage blood sugar levels Maintain or get to a healthy weight	Do both aerobic and resistance exercise Do moderate-to-vigorous aerobic exercise for approximately 150 minutes/week Start slowly, progressively increase time and intensity of exercise Check effect of exercise on blood sugar level
Taking medication daily	Lower blood sugar level Reduce risk of heart disease	Understand the purpose of medication Stick to a schedule Use a pill box Use an alarm or reminders
Taking care of feet	Avoid foot ulcers and amputation	Check feet every day for cuts, cracks, blisters, or sores Trim nails straight across Apply good skin lotion See footcare specialist when needed Appropriate footware, with room to prevent skin irritation
Accessing psychosocial resources and support	Prevent diabetes distress, anxiety, and depression	Inform family and friends on ways to support diabetes management Engage in peer support groups Build a health care team Maintain healthy daily routines and habits Mindfulness and relaxation practice

This meant integrating in closed time routines, such as morning routine or working hours, components of self-management performed every day (e.g., medication management, blood glucose monitoring), and integrating activities such as practicing new recipes or trying a new physical activity in weekly open time. Thus, a key finding of this study is that modifying existing routines is a real challenge. Diabetes self-management needs to be included in daily occupations to meet the demands of daily life, but this also requires having the support to become aware of these routines to understand the ways in which they positively or negatively influence engagement in self-management.

Behavioral Change Models

There are several models that can be used to support occupational therapy interventions aimed at changing behaviors to promote self-management of diabetes symptoms.

Self-Regulation Theory

Self-regulation describes the ability to monitor the results of one's actions and then choose a subsequent behavior.[36] Three ingredients are required for self-regulation: (1) a set of standards, goals, or ideals with meaning and relevance to the person's specific life situation; (2) the person's ability to self-monitor and determine whether anything needs to be changed to meet the his or her needs and standards; and (3) in case maintaining the desired standards is not possible, adjustments are required. A person with higher self-regulatory skills is more able to manage an impulse. However, where there are several competing demands, the person's ability to regulate might be diminished.

Goal Setting and Goal Striving Theory

One example of a self-regulation model is Goal Setting and Goal Striving.[37] A "goal" is mental image of a desired state or outcome that a person considers as the ultimate result of his or her actions. It is by setting goals that a sense of urgency and motivation to achieve these commitments is attained. If the goals are set at the level that they seem unattainable, the individual will be reluctant or less motivated to pursue his or her goals. The characteristics of the goals include how motivational orientation they are, their level of difficulty, the type of the goal, how specific the goal is (concrete or abstract), and the proximity of the end state. People tend to be involved with goal-oriented behaviors if the goals are intrinsically motivated, feasible, and harmonious with their other personal goals.[37] Achievable goals with moderate level of challenge are more likely to be approached and pursued by people.

Self-Efficacy Theory

Self-efficacy is defined as the confidence or belief that an individual has in his or her ability to execute a particular cognition or behavior.[38] Self-efficacy is a part of self-regulatory processes through which individuals shape environmental and interpersonal resources and behavior toward a desired end.[38] The concept of self-efficacy is the central tenet of Bandura's Social Learning Theory.[38] This theory emphasizes the underpinning role of personal mastery in the psychological and behavioral processes, leading to behavioral change.[39] Based on Bandura's theory, efficacy beliefs have a potent influence in self-knowledge and beliefs of self-determination, and they direct human behavior on a fundamental level.[38,40] Based on this theory, in order for individuals to make important changes in their lives to increase health outcomes, they must believe in their capability of making such changes.[40] Even if they have skills to make changes, it is possible that their poor belief in their capability result in not taking any actions.

The key concepts of Bandura's Social Cognitive Theory are listed as follows:

- *Competence mastery:* When a person practices a task and repeatedly achieves successful experiences, his or her self-confidence would improve, which will result in repeating the task over time.
- *Vicarious learning:* Observing other people's success in similar behavioral change results in the belief that the person has the ability to make a change in his or her own behavior.
- *Social persuasion:* The use of positive verbal persuasion can help influence an individual to take actions. Positive messages from others such as "great work" and "you are improving well" help the person build confidence.
- *Self-appraisal:* This involves becoming self-aware of feelings when a person is in a stressful situation. There is a need to be self-aware in order to understand feelings of anxiety or stress that may prevent us from performing the task or achieving the goal.

As self-efficacy beliefs and expectations strongly influence individual's choices, decisions, behaviors, and persistence,[41] many argue that a good self-management program should rest on a theoretical basis of changing self-efficacy.[42]

Transtheoretical Model

The Transtheoretical Model is focused on behavioral change and is articulated through the stages of change.[43] Based on this model, people generally go through several stages of changes before they can maintain the new behavior. People at *precontemplation* stage have no intention of taking any action to change their behavior. It can be because of lack of motivation, lack of information, or lack of awareness of how the changes can help them. When people are at a *contemplation* stage, they might have better awareness of importance of changes but feel ambivalent about making the necessary changes. At *preparation* stage, there is intention to take action and an action plan is in place. People at an *action* stage have modified behaviors and taken actions to make changes to their lifestyle. The *maintenance* stage is when people are maintaining their behavioral changes and become increasingly confident that they can maintain their lifestyle changes.[43]

Chronic Care Model

Wagner[44] created the Chronic Care Model (CCM), a primary care–based framework for individuals with chronic conditions. The CCM includes four essential and independent components: self-management support, delivery system design, decision support, and information technology.[45] These components function in the broader context of community and health care system. The CCM highlights the importance of productive interaction between informed, activated clients, and prepared proactive health care providers. The CCM encourages the health care providers to work collaboratively with their clients and support the management of their conditions.

Management of a chronic condition has two active parties: one is the person who needs to have knowledge and skills to manage the condition and can apply those skills to his or her life; and the other one is the health care provider who helps the person manage his or her condition by providing him or her information, encouragement, and support. This is in opposed to prescribing to the client what to do, and when and where make changes. The health care provider invites the client to have input in defining the problem, set goals, and plan to manage a certain problem. Sustained follow-up is also known as essential to self-management support.

Self-Management Education and Self-Management Support Programs

The diabetes self-management education and support (DSMES) is well known as a critical component of care for all people with diabetes. The National Standards for Diabetes Self-Management Education and Support[46] emphasizes that people with diabetes should be engaged in management and intervention plans in every stage of their condition.

Self-Management Education and Support

Self-management education is defined as the ongoing process of facilitating learning of knowledge and skills necessary for people with a chronic disease to actively engage in self-management delivered by specialized health care professionals.[35] Self-management support is an activity provided by health care professionals to assist people with chronic diseases to manage their condition on an ongoing basis.[35]

Self-management support can be peer led or provided in collaboration with social and health care professionals working in the community. Thus, self-management education comprises any educational processes that provide individuals with the knowledge and skills to inform decisions and increase their capacity and confidence to apply these skills in daily-life situations. Diabetes self-management programs should include both education and support and contain multiple strategies to help ongoing adaptation to one's condition, progressive learning, and adapted and personalized behavioral change facilitation. The expertise of professionals, but also of individuals who live with diabetes, is important because they can share with others their experiential knowledge and provide genuine and comprehensive support to others going through the same or similar adaptation process.

Chronic Disease Self-Management Program

Self-management programs are well known for improving quality of life, self-efficacy, and decreasing health care utilization in people with chronic conditions. One of the most studied evidence-based self-management programs is the Chronic Disease Self-Management Program (CDSMP) developed by Lorig et al. in 1978.[47] The generic program[48] includes 6-week sessions that are 2.5 hours each. The program is delivered by two trained and licensed facilitators. The facilitators are lay leaders, that is, a person with a chronic condition who had training for facilitating the program. During the program, the participants gain confidence and acquire skills to better manage their condition. The program is found to be effective in improving general health and lowering health care utilization.[48] The program has been used worldwide, translated to many other languages, and used for several conditions such as arthritis, diabetes, health disease, multiple sclerosis, and stroke. The program is usually presented as a group face-to-face program, but there is evidence that the online version of the program is also effective.

Team Care Approach for Diabetes Management

Client living with diabetes need the support from an interdisciplinary team who will work collaboratively to improve diabetes self-management and prevent complications. Evidence suggests that a team approach can lower the risk for diabetes complications.[49] Working with family physicians, nurses, pharmacists, nutritionists, social workers, and other health care professionals is essential to answer the multiple and constantly changing needs of clients.[50] Tricco and colleagues[51] showed, in a meta-analysis, that strategies targeting diabetes care teams led to significant improvements in clients' blood glucose, cholesterol, and blood pressure levels. However, barriers to interprofessional collaboration in primary care are frequent and are related to lack of knowledge of other professionals' role and lack of communication.[52] It is thus important to learn what everyone on the team can bring in terms of expertise (see Table 45-3), how they can help in answering clients' needs, and using good communication tools, such as the electronic medical record, to share information between team members.

Occupational Therapy for People Living with Diabetes

The focus on occupational therapy interventions in this chapter is on supporting individuals in managing diabetes. Although occupational therapists can provide interventions for complications that arise from diabetes including amputations, visual impairment, and neuropathy, the specific interventions for these health conditions are found in other chapters.

The primary role for occupational therapists working with individuals with diabetes is to support the

Table 45-3. Other Professionals' Role in Diabetes Management

PROFESSIONAL	MAIN ROLE	RELATED PATIENTS' NEEDS
Family physician	Monitoring risk factors and complications, coordinating care, and referring to specialist medical care as required	Maintaining and monitoring blood glucose levels Controlling hypertension and lipids Being aware a medical test results Knowing personal blood glucose level target Helping with smoking cessation
Kinesiologist	Supporting engagement in physical activity and healthy life habits	Doing regular physical activity Understanding effect of physical activity on blood sugar level
Nurse	Providing diabetes self-management education and foot care	Understanding diabetes and signs of hypoglycemia and hyperglycemia Knowing how to take medication and blood glucose monitoring device Knowing general diabetes self-management skills Caring for feet
Nutritionist	Supporting engagement in healthy eating and development of personalized eating plan and goals	Knowing what to eat Reading food labels Calculating carbohydrates Managing body weight
Optometrist	Vision care, conducting eye examination	Preventing eye complications
Pharmacist	Adjusting medication, preventing drug interactions, providing support for adherence to medication	Knowing how to take medication Understanding possible medication interactions
Physiotherapist	Providing rehabilitation to manage any complications (e.g., stroke, cardiac), supporting physical activity	Managing pain Doing regular physical activity
Podiatrist or foot care specialist	Supporting foot care, including nail and skin care, ensuring proper footware and orthotics	Caring for feet Wearing appropriate footware
Psychologist	Providing psychological support, monitoring symptoms of anxiety and depression	Improving and maintaining self-management motivation Receiving psychological support for self and family and friends
Social worker	Providing psychological support, connecting to community resources, supporting families	Managing costs associated with diabetes care Participating to social and group activities to support self-management Receiving psychological support for self and family and friends

individuals in the engagement in healthy lifestyles to manage diabetes.[53] Occupational therapists working with individuals with diabetes will be primarily situated in community and primary care settings, working in an interprofessional team, or a patient-centered medical homes.[54] Patient-centered medical homes provide more comprehensive and coordinated care than physician only care and thought to provide more efficient delivery of services. Within interprofessional primary care teams in Canada, one study found that the proportion of individuals with diabetes who were seen by an occupational therapist had fewer emergency department visits compared to those who were seen by a physician only.[55] With the increasing prevalence of diabetes and other chronic diseases, it is anticipated that there will be a greater emphasis on team-based primary care models.[56] Primary care continues to be an emerging area of practice for occupational therapists, and supporting individuals to live with diabetes in this setting is an important role.

Occupational Therapy Evaluation

People with diabetes often do not have the opportunity to receive occupational therapy services. However, the occupational therapist can help them recognize and act on the difficulties they encounter by taking into account all their lifestyle habits and occupations in order to better integrate self-management activities into their occupational routine and better manage the psychological and social impacts that diabetes can cause.

The occupational therapists intervention process will begin with an assessment of the client's difficulties in performing personal, leisure, and work activities, including diabetes self-management activities. The physical and emotional dimensions of the person are relevant to assess, such as pain, mobility, and the presence of **diabetes distress** or depressive symptoms. Social support is also very important to help clients engage in self-management, and occupational therapists should assess the availability and amount of social support to which the person has access. Another important aspect of the environment is resources available in the community for people living with diabetes and the person's economic situation that may influence different life habits choices. Nevertheless, the most important aspect of the occupational therapist assessment process is documenting occupational issues experienced by client that may be related to diabetes self-management activities; adaptation to the diseases and its physical, psychological, or social consequences; diabetes complications such as low vision or neuropathy; or occupational balance between self-care, work, leisure, and self-management activities.

Based on the conceptual model used by the occupational therapist, different tools can be used to conduct the assessment process and to assess the effects of the intervention. If the COPM is selected to guide the process, it can be used to help the client identify and prioritize his or her occupational issues.[57] The COPM is an individualized, client-centered outcome measure.[17] A semi-structured interview enables the client to identify areas of difficulty in the areas of self-care, productivity, and leisure. The client rates the importance of each identified issue on a scale ranging from 1 to 10 (1 = *with great difficulty or not satisfied*, 10 = *with no difficulties or completely satisfied*). Clients subsequently rate as many as five identified problems on their perceived level of performance and satisfaction with their performance on each of the five identified issues. On reassessment, clients rate their performance and satisfaction on the issues identified in the initial assessment. A change score is obtained by subtracting the post-treatment score from the initial score. The COPM has been found to be both a reliable and a valid measure across diagnostic categories and treatment settings.[58] Because many diabetes interventions are goal oriented, the COPM was felt to offer an individualized assessment that then enabled planning for targeted intervention strategies.[16] Additionally, the individual nature of the COPM was felt to support individuals in prioritizing their self-management strategies to specific functional challenges.

Occupational therapists can also complete their assessment using diabetes-specific questionnaires that can allow them to document their clients' perceptions of diabetes self-management and impacts on their quality of life. The Summary of Diabetes Self-Care Activities Measure[59] and the Diabetes Self-Management Questionnaire[60] are two questionnaires documenting five self-management domains: general diet, specific diet, exercise, blood glucose testing, and foot care. The Audit of Diabetes-Dependent Quality of Life (ADDQoL)[61] is a 19-item questionnaire assessing the impact of diabetes on 19 life domains, including physical functioning, symptoms, psychological well-being, social well-being, role activities, and personal constructs. Clients can evaluate life domains that are relevant to themselves and indicate the importance of those domains to their quality of life as well as the direct impact of diabetes on those domains.

Occupational Therapy Intervention

As described by Youngson,[62] occupational therapists can bring their unique occupation-focused perspective to support clients with diabetes and the health care team. The additional contribution of occupational therapists within the team was seen as supporting the integration of diabetes self-management into everyday activities and routines, intervening at the environmental level, empowering individuals in self-management, addressing work/life, and supporting occupational balance.[63] It is important for occupational therapists not to duplicate services already offered and rather focus of our interventions on the "how to do" instead of the "what to do."

Overall, the focus of occupational therapy interventions is to understand the challenges of self-management, support engagement in the process of change, and consider multiple occupational choices. Many people living with diabetes can benefit from occupational therapy when they experience difficulties with their self-management, work, and daily activities. Client with complications such as vision loss, neuropathic pain, or amputation can even more benefit from occupational therapists' expertise in assessing, improving, and adapting for impairment or incapacities and reducing disability.[64] For example, occupational therapy can help in using safe cooking methods, provide techniques to held adherence to medication regimen, use low-vision devices to measure insulin; teach protective techniques, and compensate for peripheral sensory loss.[64] Occupational therapists can also use cognitive–behavioral and problem-solving approaches to support clients with diabetes distress or depression to improve their occupational performance.

Resilient, Empowered, Active Living with Diabetes

The Resilient, Empowered, Active Living with Diabetes (REAL) intervention[65] is an evidence-based occupational therapy–led diabetes intervention and is an adaptation of Lifestyle Redesign intervention.[66] The REAL intervention includes seven modules that support individuals in incorporating diabetes self-management tasks into everyday routines. Topics include goal setting, living with diabetes, activity, and health (see Fig. 45-2).

The intervention is goal based, and the modules are designed to be delivered in a way to meet each individual's diabetes management goals and needs. The intervention can be delivered over a 6-month period. The REAL intervention consists of four core principles informed by multiple theoretical perspectives. The first principle recognizes that occupations take place in multiple contexts and that the interrelationships between body structures and functions and the environments influence occupation. The second principle is the importance of using narrative to understand the impact of diabetes on everyday activities. The third principal considers goal-directed and habitual actions. The fourth principal considers the individual as a complex system and, in doing so, understands previous life experiences and evolving behavioral patterns over time. Originally developed for adults, research has demonstrated that this is also a feasible intervention for young adults.[67] Although there have been no published outcome studies on the REAL intervention, REAL offers a manualized occupation-focused diabetes education program that would fit well in a primary health care or community setting.

Do-Live-Well Program

The Do-Live-Well is an occupation-focused health promotion framework that "depicts the relationship between what people do every day and their health and well-being."[68(p2)] The Do-Live-Well framework includes four sections: (a) dimensions of experience, (b) activity patterns, (c) health and well-being outcomes, and (d) forces that influence activity engagement[68] (see Fig. 45-3).

The activity patterns component of the Do-Live-Well considers not only the activities people engage in but also how they engage in them. Five elements are considered: engagement, meaning, balance, control/choice, and routine. For individuals with diabetes, these elements could be explored when examining healthy activities and how to implement these into daily life. The framework has not directly been applied to individuals with diabetes, but rather offers a broad perspective that can bring an understanding of activity patterns to support the application of diabetes self-care into

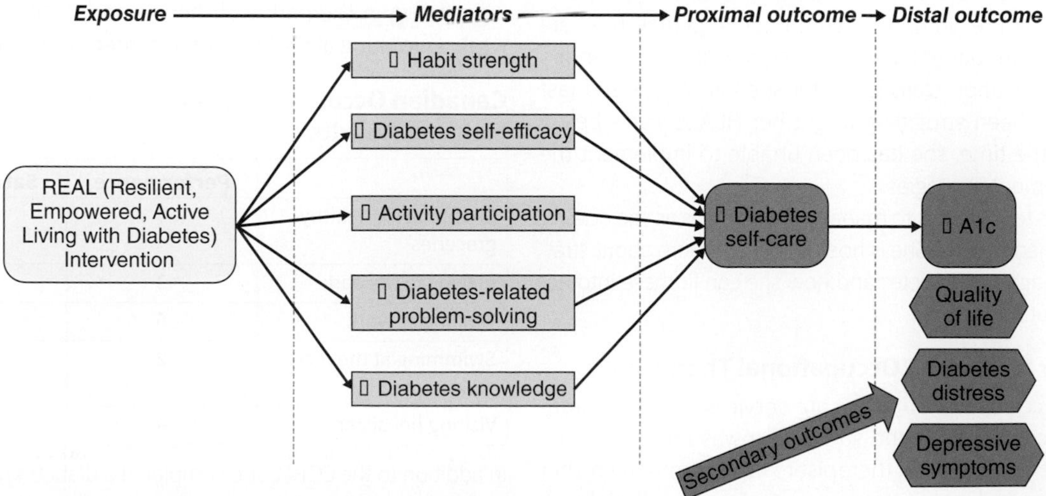

Figure 45-2. Resilient, Empowered, Active Living with Diabetes (REAL) intervention. (Reprinted with permission from Pyatak EA, Carandang K, Davis S. Developing a manualized occupational therapy diabetes management intervention: Resilient, Empowered, Active Living with Diabetes. *Occup Ther J Res.* 2015;35(3):187–194.)

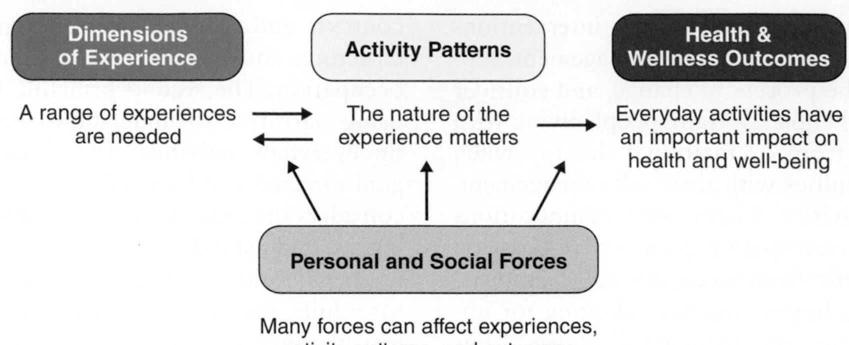

Figure 45-3. Do-Live-Well program. (Reprinted with permission from Moll SE, Gewurtz RE, Krupa TM, Law MC, Lariviere N, Levasseur M. "Do-Live-Well": a Canadian framework for promoting occupation, health, and well-being. *Can J Occup Ther.* 2015;82(1):9–23.)

daily routines. Because the Do-Live-Well is grounded in health promotion, it offers an ideal framework for occupational therapists working with individuals with diabetes to develop targeted interventions.

Conclusion

In conclusion, the occupational therapist has an important role to play in helping people with diabetes and all those with different chronic conditions. Occupational therapists can support their adaptation to this major life change and help them improve their self-management skills. Although occupational therapists are not yet considered as full members of the diabetes interdisciplinary team, their role in supporting the development of occupational balance and integration of self-management activities into daily routine work and leisure activities must be promoted.

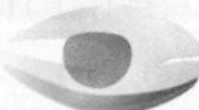

CASE STUDY

Client Information

Francisca is a 54-year-old woman who was diagnosed with type 2 diabetes 1 year ago. She has a BMI of 32 (>30 is considered obese) and also a history of hypertension. She lives with her husband and her two grandchildren in a two-bedroom apartment. Francisca is a personal support worker who works full time at a nursing home and alternates between day and afternoon shifts. She also picks up some additional shifts on the weekends to make ends meet. Her husband is not working, and she is the primary wage earner. Together, they are raising their granddaughters ages 3 and 5. Francisca attended a diabetes education class just after she was diagnosed last year and has been struggling to get her HbA1c levels below 8. With so little time, she has been unable to implement the self-management strategies.

Her goal is to find ways to manage her diabetes as she doesn't like to take medications. She is hoping to learn more about strategies to manage her diabetes and how she can fit these into her busy daily routine.

Reason for Referral to Occupational Therapy

Francisca receives her primary care services at the community health center down the street. She was referred to the primary care occupational therapist to assist in managing her daily routines and activities to improve her overall diabetes management and support a healthy lifestyle. Because of the demands of both work and caregiving for her grandchildren, Francisca has been having difficulty finding the right balance in her life.

Assessment Process and Results

Francisca's assessment was completed at the community health center in the occupational therapists office. The COPM was used to identify the problems Francisca is having in her daily activities. She identified a number of programs, and her five most important issues were shopping for healthy groceries, playing in the park with her granddaughters, walking at work, swimming at the recreation center, visiting her sister.

Canadian Occupational Performance Measure Results

	Performance	Satisfaction
Shopping for healthy groceries	5	5
Playing in the park	3	4
Walking at work	6	3
Swimming at the recreation center	2	2
Visiting her sister	4	4

In addition to the COPM, she completed a diabetes questionnaire exploring her self-management strategies. It was noted that she is currently using very few of the strategies she had been introduced to a year ago. She also had a hard time articulating her goals and

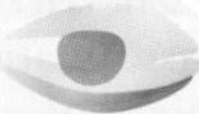

CASE STUDY (continued)

was generally overwhelmed during the assessment. At one point, she became teary when describing how she is trying to cope with her diabetes and also look after both her husband and her grandchildren. Francisca was noted to become short of breath when walking the length of the center's hallway. Francisca did not report any sensory changes in her hands or feet; however, her footware was noted to in poor condition and poorly fitting.

Occupational Therapy Problem List

- Difficulties with instrumental activities of daily living (IADLs), specifically shopping
- Decreased social engagement
- Decreased endurance impacting on walking and swimming
- Difficulties looking after and playing with her granddaughter
- Difficulties coping with diabetes management

Occupational Therapy Goal List

Long-term goal: Francisca will be able to engage in health-promoting activities, including swimming, walking, healthy eating, and playing with her grandchildren in 3 months.

Initial short-term goals:

- Francisca will be able to identify complications that are related to diabetes and describe diabetes self-management strategies.
- Francisca will be able to identify and create a daily routine that will enable her to implement self-management strategies.
- Francisca will attend aquafit at the recreation center two times per week.
- Francisca will shop for and prepare healthy meals on a daily basis.
- Francisca will play at the park with her grandchildren on the weekends.
- Francisca will be able to walk for 20 minutes with no shortness of breath.

Intervention

Francisca attended the REAL diabetes education program at the community health center. She completed each of the seven modules over 6 months and was able to schedule her appointments to fit with her work schedule. In the first module, Francisca developed two goals using the Goal Attainment Scale. These goals were used to tailor the intervention to support her in implementing strategies into her busy routine. Francisca learned more about diabetes and began to have a better understanding of the importance of managing her diabetes. She was able to describe the complications related to diabetes and established a daily routine of monitoring her blood sugars. She was also able to come up with a plan to better communicate her desire to use self-management as opposed to medications to her physician. She made arrangements to attend the diabetes clinic offered at the center on a more regular basis. A great deal of time was spent reviewing her daily routines and finding how she can better implement the self-management strategies. She worked with her employer to reduce her evening shifts so she could see her grandchildren and regularly attend aquafit. Francisca also began to plan her weekly meals and, together with her grandchildren, planned weekly shopping trips to the grocery store and farmers markets. Francisco recognized how difficult the diagnosis of diabetes was emotionally and recognized that eating junk food was something she did to manage her emotions. She attended a Choices for Change workshop given by the dietitian and was able to lose 25 lb over 6 months.

On completion of the REAL program, Francisco attends twice yearly follow-up occupational therapy appointments to ensure her strategies are fitting into her daily routines.

References

1. Bommer C, Sagalova V, Heesemann E, et al. Global economic burden of diabetes in adults: projections from 2015 to 2030. *Diabetes Care*. 2018;41(5):963–970.
2. Bilous R, Donnelly R. *Handbook of Diabetes*. 4th ed. Oxford: John Wiley & Sons; 2010.
3. American Diabetes Association. 2. Classification and diagnosis of diabetes: standards of medical care in diabetes—2018. *Diabetes Care*. 2018;41(Suppl 1):S13–S27.
4. Punthakee Z, Goldenberg R, Katz P; Diabetes Canada Clinical Practice Guidelines Expert Committee. Definition, classification and diagnosis of diabetes, prediabetes and metabolic syndrome. *Can J Diabetes*. 2018;42:S10–S15.
5. Prebtani AP, Bajaj HS, Goldenberg R, Mullan Y; Diabetes Canada Clinical Practice Guidelines Expert Committee. Reducing the risk of developing diabetes. *Can J Diabetes*. 2018;42:S20–S26.
6. Knowler WC, Barrett-Connor E, Fowler SE, et al. Reduction in the incidence of type 2 diabetes with lifestyle intervention or metformin. *N Engl J Med*. 2002;346(6):393–403.
7. Diabetes Canada. Complications. 2019; https://www.diabetes.ca/diabetes-and-you/complications. Accessed January 31, 2019.
8. Hwang JE, Truax C, Claire M, Caytap AL. Occupational therapy in diabetic care—areas of need perceived by older adults with diabetes. *Occup Ther Health Care*. 2009;23(3):173–188.
9. Fritz H. The influence of daily routines on engaging in diabetes self-management. *Scand J Occup Ther*. 2014;21(3):232–240.
10. Pyatak EA, Carandang K, Vigen CL, et al. Occupational therapy intervention improves glycemic control and quality of life among young adults with diabetes: the Resilient, Empowered, Active Living with Diabetes (REAL diabetes) randomized controlled trial. *Diabetes Care*. 2018;41(4):696–704.

11. Pansier B, Schulz PJ. School-based diabetes interventions and their outcomes: a systematic literature review. *J Public Health Res.* 2015;4(1):467.
12. Turner SL, Berg CA, Butner JE, Wiebe DJ. Attention problems as a predictor of type 1 diabetes adherence and metabolic control across adolescence. *J Pediatr Psychol.* 2018;43(1):72–82.
13. Piven E, Duran R. Reduction of non-adherent behaviour in a Mexican-American adolescent with type 2 diabetes. *Occup Ther Int.* 2014;21(1):42–51.
14. Reinehr T. Type 2 diabetes mellitus in children and adolescents. *World J Diabetes.* 2013;4(6):270–281.
15. Burda MH, van der Horst F, van den Akker M, et al. Supporting people with diabetes mellitus in applying for and participating effectively in paid work: validation of successful diabetes-related behaviors by experiential experts and professional care providers. *J Occup Environ Med.* 2012;54(12):1491–1499.
16. Marinho FS, Moram CB, Rodrigues PC, Franzoi AC, Salles GF, Cardoso CR. Profile of disabilities and their associated factors in patients with type 2 diabetes evaluated by the Canadian Occupational Performance Measure: the Rio De Janeiro type 2 diabetes cohort study. *Disabil Rehabil.* 2016;38(21):2095–2101.
17. Law M, Carswell A, Baptiste S, McColl M, Polatajko H, Pollock N. *Canadian Occupational Performance Measure Manual.* 5th ed. Ottawa, Canada: CAOT Publications ACE; 2014.
18. da Cruz Anjos DM, de Souza Moreira B, Pereira DS, et al. Impact of type-2 diabetes time since diagnosis on elderly women gait and functional status. *Physiother Res Int.* 2017;22(2):e1651.
19. Fouad RA, Hassan BH, Ibrahim AF. Quality of life and physical functioning of the diabetic middle aged and older adults. *GSTF J Nurs Health Care (JNHC).* 2014;1(2):89–100.
20. Wong EL, Woo J, Hui E, Chan C, Chan WL, Cheung AW. Primary care for diabetes mellitus: perspective from older patients. *Patient Prefer Adherence.* 2011;5:491–498.
21. Liu NF, Brown AS, Folias AE, et al. Stigma in people with type 1 or type 2 diabetes. *Clin Diabetes.* 2017;35(1):27–34.
22. Tareen RS, Tareen K. Psychosocial aspects of diabetes management: dilemma of diabetes distress. *Transl Pediatr.* 2017;6(4):383.
23. Hunt CW. Technology and diabetes self-management: an integrative review. *World J Diabetes.* 2015;6(2):225.
24. Hinshaw L, Basu A. Technology use for problem solving in adolescent type 1 diabetes. *Diabetes Technol Ther.* 2015;17(7):443–444.
25. Litchman ML, Allen NA. Real-time continuous glucose monitoring facilitates feelings of safety in older adults with type 1 diabetes: a qualitative study. *J Diabetes Sci Technol.* 2017;11(5):988–995.
26. Griggs S, Morris NS. Fatigue among adults with type 1 diabetes mellitus and implications for self-management: an integrative review. *Diabetes Educ.* 2018;44(4):325–339.
27. Kalra S, Sahay R. Diabetes fatigue syndrome. *Diabetes Ther.* 2018;9(4):1421–1429.
28. Creamer J, Attridge M, Ramsden M, Cannings-John R, Hawthorne K. Culturally appropriate health education for type 2 diabetes in ethnic minority groups: an updated Cochrane Review of randomized controlled trials. *Diabet Med.* 2016;33(2):169–183.
29. Dubouloz CJ, King J, Paterson B, Ashe B, Chevrier J, Moldoveanu M. A model of the process of transformation in primary care for people living with chronic illnesses. *Chronic Illn.* 2010;6(4):282–293.
30. Berry E, Lockhart S, Davies M, Lindsay JR, Dempster M. Diabetes distress: understanding the hidden struggles of living with diabetes and exploring intervention strategies. *Postgrad Med J.* 2015;91(1075):278–283.
31. Schmidt-Busby J, Wiles J, Exeter D, Kenealy T. Understanding "context" in the self-management of type 2 diabetes with comorbidities: a systematic review and realist evaluation. *Diabetes Res Clin Pract.* 2018;142: 321–334.
32. Miller WR, Lasiter S, Bartlett Ellis R, Buelow JM. Chronic disease self-management: a hybrid concept analysis. *Nurs Outlook.* 2015;63(2):154–161.
33. Udlis KA. Self-management in chronic illness: concept and dimensional analysis. *J Nurs Healthc Chronic Illn.* 2011;3(2):130–139.
34. American Association of Diabetes Educators. AADE7 Self-Care Behaviors. 2019; https://www.diabeteseducator.org/living-with-diabetes/aade7-self-care-behaviors. Accessed January 31, 2019.
35. Sherifali D, Bai JW, Kenny M, Warren R, Ali M. Diabetes self-management programmes in older adults: a systematic review and meta-analysis. *Diabet Med.* 2015;32(11):1404–1414.
36. Brandt CL. Study of older adults' use of self-regulation for COPD self-management informs an evidence-based patient teaching plan. *Rehabilitation Nursing.* 2013;38(1):11–23.
37. Mann T, de Ridder D, Fujita K. Self-regulation of health behavior: social psychological approaches to goal setting and goal striving. *Health Psychol.* 2013;32(5):487–498.
38. Bandura A. *Self-Efficacy: The Exercise of Control.* New York, NY: W.H. Freeman and Company; 1997.
39. Maddux JE. *Self-Efficacy, Adaptation, and Adjustment: Theory, Research, and Application.* New York, NY: Plenum Press; 1995.
40. Bandura A. Health promotion from the perspective of social cognitive theory. *PsycholHealth.* 1998;13:623–649.
41. Brekke M, Hjortdahl P, Kvien TK. Changes in self-efficacy and health status over 5 years: a longitudinal observational study of 306 patients with rheumatoid arthritis. *Arthritis Rheum.* 2003;49(3):342–348.
42. Burckhardt CS. Educating patients: self-management approaches. *Disabil Rehabil.* 2005;27(12):703–709.
43. Prochaska JO, Velicer WF. The transtheoretical model of health behavior change. *Am J Health Promot.* 1997;12(1):38–48.
44. Wagner EH. Chronic disease management: what will it take to improve care for chronic illness? *Eff Clin Pract.* 1998;1(1):2–4.
45. Wagner EH, Austin BT, Davis C, Hindmarsh M, Schaefer J, Bonomi A. Improving chronic illness care: translating evidence into action. *Health Aff.* 2001;20(6):64–78.
46. Beck J, Greenwood DA, Blanton L, et al. 2017 National standards for diabetes self-management education and support. *Diabetes Educ.* 2018;43(5):449–464.
47. Lorig K, Ritter PL, Villa FJ, Armas J. Community-based peer-led diabetes self-management: a randomized trial. *Diabetes Educ.* 2009;35(4):641–651.

48. Lorig KR, Ritter P, Stewart AL, et al. Chronic disease self-management program: 2-year health status and health care utilization outcomes. *Med Care.* 2001;39(11):1217–1223.
49. Clement M, Filteau P, Harvey B, et al. Organization of diabetes care. *Can J Diabetes.* 2018 42:S27–S35.
50. Vachon B, Huynh AT, Breton M, et al. Patients' expectations and solutions for improving primary diabetes care. *Int J Health Care Qual Assur.* 2017;30(6):554–567.
51. Tricco AC, Ivers NM, Grimshaw JM, et al. Effectiveness of quality improvement strategies on the management of diabetes: a systematic review and meta-analysis. *Lancet.* 2012;379(9833):2252–2261.
52. Supper I, Catala O, Lustman M, Chemla C, Bourgueil Y, Letrilliart L. Interprofessional collaboration in primary health care: a review of facilitators and barriers perceived by involved actors. *J Publ Health.* 2015;37(4):716–727.
53. Gardener L, Bourke-Taylor H, Ziviani J. Occupational therapy: an untapped resource for children and adolescents with type 1 diabetes. *Aus Occup Ther J.* 2017;64(1):79–82.
54. Leclaire L, Donnelly C, Hand C, Wener P, Letts L. The role of occupational therapy in primary care: a scoping review. In: World Federation of Occupational Therapists; 2018; Cape Town, South Africa.
55. Donnelly C, Green M, Birtwhistle R, French S, Tranmer J. The impact of interprofessional primary care providers on health care utilization for individuals with diabetes: a linkage study. In: North American Primary Care Group Annual Meeting; 2018; Chicago, IL.
56. Halle AD, Mroz TM, Fogelberg DJ, Leland NE. Occupational therapy and primary care: updates and trends. *Am J Occup Ther.* 2018;72(3):7203090010p1-7203090010p6.
57. Donnelly C, O'Neill C, Bauer M, Letts L. Canadian Occupational Performance Measure (COPM) in primary care: a profile of practice. *Am J Occup Ther.* 2017;71(6):1–8.
58. Parker DM, Sykes CH. A systematic review of the Canadian Occupational Performance Measure: a clinical practice perspective. *Br J Occup Ther.* 2006;69(4):150–160.
59. Toobert DJ, Hampson SE, Glasgow RE. The summary of diabetes self-care activities measure: results from 7 studies and a revised scale. *Diabetes Care.* 2000;23(7):943–950.
60. Schmitt A, Gahr A, Hermanns N, Kulzer B, Huber J, Haak T. The Diabetes Self-Management Questionnaire (DSMQ): development and evaluation of an instrument to assess diabetes self-care activities associated with glycaemic control. *Health Qual Life Outcomes.* 2013;11:138.
61. Bradley C, Todd C, Gorton T, Symonds E, Martin A, Plowright R. The development of an individualized questionnaire measure of perceived impact of diabetes on quality of life: the ADDQoL. *Qual Life Res.* 1999;8(1-2):79–91.
62. Youngson A, Wilby H, Cole F, Cox D. Conceptualising diabetes self-management as an occupation. In: College of Occupational Therapists 40th Annual Conference and Exhibition; June 28–30, 2016, 2016; Harrogate, UK.
63. Haltiwanger EP, Galindo D. Reduction of depressive symptoms in an elderly Mexican-American female with type 2 diabetes mellitus: a single-subject study. *Occup Ther Int.* 2013;20(1):35–44.
64. Sokol-McKay DA. *Occupational Therapy's Role in Diabetes Self-Management.* Bethesda, MD: American Occupational Therapy Association; 2011.
65. Pyatak EA, Carandang K, Davis S. Developing a manualized occupational therapy diabetes management intervention: resilient, empowered, active living with diabetes. *Occup Ther J Res.* 2015;35(3):187–194.
66. Jackson J, Carlson M, Mandel D, Zemke R, Clark F. Occupation in lifestyle redesign: the well elderly study occupational therapy program. *Am J Occup Ther.* 1998;52(5):326–336.
67. Carandang KM, Pyatak EA. Feasibility of a manualized occupation-based diabetes management intervention. *Am J Occup Ther.* 2018;72(2):7202345040p1-7202345040p6.
68. Moll SE, Gewurtz RE, Krupa TM, Law MC, Lariviere N, Levasseur M. "Do-Live-Well": a Canadian framework for promoting occupation, health, and well-being. *Can J Occup Ther.* 2015;82(1):9–23.

Chapter 46

Alzheimer Disease and Other Dementias

Rosanne DiZazzo-Miller

LEARNING OBJECTIVES

This chapter will allow the reader to:

1. Classify and define the various types of dementias.
2. Identify and select appropriate assessments for patients with dementia.
3. List relevant interventions for clients with dementia.
4. Describe areas of need for caregiver assessments and interventions that empower both persons with dementia and caregivers.
5. Analyze a case study and develop an intervention plan inclusive of client-centered care and occupation-based goals.

CHAPTER OUTLINE

TERMINOLOGY

Alzheimer dementia: a label that refers to the underlying disease or the entire continuum of the disease.

Alzheimer disease: the most common form of dementia, comprising approximately 60% to 80% of dementias, and involves neurological plaques and tangles responsible for cognitive deficits.

Creutzfeldt–Jakob disease: type of dementia that is rare, progressively fatal, and specifically causes memory, coordination, and behavioral impairments.

Dementia with Lewy bodies: type of dementia that results from abnormal clumps of the protein alpha-synuclein with onset typically resulting in motor and cognitive impairments.

Frontotemporal lobar degeneration: formerly called frontotemporal dementia; is a type of dementia that includes primary progressive aphasia, Pick's disease, corticobasal degeneration, and progressive supranuclear palsy.

Mild cognitive impairment (MCI): believed to be a precursor to Alzheimer dementia that affects mild thinking impairments, although activities of daily living (ADLs) remain intact.

Mixed dementia: type of dementia that exists when there is evidence of two or more causes of dementia.

Neurocognitive disorder (NCD): the newly replaced *Diagnostic and Statistical Manual of Mental Disorders, Fifth Edition (DSM-5)* term for dementia, although diagnostic information remains the same.

Parkinson disease: a neurodegenerative disease that presents with movement challenges (e.g., rigidity and tremors) and often results in dementia from accrued Lewy bodies in the cortex, along with clumps and tangles.

Preclinical dementia: occurs when brain changes are noted (e.g., cerebrospinal fluid or biomarkers) that show disease onset; however, no visible symptoms are observed or reported.

Vascular dementia: form of dementia that accounts for approximately 40% of dementias (10% present with vascular dementia alone) and occurs most commonly from blood vessel blockage.

Description of Alzheimer Disease and Other Dementias

Epidemiology

Epidemiology refers to new cases within a given time period and population. Approximately 484,000 people in the United States aged 65 years or older developed **Alzheimer dementia** in 2018.[1] As the population ages, risk increases. Approximately 66,000 new cases of Alzheimer dementia occur among people aged 65 to 74 years. This figure increases to 245,000 new cases among people aged 85 years and older (i.e., defined as the oldest old).[1–3] A person develops Alzheimer dementia in the United States every 65 seconds—a figure that will increase to every 33 seconds by 2050.[1] The estimated lifetime risk for Alzheimer dementia based on gender for women at age 65 was approximately 1 in 10, compared to approximately 1 in 20 for men.[1] As the baby-boomer generation reaches age 65, the number of people aged 65 years and older is expected to reach 7.1 million by 2025; therefore, the number of people in this age group diagnosed with Alzheimer dementia is projected to increase from 5.5 million to 13.8 million.[1] The duration of Alzheimer dementia for people aged 65 years and older is between the ages of 4 and 20 years. Alzheimer disease–related death rates have also dramatically increased for people aged 65 to 74 years.[1]

Definition

Although dementia and **Alzheimer disease** are often used interchangeably, it is important to understand each term and how both contribute to this area of clinical study. Dementia is a group of symptoms, or syndrome, that manifests from a variety of causes and in multiple ways. Several types of dementia exist, and it is common for patients to have more than one type—referred to as **mixed dementia.**[1] There are also individuals who have dementia-like symptoms without evidence of Alzheimer-related brain changes, resulting from disorders such as depression, alcohol abuse, and vitamin deficiencies.[1,4] Regardless of type or cause, common symptoms of dementia include challenges related to memory, communication, and problem-solving. Often at the root of these challenges lies neurons that have been damaged or destroyed. Alzheimer disease is a condition in which neurons have been damaged or destroyed, affecting mobility and bodily functions, and is ultimately fatal.[1]

The National Institute on Aging (NIA) and the Alzheimer's Association set forth revised guidelines in 2011 for the diagnosis of Alzheimer disease.[5] Originally, and as seen in the 1984 diagnostic criteria, diagnosis was heavily based on physician clinical judgment with feedback from family and friends. The updated guidelines continue to include physician judgment and family input, but now also include biomarker tests to measure the actual presence or absence of the disease.[1,6] Biomarker tests typically include the amount of beta-amyloid in the brain as shown on positron emission tomography (PET) scans, proteins in fluid such as tau and beta-amyloid in the cerebrospinal fluid, and glucose metabolism in the brain.[1,7] In addition to these changes, three stages of Alzheimer disease have been identified in the revised guidelines: (1) one stage with dementia (i.e., dementia due to Alzheimer disease), (2) one stage in which symptoms are present (e.g., **mild cognitive impairment** [MCI] secondary to Alzheimer disease and dementia secondary to Alzheimer disease), and (3) one stage without symptoms (e.g., **preclinical dementia**, preclinical Alzheimer disease).[1,8] Table 46-1 provides information on the three main areas included in the revised guidelines for diagnosing Alzheimer disease.

Prevalence and Background

Every 3 seconds, someone in the world develops dementia.[9] An estimated 50 million people worldwide have dementia, and this number is projected to double every 20 years.[9] With the fastest growth of older individuals in China, India, and southern Asia, the greatest number of estimated cases of people with dementia is in Asia with 22.9 million, followed by Europe at 10.5 million, the Americas at 9.4 million, and Africa with 4 million.[9] In the United States, Midwestern states on average have the lowest occurrence of Alzheimer dementia (e.g., 13.6%–20.2%) compared to western states, which range from 26.9% to 40%.[1] States with over 40% occurrence rates

Table 46-1. Terminology in 2011 Revised Guidelines for Diagnosing Alzheimer Disease

STAGE	DESCRIPTION
Dementia due to Alzheimer disease	Evidence of an Alzheimer-related biomarker in addition to challenges with behavior, memory, and thinking that impact occupational functioning
Mild cognitive impairment due to Alzheimer disease	Evidence of an Alzheimer-related biomarker in addition to challenges with cognition that is more than what is considered normal given his or her age
Preclinical Alzheimer disease	Evidence of brain changes (e.g., cerebrospinal fluid and blood), yet no noted challenges with memory. Can occur up to 20 year prior to symptom onset

Data from Alzheimer's Association[1] and Sperling et al.[8]

include Nevada, Arizona, Virginia, South Carolina, and Georgia.[1] The estimated cost of dementia in 2015 was calculated as $818 billion in the United States alone; this figure is anticipated to increase to $2 trillion worldwide by 2030.[9] There is an estimated 5.7 million cases of people with Alzheimer dementia in the United States, with about 200,000 individuals under the age of 65.[1] This number increases with age; for example, 3% of people in the 65 to 74 year age group have Alzheimer dementia—a figure that steadily increases to 80% in people aged 75 years or older.[1] Although age does not appear to have a bearing on gender, women comprise the majority of Alzheimer or other dementias at 3.4 million in the United States compared to 2 million men.[1]

Given these statistics, it is important to understand the existence of a treatment gap between high- and low-income countries, suggesting that three-quarters of people with dementia are undiagnosed and do not have access to treatment or other supports available to people with formal diagnoses.[9] This treatment gap presents many opportunities for occupational therapists since often, proper screening secondary to common occurrences such as falls and other accidents can lead to formal diagnosis and proper intervention and support.

Etiology

Researchers believe that various factors contribute to or influence the onset and progression of dementia, leaving the etiology unknown.[10] The *Diagnostic and Statistical Manual of Mental Disorders, Fifth Edition* (*DSM-5*) replaced the term dementia with **neurocognitive disorder (NCD)** in an attempt to reduce stigma related to the definition of dementia—which originated from the late 18th-century *demens*, meaning "out of one's mind."[11,12] This change has no bearing on disease description. Complex attention, executive function, learning and memory, language, perceptual-motor function, and social cognition continue to be the six cognitive domains affected in both mild and major NCD.[11] In addition, subtypes of minor and major NCD are now outlined in the *DSM-5*, including those due to Alzheimer disease, **frontotemporal dementia, dementia with Lewy bodies,** traumatic brain injury, substance/medication-induced dementia, Prion disease, **Parkinson disease,** Huntington disease, other medical conditions, multiple etiologies, and unspecified NCD.[11,12] Given the various causes of dementia, increasing age is the most important risk factor because the number of people with dementia doubles every 5 years.[5]

Lifestyle and Genetics

Age, family history (i.e., a parent, brother, sister, or child with dementia), and genetics increase risk.[13] The most probable cause of late-onset Alzheimer dementia is likely due to a combination of environmental and lifestyle factors and genetics.[5] Heart disease, stroke, and high blood pressure are believed to contribute to the development of Alzheimer disease, and therefore, proper diet, physical activity, smoking cessation, and moderating alcohol consumption may improve health and decrease disease risk.[1,5,13] Various types of infections and brain trauma, such as concussions, are also believed to play a role in the development of dementia.

One primary concern expressed by patients with dementia relates to whether they have passed on a genetic heritance to their children. Genes can have variant forms or mutations. Variant genes mixed with others account for qualities such as height. Mutations can be more harmful and may ultimately lead to a faulty gene that is inherited through generations, such as the gene responsible for Huntington disease.[13] Dementia is more likely to be caused by a mutated gene rather than a variant gene, although multigene variants have been linked to dementia in some families. Genetics play different roles in the four most common dementia types: Alzheimer disease, vascular dementia, dementia with Lewy bodies, and frontotemporal dementia.[13]

Owing to familial clustering (i.e., many close family members are affected by Alzheimer disease), researchers suggest that genetic mutations may be responsible for dementia.[13] Although no one specific gene has been found responsible for Alzheimer disease, studies have found that a mutation of one of three genes may be responsible, including amyloid precursor protein (*APP*), presenilin gene 1 (*PSEN-1*), and presenilin gene 2 (*PSEN-2*).[13] People who have one form of the apolipoprotein (E APOE) on chromosome 19 have been shown to possess increased risk.[5] Other genes that have been identified as having a role in Alzheimer disease include *CLU*, *CR1*, *PICALM*, *BIN1*, *ABCA7*, *MS4A*, *CD33*, *EPHA1*, and *CD2AP*.[13] Early-onset Alzheimer disease—defined as people aged 30 through mid-60s—is believed to be highly linked to genetics, although not all cases are. If a mother or father carries the genetic mutation seen on chromosomes 21, 14, and 1, their offspring have a 50/50 chance of inheriting the mutation and a high risk of developing early onset.[5] To put this into perspective, more than 450 families carry the *PSEN-1* gene mutation on chromosome 14, which causes 80% of early-onset familial Alzheimer disease.[5,13] The *APP* gene mutation on chromosome 21 is present in more than 100 families worldwide.[5,13] This is important because *APP* affects the production of the protein beta-amyloid, and a buildup of beta-amyloid in the brain is hypothesized to be a major contributing factor to Alzheimer disease. The mutation of *PSEN-2* on chromosome 1 is present in more than 30 families, which is thought to be responsible for late-onset Alzheimer disease.[5,13] Although these genes have been identified, only 1 in 10 have a strong family pattern of inheritance. Rather than inheriting these genes from one generation to the next, more than 20 gene variants have been identified as at-risk genes and do not show much support related to inheritance.

The second most common type of dementia after Alzheimer disease is **vascular dementia.**[1] Although no known single-gene mutations have been found for vascular dementia, mutations in *NOTCH3* and *CADASIL* appear to play a role in some rare forms of vascular dementia.[13] Additionally, *APOE* may be linked to vascular dementia, although research has not found definitive evidence. Here again, high cholesterol, high blood pressure, type 2 diabetes, and family history of stroke or heart disease can increase risk and have been shown to heighten the likelihood of developing vascular dementia in later life.[13]

Frontotemporal dementia is the main type of dementia for which genes may play the largest role because there is a strong family history in 10% to 15% of people with this dementia type and up to 30% of cases are linked to a single gene.[13] Mutations in three genes, *C9ORF72*, genes for the proteins tau (*MAPT*), and progranulin (*GRN*), can be linked to most familial frontotemporal dementia cases.[13] In fact, if someone carries *MAPT* or *GRN*, offspring have a 50/50 chance of inheriting the mutation, and nearly all who have this mutation will develop frontotemporal dementia.[13] In addition, a new gene variant, *THEM106B*, has been found to increase the risk for developing frontotemporal dementia.[13]

Unlike frontotemporal dementia, genetics regarding dementia with Lewy bodies is not well understood, and there is little research supporting any familial link toward the development of this dementia type. Therefore, no genetic mutations have been identified, although some gene variants, such as *APOE*, which plays a key role in Alzheimer disease, and glucocerebrosidase (*GBA*) and alpha-synuclein (*SNCA*), which play a role in Parkinson disease, have been shown to increase the risk for dementia with Lewy bodies.[13]

Genetic testing can be performed as a diagnostic measure for people who have already been diagnosed with dementia or as a predictive measure for relatives who are concerned that they may carry dementia-related genes based on family history. Genetic testing is available for the Huntington disease gene (*HTT*), Alzheimer-related genes (*APP*, *PSEN-1*, *PSEN-2*), and frontotemporal-related genes (*MAPT*, *GRN*, *C9ORF72*); however, testing may be offered only under specific conditions and with appropriate counseling.[13]

Dementia Course, Prognosis, Signs, and Symptoms

As can be seen, each type of dementia has differing features. Table 46-2 provides an outline of the course and prognosis, signs and symptoms, and medical management for each dementia type discussed in this chapter.

Medical Management

The medical management of Alzheimer dementia includes both pharmacological and nonpharmacological interventions to treat the spectrum of symptoms present in the various disease stages. As mentioned earlier, some diagnoses require biomarkers, although the majority of diagnoses rely heavily on the report and documentation of mental decline. Some biomarkers such as beta-amyloid and tau levels in cerebrospinal fluid, and brain changes noted through imaging via magnetic resonance imaging (MRI) or computed tomography (CT), can rule out other conditions that may cause symptoms similar to Alzheimer dementia, such as stroke, tumors, or head trauma.[13,15] PET scans of the brain can reveal the presence of amyloid plaques.[15] In fact, an imaging tracer (i.e., Pittsburgh compound B, flutemetamol F18, and florbetaben F18) can reveal amyloid plaques during PET scans.[13,16,17] Cerebrospinal fluid proteins can also be used to analyze the presence of Alzheimer-related cerebrospinal fluid proteins, as well as measurable changes in urine or blood levels with biomarkers such as tau and beta-amyloid.[15–17]

There is currently no cure for Alzheimer disease. The main purpose of intervention is to maximize activities of daily living (ADLs), memory, cognition, mood, behavior, quality of life, and social participation, as well as to ensure a safe living environment. Five Food and Drug Administration (FDA)–approved Alzheimer drugs (Aricept, Razadyne, Exelon, Namenda, and Namzaric) can slow the progression of symptoms by supporting communication of the neurons, synapses, and neurotransmitters in the brain.[18] Managing behavioral and psychological symptoms—which typically include agitation, aggression, depression, mood, and psychosis—are typically first addressed through nonpharmacological means such as minimizing challenges, and maximizing safety and comfort for the person with dementia.[18] No drugs have been FDA approved to address behavioral and psychiatric symptoms from dementia, although various psychological drugs such as antipsychotics, antidepressants, anticonvulsants, and mood stabilizers have been found helpful.[18,19]

Functional Impairment in Daily Occupation

As shown in Table 46-2, the course and symptoms of dementia vary depending on type. Cognition, behavioral and psychological changes, ADLs, and motor control are the main areas of functional impairment and are noted throughout the various stages of dementia progression. Generally, dementia is broken into three stages: early, middle or moderate, and late or severe. However, the seven-stage model based on the Global Deterioration Scale[20] uses the following criteria:

- *Stage 1:* No noted impairments.
- *Stage 2:* Very mild cognitive decline, although nothing more beyond normal aging.
- *Stage 3:* Mild cognitive decline is present and noticeable by family and friends.

Table 46-2. Dementia Type, Course and Prognosis, and Signs and Symptoms

DEMENTIA TYPE	COURSE AND PROGNOSIS	SIGNS AND SYMPTOMS
Alzheimer disease	Alzheimer disease is the most common type of dementia and can begin years before signs or symptoms develop. As a slowly progressive brain disease, the most common pathologies include accumulation of plaques and tangles inside neurons and ultimately neuron damage and death, thereby affecting their ability to transmit impulses. May live 20+ years after diagnosis.	The most common signs and symptoms of Alzheimer disease center on challenges with memory, such as recent conversations and events. Apathy and depression may develop followed later by challenges with communication, judgment, behavior, and confusion. The end stages of Alzheimer disease progress to the point of expressive aphasia, dysphagia, and mobility problems.
Vascular dementia	Vascular dementia is the second most common type of dementia and is also commonly found with people who have another type of dementia. Typically, clients with vascular dementia have evidence of some type of infarct or bleeding in the brain caused by blockage or damage of blood vessels. People typically live 5 years after symptoms are present.	Rather than challenges with memory, the most common signs and symptoms of vascular dementia include executive functions such as impaired judgment, decision-making, and organization. With progression, additional cognitive and motor challenges typically occur.
Dementia with Lewy bodies	In dementia with Lewy bodies, there are clumps present in the cortex, resulting in cognitive impairment. Dementia with Lewy bodies is often a comorbidity with Alzheimer disease, thereby leading to a mixed dementia diagnosis. People typically live 6–12 years after symptoms are present.	Most often, clients will report difficulty with sleeping early on. This is typically followed by visual hallucinations and mobility impairments, including Parkinsonian-type motions.
Frontotemporal lobar degeneration	Frontotemporal lobar degeneration previously referred to as frontotemporal dementia is often affected by nerve cells in the frontal and temporal lobe regions of the brain, resulting in atrophy of these brain structures. Layers of the cortex have abnormal proteins. Frontotemporal lobar degeneration includes a behavioral-variant form, primary progressive aphasia, Pick disease, corticobasal degeneration, and progressive supranuclear palsy.	Typically, symptoms develop with a younger onset of 45–60 years. Signs and symptoms are seen most predominantly through changes in behavior and personality as well as expressive and receptive aphasia with memory challenges present later in disease progression.
Parkinson disease	Parkinson disease begins with degeneration of nerve cells that produce dopamine. Much like dementia with Lewy bodies, Parkinson disease presents with clumps in the cortex as well as clumps and tangles in the substantia nigra.	Motor control is mostly affected including movement that is slow, rigid, with tremors present that affect mobility.
Creutzfeldt–Jakob disease	Prion, which is a misfolded protein, causes other proteins in the brain to malfunction. Etiology is unknown, although there is a possibility of a link to heredity and/or prion infection. A variant form of Creutzfeldt–Jakob disease is thought to have been caused by mad cow disease.	Rare and rapidly fatal impairment of memory and coordination with noted behavioral changes
Normal pressure hydrocephalus	Normal pressure hydrocephalus is caused by cerebrospinal fluid that is not reabsorbed and, therefore, causes a buildup of fluid and pressure in the brain. History of brain hemorrhage and meningitis may present an increased risk. Occasionally, shunts may be effective in draining the additional fluid.	Signs and symptoms include challenges with mobility and memory, and incontinence.

Data from Alzheimer's Association[1] and Dening and Sandilyan[14]

- *Stage 4:* Moderate cognitive decline to the point that neurologists can make a diagnosis. Challenges are present in short-term memory and basic arithmetic.
- *Stage 5:* Moderately severe cognitive decline is marked by challenges with ADLs coupled with confusion and disorientation, making independent living a challenge.
- *Stage 6:* Severe cognitive decline includes a worsening of all previously stated challenges in addition to the onset of personality changes and difficulty recognizing family members and friends.
- *Stage 7:* Very severe cognitive decline marks the final stage as well as the most significant impairments to memory, communication, and motor control.

Early-Stage Functional Impairments

Although stages can provide an idea of functional impairment, it is important to realize that each individual with dementia can present with different and unique symptoms. Additionally, the length of each stage can vary considerably for each client. In the early stage, or stages 1 to 3[20] using the seven-stage model, the realization that something may be wrong begins to set in. Most individuals try to mask their symptoms through various compensatory techniques such as relying more heavily on phone reminders and post-it notes. Memory lapses or momentary confusion may occur, and individuals may begin to seek help for instrumental activities of daily living (IADLs) that involve more complex tasks.

Middle-Stage Functional Impairments

In the middle stage, or stages 4 to 5,[20] memory lapses and confusion increase, and poor judgment and even wandering may begin to become areas of concern. Memory deficits begin to involve personal information, such as home addresses and phone numbers, and important dates, such as birthdays and anniversaries. In dementia with Lewy bodies, more motor-related declines are present, and in frontotemporal (behavior variant) dementia, inappropriate behaviors begin to create additional functional obstacles. Overall, ADLs such as bathing, grooming, dressing, eating, transferring, and toileting begin to require assistance. IADLs such as communication, shopping, food preparation, housekeeping, laundry, transportation, medication, and financial management begin to become challenging as well. Sleep patterns may also become disrupted. In the middle stage of dementia, family and friends notice personality changes along with psychological challenges such as fear, depression, and paranoia. It is understandable, then, that social withdrawal tends to follow. In this stage, caregivers (e.g., care partners) typically begin to feel stressed and overwhelmed and experience feelings of burden and depression.

Late-Stage Functional Impairments

In the late stage, or stages 6 to 7,[20] people with dementia experience severe decline in both cognitive and physical function. Independence in all areas of life is severely impacted, including purposeful communication, eating, swallowing, bowel and bladder control, and mobility. Agitation and irritability are intensified, and individuals typically require maximum assistance with all ADLs. In this later stage, the focus of functioning turns to comfort and quality of life for the client, and support for caregivers.

Evaluation and Intervention of Functional Skill Deficits Secondary to Alzheimer Disease and Other Dementias

Assessment and Evaluation for Dementia

Occupational therapy (OT) assessment and evaluation should, as always, be client centered and involve the person with dementia, their caregiver(s), and any family members. Although others are helpful to have present during the initial evaluation, it is critical to empower the person with dementia to have an active role in this process. Typically, the evaluation is broken down into assessments, including an occupational profile through observation and interview, followed by assessments for ADLs, cognition, and psychosocial and physical functioning. Prior to working with clients with dementia, it is critical to review their chart and identify any precautions or contraindications. In general, clients with dementia are at an increased risk for falls and are more easily overwhelmed and overstimulated. Unlike remedial techniques that are implemented when communicating with clients diagnosed with other neurological challenges such as brain injury or stroke, it is not useful or productive to argue with or attempt to orient clients with dementia who are disoriented and insist on things that are not reality based. Examples include time, date, season, and the current president. Attempts at orientation or disagreement with clients with degenerative neurological disease must be done so under extreme care because such attempts can lead to arguments that will increase anxiety, agitation, and paranoia. Assessments are invaluable in identifying these and additional areas that present challenges to people with dementia. The Assessment Table provides a selected list and description of appropriate assessments for dementia care.

Intervention Procedures for Impairments Associated with Alzheimer Dementia

Based on dementia stage, client strengths and weaknesses, and additional evaluation findings, occupational therapists develop treatment plans that address task simplification, remediation or compensation when possible, environmental modifications, health promotion, and caregiver training. The following outlines key interventions areas:

Task Simplification

Most clients with dementia are cared for in the home by family caregivers.[1] As dementia progresses, everyday tasks become more challenging, and both clients and caregivers will need to use adaptation, compensation, and task simplification. When simplifying tasks for clients with dementia and/or their caregivers, it's important to provide clear, concise verbal directions as well as visual and tactile cues when possible. Task simplification most often includes setup. For example, if engaging clients in meal preparation, therapists should arrange all food and materials in advance and in sequential order to promote function (Fig. 46-1). Similarly, if engaging clients in dressing, therapists should set up clothes in sequential order; clothing should be selected that is easiest to don, such as pullover shirts, elastic waistband pants, and slip-on shoes (Fig. 46-2). While setup is important, it is equally important to break down tasks into simple steps.[21]

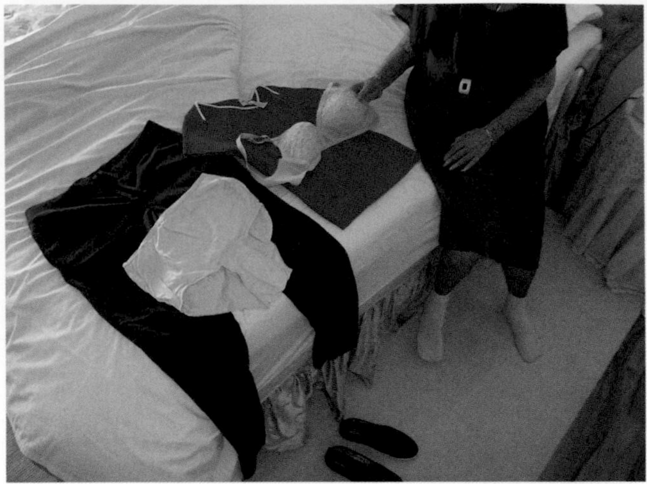

Figure 46-2. Task simplification. When engaging clients in dressing, therapists should set up clothes in sequential order; clothing should be selected that is easiest to don, such as pullover shirts, elastic waistband pants, and slip-on shoes.

Environmental Modification

Environmental modifications are often necessary with the progression of dementia secondary to increased fall risk; however, it is important to consider when making modifications that familiar surroundings most optimally promote client function. Modifications that promote safety and mobility are outlined in Table 46-3. These modifications typically include adjustments to address vision and hearing loss, confusion, and visual–spatial challenges; it is equally important, however, to consider the importance of structured, predictable daily routines.[23]

Remediation

Typically, with degenerative neurological conditions, remediation of cognitive abilities is not a focus of treatment; however, research has shown improvement in cognition and quality of life for study participants with mild-to-moderate dementia after engaging in cognitive stimulation therapy (CST) for people using money, word games, present-day famous faces, and reality orientation boards. In this study, CST compared favorably with pharmacological treatments.[24] Restoration of physical function should be addressed in terms of range of motion (ROM), strength, and overall endurance. Although remediation of physical function is possible, it is important that therapists take a gentle, structured approach and prevent overfatigue. A home program that is short and easy to follow, with appropriate and plentiful visual aids, will help facilitate goals centered on physical functioning. Home exercise programs, coupled with behavioral management training for caregivers, were shown to have significant improvements in patient physical functioning and depression, and decreased institutionalization.[25] Using client-centered tools, such as old family photo albums, and client-identified favorite music and television shows is another way to stimulate memory and discussion of past events because long-term memory remains intact longer than short-term memory. With this said, it is important to understand the degenerative nature of dementia and that although improvements can be made mentally and physically, the progressive nature of this disease will ultimately cause decline in all areas of functioning. Occupational therapists are assigned with the important role of intervening to improve and maintain daily functioning that enhances qualify of life for as long as possible.

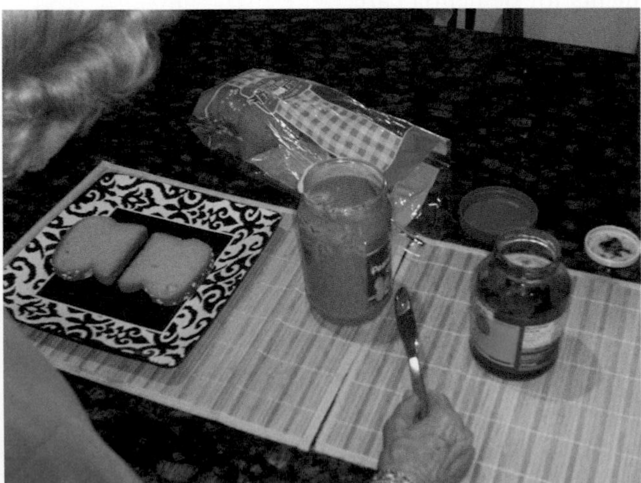

Figure 46-1. Task simplification. When engaging clients in meal preparation, therapists should arrange all food and materials in advance and in sequential order to promote function.

Compensation

While remediation, as discussed earlier, can be appropriate given each client's unique case, compensation tends to be a major focus of treatment, especially as it pertains to cognitive functioning and behavioral changes. Compensatory interventions should focus on identifying strengths and weakness of clients and caregivers; assessing levels of burden, depression, and quality of life; and developing treatment plans to

Table 46-3. Environmental Modifications that Promote Safety and Mobility

ENVIRONMENTAL MODIFICATION	DESCRIPTION
Reduce clutter	Declutter the environment by removing throw rugs, simplify and organize objects, place objects in sequence of use, and label objects when appropriate.
Improve lighting	Improve lighting during tasks and throughout walkways. Have the option of dim lighting for moments when bright lights may be overwhelming or overstimulating.
Decrease glare	Lighting can sometimes cause shadows that can be perceived to be confusing or even frightening. Check for glare throughout the home and reduce when possible.
Increase contrast	Utilize color contrast throughout all areas of the home. Toilet seats are commonly overlooked and are often white against a white background, making them appear to be the floor. Safe paint or tape can outline the seat. White coffee or tea cups are ideal along with dinner ware that is color contrasted to the table and food.
Arrange furniture	Furniture should be arranged in a manner that promotes clear and uncluttered walkways. Low stools present safety hazards.
Address wandering	Install items to deter, prevent, and monitor wandering such as disguising doors, installing open door alerts and security cameras, and implementing an ID system.
Address sound	Decrease noise that can be overstimulating, such as two televisions turned on at the same time or one turned on too loudly. Play client-preferred music softly in the background during meals and bathing to increase comfort and calmness.
Limit choices	Too many choices for meals, clothes, and so on can lead to being overwhelmed. Limit choices to two to three options both verbally and visually. Present food one item at a time. Use one- to two-step commands when cuing. Limited labeling can also provide visual cues for locating rooms and objects.
Use adaptive equipment	Use bathroom equipment such as a tub bench, toilet rail, grab bars, hand held shower, and a long-handled sponge. Tubing can be used to increase grip size of many items, such as toothbrushes, pens, combs, and utensils as well as deep plates/bowls.

Data from Fraker et al.[21] and van Hoof et al.[22]

provide education, training, and resources for modifying or adapting the identified occupations, client factors, and performance skills that impact overall occupational functioning.

Wellness and Health Promotion

Health promotion is important to address for both the care recipient and caregiver. Strengthening and maintaining health and wellness for both parties typically leads to enhanced occupational functioning. It is important to understand how clients and caregivers manage their stress in order to plan and provide appropriate training and resources. Wellness and health promotion includes examining and addressing self-management behaviors, such as good habits and routines, nutrition, and engagement in exercise and social activities.[26] Wellness and health promotion begins with awareness through proper education and resources.

Caregiver Training

More than 16 million caregivers provide informal, unpaid care for people with dementia.[1] In fact, more than half of informal, family caregivers of people with dementia help with transfers, toileting, bathing, grooming, and feeding.[1] Caregiving is an immense responsibility and can cause unhealthy levels of stress and anxiety.[27] Such anxiety, coupled with feelings of unpreparedness to deal with their loved one's newly challenging behaviors, presents uncomfortable and sometimes irritating situations. Research has shown that caregiver interventions can lead to increased ADL knowledge,[28] decreased burden, and improved quality of life.[29] The following areas of caregiver training are outlined as follows:

- Because many caregivers personalize the behavioral changes and verbal attacks of care recipients, it is critical to first educate caregivers about the neurological and physiological changes occurring in clients' brains. This will help caregivers understand that people with dementia do not have control over their behaviors. Next, it is critical to provide education and training in client ADL performance because over half of informal family caregivers provide assistance with ADLs.[1] As with all areas of functioning, it's important for caregivers to provide only assistance as needed to encourage client functioning as much as possible.

- Within caregiver training, it is also important to explain the degenerative nature of dementia and that, rather than correcting clients' incorrect statements, it is more beneficial to let such statements go to avoid confrontation. In the same manner, redirection of the client is a useful technique to avoid inappropriate or combative behaviors.
- Caregiver communication styles can influence the difference between successful and unsuccessful outcomes. In the early to early-moderate stages of dementia, clients realize their own memory challenges and often attempt to mask problems or become defensive about them. When communicating, it is critical to be positioned at eye level with the client, allow clients time to respond to questions, and help with word-finding only when it appears that assistance is welcome.
- Although bathing, grooming, and dressing are commonly performed daily, it is important to understand that bathing specifically can be extremely challenging for clients and there is no reason why this activity needs to occur more than two to three times per week. People with dementia often experience fear of water, and although physical appearance is important, cleanliness can be achieved with sponge baths. It is important to ensure privacy, a softly lighted environment, warm water temperature, setup of all supplies prior to bathing, use of adaptive equipment as appropriate, and overall safety such as locks on medicine cabinets and an environment free of nearby electrical appliances. Educate caregivers to allow bathing to be relaxing and enjoyable, rather than rushed. Bathing is also an excellent opportunity to perform skin checks for breakdown and bruising. Once in the tub or shower, shampooing may become challenging, and therefore, this task can be performed separately on another day or at a sink while clothed. Techniques such as wearing a waterproof visor to prevent soap from entering the eyes or using a handheld shower may help reduce combativeness. Grooming can be completed while clothed and seated with assistance as needed. Proper nail care should be completed after bathing; if clients possess thick or difficult-to-trim nails, professional assistance should be obtained. Good oral hygiene, including flossing, is essential, and dentists exist who specialize in dental care for people with dementia. Hair combing and brushing are tasks that can be completed hand-over-hand, which helps to engage clients as their disease progresses. Limiting dressing and grooming supplies to two to three choices can also prevent clients from feeling overwhelmed. Dressing from a seated position and arranging clothing items in the order in which they need to be donned can also help with successful task completion. It is important for caregivers to take note of clothing items that are preferred by clients as well as clothing types that are comfortable and easiest to don and doff. Loose-fitting clothes, slip-on shoes, and clothing with larger fasteners are easiest to negotiate. Dressing can be a good time to perform ROM exercises accompanied by music to create a fun and carefree experience.
- Eating and/or feeding are also important to consider. With disease progression, people with dementia may not recognize hunger or thirst and may experience difficulty with eating activities. Common helpful strategies include eating in a calm environment in which clients are able to eat at their own pace, recommending that caregivers and clients eat together, serving only one food at a time, ensuring that clients use the bathroom before and after eating, serving food in bowls instead of plates (bowls are easier to retrieve food from), precutting foods in bite-size pieces before serving, and maintaining the same eating schedule for each meal and on each day of the week. Additionally, it is important to ensure that caregivers understand the importance of keeping clients' chins in a neutral and slightly flexed position when swallowing.
- Toileting and transferring are important considerations that impact many areas of daily living. A quick check of the environment can reveal safety hazards, such as throw rugs, low furniture, insufficient lighting, and cluttered pathways. Proper transfer training is essential and should include education about body mechanics for both clients and caregivers, as well as appropriate methods to transfer from beds, chairs, car seats, toilets, and showers/tubs. Caregivers should be able to both verbally instruct and demonstrate how to safely transfer clients from all areas of the home. A tracker for incontinence is important as is a schedule for toileting every 2 hours. Important transfer considerations include proper seat height and contrast, ability to undress before bladder voiding accidents occur, and whether bathrooms are organized and well lit. Important considerations for toileting during the evening are commode placement next to beds and sufficient lighting in hallways and bathrooms. Clients who are incontinent should be regularly checked for skin breakdown and placed on a proper skin care routine.
- Education about respite services and support groups is crucial as caregivers need breaks from the ongoing, everyday support they must provide to maintain the health and safety of the person with dementia. Respite programs provide breaks for caregivers to focus on themselves and other family members and friends, whereas support groups provide a forum in which to bond with other caregivers and learn about how others cope with similar daily challenges.

CASE STUDY

Patient Information

Donna is an active, 75-year-old white woman who lives in a two-story home in the west side of Detroit along with her 52-year-old daughter who works full time as a bank security guard, and 20-year-old granddaughter who attends college nearby. Donna's husband passed away many years ago. She held various jobs while growing up in the city, but then became and worked as a nurse for the majority of her life, eventually retiring at age 65. Donna was known for her high level of joy, care, and love that she provided to her patients. Her leisure interests include reading the Bible, attending church, calligraphy, sewing, art, gardening, listening to Luciano Pavarotti, and the good company of family and friends. Donna has another daughter who lives in Georgia.

Donna is a smoker and has been her entire adult life. She has heart disease and high blood pressure for which she is being medically treated. Donna wears prescription lenses that just broke, and, in their place, she uses a magnifying glass. Her main source of income is social security, and she has Medicare along with supplemental insurance.

Reason for Occupational Therapy Referral

Donna's daughter, Carol, began noticing changes in her mother's ability to keep track of bills and appointments. Donna always prided herself on her home management and organization skills; however, in recent months, she reports noticing forgetfulness that is occurring more often and consistently, and changes in balance and overall endurance that impact her ability to perform ADLs and IADLs. More specifically, Carol reports that her mother has been experiencing difficulty getting ready in the morning, including occasional confusion between hot and cold water while bathing. Carol reports that Donna frequently becomes overwhelmed while dressing and sometimes dons inappropriate clothing for the season. Carol also reports that Donna's morning routine is taking notably longer than normal and that Donna appears exhausted afterward with an inability to make breakfast or do much of anything else. Carol also reports that her mother's personality has become somewhat inappropriate at times. Carol brought Donna to their family doctor who referred them to a neurologist. After meeting with the neurologist and based on medical history, physical examination, laboratory tests, and reported changes in thinking and daily functioning, a diagnosis of dementia was given without any specific type noted. As a result of the impact of Donna's newly diagnosed dementia on her daily living, the physician ordered an OT evaluation with recommendations for home adaptations.

Assessment Process and Results

An occupational therapist arrived at Donna's home approximately 1 month after diagnosis. Donna does not have a guardian or conservator. Prior to beginning the evaluation, the occupational therapist asked Donna whether she would like to answer the questions alone or have Carol present and contributing. Donna chose the latter, and all three sat down and began the evaluation process. The therapist used a top-down approach to begin the evaluation process and completed the Canadian Occupational Performance Measure (COPM); the Montreal Cognitive Assessment (MoCA); and functional screens for ROM, strength, and coordination. A home evaluation was also performed to ensure safety and accessibility within the home. Secondary to reported endurance and balance issues, the therapist issued the 6-Minute Walk Test (6MWT) for endurance and the Tinetti Balance and Gait Test. Findings revealed challenges consistent with Carol's reports about her mother's function.

Occupational Therapy Problem List

- **COPM**: Bathing is difficult due to confusion with hot/cold water. Dressing is overwhelming and confusing. Morning routine is exhausting and takes longer than reasonable. Donna is falling behind on mail organization, appointments, and bills. She reports being too tired for meal preparation.
- **MoCA**: Revealed moderate cognitive impairment (score = 23)
- **ROM, manual muscle test (MMT), and coordination**: ROM, MMT, and 9-Hole Pegboard assessment are within functional limits.
- **Home evaluation**: Closet is overwhelming with winter clothing mixed with summer and a great variety of choices. Bathroom is all white, has throw rugs, and is cluttered. Standard shower is present with no adaptive equipment. The rest of the home is accessible, although kitchen lights are dim and Donna has difficultly using the microwave because of small print.
- **6MWT**: Decreased endurance (score = 410 m; normal is 439–571)
- **Tinetti Balance and Gait Test**: Moderate risk for falls (score = 23)

Occupational Therapy Goal List

- Client will develop a binder/file system including mail, bills, and calendar with month-at-a-glance in order to increase independence in home management and organization skills.
- Client will perform a home exercise program focused on balance and endurance to improve physical functioning required for occupational performance.
- Client will safely and effectively distinguish the difference between the shower dial for hot and cold water.
- Client will perform 10 to 20 minutes per day of cognitive tasks along with her caregiver to provide daily cognitive stimulation.
- Client will engage in self-identified leisure tasks two to three times per week.
- Client and caregiver will demonstrate and implement energy conservation, task simplification, and environmental

(continued)

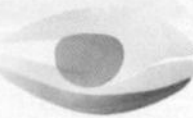

CASE STUDY *(continued)*

modifications to increase independence in ADLs and meal prep.

- Caregiver will correctly demonstrate and apply redirection techniques during communication challenges with her mom with 100% accuracy.
- Caregiver will contact the local Alzheimer's Association to receive resources, including support groups and respite care.

Intervention

1. The occupational therapist, client, and caregiver developed an effective, client-centered, and driven binder/file system so that Donna could organize her mail and bills, along with a calendar system that is visually organizing for the care recipient.
2. After client and caregiver education, Donna began a safe and efficient home exercise program for stretching, balance, and endurance.
3. The occupational therapist provided waterproof labeling on the shower dial to clearly delineate hot and cold water directions, and client education with return demonstration for safe use.
4. Donna began to perform cognitive tasks with her caregiver 10 to 20 minutes per day to provide daily cognitive stimulation, including tasks as outlined in CST guidelines (book is available for caregiver purchase, or therapists can provide tasks to perform based on CST), viewing family photos and recalling family members and events, and listening to enjoyable music such as Luciano Pavarotti. Daily cognitive stimulation activities were also used as a means to redirect smoking habits into meaningful and purposeful leisure pursuits and to implement health promotion education on smoking cessation.
5. The occupational therapist set up a small bin with client-centered leisure interests, including the Bible, the client's calligraphy set, sewing, and art and gardening supplies, to encourage leisure pursuits with her caregiver.
6. The occupational therapist provided education on energy conservation techniques, task simplification, and environmental modifications appropriate during morning ADLs and meal prep. These included setting up bathing supplies prior to bathing; limiting clothing options to two to three weather-appropriate outfits; laying out clothing in sequential order of donning; using high-contrast towels, handles, and toilet seat in her all white bathroom; having meals set up and ready to place in the oven or on the stove; clearly labeling (but not over labeling) drawers, cabinets, and refrigerator and freezer bins to decrease time spent seeking objects; identifying times of day that are more fatiguing than others; and planning structured days based on energy levels.
7. The occupational therapist provided caregiver education for and demonstration of positive, nonthreatening communication styles and redirection techniques to implement during communication challenges with her mom. Carol practiced performing these techniques during simulation opportunities with the therapist.
8. With the therapist's help, Carol contacted the local Alzheimer's Association to receive resources including information about support groups and respite care. This information is critical for Carol to have early on to address health and wellness for both herself and her mother, as well as to plan ahead for the future because she lives full time with her mother and is employed outside the home. This information will also be a source for future resources as Donna's dementia progresses and her occupational functioning declines. It will be important for Carol to plan for future systems to prevent Donna from wandering or answering the door and allowing strangers into their home.

Commonly Used Assessments in Dementia Evaluation

Instrument	Intended Purpose	Administration Time	Validity	Reliability	Sensitivity	Strengths and Weaknesses
Disability Assessment for Dementia (DAD)[34]	Interview with the caregiver about the person with dementia's ADL performance over the past 2 weeks. Measures ADLs and IADLs in community-dwelling adults with dementia.	Approximately 15 minutes	Content validity established with experts and caregivers. Criterion-related (concurrent) validity established with the Rapid Disability Rating Scale-2 ($r = -0.85$, $n = 59$) and known groups. Construct validity established with MMSE ($r = 0.54$), $n = 55$.	Test–retest reliability intraclass correlation coefficient (ICC) = 0.96 ($n = 45$). Inter-rater reliability ICC = 0.95 ($n = 31$). Internal consistency Cronbach's alpha = 0.96 ($n = 59$).	Responsiveness of the DAD over a 1-year period and therapeutic sensitivity in pharmacological studies	Strengths: Measure of actual performance in ADL over a 2-week period. Assesses client's actual performance, not estimated capability. Considers sensorimotor disturbances that may influence performance. Weaknesses: Requires a 2-week period.
Executive Function Performance Test (EFPT)[35]	The EFPT is a criterion-referenced top-down assessment of executive function skills and covers five components of executive function throughout four domains, including initiation, organization, sequencing, safety/judgment, and termination.	30–45 minutes	Concurrent validity reports high correlation with the Functional Assessment Measure for clients with acute or chronic stroke and adequate-to-high correlation with the Assessment of Motor and Process Skills (AMPS) and Short Blessed. Construct validity with known groups discriminated between clients with stroke and health controls.	High internal consistency for total score and adequate-to-high internal consistency for tasks. Inter-rater reliability was high for total score and all tasks.	Not established	Strengths: Performance-based standardized assessment of cognitive function. Top-down approach to assessment compared to many other bottom-up approaches that analyze brain function. Weaknesses: Most studies were completed in samples of people with stroke. No normative data.

(*continued*)

Commonly Used Assessments in Dementia Evaluation (*continued*)

Instrument	Intended Purpose	Administration Time	Validity	Reliability	Sensitivity	Strengths and Weaknesses
Performance Assessment of Self-Care Skills (PASS)[36]	The PASS is a performance-based criterion-referenced assessment consisting of 26 items ranging from functional mobility, personal self-care, IADLs with cognitive emphasis, and IADLs with physical emphasis. Can be given in total, alone or in combination. Two versions exist including one for home and one for clinic. Scored using a four-point (0–3) ordinal scale based on independence, safety, and adequacy.	Administration times range from 1.5 to 3 hours	Data are not available; however, the authors report content and construct validity.	Test–retest reliability for both the clinic and home version was high and ranged from ICC = 0.82–0.97) throughout independence, safety, and adequacy. Inter-rater reliability established as percentage agreement among examiners and ranged between 88% and 97% for both versions throughout independence, safety, and adequacy.	Not established	Strengths: No certification is required for administration and may be used in the home or clinic setting. Weaknesses: This test has a lengthy administration time and is not freely available.
Montreal Cognitive Assessment (MoCA)[37,38]	Designed as a rapid screening tool for mild cognitive assessment. Out of a score of 30, 26 or higher is considered normal.	Approximately 10 minutes	Concurrent validity was highly and positively correlated with the MMSE ($r = 0.867$, $p < 0.01$).	Cronbach's alpha was 0.884, high level of internal consistency. Inter-rater reliability was 0.966 ($p < 0.01$).	Detected 83% of participants with MCI and 94% with dementia	Strengths: Brief, useful screening tool to detect mild dementia and MCI. Weaknesses: Studies have had small samples with only 6-month follow-up. Conclusions are based on participants from a memory clinic.
Clinical Dementia Rating Scale (CDR)[39]	The CDR is a semi-structured interview that uses a five-point scale to assess cognitive and functional performance in the areas of memory, orientation, judgment and problem-solving, community affairs, home and hobbies, and personal care. Requires input from both the person with dementia and his or her caregiver.	Approximately 20–40 minutes. Administered to both the person with dementia and his or her caregiver.	Concurrent validity correlation was $r = 0.50$; Discriminant validity was strong.	Inter-rater reliability ranged from $r = 0.60$ –0.80.	Not available	Strengths: The CDR is noted as the best evidenced scale in a systematic review. Weaknesses: Time varies because caregiver/care recipient dyads are required for scoring.

Evidence Supporting Interventions for Clients with Dementia

Intervention	Description	Dosage	Participants	Research Design and Evidence Level	Benefit	Statistical Significance and Effect Size
A structured occupational therapy program for older adults with dementia[30]	OT program included progressive muscle relaxation (10 minutes), physical exercises (10 minutes), personal care activities and household tasks (15 minutes), and cognitive exercises and recreation activities (10 minutes). Control group did not receive intervention.	Intervention included 10 treatment sessions of 70 minutes each over 5 weeks.	Seventy-seven participants attending a memory clinic were screened for dementia and were 60+ years old (36 = treatment group; 41 = control group).	Randomized controlled trial Level I	Novel OT program provided significant improvements in participants' physical and psychological domains as measured using the World Health Organization Quality of Life—BREF, compared to control.	Treatment group reported improved physical scores ($p < 0.0001$) and psychological scores ($p < 0.0001$).
Effects of community occupational therapy on quality of life, mood, and health status in patients with dementia and their caregivers[31]	Community-based OT intervention	Ten 1-hour home-based OT sessions over 5 weeks	One hundred and thirty-five participants	Randomized controlled trial Level I	Improvement in participants' and caregivers overall quality of life was maintained 12 weeks postintervention.	People with dementia reported significantly higher quality of life ($p < 0.0001$) and general health status ($p < 0.0001$) at 6 and 12 weeks, respectively, postintervention, compared to control.
Tailored activities to manage neuropsychiatric behaviors in persons with dementia and reduce caregiver burden[32]	Tailored activity program to reduce behavioral disturbance and caregiver burden	Eight home visits by an occupational therapist. Client-centered intervention based on therapist assessment and client and caregiver feedback.	Sixty caregiver/care recipient dyads	Two-group, randomized, wait-list controlled pilot study Level I	Four months postintervention, caregivers reported reduced frequency of problem behaviors, less agitation and argumentation, and greater mastery and use of simplification techniques.	Caregivers reported a reduced frequency of behaviors ($p = 0.10$), greater activity engagement ($p = 0.029$), ability to keep busy ($p = 0.017$), less agitation ($p = 0.014$), and less argumentation ($p = 0.010$). Caregivers personally reported greater mastery ($p = 0.013$), self-efficacy, ($p = 0.011$) and use of simplification techniques ($p = 0.023$), compared to wait-list control participants.

(continued)

Evidence Supporting Interventions for Clients with Dementia (*continued*)

Intervention	Description	Dosage	Participants	Research Design and Evidence Level	Benefit	Statistical Significance and Effect Size
Exercise plus behavioral management in patients with Alzheimer disease[25]	A home-based exercise program combined with caregiver training in behavioral management techniques	Dyads were seen in their homes for 12-hour long sessions, two times per week for the first 3 weeks, followed by weekly sessions for 4 weeks, and then biweekly sessions for 4 weeks. Three follow-up sessions were conducted over 3 months.	One hundred and fifty-three community-dwelling participants who met the National Institute of Neurological and Communicative Diseases and Stroke/Alzheimer's Disease and Related Disorders Association criteria for Alzheimer disease. Caregivers were spouses or adult relatives.	Randomized controlled trial Level I	Reduced functional dependence and delayed institutionalization for the treatment group as seen 3 months postintervention with participants having significantly fewer days of restricted activity and improved scores for physical role functioning and depression.	Fewer days of restricted activity ($p < 0.001$), improved physical role functioning ($p < 0.001$), improved depression scores ($p = 0.02$), and better physical role functioning scores ($p = 0.003$) with a trend for decreased institutionalization (19% vs. 50%); at 3 and 24 months postintervention.
Efficacy of an evidence-based cognitive stimulation therapy program for people with dementia[24]	CST for money, word games, and present-day famous faces as well as reality orientation board	Fourteen session program twice per week for 45 minutes per session over 7 weeks	Two hundred and one participants (115 = intervention group; 86 = control group)	Randomized controlled trial Level I	Intervention group significantly improved on Mini-Mental State Examination (MMSE), Alzheimer's Disease Assessment Scale—Cognition, and Quality of Life Alzheimer's Disease Scale, which compare favorably with pharmacological treatments in other studies. Gains in functional outcomes, communication, and anxiety and depression were modest.	MMSE ($p = 0.044$), Alzheimer's Disease Assessment Scale—Cognition ($p = 0.014$), and Quality of Life Alzheimer's Disease Scale ($p = 0.028$)
Evidence-based occupational therapy for people with dementia and their families: What clinical practice guidelines tell us regarding implications for practice[33]	Review of literature and guideline development for effective care within the scope of OT practice for people with dementia and their families focused on ADLs, quality of life, and carer impact	Five studies including 974 participants	Dosages varied between 5 and 10 visits over 5–6 months.	Meta-analysis Level I	OT interventions that were effective included environmental assessment, problem-solving strategies, carer education, and interactive carer skills training.	Positive ADL function (standardized mean difference [SMD] 0.17, 95% confidence interval [CI]: 0.02–0.33); carer impact revealed no significant effect (SMD –0.15, 95% CI: –0.32 to 0.02); quality of life for person with dementia was significant (SMD 0.62, 95% CI: 0.43–0.81).

References

1. Alzheimer's Association. 2018 Alzheimer's disease facts and figures. *Alzheimer's Dement.* 2018;14(3):367–429. https://www.alz.org/media/HomeOffice/Facts and Figures/facts-and-figures.pdf.
2. World Health Organization. The epidemiology and impact of dementia: current state and future trends. *First WHO Minist Conference on the Global Action Against Dementia.* 2015:1–4. http://www.who.int/mental_health/neurology/dementia/thematic_briefs_dementia/en/.
3. The Swedish Council on Technology Assessment in Healthcare. *Dementia—Etiology and Epidemiology: A Systematic Review.* 2008;1(June). https://www.ncbi.nlm.nih.gov/books/NBK447961/pdf/Bookshelf_NBK447961.pdf.
4. Ridley NJ, Draper B, Withall A. Alcohol-related dementia: an update of the evidence. *Alzheimer's Res Ther.* 2013;25;5(1):3. doi:10.1186/alzrt157.
5. National Institute on Aging. Causes of Alzheimer's Disease. https://www.nia.nih.gov/health/what-causes-alzheimers-disease. Published 2017. Accessed April 27, 2018.
6. Bateman RJ, Xiong C, Benzinger TLS, et al. Clinical and biomarker changes in dominantly inherited Alzheimer's disease. *N Engl J Med.* 2012;367:795–804. doi:10.1056/NEJMoa1202753.
7. McKhann GM, Knopman DS, Chertkow H, et al. The diagnosis of dementia due to Alzheimer's disease: recommendations from the National Institute on Aging-Alzheimer's Association workgroups on diagnostic guidelines for Alzheimer's disease. *Alzheimer's Dement.* 2011;7(3):263–269. doi:10.1016/j.jalz.2011.03.005.
8. Sperling RA, Aisen PS, Beckett LA, et al. Toward defining the preclinical stages of Alzheimer's disease: recommendations from the National Institute on Aging-Alzheimer's Association workgroups on diagnostic guidelines for Alzheimer's disease. *Alzheimer's Dement.* 2011;7(3):280–292. doi:10.1016/j.jalz.2011.03.003.
9. Prince M, Comas-Herrera A, Knapp M, Guerchet M, Karagiannidou M. World Alzheimer Report 2016 Improving healthcare for people living with dementia. Coverage, Quality and costs now and in the future. *Alzheimer's Dis Int.* 2016:1–140. https://www.alz.co.uk/research/world-report-2016.
10. Crystal HA, Dickson D, Davies P, Masur D, Grober E, Lipton RB. The relative frequency of "dementia of unknown etiology" increases with age and is nearly 50% in nonagenarians. *Arch Neurol.* 2000;57(5):713–719. doi:10.1001/archneur.57.5.713.
11. American Psychiatric Association. *DSM-V.* 2013. doi:10.1176/appi.books.9780890425596.744053.
12. Alzheimer's Australia. Diagnostic criteria for dementia. *Alzheimer's Aust.* 2015:1–6. https://fightdementia.org.au/files/helpsheets/Helpsheet-DementiaQandA11-DiagnosticCriteriaForDementia_english.pdf.
13. Alzheimer's Society. *Genetics of Dementia.* Crutched Friars, London; 2018. https://www.alzheimers.org.uk/info/20010/risk_factors_and_prevention/117/genetics_of_dementia.
14. Dening T, Sandilyan MB. Dementia: definitions and types. *Nurs Stand.* 2015;29(37):37–42. doi:10.7748/ns.29.37.37.e9405.
15. Fagan AM, Holtzman DM. Cerebrospinal fluid biomarkers of Alzheimer's disease. *Biomark Med.* 2010;4(1):51–63. doi:10.2217/bmm.09.83.
16. Lowe VJ, Lundt E, Knopman D, et al. Comparison of [18F] Flutemetamol and [11C]Pittsburgh Compound-B in cognitively normal young, cognitively normal elderly, and Alzheimer's disease dementia individuals. *NeuroImage Clin.* 2017;16(July):295–302. doi:10.1016/j.nicl.2017.08.011.
17. Yeo JM, Waddell B, Khan Z, Pal S. A systematic review and meta-analysis of ^{18}F-labeled amyloid imaging in Alzheimer's disease. *Alzheimer's Dement (Amst).* 2015;1(1):5–13. doi:10.1016/j.dadm.2014.11.004.
18. Alzheimer's Association. FDA-approved treatments for Alzheimer's. https://www.alz.org/dementia/downloads/topicsheet_treatments.pdf. Published 2017.
19. Yaffe K, Fox P, Newcomer R, et al. Patient and caregiver characteristics and nursing home placement in patients with dementia. *JAMA.* 2002;287(16):2090–2097. doi:10.1001/jama.287.16.2090.
20. Reisberg B, Ferris SH, De Leon MJ, Crook T. The global deterioration scale for assessment of primary degenerative dementia. *Am J Psychiatry.* 1982;139(9):1136–1139. doi:10.1176/ajp.139.9.1136.
21. Fraker J, Kales HC, Blazek M, Kavanagh J, Gitlin LN. The role of the occupational therapist in the management of neuropsychiatric symptoms of dementia in clinical settings. *Occup Ther Heal Care.* 2014;28(1):4–20. doi:10.3109/07380577.2013.867468.
22. van Hoof J, Kort HSM, van Waarde H, Blom MM. Environmental interventions and the design of homes for older adults with dementia: an overview. *Am J Alzheimer's Dis Other Dementias.* 2010;25(3):202–232. doi:10.1177/1533317509358885.
23. Struckmeyer LR, Pickens ND. Home modifications for people with Alzheimer's disease: a scoping review. *Am J Occup Ther.* 2016;70(1):7001270020p1-9. doi:10.5014/ajot.2015.016089.
24. Spector A, Thorgrimsen L, Woods B, et al. Efficacy of an evidence-based cognitive stimulation therapy programme for people with dementia. *Br J Psychiatry.* 2003; 183(03):248–254. doi:10.1192/bjp.183.3.248.
25. Teri L, Logsdon RG, McCurry SM. Exercise interventions for dementia and cognitive impairment: the Seattle protocols. *J Nutr Heal Aging.* 2008;12(6):391–394. doi:10.1021/nl061786n.Core-Shell.
26. dal Bello-Haas VPM, O'Connell ME, Morgan DG. Maintaining health and wellness in the face of dementia: an exploratory analysis of individuals attending a rural and remote memory clinic. *Rural Remote Health.* 2014;14(3):1–17. doi:10.1123/JAPA.2013-0035.
27. Mark RE. Promote the health of dementia caregivers. *Am J Alzheimer's Dis Other Demen.* 2016;31(2):181–183. doi:10.1177/1533317515588182.
28. DiZazzo-Miller R, Winston K, Winkler SL, Donovan MA. Family caregiver training program (FCTP): a randomized controlled trial. *Am J Occup Ther.* 2017;71(5):7105190010p1–7105190010p10.doi:10.5014/ajot.2017.022459.
29. Laver K, Milte R, Dyer S, Crotty M. A systematic review and meta-analysis comparing carer focused and dyadic multicomponent interventions for carers of people with dementia. *J Aging Health.* 2017;29(8);1308–1349. doi:10.1177/0898264316660414.
30. Kumar P, Tiwari SC, Goel A, et al. Novel occupational therapy interventions may improve quality of life in older

adults with dementia. *Int Arch Med*. 2014;7(1):1–7. doi:10.1186/1755-7682-7-26.

31. Graff MJL, Vernooij-Dassen MJM, Zajec J, Olde-Rikkert MGM, Hoefnagels WHL, Dekker J. How can occupational therapy improve the daily performance and communication of an older patient with dementia and his primary caregiver?: a case study. *Dementia*. 2006;5(4):503–532. doi:10.1177/1471301206069918.
32. Gitlin LN, Winter L, Burke J, Chernett N, Dennis MP, Hauck WW. Tailored activities to manage neuropsychiatric behaviours in persons with dementia and reduce caregiver burden: a randomised pilot study. *Am J Geriatr Psychiatry*. 2008;16(3):229–239. doi:10.1097/JGP.0b013e318160da72.Tailored.
33. Laver K, Cumming R, Dyer S, et al. Evidence-based occupational therapy for people with dementia and their families: what clinical practice guidelines tell us and implications for practice. *Aust Occup Ther J*. 2017;64(1):3–10. doi:10.1111/1440-1630.12309.
34. Gélinas I, Gauthier L, McIntyre M, Gauthier S. Development of a functional measure for persons with Alzheimer's disease: the disability assessment for dementia. *Am J Occup Ther*. 1999. doi:10.5014/ajot.53.5.471.
35. Baum CM, Connor LT, Morrison T, Hahn M, Dromerick AW, Edwards DF. Reliability, validity, and clinical utility of the executive function performance test: a measure of executive function in a sample of people with stroke. *Am J Occup Ther*. 2008;62(4):446–455. doi:10.5014/ajot.62.4.446.
36. Chisholm D, Toto P, Raina K, Holm M, Rogers J. Evaluating to live independently and safely in the community: performance assessment of self-care skills. *Br J Occup Ther*. 2014;77(2):59–63. doi:10.1002/bmb.20244.DNA.
37. Bossers WJR, van der Woude LHV, Boersma F, Scherder EJA, van Heuvelen MJG. Recommended measures for the assessment of cognitive and physical performance in older patients with dementia: a systematic review. *Dement Geriatr Cogn Dis Extra*. 2012;2(1):589–609. doi:10.1159/000345038.
38. Smith T, Gildeh N, Holmes C. Validity and utility in a memory clinic setting. *Can J Psychiatry*. 2007;52(5):329–332. http://www.ncbi.nlm.nih.gov/pubmed/17542384.
39. Olde Rikkert MGM, Tona KD, Janssen L, et al. Validity, reliability, and feasibility of clinical staging scales in dementia: a systematic review. *Am J Alzheimer's Dis Other Demen*. 2011;26(5):357–365. doi:10.1177/1533317511418954.

Chapter 47

Cancer

Mary Vining Radomski, Mattie Anheluk, Ginger Carroll, and Joette Zola

LEARNING OBJECTIVES

This chapter will allow the reader to:

1. Describe general information regarding cancer incidence, categories, and care.
2. Appreciate the contribution of occupational therapy to cancer rehabilitation, survivorship, and palliative care.
3. Identify occupational therapy–specific assessment and intervention approaches with this population.
4. Advocate for the provision of occupational therapy services for persons with cancer.
5. Identify interests and potential need for professional development in this practice area.

CHAPTER OUTLINE

TERMINOLOGY

Lymphedema: a buildup of lymph fluid in the fatty tissues under the skin that causes swelling; it is often a sequela to surgery and/or radiation that involves one or more lymph nodes and remains a lifetime risk for people living with cancer.

Metastasis: occurs when cancer cells migrate into the bloodstream or lymph system, travel to other parts of the body, and form new tumors.

Palliative care: an approach that aims to improve quality of life for families and patients facing life-threatening illness. It provides relief from pain and other distressing symptoms, support to help patients live as actively as possible, and coping and bereavement assistance.

Peripheral neuropathy: refers to numbness, tingling, and/or pain caused by nerve damage.

Survivorship: the cancer journey phase that begins as patients complete medical treatment and continues throughout the remainder of the patients' lives.

Cancer: Background

Roughly 19 million Americans are expected to live with cancer by 2024 as a result of early detection, effective treatments, and a growing aging population.[1] Cancer survivors face long-term side effects and health risks as a result of both treatment and ongoing fear of recurrence.[2] These challenges may interfere with activity and role performance, necessitating the services of occupational therapists.

The term *cancer* refers to a group of diseases in which abnormal cells divide without control, can invade nearby tissues, and travel through the blood and lymph systems to other body parts.[3] Oncologists and pathologists classify cancer in order to specify a diagnosis, plan treatment, consider patient eligibility for clinical trials, and determine prognosis. For example, cancers are often classified by stage. Staging is the process of determining the severity of a person's cancer based on the degree to which a cancer has spread[4] (Table 47-1). Common elements in most staging systems consider the primary tumor site, tumor size and number, spread into lymph nodes, and the presence or absence of **metastasis.**[4]

Cancers are also classified by the body location and tissue type from which the cancer originated (also called the primary site; e.g., breast cancer). Cancers that have metastasized to different body areas are named for the locations where the cancer originated and then spread (e.g., breast cancer with metastasis to the bones). In this chapter, six cancer types are described based on body location and which reflect diagnostic groups often seen by occupational therapists. Table 47-2 summarizes diagnosis-specific problems that occupational therapists address or consider when supporting improved occupational performance.

Breast Cancer

As of 2018, there were more than 3.1 million breast cancer cases in the United States with over 260,000 new cases diagnosed each year,[5] approximately 0.9% of which are diagnosed in men.[6] Risk factors for breast cancer include age, heredity, physical inactivity, weight gain, use of hormone replacement therapy, and race.[7] Treatment for breast cancer may include surgery, chemotherapy, radiation, and/or endocrine therapy.[8]

Table 47-1 Stages of Cancer (0–IV)

STAGE	DEFINITION
0	Abnormal cells are present but have not spread to other tissues. This stage is typically highly curable.
I	Cancer that is the next least advanced; patients often have good prognosis. This is referred to as early-stage cancer because a small cancer or tumor hasn't spread to lymph nodes or other body parts.
II–III	Cancer involving more extensive disease as indicated by greater tumor size and/or cancer spread to nearby lymph nodes, but not to other body parts.
IV	Cancer that has spread to other organs or body parts. This is referred to as advanced or metastatic cancer.

Lung Cancer

The two major types of lung cancer are non–small cell and small cell.[9] Cigarette smoking is the leading cause of lung cancer, followed by environmental factors such as exposure to radon, secondhand smoke, and air pollution. Lung cancer is the deadliest form of cancer for both men and women.[10] Lung cancer tends to be diagnosed at later stages when the cancer has metastasized and the individual's daily routines are affected by symptoms.

Brain Cancer

Each year, over 22,000 adults in the United States are diagnosed with a central nervous system tumor, most of which are brain tumors.[11] Metastatic brain tumors (those resulting from cancers that have spread from other body locations) occur more frequently than primary tumors, affecting 20% to 40% of cancer patients.[12] The most common types of primary brain tumors in adults are astrocytoma, meningioma, and oligodendroglioma.[13] Glioblastoma multiforme, a type of astrocytoma, is the most common primary malignant brain tumor and the deadliest.[14] The nature of functional deficits depends on brain tumor size and location.

Table 47-2 Problems Relevant to Occupational Performance for Six Types of Cancer by Location

LOCATION	PROBLEMS THAT MAY INTERFERE WITH OCCUPATIONAL PERFORMANCE
Breast cancer	Weakness, fatigue, body-image issues, pain, lymphedema, limited range of motion (ROM), brachial plexus injury, cognitive inefficiencies
Lung cancer	Fatigue, dyspnea, weakness, limited ROM, limited endurance
Brain cancer	Cognitive problems, impaired vision and balance, decreased sensation, dysphasia, hemiparesis, impaired coordination, personality changes
Head and neck cancer	Limited cervical ROM, shoulder dysfunction, loss of scapular stability, difficulty swallowing, speech problems, stigma associated with disfigurement
Sarcoma	Possible amputation or issues associated with limb salvage, body-image issues, peripheral neuropathy, pain, fatigue, edema
Colorectal	Gastrointestinal problems (diarrhea, constipation, incontinence, bowel obstruction), physical and psychosocial challenges associated with managing an ostomy

Head and Neck Cancer

Head and neck cancer (HNC) describes malignant tumors that develop in or around the throat, larynx, nose, sinuses, and mouth. HNC accounts for about 4% of all cancers in the United States.[15] Although younger people can develop the disease, most people are older than 50 years when diagnosed.[15] The causes may include smoking, excessive alcohol use, and the human papillomavirus.[15] Treatment options include surgery, radiation therapy, chemotherapy, targeted therapy, or a combination of all—all of which may affect how a person feels, looks, talks, eats, and breathes.[16]

Sarcoma

Sarcomas are noncommon, malignant tumors that arise within bone and soft tissue. Soft-tissue sarcomas develop in fat, muscle, nerve, fibrous tissues surrounding joints, blood vessels, and deep skin tissues. Most sarcomas are found in the upper extremity (UE) and lower extremity (LE), but they can arise in any body part. Limb-sparing surgery is a common treatment for sarcoma, and amputation is now rarely needed.[17]

Colorectal Cancer

In 2018, within the United States, there were 43,030 new cases of rectal cancer and 97,220 new cases of colon cancer.[18] Incidence is similar for both men and women, with increased risk for colon cancer in those aged 50 years and older.[18] Treatment for colorectal cancer includes surgery, chemotherapy, and radiation.[19] Decreased mobility and lowered activity levels can increase gastrointestinal issue risk (such as diarrhea) and caregiver burden.[20] Some patients must learn to care for a colostomy pouching system, which may be temporarily or permanently needed as a result of colorectal cancer treatment.[21]

Phases of the Cancer Journey

Patients and providers often use metaphors to describe the cancer experience. This facilitates communication using familiar experiences to represent unfamiliar medical concepts.[22] Cancer **survivorship** is often framed as a journey, suggesting that the illness is part of a larger narrative within each person's unique path.[22]

Diagnosis

Often shocked by a cancer diagnosis,[23] patients shift their identity from a healthy to an ill person; rapidly gather information to make treatment decisions; and alter plans, activities, and roles to accommodate. The diagnosis may cause stress-related symptoms and/or emotional avoidance and withdrawal.[24]

Medical Treatment

Medical therapies for cancer typically involve surgical tumor removal, chemotherapy, radiation, and/or immunotherapy. Cancer and its treatment have the potential to interfere with patients' ability to perform activities of daily living (ADLs), instrumental activities of daily living (IADLs), and life roles (Table 47-3).[25] In addition

Table 47-3 Types of Cancer Treatment

TYPE OF CANCER TREATMENT	DESCRIPTION	SIDE/SECONDARY EFFECTS THAT MAY INTERFERE WITH FUNCTIONING
Surgery	Used to diagnose, treat, and prevent cancer	• Complications from surgery • Pain • Infection from wound site • Lymphedema
Chemotherapy	Medicines or drugs that are used to treat cancer; can be used to contain or slow tumor growth or kill cancer cells.	• Fever and chills • Nausea and vomiting • Hair loss • Fatigue • Sores in the mouth or throat • Constipation or diarrhea • Itching/rash • Muscle or joint pain • Memory changes
Radiation	The use of high-energy particles or wavelengths to kill the cancerous cells and shrink tumors	• Fatigue • Skin irritation at radiation site • Fever/chills
Immunotherapy	A type of biological therapy that uses substances made from living organisms to treat cancer	• Skin irritation at needle site • Flulike symptoms • Swelling, weight gain

Adapted from the National Cancer Institute (2017). Types of cancer treatment.

to occupational therapy, the cancer rehabilitation team includes physiatry, oncology nursing, psychosocial services, nutrition, pharmacy, pastoral care, physical therapy, speech-language pathology, lymphedema care, and fitness programs.

Survivorship

For many people, the emotional relief of completing treatment may be accompanied by disequilibrium and fear of recurrence as they reorient their lives.[26] Many patients must manage long-term health consequences of cancer treatments and lingering problems with physical functioning, fatigue, and cognition as they attempt to return to "normal" life roles. Many people demonstrate resilience and report personal growth associated with cancer. A large number of people living with cancer, however, report poor mental and physical health-related quality of life compared to adults without cancer.[27]

Palliative Care

Although most people who are diagnosed with cancer experience either a full recovery or live many years with cancer as a chronic condition,[28] those whose illness adversely affects daily functioning or is predicted to reduce life expectancy may receive **palliative care**. Palliative care is an interdisciplinary approach that optimizes quality of life and prevents or reduces suffering by addressing physical, emotional, spiritual, and social needs.[29] Palliative care is available from the time of diagnosis through cancer treatment and beyond, including the transition to end-of-life care and bereavement.[29]

Occupational Therapy Evaluation and Intervention for People Living with Cancer

Occupational therapists employ a client-centered approach that is always central to occupational therapy services while considering the unique requirements of people with cancer. Patients with cancer have complex needs and priorities that can rapidly change, depending on illness severity, treatment response, and cancer stage. Patients often experience psychosocial, emotional, or existential distress that may impact their participation in therapy and daily occupations, and prompt a reevaluation of the roles and activities from which they derive life purpose.[30,31] Especially during the treatment phase, patients tend to rely on health care providers, including occupational therapists, for information and emotional support.[32] Finally, patients' family members may have unmet needs of their own, including depression.[33] Occupational therapists revisit family members' needs for information, support, and referral at various junctures of the illness trajectory.

Occupational Therapy Evaluation Procedures and Methods

The goal of the evaluation process is to develop the intervention plan, determine whether other services are needed, and begin to develop a therapeutic partnership. In this section, these processes are considered with specific implications for patients with cancer.

Initial Assessment Preparation

When a patient with cancer is referred to occupational therapy, the therapist obtains information from the medical record regarding the cancer diagnosis, including location, stage, diagnosis date, whether the cancer is a new diagnosis or recurrence, recent or current cancer treatment and side effects, and information about any comorbid conditions (e.g., arthritis, diabetes). Additionally, precautions such as immunosuppression, thrombocytopenia, isolation, and anemia are noted. Finally, the therapist reviews related documentation from other members of the medical or rehabilitation team to avoid service duplication.

Identify Patient Priorities and Resources

At the initial occupational therapy session, the therapist begins to learn more about the patient's story. Patient priorities are identified along with the barriers, strengths, and resources that shape performance and possible progress. Therapists typically use structured interviews such as the Canadian Occupational Performance Measure[34] (COPM) to obtain information related to patients' occupation-related goals and concerns. Therapists ask patients about the composition of their social support network and allow the patients to determine whether and when to involve care partners in the evaluation process. These patient–therapist conversations are the foundation of both the assessment process and the development of therapeutic rapport.

Specify Problems and Impairments

Based on the abovementioned information, the therapist determines what if any impairment-specific assessments to administer to identify problem areas and establish baselines for progress and outcome measurement. Symptoms and impairments that are commonly assessed by occupational therapists with this population include fatigue, pain, cognitive functioning, range of motion (ROM), and physiological tolerance of activities. The examples of self-report instruments in the assessment table (at the end of this chapter) have established psychometric properties and are useful outcome measures for people with cancer. After administering symptom self-report questionnaires, therapists can then ask patients clarifying questions that will inform the intervention plan. For example, responses to a fatigue questionnaire may lead to a discussion about sleep hygiene or the impact of fatigue on home and work roles.

The evaluation approach for cognitive complaints will depend on the patient's cancer location. For example, if the patient has cognitive or visual problems after surgical brain tumor resection, the cognitive evaluation will be similar to that used for patients with acquired brain injury (see Chapters 7, 9, 10, 36, and 37). If the patient reports concerns with memory and concentration after cancer treatment, a self-report questionnaire will help elucidate specific areas of concern and the extent of the problem.

Establish Goals for the Episode of Care

Occupational therapists collaborate with patients to establish therapy goals for the episode of care, which, in some instances, may be challenging. Patients who are in the midst of shock associated with a new diagnosis or have learned of a reoccurrence may not feel ready to set therapy goals. Occupational therapists may need to collaborate with other treatment team members during such time, including the patient's family. Day-to-day performance may fluctuate due to fatigue, pain, and cancer treatment side effects, which may also lead to challenges with goal setting. Because patients' goals and priorities may change rapidly, therapists must remain aware of patient's priorities through frequent review and skilled communication.

Occupational Therapy Intervention Approaches

Occupational therapy intervention addresses a wide array of cancer-related problems (such as debility, fatigue, poor endurance, neuropathy, lymphedema, cognitive decline, UE impairment, balance, and pain)[35] and enables patients to learn to manage chronic symptoms or impairments as they resume occupational roles.[36]

Arm function

Occupational therapists address limitations in arm function that result from cancer surgeries, especially for breast cancer, including restricted ROM, arm swelling, pain, numbness, peripheral neuropathy, and weakness.[35] Occupational therapists with specialized training in **lymphedema** management use techniques such as wrapping (Fig. 47-1), garment fitting, and teaching self-management techniques to treat lymphedema. Exercise as a means to help manage lymphedema is well documented, and therapists who are trained in lymphedema management can help assure that prescribed lymphedema garments do not restrict patients' ability to effectively perform exercises.[37] An occupational therapy program for women with cancer-related lymphedema that incorporated exercise and education was found to result in improvements in UE swelling, arm ROM, quality of life, and mood.[38]

Fatigue

Cancer-related fatigue (CRF) is a distressing symptom that often impacts the quality of life of many individuals with cancer during and after treatment. CRF is more than just a feeling of being tired and interferes with all aspects of daily life.[39] CRF is defined as an upsetting and enduring sense of physical, emotional, and/or cognitive exhaustion that impedes functioning and is inconsistent with recent activity levels. Seldom a solitary symptom, CRF involves concurrent symptoms such as pain, stress, low red blood cell count, and difficulty sleeping.[40] The multifactorial nature of CRF requires therapists to partner with the entire rehabilitation team to ensure that the emotional, cognitive, physical, and social aspects of CRF are addressed.[41]

The National Comprehensive Cancer Network (NCCN) recommends referral to occupational therapy for nonpharmacological CRF intervention.[40] These interventions emphasize physical activity and psychosocial and psychoeducational therapies. Recommendations also include the following self-management strategies[40]: teaching patients to self-monitor fatigue levels, energy conservation, adaptive aide use, sleep hygiene strategies, arranging daily routines, and supporting participation in meaningful activities. Additionally, guidelines support the importance of normalizing CRF through patient and family education because symptoms can lead to fear of

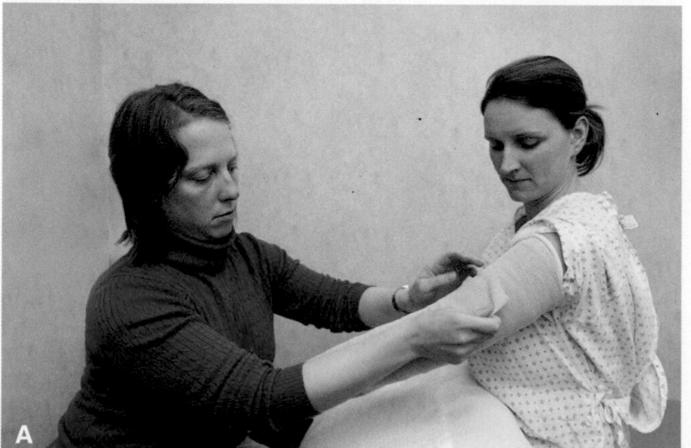

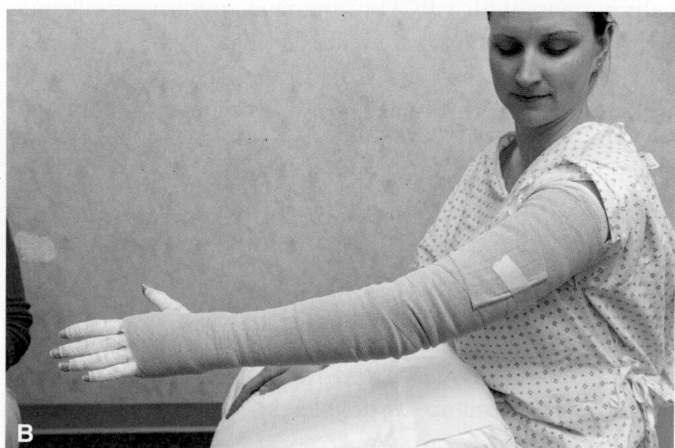

Figure 47-1. An example of an upper extremity wrapping technique for lymphedema management performed by a certified lymphedema therapist. (© Allina Health System. Used with permission.)

disease progression.[40] The occupational therapy literature further endorses the importance of exercise and other physical activity, problem-solving interventions, and cognitive–behavioral techniques for CRF.[42] Occupational therapy fatigue management interventions that were developed for patients with other chronic conditions may be applicable to CRF.[43,44]

Cognition

Cognitive changes occur in individuals with cancer as a consequence of the disease or cancer treatment. Patients with surgically resected brain tumors may experience cognitive decline similar to that of patients with other types of acquired brain injury. Occupational therapists use intervention approaches with these patients similar to those used for patients with stroke-related cognitive impairments (see Chapter 11). While patients with brain tumor experience cognitive limitations that are correlated with specific areas of brain damage, other patients (typically with breast cancer) may experience cancer-related cognitive dysfunction (CRCD; sometimes called chemobrain), which is thought to be multifactorial in origin. CRCD involves mild but disruptive changes in memory, executive functions, attention, and processing speed and has been reported in up to 30% of patients prior to any treatment and up to 75% of patients during or after treatment.[45] Possible mechanisms may be physiological (e.g., direct injury to brain tissue, oxidative stress and inflammation, cytokine dysregulation, microvascular injury) and/or psychological (e.g., styles of coping with stress, fatigue, depression).[46]

CRCD can be acute or chronic and can affect quality of life and occupational performance related to ADLs, IADLs, and life roles. Cognitive effects can endure for years and adversely affect patients' quality of life and the ability to work and contribute to society.[47] Although there is still relatively little evidence to guide CRCD management, recent research supports the benefits of cognitive strategy training. Ferguson and colleagues found that intervention combining metacognitive strategy instruction (MSI) and cognitive–behavioral therapy (CBT) is feasible and can help patients with CRCD to manage cognitive challenges (see Evidence table at the end of this chapter).[48,49] Wolf and colleagues used the Cognitive Orientation to daily Occupational Performance (CO-OP) approach, which included both global and domain-specific cognitive strategy learning. Participants experienced positive effects in subjective and objective cognitive performance and quality of life.[50] This chapter's Case Study illustrates how occupational therapists teach patients strategies to manage cognitive problems resulting from CRCD. There is no evidence to support the benefit or appropriateness of using commercial, computer-based cognitive exercises to improve everyday performance of people experiencing CRCD.

Peripheral Neuropathy

Chemotherapy-induced **peripheral neuropathy** (CIPN) describes sensory impairment of the peripheral nerves caused by neurotoxicity associated with many commonly used chemotherapy drugs. Symptoms vary depending on the severity and type of peripheral nerve involvement; people with prior neuropathy are more vulnerable. Patients report pain, numbness, and/or tingling. They may also experience cold intolerance. Motor symptoms occur less frequently and can include mild weakness and decreased reflexes. Proprioception is often affected in the LE and is associated with balance and safety problems. Rarely, autonomic functions may be impacted, resulting in constipation and urinary and sexual complications. CIPN may increase fall risk and interfere with task performance because of balance and gait impairments, weakness, and sensory loss. Occupational therapists are included among the uniquely qualified rehabilitation professionals able to address both remedial and compensatory interventions to support patients impacted by CIPN.[51]

CIPN should be addressed early through a multidisciplinary approach, which may include a preventative approach before starting chemotherapy. For example, patients whose chemotherapy regimen puts them at risk for the development of neuropathy may prevent or lessen CIPN sensory symptoms by engaging in gentle movement like shoulder circles, marching in place, wiggling their toes, and performing sensory tactile stimulation (Fig. 47-2).[52] Therapists should communicate with patients about their specific CIPN symptoms and the impact of these symptoms on daily life in order to guide interventions to improve safety, quality of life, and occupational function.[53] Therapists typically address the

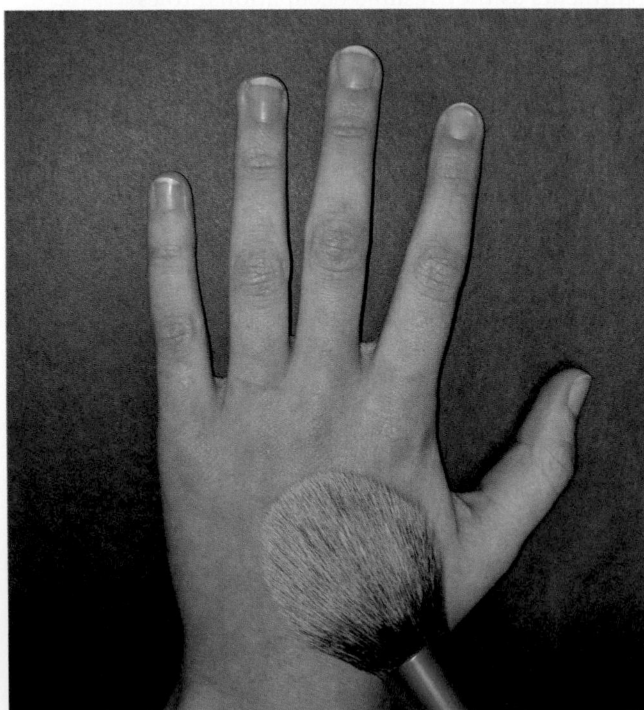

Figure 47-2. An example of sensory tactile stimulation with mental awareness of where sensation feels "normal" and where it does not.

patient's unique functional and safety concerns (including fall prevention), adaptive equipment needs, psychosocial adjustment to the effects of CIPN, and physical performance needs.

Patients with CIPN may have difficulty with buttoning, zipping, writing, cooking, sewing, home management tasks, exercising, and community mobility.[54] Occupational therapists use skill training and adaptive equipment to address these problems. Referral for driver's assessment and training may be indicated for some patients with CIPN with significant LE involvement.

Interventions targeting fall prevention commonly focus on functional mobility, ADL training, and home modification recommendations to support optimal engagement in daily-life roles. Stubblefield and colleagues proposed important home modifications and adaptive equipment needs.[55] Home modification recommendations may include maintaining clutter-free areas, removing throw rugs, using appropriate protection when handling hot and cold items, maintaining safety with sharp objects, testing water temperature with thermometers or sensory-intact body areas, setting water heaters to below 120°F (49°C), and improving stairway safety through the installation of railings and lighting. Adaptive equipment may include built-up and nonslip handles, button hooks, and bathroom aides.

Interventions to improve physical performance can include edema control, exercise, pain management techniques, modalities such as transcutaneous electrical nerve stimulation (TENS) (if not medically contraindicated), and appropriate ROM and strengthening. Psychosocial adjustment can be enhanced through relaxation training and deep breathing.[56]

Resumption of Everyday Activities and Roles

As described throughout this chapter, some patients living with cancer experience changed physical or cognitive capacities that interfere with the performance of everyday activities. Even patients with less obvious cancer-related disabilities may face challenges, resuming valued activities and roles related to exercise, work, nutrition, home and financial management, meal preparation, medication administration, and social activity.[57] Parents with cancer are typically very concerned about the welfare of their children and maintaining parenting activities.[58] Many patients worry about their ability to work; patients with cancer have lower employment rates and work fewer hours 2 to 6 years after diagnosis than adults of the same age.[59]

The ultimate goal of all occupational therapy intervention is to support patients' engagement in valued activities and roles. To recap, this is accomplished through multiple approaches:

Skills Training and Equipment

As with other diagnostic groups, occupational therapists help reduce activity limitations by providing ADL, IADL, and transfer training to persons with cancer.[35] This may involve adaptive techniques, equipment, and optimizing access within the home, particularly for individuals receiving hospice or palliative care.[60] For example, a patient, Valeria, who was paralyzed by a spinal cord tumor, was taught to use adaptive dressing techniques similar to those used by patients sustaining traumatic spinal cord injury (see Chapter 39).

Strategy Instruction

Occupational therapists help patients learn and apply strategies to manage potentially chronic conditions such as CRF, CRCD, and CIPN within the context of valued activities and roles. For example, Tom was concerned that CRF prevented him from interacting with his children at the end of a long workday. After exploring fatigue management strategies in occupational therapy, he shifted his work schedule so that he could engage in aerobic exercise (bike riding) with his daughters at the end of each workday.

Patients may also benefit from learning to use general strategies (not impairment specific) for goal setting and problem-solving, which enable them to address their own cancer-related concerns even after they have completed occupational therapy.[61,62] For example, Lyons and colleagues taught patients with breast cancer to use a behavioral activation/problem-solving (BA/PS) strategy to help improve their performance of valued activities. Each week, participants selected an important but challenging activity to which they applied the BA/PS strategy, comprised of the following steps:

1. Determining why the activity was challenging
2. Setting a relevant 1-week behavioral goal
3. Creating and implementing an action plan
4. Reflecting on the outcome of the effort

A problem-solving procedure (identify solution, evaluate pros and cons, pick a solution) was inserted in the goal-setting process when participants did not immediately know which steps to take to meet their goals. Teaching patients to use general strategies such as BA/PS contributes to goal achievement and improvement in quality of life, coping, and planning for adults with cancer (see the Evidence table at the end of this chapter).[62,63]

Interdisciplinary Rehabilitation Programs

Occupational therapists help patients resume roles and activities as part of multidisciplinary cancer rehabilitation programs, such as those designed to advance successful return to work through education (including self-care), vocational counseling (such as gradual return to work), and/or physical exercise.[64]

Supporting Wellness through Exercise

Exercise is important to long-term cancer self-management because it has beneficial effects on physical functioning, fatigue, and role and social functioning for patients actively receiving treatment for a variety of cancer types and those who have completed treatment.[65,66] People living with cancer should aim to engage in 150 minutes of moderate-intensity aerobic exercise over 3 to 5 days per week and perform resistance training that involves major muscle groups at least 2 days per week.[67] Occupational therapists help patients restart or commence new exercise regimens that are tailored to their abilities and interests.[42] Doing so involves helping patients evaluate their exercise options, and potential barriers and facilitators associated with establishing daily or weekly exercise routines. Clinicians may provide patients with a progressive walking schedule or help them explore activity options like yoga or Qigong. Patients who are severely deconditioned are often referred to specialized cancer exercise programs, but most patients engage in exercise programs in their homes or communities.

Conclusions and Recommendations

Patients benefit most from client-centered, context-informed, occupation-oriented approaches that assist them to overcome limitations posed by cancer-related impairments and to resume valued activities and roles. Occupational therapists who provide cancer rehabilitation services are privileged to share patients' uncertainty, sorrow, joy, and resilience in ways that expand and enrich their own growth and appreciation for the human experience. Beyond understanding content from this and other chapters in this textbook, occupational therapists who aspire to practice in this area must seek informal and formal ways to gain additional knowledge and expertise by, for example, reading the American Occupational Therapy Practice Guidelines for Cancer Rehabilitation[68] and/or becoming involved in the American Congress of Rehabilitation Medicine's Cancer Rehabilitation Networking Group.[69]

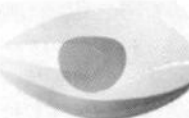

CASE STUDY

Katerina is a 42-year-old Russian American woman who was diagnosed with stage II breast cancer. Acute treatment consisted of chemotherapy, single mastectomy with lymph node biopsy, and 5 years of hormone therapy. Reconstruction surgery is pending. Diagnostic brain imaging found no metastases. Katerina is married and has two young children. Her spouse travels for work, and she is responsible for childcare and household management. Katerina works part time as a high school paraprofessional.

Occupational Therapy Referral

An occupational therapy referral was made to address cognitive complaints affecting life roles.

Assessment and Treatment

At their first session, the occupational therapist conducted an informal interview to understand Katerina's prior level of function, current concerns, and limitations. Katerina's main concern was caring for her children. Most evenings, she had difficulty initiating anything. Her family had lost their evening routines, planning meals and cooking was difficult, and bedtimes were late and inconsistent. Katerina reported attention and memory errors. She missed several appointments owing to inconsistent use of her phone calendar. She was also distracted and reported losing her keys and purse. Katerina had started making lists but left them at home. Although she reported sleep problems resulting from arm discomfort, she refused medication to ensure that she could care for her children when her spouse traveled. Once approved by her doctor, Katerina wanted to return to work but worried that cognitive problems would be noticeable by coworkers. Additionally, she worried that she would not have sufficient energy to manage work and home.

Using the COPM,[34] Katerina identified her top priorities (average total performance score 5; satisfaction score 4):

- Consistent parenting
- Consistent household management
- Consistent care of self
- Energy to manage all of her life roles
- Information management plan for home and eventually for work

Katerina identified cognition and fatigue as interfering with optimal functioning, the latter of which was being formally evaluated in physical therapy. The occupational therapist administered the Functional Assessment of Cancer Therapy – Cognitive Function (FACT-Cog)[70] to understand and measure her cognitive concerns. Katerina's total score of 42/132 indicated that she perceived a decline in her thinking that affected her quality of life.

Finally, Katerina's UE was clearly swollen and reportedly painful. Appreciating the need for specialized expertise, the occupational therapist requested doctor's orders for an evaluation by one of the department's lymphedema specialists.

Occupational Therapy Problem List

- Disrupted sleep and fatigue
- Disrupted routines
- Decreased attention and memory
- Disorganized information management

Occupational Therapy Goal List

Katerina's occupational therapy goals (that follows) centered on cognition and fatigue management to improve care of others and self, appreciating that improvements were central to longer term aspirations to return to work.

CASE STUDY (continued)

- Consistently employ bedtime routines for herself and children, evidenced by going to sleep and waking at the same time 5 of 7 days, 4 of 4 weeks.
- Effectively manage fatigue throughout the day/week by prioritizing tasks and initiating breaks using smartphone alarm cues.
- Independently and consistently manage appointments on her smartphone calendar with alarms, evidenced by no missed appointments.
- Independently support her memory with notes/lists.

Intervention

Katerina attended five additional outpatient occupational therapy sessions over a 3-month period. In the first session, the therapist explained to her that many factors were competing for her cognitive energy. The therapist asked guided questions helping Katerina determine that sleep hygiene and consistent meal preparation were key preliminary priorities. In addition to providing sleep hygiene information, the therapist helped Katerina create a bedtime checklist that included preparing for the next day, transitioning away from electronics, and maintaining consistent bedtimes for everyone. The task of cooking was manageable, but Katerina struggled due to end-of-day fatigue. She was able to see the value in advanced meal planning and shared that she had considered online grocery shopping. For her homework, Katerina agreed to implement the bedtime checklists, plan 1 weeks' worth of meals, and trial online shopping.

During her second session, Katerina discussed her strategy use over the past week. She found the bedtime routines, meal planning, and online shopping beneficial and opted to continue them. Because Katerina still struggled to manage all of her life demands, the therapist introduced the concept of an "energy budget." Katerina was able to understand that she needed to manage her energy consistently and effectively to perform optimally. She could clearly see that taking breaks throughout her day could help her more successfully manage evening tasks. Katerina was not accustomed to taking breaks and knew that she would need time to change her behavior. With guidance from her therapist, she created a weekly activity template for reoccurring tasks to pace her chores throughout the day/week and decrease fatigue. Katerina observed that she wasted time and energy worrying about possible missed appointments. She created a weekly and daily planning checklist to ensure that key tasks and family appointments were stored in her phone calendar with alarm reminders. This allowed her to observe her week in its entirety, consider her energy budget, and determine whether her plans were realistic and sustainable. Katerina's homework for the week included implementation of weekly/daily planning procedures; following her activity template with adjustments to meet her energy needs; and continued use of sleep routines, meal planning, and online shopping.

The third session started with a weekly review and discussion regarding strategy use and effectiveness. Katerina was habitually using the bedtime routines, organizational checklists, and meal planning strategies. She had made meals 5/7 days last week with positive results. The daily/weekly routine list she developed was not working, and she was unable to complete listed tasks. The therapist introduced a prioritizing strategy to help Katerina identify the tasks and appointments that needed to occur and those she could postpone or delete. As she predicted, Katerina was not good at taking breaks. She set alarms on her phone but ignored them. With cues from her occupational therapist, Katerina understood that a break could be more than a nap and generated a list of 10 possible breaks she might take (e.g., 5-minute walk, deep breathing exercises) and agreed to implement these in the coming week. Katerina was overwhelmed and requested that her next appointment be conducted in 2 weeks to provide sufficient time to use the strategies and routines.

Katerina arrived at her fourth appointment appearing well-rested. She reported consistent sleep hygiene and improved sleep quality. She also consistently completed her daily and weekly routines. Katerina had recently attended several social events in which she had difficulty following multiple conversations and remembering things when interrupted. In anticipation of her next outing, she decided to rest prior to the event and store a list of attendees in her phone to remember names. The therapist and Katerina discussed different tasks she could practice over the next 2 weeks to challenge her activity tolerance and higher level attention skills. Katerina decided to volunteer at her children's school 2 days per week for 4-hour time slots.

Session five began with a reflection of Katerina's past 2 weeks. She remained consistent in her daily/weekly routines, reported feeling more energetic and mindful of managing her energy budget, and expressed that her confidence was higher after successfully volunteering in the classroom. Katerina did note some errors when she was interrupted, prompting her therapist to introduce information about attention levels and strategies she could use to manage classroom demands. Overall, Katerina reported feeling more confident in her ability to return to work, which would be determined with her physician at an upcoming appointment. Katerina and her therapist decided to schedule a follow-up session in 1 month. Her homework included continued strategy use and intentionally increasing her activities and attention demands during the day.

Katerina attended her final occupational therapy session 1 month later at which she reported independence and confidence in care of self, her children, and home tasks. She had increased her volunteer hours at the school to 4 hours per day, 4 days per week, and was tolerating it well. Katerina felt ready to return to part-time work. Her therapist helped her anticipate challenges she might encounter at work and identify strategies she could use to ensure accurate performance. For example, Katerina created an arriving-at-work and leaving-work checklist in order to reinstate these habit sequences. She blocked her lunch hours to ensure that she had time for proper nutrition and intentional rest. The COPM was readministered, and Katerina's performance score had increased from 5 to 8; satisfaction score from 4 to 7. Her FACT-Cog had improved from 42 to 104/132. Katerina met her goals and was discharged.

Examples of Cancer-Specific Self-Report Assessments

Instrument and Reference	Intended Purpose	Administration Time	Validity	Reliability	Sensitivity	Strengths and Weaknesses
Functional Assessment of Cancer Therapy – Cognitive Function (FACT-Cog)[70]	To measure perceived cognitive issues specific to CRCD and the impact on quality of life involving four subscales: perceived cognitive impairment (PCI), impact on quality of life, comments from others, and perceived cognitive ability (PCA)	10 min	Construct validity: Breast cancer survivors rated their cognition (47%) and quality of life (53%) as greater than 1 standard deviation below that of pre-chemotherapy control group.[71] Convergent validity: PCA scores appear to be highly correlated with objective neuropsychological performance in verbal memory and executive functioning in BCS.[72]	Acceptable levels of internal consistency for English- and Chinese-speaking patients (Cronbach's alpha 0.707–0.929)[73] Acceptable test–retest reliability for English and Chinese versions (interclass correlations of 0.762 and 0.697, respectively)[73]	Minimal clinically important difference for breast cancer patients ranged from 6.9 to 10.6 points (4.7%–7.2% of the total score).[74]	Strengths: 37 items that describe functional cognitive concerns, developed for cancer population, short administration time. Limitations: Somewhat limited psychometric; variable association between self-report and performance on cognitive assessments.
National Comprehensive Cancer Network Distress Thermometer and Problem List (DTPL)[45]	To identify psychological distress	Approximately 5 min for patients to fill out; at least 10 min for provider to discuss responses with patient, if there are areas of concern	Convergent validity: Moderate positive correlation between DTPL and Brief Symptom Inventory ($r = 0.59$, $p < 0.001$)[46]	Acceptable test–retest reliability ($r = 0.800$, $p = 0.000$)[75]	77.1% sensitivity and 66.1% specificity to detect cancer-related distress; 80.9% sensitivity and 60.2% specificity to detect depression[76] A cutoff score of 3 indicates patients with clinically elevated levels of distress.[77]	Strengths: objective, structured distress screening; consistent means for prioritizing and triaging to supportive care services[78] Weaknesses: options provided in the Problem List may not encompass all critical issues experienced by patients; 0–10 scale may be too simplistic and does not give enough insight into patients' concerns[78]
Brief Fatigue Inventory (BFI)[79]	To assess the severity of fatigue, including interference in daily living	5 min	Construct validity: BFI was significantly correlated with both the Functional Assessment of Cancer Therapy (FACT) ($r = -0.88$, $p < 0.001$) and the Profile of Mood States (POMS) ($r = 0.84$, $p < 0.001$) Fatigue subscales.	High levels of internal consistency (Cronbach's alpha = 0.96)	There is evidence of BFI sensitivity as cancer patients reported a higher fatigue rating when compared to healthy control participants.	Strengths: Developed for cancer patients; short administration time; high construct validity and reliability. Weaknesses: Does not collect information such as the cognitive, affective, and somatic aspects of fatigue.

Evidence Table of Intervention Studies Supporting Occupational Therapy for Patients with Cancer

Intervention	Description	Participants	Dosage	Research Design and Evidence Level	Benefit	Statistical Significance and Effect Size
Memory and attention adaptation training (MAAT)[38]	A brief CBT approach that included education about memory, attention, relaxation training, and a variety of other compensatory strategies	Breast cancer survivors, $n = 22$ (MAAT) and $n = 13$ (control condition, support therapy); Median age = 54.6 years; No significant difference in groups' age, education, or IQ.	Participants in both conditions received 8-weekly visits, 30–45 minutes each that were delivered via videoconference. Both treatments were delivered via videoconference.	Randomized controlled trial Assessed at baseline, after treatment, 2 months later Level I	MAAT participants made significant gains in self-reported cognitive impairments and cognitive processing speed at 2-month follow-up. Anxiety related to cognitive challenges decreased. Attended treatment for cognition via video teleconferencing that they may not have attended if they had to drive.	PCI: - Trend toward statistically significant group differences in PCI at posttest ($p = 0.09$) - Statistically significant differences in PCI at 2-month follow-up ($p = 0.02$) with a medium effect size ($d = 0.52$) Anxiety about cognitive problems: - Similarly, no significant posttest group differences with respect to anxiety and cognitive problems in daily life ($p = 0.77$) - Trend toward statistically significant differences in anxiety at 2-month follow-up ($p = 0.09$) with large effect size ($d = 0.90$)
One-to-one fatigue management course for people with chronic conditions[44]	Course consists of five modules: (1) Basics of Fatigue, (2) Communication and Fatigue, (3) Body Mechanics and Making the Most of Your Environment, (4) Analyzing and Modifying Activities, and (5) Living a Balanced Lifestyle. Participants were given homework to apply the principles learned to their daily life.	$n = 49$ (35 women and 14 men) from outpatient and community-based settings Ages 35–77 years (average 56.4); diagnosis of chronic disease (71.4% had a primary diagnosis of multiple sclerosis), moderate-to-severe fatigue.	1–2 hours for 4–6 sessions until all content was covered.	One-group, pretest–posttest, follow-up design Level III	Participants demonstrated a significant decrease in fatigue and increase in self-efficacy and quality of life, except in social well-being after taking the course.	Significant within-subjects effects were found for fatigue (FACIT-FS [$p = 0.001$]), quality of life (FACT-G total score [$p = 0.021$)], and self-efficacy (SEPECSA [$p = 0.001$]). Scores on three of the four FACT-G subscales were significant: Physical Well-Being ($p = 0.002$); Emotional Well-Being ($p = 0.007$); Functional Well-Being ($p = 0.024$). No significant within-subjects effect was found for the Social Well-Being subscale ($p = 0.535$).

(continued)

36. Hunter EG, Gibson RW, Arbesman M, D'Amico M. Systematic Review of Occupational Therapy and Adult Cancer Rehabilitation: Part 2. Impact of Multidisciplinary Rehabilitation and Psychosocial, Sexuality, and Return-to-Work Interventions. *Am J Occup Ther.* 2017;71(2):7102100040p1–7102100040p8. doi:10.5014/ajot.2017.023572.
37. Hutchison NA. Diagnosis and treatment of edema and lymphedema in the cancer patient. *Rehabil Nurs.* 2018;43(4):229–242. doi:10.1097/rnj.0000000000000177.
38. McClure MK, McClure RJ, Day R, Brufsky AM. Randomized controlled trial of the Breast Cancer Recovery Program for women with breast cancer-related lymphedema. *Am J Occup Ther.* 2010;64(1): 59–72.
39. Wu HS, McSweeney M. Cancer-related fatigue: "It's so much more than just being tired." *Eur J Oncol Nurs.* 2007;11(2):117–125. doi:10.1016/j.ejon.2006.04.037.
40. Berger AM, Mooney K, Alvarez-Perez A, et al. Cancer-related fatigue, version 2.2015. *J Natl Compr Canc Netw.* 2015;13(8):1012–1039.
41. Scott JA, Lasch KE, Barsevick AM, Piault-Louis E. Patients' experiences with cancer-related fatigue: a review and synthesis of qualitative research. *Oncol Nurs Forum.* 2011;38(3):E191–E203. doi:10.1188/11.ONF.E191-E203.
42. Hunter EG, Gibson RW, Arbesman M, D'Amico M. Systematic review of occupational therapy and adult cancer rehabilitation: part 1. Impact of physical activity and symptom management interventions. *Am J Occup Ther.* 2017;71(2):7102100030p1–7102100030p11. doi:10.5014/ajot.2017.023564.
43. Toole L, Connolly D, Smith S. Impact of an occupational-based self-management programme on chronic disease management. *Aust Occup Ther J.* 2013;60(1):30–38. doi:10.1111/1440-1630.12008.
44. Van Heest KNL, Mogush AR, Mathiowetz VG. Effects of a one-to-one fatigue management course for people with chronic conditions and fatigue. *Am J Occup Ther.* 2017;71(4):7104100020p1–7104100020p9. doi:10.5014/ajot.2017.023440.
45. National Comprehensive Cancer Network. Distress management clinical practice guidelines. *J Natl Compr Care Netw.* 2003;1:344–373.
46. Hoffman BM, Zevon MA, D'Arrigo MC, Cecchini TB. Screening for distress in cancer patients: the NCCN rapid-screening measure. *Psychooncology.* 2004;13(11):792–799. doi:10.1002/pon.796.
47. Hardy SJ, Krull KR, Wefel JS, Janelsins M. Cognitive changes for cancer survivors. *Am Soc Clin Oncol Educ Book.* 2018;38:795–806.
48. Ferguson RJ, McDonald BC, Rocque MA, et al. Development of CBT for chemotherapy-related cognitive change: results of a waitlist control trial. *Psychooncology.* 2012;21(2):176–186. doi:10.1002/pon.1878.
49. Ferguson RJ, Sigmon ST, Pritchard AJ, et al. A randomized trial of videoconference-delivered cognitive behavioral therapy for survivors of breast cancer with self-reported cognitive dysfunction. *Cancer.* 2016;122(11):1782–1791. doi:10.1002/cncr.29891.
50. Wolf TJ, Doherty M, Kallogjeri D, et al. The feasibility of using metacognitive strategy training to improve cognitive performance and neural connectivity in women with chemotherapy-induced cognitive impairment. *Oncology.* 2016;91(3):143–152. doi:10.1159/000447744.
51. Stubblefield MD, Burstein HJ, Burton AW, et al. NCCN task force report: management of neuropathy in cancer. *J Natl Compr Canc Netw.* 2009;7 Suppl 5:S1–S26; quiz S7–S8.
52. Cooper C. Hand therapy for chemotherapy-induced peripheral neuropathy. In: Cooper C, ed. *Fundamentals of Hand Therapy: Clinical Reasoning and Treatment Guidelines for Common Diagnoses of the Upper Extremity.* 2nd ed. St. Louis, MO: Elsevier Mosby; 2014: 567–572.
53. Tofthagen C. Patient perceptions associated with chemotherapy-induced peripheral neuropathy. *Clin J Oncol Nurs.* 2010;14(3):E22–E28. doi:10.1188/10.CJON.E22-E28.
54. Bakitas MA. Background noise: the experience of chemotherapy-induced peripheral neuropathy. *Nurs Res.* 2007;56(5):323–331. doi:10.1097/01.NNR.0000289503.22414.79.
55. Stubblefield MD, McNeely ML, Alfano CM, Mayer DK. A prospective surveillance model for physical rehabilitation of women with breast cancer: chemotherapy-induced peripheral neuropathy. *Cancer* 2012;118(8 Suppl):2250–2260. doi:10.1002/cncr.27463.
56. Holz SC, Wininger YD, Cooper C, Smith SR. Managing neuropathy after chemotherapy in patients with cancer. *Arch Phys Med Rehabil.* 2017;98(3):605–607. doi:10.1016/j.apmr.2016.08.461.
57. Lyons KD, Svensborn IA, Kornblith AB, Hegel MT. A content analysis of functional recovery strategies of breast cancer survivors. *OTJR.* 2015;35(2):73–80. doi:10.1177/1539449214567306.
58. Semple CJ, McCance T. Experience of parents with head and neck cancer who are caring for young children. *J Adv Nurs.* 2010;66(6):1280–1290. doi:10.1111/j.1365-2648.2010.05311.x.
59. Moran JR, Short PF, Hollenbeak CS. Long-term employment effects of surviving cancer. *J Health Econ.* 2011;30(3):505–514. doi:10.1016/j.jhealeco.2011.02.001.
60. American Occupational Therapy Association. The Role of Occupational Therapy in Palliative and Hospice Care. 2015. https://www.aota.org/~/media/Corporate/Files/AboutOT/Professionals/WhatIsOT/PA/Facts/FactSheet_PalliativeCare.pdf. Accessed September 3, 2018.
61. Hegel MT, Lyons KD, Hull JG, et al. Feasibility study of a randomized controlled trial of a telephone-delivered problem-solving-occupational therapy intervention to reduce participation restrictions in rural breast cancer survivors undergoing chemotherapy. *Psychooncology.* 2011;20(10):1092–1101. doi:10.1002/pon.1830.
62. Lyons KD, Hull JG, Kaufman PA, et al. Development and initial evaluation of a telephone-delivered, behavioral activation, and problem-solving treatment program to address functional goals of breast cancer survivors. *J Psychosoc Oncol.* 2015;33(2):199–218. doi:10.1080/07347332.2014.1002659.
63. Lyons KD, Newman RM, Kaufman PA, et al. Goal attainment and goal adjustment of older adults during person-directed cancer rehabilitation. *Am J Occup Ther.* 2018;72(2):7202205110p1–7202205110p8. doi:10.5014/ajot.2018.023648.
64. de Boer AG, Taskila TK, Tamminga SJ, Feuerstein M, Frings-Dresen MH, Verbeek JH. Interventions to enhance return-to-work for cancer patients. *Cochrane Database Syst Rev.* 2015;(9):CD007569. doi:10.1002/14651858.CD007569.pub3.

65. Mishra SI, Scherer RW, Snyder C, Geigle PM, Berlanstein DR, Topaloglu O. Exercise interventions on health-related quality of life for people with cancer during active treatment. *Cochrane Database Syst Rev.* 2012;(8):CD008465. doi:10.1002/14651858.CD008465.pub2.
66. Lahart IM, Metsios GS, Nevill AM, Carmichael AR. Physical activity for women with breast cancer after adjuvant therapy. *Cochrane Database Syst Rev.* 2018;1:CD011292. doi:10.1002/14651858.CD011292.pub2.
67. Segal R, Zwaal C, Green E, et al. Exercise for people with cancer: a clinical practice guideline. *Curr Oncol.* 2017;24(1):40–46. doi:10.3747/co.24.3376.
68. Braverman B, Hunter EG. *Occupational Therapy Practice Guidelines for Cancer Rehabilitation with Adults.* Bethesda, MD: AOTA Press; 2017.
69. American Congress of Rehabilitation Medicine. Cancer rehabilitation networking group. n.d. https://acrm.org/acrm-communities/cancer/. Accessed September 25, 2018.
70. Wagner LI, Sweet J, Butt Z, Lai J-S, Cella D. Measuring patient self-reported cognitive function: development of the functional assessment of cancer therapy-cognitive function instrument. *J Support Oncol.* 2009;7:W32–W39.
71. Vardy J, Wong K, Yi QL, et al. Assessing cognitive function in cancer patients. *Support Care Cancer.* 2006;14(11):1111–1118. doi:10.1007/s00520-006-0037-6.
72. Von Ah D, Tallman EF. Perceived cognitive function in breast cancer survivors: evaluating relationships with objective cognitive performance and other symptoms using the functional assessment of cancer therapy-cognitive function instrument. *J Pain Symptom Manage.* 2015;49(4):697–706. doi:10.1016/j.jpainsymman.2014.08.012.
73. Cheung YT, Lim SR, Shwe M, Tan YP, Chan A. Psychometric properties and measurement equivalence of the English and Chinese versions of the functional assessment of cancer therapy-cognitive in Asian patients with breast cancer. *Value Health.* 2013;16(6):1001–1013. doi:10.1016/j.jval.2013.06.017.
74. Cheung YT, Foo YL, Shwe M, et al. Minimal clinically important difference (MCID) for the functional assessment of cancer therapy: cognitive function (FACT-Cog) in breast cancer patients. *J Clin Epidemiol.* 2014;67(7):811–820. doi:10.1016/j.jclinepi.2013.12.011.
75. Tang LL, Zhang YN, Pang Y, Zhang HW, Song LL. Validation and reliability of distress thermometer in Chinese cancer patients. *Chin J Cancer Res.* 2011;23(1):54–58. doi:10.1007/s11670-011-0054-y.
76. Mitchell AJ. Pooled results from 38 analyses of the accuracy of distress thermometer and other ultra-short methods of detecting cancer-related mood disorders. *J Clin Oncol.* 2007;25(29):4670–4681. doi:10.1200/JCO.2006.10.0438.
77. Cutillo A, O'Hea E, Person S, Lessard D, Harralson T, Boudreaux E. The distress thermometer: cutoff points and clinical use. *Oncol Nurs Forum.* 2017;44(3):329–36. doi:10.1188/17.ONF.329-336.
78. Hughes KL, Sargeant H, Hawkes AL. Acceptability of the Distress Thermometer and Problem List to community-based telephone cancer helpline operators, and to cancer patients and carers. *BMC Cancer.* 2011;11:46. doi:10.1186/1471-2407-11-46.
79. Mendoza TR, Wang XS, Cleeland CS, et al. The rapid assessment of fatigue severity in cancer patients: use of the Brief Fatigue Inventory. *Cancer.* 1999;85(5):1186–1196.

Acknowledgments

Cynthia Cooper, MFA, MA, OTR/L, CHT, provided expert guidance on the peripheral neuropathy section, and we are most grateful.

Chapter 48

Burn Injuries

Rebecca Ozelie

LEARNING OBJECTIVES

This chapter will allow the reader to:

1. Describe the differences between superficial, superficial partial-thickness, deep partial-thickness, and full-thickness burn injuries.
2. Explain the rationale for splinting and positioning programs for patients with burn injuries.
3. Identify occupational therapy interventions for each phase of burn recovery.
4. Describe potential complications after a burn injury and how they can impact occupational performance.
5. Discuss the effects of a burn injury on a patient's psychosocial functioning.

CHAPTER OUTLINE

TERMINOLOGY

Antideformity positions: positions opposite to common patterns of deformity used to prevent contractures.

Blanching: applying sufficient pressure to interrupt blood flow temporarily; used as an assessment of capillary flow rate.

Debriding: removing eschar and loose or necrotic tissue to prevent infection and promote healing.

Dermis: layer of skin below the epidermis that contains blood vessels, nerve endings, hair follicles, and sweat and oil glands; supports the regrowth of new epithelial tissue.

Epidermis: most superficial layer of the skin; acts as a barrier; it is continually sloughed and replaced.

Pruritus: severe itching of the skin.

Total body surface area (TBSA): assessment of the amount of injury to the skin after a burn injury.

Wound contracture: part of normal healing in which myofibroblasts in the wound bed contract to minimize the skin defect.

Z-plasty: surgical procedure in which a Z-shaped incision is made and tissue is transposed to increase tissue length.

Introduction

Approximately 486,000 burn injuries required medical treatment in the United States in 2016 and 3,275 people died from fire and smoke inhalation.[1] The ABA National Burn Repository from 2005 to 2014 reported the burn survival rate is 96.8%—the majority of burns in adults occur in males (68%); the most common cause of burns is fire/flame (43%); and most burns occur in the home (73%), followed by injuries in the workplace (8%).[2] Over 60% of patients with burn injuries are admitted to 128 regional burn centers designated by the American Burn Association; the remainder are treated at local or regional hospitals.[1] Therefore, every occupational therapist should understand the principles of care and rehabilitation of patients with burn injuries.

Burn Classification

In the past, burn depth was classified as first, second, or third degree. Today, the preferred classification terminology more accurately describes the level of cellular injury. The terms used are superficial, superficial partial-thickness, deep partial-thickness, and full-thickness (Fig. 48-1). Burns can have mixed depths, which necessitates that the burn team carefully assess the appearance and progress of each area of the wound site. Disruption of any portion of the skin has the potential to interfere with its normal functions, which include temperature regulation, fluid regulation, and its role as a physical barrier to infection.[3] Occupational therapists may treat patients with all depths of burn injuries. It is important to differentiate and understand the implications of each classification in order to plan the most effective interventions as wound healing and long-term outcomes are often determined by burn depth.

Superficial Burns

Superficial burns damage cells only in the **epidermis**[4] (see Fig. 48-1). These injuries are dry, painful, and red. With a well-nourished and intact epithelial bed at the base of the hair follicles, these injuries heal spontaneously within approximately 7 days and leave no permanent scar. Sunburn is an example of a superficial burn.

Superficial Partial-Thickness Burns

Superficial partial-thickness burns damage cells in the epidermis and the upper level of the **dermis.**[4] The most common sign of a superficial partial-thickness burn is intact blisters over the injured area.[4] Hair follicles remain intact because these are found in the deeper layers of the dermis. In addition, these injuries are painful because of the irritation of the nerve endings in the dermal layer. Superficial partial-thickness burns usually heal spontaneously within 7 to 21 days and leave minimal or no scarring.

Deep Partial-Thickness Burns

Deep partial-thickness burns cause cell injury in the epidermis and severe damage to the dermal layer.[4] These injuries appear blotchy, with areas of whitish color interspersed throughout the wound, which is the result of damage to the blood vessels in the dermal layer.[4] The injury site is painful. Spontaneous healing of deep partial-thickness burns is sluggish (3–5 weeks) because vascularity in the dermal layer is impaired. Therefore, the risk of significant scarring is increased. For this reason, deep partial-thickness burns are often grafted to expedite healing and minimize scarring.

Full-Thickness Injury Burns

In a full-thickness injury, both the epidermis and the dermal layer are destroyed.[4] These wounds appear white or waxy because of the underlying adipose tissue and are inherently insensate because of the complete destruction of the dermal nerve endings.[4] Full-thickness burns require surgical intervention, such as skin grafting, because there are no dermal elements to support the

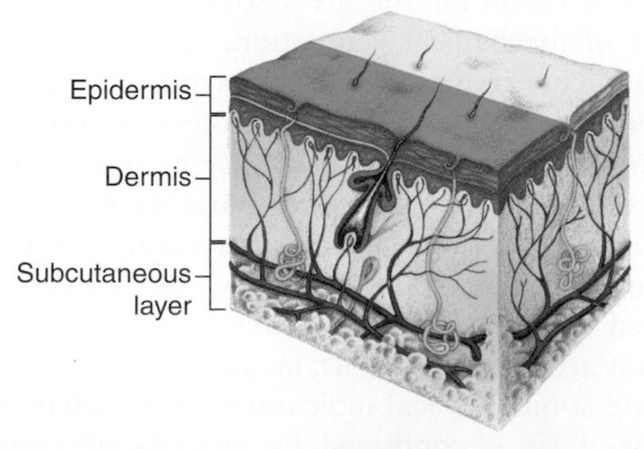

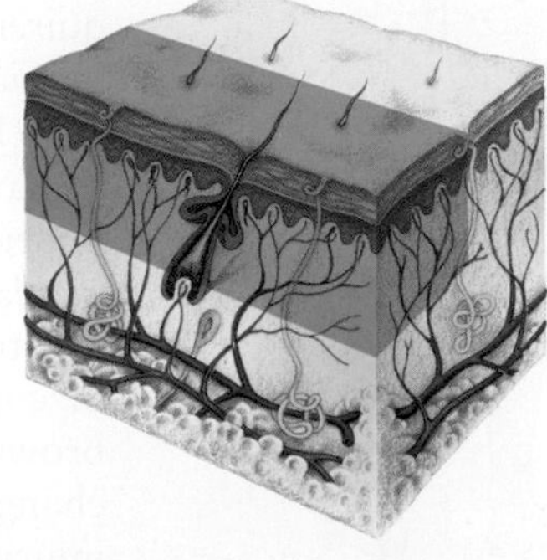

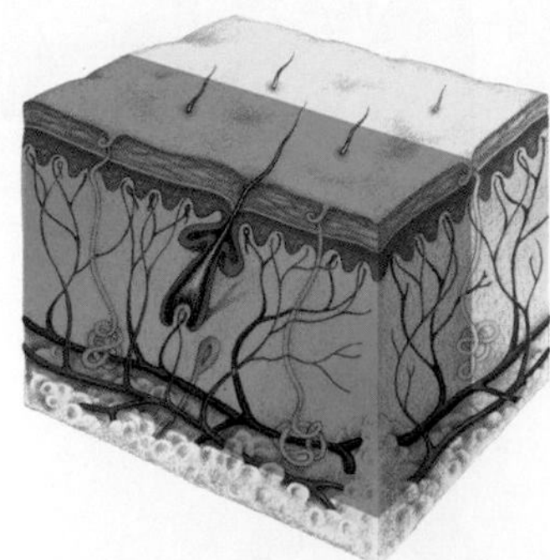

Figure 48-1. Skin anatomy status postburns.

regrowth of epithelial tissue. Some burns, such as electrical burns, may damage structures below the dermis, including subcutaneous fat, muscle, or bone.

Total Body Surface Area

An estimation of burn wound size is defined as **total body surface area (TBSA)** is critical for effective early burn management. The burn percentage TBSA is used for the following:

- Calculating nutritional and fluid requirements
- Determining level of acuity to establish the level of medical treatment needed (e.g., admission to a burn center)
- Guiding clinical treatment decisions
- Predicting mortality outcomes

There are three common methods health care providers use to estimate a burn survivor's TBSA; the "rule of nines," the "rule of palms" and the "Lund–Browder chart." The rule of nines is a commonly used technique in adults (see Fig. 48-2). For example, if an adult received a burn that included the anterior and posterior surfaces of his right arm (9%), his anterior head and neck (4.5%), and his anterior chest (18%), then his TBSA affected would be 31.5%. To determine the TBSA of a burn injury in children and infants, a modification of this technique, the Lund–Browder chart, is used. In addition, in both children and adults, the palm method is also used to estimate TBSA. The palm method estimates that the palmar surface of one's hand is approximately 1% TBSA. These current methods do have some limitations and burn injuries are often over- and underestimated.[5] This can lead to ineffective patient care and decreased burn unit efficiency. More technologically advanced methods are currently being used and studied. Recently, the use of three-dimensional imaging has been found to be superior to the rule of nines and palm method.[6]

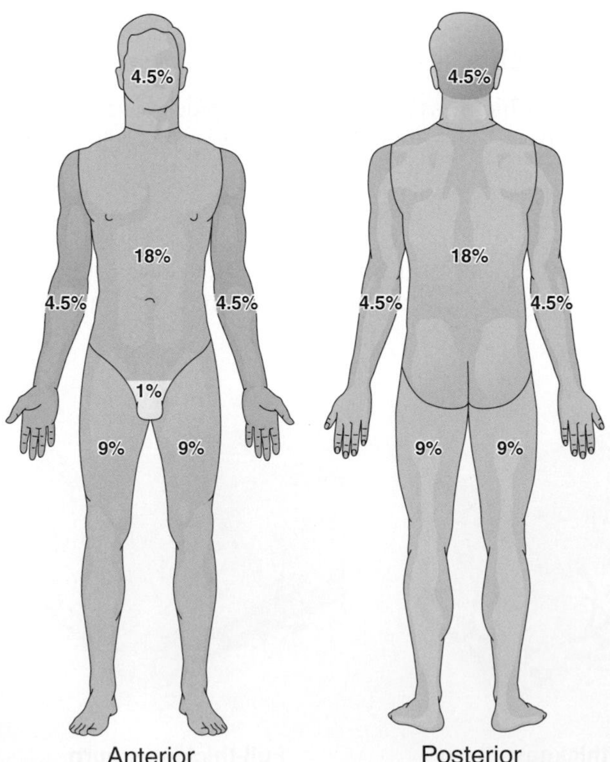

Figure 48-2. Rule of nines.

Phases of Burn Management and Rehabilitation

Identifying specific phases of burn management helps to describe the role of occupational therapy (OT) for patients with burn injuries. These include the emergent, acute, and rehabilitation phases. Each of the phases, along with accompanying OT considerations, are described.

Emergent Phase

The emergent phase of a burn injury is considered to be from initial injury to approximately 72 hours after the burn.[7]

Medical Management

During the emergent phase, the medical team attempts to stabilize the patient. This may include fluid resuscitation, establishment of adequate tissue perfusion by means of mechanical ventilation, and achievement of cardiopulmonary stability. Associated injuries, such as fractures, are also evaluated and treated during this time.

Inhalation Injury

An important consideration in the emergent phase is the possibility of an inhalation injury. An inhalation injury damages the supply of oxygen to the body due to significant edema of the upper respiratory tract, chemical irritation of the lower respiratory tract, and injuries resulting from systemic effects of carbon monoxide and cyanide.[8] Inhalation injuries are associated with the requirement of mechanical ventilation, secondary pneumonia, and acute respiratory distress syndrome.[8] About 1 in 10 patients admitted to burn centers are reported to have an inhalation injury and those with inhalation injuries experience an increase in mortality rate.[8] This increase in mortality rates makes an accurate diagnosis and treatment imperative. A history of smoke exposure in confined spaces and prolonged rescue, singed eyebrows, soot around the nostrils, facial edema, and voice changes are some physical indications of an inhalation injury. Diagnosis is confirmed by analysis of arterial blood gases, chest radiographs, and fiberoptic bronchoscopy. Medical management of an inhalation injury often includes supportive respiratory care including mechanical ventilation and bronchial hygiene.

Compartment Syndrome

Circulation can be compromised when burn injuries encircle a body segment. This is due to the inelasticity of the eschar (burned tissue) combined with increased internal pressure within fascial compartments. Local increase in pressure within the compartments of the extremities compresses blood vessels and reduces blood flow,[9] which results in what is known as compartment syndrome. If the pressure is not relieved, ischemia and necrosis may result. Symptoms of increased compartmental pressure include paresthesias, coldness, and decreased or absent pulses in the extremities. In the trunk, inelastic eschar can act as a corset, limiting lung expansion and preventing adequate respiration. Diagnosis of compartment syndrome is determined with use of Doppler ultrasound and pulse oximetry. Surgical intervention (escharotomy and/or a fasciotomy) is required to relieve the pressure and prevent tissue death (see Fig. 48-3). An escharotomy is a surgical incision through the eschar, whereas a fasciotomy is a deeper incision extending through the fascia.

Dressings

After the initial burn assessment, the medical staff will clean, debride, and dress any wound areas (see Fig. 48-4). The functions of dressings include protecting the wound against infection, maintaining a protective environment, and facilitating normal wound healing. With dressings, topical agents are used and can vary widely, although most are wide-spectrum antimicrobials. Examples include agents that contain silver (Aquacel AG), nano-crystalline silver (Acticoat), cadexomer iodine (Iodosorb), or synthetic antimicrobial (LLKKK18).[10] These antimicrobials serve to keep the level of bacterial colonization of a wound at a manageable level. It is also a common practice for wounds to be debrided or excised to remove devitalized tissue from the wound site. Debridement or excision of the wound is done by medical personnel. Debridement of blisters is controversial. Leaving blisters intact is thought to provide a positive wound healing environment, reduction in pain, and enhanced cell proliferation.[11] Those in favor of **debriding** blisters by eliminating the underlying fluid feel that the fluid can serve as a medium for bacteria.[12] The medical personnel will also make the decisions as to what dressing and topical agent is most appropriate for each patient. Although it is often the nursing staff who change the dressings, it is appropriate for occupational therapists to routinely or periodically participate in dressing removal and application as it provides opportunities to view the healing wounds. This allows the therapist to monitor healing and adjust the therapy program accordingly.

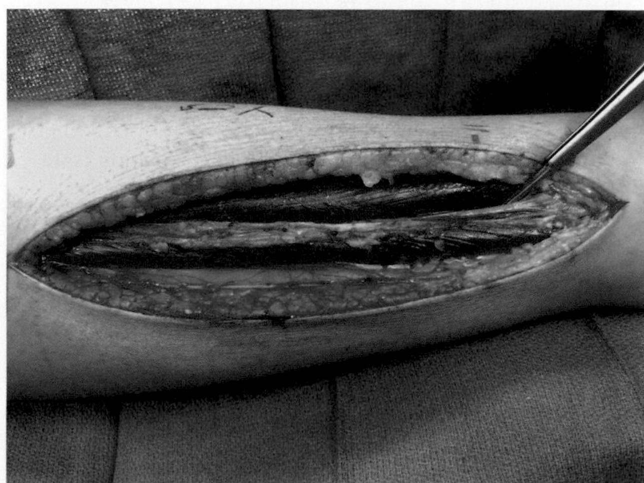

Figure 48-3. Fasciotomy.

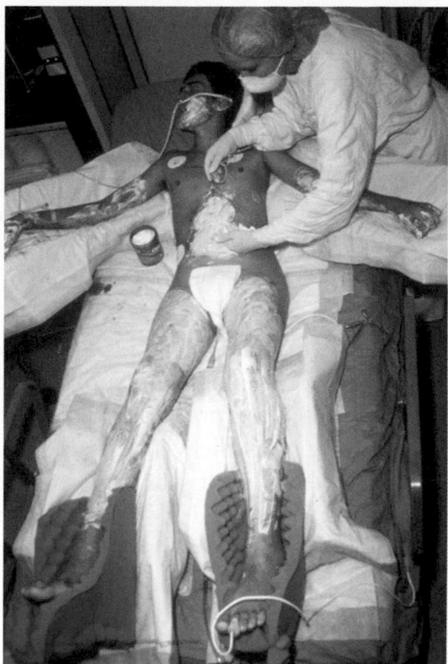

Figure 48-4. Wound cleaning and dressings.

Infection Control

One of the functions of the skin is to act as a barrier against infection.[13] Therefore, a patient with a burn injury is highly susceptible to infection, and infection is the most common cause of morbidity and mortality in patients with burns.[14] It is essential that all staff, family, and visitors adhere to strict infection control procedures. This includes washing hands frequently, using gloves when necessary, and avoiding cross-contamination through instruments and equipment.

Contracture Formation

Patients with burn injuries are at significant risk for contractures. Contractures tend to occur in predictable patterns, usually flexed, shortened positions (e.g., elbow flexion, shoulder adduction, or knee flexion) and can considerably limit the patient's ability to perform activities of daily living (ADLs). The shoulder has been found to be the most frequently contracted joint followed by the elbow, wrist, ankle, and knee.[15] In a recent Burn Model System National Database study, 33% of burn survivors developed at least one contracture with an average of three contractures per person.[15] Contractures are defined as abnormal shortening of muscle tissue, rendering the muscle highly resistant to stretching. It can be caused by fibrosis of the tissues supporting the muscle or the joint. It is important to note that **wound contracture** is a normal physiological response of the initial wound closure and healing process and subsequent scar contracture may occur as the scar matures.[16] Research of the biological principles of scar and contracture formation suggest forces applied to wounds as they heal will increase fibrosis and therefore contracture formation. Kwan and Tredget[16] advise that relieving forces to healing wounds may reduce scarring and contractures.

OT during the Emergent Phase

During the emergent phase, the occupational therapist performs an initial evaluation of the patient's needs. A full evaluation may be deferred until after the emergent phase, when the patient is more medically stable. During the screen, the therapist notes the distribution of the burn, burn type and depth, and which joints are involved. This allows the occupational therapist to establish an appropriate splinting and positioning program. It is also during this time that the therapist begins completing an occupational profile of the patient to determine preadmission functional status, roles, interests, and social supports.

OT intervention in the emergent phase focuses on the prevention of early contracture formation through the use of splints and positioning programs. It is ideal to initiate OT intervention as early as 24 to 48 hours after burn because collagen synthesis and contracture formation begin during the initial response to a thermal injury.[17]

Splinting

Ideally, splints are fabricated and applied in the initial visit, and a positioning program is established and communicated to the team. Table 48-1 describes common contracture patterns, antideformity positions, and appropriate splints. Generally, any joint involved in a superficial partial-thickness injury or worse has the potential for contracture and is usually splinted. Splint wearing times are determined by the patient's tolerance to the splint and functional ability to use the involved extremity. That is, a decrease in active movement of the involved limb indicates the need for increased splint wearing time to prevent potential contractures. For example, a heavily sedated patient cannot perform active movement and therefore requires splinting at all times,

Table 48-1 Anticontracture Positioning by Location of Burn

LOCATION OF BURN	CONTRACTURE TENDENCY	ANTICONTRACTURE POSITIONING AND/OR TYPICAL SPLINT
Anterior neck	Neck flexion	Remove pillows; use half-mattress to extend the neck; neck extension splint or collar
Axilla	Adduction	120° abduction with slight external rotation; axilla splint or positioning wedges; watch for signs of brachial plexus strain
Anterior elbow	Flexion	Elbow extension splint in 5°–10° flexion
Dorsal wrist	Wrist extension	Wrist support in neutral
Volar wrist	Wrist flexion	Wrist cock-up splint in 5°–10° extension
Hand dorsal	Claw hand deformity	Functional hand splint with MP joints 70°–90°, DIP joints fully extended, first web open, thumb in opposition (safe position; see Chapter 37)
Hand volar	Palmar contracture cupping of hand	Palm extension splint MPs in slight hyperextension
Hip-anterior	Hip flexion	Prone positioning; weights on thigh in supine; knee immobilizers
Knee	Knee flexion	Knee extension positioning and/or splints; prevent external rotation, which may cause peroneal nerve compression
Foot	Foot drop	Ankle at 90° with foot board or splint; watch for signs of heel ulcer

MP, metacarpophalangeal; DIP, distal interphalangeal.

Reprinted with permission from Pessina MA, Ellis SM. Burn management rehabilitation. *Nurs Clin North Am.* 1997;32:367.

except for therapy and dressing changes. An alert patient who can use his or her affected extremity for functional tasks, such as self-feeding or prescribed exercises, may require the use of splints only at night. Splints are applied over the burn dressing and secured with either gauze wrap or Velcro straps. Although splinting is considered the standard of care in burn treatment, there is a paucity of evidence to support its use.[18] Validation of the practice of splinting for the prevention of contracture is a research area that may be addressed by occupational therapists in the future.

Positioning

Antideformity positioning, which is used as an adjunct to splinting for prevention of contractures, can be initiated in the first visit. For example, if a patient is unable to be fitted with a custom wrist extension splint, supporting the hand on a rolled pillow can, at least temporarily, maintain appropriate joint position. Another example is removing pillows under the patient's head to limit the amount of neck flexion and potential for contracture. Positioning to elevate the upper extremities can also help to minimize upper extremity edema. Elevation can be done with foam wedges, pillows, or specialized arm troughs attached to the bed. A risk of elevating the upper extremity is the potential for brachial plexus strain.

Acute Phase

The acute phase begins after the emergent phase and continues until the wound is closed, either by spontaneous healing or skin grafts.[7] The acute phase can last several days to several months, depending on the extent of the burn and the amount of grafting required. For example, a patient with a 10% TBSA may have an acute phase of 1 week, during which the patient is mobile and undergoes one excision and grafting procedure. However, a patient with a 70% TBSA burn may be in the acute phase for several weeks, during which the patient is in an intensive care unit and undergoes many grafting procedures to close the wounds.

Support and Psychosocial Adjustment in the Acute Phase

Most patients with burn injuries report some symptoms of anxiety, depression, and even posttraumatic stress disorder after injury.[19] Several factors have been identified as risk factors for poor adjustment and postinjury onset of psychological disorders. These include preburn affective disorders, burn injury size and location, level of pain, dispositional variables, and avoidance of coping.[19] The psychosocial challenges of burn patients vary as the patient moves through each stage of physical recovery.[20] Patients in the acute stage deal with issues of depression and anxiety and may begin to exhibit signs of both acute and posttraumatic stress disorder. Also at this time, any preinjury psychopathology may become more apparent.[20]

LeDoux et al.[21] state that the burn team can foster healthy coping strategies while working with the burn patient by using the following techniques:

1. Identify strengths that each patient can emphasize, reminding him or her of the strength already involved in surviving a painful and frightening experience.
2. Validate sadness and fear.
3. Assist patient to achieve goals; this helps to show hope for the future.
4. Instill a belief that the patient can succeed.

It is also important to note that persons with burn injuries have been found to have a higher rate of mental illness before their burn injury.[22] This knowledge should cue occupational therapists working with patients with burns to critically assess for psychological needs, develop a plan of care, and work interprofessionally to meet the needs of their patient.

Team Communication

Communication with all members of the team, including the patient and the patient's family and/or support system, throughout hospitalization is essential. During this acute phase, collaboration between the occupational therapist and the burn team is essential for several reasons, including the following[23]:

1. Alerting the team to developing contractures and response to therapeutic intervention
2. Planning for perioperative splinting
3. Clarifying range-of-motion orders based on graft integrity
4. Teaching the team about environmental modifications or communication systems
5. Advocating on the patient's behalf regarding eventual outpatient needs

Medical Management

Skin grafting, which occurs primarily in the acute phase when the patient is medically stable, is required when the dermal bed is sufficiently destroyed to prevent or significantly impair spontaneous regrowth of the epithelial tissue.[24] Skin grafting is generally performed for all full-thickness burns and for large, deep partial-thickness burns. Skin grafting entails both excision of necrotic (dead) tissue and the placement of skin or a skin substitute over the wound bed.

Types of Grafts

A variety of grafting procedures are available. According to the size of the burn, availability of donor sites and medical stability of the patient, the team may opt to use one or more of the graft types described below.

- *Autografts:* Skin harvested from an unburned area of the patient is an autograft. Split-thickness autografts are considered the current gold standard.[25] Split-thickness autographs are taken at the level of the mid-dermis and allow for regeneration of epidermis. Donor sites are ideally selected for the best match of color and texture to the affected area. Donor sites may produce scarring and can be painful. Donor sites often will require scar management techniques similar to the burn site. The harvested skin can be left as a solid sheet (sheet graft) or perforated to increase the surface area (meshed graft) (see Fig. 48-5). Meshing allows the surface area of the harvested skin to cover up to one and half to nine times the original area.[26] Both sheet and meshed grafts have advantages and disadvantages. A sheet graft has the best cosmetic outcome and is thus preferred for the face and hands.[27] Infection and the development of hematoma under a sheet graft, however, can cause complete graft loss and require regrafting. A meshed graft may be less cosmetically appealing as the meshed pattern is retained permanently and can result in severe scarring.[28] The meshed graft is advantageous, however, as it covers large areas when the donor site is limited and allow drainage of blood and exudate, which prevents hematomas and improves graft adherence.[27]
- *Skin substitutes:* In cases of extensive burn injuries, where there is not sufficient donor skin to cover all of the affected area with autograft, the burn team may opt to use a variety of skin substitutes. These skin substitutes can be either biologic, such as allografts or xenografts (from cadaver and bovine skin, respectively), or synthetic, such as Biobrane comprising nylon and silastic. These dressings aid in wound management by decreasing infection, stimulating healing, preparing the wound bed for autograft skin, decreasing pain, and protecting exposed tendons, nerves, and blood vessels.[29]

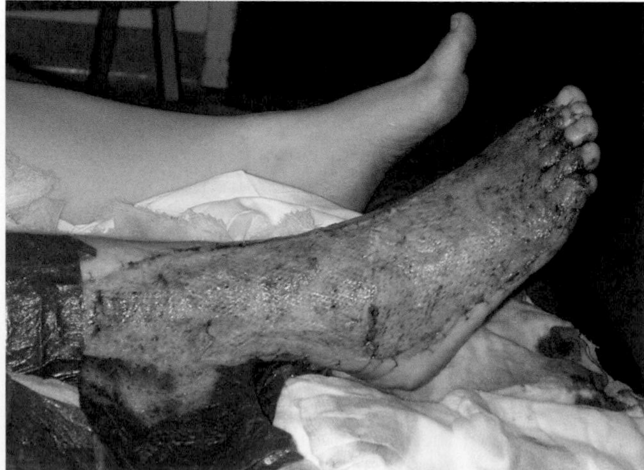

Figure 48-5. Meshed graft to lower extremity.

OT during the Acute Phase

During the acute phase, the occupational therapist performs a detailed initial evaluation. This includes a thorough chart review including a review of the past medical history. Associated diagnoses that may limit occupational performance, such as psychiatric illness, diabetes, or lung disease, are to be accounted for during OT treatment planning. Areas specifically assessed by the occupational therapist during the initial evaluation include client factors (e.g., mental functions, cognitive skills, communication and social skills, sensory functions, neuromusculoskeletal and movement-related functions, joint mobility/stability, and muscle strength/tone/endurance) and ADL and instrumental activities of daily living (IADL) performance. It is important to document specific range-of-motion (ROM) and manual muscle test (MMT) measurements for any involved joints as a baseline during the evaluation. This will allow the clinician to reassess and document progress along the course of treatment.

Evaluation can consist of standardized outcome measurements such as the Patient and Observer Scar Assessment Scale, the Disabilities of the Arm, Shoulder, and Hand Score (DASH), the Brief Burn Specific Health Scale (BSHS-B), the ICF Core Sets for Hand Conditions, the Jebsen–Taylor Hand Function (JTHF) Test, observation during task performance, and interviews with the patient and family. The potential for permanent scarring and disfigurement may cause significant anxiety and limit the patient's ability or motivation to participate in rehabilitation. Thus, early assessment of the patient's support systems allows the therapist to identify resources that may aid in early patient motivation and goal setting.

Because of the acute medical nature of many burn injuries, OT intervention in the acute phase may focus on client factors such as ROM and strength. These can be addressed through preparatory methods and tasks such as continued splinting, positioning, therapeutic exercise, and through occupations and activities. Whenever possible, activities in treatment should reflect each patient's interests and occupations. Other potential treatment activities include environmental modifications, pain remediation, and patient and family education. In the acute phase, the individual's ability to participate in treatment related to self-care and functional retraining is often limited by complex medical issues. These areas are addressed in more detail during the rehabilitation phase.

Splinting and Positioning

During the acute phase, the splinting and positioning programs established in the emergent phase are continually monitored and adjusted. Splinting schedules are adjusted according to the individual's ability to participate in activities. For example, if a patient consistently uses an affected elbow for self-feeding and ADLs during the day, decreasing the wearing time for the elbow splint to nights and rest periods is appropriate. It is imperative to check all splints often to ensure proper fit and function.[17] In addition, teaching the nursing staff and family members proper fit and application of splints can help decrease the potential for complications.

Exercise and Activity

In the acute phase, splinting and positioning are used in combination with exercise and activity.[30] Exercise is especially important to control edema, prevent muscle atrophy, tendon adherence, joint stiffness, and capsular shortening, and improve pulmonary function.[17,31] Exercise can improve muscle endurance and cardiopulmonary fitness, which are essential components of health.[32] Early incorporation of exercise and activity has also been found to reduce intensive care unit and hospital length stay, as well as improvements in ROM of joints.[33] Exercise types include passive ROM, active ROM, active assistive ROM, and functional activity. If the patient cannot participate in active exercise or activity because of poor medical status or impaired level of alertness, passive ROM is indicated. Active exercise is encouraged whenever possible,[34] and it is the role of the therapist to guide the patient toward function. Within a single treatment session, a patient may participate in all of these forms of exercise. Functional activities may be used to improve active ROM. For example, completing a meal preparation activity can be meaningful, fun, and easily adapted by changing height and distance of objects to meet upper extremity ROM goals. Contraindications to exercise include exposed tendons, recent autografts (~5–10 days), acute medical complications, and fractures.[7,17] In addition, periodic inspection of the wound by the occupational therapist is essential to determine the status of wound healing and skin integrity as related to tolerance of the exercise program.

Perioperative Care

The 5 to 10 days after a skin graft procedure is the perioperative period. A patient with a large burn injury may make many trips to the operating room for skin grafting. Each surgical procedure begins a new perioperative stage. For example, a patient needing grafting on the trunk, arms, and legs may make three trips to the operating room, with each successive area requiring proper perioperative care. The role of the occupational therapist in the perioperative period is to fabricate custom splints to immobilize the newly grafted areas in antideformity positions. Ideally, splints are fabricated immediately prior to or during surgery and applied at the conclusion of the surgery. These splints usually stay in place, along with the primary dressing, for 5 to 10 days.[7,17] During this time, ROM exercises are contraindicated to allow for graft adherence. After the primary dressing is removed, the burn team assesses the graft adherence, and a determination is made regarding the appropriateness of resuming exercise.

Pain Management

The occupational therapist must address pain issues that arise during treatment. Patients can experience both the acute feelings of pain and secondary morbidities of pain such as long-term anxiety and posttraumatic stress[35] and even delayed wound healing.[36] Many patients in intensive care cannot verbalize a subjective response to manipulation, such as during dressing changes or exercise. In these cases, the therapist monitors objective responses to pain, such as blood pressure, heart rate, and respiratory rate, and adjusts the treatment accordingly. The time of therapy sessions should be considered to allow pain medication to be administered prior to treatment. Decreased repetitions and increased rest breaks during exercise sessions may also be appropriate. Other techniques used to manage pain throughout recovery include distraction strategies, relaxation techniques, and preparatory information (informing/preparing the client regarding procedures to be performed). The use of virtual reality as a distraction has also been found to be a safe, low-cost, effective pain reduction technique.[37]

Environmental Adaptation

Beginning in the acute phase and throughout recovery, the occupational therapist may provide environmental adaptations to facilitate the patient's independence in identified occupations. Modified call buttons and bed controls, voice-activated communication systems, modifications to phones and laptops, and modified utensils (Fig. 48-6) and self-care items are examples of these environmental adaptations. These modifications can increase a patient's sense of control and independence. The development of environmental modifications is limited only by the patient's motivation and the therapist's creativity.

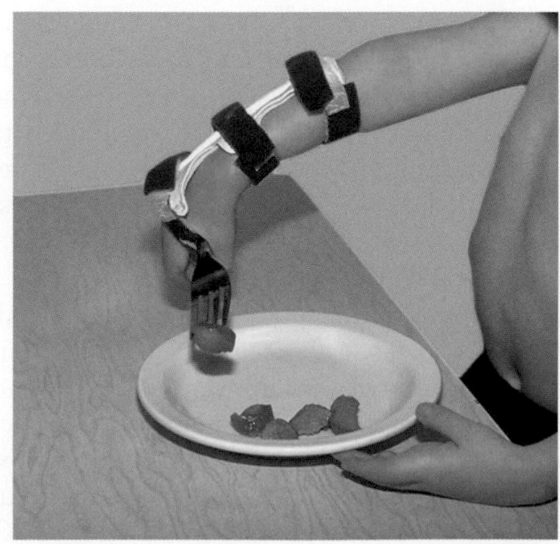

Figure 48-6. Modified utensils to facilitate independence.

Patient and Family Teaching

The occupational therapist provides members of the patient's support system with education regarding ways to interact with and support the patient during recovery. They may be encouraged to make recordings and posters or to bring in favorite music or foods. They may need to learn new ways to touch or comfort their loved one. In addition, the family and friends provide a source of information regarding the patient's roles, habits, routines, and available community resources if the patient cannot communicate this information. An educated family and/or support system can be an important asset for ensuring follow-through of the rehabilitation program.

Discharge Planning

Because hospital stays are generally short, discharge planning begins as soon as possible after admission. Many patients in the acute phase are either discharged directly home or to a rehabilitation unit. Elements to consider during discharge planning are the availability of community resources for outpatient or follow-up care, support systems available to the patient, and physical demands of the home environment. When patients who have sustained major burns cannot return to the hospital where they received acute care, it is important for the inpatient occupational therapist to establish a relationship with a therapist in the patient's community to ensure continuity of care throughout the rehabilitation phase. Whenever possible, all authorization from third-party payers should be established prior to discharge to avoid delays in the initiation of outpatient therapy. If a patient cannot be discharged directly to home, transfer to an inpatient rehabilitation facility is appropriate, and early communication with the receiving therapist is necessary to ensure continuity of care.

Rehabilitation Phase

The rehabilitation phase follows the acute phase and continues until scar maturation.[38] Scar maturation can take 6 months to 2 years.[38] It is considered complete when the scar becomes pale and the rate of collagen synthesis stabilizes.[7] The level of direct involvement of the occupational therapist during this extended time is varied. It may range from daily inpatient treatment to weekly outpatient treatment to annual clinic visits.

OT during the Rehabilitation Phase

During the rehabilitation phase, the occupational therapist continues to assess capacities and abilities such as ROM, strength, activity tolerance, sensation, and scar management. In addition, outcome measures specific to ADLs and IADLs, fine motor control, and upper extremity function are valuable in guiding treatment planning and preparing for discharge. The overall goal of OT intervention during this phase is to facilitate the patient's return to his or her previous level of occupational performance. Patients are encouraged to take increasing responsibility for their care, including collaborating to establish meaningful goals.

Range-of-Motion

In the rehabilitation stage, the patient continues to benefit from daily stretching routines established in the acute phase of care. In the early part of this phase, the rate of collagen synthesis is increased, requiring the patient to stretch frequently throughout the day. Aggressive contraction can continue for months after injury.[39] At all times, skin integrity must be monitored during stretching to prevent tearing. Massage using a non–water-based cream should precede stretching to help prevent dry skin from rupturing.[38] An appropriate stretch consists of bringing the tissue to the point of **blanching**, or becoming pale, and holding it in that position for several seconds. The patient should report tension but not pain. Overzealous stretching can result in tissue tears and edema, which increase joint stiffness. The recommended hold time of stretching exercises has been reported in the literature in varying amounts of time. One study recommends 30 to 60 seconds of hold time to be effective in improving ROM and functional recovery.[40] Another study recommended more than 3 minutes of hold time.[39] Longer hold times are thought to be potentially more beneficial but can lead to therapist fatigue, which can affect the consistency and patient's tolerance.[39] Each area of contracture is treated for at least 3 minutes per session. This yielded significant improvements in joint ROM.[39] Stretching should be initially performed by an occupational therapist. With training, the patient and/or caregiver can also be educated to complete the ROM exercises.

Strength

Resistive exercise and graded functional activities can improve strength. Patients may be taught an independent exercise program with resistive rubber ribbon or tubing, such as Theraband, to increase proximal upper body strength. Functional activities can also be graded to increase strength. For example, patients may gain strength as they perform self-care activities with increasing demands, as when progressing from sitting to standing for oral facial hygiene activities.

Activity Tolerance

A key feature of rehabilitation is mobilizing the patient as much as possible, thereby increasing his or her activity tolerance. For an inpatient, this includes increased time spent out of bed and trips to the gym and off the medical unit. With careful monitoring by the occupational therapist, activity time should be increased if there is no evidence of fatigue. Fatigue can be monitored by patient self-report and clinician observation. For inpatient and outpatient rehabilitation, this may also include facilitating patients resuming leisure activities and going on community outings.

Sensation

Newly healed skin and grafted skin may be hypersensitive, which can significantly limit functional performance. Hypersensitivity can be addressed effectively by systematic desensitization. This can be achieved by asking the patient to manipulate objects with varying textures in the environment. Initially, the patient practices holding soft textures, such as cotton balls or lambswool, and then progresses to manipulating objects with rougher textures, such as Velcro or burlap. A formal system such as the Downey desensitization program can also be used.

Coordination

Coordination can be impaired by a variety of factors, including limited ROM, strength, or sensation. Coordination can be improved through the use of selected progressive tasks designed to challenge the patient's skills. For example, a patient may be asked first to take lids off large jars and then smaller containers. The patient may also trace large letters or patterns before attempting a fine motor writing task such as working on a crossword puzzle.

Scar Management

Scar tissue formation is a natural response to wound healing.[7] It begins in the emergent phase and may take up to 2 years to mature.[41] A hypertrophic scar is an aberration of the normal healing process and presents as a red, raised, and inelastic scar[17] (Fig. 48-7). A hypertrophic scar contains an increased number of fibroblasts as compared to normal skin, and the collagen fibers are arranged in a nodular as opposed to parallel fashion.[42] The cause is thought to be a disruption in the balance between collagen synthesis and lysis.[7] The tendency for hypertrophic scarring is unique to each individual, although it tends to form over extensor joints and areas of high tension. In general, patients with large amounts of pigment in the skin and young patients are most prone to hypertrophic scarring. In addition to being cosmetically unappealing, hypertrophic scars can limit functional skills by restricting joint ROM.

Keloids are another type of scars (see Fig. 48-7). Unlike hypertrophic scars, these can appear years after the initial injury and extend beyond the site of injury.[43] Keloids are often painful, will not improve with time, most common in darker skin types, and may have a genetic predisoposition.[44] Keloids can be excised but have a high recurrence rate following surgery.[44]

Objective quantification of scars is limited and conflicting measures are used in the literature. The Patient and Observer Scar Assessment Scale and the Vancouver

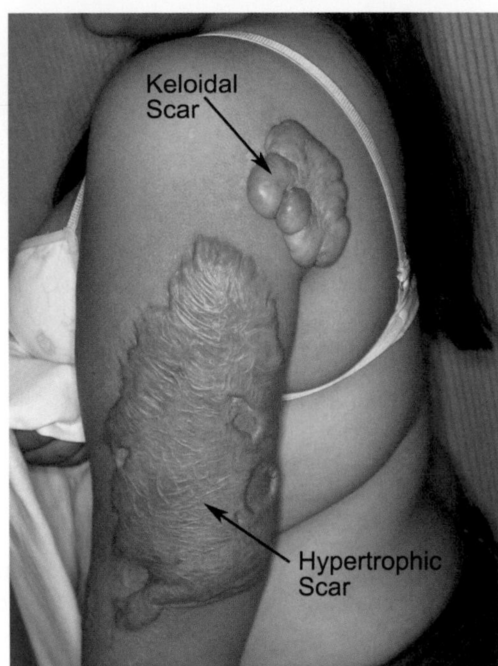

Figure 48-7. Keloid and hypertrophic scars.

Scar Scale are the most widely used scar assessment tools.[45] The Patient and Observer Scar Assessment Scale has an observer scar assessment scale and a patient scar assessment scale and the Vancouver Scar Scale is used to rate the pliability, vascularity, height, and pigmentation of scars.[46] Other assessments include the Patient and Observer Scar Assessment Scale[47] and the Matching Assessment of Scars and Photographs.[48]

The occupational therapist attempts to prevent or limit the development of hypertrophic scars. Treatment methods include a combination of techniques, including massage, pressure therapy, and the use of specialized inserts.

MASSAGE. Scar massage is frequently used to improve functional and cosmetic outcomes of scars. A systematic review found that there is preliminary evidence that scar massage may be effective in reduction of scar height, vascularity, pliability, pain, **pruritus**, and depression.[49] It is thought that scar massage causes mechanical disruption of the increased fibrotic tissue of the scar.[49] This can result in an improved cosmetic appearance and improvement in the elastic properties of the scar. Scar massage is initiated when it is determined that the burned area is closed and can withstand slight friction. Newly healed skin can be fragile and susceptible to lesions and blistering.[50] There is no set protocol for scar massage. Literature reports scar massage ranging from 10 minutes twice daily to 30 minutes twice weekly.[51] It should be applied with deep pressure (enough to blanch the scar temporarily) in either a circular pattern or perpendicular to the long axis of the scar (Fig. 48-8). Lubricant should be used during scar massage to reduce friction.

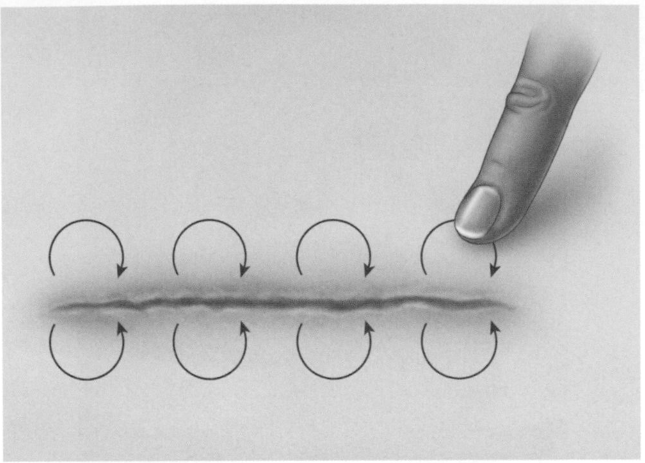

Figure 48-8. Scar massage.

Perfume-free lubricants with high water content are preferred to decrease potential irritation and provide moisture to newly healed skin. Initially, scar massage is the responsibility of the occupational therapist so that skin integrity and tolerance can be monitored. Once an established routine has been developed, the therapist should teach the patient and/or caregivers to assume responsibility for daily scar massage.

PRESSURE THERAPY. Pressure therapy has been considered a critical component of scar management since the 1970s.[52] It is thought that pressure can control collagen synthesis, facilitate scar maturation, and reduce scar redness by limiting the supply of blood, oxygen, and nutrients to the scar tissue.[53] The use of pressure therapy within a designated range of 15 to 25 mm Hg of pressure has been found to improve Vancouver Scar Scale score, pigmentation, redness, and scar brightness.[54] The occupational therapist initiates the application of gentle pressure via Tubigrip, elastic bandage wraps, Coban, or Isotoner gloves once the skin is mostly healed with no more than quarter-sized openings remaining or as indicated by the physician. Initially, pressure dressings are applied for 2-hour intervals. Wearing time is gradually increased in 2-hour increments until 23-hour wear is tolerated. Tolerance is determined by lack of blisters or new open areas. At this point, increased pressure using customized products such as Tricolast or Bioconcepts garments are indicated (Fig. 48-9). The most common amount of pressure used in practice is 15 to 25 mm Hg. Higher pressures have been found to have an increased effect, but pressures of 40 mm Hg and above induce discomfort and potential harm to the patient.[52,55] Pressure less than 15 mm Hg appear to have no or poor effect on scars.[53,56,57] Pressure garments should be worn for a minimum of 23 hours a day and for 6 to 12 months or until scar maturation.[44,58] It is customary to only remove the pressure garments for skin care, hygiene, and cleaning of garments.

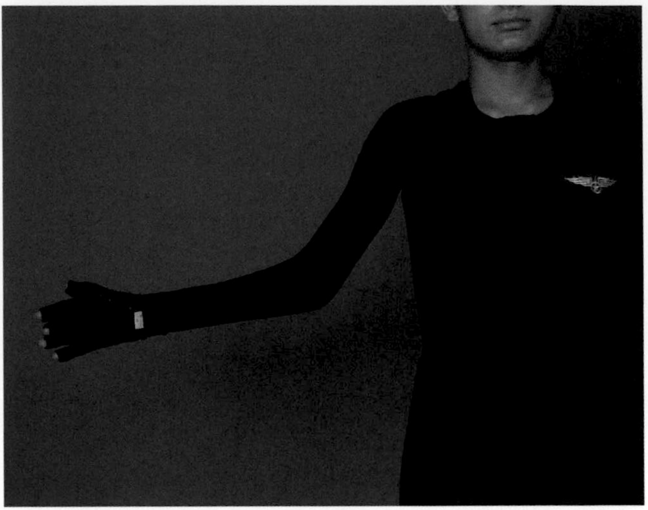

Figure 48-9. Custom pressure garments.

Custom garments cause notable shearing during application and removal and thus should be used only when the skin is healed sufficiently to withstand these forces. A skilled therapist should assist with application and removal of the garments until other staff, family, friends, and the patient have had extensive training. The therapist's role is to initiate the ordering of custom garments and oversee their use. Prolonged use of pressure therapy may results in heterotopic ossification, muscle atrophy, joint stiffness, and impaired skin perspiration.[59] Most providers of custom garments send trained personnel to measure the patient for custom fitting. For facial burns, the patient may use a transparent facial orthosis secured by elastic straps to provide even pressure distribution. These orthoses are usually fabricated by a specially trained orthotist at the request of the medical team.

Silicone products are also often used in conjunction with pressure therapy. Silicone products can include topical silicone gels, silicone gel sheets, silicone sprays, and silicone oils. It is thought that silicone reduces transepidermal water loss and can normalize the cellular process of the skin, reducing collagen production.[60,61] Silicone gel sheets are typically worn 12 to 24 hours per day and removed for bathing and skin care activities. Skin should be monitored for potential maceration or breakdown. Scar elasticity, redness, thickness, and itching have been shown to be improved after the use of silicone products.[62]

INSERTS. Inserts are also often used in conjunction with pressure garments. They may be constructed from products such as Otoform or closed cell foam (Fig. 48-10). Their purpose is to increase pressure in concave areas, such as the web spaces and the sternoclavicular depression. Silicone inserts have also been demonstrated to be effective in improving pliability, thickness, and pain in hypertrophic

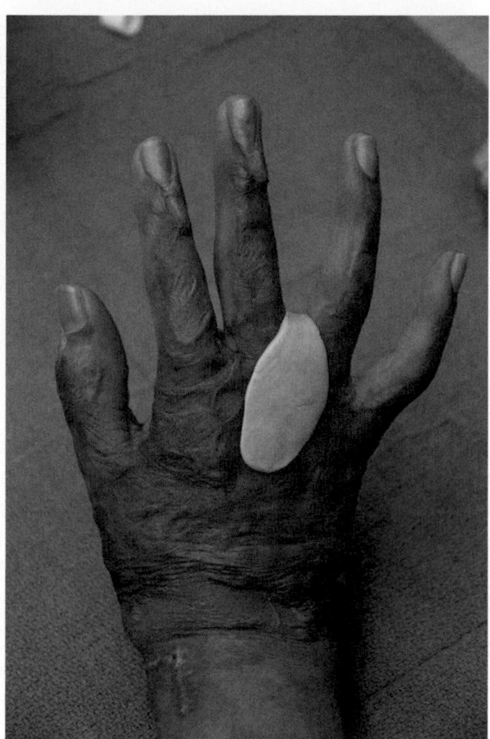

Figure 48-10. Web space inserts.

scars.[62] The design of a scar management program is determined by the available resources, careful clinical observation, and the patient's ability to comply with the program. Periodic outpatient visits to OT or an established burn clinic throughout the rehabilitation phase allow for monitoring and adjustments of the scar management program.

Self-Care and Home Management Skills

If neuromuscular limitations impede the patient's performance of functional tasks, the therapist may provide adaptive equipment, such as built-up handles for impaired grasp or long-handled utensils for decreased elbow flexion. Teaching adaptive techniques, such as performing certain activities unilaterally, may also improve independence with ADLs and IADLs.

Patient and Family Teaching

Patients and their family members should understand the rationale for each of the splints and techniques used in their care. They participate in the development of goals, so that they are invested in achieving them. Skin care is an important element in discharge teaching. Patients should practice monitoring their skin for breakdown and caring for their skin, including the daily use of a moisturizer and sunscreen. In addition, patients should have a basic understanding of wound healing and tissue response to exercise and scar management techniques.

Support and Psychosocial Adjustment during the Rehabilitation Phase

Although the patient and family typically focus on survival immediately after injury, many other issues may arise during rehabilitation. Patients face challenges related to their medical/physical wellbeing, psychological health, and functional skills and performance.[63] The increase in activity in the rehabilitation phase not only assists physical rehabilitation but also helps patients discover how their injury may affect their daily lives. Emotional reactions to the realization of loss may produce a wide range of behaviors, such as crying or expressions of anger. In addition, guilt or embarrassment regarding the injury may lead the patient to withdraw. It is also reported that burn survivors may experience posttraumatic stress disorder, depression, and social withdrawal.[64] Incidence of posttraumatic stress disorder 1 year after burn range from 18% to 45%.[63]

Evidence suggests that the psychological effects of burns may continue to increase in importance after discharge.[63] It has also been found that the process of recovery is not a simple or direct path.[63] Each burn survivor needs to be treated in a client-centered manner to provide the most appropriate care to address any psychosocial concerns.

One of the most difficult challenges for the burn therapist is caring for patients as they grieve for a functional limitation or alteration in body image.[23] The occupational therapist supports the patient by encouraging questions and verbalization of feelings about the burn injury.[23] The occupational therapist also chooses treatment activities to restore confidence and self-esteem. Group activities provide opportunities for socialization and sharing of concerns in a safe environment.[65] Given the extensive contact with the patient throughout all phases of recovery, the occupational therapist is in a unique position to identify and address psychosocial issues, but collaboration with other specialists on the burn team (e.g., nursing staff, family members, social workers, and psychologists) is essential.

Potential Complications

In addition to the potential for soft tissue contractures and loss of joint ROM, other complications may occur in any phase of burn recovery. These are listed below.

Pruritus

Pruritus (persistent itching) is a common complication after sustaining a burn injury.[66] Historically, it was thought that pruritus would improve over time as the burn injury heals. Evidence now shows that pruritus can last for several years[67,68] and can significantly affect burn survivors' quality of life.[67,68] The 5D and Leuven itch scales are two reliable and valid scales that can be used with burn survivors with pruritus.[69] The "Itch Man Scale" can be used with children and is also found to be valid and reliable.[70] The use of compression garments, scar massage, skin moisturizers, cold packs, and medications such as antihistamines or steroids may help alleviate itching.

Microstomia

Patients with facial burns in the area of the mouth are at risk for oral commissure contracture (microstomia),[38] which is tightening of the musculature around the lip area that limits mouth opening. In extreme cases, urgent surgical revision is required. This risk is exaggerated if the patient has undergone prolonged periods without eating or speaking because of intubation or respiratory compromise. In addition to daily scar massage, the therapist can teach the patient facial stretching exercises, such as yawning or grinning widely and pursing lips together. The exercises can be combined with the wearing of a microstomia splint to stretch the oral commissure. The splint may be worn as tolerated, usually starting with 10 minutes and gradually increasing to 60 minutes twice a day. These devices can be purchased commercially or fabricated by a skilled occupational therapist or in collaboration with a speech and language therapist. Additionally, the therapist can used stacked Popsicle sticks to facilitate increased vertical opening of the mouth. The cognitive level of the patient is an extremely important factor in use of a microstomia device because of the risk of an unexpected airway emergency. For example, a heavily sedated or confused patient may attempt to swallow the device.

Heterotopic Ossification

Heterotopic ossification, or myositis ossificans, is the development of new abnormal bone in soft tissues that normally do not ossify. It occurs in 0.2% to 4% of patients with major burns.[71] Burn size and depth are significant predictors of heterotopic ossificiation.[71] The most common location in the burn-injured population is the elbow, followed by the shoulder and hip.[72] Heterotopic ossification can be a debilitating complication of a burn injury and can cause pain, swelling, and rapid loss of ROM and functional use of the area impacted. Symptoms that the therapist may note include a hard-end feel when completing ROM, redness in the area, and/or the area may be warm to touch. The therapist must be aware of the symptoms and alert the team so a formal diagnosis can be determined by radiography. The medical team can then discuss the treatment of prophylaxis options and/or surgical excision. In addition, it is important to consult with the medical team to determine the recommendation for ROM. There is conflicting evidence about the effect of ROM on the progression of heterotopic ossification. Some evidence find that aggressive ROM can exacerbate heterotopic ossification and others find that heterotopic ossification progresses due to a lack of ROM.[73,74]

Heat Intolerance

Heat intolerance is caused by loss of sweating because split-thickness skin grafts typically do not contain sweat glands. To compensate for this, patients may sweat excessively in remaining unburned areas. Patients in extremely hot climates may require additional air conditioners in the home to maintain comfort.[38] The lack of sweat glands also makes healed grafts susceptible to extreme dryness[7] and patients are encouraged to use moisturizing cream often throughout the day. A heat acclimation regimen has also been found to improve heat tolerance in burn survivors.[75] Note: this should only be performed by a skilled clinician under the direction of medical personnel.

Reconstructive Surgery

An important element in burn recovery is the planning and execution of reconstructive procedures. Despite diligent efforts by the burn team and patient, contractures may develop. Reconstructive surgery can be useful in correcting these deformities. Surgery is typically performed once the scar tissue is mature; however, it may be necessary to perform reconstructive surgery before scar maturation if a severe functional deficit is present.[76] For example, an axillary contracture, which limits abduction to 80°, may significantly interfere with dressing and hygiene. A surgical procedure, a **Z-plasty**, can be performed to elongate soft tissue.[76] A skin graft to cover the deficit may be necessary once the contracture is released. Fifteen percent of patients who sustain hand injuries require reconstructive surgery.[77] Reconstructive surgery is most often performed on contractures of the little finger and web space.[77]

OT Related to Reconstructive Procedures

When results of a functional assessment or outcome measure suggest that the patient's progress toward his or her goals has ceased because of a contracture, the occupational therapist communicates this information to the burn team. Possible recommendations from the burn team may include the need for surgical release of the contracture.

Postoperatively, the occupational therapist provides a custom splint to immobilize and protect the graft in its new lengthened position. After approximately 10 to 14 days, the therapist initiates an exercise program beginning with gentle active ROM and progressing to more aggressive exercise and activity as skin integrity tolerates. Pressure therapy over the newly grafted area minimizes scarring. This includes the use of a pressure garment and an insert fabricated to match the contours of the new graft.

Return to Work

Returning to work before final scar maturation preserves function and improves the patient's self-concept.[38] However, only one-third of burn patients return to previous work roles[78] and approximately 28% will not return to any form of employment.[79] This makes it important for occupational therapists to address return to work throughout all phases of care. During the initial evaluation in the acute phase, the occupational therapist gathers information regarding the work history of the patient and specific job demands the patient previously was required to complete. With this information, the occupational therapist can guide treatment activities to prepare for return to the previous level of functioning. For example, if the patient was employed as a mechanic prior to injury, tool use should be incorporated into treatment activities as soon as possible. Patients may require job retraining if the extent of the injury renders the original job demands now unrealistic. In this case, the occupational therapist works with the patient and employer to explore appropriate job modifications.

In addition to physical limitations, burn survivors may encounter psychosocial barriers to returning to the work. These include nightmares, flashback, and concern regarding appearance and depression. Patients exhibiting these symptoms may benefit from psychological intervention that, when started early in their recovery, may enable them to return to work sooner.[80] It is also important to acknowledge if the burn injury happened at work and the effect of returning to the place of injury may have on the patient.

Special Considerations for Hand Burns

The hand is involved in more than 90% of all burns.[81] Hand burns can result in significant functional limitations and poor aesthetics. The high rate of injury to the hand is because individuals often use their hands to protect themselves or to extinguish the fire.[82] Dorsal hand burns occur more frequently than palmar injuries.[83] Significant edema frequently occurs in response to thermal injury. This pulls the hand into a position of deformity[84] characterized by thumb adduction, digital metacarpal hyperextension, interphalangeal joint flexion, and flattening of the palmar arches. If this position is maintained, the result is joint contracture and severe functional limitation; thus, it is imperative that aggressive interventions should be initiated early.[82]

Evaluation of Hand Burns

A comprehensive hand evaluation includes determination of whether ROM limitations are due to joint stiffness, intrinsic muscle tightness, extrinsic muscle tightness, or inelasticity of skin. Other factors that limit hand flexibility and decrease ROM include pain, bulky dressings, edema, exposed tendons, and the presence of eschar, which is inelastic. Once the clinician determines the cause of ROM limitations, an effective treatment plan can be devised. The Hand Burn Severity score is a simple assessment measure that has been found to be a valid and reliable measure that can assist with stratifying severity and assist with reporting outcomes.[85]

Treatment of Hand Burns

The occupational therapist must provide appropriate splinting and exercise programs to prevent contracture and expedite functional use of the burned hand. The recommended splinting position of the hand is described in Table 48-1. It is commonly referred to the intrinsic plus position. In this position, the collateral ligaments of the metacarpophalangeal (MP), proximal interphalangeal (PIP), and distal interphalangeal (DIP) joints are positioned at length, preventing ligamentous contracture so that maximum digital ROM is preserved.

Two distinct options exist for thumb position. Radial abduction maintains the first web space at maximum length. Palmar abduction is preferred, however, because this is a position of function. Hand burns are typically dorsal. When present, a deep palmar burn can lead to palmar contracture. In this case, a volar hand extension splint is appropriate. When using this position, careful monitoring of MP flexion is critical to prevent shortening of the collateral ligaments. Unfortunately, evidence is lacking regarding specific splint positions and schedules. According to Richard and Ward,[18] "Controversy about splinting in burn care is not based on the rationale for and success of splinting, but exists because of the paucity of validation of its use" (p. 392). A list of splinting options for the conditions previously discussed follows.

- ***Dynamic PIP extension splint such as LMB, or banana splints, for PIP stiffness:*** Start 10 minutes three times a day, increase wearing time as tolerated, not to exceed 60 minutes at a time.
- ***Dynamic flexion splint in which the MPs are blocked in full extension while the DIPs are passively flexed*** (for intrinsic muscle tightness): Start 10 minutes three times a day, increase wearing time as tolerated, not to exceed 60 minutes at a time.
- ***Forearm-based dynamic flexion splint that offers composite MP-DIP flexion*** (Fig. 48-11) (for

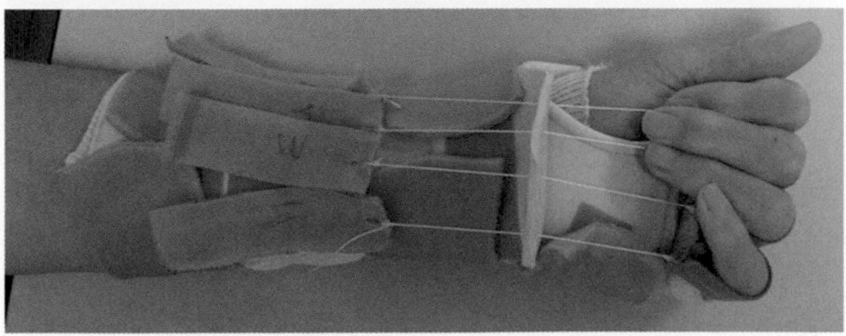

Figure 48-11. Forearm-based dynamic flexion splint.

extrinsic extensor tightness or inelastic skin that limits composite flexion): Start 10 minutes three times a day, increasing as tolerated but not to exceed 40 minutes.

- *Volar forearm-based static extension splint* (for extrinsic flexor tightness): Wear at night.
- *Forearm-based dynamic extension splint* (for extrinsic flexor tightness): Wear periodically during the day, starting with 10 minutes three times per day and progressing to 45 minutes as tolerated.

Often, individuals do not present with a single limitation; rather, a combination of factors limits the individual's ROM. The clinician must determine which factor is the primary source of dysfunction and treat accordingly. Appropriate splints are always used in conjunction with active and passive ROM, edema management, therapeutic exercises, functional activities, and scar management techniques. Splints should never be used to the extent that they limit or prevent performance of ADLs or functional activities.

Potential Complications of Hand Burns

Normal hand anatomy can be characterized by a balance of levers and pulleys that work harmoniously to achieve motion. Damage to this balanced and complex network can result in significant functional limitations.

Extensor Tendon Injury

Extensor tendon injury is often associated with dorsal hand burns because they lie superficially on the dorsal aspect of the hand. Dorsal skin is thin and flexible, which provides little mechanical protection.[86] Because of the close proximity of structures, the formation of scar tissue can greatly limit tendon excursion and create imbalance. This can result in contracture development. Boutonniere and swan-neck deformities (Fig. 48-12) are the result of extensor tendon damage.[81,87] It is recommended that customized splints are applied as soon as possible.

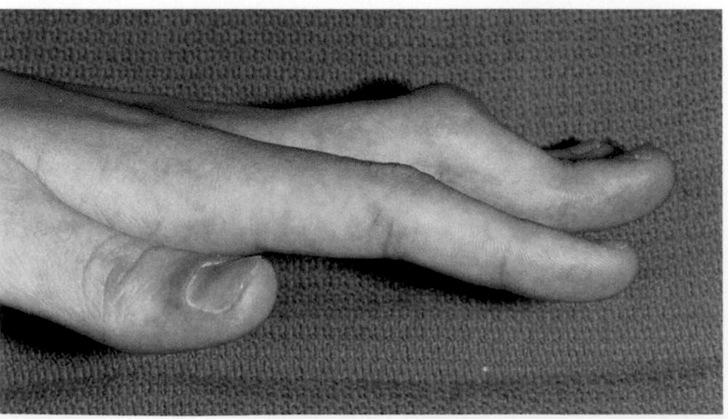

Figure 48-12. Boutonniere deformity.

Web Space Contractures

Web space contractures can be due to overgrafting of the web spaces, muscle shortening (contracture of the adductor pollicis brevis resulting in a first web space contracture), joint stiffness, or skin graft contracture in a normal response to tissue healing. Splints, scar management, and exercise are effective treatment modalities. First web space contractures (between the thumb and index finger) respond well to a web space C-splint that is lined with Otoform, a silicon gel sheet. This is usually worn at night for 6 to 8 hours. During the day, the individual performs stretching, massage, and functional activities that encourage full ROM of the affected area. For example, an individual with a first web space contracture is asked to pick up containers or game pieces of various sizes, using palmar abduction to promote full abduction of the thumb. A dynamic splint with an insert that exerts pressure over the second, third, and fourth web spaces can be appropriate for digital web space contractures. Another option is the addition of web space inserts under a pressure garment or Isotoner glove.

Future Directions

Exciting progress has occurred in regards to reconstruction techniques for the burn patient. To date, 37 successful face transplants have occurred worldwide,[88] and patients have undergone unilateral and bilateral hand transplants as well. The major goals of face and hand transplants include functional and sensory improvements; however, the potential impact they have on an individual's life satisfaction, body image, and social interaction cannot be overlooked.

The use of stem cells for wound healing is another exciting advancement in burn care. Various types of stem cells are being studied and used to treat fibrosis, scarring, and wound contractures.[10] Recently, 80% of a child's epidermis was able to be regenerated with the use of genetically modified epidermal stem cells. Two years after transplant, the child presents with high-quality functional skin.[89] The possibilities for the application of stem cells in burn care are vast and present promising solutions to wound care.

The application of 3D scanning and printing for the treatment of burn contractures is also a new advancement seen in burn care. The use of 3D scanning and printing allows for potentially increased customization, production speed, and cost effectiveness of splints.[90]

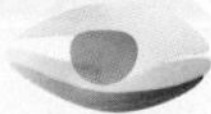

CASE STUDY

Patient Information

Nancy is a 42-year-old woman who sustained a 45% total body surface area (TBSA) burn as a result of a house fire. She presented to the emergency department with superficial and superficial partial-thickness burns to her face and neck and deep partial- and full-thickness burns to bilateral upper extremities and hands (dorsal aspect only), chest, and proximal aspect of her bilateral lower extremities. She also sustained an inhalation injury and was intubated and sedated. She was admitted to the intensive care unit. No significant medical history was reported. Split-thickness skin grafts (STSGs) were performed to her chest and upper thighs 3 days after admission. STSGs were performed to her arms and hands 10 days after admission. After skin grafting was complete, Nancy was extubated and moved to a private room. She was on a regular diet and could walk independently. She was noted to be withdrawn and was concerned regarding her ability to care for her 3-year-old daughter. Her husband and sister were present and supportive throughout her hospitalization.

Reason for OT Referral

Nancy was referred to OT during the acute phase to prevent contractures that might result in impairments in occupational functioning, to provide patient and family education, and to address psychosocial sequelae related to the burn injury.

Assessment Process and Results

The occupational therapist completed the following assessments related to Nancy's condition:

- Assessment of wound healing: Immature scar noted on bilateral forearms and dorsum of both hands
- Assessment of cognitive/social status: Awake and alert for several short periods throughout the day; also noted to appear withdrawn, not seeking social interaction
- Biomechanical assessment: ROM and MMT: Decreased elbow flexion, decreased grasp (metacarpophalangeal [MP] flexion limited), and decreased upper extremity strength bilaterally
- Role and interest assessment: Ability to care for daughter is of primary importance
- Functional assessment: Observed having difficulty using utensils, requires assistance for all ADLs, unable to use nurse call button, and observed to fatigue easily

OT Problem List

- Decreased ADL and IADL independence
- Decreased strength and ROM in bilateral upper extremities
- Withdrawn behavior
- Activity tolerance limited to 5 minutes

OT Goal List

- Participate in splinting and positioning regimen without signs of skin irritation to increase upper extremity functional use during ADLs.
- Complete bilateral upper extremity active and passive ROM exercises to increase ROM and endurance required for ADL performance.
- Increase right digit 2 to 5 MP flexion from 40° to 50° to improve ability to grasp utensils independently.
- Self-feed with modified independence and adaptive equipment as needed.
- Comb daughter's hair for 5 minutes in unsupported short sit at the edge of the bed with distant supervision.
- Participate in burn survivor support group 3 opportunities to increase knowledge of burn recovery process and address anxiety and withdrawal.

Intervention

OT provided six to seven times a week for 60 minute sessions. Bilateral elbow and hand splints were fabricated. Adaptive equipment, including a modified call button, built-up utensils, bath mitt, and modified long-handled sponge were provided. The therapist encouraged the family to bring in recordings and videos of get-well messages that Nancy could listen to. Nancy was taken to the therapy gym as much as possible and private time with her daughter was added to her daily schedule.

As the scars matured, Nancy was provided with both verbal and written instructions regarding scar management and skin care. As discharge neared, outpatient OT was arranged for three times per week with plans communicated regarding need to fit for pressure garments.

Evidence Table of Intervention Studies for Burn Injuries

Intervention	Description	Participants	Dosage	Research Design and Evidence Level	Benefit	Statistical Significance and Effect Size
Early inpatient rehabilitation on burn survivors' functional outcomes and resource utilization[91]	A burn center and an inpatient rehabilitation hospital merged. Study evaluated effect of merger on burn survivors' functional outcomes and resource utilization	About 138 burn survivors (60—transferred to rehab before merger, 78—transferred to rehab after merger)	Merger of a regional burn center and a rehabilitation hospital	Retrospective analysis of two groups, Level II	Patients who received early inpatient rehabilitation had significantly shorter burn center length of stay (LOS), shorter wait time for rehab, and improved resource utilization	Patients transferred after the merger had significantly shorter burn center LOS (28.5 $\pm$ 20.9 days vs. 38.8 $\pm$ 34.2 days, $p = 0.043$), and shorter waiting time for rehab (0.7 $\pm$ 1.1 days vs. 1.5 $\pm$ 2.3 days, $p = 0.010$) than patients transferred before the merger
Recovery of postburn hypertrophic scars in a monitored pressure therapy intervention program[92]	All subjects treated with a 6-month pressure therapy program using the Smart Pressure Monitored Suits	About 34 patients with 65 hypertrophic scars	Patients divided into early treatment group (prescribed pressure therapy within 60 days of injury) and late intervention group (prescribed pressure therapy 61 days or more after injury)	Longitudinal cohort design, Level III	Hypertrophic scars improve in appearance, pain and itch with monitored pressure therapy. Early application of pressure therapy may facilitate better outcomes as evidence by faster recovery than those in late intervention group	The early group demonstrated superior effect in improving scar lightness, yellowness ($p < 0.01$), thickness ($p < 0.01$), pigmentation score ($p < 0.05$), and pain score ($p < 0.01$) than the late group in comparison between the two groups at similar postburn timing
Effectiveness of early stretching exercises for ROM in the shoulder joint and functional recovery in patients with burns[93]	Intervention group received standardized protocol of stretching for 14 days. Control group received usual protocol	Patients with 10%–45% TBSA burns involving the axilla group were randomized into intervention ($n = 110$) and control groups ($n = 110$)	Intervention group received stretching exercises within 48–72 hours postinjury. The number of repetition was increased gradually over 3 days beginning with five reps and progressing to 20	Randomized controlled trial, Level I	Early sustained stretching exercises significantly improves the ROM and functional recovery of the shoulder joint after a severe burn injury	There is a significant beneficial difference ($p = <0.0001$) in ROM and functional recovery between the intervention and control group

ROM, range-of-motion; TBSA, total body surface area.

References

1. American Burn Association. Burn incidence and treatment in the United States. American Burn Association. 2016. http://ameriburn.org/who-we-are/media/burn-incidence-fact-sheet/. Updated 2016. Accessed September 18, 2018.
2. American Burn Association. National burn repository 2017 update. http://ameriburn.org/wp-content/uploads/2018/04/2017_aba_nbr_annual_report_summary.pdf. Updated 2017. Accessed September 18, 2018.
3. Walker NJ, Bhimji SS. *Thermal Burns*. Treasure Island, FL: StatPearls; 2018.
4. Herndon DN. *Total Burn Care*. 5th ed. Edinburgh: Elsevier; 2018:50–51.
5. Armstrong JR, Willand L, Gonzalez B, Sandhu J, Mosier MJ. Quantitative analysis of estimated burn size accuracy for transfer patients. *J Burn Care Res*. 2017;38(1):e30–e35. doi:10.1097/BCR.0000000000000460.
6. Rashaan ZM, Euser AM, van Zuijlen PPM, Breederveld RS. Three-dimensional imaging is a novel and reliable technique to measure total body surface area. *Burns*. 2018;44(4):816–822. doi:10.1016/j.burns.2017.12.008.
7. Grigsby dL, Miles W. Remodeling of scar tissue in the burned hand. *Rehabilitation of the Hand: Surgery and Therapy*. 4th ed. St. Louis, MO: Mosby; 1995:1271–1273.
8. You K, Yang HT, Kym D, et al. Inhalation injury in burn patients: establishing the link between diagnosis and prognosis. *Burns*. 2014;40(8):1470–1475. doi:10.1016/j.burns.2014.09.015.
9. de Barros MEPM, Coltro PS, Hetem CMC, Vilalva KH, Farina JA Jr. Revisiting escharotomy in patients with burns in extremities. *J Burn Care Res*. 2017;38(4):e691–e698. doi:10.1097/BCR.0000000000000476.
10. Wang Y, Beekman J, Hew J, et al. Burn injury: challenges and advances in burn wound healing, infection, pain and scarring. *Adv Drug Deliv Rev*. 2018;123:3–17. doi:10.1016/j.addr.2017.09.018.
11. Pan SC, Wu LW, Chen CL, Shieh SJ, Chiu HY. Deep partial thickness burn blister fluid promotes neovascularization in the early stage of burn wound healing. *Wound Repair Regen*. 2010;18(3):311–318. doi:10.1111/j.1524-475X.2010.00586.x.
12. Ono I, Gunji H, Zhang JZ, Maruyama K, Kaneko F. A study of cytokines in burn blister fluid related to wound healing. *Burns*. 1995;21(5):352–355. doi:10.1016/0305-4179(95)00005-4.
13. Niyonsaba F, Ogawa H. Protective roles of the skin against infection: implication of naturally occurring human antimicrobial agents beta-defensins, cathelicidin LL-37 and lysozyme. *J Dermatol Sci*. 2005;40(3):157–168. doi:10.1016/j.jdermsci.2005.07.009.
14. Gauglitz GG, Shahrokhi S, Williams FN. Burn wound infection and sepsis. *UpToDate*. 2017.
15. Goverman J, Mathews K, Goldstein R, et al. Adult contractures in burn injury: a burn model system national database study. *J Burn Care Res*. 2017;38(1):e328–e336. doi:10.1097/BCR.0000000000000380
16. Kwan PO, Tredget EE. Biological principles of scar and contracture. *Hand Clin*. 2017;33(2):277–292. doi:10.1016/j.hcl.2016.12.004.
17. Dewey WS, Richard RL, Parry IS. Positioning, splinting, and contracture management. *Phys Med Rehabil Clin N Am*. 2011;22(2):229–247. doi:10.1016/j.pmr.2011.02.001.
18. Richard R, Ward RS. Splinting strategies and controversies. *J Burn Care Rehabil*. 2005;26(5):392–396. doi:10.1097/01.bcr.0000176886.63559.8b.
19. Wiechman S, Hoyt MA, Patterson DR. Using a biopsychosocial model to understand long-term outcomes in persons with burn injuries. *Arch Phys Med Rehabil*. Epub March 2, 2018; ii: S0003-9993(18)30138-2. doi:10.1016/j.apmr.2018.01.029.
20. Wiechman SA, Patterson DR. Psychosocial aspects of burn injuries. *BMJ*. 2004;329:391–393. doi:10.1136/bmj.329.7462.391.
21. LeDoux JM, Meyer WJ, Blakeney P, Herndon D. Positive self-regard as a coping mechanism for pediatric burn survivors. *J Burn Care Rehabil*. 1996;17(5):472–476; discussion 471–472.
22. Patterson DR, Finch CP, Wiechman SA, Bonsack R, Gibran N, Heimbach D. Premorbid mental health status of adult burn patients: comparison with a normative sample. *J Burn Care Rehabil*. 2003;24(5):347–350. doi:10.1097/01.BCR.0000086070.91033.7F.
23. Pessina MA, Ellis SM. Burn management. Rehabilitation. *Nurs Clin North Am*. 1997;32:365–374.
24. Foncerrada G, Capek KD, Herndon DN, Lee JO, Sirvent RZ, Finnerty CC. The state of the art on burn wound healing. *Journal of Avid Science*. 2017:4-52. www.avidscience.com.
25. Singh M, Nuutila K, Kruse C, Robson MC, Caterson E, Eriksson E. Challenging the conventional therapy: emerging skin graft techniques for wound healing. *Plast Reconstr Surg*. 2015;136(4):524e–530e. doi:10.1097/PRS.0000000000001634.
26. MeeK CP. Successful microdermagrafting using the meek-wall microdermatome. *Am J Surg*. 1958;96(4):557–558. doi:10.1016/0002-9610(58)90975-9.
27. Hazani R, Whitney R, Wilhelmi BJ. Optimizing aesthetic results in skin grafting. *Am Surg*. 2012;78(2):151–154.
28. van der Veen VC, van der Wal MB, van Leeuwen MC, Ulrich MM, Middelkoop E. Biological background of dermal substitutes. *Burns*. 2010;36(3):305–321. doi:10.1016/j.burns.2009.07.012.
29. Halim AS, Khoo TL, Mohd Yussof SJ. Biologic and synthetic skin substitutes: an overview. *Indian J Plast Surg*. 2010;43(suppl):S23–S28. doi:10.4103/0970-0358.70712.
30. Schneider JC, Qu HD, Lowry J, Walker J, Vitale E, Zona M. Efficacy of inpatient burn rehabilitation: a prospective pilot study examining range of motion, hand function and balance. *Burns*. 2012;38(2):164–171. doi:10.1016/j.burns.2011.11.002.
31. Harden NG, Luster SH. Rehabilitation considerations in the care of the acute burn patient. *Crit Care Nurs Clin North Am*. 1991;3(2):245–253. doi:10.1016/S0899-5885(18)30734-2.
32. Wurzer P, Voigt CD, Clayton RP, et al. Long-term effects of physical exercise during rehabilitation in patients with severe burns. *Surgery*. 2016;160(3):781–788. doi:10.1016/j.surg.2016.04.028.
33. Deng H, Chen J, Li F, et al. Effects of mobility training on severe burn patients in the BICU: a retrospective cohort study. *Burns*. 2016;42(7):1404–1412. doi:10.1016/j.burns.2016.07.029.
34. Herndon DN. Prevention and treatment of deformity in burned patients. *Total Burn Care*. Philadelphia, PA: Saunders; 1996:443–454.

35. Patterson DR, Carrigan L, Questad KA, Robinson R. Post-traumatic stress disorder in hospitalized patients with burn injuries. *J Burn Care Rehabil.* 1990;11(3):181–184. doi.org/10.1097/00004630-199005000-00002.
36. Brown NJ, Kimble RM, Gramotnev G, Rodger S, Cuttle L. Predictors of re-epithelialization in pediatric burn. *Burns.* 2014;40(4):751–758. doi:10.1016/j.burns.2013.09.027.
37. Hoffman HG, Chambers GT, Meyer WJ 3rd, et al. Virtual reality as an adjunctive non-pharmacologic analgesic for acute burn pain during medical procedures. *Ann Behav Med.* 2011;41(2):183–191. doi:10.1007/s12160-010-9248-7.
38. Neistadt JM, Crepeau EB. Skin system dysfunction: burns. *Willard and Spackman's Occupational Therapy.* 9th ed. New York, NY: Lippincott; 1998:741–755.
39. Godleski M, Oeffling A, Bruflat AK, Craig E, Weitzenkamp D, Lindberg G. Treating burn-associated joint contracture: results of an inpatient rehabilitation stretching protocol. *J Burn Care Res.* 2013;34(4):420–426. doi:10.1097/BCR.0b013e3182700178.
40. Perera AD, Perera C, Karunanayake A. Effectiveness of early stretching exercises for range of motion in the shoulder joint and quality of functional recovery in patients with burns—a randomized control trial. *Int J Physiother.* 2017;4(5):302–310. doi:10.15621/ijphy/2017/v4i5/159426.
41. Jordan RB, Daher J, Wasil K. Splints and scar management for acute and reconstructive burn care. *Clin Plast Surg.* 2000;27(1):71–85.
42. Abston S. Scar reaction after thermal injury and prevention of scars and contractures. *The Art and Science of Burn Care.* Rockville, MD: Aspen; 2018:360–363.
43. Berman B, Maderal A, Raphael B. Keloids and hypertrophic scars: pathophysiology, classification, and treatment. *Dermatol Surg.* 2017;43(suppl 1):S3–S18. doi:10.1097/DSS.0000000000000819.
44. Arno AI, Gauglitz GG, Barret JP, Jeschke MG. Up-to-date approach to manage keloids and hypertrophic scars: a useful guide. *Burns.* 2014;40(7):1255–1266. doi:10.1016/j.burns.2014.02.011.
45. Bae SH, Bae YC. Analysis of frequency of use of different scar assessment scales based on the scar condition and treatment method. *Arch Plast Surg.* 2014;41(2):111–115. doi:10.5999/aps.2014.41.2.111.
46. Sulliva T, Smith J, Kermode J, McIver E, Courtemanche DJ. Rating the burn scar. *J Burn Care Rehabil.* 1990;11(3):256–260. doi:10.1097/00004630-199005000-00014.
47. Draaijers LJ, Tempelman FR, Botman YA, et al. The patient and observer scar assessment scale: a reliable and feasible tool for scar evaluation. *Plast Reconstr Surg.* 2004;113(7):1960–1965; discussion 1966–1967.
48. Masters M, McMahon M, Svens B. Reliability testing of a new scar assessment tool, matching assessment of scars and photographs (MAPS). *J Burn Care Rehabil.* 2005;26(3):273–284.
49. Ault P, Plaza A, Paratz J. Scar massage for hypertrophic burns scarring—a systematic review. *Burns.* 2018;44(1):24–38. doi:10.1016/j.burns.2017.05.006.
50. Patino O, Novick C, Merlo A, Benaim F. Massage in hypertrophic scars. *J Burn Care Rehabil.* 1999;20(3):268–271.
51. Shin TM, Bordeaux JS. The role of massage in scar management: a literature review. *Dermatol Surg.* 2012;38(3):414–423. doi:10.1111/j.1524-4725.2011.02201.x.
52. Macintyre L, Baird M. Pressure garments for use in the treatment of hypertrophic scars—a review of the problems associated with their use. *Burns.* 2006;32(1):10–15. doi:10.1016/j.burns.2004.06.018.
53. Li-Tsang CW, Zheng YP, Lau JC. A randomized clinical trial to study the effect of silicone gel dressing and pressure therapy on posttraumatic hypertrophic scars. *J Burn Care Res.* 2010;31(3):448–457. doi:10.1097/BCR.0b013e3181db52a7.
54. Ai JW, Liu JT, Pei SD, et al. The effectiveness of pressure therapy (15–25 mmHg) for hypertrophic burn scars: a systematic review and meta-analysis. *Sci Rep.* 2017;7:40185. doi:10.1038/srep40185.
55. Rappoport K, Muller R, Flores-Mir C. Dental and skeletal changes during pressure garment use in facial burns: a systematic review. *Burns.* 2008;34(1):18–23. doi:10.1016/j.burns.2007.07.003.
56. Alkhalil A, Tejiram S, Travis TE, et al. A translational animal model for scar compression therapy using an automated pressure delivery system. *Eplasty.* 2015;15:e29.
57. Candy LH, Cecilia LT, Ping ZY. Effect of different pressure magnitudes on hypertrophic scar in a Chinese population. *Burns.* 2010;36(8):1234–1241. doi:10.1016/j.burns.2010.05.008.
58. Kim S, Choi TH, Liu W, Ogawa R, Suh JS, Mustoe TA. Update on scar management: guidelines for treating Asian patients. *Plast Reconstr Surg.* 2013;132(6):1580–1589. doi:10.1097/PRS.0b013e3182a8070c.
59. Hubbard M, Masters IB, Williams GR, Chang AB. Severe obstructive sleep apnoea secondary to pressure garments used in the treatment of hypertrophic burn scars. *Eur Respir J.* 2000;16(6):1205–1207. doi:10.1034/j.1399-3003.2000.16f29.x.
60. Puri N, Talwar A. The efficacy of silicone gel for the treatment of hypertrophic scars and keloids. *J Cutan Aesthet Surg.* 2009;2(2):104–106. doi:10.4103/0974-2077.58527.
61. Mustoe TA. Evolution of silicone therapy and mechanism of action in scar management. *Aesthetic Plast Surg.* 2008;32(1):82–92. doi:10.1007/s00266-007-9030-9.
62. Anthonissen M, Daly D, Janssens T, Van den Kerckhove E. The effects of conservative treatments on burn scars: a systematic review. *Burns.* 2016;42(3):508–518. doi:10.1016/j.burns.2015.12.006.
63. McAleavey AA, Wyka K, Peskin M, Difede J. Physical, functional, and psychosocial recovery from burn injury are related and their relationship changes over time: a burn model system study. *Burns.* 2018;44(4):793–799. doi:10.1016/j.burns.2017.12.011.
64. Difede J, Cukor J, Lee F, Yurt R. Treatments for common psychiatric conditions among adults during acute, rehabilitation, and reintegration phases. *Int Rev Psychiatry.* 2009;21(6):559–569. doi:10.3109/09540260903344081.
65. Summers TM. Psychosocial support of the burned patient. *Crit Care Nurs Clin North Am.* 1991;3(2):237–244. doi:10.1016/S0899-5885(18)30733-0.
66. Nedelec B, Carrougher GJ. Pain and pruritus postburn injury. *J Burn Care Res.* 2017;38(3):142–145. doi:10.1097/BCR.0000000000000534.
67. Carrougher GJ, Martinez EM, McMullen KS, et al. Pruritus in adult burn survivors: postburn prevalence and risk factors associated with increased intensity. *J Burn Care Res.* 2013;34(1):94–101. doi:10.1097/BCR.0b013e3182644c25.

68. Gauffin E, Oster C, Gerdin B, Ekselius L. Prevalence and prediction of prolonged pruritus after severe burns. *J Burn Care Res*. 2015;36(3):405–413. doi:10.1097/BCR.0000000000000152.
69. Amtmann D, McMullen K, Kim J, et al. Psychometric properties of the modified 5-D itch scale in a burn model system sample of people with burn injury. *J Burn Care Res*. 2017;38(1): e402–e408. doi:10.1097/BCR.0000000000000404.
70. Morris V, Murphy LM, Rosenberg M, Rosenberg L, Holzer CE 3rd, Meyer WJ 3rd. Itch assessment scale for the pediatric burn survivor. *J Burn Care Res*. 2012;33(3):419–424. doi:10.1097/BCR.0b013e3182372bfa.
71. Maender C, Sahajpal D, Wright TW. Treatment of heterotopic ossification of the elbow following burn injury: recommendations for surgical excision and perioperative prophylaxis using radiation therapy. *J Shoulder Elbow Surg*. 2010;19(8):1269–1275. doi:10.1016/j.jse.2010.05.029.
72. Ranganathan K, Loder S, Agarwal S, et al. Heterotopic ossification: basic-science principles and clinical correlates. *J Bone Joint Surg Am*. 2015;97(13):1101–1111. doi:10.2106/JBJS.N.01056.
73. Coons D, Godleski M. Range of motion exercises in the setting of burn-associated heterotopic ossification at the elbow: case series and discussion. *Burns*. 2013;39(4):e34–e38. doi:10.1016/j.burns.2012.10.014
74. Holavanahalli RK, Helm PA, Parry IS, Dolezal CA, Greenhalgh DG. Select practices in management and rehabilitation of burns: a survey report. *J Burn Care Res*. 2011;32(2):210–223. doi:10.1097/BCR.0b013e31820aadd5.
75. Pearson J, Ganio MS, Schlader ZJ, et al. Post junctional sudomotor and cutaneous vascular responses in noninjured skin following heat acclimation in burn survivors. *J Burn Care Res*. 2017;38(1):e284–e292. doi:10.1097/BCR.0000000000000372.
76. Robson MC, Barnett RA, Leitch IO, Hayward PG. Prevention and treatment of postburn scars and contracture. *World J Surg*. 1992;16(1):87–96. doi:10.1007/BF02067119.
77. van der Vlies CH, de Waard S, Hop J, et al. Indications and predictors for reconstructive surgery after hand burns. *J Hand Surg Am*. 2017;42(5):351–358. doi:10.1016/j.jhsa.2017.02.006.
78. Brych SB, Engrav LH, Rivara FP, et al. Time off work and return to work rates after burns: systematic review of the literature and a large two-center series. *J Burn Care Rehabil*. 2001;22(6):401–405. doi:10.1097/00004630-200111000-00010.
79. Mason ST, Esselman P, Fraser R, Schomer K, Truitt A, Johnson K. Return to work after burn injury: a systematic review. *J Burn Care Res*. 2012;33(1):101–109. doi:10.1097/BCR.0b013e3182374439.
80. Esselman PC, Askay SW, Carrougher GJ, et al. Barriers to return to work after burn injuries. *Arch Phys Med Rehabil*. 2007;88(12 suppl 2):S50–S56. doi:10.1016/j.apmr.2007.09.009.
81. Pan BS, Vu AT, Yakuboff KP. Management of the acutely burned hand. *J Hand Surg Am*. 2015;40(7):1477–1484; quiz 1485. doi:10.1016/j.jhsa.2015.02.033.
82. Schulze SM, Weeks D, Choo J, et al. Amputation following hand escharotomy in patients with burn injury. *Eplasty*. 2016;16:e13.
83. Tanigawa MC, O'Donnell OK, Graham PL. The burned hand: a physical therapy protocol. *Phys Ther*. 1974;54(9):953–958. doi:10.1093/ptj/54.9.953.
84. Sheridan RL, Hurley J, Smith MA, et al. The acutely burned hand: management and outcome based on a ten-year experience with 1,047 acute hand burns. *J Trauma*. 1995;38(3):406–411. doi:10.1097/00005373-199503000-00022.
85. Bache SE, Fitzgerald O'Connor E, Theodorakopoulou E, Frew Q, Philp B, Dziewulski P. The hand burn severity (HABS) score: a simple tool for stratifying severity of hand burns. *Burns*. 2017;43(1):93–99. doi:10.1016/j.burns.2016.07.011.
86. Germann G. Hand reconstruction after burn injury: functional results. *Clin Plast Surg*. 2017;44(4):833–844. doi:10.1016/j.cps.2017.05.015.
87. Hunter JM, Mackin EJ, Callahan AD. *The Extensor Tendons: Anatomy and Management*. St. Louis, MO: Mosby; 1995:519–564.
88. Nizzi MC, Tasigiorgos S, Turk M, Moroni C, Bueno E, Pomahac B. Psychological outcomes in face transplant recipients: a literature review. *Curr Surg Rep*. 2017;5:26. doi:10.1007/s40137-017-0189-y.
89. Kueckelhaus M, Rothoeft T, Teig N, et al. 355 regeneration of the entire human epidermis by transgenic epidermal stem cell transplants and its implications for the treatment of burns. *J Burn Care Res*. 2018;39(suppl 1):S148. doi:10.1093/jbcr/iry006.277.
90. Visscher DO, Te Slaa S, Jaspers ME, et al. 3D printing of patient-specific neck splints for the treatment of post-burn neck contractures. *Burns Trauma*. 2018;6:15.
91. Gomez M, Tushinski M, Jeschke MG. Impact of early inpatient rehabilitation on adult burn survivors' functional outcomes and resource utilization. *J Burn Care Res*. 2017;38(1):e311–e317. doi:10.1097/BCR.0000000000000377.
92. Li P, Li-Tsang CWP, Deng X, et al. The recovery of post-burn hypertrophic scar in a monitored pressure therapy intervention programme and the timing of intervention. *Burns*. 2018;44(6):1451–1467. doi:10.1016/j.burns.2018.01.008.
93. Perera AD, Perera C, Karunanayake A. Effectiveness of early stretching exercises for range of motion in the shoulder joint and quality of functional recovery in patients with burns—a randomized control trial. *Int J Physiother*. 2017;4:262–318. doi:10.15621/ijphy/2017/v4i5/159426.

Chapter 49

Chronic Pain and Fibromyalgia

Sharon A. Gutman and Lee Ann Westover

LEARNING OBJECTIVES

This chapter will allow the reader to:

1. Understand the multifactorial and interconnected contributing factors to chronic pain syndromes.
2. Understand how chronic pain syndromes commonly affect clients' participation in desired daily life activities.
3. Understand traditional medical management of chronic pain syndromes.
4. Understand how occupational therapists evaluate functional skill deficits and occupational restrictions occurring secondary to chronic pain.
5. Understand how occupational therapists provide intervention to reduce pain and enhance participation in clients' desired daily activities.

CHAPTER OUTLINE

TERMINOLOGY

Body mechanics: the proper positioning of the body during daily activities to avoid injury and pain.

Central sensitization (CS): a central nervous system (CNS) condition that may account for the development and maintenance of chronic pain syndromes; in CS, a phenomenon referred to as wind-up occurs in which the CNS becomes highly reactive to any touch stimulus, resulting in feelings of pain from non-noxious stimuli.

Chronic pain: pain that is persistent or recurring for longer than 3 months; etiology may or may not be known.

Energy conservation: the arrangement of desired daily life activities over the day or week for the purpose of preserving patient stamina, preventing fatigue, and minimizing joint stress and pain; also involves the idea that energy expenditure can be reduced in any one activity.

Fibromyalgia (FM): widespread pain with tenderness and stiffness that is independent of a specific injury or lesion; etiology is largely unknown but may relate to CNS-processing problems.

Guarding behaviors: the adoption of dysfunctional behaviors such as bracing, posturing, and limping in an effort to protect a painful body region; commonly leads to additional musculoskeletal problems resulting from the overuse of certain muscle groups and body positions.

Low back pain (LBP): pain located between the margins of the lower ribs and crease of the buttocks; etiology may or may not be known but is commonly caused by neuroanatomical conditions, including radiculopathy, spinal stenosis, herniated spinal disks, and spinal compression and fractures.

Physical agent modalities: interventions and technologies that use force or energy to promote the healing process and reduce pain.

Work simplification: the arrangement of tools and steps in an activity to reduce pain and energy expenditure.

Chronic Pain and Fibromyalgia: Definition, Prevalence, and Background

Chronic pain and related disorders may affect as many as 20% of the global population and is attributable to 15% to 20% of physician visits worldwide.[1] The prevalence of individuals experiencing chronic pain is estimated to be as high as 36% in European households and 43% in US households.[2] In 2018, the World Health Organization (WHO) released the *International Classification of Diseases, 11th edition* (*ICD-11*), which includes a revised definition of chronic pain.[1] This revised definition is intended to better reflect the epidemiology of chronic pain than previous versions and identifies chronic pain as a global health care problem.[2] Chronic pain is now defined in the *ICD-11* as persistent or recurring pain lasting longer than 3 months.[1] This definition includes seven optional specifiers for chronic pain. *Chronic cancer pain* was introduced and can include pain from the cancer itself or related to treatment. *Chronic postsurgical and post-traumatic pain* occurs after surgical procedure or tissue injury, including burns. *Chronic neuropathic pain* is caused by injury to or disease in the somatosensory nervous system. *Chronic headache and orofacial pain* is defined as head, mouth, jaw, or face pain that occurs approximately 50% of days for 3 months. *Chronic musculoskeletal pain* includes direct pain sensation in the musculoskeletal system, but *chronic visceral pain* is often perceived as referred pain from origins in other internal organs.

The etiology of many forms of chronic pain is currently unknown; thus, the final specifier of *chronic primary pain* was newly introduced to reflect such. Chronic primary pain includes the common conditions of back pain (not otherwise attributed to musculoskeletal or neuropathic causes), fibromyalgia (FM), chronic widespread pain, and irritable bowel syndrome. Chronic primary pain is defined as occurring in one or more anatomical areas and is associated with functional impairment and emotional distress—such as difficulty with performance of activities of daily living (ADLs) and participation in life roles. Details on rheumatic pain can be found in Chapter 42. This chapter focuses primarily on chronic low back pain (LBP) and FM.

Fibromyalgia: Prevalence, Etiology, Diagnosis, and Medical Management

Prevalence

Fibromyalgia (FM) syndrome is one of the most common chronic primary pain conditions.[3] FM is defined as widespread pain with tenderness and stiffness, independent of specific injury or lesion.[3,4] Depending on diagnostic criteria and geographic location, the prevalence of FM is reported as ranging from 0.2% to 13% worldwide.[3–7] Women appear to be affected by FM significantly more than men, with as many as 2 women experiencing FM for every 0.15 men.[3,6] The prevalence also appears to increase with age, with reports of maximum occurrence over the age of 60,[6] and up to 7.4% of women over 70 experiencing FM.[3]

Etiology

The etiology of FM is largely unknown, which has contributed to difficulty diagnosing and treating the syndrome.[6–8] Abnormalities in central nervous system (CNS) pain processing are a hallmark, and as such, FM is referred to as a *centralized pain state*.[6,7] Even gentle touch is often experienced by FM patients as pain. Afferent pain signals appear to be amplified within the spinal cord, but psychosocial and environmental factors may also contribute to the amplification. These can include stressors related to acute pain, psychosocial stress, certain infections, trauma, and deployment to war. Brain regions involved in processing pain and emotion are implicated via functional magnetic resonance imaging, for instance, the amygdala, thalamus, and insula.[6] Patients who develop FM often have a personal and/or family history of chronic pain or pain syndromes.[6,7] Functional and cognitive impairments are common symptoms of FM and can include depression, anxiety, obsessive–compulsive disorder, post-traumatic stress disorder, sleep participation deficits, fatigue, headaches, paresthesia, and/or psychosis.[3,4,7]

Diagnosis

A diagnosis of FM is considered whenever widespread pain is not explained by other illness or injury.[6,7] Lab testing will not contribute to diagnosis—rather, clinicians rate sensitivity of 18 body sites, with 11 sensitive sites resulting in a diagnosis of FM; 25% of FM patients, however, do not experience the requisite tenderness in all 11 sites.[6] A psychosocial questionnaire is used in conjunction with touch sensitivity ratings to determine whether patients experience deficits in sleep participation and cognition.

Medical Management

FM is treated by combining pharmacological and nonpharmacological methods, and team-based strategy is recommended.[7] Pharmacology can be helpful, but psychosocial and functional interventions are considered central to treatment. Opioids are not effective with this population. Improved function and participation should be the primary focus for clinicians. Patients are encouraged to participate in education about the illness and importance of active participation in treatment. Diagnosis itself has proven to be helpful for many patients. Interventions should also be delivered to support sleep participation, stress management, and exercise. The strongest evidence supports education, cognitive–behavioral therapy (CBT), and exercise, but limited evidence also supports the use of alternative therapies like Tai Chi, yoga, acupuncture, myofascial release, and chiropracty. These interventions are also thought to contribute to an internal locus of control and can be implemented freely, as long as they do not cause harm to the patient.

Low Back Pain: Prevalence, Etiology, Diagnosis, and Medical Management

Prevalence

Low back pain (LBP) is the global leading cause of lost workdays due to disability.[9] Up to 540 million people, or 7.3% of the global population in 2015, were affected by LBP at any one time.[10] Rate of occurrence is estimated to be heightened in low- and middle-income countries as a result of population growth and lack of resources.[9] During the first decade of life, LBP occurrence is low. During adolescence, however, prevalence rises steeply to an estimated 37% to 40% of children ages 9 to 14.[10,11] The prevalence of LBP peaks in middle adulthood, and most adults report experiencing LBP at some point. LBP is experienced more frequently in women than in men. As people age, LBP more frequently leads to deficits in activity participation. LBP is defined by pain between the margins of the lower ribs and the crease of the buttocks.[10] As such, it is not a disease, but a symptom attributable to many possible causes.

Etiology

LBP resolves in 80% to 90% of individuals within 6 weeks. Pain that does not resolve in approximately 12 weeks is considered chronic and occurs in 5% to 10% of patients. At least one study found that back pain due to a specific pathoanatomical cause may occur in less than 1% of LBP patients in primary care.[9,10] Common identifiable conditions that cause LBP are as follows:

- *Radiculopathy* (RP) occurs with nerve-root involvement and is commonly referred to as sciatica.[12] RP is expressed as electric or shooting pain in the legs that may worsen with back pain, sneezing, straining, or coughing. RP is commonly caused by disk herniation and inflammation.
- *Spinal stenosis* is back pain or discomfort while standing still or walking that affects one or both legs.[9,12] It is frequently caused by bulging disks, narrowing of foramina or spinal canal, or other degenerative conditions (Fig. 49-1).
- *Facet joint pain or facet arthropathy* is caused by arthritis and/or inflammation in the spinal joints. This type of pain worsens with spinal extension.

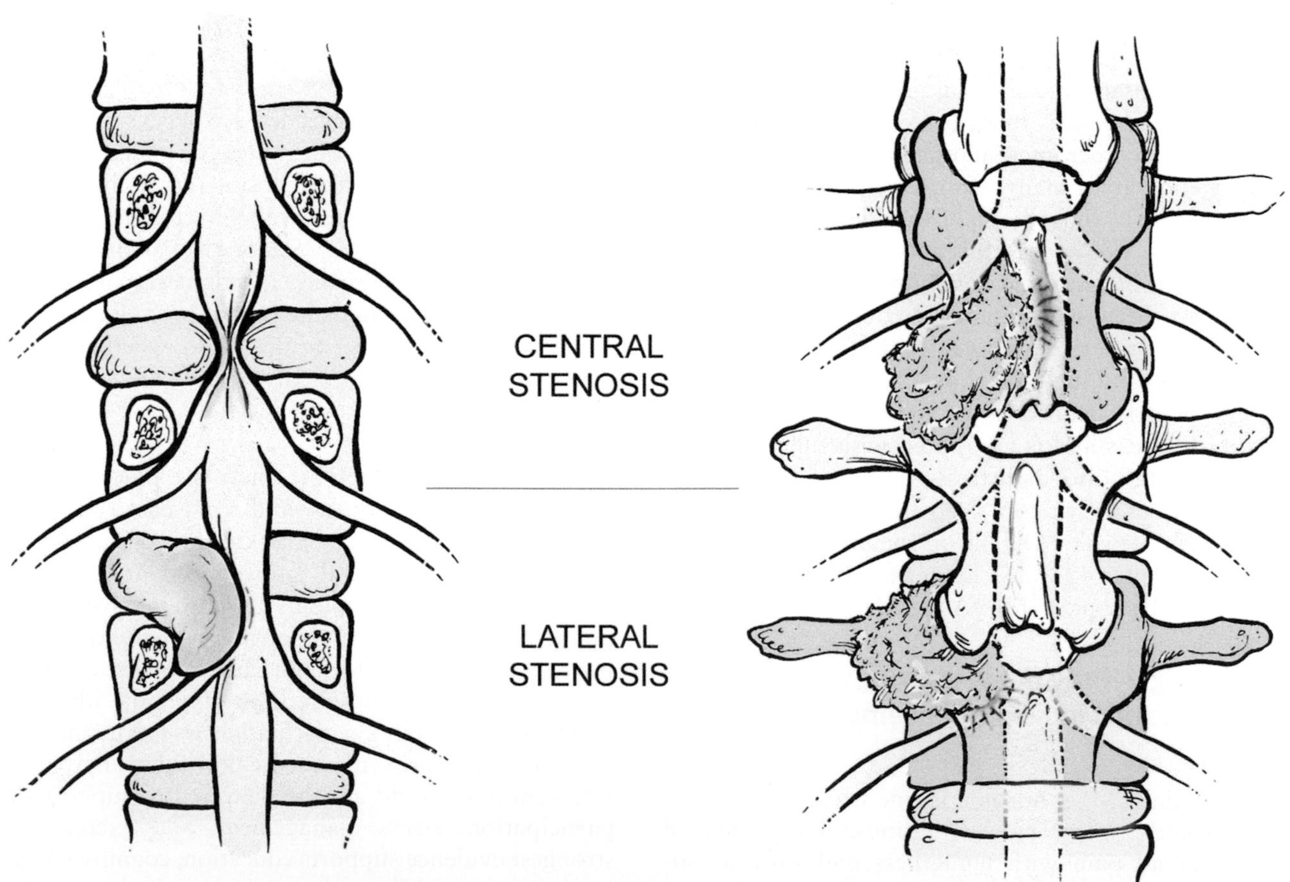

Figure 49-1. Spinal stenosis. Central stenosis (*top, left,* and *right*) usually develops at the disk level from a bulging disk with facet joint overgrowth from the inferior articular process of the lumbar vertebrae and thickening and redundancy of the ligamentum flavum. Lateral stenosis (*bottom, left,* and *right*) includes both the lateral recess and foraminal stenosis resulting from overgrowth from the superior articular process of the vertebra and other degenerative changes similar to those of central stenosis. Lateral recess stenosis affects the spinal nerve root at the disk level.

- *Spondylosis* involves age-related degenerative spinal column changes. These can include disk compression, arthritis, or osteophyte formation.
- *Spondylolisthesis* occurs when one lumbar vertebra displaces or slides over another; can lead to spinal stenosis.
- *Herniated nucleus pulposus* occurs when the outer layer of the intervertebral disk—the annulus—breaks down. This exposes the innervated inner core, the nucleus pulposus, and releases inflammatory agents that cause pain. The rupture of the annulus is often caused by stress (Fig. 49-2).
- *Compression and stress fractures* are commonly caused by arthritis, trauma, or repetitive strain (Fig. 49-3).
- *Nonspecific LBP* has no identifiable, specific cause and may represent 90% or more of LBP cases.[11]

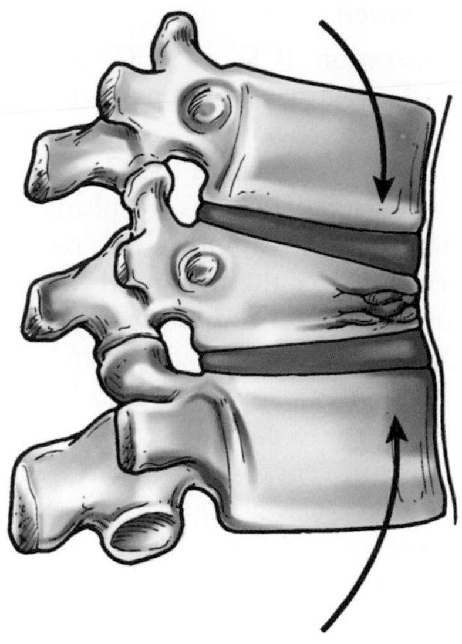

Figure 49-3. Spinal compression and fracture. Compression fracture. A compression fracture is a wedge-shaped fracture (also called wedge fracture) of the vertebral body involving the anterior column. It occurs in the thoracic and lumbar region, most often in the midthoracic and midlumbar region. Compression fractures can occur with minor trauma in older patients with osteoporosis and in younger people with significant trauma.

Risk Factors

Risk factors for all LBP include frequent physical behaviors associated with work, such as twisting, lifting, bending, repetitive motion, vibration, and static postures.[13] Psychosocial factors, such as depression, cognitive impairment, stress, and job dissatisfaction, also increase LBP risk. Smoking and obesity are also risk factors.[10]

Medical Management

Surgery for spinal conditions should be considered only when strictly necessary, because it is the most invasive treatment option with potential for complications.[14] For many conditions, however, surgery offers the most complete resolution of symptoms in the shortest amount of time.

- *Laminectomy or decompression surgery* involves the removal of the vertebral lamina, which forms the posterior of the spinal canal. This relieves pressure on the spinal cord or nerve roots in the case of stenosis.[15]
- *Spinal fusion* may be conducted in cases of degenerative disk disease, fracture, spinal instability, or herniated disk. Two or more vertebrae are permanently connected and immobilized relative to each other, often using a combination of screws, rods, and bone graft.
- *Disk dissection or discectomy* removes all or part of a damaged intervertebral disk secondary to disk herniation.
- *Vertebroplasty and kyphoplasty* are outpatient procedures in which cement is injected into vertebrae to stabilize them after a fracture.

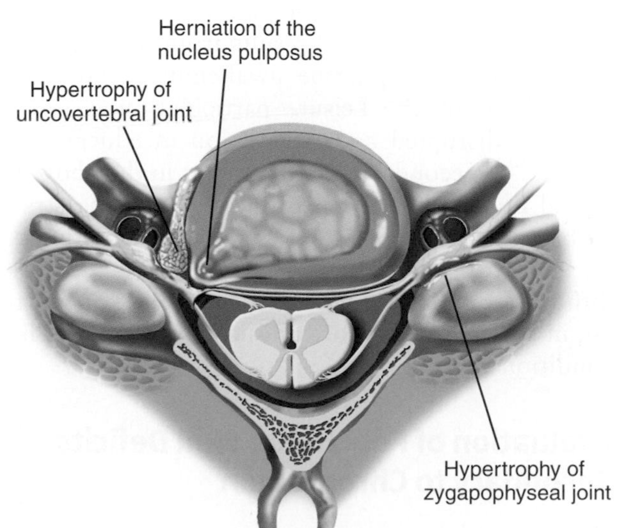

Figure 49-2. Herniated nucleus pulposus. Cross-sectional anatomy of the cervical spine depicting several pathological states: hypertrophy of the uncovertebral joints, hypertrophy of zygapophyseal joints, and herniation of the nucleus pulposus.

Medication can also be helpful in relieving LBP pain and inflammation:

- *Opioids or muscle relaxants* for pain control should be limited and used only after other medications are shown to be ineffective.[9,11,13,14,16] Opioids carry a serious risk of addiction that outweighs potential benefits.
- *Nonsteroidal anti-inflammatory drugs (NSAIDs)*,[11,13,14,17] work well with a number of back pain conditions, but are not as effective in neuropathic pain from compression or herniated disks.[16]
- *Anticonvulsant or antiseizure* medications, such as gabapentin (Neurontin), carbamazepine (Tegretol), and lamotrigine (Lamictal), are often effective against neuropathic pain. These drugs inhibit electrical signals within the CNS.

Central Sensitization

Central sensitization (CS) is a CNS condition that may account for the development and maintenance of chronic pain syndromes. In CS, a phenomenon referred to as *wind-up* occurs in which the CNS becomes highly reactive to any touch stimulus, resulting in feelings of pain from non-noxious stimuli.[18] This persistent state of CNS reactivity reduces the threshold for pain tolerance and maintains pain syndromes after anatomical injury has resolved. In CS, patients experience two primary symptoms: *hyperalgesia* and *allodynia*.[16] Hyperalgesia is increased sensitivity to painful stimuli. Allodynia is the experience of pain sensation from stimuli that should not result in pain, such as light touch. Sometimes, patients who experience CS also experience sensitivity to other sensory stimuli,[12] including sensitivity to light, odor, and sound. CS may also result in cognitive impairment, including attentional or memory deficits, and emotional distress such as anxiety.[19,20] CS may play a role in many conditions, including FM, LBP, arthritis, headaches, and neuropathic pain.[18,21,22] Up to 50 diagnoses may fall under this umbrella.[21,22] Medical management of CS targets the CNS. As such, anticonvulsant medications and antidepressants are more effective than other pain medications.[21]

Functional Impairment in Daily Occupation Secondary to Chronic Pain

The wide range of symptomatology accompanying chronic pain presents barriers to independence, role fulfillment, and occupational participation. Daily routines are interrupted, as are physical activity and even social identity.[2,10,23,24]

Activities of Daily Living

Up to one in three individuals who experience chronic pain are less able to maintain independence than those without it.[2] Pain, fatigue, and the effects of resultant depression and anxiety can impact both motivation and performance levels. Reduced ability to participate in hygiene and bathing is commonly described in the literature.[2,24] Other ADLs that are typically adversely impacted by chronic pain include dressing, functional mobility, and sexual activity.[2]

Instrumental Activities of Daily Living

Instrumental activities of daily living (IADLs)—such as meal preparation, home maintenance, shopping, driving and community mobility, work, school, and religious participation—are noted in the literature as being negatively impacted by pain caused by the same physical, cognitive, and emotional factors described earlier.[2] Performance of IADLs, care of others, care of pets, and child-rearing are often limited.[2,10,24] Health management is also identified in the literature as an area of dissatisfaction for individuals with chronic pain.[2,10] In one study, up to 39% of respondents perceived their physician to view their pain without seriousness and reported that their pain was inappropriately medically managed.[2] Numerous health care appointments and procedures, even when care is adequate, interrupt the ability to participate in desired daily activities and require functional cognitive skills, including organization, attention to detail and concentration, planning, problem-solving, and decision-making.

Work and Education

Disruption to work participation is perhaps the most widely cited deficit area in the chronic pain literature. Individuals' ability to work affects not only their own financial health, but the larger productivity of society. Up to two-thirds of people with chronic pain are less able to or cannot work outside the home.[2] One in four chronic pain patients must change jobs secondary to pain, and one in five are reported to be unemployed. Impaired job performance occurs frequently, which, in turn, may increase disruption of co-workers' performance. The incidence of job loss for individuals with chronic pain increases as much as seven times after clinical onset. Individuals who experience chronic pain are less likely to attend and complete college, and are more likely to retire early, which adversely impacts lifetime earnings.[2,10]

Other Occupational Domains

Disrupted rest and sleep is an occupational domain widely addressed in chronic pain literature, regardless of specific diagnosis, and results from pain-related fatigue, increased nighttime awakenings, and reduced total sleep time.[2–4] Leisure participation is reported to be as disrupted as participation in education and work.[2,10,24] Secondary to impairment in the abovementioned domains, social relationships become strained or broken, and participation in social activities is reduced.[2,24] Social identity changes in turn, because of difficulty fulfilling expected social roles—in particular, in societies with more physically demanding living conditions.[10]

Evaluation of Functional Skill Deficits Secondary to Chronic Pain

Occupational therapists may treat patients whose chronic pain is the primary (e.g., LBP, FM) or secondary diagnosis (e.g., pain secondary to traumatic brain injury). In many instances, chronic pain may be reported first to the occupational therapist who is treating the patient for another medical reason. When chronic pain is first detected by therapists, patients should be referred to their primary care physicians to determine, if possible, the causes and appropriate treatment. Chronic pain is multifactorial and has physical, cognitive, and psychosocial contributing factors.[25] The experience of chronic pain must be understood and assessed as a cycle in which daily stress, mood alterations, disrupted sleep, and physical activity or inactivity all interact to impact pain level.

Patient History

A number of screens and evaluations are available to assist therapists in the assessment of chronic pain syndromes. Pain should first be assessed by taking a patient history with regard to the following factors: (a) location including the site(s) of origin and whether and where radiating pain exists; (b) whether the patient can identify onset and causes (e.g., injury secondary to improper lifting); (c) whether pain is experienced as persistent or intermittent; (d) identification of pain sensory experiences, such as burning, throbbing, shooting, stabbing, tingling, or electrical (referred to as pain quality); (e) possible factors that cause pain exacerbation and relief; (f) pain intensity throughout the day and in relation to specific activities; and (g) previously attempted pain interventions.

Occupational Profile

Once the abovementioned factors are understood, chronic pain should be assessed to determine its impact on daily function using an occupational profile. Occupational profiles allow therapists to gain an understanding of the ways in which chronic pain has disrupted a patient's occupational roles and the ADLs supporting those roles. Occupational profiles also help therapists to understand how the experience of chronic pain has impacted patients' psychosocial health, daily mood, sleep patterns, daily stressors, and quality of life. It is important for therapists to understand that factors such as depression, disrupted sleep, and stress—which commonly accompany chronic pain—must be assessed and addressed in treatment for optimal effectiveness. Chapters 51 and 52 provide information regarding the assessment and treatment of depression, disrupted sleep, and stress—which must be disentangled from the physical mechanisms that may contribute to chronic pain.

Pain Diaries

Often, patients have not connected their experience of pain to sleep patterns, mood, physical activity level, stress, and diet and nutrition. In such cases, patients should be instructed to maintain a pain diary for 1 to 2 weeks in which they record:

- Pain occurrence
- Pain intensity and duration
- Pain quality
- Possible identifiable triggers
- Physical activity level
- Movement patterns used in specific activities
- Mood and stress level
- Sleep quality during the previous night
- Food intake (quality and quantity)
- Reactions to heat/cold or humid weather

This collection of data over 1 to 2 weeks allows patterns to be discerned regarding the experience of pain, and the environmental and internal stressors that may contribute to pain exacerbation or relief (see Box 49-1). Such information is critical to help patients begin to understand

Box 49-1

Pain Diary

Date	Pain Occurrence	Pain Intensity and Duration	Pain Quality (Throbbing, Aching, Stabbing, Shooting, Burning, Tingling, and Electrical)	Possible Triggers	Activity Level Preceding Pain	Movement Patterns Used in Specific Activities Preceding Pain	Sleep Quality Previous Night	Food Intake (Type and Quantity)[a]	Weather (Hot, Cold, and Humid)
Morning 6:00–11:59 am									
Afternoon 12:00–4:59 pm									
Evening 5:00–11:59 pm									
Sleep time 12:00–5:59 am									

[a] Note the intake of alcohol, caffeine, refined sugars, gluten, dairy, processed meats, corn and vegetable oils.

the interrelationship between the internal experience of pain and the external conditions that may heighten or decrease the pain experience. Without this understanding, both therapists and patients will not have sufficient knowledge to develop interventions that effectively begin to alter the pain cycle.

Visual Analog Scales

Visual Analog Scales (VASs) (also referred to as verbal or numeric rating scales) are self-report measures that allow patients to rate their pain on a continuum using numbers, qualitative descriptors, and emoticons as anchors (see Box 49-2).[26] These types of measures allow patients to document their pain level either in the present moment or as it occurred over the past week. Although VASs are easy to use, they do not allow consideration of pain with regard to changing intensity and duration—a critical factor since most patients experience chronic pain as a changing rather than stable phenomenon. VASs also do not allow for the rating of pain to be considered in relation to the internal and environmental factors noted earlier. As a result, VASs tend to oversimplify the pain experience, which then frequently leads to an oversimplification of intervention and a failure to address the multiple contributing factors of pain.

Pain Disability Index

The Pain Disability Index (PDI)[27] is a 7-item, 10-point, self-report Likert scale, where 0 = no disability and 10 = worst disability as a result of pain. The scale allows patients to rate their pain level in seven categories: family and home responsibilities, recreation and leisure activities, social activity, occupations related to work (including paid and volunteer work), sexual activity, self-care activities, and life support activities (e.g., eating, sleeping, breathing). The scale yields a total possible score ranging from 0 to 70, with higher scores indicating greater disability secondary to pain. The PDI has been found to be able to discriminate between patients having high and low pain levels[27] and possesses high test–retest reliability (intraclass correlation coefficient [ICC] = 0.83)[28] and internal consistency (alpha = 0.86).[29] The PDI allows therapists to identify activities in which patients report experiencing heightened pain in order to address those areas and document change over time.

Brief Pain Inventory

The Brief Pain Inventory (BPI) is a self-report measure that allows patients to document pain level in general life activities and is available in short (9 items) and long (17 items) versions.[30] Although initially developed for patients with pain secondary to cancer, the assessment is now commonly used for patients with chronic pain resulting from multiple causes. The scale includes the ability for patients to pinpoint their pain location on front and back anatomical diagrams. Both versions allow patients to rate their pain level from least to worst on a 10-point Likert scale in the last 24 hours and on average. Seven questions ask patients to report to what degree pain has interfered with their general activity, mood, walking ability, normal walk, relations with others, sleep, and enjoyment of life (0 = does not interfere,

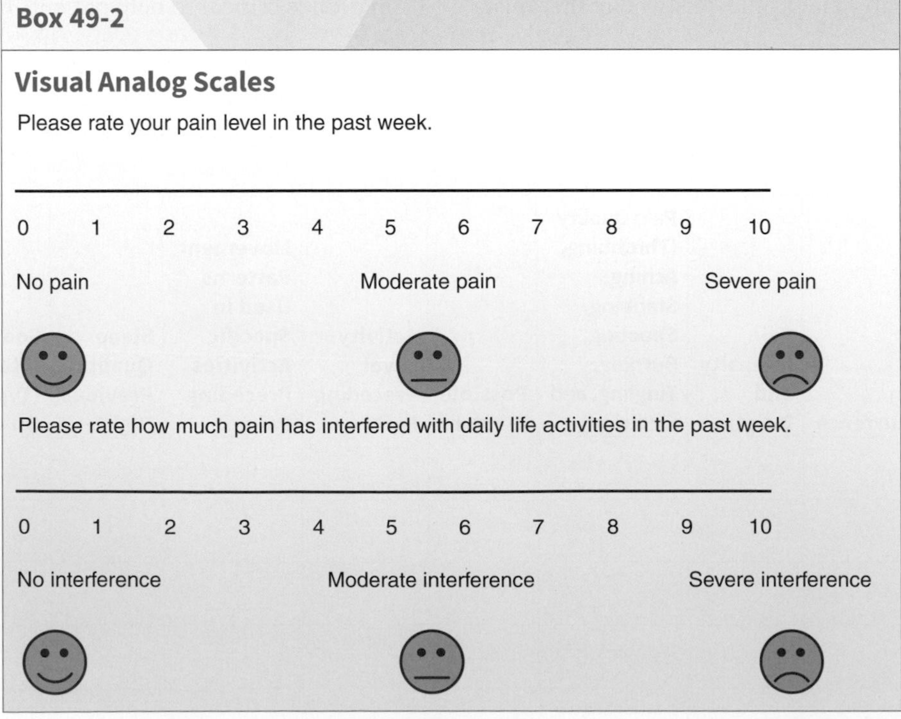

10 = completely interferes). The BPI yields two scores: a pain severity score (with a total score ranging from 0 to 40) and a pain interference score (with a total score ranging from 0 to 70). Test–retest reliability was found to be high for both pain severity and pain intensity ($r = 0.80$, respectively).[31] Internal consistency was also found to be high for both pain severity and pain intensity, with alpha coefficients ranging from 0.81 to 0.89 and 0.88 to 0.95, respectively.[32] Construct validity was also found to be high.[33] Although the BPI allows therapists to understand a patients' pain with regard to severity and interference in general life activities, it does not allow for an in-depth assessment of pain interference in the common basic ADLs and IADLs that occupational therapists typically assess.

Canadian Occupational Performance Measure

The Canadian Occupational Performance Measure (COPM) is a 5-item, 10-point rating scale (1 = most important, 10 = least important) designed to be completed conjointly by a therapist and participant and requires approximately 30 minutes to administer.[34,35] Although the scale was not designed to measure pain specifically, it can be modified to assess the patient's most important daily activities impacted by pain. Patients can be asked to identify the five most critical activities that are adversely impeded by pain in the areas of self-care, productivity (e.g., work, volunteerism, home management), and leisure. After the identification of five problems, participants are asked to rate both performance and satisfaction levels of the identified activities on a 10-point scale (1 = not satisfied; 10 = extremely satisfied). An open-ended narrative section is provided to allow therapists to record participant comments. The COPM is intended to be used pre- and postintervention to determine whether intervention impacted participants' perceived performance and satisfaction levels in identified areas. Test–retest reliability was reported to be high for both performance and satisfaction sections ($r = 0.89$, $p < 0.001$; $r = 0.88$, $p < 0.001$, respectively).[36] Inter-rater reliability was reported to be moderate for both performance and satisfaction sections (ICC = 0.67, $p < 0.05$; ICC = 0.69, $p < 0.05$, respectively).[37] Convergent validity with the Disability and Impact Profile was found to be moderate ($r = 0.74$, $p < 0.05$).[38]

Intervention of Functional Skill Deficits Secondary to Chronic Pain

Occupational therapists treat patients with chronic pain as part of an interprofessional team that includes primary care physicians, pain management specialists, nurses, physical therapists, nutritionists, and psychologists. The intervention goals of occupational therapy (OT) in the treatment of chronic pain syndromes are to help patients learn to effectively manage their pain to participate in desired ADLs. Intervention consists of education and lifestyle modification, pain reduction, and activity adaptation.

Client Education and Lifestyle Modification

As noted previously, effective pain management is best achieved when pain is understood and addressed as having multiple and interrelated physical, cognitive, and psychosocial contributing factors. It is critical to help patients understand that the experience of pain is impacted by daily stress, mood, sleep quality, physical activity, movement patterns in daily activities, and physiological reactions to heat and cold. Patients should be instructed to complete a pain diary for 1 to 2 weeks, after which therapists should help patients identify patterns between their experience of pain and the above-noted factors. Once such patterns have been identified, therapists can help patients make lifestyle changes to effectively manage pain over time.

Sleep

Poor sleep quality includes difficulty falling asleep, frequent awakenings, and insufficient total sleep time (<7–8 hours). Poor sleep quality is associated with reduced tissue repair and heightened pain levels.[39] It is important for patients with chronic pain to maintain regular sleep–wake times and attempt to gain 7 to 8 hours of sleep per night. Chapter 51 details intervention strategies that therapists can use to help patients enhance sleep quality. Therapists can also additionally help patients make changes to mattresses and sleep positions to reduce pain. For example, mattresses or mattress toppers that conform to the body and cushion bony prominences and painful regions should be adopted. Adjustable beds that can raise and lower the trunk and lower extremities can also help in pain reduction. When adjustable beds are not feasible, pillows can be used to position the body to reduce pain. For example, pillows should be evaluated to ascertain that they maintain the head and neck in a neutral aligned position that reduces rotational forces. Patients with LBP who sleep in a supine position often find that placing a pillow beneath the knees alleviates pain. Patients who sleep on their side should position a pillow between their knees to avoid internal rotation of the hips. Side-sleeping patients may also find that resting one arm across a pillow positioned at chest level reduces shoulder internal rotation and can alleviate pain.

Stress and Mood

The experience of pain activates sympathetic nervous system responses, including accelerated heart rate, increased blood pressure, and shallow respiration. Stress occurring as a result of normal ADLs commonly increases sympathetic nervous system responses, physiological inflammatory responses, and muscular tightening or guarding that can trigger pain phenomena.[40] It is critical for patients to understand the relationship between stress and pain for effective management over time. Therapists must assist patients to identify common life stressors and problem solve ways to reduce daily stress through lifestyle changes and stress reduction techniques. Lifestyle changes may involve activity simplification and pacing in daily occupations (discussed later). Stress reduction techniques can include deep breathing exercises, guided meditation and visualization, and progressive muscle relaxation. These techniques help patients to increase parasympathetic responses, including the secretion of hormones that reduce heart rate and blood pressure, and to facilitate states of emotional calmness.[41] Such techniques should become part of the patient's daily routine for effective pain management over time. Stress reduction techniques also include CBT in which patients are taught to rethink and reframe their typical thoughts to stressful situations so that such situations are no longer perceived with as great anxiety.[42] CBT is an involved practice that requires patient training over several months. Although occupational therapists can integrate CBT into sessions, patients should be referred to CBT specialists for appropriate training.

Physical Activity

Patients with chronic pain syndromes are at risk for reduced activity levels and inactivity that can commonly contribute to increased weight gain, muscle atrophy, and loss of strength and endurance needed for typical daily occupations. Because patients fear pain sensations, they commonly adopt **guarding behaviors**, such as bracing, posturing, and limping. Such dysfunctional behaviors often contribute to additional musculoskeletal problems resulting from the overuse of certain muscle groups and body positions in an attempt to avoid pain. Therapists should help patients recognize guarding behaviors and substitute their use with functional movement. Patients with chronic pain who avoid activity can learn to adopt alternative movement patterns to accomplish desired occupations (discussed in section on Body Mechanics). Patients should also be encouraged to progressively challenge their perceived physical limitations, as many patients will stop activity participation because they anticipate painful responses that may subside as more effective pain management strategies are learned. A daily routine of low-impact exercise and participation in occupations should be customized for each patient with specified dosages throughout the day. Exercise and occupational participation routines should be sufficiently gentle to avoid pain but rigorous enough to maintain joint range of motion (ROM), strength, endurance, and appropriate weight.

Responses to Climatic Changes

Many studies have documented an association between orthopedic and rheumatic pain and weather changes—particularly humidity, heat, cold, and barometric changes.[43–45] Such climatic conditions may alter fluid levels that line and lubricate joints, leading to increased inflammation. Humidity and barometric changes, in particular, may cause the tendons, ligaments, and muscles to expand, thus exacerbating inflammation and pain. There is also evidence that pain thresholds decrease in cold temperatures, causing heightened pain perception. Pain responses to humidity, heat, and cold should be part of patient education along with strategies to reduce pain when such climatic conditions occur. Strategies include (a) the use of bed and chair pads with options for heat and massage (which can be used in car, work, and home intermittently during the day and evening); (b) dressing in layers appropriate for the transition between indoor and outdoor activities throughout the day; (c) using thermal insulted gloves, hats, and shoes for cold temperatures and loose-fitting clothing of natural materials (e.g., cotton) to maintain cooler body temperatures in hot weather; (d) when possible, transferring activities from outdoor to indoor temperature-controlled environments during hot and humid weather; and (e) using over-the-counter pain patches and devices as needed.

Food Intake and Weight Control

Patients with chronic pain syndromes are at risk for gaining weight as a result of activity reduction and inactivity, and depression-related overeating. Overweight conditions exacerbate pain because of the increased demand on the musculoskeletal system.[46] Information regarding food intake and weight control should be part of client education, and patients should be assisted to understand their ideal weight, healthiest foods for weight management, portion control, and foods having inflammatory properties that should be avoided. Patients should also be assisted to develop a regular food intake schedule of well-proportioned, healthy meals. Occupational therapists can provide education regarding food intake collaboratively with nutritionists, nurses, and primary care physicians.

Body Mechanics

Body mechanics involve the proper positioning of the body during daily activities to avoid injury and pain. Patients with chronic pain syndromes should receive education regarding both the anatomy of the spine and extremities, and their proper positioning during movement to maintain health. Patient understanding of body mechanics is critical for effective long-term pain management. Patients should be provided with the opportunity to practice body mechanics within self-identified desired occupations, and relative to static and dynamic postures and transitional patterns (e.g., sit-to-stand). General principles of body mechanics involve the following:

- Maintaining a straight back and upright posture
- Carrying objects close to the body
- Lifting with the lower extremities while maintaining a wide base of support
- Avoiding rotational and compressional movements of the spine

Activities Performed in Standing

To reduce back pain for activities performed in prolonged standing—such as washing dishes at a sink and brushing teeth—patients should stand upright with their bodies facing the activity (and avoiding spinal rotation and flexion). The patient can lean against the stable counter and rest one foot on a low stool or cabinet base to achieve a posterior pelvic tilt (Fig. 49-4). Patients can also rest one upper extremity on the counter to support the spine. Patients should be instructed to turn their bodies as one unit while maintaining the spine in a neutral position. The use of an antifatigue mat may also help to reduce lower extremity and back pain.

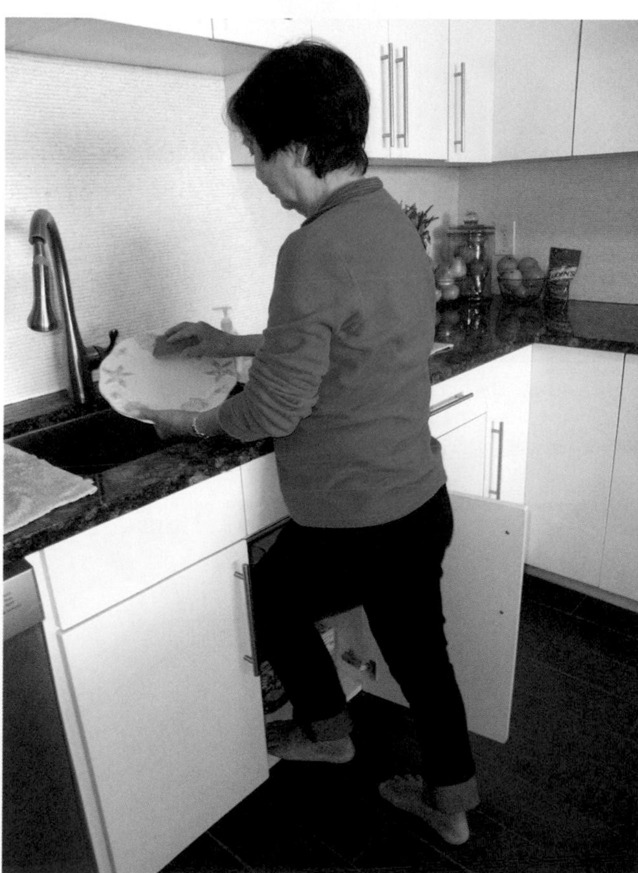

Figure 49-4. To reduce back pain for activities performed in prolonged standing—such as washing dishes at a sink and brushing teeth—patients should stand upright with their bodies facing the activity (and avoiding spinal rotation and flexion). The patient can lean against the stable counter and rest one foot on a low stool or cabinet base to achieve a posterior pelvic tilt.

Transitioning to Sit

When transitioning to sit from a standing position, patients should lower their bodies by flexing the knees and hips without bending the spine (Fig. 49-5). The patient's hands should be placed on the chair armrest to guide the descent and support the trunk. Chairs with raised seats are recommended because they require less muscular strength, which reduces spinal column stress and pain. A slightly reclined sitting posture is preferred for prolonged sitting. When seated to work at a table, patients should avoid bending over the work by moving the chair close to the work and raising or inclining the work surface as needed.

Bed Positions

When lying in bed, the ideal posture to decrease pressure on the spine is supine with the knees flexed. A pillow should be placed under the knees to maintain their flexed position (Fig. 49-6). For patients who sleep on their side, a pillow should be placed between the legs with the knees slightly flexed to reduce hip internal

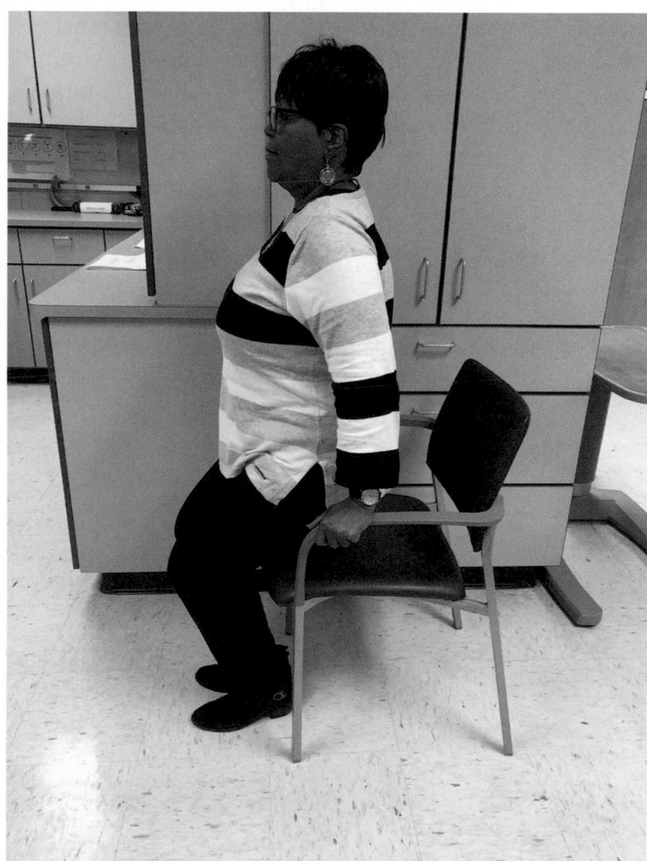

Figure 49-5. When transitioning to sit from a standing position, patients should lower their bodies by flexing the knees and hips without bending the spine. The patient's hands should be placed on the chair armrest to guide the descent and support the trunk.

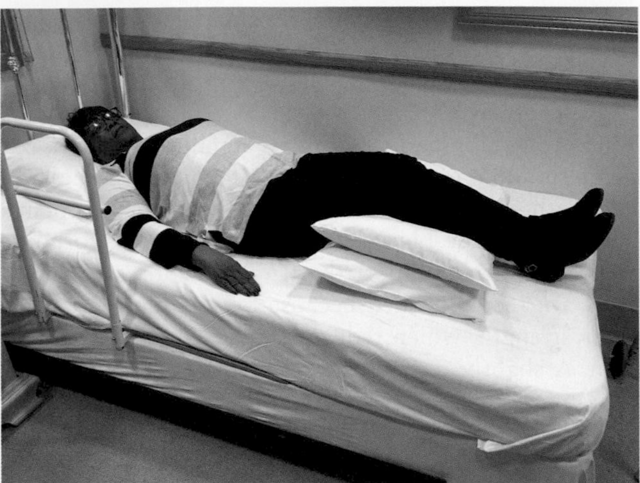

Figure 49-6. When lying in bed, the ideal posture to decrease pressure on the spine is supine with the knees flexed. A pillow should be placed under the knees to maintain their flexed position.

rotation (Fig. 49-7). A pillow can also be placed at chest level with one upper extremity draped across to prevent shoulder internal rotation. When rising from bed, patients should log roll to the edge of the bed, allow both lower extremities to descend to the floor, and use their upper extremities to support the trunk to rise to an upright seated position (Video 49-1). A small bedrail can be used for patients with decreased upper extremity strength. When entering bed, patients should maintain a straight back and use their arms as support on the bed surface (or bedrail) to lower their body to a seated position on the edge of the bed. Once seated, the patient can raise the lower extremities to the bed while lowering the trunk to a supine position (Video 49-2).

Toilet Use

The body mechanics used to sit down on a toilet seat are similar to lowering oneself to a chair. Raised toilet seats and grab bars can be used to help rise from and sit down onto toilets (Fig. 49-8). When performing hygiene tasks after toileting, patients should be taught to reach between the legs rather than rotating the spine. A long-handled tissue paper holder can be used to extend reach if needed. When flushing the toilet, patients should

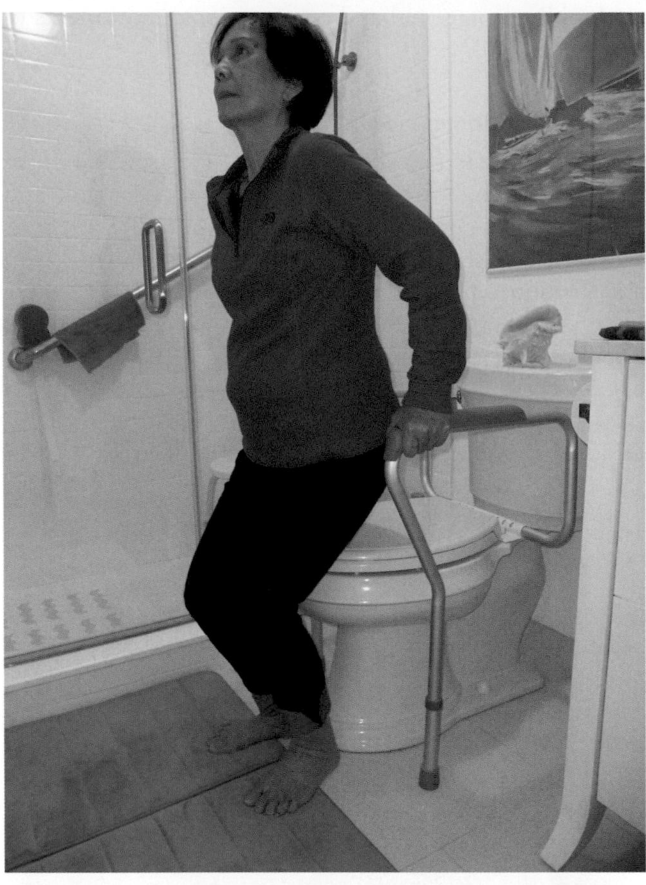

Figure 49-8. The body mechanics used to sit down on a toilet seat are similar to lowering oneself to a chair. Raised toilet seats and grab bars can be used to help rise from and sit down onto toilets.

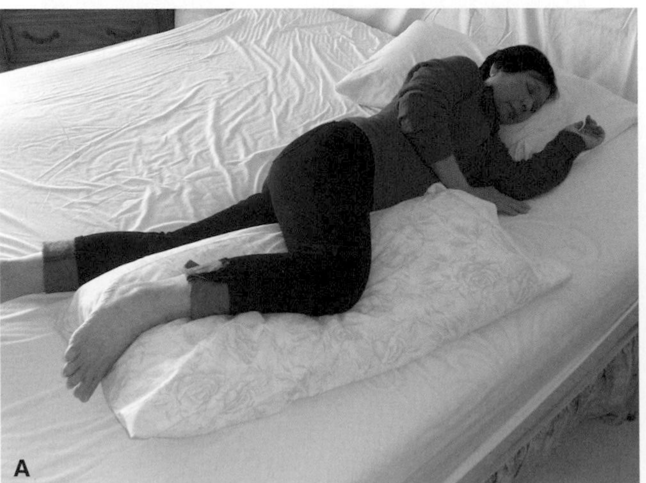

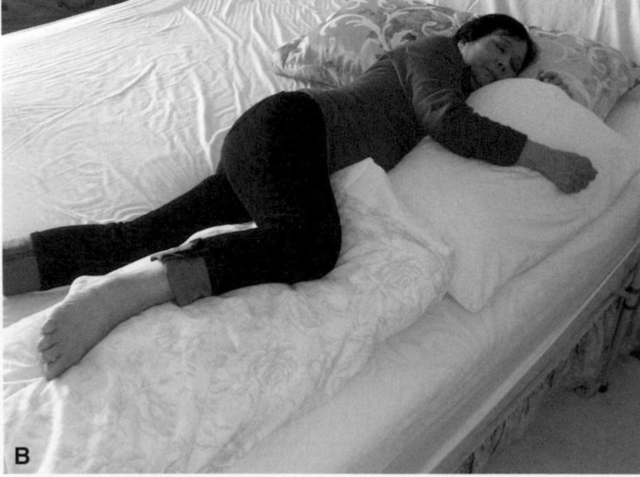

Figure 49-7. A. For patients who sleep on their side, a pillow should be placed between their legs with the knees slightly flexed to reduce hip internal rotation. **B.** A pillow can also be placed at chest level with one upper extremity draped across to prevent shoulder internal rotation.

rise from the toilet and stand, turn their bodies as a unit to face the lever (avoiding rotational trunk movement), and move as close as possible to the lever to reduce reaching. Patients can also use grab bars to support their trunk when flushing the lever (Video 49-3).

Activities Requiring Bending and Reaching: Laundry, Dressing, and Cleaning

For tasks that require excessive reaching and bending of the spine—such as sweeping, vacuuming, retrieving laundry from a machine, and reaching into a closet—patients should be taught to position the body close to the task and maintain the spine in a neutral position. For front-loading laundry machines, patients should sit on a stool facing the machine to retrieve clothing items. For top-loading laundry machines, patients should stand close to the machine and lean against it (Fig. 49-9). One upper extremity can be positioned on the machine's top surface to support the trunk, while the other extremity retrieves the clothing. If the trunk must be flexed to reach fully into the laundry basin, one leg can be extended at the hip to reduce back strain. Clothing should be retrieved in small handfuls to reduce load on the shoulders and back, and ideally placed on a 36-inch (92-cm) or higher table to fold. Folded laundry can either be carried in small bundles held close to the body or placed in rolling laundry carriers to be transported to closets and drawers. Carrying large laundry baskets should be avoided.

Dressing should be achieved through movements that maintain the back in a neutral position with avoidance of spinal flexion and rotational movements. Patients can sit in a chair to dress the trunk and upper extremities. The lower extremities can be dressed using a dressing stick, sock aid, and long-handled shoehorn. Clothing should be laid out nearby in an easy-to-reach location that does not require excessive reaching or bending.

When tools are used in activities, such as brooms and vacuums, they should be moved at short distances from the body to avoid excessive reaching that could trigger pain. Patients should move their bodies as a unit and avoid flexion and rotational spinal movements. Reachers can be used to retrieve light objects from closets and cabinets. Long-handled telescoping sponges and mops can be used to reduce bending and reaching while cleaning.

Lifting and Carrying Objects

Ideally, lifting objects from the floor should be avoided or accomplished using a reacher. When lifting objects is necessitated by work or child-rearing demands, patients

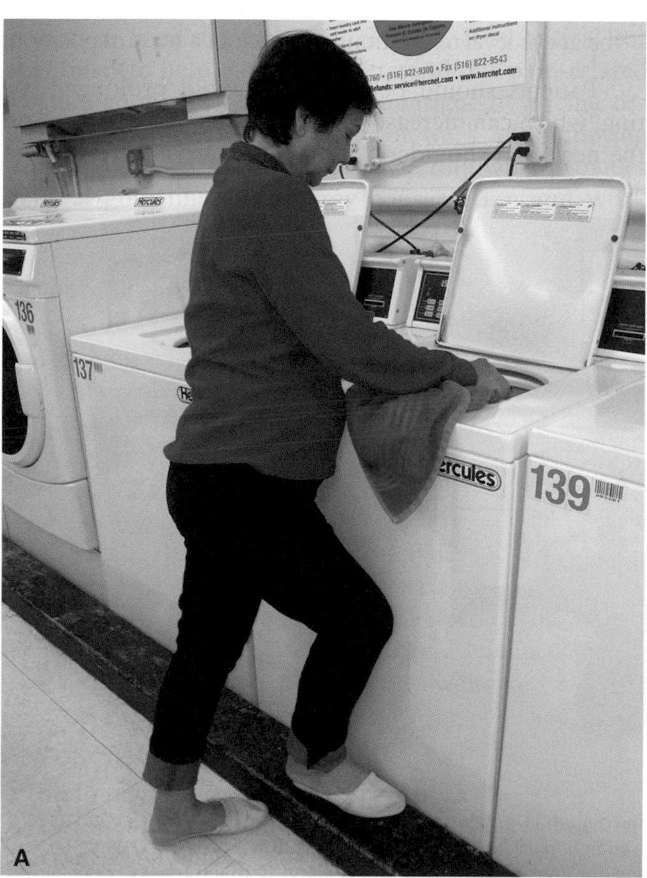

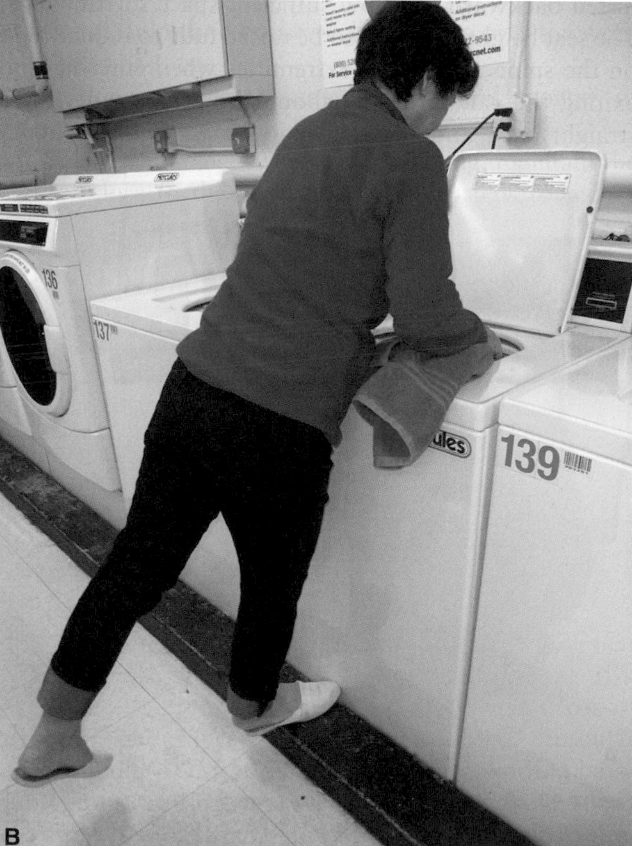

Figure 49-9. **A.** For top-loading laundry machines, patients should stand close to the machine and lean against it. One upper extremity can be positioned on the machine's top surface to support the trunk, while the other extremity retrieves the clothing. **B.** If the trunk must be flexed to reach fully into the laundry basin, one leg can be extended at the hip to reduce back strain.

pain. For these reasons, patients with chronic pain syndromes should be placed on slow, controlled, and graded strength and endurance training programs to prevent deconditioning. Interventions should begin as gentle and slow-paced activities that are initially graded to match and then gently challenge the physical and emotional abilities of each patient. Interventions should also be embedded within meaningful functional activities to each patient, such as pushing and pulling a vacuum cleaner, standing while folding laundry, and carrying weighted grocery bags. Activities can be progressively increased in time, repetitions, distances, and weight in accordance with each patient's tolerance and progress. Proper body mechanics should be emphasized in all strength and endurance training activities. Aquatic therapy is particularly beneficial for patients with chronic pain because water's buoyancy decreases gravitational forces on muscles and lessens spinal compression. Water also provides resistance helpful to build muscular strength and endurance in a gentle way over time.

Adaptive Equipment

Adaptive equipment for patients with chronic pain is recommended to reduce energy expenditure, joint strain, and spinal rotation and flexion. Chapter 42 details adaptive equipment to preserve joint integrity of patients with rheumatoid and osteoarthritis. The following are the most commonly recommended adaptive equipment and supplies for patients with FM and chronic pain secondary to orthopedic conditions:

- Shower benches, grab bars, handheld shower heads, long-handled bathing sponges and brushes
- Stools on which to sit while performing self-care at a sink, meal preparation at a kitchen counter, and household activities such as folding laundry
- Long-handled telescoping dusters, mops, and sponges
- Reachers, dressing sticks, sock aids, long-handled shoehorns, and elastic shoelaces
- Grab bars, toilet safety frames, raised toilet seats, and long-handled tissue wipes

Physical Agent Modalities

Physical agent modalities are interventions and technologies that use force or energy to promote the healing process and reduce pain. In OT, physical agents are commonly used as a precursor to interventions involving occupational participation in patient-identified desired daily activities. Physical agents can increase soft-tissue elasticity and joint flexibility and reduce painful regions in preparation for the engagement in functional activity.[49] Chapter 24 provides an exhaustive detail of available, commonly used physical agent modalities. There are several commonly used physical agents in the treatment of chronic pain (discussed later). It is important for therapists to obtain appropriate training in physical agent use and adhere to the licensing regulations of their state or municipality.

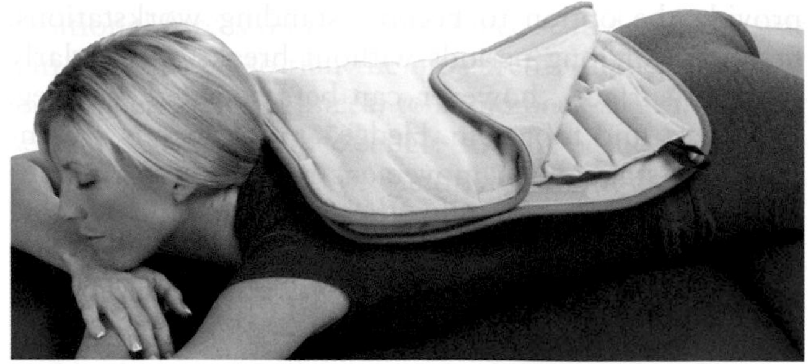

Figure 49-11. Hot packs are a form of thermotherapy that provide a moderate dose of moist heat that can be applied to a painful region. Hot packs should never be placed directly on skin; instead, dry padding should be used between hot packs and skin to avoid burns.

Hot Packs

Hot packs are a form of thermotherapy that provide a moderate dose of moist heat that can be applied to a painful region.[48,49] Hot packs are indicated for chronic conditions and should not be used for acute conditions because of heat's potential to increase inflammation. Hot packs should never be placed directly on skin; instead, dry padding should be used between hot packs and skin to avoid burns (Fig. 49-11). The patient's skin should be checked after 5 minutes of application for redness, blistering, or potential burns, and the patient asked about his or her comfort level. Generally, hot packs should be left on for 15 to 20 minutes to achieve a therapeutic effect.

Cold Packs

Cold packs are a form of cryotherapy that conduct heat out of the body and into the cooling agent.[48,50] Cold packs can be used in the management of acute inflammation and chronic pain. Some patients with chronic pain have heightened responses to cold sensations and cannot tolerate any form of cryotherapy. Dry padding should be used between cold packs and skin to avoid irritation. Therapists should monitor patients' skin and response to the modality. Cold packs should generally be applied for approximately 10 to 15 minutes.

Transcutaneous Electrical Nerve Stimulation

Transcutaneous electrical nerve stimulation (TENS) uses surface electrodes placed over the area of pain to stimulate afferent sensory nerve fibers to modulate pain perception (Fig. 49-12).[48,51] TENS can be used to

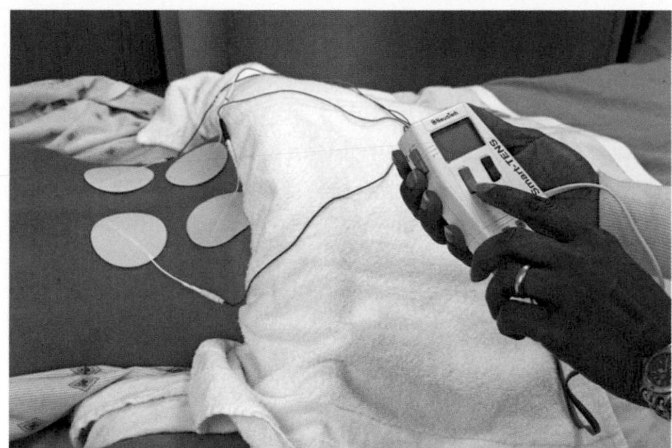

Figure 49-12. Transcutaneous electrical nerve stimulation uses surface electrodes placed over the area of pain to stimulate afferent sensory nerve fibers to modulate pain perception.

manage pain in musculoskeletal disorders, presurgically and postsurgically, and for both acute and chronic pain. Optimal electrode placement should correlate with pain structures and sources and can include dermatomes, and motor, trigger, and acupuncture points. Treatment time varies between 30 and 60 minutes. Home TENS units can be used as needed or on a three to four times daily schedule.

Biofeedback

Biofeedback uses surface electrodes and instrumentation to measure and display physiological body responses, including respiratory, cardiovascular, and neuromuscular.[48,52] The feedback provided through this technology measures activity in the neuromuscular system and can be used for motor reeducation and the retraining of functional movement to both (1) reduce pain and (2) improve functional movement in daily activities. For chronic pain, biofeedback provides information related to hyperactive muscle contraction (spasm), alerting patients to consciously relax those muscle groups. Biofeedback provides immediate feedback (auditory or visual), allowing patients to objectively measure, determine, and quantify muscle activity and track motor performance changes.

Complementary and Alternative Therapies

A range of complementary and alternative therapies are increasingly used to treat chronic pain syndromes with evidence for effectiveness. These include acupuncture,[53] acupressure,[54] Tai Chi,[55] meditation,[56] integrated yoga,[57] and energy healing[58] (e.g., Reiki, therapeutic touch, Qigong, craniosacral therapy). Most of these therapies require training, and some require certification (e.g., acupuncture). Of these therapies, occupational therapists with training could provide meditation instruction, integrated yoga and Tai Chi, and energy healing. Meditation involves a focus on deep breathing and quieting of racing thoughts in the mind that induce states of stress. A daily practice of meditation can help patients with chronic pain to reduce stress levels that may heighten muscle spasms and physiological inflammatory responses. Progressive muscle relaxation, which can be practiced as a form of meditation, directly helps patients to systematically reduce tension held in all muscle groups of the body. Other forms of mediation include visualization and guided imagery in which a narrator provides guidance to release stressful thoughts and muscle tension, often against a background of calming music. Meditation for patients with chronic pain should not be performed in the traditional lotus position (sitting cross-legged with the feet resting on the floor or thighs), but rather seated in a chair or supine with a bolster beneath the knees.

Integrated yoga is a form of yoga in which typical yoga poses are modified to reduce joint stress, maintain the spine in a neutral position (avoiding spinal flexion and rotation), and maintain the hips in positions of $<90°$ flexion. One form of integrated yoga is chair yoga in which patients perform poses while seated in a chair or in standing using the chair for support. Integrated yoga combines traditional gentle rehabilitation stretching exercises with modified yoga poses. Integrated yoga can help patients with chronic pain to maintain flexibility while using muscle groups in a gentle, low-impact manner.

Energy healing is the restoration of a patient's biofield through the channeling of what in the East is referred to as vital life force energy (i.e., Chi, Qi, and Prana). The human biofield is an electromagnetic field that surrounds and permeates living organisms.[59] Traditional Eastern biofield practitioners maintain that disease begins in the biofield as energetic imbalances. The objective of energy healing is to restore a patient's energy flow and release blockages that may impede healing processes. Such practices emphasize the idea that the body holds an innate intelligence and that the body's auto-healing response can be promoted through a practitioner's hands-on channeling of vital life force energy. A growing body of research has demonstrated support for the effectiveness of energy healing practices in various conditions, including chronic pain.

The use of complementary and alternative therapies in the treatment of chronic pain has become an important adjunct to pain medication, which, over time, has been shown to cause negative side effects, including digestive problems, liver toxicity, kidney damage, muscular atrophy, and cognitive deficits.[60]

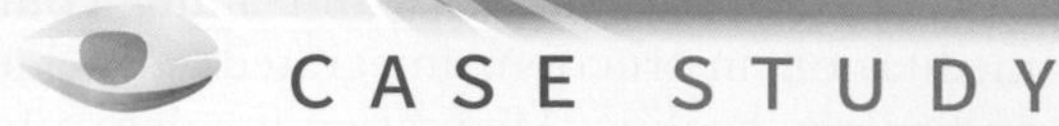

CASE STUDY

Patient Information

Nalani is a 46-year-old female of Pacific Island descent who received a diagnosis of FM 1 month ago. Symptoms include widespread musculoskeletal pain; severe fatigue, particularly after highly active days; disrupted sleep; and cognitive problems, including short-term memory deficits and difficulty concentrating. Nalani has worked full time as a nurse in a pediatric physician's practice for 12 years, but as a result of FM symptoms, has been forced to reduce her hours to part time.

Reason for Occupational Therapy Referral

Nalani was referred to OT to address pain and fatigue that have been interfering with basic ADLs and IADLs.

Assessment Process and Results

Through a patient history and the completion of a 1-week pain diary, the following information was obtained regarding Nalani's pain experience:

- Nalani experienced pain and tenderness at her cervical area, on her back across and between both scapulae, at her lumbar spine, above each iliac crest, across both sacral indentations, and at each hip and buttock area. Occasionally, pain was experienced in both knees.
- Nalani stated that pain onset began approximately 5 years ago after she sustained a car accident in which she injured her neck and, at the same time, lost her mother to cancer.
- Her pain was experienced as intermittent with worse pain reported in the early morning and after busy days at the pediatric practice. Pain was reported as aching and throbbing.
- Nalani reported that hectic days, stress, lack of sleep, and humid and cold weather exacerbated her pain level.
- Relief could sometimes be found after spending 1 to 2 days in bed.

Through an occupational profile, it was determined that many of Nalani's desired ADLs had become disrupted and difficult to complete, including showering, meal preparation, laundry, cleaning, grocery shopping, and work. Because of pain and decreased energy, she would commonly forgo laundry and cleaning for a month and then spend an entire day completing these activities, causing debilitating pain and fatigue for 2 days afterward.

COPM scores before intervention were reported as follows:

- Showering: Performance = 2, Satisfaction = 2
- Meal preparation: Performance = 3, Satisfaction = 2
- Laundry: Performance = 1, Satisfaction = 1
- Cleaning: Performance = 2, Satisfaction = 2
- Grocery shopping: Performance = 4, Satisfaction = 3
- Work: Performance = 5, Satisfaction = 5

Occupational Therapy Problem List

- Pain and tenderness in the neck, shoulders, low back, hips/buttocks, and knees that interferes with participation in desired ADLs
- Severe fatigue after showering, meal preparation, laundry, cleaning, grocery shopping, and often work
- Debilitating fatigue after overactivity, commonly resulting in 1 to 2 days of bed rest

Occupational Therapy Goal List

- Provide education about the relationship between sleep, activity level, climatic changes, and pain level.
- Provide education in and practice opportunities to use appropriate body mechanics in desired ADLs to reduce and prevent pain.
- Provide education in and practice opportunities to use energy conservation, work simplification, and adaptive equipment in desired ADLs to reduce and prevent fatigue and pain.
- Begin a slow, gentle, low-impact, progressively graded strength and endurance training program as tolerated by the patient.
- Provide education in and practice opportunities to use guided imagery and progressive muscle relaxation as forms of meditation.
- Use physical agent modalities as a precursor to occupational participation during OT intervention sessions. Provide education about hot packs and TENS units for home use.

Intervention

Intervention began by helping Nalani understand the relationships between sleep disruption, stress levels, physical exertion, and climatic conditions. Nalani was assisted to learn sleep strategies, her mattress was replaced with a softer memory foam mattress that contoured to her body and relieved pressure on bony prominences, and her pillow was replaced with one that prevented her neck from positions of flexion and rotation. A pillow was also used beneath her knees to relieve low back strain.

Nalani also received instruction in and opportunities to practice meditation in the forms of guided imagery and progressive muscle relaxation. She was given meditation videos and placed on a home meditation schedule of 5 days per week for 20-minute sessions.

The therapist and Nalani also spoke about the impact of humidity and cold on her pain levels, as she identified these as stressors. Strategies to deal with these specific weather conditions were discussed, including dress and the adoption of a dehumidifier.

Because Nalani reported that increased activity levels exacerbated pain and fatigue levels, energy conservation and work simplification strategies were taught and practiced within the specific ADLs that she identified as most important. All desired

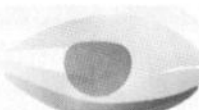

CASE STUDY *(continued)*

daily activities were scheduled over the week in intervals so that they could be slowly accomplished leaving time for rest periods. All large tasks, such as meal preparation, were broken down into smaller more manageable ones that could be paced over the day or week. Nalani was also encouraged to prepare a larger amount of food on the weekend that could be frozen and used over weekdays.

Recommended adaptive equipment and supplies to reduce fatigue and pain included (1) a shower bench and handheld shower head, shower grab bars, and long-handled bathing sponge; (2) a long-handled telescoping duster, mop, and sponge; (3) a reacher, dressing stick, sock aid, long-handled shoehorn, and elastic shoelaces; (4) grab bars at the toilet and a raised toilet seat; (5) a stool on which to perform self-care and meal preparation; and (6) lightweight cookware and dishes.

Nalani was also taught appropriate body mechanics with opportunities to practice these in the specific activities of showering, grooming at the bathroom sink, meal preparation, laundry, cleaning, and carrying grocery bags and work-related medical supplies.

A gentle, slow-paced, low-impact strength and endurance training program was begun and progressively graded in accordance with Nalani's tolerance. All training was embedded within desired daily activities, such as vacuuming; making a bed; carrying grocery bags; and retrieving, folding, and transporting laundry.

Hot packs were used at the beginning of each therapy session to loosen soft tissue and reduce pain at the low back and shoulders. Nalani also received instruction in hot pack and TENS unit for home use. Cold packs were contraindicated because Nalani reported that cold commonly induced pain and tenderness.

At the end of 3 weeks, Nalani reported that she was better able to participate in desired occupations with less pain and fatigue. She had begun to gradually increase her work hours with the support of her employer who provided work accommodations, including 10-minute rest periods each hour, the use of a wheeled cart to transport medical supplies, and the ability to use a stool while taking patient vitals.

COPM scores at intervention end were as follows:

- Showering: Performance = 5, Satisfaction = 6
- Meal preparation: Performance = 6, Satisfaction = 6
- Laundry: Performance = 5, Satisfaction = 3
- Cleaning: Performance = 7, Satisfaction = 8
- Grocery shopping: Performance = 6, Satisfaction = 6
- Work: Performance = 7, Satisfaction = 8

Evidence Table of Intervention Studies for Chronic Pain and Fibromyalgia

Intervention	Description	Participants	Dosage	Research Design and Evidence Level	Benefit	Statistical Significance and Effect Size
Lifestyle Redesign, a treatment method focused on development of healthy habits and routines for self-care[23]	Treatment includes education, self-analysis of occupation, problem-solving, development of motivation, and behavioral change. Treatment is driven by progression of modules.	Forty-five chronic pain patients (32 women, 12 men); most common diagnoses included lumbago, myalgia (e.g., FM), and complex regional pain syndrome.	Mean number of OT treatments per patient = 9.04; mode = 8 sessions; mean duration of therapy = 18 weeks	One group pretest and posttest design Level III	Significant effect on quality of life, self-efficacy, and functional abilities; no significance in pain reduction.	COPM indicated increase in performance and satisfaction of performance ($ps < 0.001$); Short form: 36 quality-of-life measure indicated increased role participation secondary to physical and mental health ($p = 0.0013$ and $p = 0.0041$) and increased social functioning ($p = 0.0004$). Pain Self-Efficacy Questionnaire indicated increased functional ability despite pain ($p = 0.0030$).
Integrated care team to reduce disability from chronic low back pain in working and private life, vs. treatment as usual[61]	In the integrated care team, a physician supervised a workplace intervention and graded activity program, including cognitive–behavioral principles. The team consisted of a physician, a medical specialist, an occupational therapist, and a physical therapist. The care team and patient shared a common goal of return to work and occupational function. They communicated closely throughout treatment via email, letters, and a conference call every 3 weeks.	Adults aged 18–65 years with LBP, had LBP for >12 weeks, were in paid work for at least 8 hours a week, and were absent or partially absent from work. These were assigned to integrated care intervention group ($n = 66$; 37 men and 29 women) and treatment as usual control group ($n = 68$; 41 men and 27 women).	Average duration of integrated care was 67 days. Median number of team consultations: physician 2.2; occupational therapist 2.4; physical therapist 6.5 individual, and 11.6 group sessions.	Randomized controlled trial Level I	Reduced time-out of work, reduced sick days, and increased occupational function for those in the integrated care group	Time before return to work was significantly shorter for integrated care group (88 days in the integrated care group and 208 days in the control group; log-rank test, $p = 0.003$). Median number of sick days in 12-month follow-up period were significantly fewer (82 in the integrated care group and 175 in the control group; Mann–Whitney U test, $p = 0.003$). After 12 months, the integrated care group experienced a significantly higher level of functional status ($p = 0.01$).

Occupational therapy interventions for adults with fibromyalgia[24]	Systematic review. Included studies were peer-reviewed and conducted between 2000 and 2014 and featured an intervention approach. Studies were not all conducted by occupational therapists, but fall within the practice domain of OT.	Forty-two articles were reviewed in the areas of cognitive–behavioral ($n = 3$), self-management ($n = 2$), relaxation and stress management ($n = 5$), and emotional disclosure ($n = 3$). Included studies featured adult populations with FM diagnosis.	Dosage varied by study.	Systematic review Level I	Strongest evidence supports physical activity to improve pain and function, moderately strong evidence supports multidisciplinary interventions for reducing pain and depression, improving function. Some evidence indicates that CBT facilitates pain reduction, and improved mood and function. Low-quality evidence supports mindfulness-based stress reduction for short-term benefits.	No statistical analysis
Yoga of awareness program to manage fibromyalgia[62]	Manualized gentle yoga poses, meditation, breathing exercises, group discussion, and study of yoga principles to develop coping skills. The program was delivered by a certified yoga teacher.	Participants were all females 21+ years old. All had diagnosis of FM for at least 1 year and had adhered to medical treatment regimen for >3 months. These were assigned to yoga intervention group ($n = 25$) and waitlist control group ($n = 28$).	Classes were conducted once a week for 8 weeks. Classes lasted 120 minutes and included 7–12 participants. Each class included 40 minutes of stretching, 25 minutes of meditation, 10 minutes of breathing techniques, 20 minutes of coping education, and 25 minutes of group discussion.	Randomized controlled trial Level I	Yoga participants experienced reduced symptoms, pain, fatigue, stiffness, depression, anxiety, tenderness, and environmental sensitivity. They also experienced improved social and activity engagement, memory, and balance.	Significant benefit for yoga group shown in pain, fatigue, stiffness, sleep, depression, memory, anxiety, tenderness, balance, and environmental sensitivity as assessed by Fibromyalgia Impact Questionnaire–Revised ($p = 0.003$). Via diary, yoga group also demonstrated significant improvement in the areas of pain ($b = -1.47$, $t = -5.90$, $p < 0.0001$), fatigue ($b = -1.68$, $t = -6.23$, $p < 0.0001$), emotional distress ($b = -1.34$, $t = -4.92$, $p < 0.0001$), vigor ($b = 0.92$, $t = 3.62$, $p = 0.0005$), success at acceptance ($b = 1.20$, $t = 5.10$, $p < 0.0001$) and relaxation ($b = 1.38$, $t = 4.36$, $p < 0.0001$).

References

1. Treede RD, Rief W, Barke A, et al. A classification of chronic pain for ICD-11. *Pain*. 2015;156(6):1003–1007. doi:10.1097/j.pain.0000000000000160.
2. International Association for the Study of Pain and European Federation of IASP Chapters. Unrelieved pain is a major global healthcare problem. https://s3.amazonaws.com/rdcms-iasp/files/production/public/Content/ContentFolders/GlobalYearAgainstPain2/20042005RighttoPainRelief/factsheet.pdf. Accessed February 7, 2019.
3. Hedari F, Afshari M, Moosazadeh M. Prevalence of fibromyalgia in general population and patients, a systematic review and meta-analysis. *Rheumatol Int*. 2017;37:1527–1539. doi:10.1007/s00296-017-3725-2.
4. Lichtenstein A, Tiosano S, Amital H. The complexities of fibromyalgia and its comorbidities. *Curr Opin Rheumatol*. 2018;30(1):94–100.doi:10.1097/BOR.0000000000000464.
5. Querioz LP. Worldwide epidemiology of fibromyalgia. *Curr Pain Headache Rep*. 2013;17(8):356–361. doi:10.1007/s11916-013-0356-5.
6. Rahman A, Underwood M, Carnes D. Clinical review: fibromyalgia. *BMJ*. 2014;348:g1224.
7. Clauw DJ. Fibromyalgia: a clinical review. *JAMA*. 2014;311(15):1547–1555. doi:10.1001/jama.2014.3266.
8. Arnold LM, Choy E, Clauw DJ, et al. Fibromyalgia and chronic pain syndromes: a white paper detailing current challenges in the field. *Clin J Pain*. 2016;32(9):737–746. doi:10.1097/AJP.0000000000000354.
9. Buchbinder R, van Tulder M, Öberg B, et al. Low back pain: a call for action. *Lancet*. 2018;391(10137):2384–2388. doi:10.1016/S0140-6736(18)30488-4.
10. Hartvigsen J, Hancock MJ, Kongsted A. What low back pain is and why we need to pay attention. *Lancet*. 2018;391(10137):2356–2367. doi:10.1016/S0140-6736(18)30480-X.
11. Maher C, Underwood M, Buchbinder R. Non-specific low back pain. *Lancet*. 2017;389(10070):736–747. doi:10.1016/S0140-6736(16)30970-9.
12. Phillips K, Clauw DJ. Central pain mechanisms in chronic pain states—maybe it is all in their head. *Best Pract Res Clin Rheumatol*. 2011;(25):141–154. doi:10.1016/j.berh.2011.02.005.
13. Chetty L. A critical review of low back pain guidelines. *Workplace Health Saf*. 2017;65(9):388–394. doi:10.1177/2165079917702384.
14. O'Connell NE, Cook CE, Wand BM, Ward SP. Clinical guidelines for low back pain: a critical review of consensus and inconsistencies across three major guidelines. *Best Pract Res Clin Rheumatol*. 2016;30(6):968–980. doi:10.1016/j.berh.2017.05.001.
15. Szpalski M, Gunzburg R, Rydevik BL, Le Heuc JL, Mayer HM, eds. *Surgery for Low Back Pain*. New York, NY: Springer; 2018.
16. Pope JE, Deer TR, eds. *Treatment of Chronic Pain Conditions: A Comprehensive Handbook*. New York, NY: Springer; 2017.
17. Foster NE, Anema JR, Chenkin D, et al. Prevention and treatment of low back pain: evidence, challenges, and promising directions. *Lancet*. 2018;391(10137):2368–2383. doi:10.1016/S0140-6736(18)30489-6.
18. Roussel NA, Nijs J, Meeus M, Mylius V, Fayt C, Oostendorp R. Central sensitization and altered central pain processing in chronic low back pain: fact or myth? *Clin J Pain*. 2013;29(7):625–638.doi:10.1097/AJP.0b013e31826f9a71.
19. Yunus MB. The role of central sensitization in symptoms beyond muscle pain, and the evaluation of a patient with widespread pain. *Best Pract Res Clin Rheumatol*. 2007;(21):481–497. doi:10.1016/j.berh.2007.03.006.
20. Curatolo M, Arendt-Nielsen L, Petersen-Felix S. Central hypersensitivity in chronic pain: mechanisms and clinical implications. *Phys Med Rehabil Clin N Am*. 2006;(17):287–302. doi:10.1016/j.pmr.2005.12.010.
21. Woolf CJ. Central sensitization: implications for the diagnosis and treatment of pain. *Pain*. 2011;152(3):S2–S15. doi:10.1016/j.pain.2010.09.030.
22. Solà JF. Central sensitization syndrome: towards the structuring of a multidisciplinary concept. *Med Clín*. 2018;2(23):68–70. doi:10.1016/j.medcle.2018.05.026.
23. Simon AU, Collins CER. Lifestyle Redesign® for chronic pain management: a retrospective clinical efficacy study. *Am J Occup Ther*. 2017;(71):7104190040. doi:10.5014/ajot.2017.025502.
24. Poole JL, Siegel P. Effectiveness of occupational therapy interventions for adults with fibromyalgia: a systematic review. *Am J Occup Ther*. 2017;71(1):7101180040p1–7101180040p10. doi:10.5014/ajot.2017.023192.
25. Ballantyne JC, Sullivan MD. Intensity of chronic pain—the wrong metric? *N Engl J Med*. 2015;373(22):2098–2099. doi:10.1056/NEJMp1507136.
26. Hawker GA, Mian S, Kendzerska T, French M. Measures of adult pain: Visual Analog Scale for Pain (VAS pain), Numeric Rating Scale for Pain (NRS pain), Mcgill Pain Questionnaire (MPQ), Short-Form Mcgill Pain Questionnaire (sf-mpq), Chronic Pain Grade Scale (CPGS), Short Form-36 Bodily Pain Scale (SF-36 BPS), and Measure of Intermittent and Constant Osteoarthritis Pain (ICOAP). *Arthritis Care Res*. 2011;63(S11):S240–S252. doi:10.1002/acr.20543.
27. Pollard CA. Preliminary validity study of the Pain Disability Index. *Percept Mot Skills*. 1984;59(3):974. doi:10.2466/pms.1984.59.3.974.
28. Grönblad M, Hupli M, Wennerstrand P, et al. Intercorrelation and test–retest reliability of the Pain Disability Index (PDI) and the Oswestry Disability Questionnaire (ODQ) and their correlation with pain intensity in low back pain patients. *Clin J Pain*. 1993;9(3):189–195.
29. Tait RC, Pollard CA, Margolis RB, Duckro PN, Krause SJ. The Pain Disability Index: psychometric and validity data. *Arch Phys Med Rehabil*. 1987;68(7):438–441. https://www.researchgate.net/profile/Raymond_Tait/publication/19556299_The_Pain_Disability_Index_Psychometric_and_validity_data/links/543c0c150cf2d6698be3640d/The-Pain-Disability-Index-Psychometric-and-validity-data.pdf
30. Cleeland CS, Ryan KM. Pain assessment: global use of the Brief Pain Inventory. *Ann Acad Med Singapore*. 1994;23(2):129–138.
31. Pelayo-Alvarez M, Perez-Hoyos S, Agra-Varela Y. Reliability and concurrent validity of the Palliative Outcome Scale, the Rotterdam Symptom Checklist, and the

Brief Pain Inventory. *J Palliat Med*. 2013;16(8):867–874. doi:10.1089/jpm.2012.0625.
32. Wu JS, Beaton D, Smith PM, Hagen NA. Patterns of pain and interference in patients with painful bone metastases: a brief pain inventory validation study. *J Pain Symptom Manage*. 2010;39(2):230–240. doi:10.1016/j.jpainsymman.2009.07.006.
33. Gjeilo KH, Stenseth R, Wahba A, Lydersen S, Klepstad P. Validation of the Brief Pain Inventory in patients six months after cardiac surgery. *J Pain Symptom Manage*. 2007;34(6):648–656. doi:10.1016/j.jpainsymman.2007.01.010.
34. Law M, Polatajko H, Pollock N, Mccoll MA, Carswell A, Baptiste S. Pilot testing of the Canadian Occupational Performance Measure: clinical and measurement issues. *Can J Occup Ther*. 1994;61(4):191–197. doi:10.1177/000841749406100403.
35. Law M, Baptiste S, Carswell A, McColl MA, Polatajko H, Pollack N. *Canadian Occupational Performance Measure*. 4th ed. Ottawa, ON: Canadian Association of Occupational Therapy; 2005.
36. Cup EH, Scholte op Reimer WJ, Thijssen MC, van Kuyk-Minis MA. Reliability and validity of the Canadian Occupational Performance Measure in stroke patients. *Clin Rehabil*. 2003;17:402–409. doi:10.1191/0269215503cr635oa.
37. Eyssen IC, Beelen A, Dedding C, Cardol M, Dekker J. The reproducibility of the Canadian Occupational Performance Measure. *Clin Rehabil*. 2005;19:888–894. doi:10.1191/0269215505cr883oa.
38. Dedding C, Cardol M, Eyssen IC, Dekker J, Beelen A. Validity of the Canadian Occupational Performance Measure: a client-centered outcome measurement. *Clin Rehabil*. 2004;18:660–667. doi:10.1191/0269215504cr746oa.
39. Boakye PA, Olechowski C, Rashiq S, et al. A critical review of neurobiological factors involved in the interactions between chronic pain, depression, and sleep disruption. *Clin J Pain*. 2016;32(4):327–336. doi:10.1097/AJP.0000000000000260.
40. Fischer S, Doerr JM, Strahler J, Mewes R, Thieme K, Nater UM. Stress exacerbates pain in the everyday lives of women with fibromyalgia syndrome—the role of cortisol and alpha-amylase. *Psychoneuroendocrinology*. 2016;63:68–77. doi:10.1016/j.psyneuen.2015.09.018.
41. Telles S, Gerbarg P, Kozasa EH. Physiological effects of mind and body practices. *BioMed Res Int*. 2015;2015:983086. doi:10.1155/2015/983086.
42. Turner JA, Anderson ML, Balderson BH, Cook AJ, Sherman KJ, Cherkin DC. Mindfulness-based stress reduction and cognitive behavioral therapy for chronic low back pain: similar effects on mindfulness, catastrophizing, self-efficacy, and acceptance in a randomized controlled trial. *Pain*. 2016;157(11):2434–2444. doi:10.1097/j.pain.0000000000000635.
43. Timmermans EJ, Schaap LA, Herbolsheimer F, et al. The influence of weather conditions on joint pain in older people with osteoarthritis: results from the European project on OSteoArthritis. *J Rheumatol*. 2015;42:1885–1892. doi:10.3899/jrheum.141594.
44. Shulman BS, Marcano AI, Davidovitch RI, Karia R, Egol KA. Nature's wrath—the effect of weather on pain following orthopaedic trauma. *Injury*. 2016;47(8):1841–1846. doi:10.1016/j.injury.2016.05.043.
45. Timmermans EJ, van der Pas S, Dennison EM, et al. The influence of weather conditions on outdoor physical activity among older people with and without osteoarthritis in 6 European countries. *J Phys Act Health*. 2016;13(12):1385–1395. doi:10.1123/jpah.2016-0040.
46. Okifuji A, Hare BD. The association between chronic pain and obesity. *J Pain Res*. 2015;8:399–408. doi:10.2147/JPR.S55598.
47. Hedge A. *Ergonomic Workplace Design for Health, Wellness and Productivity*. Boca Raton, FL: CRC Press; 2016.
48. Dailey DL, Law LA, Vance CG, et al. Perceived function and physical performance are associated with pain and fatigue in women with fibromyalgia. *Arthritis Res Ther*. 2016;18(1):68. doi:10.1186/s13075-016-0954-9.
49. Bracciano A. *Physical Agent Modalities: Theory and Application for the Occupational Therapist*. 3rd ed. Thorofare, NJ: Slack; 2019.
50. Malanga GA, Yan N, Stark J. Mechanisms and efficacy of heat and cold therapies for musculoskeletal injury. *Postgrad Med*. 2015;127(1):57–65. doi:10.1080/00325481.2015.992719.
51. Jauregui JJ, Cherian JJ, Gwam CU, et al. A meta-analysis of transcutaneous electrical nerve stimulation for chronic low back pain. *Surg Technol Int*. 2016;28:296–302. https://www.researchgate.net/profile/Jaydev_Mistry/publication/299715553_A_Meta-Analysis_of_Transcutaneous_Electrical_Nerve_Stimulation_for_Chronic_Low_Back_Pain/links/570cecba08aed31341cef997.pdf
52. Sielski R, Rief W, Glombiewski JA. Efficacy of biofeedback in chronic back pain: a meta-analysis. *Int J Behav Med*. 2017;24(1):25–41. doi:10.1007/s12529-016-9572-9.
53. Vickers AJ, Vertosick EA, Lewith G, et al. Acupuncture for chronic pain: update of an individual patient data meta-analysis. *J Pain*. 2018;19(5):455–474. doi:10.1016/j.jpain.2017.11.005.
54. Lin WC, Yeh CH, Chien LC, Morone NE, Glick RM, Albers KM. The anti-inflammatory actions of auricular point acupressure for chronic low back pain. *Evid Based Complement Alternat Med*. 2015;2015:103570. doi:10.1155/2015/103570.
55. Yu X, Lim CF, Zaslawski C, Cheng YW. Tai chi for chronic pain conditions: what does the meta-analysis tell us? *Focus Altern Complement Ther*. 2016;21(34):180–182. doi:10.1111/fct.12267.
56. Hilton L, Hempel S, Ewing BA, et al. Mindfulness meditation for chronic pain: systematic review and meta-analysis. *Ann Behav Med*. 2016;51(2):199–213. doi:10.1007/s12160-016-9844-2.
57. Cramer H, Klose P, Brinkhaus B, Michalsen A, Dobos G. Effects of yoga on chronic neck pain: a systematic review and meta-analysis. *Clin Rehabil*. 2017;31(11):1457–1465. doi:10.1177/0269215517698735
58. Marletta G, Canfora A, Roscani F, et al. The complementary medicine (CAM) for the treatment of chronic pain: scientific evidence regarding the effects of healing touch massage. *Acta Biomed*. 2015;86(2 suppl):127–133. http://www.mattioli1885journals.com/index.php/actabiomedica/article/view/4795
59. Rubik B, Muehsam D, Hammerschlag R, Jain S. Biofield science and healing: history, terminology, and concepts.

Glob Adv Health Med. 2015;4(suppl):8. doi:10.7453/gahmj.2015.038.suppl.
60. Gore M, Sadosky A, Stacey BR, Tai KS, Leslie D. The burden of chronic low back pain: clinical comorbidities, treatment patterns, and health care costs in usual care settings. *Spine.* 2012;37(11):E668–E677. doi:10.1097/BRS.0b013e318241e5de.
61. Lambeek LC, van Mechelen W, Knol DL, Loisel P, Anema JR. Randomised controlled trial of integrated care to reduce disability from chronic low back pain in working and private life. *BMJ.* 2010;340:c1035. doi:10.1136/bmj.c1035.
62. Carson JW, Carson KM, Jones KD, Bennett RM, Wright CL, Mist SD. A pilot randomized controlled trial of the Yoga of Awareness program in the management of fibromyalgia. *Pain.* 2010;151(2):530–539. doi:10.1016/j.pain.2010.08.020.

Chapter 50

Human Immunodeficiency Virus

Gayle J. Restall

LEARNING OBJECTIVES

This chapter will allow the reader to:

1. Understand the social and epidemiological history of HIV/AIDS in the United States, focusing on the populations most prevalently infected.
2. Summarize the natural history of HIV and its concomitant medical and social trajectories.
3. Extrapolate the effects of HIV/AIDS on the occupations of people living with HIV/AIDS.
4. Select tools and assessment strategies to ascertain the occupational needs of individuals living with HIV/AIDS.
5. Describe intervention strategies to maintain, restore, and promote meaningful occupations of individuals living with HIV/AIDS.

CHAPTER OUTLINE

TERMINOLOGY

Cultural safety: the creation of environments in which people feel safe and are not assaulted for who they are and what they need; it involves respect, shared meaning, knowledge, and experience[1]; to attain cultural safety, occupational therapists must understand their own positionality, and the social and historical context in which clinical encounters occur.

HAART: an acronym for highly active antiretroviral therapy, which is a combination of pharmaceutical interventions configured to act on HIV at different points of reproduction of the virus.

Health inequities: unfair and unjust systematic differences in the health status of groups of people as the result of social factors, including ethnicity, gender, education, employment, and socioeconomic status.

Opportunistic infections: infections that occur when organisms that are normally not harmful become pathogenic when the body's immune system is compromised.[2]

Retrovirus: a virus that can make copies of itself in host cells because it has an enzyme called reverse transcriptase that enables transcription of RNA to DNA.[2]

Description of Human Immunodeficiency Virus

Introduction

Human immunodeficiency virus (HIV) is a **retrovirus** that attacks the immune system and over time leads to acquired immunodeficiency syndrome (AIDS)—a condition in which progressive immune system failure allows fatal **opportunistic infections** to thrive in the human body. The symptoms associated with HIV were first described in 1981,[3–5] and later in 1993, AIDS was officially defined.[6] Surveillance systems for both HIV and AIDS have been established and revised in the United States[7,8] and internationally.[9,10] HIV/AIDS is regarded as a global pandemic because it has dramatically affected nations and populations throughout the world. Initially a fatal diagnosis, life expectancies have increased as a result of advances in medical management; HIV/AIDS is now considered a chronic disease.[11] Primary, secondary, and tertiary prevention strategies continue to be important to prevent the spread of the virus, prevent AIDS-related deaths, and support patients' ability to successfully age with HIV. The experiences and life trajectories of people aging with HIV are influenced by multiple health and social factors. The biological and physical aspects of HIV/AIDS have been systematically studied and documented, but the more variable social trajectory continues to be shaped by the sociopolitical context in which individuals experience the disease. Consequently, quality of life after diagnosis is highly contingent on resources, supports, and access to relevant treatment. Occupational therapists can provide valuable programs and services to improve the lives of people with HIV/AIDS.

Epidemiology

HIV/AIDS Globally

According to the World Health Organization (WHO), 36.7 million people were living with HIV/AIDS in 2016.[12] Of those living with HIV/AIDS, 17.8 million were women aged 15 years or older, whereas 2.1 million were children and adolescents under the age of 15. Approximately 1.8 million new HIV infections occurred in 2016, representing a decline of 16% from 2010 estimates.[12] Changes in the annual number of new infections between 2010 and 2016 varied among global regions with the steepest declines in eastern and southern Africa (29%), as compared to 60% increases in eastern Europe and central Asia. In comparison, North America and western and central Europe experienced a 9% decline in annual rates of new infections. Estimates of the extent of the global HIV/AIDS pandemic are complicated by differences in surveillance methodology. Nevertheless, annual AIDS-related deaths peaked at around 1.9 million in 2005 and fell to 1.0 million in 2016. The decline in deaths has been attributed primarily to antiretroviral therapy (ART). Despite substantial declines, AIDS-related illnesses continue to be the leading cause of death worldwide for women aged 15 to 59 years.[12]

Populations and subgroups most affected by HIV/AIDS vary greatly by country and prevailing social, economic, and political conditions; however, the WHO has identified five key populations that are at increased risk of contracting HIV: men who have sex with men, people who inject drugs, people in prisons and other closed settings, sex workers, and transgender people.[13] These populations are not mutually exclusive and often experience social contexts that increase their vulnerability

In 2014, the WHO advanced the 90-90-90 targets for ending the AIDS epidemic: (1) 90% of people with HIV know their HIV status, (2) 90% of people diagnosed with HIV receive ongoing ART, and (3) 90% of people receiving ART have viral suppression.[14] The WHO predicted that achieving these targets would prevent HIV-related illnesses, AIDS-related deaths, and new HIV infections, ending the AIDS epidemic by 2030. Acknowledging the social, political, and economic drivers of both the HIV epidemic and the response to HIV, the Joint United Nations Programme on HIV/AIDS (UNAIDS) has stressed the importance of multisectoral collaboration to address factors including inequality, poverty, education, economic growth, peace, safe cities, **cultural safety**, and healthy living.[15]

HIV/AIDS in the United States

At the end of 2015, 973,846 people were living with a diagnosis of HIV in the United States, and approximately 15% more were infected but undiagnosed.[16] Incidence rates of new infections have decreased by 8% from 2010 to 2015.[16] Despite these advances, HIV/AIDS remains a significant cause of death in the United States. In 2016, the most frequent modes of transmission for new HIV diagnoses were male-to-male sexual contact (67%), heterosexual contact (24%), injection drug use (6%), and combined male-to-male sexual contact and injection drug use (3%).[16] From 2011 to 2015, males accounted for 81% of new diagnoses.[16] At the end of 2015, 71% of males living with HIV 13 years of age and older were believed to have contracted the virus through male-to-male sexual contact. In contrast, 87% of new diagnoses for females 13 years of age and older were attributed to heterosexual contact.[16] Blacks/African Americans have the highest prevalence rates of HIV infection among racial and ethnic groups. In 2016, women accounted for 19% of new diagnoses, 61% of whom were black/African American.[17] Drug therapies administered during the perinatal period have substantially reduced transmission from mother to child. HIV infection rates among infants have diminished, with 99 new diagnoses of perinatal HIV transmission in 2016.[18]

Etiology

HIV is a retrovirus that results in a gradual deterioration of the immune system. Once the virus enters the human body, it overwhelms the CD4+ T cells that usually defend the body against viruses. HIV converts its own RNA into a form that can be recognized and replicated using the DNA of the host, a process called transcription. Once emitted into the cytoplasm of the cell, this reconfigured virus translates itself prolifically, producing new copies and long chains of viral proteins that mature into new infectious particles that are emitted into other cells. The damage to the immune system makes it increasingly difficult for the body to resist other infections and diseases, and the person becomes more susceptible to opportunistic infections.[2] HIV is transmitted through person-to-person contact with blood, semen, pre-seminal fluid, rectal fluids, vaginal fluids, and breast milk. Studies have shown that HIV does not live long outside the body and is not spread through contact with saliva, sweat, or tears, or through air or water.[19] HIV status is confirmed by blood tests such as nucleic acid tests, antigen/antibody tests, and antibody tests. Rapid screening tests, oral antibody self-tests, and home collection tests are becoming increasingly available and, if positive, need to be followed by a confirmatory test.[20] Universal screening programs have been advocated because many people living with HIV remain undiagnosed.

It is rare for health care providers to contract HIV through patient contact. In these cases, transmission is most likely to occur as a result of a piercing from a contaminated needle or other sharp item.[21] Precautions are advised if the provider is handling blood and blood products, regardless of whether HIV infection or risk status is known.[22] Universal precautions include using barriers such as gloves and masks, washing skin that comes in contact with bodily fluid, and safe and careful disposal of sharps. Special care should be taken to avoid exposing HIV-positive persons to infectious agents because their compromised immunity makes them more vulnerable to opportunistic infections that can cause serious health consequences.

Course, Prognosis, and Contextual Factors

Different strains of HIV have been identified.[23] Viral load and strength of a particular HIV strain have been associated with the rate of disease progression. HIV-1 is the most common strain in the United States and worldwide, and is associated with a more rapid progression than the HIV-2 strain found in some areas of West Africa. Some people seem to be resistant to rapid translation of the virus, and there is a minority of individuals who do not progress through clinical stages even without being on ART.[23] Concurrent diseases or poor health status before infection can increase vulnerability and complicate medical interventions. Early detection of infections and adherence to medication regimens can prevent or slow the virus from usurping the immune system in people who respond positively to medications.

Sociopolitical Context of HIV/AIDS

HIV infection is most frequently attributed to unprotected sexual intercourse. Globally, infections rates are highest among women who have sex with men. People experiencing poverty in poorly resourced countries are more vulnerable to the spread of HIV. According to 2015 data, sub-Saharan Africa represented 66% of new HIV infections worldwide, 47% of which were women aged 15 years and older.[24] In the United States, HIV is still most prevalent among men who have sex with men; however, the incidence of infection attributed to heterosexual sex is rising. HIV disproportionally affects minority groups, particularly African Americans.[17] The distribution of HIV represents an alarming health disparity globally and in the United States.

Stigma and Discrimination

HIV is a highly stigmatized health condition. In North America, men who have sex with men, people of color (Black/African American, Hispanic/Latino, and Indigenous), transgender women, injection drug users, and sex workers are overrepresented in the population of people living with HIV. People associated with socially stigmatized identities, in addition to HIV, can have compounded experiences of oppression. Crenshaw initially coined the term intersectionality to describe how being a woman and being black intersected in the experiences of oppression.[25] Since that time, intersectionality has become an important way of conceptualizing people's experiences resulting from multiple stigmatized identities. Occupational therapists need to recognize and understand the ways that people living with HIV can experience intersecting forms of stigma and discrimination. Therapists need to develop cultural humility and implement culturally safe practices to promote productive therapeutic relationships based on inclusion, trust, and respect.[26] Therapists also need to identify and respond to **health inequities** that result from historical and current injustices, diverse identities, living arrangements, and access to opportunities that promote health and well-being. Ensuring knowledge of and linkage to external health, social, and peer support services, and advocacy for fair and just policies and practices are important strategies.

Because of the risks for discrimination within the environments in which people with HIV live, work, spend leisure time, and build meaningful relationships, disclosure of HIV status can be a complex decision. The criminalization of HIV nondisclosure, in situations in which HIV transmission is likely, is embedded in laws in many jurisdictions and further compounds disclosure decision-making. Despite the lack of evidence that HIV nondisclosure laws have reduced transmission rates, and in the context of successful prevention and treatment, these laws persist.[27] People living with HIV have protections under anti-discrimination legislation, and occupational therapists should be aware of these protections and connect people with resources to help them understand their confidentiality rights. Efforts to reduce HIV-associated stigma are important to promote prevention, testing, and linkage to care.

Signs and Symptoms

Without treatment, people with HIV typically progress through stages.[19] Stage 1 is the acute infection period in which people with HIV are highly infectious. Within 2 to 4 weeks of initial exposure, most, although not all people infected with HIV experience flulike symptoms, such as fever, headache, chills, rash, sore throat, fatigue, mouth ulcers, and enlarged lymph nodes. Until the body's immune system is depleted of resources to combat the virus, the infected person may not experience further symptoms. Many people remain unaware that they have the virus.[20] Stage 2 is the chronic stage in which the virus is active but reproduces at low levels, leaving the individual with few symptoms; however, the virus can still be transmitted during this stage. For some people who are not taking medications, this stage may last up to a decade or be much shorter. For many people with HIV who take ART medications as prescribed, this stage may last several decades. In addition, with medications, people's viral load can be suppressed to very low levels with much less likelihood of virus transmission. Stage 3 is AIDS; symptoms include weakness, weight loss, chills, fevers, sweats, and swollen lymph glands. A diagnosis of AIDS is made when a person with HIV has a CD4 count less than 200 cells per mm^3 or has an AIDS-defining condition that includes opportunistic infections and life-threatening cancers.[28]

As the disease progresses, people with HIV often experience HIV-associated neurocognitive disorders (HANDs), characterized by impairment with memory, concentration, attention, and motor skills. The symptoms have been classified into three conditions according to symptom severity and functional impairment:

- Asymptomatic neurocognitive impairment (ANI)
- HIV-associated mild neurocognitive disorder (MND)
- HIV-associated dementia (HAD)[29]

People living with HIV experience higher rates of mental health conditions than the general public.[30] These conditions can include depression, anxiety, and post-traumatic stress disorder. In addition, stressful life situations, HIV infection, opportunistic infections, and/or some medicines used to treat HIV may contribute to the development of mental health conditions.

Aging with HIV

The success of current medication regimes has meant that many people with HIV are living long-term. People aged 50 years and older account for approximately 45% of Americans living with HIV and comprise two distinct groups.[31] One group consists of people newly diagnosed. In 2015, 17% of new HIV diagnoses in the United States were attributed to people aged 50 years and older.[31] The second group consists of people living long-term with HIV as the result of successful treatments that have transformed HIV into a chronic health condition. This latter group comprises the majority and will continue to increase in numbers, presenting unique and not yet fully understood challenges to HIV intervention for successful aging.

People aging with long-term HIV are at higher risk of co-occurring chronic health conditions, including cardiovascular disease, some cancers, kidney disease, liver disease, cognitive impairment, frailty, and bone disease.[32,33] These comorbid conditions tend to occur at younger ages and with greater frequency as compared to the general population and may be related to multiple social and other risk factors, in addition to the direct effect of HIV and antiretroviral treatments.[31] As people living with HIV age, co-occurring chronic health conditions can increase the risk for and experience of functional impairments that can restrict engagement in meaningful activities. Promoting physical and psychosocial well-being should be a priority with attention to early and sustained treatment; control of risk factors; addressing health disparities through health care, and health and social policy initiatives; strategies to reduce stigma and discrimination; interventions to promote health such as physical activities; and social support networks.[31] People living with HIV have identified the importance of maintaining social support networks, taking responsibility for their health, assuming a healthy lifestyle, and taking part in meaningful activities important to aging well.[34]

Medical Management

The best treatment for HIV is prevention. Prevention strategies entail raising public awareness, providing education, and promoting individual behaviors that avoid risk or minimize harm. Proper and consistent condom use during anal and vaginal sex is an important universal prevention strategy. For people who use injection drugs, harm reduction strategies have been shown to be safe and effective, and include needle and syringe exchange programs, and opioid substitution treatments.[35,36]

Pre-exposure prophylaxis (PrEP)—a combination of two antiretroviral drugs (tenofovir disoproxil fumarate and emtricitabine)—is an option for those at high risk, including HIV-negative partners in serodiscordant relationships, injection drug users who share needles, and people who frequently have unprotected sex.[37,38] For individuals who are at incidental risk for exposure to HIV, such as occupational exposure when handling blood products or after sexual assault, postexposure regimes of antiretroviral medications started as soon as possible and within 72 hours with follow-up are recommended.[39,40]

Advances in pharmaceutical interventions have increased survival and extended years of quality life. ART consists of a combination of pharmaceuticals to treat HIV and should be started as soon as possible. Currently, there are seven classes of drugs used to treat HIV, and most people take a combination of three drugs from at least two drug classes. Combination therapies, called highly active antiretroviral therapy (**HAART**), are aimed at preventing HIV from reproducing itself, thus reducing the loss of CD4 cells that have the important function of helping the body to fight infections.[41] Thus, ART medications can maintain or increase the CD4 cells in the system while reducing viral load (Fig. 50-1). Consistent use of ART medications, in many people, can suppress viral loads to levels that are essentially undetectable by HIV viral load tests.[28] In addition, there is now a convincing body of evidence that a person with sustained undetectable viral loads cannot transmit the virus through sexual contact.[42,43] Long-term use of HAART is associated with side effects, including fat redistribution, liver damage and disease, insulin resistance, osteoporosis, nervous system effects, and psychiatric disorders.[41] Despite such side effects, these medications have clear advantages for increasing life expectancy of people living with HIV and for preventing the virus' spread.

Mother-to-child transmission of HIV during pregnancy, childbirth, and breastfeeding can also be prevented. Mothers taking HIV medications throughout pregnancy, labor, and delivery; who provide HIV medications to their baby for 4 to 6 weeks; and who do not breast feed or pre-chew their baby's food, have reduced the risk of transmission to approximately 1%.[18] The Centers for Disease Control and Prevention recommend that all pregnant women be routinely tested for HIV.

Functional Impairment in Daily Occupation

The symptoms and impairments resulting from HIV and its treatments, as well as sociopolitical barriers such as poverty and discrimination, can affect many aspects of people's lives, including their ability to engage in meaningful activities and social roles. Understanding the complexity of these roles for a client with HIV is important

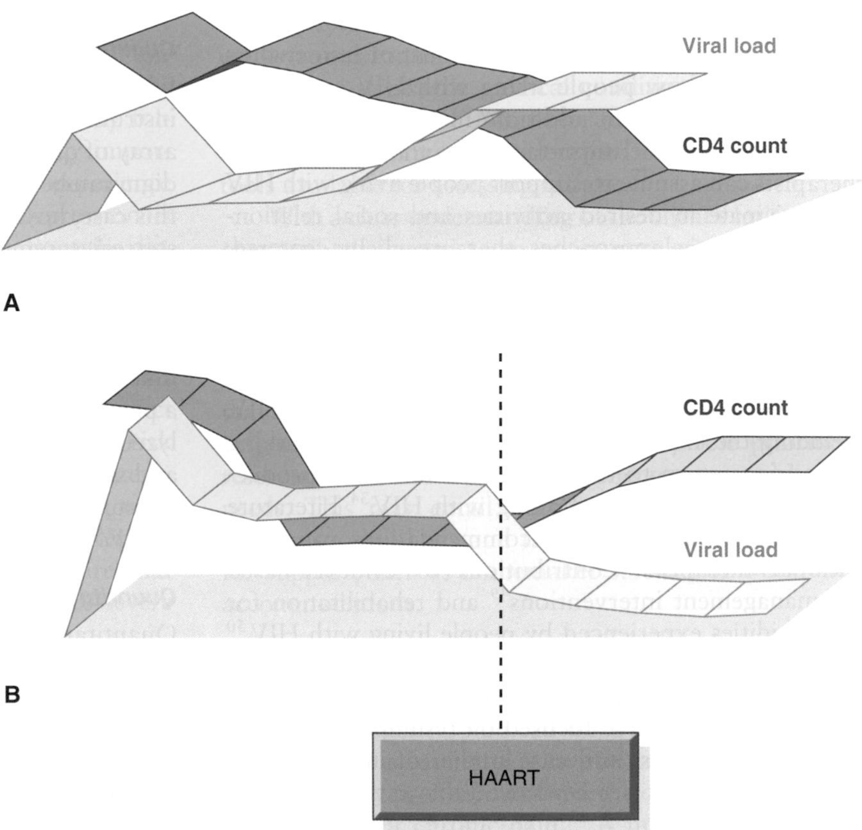

Figure 50-1. A. Natural progression of human immunodeficiency virus (HIV) infection. **B.** Progression of HIV infection with highly active antiretroviral therapy (HAART).

Evidence Table for Occupational Therapy HIV/AIDS Intervention Studies (*continued*)

Intervention	Intervention Description	Participants	Dosage	Research Design and Evidence Level	Benefit	Statistical Significance and Effect Size
A 2-year pilot program to improve balancing health, work, and daily life that combined job skills training with chronic disease self-management[54]	The job skills training program entailed daily participation to which 6-biweekly sessions were added to address disease self-management, health, vocational performance, and quality of life.	Six groups of adults ($n = 53$) participated in the program over a 2-year period, 28 females and 25 males diagnosed with HIV 4+ years. Forty-two participants contacted 3–5 months postintervention. Twenty-one percent lost to follow-up.	For 6–7 weeks, 6 hours per day. Six 1.5-hour self-management focused sessions were integrated into an existing job skills training program to facilitate transition to work. Topics included balancing work and daily life, energy conservation, and nutrition.	Nonrandomized groups (6) received the same intervention over a 2-year period with pre- and post-examination of up to 42 individuals on key outcomes as measured by 11 scales, including the Canadian Occupational Performance Measure. Level III	Fifty-two percent of retained participants were working successfully, with another 41% actively seeking employment.	Outcome was determined using paired t tests and effect sizes. Three of the 11 scales indicated moderate-to-large effect sizes upon follow-up: perceived ability to balance health, work, and daily life ($r = 0.46$); health management and work ($r = 0.61$); and perceived ability to work ($r = 0.72$). However, only perceived ability to work showed significant ($p = 0.00$) improvement after treatment, which indicated that the outcome was probably not owing to chance.
Case studies of occupational therapy interventions with three people living with HIV who had diverse comorbidities and impairments[55]	Interventions were tailored to each of the clients' goals and assessment results. Interventions primarily occurred within clients homes and included promotion of ADLs and IADLs, environmental modification for home safety, recommendations for equipment, community navigation, priority setting, problem-solving, energy conservation, planning for stable housing, and home exercise program.	Client 1 was a 57-year-old single white male who was HIV positive for 28 years. Client 2 was a 50-year-old single black male who was HIV positive for 12 years. Client 3 was a 28-year-old single black female who was HIV positive for 8 years.	Client 1 had seven home sessions and three follow-up phone calls. Client had 12 home sessions and on home follow-up appointment. Client 3 had six home sessions and one follow-up phone call.	Descriptive case reports Level NA	Client 1 had little positive change and declined in some areas. Clients 2 and 3 showed positive changes in several areas.	No statistical analysis

References

1. Williams R. Cultural safety—what does it mean for our work practice? *Aust N Z J Public Health*. 1999;23(2):213–214.
2. Porta M. *Dictionary of Epidemiology*. Oxford: Oxford University Press Incorporated; 2014. Accessed May 14, 2018.
3. Gottlieb MS, Schroff R, Schanker HM, et al. *Pneumocystis carinii* pneumonia and mucosal candidiasis in previously healthy homosexual men: evidence of a new acquired cellular immunodeficiency. *N Engl J Med*. 1981;305:1425–1431.
4. Masur H, Michelis MA, Greene JB, et al. An outbreak of community-acquired *Pneumocystis carinii* pneumonia: initial manifestation of cellular immune dysfunction. *N Engl J Med*. 1981;305:1431–1438.
5. Siegal FP, Lopez C, Hammer GS, et al. Severe acquired immunodeficiency in male homosexuals, manifested by chronic perianal ulcerative herpes simplex lesions. *N Engl J Med*. 1981;305:1439–1444.
6. Centers for Disease Control and Prevention. 1993 revised classification system for HIV infection and expanded surveillance case definition for AIDS among adolescents and adults. *MMWR Recomm Rep*. 1992;41(RR-17):1–19. https://www.cdc.gov/mmwr/preview/mmwrhtml/00018871.htm. Accessed November 9, 2018.
7. Centers for Disease Control and Prevention. CDC guidelines for national human immunodeficiency virus case surveillance, including monitoring for human immunodeficiency virus infection and acquired immunodeficiency syndrome. *MMWR Recomm Rep*. 1999;48(RR-13):1–28.
8. Nakashima AK, Fleming PL. HIV/AIDS surveillance in the United States, 1981–2001. *J Acquir Immune Defic Syndr*. 2003;32(suppl 1), S68–S85.
9. UNAIDS/WHO. Guidelines for second generation surveillance: the next decade. World Health Organization Web site. http://whqlibdoc.who.int/hq/2000/WHO_CDS_CSR_EDC_2000.5.pdf. Published 2000. Accessed May 14, 2018.
10. UNAIDS/WHO. Guidelines for second generation HIV surveillance: an update: know your epidemic. World Health Organization Web site. http://www.who.int/hiv/pub/surveillance/2013package/module1/en/. Published 2013. Accessed May 14, 2018.
11. Justice AC. HIV and aging: time for a new paradigm. *Curr HIV/AIDS Rep*. 2010;7(2):69–76. doi:10.1007/s11904-010-0041-9.
12. UNAIDS. UNAIDS data 2017. UNAIDS Web site. http://www.unaids.org/en/resources/documents/2017/2017_data_book. Published 2017. Accessed March 30, 2018.
13. World Health Organization. Consolidated guidelines on HIV prevention, diagnosis, treatment and care for key populations. WHO Web site. http://www.who.int/hiv/pub/guidelines/keypopulations/en/. Published 2014. Accessed February 20, 2018.
14. UNAIDS. 90-90-90: an ambitious treatment target to help end the AIDS epidemic. UNAIDS Web site. http://www.unaids.org/en/resources/documents/2017/90-90-90. Published 2014. Accessed February 20, 2018.
15. UNAIDS. On the fast track to end AIDS. UNAIDS Web site. http://www.unaids.org/en/resources/documents/2015/UNAIDS_PCB37_15-18. Published 2015. Accessed February 20, 2018.
16. Centers for Disease Control and Prevention. HIV surveillance report. Centers for Disease Control and Prevention Website.https://www.cdc.gov/hiv/statistics/overview/index.html. Updated May 7, 2018. Accessed May 14, 2018.
17. Centers for Disease Control and Prevention. HIV among women. Centers for Disease Control and Prevention Web site. https://www.cdc.gov/hiv/group/gender/women/index.html. Updated March 9, 2018. Accessed May 14, 2018.
18. Centers for Disease Control and Prevention. HIV among pregnant women, infants and children. Centers for Disease Control and Prevention Web site. https://www.cdc.gov/hiv/group/gender/pregnantwomen/index.html. Updated March 21, 2018. Accessed May 14, 2018.
19. Centers for Disease Control and Prevention. About HIV/AIDS. Centers for Disease Control and Prevention Web site. https://www.cdc.gov/hiv/basics/whatishiv.html. Updated March 16, 2018. Accessed May 14, 2018.
20. Centers for Disease Control and Prevention. HIV testing. Centers for Disease Control and Prevention Web site. https://www.cdc.gov/hiv/basics/testing.html. Updated March 16, 2018. Accessed May 14, 2018.
21. Centers for Disease Control and Prevention. HIV transmission. Centers for Disease Control and Prevention Web site. https://www.cdc.gov/hiv/basics/transmission.html. Updated March 16, 2018. Retrieved May 14, 2018.
22. Centers for Disease Control and Prevention. Isolation precautions. Centers for Disease Control and Prevention Web site. https://www.cdc.gov/infectioncontrol/guidelines/isolation/index.html. Updated October 31, 2017. Accessed June 1, 2018.
23. Bartlett J. The natural history and clinical features of HIV infection in adults and adolescents. In: Hirsch M, Bloom A, eds. *Up-to-date*. Waltham, MA: UpToDate; 2018.
24. World Health Organization. AIDS by the numbers. WHO Web site. http://www.unaids.org/sites/default/files/media_asset/AIDS-by-the-numbers-2016_cn.pdf. Published 2016. Accessed June 2, 2018.
25. Crenshaw K. Demarginalizing the intersection of race and sex: a black feminist critique of antidiscrimination doctrine, feminist theory and antiracist politics. *University of Chicago Legal Forum*. 1989;1(8):139–167. https://chicagounbound.uchicago.edu/uclf/vol1989/iss1/8. Accessed October 27, 2018.
26. Beagan BL. Approaches to culture and diversity: a critical synthesis of occupational therapy literature. *Can J Occup Ther*. 2015;82(5):272–282. doi:10.1177/0008417414567530.
27. Centre for HIV Law & Policy. Criminal law. Centre for HIV Law & Policy Web site. http://www.hivlawandpolicy.org/issues/criminal-law. Accessed March 20, 2018.
28. U.S. Department of Health and Human Services. HIV/AIDS glossary. NIH Web site. https://aidsinfo.nih.gov/understanding-hiv-aids/glossary. Updated June 3, 2018. Accessed June 3, 2018.
29. Price R. HIV-associated neurocognitive disorders: management. In: Bartlett J, Bloom A, eds. *Up-to-date*. Waltham, MA: UpToDate; 2018.

30. National Institute of Mental Health. HIV/AIDS and mental health. NIMH Web site. https://www.nimh.nih.gov/health/topics/hiv-aids/index.shtml. Updated November 2016. Accessed June 3, 2018.
31. Centers for Disease Control and Prevention. HIV among people aged 50 and over. Centers for Disease Control and Prevention Web site. https://www.cdc.gov/hiv/group/age/olderamericans/index.html. Updated February 12, 2018. Accessed March 30, 2018.
32. Van Epps P, Kalayjian RC. Human immunodeficiency virus and aging in the era of effective antiretroviral therapy. *Infect Dis Clin North Am*. 2017;31(4):791–810. doi:10.1016/j.idc.2017.07.007
33. Escota GV, O'Halloran JA, Powderly WG, Presti RM. Understanding mechanisms to promote successful aging in persons living with HIV. *Int J Infect Dis*. 2018;66:56–64. doi:10.1016/j.ijid.2017.11.010.
34. Solomon P, Letts L, O'Brien KK, Nixon S, Baxter L, Gervais N. "I'm still here, I'm still alive": understanding successful aging in the context of HIV. *Int J STD AIDS*. 2018;29(2):172–177. doi:10.1177/0956462417721439.
35. Wodak A, Maher L. The effectiveness of harm reduction in preventing HIV among injecting drug users. *N S W Public Health Bull*. 2010;21(3–4):69–73.
36. UNAIDS. Harm reduction. UNAIDS Web site. http://www.unaids.org/en/resources/presscentre/featurestories/2016/october/20161009_harmreduction. Published October 16, 2016. Accessed March 30, 2018.
37. Centers for Disease Control and Prevention. PrEP. Centers for Disease Control and Prevention Web site. https://www.cdc.gov/hiv/basics/prep.html. Updated March 23, 2018. Accessed May 14, 2018.
38. United States Public Health Service. Preexposure prophylaxis for the prevention of HIV infection in the United States—2017 update: a clinical practice guideline. Centers for Disease Control and Prevention Web site. https://www.cdc.gov/hiv/pdf/risk/prep/cdc-hiv-prep-guidelines-2017.pdf. Updated 2017. Accessed May 14, 2018.
39. United States Public Health Service. Updated guidelines for antiretroviral postexposure prophylaxis after sexual, injection drug use, or other nonoccupational exposure to HIV—United States, 2016. Centers for Disease Control and Prevention Web site. https://www.cdc.gov/hiv/pdf/programresources/cdc-hiv-npep-guidelines.pdf. Publication date April 18, 2016. Updated May 23, 2018. Accessed June 3, 2018.
40. Kuhar DT, Henderson DK, Struble KA, et al. Updated US Public Health Service guidelines for the management of occupational exposures to human immunodeficiency virus and recommendations for postexposure prophylaxis. *Infect Control Hosp Epidemiol*. 2013;34(9):875–892. doi:10.1086/672271.
41. U.S. Department of Health and Human Service. HIV medicines and side effects. U.S. Department of Health and Human Service, NIH Web site. https://aidsinfo.nih.gov/understanding-hiv-aids/fact-sheets/22/63/hiv-medicines-and-side-effects. Reviewed October 9, 2017. Accessed May 14, 2018.
42. Granich R, Crowley S, Vitoria M, et al. Highly active antiretroviral treatment as prevention of HIV transmission: review of scientific evidence and update. *Curr Opin HIV AIDS*. 2010;5(4):298–304. doi:10.1097/COH.0b013e32833a6c32.
43. Montaner JS, Lima VD, Harrigan PR, et al. Expansion of HAART coverage is associated with sustained decreases in HIV/AIDS morbidity, mortality and HIV transmission: the "HIV Treatment as Prevention" experience in a Canadian setting. *PLoS One*. 2014;9(2):e87872. doi:10.1371/journal.pone.0087872.
44. O'Brien KK, Hanna S, Gardner S, et al. Validation of the Episodic Disability Framework with adults living with HIV. *Disabil Rehabil*. 2014;36(4):319–329. doi:10.3109/09638288.2013.793408.
45. Restall G, Sullivan T, Carnochan T, Etcheverry E, Roger K, Roddy P. A service delivery model for addressing activity and social participation needs of people living with HIV. *Open J Occup Ther*. 2017;5(2). doi:10.15453/2168-6408.1258.
46. Beauregard C, Solomon P. Understanding the experience of HIV/AIDS for women: implications for occupational therapists. *Can J Occup Ther*. 2005;72(2):113–120. doi:10.1177/000841740507200206.
47. Barkey V, Watanabe E, Solomon P, Wilkins S. Barriers and facilitators to participation in work among Canadian women living with HIV/AIDS. *Can J Occup Ther*. 2009;76(4):269–275. doi:10.1177/000841740907600405.
48. Ledgister K, Fleming-Castaldy RP. The perceptions of persons living with human immunodeficiency virus/acquired immune deficiency syndrome about their experiences in regaining productive occupations: a Delphi study. *Occup Ther Mental Health*. 2017;33(3):235–258. doi:10.1080/0164212X.2017.1311241.
49. Bernardin KN, Toews DN, Restall GJ, Vuongphan L. Self-management interventions for people living with human immunodeficiency virus: a scoping review. *Can J Occup Ther*. 2013;80(5):314–327. doi:10.1177/0008417413512792.
50. O'Brien KK, Solomon P, Trentham B, et al. Evidence-informed recommendations for rehabilitation with older adults living with HIV: a knowledge synthesis. *BMJ Open*. 2014;4(5):e004692. doi:10.1136/bmjopen-2013-004692.
51. Kielhofner G, Braveman B, Finlayson M, Paul-Ward A, Goldbaum L, Goldstein K. Outcomes of a vocational program for persons with AIDS. *Am J Occup Ther*. 2004;58(1):64–72.
52. Kielhofner G, Braveman B, Fogg L, Levin M. A controlled study of services to enhance productive participation among people with HIV/AIDS. *Am J Occup Ther*. 2008;62(1):36–45. doi:10.5014/ajot.62.1.36.
53. Bedell G. Balancing health, work, and daily life: design and evaluation of a pilot intervention for persons with HIV/AIDS. *Work*. 2008;31(2):131–144.
54. Misko AN, Nelson DL, Duggan JM. Three case studies of community occupational therapy for individuals with human immunodeficiency virus. *Occup Ther Health Care*. 2015;29(1):11–26. doi:10.3109/07380577.2014.941452.
55. O'Brien K, Bayoumi A., Strike C, Young N, King K, Davis A. How do existing HIV-specific instruments measure up? Evaluating the ability of instruments to describe disability experienced by adults living with HIV. *Health Qual Life Outcomes*. 2010;8:88. doi:10.1186/1477-7525-8-88.

56. Worthington C, O'Brien K, Zack E, McKee E, Oliver B. Enhancing labour force participation for people living with HIV: a multi-perspective summary of the research evidence. *AIDS Behav*. 2012;16(1):231–243. doi:10.1007/s10461-011-9986-y.
57. O'Brien KK, Solomon P, Bergin C, et al. Reliability and validity of a new HIV-specific questionnaire with adults living with HIV in Canada and Ireland: the HIV Disability Questionnaire (HDQ). *Health Qual Life Outcomes*. 2015;13:124. doi:10.1186/s12955-015-0310-9.
58. Cooper V, Clatworthy J, Harding R, Whetham J; Emerge Consortium. Measuring quality of life among people living with HIV: a systematic review of reviews. *Health Qual Life Outcomes*. 2017;15(1):220. doi:10.1186/s12955-017-0778-6.
59. Kielhofner G, Mallinson T, Crawford C, et al. *The User's Manual for the Occupational Performance History Interview (Version 2.1) OPHI-II*. Chicago, IL: Model of Human Occupation Clearinghouse, Department of Occupational Therapy, College of Applied Health Sciences, University of Illinois at Chicago; 2004.
60. Baron K, Kielhofner G, Iyenger A, Goldhammer V, Wolenski J. *The Occupational Self-Assessment (OSA) (Version 2.2)*. Chicago, IL: Model of Human Occupation Clearinghouse, Department of Occupational Therapy, College of Applied Health Sciences, University of Illinois at Chicago; 2006.
61. Braveman B, Robson M, Velozo C, et al. *Worker Role Interview (WRI) (Version 10.0)*. Chicago, IL: Model of Human Occupation Clearinghouse, Department of Occupational Therapy, College of Applied Health Sciences, University of Illinois at Chicago; 2005.
62. Fisher AG. *Assessment of Motor and Process Skills*. 7th ed. Fort Collins, CO: Three Star Press; 2012.
63. Merritt B, Gahagan J, Kottorp A. HIV and disability: a pilot study exploring the use of the assessment of motor and process skills to measure daily life performance. *J Int AIDS Soc*. 2013;16:17339. doi:10.7448/IAS.16.1.17339.
64. Law M, Baptiste S, Carswell A, et al. *Canadian Occupational Performance Measure*. 5th ed. Ottawa, ON: CAOT Publications ACE; 2005.
65. Robertson K, Bayon C, Molina JM, et al. Screening for neurocognitive impairment, depression, and anxiety in HIV-infected patients in Western Europe and Canada. *AIDS Care*. 2014;26(12):1555–1561. doi:10.1080/09540121.2014.936813.
66. Nanni MG, Caruso R, Mitchell AJ, Meggiolaro E, Grassi L. Depression in HIV infected patients: a review. *Curr Psychiatry Rep*. 2015;17(1):530. doi:10.1007/s11920-014-0530-4.
67. Greene M, Hessol NA, Perissinotto C, et al. Loneliness in older adults living with HIV. *AIDS Behav*. 2018;22(5):1475–1484. doi:10.1007/s10461-017-1985-1.
68. Harris LM, Emlet CA, Pierpaoli Parker C, Furlotte C. Timing of diagnosis: understanding resilience narratives of HIV positive older adults diagnosed pre- and post-HAART. *J Gerontol Soc Work*. 2017:1–26. doi:10.1080/01634372.2017.1402841.
69. Rueda S, Law S, Rourke SB. Psychosocial, mental health, and behavioral issues of aging with HIV. *Curr Opin HIV AIDS*. 2014;9(4):325–331. doi:10.1097/COH.0000000000000071.
70. UNAIDS. Reduction of HIV-related stigma and discrimination. 2014. http://www.unaids.org/sites/default/files/media_asset/2014unaidsguidancenote_stigma_en.pdf. Accessed February 20, 2018.
71. Jong E, Oudhoff LA, Epskamp C, et al. Predictors and treatment strategies of HIV-related fatigue in the combined antiretroviral therapy era. *AIDS*. 2010;24(10):1387–1405. doi:10.1097/QAD.0b013e328339d004.
72. Bruce RD, Merlin J, Lum PJ, et al. 2017 HIV Medicine Association of Infectious Diseases Society of America clinical practice guideline for the management of chronic pain in patients living with human immunodeficiency virus. *Clin Infect Dis*. 2017;65(10):1601–1606. doi:10.1093/cid/cix848.
73. Stanos S. Focused review of interdisciplinary pain rehabilitation programs for chronic pain management. *Curr Pain Headache Rep*. 2012;16(2):147–152. doi:10.1007/s11916-012-0252-4.
74. Heaton RK, Franklin DR, Ellis RJ, et al. HIV-associated neurocognitive disorders before and during the era of combination antiretroviral therapy: differences in rates, nature, and predictors. *J Neurovirol*. 2011;17(1):3–16. doi:10.1007/s13365-010-0006-1.
75. Ranka JL, Chapparo CJ. Assessment of productivity performance in men with HIV associated neurocognitive disorder (HAND). *Work*. 2010;36(2):193–206. doi:10.3233/WOR-2010-1020.
76. Askari S, Fellows L, Brouillette MJ, Moriello C, Duracinsky M, Mayo NE. Development of an item pool reflecting cognitive concerns expressed by people with HIV. *Am J Occup Ther*. 2018;72(2):7202205070p1–7202205070p9. doi:10.5014/ajot.2018.023945.
77. Clare L, Linden DE, Woods RT, et al. Goal-oriented cognitive rehabilitation for people with early-stage Alzheimer disease: a single-blind randomized controlled trial of clinical efficacy. *Am J Geriatr Psychiatry*. 2010;18(10):928–939. doi:10.1097/JGP.0b013e3181d5792a.

Chapter **51**

Sleep Disorders Secondary to Orthopedic and Neurological Disorders

Sharon A. Gutman

LEARNING OBJECTIVES

This chapter will allow the reader to:

1. Identify and evaluate possible sleep disorders in patients receiving occupational therapy services.
2. Understand the physiology underlying sleep disorders that patients commonly experience.
3. Understand how sleep disorders can impact daily occupational activities and performance in therapy sessions.
4. Modify patient environments to promote sleep onset and maintenance.
5. Help patients establish new and modify existing routines and habits to promote sleep onset and maintenance.
6. Help patients modify daytime activity levels to promote sleep onset and maintenance.
7. Bring a nonpharmacological treatment approach to the treatment team to address patient sleep disorders.

CHAPTER OUTLINE

TERMINOLOGY

Chronic insomnia: a sleep disorder characterized by an inability to obtain sufficient quantity and quality of sleep per night that persists overtime and leads to ongoing sleep deprivation.

Circadian rhythm modulation: a 24-hour biological clock that regulates sleep, arousal, body temperature, muscle tone, blood pressure, and hormonal secretion; is located in the hypothalamus; and responds to cues of light and darkness.

Nighttime awakenings: the experience of waking during the night for a length of time often resulting from the need to void, feeling too warm, anxiety and depression, and disordered neurochemical and neurohormonal sleep regulators.

Sleep deprivation: the experience of insufficient sleep that persists overtime and leads to chronic daytime drowsiness and fatigue, poor concentration and memory, poor school and work performance, and interpersonal relationship problems.

Sleep latency onset: the amount of time required to fall asleep (also referred to as sleep initiation or induction).

Sleep maintenance: the ability to remain asleep and return to sleep if awakened, during a 7- to 8-hour time period.

Sleep Disorders: Definition, Prevalence, and Background

An estimated 50 million adults in the United States have diagnoses of **chronic insomnia** that exist independently of or occur secondary to a comorbid medical condition.[1] Approximately 70% of primary care patients[2] and 35% of assisted living residents[3] have been treated for chronic insomnia or disrupted sleep. Chronic insomnia is a sleep disorder characterized by an inability to obtain sufficient quantity and quality of sleep per night that continues overtime and leads to ongoing **sleep deprivation.**[1] Chronic insomnia can take the form of poor sleep initiation and maintenance, persistence **nighttime awakenings**, early morning awakenings, and an inability to return to sleep once awakened. Chronic insomnia that exists independently of a comorbid clinical condition is believed to result largely from neurochemical and hormonal mechanism impairment that disrupts **circadian rhythm modulation** and the regulation of sleep–wake cycles. Sleep disorders that occur secondary to medical conditions (e.g., sleep apnea, traumatic brain injury [TBI], chronic pain) may begin as secondary consequences of a physiological problem, but if left untreated, become chronic and result in circadian rhythm dysregulation.[4]

Patients with ongoing and undiagnosed sleep deprivation experience daytime drowsiness and fatigue, poor concentration and memory, irritability leading to problems in interpersonal relationships, and poor work and school performance.[4] There is substantial evidence that chronic insomnia increases the risk of hypertension, cardiopulmonary disease, diabetes, depression, anxiety, obesity, and hospital readmission.[5]

Typically, sleep disturbances are medically managed through sedative–hypnotic pharmaceuticals.[6] Although medications such as benzodiazepines (e.g., temazepam [Restoril], triazolam [Halcion], flurazepam) and non-benzodiazepine receptor agonist hypnotics (e.g., zolpidem [Ambien], zaleplon [Sonata], eszopiclone [Lunesta]) have high efficacy and are widely available, they are associated with dependence and tolerance overtime, commonly leading to morning drowsiness and memory impairment, and have been reported to cause disorders such as somnambulism (i.e., sleep walking) and sleep amnesia (i.e., engaging in behaviors that cannot be recalled upon awakening).[7] More alarmingly, the use of sedative–hypnotics in the elderly has been highly correlated with falls and resultant hip fractures.[8] As a result of these negative side effects and drug use consequences, there is a growing movement among physicians and patients to increasingly use nonpharmacological interventions in the treatment of chronic sleep disorders.[9]

Occupational therapists provide nonpharmacological sleep interventions that target modification to (a) the environment, (b) routines and habits related to the daily sleep–wake cycle, and (c) daily activity levels impacting sleep initiation and maintenance.[10] This focus contributes a unique perspective to the treatment team that, combined with medical management, can effectively ameliorate fragmented sleep commonly occurring in patients referred for occupational therapy services as a result of neurological or orthopedic conditions. This chapter describes the occupational therapy evaluation and intervention of sleep disorders resulting from disrupted circadian rhythm regulation secondary to environmental factors and/or comorbid medical conditions.

The Physiology of Sleep

Normal sleep is divided into two types, non-rapid eye movement (NREM) and rapid eye movement (REM) sleep that alternate throughout the sleep period. In the absence of sleep disorders, humans begin sleep through NREM stages 1 to 3. The first REM sleep period occurs approximately 90 minutes later and the two sleep types—REM and NREM—alternate in 90-minute periods, with each successive REM stage commonly increasing in length. NREM is divided into three distinct stages of progressive depth.[11]

Each NREM stage has distinct brain wave patterns, eye movements, and muscle activity. The initial sleep stage, NREM stage 1, commonly occurs from 1 to 7 minutes and is characterized by alpha waves marking a wakeful relaxed state. NREM stage 2 follows and occurs for 10 to 25 minutes of the initial cycle but increases in length with each successive sleep cycle. NREM stage 2 sleep constitutes approximately one half of a total sleep period and is characterized by low-voltage brain waves with sleep spindles and K-complexes that are believed to be important in learning and memory consolidation. NREM stage 3 follows and is characterized by delta brain waves consisting of slow, high-voltage waves lasting for about 20 to 40 minutes of the initial sleep cycle and constituting 10% to 15% of the total sleep period. REM stage is then entered and is characterized by low-voltage, mixed-frequency brain waves (theta and slow alpha), musculoskeletal paralysis or atonia, and REMs. REM stage sleep initially lasts for about 1 to 5 minutes but can increase to 30-minute periods as successive REM cycles occur. Dreaming commonly occurs within REM stage sleep.[11,12]

The sleep–wake cycle is largely regulated by the circadian rhythm system, which is a 24-hour "biological clock" that regulates sleep, arousal, body temperature, muscle tone, blood pressure, and hormone secretion. This system is located in the suprachiasmatic nucleus of the hypothalamus and responds to cues of light and darkness. The suprachiasmatic nucleus receives messages from brightness detector cells located in the retina that serve to daily reset the clock.[13] Researchers have suggested that the advent of industrialization, a 24-hour light availability, and access to technology with internal light sources (computers, smartphones, Kindles) have contributed to 20% of sleep disorders in Western societies.[14] The suprachiasmatic nucleus also connects to a pathway that controls the secretion of melatonin, which is a sleep-inducing hormone produced by the pineal gland primarily in the evening before bedtime. Normal sleep–wake cycles are regulated by a homeostatic balance between a drive for sleep and a drive for wakefulness. Human sleep needs accumulate during the day and early evening, peak before bedtime, and diminish during the sleep period.[15]

Several neurotransmitters play key roles in the sleep–wake cycle, including dopamine, norepinephrine, serotonin, histamine, glutamate, acetylcholine, and orexin. Many of these neurotransmitters exhibit high activity during wakefulness, diminish during NREM sleep, and are at their lowest levels during REM sleep. For example, both serotonin and histamine promote wakefulness, increase the amount of time it takes to fall asleep, and can decrease REM stage sleep. Although orexin activation facilitates wakefulness, low levels of this neurotransmitter in the evening can serve to stimulate sleep. Conversely, orexin deficiency may result in fragmented sleep characterized by dysfunctional cycles of NREM and REM stages.[16]

The neurotransmitter and neuromodulator adenosine serves to inhibit wakefulness and induce sleep. Adenosine levels build throughout the day, and, during the night, after the body has experienced sufficient NREM restorative sleep, adenosine levels decline, allowing for wakefulness.[17] Cytokines, which are small signaling protein molecules (including interleukin and interferon), contribute to this process. While cytokines are usually produced by the immune system in response to infection, they also have hypnogogic properties that induce drowsiness—perhaps to allow the body to conserve energy so that the immune system can optimally attack pathogens.[18]

As noted earlier, melatonin is a sleep hormone converted from serotonin in the pineal gland and increases in level before bedtime, causing drowsiness and lowered body temperature. Melatonin levels then increasingly rise to a normal level by the early morning. Synchronously, secretion of the stress hormone cortisol begins to increase toward the early morning in preparation for waking and is commonly capped by a 50% increase in production approximately 20 to 30 minutes after waking, referred to as the cortisol awakening response. Dysfunction in any of these neurotransmitter and neurohormonal systems, or in multiple systems, can result in sleep disorders.[16]

The Impact of Sleep Disorders on Daily Occupation

As noted earlier, chronic sleep disorders in the general population negatively impact daily participation in desired activities and result in daytime drowsiness; decreased attention, concentration, and memory; poor performance in work and school activities; and irritability that affects social interactions.[4] Chronic sleep deprivation has also been highly correlated with both auto vehicle and work-related accidents and injuries,[19] and an increased risk of systemic disease, including hypertension, cardiopulmonary disease, and diabetes.[5]

The effects of chronic insomnia are doubly consequential when they occur in patients receiving hospital and assisted care services who, as a result of sleep disorders, are more likely to have poorer health outcomes, falls, and morbidity.[20] Patients receiving occupational therapy services, who have fragmented sleep as a result of hospitalization, are commonly unable to participate fully in rehabilitation activities, have difficulty concentrating and attending to therapy services, and may be more resistant to engage in therapy-related occupations. Sleep disorders are common in many neurological and orthopedic disorders and can exacerbate symptoms, reduce restorative sleep, and increase the risk of falls.[21] In the elderly with dementia, sleep disorders adversely affect cognitive functions such as memory, increase agitation and wandering, and heighten the risk of falls with resultant fractures.[22]

Patients with TBI commonly experience disruption of the circadian rhythm cycle as a result of injury and lose normal sleep–wake cycles. This loss of normal sleep patterns can result in chronic sleep deprivation that exacerbates the executive function impairments commonly accompanying TBI. Poor concentration, reduced executive control of cognitive functions, and greater disinhibition of thoughts and verbalizations can all become pronounced with the onset of a sleep disorder. Patients may be more lethargic than normal, or conversely, more rowdy and resistant to participate in therapy.[23] Relearning basic daily living skills lost as a result of injury (e.g., self-care, grooming, cold meal preparation) commonly becomes more inefficient when patients experience chronic sleep loss. Relearning or newly learning higher level life skills (e.g., money management, hot meal preparation, public transportation use) may become more challenging and seemingly unattainable when cognitive processes are negatively impacted by chronic sleep disruption.

Sleep disorders are also common after cerebrovascular accident (stroke), and an estimated 50% of patients with stroke experience chronically disrupted sleep resulting from circadian rhythm dysfunction and/or breathing difficulties secondary to stroke. Sleep apnea, in which the upper respiratory tract becomes obstructed repeatedly during sleep, is the most common breathing disorder resulting from stroke and increases the risk of a second stroke by 20% to 40%. Sleep disorders secondary to stroke may also result from circadian rhythm impairment in which the neurotransmitters and hormones responsible for sleep induction and awakening are not functioning appropriately. In both cases, sleep deprivation adversely inhibits neural recovery after stroke and heightens cognitive and motoric deficits.[24] Patients may arrive to therapy lethargic and disengaged, or conversely, may be agitated and resistant to participate in therapy activities. Cognitive deficits secondary to stroke are commonly exacerbated by sleep loss and may inhibit new learning or relearning of daily life skills.

It is estimated that 70% of patients with spinal cord injury (SCI) experience sleep disturbance as a result of one or more of the following: hypoventilation and obstructive sleep apnea, circadian rhythm dysfunction resulting from neurochemical–hormonal disruption and body temperature dysregulation, movement disorders such as restless leg syndrome, chronic pain and paresthesia syndromes (abnormal sensations such as burning or tingling), depression and anxiety, and voiding problems. As a result, patients with SCI may feel chronically sleep deprived, experience daytime drowsiness and fatigue, have memory and concentration problems, and may feel unmotivated to participate in therapy.[25] Adults with SCI and sleep loss commonly report a high percentage of napping during the day that interferes with daily activities such as maintaining a regular weight shift schedule to reduce skin breakdown and decubiti ulcers; regularly emptying urinal leg bags and voiding, which may otherwise result in urinary tract infections, kidney damage, and autonomic dysreflexia (a life-threatening event resulting in uncontrolled hypertension); regularly inspecting skin integrity to reduce the occurrence of skin breakdown; and engaging in possible exercise and stretching to maintain available muscle strength and prevent contractures.[26]

Chronic pain syndromes (e.g., rheumatoid and osteoarthritis, low back and neck pain, fibromyalgia) account for the most common reasons that patients experience sleep disturbance, and an estimated 20% of primary care patients report sleep disruption secondary to chronic pain.[27] In several studies, 60% to 70% of patients referred to pain management programs reported chronic sleep loss with longer periods needed to fall asleep, fewer total hours asleep, more frequent nighttime awakenings, and nighttime awakenings of longer duration than that of the average population.[27,28] In another study, researchers found that pain tolerance decreased and pain perception increased as people experienced fewer hours of sleep.[29] Patients with pain were also found to experience fewer minutes in deep sleep stage 3 in which cell restoration and healing are believed to be most active.[30,31] Patients with sleep disorders secondary to chronic pain syndromes commonly avoid daily occupations that may trigger pain, or they may feel too fatigued to participate in desired occupations. Activity avoidance commonly results in diminished muscular strength and endurance that exacerbates the pain syndrome. Activity avoidance also leads to diminished or insufficient daytime activity that compounds the sleep disorder in a bidirectional manner.[31]

Occupational Therapy Evaluation and Intervention of Sleep Disorders

As noted earlier, occupational therapists provide evaluation and intervention of sleep disorders that target modification to (a) the environment, (b) routines and habits related to the daily sleep–wake cycle, and (c) daily activity levels impacting sleep initiation and maintenance. When therapists detect patient sleep disorders, they should alert other members of the treatment team or, for community-dwelling patients, encourage patients to disclose sleep disorders to primary care physicians (PCP). While occupational therapists provide nonpharmacological sleep interventions, such services may be most effective when combined with medical management including continuous positive-airway pressure (also known as CPAP) ventilators and nonpharmacological sleep inducers such as melatonin (which can be obtained over-the-counter but should be discussed first with a PCP to determine its potential interaction with other medications).

Evaluation and Intervention of the Environment

Hospital and assistive care environments have been shown to adversely affect the amount and quality of patient sleep as a result of nighttime noise, lights, patient and staff activity, and sleep interruptions because of medical tests and procedures. Additionally, hospital and assisted care environments frequently do not provide sufficient access to external cues of day and night, and as a result, patients' circadian rhythm systems desynchronize with normal day–night cycles. It is common for hospital patients to feel sleep deprivation as a result of frequent awakenings, fragmented sleep, and insufficient restorative sleep.[32] Residents of long-term care facilities, who have been exposed to these sleep reducing factors overtime, commonly experience chronic sleep deprivation that severely interferes with participation in daily occupation. Moreover, many long-term care residences are characterized by nonstimulating environments that promote excessive daytime napping that further exacerbates sleep disorders.[33] Therapists working within inpatient settings should expect that patients will likely experience sleep disruptions that may impact alertness, cognitive skills, motor function, and fatigue levels.

A number of sleep assessments, having acceptable reliability and validity, exist that can be used to measure patient sleep disturbances (e.g., Pittsburgh Sleep Quality Index[34] and General Sleep Disturbance Scale[35]); however, because these collect data about sleep in the past weeks or more, they may not be appropriate for hospitalized patients in an acute or subacute setting. Such assessments would be appropriate for use with long-term care residents and outpatients. As a general assessment, patients should be queried about their sleep amount and quality, including the following:

1. How did you sleep last night (poor, fair, good)?
2. Was your sleep restful?
3. On a scale ranging from 1 to 5 (1 = not at all fatigued, 5 = very fatigued), how fatigued do you feel today?
4. What time did you go to bed?
5. Did you have difficulty falling asleep?
6. How long did it take you to fall asleep?
7. Did you wake during the night?
   a. How many times do you remember waking up?
   b. How long were you awake before you fell back to sleep?
   c. What made you wake up during the night?
8. What time did you wake up in the morning?
9. How many hours did you sleep last night?

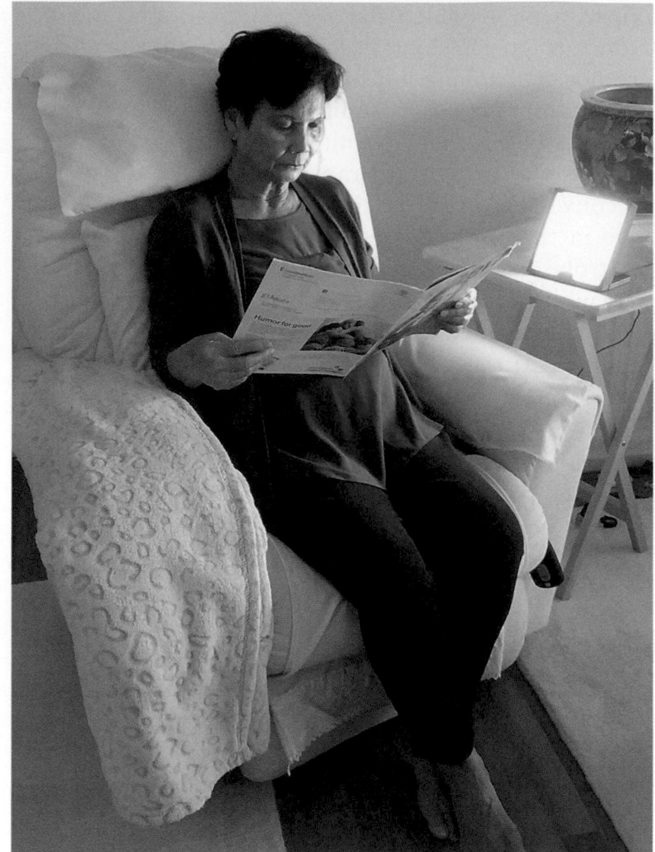
Figure 51-1. Client using light box.

Although several studies have found strong evidence that daytime light therapy improves both the quality and quantity of patient sleep, most hospital and assisted care environments do not provide sufficient exposure to daylight as a result of insufficient windows, reliance on florescent lighting, and location in regions lacking adequate sunlight. Patient rooms, resident dayrooms, and eating areas should be supplemented with artificial lighting systems that serve as an external cue to appropriately reset the circadian rhythm clock. Although the dose of light varied among studies, effectiveness was observed when artificial light systems of 2,500 to 10,000 lux were administered for 30 minutes to several hours per day (a typical room with average daylight has approximately 250 lux). Such light systems are relatively inexpensive and safe (do not emit heat or ultraviolet [UV] rays), and small light boxes can be purchased for patient rooms; larger systems can be installed in common areas. Researchers found that daytime use of external light systems in the range of 2,500 to 10,000 lux in hospitalized patients increased total sleep time, reduced nighttime awakenings, reduced sleep onset latency, and reduced nighttime wandering in the elderly with dementia.[36–39] Outpatients experiencing sleep disorders can also use light boxes each day, for a prescribed period, in their homes (see Fig. 51-1).

To further provide external light cues by which patients can reset their circadian rhythm system, patient room lighting should be dimmed in preparation for sleep 2 hours before bedtime. Eye masks and blinds or blackout shades have been shown to enhance sleep and should be used along with a cessation of noise and activity 1 hour before sleep onset (e.g., TVs turned off, patients should be undisturbed with the exception of medical necessities). One study found that the use of patient eye masks and earplugs to reduce light and noise disturbances, the dimming of facility hallway lights, and the provision of a 7-hour undisturbed sleep period enhanced sleep amount and quality in hospitalized patients and long-term care residents.[40] Outpatients' bedrooms should be evaluated to determine whether similar modifications are needed to reduce nighttime light and noise levels. Although nighttime light should be reduced to enhance sleep, it should be noted that automatically lighting nightlights should be used to prevent falls when patients awake and rise to use the bathroom or commode. Upon awakening, window blinds should be raised to allow daylight and artificial light systems described earlier should be used early in the day to provide cues by which patient circadian rhythm clocks can be reset.

Occupational therapists should also perform an ergonomic evaluation of patient beds and pillows to

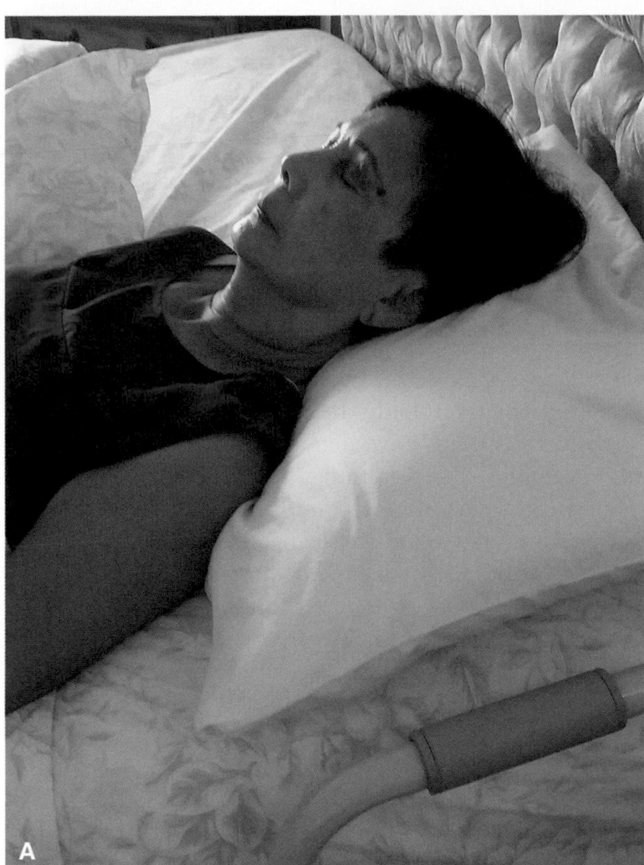

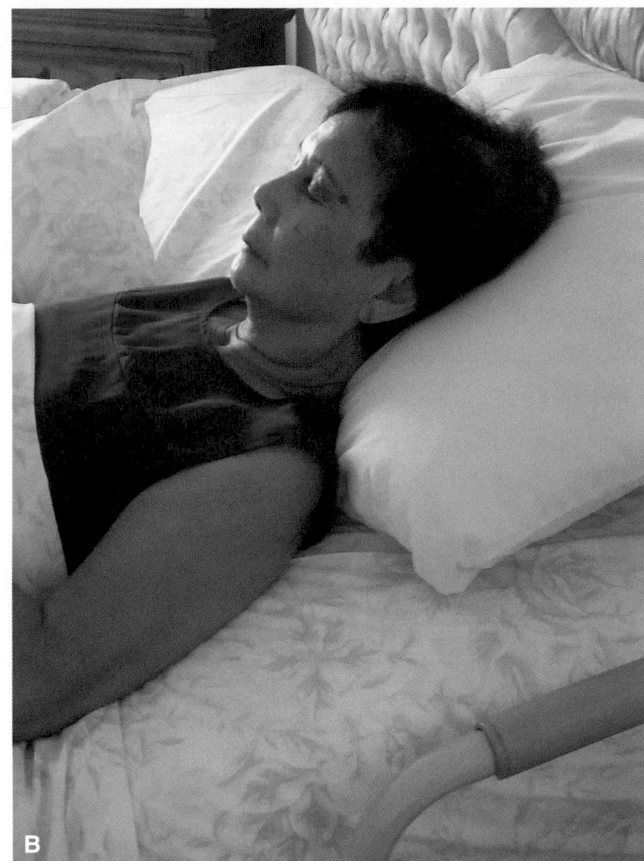

Figure 51-2. A. Pillow that appropriately supports the head and neck in neutral position. **B.** Pillow that inappropriately pushes the head and neck into forward flexion.

determine that both do not cause pain or discomfort that interferes with sleep. For side sleepers, pillows should be no higher or lower than the width between the lateral shoulder and cervical area and should allow the head to rest comfortably within a shallow depression. Pillows should maintain the head and neck in a neutral position and should not push the head and neck into flexion, extension, or rotation (see Fig. 51-2). For patients who sleep on their back or who have been positioned on their back and are immobile, pillows should maintain the head and neck in a neutral position and should not push the head into forward flexion. Pillows, wedges, and bolsters may need to be incorporated into the sleep area to accommodate patients requiring specific positioning of the spine and limbs.

Mattresses should also be evaluated to determine that they are sufficiently soft to prevent pressure on bony prominences while maintaining the spine in alignment. Conversely, mattresses that allow patient spines to settle into a flexed position will likely cause pain and discomfort that interfere with sleep. One study found a significant reduction in cervical, thoracic, and lumbar pain that enhanced patient reported sleep quality by replacing traditional hospital beds with medium soft mattresses.[41] When the replacement of mattresses is cost-prohibitive, inexpensive mattress toppers—such as memory foam toppers—can be used to modify the sleep berth.

Therapists should also assess the patient's desired room temperature at night. Because the human body experiences a 1- to 2-degree temperature reduction at night to induce sleep,[13] it is important that patient rooms remain sufficiently cool, but not cold. Because body mass index and weight affect one's temperature, patients should be individually assessed to determine appropriate nighttime room temperature. When facility thermostat settings cannot be reset, the amount and type of bedding materials should be adjusted to maintain a comfortable sleep environment temperature.

A number of studies have also demonstrated the effectiveness of aromatherapy in the promotion of sleep onset and maintenance with patients in hospital and long-term care facilities, particularly patients having coronary artery disease, dementia, and renal disease. Although all scents used demonstrated similar sleep-inducing effects, lavender oil was found to be most effective in increasing total time asleep, reducing the amount and length of nighttime awakenings, and reducing nighttime wandering, specifically in patients with dementia. Patients also reported a reduction in general anxiety. In these studies, aromatherapy was delivered through massage or dispensed from a cool mist diffuser (with an automatic safety shutoff valve) that began approximately 1 hour before bedtime and continued for a 2- to 5-hour period.[42–45]

Evaluation and Intervention of Routines and Habits Related to the Sleep–Wake Cycle

Occupational therapists also evaluate the routines and habits that affect patients' sleep–wake cycles, particularly for outpatients and long-term care residents. Sleep researchers have found a high correlation between the evening use of technology having an external light source (e.g., computers, laptops, smartphones, Kindles, televisions) and the presence of sleep disorders.[14] Such technologies impact the circadian rhythm clock by providing false cues of daylight that reduce evening melatonin production normally inducing drowsiness.[46] For this reason, the National Sleep Foundation recommends that the use of such technologies be ceased, at a minimum, 1 hour before bedtime.[47] Similarly, in hospital and assistive care facilities, televisions should be turned off 1 hour before bedtime.

It is also recommended that patients maintain consistent sleep and wake times each day and limit daytime napping to no more than 30 minutes. If patients experience sleep problems one night, they should be encouraged to maintain their normal activity level the next day and refrain from napping in an attempt to recapture lost sleep. Food intake should be restricted to 3 to 4 hours before bedtime, and foods that disrupt sleep or stimulate wakefulness—such as caffeine, spicy and hot foods, chocolate, and carbonated drinks—should be ingested no later than 6 hours before bedtime, if at all. Stimulants, such as nicotine, caffeine, and alcohol, reduce sleep induction and maintenance, and should be avoided in patients identified as having sleep disorders.[47]

The National Sleep Foundation also recommends the consistent and regular participation in sleep routines that serve as neural cues of sleep readiness. For example, patients can be taught to develop sleep routines involving the participation in calming activities directly before bedtime, such as taking a warm bath or shower (which temporarily raises body temperature and is then followed by a temperature reduction that promotes drowsiness), listening to relaxing music, reading (avoid Kindle use), or drinking noncaffeinated herbal tea. These activities, when engaged in regularly, come to be associated with sleep onset and may trigger the neurochemical and hormonal cascade of events responsible for sleep induction. Similarly, it is suggested that the bedroom area be used only for sleep (and sleep-related activities) so that an association can be made between its use and sleep onset.[47] This means that patients who are accustomed to watching television in bed, working at a desk in the bedroom, making phone calls from bed, and exercising in the bedroom area must be informed that such activities promote sleep problems. Such patients should be encouraged to reconfigure their habits so that performance of these activities occurs outside the bedroom area.

Several studies have demonstrated the effectiveness of engaging in self-calming activities directly before bed—such as meditation, mindfulness practice, and relaxing training—to induce sleep.[48] Patients can be taught the use of these strategies and can then engage in them independently or with the assistance of guided CDs and phone apps (these can be programmed to turn off automatically when completed). A number of studies have demonstrated that self-relaxation techniques used by community-dwelling clients and patients in long-term care residences improved sleep quality, reduced nighttime awakenings, and increased total time asleep.[49–51] Self-relaxation techniques were shown to be not only highly effective in sleep promotion but also decreased depression and anxiety levels that interfered with sleep. Several complementary health researchers have found that 20 to 30 minutes of meditation per day can actually reduce the need for sleep if the meditation can induce the brain wave patterns found in sleep stages 1 to 3.[52] The self-calming strategies used in the previously described studies were implemented for 20 to 45 minutes per session, 1 hour before bedtime. Self-relaxation training is a highly effective, simple, and inexpensive method of improving sleep in outpatients and long-term care residents.

Therapists should also ask community-dwelling patients with sleep disorders to complete a 2-week sleep diary in which information about sleep patterns are recorded and analyzed to determine what environmental, dietary, and physical factors may adversely impact sleep. Patients use sleep diaries to record such information as length of time needed to fall asleep, number and length of nighttime awakenings, total time asleep, reason for nighttime awakenings (e.g., bathroom use, excessive worry, warm bedroom temperature), food and drinks ingested during the previous day and evening, occurrence and length of daytime naps, use of medications, daytime activity level, daytime stress level, pre-bedtime routines, use of technology with external light sources, and amount of daylight exposure (see Fig. 51-3). Over a 2-week period, the recording of such information

	Day 1 Date _____	Day 2 Date _____	Day 3 Date _____	Day 4 Date _____	Day 5 Date _____	Day 6 Date _____	Day 7 Date _____
Time I went to bed	am/pm	am/pm	am/pm	am/pm	am/pm	am/pm	am/pm
Time I woke up	am/pm	am/pm	am/pm	am/pm	am/pm	am/pm	am/pm
Time it took to fall asleep	min/hr	min/hr	min/hr	min/hr	min/hr	min/hr	min/hr
Number of times I woke up during the night	#	#	#	#	#	#	#
Length of nighttime awakenings	min/hr	min/hr	min/hr	min/hr	min/hr	min/hr	min/hr
Reasons for nighttime awakenings (bathroom use, felt warm, heard noise, etc.)	# Reasons:	# Reasons:	# Reasons:	# Reasons:	# Reasons:	# Reasons:	# Reasons:
Level of daytime fatigue	1 = very fatigued 2 = somewhat fatigued 3 = refreshed	1 = very fatigued 2 = somewhat fatigued 3 = refreshed	1 = very fatigued 2 = somewhat fatigued 3 = refreshed	1 = very fatigued 2 = somewhat fatigued 3 = refreshed	1 = very fatigued 2 = somewhat fatigued 3 = refreshed	1 = very fatigued 2 = somewhat fatigued 3 = refreshed	1 = very fatigued 2 = somewhat fatigued 3 = refreshed
Number of caffeinated and/or alcoholic drinks	# am # pm	# am # pm	# am # pm	# am # pm	# am # pm	# am # pm	# am # pm
Time of my last meal of the day	am/pm	am/pm	am/pm	am/pm	am/pm	am/pm	am/pm
Medications taken today							
Number and length of any naps today	# min/hr	# min/hr	# min/hr	# min/hr	# min/hr	# min/hr	# min/hr
How many hours before bedtime did I use a TV, Kindle, smartphone, or computer today	# hours	# hours	# hours	# hours	# hours	# hours	# hours
Activities I did in the hour right before bed							
Activity level today	1 = not much activity 2 = moderate amount of activity 3 = high level of activity	1 = not much activity 2 = moderate amount of activity 3 = high level of activity	1 = not much activity 2 = moderate amount of activity 3 = high level of activity	1 = not much activity 2 = moderate amount of activity 3 = high level of activity	1 = not much activity 2 = moderate amount of activity 3 = high level of activity	1 = not much activity 2 = moderate amount of activity 3 = high level of activity	1 = not much activity 2 = moderate amount of activity 3 = high level of activity

Figure 51-3. Sleep diary.

can reveal factors that may disrupt sleep and that can be modified through changes to the environment, routines and habits, and daily diet. Therapists should note that lifestyle changes, even positive ones that promote sleep, are difficult for patients to make and should be undertaken in steps that allow patients to make needed adjustments at their own pace—otherwise, needed modifications may be abandoned.

Evaluation and Intervention of Daily Activity Levels Impacting Sleep Initiation and Maintenance

Multiple studies have been implemented to examine the impact of daily activity level on sleep quantity and quality in community-dwelling and long-term care clients. Although the results of this body of literature are mixed, about half found that higher daytime activity levels corresponded with greater sleep induction and maintenance.[53] Studies in which both physical and social activities were used to stimulate cognitive and motor functions—as opposed to exercise alone—had the greatest positive impact on sleep. Interventions were provided in the form of physical resistance strength training, walking, elastic band wheelchair exercises, and low-intensity Tai Chi, combined with engagement in socially stimulating activities (e.g., group discussions, games, creative arts) for 30 to 45 minutes, 3 to 5 days per week, over 7 weeks to 6 months. This body of research found that engagement in exercise alone was not sufficient to positively impact sleep behaviors, but when combined with socially stimulating activities, it significantly improved sleep induction and total sleep time and reduced nighttime awakenings.[53–56] One study also found that when residents were prevented from daytime napping and instead engaged in an occupation-based intervention, they experienced greater total nighttime sleep.[57]

When occupational therapists detect sleep disorders in community-dwelling and long-term care residents, they should evaluate the patient's daily activity level to determine whether it is sufficiently physically, cognitively, and socially stimulating. This can be achieved by having patients complete daily activity configurations or maintain daily activity logs and journals. Staff members and family can also be solicited to provide information about the patient's daily activity levels. Each patient's ability to tolerate and engage in activity will be unique, and therapists should tailor activity interventions for individual clients based on their specific abilities and impairments. Daytime napping and excessive engagement in passive activities (e.g., television viewing) should be prevented or significantly reduced and replaced with activity having a tolerable physical, cognitive, and social component. Engagement in activity should also be paced and spread throughout the day and early evening to prevent fatigue. Patients in long-term care residences should not be left to experience prolonged daytime periods (more than 1 hour) of inactivity; however, activity should be manageable and not fatiguing. Therapists should also assess sleep variables (e.g., sleep onset latency time, total sleep time, number and length of nighttime awakenings) after intervention has been provided for at least 2 weeks to determine intervention effectiveness and the need for modification. Because sleep needs tend to decrease with age, therapists should consider patients' perceived quality of sleep and reported daily fatigue level with greater importance in comparison to total sleep hours.

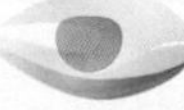

CASE STUDY

Patient Information

Angelina is an 84-year-old Philippine American woman who has returned to her assisted living residence after a 1-month rehabilitation hospitalization secondary to a fall and resultant right hip fracture. She has experienced memory loss in the past year and has been prescribed Aricept. Upon return to her long-term care residence, Angelina has been receiving both occupational and physical therapy to increase strength and endurance, but has not been making progress. She is often lethargic and cantankerous during therapy, and frequently refuses services. When she does attend therapy, she is often observed asleep in her wheelchair.

Reason for Occupational Therapy Referral

In addition to increasing strength and endurance, Angelina has been referred for occupational therapy services to increase independence in self-care and basic activities of daily living (ADLs).

Assessment Process and Results

The occupational therapist determined that Angelina's fall occurred in the middle of the night when she awoke to use the bathroom. Angelina reported that in the past year, she regularly experienced 2 to 3 awakenings per night for different reasons identified as needing to void, feeling too warm, hearing noises, and feeling pain from her fracture. She reported that she watches television until she can fall back to sleep. Because of her memory problems, her doctor decided that a sedative–hypnotic sleep medication would be contraindicated. She is presently taking Tylenol with Codeine to manage her fracture pain. Based on this information and observing Angelina fall asleep during therapy, the occupational therapist suspected a possible sleep disorder and administered the Pittsburg Sleep Quality Index. This assessment revealed that Angelina had typically slept 4 to 5 hours per night in the last month, had a

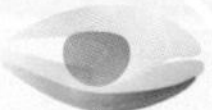

CASE STUDY *(continued)*

sleep onset latency time of 1 hour before she fell asleep, awoke three to four times each night, remained awake for 30+ minutes before falling back to sleep, and experienced a high level of daytime fatigue.

Further assessment of her daytime activity level revealed that Angelina watched television and napped most of the day. Her physical and occupational therapy sessions were scheduled back-to-back, and she reported feeling fatigued directly afterward. She stated that she remained in bed for most of the day because of pain, but noted that her mattress was not comfortable and often increased her pain level. This information prompted the therapist to evaluate Anglina's facility apartment, which is a small one-bedroom, one-bathroom unit with a kitchenette that is rarely used. Angelina reported that although she is usually a side-sleeper, she has been forced to sleep on her back after her fracture because of pain. The therapist noted that Angelina's pillow is too high and pushes her head into forward flexion. The apartment is north facing and has little sunlight. Noises from other residents and staff can readily be heard, and Angelina states that such noises keep her awake throughout the night. To reduce noise level and maintain some evening light in the apartment, Angelina reported that she keeps her bedroom television on throughout the night. No automatically lighting nightlights were observed. The apartment was noted to be warm, and Angelina stated that she liked a warm apartment because she often felt cold; however, she also reported that she sometimes woke during the night feeling too hot. The therapist additionally inquired about Angelina's dietary habits and found that she drank coffee at every meal and was reluctant to change this habit.

Occupational Therapy Problem List

- Decreased strength and endurance secondary to right hip fracture
- Decreased independence in self-care and basic ADLs
- Hip fracture pain that interferes with sleep
- Sleep disorder that may adversely impact therapy participation, memory, daytime alertness, and daytime activity level

Occupational Therapy Goal List

- Increase strength and endurance sufficient to participate in self-care and basic ADLs with minimum assistance by 2 weeks.
- Modify the bed and pillow to decrease pain interfering with sleep (from a self-reported pain level of 8 to 5 on a 10-point scale, 0 = low, 10 = high) by 1 week.
- Establish nighttime sleep routines that decrease sleep onset latency (from 1 hour to 30 minutes) and reduce nighttime awakenings (from 4 to 2) in 3 weeks.
- Establish daytime activity levels that increase total time asleep (from 5 to 7 hours) and decrease daytime fatigue levels (from a self-reported fatigue level of 8 to 5 on a 10-point scale, 0 = low, 10 = high).

Intervention

Angelina continued to receive occupational therapy services to increase strength and endurance needed to engage in bathing, grooming, and dressing with minimum assistance. She was observed to be more alert during therapy and was less resistant to participation. To make her bed more comfortable, a memory foam mattress topper was placed over her current mattress to provide greater cushioning and reduce pressure on her bony prominences, particularly at the fracture site. The pillow was also replaced with one that maintained her head and neck in a neutral position while lying supine on her back. These modifications now enabled Angelina to rest in bed with less reported pain. The therapist encouraged Angelina to use ear plugs while sleeping to reduce noise level; refrain from keeping the television on all night; and sleep with lighter, layered blankets to reduce the likelihood of waking from feeling too warm. An automatically lighting nightlight was installed to provide illumination when awakening to use the commode. Angelina also agreed to try a cool mist aromatherapy diffuser (1 hour before bedtime and continuing for 5 hours), a 10,000-lux light box each morning for 30 minutes, and a relaxation CD 30 minutes before bed.

Although she was hesitant, Angelina agreed to replace her lunch and evening coffee with herbal decaffeinated tea. The recreational therapist and case manager also helped convince her to participate in several daytime activities (such as world events and creative arts groups) instead of watching television and napping. Her occupational and physical therapy sessions were rescheduled 1 hour apart to reduce fatigue level.

In 4 weeks, Angelina reported that she was able to maintain these changes and was sleeping better. A Pittsburgh Sleep Quality Index administered at 4 weeks revealed that her total sleep time increased from 5 to 6.5 hours, sleep onset latency was reduced from 1 hour to 30 minutes, total nighttime awakenings decreased from 4 to 2, and daytime fatigue level decreased from 8 to 4. Pain level at night was also reported to decrease from 8 to 5, and Angelina additionally stated that she felt more alert and experienced less memory problems.

Evidence Table of Intervention Studies for Sleep Disorders

Intervention	Description	Participants	Dosage	Research Design and Evidence Level	Benefit	Statistical Significance and Effect Size
Reducing nighttime noise, light, and staff activity to increase sleep in hospital patients[58]	Nurse's nighttime care routines were changed to provide an uninterrupted period between 11:00 pm and 5:00 am. Noise level and activity were decreased, and light reduced to 40 lux.	Fifty-five surgical intensive care patients (28 = treatment group; 27 = control group)	Environmental changes occurred 7 days/week for 3 months from 11:00 pm to 5:00 am	Two group controlled study Level II	An undisturbed period from 11:00 am to 5:00 am and the control of nighttime noise, light, and care activities improved patients' perceived sleep quality.	Treatment group reported better perceived sleep ($t = -2.28$, $p = 0.027$) and sleep efficiency ($t = -2.03$, $p = 0.047$)
Light therapy to reduce sleep problems in adults with sleep disorders[36]	Review of the effect of light therapy on sleep problems in adults with general sleep problems, circadian rhythm sleep disorders, insomnia, and sleep disorders related to dementia	Fifty-three studies with a total of 1,154 participants were included.	Light ranging from 2,500 to 10,000 lux delivered for a mean of 18.72 days (standard deviation [SD] = 18.49) and a mean of 1.81 hours/day (SD = 1.71)	Meta-analysis Level I	Light therapy was effective for sleep problems in general, particularly for circadian rhythm and insomnia disorders.	Hedges' g effect sizes were calculated. Light therapy was found effective in the treatment of sleep problems in general ($g = 0.39$, $p < 0.01$) and for circadian rhythm sleep disorders ($g = 0.41$, $p < 0.01$), insomnia ($g = 0.47$, $p < 0.08$), and sleep problems related to dementia ($g = 0.30$, $p < 0.02$) specifically.
Comparison of (1) resistance strength training and walking (RST/W), (2) social activity (SA), (3) combined social activity and RST (RST/W + SA), and (4) usual care on sleep quality in long-term care residents[53]	RST/W received high-intensity physical resistance strength training and walking. SA group received social activity consisting of discussion, creative arts, music, and cooking groups. Control group received usual care.	One hundred sixty-five elderly residents of 13 long-term care facilities	RST/W group received intervention for 3 days/week for 45 minutes, over 7 weeks. SA group received intervention for 1 hour, 5 days/week, over 7 weeks. The combined RST/W + SA group received both interventions. Control group received usual care.	Randomized controlled trial Level I	Combined RST/W + SA significantly improved sleep in participants. The interventions by themselves had no significant effect on sleep.	Total sleep time was found to be significantly greater ($p < 0.01$, $d = 0.53$) in the combined RST/W + SA group compared to all other groups and increased 35.3 minutes. Sleep efficiency was also greater ($p < 0.05$, $d = 0.45$) in the combined RST/W + SA group compared to all other groups.

Aromatherapy to promote sleep quality in hospitalized and long-term care patients[42]	Aromatherapy was administered in the form of massage and inhalation.	Twelve studies were included in meta-analysis. Study participants ranged in number from 36 to 72 and consisted of hospitalized and elderly long-term care residents.	Seven studies administered aromatherapy before bedtime in the form of a massage; five studies provided inhalation aromatherapy 30 minutes before bedtime and continuing for 1–2 hours. Length of studies was not reported.	Meta-analysis Level I	Aromatherapy, used in the form of massage or inhalation, promoted sleep in hospitalized and long-term care patients.	Meta-analysis of the 12 studies using a random-effects model showed that aromatherapy effectively improved sleep quality (95% confidence interval [CI], 0.540–1.745; $Z = 3.716$). Subgroup analysis showed that inhalation aromatherapy (95% CI, 0.792–1.541; $Z = 6.107$) was more effective than massage therapy (95% CI, 0.128–2.166; $Z = 2.205$).
Mindfulness training to promote sleep quality in community-dwelling elderly with chronic insomnia[48]	Mindfulness training was provided in group sessions and practiced by participants independently. Control group received sleep hygiene education group.	Community-dwelling elderly with chronic insomnia were randomly assigned to mindfulness training group ($n = 24$) and sleep hygiene group ($n = 25$).	Both groups were delivered in 2-hour, weekly sessions over 6 weeks. Both groups were able to practice techniques independently on own.	Randomized controlled trial Level I	Mindfulness training group experienced improvements in **sleep latency onset**, **sleep maintenance**, and total sleep time compared to sleep hygiene group	At posttest, the mindfulness training group demonstrated a statistically significant improvement in sleep quality and efficiency compared to the sleep hygiene group (mean = 7.4 ± 1.9, $p < 0.05$, $d = 0.89$, 95% CI, 0.6–2.9).

References

1. Ford ES, Cunningham TJ, Giles WH, Croft JB. Trends in insomnia and excessive daytime sleepiness among US adults from 2002 to 2012. *Sleep Med*. 2015;16(3):372–378. doi:10.1016/j.sleep.2014.12.008.
2. Bjorvatn B, Meland E, Flo E, Mildestvedt T. High prevalence of insomnia and hypnotic use in patients visiting their general practitioner. *Fam Pract*. 2016;34(1):20–24. doi:10.1093/fampra/cmw107.
3. Li J, Grandner MA, Chang YP, Jungquist C, Porock D. Person-centered dementia care and sleep in assisted living residents with dementia: a pilot study. *Behav Sleep Med*. 2017;15(2):97–113. doi:10.1080/15402002.2015.1104686.
4. Sateia MJ, Buysse D, Krystal AD, Neubauer DN, Heald, JL. Clinical practice guideline for the pharmacologic treatment of chronic insomnia in adults: an American Academy of Sleep Medicine clinical practice guideline. *J Clin Sleep Med*. 2017;13(2):307–349. doi:10.5664/jcsm.6470.
5. McHill AW, Wright KP. Role of sleep and circadian disruption on energy expenditure and in metabolic predisposition to human obesity and metabolic disease. *Obesity Rev*. 2017;18(S1):15–24. doi:10.1111/obr.12503.
6. Sateia MJ, Sherrill WC, Winter-Rosenberg C, Heald JL. Payer perspective of the American Academy of Sleep Medicine clinical practice guideline for the pharmacologic treatment of chronic insomnia. *J Clin Sleep Med*. 2017;13(2):155–157. doi:10.5664/jcsm.6428.
7. Buysse DJ, Rush AJ, Reynolds CF. Clinical management of insomnia disorder. *JAMA*. 2017;318(20):1973–1974. doi:10.1001/jama.2017.15683.
8. Min Y, Kirkwood CK, Mays DP, Slattum PW. The effect of sleep medication use and poor sleep quality on risk of falls in community-dwelling older adults in the US: a prospective cohort study. *Drugs Aging*. 2016;33(2):151–158. https://link.springer.com/article/10.1007/s40266-015-0339-9.
9. Min Y, Nadpara PA, Slattum, P.W. The association between sleep problems, sleep medication use, and falls in community-dwelling older adults: results from the Health and Retirement Study 2010. *J Aging Res*. 2016;2016:3685789. doi:10.1155/2016/3685789.
10. Gutman SA, Gregory KA, Sadlier-Brown MM, et al. Comparative effectiveness of three occupational therapy sleep interventions: a randomized controlled study. *OTJR*. 2017;37(1):5–13. doi:10.1177/1539449216673045.
11. Nayak CS, Bhowmik A, Prasad PD, Pati S, Choudhury KK, Majumdar KK. Phase synchronization analysis of natural wake and sleep states in healthy individuals using a novel ensemble phase synchronization measure. *J Clin Neurophysiol*. 2017;34(1):77–83. doi:10.1097/WNP.0000000000000325.
12. Vyazovskiy VV, Delogu A. NREM and REM sleep: complementary roles in recovery after wakefulness. *Neuroscientist*. 2014;20(3):203–219. doi:10.1177/1073858413518152.
13. Morin LP. Neuroanatomy of the extended circadian rhythm system. *Exp Neurol*. 2013;243:4–20. doi:10.1016/j.expneurol.2012.06.026.
14. Chang AM, Aeschbach D, Duffy JF, Czeisler CA. Evening use of light-emitting eReaders negatively affects sleep, circadian timing, and next-morning alertness. *Proc Natl Acad Sci U S A*. 2015;112(4):1232–1237. doi:10.1073/pnas.1418490112.
15. Reiter RJ, Tan DX, Galano A. Melatonin: exceeding expectations. *Physiology*. 2014;29(5):325–333. doi:10.1152/physiol.00011.2014.
16. Saper CB, Fuller PM. Wake–sleep circuitry: an overview. *Curr Opin Neurobiol*. 2017;44:186–192. doi:10.1016/j.conb.2017.03.021.
17. Yuan XS, Wang L, Dong H, Li RL, Qu WM, Huang, ZL. Striatal adenosine A_{2A} receptor neurons regulate sleep behavior. *Sleep Med*. 2017;40:e359. doi:10.1016/j.sleep.2017.11.1059.
18. Verster J, van de Loo A, Mackus M, et al. Cytokines and sleep: effects on daytime sleepiness. *Sleep Med*. 2017;40:e338–e339.
19. Bioulac S, Franchi JAM, Arnaud M, et al. Risk of motor vehicle accidents related to sleepiness at the wheel: a systematic review and meta-analysis. *Sleep*. 2017;40(10):zsx134. doi:10.1093/sleep/zsx134.
20. Irwin MR, Olmstead R, Carroll JE. Sleep disturbance, sleep duration, and inflammation: a systematic review and meta-analysis of cohort studies and experimental sleep deprivation. *Biol Psychiatry*. 2016:80(1):40–52. doi:10.1016/j.biopsych.2015.05.014.
21. Wu L, Sun D. Sleep duration and falls: a systemic review and meta-analysis of observational studies. *J Sleep Res*. 2017;26(3):293–301. doi:10.1111/jsr.12505.
22. Chen PY, Chiu HT, Chiu HY. Daytime sleepiness is independently associated with falls in older adults with dementia. *Geriatr Gerontol Int*. 2016;16(7):850–855. doi:10.1111/ggi.12567.
23. Imbach LL, Büchele F, Valko PO, et al. Sleep–wake disorders persist 18 months after traumatic brain injury but remain underrecognized. *Neurology*. 2016;86(21):1945–1949. doi:10.1212/WNL.0000000000002697.
24. Jee S, Jeon H. Management of frequent sleep problem after stroke. *Brain Neurorehabil*. 2016;9(1):20–24. doi:10.12786/bn.2016.9.1.20.
25. Sankari A, Martin JL, Bascom AT, Mitchell MN, Badr MS. Identification and treatment of sleep-disordered breathing in chronic spinal cord injury. *Spinal Cord*. 2015;53(2):145–149. doi:10.1038/sc.2014.216.
26. Fogelberg DJ, Leland NE, Blanchard J, Rich TJ, Clark FA. Qualitative experience of sleep in individuals with spinal cord injury. *OTJR*. 2017;37(2):89–97. doi:10.1177/1539449217691978.
27. Alsaadi SM, McAuley JH, Hush JM, Maher CG. Prevalence of sleep disturbance in patients with low back pain. *Eur Spine J*. 2011;20(5):737–743. doi:10.1007/s00586-010-1661-x.
28. Cheatle MD, Foster S, Pinkett A, Lesneski M, Qu D, Dhingra L. Assessing and managing sleep disturbance in patients with chronic pain. *Anesthesiol Clin*. 2016;34(2):379–393. doi:10.1016/j.anclin.2016.01.007.
29. Schrimpf M, Liegl G, Boeckle M, Leitner A, Geisler P, Pieh C. The effect of sleep deprivation on pain perception in healthy subjects: a meta-analysis. *Sleep Med*. 2015;16(11):1313–1320. doi:10.1016/j.sleep.2015.07.022.
30. Choy EH. The role of sleep in pain and fibromyalgia. *Nat Rev Rheumatol*. 2015;11(9):513–520. doi:10.1038/nrrheum.2015/56.

31. Boakye PA, Olechowski C, Rashiq S, et al. A critical review of neurobiological factors involved in the interactions between chronic pain, depression, and sleep disruption. *Clin J Pain.* 2016;32(4):327–336. doi:10.1097/AJP.0000000000000260.
32. Bihari S, Doug McEvoy RD, Matheson E, Kim S, Woodman RJ, Bersten AD. Factors affecting sleep quality of patients in intensive care unit. *J Clin Sleep Med.* 2012;8(3): 301–307. doi:10.5664/jcsm.1920.
33. Ye L, Richards KC. Sleep and long-term care. *Sleep Med Clin.* 2018;13(1):117–125. doi:10.1016/j.jsmc.2017.09.011.
34. Buysse DJ, Reynolds CF, Monk TH, Berman SR, Kupfer DJ. The Pittsburgh Sleep Quality Index: a new instrument for psychiatric practice and research. *Psychiatry Res.* 1989;28(2):193–213. doi:10.1016/0165-1781(89)90047-4.
35. Lee SY. Validating the General Sleep Disturbance Scale among Chinese American parents with hospitalized infants. *J Transcult Nurs.* 2007;18(2):111–117. doi:10.1177/1043659606298502.
36. van Maanen A, Meijer AM, van der Heijden KB, Oort FJ. The effects of light therapy on sleep problems: a systematic review and meta-analysis. *Sleep Med Rev.* 2016;29:52–62. doi:10.1016/j.smrv.2015.08.009.
37. Wu MC, Sung HC, Lee WL, Smith GD. The effects of light therapy on depression and sleep disruption in older adults in a long-term care facility. *Int J Nurs Pract.* 2015;21(5):653–659. https://doi.org/10.1111/ijn.12307.
38. Figueiro MG, Plitnick BA, Lok A, et al. Tailored lighting intervention improves measures of sleep, depression, and agitation in persons with Alzheimer's disease and related dementia living in long-term care facilities. *Clin Interv Aging.* 2014;9:1527–1537. https://www.ncbi.nlm.nih.gov/pmc/articles/PMC4168854/.
39. Akyar I, Akdemir N. The effect of light therapy on the sleep quality of the elderly: an intervention study. *Aust J Adv Nurs.* 2013;31(2):31–47. https://search.informit.com.au/documentSummary;dn=285578734109039;res=IELAPA.
40. Hu RF, Jiang XY, Zeng YM, Chen XY, Zhang YH. Effects of earplugs and eye masks on nocturnal sleep, melatonin and cortisol in a simulated intensive care unit environment. *Crit Care.* 2010;14(2):R66. doi:10.1186/cc8965.
41. Ancuelle V, Zamudio R, Mendiola A, et al. Effects of an adapted mattress in musculoskeletal pain and sleep quality in institutionalized elders. *Sleep Sci.* 2015;8(3):115–120. doi:10.1016/j.slsci.2015.08.004.
42. Hwang E, Shin S. The effects of aromatherapy on sleep improvement: a systematic literature review and meta-analysis. *J Altern Complement Med.* 2015;21(2):61–68. doi:10.1089/acm.2014.0113.
43. Cho MY, Min ES, Hur MH, Lee MS. Effects of aromatherapy on the anxiety, vital signs, and sleep quality of percutaneous coronary intervention patients in intensive care units. *Evid Based Complement Alternat Med.* 2013; 381381. doi:10.1155/2013/381381.
44. Hajibagheri A, Babaii A, Adib-Hajbaghery M. Effect of Rosa damascene aromatherapy on sleep quality in cardiac patients: a randomized controlled trial. *Complement Ther Clin Pract.* 2014;20(3):159–163. doi:10.1016/j.ctcp.2014.05.001.
45. Karadag E, Samancioglu S, Ozden D, Bakir E. Effects of aromatherapy on sleep quality and anxiety of patients. *Nurs Crit Care.* 2017;22(2):105–112. doi:10.1111/nicc.12198.
46. Fonken LK, Nelson RJ. The effects of light at night on circadian clocks and metabolism. *Endocr Rev.* 2014;35(4): 648–670. https://doi.org/10.1210/er.2013-1051.
47. National Sleep Foundation. Sleep hygiene. 2018. https://sleepfoundation.org/sleep-topics/sleep-hygiene.
48. Black DS, O'Reilly GA, Olmstead R, Breen EC, Irwin MR. Mindfulness meditation and improvement in sleep quality and daytime impairment among older adults with sleep disturbances: a randomized clinical trial. *JAMA Intern Med.* 2015;175(4):494–501. doi:10.1001/jamainternmed.2014.8081. Accessed December 14, 2018.
49. Örsal Ö, Alparslan GB, Özkaraman A, Sönmez N. The effect of relaxation exercises on quality of sleep among the elderly: holistic nursing practice review copy. *Holist Nurs Pract.* 2014;28(4):265–274. doi:10.1097/HNP.0000000000000032.
50. Ong JC, Manber R, Segal Z, Xia Y, Shapiro S, Wyatt JK. A randomized controlled trial of mindfulness meditation for chronic insomnia. *Sleep.* 2014;37(9):1553–1563. doi:10.5665/sleep.4010.
51. Sun J, Kang J, Wang P, Zeng H. Self-relaxation training can improve sleep quality and cognitive functions in the older: a one-year randomised controlled trial. *J Clin Nurs.* 2013;22(9–10):1270–1280. doi:10.1111/jocn.12096.
52. Kaul P, Passafiume J, Sargent RC, O'Hara BF. Meditation acutely improves psychomotor vigilance, and may decrease sleep need. *Behav Brain Funct.* 2010;6(1):47. doi:10.1186/1744-9081-6-47.
53. Richards KC, Lambert C, Beck CK, et al. Strength training, walking, and social activity improve sleep in nursing home and assisted living residents: randomized controlled trial. *J Am Geriatr Soc.* 2011;59(2):214–223. https://doi.org/10.1111/j.1532-5415.2010.03246.x.
54. Lorenz RA, Gooneratne N, Cole CS, Kleban MH, Kalra GK, Richards KC. Exercise and social activity improve everyday function in long-term care residents. *Am J Geriatr Psychiatry.* 2012;20(6):468–476. https://doi.org/10.1097/JGP.0b013e318246b807.
55. Kuck J, Pantke M, Flick U. Effects of social activation and physical mobilization on sleep in nursing home residents. *Geriatr Nurs.* 2014;35(6):455–461. doi:10.1016/j.gerinurse.2014.08.009.
56. Taboonpong S, Puthsri N, Kong-In W, Saejew A. The effects of Tai Chi on sleep quality, well-being and physical performances among older adults. *Pac Rim Int J Nurs Res.* 2008;12(1):1–3. https://www.tcithaijo.org/index.php/PRIJNR/article/view/5887.
57. Leland NE, Fogelberg D, Sleight A, et al. Napping and nighttime sleep: findings from an occupation-based intervention. *Am J Occup Ther.* 2016;70(4):7004270010p1–7004270010p7. doi:10.5014/ajot.2016.017657.
58. Li SY, Wang TJ, Vivienne Wu SF, Liang SY, Tung HH. Efficacy of controlling night-time noise and activities to improve patients' sleep quality in a surgical intensive care unit. *J Clin Nurs.* 2011;20(3–4):396–407. doi:10.1111/j.1365-2702.2010.03507.x.

Chapter 52

Psychosocial Adaptation to Disability

Pat Precin

LEARNING OBJECTIVES

This chapter will allow the reader to:

1. Identify and evaluate possible psychosocial disorders in patients receiving occupational therapy services.
2. Understand the disability experience for the adult after experiencing disease or injury resulting in permanent disability.
3. Understand how psychosocial issues can impact daily performance and occupational activities during intervention.
4. Use different models of adjustment to disability to inform treatment.
5. Understand disability culture and the independent living movement.
6. Understand different methods that occupational therapists use to facilitate psychosocial adjustment.

CHAPTER OUTLINE

TERMINOLOGY

Adjustment to disability: a process by which individuals progressively acclimate to disability by passing through specific stages such as denial, anger, depression, and acceptance.

Cognitive–behavioral model: a psychosocial frame of reference often used to promote adjustment to disability.

Denial: a psychological defense mechanism used by certain individuals that involves not acknowledging certain aspects of reality (their disability) in order to tolerate anxiety.

Disability culture: a social movement initiated in the 1980s to recognize, understand, empower, and celebrate different lifestyles of people with disabilities.

Independent living movement: a worldwide philosophy and movement originating in the 1960s in which people with disabilities work together to advocate for decreasing barriers, equal opportunities, respect, peer support, self-respect, self-help, and self-determination.

Post-traumatic stress disorder: a psychiatric diagnosis originating from exposure to repetitive or an isolated psychological trauma and marked by persistent flashbacks of unprocessed trauma, hypervigilance, and a general feeling that the world is unsafe.

Psychodynamic model: a psychosocial frame of reference that helps patients increase participation in occupation by eliminating unconscious barriers.

Psychosocial adjustment: a process by which individuals are able to manage psychosocial issues following a disability in order to more fully participate in occupation.

Stage models: methods by which individuals can obtain psychosocial adjustment and adjustment to disability by passing through a series of linear stages predetermined by the model.

Transtheoretical change model: a model describing different stages that individuals pass through in order to make and maintain a change in their lives.

The Disability Experience

An estimated 1 billion adults or 15.3% of the adult global population have a disability.[1] Psychosocial issues are difficulties that pertain to both psychological and social areas.[2] Examples of psychosocial issues often seen in physical rehabilitation are role loss, depression, **post-traumatic stress disorder** (PTSD), and substance abuse and are addressed in this chapter. Sleep disorders are also psychosocial issues that often occur secondary to neurological and orthopedic disorders and are addressed in Chapter 51.[3] Psychosocial issues often co-occur with physical disabilities and have been shown to affect the disability experience and rehabilitation outcomes in patients with cardiac issues,[4–6] stroke,[7] spinal cord injuries,[8] cancer,[9] athletic injuries,[10] and neurological diagnoses.[11]

When an adult incurs a disease or injury in adulthood that results in permanent disability, he or she may experience a multitude of changes. These changes are not limited to the physical injury or disease process but can include psychosocial issues as well. Life roles, family position, work interactions, self-worth, and personal narrative can be affected. Disruption in any of these areas can hinder the process of adaptation. Yet, adjustments to these areas, if made in a thoughtful, careful, therapeutically guided manner, can not only aid in adapting to an illness but promote personal growth through having struggled with adversity. Occupational therapists are well equipped to assess and address issues related to these areas. Providing evidence-based interventions that foster adjustment to changes in roles, family position, work interactions, self-worth, and personal narratives can guide patients on their way to occupational, social, and community engagement.

Role loss frequently occurs in adults who have experienced disabilities as adults. After a disability, patients may no longer be able to fully participate in roles that were meaningful and necessary to them and their families. A mother may no longer be able to function in her role as the primary caretaker of her children. The loss of ability to function in previous roles can result in painful feelings, such as depression, confusion, loss of identity, and shame. These feelings can hinder adaptation by causing avoidance of taking steps to reengage in roles, especially if the steps bring awareness of limitations and difficult feelings. Therefore, the goal of trying to modify or resume roles can seem daunting to patients.

Role loss may affect the family and the patient's position in the family. A mother who can no longer assume her role as the caretaker of her children may have to relinquish this role to an in-law, changing her position in the family. Resulting feelings may include anger, helplessness, resentment, and fear that her children may grow up without experiencing her as their mother. These negative emotions can affect the mother's adaptation to disability and the family's ability to function as a healthy integrated unit. The role of the occupational therapist would be to (1) identify shifts in the patient's family position and possible areas of functional deficits that interfere with occupational engagement and (2) provide best practice interventions to the patient and family (in conjunction with the social worker if possible).

A patient who has incurred a disease in adulthood may also experience a change in work interaction. Work interaction can refer to job loss, job change, unemployment, altered work responsibilities, increased work pressure or stress, or a change in co-workers' or bosses' perceptions of the patient's new work abilities. There may also be a change in interaction with the work environment, such as requiring a different type of chair, desk, or light source. Even if a patient is able to return to work with a disability, the patient may experience new fatigue when attempting to perform job duties that were easy to perform in the past. The occupational therapist would assess the patient's work interaction and adjustment and then provide intervention that can help the patient make a smooth transition to his or her work or volunteer situation.

When a patient undergoes a disease process or injury that results in a permanent disability in adulthood followed by changes in roles, family position, and work interaction, self-worth is likely to be affected. Patients in this situation often experience a period of time when they feel distressed about themselves and their limitations. In addition, they may receive negative feedback from their social and physical environment. The physical environment is no longer as easy to negotiate. Patients are reminded of this on a daily basis. The social stigma of having a disability (being a person who is disabled, therefore not "normal") can be pervasive throughout work, social, and virtual environments[12] and is likely to affect a person's self-worth through internalization.

When patients experience a decrease in self-worth, their life narratives may also change. Life narratives are stories about how people view themselves in context.[13] Each person's narrative is unique, fluctuates overtime, and is sensitive to experiences, emotions, and personal growth. Prior to injury, a patient's life narrative may include being a businessman, father of five children, loving husband, financial provider, and avid skier who feels confident in and proud of his roles and accomplishments at the age of 37. He may be looking forward to a long productive life with many grandchildren. His narrative did not include the fact that this all changed because of a car accident, which resulted in an above the knee amputation. Four months after the accident, his narrative may sound more like this:

> I hate this. I can't do this anymore. I'm in so much pain and everything takes so long to do. I can't believe that at age 37 I'm unemployed and my wife has to find a job to support us. I'm so stressed out that we may not make our mortgage payments. I feel so inadequate…like I let everyone down. I hate myself. I wish I could undo everything and go back to the way things were. Instead, I want it all to be over.

This is a sad but typical life narrative, given this patient's circumstance. His occupational therapist could help him begin to regain control and create a new life through narrative writing and cognitive–behavioral techniques in which he would create his (1) current life narrative, (2) projected future narrative, and (3) in-between narratives that would move him toward his projected future.[14]

Adjustment to Disability

Adjustment to disability is unique to each patient; however, there are different practice models that occupational therapists can use to help understand their patients' unique experience of disability and guide them through the **psychosocial adjustment** process while providing appropriate treatment. Some of these models include adaptation to disabilities, psychodynamic, cognitive–behavioral, and transtheoretical. **Stage models** are methods by which individuals can obtain adjustment to psychosocial and physical disability by passing through a series of linear stages predetermined by the model. An example of a stage model is the adaptation to disabilities model,[15] where patients first experience, then pass through stages of **denial**, anger, depression, and acceptance in that order; the model is summarized in the subsequent sections.

Denial, Anger, Depression, and Acceptance

When patients first learn of their diagnosis or understand that they have an injury, they may use the defense mechanism of denial to ward off anxiety related to the reality of their situation. The process of rehabilitation allows patients to slowly become aware of their limitations through functional assessments and interventions directed toward improving deficits and maximizing strengths. This process helps patients move out of denial and into the second stage, anger.

Anger can be a healthy vehicle through which patients expel pent up energy and avoid initial depression (turning their anger onto themselves) and is an appropriate emotion to experience at this point in recovery. Some patients, however, never move past the anger stage, and prolonged anger can interfere with rehabilitation. An occupational therapist can help patients move out of the stage of anger by allowing them to verbally express their anger in the beginning of each session, then helping them to focus on the rehabilitation task. The patient's emotion is validated, and the patient is shown how to move through anger, or redirect the energy of the anger toward engagement in productive tasks. The patient may be better able to manage anger on his or her own after this experience. If anger is not validated, it may perpetuate and interfere with progress to the third stage, depression.

The stage of depression occurs as patients become exhausted from rehabilitation efforts, social supports and attention from visitors wanes, caregivers become emotionally and physically depleted and can no longer respond to the patient in the same supportive manner, disappointment from lack of swift progress is experienced by the patient and echoed throughout the family, and hope of return to previous functioning that may have been present in the beginning may be lost.

When a patient moves out of the depression stage, he or she moves toward acceptance. Those who achieve acceptance have come to terms with their limitations and are willing to use their strengths to accomplish new goals and roles in life. They are able to establish and engage in new occupations that hold meaning for their lives and enhance their social networks to include others who understand disability. Acceptance does not necessarily imply physical improvement. Instead, it is a lived attitude.

Psychodynamic Model, Cognitive–Behavioral Model, and Transtheoretical Change Model

The **psychodynamic model** focuses on how memories of past experiences and unconscious processes affect current behavior. The model values the symbolic nature of activities and mandates that they be selected for intrinsic meaning and relevance to the patient. This model is often used when conscious-based ego-focused interventions do not produce the desired result. For example, an occupational therapist observes that a patient in her money management group is not adhering to her budget from week-to-week, despite having learned necessary money management skills. The occupational therapist reasons that there may be a psychodynamic component involved and asks what money means to the patient. The patient informs the group that her mother used to give her a small weekly allowance, but after her mother's death, her father said that she should be financially independent. The group empathetically inquired about the mother's death, and the patient replied that she was sad but secretly angry at her father for not replacing her mother's nurturance expressed through gifting the allowance. An interpretation was made that perhaps her repressed anger toward her father inhibited her budgetary follow-through. In the next group session, the patient had followed her budget, theoretically because she had become aware of how her repressed anger and desire for nurturance (both unconscious) had been affecting her current behavior.

Rather than reflecting on how the past and unconscious material affect current maladaptive behavior, the **cognitive–behavioral models** focus on how current unhealthy thought patterns can lead to unhealthy behavior. Interventions involve developing healthy patterns of thinking that lead to targeted behavioral changes. Cognitive–behavioral therapy (CBT) is an example of a cognitive–behavioral practice model whose effects have been found to generalize to real-world settings (home, community, work).[16] Occupational therapists who use methods of CBT carefully observe, record, and examine patients' reactions to experiences and links between thinking and behaving. These therapists reward successively graded goals-shaping thoughts and behaviors that indicate successful adaptation. They point out patterns in patient narratives that suggest helplessness or negative projections about the future, helping to substitute more positive thoughts and self-statements. Treatment programs reinforce adherence and good self-care, such as wearing a splint or taking medication, and work to extinguish damaging habits, such as smoking, and socially isolating behaviors, such as aggressive outbursts. CBT treatment components may be designed for individual or group work directed toward specific symptoms, including pain, depression, or insomnia.[17] Skills for self-regulation, including assertive communication and practicing the relaxation response (RR), may also be the components of CBT.[18]

The **transtheoretical change model** is based on the observation that people make changes by advancing through an ordered series of stages: precontemplation, contemplation, preparation, action, maintenance, and termination. Patients in precontemplation are not interested in making a change in the near future (6 months) and may not be aware that change is necessary. Occupational therapists can provide patients with psychoeducation about specific healthy and unhealthy behaviors related to their issues in order to help them become aware of their unhealthy habits and progress to the contemplation stage. During contemplation, patients use their new knowledge to intend to begin a healthy behavior within 6 months. Occupational therapists can help patients evaluate pros and cons and set goals because ambivalence around change can result in procrastination. During the preparation stage, patients are ready to begin their goal for change within the next month. Occupational therapists can help patients take short-term steps to help prepare for the change (e.g., informing friends and family that they would like to change their behavior) and create a plan for change. Occupational therapists can encourage patients to think, discuss, and write narratives about what their lives will be like once they have made the change, because fear of failure is the primary barrier to moving into the stage of action. Patients have made their change within the past 6 months during the action stage, so occupational therapists can help patients focus on their goal and resist temptation to return to unhealthy behaviors. Guiding patients through the processes of substituting positive behaviors for unhealthy ones; avoiding people, places, and things that may keep them from continuing their new behavior; spending time with supportive individuals; and rewarding themselves can enhance commitment to change. Patients are considered to be in the maintenance stage if they have completed 6 months or more of their new behavior. Occupational therapists can help patients identify and avoid triggers that may result in relapse (terminating the healthy behavior or engaging in the unhealthy behavior of the past), and identify and use healthy coping mechanisms (e.g., talking to friends) to handle stress and manage emotions instead of resorting to previous unhealthy behaviors. The final stage of termination is achieved after the patient's new behavior has become part of his or her routine/lifestyle and no energy is needed to successfully maintain it. Not all patients achieve this stage.[19]

Disability Culture and the Independent Living Movement

It is important to consider social context when attempting to understand the experience of disability in patients. The **independent living movement** is a worldwide philosophy and movement originating in the 1960s in which people with disabilities work together to advocate for decreasing barriers, equal opportunities, respect, peer support, self-respect, self-help, and self-determination. This movement was successful in accomplishing some of these issues (e.g., through the Paralympics)[20] and led to what is now called **disability culture**. Disability culture is a social movement initiated in the 1980s to recognize, understand, empower, and celebrate different lifestyles of people with disabilities.[15] The disability arts movement and the Disability Pride Parade are just a few examples of the many different movements and programs developed within disability culture that continue to flourish. As occupational therapists expand their rehabilitation framework to view themselves as professionals who use occupation to promote healthy living and well-being,[21] they are better able to incorporate the independent living movement and disability culture into their interventions.

How Occupational Therapists Facilitate Psychosocial Adjustment

Occupational therapists provide evaluation of and intervention for psychosocial disorders such as role loss, depression, PTSD, and substance abuse that produce behaviors maladaptive to physical rehabilitation and the process of adaptation. When occupational therapists detect psychosocial disorders, they should notify the treatment team or persuade outpatient clients to make appointments with their primary care physicians because interdisciplinary treatment of psychosocial disorders may be the most effective type of treatment.[9,22]

Occupational Therapy Evaluation and Intervention of Role Loss

The developmental tasks of adulthood include confirming career choice, finding a partner, and parenting children. When an adult at this point in the life cycle becomes disabled, plans and conceptions about the future, which may already have been the focus of substantial effort, require reorganizing. Ongoing life satisfaction and dignity, rather than level of self-care, are becoming recognized as the most valuable measures of rehabilitation success and may be most congruent with patient and family hopes and expectations.[23,24] These measures should, therefore, be the basis of intervention concerning loss of and reassignment of roles.

The occupational therapist would begin treatment by identifying previous role functions and assessing the patient's ability, motivation, and support to resume them. The Role Checklist[25] is used to assess patients' past, current, and future roles and the amount of value patients place on each role. Occupational therapists can use this assessment to (1) identify barriers to current and future patient roles that are highly valued and (2) set goals for surmounting barriers, making accommodations within roles, and/or selecting new roles that hold value. If patients become overwhelmed with the process of redefining or selecting new roles, the Activity Card Sort[26] (see Fig. 52-1) can be administered to help patients gain insight into realistic activity preferences, which may then aid in role adjustment.

Because patients may be striving to regain their roles by merging their old and new realities, occupational therapists can help them revise and reformulate expectations. The occupational therapy (OT) treatment plan integrates psychological demands and addresses them in concert with activities of daily living (ADLs), strengthening, endurance, mobility, and prevocational training. Adapting to disability occurring at this stage may require altering vocational course, finding different leisure activities, redesigning an intimate partnership, and rebalancing parenting roles. Occupational therapists model problem-solving with realistic expectations—reconciling capacities, and working with patients' strengths toward a sense of fulfillment[27]—and helping patients reclaim personal continuity and create meaningful life narratives, which integrate their experiences of illness or injury.[28,29] Occupational therapists can reinforce patients' motivation to heal and nurture their well-being at critical turning points and in the face of what for some will be lasting physical compromise.[30]

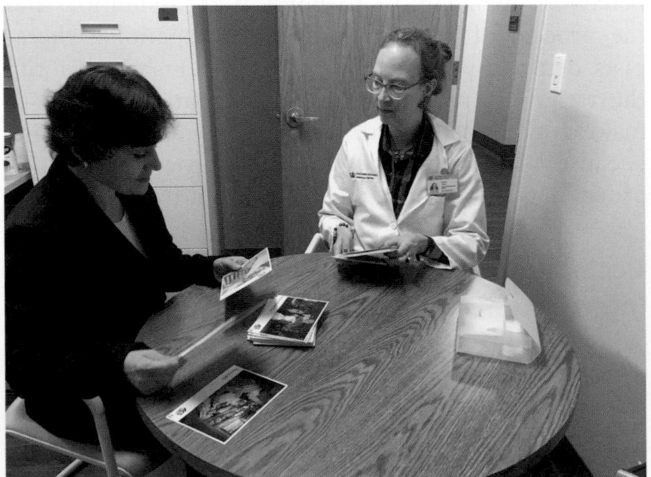
Figure 52-1. Administration of the Activity Card Sort.

As an ADL, sexual activity merits an accepting, problem-solving focus. The occupational therapist explicitly helps the disabled person by encouraging him or her to reconceptualize sexuality and sexual activity more broadly and to explore new possibilities for sexual expression. When the disabled individual has a consistent sexual partner, the therapist may offer the opportunity to include him or her in teaching or treatment sessions. The disabled person and his or her sexual partner may learn to adapt to periods of fatigue, continence timing, or requirements for special positioning (see Chapter 27).

Families as well as patients may need help reorganizing. Family reorganization requires learning and concrete problem-solving, as well as transformation within the family unit, parallel to that of the disabled person. Occupational therapists can help partners and families forge new identities among themselves and within their communities.

Occupational Therapy Evaluation and Intervention of Depression

More than 300 million people currently experience depression according to the 2018 World Health Organization report.[31] Depression may be more prevalent in patients receiving rehabilitation treatment or adapting to a disease process or injury than in individuals without disabilities.[32] Depression is the most frequently experienced psychological result of stroke.[33] Up to half of stroke survivors develop depressive signs and symptoms[34]; yet, depression is frequently underdiagnosed.[35] It is imperative that occupational therapists learn to identify symptoms, signs, and behaviors characteristic of depression in their patients during physical rehabilitation sessions.

Signs and symptoms of depression commonly observed in patients undergoing rehabilitation according to Precin[32] are listed as follows. They are meant as a guide because the etiology of depression for each patient may differ: what may cause depressive signs/symptoms in one patient may not cause depression in another patient.

Mild Depression

- Poor concentration
- Sadness
- Irritability
- Neediness
- Anger
- Depressed mood
- Indecisiveness
- Lethargy
- Intrusive thoughts
- Loneliness
- Anxiety

Moderate Depression

- Despair
- Sensitivity
- Feeling overwhelmed
- Feeling inadequate
- Despondence
- Fearful
- Decreased self-esteem
- Anguish
- Excessive guilt

Severe Depression

- Change in weight
- Change in appetite
- Sleep disturbances (narcolepsy, insomnia)
- Decreased sexual drive
- Desperation
- Feeling hopeless
- Feeling helpless
- Feeling worthless
- Suicidal ideation

These symptoms and signs may manifest in different behaviors that can be recognized by occupational therapists. Some behaviors characteristic of mild, moderate, and severe depression that frequently occur in physical rehabilitation are listed as follows.[32]

Behaviors Characteristic of Mild Depression

- Difficulty planning for the near future
- Obsessing about tasks
- Becoming frustrated easily
- Sitting alone

Behaviors Characteristic of Moderate Depression

- Reacting negatively to feedback
- Inability to make simple decisions
- Crying
- Making self-depreciating remarks
- Reporting psychosomatic symptoms
- Exhibiting overly dependent behavior
- Talking about the past, present, and/or future in a pessimistic manner
- Withdrawing socially
- Perseverating and/or ruminating on issues

Behaviors Characteristic of Severe Depression

- Staying in bed all day
- Poor hygiene
- Decreased interest in activities that used to elicit pleasure
- Suicide attempt

If occupational therapists identify any of the signs/symptoms/behaviors of depression mentioned previously, they could perform a more in-depth assessment using the following standardized, reliable, and valid instruments typically used to measure levels of depression, self-efficacy, and self-esteem: Beck Depression Inventory,[36] General Self-Efficacy Scale-6,[37] or the Rosenberg Self-Esteem Scale.[38] These are self-report assessments that can be completed in under 10 minutes. If the patient demonstrates signs, symptoms, or behaviors indicative of severe depression, the occupational therapist should make a referral to a psychiatrist and alert the treatment team. Additional referrals may be made to psychological services for chronic depression. The most important goal is patient safety.[39]

If depression is not identified during physical rehabilitation, it may go untreated and worsen, resulting in the inability to make full use of rehabilitation. When depression is treated in rehabilitative settings, treatment usually consists of medication and psychotherapy, but the effectiveness of both is questionable and may produce harmful side effects, especially in the elderly.[35] Depression post-stroke resulted in poor rehabilitation outcomes, increased caregivers' stress, cognitive and physical impairments, substance misuse, increased risk of suicide and patient death, increased utilization of medical resources, and poor treatment compliance.[40–42] Depression in cardiac rehabilitation predicted poorer outcomes[6] and greater dropout rates[5] when compared to cardiac rehabilitation patients without depression. Patients who developed depression during sports injury rehabilitation demonstrated poorer rehabilitation outcomes and less frequently returned to their sport[10] when compared to sports rehabilitation patients without depression. Depression resulted in lower return-to-work rates in cancer survivors.[9]

Several studies have demonstrated the effectiveness of engaging patients in problem-solving activities in conjunction with antidepressants to decrease depression and promote overall psychosocial adaptation during physical rehabilitation.[43,44] Occupational therapists can help patients identify several problems they are experiencing as barriers to rehabilitation and adaptation. The patient would be instructed to write a goal that would alleviate each problem and then identify three to four steps to take within a week to achieve each goal. The therapist would follow up with each of the patient's goals one-at-a-time until all steps had been taken and the goal accomplished. Problem-solving in this manner can help patients actively regain control over certain aspects of their daily life and empower them in the rehabilitation process.

Livneh and Martz[45] identified a combination of coping strategies that predicted psychosocial adaptation and decreased depression in patients with spinal cord injuries. These coping strategies were problem-solving, cognitive restructuring, planning, active acceptance, and seeking social support. Occupational therapists can engage patients in the act of cognitive restructuring (a component of CBT) by identifying patients' statements that indicate maladaptive thoughts, reality testing the validity of these thoughts during physical rehabilitation, and then readjusting thoughts to be more realistic and adaptive.

An example of how to combine cognitive restructuring, problem-solving, planning, and seeking social support follows. A patient might express that he or she cannot do something (possible maladaptive thought). The occupational therapist would then perform reality test with the patient by saying, "I think you were able to do this yesterday, isn't that so?" The patient may respond, "yes." Then, the therapist might ask, "What is making it hard for you today?" (asking the patient to identify a barrier and challenging the belief that he or she cannot perform the task in question). The occupational therapist helps the patient problem solve around the barrier in order to alleviate the problem, which allows engagement in the activity that was previously thought to be impossible. This process dispels the patient's unrealistic and maladaptive thought and serves as an example of how the patient could then follow the same process on his or her own when future maladaptive thoughts arise. If the patient still requires assistance, the occupational therapist could help the patient reach out to family members (seeking social support) to help continue this process during family visits by training the family in this process (psychoeducation).

An evidence-based review of the effectiveness of interventions for adults with psychological impairment poststroke identified problem-solving, behavioral therapy, and motivational interviewing as effective interventions for the treatment of depression.[46] The four premises of motivational interviewing are empathy, identify discrepancies, promote self-efficacy, and accept patients' resistances.[47] When using motivational interviewing, occupational therapists would demonstrate consistent empathy while pointing out differences between patients' goals and current behavior and showing their belief that goals can be achieved.

A systematic review of OT and multidisciplinary approaches for the rehabilitation of patients with cancer revealed studies that supported the use of problem-solving, cognitive-behavioral therapy, psychoeducation, life review, and expressive writing approaches[9] to decrease depression. Treatment for depression can also continue after discharge. A home leisure education program poststroke was found to be effective in the treatment of depression.[48] The goals of a leisure education program may be to (1) teach the patient the benefits of social participation and engagement in activities that lead to self-assertiveness, reengagement, and self-determination; and (2) then help them to identify and pursue new daily-life activities that are meaningful.[39]

Occupational Therapy Evaluation and Intervention of Post-Traumatic Stress Disorder

PTSD is a psychiatric diagnosis originating from exposure to repetitive or an isolated psychological trauma and marked by persistent flashbacks to unprocessed trauma, hypervigilance, and a general feeling that the world is unsafe. Individuals injured or disabled through war, natural disaster, accident, abuse, or violent crime are at high risk. For some patients, the resulting disability may constitute lifelong physical evidence of the traumatic experience, serving as a proprioceptive cue or trigger for PTSD symptoms and continuing stress reactions. Symptoms observed during physical rehabilitation can include hyperarousal, nervousness, fearfulness, nightmares, flashbacks, ruminations, emotional numbing, and dissociation.[49] Individuals showing symptoms of PTSD usually require referral to be evaluated for specialized psychotherapy and possible medication. Coordination between caregivers is critical to a positive outcome for these patients, who need a safe, predictable environment in which they can make sense of their experiences. If the occupational therapist is not sure whether or not to make a referral, he or she can administer The Primary Care PTSD Screen for DSM-5 (PC-PTSD-5),[50] a five-question screen for PTSD. If the score is 3 or greater, a referral should be made.

There are five defined stages of intervention for PTSD according to Herman,[51] including:

1. Developing a healing relationship
2. Safety
3. Recalling past memories and mourning
4. Reconnecting
5. Commonality

Occupational therapists can help individuals during each stage. In order to develop a healing relationship, the occupational therapist can empower the patient by fostering trust, autonomy, initiative, competence, and identity formation. Patients with PTSD should be an active part of their recovery. Any intervention that takes power from patients has the potential to retraumatize patients by creating a "power-over" dynamic reminiscent of past trauma and may revictimize and trigger patients. Therefore, occupational therapists should counter the dynamic of dominance in the therapeutic relationship by increasing the range of treatment choices, respecting the patient's autonomy by remaining emotionally neutral, validating feelings and narrative stories, providing psychoeducation on symptoms, using persuasion rather than coercion, using ideas rather than dogmatic interventions, and fostering mutuality rather than authoritarian control.

In stage 2, occupational therapists help patients regain safety over their minds, bodies, and environments. To regain safety over their minds, occupational therapists help patients name the problem by giving them language for the experience (diagnosis, signs, symptoms) and provide explanations for current difficulties, informing them that they are not alone, not crazy, and can expect to recover in the way others with PTSD have. Patients can be taught to keep daily logs to track their response to symptoms. Restoring ego functions includes helping the patient initiate, carry out plans, exercise independent judgment, and utilize self-soothing strategies. Control of the body includes basic health needs, regulation of bodily functions, sleep, eating, exercise, control of self-destructive behaviors, symptom management, and decreasing hyperarousal and intrusive symptoms. Control of the environment includes financial security, mobility, plans for self-protection, safe living environments, and family meetings.

During stage 3, occupational therapists help patients talk or write about their traumatic experience, helping them associate affect with factual statements of the experience while normalizing patients' responses. Next, occupational therapists help patients construct new interpretations of the traumatic experience that are no longer about shame and humiliation, but affirm dignity and value. Listening to their narratives is a very important part of the first stage of their treatment but can be disturbing; strong team support and supervision become important for all involved, such as caregivers and occupational therapists.

Occupational therapists are well equipped to help patients at stage 4 reconnect with others and find new ways of living as survivors (social action and public truth-telling can be therapeutic). During the final stage of commonality, therapy groups can be used to create a sense of belonging because trauma isolates, bear witness and affirm because trauma stigmatizes and shames, restore humanity because trauma dehumanizes, provide a sense of universality, and provide treatment for different stages. Occupational therapists use groups at this stage to help members organize their daily-life structure and enhance their ability to feel safe while participating in meaningful roles and activities in the community.[52]

Occupational Therapy Evaluation and Intervention of Substance Abuse

The use of drugs and alcohol has been associated with depression and anxiety after traumatic head injury[53] and may be prevalent in patients in vulnerable states as a result of other injuries or diseases. In response to the American Occupational Therapy Association's Evidence-Based Literature Review Project,[54] Stoffel and Moyers[55] performed an interdisciplinary systematic review of effective treatment for individuals diagnosed with substance-use disorders and found four effective treatment approaches that could be used by occupational therapists: brief interventions, CBT, motivational strategies, and 12-step programs, and are summarized as follows.

Brief interventions occur in one session that can run from 5 minutes to an hour and focus on identifying a substance abuse problem and then motivating the patient to do something about it.[55] Substance abuse occurs frequently in people with disabilities, but patients in rehabilitation may be reluctant to disclose their use even if it is problematic. Therefore, occupational therapists need to look for signs, symptoms, and behaviors of substance use that can be identified during a brief intervention. Pain medication can be very addicting, so it is important for the occupational therapist to understand patients' medication dose, frequency, and type. Signs, symptoms, and behaviors characteristic of patients who are abusing substances may include cognitive deficits, isolation, alcohol on breath, disinhibition, denial, belligerence, low frustration tolerance, inappropriate interpersonal behavior, paranoia, impaired judgment, poor boundaries, impulsivity, violence, emotional lability, thought disturbances, irritability, slurred speech, and intense emotions.[32] If some of these characteristics are observed, occupational therapists can ask patients about substance use by taking an occupational history using the following questions:

- Is the patient functioning in work or school? Is the patient maintaining relationships?
- Are any family members likely to be helpful in describing the patient's history?
- Is there any evidence that substance abuse was a primary cause of the condition?
- Might the condition have provoked substance abuse?
- Are there predisposing factors such as depression, trauma, family history, or membership in a marginalized group?
- Does evidence support need for referral?

Sometimes, it is easier for patients to report their use if a standardized assessment is used (once removed from reporting directly to the therapist). The Substance Abuse Screening Test[56] is a short self-report questionnaire that an occupational therapist could administer to identify people who abuse substances and those at risk for abuse. Brief intervention could also include the distribution of psychoeducational material to the patient and his or her family that addresses the deleterious effects of use, benefits of harm reduction or abstinence, the fact that substance abuse is a chronic disease that involves relapse and not a result of victimhood or weak character, and information on available 12-step groups with a recommendation to participate.[55] Brief interventions work well when the treatment priority is physical rehabilitation due to the reason for referral, limited time, or lack of reimbursement for substance abuse services.

CBT can be used to develop healthy skills to avoid relapse by changing maladaptive thoughts and distorted thinking that trigger substance use. Maintaining and reviewing a substance-use diary documenting the nature of use (frequency of use, time of day, who they were with, what they were feeling and thinking, where they were, what they were doing, what drug they used, where they obtained the drug) can help patients identify maladaptive thoughts and cognitively restructure them. The diary can also be used to increase awareness of patterns of use that patients can use to predict and avoid future relapses. The more insight patients have about their addiction process, the greater the chance that they will be able to progress in the recovery process. This intervention does not take a lot of time because patients keep the diary on their own. They just require instructions about how to begin. Occupational therapists review diary entries as often as possible and provide positive feedback when appropriate.

The development of time and stress management, ADLs, and social skills are important to recovery because individuals who abuse substances may have deficits in each of these areas. Substance abuse can become an occupation that takes over all aspects of the patient's life. Once the abuse is no longer an occupation, patients often need help reorganizing their day-to-day activities and relearning to manage their emotions. There are workbooks[13] with established effectiveness[57] that patients can use on their own to develop these skills. The occupational therapist can provide the patient with a workbook and then check the patients work in following sessions.

Occupational therapists can also use cognitive–behavioral methods to help patients achieve the following long-term goals:

- Improve health habits and self-care.
- Develop skills in self-regulation and impulse control.
- Develop substance-free leisure skills.
- Develop the ability to plan ahead to avoid relapse.
- Develop the ability to set realistic short-term goals related to sobriety.
- Experience group participation, learn to communicate needs, learn to give and receive support.
- Prepare for a constructive vocational role.
- Value a clean and sober identity.
- Connect with community resources such as Alcoholics Anonymous (AA) to maintain sobriety.

All of these skills promote patients' self-efficacy in their process of staying sober. It may also be helpful to guide patients in the process of comparing their lives before and after sobriety to reinforce their progress and the positive aspects of their lives so they keep moving in a forward direction.

Motivational strategies can be used to identify the patient's stage of change and then foster his or her motivation to change.[55] Motivational interviewing, as previously mentioned, is a patient-centered strategy that increases intrinsic motivation using nonconfrontational communication that reflects empathy and is an effective strategy to use when patients verbalize resistance to change.[47] Decision balancing helps patients weigh the pros and cons of using drugs so that the cons outweigh the pros. Motivational enhancement therapy can be used to keep patients involved in their change processes after initial changes have been made.[55]

The 12-step treatment programs utilize the principles of 12-step support groups, such as AA and Narcotics Anonymous. Unlike 12-step support groups, 12-step treatment programs are often lead by a professional, are nonconfrontational, accept harm reduction when full abstinence seems unattainable, and allow for the taking of prescribed medications. According to Stoffel and Moyers,[55] occupational therapists can use 12-step treatment programs to evaluate a patient's readiness for 12-step support groups, help patients develop external supports that promote sobriety, design interventions that incorporate 12-step principles, and promote continuation of healthy habits that replace unhealthy habits associated with substance use. They suggest the use of spirituality as a form of treatment to help patients identify their meaning of life and, in keeping with the 12-step tradition, to educate and reinforce that recovery from substance abuse is a lifelong commitment.

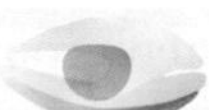

CASE STUDY

Patient Information

Leslie is a 66-year-old recently retired white female who has returned to independent living after a 5-day rehabilitation hospitalization secondary to a car accident and resultant complex fracture of the right wrist of her dominant hand. She has been prescribed oxycodone for pain. Leslie has been receiving outpatient OT at her community physical rehabilitation clinic for an exercise regime to decrease edema in her right upper extremity. However, it appears that she may not be performing her daily home exercise routine because she is unaware of how to do it in the clinic and appears lethargic and slurs her words.

Reason for Occupational Therapy Referral

In addition to decreasing edema, Leslie has been referred for OT services to increase independence in self-care and basic ADLs using her nondominant hand.

Assessment Process and Results

The occupational therapist inquired about Leslie's ability to follow through with her home exercise regime. Leslie reported being tired all the time and not being motivated to do much of anything. So, instead of conducting the OT treatment session planned for that day at the clinic, Leslie agreed to do a spontaneous home visit to determine her ability to function independently. Her home was in disarray. It was clear that she had not been doing dishes, laundry, or cleaning. She did not seem concerned about the status of her house and had no reservations about the occupational therapist noting its condition. Leslie was focused on taking her pain medication, stating that she did not want to start exercising until she had adequate pain relief. At this point, the occupational therapist suspected that Leslie may be taking too much pain medication and asked to see her medication vile. The remaining number of pills was too low for her dosage, indicating that she had taken too many. When the number of remaining pills was brought to her

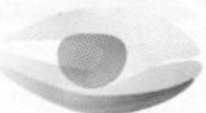

CASE STUDY *(continued)*

attention, Leslie responded that she was an alcoholic in recovery, had a high tolerance for pain medication, and needed more than an average person.

The occupational therapist administered the Substance Abuse Screening Test and took an occupational history regarding her substance use. Leslie had starting drinking in high school and continued until age 32 when her boss referred her to the Employment Opportunity Program for treatment or risk losing her job. Leslie followed through with substance abuse counseling and a 12-step program until she felt she no longer needed treatment for alcohol abuse at age 45. Prior to her retirement at age 65, Leslie had over 20 years of sobriety. After retirement, Leslie reported having nothing to do and feeling depressed and lonely because she never married, had children, and had not been in an intimate relationship for several years, stating that it was hard to find a lesbian partner at her age. To fill her time and loneliness, Leslie started drinking again. She admitted that her current car accident could have been a result of her drinking before driving and, while crying, blamed herself for her current situation. Her occupational therapist empathetically added that her current pain medication is highly addictive and may be making it harder for her to function. Leslie replied that she wants to stop drinking now but continues to drink and isolate as a result of feeling unsafe in the world after the accident.

The occupational therapist administered the Beck Depression Inventory because of Leslie's self-blame and sadness. Results indicated that Leslie is depressed, but not suicidal, and has some hope for the future. The occupational therapist administered the PC-PTSD-5 because Leslie no longer feels that the world is a safe place after her accident and isolates herself inside her home. Leslie scored a 3 on the PC-PTSD-5, indicating the need for referral for full PTSD evaluation by a psychologist.

Occupational Therapy Problem List

- Inability to use dominant arm secondary to right wrist complex fracture
- Edema in the right upper extremity
- Co-occurring pain medication and alcohol misuse
- Currently experiencing depression
- Currently experiencing symptoms of PTSD
- Isolated in home most of the time
- Fatigue
- Poor ADL and self-care skills
- Social isolation
- Noncompliant with home exercises
- Few leisure pursuits
- Loss of the role of employee

Occupational Therapy Goal List

- Increase dexterity, strength, and endurance in the left upper extremity sufficiently to participate in basic ADLs and self-care by 2 weeks.
- Comply with daily exercise routine to decrease edema in the right upper extremity (using a written exercise log noting the amount of time spent exercising, whether or not the recommended routine was completed, and if not, what barriers prevented completion).
- Decrease oxycodone use until abstinent by 1 week upon recommendation by physician (from self-report) and decrease use of alcohol until abstinent by 2 months (by counting clean days).
- Decrease level of depression as noted on the Beck Depression Scale by 2 months.
- Decrease symptoms of PTSD by decreasing her score from 3 to 2 on the PC-PTSD-5 by 3 months.
- Increase the amount of time spent in purposeful activities (leisure and therapeutic) performed outside the home and with others from 2 to 7 hours per week by 3 weeks, using a self-report calendar.
- Decrease daytime fatigue levels from 9 to 6 on a 10-point scale (0 = low, 10 = high) in 2 weeks.

Intervention

Leslie continued to receive OT services to increase independence in self-care and basic ADLs using her nondominant hand and decrease edema in her dominant upper extremity. Her physician agreed to help her taper slowly off oxycodone and replace it with Tylenol 3 for pain management after which she was observed to be more alert and motivated during therapy sessions and no longer slurring her words. Leslie agreed to resume daily AA meetings at her local LGBTQ+ (lesbian gay bisexual transgender queer/questioning) community center because she was familiar with 12-step programs and found them helpful in the past. These meetings helped her make new friends with similar lifestyles. Her feelings of safety in these meetings extended to her larger world by helping Leslie realize that her accident resulted from her drinking and that she could become sober again. She met friends who shared common leisure interests and thus felt less lonely and isolated. Leslie became motivated to take care of her home in order to invite friends over.

Leslie received education from her occupational therapist about edema, which indicated that if severe enough could cause death. As a result, she completed her prescribed daily exercise routine for her dominant upper extremity. She had more energy after decreasing her alcohol and oxycodone consumption and was thus able to complete all nondominant upper extremity exercises as per her daily exercise log.

After 3 months, Leslie reported that she was able to maintain these changes and was retested. Her Beck Depression Scale score improved. Her score on the PC-PTSD-5 improved from 3 to 2. Scores on the fatigue scale improved from 9 to 4. Leslie spent an average of 4 hours per day engaged in purposeful leisure, social, and therapeutic activities outside the home, as noted on her calendar. She was attending daily AA groups that she found very helpful and achieved her 30-day token for sobriety from alcohol and oxycodone. Through Leslie's work with her occupational therapist, she was able to redefine her role as retiree. In 3 months, she went from spending most of her time drinking to engaging in community leisure pursuits with newly acquired sober friends and participating in daily AA meetings.

Evidence Table of Intervention Studies for Psychosocial Adaptation to Disability

Intervention	Description	Participants	Dosage	Research Design and Evidence Level	Benefit	Statistical Significance and Effect Size
Occupational therapy (OT) interventions to improve occupational performance for patients with psychological impairment poststroke[46]	Six interventions were identified to treat depression, mental health quality of life, or anxiety: 1. Exercise/movement therapy 2. Behavioral therapy and stroke education 3. Behavioral therapy only 4. Care support and coordination 5. Stroke education only 6. Community-based interventions	Thirty-eight studies were included in this evidence-based review. Thirty-seven studies were Level I, one study was Level II, and one study was Level III. Study participants consisted of stroke survivors in various settings and at various amounts of time poststroke.	Intensive interdisciplinary treatment in the community consisted of six or more home visits. No other lengths of interventions were given.	Evidence-based review Level I	Problem-solving, behavioral techniques, and motivational interviewing were effective in treating depression. Interdisciplinary home programs were effective in decreasing anxiety and depression and increasing health-related quality of life poststroke.	Results listed under "Benefit" were all statistically significant, but no specific effect sizes were reported for individual studies.
Psychosocial interventions for women diagnosed with substance abuse to improve: substance use, intrapersonal functioning, health education, skill development, parenting skills, trauma, mental health (depression, anxiety, PTSD), occupation/productivity, sexuality, mindfulness/meditation, housing, and body image[58]	Interventions included education, motivational interviewing, skills based, CBT, psychotherapy, therapeutic community, experimental, peer counseling, goal setting, mindfulness/meditation, and 12-step groups. Treatment was group based ($n = 18$), individual based ($n = 14$), and combined group and individual ($n = 10$).	Forty-two studies were included in this scoping review. Study participants consisted of women diagnosed with substance abuse in various settings (inpatient $n = 13$, outpatient $n = 22$, combined inpatient/outpatient $n = 7$).	All programs varied, no specific dosages were given.	Scoping review Level I	The majority of the programs used harm reduction ($n = 32$) and multiple interventions that addressed multiple goals for psychosocial rehabilitation related to substance abuse.	No statistical significance or effect sizes were reported.

Interdisciplinary intervention and rehabilitation within OT scope of practice to maximize activity and participation in adult cancer survivors[10]	There were four categories of intervention: multidisciplinary ($n = 5$), psychosocial ($n = 29$), return-to-work ($n = 3$), and sexuality ($n = 2$).	Fifty-two studies were included in this systematic review: 45 Level I, 3 Level II, and 3 Level III. Study participants consisted of adult cancer survivors in various settings and with various types and stages of cancer	Multidisciplinary treatment programs consisted of OT, physical therapy [PT], and other health care professional interventions. Psychosocial treatments included stress management, problem-solving, life review, expressive groups, CBT, and mindfulness. Return-to-work intervention included strengthening exercises. Sexuality interventions were psychoeducation, medical, and exercise.	Systematic review Level I	Psychosocial strategies reduced anxiety and depression and multidisciplinary rehabilitation improved function and participation in adult cancer survivors regardless of their type of cancer.	Strong evidence: (1) multidisciplinary rehabilitation improved function and participation, (2) CBT and educational treatments (knowledge of illness and side effects, problem-solving) decreased anxiety longer than 3 months postintervention and depression 1–3 months postintervention.
Interdisciplinary (OT, nursing, medicine, social work, psychology, public heath, sociology) interventions for patients diagnosed with substance abuse[55]	Interventions were: brief interventions, motivational strategies, cognitive behavioral therapy (CBT), and 12-step programs	Twenty studies were included in this evidence-based review. Eight studies were Level I, five studies were Level II, one study was Level III, and six were Level V. Study participants consisted of patients diagnosed with substance abuse in various settings and at various amounts of time poststroke.	Brief intervention sessions: 5–60 minutes × 3 sessions over time, CBT included teaching coping skills used for relapse prevention or harm reduction and cognitive reframing. Motivational strategies included decision balancing, motivational interviewing, motivational enhancement therapy, and FRAMES.	Evidence-based review Level I	Brief interventions, motivational strategies, CBT, and 12-step programs were effective in improving cognitive performance and health maintenance outcomes in patients diagnosed with substance abuse.	Varied according to study
Psychosocial interventions for survivors of motor vehicle accidents diagnosed with PTSD[59]	Interventions were cognitive therapy, a self-help booklet based on CBT, or repeated assessments.	Ninety-seven survivors of motor vehicle accidents diagnosed with PTSD during the first 3 months postaccident at risk for a diagnosis of persistent PTSD	CBT delivered for a mean of 9-weekly 60-minute sessions and a mean of 2.4-monthly follow-up sessions. Self-help 64-page booklet. Repeated assessments were administered without intervention.	Randomized controlled trial Level 1	Cognitive therapy was effective in preventing chronic PTSD in patients diagnosed with recent-onset PTSD. A self-help booklet of CBT exercises was not effective.	Fewer CBT patients (3 [11%]) had PTSD than those given the self-help book (17 [61%]); odds ratio, 12.9; 95% confidence interval [CI], 3.1–53.1) or repeated assessments (16 [55%]; odds ratio, 10.3; 95% CI, 2.5–41.7).

PTSD, post-traumatic stress disorder.

References

1. World Health Organization & The World Bank. *World Report on Disability*. 2011. https://www.who.int/disabilities/world_report/2011/report.pdf.
2. Brown C, Stoffel VC. *Occupational Therapy in Mental Health: A Vision for Participation*. Philadelphia, PA: F. A. Davis Company; 2011.
3. Gutman S. Sleep disorders secondary to orthopedic and neurologic disorders. In: Radomski MV, Latham CA, eds. *Occupational Therapy for Physical Dysfunction*. 7th ed. Philadelphia, PA: Lippincott Williams & Wilkins; in press.
4. Jackson AC, Le Grande MR, Higgins RO, Rogerson M, Murphy BM. Psychosocial screening and assessment practice within cardiac rehabilitation: a survey of cardiac rehabilitation coordinators in Australia. *Hear Lung Circ*. 2017;26(1):64–72. doi:10.1016/j.hlc.2016.04.018.
5. Pardaens S, De Smedt D, De Bacquer D, Willems A-M, Verstreken S, De Sutter J. Comorbidities and psychosocial characteristics as determinants of dropout in outpatient cardiac rehabilitation. *J Cardiovasc Nurs*. 2015;32(1): 14–21. doi:10.1097/JCN.0000000000000296.
6. Shen BJ, Gau JT. Influence of depression and hostility on exercise tolerance and improvement in patients with coronary heart disease. *Int J Behav Med*. 2016;24(2):312–320. doi:10.1007/s12529-016-9598-z.
7. Pratiwi SH, Sari EA, Hernawaty T. Level of anxiety and depression in post-stroke patients at DR. Hasan Sadikin Hospital Bandung. *Jurnal Pendidikan Keperawatan Indonesia*. 2017;3(2):139–144. https://pdfs.semanticscholar.org/9424/175836b957e7a33b9a0c02693685e333534f.pdf.
8. Murphy GC, O'Hare MA. Using psychology theory to guide serious-injury vocational rehabilitation: predicting the use of job-retention interventions for those living with spinal cord injury. *Med Res Arch*. 2017;5(6):1–15. file:///C:/Users/sg2422/Downloads/1282-1-4607-1-10-20170512.pdf.
9. Hunter EG, Gibson RW, Arbesman M, D'Amico M. Systematic review of occupational therapy and adult cancer rehabilitation: part 2. Impact of multidisciplinary rehabilitation and psychosocial, sexuality, and return-to-work interventions. *Am J Occup Ther*. 2017;71(2):7102100040p1–7102100040p8. doi:10.5014/ajot.2017.023572.
10. Podlog L, Heil J, Schulte S. Psychosocial factors in sports injury rehabilitation and return to play. *Phys Med Rehabil Clin N Am*. 2014;25(4):915–930. doi:10.1016/j.pmr.2014.06.011.
11. Harris M, Thomas G, Thomas M, et al. Supporting wellbeing in motor neuron disease for patients, carers, social networks, and health professionals: a scoping review and synthesis. *Palliat Support Care*. 2018;16(2):228–237. doi:10.1017/S1478951517000700.
12. Vash CL, Crewe NM. *Psychology of Disability*. New York, NY: Springer; 2004.
13. Precin, P. *Client-Centered Reasoning: Narratives of People with Mental Illness*. Brattleboro, VT: Echo Point Books and Media; 2015.
14. Drapalski AL, Lucksted A, Perrin PB, et al. A model of internalized stigma and its effects on people with mental illness. *Psychiatr Serv*. 2013;64(3):264–269. https://ps.psychiatryonline.org/doi/pdf/10.1176/appi.ps.001322012.
15. Barnes C, Mercer G. Disability culture assimilation or inclusions? In: Albrecht GL, Seelman KD, Bury M, eds. *Handbook of Disability Studies*, Thousand Oaks, CA: Sage; 2001:515–534.
16. Stewart RE, Chambless DL. Cognitive-behavioral therapy for adult anxiety disorders in clinical practice: a meta-analysis of effectiveness studies. *J Consult Clin Psychol*. 2009;77(4):595–606. doi:10.1037/a0016032.
17. Perlis ML, Jungquist C, Smith MT, Posner D. *Cognitive Behavioral Treatment of Insomnia: A Session by Session Guide*. New York, NY: Springer, 2008.
18. Benson H, Proctor W. *Relaxation Revolution: Enhancing Your Personal Health Through Science and Genetics of Mind Body Healing*. New York, NY: Scriber; 2010.
19. Prochaska JO, Norcross JC. *Systems of Psychotherapy: A Transtheoretical Analysis*. 8th ed. Stamford, CT: Cengage Learning; 2014.
20. Kavanagh E. Affirmation through disability: one athlete's personal journey to the London Paralympic Games. *Perspect Public Health*. 2012;132(2):68–74. doi:10.1177/1757913911435757.
21. Pizzi MA, Reitz SM, Scaffa ME. Health promotion and well-being for people with physical disabilities. In: McHugh Pendleton H, Shultz-Krohn, eds. *Pedretti's Occupational Therapy-E Book: Practice Skills for Physical Dysfunction*. London: Mosby; 2001:58–70.
22. Persson E, Eklund, M, Lexell J, Rivano-Fischer M. Psychosocial coping profiles after pain rehabilitation: associations with occupational performance and patient characteristics. *Disabil Rehabil*. 2017;39(3):251–260. doi:10.3109/09638288.2016.1141243.
23. Dorset P. The importance of hope in coping with severe acquired disability. *Aust Soc Work*. 2010;63:83–102. doi:10.1080/03124070903464293.
24. Wadensten B, Ahlstrom G. The struggle for dignity by people with severe functional disabilities. *Nurs Ethics*. 2009;16:453–465. doi:10.1177/0969733009104609.
25. Oakley F, Kielhofner G, Barris R, Reichler RK. The Role Checklist: development and empirical assessment of reliability. *Occup Ther J Res*. 1986;6(3):157–169. doi:10.1177/153944928600600303.
26. Baum CM, Edwards D, Michael E. *Activity Card Sort (ACS)*. 2nd ed. Bethesda, MD: American Occupational Therapy Association Press; 2008.
27. Bontje P, Kinebanian A, Josephsson S, Tamuura Y. Occupational adaptation: the experience of older persons with physical disabilities. *Am J Occup Ther*. 2004;58:140–149. doi:10.5014/ajot.58.2.140.
28. Charon R. Narrative medicine: attention, representation, affiliation. *Narrative*. 2005;13:261–270. https://www.jstor.org/stable/20079651.
29. Charon R. *Narrative Medicine: Honoring the Stories of Illness*. New York, NY: Oxford University Press; 2006.
30. Pande N, Tewari S. Understanding coping with distress due to physical disability. *Psychol Dev Soc*. 2011;23:177–209. doi:10.1177/097133361102300203.
31. World Health Organization. Depression. World Health Organization Web site. http://www.who.int/news-room/fact-sheets/detail/depression. Published March 22, 2018. Accessed August 16, 2018.
32. Precin P. Psychosocial disorders. In: O'Sullivan SB, Schmitz, TJ, Fulk G, eds. *Physical Rehabilitation*. 6th ed. Philadelphia, PA: FA Davis Company; 2014:1175–1221.

33. Barker-Collo SL. Depression and anxiety 3 months post stroke: prevalence and correlates. *Arch Clin Neuropsychol.* 2007;22(4):519–531. doi:10.1016/j.acn.2007.03.002.
34. Carota A, Bogousslavsky J. Stroke-related psychiatric disorders. *Handbook of Clinical Neurology.* 2008;93:623–651. https://doi.org/10.1016/S0072-9752(08)93031-1.
35. Miller EL, Murray L, Richards L, et al. Comprehensive overview of nursing and interdisciplinary rehabilitation care of the stroke patient: a scientific statement from the American Heart Association. *Stroke.* 2010;41:2402–2448. https://www.ahajournals.org/doi/pdf/10.1161/str.0b013e3181e7512b.
36. Beck AT, Steer RA, Brown GK. *Beck Depression Inventory-II.* San Antonio, TX: The Psychological Corporation; 1996; 78(2):490–498.
37. Romppel M, Herrmann-Lingen C, Wachter R, et al. A short form of the General Self-Efficacy Scale (GSE-6): development, psychometric properties and validity in an intercultural non-clinical sample and a sample of patients at risk for heart failure. *Psychosoc Med.* 2013;10:Doc01. doi:10.3205/psm000091.
38. Rosenberg M. Rosenberg self-esteem scale (RSE). Acceptance and commitment therapy. *Measures Package, 61.* Wollongong, Australia: University of Wollongong; 1965;61:52. https://ueb.ro/psihologie/docs/Psihologie_pozitiva_teste_si_scale.pdf#page=61. Accessed October 9, 2018.
39. Livneh H, Antonak RF. Psychosocial adaptation to chronic illness and disability: a primer for counselors. *J Couns Dev.* 2005;83(1):12–20. doi:10.1002/j.1556-6678.2005.tb00575.x.
40. Hackett ML, Anderson CS, House A, Halteh C. Interventions for preventing depression after stroke. *Cochrane Database Syst Rev.* 2008;(3). doi:10.1002/14651858.CD003689.pub3.
41. Lenze EJ, Munin MC, Quear T, et al. Significance of poor patient participation in physical and occupational therapy for functional outcome and length of stay. *Arch Phys Med Rehabil.* 2004;85(10):1599–1601. doi:10.1016/j.apmr.2004.03.027.
42. Whyte EM, Mulsant BH, Rovner BW, Reynolds CF. Preventing depression after stroke. *Int Rev Psychiatry.* 2006;18(5):471–481. doi:10.1080/09540260600935470.
43. Mitchell PH, Veith RC, Becker KJ, et al. Brief psychosocial–behavioral intervention with antidepressant reduces poststroke depression significantly more than usual care with antidepressant: living well with stroke: randomized, controlled trial. *Stroke.* 2009;40(9):3073–3078. doi:10.1161/STROKEAHA.109.549808.
44. Robinson RG, Jorge RE, Moser DJ, et al. Escitalopram and problem-solving therapy for prevention of poststroke depression: a randomized controlled trial. *JAMA.* 2008;299(20):2391–2400. doi:10.1001/jama.299.20.2391.
45. Livneh H, Martz E. Coping strategies and resources as predictors of psychosocial adaptation among people with spinal cord injury. *Rehabil Psychol.* 2014;59(3):329–339. doi:10.1037/a0036733.
46. Hildebrand MW. Effectiveness of interventions for adults with psychological or emotional impairment after stroke: an evidence-based review. *Am J Occup Ther.* 2015;69(1):6901180050p1–6901180050p9. doi:10.5014/ajot.2015.012054.
47. Miller WR, Rollnick S. *Motivational Interviewing: Preparing People to Change Addictive Behavior.* 2nd ed. New York, NY: Guilford Press; 2002.
48. Desrosiers J, Noreau L, Rochette A, et al. Effect of a home leisure education program after stroke: a randomized controlled trial. *Arch Phys Med Rehabil.* 2007;88(9):1095–1100. doi:10.1016/j.apmr.2007.06.017.
49. Champagne T, Koomar J, Olson L. Sensory processing evaluation and intervention in mental health. *OT Practice.* 2010;15(5):CE-1–CE-7.
50. Prins A, Bovin MJ, Kimerling R, et al. *The Primary Care PTSD Screen for DSM-5 (PC-PTSD-5).* [Measurement instrument]. 2015. https://www.ptsd.va.gov/professional/assessment/documents/pc-ptsd5-screen.pdf.
51. Herman JL. *Trauma and Recovery: The Aftermath of Violence—From Domestic Abuse to Political Terror.* London: Hachette UK; 2015;18(1):131–132. doi:10.1111/j.1471-6402.1994.tb00301.x.
52. Precin, P. Occupation as therapy for trauma recovery: a case study. *Work.* 2011;38(1):77–82. doi:10.3233/WOR-2011-1106.
53. Anson K, Ponsford J. Coping style and emotional adjustment following traumatic brain injury. *J Head Trauma Rehabil.* 2006;21(3):248–259. https://journals.lww.com/headtraumarehab/Fulltext/2006/05000/Coping_and_Emotional_Adjustment_Following.5.aspx.
54. Lieberman D, Scheer J. AOTA's evidence-based literature review project: an overview. *Am J Occup Ther.* 2002;56(3):344–349. doi:10.5014/ajot.56.3.344.
55. Stoffel VC, Moyers PA. An evidence-based and occupational perspective of interventions for persons with substance-use disorders. *Am J Occup Ther.* 2004;58(5):570–586. doi:10.5014/ajot.58.5.570.
56. Hibpshman T, Larson S. *Substance Abuse Screening Test.* East Aurora, NY: Slosson Educational Publications, 1993.
57. Precin P. Efficacy of a stress management module in managing stress and clean time in dual diagnosis (mental illness and substance misuse) clients. In: Huri M, ed. *Occupational Therapy—Occupation Focused Holistic Practice in Rehabilitation.* Rijeka: Intech; 2017:67–80.
58. Leppard A, Ramsay M, Duncan A, Malachowski C, Davis JA. Interventions for women with substance abuse issues: a scoping review. *Am J Occup Ther.* 2018;72(2):7202205030p1–7202205030p8. doi:10.5014/ajot.2018.022863.
59. Ehlers A, Clark DM, Hackmann A, et al. A randomized controlled trial of cognitive therapy, a self-help booklet, and repeated assessments as early interventions for posttraumatic stress disorder. *Arch Gen Psychiatry.* 2003;60(10):1024–1032. doi:10.1001/archpsyc.60.10.1024.

Index

Note: Locators followed by '*f*' and '*t*' refers to figures and tables respectively.

A

B

C

D

E

F

G

H

I

P

Q

R

T

U

V

W

Z